HILARY WALKER

WATSON'S
Medical-Surgical Nursing and Related Physiology

Adapted for use in the United Kingdom and the Republic of Ireland by the following team of Clinical Nurses and Nurse Teachers.

General Advisers

Susan M. Hinchliff

Jacqueline M. Isard

Barbara A. Parfitt

F. Mary Wellington

Adapters

Rosamond J. Andrew

Clive Andrewes

Sally Chesson

S. José Closs

Vivien E. Coates

Joyce Wendy Hackney

Susan M. Hinchliff

Jacqueline M. Isard

Pamela A. Jackson

Evangeline Karn

Betty Kershaw

Dorothy A. Kewley

Brigid Mary Knight

Brenda E. Lamb

Susan Lomasney

Penelope J. Mawson

Barbara A. Parfitt

Lesley Pemberton

Robert J. Pratt

Margaret Rutter

Caroline Mary Shuldham

WATSON'S
Medical-Surgical Nursing and Related Physiology

THIRD EDITION

Jeannette E. Watson MScN

Professor Emeritus,
Faculty of Nursing,
University of Toronto,
Toronto, Canada

Joan R. Royle RN, MScN

Associate Professor,
Faculty of Health Sciences,
McMaster University;
Clinical Nurse Specialist,
St Joseph's Hospital,
Hamilton, Canada

Baillière Tindall
LONDON PHILADELPHIA TORONTO
SYDNEY TOKYO HONG KONG

Baillière Tindall   33 The Avenue
W. B. Saunders   Eastbourne, East Sussex BN21 3UN, England

West Washington Square
Philadelphia, PA 19105, USA

1 Goldthorne Avenue
Toronto, Ontario M8Z 5T9, Canada

ABP Australia Ltd, 44–50 Waterloo Road
North Ryde, NSW 2113, Australia

Ichibancho Central Building, 22–1 Ichibancho
Chiyoda-ku, Tokyo 102, Japan

10/fl, Inter-Continental Plaza, 94 Granville Road
Tsim Sha Tsui East, Kowloon, Hong Kong

First edition published 1972 by W. B. Saunders Company as *Medical-Surgical Nursing and
Related Physiology*, by Jeannette E. Watson.
Second edition published 1979 by W. B. Saunders Company
Third edition published 1987 by Baillière Tindall as *Watson's Medical-Surgical Nursing and
Related Physiology*, by Jeannette E. Watson and Joan Royle

Typeset by Phoenix Photosetting, Chatham
Printed and bound in Great Britain
by Mackays of Chatham Ltd

British Library Cataloguing in Publication Data

Watson, Jeannette E.
    Watson's medical-surgical nursing and related physiology.—3rd ed.
    1. Nursing
    I. Title II. Watson, Jeannette E   III. Royle, Joan. Medical–surgical nursing and
    related physiology
    610.73   RT41

ISBN 0–7020–1190–8

Contents

PART I

PART II

Contributors

M. Leslea Anderson RN, MS
Assistant Director of Nursing,
Chedoke–McMaster Hospitals,
Chedoke Hospital Division;
Associate Clinical Professor, Nursing,
Faculty of Health Sciences,
McMaster University,
Hamilton, Ontario, Canada

Patricia M. Kearns RN, MScN
Director of Education and Professional
    Standards,
St Joseph's Health Center,
Toronto, Ontario, Canada

Rose Kinash RN, MScN
Associate Professor,
College of Nursing,
University of Saskatchewan,
Saskatoon, Saskatchewan, Canada

Donna Shields-Poë RN, CNM, MSN, MScPH
Clinical Nurse Specialist,
Mount Sinai Hospital;
Clinical Associate,
Faculty of Nursing,
University of Toronto,
Toronto, Ontario, Canada

Adaptation Team

General Advisers

Susan M. Hinchliff BA, SRN, RNT
Visiting Lecturer in Nursing Studies, The Polytechnic of the South Bank

Jacqueline M. Isard MSc, BA, RGN, RM, DipN, STD, MBIM
Regional Training Officer, South East Thames Region

Barbara A. Parfitt MSc, MCommH, FamNursPract, SRN, SCM, RNT
Lecturer in Nursing, The University of Manchester

F. Mary Wellington SRN, RNT
Senior Nurse: Education, The Wolfson School of Nursing of Westminster

Adapters

Rosamond J. Andrew SRN, ONC, CNT
Clinical Teacher, The Wolfson School of Nursing of Westminster

Clive Andrewes BSc, SRN, RMN, DN (Lond)
Charge Nurse, The London Hospital

Sally Chesson RSCN, SRN
Ward Sister, Charing Cross Hospital

S. José Closs BSc, MPhil, SRN
Research Associate, University of Edinburgh

Vivien E. Coates BA, MPhil, SRN
Lecturer in Nursing, The University of Ulster

Joyce Wendy Hackney SRN, SCM
Ward Sister, Manchester Royal Infirmary

Susan M. Hinchliff BA, SRN, RNT
Visiting Lecturer in Nursing Studies, The Polytechnic of the South Bank

Jacqueline M. Isard MSc, BA, RGN, RM, DipN, STD, MBIM
Regional Training Officer, South East Thames Region

Pamela A. Jackson BSc(Hons), RGN, RHV, RCNT
Lecturer in Nursing Studies, The University of Surrey

Evangeline Karn RGN, RNT, DN(Lond), DipEd
Nurse Tutor, Charing Cross Hospital

Betty Kershaw MSc, RGN, RNT, OND, DipAdvNursStudies, RCNT
Director of Nursing Studies, The Royal Marsden Hospital

Dorothy A. Kewley SRN, SCM, HVCert
Senior Nurse, Cumberland Royal Infirmary

Brigid Mary Knight SRN, OND, DN(Lond), DipNEd
Nurse Tutor, The Wolfson School of Nursing of Westminster

Brenda E. Lamb SRN, ONC, DN(Lond)
Director of Nursing Services (Acute Unit), Basildon and Thurrock District
Health Authority

Susan Lomasney RGN
Ward Sister, Charing Cross Hospital

Penelope J. Mawson SRN
Ward Sister, Guy's Hospital

Barbara A. Parfitt MSc, MCommH, FamNursPract, SRN, SCM, RNT
Lecturer in Nursing, The University of Manchester

Lesley Pemberton SRN, RCNT, RNT, FETC, CertEd, DN(Lond)
Nurse Tutor, Oldham School of Nursing

Robert J. Pratt BA, MSc, RGN, RNT, DN(Lond)
Head of Department (Continuing Education), Charing Cross Hospital

Margaret Rutter MSc, SRN, SCM, OND, DN(Lond), DipNEd, RCNT, RNT
Senior Nurse Tutor, Chelsea Hospital for Women

Caroline Mary Shuldham SRN, RCNT, RNT, DN(Lond), PGCEA
Senior Nurse Tutor, South West Surrey Health Authority

Preface

The objective in the writing of this edition has been to have the content and the format in which it is presented reflect:

1   The expanding body of knowledge in the health-care field, as applicable to adults who come within the scope of medical–surgical nursing.
2   The changes and increasing responsibilities in the nurse's role.

The planning and writing also have taken into consideration the helpful suggestions made by readers of the second edition and the comments submitted by reviewers of chapters as the project proceeded. The authors are grateful for the suggestions, and when there was a consensus and they were within the scope of this textbook efforts were made to comply.

The book is divided into two parts. In Part I, Chapter 1 has been revised and emphasizes the components of the nursing process (assessment, identification of patient problems, nursing intervention and evaluation). An additional chapter (Chapter 2) addresses patient teaching, which is an integral part of all nursing. The remaining chapters in Part I are not specific to medical–surgical nursing; patient's responses are presented that are common to most clinical areas.

Part II relates to common specific disorders that involve medical and/or surgical management. As well as extensive revision of chapters from the second edition, this section includes a new chapter (Chapter 19) on nutrition and metabolism. The separate chapter on nursing in disorders of the pancreas has been deleted; Chapter 18 now includes a discussion of the exocrine pancreas, while the endocrine role and disorders are included in the chapter on nursing in disorders of the endocrine system (Chapter 20).

In order to assume their responsibilities safely and effectively, nurses require an understanding of normal body functioning, the pathophysiology and the impact on the family of dysfunction and disease. Such knowledge is basic to the assessment of patients, the identification (diagnosis) of existing and potential physiological, physical and psychosocial problems that are amenable to nursing intervention, as well as to the implementation of appropriate effective nursing intervention. An understanding of the rationale of the medical therapeutic measures is also important in order to assess and assist with the patient's responses to treatment.

Where appropriate, a review of normal structure and physiology is presented at the beginning of the chapters. Content following this review provides information about common disorders and applies the nursing process in most instances. The reader is reminded that the nursing process is presented as a guide or framework. It is always necessary to modify or adapt the suggested nursing intervention to individual patient's and family's responses to the disorder and treatment, which are identified by careful assessment.

The authors gratefully acknowledge the contributions made to the manuscript by Leslea Anderson, Patricia Kearns, Rose Kinash and Donna Shields-Poë. The suggestions and comments made by the consultants (selected because of their expertise) were very helpful and appreciated.

In order to make the content more meaningful and useful to students and practising nurses in the United Kingdom and the Republic of Ireland, changes have been made in terms, procedures and medications contained in the manuscript. The adaptation of the content has been made by expert practitioners in the United Kingdom under the direction of Miss R. Milton-Thompson, Associate Nursing Editor of Baillière Tindall. The authors are grateful to those who participated in the adaptation. The encouragement and cooperation of Miss Milton-Thompson and Mr David Inglis (Publishing Director) and the work done by Miss Carrie Bennett have been greatly appreciated, as well as the editing by Miss Debbie Harris.

Jeannette E. Watson
Joan R. Royle

Acknowledgements

Some of the figures and tables in this book are based on material published elsewhere. The sources are as follows.

Fig. 24.3: American Cancer Society, New York.

Fig. 24.5: American Cancer Society. *Help Yourself to Recovery*.

Fig. 24.12C: *Am. J. Cardiol.* (1984) Vol. 34 No. 487.

Fig. 25.20: Banerjee (1982) *Rehabilitation Management of Amputees*. Baltimore, MD: Williams and Wilkins. p. 375.

Fig. 16.6: Bates (1983) *A Guide to Physical Examination*, 3rd ed. Philadelphia: JB Lippincott. p. 138.

Table 16.9: Bauwens EE & Anderson SV (1981) *Chronic Health Problems*. St Louis: CV Mosby. pp. 177–179.

Table 12.1: Behrman RE & Vaughan VC (1983) *Nelson's Textbook of Pediatrics*, 12th ed. Philadelphia: WB Saunders. p. 1207.

Fig. 23.18: Bleier I (1971) *Maternity Nursing*, 3rd ed. Philadelphia: WB Saunders. p. 188.

Tables 14.4 & 14.5: Braunwald E (1984) *Heart Disease: A Textbook of Cardiovascular Medicine*. Philadelphia: WB Saunders. p. 287.

Fig. 9.1: Canadian Cancer Society, Toronto (1985). *Cancer Can be Beaten. The Facts*. pp. 28 & 29.

Figs. 23.15, 23.16 & 23.17: Cavanagh D (1969) The vaginal examination. *Hosp. Med.*, Vol. 5. pp. 35–51.

Table 26.7: Chedoke–McMaster Hospital (The Physiotherapy Department), Ontario, Canada.

Fig. 24.2: de Graaff KM (1984) *Human Anatomy*. Iowa: Wm C Brown, p. 649.

Fig. 25.23A: Engstom B & Van de Ven C (1985) *Physiotherapy for Amputees (The Roehampton Approach)*, Edinburgh: Churchill Livingstone.

Table 26.1: Fields WL & McGinn-Campbell KM (1983) *Introduction to Health Assessment*. Reston, Virginia: Reston Publishing. pp. 285–286.

Fig. 25.4, 25.16 & 26.2: Gartland JJ (1974) *Fundamentals of Orthopedics*, 2nd ed. Philadelphia: WB Saunders. pp. 31, 349–350 & 363.

Fig. 1.5: Greene E, Montemuro M & Royle J. *The Nursing Assessment*. Department of Nursing, St John's Hospital, Ontario, Canada.

Table 4.2 & Fig. 4.5: Gurevich I & Tafuro P (1985) Nursing measures for the prevention of infection in the compromised host. *Nurs. Clin. N. Am.*, Vol. 20 No. 1. p. 156.

Table 22.2: Guyton AC (1981) *Human Physiology and Mechanisms of Disease*, 3rd ed. Philadelphia: WB Saunders. p. 431.

Figs. 14.15 & 22.9: Guyton AC (1984) *Physiology of the Human Body*, 6th ed. Philadelphia: WB Saunders. pp. 284 & 212.

Figs. 8.2, 14.8 & 21.4: Guyton AC (1986) *Textbook of Medical Physiology*, 6th ed. Philadelphia: WB Saunders. pp. 595, 177 & 415.

Fig. 23.10: Hatcher RA et al (1981) *Contraceptive Technology*. New York: Irvington Publishers. p. 10.

Figs. 16.2, 22.1, 22.3 & 22.7: Jacob SW, Francone CA & Lossow WJ (1982) *Structure and Function in Man*, 5th ed. Philadelphia: WB Saunders. pp. 451, 235, 239 & 255.

Fig. 22.8: Jung & Hassler (1960) *Handbook of Physiology*. Baltimore, MD: Williams & Wilkins. Section I, Vol. II (© American Physiology Society).

Tables 23.2 & 23.3: Katchadourian HA & Lunde DT (1975) *Fundamentals of Human Sexuality*, 2nd ed. New York: Holt, Rinehart & Winston. pp. 82 & 83.

Table 27.1: Kim MJ, McFarland GK & McLane AM (1984) *Pocket Guide to Nursing Diagnoses*. pp. 53–54.

Fig. 16.7: Leifer G (1977) *Principles and Techniques in Pediatric Nursing*, 3rd ed. Philadelphia: WB Saunders. p. 138.

Table 25.2: Lentz M (1981) Selected aspects of deconditioning secondary to immobilization. *Nurs. Clin. N. Am.*, Vol. 16 No. 4. p. 735.

Fig. 23.26: Lerner J & Khan Z (1982) *Mosby's Manual of Urologic Nursing*, 3rd ed. St Louis: CV Mosby. p. 43.

Fig. 21.8: Lewis SM (1981) Pathophysiology of chronic renal failure. *Nurs. Clin. N. Am.*, Vol. 16 No. 3. p. 504.

Figs 17.8 & 22.24: Luckman J & Sorenson (1980) *Medical–Surgical Nursing: A Psychophysiologic Approach*, 2nd ed. Philadelphia: WB Saunders. pp. 1415 & 530.

Fig. 18.4: Mount Sinai Hospital, Toronto, Canada.

Fig. 20.3: MacLeod J (ed) (1984) *Davidson's Principles and Practice of Medicine*, 14th ed. Edinburgh: Churchill Livingstone. Chapter 12.

Figs 23.14 A & B: Masters WH & Johnson VE (1966) *Human Sexual Response*. Boston, MA: Little, Brown. p. 183.

Fig. 23.12: Matsumoto S et al (1968) Environmental anovulatory cycles. *Int. J. Fertility*, Vol. 13 No. 1. pp. 15–23.

Fig. 27.5: Mendelsohn S, Maelor Hospital, Wrexham, United Kingdom.

Table 22.5: Mitchell PH & Irvin NJ (1977) Neurological examination for nursing purposes *J. Neurosurg. Nurs.*, Vol. 9 No. 25.

Figs 28.5, 28.6 & 28.7: Nave CC & Nave BC (1980) *Physics for the Health Sciences*, 2nd ed. Philadelphia: WB Saunders. pp. 283, 287 & 285.

Fig. 20.7: Notkins AL (1979) The causes of diabetes. *Sci. Am.*, Vol. 241 No. 5. pp. 62–73.

Table 27.3: Norton D, McLaren R & Exton-Smith AN (1975) *An Investigation of Geriatric Nursing Problems in Hospital*. Edinburgh: Churchill Livingstone.

Table 18.3: Patton F (1981) Hepatitis: current concepts. *Crit. Care Nurs.*, Vol. 1 No. 3. p. 24. (© Critical Care Nursing Association).

Fig. 8.3: Raiman J, *London Hospital Pain Chart*. London Hospital Medical College.

Fig. 26.5: *Rheumatic Disease: Occupational Therapy and Rehabilitation* (1977) Philadelphia: FA Davis.

Figs. 15.1, 15.2, 15.3 & 15.4: Rice V (1981) Shock: a clinical syndrome. Part II: The stages of shock. *Crit. Care Nurs.*, Vol. 1 No. 4. pp. 5–9. (© Critical Care Nursing Association).

Table 6.5: Rice V (1984) Shock management. Part I: Fluid volume replacement. *Crit. Care Nurs.*, Nov/Dec. pp. 71–73.

Table 13.16: Royle J & Green E (1985) Right atrial catheters: a patient and family education program. *Can. Nurs.*, Vol. 81 No. 3. p. 52.

Fig. 24.4: Rubin P (ed) (1983) Clinical Oncology. *A Multidisciplinary Approach*, 6th ed. New York: American Cancer Society. p. 123.

Fig. 21.17: Sabiston DC Jr (ed) (1981) *Davis–Christopher Textbook of Surgery*, Philadelphia: WB Saunders. p. 1749.

Figs 13.2 & 13.3: St John's Hospital (Department of Nursing), Ontario, Canada.

Fig. 16.14: Secor (1969) *Patient Care in Respiratory Problems*. Philadelphia: WB Saunders. p. 131. (Courtesy of the Harris Calorific Co., Cleveland, Ohio.)

Fig. 29.7: Shah N. In patient booklet—*Glue Ear*. Royal National ENT Hospital, Grays Inn Road, London.

Fig. 19.1: Sherwin R & Felig P (1978) *Med. Clin. N. Am.*, Vol. 62 No. 695.

Table 23.1: Shields-Pöe DA (1981) Unpublished Master's Thesis, University of Toronto, Department of Preventive Medicine and Biostatistics, Toronto, Canada.

Table 26.2: Simpson CT (1983) Adult arthritis: heat, cold or both? *Am. J. Nurs.*, Vol. 83 No. 2. p. 272.

Fig. 17.3: Sleisenger MH & Fordtran JS (eds) (1978) *Gastrointestinal Disease*, 2nd ed. Philadelphia: WB Saunders.

Fig. 21.3: Smith K (1980) *Fluids and Electrolytes: a Conceptual Approach*. Edinburgh: Churchill Livingstone. p. 63.

Fig. 28.9: Smith and Nephew Ltd, Hessle Road, Hull. (Booklet—*Understanding Cataract*.)

Tables 20.6 & 13.18: Smith LH & Thier SO (1985) *Pathophysiology*, 2nd ed. Philadelphia: WB Saunders. pp. 379 & 279.

Fig. 24.1: Soterakos M (1981) Nursing care of the patient with breast cancer. In: Bouchard-Kurtz & Speese-Owens, *Nursing Care of the Cancer Patient*, 4th ed. St Louis: CV Mosby. p. 160.

Fig. 23.11: Speroff L, Glass RH & Kase N (1983) *Clinical Gynecologic Endocrinology and Intertility*, 3rd ed. Baltimore, MD: Williams & Wilkins. p. 81.

Fig. 25.5C: Steer-Nicholson (1984) The Belfast Fixator. *Nurs. Times*, Feb. 22nd.

Fig. 25.5 A & B: Stewart & Hallet (1986) *Traction and Orthopaedic Appliances*. Edinburgh: Churchill Livingstone.

Fig. 17.13: Sunnybrook Medical Center (The Medical Photography Department), Toronto, Canada.

Fig. 17.4: Trier JS & Rubin CE (1965) *Gastroenterology*, Vol. 49 No. 574.

1
The Science of Nursing

PART I

Nursing as a Practice Discipline

Nursing is concerned with the health of patients and clients thoughout their life. It focuses on an individual's mental and physical health as he interacts with his environment and which is expressed through an individual's functional competence. It is called a practice discipline because relevant knowledge from the physical, biological, behavioural, social and medical sciences is organized and used by nurses, and systematically applied to practice. Nursing knowledge also derives from nursing practice, clinical nursing research and an understanding of what happens to patients in health and illness. All this contributes to a scientific basis for the nursing care of patients.

Over the past 20 years, several theories have emerged which organize nursing in ways that are useful to practice. While components of these theoretical models may be organized in different ways by different theorists, all agree that concepts concerned with the individual, the environment and health and the interrelationships between these are important in planning and implementing nursing care. While the focus of nursing may vary among theorists, all agree that any application must be systematic, goal-directed and must consistently use the nursing process.

Concepts Central to Nursing

(See Fig. 1.1).

THE INDIVIDUAL

An understanding of the patient or client is basic to nursing. He is viewed in the context of a human being and as a unique person with his particular make-up, experiences and responses. The person has a distinct identity, in addition to being a member of a family and community. He is in constant interaction with his environment. His interactions and responses are influenced by his sociocultural background, life-style, set of values, capabilities, interests, past experiences and the patterns of behaviour laid down as a result of those experiences; these factors contribute to his uniqueness. Each person is regarded as having worth, dignity and the right to pursue health, happiness, love, security, purpose and freedom.

When data about a patient and his health problem are being collected, the patient should be viewed as a biological, psychological, social, cultural and spiritual being. These features are interrelated and integrated to comprise the person as a total (holistic) entity. Information relating to each aspect is analysed and organized and, in making decisions about the significance of this data, the nurse considers the individual holistically by looking at the implications for the total person and not merely his component parts.

There is a consensus among nursing theorists that the recipient of care should be informed about his health status, make informed decisions compatible with personal beliefs and values and actively participate (within his potential) in the care process. All persons have essential basic human needs; nursing intervention may be indicated when the individual cannot independently satisfy these needs. Basic biological needs include an intake of oxygen, fluids, food, elimination of wastes, rest, sleep, some activity, change of position and maintenance of body temperature within a definite range. Significant psychosocial needs of each person include: a sense of security, the maintenance of an identity as an individual, acceptance, a sense of being wanted and belonging, the opportunity for socialization, independence and at times dependence and interdependence, freedom to make decisions; and opportunities to develop and use his potential. He should have interests and goals, and the opportunity to feel self-respect. He needs to feel useful and to have a sense of achievement.

Environment

The relationship between an individual and his environment is very dynamic and influences his health as well as his life-style. When we consider the internal and external environments of man within the context of nursing, the internal environment is comprised of everything within the skin and mucous membranes of the body. It encompasses all structural and physiological aspects of the human body and may be modified by assimilated psychological and sociocultural experiences. The external environment includes physical surroundings, patterns of relation-

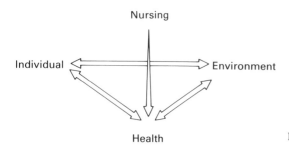

Fig. 1.1 Concepts central to nursing.

ships and interactions with family and society, external resources, and the ways in which the individual has contact with a health-care delivery system.

Nursing is directed towards managing the way in which the patient or client interacts with the environment, promoting health, preventing disease and delivering care in illness. Specific strategies and actions enabling the nurse to direct or manage that interaction vary according to the individual, his environment and his health problem.

Health

Health is a goal to be attained and maintained. The two major components of health are the subjective or feeling aspect and the objective or functional component. The subjective aspect relates to the individual's feelings of being well, while the objective component refers to the physiological and psychological ability to function or carry out actions and interactions necessary for daily living and the individual's life-style.

There are varying levels of health as it fluctuates in relation to situations and events. How health is perceived is influenced by cultural and educational background and past experiences. An individual's health is measured against some yard-stick or set of standards. The standard used may be absolute; for example, it may be the presence or absence of disease or the ability or inability to function as a contributing, independent member of society. Other measurements may be relative and give greater consideration to subjective components such as the sense of well-being and quality of life. As well as the physiological and functional aspects of health, nursing is concerned with subjective factors contributing to this quality of life and the opportunity the individual has to realize his potential. Effects of the internal environment on functioning, well-being and life-style are readily apparent. The effects of unfavourable external environmental factors significant to health, such as polluted air, water, noise, and adverse living conditions are complex and more difficult to identify and change. Other factors related to an individual's life-style, such as the amount of physical exercise he takes, his dietary and smoking habits, his levels of stress and the relationships he

has with others, can also affect health. These factors should be identified and, perhaps, modified.

Nursing

The role of nursing evolves in response to the needs of society and an expanding body of nursing knowledge. Consequently, definitions change. Nursing has its roots in nurturing and caring; it remains patient- or client-centred and results are measured in terms of patient outcomes.

Reviews of various definitions of nursing indicate how they have expanded in scope.[1] Henderson describes the nurses' unique function as:

'assisting the individual, sick or well, in the performance of those activities contributing to health or its recovery (or to a peaceful death) that he would perform unaided if he had the necessary strength, will, or knowledge.'[2]

Similarly, nursing is defined by Wiedenbach as:

'facilitating the efforts of the individual to overcome the obstacles which currently interfere with his ability to respond capably to demands made of him by his condition, environment, situation and time.'[3]

These earlier definitions describe the art of nursing and illustrate the nurturing and comforting themes. Later definitions broaden the scope of nursing to reflect the scientific base which uses a systematic approach, giving consideration to family and community as well as to the individual. King states that using a systematic process facilitates the organization and selection of knowledge for nursing practice.[4]

Current definitions of nursing include the components of nurse–patient interaction, a systematic approach and a concern with the concepts of the whole man, environment and the goal of health, as

---

[1] Greene (1979), pp. 57–64.
[2] Henderson (1966), p. 15.
[3] Wiedenbach (1964), pp. 14–15.
[4] King (1971).

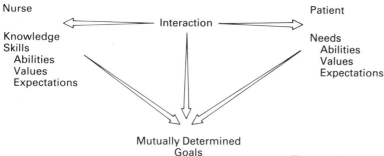

Fig. 1.2 Nurse–patient relationship.

well as with the caring and nurturing themes. McGee defines nursing as:

'a situationally derived system of nurse–client (individual, family or community) interaction that is based on the assessment of function and need and is designed to optimize the client's functional competence through (1) environmental modification, (2) behavioral modification and/or reinforcement, and (3) biological care and maintenance using strategies of nursing care in appropriate dosage.'[5]

Goals of nursing

In recent years nursing has shifted from pre-occupation with illness and disease processes to focus on health. Greater consideration is given to factors which contribute to health and to the impact of illness and disease on the functioning and lifestyle of the individual and family. The goals of nursing are to promote, maintain and restore health, as well as to support the individual and family through stressful events, which may include death and bereavement.

Nurse–patient relationship

The nurse–patient relationship is of great importance in all phases of nursing. A professional or therapeutic relationship differs from a social relationship in that it is collaborative and is directed towards meeting the client's or patient's goals (see Fig. 1.2). It may be time-limited and take place within a structured and designated setting (such as a hospital). People tend to have preconceived ideas about the nurse as well as about how they themselves should behave as patients. Clarification of these perceptions may be necessary before an effective rapport can develop. The professional purpose of the relationship gives direction to the role assumed by the nurse and to the way in which she applies her knowledge and skills. The nurse brings to the relationship respect for the person's uniqueness and integrity and an appreciation of the patient's right to participate in or receive

care. The patient, as an active participant, brings certain abilities and values, as well as his own background of culture, education, experiences and needs, with the right to demonstrate and apply these in decisions and the care process. Mutual acceptance is fundamental to the effectiveness of the nurse–patient relationship.

As the nurse develops empathy with the patient or client, so he should develop trust and confidence in the nurse. With each patient encounter, the nurse's role is mutually agreed by the nurse and patient. A sincere interest and willingness to help may be demonstrated by the nurse being non-judgemental, accepting the patient, demonstrating thoughtfulness, anticipating needs, showing concern, and by being ready to listen to the patient and answer questions. Frequently, an appropriate, light touch of the nurse's hand conveys acknowledgement and understanding of problems and anxieties, as well as caring.

Recognition of identity by addressing the patient by name, respect for personal preferences and demonstrating flexibility contribute to a satisfactory relationship. Appreciation of the family's concerns and its members' need for an interpretation of what is happening to the patient fosters trust and confidence. Expressing and sharing information with them may prove therapeutic.

During the total nurse–patient relationship, the nurse's responsibilities include that of being the patient's advocate. When acting on behalf of the patient, attempts are made to assess carefully the situation from the patient's point of view, rather than simply deciding what is 'good for' the patient on the basis of past nursing experience.

Confidentiality must be respected; it is an important factor in establishing good nurse–patient relationships. When information must be shared with other members of the care team, the patient should be advised of the reasons and the advantages of communicating it to others.

When necessary, the nurse should provide information to assist the patient and/or his family to make informed decisions about the individual's health care (e.g. about a procedure, a form of therapy or a change in circumstances).

[5] McGee (1975), p. 127.

While the nurse is under an obligation to attend anyone in her care regardless of race, nationality, politics or creed, there may be practical situations where the patient's choice is in conflict with the nurse's personal values and beliefs. In such cases, the nurse may feel morally and ethically obliged to withdraw from the situation. However, the nurse must ensure continuity of care by someone who is comfortable with the patient's choice. Resolution of ethical dilemmas is very difficult. The United Kingdom Central Council provides guidelines in its *Code of Professional Conduct* and recognizes that the patient has the right to make decisions and choices.

The development of the nurse–patient relationship occurs in three distinct phases:

1 Orientation phase
2 Working phase
3 Termination phase

The length and scope of each phase is determined by its purpose and the situation in which it occurs. In a brief encounter with a critically ill patient in an emergency department, the relationship is based on efforts directed towards meeting life-threatening needs and is usually terminated in a short time. In long-term or community health settings when the patient presents with multiple and complex problems, the interaction may extend over several weeks, months or years and the relationship is challenging for all concerned. The patient and family may need help in adjusting to chronic disability or to prepare for impending death.

The *orientation phase* includes introduction to the patient, the creation of an atmosphere conducive to learning and establishment of a mutual contract for nursing activity. The initial interview is structured by the nurse to establish a rapport with the patient, obtain pertinent clinical data, and make plans for care. During this phase, initial roles are defined and the patient's reasons for being in this situation and his expectations of care are explored.

The *working phase* involves providing information and nursing actions that are directed towards assisting the patient to alleviate his problems, make informed choices, set goals and participate in care. The nurse provides direct intervention when the patient is unable to undertake self-care. Goals are reviewed frequently and are redefined as the patient's situation and condition change.

The *termination phase* requires planning and is built into the relationship from the beginning. It is directed by the purpose and goals of the relationship. The nurse supports the patient in assuming independence, makes referrals and identifies resources to assist the patient in moving towards self-management. The ease or difficulty with which this is accomplished depends on the effectiveness of the nurse–patient relationship throughout the three phases. The patient and nurse evaluate the outcomes in relation to how far defined goals have been achieved.

Nursing Process

The nursing process is the systematic approach used in carrying out nursing activities with and for the patient (see Fig. 1.3). It is purposeful and interactive

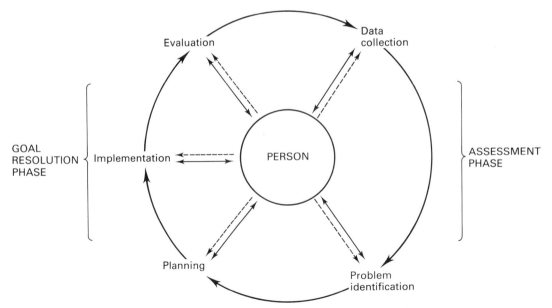

Fig. 1.3 Nursing process model.

in nature, and involves both intellectual and physical activities. The process consists of five logical, interrelated steps of:
1 Assessment or data collection
2 Identification of patient problems (nursing diagnosis)
3 Planning
4 Implementation
5 Evaluation

ASSESSMENT

Use of the nursing process enables the nurse to organize knowledge systematically and to make decisions that are patient-centred and goal-directed. The nurse must decide what data will be significant and what information is to be collected. Findings are analysed on the basis of the bio-psycho-social sciences, as applied to the behaviour of man and the goals of nursing practice. Actual and potential health problems are identified and goals and priorities set for both immediate and long-term care. Plans for nursing intervention are made, taking into consideration the uniqueness of the individual, his goals and contributions that can be made by his family and other members of the health-care team. Nursing interventions are evaluated in terms of how effectively the defined patient goals and ongoing adjustments have been achieved relative to the individual's changing health status.

DATA COLLECTION

Knowledge of the basic sciences and models and theories of nursing provide a framework for the selection and organization of data. Nursing history tools and forms for organizing and documenting a physical assessment are available to assist in collecting and documenting significant data. These tools help the nurse to systematically collect, document and communicate data obtained. Initial data collection is determined by the severity of his presenting illness and such circumstances as the patient's level of fatigue, pain, or any assessment taken recently by other health-care professionals. Identification of causative factors gives direction to nursing intervention. Documentation of base-line observations with which to compare further changes in the patient's health status, is essential. For example the location, size and depth, colour and drainage associated with a pressure sore are documented and used to evaluate results of treatment.

Data collection for a comprehensive profile of the patient's health includes past and present biological, psychological and social functioning, and environmental and life-style factors that may affect health.

Assessment of the patient requires data on: physiological functioning; the onset, nature, severity and duration of dysfunctional problems; the use and effectiveness of physiological compensatory mechanisms; and perceived and actual effects of any disruption of activities of daily living and life-style.

Psychosocial assessment requires data on: the daily activities and life-style of the patient; the family situation; home environment; occupation; economic status; community environment; past patterns of coping; recent events or changes that have altered the patient's life; and the patient's perceptions of the effects of the present health problem on life-style, roles and relationships. The data collection must also include environmental and other variables related to health problems (see Fig. 1.4).

Data may be classified as subjective or objective:
- *Subjective* information is obtained from the patient, friends or relatives regarding the patient's feelings and perception of the situation. Feelings such as fear, pain and itching are examples of subjective data.
- *Objective* information is obtained about the patient by means of observation, physical examination and laboratory reports. Vital signs, blood cell counts and description of sputum are examples of objective data. These facts are measurable and can be confirmed by others.

Sources of data
The patient is the primary source of data. Secondary sources include family members, friends, other members of the health team, the patient's records and other relevant written records.

Methods of data collection
The nurse uses various techniques and approaches in data collection. Interviewing and physical examination are used directly with the patient. A structured assessment interview provides subjective information on the patient's background, perception and feelings about the situation. Objective data are obtained by the physical examination techniques of inspection, palpation, percussion and auscultation. Assessment data specific to various body systems are outlined in relevant chapters.

No one source of data or method of collection is adequate. Validation of data and assumptions made are essential to ensure that messages conveyed by the patient are being received and interpreted accurately by the nurse. This is achieved by comparing data collected from several sources and by confirming with the patient that the needs and goals are as stated. Data collected from the patient may be elaborated and validated by the patient's family, health records and other health professionals. Results of diagnostic tests, medical care plans and the assessments and plans of other health professionals are obtained from the patient's notes and from discussion with other members of the health-care team. Review of the literature assists the nurse in identifying and interpreting significant and relevant data.

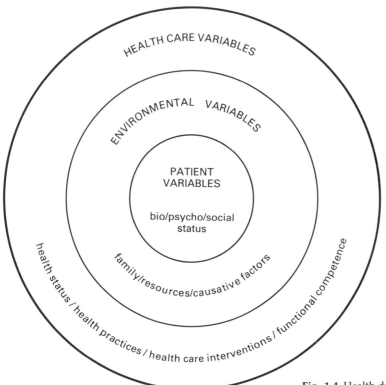

Fig. 1.4 Health data.

IDENTIFICATION OF PATIENT PROBLEMS

The nurse will need to make a judgement about the effects of the patient's condition and the actual or potential problems he faces as a result. This identification of patient's problems, which should be made on the basis of observing, assessing and talking to the patient is sometimes referred to as a 'nursing diagnosis'[6] (see Fig. 1.5). The nurse will be able to give a concise statement of the patient's response to a situation or event which is actually or potentially unhealthy and includes the causative factors requiring intervention. The health problems that fall into the realm of nursing are identified. Descriptions that may be included in the diagnostic statement may specify the degree and duration of the problem.

While collecting the data, the meaning and relevance of the information elicited are continuously questioned. Data are sorted, patterns are identified and diagnoses are made. Both the assessment and the diagnostic process are continuous. The emergence of specific patterns or cues from the data, combined with the nurse's existing knowledge base, identifies actual or potential problems and gives direction for more specific data collection that will confirm or rule out problems (see Fig. 1.4). Classifi-

cation systems are being developed to assist in the accurate communication of patient problems and needs from one nurse to another. Progress is also being made in identifying characteristics and essential criteria for each diagnostic category. The reader is referred to the writing of Jones and the National Group for Classification of Nursing Diagnoses.[7,8]

PLANNING

The planning phase of the nursing process consists of setting priorities, identifying goals, proposing interventions, weighing alternatives and predicting outcomes.

PRIORITY SETTING

Once patient problems (potential and actual) have been identified, priorities are set to provide direction for nursing interventions. Knowledge, experience and, in some critical situations, intuition are applied in priority setting. If the situation is life-threatening, support systems immediately assume priority. In many situations, priority setting involves patient

---

[6] Miller & Keane (1983), p. 318.

[7] Jones (1979), pp. 65–72.
[8] Kim, McFarland & McLane (1984).

Diagnostic Process

Example

Mrs A, a 58-year-old female patient, during the early postoperative period following a hysterectomy, has an indwelling urinary catheter

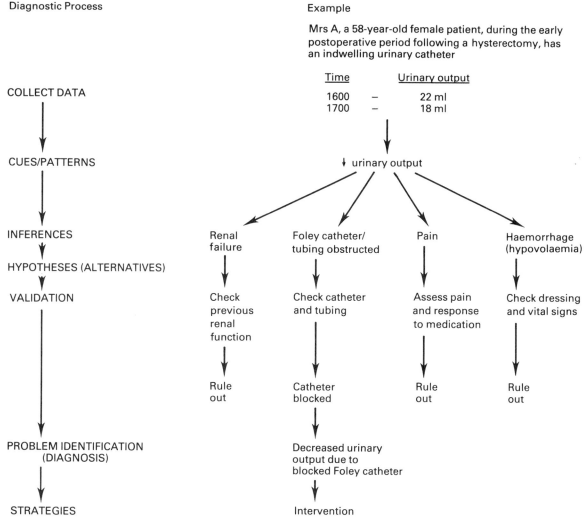

Fig. 1.5 Diagnostic process.

and family participation to prevent conflicts arising and to enhance active cooperation in care activities.

There is no one tool or framework available that assists in making decisions on priorities of patient care in all situations. Emergency and life-threatening circumstances readily dictate priorities for intervention; other situations may require more consideration. Maslow's framework, which presents an ordered classification of human needs, may be helpful to rank patient problems.[9] It is based on motivation theory and implies that the client contributes to the decision. Physiological needs (for oxygen, water, food) are ranked as top priorities, followed by safety and security, love and belonging, self-esteem and self-actualization. Communicating the reasons for priorities helps in establishing mutual goals;

failure to consider what is important to the patient may create conflict and delay in achieving health goals.

SETTING GOALS AND PREDICTING OUTCOMES

The goals emerge from the identification of patient problems and are directed towards promotion, maintenance and restoration of health, the alleviation of suffering and giving support to the dying when death is inevitable.

Predicted outcomes are expressed in terms of measureable patient behaviour that may be expected as a result of nursing intervention. Each outcome describes the anticipated change of understanding and behaviour as well as the time-scale during which it should be expected to occur. Some expectations are therefore immediate, whilst others are long term.

[9] Maslow (1970).

In the clinical situation described in Table 1.1, the goal for nursing intervention for Mrs A would be 'to prevent postoperative respiratory complications'. The expected outcome would read as follows.

Mrs A:

1 States the reasons for carrying out deep-breathing exercises and coughing
2 Practises deep breathing and coughing with guidance
3 Independently performs deep breathing and coughing as often as the prescribed frequency throughout the day and evening for the first 3–5 postoperative days
4 Demonstrates regular rhythmic respirations and the presence of vesicular breath sounds on auscultation of her lungs.

The setting of goals and expected outcome serves to provide a time-scale, direction and criteria for evaluating nursing interventions as well as giving a sense of purpose.

Table 1.1 Application of the diagnostic process.

Situation: The nurse caring for Mrs A, a 45-year-old woman who has had a cholecystectomy the previous morning was informed that she had not been doing the prescribed deep-breathing and coughing exercises.

Questions to guide decision making	Application to clinical situation
1 Is this patient normally able to meet her own needs?	Prior to hospitalization, Mrs A was a healthy active wife, mother and member of her community. She was able to meet her basic needs within her family and community
2 What is this patient's present problem?	Mrs A underwent abdominal surgery for removal of her gallbladder within the past 24 hours. Information indicates that she has not carried out the prescribed deep-breathing and coughing exercises
3 Is this a nursing problem?	Yes. Maintenance of respiratory functioning and prevention of complications fall within the domain of nursing
4 What information is needed?	Information is needed about: (a) Mrs A's actual respiratory functioning (b) Factors contributing to her behaviour in not carrying out the exercises
5 What knowledge is needed?	Knowledge of: (a) normal respiratory functioning (b) the effects of anaesthetic agents on the respiratory tract (c) the effects of a high abdominal incision and abdominal pain on thoracic movement (d) human behaviour and response to hospitalization and surgery
6 Is the data base for both nurse and patient sufficient and accurate?	No. (a) The consequences of failure to carry out the exercises have not been discussed with Mrs A (b) Mrs A's actual respiratory status needs to be assessed (c) The severity and effects of incisional pain have not been assessed
7 What patterns emerge from the data and knowledge base?	Respiratory complications are a potential problem, so the patient needs assistance in keeping respiratory passages clear of secretions
8 Are there alternative explanations to the interpretation of the data?	There are several possible reasons why Mrs A did not perform the breathing and coughing exercises: (a) Was she taught the exercises? (b) Is pain or abdominal muscle weakness interfering? (c) Are there associated problems interfering with her ability to comprehend instructions (e.g. visual or hearing loss, motivation, anxiety)?
9 Can a nursing diagnosis be formulated?	Yes. (a) Potential (or actual) impaired ventilation due to inadequate airway clearance (b) Knowledge deficit secondary to lack of instruction on deep-breathing and coughing exercises
10 Is further information necessary to confirm the diagnoses?	Assessment of respiratory status should be based on objective measurements. Identification of reasons for not carrying out deep-breathing and coughing exercises would need to be confirmed with Mrs A

DEVELOPING THE PLAN OF ACTION

Actions to be carried out by the nurse and/or patient are selected on the basis of the predictable outcomes and are consistent with the identified goals. The plan of action is confirmed with the patient and is then recorded on the patient's notes and/or nursing care plan. Medical orders and the plans developed by the physiotherapist, social worker, speech therapist or other health professionals are integrated with the planned nursing actions to develop an overall schedule for patient care. When problems are identified by the nurse that are outside the realm of nursing, a referral is made to the appropriate member of the health-care team. Similarly, when patient problems are identified that are beyond the expertise of one particular nurse, referrals are made to qualified nursing colleagues. These may be clinical nurse specialists, nurses practising in a special care area or speciality, or community nurses. Cooperation and sharing of knowledge and skills provide quality and continuity of care. The patient is made aware of and agrees to the expectations and plans.

IMPLEMENTATION

Implementation (or nursing intervention) is the actual carrying out of the nursing care proposed in the patient care plan. The scope of nursing action includes:

- Supportive measures that are designed to assist the patient with activities he is unable to perform and to reinforce coping mechanisms
- Therapeutic measures
- Continuous data collection and monitoring of the patient's condition
- Health promotion and health maintenance activities such as teaching
- Coordination of care by other members of the health-care team
- Reporting, recording and consultation

Examples of nursing intervention for Mrs A in the previous illustration might include:
- Explaining the reasons for deep breathing and coughing
- Demonstrating the technique
- Observing Mrs A deep breathing and coughing
- Splinting Mrs A's abdomen with a pillow and hand as support while she breathes deeply and coughs
- Continuous assessment of her respiratory status

EVALUATION

Evaluation is the interpretation of the effectiveness of the intervention based on the *expected outcomes.* For example, the goal 'to prevent postoperative respiratory complications' for Mrs A is achieved if she demonstrates the behaviour identified in the expected outcome. Evaluation data are collected during and following nursing intervention and are then compared with the expected outcomes. When the patient behaviour indicates that the goals have been achieved, the nurse and patient either move to the next level of expectations or the relationship is terminated. If the expected outcomes are not met, the nurse explores the reasons why by questioning. For example: Were the goals realistic? Were the expected outcomes stated in measurable terms? Were the actions inappropriate, or did the patient's situation alter? Goals are then re-examined, modified if necessary and priorities are re-established in relation to the patient's level of achievement and/or change in health status.

DOCUMENTATION

The patient's health record can be used as a legal document. The nurse is accountable for ensuring that information recorded in the notes is accurate, clear, concise, factual, and complete. Data collection, identification of patient problems, plan of care, interventions and results of the interventions and evaluation of expected outcomes are recorded.

All members of the health-care team should share the patient's record. It thus becomes a means of providing information about the patient's condition, the health professionals' care plans and also contributes to continuity of care. Accurate and comprehensive written documentation facilitates collaboration and cooperation among members of various health-care professions to ensure optimum use of resources on the patient's behalf. The record is a confidential document; it is only available to those participating in the care by permission of the patient and health authority.

References and Further Reading

BOOKS

Adam E (1980) *To be a Nurse.* Philadelphia: WB Saunders.

Carison JH, Craft CA & McGuire AD (1982) *Nursing Diagnosis.* Philadelphia: WB Saunders.

Carpenito LJ (1983) *Nursing Diagnosis: Application to Clinical Practice.* St Louis: JB Lippincott.

Faulkner A (1985) *Nursing, A Creative Approach.* Eastbourne: Baillière Tindall.

Fitzpatrick J & Whall A (1983) *Conceptual Models of Nursing.* Bowie, MD: Robert J Brady.

Gordon M (1982) *Nursing Diagnosis: Process and Application.* New York: McGraw-Hill.

Hall JE & Weaver BR (1974) *Families in Crisis.* Philadelphia: JB Lippincott. Chapter 2.

Henderson V (1966) *The Nature of Nursing.* New York: Macmillan.

Kim MJ, McFarland GK & McLane AM (1984) *Classification of Nursing Diagnoses.* St Louis: CV Mosby.

King I (1971) *Toward a Theory of Nursing.* New York: John Wiley & Sons.

McFarlane JK & Castledine G (1982) *The Practice of Nursing Using the Nursing Process*. London: CV Mosby.

McGee M (1975) *Determination of Family Decision-Making Capacity by Community Health Nurses and a Measurement of Nursing Impact in Development and Use of Indicators in Nursing Research*. Proceedings of the 1975 National Conference on Nursing Research. Edmonton.

Marriner A (1983) *The Nursing Process: A Scientific Approach to Nursing Care*, 3rd ed. St Louis: CV Mosby.

Maslow A (1970) *Motivation and Personality*, 2nd ed. New York: Harper & Row.

Miller BF & Keane CB (1983) *Encyclopedia and Dictionary of Medicine, Nursing and Allied Health*, 3rd ed. Philadelphia: WB Saunders.

Orem DE (1980) *Nursing Concepts of Practice*, 2nd ed. New York: McGraw-Hill.

Orem DE (1979) *Concept Formulization in Nursing by Nursing Development Conference Group*. Boston: Little, Brown.

Parsee RR (1981) *Man-Living-Health: A Theory of Nursing*. New York: John Wiley.

Pearson A & Vaughan B (1986) *Nursing Models in Practice*. London: Heinemann.

Riehl JP & Roy C (1980) *Conceptual Models for Nursing Practice*, 2nd ed. New York: Appleton-Century-Crofts.

Rogers M (1970) *An Introduction to the Theoretical Basis of Nursing*. Philadelphia: FA Davis.

Roper N, Logan W & Tierney A (1983) *Using a Model of Nursing*. Edinburgh: Churchill Livingstone.

Roy C (1976) *Introduction to Nursing: An Adaptation Model*. Englewood Cliffs, NJ: Prentice–Hall.

Stevens BJ (1979) *Nursing Theory: Analysis, Application, Evaluation*. Boston: Little, Brown.

Sundeen SJ, Stuart GW, Rankin ED & Cohen SA (1981) *Nurse–Client Interaction*. St Louis: CV Mosby.

UKCC (United Kingdom Central Council for Nursing, Midwifery and Health Visiting) (1984) *Code of Professional Conduct for the Nurse, Midwife and Health Visitor*, 2nd ed. London: UKCC.

Weller BF (1987) *Baillière's Encyclopaedic Dictionary of Nursing and Health Care*. Eastbourne: Baillière Tindall.

Wiedenbach E (1964) *Clinical Nursing*: A Helping Art. New York: Springer.

Wilson HS & Kneisl CR (1979) *Psychiatric Nursing*. Menlo Park, California: Addison–Wesley. Chapter 6

PERIODICALS

Aggleton P & Chalmers H (1984) Models and theories: defining the terms. *Nurs. Times*, Vol. 80 No. 36, pp. 24–28.

Aggleton P & Chalmers H (1984) Models and theories: 2 the Roy adaptation model. *Nurs. Times*, Vol. 80 No. 40, pp. 45–48.

Aggleton P & Chalmers H (1984) Models and theories: 3 the Riehl interaction model. *Nurs. Times*, Vol. 80 No. 45, pp. 58–61.

Aggleton P & Chalmers H (1984) Models and theories: 4 Rogers' unitary field model. *Nurs. Times*, Vol. 80 No. 50, pp. 35–39.

Aggleton P & Chalmers H (1985) Models and theories: 5 Orem's self care model. *Nurs. Times*, Vol. 81 No. 1, pp. 36–39.

Aggleton P & Chalmers H (1985) Models and theories: 6 Roper's activities of living model. *Nurs. Times*, Vol. 81 No. 7, pp. 59–61.

Aggleton P & Chalmers H (1985) Models and theories: 7 Henderson's model. *Nurs. Times*, Vol. 81 No. 10, pp. 33–35.

Aggleton P & Chalmers H (1985) Models and theories: 8 critical examination. *Nurs. Times*, Vol. 81 No. 14, pp. 38–39.

Andreoli KG & Thompson CE (1977) The nature of science in nursing. *Image*, Vol. 9 No. 2, pp. 32–37.

Bramwell L (1985) Nursing science: retrospect and prospect. *Cancer Nurs.*, Vol. 81 No. 3, pp. 45–48.

Carper BA (1979) The ethics of caring. *Adv. Nurs. Sci.*, Vol. 1 No. 3, pp. 11–19.

Curtin LL (1979) The nurse as advocate: a philosophical foundation for nursing. *Adv. Nurs. Sci.*, Vol. 1 No. 3, pp. 1–10.

Dossey B & Guzzetta CE (1981) Nursing diagnosis. *Nurs. '81*, Vol. 11 No. 6, pp. 34–38.

Flaskerud JH & Halloran EJ (1980) Areas of agreement in nursing theory development. *Adv. Nurs. Sci.*, Vol. 3 No. 1, pp. 1–7.

Gortner SR (1980) Nursing science in transition. *Nurs. Res.*, Vol. 29, No. 3, pp. 180–183.

Greene JA (1979) Science, nursing and nursing science: a conceptual analysis. *Adv. Nurs. Sci.*, Vol. 2 No. 1, pp. 57–64.

Inzer F & Aspinall MJ (1981) Evaluating patient outcomes. *Nurs. Outlook*, Vol. 29 No. 3, pp. 178–181.

Jones PE (1979) A terminology for nursing diagnosis. *Adv. Nurs. Sci.*, Vol. 2 No. 1, pp. 65–72.

Keller JJ (1981) Toward a definition of health. *Adv. Nurs. Sci.*, Vol. 4, No. 1, pp. 43–64.

Radotovich Price M (1980) Nursing diagnosis: making a concept come alive. *Am. J. Nurs.*, Vol. 80 No. 4, pp. 668–671.

Sigman P (1979) Ethical choice in nursing. *Adv. Nurs. Sci.*, Vol. 1 No. 3, pp. 37–52.

Smith JA (1981) The idea of health: a philosophical inquiry. *Adv. Nurs. Sci.*, Vol. 3 No. 3, pp. 43–50.

Stainton M (1982) The birth of nursing science. *Cancer Nurs.*, Vol. 78 No. 10, pp. 24–28.

Terris M (1975) Approaches to an epidemiology of health. *Am. J. Public Health*, Vol. 65 No. 10, pp. 1037–1044.

Whall AL (1980) Congruence between existing theories of family functioning and nursing theories. *Adv. Nurs. Sci.*, Vol. 3 No. 1, pp. 59–67.

Williamson JA (1981) Mutual interaction: a model of nursing practice. *Nurs. Outlook*, Vol. 29 No. 2, pp. 104–107.

2
Patient Education in Health Promotion

Health Promotion

Health-promoting activities have long been an integral part of nursing. Florence Nightingale in 1859 stated that nursing:

'has been limited to signify little more than the administration of medicines and the application of poultices. It ought to signify the proper use of fresh air, light, warmth, cleanliness, quiet, and the proper selection and administration of diet.'[1]

Today, nursing is defined as more than the care and nurture of individuals when they are ill; the primary goal is recognized as being health promotion, and the primary focus is seen as assisting individuals to achieve a positive state of health, well-being and improved quality of life. Health promotion is defined by Pender as 'activities directed towards sustaining or increasing the level of well-being, self-actualization and personal fulfilment of a given individual or group.'[2]

Health promotion can be applied at any level. For an individual who is unwell, activities are directed first to restoring health or to helping achieve an improved state of functioning and well-being. Promotion is concerned with helping individuals to positively change their behaviour and to alter lifestyle to improve their health. Those with long-term health problems may never feel really well but they have a right to obtain the knowledge, skills and resources needed to improve health, to achieve a level of functioning that is maximal for them and to have an improved quality of life.

Patient teaching is generally accepted as a professional responsibility of nurses but it is argued that this activity does not take place as often or as effectively as it should. However, where it is genuinely acknowledged that the patient has a right to make his own decisions and assume responsibility for his own health (and where more than lip service is paid to this notion), effective patient education should follow as a natural sequence of events.

Health Education and Patient Education

The terms health education and patient education are not synonymous although both have the common goals of achieving optimum health and quality of life. *Health education* is broader in scope and may be defined as planned combinations of learning activities directed towards helping the individual, family and/or community behave in ways that are most likely to promote health. The *aim* of health education differs with circumstances. It may be:
1 Education directed towards modifying an otherwise healthy person's behaviour so that he attains a higher quality of health and life
2 Education directed towards altering the individual's behaviour and life-style in order to prevent disease and maintain a stable state of health
3 To improve function in those who are, or who have been, ill.

Health is a dynamic process and such aims may merge and alter as change and growth occur.

Patient education could be said to be a component part of health education. Patient education refers to planned combinations of learning activities designed to assist people who are having, or have had, experience of illness or disease to make changes in their behaviour that are conducive to health.[3]

The Nurse as an Educator

Nurses, by their commitment to the health of individuals, families and the community, are responsible for health teaching in order to achieve any of the health education aims cited above, in any area of health care. This chapter will, however, focus primarily on patient education for those who are ill, or have recently experienced illness.

In such situations, the patient should be provided with opportunities to acquire the necessary knowledge, skills and resources to achieve the best possible level of functioning, make informed decisions

---

[1] Nightingale (1970).
[2] Pender (1982), p. 42.

[3] Green, Kreuter, Partridge & Dieds (1979), p. 7.

about care and be an active participant in that care. The nurse's role includes sharing her professional knowledge and skills so that she can help the patient do as much as he can for himself. How far he can take responsibility for this will vary according to circumstances and his state of health. Teaching may initially have a low priority in acute care settings due to the patient's critical or life-threatening condition and, while unable to carry out his own care, support and help will be provided for him. Even at this stage, however, the nurse can provide advice and encouragement in health education matters and this becomes an important part of the nursing process as he improves.

For effective patient education, the nurse requires:

- Knowledge of the principles of learning and methods of teaching
- Knowledge and skills in the area to be taught
- An understanding of human behaviour and the effects of health on behaviour
- Communication skills, which include interviewing skills, group-process skills and an ability to be an active listener in order to identify, clarify and validate non-verbal, as well as verbal, messages
- Skill in the use of educational materials and resources
- An ability to work collaboratively with others
- A sincere interest in patients
- Respect for patient's rights
- An awareness of the professional responsibility for patient teaching
- An awareness of her own personal strengths and weaknesses

The Patient Educator's Role

Both formal and informal teaching may be provided by several nurses and members of other health-care disciplines (e.g. doctor, physiotherapist, pharmacist, dietitian). Learning may be enhanced when each contributes his unique knowledge and skills. In order to prevent confusing or, sometimes, conflicting information, teaching must be planned, coordinated and documented. Health education should be a collaborative effort of all members of the health-care team with the patient as the central focus. The use of a teaching plan involving all the health professionals concerned provides a means of communication and a record of the patient's and family's educational needs, what must be taught, teaching methods and evaluation of how well each component part of the teaching has been understood. Written teaching plans promote consistency of content, continuity and are thus more logical to the patient.

The Patient's Role in the Education Process

For effective health education the patient should be an active participant. He is ultimately responsible for his health and for altering his life-style if appropriate, in order to improve or maintain his own health. Emphasis is placed on the need and right of patients to be fully informed about their own health care. Patient-centred teaching is an interactive process between the patient and the nurse or other knowledgeable and skilled professionals. Involvement of the patient throughout the process increases the likelihood of successful learning, the development of skills necessary to adapt to future changes in health and less hesitancy in seeking information and resources.

Principles of Learning as Guidelines for Patient Teaching

Principles of learning serve as guides to action; the nurse who is familiar with the basic principles of adult education creates conditions conducive to learning (see Table 2.1). Teaching should be goal-directed and should start where the learner is in order to be relevant and to make sense to each individual patient. Tasks and information should be broken down into small steps or segments to facilitate understanding. Repetition reinforces learning. Success enhances motivation, so feedback is essential to the learning process and should be continuous and frequent.

In many instances, learning can be uncomfortable. It may involve giving up old, familiar ways of doing things and changing values and ways of thinking. Mild anxiety on the part of the learner is beneficial and is motivating; however, severe anxiety immobilizes and interferes with learning. Patients need time to test new information and skills and to compare results with old methods and habits. They will make mistakes and may go back instead of making progress forward. Support and encouragement are needed, and acceptance of their discomfort and setbacks, as well as acknowledging their success, is important.

The Process of Patient Education

The process of patient education parallels the steps of the nursing process and includes data collection

Table 2.1 Education of adults.*

Principles of learning	Teaching activities
'Adults tend to have a fairly well-developed self-concept which allows them to act independently. Also, learning needs are related to current life situations.'[1]	**1** To facilitate learning in adults, one begins by assessing where the learner is starting. An assessment is conducted of: the learner's expectations about what to learn, how much time will be devoted to learning, his/her questions, concerns and resources
'Learners learn best when they are involved in developing learning objectives for themselves which are congruent with their current and idealized self-concept.'[2,3,4]	**2a** The learner must be encouraged to play an active role in goal setting and the periodic review of goal attainment and/or goal revision **2b** Goals must begin at the learner's perceived level of need **2c** Goal setting is an interactive process between the learner and expert (or facilitator) **2d** To keep goals relevant to the learner, objectives need to be modified as the learner grows and his needs change
Adults are busy and 'are expected to be productive'.[1,5,6]	**3** Adults need to know what they will learn or gain in any educational experience. Goal setting is an important component in any educational programme for adults
'Learning involves change. Adults experience a constant push (to change) and pull (to return to the status quo). Both forces are important. "Change stimuli" evolve as we experience new things that we cannot explain or understand with our existing knowledge. Forces to remain the same provide us with stability in our lives.'[1]	**4a** 'Change stimuli' should be assessed: What forces exist in the learner's life that are moving him/her towards change, learning, growth? **4b** Resistance to changes should be assessed: What forces (physical, emotional, cognitive) are impeding movement and blocking learning? Are some old beliefs or knowledge inconsistent with new ideas, behaviours or knowledge?
'Adults need a learning environment which does not threaten them and which supports and encourages them.'[5,7,8,9]	**5** A safe, and non-threatening, learning environment should be created. It is important to encourage the patient (building on strengths, recognition of positive steps, permission of risk); the nurse's manner with the learner should be non-judgemental, open and based on respect
'Adults have already developed organized ways of focusing on, taking in, and processing information. These are referred to as cognitive styles and are assumed to remain relatively constant and consistent throughout adulthood.'[10,11,12,13]	**6** The learner's previous experiences should be reviewed in order to seek his/her preferred learning approaches. Alternative ways to learn information should be identified. The nurse should try to provide material in several formats or use a variety of media.
'Adults process information at different rates and deal with information overload by selecting, deleting, distorting, oversimplifying and overgeneralizing.'[14,15,16,17]	**7** In working with adults it is useful to: (a) ask the learner what information he or she has heard (b) repeat information in different ways (c) use examples (d) relate information to goals Too much information should not be given at any one time
'Learners react to a learning experience out of an organized whole self-concept and perceive the experience as an integrated whole.'[5,18]	**8** Learning activities that help learners to organize and integrate information should be used. For example: (a) discussion of new information (b) flow charts, models, diagrams (c) exploration of examples, uses, implications of new information
'Role learning is not carried out through formal, logical or sequential processes but through interpersonal interactions, modelling, and experimenting.'[19]	**9** If new learning involves adoption, and learning about a new role, adults must be given opportunities to: (a) observe role behaviours (b) interact with 'role models' (c) try out new behaviours in a safe environment
'Basically, there are two types of needs, "deficit needs" (for survival and security tendencies) and growth or being needs (belonging, self-esteem, self-actualization).'[20]	**10a** If the learning need is a deficit need (which patient education needs often are), the learner may require considerable structure and help in finding his or her own direction. He/she may need prolonged support and frequent feedback from the expert or facilitator **10b** Individuals who have growth or being needs may be able to plan and conduct their own educational experience

*Mitchell (1974).

[1] Brundage & MacKeracher (1980); [2] Tough (1971); [3] Rubin (1969); [4] Smith (1976); [5] Kidd (1973); [6] McKenzie (1977); [7] Knowles (1970); [8] McClusky (1970); [9] Combs (1974); [10] Cawley et al (1976); [11] McKenney & Keen (1974); [12] Kolb & Fry (1975); [13] McLaren (1975); [14] Toffler (1970); [15] Katz & Kahn (1979); [16] Bandler & Grinder (1975); [17] Cropley (1977); [18] Brim (1966); [19] Goslin (1969); [20] Maslow (1970).

and assessment, identification of learning needs, goal setting and planning, implementation and evaluation. The discussion of each step of the process involves collaboration between the nurse and patient. Documentation is an essential component of each step. Table 2.2 outlines a framework for collection of the data that is relevant to the patient's educational needs.

Table 2.2 Assessment of patients' educational needs.

Patient characteristics

Attitudes to health
Past experiences with illness
Physical condition
Emotional state
Intellectual ability
Support systems
Preferred methods of learning

Other factors influencing learning

Patient/family perceptions of learning needs
Patient goals
Factors facilitating learning
Barriers to learning
Learning needs identified by health professionals ⎱ Validated with patient/family

ASSESSMENT

Assessment begins with identifying those patient characteristics that influence learning. Biographical data, results of diagnostic studies and the medical plan of care can be obtained from the patient's notes. Much information about the individual is obtained during any physical examination and when giving care. Factors which are assessed and which influence patient education processes include the following:

Attitudes to health and customs. The patient's attitudes to health and how far he believes himself to be responsible for his own health will influence learning. Religious and cultural beliefs influence eating habits, life-style and receptiveness to health care and prescribed therapy. This information is also useful to the nurse in helping the patient make decisions about his care.

Past experience with illness. Information about his past health history should be collected, including how he coped with illness and what changes in health habits and life-style followed as a result.

Physical condition. The patient's general feeling of well-being or illness influences his capacity and readiness to learn. His ability to carry out activities of daily living and to manage tasks and procedures necessary for self-care is assessed. Vision, hearing and touch, as well as manual dexterity and mobility, are assessed since they are important in physical functioning.

Emotional state. Emotions affect an individual's readiness to learn and response to teaching. In illness, and when there is a permanent loss of function, patients may progress through stages of adaptation or grieving. These stages include *denial, anger* and *resentment, recognition* and *acceptance*. With acceptance, hopefully, the patient begins to participate in decision making and develops independence.

Intellectual ability. As well as a willingness and desire to learn, the patient's ability to understand his condition and solve related problems will contribute to effective learning. The length of the individual's attention span, basic knowledge and fluency in the language being used should be kept in mind when considering comprehension and learning.

Support Systems. The responses of family and friends to the patient's situation can play an important part in the patient's education. If supportive, they facilitate learning and provide reinforcement for positive changes in behaviour.

Barriers to learning. Individual deterrents to learning include sensory deficits, decreased ability to comprehend, lack of orientation to time, place and person, decreased manual dexterity and loss of physical mobility. Learning is also inhibited by lack of motivation and readiness to learn on the part of the patient.

Severe anxiety can interfere with learning, so worry about lack of social and financial support and resources may inhibit effective patient education. If the language or form of words used by those teaching is unfamiliar or too technical (or perhaps too patronizing) that, too, can act as a barrier to understanding.

IDENTIFICATION OF LEARNING NEEDS

A learning need is the educational gap between the present and desired or required level of competence. It is mutually identified by the nurse and the patient from analysis of the data collected and the needs expressed by the patient. The identification of learning needs should include a description of what the patient should know or be able to do and the factors influencing it. Health professionals have the necessary knowledge, experience and information about the patient's health problem and its management to plan a comprehensive teaching programme, bearing in mind the individual's particular needs. The nurse caring for a patient who has been recently diagnosed as having insulin-dependent diabetes mellitus uses her knowledge of diabetes and its management to identify the patient's need for: information about diabetes; skill in administering insulin; knowledge and skill in dietary management; changes in daily routine; and information about the special care of feet and skin. The patient may not perceive the needs identified by health care personnel as essential nor may he wish to acquire the knowledge and skills required.

It is necessary that the learning needs identified by professionals are discussed with the patient and his family and an explanation should be given as to why these needs are relevant to the patient's health.

The family should receive teaching on how they can best assist with the daily activities that the patient cannot carry out for himself and what resources and environmental changes can be provided to promote patient self-care.

The patient's preferred method of learning. Certain methods of teaching and learning work better than others with different patients. Past educational experience will influence the effectiveness of various teaching methods and learning patterns. It is useful to identify whether the patient learns best by reading, viewing an audio-visual programme or carrying out a learning activity, and whether he prefers one-to-one or group teaching or indeed a combination of several methods. This knowledge assists in selecting learning strategies that are meaningful and preferred by the patient and are therefore more likely to be effective.

Patient/family perceptions. Identifying educational needs and setting priorities requires assessing the patient's and his family's present knowledge, how they see his present level of functioning and what the desired level of competence may be. It is important to know if they are able to look at the long-term implications or are only able to focus on what is happening today. This sort of assessment must be a continuous process as changes occur once the patient has achieved the initial goals, coped with the impact of illness and begun to accept the changes to his life.

Patient goals. The patient's goals and priorities for present and future functioning should be determined. His motivation and readiness to assume responsibility for his health care are assessed. The assessment may reveal that the patient's goals differ from those of health professionals and of relatives, resulting in conflicts and confusion which hinder learning.

PLANNING

Setting goals

Once learning needs have been identified, the nurse works with the patient to establish goals for learning, to determine priorities for teaching content and to select methods of teaching. Learning goals are usually divided into *short-term goals* for immediate learning needs and *long-term objectives* which define the eventual expected outcomes. The learner may be a patient or a family member, a group of patients or a group of patients and family members. The knowledge or skill to be achieved is defined and the expected level or degree to which it will be met is stated. The final component of objective-setting is defining the time in which the desired change is expected to occur. Behavioural objectives are worded in simple, basic terms that are clear to the patient and all members of the health-care team. Action verbs such as 'state', 'describe', 'demonstrate', and 'perform safely' identify what is expected of the patient and give direction for designing the content and process of the learning experiences. Objectives may include all three categories of learning:

1 Cognitive (knowledge)
2 Psychomotor skills
3 Attitudes

Objectives break learning tasks into small, sequential steps that can be achieved independently before the total goal is mastered. The patient knows what is expected of him at each point, as well as the overall goal.

Again, using the diabetic patient as an example, behavioural objectives for the patient might be to:

1 *State* the action of insulin.
2 *Demonstrate* the technique of drawing up the prescribed amount of insulin into a syringe.
3 *Verbalize* his feelings related to giving his own injection of insulin.

PRIORITY SETTING

Priority is given to what the patient perceives as important and is ready to learn. If conflicts arise between what the nurse perceives as important and what the patient needs to know, negotiation and compromise become necessary to facilitate learning and compliance. The nurse can influence the patient's receptiveness to learn by providing the information the patient requires to make a decision. The first priority is the learning of survival skills so that the patient can provide safe self-care. For example, the patient learns about his diabetes, prescribed diet and how to administer his insulin. Following this, priority is given to other details of his therapeutic regimen (e.g. dietary exchanges, activity, etc.). Last, knowledge that would be helpful and which the patient wants to know, but could be gained from pamphlets, books and sources such as the Diabetic Association, is given.

Planning patient teaching

SELECTION OF METHODS OF PRESENTATION

Planning teaching requires the selection of appropriate approaches and methods of presenting information to the patient. Teaching strategies are selected to meet the unique characteristics of the patient and to involve as many senses as possible. If the family is supportive, members are included as active participants in the plan. If the patient has a physical and/or sensory defect, a teaching method is planned that will compensate for it. For example, in the case of a physical handicap, aids and equipment are made available to facilitate manual functioning and dexterity; auditory resource material is used with the blind, and colours that are difficult for the elderly to see are avoided. (Table 12.3, see p. 230, lists factors influencing learning in the elderly and teaching strategies that are useful.)

Organized teaching can be effective as has been shown in studies validated by pulmonary function tests, which demonstrate that structured preoperative instruction significantly improves a patient's ability to carry out deep-breathing and coughing exercises postoperatively.[4,5]

The teaching content in patient education may relate to a patient's present illness, the general health habits of the patient and/or family, or to a specific health problem of a family member. Teaching content must be accurate, expressed in terms and language understandable to the learner(s) and adapted to age, cognitive ability, education and culture. Time and opportunities for questions, correction and repetition should be given consideration when planning teaching programmes.

Uninterrupted periods for instruction should be planned for times when the patient is most likely to be comfortable and rested. Periods of teaching should be relatively short, as offering too much information at one time may defeat the purpose and leave the patient feeling confused and discouraged.

Practical procedures should be broken down into a logical sequence of steps. First, the procedure should be demonstrated as a whole so that the patient is provided with an overview; then each step should be shown slowly and in detail. Time and opportunity should be allowed for practising the technique as soon as possible after the demonstration. Repetition and receptiveness to questions reinforces learning.

Sometimes group instruction may be more effective than individual instruction and some studies have shown that increased structure of the content and presentation enhances learning.[6] It is all the more important, therefore, that the nurse finds out from the patient what his preferred method of learning is. Table 2.3 lists various methods of presentation and summarizes some benefits and disadvantages of each. Using a combination of methods that actively involve the patient in the education process is most likely to produce positive results.

---

[4] Lindeman & Van Aernam (1971), p. 332.
[5] King & Tarsizano (1982), p. 324.
[6] Cohen (1981), p. 15.

DOCUMENTATION OF THE TEACHING PLAN

The written teaching plan lists the patient's goals, expected outcomes, teaching content, learning aids, resources and teaching methods to be used. The patient should be given a copy to reinforce his participation in the process and a copy should be available to all members of the health-care team.

Learning contracts

The learning objectives and teaching plan are validated by the patient and a formal or informal agreement is reached. The contract is based on the belief that the teacher and learner are partners and incorporates the principle of positive reinforcement. The nurse and patient mutually identify the learning goals and objectives and discuss their expectations of each other. The verbal or written contract outlines how responsibility for achieving each goal or objective will be divided. The patient has a clear understanding of what is expected of him and the likely consequences of not meeting these expectations. Contracts are developed so that the patient can and will achieve learning, while the nurse agrees to meet the commitment of providing information, appropriate instructional resources, demonstrations, supervision of practice sessions and feedback, and coordinates the contract with others involved in the patient's care. Verbal or written contracts are explicit, include time-scales for evaluation and allow for flexibility.

Following evaluation, the contract is redefined, or if all of the goals have been met the contract is discharged. A contract may be used in relation to one specific task or it may specify a commitment for one day or for extended periods of time. Complex behaviours are broken down and each component is evaluated as achieved (or not). A contract of learning generally saves time because expectations are clear and easily communicated; it promotes development of the nurse–patient relationship, and actively involves the patient in decision making about his health care.

IMPLEMENTATION

The actual carrying out of the teaching plan follows the guidelines developed during the planning phase and incorporates principles of learning. Many learning activities can be incorporated into patient care. For example, the nurse can provide information about drugs when they are being given; then later, she can ask the patient to state what he understands about the action of each drug. An explanation may be given each time a procedure is performed and the patient may be expected to assume responsibility gradually for parts of the task and eventually be able to complete the procedure. Some learning activities require rescheduling to involve family members or a

Table 2.3 Methods of teaching patients.*

Method	Benefits	Disadvantages
Person to person (one to one) A teacher/learner interaction that is responsive to the learning needs of the learner. It may be spontaneous or planned	—Ultimate in flexibility —Individualized (in pace and content) —Promotes learning of facts, attitudes, skills —Responsive to learner's feelings	—One of the two needs to assume leadership —Requires rapport between the two —Expensive
Discussion (patient groups and/or support groups) A flexible strategy used with groups of any size but usually in small groups with or without a designated leader. The learner is an active participant, asking questions, sharing experiences and mutually solving problems	—A broader range of problems can be identified and strategies discussed —Patients help patients —Strategies suggested by other patients may be more credible —Promotes self-awareness, changes in attitude, problem-solving	—Requires a skilled group-facilitator —Takes time for group members to develop trust and become cohesive —Some individuals are uncomfortable in a group situation —May digress from topic
Demonstration Used to teach a skill or procedure step by step. Learner may be an active or passive participant	—Can be done for 1–30 patients for skill-orientated learning —Good for initiating new behaviours. Safer when patient takes over	—Requires skilled demonstrator —Components of new skill need to be separated which is time-consuming in planning and demonstrating
Role-play The learner responds spontaneously to a planned event. He acts out a real or hypothetical situation and is able to experience responses, and select and practise alternative, new behaviours	—Allows learner to practise new responses and behaviours in a safe environment — Develops self-awareness; individual becomes sensitive to stresses, tensions, and helps work through these —Brings about attitude changes	—Many find role-playing uncomfortable —Needs a skilled facilitator
Lecture A structured presentation by a qualified person or expert to a group that may be small or large	—Efficient way to convey knowledge —Highly credible; lecturer can broaden the way people see a situation —Can be inspirational and/or entertaining —Is structured and precisely timed —Can reach a large number of people	—Learner often very passive and uninvolved. —Lecture may not cover learner's needs —Requires a prolonged span of attention by the learner
Reading material Appropriate printed information is supplied in the form of pamphlets, articles, books which may contain illustrations	—Efficient —Can be easily prepared —Easy to reproduce and revise —Can combine visual (i.e. diagrams, pictures) with printed material —Can be used independently and retained for future reference	—Requires reading skills —Non-interactive when used on its own —May not address patient's questions —Learning tends to be fact-oriented
Tape/slide Slides are used to present visual material which is synchronized with a prepared and taped audio presentation, lecture or discussion	—Can provide a concise summary of knowledge, skills —Can be used individually or in a small or large group (by projection) —Can be repeated as often as necessary at little cost —Slides can be updated —Can be used independently	—Relatively high development costs —Must be focused and short —Requires appropriate hardware (synchronized tape–slide unit) —Requires hearing and visual acuity
Videotape/cassettes Material is recorded and filmed; sound and visual material are presented concurrently	—Television media familiar to most —Can present facts, demonstrate skills —Can be repeated as often as necessary at little cost —Can be used individually and for small groups —Can operate independently	—High development costs —Updating portions difficult —Requires hardware (video playback equipment) —Requires hearing and visual acuity

*Mitchell (1974).

group of patients. Having learning resources (e.g. pamphlets, books, insulin syringe and needle) available for use by the patient is very helpful and frequently initiates questions and problem-solving sessions.

All teaching activities should be documented on the patients' record with a description of the patient's response and progress.

EVALUATION

Evaluation of the teaching programme and the patient's learning should be continuous. Revisions are made as indicated and in some instances are made on the spot if the patient is not responding positively to the planned strategy. Information may be repeated and examples to which he can relate are used. Outcomes of teaching are assessed—what effect the teaching had, whether the objectives have been met, and whether the patient has acquired the knowledge and skills he needs. Is his anxiety and uncertainty reduced? Is he becoming more involved in decision making and in his care? In a few instances, tools such as paper and pencil tests may be used to evaluate knowledge. Role-playing or simulation may be used to assess changes in the patient's behavioural responses and in his ability to apply knowledge to real-life situations. The patient must also be an active participant in the ongoing and final evaluation of the educational plan. Observation and feedback are the primary ways in which the nurse determines if behavioural change has occurred.

Achievement, or lack of it, in meeting the expected outcomes is documented on the health record. If the objectives have not been met, the nurse and patient reassess learning needs, identify factors hindering learning and develop a revised plan to meet the deficit. If the objectives have been met, new learning objectives may be developed that build on the level of knowledge and skills acquired.

Discharge Planning

Learning health-care and health-management skills requires time for assimilation and practice. It also requires a period of testing in the home and community where the new behaviour is applied and integrated into the patient's daily routine and life-style. One learning programme in one health-care setting rarely provides the patient and family with the opportunity to achieve fully their established goals. When the patient leaves the hospital, referrals may be made to community health services who can provide further information and resources necessary for the patient and family. The patient may also be introduced to relevant self-help groups and organizations in the community. Written information and instruc-

tions are given to the patient for future reference which will reinforce what he has been taught.

References and Further Reading

BOOKS

Bandler R & Grinder J (1975) *The Structure of Magic*, Volumes I & II. Palo Alto, CA: Science and Behavior Books.

Boore JRP (1978) *Prescription for Recovery*. London: Royal College of Nursing.

Brim OG Jr & Wheeler S (1966) *Socialization After Childhood: Two Essays*. New York: John Wiley.

Brundage DH & Mackeracher D (1980) *Adult Learning Principles and Their Application to Program Planning*. Toronto, Ontario: Ministry of Health.

Chatham MAH & Knapp BL (1982) *Patient Education Handbook*. Bowie, MD: Robert J Brady.

Combs AW (1974) Humanistic approach to learning in adults. In RW Bortner (ed.), *Adults as Learners*. Proceedings of a conference held at the Institute for the Study of Human Development, Pennsylvania State University, University Park.

Cropley AJ (1977) *Lifelong Education: A Psychological Analysis*. Publication of the Unesco Institute of Education. Toronto: Pergamon Press.

Doak C, Doak L & Root, LH (1985) *Teaching Patients with Low Literacy Skills*. London: JB Lipincott.

Elwes L & Simnett I (1985) *Promoting Health, A Practical Guide to Health Education*. Chichester: John Wiley.

Freedman CR (1978) *Teaching Patients*. San Diego: Coursware.

Goslin DA (ed) (1969) *Handbook of Socialization Theory and Research*. Chicago: Rand McNally.

Green LW, Kreuter M, Partridge KB, & Dieds SG (1979) *Health Education Planning: A Diagnostic Approach*. Palo Alto, CA: Mayfield.

Hayward J (1975) *Information: A Prescription Against Pain*. London: Royal College of Nursing.

Health Education Council (1980) *Helping People to Stop Smoking, A Guide for Hospital and Community Nurses*. London: Health Education Council.

Henley A (1979) *Asian Patients in Hospital and at Home*. The King's Fund.

Katz D & Kahn RL (1970) Communication: the flow of information. In JH Campbell & HW Helper (eds), *Dimensions in Communication: Readings*, 2nd ed. Belmont, CA: Wadsworth.

Kidd, JR (1973) *How adults learn*, Revised ed. New York: Association Press.

Knowles MS (1970) The Modern Practice of Adult Education. New York: Association Press.

Knowles M (1975) *Self-Directed Learning*. New York: Association Press.

Kolb DA & Fry R (1975) Towards an applied theory of experiential learning. In CL Cooper (ed.), *Theories of Group Processes*. London: John Wiley.

Maslow A (1970) *The Farther Reaches of Human Nature*. New York: Viking.

McClusky HY (1970) An approach of a differential psychology of the adult potential. In SM Grabowski (ed.), *Adult Learning and Instruction*. Syracuse, NY: ERIC Clearinghouse on Adult Education.

McLaren JA (1975) *Preference for Structure in Adult Learning Situations as a Function of Conceptual Level*. Unpublished master's thesis, University of Toronto.

Megenity JS & Megenity J (1982) *Patient Teaching: Theories, Techniques and Strategies*. Bowie, MD: Robert J. Brady.

Mice PR & Roso HS (1975) *Health Education and Behavioural Science*. Oakland, CA: Third Party Association.

Mitchell DLM (1974) *Development of Patient Education Programs*. Proceedings of the Canadian Congress of Rehabilitation, March 1974.

Narrow BW (1979) *Patient Teaching in Nursing Practice*. New York: John Wiley.

Nightingale F (1970) *Notes on Nursing: What It Is About and What It Is Not*. London: Gerald Duckworth. (First published by Harrison & Sons, 1859).

Pender NJ (1982) *Health Promotion in Nursing Practice*, Norwalk, CT: Appleton-Century-Croft.

Redman BK (1982) *The Process of Patient Education*, 5th ed. St Louis: CV Mosby.

Rogers J (1977) *Adults Learning*, 2nd ed. Milton Keynes: Open University Press.

Rubin LJ (1969) *A Study on the Continuing Education of Teachers*. Santa Barbara, CA: Center for Coordinated Education, University of California. Also available as ED 036 487.

Satow A & Evans M (1985) *Working with Groups*, Health Education Council/Tacade Publications.

Simpson JEP & Levitt R (eds) (1981) *Going Home*. Edinburgh: Churchill Livingstone.

Smith RM (1976) *Learning How to Learn in Adult Education*, Information Series no. 10. De Kalb, IL ERIC Clearinghouse in Career Education. Also available as ED 132 245.

Squyres WD (ed.) (1980) *Patient Education: An Inquiry into the State of the Art*. New York: Springer.

Toffler A (1970) *Future shock*. New York: Random House.

Tough AM (1971) *The Adult's Learning Projects*. Toronto: Ontario Institute for Studies in Education.

Training in Health and Race (1985) *Black Women and the Maternity Services*. Training in Health and Race.

Wilson-Barnett J (ed) (1983) *Patient Training*. Edinburgh: Churchill Livingstone.

PERIODICALS

Bream S (1985) Teaching the elderly about drugs. *Nurs. Times*, 17 July.

Brubacker BH (1983) Health promotion: a linguistic analysis. *Adv. Nurs. Sci.*, Vol. 5 No. 3, pp. 1–14.

Bruhn JG, Cordova D, Williams JA & Fuenter RG (1979) The wellness process. *J. Community Health*, Vol. 2, No. 3, pp. 209–221.

Cawley R et al (1976) Cognitive styles and the adult learner. *Adult Educ.*, Vol. 26 No. 2, pp. 101–116.

Cooke J (1986) Lip service. *Nurs. Times*, 1 January.

Cohen NH (1980) Three steps to better patients. *Nurs. '80*, Vol. 10 No. 2, pp. 72–74.

Cohen SA (1981) Patient education: a review of the literature. *J. Adv. Nurs.*, Vol. 6 No. 1, pp. 11–18.

Corkadel L & McGlashan RN (1982) A practical approach to patient teaching. *J. Cont. Educ. Nurs.*, Vol. 14 No. 1, pp. 9–15.

De Haes WFM (1982) Patient education: a component of health education. *Patient Couns. Health Educ.*, Vol. 4 No. 2, pp. 95–102.

Dodge JS (1972) What patients should be told: patients' and nurses' beliefs. *Am. J. Nurs.*, pp. 1852–1854.

Flynn JB & Griffin PA (1984) Health promotion in acute care settings. *Nurs. Clin. N. Am.*, Vol. 19 No. 2, pp. 239–250.

Garraway WM, Akhtar AJ, Hockey L & Prescott RJ (1980) Management of acute stroke in the elderly: follow-up of a controlled trial. *Br. Med. J.* Vol. 281, pp. 827–829.

Gould D (1984) Time to explain. *Nurs. Mirr.* 22 February.

Hopps L (1983) A case for patient teaching. *Nurs. Times*, 7 December.

Jang, NK & Becker MH (1984) Contingency contracting to enhance patient compliance: a review. *Patient Educ. Couns.*, Vol 5 No. 4, pp. 165–177.

Jenny J (1978) A strategy for patient teaching. *J. Adv. Nurs.*, Vol. 3 No. 4, pp. 341–348.

Johnson J (1982) The effects of a patient education course on persons with a chronic illness, *Cancer Nurs.*, Vol. 5 No. 2, pp. 117–123.

King I & Tarisitano B (1982) The effect of structured and unstructured preoperative teaching: a replication. *Nurs. Res.*, Vol. 31 No. 6, pp. 324–329.

Kogan HN & Betrus PA (1984) Self-management: a nursing mode of therapeutic influence. *Adv. Nurs. Sci.*, Vol. 6 No. 4, pp. 55–73.

Lindeman CA & Van Aernam B (1971) Nursing interventions with the presurgical patient: the effects of structured and unstructured preoperative teaching. *Nurs. Res.*, Vol. 20 No. 4, pp. 319–327.

Logan M (1984) Health contracting: the client's perspective. *Cancer Nurs.*, Vol. 80 No. 4, pp. 27–29.

McKenney JL & Keen PGW (1974) How managers' minds work. *Harvard Business Rev.*, Vol. 52 No. 3, pp. 79–90.

McKenzie L (1977) The issue of andragogy. *Adult Educ.*, Vol. 27 No. 4, pp. 225–229.

Macleod C Jill & Webb P (1985) Health education—a basis for professional nursing practice. *Nurs. Educ. Today*, Vol. 5, pp. 210–214.

Moore PV & Williamson GC (1981) Health promotion: evaluation of a concept. *Nurs. Clin. N. Am.*, Vol. 19 No. 2, pp. 195–206.

Roberts CS (1982) Identifying the real patient problems. *Nurs. Clin. N. Am.*, Vol. 17 No. 3, pp. 481–489.

Sloan PJM (1984) Survey of patient information booklets. *Br. Med. J.*, Vol. 288 No. 6421, pp. 915–919.

Smith JP (1979) The challenge of health education for nurses in the 1980s, *J Adv. Nurs.*, Vol. 4 No. 5, pp. 531–543.

Stanton M (1983) A conceptual model for the implementation of patient education in the general short-term hospital. *Patient Educ. Couns.*, Vol. 5 No. 3, pp. 130–134.

Steckel SB (1982) Predicting, measuring, implementing and following up on patient compliance. *Nurs. Clin. N. Am.*, Vol. 17 No. 3, pp. 491–498.

Walsh PL (1982) Design considerations for adult patient education, *Patient Couns. Health Educ.*, Vol.4 No. 5, pp. 84–88.

Wilson-Barnett J (1981) Keeping patients informed. *Nursing*, Vol. 31, November.

Wilson–Barnett J & Osborne J (1983) Studies evaluating patient teaching: implications for practice. *Int. J. Nurs. Stud.*, Vol. 20 No. 1, pp. 33–44.

Wise PS (1979) Barriers (or enhancers) to adult patient education. *J. Cont. Ed. Nurs.*, Vol. 10 No. 6, pp. 11–16.

Zangari ME & Duffy P (1980) Contracting with patients in day-to-day practice. *Am. J. Nurs.*, Vol. 80 No. 3, pp. 451–455.

Zemble S (1983) Teaching people to manage their health. *Nurs. Manage.*, Vol. 14 No. 3, pp. 36–38.

3
The Nurse and Rehabilitation

Rehabilitation is a developing concept in health care. It is defined as that set of processes whereby an individual is assisted, through direct care and learning activities, to achieve the level of physical, mental, social and occupational functioning which will provide both a satisfactory and fulfilling life. In the presence of major disability, rehabilitation requires the participation of many health disciplines, the patient and those most important to him.

The multidisciplinary team consists of a group of individuals who will work together towards a common goal—the rehabilitation of the patient. The multidisciplinary team most usually includes nurses, doctors, occupational therapists, physiotherapists, medical social workers and, depending on the individual requirements of the patient, may include speech therapists, psychologists, dietitians, surgical appliance fitters, pharmacists and the disablement resettlement officer. The most important members of the multidisciplinary team are the patient and his family.

The nurse involved in helping the patient to achieve the goal of a satisfactory and fulfilling life, directs her efforts to four areas:
1 The practice of nursing care
2 Teaching of skills and concepts
3 Coordination of certain activities of the patient's programme
4 Representing her discipline on the multidisciplinary team

Practice of Nursing Care

Nursing care is the term used to describe the types of activities undertaken on behalf of the patient. It includes not only practical skills but also interpersonal and teaching skills. Initially, the nursing care is directed towards those necessary human activities which the patient can no longer perform for himself. Hygiene, nutrition, elimination, the prevention of decubitus ulcers, and personal safety are high on the list of priorities. As the nurse assesses the patient to determine where his needs lie in relation to these areas, she also determines the strengths and capabilities that the patient possesses so that these can be incorporated in the care plan. Those persons closest to the patient are included in the assessment so that they can be supported and assisted along with the patient.

The nurse uses her knowledge about the injury or disease process affecting the patient to assist her in planning the patient's care. In conjunction with her practical and technical nursing skills, the nurse will have to use all her communication skills to assist and support patients and families who are struggling with new, bewildering and often frightening situations.

It may be argued that the rehabilitation nurse's role is no different from that of nurses in other areas of health care. What is different though is the order of priorities set. A move is made from the life-saving activities necessary in the acute phase of the illness to the life-style and learning considerations required because of the loss of function.

Teaching

Teaching activities are an integral part of the nurse's role in rehabilitation. The patient's attainment of a satisfactory and fulfilling life-style is not only based upon excellent physical care, but also on the learning of new approaches to self-care. If complete self-care is an unattainable goal because of the nature of the disability then the patient requires sufficient knowledge about his planned care to direct others in the provision of it; teaching and learning are therefore necessary in rehabilitation programmes. Through both formal and informal teaching–learning sessions, patients, their families or friends should gradually be able to assume responsibility for the patient's everyday care, to understand the reasons for this care and to recognize when the patient may require professional support.

Preparation for teaching patients, families and friends how to give planned care begins with an assessment of their learning needs, their understanding of normal body functions, what is involved in the presenting disabilities and why, their understanding of their role in providing care, and any experience they may have had in caring for other disabled or ill persons. Formal assessment using an outline or guide is recommended. This assumes that all the important areas are assessed and helps to avoid making assumptions about any learner's knowledge or skill.

Once the assessment is done, the nurse, together with the patient and his family, defines clear, measurable goals, including what is to be learned, the methods to be used and what outcomes can be expected. Once the goals have been set the content to be taught can be organized and a timetable established which will ensure participation by all.

The nurse uses care plans to document the mutually determined goals. She ensures that these are regularly evaluated and updated as progress is made. A summary of the learner's newly acquired knowledge and skills is important to show that the set goals are relevant to the disability and the learner's needs, that the material presented was understood and that the learners demonstrated their skill in providing or directing care. Care plans also allow other nurses and members of the multidisciplinary team to know what learning is required and how it is to be presented. They also provide a plan which allows for continuity of input.

Throughout this process the nurse should be aware that the patient, together with his family or friends, may encounter difficulties in putting the learning into practice after the patient's discharge. Different facilities, anxiety or a belief that certain practices are required only in hospital or rehabilitation settings are factors contributing to practice breakdown. The nurse may prevent unnecessary hospitalization for the patient if the patient, family or friends are provided with a list of names, addresses and telephone numbers to be contacted if, and when, questions or difficulties arise.

In summary, the teaching process involves:
- Assessment of learning needs
- Negotiation of learning goals with the learners
- Development of content and methods for teaching
- Presentation of material
- Evaluation of learning
- Plans for follow up (as required)

Coordination of the Rehabilitation Programme

The rehabilitation programme for the patient is planned and implemented by members of several disciplines. The nurse coordinates these activities, ensuring that all members of the multidisciplinary team are aware of one another's activities and the patient's mental and physical status. While it appears as a simple task on the surface, the nurse has responsibility for more than one patient, and in any given day may need to communicate with and coordinate up to 20 or 30 people. Well-developed communication and organizational skills are essential.

Since the coordination of activities involves the patient and family as well as the team members providing treatment, it is essential that communication with the nurse takes place on a regular basis. The nurse needs to know not only where and at what time treatments are being given, but also what stage of treatment and learning the patient has reached. This information allows the nursing team to reinforce skills learned by the patient, alter the patient care plan to reflect these skills and help the family understand the patient's progress. Ideally, the nurse's coordination will result in the patient being in the right place at the right time with all the necessary people being aware of what is happening or not happening, and providing the patient with both appropriate encouragement and support to ensure full benefit from the rehabilitation programme.

Representation of all the Multidisciplinary Team

The nurse's role as a member of the multidisciplinary team is of great importance. Her continual contact with the patient throughout the 24 hours provides the opportunity for a greater understanding of the patient's physical and mental needs and progress, which she can communicate to her colleagues in the multidisciplinary team responsible for the individual patient's programme.

PLANNING PATIENT CARE

THE ACUTE PHASE

Primary goals for patients during the acute phase of the illness are directed towards their survival and recovery—but, at the same time, towards the prevention of complications arising as a result of the illness or injury or resultant immobility, so that recovery can be achieved with a minimum of dysfunction or complications.

The risk of complications exists for all acutely ill patients. This risk is increased in the presence of neurological damage resulting in alterations in motor and/or sensory function or levels of consciousness and in enforced immobilization as part of treatment. Any invasive procedure or treatment also increases the risk of complications.

Assessment

To plan effective nursing care the nurse needs to be able to assess the patient's present needs. Information is needed not only about present needs, but also about the patient's previous physiological, psychological, occupational and social functioning which may affect long-range goals.

The care plan must also include measures to prevent potential problems: for example skin breakdown, muscle and tendon contracture and reduced joint movement, alteration in elimination, alteration in breathing pattern, and the potential for infection.

Potential patient problems (see Table 3.1)

The potential patient problems are listed below, and the planning and implementation of nursing care are discussed.

Table 3.1 Nursing diagnoses and goals in the acute phase of an illness/injury.

Potential patient problems	Goal
1 Potential for skin breakdown	Skin is clean, supple and intact
2 Potential for muscle contractures and joint ankyloses	Muscles are free from contractures; joints mobile
3 Alteration in elimination (bowel and bladder)	An acceptable pattern of elimination is established and/or maintained
4 Potential for alteration in breathing pattern	Adequate O$_2$ intake is maintained
5 Potential for infection	Patient is infection free. If infections develop, they should be identified and treated promptly

1. POTENTIAL FOR SKIN BREAKDOWN

There is a potential for skin breakdown due to prolonged pressure over bony prominences. The *goal* is that the patient's skin remains intact.

Prolonged pressure, particularly over bony prominences, compresses the blood vessels bringing nourishment to the skin. This results in necrosis and sloughing of the tissues in that area (decubitus ulcer/pressure sore[1]). Turning and repositioning the patient every 1–2 hours allows for normal blood flow and prevents ulcer formation. When turning the patient the nurse examines the skin over the bony prominences for redness or other damage. The use of pressure-relieving devices (e.g. ripple mattresses, water beds or low air loss beds) is helpful in preventing tissue breakdown. It is important to remember that special mattresses designed to relieve pressure are not sufficient alone to prevent skin breakdown but may allow for an extension in the time between turning. If the patient is experiencing muscle spasm, the use of fleece-lined elbow and heel protectors assists in preventing tissue breakdown from the resulting friction. Attention will also need to be directed towards hydration and nutritional levels which will contribute towards the integrity of the patient's skin. (For more detailed information on decubitis ulcers see pp. 1041–1044.)

2. POTENTIAL FOR REDUCED JOINT MOVEMENT

Muscle contractures may develop due to neuromuscular pathology or maintenance of one position over

[1] Dinsdale (1974), p. 151.

an extended period of time. The *goal* is that the patient is free of contractures.

Prolonged immobility, with or without spasticity, results in contracture and joint stiffness. Passive range of movement exercises (under the supervision of a physiotherapist) contribute to the prevention of contracture. Positioning of the patient to break down existing spasticity helps to reduce the risk of contracture formation. Persons who have had strokes are at great risk of developing contractures. Positioning for these patients is very important; efforts are directed toward the following objectives:

- Encouraging awareness of the affected side
- Providing as near normal sensory input as possible
- Encouraging relaxation of spastic limbs by breaking up spastic patterns
- Providing support for paralysed limbs to prevent stretching of soft tissue structures (tendons and ligaments), when muscular support and sensation have been lost
- Encouraging positions which will not facilitate or reinforce the typical patterns of spasticity
- Relieving pain and providing maximum comfort for the patient
- Preventing tissue breakdown and the development of decubitus ulcers

Bed positioning
This includes back- and side-lying. The bed should have a firm base.

Back-lying. To create sensory input and facilitate bilateral body awareness, the nurse should ensure that the patient's head is tilted to the midline and that his shoulders are aligned with the pelvis. The head should be supported on one pillow with the shoulders on the mattress (see Fig. 3.1); this counteracts the tendency for the head to tilt and breaks up extensor spasm. If the patient has cardiac or respiratory problems, more than one pillow may be necessary under the head and shoulders. The main consideration when positioning the arm is to give adequate support for weak muscles and to break up spastic patterns. One small pillow is placed under the shoulder to support the scapula and one lengthwise under the extended arm. The arm is in slight elevation and abduction with the hand facing the body, the fingers loosely spread on the pillow and the thumb away from the palm. If problems with pain or spasticity are present, this arm position can be altered to fit the needs of the patient, e.g. slight flexion of the elbow or pronation of the arm.

The shoulders and pelvis should be aligned, with no undue trunk side flexion. Positioning the affected leg follows the same principles as with the arm. Weak muscles should be supported and strong spastic patterns broken up, while appropriate sensory stimulation is provided to facilitate awareness. With a flaccid or slightly spastic leg, a pillow is placed lengthwise under the leg, putting it in slight abduction with the knee in flexion. A trochanteric roll on the outside of the thigh may be used if external rotation is not prevented by one pillow. If the affected hip is painful, then a small pillow may be placed under it, raising it slightly and giving it support. With severe spasticity, a few degrees of knee flexion are not enough. A wedge may be placed under the knee, but care must be taken that there is no outward rotation of the leg. In this position, a special point to remember is that the feet should not be touching the footboard as this increases any spasticity already present in the leg. A space should remain between the mattress and the footboard to keep the heel on the unaffected side free from pressure. While the use of two pillows under the knees can help to prevent pressure on the heel of the affected foot, the heel should be checked frequently for redness. If redness does occur, a heel protector is used.

Side-lying. Side-lying should be alternated with back-lying; normal rolling into the position is encouraged, turning head and shoulders first and then the knees. During the early acute phase of the patient's treatment when sensory loss and flaccidity are most marked, lying on the affected side is discouraged as this places a stretch on the soft tissues around the shoulders, often resulting in pain. With the patient lying on the unaffected side, the affected arm is brought forward into the patient's visual field to encourage awareness of the arm and its position in relation to the rest of the body. The patient's head should be positioned on one pillow with the shoulder on the mattress. The unaffected arm can be

placed in one of three positions in front of the patient: two positions with the arm flexed, and one with the arm extended (see Fig. 3.2). The extended position is not often used as it is awkward in a single bed. The shoulder is brought forward and the arm flexed, and placed with the palm resting downward. The first of the two flexed positions is with the palms together, the thumbs and fingers extended and placed under the face and the elbow supported by a pillow. This promotes awareness of the affected hand because it can be felt against the face. Some patients may find it more comfortable to use the second flexed position, which is to rest the affected forearm on the pillow in front of the face. A single thickness of pillow is required but should be thick enough to prevent excessive adduction of the arm. Again, the fingers are extended with the thumb away from the palm and within the patient's field of vision.

When positioning the lower extremities, the affected leg is flexed and supported with one pillow which prevents excessive adduction of that leg and stretching of the muscles around the hip. The unaffected leg is positioned behind the affected leg and is slightly flexed. Ankles are in a neutral position. Care is taken to relieve pressure on the external malleolus of the unaffected leg. The trunk is rotated slightly forward. A pillow can be used to support the small of the back for stability. The patient may find side-lying difficult to maintain because of a lack of balance, equilibrium reaction, and loss of depth perception.[2]

---

[2] Van Hullenaar (1982).

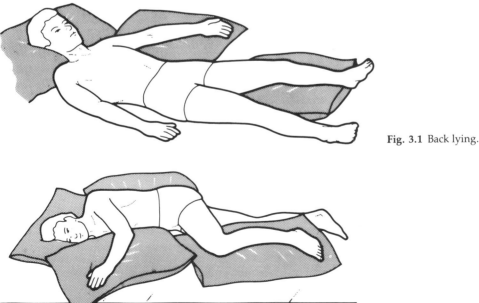

Fig. 3.1 Back lying.

Fig. 3.2 Side lying.

While these positions are directed towards patients with strokes the principles involved are relevant for any patient with muscle spasticity.

In some situations (e.g. severe head injury), splinting of the extremities may be required because of severe spasticity. This intervention, and the prescribing of antispasmodics are carried out on orders from the medical staff.

3. POTENTIAL FOR ALTERATIONS IN ELIMINATION

Alterations in elimination (bowel and bladder) may be due to neuromuscular pathology, alterations in level of consciousness, immobility or dietary/fluid intake alterations. The *goal* is to maintain bowel and bladder elimination.

Bladder elimination
Neurogenic shock (see p. 386), systemic shock or sudden changes in fluid intake and activity level are some of the causes of interference in urinary elimination. Patients in a state of systemic shock should be carefully observed for renal impairment. The medical staff must be notified immediately if the urinary output is less than 35 ml per hour.

Neurogenic shock depresses the neuromuscular responses of the urinary bladder and pelvic floor; musculature becomes flaccid and urine is retained, often in large quantities. This retention, with or without overflow, can increase blood pressure, often rapidly, to hazardous levels. Prolonged distension of the bladder may damage the nerve responses (both somatic and autonomic) in the bladder walls producing long-term difficulties in bladder contractions. Introduction of an indwelling catheter or intermittent catheterization (the latter is preferable) ensures emptying of the bladder and reduces the risk of complications. An accurate record of fluid intake and urine output identifies changes in urinary output.

Prolonged use of an indwelling catheter may be responsible for the development of serious long-term urinary tract problems, including bladder calculi, infection, urethral irritation or erosion. Minimal disruption of the drainage system, meticulous perineal and catheter hygiene, adequate fluid intake and removal of the catheter as soon as possible are ways of reducing the risk of urinary tract dysfunction. The use of intermittent catheterization, to ensure urinary elimination with the fewest problems, is decided upon after assessment of the patient's total physical condition has been carried out. If excessive agitation or movement of injured limbs is involved, an indwelling catheter may be the best approach (see Chapter 21).

Bowel elimination
Spontaneous evacuation of the bowels does not occur if the patient is in spinal shock; the bowel is atonic during this phase and impaction readily develops. A full bowel affects blood pressure in the same way as a distended bladder; consequently a routine of bowel evacuation using enemas or suppositories should be established. An awareness of the patient's previous bowel habits assists in establishing the usual time for this activity. Enemata are discontinued when the neurogenic shock resolves; an appropriate routine using less harsh methods is then established.

Immobility, alterations in the usual fluid and nutritional intake and medications also contribute to alterations in normal bowel function. Constipation is the most common complication in these instances and should be addressed as described on page 519. Suppositories are often the most helpful intervention; the action time of such medication should be noted so that the nurse ensures that the bed is prepared and, if possible, the patient should be positioned to minimize effort, discomfort and soiling.

If bowel retraining is required, the establishment of a specific time for this process is as important as the selection of the type of routine used (see p. 519).

4. POTENTIAL FOR ALTERATION IN BREATHING PATTERN

Alteration in breathing pattern may develop due to neuromuscular impairment, enforced immobility and/or altered level of consciousness. The *goal* is to maintain adequate oxygen intake and carbon dioxide expiration.

Patients with no apparent respiratory problems still need to be assessed frequently for changes in respiration, including dyspnoea, use of accessory muscles, altered chest expansion, ability to cough, persistent cough, respiratory depth changes and the presence of crackles and wheezes. Unless contraindicated by the treatment or illness/injury, the patient is positioned to facilitate unobstructed air entry and maximum lung expansion. If crackles and wheezes develop, a routine is established which involves percussion to loosen secretions which are removed by suctioning or expectoration. Those persons with a history of lung disease or neuromuscular impairment are at the greatest risk (see Chapter 16).

5. POTENTIAL FOR INFECTION

There is a potential for infection due to invasive lines (i.e. arterial, venous and urinary catheters), existing pathology or immobility. The *goal* is that the patient remains infection free or if infection develops, it is promptly treated.

Arterial and venous lines, urinary catheters, suction and drainage tubing are commonly used when the patient requires acute care. These are major risk factors for infection. The risk of infection can be reduced by:

- Maintenance of strict aseptic techniques in the management of all peripheral lines
- Coordination of entry into lines to keep the number of entries to the minimum
- Prompt identification and reporting of signs and symptoms of infection (see Chapter 5).
- Compliance with existing treatment regimens

The above diagnosis may be far down the list of the nurse's priorities for providing care to acutely ill patients because of the need for those activities directed towards stabilizing, treating and diagnosing the patient. If potential problems are not addressed, patients may acquire a problem, such as infection, which adds to their life-threatening situation and discomfort and which will extend their hospital stay.

REHABILITATION PHASE

The preceding discussion relates to nursing actions which may prevent or relieve additional physical problems beyond those resulting from the patient's primary illness or injury. Priorities set during the rehabilitation phase of care are directed towards maintaining life and the integrity of basic bodily functions. Once the patient's condition has stabilized, the priorities shift towards increasing the patient's control over his care. Depending on the severity of the disability, this control may involve knowing what needs to be done to ensure personal care is properly carried out and being able to direct others in the care or it may involve re-establishing independence in caring for one's self.

A satisfactory life-style is not something that can be achieved by learning a few techniques in hospital, nor is there a magical period of time in which success can be guaranteed. Careful planning and negotiating with the rehabilitation team and the patient's family are required to establish long- and short-term goals.

The health-care team establishes with the family and patient what the patient's actual problems are, the implications of these problems and what can be expected for future functioning. This is a difficult time for the patient and family; often the patient has just survived a major illness. The question of whether or not the patient would live has been the most important concern for all involved. When it is learned that the person is indeed going to live, relief is felt in terms of what people already know and have experienced. Life to them may mean the life and function that the patient had before the illness or injury. For those with spinal cord injury, severe head injury, stroke and other severely debilitating problems, previous functional ability may not be possible. Varying periods of time are required for realization of both the immediate effects on the patient and his family and the possible outcomes of rehabilitation.

Assessment

Admission to a rehabilitation programme does not mean that portions of the care plan used when the individual was receiving care in an acute setting are no longer relevant. Ideally, on transfer to another ward the care plan from the acute setting is sent with the patient, so the nurses in the rehabilitation setting quickly acquire a picture of specific problems the patient has experienced and how they were dealt with. This not only provides continuity of care and a firm basis for evaluation of that care, but also gives the patient a sense of confidence as he sees that his needs are known and are being addressed in a familiar manner.

Certain problems can be expected to continue when the patient enters a rehabilitation programme: potential for skin breakdown, potential for contractures, alteration in elimination, and potential for infection are to be expected in the patient with neurological disabilities. To a lesser degree, one may expect a potential for alterations in breathing pattern, particularly if the disease or injury has affected the motor function of the chest muscles and/or the diaphragm. Actual nursing care problems or diagnoses are identified as the nurse assesses the patient.

Since the patient's present function, as well as his potential for future functioning, is important for the development of a care plan, the nurse requires an understanding of the anatomy and physiology of the nervous system, the musculoskeletal system and the urinary tract. This allows the nurse to deal with the patient's condition and to predict possible function.

Potential patient problems (see Table 3.2)

Table 3.2 Nursing diagnoses and goals in the rehabilitation phase

Potential patient problems	Goal
1 Impaired physical mobility	Attainment of maximum mobility possible
2 Lack of knowledge	Can describe the implications of the illness or injury to life activities. Demonstrates ability to perform necessary activities or direct others to do so
3 Inability to perform self-care	The patient has the skills and processes necessary to carry out self-care activities or direct others to do so
4 Alterations in cognition	The patient is aware of who he is, where he is and why
5 Fear, anxiety, grieving	The patient can discuss with others the meaning of illness or injury to his life. The patient begins to plan for life outside the treatment setting
6 Impaired verbal communication	The patient is able to communicate with others

1. IMPAIRED PHYSICAL MOBILITY

Physical immobility can result from injury, illness or enforced bed rest. Improvement in or total return of functional mobility is the main objective of the patient and his family. The attainment of this *goal* is dependent upon the cause and extent of the impairment, as well as the patient's compliance with exercises and routines developed by the multidisciplinary team. The nurse is involved in several activities as the patient moves through the rehabilitation and treatment plan. The patient's immediate environment is arranged for safety; items such as call-bell, drinks, radio or television switches are placed so they can be seen and reached safely. Touch-sensitive controls may be used if there is debility of the patient's upper extremities. These controls provide independence in operating, for example, call-bells, telephones, audiovisual equipment, lights and typewriters.

The nurse, occupational therapist and physiotherapist cooperate in cooordinating those activities which lead to improved mobility, such as exercise programmes, turning and positioning, transferring (i.e. from bed to chair, chair to toilet, etc.) and the use of frames, crutches and walking sticks. The nurse should be aware of each patient's particular programme so that she can carry out specific activities for the patient, provide supervision and encourage independence according to the stage the patient has achieved in his recovery.

Outcomes for most of the components of an individual's rehabilitation programme are dependent upon the level of mobility which can be achieved. The greater the loss of mobility, the more support systems the patient requires, for example environmental controls, electric or manual wheelchairs, crutches, walking sticks, attendants and periodic supervision.

The patient's goal for total return to independent mobility may be unattainable. In this instance the nurse should provide support to help the patient adjust his goals as he adapts to new means of mobility.

2. LACK OF KNOWLEDGE

The *goal* is for the patient to acquire the knowledge necessary to direct or perform self-care and to begin to build a satisfactory life-style.

The major component of any rehabilitation programme is learning new ways to perform life-activities. The patient and family are taught what to expect as a result of the disease or injury as well as the knowledge and skills required to cope with it. This includes functional skills, the action of drug therapy, availability and use of community resources (supportive, occupational and recreational) and the signs and symptoms which signal the need for medical assistance.

What has to be learned depends upon the presence of other nursing diagnoses. These are discussed briefly below in conjunction with more functional considerations.

If we accept that the outcome of rehabilitation is ideally the establishment of a satisfying and fulfilling life-style, then we must be aware that the patient is unlikely to be able to define what this will be as he moves into his rehabilitation programme. The nurse who is acquainted with the stages experienced in acceptance of loss will be better able to assist patients as they move through denial to acceptance. It is well to remember that there is no defined time-scale for this process; all patients may not experience all the identified stages or may not complete the process before discharge from the rehabilitation programme. It is also important to be aware that the nurse's perception of the severity of an individual's disability is not necessarily how the patient perceives it. These are major points to be considered when learning programmes are planned for a patient's rehabilitation. Negotiation of objectives should be done very carefully as the learner may not understand what he needs to know and may have some unrealistic expectations of what he will be able to accomplish. This includes the patient underestimating as well as overestimating his abilities. The nurse, as a member of the multidisciplinary team, needs to be aware of the need to evaluate and renegotiate the learning plan so that objectives can be deleted or added without the patient feeling unnecessary failure.

3. INABILITY TO PERFORM SELF-CARE

Inability to perform self-care is related to (1) feeding, (2) bathing and general hygiene, (3) dressing/grooming and (4) toileting. Addressing this diagnosis involves teaching patients new ways of performing activities of dailing living (ADL) and is the responsibility of all members of the rehabilitation team.

ADL are those acts performed by all healthy adults as they begin and move through their day. Activities such as turning off the alarm clock, getting out of bed, going to the bathroom and dressing are so fundamental to our lives that we perform them without thinking about their performance. For those who have severe motor loss, these activities must be totally relearned. Relearning basic self-care skills is not particularly interesting and frequently provides a constant reminder of the losses experienced by the patient. However, without these skills, learning new approaches to mobility or new vocational skills is useless.

The self-care diagnosis as defined above needs to be broken down into component parts for comprehensive planning.

Inability to feed oneself

The *goal* is for the patient to be able to eat independently with or without mechanical aids. Patients who have lost full use of one or both arms will have this diagnosis. Determining factors include difficulty in managing cutlery, inability to grasp utensils and move the hand to the mouth. The nurse and the occupational therapist work together to identify the intervention required and what assistive devices may help the patient regain independence in feeding. In many instances the physiotherapist provides an exercise programme which increases the patient's ability to perform this task. The nurse's responsibilities include recognizing the problem, acquiring the relevant resources, and implementing the mutually planned intervention.

Meal-times are social times in western culture. The relearning of feeding skills is often messy and this may be unappetizing to the patient and those around him. Practice time is required to master the equipment and the new approach to feeding (e.g. moving from the dominant hand to the non-dominant; the use of padded or reshaped utensils). During the learning period the patient needs encouragement that he can succeed in feeding himself both effectively and in a socially acceptable way.

Inability to wash and bathe

The *goal* is to establish a procedure which the patient can follow or direct others to follow, which ensures efficient hygiene in a safe manner. The procedure is tailored so that it can be done easily in the patient's own environment.

The nurse, occupational therapist and physiotherapist coordinate their efforts to help patients relearn this function. Exercises to help the patient get in and out of the bath or shower go hand-in-hand with devices such as bath seats and back brushes with long or curved handles. Supervision of patients as they bathe ensures safety, allows for repetition of directions if necessary and for positive feedback.

It is important for those patients who cannot achieve independence in bathing to have sufficient knowledge to direct others in peforming this task. Specific positioning, how to obtain the correct water temperature and the use of any special equipment such as shower chairs should be demonstrated to the patient. Family members or those people who will be providing the patient's supportive care are taught and supervised in bathing activities.

Bathing is of course only one portion of daily hygiene; hair care, shaving, cleaning of teeth and the care of nails are all included and may require approaches different from the ones previously used and especially adapted equipment may be needed. For example, a universal cuff may be used; this is a strap which fits around the patient's hand and which has a small pocket into which a comb, toothbrush or other device may be fitted. This allows a patient who is capable of gross movements only to perform tasks requiring more defined movements.

Inability to dress

The *goal* is for the patient to be able to dress himself or direct others to perform this activity. The learning of dressing techniques in combination with clothing adaptations allows many patients to become independent in dressing. Teaching of these techniques and the clothing alterations are done collaboratively among nurses, occupational therapists and physiotherapists. As with the relearning of all physical skills, physiotherapy is essential. Without the strength to perform the task the patient will fail and may believe that he has lost the ability to perform this activity. Planning for these activities should thus include time to gain this strength, as well as to learn to perform the actual activities themselves.

Inability to use the toilet

The *goal* is for the patient to be able to perform these activities or direct others to do so.

The patient is helped to achieve transferring to and from the toilet, the manipulation of clothing and performing of hygiene measures. Again, nurses and other disciplines cooperate in timing and teaching the necessary skills. The place for these activities in the overall planning is important; it is appropriate to begin the teaching and practice for toileting after the patient has learned to transfer from bed to wheelchair.

Patients who are learning to walk using devices such as crutches, walking sticks, callipers or braces should have demonstrated good balance and management of these devices before beginning independence in toileting. Other considerations may be necessary for those with alterations in elimination (see bowel and bladder retraining, pp. 519 & 763).

These diagnoses address the basic issues related to activities of daily living but do not by any means include all problems patients present with, nor state how the priorities should be set. The patient's ability to participate in an ADL programme may depend on his cognitive level (i.e. his orientation to time, place and person), his ability to concentrate and his ability to learn. While for some this may relate to how he was before his illness or injury most *alterations in cognition* are a result of it.

4. ALTERATION IN COGNITION

Alteration in cognition may be due to brain damage (stroke, head injury) or drug side-effects. The *goal* is for the patient to be oriented to time, place and person. The patient should understand the goals for his/her rehabilitation.

Some patients with severe head injury or dementia may have permanent losses which cannot be recovered, but most can achieve acceptable cognitive functioning.

The elderly who have moved from the acute setting to a rehabilitation programme may appear 'confused' for several reasons, including change of surroundings and routine. A person who has had a stroke or who has received sedation may be attempting to function through the mental haze which may have developed. A careful review of the patient's medications with the doctor and pharmacist on admission and frequently throughout the patient's hospital stay ensures that those required are provided in appropriate dosage. Side-effects should be known and the patient monitored for these; frequently it is the cognitive level that is adversely affected by the drugs being administered.

Consistent repetition of who the patient is, where he is, why he is there and who is speaking to him is a process which helps keep him oriented to reality. Family members should be informed of these activities and why they are being used, since they may be upset when they hear staff constantly saying the same thing, asking the same questions and speaking in ways which they interpret as 'talking down' to their loved one. An explanation as to why this is being done, as well as explaining that complex conversation and activity often causes an increase in the patient's confusion and anxiety, may be sufficient to help families understand. Many who are confused on admission improve rapidly and are oriented to time, place and person within a few days. Persons with severe head injuries may not respond as readily and will require carefully planned approaches usually developed by the team as a whole (see Chapter 10).

5. FEAR, ANXIETY, GRIEVING AND DISTURBED BODY IMAGE

Fear, anxiety, grieving and disturbed body image may occur due to loss of function and lack of understanding of the implications of the loss. The *goal* is for the patient to begin to resolve grief, reduce anxiety and identify personal strengths which can be used in re-establishing independence. The responses—fear, anxiety, etc.—are normal and the patient may experience a combination of these. The nurse, in cooperation with other team members (e.g. social workers, psychologists), works towards helping him to achieve this goal.

- Fear is a specific response to a situation and can be identified by the patient
- Causes of anxiety are often non-specific; the patient may only be able to describe feelings of uneasiness, tension or uncertainty
- Grief is a response to loss. Loss of function may trigger the loss of other things valued by the patient such as career, favourite activities or the companionship of loved ones
- Alteration in body image can occur as a result of functional loss, loss of a limb or body part or an alteration in physical appearance

The intensity of the reaction depends upon the value the patient placed on what has been lost.

It may be difficult or impossible for the nurse to pinpoint the reactions of the patient which define the above diagnoses, and initially these diagnoses may have to be dealt with together.

The nurse's ability and skill in interviewing, listening, supporting and reporting findings accurately are required if the patient's needs and concerns are to be identified, managed expediently and effectively. Expected outcomes include the patient's ability to:

- Identify and discuss his/her fears
- Begin to identify the meaning of the loss(es) to him/her
- Begin to plan in collaboration with the team and family members the care and activities to follow discharge
- Identify strengths which will assist in a meaningful and fulfilling life-style
- Participate fully in the rehabilitation programme

6. IMPAIRED VERBAL COMMUNICATION

Impaired verbal communication may occur in brain damage (stroke, head injury). The *goal* is to establish a communication system which will allow the patient to communicate with others.

When providing care for a patient with an impaired ability to communicate, immediate efforts are made to establish a means of communicating at least some basic concepts. The nurse works cooperatively with the speech therapist as the latter identifies the patient's specific communication deficits and plans a treatment programme. Familiarity with the patient's treatment allows for appropriate reinforcement for the patient and provides for continuity of care.

The speech therapist provides answers to questions such as: 'Is the patient able to understand?'; 'Are there certain words or phrases which the patient can say?'; 'Can the patient read and/or write?'; 'Does the impairment involve the patient's primary language or only secondary ones?'; 'Can the patient recognize objects and pictures?' and; 'Are there particular symbols or gestures which the patient should be encouraged to use?' The nurse uses the answers to these questions when establishing the patient's care plan.

The patient's family and friends are made aware of the communication techniques being used by the rehabilitation team. Prompt introduction of these measures develops communication between patient, family and nursing staff before the patient feels totally cut off from those around him.

Patients with impaired communication may best respond when spoken to in short, simple sentences and in a normal tone of voice. Complex questions are avoided. If perseveration (the automatic repetition of a word or phrase in response to varied stimuli) occurs the patient should be stopped. If the word is an appropriate one (e.g. yes or no) then once the flow of words has stopped the patient is encouraged to respond once and appropriate action is then taken on the request or decision.

Initially, profanity may be the only language a patient can use. It is not understood why this happens but it does not necessarily reflect the person's usual language pattern. The patient who experiences this phenomenon may be distressed by his uncontrolled response and needs reassurance that the nurse does not see him as profane. The nurse informs the patient's family and visitors of the patient's response. This allows them to reinforce positive language patterns and appropriately discourage inappropriate habits. Also, family members and visitors may feel more comfortable about visiting and may spend more time with the patient; feelings of isolation and of being abandoned, which many people with communication loss experience, may, in turn, be lessened.

Summary

Rehabilitation is a process whereby individuals with alterations in their ability to function are assisted in acquiring skills and knowledge that will allow the development of a satisfactory and fulfilling life-style. The ideal outcome of this process is that patients regain or attain independence. If the nature of the patient's illness or injury makes this goal unattainable, then patients are encouraged to use their knowledge to direct others in providing care for them.

Family members and friends of persons with functional loss are included in teaching–learning activities related to techniques of care.

The nursing diagnoses discussed above represent some of the more common patient-care problems related to rehabilitation; it is by no means an all inclusive list. Frequent patient assessment is required to ensure that patients' nursing care problems, both potential and actual, are identified, planned for, implemented and evaluated.

Rehabilitation is not complete when patients are discharged from the rehabilitation setting; rather, they should have received only the knowledge and skills necessary to *begin* to cope with the real world.

References and Further Reading

BOOKS

Anderson ML (1983) *Rehabilitation Nursing: Can We Get There From Here?* Proceedings of the First Canadian Congress of Rehabilitation. Ottawa, Ontario.

Basmajian JV & Kirby RL (1984) *Medical Rehabilitation*. Baltimore: Williams & Wilkins.

Bishop DS (1980) *Behaviour Problems and the Disabled*. Baltimore: Williams & Wilkins.

Evans CD (1981) *Rehabilitation After Severe Head Injury*. Edinburgh: Churchill Livingstone.

Frazer FW (ed.) (1982) *Rehabilitation Within the Community*. London: Faber and Faber.

Levin LS, Katz AH & Holst E (1979) *Self-Care: Lay Initiatives in Health*. New York: Prodist.

Mattingly S (ed.) (1977) *Rehabilitation Today*. London: Update Publications.

Morrissey AB (1957) *The Professional Nurse on the Rehabilitation Team, The Handicapped and their Rehabilitation*, ed. Harry A Pattison. Springfield, Ill: Charles C Thomas.

Mulley GP (1985) *Practical Management of Stroke*. London: Croom Helm.

Pohl ML (1968) *The Teaching Function of the Nursing Practitioner*. Debuque, IA: WC Brown.

Storch J (1982) *Patients' Rights*. Toronto: McGraw-Hill Ryerson.

Van Hullenaar S (1982) Positioning Techniques for the Hemiplegic Patient in Bed and Wheelchair. Paper presented at Stroke Seminar, Hamilton, Ontario, (unpublished).

Werner-Beland JA (1980) *Grief Responses to Long-Term Illness and Disability*. Reston, VA: Reston Publishing.

PERIODICALS

Barkin M, Dolfin D, Herschorn S et al (1983) The urologic care of the spinal cord injury patient. *J. Urol.*, Vol. 129 No. 2, pp. 135–139.

Barry K (1983) A discharge planning protocol conceptualized by a clinical nurse specialist . . . rehabilitative planning. *J. Rehabil. Nurs.*, Vol. 8 No. 5, pp. 27–30.

Brown JW, Leader BJ & Blum CS (1983) Hemiplegic writing in severe aphasia. *Brain Lang.*, Vol. 19 No. 2, pp. 204–205.

Callahan ME (1984) Caring for a stroke patient like me. *Nursing (Horsham)*, Vol. 14 No. 5, pp. 65–67.

Cammermeyer M (1983) A growth model of self-care for neurologically impaired people. *J. Neurosurg. Nurs.*, Vol. 15 No. 5, pp. 299–305.

Clough DH & Mauring JT. (1982) ROM Versus NRx, *J. Gerontol Nurs.*, Vol. 5, pp. 278–286.

Dinsdale SM (1974) Decubitus ulcers: role of pressure and friction in causation, *Arch. Phys. Med Rehabil.*, Vol. 55 No. 4, pp. 147–152.

Dudas S & Stevens KA (1984) Central cord injury: implications for nursing. *J. Neurosurg. Nurs.*, Vol 16 No. 2, pp. 84–88.

Elliott FC (1983) A nursing protocol for anxiety following catastrophic injury. *Rehabil. Nurs.*, Vol. 8 No. 3, pp. 18–20, 38.

Gans JS (1983) Hate in the rehabilitation setting. *Arch. Phys. Med. Rehabil.*, Vol. 64 No. 4, pp. 176–179.

Garber SL et al (1983) Trochanteric pressure in spinal cord injury. *Arch. Phys. Med. Rehabil.*, Vol. 63 No. 11, pp. 549–552.

Goodman-Smith R & Turnbull J (1983) A behavioural approach to the rehabilitation of severely brain-injured adults. *Physiotherapy*, Vol. 69 No. 11, pp. 393–396.

Gruskin AK, Abitante SM, Gorski AT (1983) Auditory feedback device in a patient with left-side neglect. *Arch. Phys. Med. Rehabil.*, Vol. 64 No. 12, pp. 606–607.

Haberman B (1982) Cognitive dysfunction and social rehabilitation in the severely head-injured patient. *J. Neurosurg. Nurs.*, Vol. 14 No. 5, pp. 220–224.

Hamrin E (1982) Early activation in stroke: does it make a difference? *Scand. J. Rehabil. Med.*, Vol. 14 No. 3, pp. 101–109.

Hart G (1983) Strokes causing left vs right hemiplegia: different effects and nursing implications. *Geriatric Nurs.*, Vol. 4 No. 1, pp. 39–43.

Ingram N (1983) Mastering left hemiplegia. *Geriatric Nurs.*, Vol 4 No. 1, p. 42.

Kasmarik PE (1982) The stroke patient: an individual challenge! *J. Gerontol. Nurs.*, Vol. 8 No. 11, pp. 624–629, 661.

Knust SJ & Quarn JM (1983) Integration of self-care theory with rehabilitation nursing. *Rehabil. Nurs.*, Vol. 8 No. 4, pp. 26–28.

Kussofsky A, Wadell I & Nilsson BY (1982) The relationship between sensory impairment and motor recovery in patients with hemiplegia. *Scand. J. Rehabil. Med.*, Vol 14 No. 1, pp. 27–32.

Madorsky JG & Madorsky A (1983) Wheelchair Racing: an important modality in acute rehabilitation after paraplegia. *Arch. Phys. Med. Rehabil.*, Vol. 64 No. 4, pp. 186–187.

Morse HA (1982) 90 Days: a patient shares his perspectives, his humour and his thanks. *Nurs. Manage.*, Vol. 13 No. 9, pp. 34–36.

Newcombe F (1982) The physiological consequences of closed head injury; assessment and rehabilitation. *Injury*, Vol. 14 No. 2, pp. 111–136.

Pinkerton AC & Griffin ML (1983) Rehabilitation outcomes in females with spinal cord injury: a follow-up study. *Paraplegia*, Vol. 21 No. 3, pp. 166–175.

Rinehart MA (1963) Considerations for functional training in adults after head injury. *Phys. Ther.*, Vol. 63 No. 12, pp. 1975–1982.

Rogers JC (1982) The spirit of independence: the evolution of a philosophy. *Am. J. Occup. Ther.*, Vol. 36 No. 2, pp. 709–715.

Solomon J (1982) Sex and the spinal cord injured patient. *J. Neurosurg. Nurs.*, Vol. 14 No. 3, pp. 125–127.

Talmage EW & Collins GR (1983) Physical abilities after head injury: a restrospective study. *Phys. Ther.*, Vol. 63 No. 12, pp. 2010–2017.

Tilton CN & Maloof M (1982) Diagnosing the problems in stroke. *Am. J. Nurs.*, Vol. 82 No. 4, pp. 596–601.

Torrance M (1983) Back on their feet: to do or not to do . . . how rehabilitation begins. *Nurs. Times.*, Vol. 79 No. 43, pp. 24–25.

Weinberg JS (1983) Human sexuality and spinal cord injury. *Nurs. Clin. N. Am.*, Vol. 17 No. 3, pp. 407–419.

Wilcox AC & Oi CW (1984) The unconscious patient: total patient care. *Nursing (Oxford)*, Vol. 2 No. 23, pp. 675–678.

4

Disease: Causes and Tissue Responses

THE NORMAL CELL

The material of which all living matter is composed is referred to as protoplasm. It is organized in discrete microscopic units called cells. There are many different types of cells in the human body; they vary in size, shape, composition and function and are derived from pre-existing cells. They all have certain common characteristics in structure and activity. All body tissues are composed of cells and cellular products.

A knowledge of the organization of the basic structural and functional unit contributes to an understanding of the structure and functions of the body and its component parts. An appreciation of the normal is necessary for recognition of the abnormal as well as for an awareness of the effects of disease and the necessary supportive measures.

Structural Features of a Cell

All cells have three main structural parts at some time in their life cycle: a surface membrane, cytoplasm and a nucleus (see Fig. 4.1).

CELL MEMBRANE

The cell is enveloped by a very thin membranous structure which gives delineation, support and protection to the cell substance, and provides the interface between the cell content and interstitial fluid. The cell or unit membrane is a porous, trilaminar structure composed of lipid and protein molecules. Its semipermeability allows for the selective transfer of water and small molecular solutes in and out of the cell. The unit membrane also plays important roles in the constant movement of the cell surface and the

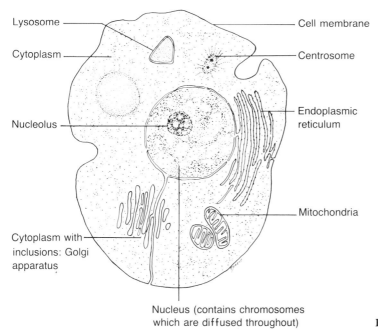

Lysosome — Cell membrane
Cytoplasm — Centrosome
Nucleolus
Endoplasmic reticulum
Mitochondria
Cytoplasm with inclusions: Golgi apparatus
Nucleus (contains chromosomes which are diffused throughout)

Fig. 4.1 Diagram of a typical cell.

entrapment of substances. The adhesive properties of the cell coat or outer surface function to hold the cells together to form tissues. It is also suggested that the cell membrane is capable of differentiating between the body's own cells and alien cells.

CYTOPLASM

Cytoplasm forms the bulk of the cell. Its composition varies according to the specialized function of the cell. For example, the cytoplasm of mature red blood cells contains the haematin–protein compound haemoglobin for the purpose of transporting oxygen; muscle cell cytoplasm has compounds responsible for chemical reactions that bring about a thickening and shortening of the cell (contraction). There is a relatively high concentration of protein, potassium, magnesium, and phosphate in the cytoplasm; this is in contrast with fluid outside the cell where sodium, chloride, and bicarbonate are the predominant electrolytes.

Cytoplasm is in a fluid state, consisting largely of water, and contains several functional structures or organelles—the endoplasmic reticulum, Golgi apparatus, mitochondria, lysosomes and centrioles.

The endoplasmic reticulum is a network of tubules and vesicles that are connected with the nuclear and cell membrane. The channels serve to transfer materials from one part of the cell to another. On the outer surfaces of many parts of the tubules are small granular particles called ribosomes which consist of ribonucleic acid (RNA) and protein. The ribosomes are considered to be responsible for the synthesis of protein substances characteristic of the particular type of cell. The products may be for cell use (e.g. enzymes, structural components) or for secretion.

The Golgi apparatus is a series of small vesicles associated with the endoplasmic reticulum. It is prominent in cells which are involved with secretion; secretions formed by the ribosomes are collected in these vesicles.

The mitochondria are small, oval bodies which vary in number in different cell types according to the level of cell activity. They contain oxidative enzymes to catalyse reactions that liberate energy which is needed for cellular functions. The cells that are high energy producers (e.g. muscle cells) contain more mitochondria than low energy producing cells (e.g. connective tissue cells).

Lysosomes contain hydrolytic enzymes that break down particles that are useless or harmful to the cell. Leucocytes contain an unusual number of these minute bodies in order to destroy organisms and other foreign substances taken into the cells by phagocytosis.

Two cylindrical centrioles situated close to the nucleus play an important role in cell division.

NUCLEUS

The nucleus is a spherical or ovoid body enclosed in a membrane and, in most cells, lies centrally within the cytoplasm. This structure is the vital control centre of the cell; without it the cell cannot reproduce, and its activities cease. An exception to the latter point is the erythrocyte produced by bone marrow cells; as the red blood cell matures, its nucleus is extruded, haemoglobin is formed, and the cell is released into the circulation where it functions as a transport for oxygen for approximately 100–120 days.

The nucleus contains the chromosomes, which determine cell characteristics and transmit the heredity of the cell and the organism from one generation to the next. All human somatic cells contain 23 pairs of chromosomes. When the cell is not in the reproductive phase the chromosomes are scattered throughout the nucleus as long, drawn-out threads. They are readily stainable and may be referred to as chromatin material. Each chromosome consists of a chain of units called genes. The gene is a large, complex molecule of a protein compound known as deoxyribonucleic acid (DNA) which is capable of self-duplication. Each gene has a specific location on a particular chromosome. The DNA of each gene is made up of the same component elements, but the structural arrangement of these varies from one gene to another. The specific sequence of amino acids determines the specific genetic information. The genes contain information necessary for controlling the development and activity of the cells. They do this through directing specific protein synthesis by the cytoplasm. In other words, the DNA determines the cell properties by directing the essential cytoplasmic composition associated with the cell's particular functions. It is suggested that each gene is responsible for the formation and nature of one enzyme which acts as a catalyst.

A second protein found in the nucleus is ribonucleic acid (RNA). It is produced by the DNA and transmits the encoded information of the genes to the ribosomes of the cytoplasm. Within the nuclear material, minute spherical bodies called nucleoli appear. They contain RNA and other proteins concerned with the synthesis of RNA. Three types of RNA molecules have been identified as having important roles in protein synthesis (mRNA functioning as a messenger, tRNA which transports and rRNA which is situated on the ribosomes).[1]

Physiological Activities of the Cell

METABOLISM

Intracellular activites are chemical reactions which are referred to collectively as metabolism. The metabolic processes are of two types. *Catabolism* refers to

---

[1] Guyton (1986) pp. 31–32.

reactions in which there is a chemical breakdown of compounds into simpler compounds or atoms; this breakdown is initiated by enzymes in which glucose, fatty acids and amino acids react with oxygen to release energy. This energy is used to form adenosine triphosphate (ATP) which functions in membrane transport, protein synthesis by the cell and in supplying the energy needed for muscle contraction. New compounds are synthesized from simpler substances during the anabolic process, or *anabolism*. Both types of processes occur to some extent at all times to maintain the cells and perform the functions that contribute to the overall activities and maintenance of the body as a whole. At times the rate of anabolism may exceed that of catabolism and cell substances accumulate; at times of increased body activity, catabolism proceeds more rapidly and cell substances may be markedly reduced.

A requisite to cellular health and normal functioning is the provision of adequate amounts of essential nutrients such as proteins, carbohydrates, minerals and vitamins. The substances used in metabolism are taken into the cell from the immediate extracellular fluid environment. A constant supply of oxygen is necessary for metabolism. Cellular activities cannot be sustained without the products of oxidative processes. The catabolism of many compounds to release energy results in the production of carbon dioxide, which is eliminated from the cell; this elimination of carbon dioxide and the absorption of oxygen comprise cellular respiration. In addition to carbon dioxide, various substances may be formed during metabolism which are of no use to the cell and, if retained, inhibit cellular functions. These waste products are passed out of the cell and are eliminated from the body through an excretory channel. Substances called secretions are formed by some cells to serve a specific useful purpose when discharged. For example, some cells secrete mucus to protect cells from irritating materials; cells of the thyroid secrete thyroxin, which influences the rate of metabolism, particularly the oxidative process, of practically all cells in the body.

The cellular chemical reactions are catalysed by enzymes that are produced by the ribosomes under the direction of the genes via RNA. These catalytic protein compounds are specific; that is, there is a particular enzyme for each type of chemical reaction. The reaction may be to break down a compound, transfer an atom or molecule from one compound to another or rearrange component atoms within a molecule. The breakdown of a complex compound involves a series of reactions and a specific enzyme for each reaction. If one enzyme is lacking, the normal metabolism of the substance is arrested at that level. For example, a specific enzyme is necessary to convert galactose to glucose so that it can be catabolized to carbon dioxide and water and release required energy. If the gene that directs the production of the necessary enzyme is abnormal or absent, the galactose accumulates, resulting in an abnormally low blood sugar level, weakness due to the lack of energy production and mental deficiency as a result of an inadequate supply of glucose to the brain cells. The condition is known as galactosaemia and is classified as an inborn error of metabolism; this implies an inherited enzyme abnormality or deficiency. Similarly, the condition known as phenylketonuria is due to a congenital deficiency of the enzyme that promotes a reaction to convert the amino acid phenylalanine (a component of many proteins) to tyrosine. Phenylalanine accumulates in the blood and spinal fluid and is damaging to the brain, resulting in mental retardation. The absence of the enzyme is detected through its excretion in the urine as phenylpyruvic acid—hence, the name phenylketonuria. If detected soon after birth, a diet low in proteins containing phenylalanine may prevent mental deficiency.

CELLULAR MOVEMENT

Cytoplasm is fluid. Movement of the whole or a part of a cell may occur by the flow of cytoplasm from one part to another in a manner similar to that observed in the amoeba. Leucocytes move in this way in their migration out of the blood stream into extracellular spaces and when they surround and engulf an organism or particle. The movement of a muscle cell (contraction) is achieved by shortening of the cell with a corresponding increase in the thickness; this action is the result of a series of chemical reactions within the cytoplasm. Some cells have cilia, which are fine, hair-like processes of the cytoplasm which quickly swing in one direction and then slowly resume their former position. They move particles along a surface in the direction of their initial lashing motion. Organized movement of definite parts of the cell occurs as the cell proceeds through the reproductive process.

IRRITABILITY

Cells are sensitive and will react to changes in their immediate environment. A change which will initiate a cellular response is referred to as a stimulus. The type of reaction or response of the cell will vary with the type of stimulus and the characteristics of the particular type of cell. Cells may be more irritable to a specific type of stimulus than to others.

REPRODUCTION

New cells are necessary for growth of the organism and for replacement of worn-out cells. They are produced by a cell dividing into two cells, each having a nucleus with 23 pairs of chromosomes as well as cytoplasm with the same properties as those of the parent cell. This process of cell division is referred to as *mitosis*, and it involves a series of changes in which there is a rearrangement of the centrioles and chromosomes and a subsequent division of the nucleus and the whole cell.

The interval between the end of one mitosis and the beginning of the next is referred to as the interphase, or the amitotic or intermitotic phase. The changes characteristic of cell reproduction are described as they occur in the following four phases (Fig. 4.2).

1 *Prophase*. Preceding this initial phase, cell substance is increased, and the DNA duplicates itself. Each chromosome divides longitudinally into two chromatids which remain attached by a centromere. The chromosomes coil spirally becoming shorter and thicker, and appear as distinct entities. The two centrioles move away from each other to opposite poles of the cell and develop fibrils stretching out between them to form a spindle. The nucleoli and nuclear membrane disappear.

2 *Metaphase*. The fibrils of the centrioles grow into the nuclear region to become attached to the centromeres of the chromosomes, which arrange themselves in a line between the two centrioles.

3 *Anaphase*. The two chromatids of each chromosome separate at their centromere; each is attracted by a fibril toward the opposite centriole. This results in an equal number of chromatids— corresponding to the original number of chromosomes (46)—being located in either half of the cell.

4 *Telophase*. The final phase involves nuclear reformation in order to enclose each group of chromatids and constriction of the cytoplasm by indentation of the cell membrane through the centre. The spindle formed by the fibrils disappears, a typical nucleus forms in each half of the cell, and the chromatids lengthen (uncoil) and diffuse irregularly throughout the nucleus. Each pair of centrioles replicates, and final division of the cytoplasm produces two separate cells which are identical in structure to the original parent cell.

Normally, cell reproduction is controlled to meet the tissue needs of the organism; during the growth period and as cells wear out or are destroyed they are produced in a number sufficient to produce or maintain normal tissue mass. Unfortunately, the substance or mechanism by which the rate of cell reproduction is controlled has not yet been identified. In certain disease conditions, such as cancer, this control is lost by some cells and they are produced in excess.

MEIOSIS (REDUCTION DIVISION)

A new organism is conceived by the union of a female gamete (ovum) and a male gamete (sperm). The union forms a single cell from which all the cells of the body are derived. Obviously, the characteristic number of chromosomes (46) must be established in the initial single cell.

Initially, when both the female and male germ cells are produced by the sex glands they contain 23 pairs of chromosomes. During a maturation process, a special type of cell division takes place in which the number of chromosomes is reduced to half. This cell division process is referred to as meiosis, or reduction division. In meiotic cell division, one of each pair of chromosomes passes to an opposite end of the cell. When the two halves separate each daughter cell contains only 23 *single* chromosomes (the haploid number of chromosomes). At conception, the union of the sperm with haploid chromosomes and an ovum with a corresponding number establishes the distinctive 23 *pairs* of chromosomes. The resulting

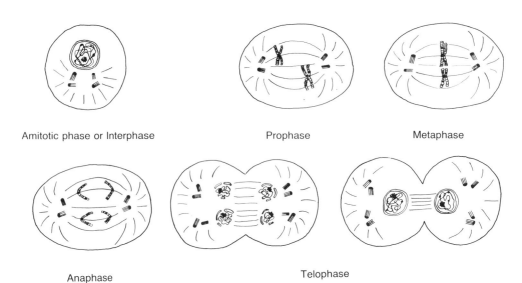

Amitotic phase or Interphase   Prophase   Metaphase

Anaphase   Telophase

Fig. 4.2 Phases of mitosis.

cell rapidly reproduces by mitosis, which continues in order to form the new organism.

MOVEMENT OF SUBSTANCES ACROSS THE CELL MEMBRANE

There is a continuous movement of substances in and out of the cells by physical passive processes and by cellular action. The extracellular fluid, which includes both the interstitial and vascular fluids, is the source of nutrients and other substances that enter the cell. Variations in composition of extracellular and intracellular fluids are essential to the life and functioning of the cell and are selectively maintained by the transport processes of diffusion and active transport.

Active transport involves the chemical combination of a substance with a carrier and requires energy to effect the movement. For example, a much higher concentration of potassium is required within the cells than in the extracellular fluid; however, the reverse is true of sodium. In order to maintain these conditions, the cells actively transport potassium in and sodium out. The active movement of sodium out of the cell and potassium into the cell is called the sodium–potassium pump.[2] The carrier which functions in this process is also able to split the ATP molecule, releasing energy that is necessary to overcome the pressure gradient. Calcium, magnesium and other ions are actively transported by a similar method. The active transport of some substances across membranes is facilitated by a chemical reaction and/or a 'carrier system', details of which in most instances remain unknown.

A method of active transport used with large molecular substances such as protein and fat is pinocytosis. This process involves invagination of the cell membrane at the site of contact with the particle. The molecule sinks into the invaginated area and is surrounded by the membrane. A vesicle is formed which separates from the membrane and is moved into the cytoplasm where it disappears, releasing its contents.

The physical processes concerned with the movement of substances in and out of the cell are diffusion and osmosis.

Diffusion is the continual, spontaneous movement and intermingling of molecules or ions in liquids or gases. The tendency is for the particles to disperse throughout the space in which the solution or gas is contained so as to produce a uniform concentration. Random movement continues when uniformity is achieved. Water, gases and some solutes diffuse readily through a semi-permeable membrane; if the distribution is equal on both sides, the constant random motion of particles results in the movement

of as many particles in one direction as the other. The diffusion of more molecules of a substance in one direction than in the opposite is dependent upon a concentration gradient. Large particles diffuse more slowly than smaller ones.

Diffusion is responsible for the movement of gases between the alveolar air of the lungs and the blood and between the blood and the cells. Similarly, many substances absorbed from the intestine create a pressure gradient between the blood and the interstitial fluid and between the interstitial fluid and the intracellular content; this results in the diffusion of these substances from the blood to the interstitial fluid and on into the cells. In the opposite direction, products of metabolism diffuse from the cells into the interstitial fluid and then into the blood.

Osmosis is the movement of water through a semipermeable membrane from a solution of lesser solute concentration to one of greater concentration. It occurs only when two solutions with different concentrations of solutes are separated by a semipermeable membrane through which the solutes do not readily diffuse. The volume of water that is retained by the solution of greater concentration is dependent upon the osmotic pressure exerted by the solute of that solution. Solutes in a solution tend to hold or attract water; this affinity or drawing power is referred to as osmotic pressure.

Osmosis is illustrated in Fig. 4.3. Fig. 4.3A represents a 5% aqueous solution in compartment X and a 15% aqueous solution in compartment Y, which are separated by a semipermeable membrane. The latter is permeable to the solvent and this particular solute, with the result indicated in A_2. Diffusion of water and the solute occurs, and eventually an equal volume of a homogeneous solution is found in both X and Y compartments.

In Fig. 4.3B the 5% aqueous solution in compartment X is separated from the 15% aqueous solution by a semipermeable membrane that permits the solvent to pass from one compartment to the other (i.e diffuse in both directions), but is impermeable to the solute particles in both solutions. Although the membrane is permeable to the solvent on both sides, the osmotic pressure (drawing power) of the greater number of solute particles in compartment Y results in a net gain in the volume of solvent in that compartment. The water diffusing from X to Y continues to be retained in compartment Y until the hydrostatic pressure created by the solution counteracts the osmotic pressure. The fluid pressure in Y reaches a point that opposes diffusion of water molecules from X to Y.

The degree of osmotic pressure of a solution is proportional to the number of particles of solute. Because the molecular weight of the molecules or ions of the solute does not influence the osmotic pressure, the unit used to quantify osmotic pressure or indicate the concentration according to the

---

[2] Guyton (1986), p. 97.

A   MEMBRANE PERMEABLE TO BOTH SOLUTE AND WATER

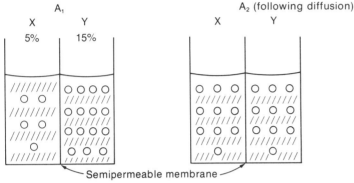

O = Solute particle
/ = Water

B   MEMBRANE PERMEABLE ONLY TO SOLVENT

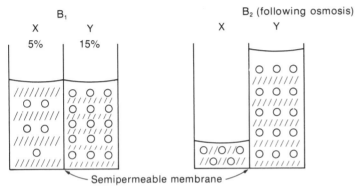

O = Solute particle
/ = Water

Fig. 4.3 Osmosis: see text for explanation.

numbers of particles is the osmole (SI unit, *osmol*) or milliosmole (SI unit, *mosmol*). *The osmolality* of a solution refers to the number of solute particles in a solution per unit of solvent; the greater the number of particles, the greater the osmolality of that solution. In a solution of sodium chloride (NaCl) each molecule of the solute dissociates and forms two osmotically active particles, Na^+ and Cl^-. In a solution of glucose the molecules of the solute do not dissociate into component ions, so that one molecule of glucose represents only one osmotically active particle or 1 osmol.

The term *osmolarity* indicates the number of osmoles or milliosmoles in 1 litre of solution.

A greater concentration of potassium, phosphate, magnesium and protein exists within the cells as compared to that of the extracellular fluid. Sodium, bicarbonate and chloride are found in higher concentration outside the cell than within. Normally the osmotic pressure created by the solutes remains relatively constant on both sides of the cell membrane, and water diffuses in and out of the cell without a net loss or gain on either side of the membrane. Under such circumstances, the fluids are said to be isotonic; that is, the fluid on each side of the membrane has the same osmotic pressure.

When the osmotic pressure within the cell becomes greater than that of the interstitial fluid, osmotic equilibrium is quickly restored by the movement of water into the cell. Conversely, when the solutes of the extracellular fluid become concentrated, water passes out of the cell. This latter situation may occur in dehydration, which may be due to an excessive loss of extracellular fluid from the body or to an inadequate fluid intake. Unless the extracellular fluid volume is restored, the loss of water from the cells may interfere with normal cell functioning.

Solutions administered intravenously may be classified as isotonic, hypertonic or hypotonic. An *isotonic* solution has the same osmotic pressure as the plasma.

A *hypertonic* solution has a greater number of solute particles than the plasma. When such a solution is given intravenously, the increased osmotic pressure of the plasma causes water to pass out of the blood cells and from the interstitial spaces across the capillary membranes. A hypertonic solution of glucose or a preparation of urea may be given to a patient with cerebral oedema. The increased osmotic pressure of the blood draws fluid into the capillaries in the brain, thus reducing the oedema.

A *hypotonic* solution has a lower osmotic pressure than the plasma. When given intravenously it reduces the plasma osmotic pressure, and water passes into the blood cells, causing them to swell and burst (haemolysis).

General Organization of the Body

Going from the simplest to the more complex, the structural units of the body are the cells, tissues, organs and systems.

TISSUES

As cited previously, the cell is the basic structural and functional unit of the body. Those similar in structure and function are held together by intercellular substances to form a tissue. The distinctive features of a tissue are determined by the special characteristics of the constituent cells and intercellular substance. Just as the cells of one type of tissue vary in composition, size, shape and arrangement from those of another, the intercellular substance varies in nature and amount. It may be dense and hard, fluid or gel, or it may occur in the form of fibres. It may be rigid or pliable, elastic or non-extensible, and tough or fragile. In certain tissues (e.g. epithelium), the intercellular substance is minimal; in these cases the cells provide the bulk and the particular function of the tissue. In other tissues (e.g. bone) there is more intercellular substance which plays a major role.

There are four major types of tissues: epithelial, connective, muscular and nervous. Variations occur in the tissues of these major categories as the cells and intercellular substance are adapted to meet the various needs of the body.

Epithelial tissues function in protection, secretion, absorption, filtration and excretion. They are found covering all external and internal surfaces as well as in secreting structures and consist mainly of cells with a minimal amount of intercellular substance. The cells reproduce readily, which is essential to the maintenance of surface and lining tissues. Examples of epithelial tissues are the skin, mucous and serous membranes, and the endothelial lining of the blood and lymph vessels and heart chambers.

Connective tissues are concerned mainly with the physical form and the mechanical activities of the body rather than with its physiological activities. They provide an internal supporting framework, protection for other structures and connections between parts of the body so they become a functional unit. The intercellular substance predominates in connective tissues and gives these tissues their special characteristics. Examples are bones, tendons, ligaments, cartilage, fascia and adipose tissue. Blood is classified as a connective tissue; in this instance the cells have an equally significant role as that of the intercellular substance, plasma.

Muscular tissue is responsible for all movements of the body and its organs. The elongated cells (fibres) with their contractile property are important functional units; the relatively small amount of intercellular substance serves only as retaining material. The cytoplasm of muscle cells is called sarcoplasm. Muscle fibres, with the exception of those of visceral muscle, are not capable of cell reproduction; when severely damaged they degenerate and are replaced by connective tissue.

Nervous tissues form the brain, spinal cord and the network of nerve fibres throughout the body. There are two types. One type consists of specialized cells (neurons) which initiate and transmit impulses to control and coordinate the physical and mental activities by which the body adapts itself to changes in its external environment. The neurons are incapable of cell division; if a cell process (nerve fibre) outside the brain or cord is injured, it may regenerate only if the cell body is uninjured (see Chapter 22). The other type of nervous tissue is made up of neuroglial cells and is found in the brain and spinal cord. It serves to support and protect the nervous tissue proper.

ORGANS

A combination of different types of tissues which are arranged to work in conjunction with one another forms an organ, such as the heart, liver or stomach. Each organ has a definite form and location in the body and performs specialized activities which are dependent upon the functional contribution of each constituent tissue.

SYSTEMS

Several organs are arranged and correlated to form a system, which performs an overall major body function. For example, the digestion of food is dependent upon the coordinated activity of the alimentary tract and accessory organs of the digestive system. The skeletal, muscular, circulatory, respiratory, digestive, excretory, nervous, endocrine and reproductive systems compose the major complex structural units. Total body functioning is dependent upon the coordinated activities of its various systems. No system functions independently of the others.

HEALTH AND DISEASE

Introduction

Health and disease are relative terms which are difficult to define precisely. The condition of the organism is the composite result of interaction between the cells within the body, and between the body and its environment. The organism demonstrates an amazing ability to adapt to internal and external environmental changes, and to repair or compensate for stress and damage that it experiences. As long as the interaction and adaptive mechanisms can maintain normal structure and optimum function is accompanied by a sense of well-being and achievement of a life that is personally satisfying, the individual is said to be healthy. Disease adversely affects health through an interruption or disorder of function.

Health and illness may be influenced by factors in the individual's external and internal environments. *External* variables include: physical environmental conditions such as the quality and availability of water, food, air, sanitation and housing; sociocultural factors such as family structure, customs and relationships, education and financial resources; and the quality and availability of health care services. *Internal* factors which influence health include: the individual's genetic, physical, physiological, biochemical and psychological traits; growth and development; the effectiveness of the body's regulatory and adaptive mechanisms in maintaining a relative constancy in the internal environment in response to internal and external changes; the ability of cells and tissues to respond to trauma and disease; and biological rhythms or 'inner clocks' which account for daily, weekly and monthly changes in body functioning. For example, body temperature, blood pressure and pulse rate are cyclic in nature and are normally lower at night and during sleep and higher in late afternoon.

There are varying degrees of departure from normal; they may be severe enough to incapacitate the individual, or may be less serious, allowing the individual to remain active but without a sense of well-being. On the other hand, people with some disorders adjust their life-style to prescribed therapy and optimum activity, achieving functional competence and a quality of life within the definition of health. The insulin-dependent diabetic may fall into this group.

Causes of Disease

The cause of some disease is unknown and research continues to search for the aetiological factors in such conditions as cancer, multiple sclerosis, rheumatoid arthritis, leukaemia and psychosis. In some diseases, predisposing and perpetuating factors have been recognized even though the primary causative factor has not been identified. Such information contributes to preventive care. When the cause is unknown, care and therapy are based principally on the signs and symptoms.

Recognized causes of disease include the following:

HEREDITY

When an ovum is fertilized by a spermatozoon, each contributes 23 chromosomes which combine to form the nucleus of the single cell that is the origin of a new being. The chromosomes of the gametes transmit traits and characteristics from one generation to the next by their genes' influence on the biochemical activity of the cells of the new organism.

The number of abnormal conditions attributed to chromosomal aberrations seems to increase progressively as more research is carried out in this clinical area. Hereditary disease may be transmitted from one generation to another by a genetic or chromosomal disorder in one or both gametes. Abnormal cellular development and activity may result from an irregularity in chromosomal number or structure. As a result of non-disjunction in meiosis, the cells may have more or fewer than the normal number of chromosomes. Down's syndrome, a relatively common inherited disease, is characterized by an extra chromosome; the cells contain a total of 47 rather than 46. The cells in Turner's syndrome manifest a deficiency of chromosomes—one sex chromosome is missing.

Structural aberrations result from the abnormality of one or more genes of a chromosome. The patterns of these defects vary and include: (1) the separation of a chromosomal fragment or gene and its attachment to another chromosome (translocation); (2) the exchange of places by two genes from different chromosomes (reciprocal translocation); (3) omission of a gene or segment of a chromosome (deletion); or (4) breaks along the chromosome and ensuing realignment and change of gene locus.

The abnormality resulting from a change in a chromosome or gene is known as a mutation. The cause is unknown, but mutation can be induced experimentally by radiation and some chemicals. If the mutation is present in a gamete, the abnormal trait is passed on to the offspring and may be expressed as an hereditary disease, depending upon the gene dominance. The mutant gene may be carried by one of the autosomes, which are the 22 pairs of chromosomes not involved in sex determination. The mutation, then, is referred to as autosomal. If the mutation is in a chromosome of the 23rd pair, which is concerned with sex determination, it is known as a sex-linked mutation. Mutant genes in sex-linked inherited disease are carried by the X chromosomes. If the mutant gene is recessive in penetrance, the disease will not be expressed in a female who has two X chromosomes unless both genes for that particular trait are mutant. In the case of a male, the disease will be expressed, since the 23rd pair of chromosomes is X and Y. There is no gene on the Y chromosome corresponding to the mutant gene on the X chromosome, so the mutation is fully expressed whether or not the mutant gene is dominant or recessive.

The expression or actual development of some diseases classified as hereditary is dependent upon the combined effects of genetic and environmental factors. An individual may carry a mutant gene which predisposes him to a particular disorder that does not develop unless the cells are subjected to certain circumstances. Non-insulin dependent diabetes mellitus is an example of such a disorder; obesity provides the circumstance that is favourable for expression of the disease.

A gene for each trait is received from each parent; in some instances, the new organism may receive only one defective gene, and the manifestation of disturbance will depend on whether the gene is dominant or recessive. If it is dominant, the abnormality will be expressed, but if it is recessive the normal gene will dominate, resulting in normal structure and functioning. If each parent contributes a defective recessive gene for a particular trait, the abnormality is expressed as an hereditary disease.

DEVELOPMENT DEFECTS

Some abnormal structural and functional defects that are present at birth are due to a failure or an abnormality in the developmental process during the embryonic or fetal stage. The cause in most cases is unknown. Developmental defects are seen in some infants born to mothers who have had a viral infection during the first trimester of pregnancy. It is suggested that the virus may pass through the placenta and into the developing tissues of the embryo, thus interfering with normal tissue development. Toxic chemicals taken during pregnancy, such as the drug thalidomide, may disturb normal fetal development. Lysergic acid diethylamide (LSD) and radiation are also suspects for causing abnormal development, as is excessive alcohol.

BIOLOGICAL AGENTS

One of the commonest causes of disease is the invasion of the body by bacteria, viruses, fungi or parasites. They harm or destroy the tissues by their direct action on the cells or by the toxins they produce. The disease is referred to as an infection, which is discussed in the next chapter.

PHYSICAL AGENTS

Tissues may suffer injury or destruction as a result of external forces in the environment. These include pressure, blows, falls, lacerations and the entry of foreign bodies, such as bullets.

Cells may be destroyed when subjected to extreme heat or cold. Exposure to excessive sun rays and to radiation from x-rays or radioactive material may alter cell structure and activity or may actually cause destruction of the cells.

CHEMICALS

When some chemicals are introduced into the body they have an injurious effect on tissue cells. The chemical may disrupt normal cellular chemical reactions either by forming incompatible compounds or by interfering with normal enzymatic action within the cells.

DEFICIENCIES AND EXCESSES

An inadequate supply of materials essential to normal tissue structure and activity may cause a variety of diseases. The deficiency may be due to an insufficient intake of nutritional substances or a specific element, lack of absorption from the intestine, or an interference in the delivery of the essential substances to the cells by the circulatory system.

The lack of a normal oxygen supply to any tissue seriously impairs its function. If the supply is completely cut off, the cells quickly die. The deficiency may be local or general; local hypoxia may be due to a blockage of the vessels supplying the affected area. General oxygen deprivation may be due to respiratory insufficiency or a disturbance in the oxygen-carrying or delivery mechanisms.

An excess of nutrients may also create problems, such as increased demands on body function and the storage of excess fat. Morbidity statistics indicate a higher incidence of hypertension, cardiovascular diseases and diabetes in obese persons.

EMOTIONS

Psychological reactions to stressful situations may influence a person's autonomic nervous system and alter its control of visceral activities. Changes in autonomic innervation may increase or decrease the function of certain structures; this may have marked effects on total body functioning.

TISSUE RESPONSES

Illness may be caused by the responses or reaction of

tissues to an injury or irritation. Examples of this are inflammation and allergic reaction, both of which are discussed in ensuing sections of this chapter.

Homeostasis

A state of homeostasis, which is the maintenance of relatively constant conditions in the internal environment, is required for normal cell functioning. This necessitates the continuous intake of certain substances into the internal environment and the elimination of substances which would be harmful if retained. Coordination of many body mechanisms is required to maintain constancy in the internal environment.

Nutrients are absorbed into the body through the gastrointestinal system and gases enter through the respiratory system. The circulatory system transports these nutrients and gases to the cells and transports wastes which are eliminated through the intestinal system, kidneys and lungs. Homeostasis does not refer to a state of absolute constancy but rather to a dynamic balance that varies within narrow limits. Derangements beyond these limits are not compatible with normal cell functioning. The internal interstitial environment must be maintained within a definite temperature and pH range; it must be capable of supplying the cells with oxygen and other essential materials, as well as removing their secretions and waste products. Cellular activities tend to produce changes, but under normal conditions body mechanisms operate continuously to restore and maintain a suitable environment. To quote Guyton: 'Essentially all the organs and tissues of the body perform functions that help to maintain these constant conditions.'[3]

Homeostasis as applied in a physiological context may be broadened to include psychosocial and sociocultural stability and balance. Psychosocial and cultural factors influence the physiological responses of an integrated being. Thus, homeostasis may be viewed as stability and balance of the total individual.

To maintain homeostasis, internal mechanisms must exist to compensate for changes in the external and internal environment. A decrease in oxygen may be caused by external factors such as a decrease in oxygen concentration in the external environment at high altitudes or from internal respiratory disturbances. The body responds initially by increasing the heart and respiratory rates to ensure that the body's demands for oxygen are met. Long-term compensatory mechanisms include the increased production of red blood cells to increase the oxygen-carrying capacity of the blood and facilitate oxygen uptake.

[3] Guyton (1986), p. 3.

Injury to the skin or mucous membranes interrupts the body's defensive barrier against invasion of foreign substances. The internal inflammatory and immune mechanisms provide the next line of defence against the foreign substances and also respond to internal conditions which cause cell damage or death (e.g. myocardial infarction, neoplasms). Maintenance of homeostasis is dependent upon protective and reparative mechanisms such as inflammation, tissue repair and immunity.

BODY RESPONSES TO DISEASE AGENTS

Body responses and manifestation patterns are frequently similar for different disease agents. Examples of reactions common to many primary causative factors include changes in body temperature, pulse, respiration, physical ability, body comfort and food tolerance. Pathological agents initiate non-specific as well as specific reactions. In many instances the reaction is produced as a defence mechanism but may be more damaging and stressful than the primary disease agent. The effects of disease vary not only with the type of primary agent but also with the particular individual and his responses. Defensive and adaptive capacities vary among persons; they are influenced by the individual's inherited constitution, environmental circumstances, total life-style and sum total of past experiences.

When tissue cells are subjected to adverse conditions they may exhibit one or more of the following: inflammation, regeneration and repair, degeneration, necrosis, atrophy, hypertrophy, hyperplasia, metaplasia, neoplasia or the immune response.

Inflammation

The process of inflammation is a local tissue reaction to injury or irritation. It is designed to remove or destroy the injurious agent, keep the injury localized and repair the damage (see Fig. 4.4).

Agents which cause inflammation are:
- Physical
  - (a) mechanical (e.g. trauma, pressure)
  - (b) thermal (e.g. extreme heat and cold, radiant energy)
- Chemical (e.g. strong acids and alkalis, irritating gases, poisons, products of necrotic tissue, products of altered metabolism)
- Biological (e.g. microorganisms)
- Immunological (e.g. antigen–antibody and autoimmune reactions)

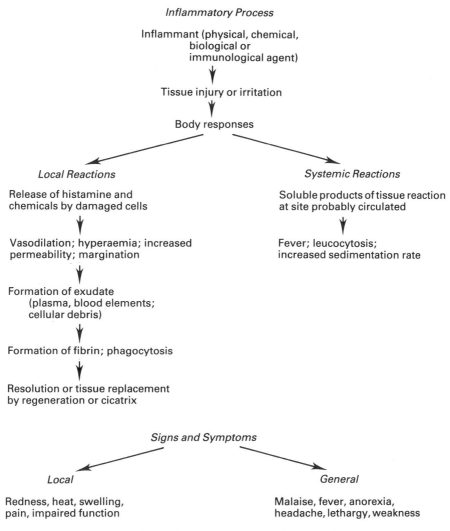

Inflammatory Process

Inflammant (physical, chemical,
biological or
immunological agent)

Tissue injury or irritation

Body responses

Local Reactions

Release of histamine and
chemicals by damaged cells

Vasodilation; hyperaemia; increased
permeability; margination

Formation of exudate
(plasma, blood elements;
cellular debris)

Formation of fibrin; phagocytosis

Resolution or tissue replacement
by regeneration or cicatrix

Systemic Reactions

Soluble products of tissue reaction
at site probably circulated

Fever; leucocytosis;
increased sedimentation rate

Signs and Symptoms

Local

Redness, heat, swelling,
pain, impaired function

General

Malaise, fever, anorexia,
headache, lethargy, weakness

Fig. 4.4 The inflammatory process and signs and symptoms.

The intensity of the reaction depends on the nature and severity of the causative factor and on the reactive capacity of the individual.

LOCAL RESPONSES

Cellular injury results in an acute local reaction characterized by an immediate vascular response with an accumulation of plasma fluids and proteins. This is followed by white blood cell activity and the formation of exudate at the site of injury.

Vascular Reponses
In the initial phase, there is a momentary constriction of the blood vessels at the site of injury. This is immediately followed by dilation, an increased local blood supply (hyperaemia) and a marked increase in vascular permeability. These changes result in the escape of relatively large amounts of plasma and some cells into the interstitial spaces. Histamine, released by injured or irritated cells, is the major mediator of this initial response. Other chemicals of the kinin[4] and the complement[5] systems also function as mediators in initiating and sustaining the vascular responses.

Local manifestations of the vascular response are: redness and heat of the affected area as a result of the hyperaemia; swelling and firmness due to the accumulation of the fluid and cells in the interstitial

---

[4] *Kinin system* is a group of endogenous amino acid compounds that act on smooth muscle tissue as found in the vascular system.

[5] *Complement system* comprises a series of enzymes which are composed of amino acids and are present in normal serum. They interact with the defensive antibody–antigen reaction.

spaces; pain caused by the pressure of the fluid on nerve endings as well as by chemical irritation of the substances released from the injured cells; and impaired function of the area.

Cellular Responses

As plasma and some blood cells escape into the interstitial spaces, the intravascular volume is reduced and the rate of blood flow through the dilated vessels is decreased. The blood cells, especially the leucocytes, move out of the central portion of the stream and collect along the vessel walls; this process is referred to as margination or pavementing. The leucocytes, along with macrophages,[6] migrate through the capillary walls to the inflammatory site, where they attack the offending agent and assist in disposing of the cellular debris by phagocytosis. The leucocytes, which at this stage are principally neutrophils, and macrophages are attracted to the site of injury by chemicals released from the damaged cells. The number of neutrophils available for migration may be increased rapidly. The reacting tissues may release a globulin substance, referred to as the leucocytosis-promoting factor, which is carried from the area and eventually reaches the bone marrow via the blood. It stimulates the release of white blood cells, especially neutrophils, by the marrow. If the initiating factor involves an antigen, antibodies are brought to the site in the escaping plasma, which make the offending agent more susceptible to phagocytosis or which may neutralize toxins liberated by the agent.

If the causative agent is not checked in these early responses, an increased number of macrophages are produced through the release of increased numbers of lymphocytes and monocytes by reticuloendothelial tissues (e.g. lymph glands, spleen). These leucocytes become larger, more motile and more capable of phagocytosis as they are attracted to the affected tissues by chemotaxis.

The causative agent is removed or destroyed by phagocytosis. Localization of the injury is promoted by the aggregation of white blood cells around the agent and by the formation of a fibrin network from fibrinogen, a normal protein component of the blood. The fine insoluble fibres form an interlacing network that walls off the affected area.

The inflammatory exudate

The fluid and blood elements that escape from the intravascular compartment, the products released by the injured and dead tissue cells, and the causative agent, if it is invasive or endogenous, comprise the inflammatory exudate. The nature and amount of the exudate depend upon the intensity and nature of the cause and the tissues involved.

---

[6] *Macrophages* are large wandering phagocytic cells capable of engulfing large particles. Monocytes comprise the majority of these cells.

A *serous exudate* consists chiefly of fluid with few cells and little or no fibrin. It is seen in the early stages of inflammation or when the injury is mild. An example is the fluid in a blister or that which accumulates when a serous membrane, such as the pleura or the peritoneum, is irritated.

Purulent exudate, or pus, is a thick fluid made up of leucocytes, dead and living microorganisms which caused the injury, liquefied dead tissue cells, and the fluid and blood elements that escaped from the vessels. The formation of pus may be referred to as suppuration, and organisms that cause it are classified as pyogenic. A localized collection of purulent exudate is called an abscess. The localization is maintained by surrounding the area with leucocytes and fibrin. If the organisms migrate through the barrier to surrounding tissues, the infection spreads and is called *cellulitis*.

Catarrhal exudate is produced by mucous membranes and mucus-secreting cells. It is a clear fluid containing mucoid material and white blood cells. An example is the nasal secretions produced with the common cold.

Fibrinous exudate indicates a vascular permeability that allows a greater amount of fibrinogen to leak into the interstitial area. The protein is precipitated by tissue extract (thromboplastin), which is released by injured cells and blood platelets and forms fibrin. An excessive amount of fibrin may form a membranous coating over a tissue surface, and its stickiness may cause the surfaces to adhere. The fibrin may be replaced by fibrous tissue, and bands of fibrous adhesions may form between two surfaces. Adhesions develop most frequently on serous surfaces such as the pleura, pericardium and the intestines.

A *haemorrhagic exudate* contains a large number of erythrocytes and may be described as sanguineous.

The exudate in the inflammatory process functions to neutralize the irritants and toxins by dilution, and to transport antibodies to the site of injury.

SYSTEMIC RESPONSES

In many inflammatory conditions, especially in those caused by invasive microorganisms, an examination of the blood reveals a greater than normal number of leucocytes. This is referred to as leucocytosis. The mechanism by which this is initiated was mentioned earlier. An increase in the blood sedimentation rate also occurs. (This is the rate at which the erythrocytes settle out of a given volume of blood in 1 hour.) If the inflammation is caused by microorganisms, a serum titre may demonstrate a significant increase in antibodies.

Soluble products of the tissue reaction may diffuse into the bloodstream or be delivered via the lymph stream to be circulated throughout the body, causing general body irritation and responses. These produce non-specific responses which are manifested as the general signs and symptoms. These include general malaise, loss of appetite, headache, lethargy, weakness and discomfort. The severity of general responses depends upon the amount and toxicity of the absorbed inflammatory products, which in turn are determined by the nature and intensity of the offending agent.

Fever is common, especially if the inflammatory process is caused by invasive microorganisms or by considerable destruction of tissue cells. If the process is associated with poor nutrition tissue protein catabolism takes place and the patient may become severely debilitated.

REPARATIVE PHASE

Once the causative agent has been overcome and the debris cleared away by the leucocytes, macrophages and lymph drainage, the affected area returns to normal or, if necessary, is filled in by regeneration of the respective tissue cells or fibrous scar tissue, or by a combination of the two.

When the injury is slight, cell changes may be reversible, and complete recovery occurs. If the irritant caused the inflammatory response without cellular necrosis, the exudate is removed and the area returns to normal; this result is called *resolution*.

In the case of a more severe injury, the damage to some cells may be irreversible and they die. The area is healed by replacement of the destroyed tissue with living cells. The healing is by *regeneration* if the new cells produced by the surrounding cells are similar in structure and function to the cells being replaced. The ability to reproduce cells varies greatly from one type of tissue to another. Nervous, muscular and elastic tissues have very little or no regenerative capacity after structural growth is completed. Epithelial, fibrous, bone, lymphoid and bone marrow tissues exhibit a much greater ability to reproduce like cells.

When regeneration is not possible, repair occurs by replacing the lost tissue with fibrous tissue. The fibrin of the inflammatory exudate, which was formed in response to the injury, provides a framework in which granulation tissue develops. The latter is formed by the ingrowth of capillaries from surrounding vessels and by fibroblasts from marginal connective tissue. The formation of granulation tissue in an injured area is sometimes referred to as 'organization'. At this stage, the tissue appears as a very soft, gelatinous-like red mass because of its many newly-formed capillaries and large immature fibroblasts around which collagen fibres develop. As the fibroblasts and collagen fibres mature, the tissue shrinks, many capillaries are constricted and obliterated, and an area of firm fibrous tissue remains, known as a *cicatrix*, or *scar*. Marginal surface epithelium (e.g. skin) proliferates to form a surface covering.

The fibrous tissue substitution for the original specialized cells may reduce the functional capacity of the affected structure or may cause mechanical interference because of its firm, constricting nature, such as is seen when a peptic ulcer heals and subsequently causes pyloric stenosis.

CLASSIFICATION OF INFLAMMATION

Inflammation may be classified:

1 *According to the duration of the reaction*. It may be termed *acute* if it has a sudden onset and progresses quickly to recovery, permanent injury or death. *Chronic* inflammation usually has an insidious onset and persists over a period of months to years. It is characterized by the presence of repair and healing, along with advancing and continuous inflammation and cellular destruction. There is extensive granulation and scar tissue formation. A *subacute* inflammatory process is usually considered intermediary to the foregoing types in both severity and duration.

2 *According to the structure affected*. The suffix -*itis* is used to denote inflammation of the particular tissue or structure indicated by the preceding part of the word. For example: myocarditis implies inflammation of the muscle fibres of the heart, pneumonitis, inflammation of the lung tissue; laryngitis, inflammation of the larynx; peritonitis, inflammation of the peritoneum; and so on.

3 *According to the nature of the exudate*. Fibrinous inflammation indicates that a relatively large amount of fibrin is formed. Purulent inflammation implies suppuration.

4 *According to the causative agent*. Another basis of classification that may be used occasionally relates to the nature of the inflammatory agent. The terms traumatic, chemical, bacterial or allergic may be used as descriptive terms.

NURSING PROCESS

The nurse caring for a patient with an inflammation follows the steps of the nursing process to collect data on the patient's response to the injury and the factors causing the inflammatory response. Data are analysed (i.e. an assessment is made) potential and actual patient problems are identified. Nursing intervention is planned, and expected outcomes to measure the effectiveness of the intervention are stated.

Assessment

Clinical manifestations of inflammation presented by a patient will vary according to the characteristics of the causative agent, the age and general health status of the patient and the site of injury. Data collection by the nurse is facilitated when the site of injury can be directly observed. When direct observation is not possible, several objective and subjective indicators of the severity of the response can be measured. Table 4.1 lists objective and subjective data to be collected when a patient has an inflammation.

FACTORS INFLUENCING THE INFLAMMATORY RESPONSE AND HEALING

Identification of the causative agent and of factors which affect the inflammatory response and repair is necessary if the nurse is to plan nursing intervention that is purposeful and relevant to the individual patient.

Causative agent factors. Agent-related variables which influence the severity and degree of tissue destruction include the amount and potency of the agent and the duration of contact.

Patient-related factors
Local factors which influence the inflammatory–reparative response include:
- The type of tissue affected. Some tissues have a greater ability to reproduce cells than others; for example, epithelial tissue cells can reproduce rapidly, muscular tissue cells reproduce much more slowly and nerve cells do not reproduce at all. A good blood supply to the damaged tissue plays an important role in the reparative process.
- Tissue trauma and a reduced blood supply. The more serious the tissue injury and the greater the interference with the blood supply to the affected area, the longer will be the period required to replace the destroyed tissue.
- Infection. Invasion of the wound by micro-organisms may increase tissue destruction and impede the formation of granulation tissue.
- Mechanical factors. Friction on a wound destroys the soft granulation tissue. The presence of a foreign body or tissue movement prevents or interferes with the apposition of the wound edges.

Systemic factors that influence the individual's response to causative agents are:
- The age of the patient. Immunocompetence and vascular integrity are less effective in the newborn and the elderly.
- Nutritional status. A deficient intake of protein results in a lack of the essential amino acids from which new tissue is constructed. An insufficient supply of vitamin C (ascorbic acid) prevents the formation of collagen fibres that support the developing fibrous tissue.
- Hormonal imbalance. Excessive glucocorticoids inhibit inflammation and healing.

STAGES OF HEALING

Healing takes place in three overlapping phases:
1 The lag or catabolic stage is identified by the signs of the acute inflammatory response which brings materials that are essential for tissue repair to the site of injury. A fibrin network bridges the area and a scab may be seen in superficial wounds.
2 The reconstructive phase begins at 4–5 days and is characterized by the formation of collagen and granulation. The wound appears as an irregular, raised, red, immature scar.
3 The maturation or reorientation phase can last for up to 2 years. The scar fades and contracts and will vary in size and appearance from a barely visible thickened line under the surface skin to an irregularly shaped, large, indented and contracted area of scar tissue.

Identification of patient problems

Interpretation of the data collected by the nurse will identify the problems and the factors that influence the inflammatory and reparative processes. Nursing intervention is then planned and implemented to meet the specific needs of the individual.

Table 4.1 Assessment of the patient with an acute inflammation.

Local response	Exudate	Systemic responses
Objective data	*Objective data*	*Objective data*
Redness	Amount of exudate	Elevated body temperature
Heat	Consistency	Increased white blood count (WBC)
Oedema	Colour	Increased erythrocyte sedimentation rate (ESR)
Impaired function	Odour	Growth of pathogens in blood culture
	Growth of organisms on culture	
Subjective data		*Subjective data*
Pain and discomfort		General malaise
		Loss of appetite
		Headache
		Lethargy
		Weakness
		Discomfort

Nursing intervention

1 *Prevention of further injury*
- The inflammatory agent should be removed or minimized depending on the specific patient situation. This may require medical or surgical intervention as well as nursing action. External agents should be removed immediately being careful to minimize manipulation of the affected part. Pressure, thermal agents and penetrating objects require immediate removal. External chemical agents are diluted and the area irrigated with water or normal saline. Tissue and/or blood cultures are taken to identify microorganisms.

  With some internal inflammatory responses such as myocarditis, the most appropriate intervention may be directed towards removing the cause, preventing further injury and minimizing the effects of the event.
- The patient should be positioned to eliminate pressure on the affected area. If a limb or joint is affected good alignment and gentle passive and/or active movement are important considerations to avoid permanent deformity and impairment of function.
- Dressings should be applied to open lesions to protect them from trauma, airborne contaminants and, in some instances, to prevent the spread of infection to others.
- Basic aseptic techniques should be practised, such as frequent hand-washing and careful disposal of contaminated dressings.

2 *Promote healing and tissue repair*
- The affected part should be placed at rest to decrease energy demands, prevent further trauma and lessen the pain.
- The affected part should be elevated to encourage venous and lymphatic drainage; this reduces swelling, lessens pain and increases the flow of fresh blood into the area. Fresh blood carries more elements to combat the offending agent and facilitate repair.
- Heat or cold should be applied to the area. Heat relaxes the muscle tissue and facilitates an increased blood flow. Cold causes constriction of vessels, reducing the volume of exudate and the degree of swelling. It reduces the sensitivity of the nerve endings, thereby lessening pain, and also retards the multiplication of bacteria when they are the causative agent.
- The nurse should promote and/or maintain the nutritional status of the patient. Fluid intake is increased to promote dilution and elimination of toxic products. Caloric intake should be adequate to meet the increased energy demands and tissue breakdown. Protein is required to provide the essential amino acids necessary for new tissue construction. Vitamin C is needed for the formation of collagen fibres that support the developing fibrous tissue.

- Physical rest, comfort and relaxation should be promoted to decrease the energy being expended by the patient.
- Prescribed medications should be administered, which may be an antimicrobial preparation such as an antibiotic, sulphonamide or antitoxin and/or an antiinflammatory drug such as aspirin or a corticosteroid preparation.
- When there is an open lesion the exudate and necrotic tissue should be removed to promote healing. This may be achieved by the use of packing to act as a wick, absorbent dressings, or vacuum (suction) drainage, as well as by physical or chemical *debridement.*[7]

Expected outcomes

The effectiveness of nursing intervention in inflammation may be determined by identification of the following:
- Reduction and eventual absence of redness, heat, oedema, pain and impaired function
- Reduction or absence of exudate
- Return of body temperature, white blood cell count and erythrocyte sedimentation rate (ESR) to normal levels
- Absence of growth of pathogens on culture
- Ability to resume usual activities
- Clean, intact, viable tissue at the site of injury

Tissue Degeneration

Degeneration is characterized by oedema of the cells, changes in the chemical reactions and composition of the cytoplasm and disturbances in cell function. The degeneration is named in accordance with the changes observed in the composition and appearance of the cells. These terms include: fatty, cloudy, oedema, hyaline (translucent), amyloid (waxy, starch-like), and mucoid.

Necrosis

Necrosis is degeneration that has proceeded to the death of cells, tissues or organs within a living organism. It may be caused by:
- Interference with nutrition to the part
- Mechanical injury
- Extreme heat or cold
- Chemical or bacterial poisons
- Radiation
- Loss of nerve supply

---

[7] *Debridement* is the removal of devitalized tissue and contaminated and foreign material from a lesion.

Types of necrosis include:
- Liquefaction necrosis, which occurs when cellular enzymes liquefy the dead cells
- Coagulation necrosis, caused when proteins coagulate to form a firm, dry mass
- Caseous necrosis, resulting in the formation of soft, greyish-white cheesy material
- Fat necrosis, which occurs when pancreatic juices are released into the retroperitoneal area, resulting in digestion of fat.

Gangrene is the death of a relatively large area of tissue; it may involve a part or the whole of an organ or limb. *Infarction* is a term used to denote necrosis of an area of tissue caused by ischaemia (inadequate blood supply to the part).

Disturbances in Proliferation and Differentiation of Cells and Tissue

These disturbances include atrophy, hypertrophy, hyperplasia, metaplasia and neoplasia.

ATROPHY

Atrophy is a decrease in the size of tissues or organs, that were previously of normal size, due to a decrease in the size or number of constituent cells. The causes of atrophy may be:
- Nutritional deficiency
- Disuse
- Interruption of the nerve supply
- Pressure on the part
- Lack of endocrine stimulation.

An example of the latter cause is atrophy of the uterus and breasts after menopause, which results from a decrease in the concentration of sex hormones.

HYPERTROPHY AND HYPERPLASIA

A frequent response of a tissue to the increased demands placed upon it is hypertrophy, which is achieved by an increase in the *size* of the individual cells. This may be observed in the enlargement of skeletal muscle fibres which occurs with increased work and exercise.

An increase in the volume of tissue due to an increased *number* of cells is called hyperplasia.

Hypertrophy and hyperplasia are beneficial when an increase in function is necessary. The heart, for example, may compensate for increased resistance to the flow of blood from a chamber by the hypertrophy of the myocardial fibres of the walls of that chamber. Hyperplasia of the bone marrow and lymphoid tissues increases the number of leucocytes and is helpful in severe infection. In other instances, an increase in the size of a structure may be harmful. Hypertrophy of the heart muscle may require a greater blood supply than the coronary arteries can supply. An enlarged organ may cause pressure or obstruction in some situations. A frequent example of this is hyperplasia of the prostate gland; the enlarged gland imposes upon the urethra, causing retention of urine.

METAPLASIA

This tissue response to adverse conditions is the replacement of tissue by cells that are different from their predecessors. The replaced cells are normal but are located in an area of the tissue where they are not usually found. For example, following repeated injury and irritation, the normal, ciliated, mucus-secreting epithelial lining of the respiratory tract may be replaced by a thicker, non-secreting squamous epithelium. This substitution reduces the normal, protective cleansing mechanisms and predisposes to infection.

NEOPLASIA

This term means new formation or growth. Normally, the production of cells is a regulated process allowing for growth of the organism in early life and for replacement of worn-out or damaged cells throughout the total life span. Occasionally, the control of cell reproduction is lost in some tissue and an excessive production occurs. The cells are usually atypical, serve no useful purpose, develop at the expense of surrounding tissues and continue their characteristics through successive generations of cells. The resulting mass is referred to as a *newgrowth* or *neoplasm*.

When the neoplasm produces an evident swelling, it may be called a tumour. If it remains localized and the rate of growth of the cells is relatively slow, the new growth is said to be *benign*. *Malignant neoplasms* (cancers) grow more rapidly and spread into surrounding tissues. Some of their cells may be carried from the site of their origin and may set up colonies of the malignant cells (metastases) in other areas of the body. The proliferative growth of malignant cells, with their invasion and destruction of normal tissue, may result in death of the patient. Cancer is discussed in Chapter 9.

The Immune Response

The immune response is a physiological reaction of the body to factors that it considers threatening and foreign to it. A factor which evokes the immune response is referred to as an *antigen* (immunogen), which may be a foreign protein, polysaccharide or lipoprotein complex in the form of bacteria, viruses, toxins or tissue cells from another organism. The response is initiated by the body's ability to recognize what is foreign to it, what is self and non-self and what is threatening. The inflammatory or phagocytic system which produces a non-specific response to infection or injury, is the body's first line of defence. The immune system produces very specific responses through a sequence of events that results in the production of special, sensitized cells (immune bodies), which are capable of inhibiting and overcoming the offending agent and providing protection for the individual against the antigen. This type of protection against pathogens (disease-producing agents) is called *immunity*. The immune bodies may be antibodies produced by the humoral response, or sensitized lymphocytes, produced by the cellular immune response (see Fig. 4.5).

Antigens are usually exogenous (from outside the body). Occasionally the body may object to and react with some of its own cellular products, which are then referred to as *endogenous antigens* or *autoantigens*. The immune response to the latter antigens is known as an *autoimmune reaction*.

Two mechanisms are involved in the immune response; one is referred to as humoral immunity and the other as cell-mediated immunity. The *humoral immune response* entails the development and circulation of molecules of gamma globulin when antigens invade the body. These globulin molecules are known as immunoglobulins or antibodies, and

are formed by plasma cells.[8] Guyton indicates that these particular plasma cells are dormant until exposed to an antigen. They then multiply rapidly and produce immunoglobulins.[9]

Immunoglobulins (Ig) or antibodies have been classified and may be designated as belonging to one of the following groups: IgG, IgA, IgM, IgD or IgE.

The IgG type is found to be in greatest concentration, normally composing about 75% of the total. IgD and IgE normally occur in very small serum concentrations. In identifying the class to which the various antibodies belong, information has been determined about their molecular structure, concentration and distribution, movement through capillary walls, movement across the placenta into fetal circulation, and reaction with antigens.

The *cellular immune reaction* is mediated by sensitized lymphocytes, sometimes referred to as T lymphocytes because of their original association with and conditioning by the thymus gland.[10] It is suggested that these lymphocytes develop antibodies within, or 'antibody-like receptors' on their surfaces.

---

[8] *Plasma cells* are produced chiefly by reticulum cells in the lymphoid tissue in lymph nodes, spleen and gastrointestinal tract.

[9] Guyton (1986), p. 57.

[10] The *thymus* is a bilobed lymphoid gland situated in the thoracic cavity, posterior to the upper part of the sternum. It is larger and more active during the first few weeks of life, gradually declining and becoming less active during childhood.

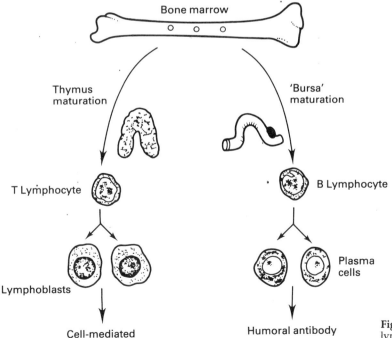

Bone marrow

Thymus
maturation

'Bursa'
maturation

T Lymphocyte

B Lymphocyte

Lymphoblasts

Plasma
cells

Cell-mediated

Humoral antibody

Fig. 4.5 Maturation processes of T and B lymphocytes.

The original lymphocytes capable of becoming sensitized are considered to be produced or processed within the thymus gland very early in life and distributed to lymphoid tissues throughout the body.[11] Table 4.2 compares the function of the T and B lymphocytes.

Table 4.2 Comparative functions of the T and B lymphocytes.*

B lymphocytes, short-lived	T lymphocytes long-lived
Humoral immunity	Cell-mediated immunity
Specific antigen recognition	Specific antigen recognition
Synthesis of antibody. Most effective in pyogenic infections and toxic reactions	Macrophage stimulation, complement activation, destruction of intracellular pathogens. Graft rejection. Immunological surveillance. Stimulation of B cell antibody production by helper cells
Immediate hypersensitivity reaction (allergy)	Delayed hypersensitivity reactions (skin test to antigens)
Transferable by plasma	Transfer uncommon, occurs only via cells
Mostly in blood	Mostly in lymph tissue

*Gurevich and Tafuro (1985).

ANTIGEN–ANTIBODY REACTION

Immune bodies, whether antibodies or T lymphocytes, are specific for each antigen—that is, they are capable of opposing only the antigen which initiated their formation. For example, diphtheria antibodies will not be effective if the invaders are typhoid bacilli.

Antibodies react with antigens in three different ways:
1 By direct attack on the antigens
2 By activation of the complement system to destroy the antigens
3 By activation of the anaphylactic system to alter the environment surrounding the antigen

Antibody reactions which act directly on the antigens include
1 *Precipitation* of the antigens from their fluid medium
2 *Lysis*, which results in dissolution of the antigens
3 *Agglutination*, in which the antigens are clumped together, thus rendering them ineffective
4 *Neutralization* in which the antibody neutralizes the toxic products of the antigens.

A group of at least nine enzyme precursors have been recognized as playing an important role in some antigen–antibody reactions. They are referred to collectively as the complement system. They are classically numbered according to the order in which they were originally believed to enter the reaction.

The sequential order in which they enter the reaction is C1, C4, C2, C3, C5, C6, C7, C8 and C9. Some enzyme precursors have sub-components indicated by a letter (e.g. C3a, C4b). The enzyme precursors promote vascular permeability, phagocytosis and cellular lysis; they do not act directly on the antigen but combine with the antibody after it attaches to the antigen. This interaction activates the complement, which then initiates a sequence of enzymic reactions that cause disruptions of areas of cell membranes and eventual irreversible destruction of the cells.

Guyton lists the more important reactions of these enzyme precursors as:
- *Opsonization*, a process that facilitates phagocytosis of the antigen
- *Lysis*, which results in digestion of portions of the cell membrane and rupture of the cell
- *Agglutinization*, or clumping, of the antigens
- *Neutralization* of viruses
- *Chemotaxis*, which results in an increased number of neutrophils and macrophages to the area
- *Activation* of mast cells and basophils
- *Inflammatory* reactions to localize the antigens.[12]

The IgE antibodies attach to the membranes of some body cells, sensitizing these cells to the antigen and causing an allergic or anaphylactic response. When the antigen attaches to a sensitized cell, histamine, chemotaxic factor and lysosomal enzymes are released from the cell causing an inflammatory response which helps to localize the antigen. Anaphylactic reactions can also be harmful to the body.

When an antigen is present for the first time, the antibody concentration (titre) is not significant until about the 6th or 7th day, when the immune bodies rapidly increase. As a result of the lag, the host develops the disease. When the antigen is eliminated, the immune bodies gradually decline over a period of several weeks. The period of immunity developed following the invasion by some antigens may be brief and transient, such as that which occurs with the common cold and pneumonia. With other diseases the immunity lasts for long periods, even for life (e.g. measles and diphtheria). In the latter case a phenomenon referred to as 'memory' by immunologists remains in the dormant plasma cells and lymphoblasts in lymphoid tissues. On re-exposure to the same antigen, production of the special immune bodies promptly occurs; the number increases rapidly enough to overcome the antigens before the disease develops, thus providing the individual with immunity. This recognition of the antigen by the body, and the effective response, is the basis of the single booster doses of immune-producing preparations. Initially, in artificially induced immunization, administration of a series of antigen doses is necessary to evoke immune body production and establish the 'memory' by which the

---

[11] Guyton (1986), p. 61–62.

[12] Guyton (1986), p. 65.

tissues recognise the antigen. After that only a small amount of the antigen is necessary to maintain effective protection.

Antigen–T lymphocyte reaction

The sensitized lymphocytes of the cellular immune system act by binding with antigens in the membranes of invading cells and releasing cytotoxic substances, mainly lysosomal enzymes which attack the cell directly. Release of lymphokinins and other substances provides for indirect attack on the invading cell. These substances include

- *Chemotaxic factor*, which causes macrophages to enter the area
- *Migratory inhibition factor*, which stops migration of macrophages and lymphocytes from the area
- A substance that increases the *phagocytic* activity of macrophages
- *Transfer factor*, which sensitizes other lymphocytes in the tissue[13]
- *Immune interferons*, which inhibit viruses.[14]

Sensitized lymphocytes can exist for as long as 10 years and form 'memory cells' in much the same way as the humoral antibody system. The cellular immune response is a factor in immunity to all infections, but is particularly important in response to slow-growing bacteria such as the tubercle bacilli, cancer cells, cells of transplanted organs, fungi and some viruses.

Natural immunity

Immunity to some diseases occurs naturally and congenitally, and is dependent upon certain substances occurring normally in the blood. Examples of substances which react with antigens include; phagocytic cells (e.g. leucocytes); lysozyme, which breaks down microorganisms; some polypeptides, which react with certain types of bacteria; properdin, which in association with a complement reacts with gram-negative bacteria; and certain naturally occurring antibodies in the blood. Other forms of natural immunity include the acid secretion and digestive enzymes of the stomach, which destroy ingested organisms; and the resistance of the skin to invasion by organisms.[15]

Natural immunity varies with species, races and individuals. A species of animal may be very susceptible to a certain antigen which is incapable of producing disease in humans. An example is the high susceptibility of cats and dogs to distemper and the natural immunity to the causative agent possessed by humans. Persons of the negro race exhibit a poor resistance to tuberculosis as compared with that of caucasians, but the exact reverse is apparent in relation to malaria. Natural resistance or immunity to certain antigenic microorganisms may be present in some individuals but absent in others; this is evident when a family or group is exposed equally for the first time to a specific antigen and all but one or two become ill. In addition to the protective substances normally present in the blood, age is considered to be a factor in natural immunity; certain infections have a higher incidence in children and rarely occur in adults.

Acquired immunity

This type of immunity may be active or passive. Actively acquired immunity develops when the host forms his own antibodies in response to an antigen. An individual may acquire this immunity by having had the disease, or it may be produced artificially by a series of injections of the antigen. The length of time active immunity lasts varies; it may be very brief for some antigens, while for others it may be lifelong because of the established ability of the tissues to recognize the antigen promptly and produce the appropriate immune bodies rapidly.

Passive acquired immunity may be natural or artificially induced. Natural passive immunity occurs in the newborn infant. This type is passive because the antibodies were developed by the mother and passed through the placenta to the fetus or the colostrum to the infant. These maternal antibodies provide a temporary immunity, protecting the infant only through the first few months of life.

Artificial passive immunity is conferred by injecting serum taken from another organism, usually an animal, which has actively produced immune bodies, e.g. human tetanus antitoxin or human immune globulin. This type of immunity is rapidly established but is of short duration. The antibodies are foreign to the recipient and are destroyed in a relatively short period. As previously indicated, it takes time to produce antibodies upon first exposure; serum that contains specific immune bodies is administered only to those who already have the disease or who are known to have been exposed to the antigen. The foreign antibodies provide an immediate defence during the period in which the recipient is forming his own antibodies.

DISORDERS OF THE IMMUNE RESPONSE

'More than ever it has become apparent that dependent as man is for his survival on the immune system, so vulnerable is he to the wide-ranging disorders in its function.'[16] Normally, the immune response is a physiological defence mechanism, but it may fail as such as a result of a deficiency in the necessary elements, or because of an exaggerated, altered or inappropriate reaction, referred to as

---

[13] Guyton (1986), pp. 65–66.
[14] Fudenberg, Stittes, Caldwell & Wells (1980), p. 268.
[15] Guyton (1986) p. 60.

[16] Robbins, Angell & Kumar (1981).

hypersensitivity or allergy. The severity of the disorders varies greatly, ranging from slightly to totally incapacitating and life-threatening.

Immune deficiency disease

An immune deficiency state may be the result of dysfunction within the humoral-mediated immune system, the cell-mediated (T cell) immune system, or both.

IMMUNOGLOBULIN DEFICIENCY SYNDROMES

Deficiency in the humoral immune system is manifested by susceptibility to infections, especially those of bacterial origin. Inadequate amounts of the gamma fraction of serum globulin results in a failure in antibody formation. Hypo- or agammaglobulinaemia may be primary or secondary. Primary deficiency in immunoglobulins is congenital and is thought to have·a sex-linked (X chromosome) recessive hereditary basis.

Evidence now suggests that there are two forms of the disease, as most affected males have few immunoglobulin-bearing B lymphocytes, while others have been found to have a normal number of B lymphocytes which fail to differentiate into plasma cells.[17] The congenital deficit may not show up in the first few months of life because of the infant's passive immunity acquired from the mother in utero. Immunologists suggest that a selective deficiency may occur within the immunoglobulins i.e. only one of the classes (IgG, IgM, IgA, IgD, IgE) of antibodies may be lacking. IgA is cited as being the one that is most frequently decreased or absent. Individuals with hypogammaglobulinaemia experience recurrent upper respiratory infections and also show a higher incidence of autoimmune diseases.[18,19]

Secondary immunodeficiencies are associated with malnutrition, malignant disease, extensive radiation exposure and certain drugs such as some antibiotics, cytotoxic drugs and corticosteroids which interfere with the functioning and cell production of the lymphatic system. Acquired deficiencies may also be secondary to disease affecting the reticuloendothelial tissues (e.g. Hodgkin's disease, leukaemia) or it may develop as a result of an excessive loss of blood protein, as occurs with the nephrotic syndrome and some intestinal disturbances.

CELL-MEDIATED IMMUNE DEFICIENCY

Individuals with this type of deficiency are particularly susceptible to viral infections. There is a diminished production of the special, sensitized small lymphocytes (T cells). Primary deficiency in the cell-mediated immune mechanism is usually accounted for by failure in the development of the thymus (thymic aplasia or dysplasia). The diminished protection shows up early in life; individuals do not usually survive beyond the first two or three years of life. Cell-mediated immune deficiency may be secondary to Hodgkins's disease, leucopenia, severe stress incurred by trauma or acute infection, or excessive corticoid blood levels.[20]

Acquired immune deficiency syndrome (AIDS)

AIDS is a serious infectious health problem in which there is impaired functioning of the body's immune system.[21,22,23,24,25]

CAUSE

AIDS is caused by the human immunodeficiency viruses (HIV), which attack and may destroy T4 lymphocytes (helper T cells). The major effect is on cell-mediated immunity, resulting in the individual's predisposition to serious infections and rare forms of malignant diseases, such as Kaposi's sarcoma. Lymphopenia (decrease in the number of lymphocytes in the blood), a T lymphocyte deficiency and a failure to respond to antigens develop.

The virus may be found in blood, semen, saliva, tears and breast milk of an infected person.

TRANSMISSION OF AIDS

The AIDS virus may be transmitted by intimate sexual contact, open-mouth kissing, transfusion of infected blood or blood products, the sharing of contaminated needles or syringes, and by an infected mother to her infant (in utero or in breast feeding).

There is no evidence of person-to-person transmission by ordinary casual contact (such as in school or the work place), nor of airborne or food transmission.

When an individual becomes infected, he may develop some minor symptoms but is able to live an active independent life. This person can infect others. Those who are infected may go on to fully develop the acquired immune deficiency syndrome. It is suggested that probably genetically determined factors and the health status of the host may influence the development of AIDS in the infected person.

---

[17] Braunwald et al (1987), p. 1390.
[18] Braunwald et al (1987), p. 1390.
[19] Wyngaarden & Smith (1985), pp. 1855–1866.
[20] *Adrenocortical secretions* depress lymphoid tissue activity and the production of lymphocytes.
[21] Advisory Committee—American Hospital Association (1984), p. 242–248.
[22] Bennett (1985).
[23] Korcok (1985), pp. 1241–1248.
[24] Laurence (1985), p. 92.
[25] Turner & Pryor (1985), pp. 25–37.

Persons at high risk of developing AIDS are all sexually active individuals outside of monogamous relationships and intravenous drug users. Other high-risk groups include recipients of multiple transfusions of whole blood products and infants of infected mothers.

The increasing incidence of AIDS is mainly within the high-risk groups and not in the general population. However, HIV infection is now moving slowly into the general population due to HIV infections in 'bridging groups', e.g. intravenous drug users, bisexuals and prostitutes. The infection may develop at any age but currently the incidence is highest in young and middle-aged males.

MANIFESTATIONS

When an individual becomes infected, he may develop some subclinical response or minor symptoms. These minor symptoms in a person whose blood is positive for the HIV antibody are referred to in the literature as AIDS-related complex (ARC). Other infected persons may go on to develop AIDS.

AIDS is characterized by a wide variety of signs and symptoms. Early manifestations include lymphadenopathy (swollen glands), fever, night sweats, malaise, fatigue, loss of strength, loss of weight, and persisting cough. Thrombocytopenic purpura and diarrhoea may also develop. Mental incompetence may gradually be manifested.

Opportunistic infections develop; these may be herpes simplex, respiratory infection, candidiasis (a fungal infection of the oral mucosa which may extend into the oesophagus and/or the respiratory tract), Pneumocystis carinii interstitial pneumonia (a protozoan infection), cryptococcal meningitis, lymphadenopathic toxoplasmosis (a sporozoan parasitic disease), or disseminated cytomegalovirus.

The malignant disease most commonly seen in AIDS patients is Kaposi's sarcoma. This is a particularly rare and metastasizing form of newgrowth which may be multifocal but primarily involves the skin. In individuals with AIDS, Kaposi's sarcoma involves most of the internal organs of the body, producing a wide range of symptoms.

Laboratory reports show lymphopenia (decrease in the number of lymphocytes in the blood), T cell deficiency and thrombocytopenia (platelet deficiency).

DIAGNOSIS

Tests which are used to confirm infection by the AIDS virus include: the blood serum test for specific antibodies to the HIV organism, the Western blot test which identifies antibodies to viral protein and the enzyme-linked immunoadsorbent assay (ELISA).

A positive test for HIV antibodies means two things: (1) the individual has been infected with HIV and (2) as far as we know, will remain infected and infectious for life. Antibodies for HIV are non-neutralizing, hence are only a marker of infection; it is not thought that they are 'containing' the infection. Most scientific evidence to date indicates that perhaps all individuals infected with HIV will eventually (i.e. over a 20 year time-span) develop some indicators of ill-health as a result of infection.

A problem is that a negative initial test does not necessarily indicate that the person is not infected; the test for specific antibodies may not be positive for several months following infection. Also, some individuals infected with HIV fail to mount an antibody response that can be detected by current screening tests.

If the person is in a high-risk group or is known to have been exposed to a person who has AIDS, the tests are repeated, at least three times. The incubation period for seroconversion (i.e. the time from virus entry to when there are enough antibodies to produce a positive test) may be up to 6 months (average is up to 3 months). Although the antibody test is negative before seroconversion, the person is infectious. The incubation period for AIDS (i.e. from infection to the development of symptoms) has not been identified. Data are non-conclusive; references indicate that the incubation period may range from weeks to years, being influenced by dosage, virulence, and pathogenicity of the causative virus, mode of transmission and the overall condition of the host.

TREATMENT

Management of the patient with AIDS involves the prevention of the spread of the disease as well as treatment and care of the person with the infection.

Considerable research has been undertaken to generate greater knowledge of the pathology of AIDS and find successful forms of prevention and treatment. To date, no specific curative therapy has been found and the prognosis for patients who have developed AIDS is poor. Life expectancy following the development of opportunistic infection(s) and/or a malignant disease is relatively short. Treatment is directed toward the infections and malignant disease that are serious complications of the disorder.

The patient may remain ambulatory for a period of time and be capable of continuing employment and living a normal life-style. He is followed closely by frequent visits to the clinic or doctor. It is important to inform him about his disease, the importance of preventing infections and maintaining a healthy lifestyle (e.g. adequate nutrition, rest, moderate exercise) and his role in the protection of others. The progressive complexity of the sequelae in AIDS necessitates frequent and prolonged hospitalization.

NURSING INTERVENTION

The nurse caring for the patient with AIDS requires an understanding of the disorder in order to appreciate the patient's and family's concerns and to assist in providing the necessary support. In addition, the nurse has an important role to play in the prevention of the spread of AIDS in practice and by providing information.

PATIENT CARE

When caring for a patient with AIDS, risk-containment measures are a part of the nursing care plan. Precautionary measures cited on p. 53 are applicable.

As with treatment, the identification of patient problems largely depends on the nature of the complications. For example, patients with AIDS commonly develop Pneumocystis carinii pneumonia. Nursing intervention would therefore be similar to that cited in Chapter 16. If severe candidiasis developed, both respiration and the taking of food might be involved because of extension of the secondary infection into the oesophagus and respiratory tract. Respiratory assistance (e.g. suctioning, intubation) and the use of other channels for the provision of fluids and nutrients might become necessary.

It is important to consider the implications of this disorder for the patient and his family and friends. The patient is faced with the diagnosis of an incapacitating, incurable disease. Psychosocial and probably economic problems are incurred as well as physical disability and suffering, fear and anxiety. Because it is frequently sexually transmitted, a stigma may be attached to the diagnosis by some persons which may lead to isolation and rejection of the patient.

The nurse should assess the patient's and family's reactions and attitudes and should make an effort to promote open communication and a supportive relationship. There should be no reluctance on the part of health-care workers to provide the care and support required by the patient.

The nurse should encourage the patient and family to freely express their concerns, listen willingly and take time to answer their questions. The patient should be assisted to identify his remaining strengths for coping and is allowed, as much as possible, to participate in decisions in order to preserve his personal control, independence and self-esteem. Reference to a counselling or chaplaincy service may be recommended as a source of assistance.

Excellent hygienic care, frequent positioning, back rubs, assistance as required in taking nourishment, turning, and when toileting and ambulating, and prompt response to call button, indicate thoughtfulness and caring as well as provide physical comfort to the patient.

It should be remembered that the patient's defective immune system places him at high risk of infec-

tion. He should not be exposed to health-care personnel who have an infection such as upper respiratory infection.

PATIENT EDUCATION

The Department of Health and Social Security, the Royal College of Nursing, the voluntary agencies and hospital infection control committees have issued information about AIDS and guidelines for persons with AIDS, high-risk groups, health-care personnel and the general public.

As cited before, the person with HIV infection may be well enough for a period of time to live a free independent life at home. He must be alerted to his responsibilities in relation to preventing the spread of his infection to others.

Patient and family education includes the following considerations.

1 Information about the nature of the infection, the modes of transmission and signs and symptoms which should prompt the contacting of the clinic or doctor.

2 Detailed instruction and discussions of preventive measures are necessary. The patient and family may be given a written outline of the important precautionary measures, which include the following:
a) Blood, organ or tissue donation should not be made.
b) You should inform your sex partner of your infection and should encourage her/him to see a doctor.
c) Multiple sexual contacts should be avoided.
d) A condom should be worn during intercourse.
e) Oral–genital contact and open-mouth kissing should be avoided.
f) During menstruation the infected female should not participate in any sexual activities that would place her partner at risk of exposure to blood. Sanitary towels and tampons should be carefully wrapped and disposed of in an impervious receptacle.
   Pregnancy should be avoided. Infants may become infected in utero or postnatally through breast feeding.
g) Sharing of parenteral needles and personal hygiene articles such as razor or toothbrush should be avoided.
h) Electrolysis, ear piercing, tattooing and any activity that could contaminate equipment and expose others to infection should be avoided.
i) Any person providing a service which might expose them to your body fluids or secretions (dentists, doctors, nurse, chiropodist) should be advised of your infection.
j) Articles accidentally contaminated with body fluid or blood should be cleansed promptly with a 1–10 solution of sodium hypochlorite 5.25% (household bleach) in water.

k) Good hygienic care should be practised (frequent washing of hands, bathing and mouth care).

PRECAUTIONARY MEASURES FOR HEALTH-CARE PERSONNEL

1 Hands should be washed thoroughly before and after patient care procedures.
2 Gloves should be worn if there is potential contact with blood, blood products, body fluids, secretions, or excretions of the infected person.
3 Strict precautionary care is necessary when handling needles or sharp instruments contaminated by the patient's blood. Needles should be disposed of in a puncture-proof container and should not be re-sheathed or bent to reduce the risk to the handler.
4 Specimens from a patient with AIDS should be placed in a special second container and clearly labelled Biohazard or Risk of Infection.
5 A contaminated surface should be cleansed promptly with a 1–10 hypochlorite solution 5.25% (household bleach) in water.
6 If there is a possibility of contamination of the health-care worker's clothing during care procedures, a gown should be worn.
7 A mask may be worn when caring for the AIDS patient who is coughing and has a respiratory infection.

If a health-care worker becomes accidentally exposed to the blood or body fluid by a needle-stick, scratch or laceration, the area should be cleansed thoroughly and an antiseptic applied immediately. The incident should be reported promptly to a doctor and the employer. The worker's condition should be observed for several months.

Hypersensitivity (allergy)

The term hypersensitivity or allergy implies an altered state of tissue reactivity related to the immune system. Some persons have an unusual sensitivity to certain substances and, upon contact with them, manifest an adverse reaction which is not seen in most people. The substance may be referred to as an *allergen* or an *antigen* since it causes an immune response.

The allergen is usually a protein. In the few exceptions in which it is non-protein, it becomes linked to a protein in the body and forms a compound to which the tissues are sensitive. The reaction-producing substance is specific to the individual and may be a food, an animal or plant emanation (e.g. horse dander, pollen), a chemical (e.g. dye) or a drug. It may reach the tissues by inhalation, ingestion, parenteral injection, or by direct contact with the skin. In the case of ingestion, the allergen may have a local effect upon the gastrointestinal tissues, or may be absorbed unchanged and carried by the blood to sensitive tissues.

Immune responses are usually beneficial, but in hypersensitive persons they become adverse and harmful in response to certain antigens. The first contact with the allergen may not produce manifestations of hypersensitivity, but subsequent contacts produce an inappropriate and exaggerated response that injures tissue cells and may result in the release of harmful chemical substances which are circulated, producing adverse effects on other tissues. The inflammatory process may develop at the site of the injured cells.

Common immunological disorders attributed to exogenous allergens include hay fever, asthma, eczema, urticaria, dermatitis, specific drug sensitivity (e.g. penicillin, sulphonamide preparations, aspirin, foreign serum) and specific food sensitivity (e.g. milk, wheat, eggs, shellfish, mushrooms). There is an increasing awareness of the possibility that hypersensitivity to unknown foreign or endogenous materials may account for a wide variety of pathological conditions. A hypersensitive reaction is considered to be the causative factor in rheumatic fever and glomerulonephritis. Currently there are an increasing number of references suggesting a similar aetiological basis for rheumatoid arthritis and collagen diseases such as lupus erythematosus, polyarteritis and scleroderma.

Cells in which a sensitivity is most frequently manifested appear to be those of the epithelial, connective and smooth muscle tissues. Areas of the body most frequently involved are the respiratory tract, skin and gastrointestinal tract. Reactions may take the form of: (1) itching, excessive secretion and oedema of the nasal pharyngeal mucous membrane (hay fever); (2) spasmodic constriction of the muscle tissue of the bronchial tubes and swelling and oedema of their mucosa (asthma); (3) erythematous, vesicular and inflammatory eruptions of the skin (urticaria, eczema, dermatitis); (4) vomiting and diarrhoea (food sensitivity); (5) increased permeability of blood vessels and generalized oedema (angioneurotic) or (6) vasodilation leading to circulatory failure, manifested by a weak pulse, sharp fall in blood pressure and collapse (anaphylaxis). Combinations of these may occur in the same patient. One allergen may cause a reaction in more than one area of the body. For example, a person with hypersensitivity to a particular food may develop both gastrointestinal and skin reactions, or may develop asthma and a gastrointestinal reaction. The reaction varies in different persons, depending upon their tissue sensitivity.

Genetic factors are of significance in allergic reactions; it is thought that the capacity to develop a hypersensitivity can be inherited. Abnormal immune reactions tend to occur in families. The disorder may differ from one family member to another—one may exhibit a skin reaction; another may suffer from asthma. At the same time, siblings or offspring of the affected person may not manifest any hypersensitivity. When there is a history of an allergy on both the maternal and paternal sides, a greater number of the offspring become affected and reactions appear at an earlier age.

TYPES OF HYPERSENSITIVITY

Abnormal and harmful immune reactions to antigens may be classified as immediate or delayed, and according to the mechanism or nature of the response.

Immediate hypersensitive states develop as the result of antigen–antibody interaction. This classification includes those abnormal-immune reactions characterized by the rapid appearance of manifestations, usually within 5–15 minutes of antigen–antibody contact.

Delayed hypersensitive reaction is brought about by the interaction of an antigen and sensitized T lymphocytes. The first signs and symptoms appear within approximately 12 hours and become progressively more intense, reaching a peak in 2–4 days.

The most widely accepted categorization of hypersensitivity reactions, that of Gell and Coombs,[26] indicates three immediate reactions; anaphylactic or type 1 reaction, cytotoxic or type 2 reaction, and immune complex or type 3. The delayed reaction is referred to as the T cell-mediated hypersensitivity or type 4. Irvine cites two other reactions: stimulating antibody reaction, type 5 (humoral) and lymphoid (K) cell-dependent antibody-mediated cytotoxicity, type 6 (cellular).[27]

Anaphylactic immediate hypersensitivity (type 1).
Until recently, anaphylaxis always implied a very severe life-threatening allergic reaction which caused severe shock. Currently, it has a broader concept and refers to a particular immune mechanism rather than to the severity of the response. Anaphylactic reactions vary from mild to severe and occur in individuals previously sensitized to a certain antigen.

This type of reactivity results from the reaction of an antigen with IgE antibodies. The antigen and antibodies become 'fixed' to the surface of mast cells in tissues and to basophils in the circulation.[28] Following the first exposure to the antigen, the individual is sensitized to the antigen. Second exposure to the antigen triggers an antigen–antibody interaction and the release of chemicals from the mast cells. The chemically active mediators that are released include histamine, serotonin and a slow-reactive substance (SRF). These chemicals cause an increase in capillary permeability and the contraction of smooth muscle, particularly in the smooth muscle of the lungs, bronchial tubes and vascular endothelium. Secondary chemical factors released by the cells include eosinophil chemotaxic factor, and bradykinin which exert their effects upon adjacent tissues.

The severity of the hypersensitive response is dependent upon the concentration of chemical mediators and the tissues and structures they affect.

The anaphylactic reaction may be local or systemic, depending upon the portal of entry of the antigen. Local reactions occur when the antigen–antibody reaction is on cells in target organs such as the gastrointestinal tract, respiratory mucosa or the skin. In respiratory reactions, the commonest allergens are airborne particles of dust, pollen, moulds and animal dander. The individual experiences the sneezing, nasal congestion, and increased secretion, itching and 'watering' of the eyes characteristic of allergic rhinitis (hay fever). If the antigen is inhaled, bronchospasm (asthma) and/or laryngeal oedema may cause respiratory distress. The intestinal mucosa in a sensitized person may react locally to the antigen causing crampy pain, vomiting and diarrhoea. If the antigen is absorbed, a combined systemic and local reaction may develop. The *systemic form* of anaphylaxis is likely to be severe and potentially fatal, and may be called *anaphylactic shock*. It nearly always develops very rapidly following parenteral injection of the antigen, but may occur rarely after the ingestion of food or drug allergens. The commonest antigens in anaphylactic shock are foreign serum (e.g. tetanus antitoxin), some drugs such as penicillin and streptomycin, contrast medium used in intravenous pyelograms, and bee venom from a sting.

The signs and symptoms of systemic anaphylaxis appear rapidly. The first may be a diffuse erythema and urticaria, sneezing and coughing. The patient may complain of diffuse pruritus and/or tightness in the chest which is followed by sneezing, dyspnoea and cyanosis. Localized tissue swelling of the eyelids, lips, tongue, hands, feet, genitalia and larynx develops within minutes. Laryngeal oedema and bronchospasm result in severe respiratory distress and insufficiency. Gastrointestinal disturbance may be manifested by nausea, vomiting, colicky pain and diarrhoea. There is a sharp decrease in blood pressure as vascular collapse develops; the pulse is rapid and weak and may quickly become imperceptible. The skin becomes pale and cold, pupils dilate and the patient may lose consciousness. The picture is one of cardiorespiratory failure and severe shock.

Nursing process in anaphylactic shock. Urgent intervention by the nurse and doctor is necessary to prevent the reaction from proving fatal.

Planning. Goals of intervention are to:
● Maintain ventilation

---

[26] Gell, Coombs & Lachman (1975), p. 764.
[27] Irvine (1984), Chapter 14.
[28] *Mast cells* are wandering cells that are found in most tissues and are especially abundant in connective tissues.

- Support the cardiovascular system
- Decrease the hypersensitivity response
- Alleviate the psychological distress caused by the experience
- Prevent future reactions
- Initiate prompt treatment of any future reactions

Nursing intervention. Measures to achieve these goals include:

1 *Maintenance of an airway and adequate oxygen intake.* The patient is placed in the recumbent position, with the neck extended. It may be necessary to introduce an oropharyngeal airway if the patient loses consciousness and the tongue and jaw are blocking passage of air. Suction is used to remove secretions and fluid. If the respiratory distress is unrelieved, and laryngeal spasm and oedema are suspected, an endotracheal tube may be used or a tracheostomy may be necessary to establish an airway.

Forty per cent oxygen is administered to decrease the hypoxia resulting from respiratory insufficiency. The method of administration used will depend on whether the patient is intubated or has a tracheostomy.

Vascular collapse leading to cardiorespiratory failure necessitates cardiopulmonary resuscitation (see p. 354).

If the patient experiences severe bronchospasm (asthma) without vascular collapse and shock, aminophylline, 250–500 mg, may be given very slowly over 15–30 minutes intravenously to promote bronchial dilation.

2 *Circulatory support.* The patient is positioned with the lower body elevated and constrictive clothing is loosened or removed. An intravenous infusion (usually 5% dextrose in water) is started to increase the intravascular volume and provide a vehicle for the administration of drugs.

An antihypotensive drug such as noradrenaline acid tartrate (Levophed), 8–12 μg/min; dopamine (Inotropin), 2–5 μg/kg/min or metaraminol (Aramine), 15–100 mg may be administered by intravenous infusion. The rate of flow is prescribed according to blood pressure, which is monitored every 2–5 minutes initially and then every 5–10 minutes.

The patient requires constant nursing observation. Vital signs are checked and recorded at intervals of 10–15 minutes; the intervals are gradually lengthened as the patient shows improvement. The patient usually has a cardiac monitor to ensure prompt identification of a cardiac arrhythmia.

3 *Decreasing the hypersensitivity reaction.* If the injection of the antigen has been made in a limb, a tourniquet is applied above the site to decrease circulation of the antigen. The tourniquet is released every 15 minutes for 3–5 minutes. Adrenaline, a 1:1000 solution 1 mg/ml, 0.1–0.5 ml is prescribed to be given immediately subcutaneously or intramuscularly. It is generally given in small repeated doses to relax bronchial and laryngeal spasm if respiratory distress persists. An injection of 0.1–0.3 ml may also be made at the site of injection, but generally 2 ml given over 5 minutes is the maximum that should be given.

A corticosteroid preparation such as hydrocortisone sodium succinate (Solu-Cortef) or methylprednisolone sodium succinate (Solu-Medrone) may be given intravenously to reduce tissue sensitivity. A corticosteroid preparation (e.g. prednisone) is usually administered orally for seven days following recovery from the critical phase of the reaction.

4 *Psychological support.* Systemic anaphylactic reaction is a frightening experience. The seriousness of the situation is readily sensed by the patient and family and some explanation of what is occurring is necessary, as is reassurance that everything possible is being done. It is helpful if someone is able to devote her full attention to reducing the patient's fears and providing the much needed support, and to meet the patient's requests, such as notification of a family member. This arrangement prevents possible interruption and delay of the therapeutic team.

5 *Prevention of future reactions.* The patient and family should be told the cause of the anaphylactic reaction and should be helped to make plans to avoid further contact with the allergen. Awareness of the cause helps the patient to avoid further exposure by informing health professionals of drug allergies or by avoiding situations where the agent (e.g. insect) might be present.

6 *Prompt treatment of any future reactions.* This is facilitated by the patient carrying a card and wearing an 'alert' bracelet or tag which identifies the allergen and the allergic response. If future exposure to the allergen is likely, it is recommended that the patient carries a commercially prepared, preloaded syringe of adrenaline. Family members, as well as the patient, should be taught to administer the adrenaline subcutaneously and to apply a tourniquet if the allergen enters an extremity. They must be made aware of the importance of getting the patient to a doctor or an accident and emergency department immediately.

Cytolytic immediate hypersensitivity (type 2)
This type of reaction, which may also be called cytotoxic, is destructive to the sensitized tissue cells that are attacked by antibodies. The cells have an antigenic component, which may be an integral part of the cells, or an exogenous substance such as a drug that has become firmly attached to the cells. The interaction with the antibodies, which are usually of the IgG class or occasionally the IgM class, may produce agglutination, lysis and cell destruction. Factors in the complement system facilitate the adverse

antigen–antibody reactions and subsequent dissolution of the cell.

Examples of the cytotoxic hypersensitive response include incompatible blood transfusion reaction, haemolytic anaemia, drug-induced leucopenia and possibly, glomerulonephritis.

Immune complex immediate hypersensitivity (type 3)

Two types of disorders fall into this category of hypersensitivity: the *Arthus reaction*, which produces localized lesions, and *serum sickness*, which is more systemic and diffuse. The offending immunoglobulin is most often of the IgG group, but in some instances similar reactions occur if the individual has a high level of circulating IgE antibodies. The antigen–antibody precipitates and holds complement-forming complexes that are deposited in certain tissues. The complement initiates a sequence of reactions and polymorphonuclear leucocytes are attracted to the sites. Inflammation is induced in the tissues by the interactions and release of enzymes.

The Arthus reaction occurs at the site of injection of the antigen. The complex formed in this type of hypersensitivity has a predilection for the small blood vessels; vasculitis develops and may progress to irreversible vascular damage or occlusion of the vessels, leading to interference with the blood supply to some tissues and ensuing necrosis.

Serum sickness may follow the administration of a foreign serum, such as diphtheria antitoxin and tetanus antitoxin, or the giving of some drugs such as sulphonamide, penicillin or streptomycin. The area affected by the antigen–antibody complex is not confined to the site of injection. Deposition of the antigen–antibodies and subsequent inflammatory reaction may be in: (1) the joints, causing swelling, reduced mobility and pain; (2) the kidneys, resulting in glomerulonephritis; or (3) the respiratory system, giving rise to laryngeal oedema, bronchospasm or interstitial pneumonitis. Involvement of diffuse skin areas may be manifested by rashes or urticaria.

Cell-mediated delayed hypersensitivity (type 4)

This type of hypersensitivity is cell-mediated and is most commonly induced by infectious agents such as the viruses that cause measles, herpes, smallpox, mumps, and bacteria, such as the tubercle bacilli, *Treponema pallidum*, streptococcus and salmonellae. The reaction may also occur in the form of contact dermatitis in individuals who become allergic to chromium, nickel, primula plants and poison ivy. These substances become antigenic by combining with proteins in the skin. The dermatitis is manifested by redness, swelling, vesicles (blisters), exudation ('weeping') and scaling. The cell-mediated allergic response is also involved in the rejection process that may follow tissue or organ transplantation (see p. 59) and in several autoimmune diseases such

as rheumatoid arthritis and systemic lupus erythematosus.

The example most often used to illustrate this delayed immune response is the reaction to an intradermal injection of tuberculin[29] which is used as a test for sensitivity to tubercle bacilli. The individual who has been sensitized by previous entry of the tubercle bacilli into the body produces an inflamed, indurated area at the site of the injection gradually over 18–48 hours. The delayed hypersensitive reaction is not brought about by circulating immunoglobulins but by specially sensitized lymphocytes (T cells). The site of 'attack' by the antigen becomes infiltrated with a large number of reticuloendothelial cells, mainly lymphocytes. In interacting with the antigen, the lymphocytes release substances currently referred to as lymphokines, which have varied effects—some have a chemotactic effect, which attracts still more lymphocytes to the site, and others are toxic to tissue cells. One type is said to suppress the migration of macrophages, and is referred to as the migration inhibitory factor (MIF). Immunologists indicate that there is still much to be determined concerning the mechanism of cell-mediated hypersensitivity.

Stimulating antibody reaction (type 5)

It is suggested that in this type of allergic reaction, certain IgG immunoglobulins have the ability to stimulate the tissue cells involved in the reaction rather than damage them. Some cases of thyrotoxicosis, and especially neonatal hyperthyroidism, are attributed to this class of hypersensitivity.[30]

Lymphoid (K) cell-dependent antibody-mediated cytotoxicity reaction (type 6)

Irvine attributes this hypersensitivity to lymphocytes which are not of the type usually involved in immune responses. These cells react with an immunoglobulin–antigen 'fixed' by complement on the surface of the sensitive tissue cells. As a result of the interaction, the lymphocytes have a toxic effect on the tissue cells, causing inflammation or degenerative changes. It is suggested that these cells are active in autoimmune thyroid disease (Hashimoto's thyroiditis).[31]

ASSESSMENT

Identification of allergens

The most important factor in the care of the hypersensitive person is avoidance of the allergen (antigen). Identification of the offending factor becomes paramount.

---

[29] The solution used is a purified protein extract from cultures of tubercle bacilli. It is available in 1:100, 1:1000, and 1:10000 dilutions.
[30] Irvine (1984), pp. 28–29.
[31] Irvine (1984), pp. 28–29.

History. An effort is made to learn of any allergic disorders in the family and a detailed history is taken of the patient's past illnesses, current complaint(s), personal activities, occupation and environment. The allergen may be recognized readily by the patient, family or nurse when repeated reactions are associated with the inhalation, ingestion or injection of a certain substance. For example, the individual may become ill each time he eats a particular food or may develop a rash following the wearing of a particular article of clothing, or the nurse may note that certain signs or symptoms are manifested whenever he receives a certain drug.

Physicians and institutions concerned with the investigation of hypersensitivity usually have an especially constructed history form on which relevant information is recorded. Detailed questions are presented under major headings such as: Present illness and presenting symptoms; Past illnesses; Family allergic disorders; Drugs; Immunization; Occupation; Recreation, Responses to weather; Foods; Skin applications; Contact with animals; Contact with plants; Environments (home, occupation, others); Patient's observations and comments (suspected allergen).

Sensitivity tests. Sensitivity to a substance may be detected by an intradermal or scratch skin test in which extracts of common allergens (dust, moulds, feathers, animal danders, pollens, cosmetics, dyes, wool, synthetic clothing material and various foods and drugs) are used. The intradermal method involves the injection of a minute dose of each extract into the superficial layers of the skin. A small amount of normal saline is injected as a control or comparison. In the scratch test, a drop of each allergen is applied at areas along a superficial scratch. A small mark is made at the exact site of the allergen injection or application so that the size of the local response can be measured.

The arm or the upper back may be the site used for the test; the former is preferable so that at early signs of a reaction a tourniquet can be applied to slow absorption and prevent anaphylaxis. Emergency equipment and drugs that are used in the treatment of anaphylactic shock (see p. 55) should be readily available for immediate use.

The sites are observed 15–30 minutes after the administration of the allergens. A positive reaction is indicated by itching and the appearance of erythema and a wheal (a blanched elevation surrounded by redness). The area of reaction is measured and recorded in centimetres, which the doctor then interprets as positive—1+, 2+, 3+, etc. The patient may be very apprehensive about the many injections or scratch areas and evident positive reactions. Before the allergens are administered he should be given an explanation of the nature and purpose of the tests.

During investigation of an immunological disorder, blood serum studies may be performed to determine the concentration of gamma globulin, antibodies and the various immunoglobulin classes. Tests may also be made to detect autoimmune antibodies, as well as complement fixations in antigen–antibody reactions (complement fixation test). A differential leucocyte count may be done, since eosinophils and lymphocytes may be increased in certain allergic disorders.

POTENTIAL PATIENT PROBLEMS

The nurse should be aware of the potential problems that may develop as a result of the patient's altered immune response.

PLANNING

The goals in hypersensitivity are to:
- Decrease or eliminate exposure to allergens
- Decrease the hypersensitivity response
- Increase resistance to specific antigens
- Develop an understanding of health care hypersensitivity in the patient and family with hypersensitivity problems
- Minimize the patient's psychological problems

NURSING INTERVENTION

1 *Avoidance of the allergen.* Once the allergen has been identified, it is essential that the nurse, patient and family are made aware of its source and the mode of contact or entry into the body. Avoidance of the allergen may involve such things as the elimination of a particular food from the diet, the use of foam-rubber pillows instead of those filled with feathers, the use of non-allergic cosmetics, avoidance of clothing made of certain materials, or the removal of certain pets from the environment. Air conditioning to reduce pollen and dust inhalation may be necessary, or in extreme cases, moving to another geographical area or changing jobs.

2 *Decrease the hypersensitivity response.*[32] Drugs commonly used to decrease the immune response include the following:
   (a) antihistamine preparations, such as chlorpheniramine maleate (Piriton), diphenhydramine hydrochloride (Benadryl).
   (b) cortisone (prednisolone, prednisone).
   (c) adrenaline, used in severe reactions, especially bronchospasm.
   (d) isoprenaline may be nebulized and inhaled to promote bronchial dilation. Phenylephrine hydrochloride (Neophryn) may be used locally in spray form to relieve nasal congestion in allergic rhinitis (hay fever).
   (e) In skin reactions, examples of topical applications that may be prescribed are adrenocorticoid cream or ointment (hydrocortisone cream

---

[32] For care in anaphylactic shock see pp. 54–55.

or ointment, 0.5 or 1%) and calamine lotion. If the skin allergic response is generalized, oatmeal or hydrolyzed starch baths may reduce pruritus.

3 *Minimize and/or prevent future reactions.*

(a) Observation of the following precautions may avert a serious reaction in some instances. Patients should be questioned as to allergy and drug and food sensitivity upon admission to hospital and clinic, and also when an initial home visit is made. If any such sensitivity is indicated, it should be reported to the doctor and it should also be clearly and conspicuously marked on the front of the patient's chart and patient care plan. The patient should carry a notice of his allergic problem in his wallet or pocket, or wear an 'alert' tag or bracelet to ensure that he is given prompt treatment if a reaction occurs in the future.

(b) Before administering the first dose of a drug that is known to be a common allergen, it is advisable to ask the person if he has ever taken it before; this may elicit a history of a previous reaction. The patient is observed closely after the first two or three doses of any of these drugs for signs of an untoward reaction. Common offenders include penicillin, streptomycin, animal serum (e.g. tetanus antitoxin), acetylsalicylic acid and iodide preparations used as contrast media in x-rays. Penicillin, radiopaque contrast media and sera are responsible for the greatest incidence of anaphylaxis. Before giving the initial dose of either of these, a small test dose should be given intradermally. A sensitivity reaction is manifested by the appearance of itching, erythema and a wheal at the site of administration within 15–20 minutes. When the initial dose of a drug known to cause adverse reactions is given in a clinic or doctor's office, the patient is asked to remain for 20–30 minutes.

An emergency tray or trolley should be kept fully equipped and should be quickly available. Its location and the equipment it contains should be familiar to all staff, in the event of a serious reaction. Minimal equipment on such a tray would be tourniquets, nasopharyngeal airway, endotracheal tube and laryngoscope, sterile syringes and needles, alcohol wipes, and a drug box containing ampules of adrenaline 1:1000 (aqueous), normal saline, and diphenhydramine hydrochloride (Benadryl).

Early signs of anaphylaxis are redness and itching at the site of injection, repeated sneezing, pallor, and complaints of a peculiar sensation in the throat, a tightness of the chest or faintness.

(c) *Hyposensitization.* This consists of a series of subcutaneous injections of the specific allergens to which the patient showed a positive reaction in sensitivity tests. The first few doses are very small, and are then progressively increased over an extended period of time. The exact mechanism by which this procedure reduces the patient's hypersensitivity is not understood clearly. It is suggested that with the resulting increase in antibodies, a larger amount of the allergen is required to elicit a reaction, or that the antibodies are so increased that they block the access of the allergen to the sensitive tissue cells.

It must be remembered that with the administration of any allergen there is the possibility of an immediate anaphylactic reaction. Equipment and medications used in anaphylaxis should be at hand in the event of such an emergency (see above). If the antigen injection is given in an outpatient clinic or doctor's surgery the patient is asked to remain for 20–30 minutes for observation.

4 *Develop an understanding of health care in the patient and family with hypersensitivity problems.* The nurse may play an important role in helping the patient and family to understand and accept the condition, imposed limitations and necessary adjustments and treatment. Considerable planning, teaching and direction are necessary to prepare the patient for self-care and the prevention of hypersensitive reactions. (Chapter 2 provides a guide for developing teaching strategies.)

The teaching programme should include identification of ways in which the patient may decrease or avoid exposure to the antigen.

If the antigen is a food, the patient is advised as to what foods should be eliminated from his diet. Substitutions are outlined to ensure that nutritional requirements are met. The patient's cultural and religious practices must also receive consideration in recommending plans. When the provoking substance is an inhalant, the patient's living environment is assessed and the patient and family are helped to make plans for effective environmental control. Procedures for reducing pollens, moulds, feathers and dander are discussed. The ideal solution is, of course, a mechanical system of air filtration and conditioning in the home and place of work, but this may not be economically feasible. Practical procedures include the removal of pets, damp dusting and vacuum cleaning, the replacement of feather pillows and cushions with foam rubber or a synthetic, the enclosure of mattresses in plastic, and the removal of rugs, curtains and other 'dust catchers'.

The patient and family are made familiar with the early signs and symptoms of a reaction and instructed as to the appropriate action. Prescribed medications are discussed with them; the purpose, dosage, times at which they should be taken and possible side-effects are outlined. For example, in relation to side-effects, if the patient is taking an antihistamine he is alerted to the possibility of drowsiness and the associated risk in driving; timing of taking the drug may require adjustment in accord with his activities. Corticosteroids used to reduce sensitivity may result in the development of moon face, acne and lowered resistance to infection. The importance of avoidance of self-medication and non-prescribed drugs is stressed.

The importance of maintaining resistance to prevent recurrence of the allergic disorder is cited; adequate nutrition and rest, avoidance of chilling and physical and mental exhaustion, appropriate recreation and personal habits are reviewed. Allergic responses may be readily aggravated by emotional stress. The immune disorder may create emotional stress which in turn exacerbates the disorder, setting up a vicious circle. If the patient is known to be allergic to insect bites (e.g. bee sting) he is warned that he should avoid areas where he may be exposed and that he should always carry a tourniquet and emergency drugs.

5 *Psychological support.* The imposed limitations and essential adjustments may entail sacrifice on the part of the patient and family. A change of residence, occupation, and forms of recreation, and the giving up of a pet, certain foods, cosmetics and/or other things may be necessary. The proposed therapeutic change in the individual's accustomed way of life is likely to cause some emotional distress. The patient may become depressed and angry, and signify non-acceptance of the restriction. Family members may show some resentment, blaming him for any adjustments that are required of them.

The nurse, realizing that the patient and family require time to work through the prescribed therapeutic regime, should convey an appreciation of the demands. A willingness to listen to the patient's and family's concerns encourages them to talk about their problems and feelings, making it possible to help them make plans and set priorities that are realistic and feasible for them. Efforts are made to explore possible solutions with them. The need for various types of assistance (e.g. socioeconomic, educational) may be recognized, and a referral made to a social service agency.

EXPECTED OUTCOMES

Effectiveness of nursing intervention may be determined by evidence of the following:
- The patient and family make plans for appropriate adaptations in the patient's living environment so that environmental allergens can be avoided.
- Fewer and/or less severe hypersensitivity reactions occur.
- The patient and family demonstrate knowledge of daily health management.
- The patient and family demonstrate the necessary

knowledge and skills required for care when a reaction occurs. This knowledge may be shown verbally or by implementing the plan during a reaction.

AUTOIMMUNE DISEASE

The body differentiates between its own body constituents and exogenous or foreign protein. Generally, immune bodies are formed only in response to an exogenous antigen. Occasionally, an antigen may be developed within a person (autoantigen) which stimulates the formation of antibodies (autoantibodies). The antigen may be produced by the entrance of a foreign non-antigenic substance which combines with an endogenous protein, altering it and making it antigenic. The formation of immune bodies by the body against its own protein is known as autoimmunization. The antigen–antibody combination may cause a reaction, and the resulting disease is classified as autoimmune.

Tissue transplantation
The transplantation of tissue or an organ from one person to the body of another has recently received a great deal of attention. Some degree of success has been achieved in the transplantation of a kidney from one person to another, but allograft[33] rejection still poses a serious problem. Rejection of the graft by the recipient is an immune response. Laboratory research and experimentation continue to search for a means whereby the rejection process can be controlled so that a healthy organ may be transplanted from one person to another and be accepted.

Foreign tissue is treated as antigenic and the body rejects it by producing immune bodies which attack it. All tissue cells contain antigens which differ from one individual to another (except identical twins, in which case there is histocompatibility because they are genetically identical). Although there are many tissue antigens, some are stronger than others and are more likely to be effective in causing the immune response that comprises rejection. The major antigens have been designated as belonging to the HLA system.

In selecting donor tissue the search is for tissue that has similar major antigenic components, or one that has at least very few differences. In other words, it is the extent of the 'major' antigenic differences between the donor and the recipient that determines the fate of the graft. The antigens of the HLA system occur in almost all tissue cell except red blood cells. Erythrocytes contain antigens which belong to the

---

[33] An *allograft* or *homotransplant* is the transfer of tissue or an organ from one person to another with a different genetic constitution. A *syngeneric graft* or *syngraft* is the transfer of tissue or an organ from one person to another who is genetically the same; the donor and recipient are identical twins.

blood grouping (ABO) system. Leucocytes contain all the antigens of the HLA sytstem and are used in tissue typing and in identifying a histocompatible graft. The tissue donor must also be of the same blood type as the recipient. The closer the relationship between the donor and recipient, the greater is the chance for success.

The rejection process is considered to be a cell-mediated delayed immune (type 4) reaction. In an effort to prevent rejection following an allograft several different measures may be used to suppress the immune response. These include the administration of immunosuppressive drugs such as cyclosporin, azathioprine (Imuran), corticosteroid preparations (e.g. prednisone), and antilymphocytic globulin and, rarely, body irradiation. Unfortunately, the side-effects of these 'preventive' measures are severe and may be life-threatening as a result of their toxicity or their effect of decreasing resistance to infection.

Further reference is made to organ transplant (kidney, cornea) in the respective ensuing chapters.

References and Further Reading

BOOKS

Braunwald E et al (eds) (1986) Harrison's Principles of Internal Medicine, 11th ed. New York: McGraw-Hill. Chapters 256–259.
DHSS (1986) Acquired Immune Deficiency Syndrome—AIDS—Booklet 3. Guidance for surgeons, anaesthetists, dentists and their teams in dealing with patients infected with HTLV III, CMO(86) 7, London.
Fudenberg HH, Stittes DP, Caldwell JL and Wells JV (eds) (1980) Basic and Clinical Immunology. Los Altos, CA: Lange. Section 1.
Gell PGH, Coombs RRA & Lachman PJ (eds) (1975) Clinical Aspects of Immunology, 3rd ed. Oxford: Blackwell Scientific, p. 764.
Guyton AD (1986) Textbook of Medical Physiology, 7th ed. Philadelphia: WB Saunders. Chapter 1–9 inclusive.
Ham AW & Cormack DH (1979) Histology, 8th ed. Philadelphia: JB Lippincott. Part 2.
Hart LK, Reese JL & Fearing MC (eds) (1981) Concepts Common to Acute Illness. St Louis: CV Mosby. Chapter 10.
Irvine WJ (ed.) (1979) Medical Immunology. Edinburgh: Teviot Scientific. p.50.
Irvine WJ (1984) Immunological factors in disease. In J Macleod (ed.), Davidson's Principles and Practice of Medicine, 14th ed. Edinburgh: Churchill Livingstone.
Jones P (1986) Proceedings of the AIDS Conference 1986 at Newcastle-upon-Tyne, UK, London: Intercept Publishers.
Muir BL (1980) Pathophysiology: An Introduction to the Mechanisms of Disease. New York: John Wiley & Sons. Chapters 8 and 10.
Pratt RJ (1986) AIDS—A Strategy for Nursing Care. London: Edward Arnold.

Report of the RCN AIDS Working Party (1986) Nursing Guidelines on the Management of Patients in Hospital and the Community Suffering from AIDS. London: Royal College of Nursing.
Robbins SL, Angell M & Kumar V (1981) Basic Pathology, 3rd ed. Philadelphia: WB Saunders. Chapters 1, 2 & 6.
Smith AL (1980) Microbiology and Pathology, 12th ed. St Louis: CV Mosby. Chapters 10, 11, 12 & 42.
Smith LH & Thier SO (1985) The Biological Principles of Disease, 2nd ed. Philadelphia: WB Saunders. Chapters 1 & 3.
Vander AJ, Sherman JH & Luciano DS (1985) Human Physiology: The Mechanisms of Body Function, 4th ed. New York: McGraw-Hill, pp. 599–640.
Wyngaard JB & Smith LH (eds) (1985) Cecil Textbook of Medicine, 17th ed. Philadelphia: WB Saunders, pp. 1469–1890.

PERIODICALS

Advisory Committee—American Hospital Association (1984) A hospital-wide approach to AIDS. Infection Control, Vol. 5 No. 5, pp. 242–248.
Batten C & Tabor R (1983) Nursing the patient with AIDS. Cancer Nurs., Vol. 79 No. 10, pp. 19–22.
Bennett J (1985) HTLV–III AIDS link. Am. J. Nurs., Vol. 85 No. 11, pp. 1086–1089.
Bruno P (1979) The nature of wound healing: implications for nursing practice. Nurs. Clin. N. Am., Vol 14 No. 4, pp. 667–682.
Cianci J & Lamb J (1981) Organ transplantation: matching organ donors and recipients. Am. J. Nurs., Vol. 81 No. 3, pp. 544–545.
Ern M (1980) Programmed instruction: cancer care immunology: bone marrow transplantation. Cancer Nurs., Vol. 3 No. 5, pp. 387–400.
Frances MJ & Lancaster LE (1983) The inflammatory immune response: the body's defence against invasion. Crit. Care Nurs., Vol. 3 No. 5, pp. 64–86.
Griffin JP (1983) Acquired immune deficiency syndrome: a new epidemic. Crit. Care Nurs., Vol. 3 No. 2, pp. 21–24, 28.
Grossberg SE (1981) Interferon: what lies ahead. Diagn. Med., Vol. 4 No. 3, pp. 73–77.
Gurevich I (1985) Symposium on infection in the compromised host: the competent internal immune system. Nurs. Clin. N. Am. Vol. 20 No. 1, pp. 151–161.
Gurevich I & Tafuro P (1985) Nursing measures for the prevention of infection in the compromised host. Nurs. Clin. N. Am., Vol. 20 No. 1, pp. 257–260.
Howes AC (1984) Nursing diagnoses and care plans for ambulatory patients with AIDS. Top. Clin. Nurs., Vol. 6 No. 2, pp. 61–66.
Korcok M (1985) AIDS Hysteria—a contagious side-effect, Can. Med. Assoc. J., Vol. 133 No. 12, pp. 1241–1248.
La Camera DJ, Masur H & Henderson DK (1985) Symposium on infection in the compromised host: immunodeficiency syndrome. Nurs. Clin. N. Am., Vol. 20 No. 1, pp. 241–256.
Laurence J (1985) The immune system in AIDS. Sci. Am., Vol. 253 No. 6, pp. 84–93.
Lind M (1980) The immunologic assessment: a nursing focus. Heart Lung, Vol. 9 No. 4, pp. 658–661.
Lodishj HF & Rothman JE (1979) The assembly of cell membranes. Sci. Am., Vol. 240 No. 1, pp. 48–63.
Scholl K (1983) Understanding AIDS. Cancer Nurs., Vol. 79 No. 10, pp. 16–18.

Theofilopoulos AN & Dixon FJ (1980) Detection of immune complexes: techniques and implications. *Hosp. Pract.,* Vol. 15 No. 5, pp. 107–121.

Turner JG & Pryor ER (1985) AIDS Epidemic risk containment for home health-care providers. *Fam. Community Health*, Vol. 8 No. 3, pp. 25–37.

5
Infection

The term infection implies entrance into the body of pathogenic (disease-producing) organisms. The invasion may not always produce a disease state. The development of infection depends on the ability of the microorganism to invade body tissue and to multiply there producing a response in the host. The reader is referred to Chapter 4 for discussion of inflammation and immunity which serve to prevent infection in the body.

Much progress has been made in recent decades in the fields of microbiology and epidemiology,[1] which has resulted in a marked decrease in the incidence of many infectious diseases (e.g. measles, mumps, diphtheria, typhoid fever, smallpox, poliomyelitis). Knowledge of the chain of infection has led to more effective preventive measures such as immunization, health education and improved sanitation. Worldwide control of smallpox illustrates the effectiveness of preventive programmes. Although the discovery of new antibacterial drugs has contributed to a reduction in deaths as a result of invasion by microorganisms, much absenteeism and illness can still be attributed to infections.

Concern is being expressed that the number of children being immunized in the United Kingdom is decreasing as the community becomes complacent in the face of disease control. The incidence of many sexually transmitted diseases continues to rise in the United Kingdom. Continued progress in the control and eradication of infectious diseases requires ongoing and effective health education programmes for the promotion of health as well as disease prevention.

Infection affecting specific body systems is discussed in the ensuing respective chapters. This chapter presents some information relevant to infection in general.

The Chain of Infection

Infections develop as a result of a chain of events which link the infectious agent with a susceptible host. The links in the chain include the *causative agent*, a *reservoir* for the agent to grow and multiply, a

[1] *Epidemiology* is the study of the occurrence and distribution of a disease.

mode of escape from the reservoir, a *mode of transmission*, a *mode of entry* and a *susceptible host*. All links in the chain must be present for infection to occur. If the chain is incomplete, infection does not develop. Intervention directed at any link in the chain can prevent the development of infection. Fig. 5.1 illustrates the links that must be present for infection to occur and the factors which influence the process.

CAUSATIVE AGENTS

The organisms capable of producing infection include bacteria, viruses, fungi, protozoa and parasitic worms.

Bacteria are forms of plant life which are microscopically visible and are broadly classified according to their shape as cocci (spherical), bacilli (rod-shaped) or spirochetes (spiral). They may be found almost anywhere. They are present in the soil, air, water, food and refuse and are also found in some body cavities and on the body surface.

Bacteria are a major cause of disease. Examples of bacterial diseases are diphtheria, streptococcal infection, staphylococcal infection, typhoid fever and tetanus. Many types are non-pathogenic; some species normally inhabit a particular area of the body without causing disease and are referred to as the normal bacterial flora of that area (or commensals). For example: the skin is a normal habitat of staphylococci; colon bacilli are always present in the intestine; and lactobacilli inhabit the vagina. Commensals may play an essential role in the body; for instance, a main source of vitamin K, which is necessary for bloodclotting, is the bacterial action in the intestine. The bacterial flora may be potential pathogens if they gain access to other areas of the body.

Viruses are the smallest pathogenic organisms and may only be seen under electronmicroscopic magnification. They produce disease by entering the host's cells where they may cause proliferation, degeneration or destruction. When viruses invade the body cells they may be destroyed by the host's defence mechanisms, or may survive and become established indefinitely. The initial clinical effect of the invasion may disappear but the virus may remain dormant within the host's cells, only to cause further trouble later as a result of some stimulus. When the entrance of a virus into tissue cells stimulates cell reproduction (proliferation) the new cells contain the virus. There are many varieties or strains, and their intracellular location within the hosts has made

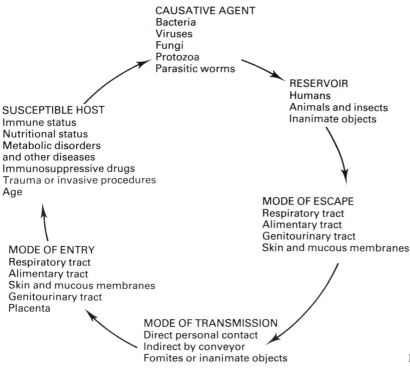

Fig. 5.1 The chain of infection.

effective therapy and control more difficult. Examples of viral diseases are the common cold, influenza, measles, mumps and poliomyelitis. There is also accumulating evidence that viruses are associated with the development of some malignant diseases.

Fungi are multicellular, mould-like organisms which produce interlacing filaments or chains. A disease caused by a fungus is called a mycosis, or it may be indicated by the suffix *-osis* preceded by the name of the causative fungus. Thrush, ringworm and histoplasmosis are examples of mycotic disease.

Protozoa are single-celled organisms that belong to the animal kingdom and are more complex in structure and activity than bacteria. Diseases that are caused by protozoa include malaria, sleeping sickness, amoebic dysentery and trichomoniasis.

Infection may be caused by *parasitic worms*, which may be referred to as helminths. The helminthic infections most commonly seen are those caused by the roundworm, pinworm. tapeworm and *Trichinella spiralis*. The latter causes trichinosis. The filarial worm (fluke), which causes filariasis or elephantiasis, and the hookworm are more prevalent in tropical areas.

CHARACTERISTICS OF THE CAUSATIVE AGENT

Virulence refers to the capacity of organisms to survive, multiply and injure the host's tissues. Virulence differs among species and among members of the same species. It is affected by the source of the organism, the rapidity of transfer and the specific characteristics of the organism. The size, shape and structure of the organisms influence their ability to survive and multiply. Some bacteria have capsules, others produce spores and viruses possess a protective protein coat which also has an affinity for receptor sites on the surface of susceptible cells. Organisms also vary as to the nutrients, temperature and other environmental factors required for growth. The virulence of pathogenic organisms is related to their ability to produce and release harmful chemical substances called toxins. The toxins may be liberated by the organisms while they are alive (exotoxins), or they may be released with the disintegration of the organisms (endotoxins). Toxins may injure the cells at the site of their release and may also be absorbed into the blood and affect other structures throughout the body. In most instances the toxin is specific as to the tissues it affects.

Many microorganisms have an affinity for certain tissues and organs. For example, the virus that causes mumps has a predilection for the parotid glands. Similarly the pneumococcus readily affects the lungs and the meningococcus prefers the meninges.

The reservoir

Microorganisms that cause infection in humans need a reservoir in which to grow and multiply. They may come from sources external to the human body or may be normal inhabitants of the body. The normal flora of the body cause disease when the host's resistance is lowered, or when the organisms are transferred to another area of the body where they are not normally found.

External reservoirs of infectious agents may be other humans, animals, insects or inanimate objects. These sources provide reservoirs where the organisms can live and propagate and from which they are transferred to the host.

The most common reservoir is a human who may be in the incubation period, acute stage or convalescence of the disease, or who may be a carrier (vector). The latter may appear healthy but harbour pathogenic organisms which can be transmitted to others.

Tuberculosis and brucellosis (undulant fever) are examples of infections that may be contracted from cows. Animals infested with parasites may be a source of disease if they are used as meat. Rabies is acquired from rabid dogs, cats or other infected animals. The source of psittacosis in man is usually a parrot, and the tsetse fly is usually the source of trypanosomiasis (sleeping sickness).

The most common inanimate reservoirs are soil and decaying animal and vegetable matter. Tetanus usually develops as a result of soil contamination of a wound. Soil may also be a source of some pathogenic fungi.

Mode of escape

Infectious agents require a means of escaping from the reservoir. Exit from human reservoirs may be by the respiratory, alimentary or genitourinary tracts or from open lesions on the skin or mucous membranes.

Mode of transmission

Pathogenic agents may be transmitted from their source by direct or indirect contact. In direct spread the infecting agent is transferred directly from the reservoir to the person. Indirect transmission implies an intermediary contaminated conveyor or object. Conveyors frequently support the life and growth of the organisms. Transmission of the disease-producing organism by indirect contact occurs in airborne infections (e.g. respiratory diseases) and water and food infections (e.g. food poisoning, typhoid fever). *Fomites* is a term applied to inanimate objects that spread infection; examples are bedding, towels, dishes, instruments and furniture.

Mode of entry

The infecting agents may enter the host through the respiratory tract, the alimentary tract, a break in the skin or the genitourinary tract. A fetus may become infected by transplacental transmission. Normally the placenta is an effective barrier, but certain organisms, such as the spirochete that causes syphilis and viruses if present in the mother, are likely to cross the placenta and enter the fetus.

Susceptible host

The development of infection after the infectious agent has entered the body depends on the characteristics of the microorganism and on the nature of the local tissue and defences of the host.

DEFENCES

Defences against pathogens are natural (innate) or acquired.

Innate defences
Normal body structure and activities provide the individual with considerable protection against infection. Externally, the skin is an effective barrier against the entry of organisms as long as it remains intact. The acidity and fatty acid content of its glandular secretions tend to destroy or inhibit the growth of many pathogens.

The mucous membrane of the respiratory tract plays an important protective role. Its secretion traps and carries away organisms; the cilia filter the air and sweep out offenders. The mucus may also induce coughing, which forcefully expels material bearing organisms from the tract. Drying of the membrane, destruction of the cilia and loss of the cough reflex reduce the protective mechanism.

The mucus secreted in the gastrointestinal tract protects the mucous membrane lining from the hydrochloric acid and digestive enzymes. Absence of the mucus could result in ulceration that would permit the entrance of pathogens. The acidity of the gastric secretion destroys many organisms that are ingested.

The microorganisms that are normal inhabitants of some areas of the body may play a defensive role. For example, the reaction of the natural flora of the secretions of the vaginal mucosa produces an acidity that creates a resistance to infective agents.

Another important natural defence mechanism is phagocytosis; pathogens that invade the body may be engulfed and destroyed by leucocytes and macrophages. In many infections the number of leucocytes in circulation is rapidly increased, and they migrate to the site of invasion. Changes in the proportion of different types of leucocytes are characteristic of infection by certain types of organisms. Lymph nodes are strategically situated along the course of the lymphatics and filter out bacteria to be destroyed by phagocytosis.

The inflammatory process is a protective mechanism and is described on p. 40–43.

Body fluids contain some substances that are antibacterial. One of these is an enzyme (lysozyme) that destroys bacteria by breaking down their cell walls. Plasma contains gamma globulin which forms antibodies in response to infective agents or their toxins.

Good health habits such as optimal nutrition and hydration, adequate rest and exercise, and the avoidance of fatigue and stress promote the body's natural resistance to infection.

Some persons have what is referred to as a natural immunity to certain diseases. Immunity may be defined as the resistance of the body to pathogenic organisms. Natural immunity to certain pathogens varies with species, races, individuals and with age. Natural immunity is discussed in more detail on p. 49.

Acquired defences
Immunity to an infection may be acquired by an individual as a result of contact with the infecting agent or its products. The host develops an immunity by forming antibodies or sensitized T lymphocytes. Artificially induced active immunity for certain diseases is recommended for every person. Immunity is discussed in the preceding chapter under 'The Immune Response'.

Factors Predisposing to Infection

Factors that influence the host's resistance and susceptibility to infection include the following:

Nutrition. Poorly nourished persons have an increased susceptibility to infection, particularly if their diet has been deficient in protein and vitamins. Their natural tissue resistance and ability to form antibodies are reduced.

Age. Infants, children and elderly persons are less able to resist infection.

Occupation. Certain occupations provide increased exposure to infecting agents or may reduce the efficiency of one's protective mechanisms. For example, persons working with cattle may be exposed to undulant fever; those working in mines are more susceptible to tuberculosis.

Exposure to cold. A lowering of the body temperature below normal is thought to decrease the ciliary movement in the respiratory tract, reduce the blood supply to superficial tissues and suppress antibody formation, all of which are natural defence mechanisms.

Exposure to radiation. Exposure to large doses of radiation, particularly total body irradiation, reduces the patient's defence mechanisms. Leucocyte and anti-body production are suppressed. Bone marrow and the mucosa of the gastrointestinal tract are the two types of tissue most affected by radiation.

Metabolic disturbances and other diseases. The person who already has some abnormality in function within the body is less able to resist or cope with an infection. For instance, the diabetic is believed to be more prone to infection because phagocytosis, chemotaxis and the bactericidal function of neutrophils are diminished when hyperglycaemia or ketoacidosis is present.[2]

Immunosuppressive therapy. The patient receiving immunosuppressive drugs such as corticosteroids, antibiotics or cytotoxic drugs exhibits a marked susceptibility to infection. These drugs suppress the protective inflammatory response and the production of lymphocytes and antibodies.

The Course of the Infectious Disease

The course of most infectious diseases extends over the following phases:

Incubation period. This is the interval between the time the organism enters the body and the initial clinical manifestations of an infection. During this stage the organisms multiply. The length of the incubation period varies with different organisms; for example, the incubation period for streptococcal infection is about 1–3 days, and for measles about 8–15 days.

Acute illness is the stage in which the disease reaches its full intensity. The length of the period of acute illness varies from a few hours to weeks. It is generally predictable for the specific disease.

Convalescence is the stage during which the clinical manifestations subside. Many infectious diseases are self-limiting and recovery takes place over a short, defined period of time. The development of complications or of residual manifestations of the disease, such as paralysis due to poliomyelitis, may prolong recovery. Death is also a possibility from some highly virulent diseases or as a result of complications.

Types of Infections

Certain terms may be used to describe infection. *Local* means the infection remains confined to one area. A *generalized systemic* infection is one in which

---

[2] Donohue-Porter (1985), p. 191.

the organisms are disseminated throughout the body.

A *focal* infection occurs when the infection spreads from a confined area to other parts of the body.

A *mixed* infection is due to more than one type of pathogen. If a person becomes infected by another type of organism during the course of an infection, it is termed a *secondary* infection, and the initial one is referred to as *primary*. An infection may be *acute* or *chronic*.

The presence of bacteria in the blood produces *bacteraemia*. *Septicaemia* means organisms have entered the bloodstream and are actively multiplying and producing toxins. Toxaemia implies a concentration of bacterial toxins in the blood. *Pyaemia* is a type of septicaemia in which the organisms are clumped together or incorporated into small thrombi. The clumps or thrombi may become deposited at various sites throughout the body and may cause small, scattered abscesses.

Nosocomial infection. Hospital-acquired or *nosocomial* infections are infections which occur in hospitalized patients that were not present or incubating at the time of admission. The infection may result from endogenous organisms carried by the patient or originate from the animate or inanimate environment of the hospital. The latter are potentially preventable infections. Hand-washing is the simplest and most effective preventive measure. Nosocomial infections result in prolonged hospitalization, increasing the cost of treatment as well as causing discomfort and inconvenience for the patient

Nursing Process

ASSESSMENT

DATA COLLECTION

Health history. Specific factors from the patient's health history that are relevant to infections include: age; immunization history, including dates and type of immunization received; childhood communicable diseases; history of metabolic and chronic diseases; medication history, particularly in relation to immunosuppressive drug therapy and cortico-steroids; general nutritional status; exposure to radiation; occupational and home environments and history of recent travel; and information about recent crises and changes in life-style (marriage, deaths, new baby, etc.), as well as subjective symptoms of infectious diseases (headache, chills, anorexia, nausea, apathy, fatigue, joint and muscle pain and general malaise).

Physical assessment. Assessment of the patient for objective signs of infection includes: the recording of vital signs (temperature, and pulse and respiratory rates) and observing his overall appearance (e.g. for flushing of the skin and perspiration, general posture and body positioning). The patient should be observed for a tendency to splint, guard or failure to use certain body parts. The skin is examined for rash, lesions, warmth and moisture. Lymph nodes are palpated to see if they are enlarged or tender and the chest is auscultated for râles.

DIAGNOSTIC PROCEDURES USED IN INFECTIONS

Leucocyte count and differential
Some infections cause an increase in the white blood cells well above the normal, while in others there may be a decrease below the normal. An increase in a particular type of leucocyte is recognized as being characteristic of certain infections (see Table 5.1).

Erythrocyte sedimentation rate
The rate at which the red blood cells settle in a specimen of blood is increased in infection and inflammation.
> Normal:
>> Westergren method—male, 0 to 15mm in 1 hour: female, 0 to 20mm in 1 hour
>> Wintrobe method—male, 0 to 9mm in 1 hour; female, 0 to 15mm in 1 hour
>> Cutter method—male, 0 to 8mm in 1 hour; female, 0 to 10mm in 1 hour.

Antibody tests
A specimen of blood may be examined to determine the concentration of antibodies present: this is referred to as an antibody titre. Microorganisms act as antigens, stimulating the production of antibodies. Tests may also be done to detect the presence of certain antigens or antibodies; a known antibody may be used to determine the presence of an antigen, or a known antigen may be used to detect antibodies.

Identification of the causative organism
Identification of the causative agent involves the isolation of the organism from the body tissue or secretion in which it is located. This is done by the following methods:
Direct examination involves a specimen of sputum, blood, spinal fluid, urine, faeces, or the discharge or scrapings from a lesion being stained and examined under the microscope for organisms. Appearance, shape and certain staining characteristics assist in identifying different organisms.
Cultural growth involves the sterile collection of suspect material from the patient and introduction of this material to a nutrient culture media, chick embryo or tissue culture media. The media are observed for a period of time for the growth of organisms. The material to be cultured may be sputum, nasal or throat secretions, blood, urine, faeces, wound discharge or spinal fluid.

Table 5.1 The white cell differential count in infectious processes.*

Cell type	Number	Per cent of total	Functions/changes
Leucocytes	4.0–11.0	100	—
Neutrophils	2.5–7.5	40–75	Non-specific Responsible for Phagocytosis Increased leucocytosis in infection = shift to the left Decrease Leucopenia in some viral infections
Juvenile neutrophils (bands)	0–0.006	0–10	Increased in infection = shift to the left
Lymphocytes	1.50–4.0	20–50	Increased lymphocytosis in viral and tuberculous infection Decrease lymphopenia in AIDS and chronic TB
Monocytes	0.20–0.8	2–10	Increased in TB, rickettsial and some viral infections, and malaria
Eosinophils	0.04–0.4	1–6	Increase eosinophilia in parasite infections and allergy
Basophils	0.01–0.1	<1	Not affected by infections

*Hoffbrand & Pettit (1984)

Animal inoculation may be used for the identification of the organism of a few diseases such as tuberculosis and mycotic infections. Appropriate material from the patient is injected into a laboratory animal. The animal is killed after a certain period and examined for evidence of the suspected disease.

All specimens collected to determine the presence and type of pathogenic organism must be collected with sterile equipment and placed in a sterile container. Special sterile containers are usually provided by the laboratory for particular specimen materials, along with directions as to the necessary precautions to be observed in the collection. The specimen should be delivered promptly to the laboratory to avoid drying; if this is not possible, it is recommended that it be stored in the refrigerator until it can be cultured or examined.

Some anti-infective drugs are only effective in infection caused by certain organisms, while others can be used for a much greater variety of infections. In order to select an antimicrobial drug, the doctor may ask for an *organism sensitivity test*. When the infecting organism is identified, a culture of it is tested with several antimicrobial drugs, such as different antibiotics, to identify which drug is most effective in destroying the organism.

Skin tests
Two skin tests are the tuberculin and Schick tests. In the tuberculin test, a small dose of old tuberculin or purified protein derivative tuberculin is injected intradermally on the flexor surface of the forearm. A positive reaction is indicated by swelling and oedema at the site of injection and a surrounding redness in 2–3 days; this result means the individual has or has had an infection by tubercle bacilli, acquired either naturally or following a BCG. The test is considered negative if there is no reaction. If the first test is negative, the test may be repeated with a larger dose of tuberculin.

The Schick test which is less frequently used, determines susceptibility to diphtheria. A small dose of diphtheria toxin standard dilute (0.1 ml) is administered intradermally into a forearm, and a dose of inactivated toxin is given intradermally in the opposite arm. The latter is used as the comparative control. In a positive reaction, the site of the active toxin injection manifests redness in 48 hours which persists for 1–2 weeks. The control shows no reaction. A positive reaction indicates that the recipient of the toxin does not have antibodies to neutralize the toxin and is considered susceptible. A negative Schick test shows no reaction on either arm and indicates the person has sufficient antitoxin antibodies to protect him.

CLINICAL MANIFESTATIONS OF INFECTION

During the incubation period, symptoms of infection are usually general and include headache and malaise. Manifestations common to many infections during the acute stage include the following systemic and local symptoms: fever, which may be preceded by chills; an increase in the pulse and respiratory rates; anorexia; nausea and vomiting; headache; apathy and fatigue; joint and muscle pain; and general malaise. The patient may appear hot and flushed, and the tongue is frequently furred and dry. There may be enlargement and tenderness of the lymph nodes that receive the lymph from the site of infection.

If the infection is local, the classic symptoms are that the area becomes red (rubric) and hot (hyperthermic) due to the vasodilation, swollen (oedema) due to the increased vascular permeability, and painful (dolor) as a result of the release of chemical mediators and pressure from the increased fluid. These symptoms are also seen in inflammatory responses described in Chapter 4. Inflammation is always present with infection unless the patient's immune system is severely impaired. Infection, on the other hand, is not always present with inflammation as inflammation may be caused by heat, radiation or trauma, as well as by microorganisms.

In addition to the common signs and symptoms described above, specific features characteristic of a specific infection may be present and may play an important role in the diagnosis. For example, certain infections cause a rash, while others may give rise to a marked increase in a particular type of leucocyte. (See Table 5.2 for information relating to common communicable diseases.)

POTENTIAL PATIENT PROBLEMS

Analysis of the data collected from the patient's history, by physical examination and specific diagnostic tests will lead to the identification of potential patient problems (for the patient with an increased risk of infection) or to actual patient problems (for the patient with an actual infection).

Increased potential for infection may be related to breakdown in any link of the infectious chain resulting in the individual being exposed to the infectious agent or to factors in the individual which increase susceptibility to infection once the organism has been transmitted. These factors include inadequate acquired or innate immunity, poor nutritional status, age, metabolic disturbances or other diseases and immunosuppression.

The following patient problems relate to most individuals with infectious diseases:

1 Physical and social isolation associated with limitations imposed by the potential for transmission of infectious agents and the resulting infection control measures
2 Alterations in nutrition, as the patient's intake may be less than his body requirements in fever (increased energy expenditure)
3 Alterations in comfort associated with the inflammatory process
4 Alterations in certain body functions related to the manifestations of specific infectious diseases (e.g. altered bowel function with diarrhoea or ineffective airway clearance related to increased respiratory secretions)
5 Alterations in self-management related to functional loss resulting from sequelae or complications of the infection

PLANNING

Nursing goals are to:
1 Provide a safe environment
2 Control the sources of infection
3 Prevent transmission of infectious agents
4 Protect the patient with an increased susceptibility to infection
5 Support the functioning of the individual with an infection

Goals for the patient with an infection are to:
1 Minimize the impact of physical and social isolation
2 Maintain adequate fluid and nutritional status
3 Prevent and/or alleviate discomfort
4 Maintain body functioning
5 Maintain and/or promote functional competence

Prevention and control of infection

COMMUNITY MEASURES

Environmental control measures in the community for the control of infectious diseases are directed at various links in the chain of infection. Organisms are destroyed through chemical spraying of specific environments. Adequate sewage disposal and the provision of a safe water supply destroy one of the major links in the chain by removing major reservoirs for microorganisms. These are major factors to consider in underdeveloped areas in Europe and the rest of the world. Control of diseases such as typhoid fever and many gastrointestinal infections in children is dependent on these two factors. The control of insects is one method of decreasing the likelihood of transmission of infectious agents as are isolation measures to control the transfer of organisms from infected individuals. Immunization programmes are directed at increasing the immunity of susceptible people.

Many measures to control infectious diseases in the community are controlled by legislation and are monitored by international, EEC, national and environmental health departments of local government authorities. The World Health Organization (WHO), an agency of the United Nations, monitors outbreaks of infectious diseases throughout the world and institutes appropriate preventive and control measures. The Communicable Disease Surveillance Centre (CDSC) is an agency of the Public Health Laboratory Services which monitors infectious diseases on a national level. This centre provides epidemiological, laboratory, consultative and other services for the identification of communicable diseases, and intervenes to control outbreaks of communicable diseases. The CDSC provides guidelines for infection control in hospitals and the community.

Immunization programmes. These programmes provide artificially induced active immunity for certain diseases. Immunization programmes have made a major contribution to the dramatic decline in the incidence of diseases such as poliomyelitis and the eradication of smallpox. An immunization regimen is recommended for all infants and children. Parents are instructed that immunization should begin when the infant is 2 or 3 months of age and informed of the various resources (family doctor, paediatrician, community health centres).

Immunization schedules and practices vary in different countries and in different areas. This service is generally available through local health authorities or agencies and therefore is accessible to most individuals without concern for cost.

Routine immunization is generally provided for diphtheria toxoid, pertussis (whooping cough), tetanus, rubella (German measles), mumps, measles and poliomyelitis. Smallpox vaccine is no longer used in routine immunization programmes but may be given to individuals in specific circumstances.

Artificially induced immunity becomes weaker over a period of months to years; it varies in relation to the different diseases. As a result, reinforcing doses of some immunizing agents are necessary. Records of immunization received and the date it was obtained should be kept by each individual for future reference.

For individuals who have been exposed to certain pathogenic organisms, prophylactic measures include: the administration of booster or recall doses of toxoid (e.g. diphtheria toxoid, tetanus toxoid) to enhance existing immunity; human immune serum globulins and antitoxins to provide passive immunity; or antibiotics to augment body defences in combating the organisms.

In the UK, some diseases are notifiable by law to the Medical Officer for Environmental Health; the doctor who diagnoses the infection is responsible for the notification. Examples include measles, tuberculosis and whooping cough. Tests are carried out to determine whether they have the disease or should have prophylactic treatment.

Nursing responsibilities include informing individuals of the importance of receiving prophylactic treatment when relevant and ensuring that they are aware that prophylactic preparations for active or passive immunization can be obtained from general practitioners or health centres.

Individuals travelling to countries where there is an incidence of infectious diseases not common in their community, should consult their general practitioners about immunization requirements for their protection.

Nurses have an important role to play in teaching individuals measures to prevent infection. The nurse assesses if the individual family and/or community have safe water to drink and adequate toilet facilities. Individuals travelling to other countries or other areas of their own country, can be helped by the nurse to assess the environment they will be in for safe water and housing, sewage disposal and the availability of health services.

INFECTION CONTROL IN HOSPITALS

The hospital environment presents a high risk for infection, especially for patients with debilitating diseases. Nosocomial infections are acquired in hospital and were not present at the time of admission.

Many patients with different infections are potential sources. Unless precautions are taken and strict medical asepsis is observed, infection may be transmitted from one patient to another. Hand-washing is the most important precaution to be taken.

Hospital personnel may harbour organisms without manifesting illness themselves. But, unfortunately, if these infective agents are transmitted to patients, whose defence mechanisms are less effective because of their illness, the infection can be a serious complication and may be life-threatening and prolong their hospitalization.

The nurse has a responsibility in any situation where infection is known to exist, or where there is the possibility of infection, to practise and promote measures that will confine the organisms and prevent their spread to other persons.

Measures to prevent hospital-acquired infections include:

- Recognition of the possible risk of infection among hospitalized patients
- Questioning the use of invasive procedures and implementing these procedures only when necessary
- Following strict surgical aseptic techniques when carrying out invasive procedures (e.g. urinary catheterization, intravenous infusion)
- Instruction of patients and visitors in measures to prevent spread of organisms (e.g. hand-washing, covering nose and mouth with tissues when coughing, not sharing personal objects and not visiting if an infection is suspected)
- Prompt identification and treatment of infections in hospital personnel
- Implementation of isolation procedures for certain infected patients
- The practice of hand-washing under running water with soap and friction before and after provision of care for a patient and/or following the handling of patient articles
- Efficient domestic cleaning of wards, isolation rooms and other areas of the hospital (e.g. damp mopping to decrease dust and the use of approved hospital disinfectants)

Control of infection by isolation
When an individual has an infection, measures must be instituted to protect others in the home or hospital environment from the infected persons's pathogens. The specific protective measures instituted will be determined by (1) the virulence of the organism present, (2) the source of the organism (e.g. respiratory secretions, faeces, urine, wounds and skin and/or blood), (3) the mode of transmission of the organisms (direct or indirect contact or fomites), (4) the mode of entry of the organism, (5) the susceptibility of the host and (6) the institutional policies. In the home, as in the hospital, consideration must be given to the age and susceptibility of other individuals who are in contact with the patient and to the

Table 5.2 Common communicable diseases*

Communicable disease	Causative agent	Source(s) and transmission	Portal of entry	Incubation period	Isolation	Immunization	Comments
Chickenpox (varicella)	Virus (varicella zoster virus)	Infected persons; articles contaminated by discharge from vesicles and mucous membranes Transmitted by direct contact with infected person—respiratory droplets, crusts of lesions; indirect via articles contaminated with respiratory discharge or discharge of lesions	Nasopharynx suggested	10–21 days	Patient isolated until all lesions have crusted	Active: by disease Passive: by human zoster immune plasma, or by zoster immune globulin (if available)	Virus can infect adults who were infected with chickenpox earlier and cause herpes zoster (shingles)
Common cold	Numerous viruses	Respiratory droplets of infected persons Transmitted by direct contact with infected person	Nasopharynx	1–4 days	Precautions to prevent spread of respiratory droplets and secretions of infected persons	None	
Diphtheria	Diphtheria bacillus (*Corynebacterium diphtheriae*)	Respiratory secretions and saliva of infected persons or carriers; food Transmitted by direct or indirect contact	Nasopharynx	2–6 days	Strict isolation until several (usually six) successive, daily negative throat and nasal cultures are obtained	Active: 1 by disease 2 toxoid Passive: Diphtheria antitoxin. An antibiotic is usually given in conjunction with the antitoxin	Schick test may be made to determine the presence or absence of specific antibodies; immunized persons can become carriers of the infective organism
Encephalitis	Viruses	Bite from infected mosquito or contact with infected birds or rodents	Skin	4–21 days	None; not transmitted from man to man	Formalinized virus vaccines for high-risk persons	Prophylactic measures are directed toward eradication of the mosquito
Gas gangrene	Clostridia (anaerobic spore forms)	Soil and human intestinal tract Transmitted by soil or soil-contaminated articles; faeces	Deep wounds	1–4 days	Modified; strict precautionary measures to prevent spread by wound drainage	Passive: gas gangrene antitoxin	Early extensive débridement of deep macerated wounds; patient receives antibiotics and a high concentration of oxygen; the latter is administered in a hyperbaric oxygen chamber
Gonorrhoea	Gonococcus (*Neisseria gonorrhoeae*)	Urethral or vaginal secretions of infected persons Transmitted by sexual intercourse	Urethral or vaginal mucosa; eyes, anal canal, and throat may also be portals of entry	3–8 days	Careful handling and disposal of articles contaminated by discharge	None	Treatment is administration of penicillin; efforts are made to identify and treat contacts
Hepatitis (infectious type A)	Hepatitis A virus	Faeces and blood of infected persons Transmitted by contaminated food and water	Gastrointestinal tract	15–50 days	Modified; use of gown when giving direct patient care; careful handling and disposal of emesis and faecal discharge	Passive: human immune serum globulin	
Hepatitis (serum type B)	Hepatitis B virus	Blood or semen from infected persons or carriers Transmitted by parenteral injection or by sexual intercourse	Skin and blood vessels	6 weeks to 6 months	Modified; careful handling and disposal of blood, wound discharges and excreta	Passive: Human immune serum globulin or hepatitis B immune globulin Active: hepatitis B vaccine	Prophylactic measures include careful selection of blood donors and adequate sterilization of equipment used in parenteral injections
Herpes simplex	Herpes simplex virus: type I (herpes labialis), type II (herpes genitalia)	Direct contact with saliva or lesions of infected person and by sexual contact	Mouth, skin and genitalia	up to 14 days	Careful handling and disposal of articles contaminated by lesions	None	Recurrences are common

Table 5.2—*continued*

Communicable disease	Causative agent	Source(s) and transmission	Portal of entry	Incubation period	Isolation	Immunization	Comments
Influenza	Numerous viruses (types A, B, C)	Respiratory secretions of infected persons Transmitted by direct contact; respiratory droplets, possibly airborne	Nose or mouth	1–4 days	Avoid direct contact	Polyvalent influenza virus vaccines	Amantadine hydrochloride (Symmetrel) may be used for prophylaxis against type A influenza for high risk individuals
Legionnaires' disease (Legionella pneumonia)	*Legionella pneumophila*	Soil and water, dust No evidence of transmission from patient to contacts	Nasopharynx	2–10 days	None	None	Treat with erythromycin; assisted ventilation and shock management are essential
Malaria	*Plasmodium* protozoa	Mosquitoes and blood of infected persons Transmitted by bite from infected mosquito	Skin	6–37 days	Careful handling and disposal of articles contaminated by blood of infected persons	None	Prophylactic measures include antimalarial drugs for persons exposed to infected mosquitoes and programmes to eradicate mosquitoes
Measles (rubeola)	Rubeola virus	Nose and throat secretions, blood and urine of infected persons Transmitted usually by droplet spread	Respiratory tract	8–15 days	Isolate from 7 days after exposure to 5 days after rash appears	Active: 1 by disease 2 vaccine (a) live attenuated measles virus vaccine (b) inactive measles virus vaccine Passive: Human immune serum globulin	
Meningitis	Meningococcus; numerous viruses and other organisms such as streptococcus tubercle bacillus	Respiratory secretions from infected persons or carriers Transmitted by respiratory droplets	Nose and mouth	Varies with causative agent	Strict isolation with meningococcal meningitis; careful handling and disposal of articles contaminated by respiratory secretions	Active: vaccine for types A and C meningococci	The prophylactic measure is to administer antibiotics such as rifampicin and sulphadiazine to eliminate carriage and for contacts
Mumps (epidemic parotitis)	Myxovirus mumps	Saliva of infected persons Transmitted by direct contact with infected persons, respiratory droplets and oral secretions	Nose and mouth	14–21 days	Isolation from onset of swelling until swelling subsides	Active: 1 by disease 2 live attenuated mumps vaccine	Passive immunization with human mumps immune globulin is of unproven value in adults and is not recommended in children
Paratyphoid fevers	Salmonella species of organisms	Urine and faeces of infected persons Transmitted by ingestion of contaminated water and food	Gastrointestinal tract	7–21 days	Modified; use of gown when giving direct patient care; thorough disinfection of articles contaminated with urine and faeces	Paratyphoid A and B vaccine (combined with typhoid vaccine)	An important prophylactic measure is strict sanitary precautions in the handling of food and water
Pertussis (whooping cough)	Bordetella (*Haemophilus pertussis*)	Respiratory secretions of infected persons Transmitted by droplet spread	Respiratory tract	7–21 days	Modified; measures to prevent spread of respiratory secretions; disinfect soiled articles	Active: 1 by disease 2 pertussis vaccine	Passive immunization with human pertussis immune globulin has not been shown to be effective and is not recommended
Poliomyelitis	Polioviruses (3 types)	Gastrointestinal tract of infected persons and carriers Transmitted by direct contact with nasopharyngeal secretions of infected persons, vomitus and stools	Gastrointestinal tract	5–21 days	Strict isolation until temperature returns to normal; careful handling and disposal of respiratory secretions, emesis and faeces during the acute stage	Active: 1 by disease 2 trivalent oral polio vaccine or inactivated polio vaccine (Salk type)	

Table 5.2—*continued*

Communicable disease	Causative agent	Source(s) and transmission	Portal of entry	Incubation period	Isolation	Immunization	Comments
Rabies	Virus	Saliva of infected animals and persons Transmitted by bite from rabid animal	Skin	10 days to 2 years	Strict isolation	Active: (a) duck embryo rabies vaccine given in 23 doses over 2 weeks *or* (b) nerve tissue rabies vaccine (Semple method) 14 daily doses *or* human diploid rabies vaccine given in 5 doses (use of this vaccine is preferable when it is available) Passive: human rabies immune globulin	Following exposure to rabies, a combination of active and passive immunization should be used
Rubella (German measles)	Rubella virus	Infected persons Transmission by direct contact or droplet spread of nasopharyngeal secretions	Respiratory tract	14–21 days	None	Active: 1 by disease 2 live attenuated rubella virus vaccine Passive: human immune serum globulin	Pregnant women should avoid any possible contact with infected persons; congenital anomalies result from infection in first trimester of pregnancy
Streptococcal diseases (sore throat, scarlet fever, impetigo, erysipelas)	ß-Haemolytic streptococci group A	Respiratory secretions of infected persons or carriers and through contaminated articles, milk and foods	Nasopharynx and skin	1–3 days	Precautions to prevent spread of respiratory droplets and secretions of infected persons; careful handling and disposal of contaminated articles	None	Prophylactic treatment with penicillin G to prevent recurrence in high-risk persons
Syphilis	Treponema pallidum	Exudate and blood of infected persons Transmitted by sexual intercourse; contact with open lesions; blood transfusion	External genitalia, mucosal surfaces, bloodstream	14–90 days	Careful handling and disposal of articles contaminated by discharge from lesions	None	Careful screening of donor blood before use
Tetanus (lockjaw)	Tetanus bacillus (*Clostridium tetani*)	Animal faeces and soil	Deep macerated wounds	5–21 days	None	Active: tetanus toxoid Passive: human tetanus immunoglobulin; tetanus antitoxin	If a patient has not received tetanus toxoid and receives an injury, tetanus immune globulin is prescribed as a prophylactic measure; Tetanus antitoxin is only used if tetanus immune globulin is not available
Toxic shock syndrome	*Staphylococcus aureus*	Organisms have been found in throat, cervix, vagina and rectum. Toxins have been found in blood and breast milk	Vagina and unknown	2–5 days, usually post onset of menstruation or postsurgery	Evidence exists of transmission to other patients in hospital and to spouses, therefore strict isolation is recommended	None	Treat with antistaphylococcal antibiotic drugs. Incidence is highest in the postmenstrual period in women who use extra absorbent tampons and in both men and women post surgery
Tuberculosis	Tubercle bacillus	Sputum from infected persons; milk from infected cows Transmission by droplet spread; ingestion of contaminated milk and contaminated articles	Respiratory or gastrointestinal tract	Varies	Careful handing and disposal of articles contaminated by secretions	Active: 1 infection not absolute immunity, but individual is less likely to develop disease on subsequent exposure to disease	Chemoprophylactic drugs may be administered to persons who are known to be infected

Table 5.2—*continued*

Communicable disease	Causative agent	Source(s) and transmission	Portal of entry	Incubation period	Isolation	Immunization	Comments
						2 BCG vaccine given to persons showing negative tuberculin tests and living in areas of high tuberculin prevalence	
Typhoid fever	*Salmonella typhi*	Excreta of infected persons and carriers. Transmitted by contaminated food and water	Gastrointestin-al tract	7–21 days	Strict isolation until stool tests are repeatedly negative	Active: 1 by disease 2 typhoid vaccine	

*Information compiled from: Bader (1979); Ontario Medical Association; The Hospital for Sick Children, Toronto; Ontario Ministry of Health (1980).

physical resources. Ideally, a private bedroom should be used for the infected individual.

Categories of isolation. The Communicable Disease Surveillance Centre provides guidelines for isolation precautions in hospitals. Most hospitals in Europe utilize these guidelines, making changes to meet their specific needs. The standard isolation precaution categories have included strict isolation and respiratory, enteric, protective, wound or blood precautions. The revised categories are disease-specific and handle each condition separately, as well as retaining the previous list of infective material (secretions, excretions, body fluids and tissues). This knowledge permits hospital personnel to determine what control measures to institute. Categories include strict, contact, respiratory, tuberculosis isolation, enteric, drainage/secretion and blood/body fluid precautions.[3]

- *Strict isolation* is the most restrictive method for the patient. It is implemented when a patient has an infectious disease which can be transmitted by both direct contact and airborne routes. Varicella (chicken pox) and pharyngeal diphtheria are examples of infectious conditions requiring strict isolation. The patient and all articles in the room are considered to be contaminated with the infected organisms. A private room with a closed door is essential. Protective measures include: the use of gowns, masks and gloves when in the patient's room; the use of disposable meal-trays and equipment, the proper labelling and double bagging of laundry, laboratory specimens and waste; and disinfection of the room and its contents after use. Hands must be washed on entering and before leaving the room.
- *Contact isolation* is a new category used for diseases that are highly transmissible or for organisms that are highly resistant or have other unique characteristics. These patients do not require strict isolation but precautions must be taken during

any contact with the patient or his immediate environment. Precautions include hand-washing before and after contact and the use of gloves and gowns during contact.
- *Respiratory isolation* is instituted for infections spread by the airborne route and by respiratory secretions. Measles, mumps and meningococcal meningitis are examples of infectious diseases spread by respiratory secretions and airborne droplets. Hands should be washed on entering the room and before leaving. Masks should be worn and articles contaminated with secretions must be disinfected or disposed of in special containers and labelled.
- *Tuberculosis isolation* (acid-fast bacilli (AFB) isolation) is a new category for adults with sputum smears positive for acid-fast bacilli or a chest x-ray suggesting pulmonary tuberculosis.[4] Precautions for respiratory isolation are followed until three successive sputum cultures are negative for acid-fast bacilli.
- *Enteric precautions* are instituted for patients with infections transmitted through the gastrointestinal tract. Patients with typhoid fever, viral hepatitis type A and gastroenteritis caused by Salmonella, *Shigella dysenteriae*, enterotoxic *Escherichia coli (E. coli)* are cared for using enteric precautions. Protective measures are designed to prevent transmission of organisms from infected faeces. If soiling is likely, gowns and gloves should be worn. Stool specimens require protective packaging and proper labelling, and soiled linen, equipment or supplies must be properly handled.
- *Drainage/secretion precautions* are used for patients with infections where the organisms are present in wounds or wound drainage (e.g. herpes simplex) or body secretions such as saliva or tears. Precautions include hand-washing and the use of gowns and gloves when direct contact with secretions occurs.
- *Blood-body fluid precautions* are instituted when the

---

[3] Jackson (1984), p. 210.

[4] Jackson (1984), p. 211.

pathogen is present in the blood and body fluids, as with hepatitis (types B and non-A, non-B), malaria and arthropod-borne viral fever. Acquired immune deficiency syndrome (AIDS) is included in this category. Disposable needles and syringes are used to take blood specimens which should then be placed in a bag and prominently labelled with the patient's diagnosis to alert laboratory workers. Used intravenous equipment, needles and syringes are placed in containers which are closed and labelled to protect handlers. It is important not to re-sheathe needles after use.

INFECTION CONTROL PRACTITIONER

Most large hospitals employ an infection control nurse. This individual is responsible for the implementation and monitoring of infection control policies, for collecting data on hospital infections, conducting epidemiological studies to identify the existence and extent of a problem, and recommending interventions and evaluating the effectiveness of infection control programmes. The infection control nurse acts as a consultant to hospital personnel, teaches staff and reinforces policies and procedures. The infection control nurse is a member of the hospital infection control committee and works cooperatively with the local environmental health department and other community agencies.

NURSING INTERVENTION

Five potential problems are relevant to most patients with infections. A care plan developed for an individual patient would be more specific and comprehensive by including additional diagnoses relevant to the individual patient's situation.

1. PHYSICAL AND SOCIAL ISOLATION

The *goal* is to minimize the impact of physical and social isolation.

Infection control measures are implemented to isolate the organisms, not the patient. The nurse should assess how the patient perceives the situation in order to provide meaningful support and to decrease concerns and anxiety. Isolation may have negative and frightening connotations for the patient and family. Feelings of rejection, or guilt or of being punished are not uncommon. Explanations should be given to the patient and family as to the reasons for the protective measures. Specific details as to what these measures involve for the patient, visitors and hospital personnel and the expected length of the period of isolation are outlined. The nurse should not assume that explanations made on admission will be fully comprehended, because at that time the individual was probably very anxious. Repetition of

explanations and assessment of the patient's perceptions and understanding should be on-going.

The patient, family and nurse should take time to explore feelings and to develop plans to compensate for the physical and social isolation that the patient in isolation may experience. Interests and leisure activities can be elicited which may help the patient to make plans that are realistic for the situation and meaningful to him. Books, radios, television sets, telephones, family pictures and craft articles may be made available or brought in by the family if appropriate to the patient's interest and current condition. Sedentary activities are usually preferable because of the patient's need for rest. Visitors are encouraged within the isolation limitations. The patient and family are expected to participate in the planning and carrying out of care within the limits of their interest and abilities.

When the patient is being cared for at home, the nurse helps the family to plan patient care so there will be minimal disruption of family routine and to enable the patient to participate in decisions and important family activities.

2. ALTERATIONS IN NUTRITION

The *goal* is to maintain adequate fluid and nutritional status.

Fluids. Fluids promote the dilution and excretion of toxins and are also necessary because of fever that is characteristic of many infections. They also prevent dehydration which can occur because of diaphoresis.

Patient assessment involves monitoring of body temperature, the presence of chills and signs of dehydration. Chills occur when the body attempts to raise its temperature. Body temperature should be measured following each episode of chills. Signs of dehydration include: loss of skin turgor, as determined by gently raising and pinching a fold of skin and observing the time it takes to return to its original shape; a decrease in urinary output (fluid intake and output should be accurately monitored); change of shape of eyeballs, which appear sunken; depression of the fontanels in young children when palpated; and subjective sensations of thirst and dryness.

The patient's fluid intake should be increased to a minimum of 2500–3000 ml unless contraindicated by cardiovascular or renal impairment.

Nutrition. A high caloric, high protein and high vitamin diet (especially vitamin C), is important for the patient with an infection. The metabolic rate increases as the body temperature rises, resulting in increased energy expenditure. Extra calories should be given to prevent the breakdown of body tissue and to meet the increased energy demands. Proteins and vitamins play important roles in the formation of antibodies and tissue repair. Anorexia may be a problem; frequent small amounts of nourishing foods may be necessary.

Increased rest should be planned for the patient in order to conserve energy and decrease the caloric demands of the body. Treatments and care activities are planned so that uninterrupted periods are possible. For example, when the patient must be disturbed for the administration of an anti-infective drug, other therapeutic and supportive measures are carried out at that time if at all possible.

3. ALTERATIONS IN COMFORT

The *goal* is to prevent and/or alleviate discomfort.

Various nursing measures may be necessary to provide symptomatic relief. In the early stages of the infection, the patient may complain of chilliness; extra bedcovers and warmth should be provided. When the patient develops a fever, tepid sponges may be used to reduce the temperature, the bedcovers are reduced to a minimum, and efforts are made to maintain a cool environment. Cold compresses or an ice bag may provide some relief for the headache that often is experienced during infection. Frequent changes of position, massage of the back and turning of the pillows, often help the patient to rest.

The dry mouth, coated tongue and sordes that frequently accompany infectious disease and fever are a source of discomfort. Regular cleaning of the teeth, frequent mouth rinses and the application of a cream or oil to the lips as well as increased fluid intake are used to promote comfort.

Skin care is important for the patient with a rash, dry itching skin or who is sweating excessively. The skin should be bathed with warm water, using a soft cloth, and patted dry. Soaps and perfumed skin preparations should be avoided as they tend to dry and irritate the skin. If soap is required, a superfatted soap preparation should be used.

The patient may experience pain in the infected area; a bed-cradle over the area to take the weight of the bedding may help. Analgesics for the relief of pain are administered as prescribed.

An important nursing measure that contributes to the patient's comfort is the relief of anxiety and apprehension that are common in any illness. The patient and family are kept informed of his progress, treatment and anticipated results. They are encouraged to participate in planning and in implementing care activities. The nurse assesses the patient's responses to illness and treatment and provides opportunity for the patient to discuss perceptions and concerns, to ask questions and express feelings.

4. ALTERATIONS IN CERTAIN BODY FUNCTIONS

The *goal* is to maintain body functioning.

Assessment of physiological responses to infection is continuous and directed by the expected manifestations of the disease and potential complications. Bowel function is carefully monitored when the patient has an infection of the gastrointestinal tract and in children who frequently manifest gastrointestinal symptoms with a fever. Urine output is monitored with acute systemic infection caused by toxin-producing bacteria in the elderly, and in patients with cardiovascular or renal disorders. Respiratory status is assessed for all patients with respiratory infections or who have restricted mobility. Ear infections, meningitis and encephalitis are complications that can develop with measles. Changes in pain or discomfort, neurological and mental status should be observed and reported promptly. Vital signs are recorded at frequent intervals and the patient should be observed closely and examined for changes that might indicate spread of the infection or complications. For example, if there is infection in a foot, the complete limb should be examined for redness, tenderness, and swelling and the lymph nodes in the groin checked for tenderness and swelling.

Administration of anti-infective agents. Anti-infective agents are prescribed to destroy or control the causative organisms and thus limit the disease process and decrease the incidence of complications.

Prior to the administration of an antiinfective agent, the patient is questioned about any known allergies or drug reactions. The nurse must be familiar with the possible side-effects of the drug being used and must be alert for very early signs of untoward reactions. Side-effects vary with the specific drug but generally include skin rashes, nausea, vomiting and diarrhoea.

When administering antimicrobial drugs it is important to provide adequate constant serum and tissue levels of the antimicrobial agent. To achieve this, the nurse must administer the medications on time and if given intravenously, administer in the prescribed time interval (e.g. 20 minutes). Aminoglycoside preparations pose the greatest potential for such problems. If they are given too early, the blood levels become excessive and toxicity develops. If administered late, prolonged periods with subtherapeutic levels decrease their effectiveness. The administration of intravenous aminoglycosides is usually planned over a 30–60 minute period to provide optimum levels. Similar precautions should be taken with other antibiotics. The nurse must also be alert to the fact that penicillin has the potential of inactivating aminoglycosides. It is important to space the administration of different antimicrobial agents so that a constant serum level of the specific drug is maintained and so that incompatible drugs are not mixed together. Different intravenous lines are used or the drugs are given by different routes. Knowledge of the patient's serum levels for antimicrobial agents assists the nurse in monitoring for signs of toxicity and for therapeutic effects of the medications.

When the patient is taking antimicrobial drugs at home or is being discharged from hospital with a prescription for these agents, it is important that the nurse instruct the patient to complete the full course of the prescribed medication and give specific instructions as to when drugs are to be taken. Times are determined by assessing the patient's daily lifestyle. The nurse should explain that antimicrobial therapy should not be stopped when the patient feels better and that medications prescribed for a previous illness should not be substituted.

5. ALTERATION IN SELF-MANAGEMENT

The *goal* is to maintain and/or promote functional competence.

The incidence of major communicable diseases has been greatly reduced as a result of improved socioeconomic and environmental conditions, worldwide immunization programmes and advances in microbiology and epidemiology. Medical advances have contributed to improved management of the patient with an infectious disease and a decrease in the incidence and severity of residual effects and complications from the disease. The elderly, very young and those with debilitating diseases whose body defences are decreased, show a greater incidence of sequelae.

Specific nursing interventions for the patient with functional loss or other complications of infectious diseases will depend on the nature and severity of the impairment. The reader is referred to p. 235 onwards for information on nursing management of the respective disorder.

The patient and family can be helped to cope with functional loss or impending death by first identifying how they are perceiving the situation. Knowledge of the home situation, family and community resources as well as the socioeconomic status helps the patient, family and nurse to develop realistic plans for follow-up care and rehabilitation. Patient and family instruction includes knowledge of the disease, its signs and symptoms and the possibility of recurrence, as with infections such as tuberculosis and malaria. Manifestations of recurrence and the action to take are stressed. Self-care skills are taught and community resources outlined. Necessary referrals are made if continuity of care and supervision are needed. Plans for rehabilitation are made to promote optimal return of activity and independence. The family and patient should be told of the anticipated outcomes and helped to recognize and deal with the consequences of any permanent impairment. They may require considerable support and counselling to help them accept an impairment and its implications, and to make realistic plans to deal with the temporary or permanent impairment or with death.

EXPECTED OUTCOMES

The patient:
1 States the reasons for protective measures.
2 Carries out the recommended infection control measures.
3 Verbalizes his feelings and concerns about restrictions imposed by illness and isolation.
4 Demonstrates decreased manifestations of the infection: skin turgor is normal, urine output is normal; body temperature decreases to normal; leucocyte count and erythrocyte sedimentation rate return to normal; bowel elimination is regular and normal for the patient.
5 Maintains body weight within 2 kg of usual weight.
6 Verbalizes absence of or minimal discomfort.
7 Increasingly participates in and assumes responsibility for personal care.
8 Follows the prescribed therapeutic regimen.
9 States the signs and symptoms of recurrence of the disease and actions to take if these occur.
10 Describes plans for rehabilitation if necessary.
11 Describes plans for follow-up care.

References and Further Reading

BOOKS

Axnick KJ & Yarborough M (eds) (1984) *Infection Control*. St Louis: CV Mosby.
Ayliffe GAJ, Geddes AM & Williams JD (1981) *Control of Hospital Infection*, 2nd ed. London: Chapman & Hall.
Benson AS (ed.) (1980) *Control of Communicable Diseases in Man*. Washington DC: The American Public Health Association.
Braunwald E et al (eds) (1986) *Harrison's Principles of Internal Medicine*, 11th ed. New York: McGraw-Hill. Part 3. Chapters 8 & 9.
Hoffbrand AV & Pettit JE (1984) *Essential Haematology*, 2nd ed. Oxford: Blackwell Scientific.
Howe PS (1981) *Basic Nutrition in Health and Disease*, 7th ed. Philadelphia: WB Saunders. Chapter 20.
Krupp MA & Chatton JJ (eds) (1983) *Current Medical Diagnosis and Treatment*. Los Altos, CA: Lange. Chapters 21–28.
Ontario Medical Association (1980) *Immunization and Related Procedures: A Guide for Physicians in Ontario*. The Hospital for Sick Children, Toronto: Ontario Ministry of Health.
Palmer MB (1984) *Infection Control: A Policy and Procedure Manual*. Philadelphia: WB Saunders.
Parker MJ & Stucke VA (1982) *Microbiology for Nurses*. London: Baillière Tindall.
Smith AL (1980) *Microbiology and Pathology*, 12th ed. St Louis: CV Mosby.
Swonger AL (1978) *Nursing Pharmacology*. Boston: Little, Brown. Chapter 9.
Wehrle PF & Top FH Sr (eds) (1981) *Communicable and Infectious Diseases*, 9th ed. St Louis: CV Mosby.
Wellington FM et al (1987) *Baillière's Pharmacology and Drug*

Information for Nurses. Eastbourne: Baillière Tindall. Section 7.

Wistreich GA & Lechtman MD (1980) *Microbiology*, 3rd ed. Encino, CA: Glencoe.

PERIODICALS

Arking L & Saravolatz L (1980) Antimicrobial treatment: a coordination challenge for nursing. *Nurs. Clin. N. Am.*, Vol. 15 No. 4, pp. 689–701.

Bader M (1979) Infection control: immunization. *Top. Clin. Nurs.* Vol. 1. No. 2, pp. 7–21.

Donohue-Porter P (1985) 'Insulin-dependent diabetes mellitus. *Nurs. Clin. N. Am.*, Vol. 20 No. 1, p. 191.

Fekety R (1981) Prevention and treatment of viral infections. *Postgrad. Med.* Vol. 69 No. 1, pp. 133–141.

Ferguson CK & Roll LJ (1981) Human rabies. *Am. J. Nurs.* Vol. 81 No. 6, pp. 1174–1179.

Gelluci BB & Reheis CE (1979) Infection, nutrition and the compromised patient. *Top. Clin. Nurs.*, Vol. 1 No. 2, pp. 23–33.

Hargiss CO (1980) The patient's environment: haven or hazard. *Nurs. Clin. N. Am.*, Vol. 15 No. 4, p. 671–688.

Hargiss CO & Larson E (1981) Infection control, guidelines for prevention of hospital acquired infection *Am. J. Nurs.*, Vol. 81 No. 12, pp. 2175–2183.

Jackson MM & Lynch P (1984) Infection control: too much or too little. *Am. J. Nurs.*, Vol. 84 No. 2, pp. 208–211.

Kellerhals SA (1979) Isolation for person–environment protection: rationale and utilization. *Top. Clin. Nurs.*, Vol. 1 No. 2, pp. 67–75.

Krause SL & Poppas SA (1979) The nurse epidemiologist: role and responsibilities. *Top. Clin. Nurs.*, Vol. 1 No. 2, pp. 1–6.

Langslet J & Habel ML (1981) The aminoglycoside antibiotics. *Am. J. Nurs.*, Vol 81 No. 6, pp. 1144–1146.

Larson E (1979) Hands: the healers and killers. *Top. Clin. Nurs.*, Vol. 1 No. 2, pp. 59–65.

McArthur BJ (1980) Microbiology: a concern for nursing. *Nurs. Clin. N. Am.*, Vol. 15 No. 4, pp. 655–669.

Messner RL (1985) Targets for infection: institutionalized elderly. *Cancer Nurs.*, Vol. 81 No. 8, pp. 24–26.

Pfaff SJ & Terry BA (1980) Discharge planning: infection prevention and control in the home. *Nurs. Clin. N. Am.*, Vol. 15 No. 4, pp. 893–908.

Selekman J (1980) Immunization: what's it all about? *Am. J. Nurs.*, Vol. 80 No. 8, pp. 1440–1445.

Swartz MN (1979) Clinical aspects of legionnaires' disease. *Ann. Intern. Med.*, Vol. 90 No. 4, pp. 492–495.

6

Fluid and Electrolyte Balance; Acid–Base Balance

Fluid and Electrolyte Balance

Normal body functioning demands a relatively constant volume of water and definite concentrations of certain chemical compounds known as electrolytes. The distribution of certain proportions of total body water and certain electrolytes in the various fluid compartments is also important.

The body fluid and electrolytes are balanced when water and the various electrolytes are present in normal amounts in the major fluid compartments of the body. The relative constancy or balance is maintained by a number of regulatory processes that involve the cardiovascular and urinary systems.

BODY WATER

Water is essential for all body processes; it transports substances to and from the cells, promotes necessary chemical activities, and maintains a physiochemical constancy that is important in normal cellular functions.

Approximately 60–65% of the total body weight of an average adult is water, and represents about 40–45 litres in a man weighing 70 kg. The proportion of body weight that is water varies with age, sex and the amount of fatty tissue. In the newborn infant, water comprises about 75% of the body weight but progressively decreases with age to adult levels. After 3–5 years of age the percentages of extracellular fluid are the same as for adults. This level is maintained until early senescence, when a gradual decrease again begins. Since fatty tissue is practically free of water, the proportion of water to body weight is less in an obese individual and in females, who have more body fat than males.

Distribution of body water

Body water is contained within two major physiological reservoirs—the intracellular and extracellular compartments. Intracellular fluid comprises about 40% of body weight. The extracellular fluid, which is about 20% of the total body weight, is subdivided into the intravascular and interstitial fluids (see Fig. 6.1). The intravascular fluid is that contained within the blood vessels and refers to the plasma component of the blood. The interstitial fluid is that contained in the tissue spaces between the blood vessels and the cells and includes that found within the lymph vessels. The latter provides an internal environment for all cells as well as an exchange medium between the blood and the cells. These major fluid compartments are separated by semipermeable membranes.

Another compartment of fluid has recently been referred to as the transcellular fluid. This represents a much smaller proportion of total body water and is of less clinical significance in assessing the patient's hydrational status and maintaining the normal fluid balance. The transcellular fluid includes gastrointestinal secretions, cerebrospinal fluid, intraocular fluid, and pleural, peritoneal and synovial secretions.

Normally, body water is in a dynamic state; there is constant loss and replacement, and changes in location and volume. Water enters the body through the intestinal tract via the mouth and leaves the body through the skin, lungs, intestines and kidneys.

Solutes in body water

Solutes are minute particles dissolved in the body fluid and may be molecules or fragments of molecules. They include inorganic and organic substances which are important for their impact on

| Intracellular fluid | Extracellular fluid | |
	Interstitial fluid	Plasma
25 litres	15 litres	5 litres
40% Body weight	20% Body weight	

Fig. 6.1 Distribution of body water in adults.

the electrochemical and osmotic activity within each fluid compartment. When the inorganic solutes dissolve in water they dissociate into separate electrically charged atoms or radicals called ions. These charged particles are called electrolytes and act as conductors of electrical current in the solution. For example: sodium chloride (NaCl) in solution forms sodium ions (Na$^+$) and chloride ions (Cl$^-$); sodium bicarbonate (NaHCO$_3$) breaks up into sodium ions (Na$^+$) and hydrogen carbonate ions (HCO$_3^-$); and calcium chloride (CaCl$_2$) yields a calcium ion (Ca^{2+}) and two chloride ions (Cl$^-$) for each calcium ion, because calcium is a bivalent ion. The ions that have given up an electron are positively charged and are called cations and those that have gained an electron are negatively charged and called anions.

The organic solutes are of both large and small molecular size. The smaller organic solutes (e.g. amino acids, urea) diffuse across semipermeable membranes and are less important in the distribution of water, but if present in excessive amounts they may promote the retention of water. The large molecular organic substances are the blood proteins (albumin, globulin, fibrinogen), which have a major influence on the movement of fluid between the intravascular and interstitial compartments. The size of the molecules inhibits free diffusion of the blood proteins across the capillary membrane.

Electrolyte composition of the fluids

Although the extracellular and intracellular fluids are separated by the cellular semipermeable membrane, marked differences exist between the electrolyte concentrations in the two compartments. The difference is maintained by the cells, which actively reject certain electrolytes and retain others. For example, sodium is in much higher concentration in the extracellular fluid; the difference is maintained by cellular action referred to as the sodium pump, which ejects sodium from the cells.

The major ions of cellular fluid in order of their quantity are potassium (K$^+$), phosphate (HPO$_4^{2-}$), magnesium (Mg^{2+}) and protein (Pr$^-$). Much lesser amounts of sodium (Na$^+$), sulphate (SO$_4^{2-}$), hydrogen carbonate (HCO$_3^-$), chloride (Cl$^-$) and calcium (Ca^{2+}) are also present.

In the extracellular compartments sodium (Na$^+$), chloride (Cl$^-$) and hydrogen carbonate (HCO$_3^-$) are in highest concentrations; protein (Pr$^-$), calcium (Ca^{2+}), potassium (K$^+$), magnesium (Mg^{2+}), phosphate (HPO$_4^{2-}$) and sulphate (SO$_4^{2-}$) occur in much lesser amounts. A significant difference between the intravascular and interstitial fluids is the greater quantity of large molecular protein in the former. The other electrolytes diffuse readily between the two compartments, but the large particles of protein are unable to pass through the capillary membrane (see Table 6.1).

Table 6.1 Electrolytes in body fluids.

Intracellular	Extracellular
Potassium (K$^+$)	Sodium (Na$^+$)
Phosphate (HPO$_4^{2-}$)	Chloride (Cl$^-$)
Magnesium (Mg^{2+})	Bicarbonate (HCO$_3^-$)
Protein (Pr$^-$)	Protein (Pr$^-$)*
Sodium (Na$^+$)*	Calcium (Ca^{2+})*
Bicarbonate (HCO$_3^-$)*	Potassium (K$^+$)*
Sulphate (SO$_4^{2-}$)*	Phosphate (HPO$_4^{2-}$)*
Chloride (Cl$^-$)*	Magnesium (Mg^{2+})*
Calcium (Ca^{2+})*	Sulphate (SO$_4^{2-}$)*

*Occur in much lesser amounts.

Measurement of electrolyte concentration and osmotic activity

Electrolyte concentration

The presence of certain electrolytes in relatively definite concentrations in each fluid compartment of the body is necessary to maintain the volume and location of body fluid; therefore it is clinically important to be able to measure these. Since cellular and interstitial fluid are not readily accessible for examination, clinically, measurements are made of the plasma. The concentration of plasma electrolytes may be measured in *millimoles per litre (mmol/l)*. A *mole* refers to the number of particles of a substance in a solution rather than to the mass or molecular weight of the substance. One mole of a substance contains the same number of elementary particles as there are atoms in 12 g of carbon. The particles may be atoms, molecules or ions [e.g. 1 mole of sodium ions (Na$^+$) = 23 g; 1 mole of hydrogen carbonate (HCO$_3^-$) = 61 g]. Substances in biological systems frequently are fractions of moles (mol) and are expressed as *millimoles* (mmol), *micromoles* (μmol), *nanomoles* (nmol) or *picomoles* (pmol) (1 mmol is one thousandth or 10^{-3} of a mole; 1 μmol is one millionth or 10^{-6} of a mole; 1 nmol is one thousand millionth or 10^{-9} of a mole; 1 pmol is one billionth or 10^{-12} of a mole).

A second unit of measurement of electrolyte concentration in body fluids that is frequently used is the milliequivalent. When chemicals react or combine, each does so in a certain definite, unvarying proportion. An *equivalent* represents a unit of chemical activity or the combining power of a substance.[1] In clinical application, the amounts of active substances in equivalents are fractional, so the concentrations are expressed in milliequivalents. One *milliequivalent* (mEq) is one thousandth of an equivalent.

Information as to the number of units available for physiological chemical activity is more meaningful than a statement of the weight of a substance in milligrams or grams per cent. Table 6.2 lists the normal range of electrolyte concentrations in plasma.

---

[1] A chemical *equivalent* may be defined as the amount of a substance (in grams) that will react with one mole of hydrogen.

Table 6.2 Millimoles and milliequivalents per litre of electrolytes in serum.

Electrolyte	mEq/l	mmol/l
Hydrogen carbonate (HCO_3^-)	24–28	24–28
Calcium (Ca^{2+})	4.5–5.5	2.2–2.6
Chlorine (Cl^-)	100–106	100–106
Magnesium (Mg^{2+})	1.5–2.5	0.8–1.3
Phosphate (HPO_4^{2-})	1.0–1.5	0.8–1.5
Potassium (K^+)	3.5–5.5	3.5–5.5
Sodium (Na^+)	135–145	135–145

Osmotic activity

When two solutions of differing concentrations are separated by a semipermeable membrane, the solvent passes from the least concentrated solution to the greatest, in order to equalize the solute concentration on both sides of the membrane. This process is referred to as *osmosis*. The direction and degree of osmotic activity is proportional to the number of solute particles and is not influenced by the molecular weight of the particles. As the concentrations of solute in the two solutions approach equalization, pressure develops which decreases the flow of solvent across the membrane. This pressure is referred to as *osmotic pressure*. The *osmole* (osmol) is the unit of measurement of osmotic pressure. One milliosmole (mosmol) is one thousandth of an osmole. The osmotic activity of solutions is influenced by the extent to which the solutes ionize. An increase in the number of particles from ionization of the molecules of solute increases the osmotic pressure. A solute that does not ionize, such as glucose, produces less osmotic pressure. One mole of a substance that does not dissociate into ions is equal to 1 osmol. One mole of sodium chloride, which dissociates almost completely into sodium ions and chloride ions, equals 2 osmols. For example, 1 litre of a solution with 60 mmol of sodium chloride dissolved in it, contains 120 mosmol per litre of the solution.

Osmole concentration of the body fluids plays an important role in the distribution and exchange between compartments of water and dissolved substances. The osmotic activity is a result of the combined osmotic pressure of several solutes. *Osmolality* is the osmole concentration per unit of solvent. *Osmolarity* refers to the concentration of active particles per unit of solution. Since a litre of plasma contains about 90% water and 10% solids, such as proteins, lipids, urea and glucose, the osmolality of the solution is the more accurate measurement.[2] The osmolality refers to the number of active particles in the volume of water, while the osmolarity measures the number of active particles in the total litre of plasma. The term *tonicity* refers to the effective osmolality of a solution. Isotonic solutions have an osmolality of 285 mosmol, which is the same as for body fluids. A hypotonic or hypo-osmolar solution has an osmolality of less than 285 mosmol per litre and a hypertonic or hyperosmolar solution has an effective osmolality greater than 285 mosmol.

EXCHANGES BETWEEN COMPARTMENTS

Movement of water between fluid compartments

A continuous exchange of water takes place between the intravascular and interstitial fluids and between the cellular and interstitial fluids. Water diffuses readily through the semipermeable membranes which separate the compartments. But the net exchange of water is dependent on two principal forces: the osmotic pressure created by the electrolytes and the blood proteins, and the hydrostatic pressure of the blood. When the osmotic pressure changes in one compartment, water moves across the semipermeable membrane from the area of lesser osmotic pressure to that of the greater until an equilibrium is established. The hydrostatic pressure created by the volume of blood flowing through the vessels is the driving force that causes filtration of fluid through the semi-permeable membranes of the capillaries.

Exchange between intravascular and interstitial compartments

The total volume of fluid that moves across the capillary membranes is enormous because of the vast number of capillaries, but the net exchange between the intravascular and interstitial compartments is very small. Fluid moves out at the arterial end of the capillary and moves back in at the venous end.

Two opposing forces exist within the vascular compartment: the hydrostatic pressure of the blood, which forces fluid out through the semipermeable membrane, and the osmotic pressure of the blood proteins, which is a holding or pulling force opposing the flow of fluid across the vascular membrane. The volume and direction of movement of fluid depends on the difference between these two opposing forces. When the blood enters the arterial end of the capillaries the hydrostatic pressure is greater than the protein osmotic pressure, and fluid filters out of the vessels, taking with it diffusible solutes. The movement of fluid out of vessels is facilitated also by the negative hydrostatic pressure and the osmotic pressure in the interstitial spaces. As a result, the force which promotes the movement of fluid through the capillary membrane is the sum of the positive outward pressure from within the capillaries and the negative hydrostatic pressure[3] and the osmotic pressure in the interstitial spaces.[4]

---

[2] Smith (1980), p. 19.

[3] The *hydrostatic pressure* within the interstitial spaces remains negative due to the continuous lymphatic drainage.

[4] Guyton, (1986), p. 358.

This fluid movement may be expressed as follows:

Intracapillary hydrostatic pressure (CHP) − [plasma osmotic pressure (POP) + negative interstitial hydrostatic pressure (Int.HP)] + interstitial osmotic pressure (Int.OP) = net outward force.

For example, when CHP = 30 mmHg, POP = 28 mmHg, Int.HP = 5.3 mmHg, and Int.OP = 6 mmHg the equation is as follows:

$30 − [(28) + (−5.3)] + 6 = 13.3$
i.e. in this example *net outward force* = 13.3 mmHg

The blood hydrostatic pressure is reduced as the blood flows through the capillaries and becomes less than the plasma osmotic pressure. As a result, fluid is drawn into the vascular compartment from the interstitial spaces at the venous end of the capillaries. The pressure that results in this reverse direction of flow at the venous ends of the capillaries may be expressed in the following equation:

Plasma osmotic pressure (POP) − [capillary hydrostatic pressure (CHP) − negative interstitial hydrostatic pressure (Int.HP)] − interstitial osmotic pressure (Int.OP) = net inward force.[5]

For example, when POP = 28 mmHg, CHP = 10 mmHg, Int.HP = 5.3 mmHg and Int.OP = 6 mmHg, the *net inward force* = 6.7 mmHg.
i.e. $28 − [(10) − (−5.3)] − 6 = 6.7$

The effective forces operating in fluid movement through the capillary membrane are also outlined in Fig. 6.2.

---

[5] Guyton (1986), p. 358.

Exchange between extracellular and intracellular compartments

The net exchange of water between the cellular and interstitial fluids is governed by differences in the osmotic pressure in the two compartments (Fig. 6.3). In the extracellular fluid, the principal osmotic forces are exerted by the sodium and chloride ions. Potassium, magnesium and phosphate are mainly responsible for the osmotic pressure within the cells. Normal electrolyte concentrations maintain equal osmotic pressures in both compartments, and water diffuses freely between the compartments without net gain or loss in either. A decrease in the volume of extracellular water causes an increase in the concentration of ions and a corresponding increase in the osmotic pressure. This results in the movement of water from the cellular compartment into the interstitial space to establish an equilibrium. Conversely, if the osmotic pressure within the cells exceeds that of the interstitial fluid, water moves into the cells.

Movements of solutes between fluid compartments

The principal mechanisms responsible for the movement of solute particles across the semipermeable membranes are diffusion, filtration, solvent drag and active transport by cell membranes.

Only small molecular solutes *diffuse* through the membranes. Although their continuous random movement results in their transfer in both directions, the net movement tends to be to the compartment having the lower solute concentration. The diffusion of solutes through the membranes occurs at a much slower rate than water. Diffusion is also influenced by the electrical charges of the solute ions. When

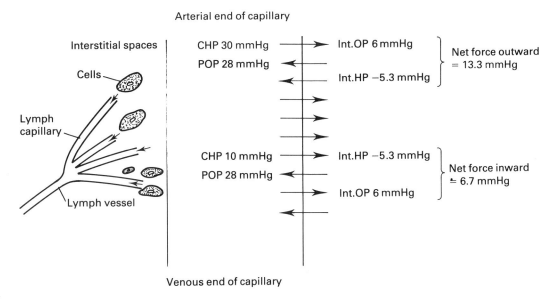

Fig. 6.2 Exchange of water between intravascular and interstitial compartments.

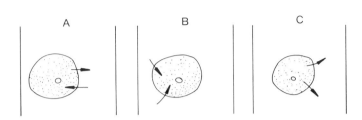

Fig. 6.3 Exchange of water between cellular and interstitial compartments. *A*, Osmotic pressure of interstitial fluid is equal to that within the cell. Water passes freely between the compartments without net gain or loss. *B*, Osmotic pressure of interstitial fluid is less than that within the cell. Water passes into the cell. *C*, Osmotic pressure of interstitial fluid is greater than that within the cell. Water passes out of the cell.

there is a difference in potential between two compartments the ions move, attempting to equilibrate the positively and negatively charged ions; positive ions move to the area that is negatively charged and negative ions move in the opposite direction.

The *filtration* process involves the forcing of water and small molecular solutes through the semipermeable membranes. The force is created by a difference in hydrostatic pressure on the two sides of a membrane. Filtration operates across the capillary walls, promoting the movement of water and small molecular solutes in the plasma into the interstitial compartment.

Solvent drag refers to the molecules of solutes that tend to flow with the water across the membranes. The amount is not great, but a small amount always moves with the solvent in such a dynamic situation.

Active transport by the cell was referred to in Chapter 4. The cell actively engages in the transport of sodium out to maintain a low sodium concentration in the intracellular compartment. At the same time it actively transports potassium into the cell and retains it to maintain a high potassium concentration within. Both sodium and potassium ions diffuse readily through the semipermeable membranes but are prevented from establishing equal concentrations within the intracellular and extracellular compartments by the sodium–potassium pump within the cells.

Active transport in the form of pinocytosis and phagocytosis also occurs. These processes take substances into the cell and are important in the movement of larger, non-diffusible molecules. Conversely many substances, such as wastes and

hormones, must be moved out of cells. This process may be referred to as exocytosis, or reverse pinocytosis.

FLUID BALANCE

A minimum daily intake equal to certain obligatory fluid losses is necessary to maintain the optimum volume and distribution of body fluid. The daily obligatory losses total approximately 1300 ml, which include the water evaporated from the skin and lungs and the minimum volume required by the kidneys to excrete the solid metabolic wastes. Approximately 900 ml are lost in sweat and respiration, and 400 ml is considered the minimum quantity required by normal kidneys to eliminate the metabolic wastes (see Table 6.3).

Sources of body fluid are the ingested fluid and foods and the cellular oxidation processes. The average fluid and food intake by healthy persons usually provides a volume well in excess of the obligatory losses.

A balance is maintained between the intake and output by certain mechanisms in order to preserve a constancy in fluid volume. When the intake is reduced or if there is an excessive loss, as in vomiting or diarrhoea, the urinary output is decreased and one is prompted to increase the intake by the sensation of thirst that usually develops. Conversely, if there is an increase in the intake, a corresponding increase in the urinary output occurs.

When the intake volume does not equal that of the obligatory loss, body fluid is drawn upon, and the normal volume is reduced. One then develops a *negative fluid balance (dehydration)* which may seriously affect body functioning if not corrected

Table 6.3 An average daily water intake and output

Intake		Output	
Fluid ingested	1300 ml	Urine	1500 ml
Water content of ingested food	1000 ml	Faeces	150 ml
Water of oxidation	250 ml	Via lungs and skin	900 ml
Total intake	2550 ml	Total output	2550 ml

promptly. Electrolyte concentrations and osmotic pressures are altered, resulting in abnormal fluid shifts between compartments. Faulty excretion with a continued intake may result in an excessive volume in the fluid compartments, producing a *positive fluid balance*. Electrolyte concentrations are changed, and harmful excesses and wastes are retained.

Regulation of the fluid intake and output to preserve constancy in the internal environment occurs through the sensation of thirst, neural and hormonal mechanisms, and renal activity.

Thirst
This is a sensation which one interprets as a need for fluid. The fluid may be needed to cover a loss or to reduce an elevated osmotic pressure of the extracellular fluid which may be due to an excessive sodium or protein intake.

The thirst centre in the hypothalamus is sensitive to an increase in the osmotic pressure, a decrease in perfusion pressure of the extracellular fluid, and to angiotension II. When osmolality rises and the intravascular volume decreases, as in haemorrhage, the cells of the hypothalamus are stimulated and the person experiences the sensation of thirst and seeks water. When osmolality falls, thirst is inhibited. Dryness of the oral and pharyngeal mucous membrane also initiates the thirst sensation.

Adjustment of kidney output
The kidneys perform the most important role in regulating the volume and chemical composition of body fluids. Certain factors from outside the kidneys influence them in the amount of fluid and electrolytes they should reabsorb or eliminate in the urine to preserve homeostasis.

A large amount of water and solutes is filtered out of the blood into the renal tubules. The production of the filtrate depends upon the hydrostatic pressure of the blood; if there is a fall in blood pressure, there is a corresponding decrease in the volume of filtrate. About 80% of the filtrate is quickly reabsorbed in the proximal portion of the renal tubules. Absorption of water and salts in the distal portion of the tubules is adjusted to the amount necessary to maintain normal volume and osmotic pressure of the body fluids.

The tubules are governed as to how much water to reabsorb by the antidiuretic hormone (ADH). This hormone is secreted by the hypothalamus and is delivered to the posterior lobe of the pituitary gland (neurohypophysis) where it is stored and released as required. Within the hypothalamus are cells (osmoreceptors) that are sensitive to variations in the osmotic pressure of the extracellular fluid. An increase in the osmolality of the extracellular fluid results in impulses being delivered to the posterior pituitary lobe, which bring about the release of ADH. The release of ADH is stimulated by the action of angiotension II (see Chapter 21). The increased osmotic pressure may be due to a water deficit, an increased intake of sodium chloride or an excessive amount of glucose. The hormone stimulates the wall of the collecting ducts of the renal tubules, making them permeable to water. Water is thus removed from the collecting ducts, causing an increase in the volume and a decrease in the osmolality of the extracellular fluid; this results in a decrease in the volume and an increase in the concentration of urine. Conversely, a fluid intake that lowers the osmotic pressure results in ADH being withheld, and the kidneys then allow a greater loss of water.

A second hormone that indirectly influences water balance is aldosterone, which is secreted by the adrenal cortex. It stimulates the renal cortical collecting ducts and distal tubules to reabsorb sodium and excrete potassium and hydrogen. Sodium is chiefly responsible for the osmotic pressure of the extracellular fluid; an increased absorption brings about the release of ADH and a resulting decrease in the water loss.

Aldosterone is the primary regulator of sodium reabsorption in the renal distal tubules. A less significant action of the hormone is on sodium transport in the colon and sweat glands. The secretion of aldosterone is influenced by the concentration of sodium and potassium in the extracellular fluid, angiotensin II and adrenocorticotrophic hormone (ACTH) (see pp. 690–691).

The renin–angiotensin mechanism plays a major role in the regulation of fluid volume. This mechanism is initiated by a decrease in blood pressure or flow in the afferent renal arteriole and by nerve stimulation which causes the juxtaglomerular apparatus in the wall of the afferent renal arteriole to release renin (see p. 690). Renin acts on a plasma substrate to form angiotensin II by a plasma enzyme. Angiotensin II raises the blood pressure by increasing peripheral resistance, stimulating synthesis of aldosterone by the adrenal cortex, inducing thirst and stimulating the release of the ADH by the pituitary gland (see p. 631).[7]

Water loss via the kidneys is also affected by the load of solid wastes they are required to eliminate. There is always a certain amount of solid metabolic wastes to be excreted, but it may vary with diet and cellular activities. If there is an increased amount, the kidneys may require more water to eliminate them. An example of this is seen when the blood sugar exceeds the normal; a greater volume of water is excreted in order to eliminate the excess sugar. This accounts for the increased urinary output and excessive thirst which are characteristic of diabetes mellitus.

DISTURBANCES IN FLUID BALANCE

Fluid deficit (dehydration)

A fluid deficit is a negative fluid balance; the fluid loss exceeds the intake and there is a reduction in the normal volume of body fluid. The reduction may be due to an actual loss of fluids, failure of regulatory mechanisms or a decreased intake of fluid. A negative water balance not only implies changes in the water volume, but involves changes in electrolyte concentrations.

Extracellular fluid is depleted first and is followed by changes in the intracellular fluid volume. The osmolality of the extracellular compartment is increased (hyperosmolar state); the fluid becomes hypertonic and causes water to move out of the cells. Cellular dehydration alters cellular concentrations and eventually disrupts normal cellular activities. The movement of water from the intracellular compartment helps to maintain intravascular fluid within near normal limits, and blood pressure, pulse volume and the haematocrit may remain within normal range for a period of time. If the fluid deficit is not corrected, the intravascular fluid is eventually depleted and is reflected in a fall in blood pressure, progressive weakening of the pulse and a rise in the haematocrit. Blood flow through the kidneys is reduced and the urinary output falls below the obligatory output. This leads to the retention of metabolic wastes and acidosis.

A deficit of water is usually accompanied by a loss of potassium ions, mainly from the cells. They are excreted by the kidneys or retained in the extracellular fluid in higher than normal concentration. The loss of potassium from the cells lowers the osmotic pressure of the intracellular fluid. As a result more cellular water is lost to the extracellular fluid.

In order to offset the fluid deficit, there is an increase in the secretion of ADH as a result of the hyperosmolality and decreased volume of the extracellular fluid. The increased reabsorption of water by the renal tubules minimizes the loss of body water.

In diabetes insipidus, with a deficit in ADH production and/or renal insensitivity to ADH, excessive amounts of dilute urine are excreted. The patient ingests large quantities of water and continues to excrete fluid in excess of intake. The hypotonic fluid loss results in a *hyperosmolar state*.

Water and solutes may be lost in equal proportions, as seen in haemorrhage, severe diarrhoea, burns and shifts of large volumes of fluid with intestinal obstructions or paralytic ileus. The loss from the extracellular volume is followed by a compensatory loss from the intracellular volume. The osmolality in both compartments is in equilibrium. This type of fluid loss may be referred to as an *isotonic fluid loss*. The decreased extracellular fluid volume stimulates the renin–angiotensin–aldosterone mechanisms resulting in retention of sodium and water by the kidneys. With continued loss of extracellular fluids the homeostatic mechanisms to replace volume will exceed the body's ability to replace solutes and a hypo-osmolar state will develop as the concentration of sodium decreases in proportion to the water replacement.

A hypo-osmolar state results when the solute loss exceeds the water excretion and the urine output is excessively hypertonic. Causes of fluid output with excessive electrolyte loss include the overuse of diuretics and loss of gastrointestinal secretions. Serum sodium and serum osmolarity are decreased. Water moves from the extracellular compartment into the area of higher osmolality in the intracellular compartment. Normal cell structure and function may be altered with serious effects. For example, intracranial pressure increases with cellular 'swelling', affecting many activities. The reduction in the extracellular fluid as it moves into the cells results in an increase in the serum haematocrit[8] and the blood urea nitrogen (BUN) concentration; there is a decrease in kidney perfusion, which stimulates the release of ADH to bring about a retention of sodium and water in an attempt to restore normal fluid volumes and electrolyte concentrations. This compensatory mechanism will not function if the initial cause is related to renal disease or ADH insufficiency.

Effects and manifestations of fluid depletion
The effects of dehydration depend on the volume of the fluid deficit, the type of fluid lost and the rate at which the loss develops. Effects are more acute when it develops rapidly, when the patient is an infant, a young child or an elderly person, and if the patient is debilitated.

The manifestations depend on the severity of the fluid deficit. The sensation of thirst is usually the first

---

[7] Leaf & Cotram (1980), p. 64.

[8] The *haematocrit* represents the volume percentage of erythrocytes in whole blood. The normal range for women is 37–47%, for men 40–50%.

symptom. It is suggested that this occurs when water loss is equal to about 2% of body weight (approximately a loss of 1–1.5 kg). There is a loss of weight proportional to the degree of the fluid deficit.

The skin becomes dry, as sweat secretion decreases, and loses its turgor. Salivary secretion is reduced; the mouth, pharynx and tongue become dry and a source of discomfort to the patient. Swallowing of solid food is difficult and the dryness of the mucous membranes may interfere with clarity of speech. The eyes appear sunken and the eyeballs become soft as intraocular fluid is reduced.

Blood pressure and pulse volume remain normal in the early stage of dehydration as the intracellular water moves out to replace the extracellular loss. However, if the fluid deficit is not corrected, the intravascular volume is eventually depleted; the blood pressure falls, the ·pulse becomes progressively weaker and the patient presents a picture of shock.

Urinary output is decreased (oliguria), which leads to the retention of metabolic wastes and acidosis. The patient is constipated and the hard, dry stool may cause impaction and considerable discomfort.

An elevation of temperature develops as a result of the decreased evaporation of sweat from the body surface, which normally is an important temperature control mechanism.

Laboratory data reveal changes, dependent upon the extent and type of the fluid loss. Reduction in the plasma volume and the resulting haemoconcentration is reflected in an elevated haemoglobin (normal: women 12–15 g/dl: men 13–18 g/dl) and haematocrit. Serum electrolyte levels are determined, as concentration and osmolality changes are likely to occur, and serve as a guide in fluid replacement. Urinalysis shows an increased concentration of solid wastes by an increase in specific gravity (normal range: 1.003–1.030). Estimations of the excretion of particular solids may also be made; for example, a high sodium loss may be incurred in an effort to reduce the osmolality of the extracellular fluid.

At the onset of dehydration, the patient experiences a loss of strength and manifests apathy. Disturbances in cellular function are most apparent in the brain and nervous system. Headache, hyperactivity, tremors, twitching, delirium, disorientation, incoordination and convulsions may develop when the intracellular volume is decreased. The patient may eventually lapse into coma, and death may ensue.

NURSING PROCESS

Assessment
The reader is referred to Table 6.4 for the objective and subjective data that the nurse should collect about a patient with a fluid volume deficit. Potential and actual patient problems are identified as well as causative factors. Information is obtained about risk factors to enable the nurse to identify patients at risk of developing fluid deficits and to take measures to prevent their occurrence.

Nursing intervention
The *goals* are to:
1 Prevent fluid deficit
2 Replenish fluid volume and electrolytes
3 Promote comfort and prevent further complications
4 Prevent mechanical injury which may occur as a result of confusion, disorientation and incoordination
5 Minimize the impact of undesirable physiological, psychological and environmental changes

1. Prevention of fluid deficit. Nursing activities to prevent dehydration include:
● The identification of risk factors.
● Assurance that an adequate supply of acceptable fluids is available and within reach of patient. Patients with a potential for dehydration should be reminded to drink fluids and assistance with drinking provided when needed.
● Identification of factors influencing a patient's ability to meet fluid needs, and the development of a schedule with the patient and family to meet fluid needs on a daily basis, both in hospital and at home.
● The evaluation of the patient's and family's understanding of the actions and recognizable side-effects of diuretics and the prescribed therapeutic regimen.
● Instruction as to the purpose, action, side-effects and prescribed administration schedule of diuretic therapy.
● Referring the patient to community services for continuous supervision and further teaching as needed.

2. Fluid and electrolyte replacement. The necessity to restore normal hydration and electrolyte concentrations is urgent in order to restore normal metabolism, circulation and renal function. The method used for the administration of replacement fluids will depend on the patient's condition. Intravenous infusion is used to re-establish a satisfactory balance quickly. When ordering the quantity and type of solution to be given the doctor considers the cause, source and volume of the losses and excesses as well as the general condition of the patient. Blood chemistry studies are done to determine possible electrolyte and acid–base imbalances. The choice of solution is an individual matter based on each patient's needs (see Table 6.5). The site of the infusion should be chosen with care so that there is as little interference as possible with the patient's activities of living.

Table 6.4 Assessment of fluid volume deficits.

Fluid deficit:	Potential*	Isotonic	Hyperosmolar	Hypo-osmolar
Objective data				
Integument		Dry, pale skin and mucous membranes ↓ Skin turgor Furred tongue	Dry skin and mucous membranes ↓ Skin turgor	Dry skin and mucous membranes Cold clammy skin ↓ Skin turgor
Cardiovascular system		↑ Heart rate Pulse irregular and thready ↓ BP on standing ↑ Haematocrit (except with haemorrhage) Serum electrolytes within normal range Shock (with excessive, sudden loss)	Pulse irregular and thready ↑ Serum sodium ↑ Serum bicarbonate ↑ Plasma osmolality ↑ Haemoglobin ↑ Haematocrit	↑ Heart rate Pulse irregular and thready ↓ BP on standing ↑ Haematocrit ↓ Serum sodium ↓ Serum osmolality Shock (if severe) ↑ Blood urea nitrogen
Respiratory system		↑ Respiratory rate	↑ Respiratory rate	↑ Respiratory rate
Renal system	↑ Urinary output Urinary frequency	↓ Urinary output ↑ Specific gravity of urine ↓ Urine sodium	↓ Urine output ↑ Specific gravity of urine (if due to renal disease or diabetes insipidus patient may have ↑ urine output and ↓ specific gravity)	↓ Urine output ↑ Specific gravity
Gastrointestinal system and abdomen	↓ Fluid intake	↑ Abdominal girth and altered bowel sounds (if due to fluid shift into abdomen)		
Neuromuscular system		Lethargy Restlessness	Hyperreflexia ↑ muscle tone tremors and twitching hyperactivity	↓ Level of consciousness, disorientation Incoordination, headaches Convulsions, Coma (if severe)
Other	Sudden weight loss	↓ Weight	↑ Temperature ↓ Weight	
Subjective data	Thirst	Thirst, lethargy, weakness and restlessness	Thirst, delirium, disorientation Fear and anxiety	Lethargy, weakness Confusion, dizziness and headaches
Causes	High risk factors include: extremes of age, extremes of weight, excessive losses through normal routes, (e.g. diarrhoea), loss of fluid through abnormal routes (e.g. indwelling tubes), deviations affecting access to intake or absorption of fluids (e.g. physical immobility), lack of knowledge of importance of fluids or medications (e.g. diuretics)	Loss of water and solutes in equal proportions related to: haemorrhage, severe burns, severe diarrhoea, vomiting, intestinal obstruction, paralytic ileus or abdominal fistula	A greater amount of water is lost than solutes. The extracellular loss leads to an intracellular deficit. May be due to: severe diaphoresis, burns, diabetes insipidus, ADH deficiency, failure of kidneys to respond to ADH (tubular necrosis), fever with increased respirations, unavailability of water or failure to drink fluids	Water loss with a greater proportional loss of electrolytes leading to intracellular water intoxication. May be secondary to isotonic fluid loss or due to excessive diuretic therapy, chronic renal disease with excessive sodium loss, Addison's disease, or loss of gastro-intestinal secretions.

*Kim and Moretz (1982).

When the fluid loss is isotonic, both fluid and electrolytes are administered. Normal (isotonic) saline solution is usually the solution of choice. With a hypo-osmolar loss, either isotonic or hypotonic solutions (e.g. 0.45% NaCl or 5% dextrose in water) may be given. A hypertonic solution (e.g. 3%–5% NaCl) is administered to decrease the intracellular fluid volume and cerebral oedema. Whole blood, plasma and plasma expanders are administered to correct vascular volume deficits.

Before the intravenous infusion is started, the nurse should explain the purpose and expectations of the procedure to the patient and advise him of his role. It may be necessary to splint the limb that is used or provide some form of restraint in order to prevent dislocation of the needle and maintain the flow of solution into the vein. Displacement of the needle by withdrawal from the vein or secondary puncture results in solution running into the interstitial spaces. This causes swelling and discomfort at the site of injection.

Once the intravenous infusion is started, the nurse is responsible for maintaining the desired rate of flow, detecting any difficulties and noting the patient's reactions. If the patient is an infant, young child, an elderly person or a patient with a cardiac or pulmonary condition, the rate of flow must be carefully controlled. Too rapid infusion may overload the circulatory system and lead to pulmonary oedema and possible cardiac failure.

The doctor who orders the intravenous infusion indicates the duration of time over which a given volume of fluid should be infused. Because the size of the drop delivered may vary with different makes

Table 6.5 Guide to parenteral fluids.*

Type	Description	Composition	Uses/indications	Advantages	Disadvantages	Special considerations
Blood and blood products						
Whole blood	500 ml Unit of complete blood	Red blood cells Leucocytes Plasma Platelets Clotting factors*	To replace blood volume and maintain haemoglobin (Hb) at 12–14 gm %	Provides intravascular volume Increases the oxygen carrying capacity of the blood	Possibility of limited supply Potential associated risks of hepatitis and allergic reactions Delayed administration because of necessary typing and crossmatching Possibility of type and crossmatch errors	Whole blood should be stored at 0–10°C but warmed at least 20–30 minutes before administration (never infuse cold blood) Use *fresh* whole blood whenever possible to avoid adverse metabolic changes related to stored blood

*The concentration and state of preservation of clotting factors in whole blood depends on the duration of storage and other variables.

Type	Description	Composition	Uses/indications	Advantages	Disadvantages	Special considerations
Red blood cells (packed concentrate) Fresh Frozen (also called leucocyte-poor)	300 ml Unit of whole blood minus 80% of plasma (haematocrit 70%) 200–250 ml unit with 85–90% of red blood cell mass contained in one unit of whole blood	Red blood cells 20% plasma Some leucocytes and platelets Red blood cells No plasma Almost no leucocytes or platelets	To increase the haematocrit to a minimum level of 30% To correct red blood cell deficiency and improve the oxygen carrying capacity of the blood Used in anaemia and for modest blood loss (when haematocrit is below 25–30%)	Concentrate form helps to prevent excess fluid administration in patients with cardiogenic shock (increases the oxygen carrying capacity with less volume loading) Associated with fewer risks of metabolic complications when compared to stored whole blood (decreased amount of transfused antibodies, electrolytes, etc.) Provides economic use of blood as a resource; frees other blood components, such as platelets and clotting factors, to be concentrated and stored	Slow infusion rate because of increased viscosity Decreased content of plasma proteins and coagulation factors when compared to whole blood Inadequate (alone) for volume replacement and correction of hypovolaemia Altered blood clotting with administration of more than 20 units; for every four units of red blood cells over 20, one unit of fresh frozen plasma should be administered to replenish clotting factors. High cost of frozen (thawed) red blood cells	Administer via Y-connector tubing with normal saline to increase infusion flow rate Washed red blood cells (resuspended in saline) can be given in shock to decrease red cell adhesiveness (washing decreases the cell's fibrinogen coating)
Human plasma (fresh, frozen, or dried)	200 ml Unit of uncoagulated, unconcentrated plasma (separated from one unit of whole blood)	Plasma All plasma proteins, including albumin Clotting factors (no red cells, leucocytes or platelets)	To restore plasma volume in hypovolaemic shock without increasing the haematocrit To restore clotting factors (except platelets)	Effective for rapid volume replacement Contains clotting factors	Expensive Deficient of red blood cells	Human plasma carries the risk of viral hepatitis and allergic reactions Administer fresh frozen plasma promptly after thawing to prevent deterioration of clotting factors V and VIII
Platelets	Platelet sediment from platelet-rich plasma, resuspended in 30–50 ml of plasma	Platelets Lymphocytes Some plasma	To control bleeding due to thrombocytopenia To maintain normal blood coagulability		Deficient of other coagulation factors	
Plasma protein fraction	250 ml and 500 ml units of a solution of human plasma proteins in normal saline	Albumin 44 g/l Alpha and beta globulins 6 gm/l Sodium 130–160 mEq/l Potassium 2 mEq/l Osmolality 290 mosmol/l pH 6.7–7.3	To expand plasma volume in hypovolaemic shock (while crossmatching is being completed) To increase the serum colloid osmotic pressure	Can be used interchangeably with 5% human serum albumin Osmotically equivalent to plasma Associated with low risk of hepatitis	Expensive Deficient of clotting factors Associated with larger number of side-effects such as hypotension, and hypersensitivity, than those reported with 5% albumin (due to presence of globulins) Hypotension induced by rapid intravenous administration (greater than 10 ml/min)	Plasma protein fraction as prepared from pooled plasma heated to 60°C for 10 hours (This procedure reduces the risk of transmission of hepatitis viruses) Rapid administration of large dosages can alter blood coagulation This solution should be used cautiously in patients with congestive heart failure (due to added fluid and rapid plasma volume expansion) and in patients with renal failure (due to added proteins)

Table 6.5—*continued*

Type	Description	Composition	Uses/indications	Advantages	Disadvantages	Special Considerations
Albumin	Aqueous fraction of pooled plasma prepared from whole blood in buffered normal saline		To increase the plasma colloid osmotic pressure To rapidly expand the plasma volume	Rare allergic reactions (less than 0.011% in all albumin solutions combined) Rare transmission of hepatitis virus due to heating process (transmission only occurs secondary to accidents in its preparation)	Potential leakage from capillaries in shock states associated with increased capillary permeability Possible precipitation of congestive heart failure following rapid infusion in patients with circulatory overload and compromised cardiovascular function	Albumin does not contain preservatives; therefore each opened bottle should be used at once The rate of administration of 5% albumin should not exceed 4 ml/min The rate of administration of 25% albumin should not exceed 1 ml min 25% Albumin is reserved for use in patients with pulmonary or peripheral oedema and hypoproteinaemia. Administer with a diuretic to ensure diuresis
5%	250 and 500 ml units	Albumin 50 g/l Sodium 130–160 mEql/l Potassium 1 mEq/l Osmolality 300 mosmol/l Colloid osmotic pressure 20 mmHg pH 6.4–7.4				
25% (salt poor)*	25 ml, 50 ml and 100 ml units	Albumin 240 g/l Globulins 10 g/l Sodium 130–160 mEq/l Osmolality 1500 mosmol/l pH 6.4.–7.4				

*The term salt-poor designates the 25% albumin concentration and is a carry-over from the days when acetyltryptophan replaced a 1.8% salt solution to increase the thermal stability of the product. The term salt-poor is erroneous because both concentrations of albumin contain sodium carbonate or sodium bicarbonate to adjust the pH and sodium caprylate and sodium acetyltryptophan as stabilizers.

Pharmaceutical plasma expanders						
Dextran	Biosynthesized, water soluble, large polysaccharide polymer of glucose		To rapidly expand plasma volume	All dextrans—associated with low incidence of anaphylactic reactions (<0.01%) less expensive than protein solutions LMWD—associated with fewer allergic reactions than HMWD LMWD—facilitates blood flow by decreasing red blood cell adhesiveness HMWD—leaks from the capillaries less readily than LMWD; can effectively increase plasma volume for up to 24 hours	LMWD—70% excreted unchanged in the urine, so the urine osmolality and specific gravity are altered LMWD—potential osmotic-nephrosis and renal tubular shut-down LMWD—possible bleeding from raw surfaces due to decreased platelet adhesiveness; side-effects include decreased haemoglobin haematocrit, fibrinogen, and clotting factors V, VIII, and IX HMWD—50% excreted unchanged in the urine, so the urine osmolality and specific gravity are altered HMWD—higher incidence of allergic reactions when compared to LMWD HMWD—increases blood viscosity and platelet adhesiveness	Avoid the use of dextran in patients with active haemorrhage, haemorrhagic shock, coagulation disorders, and thrombocytopenia Bleeding times can be prolonged when the correct dose of dextran 70 (1.2 g/kg/day) or dextran 40 (2 g/kg/day) are exceeded Administer dextran in dextrose solutions to patients with sodium restriction Dextran administration can interfere with typing and crossmatching of blood when the older (outdated) enzyme method is used
Low molecular weight dextran (LMWD) (dextran 40) (Rheomacrodex)	500 ml unit of solution which contains 10% dextran in either normal saline or 5% dextrose in water	Glucose polysaccharides with average molecular weight of 40 000				
High molecular weight dextran (HMWD) (dextran 70) (Macrodex)	500 ml Unit of solution which contains 6% dextran in either normal saline or 5% dextrose in water	Glucose polysaccharides with average molecular weight of 70 000				
Hetastarch	500 ml unit of a 6% solution containing a synthetic polymer of hydroxyethyl starch in normal saline	Globular and branched chain hydroxyethyl starch prepared from amylopectin Average molecular weight 69 000–70 000 Sodium 154 mEq/l Chloride 154 mEq/l Osmolality 310 mosmol/l Colloid osmotic pressure 30–35 mmHg	To expand plasma volume	Same volume expansion characteristics of albumin but with a longer duration of action (up to 36 hours) Associated with low risk of allergic and anaphylactic reactions (0.085%) Cost of hetastarch is about one-half that of plasma protein fraction and albumin Non-antigenic No danger of transmission of hepatitis virus	Potential dilution of plasma proteins and decreased plasma colloid osmotic pressure Potential dilution of clotting factors with resultant coagulation changes Potential circulatory overload in patients with severe congestive heart failure and compromised renal function Increased serum anylase level (>200 mg%), peaking within	Do not use if the solution is cloudy or deep brown or if it contains crystals Monitor clotting studies and platelet counts, observing for prolonged prothrombin and partial thromboplastin times and thrombocytopenia The safety and compatibility of additives with hetastarch have not been established; the manufacturer recommends infusing

Table 6.5—*continued*

Type	Description	Composition	Uses/indications	Advantages	Disadvantages	Special considerations
				one hour of intravenous administration of hetastarch and persisting for three to four days (due to action of amylase in hetastarch degradation)		hetastarch through a separate line, when possible, or piggy-backing the second drug The maximum infusion rate in acute haemorrhagic shock is 20 ml/kg/hour Monitor serum albumin; if it falls below 2 g%, consider substituting albumin for hetastarch
Mannitol (osmitrol)	Solution of mannitol in water or normal saline	Mannitol (inert form of sugar manose)	To raise intravascular volume To reduce interstitial and intracellular oedema To promote osmotic diuresis	Reduces intracellular swelling Increases urinary output	Potential circulatory overload in patients with congestive heart failure, pulmonary congestion, and renal dysfunction	
Crystalloid solutions (isotonic)						
Normal saline	0.9% Sodium chloride in water	Sodium 154 mEq/l Chloride 154 mEq/l Osmolality 308 mEq/l	To raise plasma volume when red blood cell mass is adequate To replace body fluid	Considered by some to be the single most important salt for maintaining and replacing extracellular fluid Increases plasma volume without altering normal sodium concentration or serum osmolality	Potential fluid retention and circulatory overload due to sodium content	
Lactated Ringer's solution (Hartman's solution)	0.9% Sodium chloride in water with added electrolytes and buffers	Sodium 130 mEq/l Potassium 4 mEq/l Calcium 2.7 mEq/l Chloride 109 mEq/l Lactate 27 mEq/l pH 6.5	To replace body fluid To buffer acidosis	Lactate is converted to bicarbonate (in the liver) which buffers acidosis Lactate replaces bicarbonate, preventing precipitation of calcium bicarbonate and calcium carbonate Lactate is more stable than bicarbonate and more compatible with ions present in the solution	Increased lactic acidosis in shock due to lactate Fluid retention and circulatory overload due to sodium content	Lactate conversion requires aerobic metabolism; therefore, it should be used cautiously in shock and other hypoperfusion states
Ringer's solution	0.9% Sodium chloride in water with added potassium and calcium	Sodium 147 mEq/l Potassium 4 mEq/l Calcium 5 mEq/l Chloride 156 mEq/l	To replace body fluid To provide additional potassium and calcium	Does not contain lactate, so can be given to patients with hypoperfusion	Potential hyperchloraemic metabolic acidosis due to high chloride concentration Potential fluid retention and circulatory overload due to sodium content	
(Hypotonic)						
½ Normal saline	0.45% Sodium chloride in water	Sodium 77 mEq/l Chloride 77 mEq/l	To raise total fluid volume		Potential interstitial and intracellular oedema due to rapid movement of this fluid from the vascular space Dilution of plasma proteins and electrolytes	
5% Dextrose (DSW)	5% Dextrose in water		To raise total fluid volume To provide calories for energy (200 kcal/l)	Distributed evenly in every body compartment (acts like free water) Reverses dehydration Prevents hyperosmolar state Maintains adequate renal tubular flow (facilitates water secretion)	Dilution of plasma proteins and electrolytes due to rapid metabolism of glucose and resultant free water	

*Rice V (1984).

of giving set, the instructions should be checked to determine the number of drops that will deliver a millilitre. The flow is monitored frequently, since the rate may change as the volume in the solution container lessens or if the needle shifts or is partially or totally blocked.

The site of injection and the vein pathway are examined for possible interstitial infusion and irritation of the vein by the solution. The patient's pulse and respirations are also assessed frequently; dyspnoea and unfavourable changes in the pulse should be reported promptly. The usual procedure when untoward reactions are suspected is to slow the rate of flow and consult the doctor immediately.

An intravenous infusion need not interfere with the care of the patient if the needle and distal portion of the tube are anchored securely with adhesive tape. The patient may be turned at regular intervals or encouraged to move about himself if he is able.

Re-evaluation of the serum electrolytes and reassessment of the individual's hydrational status are necessary. Volume and electrolyte composition of the solution are adjusted according to the results.

If the patient is permitted oral fluids, some persuasion and resourcefulness may be necessary on the part of the nurse. The patient's cooperation is sought by advising him of the importance and role of fluids in his recovery and in health. Small amounts are given at frequent intervals. Preferences for certain fluids should be ascertained and respected if possible, and the necessary assistance in taking a drink should be provided. The patient may be too sick or too weak to reach out and take the fluid himself; holding the glass and elevating his head will prove more effective than simply placing the fluid at the bedside and instructing the patient to take it.

The patient's daily fluid intake and output should be monitored and recorded. The volume, type and method of administration of the fluid intake are noted as well as the amount, type and source of fluid loss. Urine, emesis, suction drainage, wound drainage, blood loss, sweat and stools are all sources of fluid loss. Accurate measurements should be made and recorded when possible. Estimates are made for losses by sweating and respiratory evaporation which cannot be accurately measured. The patient is weighed daily, as losses or gains help the nurse assess the deficit as well as providing a guide for fluid replacement. The individual should be weighed at the same time each day, on the same scale with an empty bladder and with the same weight of clothing.

3. *Promotion of comfort.* To promote patient comfort the nurse should be aware of the following and give care as necessary:

- Mouth care. The mouth requires frequent cleansing and rinsing. Oil, petroleum jelly or cold cream may be applied to the lips to relieve dryness and prevent cracking.
- Skin care. Frequent bathing or sponging with tepid water may help to reduce the fever that may develop, as well as provide comfort for the patient. The amount of bedding and the room temperature should be adjusted to the patient's temperature as far as possible, without interfering with the comfort of other patients. Because the skin is dry, the use of soaps is restricted. Creams are applied to the skin to supply moisture and promote comfort.

  Observation of the skin for dryness and decrease in turgor provides information about the patient's hydrational status. Changes in turgor are best assessed over a bony prominence such as the forehead or back of the hand. Skin turgor may be difficult to assess in the elderly because of the loss of skin elasticity with age.
- Headache. Cold compresses to the forehead and a quiet environment with subdued lighting may relieve the patient's headache to some extent.
- Rest. The patient is encouraged to rest as much as possible in order to lessen the demand on cellular activities. Nursing care is planned so that the patient will be disturbed as little as possible.

4. *Prevention of injury.* Cot-sides or rails and close observation are necessary to protect the patient if there are indications of confusion and disorientation. The patient's call-bell and any personal requirements should be left where they can be readily reached by the patient. Physical restraints should be avoided if possible as they may further increase the patient's fear and anxiety.

5. *Emotional support.* The patient with alterations in intracellular fluid volume usually experiences anxiety, fear and restlessness. Repeated explanations of the treatments and situation are necessary to reassure the patient and increase his confidence. Family members should also be reassured as to the cause of the patient's behaviour change, what is being done to correct it and that it is usually a temporary state. Relatives are encouraged to remain with the patient as much as possible. The presence of familiar objects and family beside the patient's bed may be helpful in promoting orientation and decreasing confusion.

Expected outcomes
The expected outcomes for assessing intervention in fluid and electrolyte deficits are as follows.
1 The patient's weight increases to normal.
2 Fluid intake and output balance is normal.
3 Muscle tone and strength are normal for the particular patient.
4 The respiratory rate is normal for the patient.
5 Skin and mucous membranes are moist and warm.

6 The blood pressure returns to normal.
7 The pulse is normal in rate and volume.
8 Laboratory reports indicate that the levels of serum electrolytes, haematocrit and osmolality are within normal ranges.
9 The specific gravity of the urine and electrolyte concentrations are within normal ranges.
10 Coordination, concentration and thought processes return to normal.

Fluid excess

An increased volume of body fluid can result from excessive water intake, retention of fluid with normal or isotonic proportions of water and electrolytes, or from an excessive ingestion of sodium or other solutes such as protein and glucose.

Water intoxication. Excessive water intake results in a hypo-osmolar state with an increase in the volume of body fluid and a decrease in the concentration of solutes. When extreme, this state is referred to as water intoxication. The osmotic pressure of the extracellular fluid is less than that of the intracellular fluid. As a result, water leaves the interstitial spaces and enters the cells, disturbing their normal concentrations and activities. The amount the cells will hold is limited, so an excess may also remain in the interstitial spaces.

The cause of water intoxication is a decreased urinary output with a continuing intake of water, or an excessive intake of water without salt.

Adaptive physiological mechanisms to restore fluid balance include the inhibition of ADH secretion, which promotes water excretion by the kidneys. The decrease in serum sodium concentration in the extracellular fluid stimulates aldosterone release and conservation of sodium by the kidneys. When the cause is related to renal disease or excessive ADH secretion, these mechanisms may fail to respond.

The signs and symptoms are similar to those seen in the person with sodium deficiency. The patient experiences headache, muscle cramps, nausea and vomiting, and excessive sweating. Cerebral disturbances are manifested in drowsiness, confusion and loss of coordination. Convulsions and coma may develop if the condition is not corrected in the early stages.

Water intoxication is treated by restriction of the fluid intake and the administration of a diuretic. If the serum sodium level is below normal, a small volume of hypertonic sodium chloride solution (3% or 5%) may be given intravenously. This increases extracellular osmolarity and promotes the movement of excess water out of the cells.

Isotonic fluid excess. Where the net gain in fluid is accompanied by electrolyte gains in isotonic proportions, expansion of volume in both the extracellular and intracellular compartments occurs. Causative factors include: congestive heart failure, acute renal failure, cirrhosis of the liver, nephrotic syndrome, hyperaldosteronism, steroid therapy and excessive intravenous infusions of isotonic solutions.

Regulatory responses include (1) the suppression of ADH release in response to the increased extracellular volume, which results in increased water excretion by the kidneys and (2) increased renal perfusion as a result of the increased blood volume and thus inhibition of the renin–angiotensin–aldosterone mechanisms. In the presence of renal failure, these mechanisms fail to function. Congestive heart failure and cirrhosis of the liver also interfere with the adaptive mechanisms; in the former condition, the decreased cardiac output will result in decreased renal perfusion.

The signs and symptoms of isotonic volume excess include weight gain and oedema[9]; the blood pressure is elevated, neck veins are distended and the pulse volume is increased. Pulmonary oedema may develop due to increased pulmonary capillary hydrostatic pressure. Orthopnoea[10] and frothy sputum are signs of pulmonary oedema.

Serum electrolyte concentrations remain within normal limits; haematocrit levels and plasma proteins decrease as a result of dilution. The urinary output is increased if regulatory mechanisms are effective, but may be normal or decreased if the causative disturbance affects the kidneys' ability to remove the excess volume.

Manifestations of increased intracellular volume begin with restlessness, forgetfulness and irritability. If water intoxication develops, these symptoms become more severe and progress to convulsions and possibly coma.

Treatment of isotonic fluid excess includes the administration of a diuretic and the restriction of salt and water intake. In some instances, renal dialysis may be necessary.

Hyperosmolar volume excess. Hyperosmolar volume excess results in an extracellular volume excess and an intracellular fluid deficit. Sodium or other solutes such as protein and glucose are present in greater proportion than normal. The increased hyperosmolality of the extracellular fluid draws water out of the cells. The causes include: excessive sodium or protein intake without sufficient water (frequently seen in patients receiving nasogastric feeds); excessive intravenous administration of sodium bicarbonate; and hyperglycaemic states. The physiological response is increased renal excretion of sodium and water.

Signs and symptoms of hyperosmolar fluid

---

[9] *Oedema* may be defined as an abnormal accumulation of fluid in the extracellular spaces.
[10] *Orthopnoea* manifests as the ability to breathe more comfortably in a sitting or upright position.

volume and solute excess include a high serum sodium level, high serum osmolality, elevated temperature and increased urinary output with elevated sodium levels in the urine. The shift of fluid from the interstitial spaces leads to cellular dysfunctions manifested by anxiety, apprehension, hyperactivity, tremors, twitching, delirium, disorientation and loss of coordination. Treatment includes restriction of sodium intake and treatment of the cause, for example administration of insulin if the cause is hyperglycaemia.

Development of oedema
Oedema may be defined as an accumulation of interstitial fluid volume in excess of the normal. It may be local or generalized and may be associated with either an increase or a decrease in intravascular volume. Table 6.6 lists the physiological factors and associated disturbances which may lead to increased interstitial fluid volume.

When the intravascular volume expands, the net outward force is increased. More fluid moves from the intravascular compartment resulting in excess interstitial fluid. The decreased plasma volume results in reduced renal perfusion and stimulates the release of renin, angiotensin and aldosterone by the kidneys. This leads to the reabsorption of sodium and water by the kidneys. The resulting increase in the volume of body water and sodium concentration exacerbates oedema.

Normally, intravascular osmotic pressure promotes the movement of fluid into the vascular compartment at the venous ends of the capillaries. When this osmotic pressure is reduced, the normal amount of fluid does not pass from the interstitial spaces back into the vascular compartment. This reduces plasma volume and renal perfusion; the regulatory mechanisms lead to the retention of sodium and water in an effort to compensate.

Increased capillary permeability leads to local oedema. Local trauma and inflammation results in a shift of fluid into the interstitial space and a loss of vascular volume.

Oedema may be associated with any one of the three physiological circumstances already described or from any combination of these circumstances. In generalized oedema, the interstitial fluid volume and the amount of total body sodium are increased.

The interstitial fluid volume does not increase as long as the interstitial fluid pressure remains negative (normal, -5.3 mmHg).[11] When interstitial fluid pressure exceeds 0 mmHg the interstitial fluid volume increases precipitously.

Increased lymph flow assists in preventing oedema during the initial phase when the interstitial fluid pressure is still within the negative range. The increased flow also 'washes out' most of the proteins from the interstitial spaces and decreases the interstitial osmotic pressure by about 5 mmHg.[12] The removal of fluid and the decrease in osmotic pressure function to retain the interstitial free fluid pressure within the negative range. Once positive pressure is reached the interstitial fluid volume expands rapidly, the tissue spaces stretch and oedema results.

NURSING PROCESS

Assessment
Table 6.7 outlines objective and subjective data that should be collected in assessing fluid volume excess. Patient problems and associated causative factors are indicated.

Nursing intervention
The *goals* are to:
1 Prevent fluid volume overload

[11] Guyton (1986), p. 368.
[12] Guyton (1986), p. 368.

Table 6.6 Factors influencing oedema formation.

Physiological factors	Associated disturbances
Increased hydrostatic pressure	Venous obstruction Lymphatic obstruction Congestive heart failure Constrictive pericarditis Sodium intake in excess of renal capacity for excretion Cirrhosis of liver
Reduced osmotic pressure	Nephrosis Decreased albumin synthesis Increased albumin loss with burns Nutritional protein deficiency
Increased capillary permeability	Local trauma Inflammation Severe hypersensitivity reactions Burns

Table 6.7 Assessment of fluid volume excess.

Problem: fluid excess			
	Osmotic equilibrium (isotonic)	Hypo-osmolar (water intoxication)	Hyperosmolar (solute excess)
Objective data Integument	Oedema-pitting on pressure Mucous membranes moist	Oedema-pitting on pressure Mucous membranes moist	Oedema-pitting on pressure Mucous membranes moist
Blood and cardiovascular system	↑ Heart rate ↑ BP Venous distension (neck veins) Serum electrolytes within normal range ↓ Haematocrit ↓ Plasma proteins ↑ Blood urea nitrogen ↑ Serum creatinine	↑ Heart rate ↑ BP Venous distension (neck veins) ↓ Serum sodium ↓ Haemoglobin Haematocrit normal range ↑ Mean corpuscular volume (MCV) ↓ Serum osmolality	↑ Heart rate ↑ BP ↑ Serum sodium ↑ Serum osmolality
Respiratory system	↑ Respiratory rate Crackles present Dyspnoea Frothy sputum	↑ Respiratory rate Crackles Dyspnoea Frothy sputum	↑ Respiratory rate
Renal system	Normal, decreased or increased urinary output depending on underlying cause	↓ Urinary output ↓ Specific gravity of urine ↓ Sodium in urine	↑ Urinary output ↑ Sodium in urine
Gastrointestinal system and abdomen	↑ Abdominal girth (with cirrhosis of liver)	Anorexia Abdominal cramps Diarrhoea	
Neuromuscular system	Twitching	Muscular twitching Hyporeflexia Confusion Incoordination Coma Papilloedema	Hyperactivity Confusion Incoordination
Other	↑ Weight	↑ Weight	↑ Temperature ↑ Weight
Subjective data	Restlessness, fatigue, forgetfulness, irritability	Weakness, tiredness, confusion, apprehension	Anxiety, fatigue, restlessness, delirium

Causes	Increase in water and solutes in isotonic proportions related to:
	  Congestive heart failure
	  Cirrhosis of liver
	  Acute renal failure
	  Hyperaldosteronism
	  Steroid therapy
	  Rapid intravenous infusions of isotonic saline solutions
	  Nephrotic syndrome
		A gain in water in proportion to the solutes in the extracellular fluid leading to movement of water from the intercellular spaces due to:
		  Excessive ADH secretion resulting from stress, tumours (lung), administration of drugs that stimulate ADH production
		  Chronic caloric starvation
		  Repeated irrigation of gastric tubes with water instead of normal saline
			A gain of water with an excessive gain in solutes such as sodium, protein or glucose, in the extracellular compartments related to:
			  Excessive sodium or protein intake without sufficient water (especially with tube feeding)
			  Excessive administration of sodium bicarbonate.
			  Hyperglycaemia with diabetes or other causes

2 Decrease fluid overload and achieve fluid balance
3 Maintain skin integrity
4 Maintain normal pulmonary function
5 Minimize the stress caused by physiological, psychological and environmental changes.

1. Prevention of fluid volume overload. The prevention of fluid volume overload involves the following:

- The use of giving sets which prevent accidental excessive administration of fluids and which enable close monitoring of fluid administration throughout.
- Identification of the patient's and family's understanding of dietary restrictions and medication routine.
- Instruction as to the prescribed diet and medications.
- Patient teaching about the signs and symptoms of excessive fluid accumulation.
- Assisting the patient to utilize health-care resources for the diagnosis, treatment and continuous management of associated diseases.

2. Decreasing fluid overload. The following are important in decreasing fluid overload and achieving fluid balances.

- An accurate record is made of the fluid intake and loss. The patient should be weighed daily or every other day if possible. This should be done at the same time each day, following emptying of the bladder, with the patient wearing the same amount of clothing, and on the same weighing scale each time.
- Specific orders should be received from the doctor as to the patient's fluid and salt intake. Salt is usually restricted except in localized oedema. Fluid restrictions are governed by the patient's circulatory status and urinary output. Fluids may be restricted in renal failure to as little as 500 ml a day.
- Diuretics inhibit reabsorption of water and electrolytes within the renal tubules. Serum electrolyte levels are determined, as an excessive loss may be incurred with the diuresis. The nurse should be familiar with the method of administration and peak action time of the diuretic to ensure that patient activities are planned to promote maximum rest and privacy. Diuretics administered prior to social activities may be disturbing or embarrassing to the patient. Evening administration should occur sufficiently in advance of the patient's bedtime so as not to interfere with sleep.

  If a diuretic is ordered, an accurate record should be made of the volume of urine excreted. If the patient is ambulatory, he should be close to a toilet. Frequent use of a urinal or commode will be necessary for the bed patient. He should not be kept waiting for a urinal or commode or receive an impression that his demands are excessive. The frequent voiding can be exhausting for the patient;

necessary assistance in getting on and off the commode and allowing the patient to rest undisturbed between voidings help to conserve his energy.

3. Maintenance of skin integrity. The skin requires special attention, since oedematous tissue is poorly nourished and susceptible to breakdown. The patient's position should be changed frequently and vulnerable pressure areas examined. A ripple mattress or a sheepskin may be used to protect the skin by decreasing pressure and friction. The patient should be handled gently to prevent mechanical injury. Excesses of heat and cold should be avoided as sensitivity to temperature changes may be decreased.

4. Maintaining pulmonary function. The patient's respiratory status should be monitored frequently. Wheezing, dyspnoea and the use of accessory muscles in respiration are noted. The doctor may use auscultation to determine the presence of crackles and wheezes.

In the case of pulmonary oedema, the patient is usually placed in the semirecumbent position. This helps to decrease the venous return to the heart and lungs and may reduce the pulmonary oedema.

5. Emotional support. Changes in intracellular fluid volume lead to anxiety, apprehension, irritability and confusion. Repeated explanations should be given to the patient about the reasons for the behavioural changes and what is being done to correct the situation. Family members are encouraged to stay with the patient. Safety precautions such as the use of cot-sides may be necessary. The patient is observed frequently and is reminded each time of the nurse's presence and availability.

Expected outcomes
1 The patient's weight decreases
2 Fluid intake and output are balanced and are within normal ranges.
3 The skin is warm, dry and intact.
4 Blood pressure is normal for the particular patient.
5 The pulse is normal in rate and volume.
6 Levels of serum electrolytes, haematocrit, and osmolality are within normal ranges.
7 The respiratory rate and sounds are normal and the lungs are clear of fluid.
8 Specific gravity of the urine and electrolyte concentrations are within the normal range.
9 Coordination, concentration and thought processes return to normal.

SPECIFIC ELECTROLYTES AND IMBALANCES

Sodium (Na⁺)

Sodium is the major cation found in the extracellular fluids. Its concentration is maintained relatively constant within a narrow range (135–145 mmol/l or 135–145 mEq/l), although the amount ingested varies greatly from day to day, and between individuals.

Functions
Sodium plays an important role in fluid balance by maintaining the normal osmolality of the extracellular fluids. The osmotic pressure created by sodium is the principal factor in the movement and volume of body water. A normal concentration of sodium in the interstitial and intravascular fluids prevents excessive fluid retention or fluid loss.

Sodium contributes to normal muscular irritability or excitability. It is essential in the transmission of electrochemical impulses along nerve and muscle cellular membranes.

Cell permeability is affected by the sodium concentration; it is considered essential in the movement of some substances across the cell membrane.

Sodium ions are also important in conjunction with chloride ions and hydrogen carbonate in acid–base regulation.

Requirement, sources, metabolism
The average diet contains sodium well in excess of the suggested body requirement of 2 g (5 g of sodium chloride). Sodium occurs naturally in unprocessed foods, and much is added in the form of sodium chloride in the preparation and preservation of foods.

Ninety-five per cent of the sodium removed from the body is excreted in the urine, with the remainder leaving the body in sweat and faeces. The adrenocortical secretions, especially aldosterone, influence the metabolism of sodium. The steroid secretions promote reabsorption of sodium by the renal tubules. A deficiency of the cortical secretions (Addison's disease) causes an increase in sodium excretion in the urine and a lower serum sodium level.

Since sodium plays a major role in the regulation of the extracellular fluid volume, changes in the concentration of sodium result in changes in fluid volume. The reader is referred to Tables 6.6 and 6.7.

Hyponatraemia (sodium depletion)
Since normal kidneys are very efficient in conserving sodium when the intake is reduced, an adequate concentration for normal body functioning is usually maintained. Depletion of sodium ions in the extracellular fluid most often results from an excessive loss rather than a deficient intake. A low serum sodium level may also occur because of fluid retention; excessive fluid volume causes dilution of the sodium. This is referred to as dilutional hyponatraemia.

The *causes* of hyponatraemia, outlined in Table 6.8, include:
1 Sodium loss
2 Water gain or dilutional hyponatraemia in which a low serum sodium level develops because of dilution of the sodium by a disproportionate increase in extracellular fluid. This may follow the ingestion of a large volume of water, an abnormally high secretion of ADH, a loss of sodium without a corresponding loss of water, or an intravenous infusion of a non-electrolyte solution. The increase in ADH may occur with a cerebral injury, disease or tumour. Rarely, a decreased intake of sodium may account for a deficit as a result of a prolonged low sodium therapeutic diet.

Normally, a lowered concentration of extracellular sodium initiates a decrease in the release of ADH and an ensuing increase in the volume of water excreted in the urine. This response is made in an effort to restore normal osmolality of the extracellular compartments, but it sacrifices fluid volume. Some extracellular fluid also moves into the cells; the cells become swollen, normal cellular electrolyte concentrations are altered and cell activities may be impaired. If the sodium deficit is severe, depletion of the extracellular fluid results in the development of dehydration and its manifestations.

The movement of water into cells and the excessive loss of water are considered responsible for the *symptoms* of sodium deficit outlined in Table 6.8. If the sodium deficiency persists, complicated by a marked reduction in total extracellular fluid, the individual lapses into unconsciousness and manifests circulatory failure and shock.

A sodium deficit is not uncommon in those working in a high environmental temperature in industry, or for prolonged periods in the hot sun. The increased sweating causes an excessive loss of water and sodium; the individual experiences thirst and may drink large amounts of water without replacing the salt lost. In such situations the problem should be anticipated and sodium chloride tablets provided, which the workers are advised to take to prevent sodium deficiency.

Nursing intervention[13] *and treatment* of hyponatraemia consists of the administration of a salt-containing solution or, if necessary, an intravenous infusion of an isotonic sodium chloride solution (0.9%). The volume and additional electrolytes that may be needed are determined by the presenting symptoms, pulse rate and volume, blood pressure, urinary output, and laboratory reports of serum electrolytes. While receiving the intravenous infusion of sodium chloride, the patient should be observed closely for the disappearance of the symptoms manifested and the appearance of other changes. The rate of administration of the infusion is usually reduced after the first litre has been given. A rapid increase in extracellular sodium and osmolality may induce the

---

[13] Nursing interventions related to the nursing diagnoses identified for each electrolyte imbalance are discussed in detail in subsequent chapters.

Table 6.8 Sodium imbalance.

Sodium imbalance	Cause	Signs and symptoms	Problem
Sodium deficiency (hyponatraemia)	Sodium restricted diet Sodium loss by: (a) diaphoresis in fever or high environmental temperature (b) loss of gastrointestinal fluids with vomiting, suction, diarrhoea or fistula (c) a deficiency of adrenocortical secretions (d) renal disease (e) intracellular shift with potassium deficiency Water gain through: (a) ingestion of large volumes of water (b) increase in ADH (c) no excretion without corresponding fluid loss (d) intravenous infusion of non-electrolyte solution	Serum sodium <135 mmol/l (135 mEq/l) Apprehension Lethargy Headache Muscular and abdominal cramps and weakness Nausea and vomiting Diarrhoea Decreased urinary output followed by oliguria Twitching, convulsions Loss of consciousness Hypotension	Lack of knowledge related to dietary and fluid regimens Alterations in nutrition: less than body requirements related to inadequate sodium intake Alterations in thought processes Alterations in bowel elimination: diarrhoea Fluid volume deficit associated with fluid and sodium losses
Sodium excess (hypernatraemia)	Excessive sodium intake Inadequate water intake Loss of water and sodium ADH deficiency Adrenal hyperactivity Corticosteroid therapy Renal disease Intravenous administration of excessive sodium bicarbonate	Serum sodium >145 mmol/l (145 mEq/l) Mucous membranes dry and sticky Tongue dry and rough Thirst Decreased reflexes Restlessness Hypertension Lethargy Confusion Loss of consciousness	Lack of knowledge of dietary restrictions of sodium and of fluid requirements Alterations in nutrition more than body requirements related to excessive sodium intake Fluid volume deficit associated with inadequate fluid intake Alterations in thought processes Alterations in patterns of urinary elimination related to renal failure, ADH deficiency, corticosteroid treatment

movement of an excessive amount of water from within the cells to the interstitial compartment. If the low serum sodium level is due to dilution, the intake of water is restricted and diuresis may be initiated by the administration of a diuretic, such as frusemide (Lasix).

The individual at risk of developing hyponatraemia is taught to replace body fluid losses with electrolytes as well as water. Saline solutions or sodium chloride tablets may be taken when fluid loss is excessive.

Hypernatraemia (excess sodium)
An excess of sodium in extracellular fluid and consequent hyperosmolality may develop as a result of an excessive ingestion of sodium chloride, an inadequate water intake, or water loss without a corresponding excretion of sodium. Hypernatraemia may be associated with intracranial injury or disease that causes disturbance in the hypothalamic response to

changes in the osmolality of extracellular fluid; the disorder may result from a deficiency of ADH (e.g. diabetes insipidus). Decreased excretion of sodium by the kidneys may be caused by hyperactivity of the adrenal cortices, as in Cushing's disease, or by the administration of corticoid preparations which may promote reabsorption of sodium ions by the renal tubules. Retention of sodium may also occur in renal insufficiency, especially if the sodium intake is not reduced.

Normally, the responses to an increase in the osmolality of the extracellular fluids above normal include an increased release of ADH, thirst, decrease in sweating and movement of water out of the cells.

The *signs and symptoms* of an elevated serum sodium are listed in Table 6.8.

Nursing intervention and treatment. The disorder is *treated* by giving water orally and/or by the administration of glucose 5% in water by intravenous infusion. The underlying cause must also be investigated and treated. A low sodium diet is prescribed; depending on the cause of the hypernatraemia, the restriction may vary from 'No added salt' (2–3 g) to the more severe restriction of being permitted only 500 mg per day.

The patient is taught to prevent hypernatraemia by following prescribed dietary restrictions of sodium and maintaining an adequate fluid intake.

Expected outcomes
1 The patient is alert and oriented to time, place and person.
2 Urinary output is within normal limits.
3 Stools are formed and bowel elimination is within the usual pattern of frequency.
4 The patient's weight is stable and within the usual range.
5 The skin is warm and dry with normal turgor.
6 The oral mucosa is moist.
7 Blood pressure, pulse rate and volume are within the normal range for the patient.
8 The serum sodium level is 135–145 mmol/l (or 135–145 mEq/l).
9 The patient states actions to take to prevent fluid and electrolyte losses or excesses.

Potassium (K$^+$)

Potassium is the major cation found in the intracellular fluids and, to maintain homeostasis, the amount in the body is kept relatively constant within a range of 3.5–5.5 mmol/l or 3.5–5.5 mEq/l) of blood serum. The amount of total body potassium is about twice that of sodium. It is present only in small amounts in the extracellular fluids but is especially abundant and active within the cells.

Functions
Within the cells, potassium plays a significant role in creating the osmotic pressure that is important in preserving normal cellular fluid content. Normal volume of water, in turn, contributes to the maintenance of normal electrolyte concentrations. Potassium also influences the acid–base balance.

Potassium ions in the extracellular fluids are essential for the normal functioning of all muscle tissue, and are especially important in cardiac muscle activity. In conjunction with sodium and calcium, potassium regulates neuromuscular excitability and stimulation and is necessary for the transmission of the nerve impulses that prompt contraction of muscle fibres.

Potassium is also active in carbohydrate metabolism. It is required in the conversion of glucose to glycogen and in its subsequent storage. This element is also used in fairly large amounts in the synthesis of muscle protein.

Requirement, sources, metabolism
Potassium is widely distributed in foods; a deficiency

is unlikely if there is an adequate intake of food, since the average daily diet contains 2–4 g. Meats, whole grains, bananas, oranges, apricots, prunes, tomatoes, legumes and broccoli have a high potassium content. Potassium is readily absorbed from the small intestine. The digestive secretions contain potassium but this portion, as well as much of that found in digested foods, is normally reabsorbed.

Kidney activity is the chief regulatory mechanism for potassium; reabsorption, secretion and excretion of potassium ions by the tubular cells operate to maintain an optimum serum concentration. The kidneys can readily increase the excretion of potassium if the intake is high. The excretion of the ions is influenced by changes in the acid–base balance; the serum potassium level is higher in acidosis and lower in alkalosis. The serum level may also be influenced by the adrenocortical secretion, aldosterone. The latter promotes renal excretion of potassium ions and the conservation of sodium.

Abnormal levels
Even small variations outside the narrow normal range should receive prompt attention because of possible serious effects on cardiac activity. Slight variations in extracellular fluids are readily reflected in electrocardiographic changes.

Hypokalaemia (potassium depletion)
The *causes* of a potassium deficit are listed in Table 6.9.

When the potassium concentration of the extracellular fluid is depleted, potassium tends to move out of the cells, creating an intracellular deficit. The cells retain more sodium and hydrogen ions in an effort to establish an ionic balance. These ionic shifts seriously affect normal cell functioning, and the normal alkalinity of the extracellular fluid is altered because of its loss of hydrogen and sodium ions.

Signs and symptoms of hypokalaemia are also listed in Table 6.9. Cardiac muscle disturbance is manifested by dysrhythmias, electrocardiographic changes and increased sensitivity to digitalis that may lead to digitalis toxicity. ECG changes include a flattening of T waves, depressed ST segments and the presence of supraventricular and ventricular ectopic beats. The disturbance in myocardial functioning may progress to cardiac arrest. If the potassium deficiency becomes progressively greater, paralysis of the arms, legs and respiratory muscles may develop. Alkalosis may develop; the kidney tubules secrete hydrogen ions in excess and reabsorb hydrogen carbonate. Less water is reabsorbed, so the patient experiences polyuria.

Nursing intervention and treatment. Hypokalaemia may be *prevented* in patients known to be predisposed to it because of their receiving diuretic or steroid therapy by increasing foods high in potassium in their diet, and by taking a supplementary

Table 6.9 Potassium imbalance.

Potassium imbalance	Cause	Signs and symptoms	Problem
Potassium deficiency (hypokalaemia)	Inadequate potassium intake Excessive urinary loss with renal tubular disease, uncontrolled diabetes mellitus, increased adrenocortical secretion, steroid therapy Gastrointestinal loss with diarrhoea, intestinal fistula, vomiting, nasogastric aspiration Intracellular shift with alkalosis, intravenous administration of glucose or insulin	Serum potassium < 3.5 mmol/l (3.5 mEq/l) Muscle weakness and decreased tone Numbness Decreased reflexes Cardiac dysrhythmias ECG changes Cardiac/respiratory arrest Hypotension Muscular paralysis Abdominal distension Nausea and vomiting Decreased or absent bowel sounds Increased urine output	Lack of knowledge of dietary measures and actions of diuretics and digitalis Alterations in nutrition less than body requirements related to potassium intake Alterations in patterns of urinary elimination Alterations in bowel elimination: constipation Alteration in tissue perfusion Activity intolerance Ineffective breathing pattern
Potassium excess (hyperkalaemia)	Decreased renal excretion with renal failure, oliguria caused by dehydration or adrenocortical insufficiency Extracellular shift with tissue destruction from crush injuries or burns and metabolic acidoses Excessive intake with rapid intravenous administration	Serum potassium >5.5 mmol/l (5.5 mEq/l) Muscle weakness Paralysis Decreased reflexes Lethargy Confusion ECG changes Cardiac dysrhythmias Cardiac arrest Abdominal cramps Diarrhoea	Lack of knowledge of dietary restrictions for patients with renal failure Alterations in patterns of urinary elimination Alterations in bowel elimination: diarrhoea Activity intolerance Ineffective breathing pattern

preparation. Patients receiving digitalis should be followed-up closely and observed for early symptoms of potassium depletion. Even a slightly below normal serum level may precipitate digitalis toxicity, manifested by bradycardia (slow pulse), irregular pulse, anorexia, vomiting and/or diarrhoea and yellow vision. Patients are taught to include foods high in potassium, such as citrus fruits, yeast extract and bananas, in their diets. Instruction should be given on the actions of prescribed diuretics and the relationship between digitalis toxicity and a potassium deficit. The patient is taught to observe for signs and symptoms of potassium deficiency and of digitalis toxicity.

Treatment of hypokalaemia involves the administration of potassium orally or by intravenous infusion. If the patient's condition permits, oral administration is preferred because the low normal concentration can readily be exceeded and the problem may become one of hyperkalaemia. Potassium-rich foods are given, and potassium chloride may be prescribed in liquid or tablet form. If a liquid preparation (usually 10%) is prescribed, each dose is diluted in orange or grape juice and given immediately following a meal to avoid nausea and gastric irritation. The tablet preparation (e.g. Slow-K) is enteric-coated to prevent gastric distress.

Considerable caution is necessary if the patient is receiving potassium by intravenous infusion. It is necessary to note what the patient's urinary output has been and to keep a close record of it during and following the infusion. Potassium is not usually prescribed if the patient has oliguria or if there is any question about the adequacy of renal function, since it is the major channel by which excess is eliminated. The rate of administration of a solution with potassium is generally kept within the range of 8–10 mEq/h, depending upon the severity of the deficit, and is usually given in normal saline rather than glucose 5% since the latter may result in still further decrease in the serum level. Glucose promotes movement of potassium into the cells, thereby decreasing serum levels. Adequate dilution of potassium is essential to decrease irritation and prevent thrombophlebitis.

Close observation is made of the individual receiving potassium by infusion. The pulse should be checked at 15- to 30-minute intervals or may be continuously monitored by electrocardiogram. It is necessary to be familiar with the changes that may indicate hyperkalaemia. Laboratory assessment of the serum potassium level is made at frequent intervals.

Hyperkalaemia (excess serum potassium)
An excessive concentration of serum potassium may be the result of decreased renal excretion, increased

catabolism or the administration of excessive amounts (see Table 6.9). The destruction of tissue causes the release of intracellular potassium into the extracellular fluid. Metabolic acidosis also causes hyperkalaemia as potassium shifts from the cells. The disorder rarely occurs as a result of an excessive intake if renal function is normal.

Manifestations of high serum potassium levels resemble those of low levels in many respects (see Table 6.9).

Nursing intervention and treatment. Myocardial contractions and the conduction of cardiac impulses are impaired in hyperkalaemia. The ECG shows tall peaked T waves and a prolonged PR interval. Disordered cardiac function may progress to ventricular fibrillation (rapid, irregular, weak and ineffective contractions) and cardiac arrest.

It is important to recognize the possibility of hyperkalaemia developing in patients with impaired kidney function and oliguria. The serum level should be checked, the intake controlled and observations made of early indications of increased extracellular potassium.

Treatment of hyperkalaemia involves measures to restrict the intake of potassium, antagonize the effects of the high concentration of potassium, move potassium into the cells and increase the excretion of potassium.

Medication containing potassium and foods high in potassium are restricted. Intravenous therapy should not include any potassium-containing solution.

A slow intravenous injection of a calcium solution (calcium gluconate or chloride) may be given by the doctor to counteract the effects of the potassium on the heart. Calcium preparations are not given if the patient is receiving digitalis as they act synergistically to increase both the therapeutic and toxic effects of digitalis.[14]

Glucose and regular insulin may be given intravenously to promote the movement of potassium ions into the cells. If there is no oedema or cardiovascular overload, a solution of sodium bicarbonate may be added to the glucose or administered separately intravenously to enhance the shift of potassium into the cells, especially if the ECG reflects serious cardiac disturbance.

Potassium ions may be removed from the body by giving a cation-exchange resin such as calcium resonium. It may be prescribed to be given orally (20–50 g) or by rectum (50 g dissolved in 200 ml of water and given as a retention enema). When oliguria is present, haemodialysis or peritoneal dialysis (see pp. 714–722) may be used to reduce extracellular potassium ions.

Expected outcomes
1 The patient will assume usual daily activities.
2 Urinary output is within the normal pattern and amount.
3 Bowel elimination is within the patient's usual pattern.
4 Blood pressure, pulse rate and rhythm are within the normal range for the patient.
5 Serum potassium is 3.5–5.5 mmol/l (3.5–5.5 mEq/l).
6 The ECG is normal for the patient.
7 Muscle tone is normal.
8 Muscular strength is normal for the particular patient.

Calcium (Ca^{2+})

Calcium is present in the body in a greater amount than any other mineral. It comprises about 2% of the body weight and most of it (approximately 99%) is in the bones and teeth in the form of calcium phosphate. A relatively small amount is present and essential in the body fluids. Normal total serum calcium is within the range of 2.2–2.6 mmol/l (4.5–5.5 mEq/l or 11 mg/dl). About half of this calcium is in the form of free diffusible calcium ions (1.1–1.3 mmol/l or 2.3–2.8 mEq/l or 4.5–5.6 mg/dl) and the remainder is bound with plasma proteins or occurs as part of other compounds. The degree of protein binding decreases with acidosis and increases with alkalosis.

Functions
In addition to being the major inorganic constituent of bone tissue, calcium has an essential role in the blood clotting process, normal muscle contraction and relaxation, and nerve impulse transmission. It influences cellular permeability and is necessary for the activation of some enzymes; for example, it activates adenosine/triphosphatase in the release of energy for muscle fibre contraction.

Requirement, sources, metabolism
The minimum daily requirement of an adult is estimated to be 600–800 mg; the latter is equivalent to about three 224-ml glasses of milk. Demands are greater during the growth period and during pregnancy and lactation. It is currently being recommended that adult women require a daily calcium intake of 1200–1500 mg.[15] Calcium absorption is reduced with decreased oestrogen production in the menopause and renal calcium reabsorption is less efficient.

Dairy products are the richest source of calcium. Other sources, although they contribute much less, include egg yolks, fish, nuts, green leafy vegetables, legumes, and whole grains.

Absorption of calcium from the intestine is largely

---

[14] Meyers, Jawetz & Goldfien (1976), p. 141.

[15] Heaney, Gallagher, Johnstone & Neer (1982).

dependent upon the presence of vitamin D. It is also influenced by contents of the diet; a high phosphate concentration tends to reduce absorption, and free fatty acids may cause the formation of insoluble, non-absorbable calcium salts. An increased pH (increased alkalinity) of intestinal fluid reduces absorption. Serum calcium ion concentration also affects calcium absorption; even a slight decrease promotes increased absorption.

The principal regulator of calcium concentration in the body fluids is the parathyroid hormone (parathormone), which is secreted by the parathyroid glands. A decrease in serum ionized calcium stimulates the secretion of parathyroid hormone, which in the presence of vitamin D causes a withdrawal from the stores of calcium within bone tissue, decreased excretion by the kidneys and probably increased absorption of the mineral from the intestine. When the serum level of calcium is increased above normal, parathyroid hormone is not released, less calcium is added to the body fluids and more is excreted by the kidneys. Calcitonin, secreted by the parathyroid glands, functions to decrease blood calcium ion concentration. Its effect on plasma calcium is transient, but it produces a prolonged effect by decreasing the rate of bone remodelling and increasing the amount of calcium salts deposited in bone.[16] Urinary excretion is the principal mechanism by which excess serum calcium is eliminated from the body. A small amount is also excreted with the intestinal digestive secretions, especially bile. Unabsorbed dietary calcium is excreted by the intestinal tract.

A reciprocal relationship exists between phosphorus and calcium levels in the extracellular fluids. An elevation in one accompanies a decrease in the other, but their functions are not comparable.

Hypocalcaemia (calcium deficit)
Causes of a deficiency of ionized calcium are listed in Table 6.10.

Calcium is the mineral most likely to be deficient in the human diet because of its relatively limited sources. Decreased intestinal absorption may result from a deficiency of vitamin D, increased alkaline or fatty acid intestinal content, or disease of the intestine. Absorption may also be reduced if the content is hurried through the small intestine and eliminated, as in diarrhoea, or if it is lost in the drainage of an intestinal fistula.

A decrease in parathyroid hormone secretion produces an abnormally low concentration of calcium. This may occur as a result of a new growth in the parathyroid glands or of trauma during a surgical procedure, such as thyroidectomy.

Calcium depletion may also develop in chronic renal disease because of impaired reabsorption of the ions from the filtrate or because abnormal amounts

of phosphate are being retained, resulting in a compensatory decrease in calcium.

Lowered serum calcium produces *manifestations* of disturbed neuromuscular function. In more severe deficits, painful tonic spasms of skeletal muscles occur beginning in the hands, and may be followed by convulsions. Spasm of the larynx and respiratory muscles may interfere with breathing. Hypocalcaemia may also inhibit blood coagulation; bleeding from the mucous membranes or into the tissues, or excessive bleeding of a wound may result. Calcium ions are necessary in the conversion of prothrombin to thrombin in the blood clotting process.

Nursing intervention and treatment. Treatment depends on the cause; the deficiency, especially the acute form which is quickly and recently developed, may be rapidly corrected by the intravenous administration of a calcium solution (e.g. calcium gluconate 10% or calcium chloride 5%). The solution is given slowly. Following the initial administration of 10–30 ml a continuous infusion of a weaker solution may be given to maintain a satisfactory calcium concentration. Laboratory assessment of the serum level is made at intervals and the individual observed for positive changes or increasing severity of symptoms. Oral calcium supplements should be given if the condition permits. If the patient is allowed foods, those with high phosphorus content are omitted to promote maximum calcium absorption. Vitamin D, 100 000–200 000 units (2.5–5.0 mg) per day for 3–4 days, may be prescribed if the deficit is severe; the dosage is reduced in 2–3 days since the drug is accumulative.

If the cause is hypoparathyroidism and is not readily corrected by intravenous calcium, parathyroid extract in doses of 100–200 units may be prescribed for all patients. Environmental stimuli should be minimized to decrease the likelihood and effects of seizures.

Patients should be instructed as to the recommended daily requirements for calcium. Calcium supplements may be recommended for older women. The patient should also be informed that caffeine in coffee and cigarette smoking interfere with calcium absorption. Calcium absorption is best if tablets are taken between meals or in the evening.

Hypercalcaemia (excess serum calcium)
Causes of an excess of calcium in the extracellular fluid are listed in Table 6.10.

Manifestations of hypercalcaemia are also listed in Table 6.10. The high urinary content of calcium may lead to the formation of kidney or bladder calculi. The individual may also experience pain in bones as their structure is weakened by the withdrawal of calcium.

Nursing intervention and treatment. Treatment is directed to the primary cause, and to prompt

---

[16] Guyton (1986), p. 947.

Table 6.10 Calcium imbalance.

Calcium imbalance	Cause	Signs and symptoms	Problem
Calcium deficiency (hypocalcaemia)	Inadequate calcium intake Decreased intestinal absorption Hypoparathyroidism Impaired renal function	Serum calcium <2.2 mmol/l (4.5 mEq/l) Muscular irritability Tetany Numbness and 'pins and needles' in extremities Twitching of facial muscles Painful muscular spasms Convulsions Diplopia Abdominal cramps Urinary frequency Increased tendency to bleed	Lack of knowledge of calcium requirements and dietary sources and absorption of calcium Alterations in comfort: muscle spasm and cramps Alterations in bowel elimination: diarrhoea Alterations in patterns of urinary elimination Increased potential for injury (bleeding)
Calcium excess (hypercalcaemia)	Excessive vitamin D intake Excessive intake of calcium Hyperparathyroidism Thyrotoxicosis Prolonged immobility Malignant disease Impaired renal function	Serum calcium >2.6 mmol/l (5.5 mEq/l) Anorexia Nausea and vomiting Loss of muscle tone Weakness Constipation Increased urinary output Thirst Dehydration Mental dullness Confusion Coma Bone pain	Alterations in comfort related to bone pain Alterations in bowel elimination: constipation Alterations in patterns of urinary elimination Alterations in thought processes Activity intolerance Increased potential for injury (bone fractures)

lowering of the serum calcium level because of the serious, adverse effects on neuromuscular functions. Since renal sodium excretion is accompanied by calcium excretion, an intravenous infusion of saline is given. A diuretic such as frusemide (Lasix) may also be prescribed to promote sodium excretion. Serum levels of the electrolytes sodium, potassium and calcium are determined at intervals to ascertain progress and to determine whether serum sodium and potassium are being depleted by the diuresis.

If the hypercalcaemia is secondary to sarcoidosis (a collagen disease) or new growth, a corticosteroid preparation such as prednisone may be given, which is thought to decrease intestinal absorption and renal tubular reabsorption from the glomerular filtrate. The level of serum sodium is monitored in case hypernatraemia develops.

If the increased serum calcium is the result of malignant neoplasm in bone tissue mithramycin, a cytotoxic chemotherapeutic agent used in malignant disease, is very occasionally administered intravenously because of its side-effect of hypocalcaemia. If given, the nurse should observe the patient for other possible side-effects, which include bleeding as a result of a decrease in thrombocytes and impaired renal function.

If hypercalcaemia is associated with immobility, a regimen of full passive and active physiotherapy exercises should be carried out; a tilt table may be used to permit weight on the long bones; or ambulation is promoted to decrease calcium loss from the bones. Fluid intake should be increased to 3000–4000 ml daily if the patient's cardiovascular system will tolerate that volume. The increased fluids serve to minimize the precipitation of the calcium in the renal tubules.

Dietary intake of foods with high calcium content is restricted. Care of the patient involves precautions against falls and heavy lifting because of the weakened bone structure and the predisposition to fractures.

Other disorders associated with calcium metabolism include osteoporosis, osteomalacia and rickets, discussed in Chapter 25.

Expected outcomes
1 The patient will participate in usual daily activities or an active or passive exercise regimen will be followed.
2 Urinary output is within the normal volume.
3 Bowel elimination is within the patient's usual pattern.
4 Serum calcium is 2.2–2.6 mmol/l or 4.5–5.5 mEq/l.
5 Bone fractures or episodes of bleeding do not occur.
6 Muscle tone and strength are normal for the patient.
7 Bone pain and muscular discomfort are absent.

Phosphorus (Phosphate; HPO_4^{2-})

Phosphorus is closely associated with calcium in the body and occurs mainly in the form of phosphate. Monohydrogen phosphate (HPO_4^{2-}) occurs in a ratio of $4:1$ with dihydrogen phosphate ($H_2PO_4^-$) when the pH is normal and decreases proportionately as the pH decreases. About 80–85% of the total phosphorus is combined with calcium in the bones and teeth. The remainder is combined with protein, lipid and carbohydrate compounds, and with enzymes and other substances throughout all body cells. The normal serum level is 0.8–1.5 mmol/l (0.8–1.5 mEq/l, or 3–4.5 mg/dl).

Functions
Phosphate functions as a component in the structure of bone tissue and teeth. It is essential in the metabolism of almost all cells and is especially important in the absorption process of glucose and glycerol in the intestine, and in the formation of many enzymes essential to the intracellular oxidation process and production of energy. As part of the buffer system, it is active in maintaining acid–base balance. Through its combination with fatty acids and the formation of phospholipids it prevents an excess of free fatty acids. Monohydrogen phosphate acts as a urinary buffer by taking up hydrogen ions and is then excreted as dihydrogen phosphate in the urine.

Requirement, sources, metabolism
The requirement is comparable to that of calcium (800 mg daily) and, since phosphorus is present in nearly all foods, a dietary deficiency is not likely to occur. Dairy products and lean meats have a high phosphate content.

The metabolism is closely associated with that of calcium as mentioned in the previous discussion. Vitamin D facilitates the absorption of phosphorus from the intestine but is not actually essential for its transfer. The kidneys regulate the serum phosphorus level by their tubular excretion and reabsorption mechanisms. This regulation is influenced by the parathyroid hormone. With an increase above normal in the serum phosphate level, the parathyroid hormone is released to block renal tubular reabsorption of phosphorus from the glomerular filtrate, with an ensuing increase in the amount excreted in the urine. Conversely, a decrease below the normal serum level results in increased reabsorption in the renal tubules.

Hypophosphataemia (phosphate deficit) (see Table 6.11). Phosphorus may be depleted as a result of impaired intestinal absorption, hyperparathyroidism and osteomalacia, in which there is an imbalance of calcium and phosphorus. The main *symptoms* of phosphorus deficit are lethargy and muscle weakness as a result of decreased energy production caused by defective enzyme systems and metabolism. The primary disease that leads to the phosphorus deficit is treated.

Nursing intervention and treatment. The patient should be instructed to avoid excessive use of phosphate-binding medications such as aluminium hydroxide gels (Aludrox). Foods high in phosphorus, such as milk, cheeses, whole grain cereals and nuts, are increased in the diet.

Hyperphosphataemia (excess phosphate)
A serum phosphate level above normal may occur because of renal failure or hypoparathyroidism. Serum calcium falls and the patient may manifest the effects of hypocalcaemia.

Nursing intervention and treatment. Correction of the hyperphosphataemia is aimed at the primary causative condition. Phosphate-binding medications (aluminium hydroxide gels) are administered. Constipation is a side-effect of this medication. Calcium supplements and vitamin D are administered to lower the serum phosphate level.

Table 6.11 Phosphorus imbalance.

Phosphorus imbalance	Cause	Signs and symptoms	Problem
Phosphate deficiency (hypophosphataemia)	Malabsorption disorders (coeliac disease, sprue) Hypoparathyroidism Osteomalacia Excessive use of phosphate binding gels, e.g. aluminium hydroxide (Aludrox) Alcoholism	Serum phosphate <0.8 mmol/l (<0.8 mEq/l) Lethargy Muscle weakness and wasting Anorexia Hypoxia	Activity intolerance Lack of knowledge of adverse effects of phosphate binders Alterations in nutrition less than body requirements
Phosphate excess (hyperphosphataemia)	Renal failure Hypoparathyroidism Hypomagnesaemia	Serum phosphate >1.5 mmol/l (>1.5 mEq/l) Metastatic calcifications Signs of hypocalcaemia (cramps, tetany, convulsions), usually asymptomatic	Alterations in nutrition more than body requirements

Expected outcomes

1 The serum phosphate level is 0.8–1.5 mmol/l or 0.8–1.5 mEq/l.

2 The patient states the side-effects of phosphate-binding medications.

3 The patient expresses an understanding of a plan for medical management of the underlying cause of the phosphorus imbalance.

4 The patient is able to perform usual activities of daily living.

Magnesium (Mg^{2+})

The adult contains about 20–21 g of magnesium; 50–60% is insoluble and in combination with calcium and phosphorus in bone tissue. The remainder is found in soft tissue and in body fluids. The normal serum level of magnesium is within the range of (0.8–1.3 mmol/l (1.5–2.5 mEq/l or 2–3 mg/dl).

Functions
Magnesium is essential in the function of many enzyme systems, especially those involved with carbohydrate metabolism and protein synthesis. It also influences neuromuscular activity, the maintenance of normal ionic balance, osmotic pressure and bone metabolism.

Requirement, sources, metabolism
The suggested daily requirement for an adult is 300–350 mg. The main food sources are whole grains, legumes, seafood, soy beans, cocoa and milk. The metabolism of magnesium is similar to that of calcium.

Hypomagnesaemia (magnesium deficit)
Causes of magnesium deficiency are listed in Table 6.12.

Signs and symptoms of a magnesium deficit are frequently difficult to identify as such because the deficiency is likely to be compounded by other electrolyte deficiencies. The manifestations are predominantly neuromuscular disturbances. Nystagmus (rhythmic lateral, vertical or rolling movement of the eyes) may be observed. The patient may be restless and disoriented. Hypertension and cardiac arrhythmias may develop.

Nursing intervention and treatment. The serum level is determined and the deficit corrected by increased intake of foods high in magnesium, such as green vegetables, meat, milk and fruits or by intravenous administration of a magnesium sulphate or chloride preparation (e.g. 50 mEq of MgSO$_4$ in glucose 5% or in normal saline). The solution is given very slowly over 12–24 hours because it is a strong central nervous system depressant. This may be repeated daily until the serum concentration returns to nearly normal levels.

Hypermagnesaemia (excess serum magnesium)
An excessive concentration of serum magnesium is usually associated with renal insufficiency. Signs of magnesium excess are listed in Table 6.12.

Nursing intervention and treatment. Treatment is directed toward promoting urinary output; haemodialysis or peritoneal dialysis may be used. Magnesium-rich foods should be decreased in the diet. Antacids with magnesium, such as magnesium hydroxide gels (Maalox), are avoided.

Expected outcomes
1 The serum magnesium level is 0.8–1.3 mmol/l or 1.5–2.5 mEq/l.

Table 6.12 Magnesium imbalance.

Magnesium imbalance	Cause	Signs and symptoms	Problem
Magnesium deficiency (hypomagnesaemia)	Gastric loss through vomiting, diarrhoea, suctioning Starvation Hypoparathyroidism Alcoholism Prolonged intravenous therapy without magnesium supplementation Malabsorption disorders	Serum magnesium <0.8 mmol/l (1.5 mEq/l) Muscular weakness Muscular twitching and tremors Convulsions Nystagmus Restlessness Confusion Hypertension Cardiac arrhythmias	Alterations in nutrition less than body requirements Activity intolerance Alterations in thought processes
Magnesium excess (hypermagnesaemia)	Renal insufficiency	Serum magnesium >1.3 mmol/l (2.5 mEq/l) Bradycardia Decreased reflexes Drowsiness Weakness Coma Respiratory and cardiac arrest	Activity intolerance Alterations in thought processes Alterations in tissue perfusion Breathing pattern ineffective Lack of knowledge of side-effects of antacids with magnesium

2 The patient states adverse effects of antacids with magnesium.
3 The patient is able to perform usual daily activities.
4 The patient is alert and oriented to time, place and person.

Chlorine (Cl⁻)

Chlorine is a vital electrolyte for the maintenance of homeostasis, and occurs in the body as the chloride ion. It is found in greatest concentration in extracellular fluids; it is the major anion in the extracellular compartment.

Functions
Chloride ions, along with sodium, help to maintain normal extracellular osmotic pressure and regulate water balance. Chloride is important in the chloride shift that occurs between red blood cells and plasma (see p. 108). In this latter function it contributes to acid–base equilibrium. Chloride ions are also essential for the production of hydrochloric acid by gastric mucosal cells to provide the necessary acid medium for normal gastric digestion.

Requirement, sources, metabolism
No actual requirement for chlorine has been established. The intake is satisfactory if the sodium intake is adequate. Both intake and output are inseparable from those of sodium. Chloride is almost completely absorbed from the intestine; only an insignificant amount is lost in faeces. It is excreted by the kidneys according to the need to maintain acid–base balance. The reabsorption of chloride ions, as with sodium, is promoted by adrenocorticoid secretion, especially aldosterone.

Disorders of chloride metabolism generally are associated with disorders of sodium; excessive sodium losses, as in Addison's disease (adrenocortical insufficiency), diaphoresis and diarrhoea, are accompanied by chloride depletion.

A loss of chloride ions in excess of sodium may occur with the loss of gastric secretions incurred by prolonged vomiting, prolonged gastric aspiration or suction, or pyloric or duodenal obstruction, causing hypochloraemia. As a result of the chloride deficit there is an increase in bicarbonate ions, and alkalosis develops.

Acid-Base Balance

Normal cellular activities require that the concentration of hydrogen ions (H^+) in body fluids be maintained within a very limited range.

The acidity or alkalinity of a solution depends upon the concentration of hydrogen ions (H^+). When these are in excess of those contained in a neutral solution, the chemical reaction is *acid*; if fewer, it is *alkaline*. Normally body fluids are slightly alkaline; slight deviations in hydrogen ion concentration results in an imbalance that is disturbing and threatening to body metabolism.

Acids are substances which contain hydrogen ions that can be freed or donated by chemical reaction to other substances. Conversely, *bases* are chemical substances that can combine with hydrogen ions in a chemical reaction. A compound that completely dissociates its hydrogen ions is referred to as a strong acid; for example, hydrochloric acid, which completely dissociates when placed in water, is a strong acid ($HCl \rightarrow H^+ Cl^-$). One that only partially frees its hydrogen ions is referred to as a weak acid; for example, a molecule of carbonic acid dissociates into one hydrogen ion and a hydrogen carbonate ion ($H_2CO_3 \rightarrow H^+ HCO_3^-$), and therefore is termed a weak acid.

Hydrogen ion concentration ($[H^+]$) is measured in nanomoles per litre; the normal concentration in extracellular fluid is 40 nmol/l. An increase in the hydrogen ion concentration above 40 nmol/l indicates acidity while a decrease in the concentration of hydrogen ions indicates alkalinity.

Traditionally, hydrogen ion concentration has been measured by the pH scale. The symbol pH is used to express the hydrogen ion concentration, or the degree to which a solution is acidic or alkaline. It represents the negative logarithm of the hydrogen ion concentration. For example, a neutral solution, such as water, with a pH of 7 contains 10^{-7} or $\frac{1}{10\ 000\ 000}$ or 0.0000001 g of hydrogen ions per litre. A solution with a pH of 6 contains 10^{-6} or $\frac{1}{1\ 000\ 000}$ or 0.000001 g of hydrogen ions per litre; it contains 10 times as many hydrogen ions as a solution with a pH of 7. A pH of 8 indicates a hydrogen ion concentration per litre of 10^{-8} or $\frac{1}{100\ 000\ 000}$ or 0.00000001 g. Since a solution of pH 7 is neutral, as the pH decreases below 7 the hydrogen ion concentration increases, and the solution becomes acidic. Conversely, as the pH increases above 7 and the hydrogen ion concentration decreases, the solution becomes alkaline. In other words, a pH of 7 denotes neutrality. A pH of less than 7 indicates acidity, and the smaller the figure, the greater the degree of acidity; a pH greater than 7 denotes alkalinity, and the greater the figure, the greater the degree of alkalinity.

Obviously the use of the symbol pH or nanomoles per litre is less cumbersome than the expression of the hydrogen ion concentration by fraction or decimal.

ACID–BASE REGULATION

Blood normally has a hydrogen ion concentration of 35–45 nmol/l or a pH of 7.35–7.45. Certain mechanisms operate to maintain the hydrogen ion concentration within this very narrow range.

An arterial blood hydrogen ion concentration below 20 nmol/l or over 120 nmol/l (or a pH below 6.8 or over 7.8) is considered incompatible with normal cellular activity and life.

Cellular chemical processes produce relatively large amounts of acids, but the body is equipped with control mechanisms that maintain the required normal alkalinity.

The chief acid resulting from metabolism is carbonic acid, which is formed by the chemical combination of water and carbon dioxide ($H_2O + CO_2 \rightarrow H_2CO_3$). The combination is promoted by the enzyme carbonic anhydrase within the cells. In addition to carbonic acid, cellular activity produces a substantial quantity of stronger acids such as sulphuric, phosphoric, lactic, uric, acetoacetic, ß-hydroxybutyric and hydrochloric acid. The acids must be rapidly neutralized or weakened by chemical reactions and, since their production is continuous, there must be a constant elimination of them from the body. The volatile carbonic acid is removed via the lungs by eliminating carbon dioxide; the non-volatile acids are excreted by the kidneys.

Control mechanisms

The optimum pH of body fluids is maintained by acid–base buffer systems in the body fluids, respiratory excretion of carbon dioxide, and selective excretion of hydrogen ions or bases by the kidneys.

Buffer systems
Buffers are substances which tend to stabilize or maintain the constancy of the pH of a solution when an acid or a base is added to it. They do this by rapidly converting a strong acid or base to a weaker one which does not dissociate as rapidly.

A buffer system consists of two substances—a weak acid and a salt of that acid. The buffer systems of body fluids include the following pairs:

carbonic acid	H_2CO_3
sodium (or potassium) bicarbonate	$NaHCO_3$ (or $KHCO_3$)
acid phosphate	NaH_2PO_4
alkaline phosphate	Na_2HPO_4
acid plasma protein	HPr
proteinate	Na proteinate
haemoglobin	Hb
potassium haemoglobinate	KHb
oxyhaemoglobin	$H \cdot HbO_2$
potassium oxyhaemoglobinate	$KHbO_2$

Bicarbonate buffer system. The principal buffer pair of the plasma is the carbonic acid–sodium bicarbonate system. Maintenance of a normal pH is greatly dependent upon the ratio of carbonic acid concentration to that of sodium bicarbonate, which normally occurs as 1:20. *As long as there are 20 hydrogen carbonate ions to one carbonic acid molecule, the pH will remain within the normal range regardless of the actual amounts of the two substances.*

When a strong acid is added to a fluid that contains the carbonic acid–sodium bicarbonate system, it combines with the hydrogen carbonate ion to form carbonic acid. Thus, the strong acid which dissociates readily to yield many hydrogen ions is replaced by a weaker acid which frees fewer hydrogen ions. This reaction may be illustrated by the following equations: hydrochloric acid + sodium bicarbonate yields carbonic acid + sodium chloride (HCL + $NaHCO_3 \rightarrow H_2CO_3$ + NaCl); lactic acid + sodium bicarbonate yields carbonic acid + sodium lactate (HLa + $NaHCO_3 \rightarrow H_2CO_3$ + NaLa). If a strong base is added to a fluid containing this buffer system, the base combines with the carbonic acid to form bicarbonate (weaker base) and water as shown in the following: sodium hydroxide + carbonic acid yields sodium bicarbonate + water (NaOH + $H_2CO_3 \rightarrow$ $NaHCO_3 + H_2O$).

Phosphate buffer system. When an acid is added to a solution with the acid phosphate–alkaline phosphate system, it combines with the alkaline phosphate to form acid phosphate, a weaker acid. To illustrate, hydrochloric acid + sodium alkaline phosphate yields sodium acid phosphate and sodium chloride (HCl + $Na_2HPO_4 \rightarrow NaH_2PO_4$ + NaCl); and carbonic acid + sodium alkaline phosphate yields sodium acid phosphate and sodium bicarbonate ($H_2CO_3 + Na_2HPO_4 \rightarrow NaH_2PO_4 + NaHCO_3$). If a strong base is added to the phosphate buffer system, a weak base is formed as shown in the following: sodium hydroxide + sodium acid phosphate yields sodium alkaline phosphate + water (NaOH + $NaH_2PO_4 \rightarrow Na_2HPO_4 + H_2O$). The phosphate system is especially active in the kidneys where the acid phosphate that has been formed is eliminated. It is also important in the intracellular fluids which have higher concentrations of phosphate than found in the extracellular fluids.

Protein buffer system. Oxyhaemoglobin and reduced haemoglobin act as the acids of buffer pairs in the erythrocytes, and the potassium salt of the haemoglobin forms the other part of the system. Oxyhaemoglobin is a stronger acid (i.e. it dissociates its hydrogen ions more freely) than reduced haemoglobin and carbonic acid, and the latter is a stronger acid than reduced haemoglobin. When carbon dioxide diffuses into the red blood cells carbonic acid is formed:

$$CO_2 + H_2O \xrightarrow{\text{carbonic anhydrase}} H_2CO_3$$

This is also a reversible reaction. The carbonic acid is buffered by potassium haemoglobinate to form the weak acid haemoglobin and potassium bicarbonate ($H_2CO_3 + KHb \rightarrow HHb + KHCO_3$). When the acid haemoglobin is oxygenated to oxyhaemoglobin in the lungs it becomes a stronger acid and is rapidly buffered by potassium bicarbonate to form potassium oxyhaemoglobinate and carbonic acid ($HHbO_2 + KHCO_3 \rightarrow KHbO_2 + H_2CO_3$). Carbonic anhydrase reverses its action and the carbonic acid is broken down into carbon dioxide and water; the carbon dioxide diffuses out of the cells into the blood and into the alveoli of the lungs (see Fig. 6.4)

Intracellular buffering affects the movement of other ions, notably chloride, sodium and potassium. When hydrogen carbonate and hydrogen ions are formed from carbonic acid, some of the hydrogen carbonate diffuses out of the red blood cells into the plasma in exchange for another negatively charged ion, chloride. This movement is called the chloride shift. The remainder of the hydrogen carbonate remains in the red cells where it attaches to the intracellular potassium.

When hydrogen ion concentration is decreased extracellularly, some of the hydrogen ions released from the carbonic acid, move to the extracellular fluid in exchange for either potassium or sodium ions from the extracellular fluid. Conversely, if the extracellular hydrogen ion concentration is high, hydrogen ions will move into the cells in exchange for intracellular potassium or sodium.

Although the function of each buffer system has been discussed separately, within the body they work together in complementary and interchangeable reactions. Guyton emphasizes that any condition that changes the balance of any one of the buffer systems also changes the balance of all the others, for the buffer systems also buffer each other.[17]

Respiratory regulation

A second important factor in the maintenance of the normal pH of body fluids is the elimination of carbon dioxide in respiration. Carbon dioxide is constantly produced in cellular metabolism and diffuses from the cells into the blood and erythrocytes. As a result, carbon dioxide is in greater concentration in the blood when it enters the pulmonary capillaries than in the air in the alveoli of the lungs. The pressure gradient results in some carbon dioxide diffusing from the blood into the alveoli from which it is exhaled. This reduces the amount available to form carbonic acid in the body fluids.

The neurons of the respiratory control centre in the medulla are extremely sensitive to the concentration of carbon dioxide and hydrogen ions in body fluids. An increase in either stimulates the centre to increase the rate and volume of respirations so more carbon dioxide may be eliminated. Conversely, a decrease in

[17] Guyton (1986), p. 442.

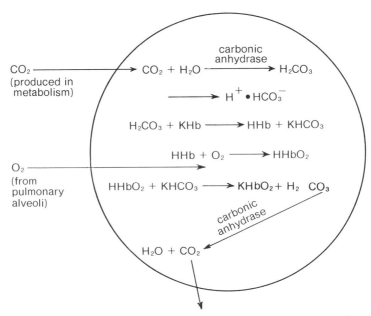

Fig. 6.4 Role of the red blood cell in pH regulation.

the concentration of carbon dioxide or hydrogen ions below the normal results in slower shallow respirations so that carbon dioxide is retained to form carbonic acid.

Obviously any condition that impairs the capacity of the lungs to eliminate carbon dioxide from the body predisposes to an increase in the carbonic acid level and a decrease in the pH of body fluids; on the other hand, increased pulmonary ventilation may increase the pH of the body fluids by the excessive loss of carbon dioxide.

Kidney regulation

The kidneys play an important role in maintaining the acid–base balance by excreting hydrogen ions and forming hydrogen carbonate in amounts as indicated by the pH of the blood. The cells of the distal portion of the renal tubules are sensitive to changes in the pH; when there is a decrease below the normal, hydrogen ions are excreted and hydrogen carbonate is formed and retained. Conversely, when there is an increased alkalinity above the normal, hydrogen ions are conserved and base-forming ions are excreted. In other words, the kidneys may excrete many or few hydrogen ions and form more or less hydrogen carbonate according to the need.

Renal regulation of hydrogen ion secretion involves three major processes: the reabsorption of hydrogen carbonate, the titration of urinary buffers, and the excretion of ammonium ions.

1 Reabsorption of hydrogen carbonate.
   (a) Within the renal tubular cells, carbon dioxide and water form carbonic acid

$$(CO_2 + H_2O \xrightarrow{\text{carbonic anhydrase}} H_2CO_3)$$

which ionizes to release hydrogen and hydrogen carbonate ions (H^+ HCO_3^-). Hydrogen ions move out into the renal tubule.

(b) Sodium bicarbonate is filtered by the glomerulus into the renal tubules and dissociates into sodium and hydrogen carbonate ions. The sodium ion moves into the tubular cell in exchange for the hydrogen ion. The sodium ion then moves by active transport into the extracellular fluid where it combines with the bicarbonate to form sodium bicarbonate.

(c) The bicarbonate in the renal tubules combines with a hydrogen ion from the tubular cells to form carbonic acid. The carbonic acid is acted upon by carbonic anhydrase from the lumenal surface to form carbon dioxide and water. The water is excreted by the tubules while the carbon dioxide diffuses through the cellular membranes into the cells and into the capillaries where it combines with water to form new hydrogen carbonate. This process serves to remove hydrogen from the tubular lumen and to return sodium to the capillaries with the hydrogen carbonate (see Fig. 6.5).

2 Urinary buffers. When excess hydrogen ions are secreted into the tubules they combine with buffers in the tubular fluid. The phosphate buffer plays an important role in acid excretion.

(a) The alkaline sodium phosphate (Na_2HPO_4) in the tubular fluid is converted to acid sodium phosphate (NaH_2PO_4) by accepting a hydrogen ion and releasing a sodium ion (Na^+). The acid sodium phosphate is excreted in the urine.

(b) The sodium ion passes into the tubular cell in exchange for the hydrogen ion that moved out. It moves by active transport into the capillary and combines with the hydrogen carbonate ion to form sodium bicarbonate ($NaHCO_3$).

3 Ammonia production. Additional hydrogen ions may be eliminated by the kidneys to form ammonia which is eliminated as an acid salt.

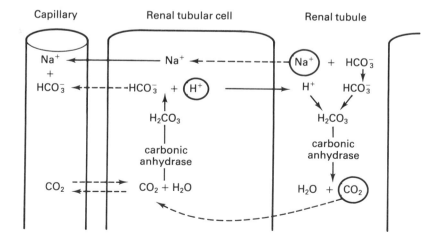

Fig. 6.5 Renal reabsorption of hydrogen carbonate.

Within the tubular cells, the amino acid glutamine is broken down, and ammonia (NH_3) is released into the tubule. Sodium chloride in the tubular fluid ionizes ($NaCl \rightarrow Na^+Cl^-$); the ammonia combines with a hydrogen ion and a chlorine ion to form ammonium chloride ($NH_3 + H^+ + Cl^- \rightarrow NH_4Cl$), which is eliminated in the urine. The sodium ion passes into the tubular cell and into the capillaries and combines with hydrogen carbonate to form sodium bicarbonate (see Fig. 6.6).

In summary, to preserve the normal pH, the kidneys reabsorb hydrogen carbonate and sodium ions in exchange for hydrogen ions. The phosphate and ammonia buffer systems result in increased sodium bicarbonate concentrations in the extracellular fluid. Hydrogen ions are secreted in the form of water, acid and as ammonium.

Acid–Base Imbalance

Normally the hydrogen ion concentration of blood is maintained within the narrow range of 35–45 nmol/l or a pH of 7.35–7.45. Acidosis or acidaemia is present when the hydrogen ion concentration is greater than 45 nmol/l or the pH is less than 7.35. Alkalosis or alkalaemia exists when the hydrogen ion concentration is less than 35 nmol/l or the pH is greater than 7.45

Tests for acid–base imbalance

Significant blood tests used in determining an acid–base imbalance include the following:
1 *Blood gases.* An estimation is made of the carbon dioxide and oxygen concentrations of the blood. These may be expressed in volumes per cent, or as mmHg partial pressure. The normal values for the oxygen in arterial blood are 17–21 volumes per cent, or a tension of 80–100 mmHg (10.6–13.3 kPa). The latter is recorded as Pao_2 80–100 mmHg. If a sample of venous blood is used, the normal value is 10–16 volumes per cent— Po_2 10–16 volumes per cent).

The normal value for carbon dioxide in arterial blood is in the range of 35–45 mmHg (4.6–6.0 kPa). Plasma normally contains 21–30 mEq/l, or 50–70 volumes per cent of carbon dioxide. This represents the carbon dioxide in the blood as carbonic acid and bicarbonate, as well as that free in solution.

Arterial blood values for blood gases are used clinically more often than venous estimations. The

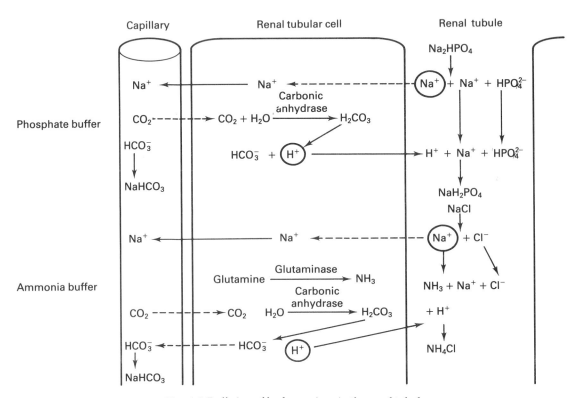

Fig. 6.6 Buffering of hydrogen ions in the renal tubule.

collection of arterial blood samples for the evaluation of blood gases involves certain measures to prevent exposure of the specimen to the air. True values cannot be obtained if air contacts the blood sample.

A readily accessible artery, such as the brachial at the antecubital space, the radial or femoral, is used. The site is cleansed with an antiseptic. A solution of heparin is drawn up into the syringe to be used to rinse the inner surface, and is then discarded. All air must be excluded from the syringe and needle.

When the needle is passed through the arterial wall, the patient is likely to experience deep sharp pain; the patient is advised of this during the preparation for the procedure and asked not to move the limb. Anticipating this possibility, the assisting nurse provides the necessary support. If arterial blood gases are to be taken frequently, an arterial line may be inserted.

Blood flows readily into the syringe because of the arterial blood pressure and pulsations. When the needle is withdrawn it is quickly inserted into the rubber stopper or capped to prevent the entry of air. The syringe is placed in an insulated container or a container of crushed ice, labelled and, with the requisition, is delivered immediately to the laboratory. If the analysis is delayed, true values are altered.

Pressure should be applied to the arterial puncture site for at least 5 minutes. When the nurse is assured that there is no bleeding, a sterile dressing is applied. The area and the area directly beneath it are checked at 15 minute and then half-hourly intervals for 2–3 hours for possible bleeding.

2 *Carbon dioxide combining power.* This provides information as to the amount of carbon dioxide carried in the blood in the form of bicarbonate. The normal is expressed as 50–65 volumes per cent, or 24–28 mEq/l (24–28 mmol/l).

3 *Hydrogen ion concentration and pH.* The normal hydrogen ion concentration is determined by an estimation of the pH. The normal value is 7.35–7.45.

4 *Serum electrolytes.* It is necessary to determine the serum concentration of various electrolytes, especially sodium, bicarbonate and potassium. See p. 80 for normal levels.

5 *Anion gap.* In body fluids anions and cations must be present in equal concentrations. Laboratory estimates of electrolyte concentrations are usually done on the major electrolytes. The anion gap is a determination of the difference between the unmeasured anions in the plasma and the unmeasured cations. Since changes in the concentrations of unmeasured ions will affect the concentrations of measured ions, the anion gap is calculated by determining the difference between the sum of the two largest cation values (sodium and potassium) and the sum of the two largest anion

values (chloride and hydrogen carbonate). Since the potassium measurement is so small, it is usually excluded from the calculation.
Cations: Na^+ 140 mmol + K^+ 0 mmol = 140 mmol
Anions: Cl^- 102 mm + HCO_3^- 26 mmol = 128 mmol
Difference = 12 mmol
Anion gap = 12 mmol/l

6 Urinalysis. Analysis of the urine may also provide useful information. Significant factors are:
(a) The pH of the urine. The normal range is 5–8, depending upon the diet and drug therapy.
(b) Total volume. Normally a minimum of 1000–1500 ml are excreted in 24 hours.
(c) Amounts of various solids, ammonia, bicarbonate, calcium, chloride, ketones and potassium.

Acidosis

When the hydrogen ion concentration is increased in body fluids, the three control mechanisms (buffer systems, respiration, and kidney activity) endeavour to re-establish a normal pH. If the carbonic acid–bicarbonate ratio can be kept normal by increased respiratory elimination of carbon dioxide and by increased kidney elimination of hydrogen ions and formation of sodium bicarbonate, the pH (and hydrogen ion concentration) is kept within normal range. The condition is then said to be *compensated acidosis.* If the mechanisms cannot compensate adequately, a decrease in the carbonic acid–bicarbonate ratio develops, the pH falls below normal (i.e. the hydrogen ion concentration rises), and a state of uncompensated acidosis exists.

TYPES OF ACIDOSIS

Acidosis may be classified according to the cause as respiratory or metabolic.

Respiratory acidosis
This condition develops as a result of hypoventilation; the elimination of carbon dioxide does not keep pace with its production. The $Paco_2$ level is elevated and the condition may be referred to as hypercapnia. The level of serum carbonic acid rises above normal and the pH of body fluids decreases. Impaired carbon dioxide excretion by the lungs is usually accompanied by reduced Pao_2 (hypoxia) because of the decreased alveolar gas exchange. Since respiratory impairment is the cause of the acidosis, the primary adaptive response is increased renal excretion of acid.

The kidneys respond to the increased level of carbon dioxide by secreting an excess of hydrogen ions, resulting in an increase in sodium bicarbonate in the extracellular fluid. The kidneys also increase their formation and excretion of ammonia, which uses more hydrogen ions and results in hydrogen carbonate production. The serum bicarbonate concentration increases, correcting the carbonic acid–hydrogen carbonate ion ratio, and the pH moves towards normal. These renal compensatory responses require one or more days to be effective provided that there is adequate blood circulation. The compensation is of greater value in acidosis associated with chronic respiratory diseases, such as emphysema and bronchiectasis.

Manifestations. The retention of carbon dioxide and the decreased pH cause a depression of the central nervous system. The patient becomes restless and apprehensive and may complain of headache at the onset; gradually his mental responses become slow and dulled. If ventilation does not improve he may become disoriented and eventually lapse into coma. Peripheral vasodilation and a rapid pulse may be associated with acute respiratory acidosis. If the acidosis is caused by chronic respiratory disease, the individual's respirations are laboured and the expiratory phase is prolonged.

Treatment. Treatment is directed toward relieving the respiratory insufficiency. Tracheal intubation or a tracheostomy with the use of a mechanical ventilator may be necessary. An infusion of an alkali preparation is given if the acidosis results from cardiopulmonary arrest. If the respiratory centre has been depressed by a drug, the appropriate antidote is prescribed. For further details of the care required in respiratory insufficiency see Chapter 16.

Metabolic acidosis
This occurs as a result of an excessive production or ingestion of acid, the retention of non-volatile acid or depletion of the hydrogen carbonate base.

Metabolic acidosis may also be classified as hyperchloraemic or anion gap, based on the serum electrolyte concentrations. The anion gap is calculated by determining the difference between the sum of the major cations (sodium and potassium) and the sum of the major anions (chloride and bicarbonate). Changes in the major ions reflect changes in the concentrations of unmeasured electrolytes, since the body maintains a balance between anions and cations. As metabolic acidosis develops, hydrogen carbonate is used in the buffering of the hydrogen ions causing a decrease in the hydrogen carbonate concentration in the extracellular fluid. If the hydrogen carbonate is used in buffering an organic acid to form an anion which remains in the serum, the hydrogen carbonate level falls and the unmeasured anions of the organic acid increase. In this situation, the anion gap increases: e.g. $(Na^+ + K^+) - (\downarrow HCO_3^- + Cl^-) \rightarrow$ an anion gap greater than 15 mmol/l.

In conditions such as diarrhoea, intestinal fistula and renal dysfunction and when a patient receives a carbonic anhydrase inhibiting drug (e.g. acetazola-

mide) or an acidifying drug (e.g. ammonium chloride), the metabolic acidosis is due to hydrogen carbonate loss; the pH falls and the chloride may increase to fill the anion gap. When the serum chloride concentration is equivalent to the hydrogen carbonate loss, the anion gap does not change: e.g. $(Na^+ + K^+) - (\uparrow Cl^- + \downarrow HCO_3^-) = 12$ mmol/l. This situation is referred to as a hyperchloraemic acidosis.

An adaptive response to the increased hydrogen ion concentration is to increase pulmonary ventilation. Respirations are increased in rate and volume to promote carbon dioxide elimination. The serum hydrogen carbonate concentration is reduced and is insufficient to buffer the increased non-volatile acids. The kidneys increase hydrogen ion secretion into the distal portion of the tubules for elimination in the urine.

Manifestations. The patient complains of headache, fatigue and drowsiness. The decreased pH causes a depression of the central nervous system; mental responses are slow and dulled and, if the acidosis is not corrected, the patient may become disoriented and eventually comatose. Anorexia, nausea and vomiting are common. Respirations increase in rate and volume (hyperpnoea). The urinary output is increased; dehydration develops rapidly as a result of the vomiting, diuresis and decreased intake. The serum hydrogen carbonate level is reduced and disturbances in the concentration of other electrolytes develop. Buffering of the increased fixed (non-volatile) acids results in the movement of potassium out of the cells; the serum potassium level rises. This may necessitate treatment for hyperkalaemia (see p. 99). The elimination of potassium in the urine will be increased. Later, when the acidosis is corrected, potassium ions move back into the cells and may cause a potassium deficit (see p. 98).

Treatment. The primary cause is treated and, if renal function is not impaired, fluid and the indicated electrolyte deficits are replaced by intravenous infusion. If acidosis has developed as a result of renal insufficiency, haemodialysis or peritoneal dialysis may be necessary.

Alkalosis

This is an acid–base imbalance in which there is a decrease in the hydrogen ion concentration below 35 mmol/l and an increase in the pH in excess of 7.45 due to a carbonic acid deficit or an excessive amount of bicarbonate. It may be classified as respiratory or metabolic.

TYPES OF ALKALOSIS

Respiratory alkalosis
This disorder is due to an excessive loss of carbonic

acid by hyperventilation. Carbon dioxide is being excreted by the lungs in excess of its production.

Effects and manifestations. The pH of the blood and the ratio of carbonic acid to bicarbonate are increased. If the condition is prolonged, large amounts of base are excreted by the kidneys, resulting in increased losses of sodium and potassium. There is a corresponding decrease in the excretion of chloride and hydrogen ions.

The patient frequently complains of dizziness. Tetany may develop as a result of increased neuromuscular irritability; signs and symptoms of this are tingling in the distal portions of the extremities, cramps, and tonic spasms of muscles which may progress to convulsions or carpopedal spasm.

Metabolic alkalosis
This decrease in hydrogen ion concentration and increase in pH may develop as the result of an abnormal loss of hydrochloric acid from the stomach in vomiting or gastric suctioning, excessive ingestion of alkaline substances (e.g. sodium bicarbonate) or a potassium deficit. The plasma concentration of bicarbonate is elevated with a corresponding increase in the pH and carbonic acid–bicarbonate ratio.

Effects and manifestations. Respirations become slow and shallow in an effort to increase the carbonic acid content of the blood. If the hypopnoea is prolonged, it may produce an oxygen deficiency and the patient becomes cyanotic.

Kidney compensation is by conservation of hydrogen and chloride ions and by increased excretion of hydrogen carbonate. If the alkalosis is caused by vomiting, there is likely to be an associated dehydration which leads to decreased urinary output and reduced renal compensation.

The patient is restless and apprehensive; tremors and twitching may be observed and tetany may ensue. Nausea, vomiting and diarrhoea may be present.

NURSING PROCESS

Assessment

Table 6.13 lists the objective and subjective data the nurse should consider when assessing a patient with an actual or potential acid–base imbalance. Aetiological factors are listed for the major acid and base disturbances.

Other factors which influence the development and the patient's ability to respond to disturbances in acid–base balance include the rate, severity and circumstances of the onset, pre-existing conditions which may interfere with adaptive responses and the individual's age. The rate of onset is particularly important because of the rapidity of events which follow acute respiratory disturbances. When the onset is severe and sudden, the body's compensatory mechanisms may not be able to respond adequately. Renal responses require one or more days to effectively compensate for acute acid–base changes. When the disturbance is long-term in nature, such as occurs in individuals living in high altitudes or those with chronic obstructive lung disease or chronic renal disease, compensatory mechanisms play a major role in minimizing the effects. On the other hand, chronic disease states may result in decreased reserves and decreased ability to respond to further disturbances. The risk of functional and structural damage from acid–base imbalances is greatest in young children and the elderly.

Potential patient problems

Potential patient problems relevant to the patient with an acid–base imbalance include:
1 Breathing pattern ineffective
2 Alterations in tissue perfusion
3 Thought processes impaired
4 Alterations in pattern of urinary elimination
5 Alterations in bowel elimination: diarrhoea
6 Lack of knowledge related to the disease process, treatment regimen, dietary plan, signs and symptoms of acid or base imbalance and actions to take if symptoms develop
7 Anxiety related to the illness

Nursing intervention specific for these problems are discussed in detail in subsequent chapters of the text—specifically Chapters 10, 15, 16, 17 and 21.

Nursing intervention

The *goals* are to:
1 Prevent acid–base imbalance and maintain optimal function
2 Promote the return of acid–base balance to normal or a compensated level
3 Promote comfort and prevent further complications
4 Minimize the impact of undesirable physiological, psychological and environmental changes

1. Prevention of acid–base imbalance and maintenance of optimal function
The nurse has an important role in the identification of risk factors. These include fluid and electrolyte imbalance, vomiting and diarrhoea, gastrointestinal drainage, renal dysfunction and metabolic disease such as diabetes mellitus. Patients with chronic health problems that may lead to acid–base imbalance require knowledge and skill to monitor their status, prevent the development of complications and maintain an optimal level of functioning. When narcotics are administered, the patient's respirations should be closely monitored and deep breathing and coughing should be performed at regular intervals to

Table 6.13 Assessment of acid–base imbalance.

	Acid–base imbalance			
	Respiratory acidosis	Metabolic acidosis	Respiratory alkalosis	Metabolic alkalosis
Objective data				
Blood and cardiovascular system	Serum pH <7.35 Serum [H$^+$] >45 nmol/l ↑ Serum bicarbonate ↑ Serum potassium	Serum pH <7.35 Serum [H$^+$] >45 nmol/l ↓ Serum bicarbonate ↑ Serum potassium ↑ Anion gap (or normal)	Serum pH >7.44 Serum [H$^+$] <35 nmol/l ↓ Serum bicarbonate ↓ Serum potassium Cardiac arrhythmias	Serum pH >7.44 Serum [H$^+$] <35 nmol/l ↑ Serum bicarbonate ↓ Serum potassium Cardiac arrhythmias
Respiratory system	Hypoventilation Respirations laboured; the use of accessory muscles Prolonged expiration ↑ Paco$_2$ ↓ Pao$_2$	Hyperventilation ↑ Rate and depth of respirations ↓ Paco$_2$ Pao$_2$ normal	Hyperventilation ↑ Rate and depth of respirations ↓ Paco$_2$	Hypoventilation Slow, shallow respirations ↑ Paco$_2$ (or normal) ↓ Pao$_2$ (if alkalosis is prolonged)
Renal system	Urine { ↑ acidity ↑ ammonia ↓ pH	Urine { ↑ acidity ↑ ammonium ↓ pH ↑ potassium ↑ output	Urine { ↑ sodium and potassium excretion ↓ chloride and hydrogen excretion	Urine { ↑ sodium and potassium excretion ↓ chloride and hydrogen excretion
Neuromuscular system	Restlessness, weakness, headache and apprehension; may progress to dullness, slow responses, disorientation and coma	Headache, weakness, drowsiness followed by slow, dulled responses, disorientation and coma	Dizziness, tetany, tonic muscle spasms, cramps, tingling in extremities, convulsions	Dizziness, tremors, twitching, tetany, cramps, tingling in extremities, convulsions
Other		Nausea and vomiting		Nausea, vomiting, diarrhoea
Subjective data	Restlessness, weakness, headache, confusion	Headache, weakness, drowsiness, confusion and nausea	Dizziness, panic	Dizziness, apprehension, panic, nausea

Causes	Hypoventilation related to:
	  Acute or chronic respiratory disease (e.g. pneumonia, chronic airway limitation)
	  Circulatory failure
	  Impaired alveolar perfusion
	  Depression of respiratory centre by drugs or cerebral disease
	  Neuromuscular disturbances e.g. Guillain–Barré syndrome, poliomyelitis, myasthenia gravis, hypo- or hyperkalaemia
		Increased acid production or ingestion related to:
		  Uncontrolled diabetes mellitus
		  Starvation with an increased catabolism of fat
		  Alcoholism
		  Lactic acidosis
		  Excessive administration of ammonium chloride or acetylsalicylic acid
		Decreased urinary output due to renal disease, severe dehydration or shock and decreased excretion of hydrogen ions with hyperkalaemia and renal failure
		Depletion of bicarbonate base associated with severe diarrhoea, vomiting, intestinal fistula or suction of fluids from the intestine or with administration of carbonic anhydrase inhibitors such as acetazolamide (Diamox)
			Hyperventilation related to:
			  Anxiety states, hysteria or central nervous system disease which produces over-stimulation of the respiratory centre
			  High fever
			  Hypoxia
			  Severe pain
			  High altitude
			  Excessive mechanical ventilation
				Abnormal loss of acid associated with vomiting or gastric suction, use of diuretics and mineralocorticoid excess and hypokalaemia
				Excessive ingestion of alkaline substances (e.g. sodium bicarbonate) is a contributing factor and not usually a primary cause

promote removal of respiratory secretions and adequate gas exchange. Although the patient with chronic airflow limitation presents with respiratory distress, the administration of oxygen promotes further retention of carbon dioxide and respiratory acidosis (see p. 109). A higher concentration of oxygen slows the respirations and less carbon dioxide is eliminated.

Diuretic therapy increases the risk of acid–base disturbances because of fluid and electrolyte depletion. The specific action(s) and potential side-effects of the diuretic being administered should be familiar to nurses and the patient.

Patient education. When a patient has a chronic health problem, both the patient and family should be taught:
- The manifestations of the disease
- The complications that can occur
- The specific plan for management of the health problem
- The actions and side-effects of medications

- The content and preparation of prescribed diets
- The signs and symptoms of the specific type of acid or base imbalance the patient is at risk of developing
- Actions to take should symptoms develop
- What health-care resources are available in the community

For example, patients with chronic respiratory disease are taught deep-breathing and coughing techniques. Patients with diabetes and renal disease are taught to regulate their diets, administer drugs and modify living habits to prevent the development of acidosis. More specific information on prevention and maintenance measures for patients with specific health problems will be found in later chapters.

2. Promotion of normal or compensated acid–base balance
Nursing interventions directed toward promoting the return of acid–base balance to normal or a compensated steady state include: (a) continuous assessment of changes in the patient's status; (b) communication of changes in the patient's condition to other members of the health team so that necessary adjustments or changes in the treatment can be made promptly; and (c) implementation of the nursing and medical plans of care.

Observations. Close observation of the patient with acidosis is important because the patient is critically ill; respiratory changes, either as a causative factor or as a compensatory response, may result in sudden changes in the individual's general condition.

The nurse should observe the vital signs, fluid balance, orientation and level of consciousness. Frequent collection of urine specimens may be required and may necessitate the use of a retention catheter. Blood specimens are taken at frequent intervals for serum hydrogen ion and electrolyte concentrations and pH estimations. Arterial blood gas determination will be done regularly and following any sudden changes in the patient's condition. The nurse should be alert for signs and symptoms of specific electrolyte deficits and excesses, especially potassium.

Early signs of disturbed neuromuscular functioning and tetany (e.g. muscle spasm and twitching) are noted and reported promptly. Trousseau's sign, which is characteristic of the onset of tetany, may be positive; it involves carpal spasm, which can be elicited by compression of the upper arm.

Fluids. If the patient is conscious, he should be encouraged to drink fluids. The fluids permitted vary with the cause of the acidosis or alkalosis. Parenteral fluids are usually administered to patients with acidosis or metabolic alkalosis. The solutions given are based on the blood chemistry reports and kidney function. The rate of flow is defined by the doctor. The patient with alkalosis may require potassium replacement either orally or intravenously if the

serum potassium concentration is low. When potassium is added to an intravenous infusion, the rate of flow is very carefully regulated; it must be administered slowly and well diluted, with the dilution being specified by the doctor. Close observation for signs of hyperkalaemia is necessary; these include a slow weak pulse, restlessness and muscular weakness. An intravenous infusion of ammonium chloride may be prescribed if the alkalosis is due to vomiting which depletes chloride ions. Precautions similar to those mentioned above in relation to parenteral potassium administration are necessary if ammonium chloride is given intravenously.

Oxygen–carbon dioxide administration. The rate, depth and characteristics of the patient's respirations should be observed closely. Oxygen may be administered to treat hypoxia, especially if the underlying cause is of respiratory origin. Oxygen is not administered to patients with hypercapnia due to chronic obstructive airways disease.

The patient with respiratory alkalosis related to hyperventilation is directed to rebreathe his own carbon dioxide by breathing into a paper bag. Inhalation of 5% carbon dioxide in oxygen may be ordered.

3. Promotion of comfort and prevention of complications
(a) *Mouth care*. Frequent mouth care is especially important because of hyperpnoea, mouth breathing, vomiting and dehydration that frequently accompany acid–base imbalances.
(b) *Safety*. Safety precautions are necessary if the patient manifests disorientation or confusion. If comatose, nursing measures applicable to an unconscious patient are required (see Chapter 10).

4. Emotional support
The patient and family require support and reassurance that everything necessary is being done. They should be kept informed about the patient's progress and advised of treatment procedures. Time is taken to listen to their concerns and to answer their questions. The patient who has a chronic health problem in which an acid–base imbalance is a potential complication receives instruction so that early signs and symptoms of imbalance may be recognized and appropriate therapeutic measures initiated should the problem arise. Preventive measures should be stressed and the importance of following the prescribed treatment plan explained.

Expected outcomes

1 The respiratory rate, rhythm and depth are normal.
2 The cardiac rate and rhythm are normal for the particular patient.
3 Serum hydrogen ion concentration, pH, $Pa\text{co}_2$

and hydrogen carbonate and potassium concentrations are within the normal range or are at a level of compensation.

4 The urine pH and electrolyte concentrations are within normal ranges.

5 Muscle tone and strength are normal for the patient.

6 Headache and disorientation or dizziness are relieved.

References and Further Reading

BOOKS

Beeson PB, McDermott W & Wyngaarden JB (eds) (1979) *Textbook of Medicine*, 15th ed. Philadelphia: WB Saunders. pp. 1950–1969.

Burke SR (1980) *The Composition and Function of Body Fluids*, 3rd ed. St Louis: CV Mosby.

Ganong WF (1985) *Review of Medical Physiology*, 11th ed. San Francisco: Lange.

Groer MW (1981) *Physiology and Pathophysiology of Body Fluids*. St Louis: CV Mosby.

Guyton AC (1986) *Textbook of Medical Physiology*, 7th ed. Philadelphia: WB Saunders. Chapters 30, 31, 32 and 33.

Harper HA, Rodwell UW & Mayes PA (eds) (1979) *Review of Physiological Chemistry*, 17th ed. Los Altos, CA: Lange. Chapters 2, 3, & 6.

Hart LK, Reese JL & Fearing MO (1981) *Concepts Common to Acute Illness*. St Louis: CV Mosby. Chapters 11 & 12.

Holloway NM (1984) *Nursing the Critically Ill Adult*, 2nd ed. Menlo Park; CA: Addison–Wesley. pp. 308–348.

Howe PS (1981) *Basic Nutrition in Health and Disease*. Philadelphia: WB Saunders. Chapters 7 & 9.

Kenney MR, Dear CB, Packa DR, & Voorman DM (eds) (1981) *AACN's Clinical Reference for Critical Care Nursing*. New York: McGraw-Hill. Chapter 20.

Kim MJ & Moretz DA (1982) *Classification of Nursing Diagnoses: Proceedings of 3rd and 4th National Conferences*. New York: McGraw-Hill.

Krupp MA & Chatton MJ (eds) (1983) *Current Medical Diagnosis and Treatment*. Los Altos, CA: Lange. Chapter 2.

Leaf A & Cotram RS (1980) *Renal Physiology*, 2nd ed. New York: Oxford University Press. Chapters 3 & 4.

Meyers FH, Jawetz E & Goldfien A (1976) *Review of Medical Pharmacology* 5th ed. Los Altos, CA: Lange. pp. 452–462.

Sabiston DC (ed) (1986) *Davis–Christopher Textbook of Surgery*, 13th ed. Philadelphia: WB Saunders. Chapter 4.

Smith K (1980) *Fluids and Electrolytes: A Conceptual Approach*. New York: Churchill Livingstone.

Smith LH & Thier SO (1985) *Pathophysiology: The Biological Principles of Disease*, 2nd ed. Philadelphia: WB Saunders. Section 10.

Wyngaarden JB & Smith LH (eds) (1985) *Cecil Textbook of Medicine*, 17th ed. Philadelphia: WB Saunders. pp. 515–544.

PERIODICALS

Clough DH & Higgins PG (1981) Discrepancies in estimating blood loss. *Am. J. Nurs.*, Vol. 81 No. 2, pp. 331–333.

Felver L (1980) Understanding the electrolyte maze. *Am. J. Nurs.*, Vol. 80 No. 9, pp. 1591–1595.

Flomenbaum N (1980) Acid–base disturbances. *Emerg. Med.*, Vol. 12 No. 17, pp. 24–25.

Folk-Lighty M (1984) Solving the puzzles of patients' fluid imbalances. *Nurs. '84*, Vol. 14 No. 2, pp. 34–41.

Goldstein B (1980) Guidelines to drug incompatibilities in large volume parenterals. *Nurs. Drug Alert*, Vol. 4 No. 8, pp. 57–60.

Heaney RP, Gallagher JC, Johnstone CC et al (1982) Calcium nutrition and bone health in the elderly. *Am. J. Clin. Nutr.*, Vol. 36, No. 5, pp. 986–1013.

Kassirer JP & Madias NE (1980) Respiratory acid–base disorders. *Hosp. Pract.*, Vol. 15 No. 12, pp. 57–71.

Keithley JK & Fraulini KE (1982) What's behind that IV line? *Nurs. '82*, Vol. 12 No. 3, pp. 33–45.

Langford A (1981) Name that acid–base. *Crit. Care Nurs.*, Vol. 1 No. 3, pp. 10–12.

Laschinger H K (1984) Demystifying arterial blood gases. *Cancer Nurs.*, Vol. 80 No. 10, pp. 45–47.

Lindshaw M (1980) When serum sodium sinks. *Emerg. Med.*, Vol. 12 No. 4, pp. 24–42.

Martof M (1985) Part I: fluid balance. *J. Neph. Nurs.*, Vol. 2 No. 1, pp. 10–18.

Martof M (1985) Part II: Electrolyte balance. *J. Neph. Nurs.*, Vol. 2 No. 2, pp. 49–55.

Martof M (1985) Part III Acid–Base Balance. *J. Neph. Nurs.*, Vol. 2 No. 3, pp. 105–112.

Menzel LK (1980) Clinical problems of fluid balance. *Nurs. Clin. N. Am.*, Vol. 15 No. 3, pp. 549–558.

Menzel LK (1980) Clinical problems of electrolyte balance. *Nurs. Clin. N. Am.*, Vol. 15 No. 3, pp. 559–575.

Miller WC (1980) The ABC's of blood gases. *Emerg. Med.*, Vol. 12, No. 5, pp. 24–37.

Nielsen L (1980) Interpreting arterial blood gases. *Am. J. Nurs.*, Vol. 80 No. 12, pp. 2197–2201.

Rector LC & Cogan MG (1980) The renal acidoses. *Hosp. Prac.*, Vol. 15 No. 4, pp. 99–111.

Rice V (1982) The role of potassium in health and disease. *Crit. Care Nurs.*, Vol. 2 No. 3, pp. 54–74.

Rice V (1983) Magnesium, phosphate and calcium imbalances; their clinical significance. *Crit. Care Nurs.*, Vol. 3 No. 3, pp. 88–112.

Rice V (1984) Shock management part 1. Fluid volume replacement. *Crit. Care Nurs.*, Vol. 4 No. 6, pp. 69–82.

Shrake K (1979) The ABC's of how to interpret a blood gas volume. *Nurs. '79*, Vol. 9 No. 9, pp. 26–33.

Stark JL & Hunt V (1984) Managing electrolyte imbalances. *Nurs. '84*, Vol. 14 No. 7, pp. 57–63.

Urrows ST (1980) Physiology of body fluids, *Nurs. Clin. N. Am.*, Vol. 15 No. 3, pp. 537–547.

Williams V & Perkins L (1984) Continuous ultrafiltration: a new ICU procedure for the treatment of fluid overload. *Crit. Care Nurs.*, Vol. 4 No. 4, pp. 44–49.

7

Body Temperature

Introduction

Accurate monitoring of body temperature is an important nursing measure. Temperature reflects the heat content of the body, and may provide information during an illness or following an injury that contributes to making the diagnosis and decisions as to the necessary therapeutic care. It may signal a change in the patient's condition that indicates the need for immediate action. Normally, the *internal* or *core body temperature* is maintained within narrow limits. The temperature of the skin and subcutaneous tissues is referred to as the *surface temperature*. The latter may vary with the temperature of the environment.

Body temperature results from the balance between the heat produced and acquired by the body and the amount lost. Normally, the body maintains a relatively constant core temperature within the range of 36–37°C. (97–98.6°F) regardless of the environmental temperature (Fig. 7.1). For this reason, man is classified as homothermic or warm-blooded as opposed to the poikilothermic or cold-blooded species whose body temperature fluctuates with variations in the environmental temperature.

HEAT PRODUCTION AND DISSIPATION

Constancy of a temperature of 36–37°C, which favours normal cellular activity, is maintained by physiological processes that preserve a balance between heat production and heat dissipation. An increased production of heat is compensated by increasing the loss; conversely, a decrease below normal body temperature initiates a decrease in the heat loss as well as an increase in the production of heat.

Heat is generated in the body by chemical reactions within the cells. The more active the tissue, the greater is its production of heat; as a result, especially large amounts of heat are produced by the muscles and liver. A small amount may be acquired from external sources by radiation and conduction. Heat production is dependent upon cellular activity, and biochemical reactions (metabolism) increase as body temperature increases. A decrease in body temperature slows the rate of cellular activity, decreasing heat production. Body temperature may

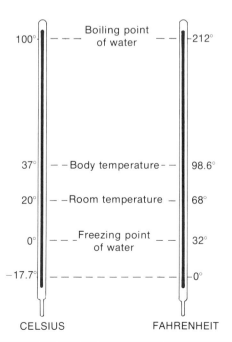

CELSIUS   FAHRENHEIT

Fig. 7.1 Two temperature scales: Fahrenheit and centigrade.

also be increased by the hormones thyroxine, adrenaline, noradrenaline and progesterone.

Normally, an excess of heat is produced within the body and must be eliminated to maintain a normal temperature. The excess is dissipated by the physical processes of radiation, conduction, convection and evaporation. Most of it is lost through the skin and the remainder is eliminated in respirations and excreta.

Radiation is the process by which radiant energy is transmitted from one object to another without direct contact. Conduction is the transfer of heat between two objects that are in contact. Convection is the process by which heat is carried away from a surface by air currents passing over it, such as occurs when a fan is used. Evaporation of 1 g of water from the surface of the skin and respiratory tract utilizes about 0.58 kcal (2.43 kJ). The sweat glands pour their secretion onto the skin surface; the heat of the blood in peripheral vessels is utilized in evaporating the secretion. Some vaporization takes place constantly, but the amount taking place on the skin varies. If there is a need to increase the heat loss, the sweat glands increase their secretion and peripheral vasodilation occurs, resulting in increased vaporization. If there is a need to conserve body heat, less moisture is released onto the skin surface and vasoconstriction reduces circulation to the periphery.

Heat loss by radiation, conduction and convection depends on a temperature gradient. If the environmental temperature is equal to or greater than that of the body, these processes are ineffective and heat dissipation becomes completely dependent on the evaporation process.

TEMPERATURE REGULATION

Temperature-regulating mechanisms are essential to prevent the damaging effects on body tissues by extremes of heat and cold.

Regulation of body temperature is coordinated by the hypothalamic *thermostat*. Responses to changes in body temperature are evoked by sensory nerve impulses that originate in temperature receptors in the skin and by the direct effect of the blood temperature on the preoptic area of the hypothalamus and possibly from other receptors in the body core.

Receptor cells that are sensitive to heat and cold are located in the skin. Guyton suggests that since there are far more cold receptors than heat receptors, peripheral detection of temperature mainly concerns detection of cold.[1] When changes in the cutaneous temperature occur, the receptors give rise to nerve impulses that are delivered to the cerebral cortex and hypothalamus of the brain. Those that reach the cerebral cortex make the individual conscious of the temperature change. He may then produce

behavioural responses to aid in correcting the change. For example, if he experiences the sensation of cold, he may voluntarily increase muscle activity to generate more heat, seek a warmer environment and add clothing to reduce the heat loss. In a hot environment, the behavioural responses might be to decrease activity in order to lower the heat production and to change to lighter clothing to permit more radiation.

In the anterior portion of the hypothalamus is a group of neurons that is referred to as the thermostatic or heat-regulating centre. This centre responds to cutaneous temperature impulses and to changes in the temperature of the blood. When the body temperature rises above normal, noradrenergic impulses responsible for peripheral vasoconstriction are reduced, resulting in passive dilation of the cutaneous blood vessels; pseudomotor nerves stimulate the sweat glands. Heat loss is increased by evaporation of the additional sweat as well as by radiation from the larger volume of blood brought to the surface.

If the normal body temperature is threatened by a reduction in body heat, the centre initiates impulses which reduce heat loss and increase the production of heat. Superficial blood vessels constrict, secretion by the sweat glands is inhibited, shivering and non-shivering thermogenesis occur (see Table 7.1).

MONITORING BODY TEMPERATURE

The thermometers for measuring body temperature may be scaled in Fahrenheit (F) or Celsius (C centigrade) and it may be necessary at times to know the equivalent of one in the other system.

The difference between the freezing point (0 °C) and the boiling point (100 °C) of water on the Celsius scale is 100 degrees; on the Fahrenheit scale the difference is 180 degrees (32 °F = freezing point; 212 °F = boiling point). This indicates that 100 Celsius degrees equal 180 Fahrenheit degrees, or one Fahrenheit degree equals $\frac{5}{9}$ of a Celsius degree. The freezing point on the Fahrenheit scale is 32 degrees, but on the Celsius scale it is 0 degrees; therefore, when converting to Celsius the 32 must first be subtracted in order to find the number of degrees to be converted. When converting to Fahrenheit the 32 must be added to the product so that the result will be adjusted for the Fahrenheit scale. The following formulae may be used when conversion from one system to the other is necessary.

The formula to convert Fahrenheit degrees to Celsius is

$$(F \text{ degrees} - 32) \times \frac{5}{9} = C \text{ degrees}$$

Example: The conversion of 100 °F to C degrees.

$$(100 °F - 32) \times \frac{5}{9} = 37.7 °C$$

The formula to convert Celsius degrees to Fahrenheit is:

[1] Guyton (1986), p. 854.

Table 7.1 Summary of temperature regulation.

	Heat loss	Heat production

Responses to cold	Heat loss is decreased by:
	  Seeking a warmer environment
	  Adding warmer clothing
	  Changing posture to decrease
	  effective surface area of body
	  Vasoconstriction of cutaneous blood
	  vessels
		Heat production is increased by:
		  Increased muscle activity (shivering
		  and voluntary activity)
		  Increased secretion of thyroxine,
		  adrenaline, noradrenaline and
		  progesterone

Response to heat	Heat loss is increased by:
	  Wearing lighter clothing
	  Seeking cooler environment
	  Use of fans
	  Vasodilation of cutaneous blood
	  vessels
	  Increased sweating
		Heat production is decreased by:
		  Decreased physical activity
		  Decreased muscle tone
		  Decreased production of thyroxine,
		  adrenaline, noradrenaline and
		  progesterone

$$(C \text{ degrees} \times \tfrac{9}{5}) + 32 = F \text{ degrees}$$

Example: The conversion of 39°C to F degrees.

$$(39°C \times \tfrac{9}{5}) + 32 = 102.2°F$$

Body temperature may be measured by placing a clinical thermometer in the sublingual area of the oral cavity, the rectum or the axilla. The site used depends upon the patient's mental state, age, and local conditions which would preclude accuracy (e.g. recent food or fluid ingestion or smoking, inflammatory disease in the site). The results of several studies indicate that 'for ordinary, regular assessment, the most accurate reflection of the body's core temperature is obtained by using the sublingual pocket.'[2] In oral monitoring, the proximity of the thermometer to the lingual and sublingual arteries provides for greater accuracy. A period of 15 minutes should elapse following the ingestion of hot or cold fluids, or smoking before taking the oral temperature.

Studies have also suggested the optimum period of time that the mercury thermometer should remain in each of the sites in order to have the maximum temperature recording.[3] These are: for oral recording, 7 minutes; for rectal recording, 3 minutes; and when the axilla is used, 10-minute placement is suggested. Electronic digital thermometers give almost instant recordings and signal when the maximum temperature has been reached.

If the body temperature shows a progressive increase towards dangerously high levels, or if a patient's condition is likely to produce fluctuations, establishing a system of continuous recording is preferable to very frequent monitoring by the usual method. It is less anxiety-producing and less disturbing for the patient, as well as more convenient for the nursing staff.

Continuous monitoring is possible with an electric thermometer, which operates on the principle that heat alters the resistance of a conductor to the flow of an electric current. Depending upon the material used as the conductor, the resistance may be increased or decreased. In continuous recording of body temperature, a temperature sensor (probe) in which a conductive material is encased may be placed in the oesophagus or rectum. A small electrical current of constant voltage is directed through the conductor. The resistance is proportional to temperature, and the voltage of the current conducted through the probe is calibrated in terms of temperature. The temperature may be determined from the position of the pointer on a Fahrenheit or Celsius scale, or the model being used may be equipped with an automatic chart recorder.[4] The temperature gradient between the core and the great toe, measured by means of an electronic probe, has been demonstrated to be a reliable prognostic indicator for patients with myocardial infarction, bacteraemia or blood and fluid loss.[5]

A study by Erickson to determine differences in oral temperature measurements using three brands of electronic and mercury thermometers demonstrated that actual temperature values differed with the sites used, as well as between electronic and mercury thermometers. The researcher emphasized the importance of using the posterior sublingual pocket as the site for oral temperature measurement and the value of using the same instrument to obtain repeated comparable measurements.[6]

Takacs and Valenti in studying the factors associated with temperature measurement in a clinical setting found wide variations in the times glass thermometers were left in place. They suggest that electronic thermometers present an advantage in clinical practice because the shorter placement time

[2] Blainey (1974), p. 1861.
[3] Nichols & Verhonick (1969), pp. 2304–2306.

[4] Nave & Nave (1985).
[5] Editor (1980), pp. 101–104.
[6] Erickson (1980), pp. 157–164.

allows nurses more time for patient interaction and result in increased patient safety and comfort.[7]

VARIABLES WITHIN THE NORMAL

The body temperature shows slight variations within the normal range from one individual to another and under certain circumstances. Variations within the normal may have several causes.

Time of day

As with many biological activities, there is an evident diurnal pattern of change in body temperature. It decreases between 2 and 6 a.m. and slowly rises throughout the day, reaching a peak between 6 and 10 p.m. This rhythm is not directly related to activity, but its pattern may be altered in persons who are active during the night and sleep during the day.

Physical activity and exposure to heat produce a transient elevation in body temperature which normally is readily dissipated by the skin and lungs.

The fever associated with illness tends to follow the normal circadian rhythm; the fever is greatest in the evening and lower through the night unless the disorder involves the temperature-regulating centre and mechanism.

Age

Infants have a higher normal temperature. Their heat production is greater owing to the higher metabolic rate associated with their growth and activity. Also, the ability to regulate heat loss and production is not sufficiently developed in the early years to regulate a constancy of temperature efficiently.

Older people have a somewhat lower normal temperature because of their slower metabolic rate and reduced muscular activity. Their mechanisms of heat production, conservation and dissipation are less efficient.

Exercise

Strenuous exercise may cause an elevation to 40°C core temperature, but it quickly returns to normal when the activity ceases. Women in labour frequently show an increase in temperature, attributed to their increased muscular activity.

Menstrual cycle

A variation in temperature is characteristic of certain phases of the menstrual cycle. There is an increase of 0.3–0.5°C when ovulation occurs, which is usually about the middle of the cycle. This is attributed to the increased activities of the endometrial cells, initiated by the secretion of progesterone. The slight increase is maintained until a day or two before the onset of menstruation, when it falls to the previous normal level.

Pregnancy

A slight increase in temperature occurs in the first 3–4 months of pregnancy and is followed by a gradual fall of 0.5–1°C. The lower temperature continues to full term and returns to the individual's normal level after parturition.

Environment

Extremes of heat and cold in the environment affect body temperature. Adjustment to cold is achieved by insulation of the body with layers of protective clothing and raising the environmental temperatures with heating devices. The body acclimatizes to cold through adaptive changes including increased thyroid activity and metabolism, and reduction in visible shivering. Heat acclimatization is achieved through increased effectiveness of the sweat mechanism.

Abnormal Body Temperature

FEVER

Fever, or pyrexia, is an elevation of the body temperature above normal. It is a manifestation of tissue injury or a disorder that results in an increase in heat production in excess of the rate of dissipation, or in an impairment of the heat-dissipating or control mechanisms.

CAUSES OF FEVER

The imbalance in body heat content may be caused by malfunction of the temperature-regulating centre, the response of the centre to a pyrogen, exposure to a very high environmental temperature, or impaired dissipation.

Disturbance in regulation by the centre may be the result of the direct action of brain disease or increased intracranial pressure, or by the action of a substance that is released into the blood at the site of tissue injury or disintegration anywhere in the body. The substance, which may be referred to as a pyrogen, reacts first with leucocytes to form a second substance called endogenous pyrogen.[8]

Stimulation of the hypothalamic heat centre by endogenous pyrogen is analogous to the setting of the thermostat of an automatic heating system to a higher level; heat is produced until the set level of temperature is achieved. The higher temperature is maintained as long as the pyrogen is present. As the concentration of the pyrogen is reduced, the level of the thermostat is lowered, and there is a corresponding decrease in the fever by activation of the heat-

---

[7] Takacs & Valenti (1982), p. 370.

[8] Guyton (1986), p. 858.

dissipating responses, peripheral vasodilation and sweating.

In the case of fever due to exposure to a high temperature, the body cannot dissipate heat as fast as it is being received from the exterior.

Fever occurring because of the inefficient heat-dissipating mechanisms is seen most often when severe dehydration develops. The secretion of sweat is reduced, resulting in a marked decrease in heat loss by evaporation.

MANIFESTATIONS AND EFFECTS OF FEVER

The onset of fever may be sudden and rapid, or the rise in body heat may develop gradually without the individual being aware of it. The initial manifestations of fever vary with the degree of disturbance in the thermostatic centre. If the elevation is moderate and gradual, the patient may experience slight chilliness for a brief period, general malaise, headache and anorexia. With a sudden and greater degree of stimulation of the centre, the patient has a chill in which he shivers and feels very cold, even though his temperature may already be above normal. Adrenaline is released which accelerates metabolism, increasing heat production. In turn, the rise in temperature further accelerates the metabolic rate and heat production. The skin becomes pale and is cold to the touch because of peripheral vasoconstriction. The shivering is increased muscular activity for the purpose of producing heat; it may be severe enough to cause chattering of the teeth and shaking of the whole body. Small elevations of skin (gooseflesh) appear and the small fine hairs become erect owing to the contraction of small muscles attached to the hair follicles. The chill lasts until the temperature reaches the level set by the stimulated thermostatic centre in the hypothalamus. Then, as long as the pyrogen is effective, a balance between the heat production and dissipation maintains the temperature at approximately this higher level.

Frequently the onset of fever in infants and young children is accompanied by a convulsion which is due to the immaturity and instability of their nervous systems.

With subsidence of the chill, the patient's skin becomes hot and flushed, and he complains of feeling hot. Disorientation and delirium are not uncommon when the fever is high, especially in older persons.

The basal metabolic rate is increased in proportion to the elevation of temperature. With a fever of 40.5°C (105°F) there is an increase in metabolic rate of approximately 50%. A negative nitrogen balance develops with the increased destruction of body protein in metabolism, and there is a loss of weight. Respirations and the heart rate are accelerated. There is a greater loss of fluid by evaporation from the hot skin and in the increased respirations.

If the temperature rises above approximately 40.5°C (105°F), there is danger of cellular damage. The hypothalamus may lose its capacity for temperature regulation, resulting in a progressive increase in fever until death occurs. The limit to which the temperature may rise before causing death is about 43.3–44.4°C (110–112°F).

When the pyrogenic factor is suddenly removed, the mechanisms that contribute to heat loss are set in operation. There is marked peripheral vasodilation and profuse sweating (diaphoresis); heat is lost rapidly by radiation and vaporization. This sudden lowering of the temperature is referred to as the *crisis of fever*. If the temperature returns to normal gradually over a period of several days, the process is known as *lysis*.

Fever is thought to serve a useful purpose in some infections. A high temperature will destroy a large number of causative organisms in gonorrhoea and neurosyphilis. Other pathogenic organisms may be made less virulent by a high fever. It is also suggested that the increased metabolism supports an increased production of antibodies, since patients who fail to develop a marked febrile response in a severe infection usually do less well.

TYPES OF FEVER

Fever may be classified according to its variation within 24 hours or 2–3 days. An intermittent fever is one in which the temperature falls to normal and rises again within the 24-hour period; a remittent fever manifests a variation of 1 or 2 degrees, but does not reach normal within the 24 hours. A relapsing fever occurs when there are alternating periods of one or several days of normal and elevated temperature.

HEAT STROKE

A heat stroke occurs with relatively long exposure to extreme heat. At first the individual may experience headache, visual disturbances, nausea and vomiting. Weakness, flaccidity of the muscles, a rapid bounding pulse and rapid respirations are manifested. The individual becomes delirious, collapses, and lapses into coma. The skin is hot and dry, and there is an absence of sweating due to dehydration and central nervous system damage. The temperature progressively rises to 40.6–43.3°C (105–110°F).

Unless the condition is discovered in the early stages and the body is rapidly cooled, circulatory failure develops and the patient dies. The patient may be immersed in a cold bath or given a cold sponge bath followed by the application of ice bags; or a cooling blanket that is used to induce hypothermia may be applied.

The prevention of recurrence of heat stroke involves patient teaching as to its cause. The hazards of a long period of exposure to extreme heat should be explained. Environmental humidity and physical activity increase the possibility of a heat stroke. Early signs and symptoms are outlined. The individual is advised that if exposure to a high temperature is necessary, certain acclimatization measures should be used. Individuals will develop increased tolerance to hot and humid conditions through gradually increasing exposures and moderate work activity. Acclimatization results in an increased rate and effectiveness of sweating, retention of sodium and increased plasma volume.

Nursing process

ASSESSMENT

Characteristics of a patient with an elevated body temperature are listed in Table 7.2 and serve as a guide to patient assessment. Nursing interventions relevant to the patient problems listed are discussed below.

NURSING INTERVENTION

The *goals* are to:
1 Decrease heat production
2 Promote heat loss
3 Support and maintain body functions
4 Promote comfort

1. Decrease heat production
Fever produces an increased metabolic rate, so the patient is advised to decrease his activity. With an elevation of 37.7°C (100°F) or higher, bed rest is usually recommended. Anticipation of the patient's needs is important in order to avoid activity on his part and unnecessary expenditure of energy. Information about his condition and treatment should be given to reduce the patient's apprehension and level of anxiety. Concern and fear may stimulate the release of adrenaline, which accelerates cellular metabolism and heat production.

2. Promotion of heat loss
Care of the feverish patient may include cooling measures to prevent the temperature reaching the level at which tissue damage may occur. The various procedures used may be classified as external surface cooling, internal surface cooling, or extracorporeal cooling.

External surface cooling is the method most often employed and may be achieved by a variety of measures. An increase in the loss of body heat by radiation and convection may be promoted by reducing the covers to a minimum, lowering room temperature, and directing air currents from electric fans over the patient. Cooling may be induced by sponging the body with tepid water.

The use of extracorporeal cooling is generally reserved for reducing body temperature during cardiac, vascular and brain surgery that necessitates interference with normal circulation, resulting in a reduced oxygen supply to the tissues. This cooling procedure involves diversion of the blood from a large vessel to outside the body where it is pumped through the heart–lung machine. While passing through the machine, the blood is cooled to a 'set' temperature and then returned to the body. The cooled blood lowers body temperature, which in turn reduces the metabolic rate and cellular requirements. The latter decreases the oxygen need, reducing possible tissue damage as a result of oxygen deficiency.

Table 7.2 Assessment of the patient with an elevated body temperature (hyperthermia).

Cause	Signs and symptoms	Problem
Increased body heat production in excess of heat loss	*Objective data:* Body temperature > 37°C (98.6°F) Skin pale, 'gooseflesh', and cold to touch followed by hot and flushed	Anxiety related to illness and fear of the unknown Alterations in thought processes
Impairment of body regulating mechanisms	Heart rate increased, pulse bounding Respiratory rate increased	Alterations in comfort Alterations in nutrition: less than body requirements
Exposure to extreme heat	Shaking of body (shivers) Chattering of teeth Fine hairs on body surface erect Convulsions (infant) Disorientation	Fluid volume deficit Potential for impairment of skin integrity Alterations in bowel elimination: constipation
	Subjective data: General malaise Anorexia and nausea Headache Sensation of cold followed by sensation of warmth Visual disturbances Confusion and delirium	

In all cooling procedures shivering is to be avoided, since it is muscular activity that increases heat production. If the patient develops shivering, a drug to depress the heat-regulating centre and prevent the shivering response may be prescribed.

Medications. If the temperature approaches dangerous levels, a drug that lowers the sensitivity of the heat-regulating centre and produces diaphoresis may be ordered. The antipyretic drug most commonly used is acetylsalicylic acid (aspirin) in doses of 0.3–0.6 g for an adult every 3–4 hours, or paracetamol 120 mg 4-hourly for children.

3. Support and maintenance measures

Assessment. The temperature, pulse and respirations are usually noted every 4 hours; they may be checked more often in high fever and when these vital signs may indicate complications. For example, when caring for a patient with brain disease or trauma, it may be necessary to record the temperature, pulse and respirations at least hourly. An increase in temperature and a decrease in pulse and respirations may indicate an elevation in intracranial pressure. Frequent monitoring may create anxiety, and a judicious explanation with reassurance will be necessary. The degree of concern aroused by the repeated checking may necessitate continuous recording using an electric thermometer.

Observations are made of the individual's nutritional status and state of hydration, since fever tends to be very debilitating and dehydrating. There is generally a corresponding increasing weakness with increasing fever. A record should be made of the colour of the skin and whether it is moist or dry. If the skin is pale rather than flushed and dry, heat dissipation will be inefficient as a result of poor surface flow. Patient responses and orientation should be noted, especially if the temperature rises to the levels of hyperpyrexia.[9] Cerebral disturbance may develop as less oxygen becomes available to the brain cells.

If the fever is of unknown origin, the nurse should observe the patient closely for the development of signs and symptoms which may be helpful to the doctor in making a diagnosis.

Care during a chill. If the patient experiences a chill at the onset of the fever, several light covers are used and tucked in closely to the body to prevent heat loss. If heat applications in the form of hot water bottles or an electric blanket or heating pad are employed, extreme precautions are necessary to avoid burning the patient. As soon as the chill is over, heat applications should be removed and covers reduced to prevent loss of body fluid and sodium by excessive sweating.

Fluids and food. Unless contraindicated by the patient's disease, the fluid intake in fever is increased to a minimum of 2500–3000 ml for an adult because more fluid is lost by evaporation from the skin and in the increased respirations. The inclusion of soups is recommended because of their salt content. A record should be made of the fluid intake and output.

Since fever is accompanied by an increase in metabolism and destruction of body protein, an increase in the caloric and protein intake is necessary. This may be difficult during the acute stage owing to anorexia and the patient's condition, but an increased intake should be put into effect as soon as possible. When the patient's intake consists mainly of fluids, calories and protein may be increased by giving milk drinks or eggnogs, and by adding cream, glucose or lactose to a commercial nutritional supplement.

4. Promotion of comfort

The mouth becomes very dry and a source of discomfort to the feverish patient. Sordes, an offensive accumulation of secretions, epithelial cells and organisms, tends to collect on the lips and teeth. The mouth should be cleansed and rinsed with a mild antiseptic solution every 2 hours. Petroleum jelly, oil or cold cream may be applied to the lips to prevent cracking.

Herpes simplex (cold sore) may develop around the lips. The lesion appears first as a sore, burning and itchy papule; then a vesicle forms, followed by encrustation and scab formation. It is due to a virus which has probably been latent in the cells and becomes activated by the higher body temperature. An antiviral ointment may be prescribed to inhibit the spread and soften the encrustation. If the lesions occur within the mouth, they may discourage the taking of fluids and nourishment; a mouthwash containing a topical anaesthetic may be ordered.

Frequent back rubs, changes of position and changes of linen may help to reduce the patient's discomfort. Frequent bathing is necessary because of the increased perspiration.

EXPECTED OUTCOMES

1 Body temperature is maintained at the normal level (37°C or 98.6°F orally)
2 Heart and respiratory rates are normal for the patient.
3 Skin is normal in colour, warmth and moisture.
4 The patient carries out usual daily living activities.

HYPOTHERMIA

Hypothermia means a subnormal body temperature and is encountered much less frequently than fever. The causes are listed in Table 7.3. Clinically, the term hypothermia is used most often to indicate deliberate cooling of a patient for therapeutic purposes.

---

[9] *Hyperpyrexia* and *hyperthermia* are terms used to indicate fever when the temperature is over 40°C (104°F).

Table 7.3 Assessment of the patient with hypothermia.

Cause	Signs and symptoms	Problem
Prolonged exposure to cold	*Objective data:*	Alterations in comfort
	Body temperature <35°C (95°F)	Alterations in thought processes
Decreased heat production related to	Skin pale, dry	Potential for impairment of skin integrity
reduced metabolism as in	Heart rate increased, pulse irregular	altered
hypothyroidism, circulatory failure,	Respiratory rate increased initially and	Altered peripheral tissue perfusion
starvation and immobility	then decreased	Impaired gas exchange
	Shivering followed by decreased reflexes	Potential for decreased cardiac output
Impairment of the	and rigidity	Potential for fluid volume deficit
temperature-regulating mechanisms	Increased urinary output	
by intracranial lesions, alcohol	Disorientation	
intoxication or heavy sedation	Coma	
	Respiratory and circulatory failure	
Therapeutically induced		
	Subjective data:	
	Drowsiness	
	Confusion	
	Sensation of cold	

PROLONGED EXPOSURE TO COLD

When an individual is accidentally exposed to extreme climatic cold, the first physiological responses are peripheral vasoconstriction, increased heat production by shivering and accelerated metabolism, and an increase in the pulse and respiratory rates. With continued exposure, the internal body temperature is gradually lowered. The cooling of the brain results in a depression of the heat-regulating centre in the hypothalamus, and the ability to protect the body temperature is lost. There is a progressive depression of metabolism and a slowing of mental and muscular responses. The individual becomes drowsy, eventually lapses into a coma, and may develop respiratory and circulatory failure.

The patient suffering cold exposure is treated by immersion in a warm bath of 42–43°C (107–110°F) for 10–20 minutes; this warms the peripheral blood and tissues. It is not prolonged since superficial vasodilation would reduce the blood supply to the vital centres. Rewarming is then continued at normal room temperature. Some instability in body temperature control is likely for 7–10 days, so the patient is usually kept at rest and under observation during that period.

INDUCED HYPOTHERMIA

Purpose and effects. Hypothermia may be intentionally produced to decrease the rate of metabolism and oxygen utilization. The low temperature may be maintained for an hour to several days, depending on the purpose and the patient's condition. It may be employed during surgery on the heart, large blood vessels or brain which necessitates a temporary interruption of the blood flow in the area. It may also be used following cerebral surgery or severe head injuries in order to prevent or reduce severe cerebral oedema or hyperthermia. Cooling of the cells reduces their activity and prevents the damage that would normally ensue with a decreased oxygen supply. Induced hypothermia may also be used in treating the patient with a high fever who does not respond to the simpler cooling measures. For example, a patient with a heat stroke or thyroid crisis usually requires hypothermic measures.

The temperature most frequently used in induced hypothermia is within the range of 32–26°C (89.6–78.8°F). The decrease in cellular activity and oxygen requirement is proportional to the decrease in temperature. A decline to 30–28°C reduces metabolism by approximately 50%. The pulse and respiratory rates are slowed and are usually accompanied by a fall in blood pressure. The patient becomes stuporous and may lose consciousness with lower hypothermic levels. There is a loss of the gag reflex and corneal and pupillary reactions, and the response to pain is diminished. The viscosity of the blood increases. The urinary output may not be markedly reduced at first, but it progressively decreases and has a low specific gravity.

Methods of induction. Hypothermia may be produced by the application of cold to the surface of the body or by extracorporeal cooling of the blood.

Surface cooling methods include immersion in an ice water bath, enclosure of the patient in large plastic sheets filled with crushed ice, placing the patient between electrically controlled blankets with coils through which a cold fluid is circulated, and the application of ice bags over the body surface. The latter may be combined with the circulation of cool air over the body by fans.

The blanket method is the most satisfactory and the one in current use; it is simpler and provides better control. The temperature of the fluid flowing through the coils is maintained at the level at which the gauge on the accompanying refrigerating unit is set. The blankets may also be used to rewarm the patient following hypothermia by adjusting the temperature controls on the machine.

The extracorporeal method of cooling is used during surgery. The blood is diverted from a large vessel, circulated through a cooling coil outside the body, and returned to another blood vessel. The heart–lung machine (pump-oxygenator), which is used in cardiac and vascular surgery as a mechanical pump to maintain circulation and to add oxygen to the blood, is also equipped with a heat exchanger that may be used to either cool or warm the blood. The extracorporeal circulation of the blood through a heat exchanger has certain advantages; the patient may be cooled more quickly, better control of the body temperature is provided, and the patient may be quickly rewarmed on completion of the surgical procedure.

Reduction of the body temperature can only take place when heat production does not compensate for heat loss. Before hypothermia induction is commenced, the patient receives a drug that depresses the heat-regulating centre and prevents the shivering response. Shivering must be avoided because of the associated heat production and the marked increase in the utilization of oxygen. The sedative effect of the drug also reduces the unpleasantness of the cooling for the conscious patient. Examples of the drugs used are chlorpromazine (Largactil) and promethazine hydrochloride (Phenergan), each of which may be administered intramuscularly or intravenously.

The core body temperature is monitored continuously during hypothermia by special electric thermometers. Probes which record the temperature are placed in the oesophagus or rectum. These are connected to a transducer that converts the heat energy to electrical energy, which is registered on a scale. When the temperature is within 1 or 2 degrees of the desired level, the cooling procedure is discontinued or reduced, and a downward drift of 1 or 2 degrees will continue. Obese persons cool more slowly and manifest a greater tendency to experience temperature drift.

Rewarming. Following surgery, the patient may be rewarmed before leaving the operating room. As cited above, if extracorporeal cooling is used, the heat exchanger of the heart–lung machine may be used to rewarm the patient. If the blanket method is used, warm water may be circulated through the coils. In many instances, the patient is simply covered with blankets and allowed to rewarm at his own rate.

Nursing process

ASSESSMENT

Table 7.3 lists causative factors and signs and symptoms to be assessed in the patient with accidental or therapeutically induced hypothermia. Problems are identified for the patient with hypothermia. Nursing interventions specific to these problems are discussed in subsequent chapters, especially Chapters 8, 10, 14, 15, 16 and 24.

NURSING INTERVENTION

The goals are that:
1 The patient and/or family understand the reasons for and implications of hypothermia
2 The patient's temperature is reduced to the prescribed therapeutic level
3 Changes in the patient's condition are identified promptly
4 Injury and complications do not occur

Preparation. The conscious patient and the patient's family may have considerable apprehension when advised that hypothermia is to be used. The purpose and method to be used should be explained, and their questions answered to reduce their anxiety.

If surface cooling is to be used, the skin should be clean and inspected for discoloured areas and lesions. If the hypothermia is to be prolonged, a light protective application of oil or lanolin is usually made to the entire body surface.

Collapse of the peripheral veins occurs with the cooling; for this reason, an intravenous infusion is started prior to induction so fluid, electrolytes and medications may be administered during the treatment. An indwelling catheter is inserted so that renal function and the fluid output may be assessed.

The preinduction medication is given as ordered, and the patient's blood pressure, pulse, respiratory rate, level of consciousness and responses are noted for a comparative base-line later. An electric thermometer is inserted in the oesophagus or rectum for continuous temperature recording.

Emergency equipment that should be assembled and readily available includes an intermittent positive pressure ventilator, oxygen, tracheostomy set and an emergency drug tray with vasopressors and cardiac and respiratory stimulants.

Care during hypothermia. A nurse should remain in constant attendance. Frequent observations and recording (usually at 15–30-minute intervals) are made of the pulse rate and rhythm, respirations and blood pressure. Continuous cardiac monitoring is instituted since cardiac irritability may increase with cooling and fibrillation may develop. Changes in the colour of the skin, lips or nail beds are noted. A continuous monitoring of the temperature is necessary;

any change in the level or indication of shivering should be reported promptly. There is danger of cardiac arrest and permanent tissue damage if the temperature falls too low.

The patient is turned or moved hourly to prevent frostbite and fat necrosis, especially in areas where skin over bony prominences may be in prolonged contact with the hypothermia blanket. The skin is carefully inspected every 1–2 hours; discoloured or firm immovable areas may indicate fat necrosis or frostbite, in which there is a crystallization of the tissue fluid. If pillows are used, the nurse makes sure they are placed under the lower blanket. In prolonged hypothermia, the light application of oil or lanolin is repeated to protect the skin. Good body alignment is kept in mind when positioning the patient in order to prevent contractures and hyper-extensions; if his condition permits, passive range of motion exercises are used during prolonged hypothermia to preserve normal joint movement and prevent circulatory stasis. Support hose may be used to prevent venous stasis.

The fluid intake and output should be accurately recorded; the fluid intake is determined by the 24-hour output. The hourly urinary output is noted, and frequent specimens are collected for analysis.

The conscious patient is encouraged and given the necessary support to breathe deeply and cough hourly. This is done at the same time the position is changed in order to keep the essential disturbances to a minimum. Since the cough and gag reflex are usually depressed, he may not be successful in coughing.

Carbon dioxide accumulation and respiratory acidosis may develop with the decreased ventilation. Blood gases are monitored frequently.

The mouth is cleansed and moistened every 2–3 hours, and the nasal passages are kept clear of secretions. The patient's head is turned to the side when cleansing the mouth to avoid fluid aspiration because of the associated depression of reflexes.

Since the corneal reflex may be absent and normal secretions are diminished, an artificial tear solution (methyl cellulose) may be instilled in the eyes.

Rewarming. Rewarming is done slowly over about 6 hours. During this period, constant observation of the patient is just as important as during the hypothermic phase. As the temperature approaches normal, the extra blankets used in rewarming are gradually removed to prevent it from rising above the normal level. Frequent checking of the pulse, respirations and blood pressure is still necessary. If medications were administered during hypothermia or the rewarming period, the nurse must be alert for possible accumulative effects of the drug(s).

After the patient is rewarmed, the special thermometer probes are removed, but recording of the temperature every 3 or 4 hours continues for 2 or 3 days, as there may be some instability of the hypothalamic heat-regulating centre, especially in the young and aged. Frequent checking of the pulse continues for the first 24 to 48 hours since the patient may still develop cardiac irregularity or fibrillation.

The indwelling catheter is removed when a normal urinary output is established. Oral fluids are administered in small amounts and progressively increased as tolerated.

EXPECTED OUTCOMES

1 The patient's body temperature is within normal limits.
2 The patient or family state reasons for and methods used to induce hypothermia.
3 The skin is clean and intact.
4 Blood pressure, pulse rate and respiratory rate are within the normal range.
5 Arterial blood gases are within the normal range.
6 Fluid intake and urinary output are in balance with normal volumes.
7 The patient is alert and oriented to time, place and person.
8 The patient is able to resume usual daily activities.

References and Further Reading

BOOKS

Braunwald E et al (eds) (1986) *Harrison's Principles of Internal Medicine*, 11th ed. New York: McGraw-Hill.

Guyton AC (1986) *Textbook of Medical Physiology*, 7th ed. Philadelphia: WB Saunders. Chapter 72.

Holloway NM (1984), Nursing the Critically Ill Adult, 2nd ed. Menlo Park, CA: Addison Wesley. pp. 348–356.

Kinney MR, Dear CG, Packa DR & Voorman DMN (1981) *AACN's Clinical Reference for Critical Care Nursing*. New York: McGraw-Hill. Chapter 41.

Muir BL (1981) *Pathophysiology: An Introduction to the Mechanisms of Disease*. New York: John Wiley. Chapter 24.

Nave CR & Nave BC (1985) *Physics for the Health Sciences*, 3rd ed. Philadelphia; WB Saunders. Chapter 15.

Sabiston DC Jr (ed.) (1986) *Davis–Christopher Textbook of Surgery*, 13th ed. Philadelphia: WB Saunders. Chapter 9.

Sorensen KC & Luckmann J (1986) *Basic Nursing: A Psychophysiologic Approach*, 2nd ed. Philadelphia: WB Saunders. Chapter 29.

Vander AJ, Sherman JH & Luciano DS (1985) *Human Physiology*, 4th ed. New York: McGraw-Hill. pp. 542–550.

PERIODICALS

Angerami ELS (1980) Epidemiological study of body temperature in patients in a teaching hospital. *Int. J. Nurs. Stud.* Vol. 17 No. 2, pp. 91–99.

Biddle C (1985) Hypothermia: implications for the critical care nurse. *Crit. Care Nurs.*, Vol. 5 No. 2, pp. 34–38.

Blainey CG (1974) Site selection in taking body temperature. *Am. J. Nurs.*, Vol. 74 No. 10, pp. 1859–1861.

Borchardt AC & Trauline KE (1982) Hypothermia in the postanaesthetic patient. *AORN J.*, Vol. 36 No. 4, pp. 648, 656–7.

Cunha BA, Digamon-Beltram M & Gobbo PN (1984) Implications of fever in the critical care setting. *Heart & Lung*, Vol. 13 No. 5, pp. 460–465.

DeLapp TD (1983) Accidental hypothermia. *Am. J. Nurs.*, Vol. 83 No. 1, pp. 62–67.

Editor (1980) The temperature of things to come. *Emerg. Med.*, Vol. 12 No. 1, pp. 101–104.

Erickson R (1980) Oral temperature differences in relation to thermometer and technique. *Nurs. Res.*, Vol. 29 No. 3, pp. 157–164.

Francis B (1982) Hot and cold therapy, *J. Nurs. Care*, Vol. 15 No. 2, pp. 18–20.

Greaves RD & Markarian MF (1980) Three-minute time interval when using an oral mercury-in-glass thermometer with or without J-temp sheaths. *Nurs. Res.*, Vol. 29 No. 5, pp. 323–324.

Kurtz KJ (1982) Hypothermia in the elderly: the cold facts. *Geriatrics*, Vol. 37 No. 1, pp. 85–93.

Nichols GA & Kucha DH (1973) Taking adult temperatures: oral measurements. *Nurs. Res.*, Vol. 22 p. 93.

Nichols GA & Verhonick PJ (1969) Time and temperature. *Am. J. Nursing.*, Vol. 69 No. 11, pp. 2304–2306.

Takacs KM & Valenti WM (1982) Temperature measurement in a clinical setting. *Nurs. Res.*, Vol. 31 No. 6, pp. 368–701.

8
The Patient with Pain

Pain

Pain is a complex, distressing experience involving sensory, emotional and cognitive components. It is generated by a stimulus which causes, or has the potential to cause, tissue damage. The quality and intensity of the pain experience vary with the individual and are influenced by psychological and sociocultural factors. Pain plays an important protective role; one progressively learns from early childhood to avoid and correct the situations which cause pain. When the sensation is lost in an area of the body as it is in spinal cord injury or leprosy, the lack of awareness of injury and the absence of normal protective responses may lead to extensive tissue damage. Pain is one of the most impelling symptoms that prompt a person to seek medical advice. It also provides information that aids the doctor in making a diagnosis. It should be remembered, however, that there are serious diseases, such as cancer and heart disease, which may be painless at the onset; as a result, persons may delay seeing a physician until the disease is in an advanced stage.

PAIN MECHANISM

The structures essential for the pain sensation are receptors that are sensitive to pain stimuli, impulse pathways to and within the central nervous system (brain and spinal cord), and areas within the brain for perception, interpretation and the initiation of responses. There is also an analgesic system for pain modulation and control.

Pain receptors

Stimuli that cause pain sensation are received by freely branching bare nerve endings which form a diffuse network in the tissue. The concentration of these receptors varies throughout the body; they are abundant in the skin and on joint surfaces, but there are relatively fewer in the deeper tissues and viscera.

Pain stimuli

A wide variety of stimuli evoke pain; these stimuli include mechanical agents (e.g., cutting, blow, friction, distension, thermal agents (extremes of heat and cold), chemicals (e.g. chemicals released by injured cells or microorganisms), electric current, ischaemia and sustained muscle contraction. Many are non-specific but elicit pain through their intensity. For instance, light pressure produces an awareness of touch, but increasing the intensity of the pressure causes pain. Similarly, heat and cold must reach a certain intensity to stimulate pain receptors.

Pain impulse pathways

The sensory, or afferent,[1] nerve fibres, whose bare terminal branches form the pain receptors, provide a peripheral pathway to conduct the impulses into the spinal cord or brain stem. These sensory nerve fibres are of two types; some are larger, have a fatty insulating sheath (myelin) and are classified as A delta fibres; the others are smaller, non-myelinated and designated C fibres. The myelinated fibres transmit the impulses very rapidly. A sudden, pain-producing stimulus causes two pain sensations. The impulses transmitted by the myelinated fibres produce the sharp, pricking, localized pain that is felt immediately when the injury occurs. The non-myelinated fibres conduct more slowly and are responsible for the more diffuse, throbbing, burning type of pain or ache that follows the immediate sharp pain associated with the initial injury.

Various theories have been presented to explain the physiology of pain, none of which has proved entirely satisfactory. The specificity theory and the gate control theory are the more prominent theories.

The *specificity theory of pain* proposes that there are specific structures (afferent nerve fibres and central nervous system pathways and neurons) concerned with the pain sensation. Pain impulses are transmitted by specific sensory nerve fibres from the stimulus site and enter the spinal cord via the posterior root ganglia to neurons within the posterior column or horn of grey matter. Some impulses may be passed to motor neurons to initiate impulses that are carried out of the cord along motor or efferent nerve fibres to skeletal muscles (see Fig. 8.1). These motor impulses produce a reflex response, such as withdrawal of the injured part from the object producing the pain stimulus (as seen in the withdrawal of the finger

---

[1] *Sensory*, or *afferent*, nerve fibres carry impulses toward the central nervous system (brain and spinal cord). *Motor*, or *efferent*, nerve fibres transmit impulses away from the central nervous system to peripheral structures.

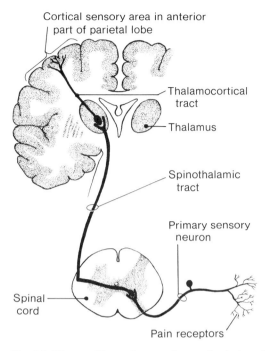

Cortical sensory area in anterior part of parietal lobe

Thalamocortical tract

Thalamus

Spinothalamic tract

Primary sensory neuron

Spinal cord

Pain receptors

Fig. 8.1 Diagram illustrating a pathway of pain impulses.

that receives a pin prick or touches a very hot object). The other pain impulses cross to the other side of the cord and ascend the anterolateral spinothalamic pathway. As the pain pathways enter the brain they separate into the pricking pain pathway and the burning pain pathway (see Fig. 8.2). The pricking pain pathway, which is composed of myelinated fibres (type A), terminates in the ventrobasal complex of the brain. From here, signals are relayed to other areas of the thalamus and to the somatic sensory cortex. The burning pain fibres, which are composed mostly of unmyelinated slow-transmitting fibres (type C), terminate in two areas of the reticular activating system, the reticular area of the brain stem and the thalamus.

The individual becomes aware of the pain when the impulses reach the thalamus and other lower centres of the brain. Interpretation of the site of the stimulus and the quality and intensity of pain is made at the cortical level. Localization of the sensation is fairly specific for the pricking type of pain; stimulation of tactile receptors is believed to play a major role in this. Burning and aching types of pain are poorly localized since their termination is more diffuse in the hindbrain and thalamus. For example, the pain may be interpreted as being in a limb rather than in a specific area of the limb.

Recognition of the specific pain pathways inherent in the specificity theory provides the basis for surgery in intractable pain. The procedure interrupts the pain pathway and impulses do not reach conscious level.

The *gate control theory* advanced by Melzack and Wall proposes that pain impulses can be regulated, modified or blocked by certain cells within the central nervous system. It is thought that impulses can be prevented from reaching the transmission cells of the posterior column by the action of the substantia gelatinosa[2] cells, which are said to 'close the gate.' Whether or not the gate is open to permit the conduction of impulses through the posterior horn cells and hence to higher levels is dependent upon the nature of the impulses delivered to the substantia gelatinosa. Siegele indicates that when cutaneous impulses aroused by such stimuli as vibration, scratching, cold and heat are transmitted by large fibres in the afferent nerve they can negate the input of the fibres of smaller diameter. That is, they close the gate. It remains open to impulses transmitted by small fibres if there is 'relatively little activity in the large fibres.'[3] The activity of the gating mechanism may also be affected by emotion and impulses in descending tracts from areas of the brain (brain stem, thalamus and cerebral cortex).[4]

The gate control theory establishes a basis for the following procedures in lessening pain and suffering: (1) distraction; (2) reducing fear and lowering the

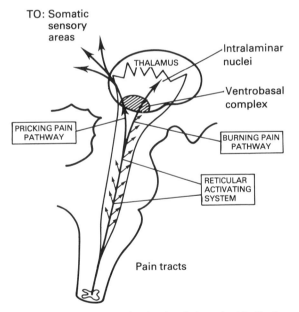

TO: Somatic sensory areas

THALAMUS

Intralaminar nuclei

Ventrobasal complex

PRICKING PAIN PATHWAY

BURNING PAIN PATHWAY

RETICULAR ACTIVATING SYSTEM

Pain tracts

Fig. 8.2 Transmission of pain signals into the hindbrain, thalamus, and cortex via the 'pricking pain' pathway and the 'burning pain' pathway. From Guyton (1986).

---

[2] The *substantia gelatinosa* is an area of special neurons located close to each posterior column of grey matter and extending the length of the spinal cord.
[3] Siegele (1974), pp. 449–450.
[4] Ganong (1985).

level of anxiety; (3) analysis of the pain and reactions by the individual, and participation in the planning to cope; (4) local counterirritants, massage and heat applications; (5) electrical stimulation; and (6) acupuncture.

Pain control mechanism

Current research supports the concept of gating and has provided new information on the mechanisms of pain modulation and control.[5]

Guyton indicates that a pain control or analgesic system exists within the brain and spinal cord. Stimulation of large sensory fibres from peripheral tactile receptors depresses the transmission of pain signals at the cord level.[6] This mechanism and simultaneous psychological effects explain the basis of pain relief by tactile stimulation, electrical stimulation and acupuncture. The theory is that descending pathways exist which inhibit the transmission of pain impulses through the posterior horns of the spinal cord and probably at points in the cerebral pathways.

It is believed that activation of the pain receptors and ascending fibres by a harmful stimulus activates the pain control or analgesic system. This involves special receptors referred to as opiate receptors, which are found throughout the nervous system but in greater concentration along the slow-conducting pain pathways and in the posterior horns of the spinal cord. Morphine and opiate derivatives are believed to produce analgesia by acting on the opiate receptors.

The brain produces endogenous analgesics in the form of enkephalins and endorphins which possess morphine-like action. The enkephalins, like the opiate receptors, are found mainly in the areas of the brain and spinal cord associated with pain control. The endorphins have been isolated from the pituitary gland and the hypothalamus. Guyton states that the enkephalins and the endorphins are presumed to function as excitatory transmitter substances that activate portions of the brain's analgesic system.[6] The concentrations of enkephalins and endorphins increase following electrical stimulation of the brain stem.

Other neurotransmitters, especially serotonin and dopamine, play important roles in pain biochemistry. Serotonin has an inhibiting effect on pain perception and probably functions as a transmitter of descending inhibitory pathways. Dopamine is believed to enhance opiate analgesia, and brain stem stimulation, and to function as a transmitter in the inhibitory pathways.[7]

Knowledge of the opiate receptors, the endogenous analgesics and other neurotransmitters in the nervous system provides direction for more effective pharmacological control of pain and provides rationale for physiological and psychological techniques of pain management.

The pain sensation has two components: perception and reactions.

PAIN PERCEPTION

Perception is the awareness or feeling of pain. The severity of the pain perceived depends upon the intensity and frequency of the pain impulses. Qualifying the type of pain and relating it to various stimuli are learned experiences. The child gradually learns to associate the unpleasant feeling with objects and situations that cause pain.

Pain threshold

The point at which a stimulus first elicits the awareness of pain is referred to as the pain threshold. The threshold is considered fairly constant and uniform for all persons and differences occur mainly in the responses.[8] The threshold may be elevated by such things as distraction, strong stimuli in other parts of the body (e.g. pain in one part of the body raises the threshold in other parts) and pathological conditions which involve the pain receptors, impulse pathways or cortical sensory areas. Depressed activity of the cerebral cortex due to certain drugs, alcohol, shock or debilitation may also raise the threshold.

A lowering of the pain threshold (hyperalgesia) may occur with inflammation or injury of structures concerned with the pain sensation or of neighbouring tissues to such structures. Tissue damage results in the release of chemical substances such as prostaglandins which lower the pain threshold. The pain threshold may also be lowered by a reduction of other stimuli. The latter accounts for a patient's increased pain during the night when ordinary stimuli are at a minimum.

Pain tolerance refers to the intensity and duration of a stimulus above the pain threshold that a person can experience or is willing to endure before responding.

PAIN REACTIONS

The reaction component of pain is composed of all the psychological, physical, voluntary and involuntary responses that are made when pain is perceived.

The physical reactions include those of skeletal muscles and the involuntary physiological responses implemented through the release of adrenaline and stimulation of the autonomic nervous system.

Muscle responses

Skeletal muscle reaction may be the immediate withdrawal reflex (cited previously), involuntary contrac-

[5] Melzack (1980), p. 96.
[6] Guyton (1986), p. 597.
[7] Wyngaarden & Smith (1985), p. 92.

[8] Guyton (1986), p. 593.

tion, or increased tone in an attempt to splint or immobilize the affected part (e.g. rigidity of the abdomen). The individual may support or rub the part, change position frequently, clench his fists, rock or pace back and forth or toss about. Voluntary muscle activity may also be involved in correcting the situation when the individual removes the offending object, treats the site or seeks assistance.

Autonomic nervous system responses

The physiological responses seen most commonly are mediated by sympathetic innervation and the secretion of adrenaline. Superficial vasoconstriction occurs; the blood supply to the skeletal muscles and brain is increased as a defence mechanism; the blood pressure, pulse and respirations increase; salivary secretion and gastrointestinal activity decrease; perspiration increases, and the pupils dilate. The individual manifests pallor, cold clammy skin and dry lips and mouth.

If the pain is deep, severe and prolonged, the above reactions may not develop and the patient may exhibit shock and extreme weakness; the blood pressure falls, the pulse weakens and nausea and vomiting may occur.

Psychological responses

Even when the intensity and the nature of the pain stimulus are the same for several persons, the type and degree of reactions are likely to vary considerably because of individual differences in psychological makeup. The nature of a person's psychological reactions is determined, to a large extent, by his past experiences and the degree of threat and frustration inherent in the pain for him. Some may audibly complain by moaning, crying or verbal expression of suffering and fear and may further indicate their distress by restlessness and purposeless movements. Others may be very stoical, remain still and suffer in silence.

Factors which may influence patients' responses include the following:

1 *Sociocultural background*. An individual's responses become conditioned by social and cultural attitudes to pain. Some learn from those around them that pain is to be endured without obvious emotional reactions. If others have been accustomed to persons in pain exhibiting outward responses which are accepted and which receive attention, they consciously or unconsciously develop a similar pattern of response.
2 *Emotional state*. If the patient is in an emotional state to begin with, his evaluation of pain is likely to be exaggerated. If the illness has disrupted plans or created financial or home problems, or the origin of the pain is the heart or a common site of cancer, the patient is threatened to a greater degree and is more fearful.
3 *Physical condition*. Psychological reactions are usually greater in weak and fatigued persons. For instance, the obstetric patient whose labour is prolonged may be quite calm and uncomplaining at first, but as she becomes fatigued and fearful that something is wrong, her pain becomes less tolerable.
4 *Previous pain experience*. Responses may be either increased or decreased by the memory of previous pain. Fear of a repetition of former severe suffering may produce marked outward reactions. With some, a greater tolerance and resignation may develop.
5 *Significance of the pain*. Apprehension is always greater when a situation is not understood or when one does not know what to expect. The patient who fears he has cancer may manifest greater pain reaction until he learns that the biopsy report is negative for malignancy.

To children, pain is a new, unpleasant and frightening experience which they cannot understand; overt expressions may be expected. The patient who has been prepared during her pregnancy by explanations of the source and purpose of the labour pains is less anxious and calmer than the unprepared patient.
6 *Distraction*. Reactions as well as perception are influenced by the amount of the patient's attention that is focused on the pain. If a situation commands considerable concentration on the part of the individual or creates pleasurable emotion, pain responses are minimized. The person actively engaged in competitive sport may not even be aware of the pain of an injury received. But if the patient focuses his whole attention on the discomfort, reactions are more pronounced.
7 *Intensity and duration of pain*. If the pain stimulus is very intense, the individual feels more threatened. He may find it difficult to control his emotional responses and may even become quite disorganized. Similarly, pain of long duration is wearying and may initiate more overt reactions; on the other hand, the patient may become more resigned to the pain and take the attitude that he has to live with it.

Interdependence of physiological and psychological reactions to pain

The emotional components of pain are interdependent with the physiological mechanisms of pain transmission and control. Both aggravate the pain and increase the complexity and intensity of the responses. Anxiety can result from pain and in turn anxiety may intensify the pain and a vicious circle develops. Physical and social functioning may be altered by the pain experience, leading to feelings of helplessness, isolation, fear and anxiety. Unless the cycle is interrupted these factors, singly or collectively, will continue to increase pain perception and intensity.

Chronic pain leads to endorphin depletion, which results in a decrease in the pain perception threshold and the tolerance threshold. Persistent pain also causes loss of sleep and appetite leading to general fatigue and disability. Uncontrolled pain frequently leads to disruptions in the family, social life and work; physiological changes lead to inefficient function and increased psychological responses to pain experience.

TYPES OF PAIN

Some of the more common terms used to classify pain are as follows:

Acute pain is time-limited and generally has a defined cause and purpose. It may be mild, moderate or severe in nature and is usually sudden in onset.

Chronic pain is a complex physiological and psychological phenomenon that causes varying degrees of disability in a large portion of the population. It may begin as acute pain but it persists over an extended period of time. The pain may be mild, moderate or severe and may be intermittent or continuous. The cause may be unknown or if identified cannot be eliminated. The associated disruption in the individual's functions and life-style frequently leads to extreme fears, depression and debilitation.

Superficial pain occurs when the receptors in surface tissues are stimulated. Conversely, *deep pain* arises from deeper tissues. Deep pain is divided anatomically into *splanchnic*, which refers to pain in the viscera, and deep *somatic* referring to pain in deep structures other than the viscera such as muscles, tendons, joints and periosteum.

Localized pain arises directly from the site of the disturbance. *Referred pain* is that which is felt in a part of the body which is remote from the actual point of stimulation. The impulses usually arise in an organ, but the pain is projected to a surface area of the body. A classic example of referred pain is that associated with angina pectoris; the pain originates in the heart muscle as a result of ischaemia, but it may be experienced in the midsternal region, the base of the neck and down the left arm. Pain arising in the gallbladder or bile ducts may be referred to the epigastrium and the right scapular region. Referred pain may also be secondary to reflex muscular spasm. The muscle spasm originates as a reflex response to pain signals elsewhere in the body, as seen when lumbar muscles go into spasm as a result of severe ureteral pain.

It is suggested that the fibres carrying the pain impulses from the viscera and those from peripheral tissues converge upon the same neuron within the spinal cord. The impulses are then interpreted as coming from the superficial area because of previous pain experience.

Projected pain occurs when impulses are set up at some point along the pain pathway beyond the peripheral pain receptors. The pain is perceived as arising at the site of the pain receptors served by the pathway in which the pain originated. A person who has had an amputation may experience what is referred to as *phantom limb pain*. Stimuli arising from the stump may be localized on the basis of the previously established body image, and as a result the pain is projected to the portion of the limb that was removed.

Persistent, severe pain that cannot be effectively controlled by the usual medications is referred to as *intractable pain*.

Headache is a frequent discomfort experienced by many persons, and applies to the pain sensation that is perceived as being in the cranial vault (i.e. facial pain, toothache and earache are excluded). Headache is a common complaint in many illnesses in which the primary disturbance is quite remote from the head.

The pain receptors within the cranium occur in the walls of the arteries and in the meninges. The actual brain tissue is devoid of pain receptors. Headache may originate with tension or spasm of associated muscles at the back of the neck. Extracranial pain is usually well localized to the area where superficial pain receptors are being stimulated.

Psychogenic pain is that experienced when there is no detectable organic lesion or peripheral stimulation. It is thought that the pain is the conversion and physical expression of a distressing psychic disturbance or problem. It must be remembered that the discomfort is very real to the individual and that efforts must be made to provide relief.

Nursing Process

INTRODUCTION

The nurse plays an important role in the identification of pain and in influencing the frequency and severity of pain. Kim emphasizes that:

'nursing practices should be directed as much on the pre- and post-experience phase as on the painful experience phase because nursing care during the anticipation of pain can influence psychological variables such as anxiety and in turn alleviate actual experience of pain. Aftermath nursing care may debrief painful experience and in turn alleviate future pain experience'.[9]

Similar research has been undertaken by Hayward in Great Britain.[10]

Advances in knowledge of the physiological and psychological dimensions of pain provide a challenge for the nurse to critically examine nursing practices in pain assessment and management. McCaffery identifies several misconceptions that

---

[9] Kim (1980), p. 57.
[10] Hayward (1975).

hamper assessment of the patient with pain. Awareness of these misconceptions and of the facts as presently understood provide guidelines which promote effective comprehensive care of the patient with pain. The facts to keep in mind when dealing with pain as listed by McCaffery are:[11]

1 The patient is the authority on his pain. Pain is whatever the experiencing person says it is, existing whenever he says it does. The patient is believed.
2 The patient who uses his pain to his own advantage may still hurt as much as he says he does.
3 Physiological and behavioural adaptation occur, leading to periods of little or no signs of pain. Lack of pain expression does not mean lack of pain.
4 Not all physical causes of pain can be identified. All pain is real, regardless of its cause. Calling pain imaginary does not make it go away.
5 A localized sensation does exist in psychogenic pain.
6 There is no direct and invariant relationship between any stimulus and the perception of pain.
7 Pain tolerance is the individual's unique response, varying between patients and in the same patient from one situation to another.
8 Health team members tend to infer less pain than the patient experiences.'

ASSESSMENT

Assessment of the pain experience is essential for diagnosis and for evaluation of pain control measures. It must include the three major dimensions of pain which are physical, emotional and perceptive. Pain is difficult to measure because it is a subjective phenomenon. Only the person experiencing the pain knows its nature, intensity, location and what it means to them.
1 Physical examination. Table 8.1 lists observable signs and symptoms of pain that may be present.
2 Location. The patient should try to be as specific as possible as to the location of the pain. For example, abdominal pain may be localized to the lower or upper right or left quadrant, epigastrium or mid-abdomen. The site may be well defined or diffuse or the path may radiate, involving a wide area.
3 Characteristics of the pain. Information collected about the nature of the pain includes the following:
  (a) *Type*: crampy; stabbing; sharp; dull; throbbing; burning; aching; boring.
  (b) *Intensity*: mild; severe; excruciating.
  (c) *Onset*: sudden or gradual. The time it began is noted and the circumstances surrounding the onset and any pre-pain experience are described.
  (d) *Duration*: persistent; intermittent. What the patient thinks would help him is considered as well.
The nurse should also take note of:
  (e) *Changes in the site*: tenderness; swelling; discoloration; firmness; rigidity.
4 Associated symptoms: nausea and vomiting; profuse perspiration; fainting; inability to perform usual functions; dulling of senses; apathy; clouding of consciousness; disorientation; inability to rest and sleep.

Pain questionnaires such as the McGill–Melzack questionnaire are useful as diagnostic techniques and for evaluation of pain control measures.

Pain assessment/observation charts are a valuable aid to the nurse and the patient. A simple linear scale may be used to denote whether pain is non-existent or excruciating, or rated in between the two extremes. The more detailed London Hospital Pain Observation Chart (see Fig. 8.3) is intended to be used by both the patient and those involved with his care. The site and severity of pain are noted on a body diagram. Analgesics and other measures taken to relieve the pain can be charted, and any additional comments may be added. This type of chart is useful in passing on information and in evaluating the management of the patient's pain.

Table 8.1 Assessment of patient's responses to pain.

Initial sympathetic responses to pain of low–moderate intensity or superficial pain	Parasympathetic responses to intense pain or chronic pain	Verbal responses	Muscular and postural responses
Increased blood pressure	Decreased blood pressure	Crying	Increased muscle tone
Increased heart rate	Decreased heart rate	Moaning	Immobilization of affected part
Increased respiratory rate	Weak pulse	Gasping	Rubbing movements
Decreased salivation and	Increased gastrointestinal activity	Screaming	Rocking movements
gastrointestinal activity	Nausea and vomiting	Silence	Drawing up of knees
Dilated pupils	Weakness		Pacing of floor
Increased perspiration	Decreased alertness		Thrashing movements and
Pallor	Shock		restlessness
Cold, clammy skin			Facial grimaces
Dry lips and mouth			Withdrawal of affected part
			Removal of offending object

[11] McCaffery (1979a), p. 21.

TO USE THIS CHART ask the patient to mark all his or her pains on the body diagram below. Label each site of pain with a letter (i.e. A, B, C etc.)

Then at each observation time ask the patient to assess:

1 the pain in each separate site since the last observation. Use the scale above the body diagram, and enter the number or letter in the appropriate column.
2 the pain overall since the last observation. Use the same scale and enter in the column marked OVERALL.

Next record what has been done to relieve the pain:

3 note any analgesic given since the last observation — stating name, dose, route, and time given.
4 tick any other nursing care or action taken to ease pain.

Finally, note any comment on pain from patient or nurse (use the back of the chart as well, if necessary) and initial the record.

Excruciating	5
Very severe	4
Severe	3
Moderate	2
Just noticeable	1
No pain at all	0
Patient sleeping	S

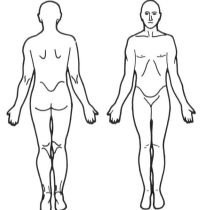

| TIME | PAIN RATING | | | MEASURES TO RELIEVE PAIN | Specify where starred | |
	BY SITES A|B|C|D|E|F|G|H	OVERALL	ANALGESIC GIVEN (Name, dose, route, time)	Lifting	Turning	Massage	Distracting activities	Position change*	Additional aids*	Other*	COMMENTS FROM PATIENTS AND/OR STAFF	Initials

Fig. 8.3 The London Hospital Pain Chart. From the London Hospital.

5 The meaning of pain. The nurse cannot assume that the patient who does not talk about pain is comfortable or that the patient who claims to be 'uncomfortable', 'miserable' or 'suffering' is referring to pain. It is important to have the patient clarify the meaning of the terms used.

A nursing history identifies social, cultural and religious beliefs that may influence responses to pain, past experiences with pain, how the pain has changed social and physical functioning of daily living, and perceptions of future implications of the pain. The medical diagnosis and its meaning to the patient should also be determined.

With chronic pain, patients' responses to pain will change depending on the stage of their disease and with the development of different patterns of coping. During the initial stages of a disease process patients may talk freely of their pain and discomfort, but with time and progression of the disease they may refrain from discussing it either as a result of coping with their prognosis or in response to social pressure from others who stop listening to repeated descriptions.

6 Coping patterns. Information should be collected on how the patient is coping with the present pain experience and how the individual has coped with past pain experiences. It is important for the nurse to know what measures have worked for this patient and if any measures have been taken that have not been effective in relieving pain.

7 Patient goals. Identification of the expectations and goals of the patient for pain management and

control is necessary before effective patient-care can be planned. Does the patient with chronic pain want to change his behaviour? What are the expectations for present and future functioning? Does the patient want to know about the pain associated with planned procedures? Is the patient motivated to acquire the knowledge, skills and changes in behaviour necessary for self-management of pain?

POTENTIAL PATIENT PROBLEMS

Factors which may affect the patient's comfort and cause pain include: injurious agents that may be physical (e.g. accidents, surgery, invasive procedures, immobility, overactivity, internal or external pressure), biological (e.g. infections), chemical (e.g. burns) and psychological (e.g. anticipatory pain).

NURSING INTERVENTION

The patient goals are to:
1 Understand the significance and meaning of the pain experience
2 Alter perception of pain
3 Alter sensory input
4 Develop skills in self-management of the pain experience

1. KNOWLEDGE OF THE PURPOSE AND MEANING OF PAIN EXPERIENCE

The nurse should provide information about the patient's actual and anticipated pain experiences and his physical condition and safety. Discussing this with the patient decreases anxiety, alleviates the actual pain experience, and alters its influence on future pain experiences. These factors promote the individual's wellbeing and security.

Table 8.2 outlines objectives, rationale and possible content areas that the nurse should include in teaching patients about the significance and meaning of pain experiences. Teaching strategies include identification of the meaning and significance of actual and anticipated events with the patient, exploration of the patient's feelings, and providing the patient with specific information. Assessment of the patient's level of anxiety and attention-span enable the nurse to provide the needed information in simple, concise terms, the content being relevant to the patient at that time. Information provided during the pre-pain experience may need to be repeated during the painful event and reviewed again during the post-pain experience.

2. ALTERATIONS OF PERCEPTION OF PAIN

Perception of pain and the anxiety associated with it are useful reactions to acute pain. They serve to pro-

tect the patient from further injury, motivate the person to seek health care and facilitate the diagnosis of the cause of pain. The goal is to reduce the pain responses to tolerable levels. Anxiety associated with chronic pain increases the pain responses, so the goal is to decrease the perception of the pain and the distress associated with it.

Measures taken to alter perception of pain and related anxiety are directed towards supporting the body's natural pain control mechanisms by stimulating endorphin release and modifying variables that influence the individual's tolerance to pain. During the pre-pain experience, nursing care is directed towards decreasing the anxiety associated with anticipation of pain. Prevention and control of pain are the goals during the pain experience, while alleviation of future pain is the aim afterwards.

Measures used to alter the perception of pain include the following:

Knowledge
Johnson and Rice have demonstrated that patients who have been given information about the type of sensations that they can expect to experience during a procedure, have less fear and anxiety during the procedure.[12] Information about anticipated pain sensations and what will be done to prevent or alleviate the pain, alters perception of pain although the pain stimuli remain the same.

Relaxation
Pain perception may be modified by relaxation, which decreases secondary sources of pain such as muscle tension and fatigue. Relaxation techniques include: selective alternate tightening and relaxation of specific groups of muscles; breathing techniques;[13] meditation; yoga; and biofeedback techniques.[14] Muscular relaxation may also be promoted by back rubs, warm baths, ice packs, comfortable room temperature and quiet relaxing music for some persons. Knowledge of what has worked for the individual patient in the past helps the nurse and patient to select relaxation measures that are meaningful and effective.

Rest and sleep
Fatigue slows mental processes and decreases the energy available for coping strategies and repair processes. Relaxation techniques and sedatives are helpful in promoting rest and sleep.

Care should be planned so that the patient is disturbed as little as possible. Consideration is given to the location of the patient in the ward, and noise in

---

[12] Johnson & Rice (1974), p. 203.
[13] *Breathing* exercises such as those taught in preparation for childbirth.
[14] *Biofeedback* techniques provide the individual with sensory evidence, usually visual or auditory, of a body function.

Table 8.2 Patient-teaching: the purpose and meaning of pain.

Objective	Rationale	Content
To promote patient safety and prevent further injury and pain	Pain has a protective purpose in signalling tissue damage. Prompt medical treatment may be life-saving for the patient with an acute myocardial infarction. Preventive measures can avert further tissue damage for the patient with rheumatoid arthritis who learns to minimize and prevent stress on affected joints	Factors precipitating the onset of pain The purpose and origin of the pain What the pain does not involve, e.g. bleeding, spread of disease Specific techniques and measures to take to prevent pain, e.g. proper body mechanics, avoiding and/or controlling emotional and physical stress Actions to take when pain occurs Available resources for emergency and preventive care
To enable the patient to assume some control over the pain experience	Anticipation of the unknown leads to feelings of helplessness, isolation and fear Patient communication and participation promotes understanding of the meaning of pain experience for the individual patient	What activities and situations are going to happen What the activities involve What will be expected of the patient What the patient can expect from the nurse and others What pain control measures are available to the patient The importance of communication of onset of pain and requesting intervention before the pain is intense Exploration of the patient's expectations, fears, anxieties and perceptions of anticipated events
To decrease anxiety	Prior knowledge of sensory experiences decreases fear and anxiety during the procedure Decreasing anxiety is thought to promote endorphin release, thus decreasing pain	Type and duration of sensations the patient may experience during procedures What will be expected of the patient What will be done to prevent and alleviate pain
To alter the impact of pain on future pain experience	Past experience with pain is known to influence individual responses to actual and anticipated pain	The cause and purpose of the pain The patient's actual reaction to the pain Measures which were effective and not effective in alleviating the pain Patient's feelings about the experience

the environment is kept to a minimum; the more the patient is alerted, the more acutely he is aware of pain.

The bedtime routine to which the patient is accustomed should be followed as closely as possible to promote night sleep. Rituals such as brushing the teeth, bedtime nourishments, warm baths are identified and encouraged.

Listening and personal contact
The patient in pain may feel isolated and cut off from the world around. The physical presence of the nurse can be reassuring and convey caring and understanding. Sitting quietly with the patient can be therapeutic; if the nurse cannot be physically present for extended periods of time, family members or friends are encouraged to be with the patient. The nurse can also assure the patient of frequent return visits and encourage the use of the call-bell to summon help.

Listening to the patient allows him to verbalize and share his fears and to offer suggestions and participate in care planning and management. The effectiveness of listening and personal contact in decreasing pain perception depends on the quality of the nurse–patient relationship. Patients in acute pain may not have the energy to talk about it but may wish to do so following the pain experience. Some patients such as those with migraine headaches may benefit most from quiet and isolation. The need for and effectiveness of each technique should be assessed on a continuous basis.

Suggestion
Positive statements regarding the action and effectiveness of medications enhance cognitive control over pain perception, as demonstrated by the effectiveness of placebos in relieving pain in some situations. Nursing statements can influence a patient's subjective assessment of an experience.

Hypnosis is a technique which uses positive suggestions to alter pain perception; it may be used for anaesthesia and for the treatment of pain of psychogenic origin.

Distraction and diversion
Depending on the nature of the illness and on the particular individual, some diversion which is acceptable to the patient provides distraction that may reduce his concentration on the pain or 'close the gate'. A brief visit and chat with someone, a few moments with his religious adviser, reading or listening to a radio may prove beneficial.

Distraction by guided imagery may focus the patient's thoughts on pleasant sensations and experiences and may be used to enhance the effects of relaxation measures and analgesic medication.

Analgesics
The drugs used to relieve pain include those that depress pain perception, reduce the patient's response to pain or relax muscle spasm.

It is important that the nurse be familiar with the action of the prescribed drug, the usual dosage, factors that influence the dosage and effectiveness of the drug, the frequency with which it may be given and the possible side-effects. A knowledge of the condition of the patient who is to receive the analgesic is also necessary. The administration may be left to the discretion of the nurse when the prescription states 'give when required' (PRN). The doctor may denote the frequency in addition, e.g. 4–6 hourly. The prescribed analgesic should be used judiciously and under conditions that will contribute to maximum benefit for the patient. Treatments and nursing measures are carried out before or immediately following the administration of the drug so the patient may remain undisturbed as much as possible. An exception is when the analgesic is given specifically prior to a painful procedure, when time must be allowed for the drug to take effect. The administration of the drug should not be withheld unnecessarily since pain may initiate harmful physiological responses and may contribute to shock. Also, the longer the patient suffers, the more fearful and apprehensive he becomes, making it more difficult to achieve relief. In other words, pain is easier to control if it is prevented or if it can be relieved soon after the onset. When persistent, severe pain, such as that often associated with terminal malignancy, is being experienced, the patient is observed closely to determine whether the drug is effective and the duration of the effect of an analgesic; the nurse's observations are then discussed with the doctor and the patient. Plans are made to administer the analgesics at more frequent and regular intervals, or to change to another drug, to prevent the pain from reaching severe intensity.

At no time should an analgesic replace nursing measures that, in many instances of less severe pain, may provide relief. Analgesics are administered in conjunction with other pain control measures that enhance the body's pain control mechanisms; analgesics interfere with endorphin production.

A great variety of drugs are used as analgesics; they range from mild acetylsalicylic acid (aspirin) to strong opiates and synthetic preparations.

Non-narcotic drugs relieve pain by acting peripherally where they block the pain chemoreceptors and relieve inflammation. They may also exert some action on the central nervous system. Narcotics act primarily on the brain and spinal cord. The combined administration of non-narcotic and narcotic preparations provides pain relief through both peripheral and central nervous system mechanisms and will reduce the amount of the narcotic required to relieve pain. Examples of non-narcotic analgesics are acetylsalicylic acid (aspirin), aspirin compounds (aspirin, phenacetin and caffeine) and paracetamol. Weak narcotic medications include dextropropoxyphene hydrochloride plus paracetamol (Distalgesic). Narcotics used as stronger analgesics include morphine, codeine, pethidine and papaveretum (Omnopon).

If the patient is apprehensive a tranquillizer, such as diazepam (Valium), may be ordered as an adjunct to an analgesic in order to decrease the patient's fear and tension and reduce his pain responses.

Antidepressant drugs such as amitriptyline (Tryptizol) and imipramine (Tofranil) have been shown to provide an analgesic effect and to enhance morphine analgesia. Phenothiazines such as chlorpromazine (Largactil) and haloperidol (Haldol) enhance the effects of morphine with their antiemetic and antipsychotic actions. These drugs are usually used in conjunction with narcotics for patients with cancer pain.

When the cause of pain is known to be muscle spasm, a preparation that produces relaxation of the muscle tissue may be prescribed. For example, spasm of the smooth muscle tissue of the gastrointestinal tract, the urinary tract and biliary tract may be relieved by antispasmodic preparations, such as hyoscine butylbromide (Buscopan), atropine sulphate and propantheline bromide (Pro-Banthine). These drugs produce their effect by reducing the parasympathetic impulses to the visceral muscle.

The analgesic drugs may produce side-effects, the incidence and nature of which vary from one patient to another. Nausea and vomiting are two of the most common reactions. The time relationship between the administration of the drug and the onset of the nausea or vomiting should be noted. Patients who are upset by morphine and codeine may tolerate meptazinol (Meptid).

The more potent analgesics, such as opiates, cause some depression of the respiratory centre. The rate and volume of respirations should be noted following the administration of these drugs, particularly in the cases of older patients and those known to have respiratory dysfunction.

The possibility of addiction when a patient is receiving repeated doses of analgesics or sedatives is largely overestimated. Repeated doses of narcotic analgesics, over 10 days, probably account for less than 1% of patients becoming addicted. Myths also abound with regard to prolonged use of narcotic analgesics in patients with chronic pain. These patients are more likely to make repeated requests for analgesia if inadequate doses are given. Long-term use of analgesics may lead to a decreasing response to the prescribed dose. The use of tranquillizers and sedatives, in addition to an analgesic, is debatable. Many of these drugs probably act by decreasing the patient's awareness, some can actually have an anti-analgesic effect (e.g. promethazine) and some may have analgesic properties (e.g. chlorpromazine). However these drugs are often used in helping to control pain.[15,16,17]

Constipation, dry mouth, impaired ability to make decisions and occasionally disorientation are also side-effects of analgesics that may occur and for which the nurse must be alert.

3. ALTERATION OF SENSORY INPUT

Removal of the cause
Removal of the cause of the pain is the most effective means of altering the sensory input. Physical removal of a splinter, or the removal of distending gas by means of a rectal tube may be the only measures necessary in some situations.

Analgesics and antiinflammatory agents
Non-narcotic analgesics and some antiinflammatory agents function at the cellular level to decrease irritation to the small diameter fibres which transmit pain impulses.

Positioning
A change of position may provide some relief for the patient by reducing the pressure and tension on the affected area. Venous and lymphatic drainage are promoted in order to decrease the accumulation of fluid in the tissue and thereby relieve pain. Adequate assistance and extreme gentleness are necessary when turning or moving the patient. The patient should be moved slowly, and support provided for the painful area. It is often helpful to ask the patient how the movement can be made least distressing for him. Good body alignment contributes to comfort by eliminating tension and hyperextension. Support and elevation of a painful limb on a pillow may be helpful. Immobilization and support by mechanical

devices may ease the patient's pain and lessen the discomfort associated with moving. Examples of such devices are a fracture board, firm mattress, a splint applied to a limb, an abdominal or chest binder and a Stryker bed (turning frame).

Cutaneous stimulation
Cutaneous stimulation activates large fibre transmission and depresses transmission of pain impulses along the small fibres, probably through the release of endorphins. Measures such as massage and the local application of a counterirritant, as well as acupuncture and electrical stimulation, enhance the body's natural mechanisms for pain modulation and control. The degree and duration of relief obtained by cutaneous stimulation varies; when selecting a specific technique consideration should be given to the individual patient as well to the convenience.

Massage. Rubbing a painful part occurs instinctively. The immediate response to striking an elbow is to hold it and rub the part. The nurse can effectively utilize this technique to alleviate a patient's pain and teach the technique to the patient and family. Massage may involve a local area such as the elbow or cover large areas of skin such as the back. Techniques include long, smooth, firm strokes or circular motions, or light, brisk movements. The hands should be warm and a lubricant used to facilitate movement. Massage is contraindicated for abdominal pain, over open skin lesions and when a thrombus is suspected such as in phlebitis.

Pressure. The application of pressure over the injury or at acupuncture points produces a numbing effect as well as decreasing the blood supply to the area. Pressure may be applied using the hand, firm objects or using the thumb and fingers to apply pressure and massage over acupuncture points.

Vibration. Vibration stimulates large fibre activity; it is most often used by patients at home or in conjunction with other methods of pain relief. Electric- and battery-operated pillows and hand vibrators are available in many shapes and sizes. Their effectiveness is greatest for acute pain.

Thermal applications. The application of moist or dry heat or cold may produce relief of pain. The effects of heat are the relaxation of muscle tension or spasm and the increased rate of blood flow through the area. Precautions should be taken to prevent burning, since the patient in pain may be less sensitive to excessive heat.

Cold applications stimulate constriction of the local blood vessels and reduce the amount of blood in the area and the accumulation of tissue fluid (lymph). This diminishes the painful swelling and congestion in the affected area. Cold also reduces the sensitivity of the pain receptors.

---

[15] Marks & Sachar (1973), pp. 173–181.
[16] Twycross (1974), pp. 184–198.
[17] McCaffery (1979b).

Topical analgesics. Applications which cause irritation of skin (counterirritants) may provide relief (see discussion of gate control theory). Examples of applications used are menthol and methyl salicylate ointment preparations and benzydamine hydrochloride (Difflam).

Electrical stimulation. Electrical stimulation of peripheral nerves is used for the relief of phantom pain and the pain associated with degenerative spinal conditions and arthritis. This is referred to as TENS (transcutaneous electrical nerve stimulation). Electrodes are applied to the surface of the skin or implanted in an area of contact with a major sensory pathway. An electric current is discharged into the electrode and produces stimulation of large afferent nerve fibres. Endorphin release is activated and small fibre transmission is blocked. Most of these units are designed to be operated by the patient, giving him control over his pain and its management.

Electrical stimulation may be used for relief of chronic pain by implanting the electrode in the spine so that the impulses enter the posterior column directly. The operative procedure for implanting the electrode of the posterior column stimulator involves open surgery and a laminectomy.

Acupuncture. Acupuncture, a very old Chinese medical procedure, has received considerable attention recently. It is currently being used to induce analgesia in some pain clinics for patients experiencing chronic and intractable pain.

The procedure involves the insertion of several long fine probes to varying depths at selected points. The sites for insertion depend upon the patient's particular problem. The probes are rotated as they are introduced and after they are in place; this enhances the stimulation. The practice sometimes involves applying electrical stimulation through the probes following their insertion.

The physiology of acupuncture, and the reason for its effectiveness in relieving pain, are not clearly understood. No one theory explains all the effects of acupuncture. Currently its effectiveness is explained on the basis of the gate control theory of pain. It is thought that insertion of the needles stimulates the pain inhibitory nerve fibres, thus stopping the impulses from reaching the brain. In addition, acupuncture increases the body levels of endorphins and this also has a pain relieving effect.

Neurosurgery to relieve pain. In some instances, *intractable pain* which cannot be effectively controlled by analgesics is relieved by surgical interruption of the pain impulse pathway either outside or within the central nervous system. The procedure is usually reserved for patients with an incurable disease or cancer and those who suffer the excruciating pain of tic douloureux (trigeminal neuralgia).

When the source of the pain is localized to a relatively small area of the body a neurectomy may be done. This involves severing or crushing the peripheral sensory nerve fibres to the affected area.

A second neurosurgical procedure used is a rhizotomy, in which the sensory pathway which carries impulses from the affected area is interrupted just before it enters the spinal cord. (The area of fibres that is severed or crushed lies between the associated posterior root ganglion and the cord.) The disadvantage of a rhizotomy is that it causes the loss of the sense of touch and position in the area, so it is used principally to relieve pain in the upper part of the trunk.

When intractable pain is in the lower part of the trunk and the lower limbs or if it involves a large part of the body which is supplied by several spinal nerves, the pain pathways in the spinal cord and, rarely, in the brain stem or thalamus are interrupted.

One procedure in use is *cordotomy*—division of sensory fibres in the lateral spinothalamic tract. A *tractotomy* may be done by severing the pain impulse-conducting pathway in the medulla and midbrain. This operative procedure is used less often because it is associated with severe side-effects.

Stereotactic surgery is used to interrupt pain pathways in the brain. *Stereotactic thalamotomy* results in interruption of the spinothalamic tract at the level of the thalamus. General anaesthesia is not required. An electrode is introduced into an area of the thalamus and either coagulation or freezing is used to interrupt the pain pathway. Pain relief diminishes gradually. Side-effects include ataxia and rarely apathy.

Interruption of these pathways causes permanent loss of the temperature sensation, as well as that of pain below the level of the interruption. Loss of these sensations eliminates natural body defences. Precautions are necessary to avoid burns, ischaemic sores from pressure, and injury. An explanation is given to the patient and instructions given as to how to avoid prolonged periods of pressure and injuries.

4. MANAGEMENT OF ONE'S OWN EXPERIENCE OF PAIN

The patient with acute pain. The patient with acute pain can influence the course of management and participate in the planning, implementation and evaluation of specific pain control measures. Knowledge of planned procedures and pain control measures, and the sensations anticipated during and after the procedures, not only decreases the patient's anxiety but also decreases the sense of helplessness and loss of control such situations present. Patients can influence management by communicating pain responses and informing carers of measures which have worked for them in the past and what has not been effective. Patients should be encouraged to participate in planning pain control measures and to evaluate the effect of these.

The Patient with chronic pain. When the cause of the pain cannot be removed, the goal becomes control of the pain experience. The patient should learn to regulate, manipulate, and generally influence pain management. Chronic pain frequently leads to major disruptions in all aspects of the individual's life. To effectively manage chronic pain, patients require knowledge of the pain, skills of coping and continuous feedback. Since many pain responses are learned behaviours, most patients can change their behavioural responses and develop new coping skills. Pain management, to be effective, must be multidimensional in approach. It is concerned with all aspects of the patient's responses to pain and the effects of these responses on the individual's well-being and life-style. The participation of family members and significant friends or relatives is essential for long-term effectiveness of behavioural change. Relatives need to learn how to interact with the patient so that they can reinforce actions conducive to improved healthy behaviour.

A teaching plan may be developed for the patient; selection of the content depends on the assessment of the patient, his goals, and his ability and willingness to participate. Examples of the content of the teaching plan and teaching–learning approaches follow.

1 Knowledge that the patient should receive:

Pain
- Characteristics of the pain experience including the onset, duration, location, quality and intensity of the pain
- Factors that precipitate pain
- Patterns of pain
- Behavioural responses to pain
- Effects of the pain and pain responses on daily life and functioning
- The meaning of the pain, including recognition that the existence of chronic pain and impairment of bodily functions do not necessarily prevent the individual from living a meaningful and self-fulfilling life
- What the pain does not mean, e.g. progression of disease, development of complications

Pain relief
- The technique and mode of action of various pain relief measures including medications, relaxation techniques, massage, biofeedback or electrical stimulation
- Alternative relief measures available
- The purpose of and expectations related to the psychological aspects of treatment
- The specific plan for pain relief developed for the patient
- Resources available to faciliate implementation of the plan
- Roles and responsibilities of health-care professionals

- Expectations and responsibilities of the patient in implementing the plan

Nutrition
- Daily food requirements
- Plan to alter the patient's diet to ensure adequate nutrition and to eliminate the excessive use of food substances (such as caffeine or sugar) which may have a detrimental effect
- If appropriate, the effects of smoking on health and well-being

Rest and sleep
- The importance of receiving adequate rest and sleep
- Individualized plan to promote rest and establish or maintain a pattern for night sleep

Physical activity
- The benefits of increasing physical activity
- Specific physical activities to be increased
- Physical activities to be decreased and avoided

Information may be provided to individuals or groups of patients. Group teaching is directed to patients with pain of similar aetiology and manifestations. Patients being taught in a group may share experiences and learn from others with similar problems. Individual sessions are also necessary for those participating in group classes to provide an opportunity to make the information applicable to the particular patient and situation, to discuss feelings, answer questions and set goals. Teaching methods utilize various forms of sensory input; sessions should be short and plans should be made for repetition and further discussions.

2 Skills
Many patients with chronic pain need to develop skill and dexterity in carrying out the planned pain relief techniques and to implement changes in their eating and sleeping habits and physical activity. The environment should facilitate social interaction and opportunity for self-management of the activities of daily living. Vocational assessment may be necessary and plans made for retraining. Teaching includes demonstration and supervised practice sessions (e.g. self-administration of medications, physical activities).

The patient's daily regime should be structured and focused on one step at a time. When one step has been successfully completed, the patient contracts for the next skill or behaviour to be achieved. Goals and expectations for each step are determined by the patient with mutual agreement of the health team. Active physical participation may not be possible or appropriate for some patients. Goals must be realistic and recognize priorities to conserve the patient's energy and enhance his quality of life.

3 Feedback and reinforcement
Positive relationships between the patient and the nurse, the patient and other members of the health team, and within the health team promote an

environment of trust, caring and openness that is essential for the development and reinforcement of positive coping behaviours by the patient. The patient's rights to make decisions, whether one approves of the decisions or not, must be respected. The person who regains some control over his daily activities usually is more motivated to exert some control over his pain.

Carrying out suggestions made by the patient, such as how to turn him so as to minimize pain, reinforces patient participation and control. On-going feedback and support are provided as the patient takes the initiative to learn new skills, increase activity and increase social interaction. Awareness of the patient's existing behaviour and its pattern and frequency of occurrence is necessary. A negative response to pain may be decreased by removing positive reinforcements for that behaviour; situations and actions that are associated with the response should be avoided. Effective changes in behaviour are accepted and reinforced. Behaviour modification techniques that provide a reward, such as praise, when a desired behaviour occurs are effective in changing behaviour but must be used with other approaches to promote change on a long-term basis. The long-term treatment programme must include opportunities for the patient to practise constructive behaviours in his home and work environment.

Family members and relatives play an important role in reinforcing and strengthening behaviour conducive to improvement in daily functioning. They are taught how to interact effectively with the patient with chronic pain, to avoid actions that lead to or reinforce pain behaviour and to give on-going feedback and support for positive behaviour.

Behaviour change is more likely to occur when goals are achievable in a short time. Long-term patient goals should be broken down into simple, graduated steps that are realistic for the patient to achieve. As the patient successfully completes one step, the achievement is acknowledged and the next step initiated.

Physiological monitoring equipment used in biofeedback is another means of providing the patient with instant feedback.

Individual and/or group therapy provides the patient with support, insight into pain behaviour, reinforcement for change and opportunity to develop self-reliance. Group therapy is useful for ensuring long-term support following discharge from hospital or a pain treatment centre.

EXPECTED OUTCOMES

1 The patient verbalizes the purpose and/or meaning of pain.
2 The patient outlines appropriate action to take when pain occurs.
3 Responses to pain decrease, as evidenced by:
   (a) heart, respiratory rates and blood pressure are within normal ranges for the patient
   (b) relaxation of skeletal muscles
   (c) absence of body postures associated with pain
   (d) absence of verbal responses such as crying, moaning or silence.
4 Verbalizaton indicates an absence of physical pain or a decrease in pain intensity.
5 The use of descriptions of emotional pain is decreased.
6 The patient is able to rest, relax and sleep.
7 The patient's attention span is increased.
8 Physical and social activities are increased.
9 The patient is able to direct and/or carry out measures for pain control.
10 The patient realistically evaluates the effectiveness of pain control measures.

References and Further Reading

BOOKS

Bonica JJ, Lindblom U & Iggo A (eds) (1981) *Advances in Pain Research and Therapy, Vol. 5: Proceedings of the Third World Congress on Pain.* New York; Raven Press.
Collins S & Parker E (1983) *The Essentials of Nursing—An Introduction to Nursing,* Chapter 5, (contributed by Raiman JA) London: Macmillan.
Ganong WF (1985) *Review of Medical Physiology,* 12th ed. San Francisco: Lange.
Guyton AC (1986) *Textbook of Medical Physiology,* 7th ed. Philadelphia: WB Saunders. Chapter 50.
Hart LK, Feese JL & Fearing MO (1981) *Concepts Common to Acute Illness.* St Louis: CV Mosby. Chapter 9.
Hayward J (1975) *Information—A Prescription Against Pain, The Study of Nursing Care Project Reports, Series 2 No 5.* London: Royal College of Nursing.
Hendler N (1981) *Diagnosis and Non-surgical Management of Chronic Pain.* New York: Raven Press.
Jacox AK (1979) Pain: *A Source Book for Nurses and Other Health Professionals.* Boston: Little, Brown.
McCaffery M (1979a) *Nursing Management of the Patient with Pain,* 2nd ed. Philadelphia: JB Lippincott.
McCaffery M (1979b) (Adapted for the UK by Sofaer B) *Nursing the Patient in Pain,* Lippincott Nursing Series. London: Harper & Row.
Melzack R (1980) Current concept of pain. In I Ajemian and B Mount (eds), *The RVH Manual of Palliative Hospice Care.* New York: Arno Press.
Melzack R & Wall PD (1982) *The Challenge of Pain.* Harmondsworth: Penguin.
Meinhart NT & McCaffery M (1983) *Pain: A Nursing Approach to Assessment and Analysis.* Norwalk, CT: Appleton-Century-Crofts.
Ng LKY & Bonica JJ (eds) (1980) *Pain, Discomfort and Humanitarian Care,* Vol. 4. New York: Elsevier.
Smith LH & Thier SO (1985) *Pathophysiology, The Biological Principles of Disease,* 2nd ed. Philadelphia: WB Saunders. Section 13.
Sternbach RA (ed.) (1978) *The Psychology of Pain.* New York: Raven Press.

Twycross RG & Lack SA (1983) *Symptom Control in Far Advanced Cancer: Pain Relief*. London: Pitman.

Wyngaarden JB & Smith LH (eds) (1985) *Cecil Textbook of Medicine*, 17th ed. Philadelphia: WB Saunders. pp. 92, 2047–2064.

PERIODICALS

Achong MR (1979) Clinical pharmacology of analgesic drugs. *Can. Fam. Physician*, Vol. 25, pp. 179–182.

Boguslawski M (1980) Therapeutic touch: a facilitator of pain relief. *Top. Clin. Nurs.*, Vol. 2 No. 1, pp. 27–37.

Bourbonnais F (1981) Pain assessment: development of a tool for the nurse and the patient. *J Adv. Nurs.*, Vol. 6, No. 4, pp. 277–282.

Brena SF & Chapman SL (1981) The learned pain syndrome. *Postgrad. Med.*, Vol. 69, No. 1, pp. 55–61.

Goldberg-Sklar C (1984) Chronic pain management: a research focus. *J. Neurosurg. Nurs.*, Vol. 16 No. 1, pp. 10–14.

Hedlin A & Dostrovsky J (1979) Understanding the physiology of pain. *Can. Nurs.*, Vol. 75 No. 2, pp. 28–30.

Heidrich G & Perry S (1982) Helping the patient in pain. *Am. J. Nurs.*, Vol. 82 No. 12, pp. 1828–1833.

Johnson JE & Rice VH (1974) Sensory and distress components of pain. *Nurs. Res.*, Vol. 23 No. 3, p. 203.

Kim S (1980) Pain, theory, research and nursing practice. *Adv. Nurs. Sci.*, Vol. 2 No. 2, pp. 43–59.

Kremer EF & Block A (1981) Behavioural approaches to treatment of chronic pain; the inaccuracy of patient self-report measures. *Arch. Phys. Med. Rehab.*, Vol. 62 No. 4, pp. 188–191.

Lovejoy NC (1980) Biofeedback: a growing role in holistic health. *Adv. in Nurs. Science.*, Vol. 2 No. 4, pp. 83–93.

Malec J, Cayner JJ, Harvey RF & Timming RC (1981) Pain management: long term follow-up of an in-patient program. *Arch. Phys. Med. Rehab.*, Vol. 62 No. 8, pp. 369–372.

Marks RM & Sachar EJ (1973) Undertreatment of medical inpatients with narcotic analgesics. *Ann. Intern. Med.*, Vol. 78, pp. 173–181.

McCaffery M (1980) Understanding your patient's pain. *Nurs. '80*, Vol. 10 No. 9, pp. 26–31.

McCaffery M (1980) Patients shouldn't have to suffer—how to relieve pain with injectable narcotics. *Nurs. '80*, Vol. 10 No. 10, pp. 34–39.

McCaffery M (1980) How to relieve your patient's pain fast and effectively with oral analgesics. *Nurs. '80*, Vol. 10, No. 11, pp. 58–63.

McCaffery M (1980) Relieving pain with non-invasive techniques. *Nurs. '80*, Vol. 10 No. 12, pp. 55–57.

McCaffery M (1981) When your patient's still in pain don't just do something: sit there. *Nurs. '81*, Vol. 11 No. 6, pp. 58–61.

McGuire DB (1984) Assessment of pain in cancer inpatients using the McGill pain questionnaire. *Oncology Nurs. Forum*, Vol. 11 No. 6, pp. 32–37.

McGuire DB (1984) The measurement of clinical pain. *Nurs. Res.*, Vol. 33 No. 3, pp. 152–156.

McGuire L (1981) A short, simple tool for assessing your patient's pain. *Nurs '81*, Vol. 11 No. 3, pp. 48–49.

Meissner JE (1980) McGill–Melzack pain questionnaire. *Nurs. '80*, Vol. 10 No. 1, pp. 50–51.

Moore DE & Blacker HM (1983) How effective is TENS for chronic pain? *Am. J. Nurs.*, Vol. 63 No. 8, pp. 1175–1177.

Moore ME, Berk SN & Nypaver A (1984) Chronic pain: inpatient treatment with small group effects. *Arch. Phys. Med. Rehabil.*, Vol. 65 No. 7, pp. 356–361.

Morgan J, Wells N & Robertson E (1985) Effects of preoperative teaching on postoperative pain: a replication and expansion. *Int. J. Nurs. Stud.*, Vol. 22 No. 3, pp. 269–280.

Peric-Knowlton W (1984) The understanding and management of acute pain in adults: the nursing contribution. *Int. J. Nurs. Stud.*, Vol. 21 No. 2, pp. 131–143.

Raiman JA (1981) Responding to pain. *Nursing* (Oxford), Vol. 1 No. 31, pp. 1362–1365.

Shealy NC (1980) Holistic management of chronic pain. *Top. Clin. Nurs.*, Vol. 2 No. 1, pp. 1–8.

Siegele DS (1974) The gate control theory. *Am. J. Nurs.*, Vol. 74 No. 3, pp. 449–450.

Terzian MP (1980) Neurological intervention for management of chronic intractable pain. *Top. Clin. Nurs.*, Vol. 2 No. 1, pp. 75–88.

Twycross RG (1974) Clinical experience with diamorphine in advanced malignant disease. *Int. J. Clin. Pharmacol.*, Vol. 9, pp. 184–198.

Voshall B (1980) The effects of preoperative teaching on postoperative pain. *Top. Clin. Nurs.*, Vol. 2 no. 1, pp. 39–43.

Wells N (1984) Responses to acute pain and the nursing implications. *J. Adv. Nurs.*, Vol. 9 No. 1, pp. 51–58.

West BA (1981) Understanding endorphins: our natural pain relief system. *Nurs. '81*, Vol. 11 No. 2, pp. 50–53.

Wilson RW & Elmassian BJ (1981) Endorphins. *Am. J. Nurs.*, Vol. 81 No. 4, pp. 722–725.

Wolf ZR (1980) Pain theories: an overview. *Top. Clin. Nurs.*, Vol. 2 No. 1, pp. 9–18.

9

The Patient with Oncological Disease

Neoplasms

This chapter addresses abnormal cell growth, the prevention and diagnosis of the disorder and the treatment and post-treatment of the patient with oncological disease.

Normally, the production of cells is a regulated process which allows for growth in early life and for the replacement of worn-out or damaged cells throughout life. The mechanisms for the initiation of cell reproduction, when tissue cells increase or replacement is needed, and the control of that reproduction so that it does not exceed the needs of the organism are not understood. Occasionally the control of cell reproduction is lost in some cells in a particular area of the body and an excessive production occurs, forming an abnormal mass that is referred to as a *neoplasm* or *newgrowth*. The cells of the neoplasm serve no useful purpose and use nutrients and oxygen, causing deprivation in the hosts's normal tissues. Oncology refers to the study of all newgrowths which may be benign or malignant.

Benign neoplasms

A benign neoplasm is considered much less of a threat to the host's life because it does not spread to other sites. It is usually possible to cure benign neoplastic disease by surgical removal of the mass.

Growth of a benign neoplasm is slow and tends to be expansive rather than invasive; the mass remains localized, frequently is encapsulated, and the cells may show little abnormality compared with those of the normal tissue from which they originated. When excised, it rarely recurs. Since a benign neoplasm is a space-occupying lesion, it may cause serious effects on neighbouring structures, depending on its size and location, in some instances it may obstruct blood vessels or a passageway or may cause pressure on vital tissues leading to serious malfunction. Some benign lesions tend to become malignant if left untreated; examples are polyps in the stomach and intestine, papillomas of the bladder and larynx, and pigmented moles.

Malignant neoplasms

A malignant neoplasm is a distinct threat to life by virtue of its ability to proliferate destructively into surrounding tissue and to other parts of the body. Some of the cells become detached from the primary mass and are carried via the blood or lymph to a distant area of the body, where they set up colonies of the malignant cells (metastases). The neoplastic cells tend to grow and reproduce rapidly and change in structure and activity in varying degrees. They lack normal cellular differentiation and are atypical in size, shape and staining properties (see Table 9.1).

In addition to being classified as malignant or benign, a neoplasm is also named according to the type of tissue involved. Classification of the more common neoplasms is found in Table 9.2

Neoplastic disease is discussed as it relates to specific organs in the respective ensuing chapters. In this chapter, certain features and problems common to malignant newgrowths are presented to give this major health problem special emphasis.

CANCER

Cancer is a term commonly used to designate any disease that is a malignant neoplasm; it is not one specific disease but a group of diseases. As cited previously, malignant neoplasms have certain common characteristics, but there are also marked differences from one type to another because of the type of tissue involved, the location, and the degree of departure from normal of the cells of the neoplasm. They differ as to signs and symptoms, effects on the host, rate of growth, metastasis, form of treatment used and their response to treatment.

Cancer begins as a localized disease, known as *carcinoma in situ* (cancer in its original site). When the cells commence invasion of surrounding tissues it may be referred to as *invasive cancer*. In the more advanced stages of the disease, cells become detached from the neoplasm and are carried by lymph or blood vessels to other parts of the body, where more cancer develops. Malignant cells may also spread by implantation or seeding within a body cavity. The serous fluid in the pleural or peritoneal cavities carries the tumour cells through the cavity. This process, as mentioned earlier, is described as *metastasizing*. Some tumours such as basal cell carcinomas and gliomas rarely metastasize while others such as melanomas and lung carcinomas metastasize widely and are less invasive. The cells carried in the lymph may be trapped in lymph nodes near the original site, producing disease in the nodes and causing what is known as *regional involvement*. Eventually

Table 9.1 Differences in benign and malignant neoplasms.

	Benign	Malignant
Cells	Relatively normal and mature	Little resemblance to normal; poorly differentiated, atypical in size and shape, non-uniform, and immature
Growth	Slow and restricted. Non-invasive of surrounding tissue; expansive, pushing aside normal tissue	Usually rapid and unrestricted. Invasive of surrounding tissue
Spread	Remains localized. Usually encapsulated	Metastasizes via blood and lymph streams
Recurrence	Rarely recurs	Frequently recurs
Threat to host	Prognosis favourable. The effect depends on size and location. May cause pressure on vital organs or obstruct a passageway, which is usually corrected by surgical excision of neoplasm	Threatens life by reason of its local destructive proliferation and formation of secondary neoplasms in other structures. Prognosis more favourable with early diagnosis and treatment, when cells show less departure from the normal and there is no metastasis

these areas of disease disseminate cancer cells to other parts.

Certain areas are known to be the most frequent sites of metastases from certain organs. For example, in breast cancer, when the disease is advanced beyond regional involvement, frequent sites of metastases are the lungs, brain and bones. In cancer of the stomach, the most common site of metastasis is the liver.

Malignant neoplasms are *graded* according to the degree of differentiation of the tumour cells and the estimated rate of growth of the tumour. Grades are designated by Roman numerals I to IV, with the higher numbers indicating a greater degree of undifferentiation and a greater degree of malignancy.

Staging refers to clinical evaluation of the extent of the cancer and is used as a basis for determining the treatment of choice. The system is referred to as TNM: the T designating the size of the tumour. Cancer in situ is indicated by T/S: T1 to T4 indicate increasing size. N0, N1, N2 and N3 indicate the extent of involvement of regional lymph nodes, while M0, M1, M2 and M3 show the extent of metastases.

INCIDENCE AND TRENDS

Cancer diseases account for a large number of deaths each year. They are second only to heart disease as a killer in the United Kingdom and it is estimated that one out of every four persons develops cancer. In 1979 (the latest year for which detailed registration statistics have been published), almost 190 000 people in England and Wales were newly registered as having cancer.[1] Statistics indicate that in recent years cancer has accounted for an increasing number of deaths. Factors which have probably contributed to the increase include: (1) a greater number of persons living to an older age, which increases cancer susceptibility; (2) the increased risk of developing certain cancers because of greater exposure to specific carcinogens (e.g. cigarette smoking); (3) new and improved diagnostic procedures; and (4) a decrease in deaths from diseases such as pneumonia, scarlet fever and other acute infections.

Statistics also show a significant change in the incidence of cancer between the two sexes over the past two decades. The mortality rate for females has decreased, owing mainly to a lesser incidence of uterine, gastric and intestinal malignant neoplasia. The death rate for males has increased, which may be attributed mainly to the greater occurrence of cancer of the lung and prostate. Fig. 9.1 shows the distribution of different types of cancer.

Statistics of the incidence of certain types of cancer may provide clues to predisposing factors and causes in relation to environment, occupations, health habits and customs, and may also indicate the value of preventive and early detection programmes. For instance, in the United States, the decrease in uterine cancer may be correlated with the increasing practice of an annual Papanicolaou vaginal smear (Pap test). The increase in cancer of the respiratory tract, particularly the lungs, is attributed to increased cigarette smoking in both sexes.

The incidence of cancer varies with age. It occurs in infants and children as well as adults but increases with advancing age. Leukaemia and neoplasms of the central nervous system account for many of the malignancies occurring in children up to 5 years of age. Between the ages of 5 and 15 years there is a lesser incidence, but from 15 on there is a steady increase.

Although the overall incidence of cancer has

---

[1] Office of Population Censuses and Surveys (1979).

Table 9.2 Classification of malignant and benign neoplasms.

Tissue of origin	Benign neoplasms	Malignant neoplasms
Epithelium		
Surface epithelium	Papilloma	Carcinoma
		Epithelioma (squamous or basal cell carcinoma)
Glandular epithelium	Adenoma	Adenocarcinoma
	Papilloma	Papillary carcinoma
	Polyp	Papillary adenocarcinoma
Melanocytes (cells that synthesize the pigment melanin)	Naevus	
	Melanoma	Malignant melanoma
Connective tissue		Sarcoma
Fibrous tissue	Fibroma	Fibrosarcoma
Embryonic fibrous tissue	Myxoma	Myxosarcoma
Bone	Osteoma	Osteosarcoma
Cartilage	Chondroma	Chondrosarcoma
Fatty tissue	Lipoma	Liposarcoma
Muscle tissue		
Smooth muscle	Leiomyoma	Leiomyosarcoma
Skeletal muscle	Rhabdomyoma	Rhabdomyosarcoma
Endothelial tissue		
Blood vessels	Haemangioma	Haemangiosarcoma (angiosarcoma)
		Haemangioendothelioma
Lymph vessels	Lymphangioma	Lymphangiosarcoma
		Lymphangioendotheliosarcoma
Haematopoietic and reticuloendothelial tissues		
Bone marrow		Myelogenous leukaemia
		Multiple myeloma
		Ewing's sarcoma (endotheliosarcoma)
Lymphoid tissue		Hodgkin's disease
		Lymphocytic leukaemia
		Lymphosarcoma
		Lymphoma
Nerve tissue		
Nerve	Neuroma	Neurogenic sarcoma
	Neurofibroma	
Ganglion	Ganglioneuroma	Neuroblastoma
Brain	Glioma	Glioblastoma
		Astrocytoma
		Medulloblastoma
Meninges	Meningioma	Malignant meningioma
Placental tissue	Hydatid mole	Choriocarcinoma
Adrenal medulla	Phaeochromocytoma	Malignant phaeochromocytoma
More than one tissue (mixed)		
Gonads	Teratoma (e.g. dermoid cyst of ovary)	Malignant teratoma (e.g., Wilms' tumour or embryonal carcinosarcoma)

increased, the survival rate of individuals diagnosed as having cancer has also increased over the past 20 years. This increase in survival of 5 years following diagnosis is attributed primarily to improved treatment and management of patients and to early diagnosis of the cancer.

CAUSATIVE FACTORS

A great deal of effort on the part of microbiologists and medical research scientists has been directed toward identification of a specific cause and treatment of cancer. Much information has been

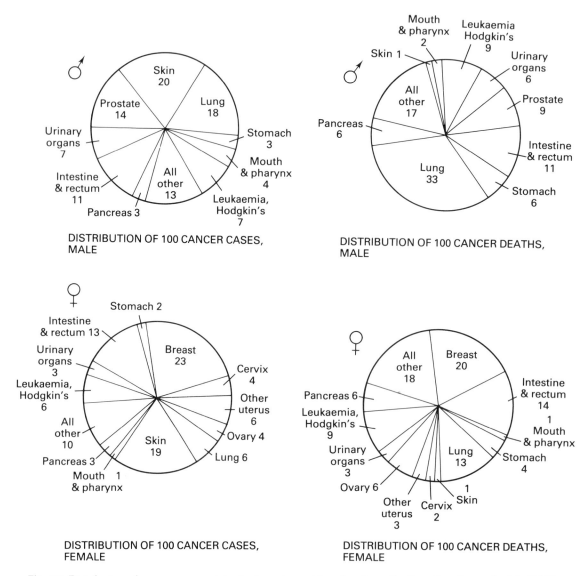

Fig. 9.1 Distribution of cancer cases and deaths in males and females. From the Canadian Cancer Society (1985).

obtained about cancerous diseases, and new and improved therapeutic measures have resulted in an increase in survival rates. Intensive study of cancer cells has led to the conclusion that the uncontrolled multiplication of atypical cells characteristic of cancer is due to a change in the structure of the deoxyribonucleic acid (DNA) in the nucleus of a cell. Once these atypical cells develop, the abnormal characteristics are continued in the cells that result from their mitosis. Certain chemical and physical agents appear to act as catalysts in causing some cancers, but a common specific causative factor that initiates and promotes the transformation of a normal cell into a malignant one remains obscure.

It has become apparent that a number of factors, both intrinsic and extrinsic, play a role in the development of the disease. Agents that incite malignant changes in cells are referred to as *carcinogens*.

Intrinsic factors

Contributory or controlling factors within the individual are considered to be his genetic make-up, hormonal balance and immunological response.

Three types of *genetic factors* exist which may influence the development of cancer. Smith and Thier indicate one factor as being chromosomal disorders involving the absence, duplication or rearrangement of long segments of genetic material. For example, the risk of leukaemia is 11 times greater in individuals with Down's syndrome (each cell contains an extra chromosome). The incidence of retinoblastoma is greater in children born with the absence of part of a chromosome. Single-gene disorders are known to predispose to neoplasia of the haematopoietic and lymphoreticular system. Another factor is that of polygenic abnormalities, in which multiple genes interact with environmental conditions or agents.[2] Studies of twins and of the familial incidence of cancers further demonstrate the influence of genetic factors on susceptibility.

Research on oncogenes, which have the potential to cause cancer when activated, and the discovery of movable genes, which are presumed to activate the oncogene by disruption of the DNA, hopefully will provide answers on the aetiology of cancer and lead to more effective, preventive, diagnostic and treatment techniques.

An *excessive concentration of certain hormones* appears to influence the change of some normal cells to malignant ones, with subsequent uncontrolled growth. Such cancers are said to be hormone dependent and manifest changes in growth activity when the concentration of certain hormones is altered. For instance, oestrone and oestradiol (ovarian oestrogenic hormones) favour the growth of some breast cancers, while androgens (male hormones) tend to suppress their progress. Cancer has been produced experimentally in mice by the injection of oestrogen. Whether the hormone is the primary incitant in hormone-supported cancer in humans or whether it simply produces a tissue susceptibility to viral, chemical or physical carcinogens is not known. There are striking differences in the incidence of some cancers in males and females. The fact that breast cancer is frequent in females and rare in males may be explained on the basis of hormonal differences. But the reason for the much higher incidence of cancer of the stomach and urinary system in males than in females is not understood.

In the last decade there has been renewed interest in *cancer immunology*. Considerable attention and support are being given to the concept that the abnormal cells of the neoplasm contain substances that are foreign to the host's normal body cells and are therefore antigenic. The neoplastic antigens prompt an immune response in the host that controls the development, growth and spread of the disease. There is evidence that spontaneous regression and disappearance of the neoplasm have occurred when the host's immune mechanisms have destroyed the neoplastic cells. If the host's immune response is deficient the abnormal cells multiply rapidly, invade surrounding tissues and spread to distant areas. It has been observed that there is a higher incidence of cancer in persons with an inadequate immune response, which may be due to primary immu-

nodeficiency disease, immunosuppressive drugs, radiation exposure, or the ageing process.[3,4]

Sabiston suggests that tumour immunity is mediated by a variety of immune mechanisms, including: humoral antibodies; T and B lymphocytes; killer (K) lymphoid cells, which are antibody dependent; natural killer (NK) lymphoid cells, which can act on tumour cells without specific immunization; and macrophages.[5]

Investigation of immune factors in cancer continues with the hope of determining why the patient's defence mechanisms fail. Immunoprevention of cancer by administering vaccines to individuals at risk from exposure to physical or chemical carcinogens is a possibility for the future. Researchers hope to find a safe antigenic preparation that will stimulate immune mechanisms specific to cancer cells (active immunity), or a serum that will transfer immunity (passive immunity) to destroy the neoplastic cells or confine them locally.

Extrinsic factors

It has been well established that the development of most cancer diseases is due to or enhanced by some factors in the environment. These include certain chemicals, physical agents and viruses. Certain *chemical and physical agents* and some *viruses* are recognized as having a causative role. Many chemicals in the environment are being studied as possible carcinogens and a number have been determined to be offenders. The latter include asbestos, hydrocarbons (coal-tar products), aniline dyes, chromates, nickel and arsenic. Many of these have been recognized through the high incidence of cancer associated with occupational exposure to the specific chemical. For example, persons working with an aniline dye, which may be absorbed through the skin and excreted in the urine, show a high incidence of urinary bladder cancer. A causative relationship has also been established between asbestos and lung cancer. Insecticides and herbicides are highly suspect, and animal growth-stimulating hormones and some food additives are being investigated as potential carcinogens. Cigarette smoking as a cause of cancer of the respiratory tract and the bladder has been well documented. Air pollutants are also suspect, especially in relation to lung cancer. Research has indicated that there is usually a relatively long latent period between exposure to chemical carcinogens and cancer development.

Significant physical carcinogens include excessive exposure to the sun's rays, radiation and chronic irritation. A large percentage of skin cancers are attributed to excessive exposure to the sun's rays. Fair-skinned individuals with less natural pigmen-

---

[2] Smith & Thier (1985), p. 272.

[3] Smith & Thier (1985), p. 272.
[4] Sabiston (1986), p. 450.
[5] Sabiston (1986), p. 509.

tation of the skin, and those whose occupation keeps them outdoors (e.g. farmers), appear to be more susceptible to neoplastic changes in the dermal cells as a result of excessive sun exposure. X-rays and radioactive substances have proved beneficial in the diagnosis and treatment of some diseases, but repeated and heavy radiation may lead to malignant neoplasia. The adverse effects may not be seen for quite a long period following irradiation, since the effects can be cumulative. Repeated exposures to an amount that is considered harmless may eventually be of pathological significance. This was unfortunately found to be the case with personnel working with x-ray equipment before the need for more adequate shielding was recognized; many developed leukaemia or cancer of the skin.

Chronic irritation of an area and repeated tissue destruction and repair are thought to be contributory factors in the development of cancer. For example, the incidence of cancer of the lip is greater in pipe smokers; similarly, cancer of the cervix is more prevalent in women with unrepaired cervical ulcerations.

Scientists have established that various types of RNA and DNA tumour viruses produce some forms of malignant neoplasia in experimental animals. As a result, intensive research is being conducted in an effort to identify viruses as a cause of cancer in man. Viral aetiology is particularly suspect in leukaemia, lymphomas and breast cancer. Viruses are known to cause warts and mucosal papillomas in man, and herpes simplex virus has been associated with cancer of the cervix. The successful isolation of human viruses in some patients with leukaemia and from breast cancerous tissue strongly supports the aetiological role of viruses in malignant disease but the exact viral action in producing cancer is not known.

Management of the Oncological Patient

PREVENTION AND EARLY DETECTION OF CANCER

Oncological nursing is directed towards the prevention and early detection of neoplasms as well as the care of the patient in the diagnostic, therapeutic and post-treatment phases, including remission and recovery or the advanced stage of cancer. It is important to consider the patient's family and friends in all nursing care plans. Responsibilities include educating the patient and his family in the prevention and early diagnosis of oncological disease and in early effective management of the patient.

IDENTIFICATION OF THE PATIENT'S PROBLEM AND NURSING INTERVENTION

One problem is the public's *lack of information*, which

impedes the prevention and early detection of cancer.

At present it is not possible to prevent all types of cancer, but some types can be prevented by avoidance of recognized carcinogens. The public needs to understand the cancer problem more thoroughly, and every nurse has an obligation to participate in disseminating the necessary knowledge. Every opportunity should be taken to advise uninformed persons of the importance of avoiding exposure to carcinogenic agents and the role of early detection and treatment. Many need help in forming more hopeful and constructive attitudes because of their abnormal fear and fatalistic point of view of cancer. Many do not realize that several types of cancer can be detected in an asymptomatic phase by certain examinations (e.g. cervical smear test), and that some cancers can be cured if treated in the early stage. Improved 5-year survival rates in patients with cancer are attributed to early detection, staging and treatment advances.[6]

A person with an early sign may delay a visit to the doctor or clinic because of fear of being told that he has cancer. Malignant neoplasm begins as a localized disease; if all the cancer cells are confined to their source of origin, most cancers may be successfully treated. Delay in detection and treatment diminishes chances of cure and survival, since it permits the growing neoplasm to invade surrounding tissues, with cells becoming detached and carried to other body areas (metastases). Important early symptoms that are stressed in public education are:

- Unusual bleeding or discharge from any body orifice
- A lump or thickening in the breast or elsewhere
- A sore that does not heal
- A persistent change in bowel or bladder habits
- A persistent cough or hoarseness
- Indigestion or difficulty in swallowing
- An obvious change in a wart or mole

In many instances, on investigation of early symptoms, the findings are negative and the individual who has put off the visit to the doctor because of fear has experienced much needless anxiety.

The Health Education Council and cancer societies have instituted intensive campaigns to alert the public to potential sources of cancer, high risk factors, early detection and the fact that 'cancer can be beaten'. When more people have been informed, a more positive, hopeful attitude to the disease will develop. As part of public education, organizations advocate the following precautions:

1 Have a medical and dental checkup.
2 Watch for any change in your normal state of health.
3 Find out about any lump or sore that does not heal.
4 Protect yourself against too much sunlight.

---

[6] Woods & Kowalski (1982), p. 535.

5 Do not smoke.
6 Have a cervical smear test *at least* every 3 years.
7 Do a monthly breast self-examination.

Emphasis is placed on the role of regular periodical examinations. The nurse has many opportunities to discuss with her patients and friends the importance of regular self-examination of the breasts and the three-yearly cervical smear test (see section in this chapter on Exfoliative Cytological Tests). The breast self-examination procedure should be explained and the excellent pamphlets published by the Mastectomy Association, which clearly outline and illustrate the examination steps, should be made available. Many persons also require information regarding the significance of avoiding excessive exposure of the skin to the sun's rays.

The nurse should inform people that cigarette smoking causes lung cancer and help them to break the habit. (The Health Education Council produce excellent leaflets on this topic). The nurse who continues to smoke is setting a very poor example and is contributing to defeat in the battle against smoking.

In some occupations the employees may be brought in direct contact with a carcinogenic substance at work. Industrial regulations are necessary to protect employees and communities from carcinogenic hazards. In addition to protective measures for those in a high-risk work situation, the workers require an understanding of the risk and the significance of conscientious respect for the precautions. They should be advised of early symptoms that must be reported promptly, and should receive frequent regular examinations. Some industries may disseminate offending substances that could affect many citizens in the community. Governments are becoming more aware of such hazards and are requiring protective measures.

All industries, as well as those cited above, should be encouraged by their occupational health department to provide cancer education. An attempt should be made to identify high-risk individuals such as heavy smokers and those with a family history of the disease, and appropriate measures for early detection established.

In order to assume the expected role in cancer prevention and an early detection programme, the nurse must keep informed about the trends in the incidence of cancer and current advances being made. The work and the publications of the relevant organizations (such as BACUP or the Marie Curie Memorial Foundation) should be familiar to the nurse. An important contribution can be made by advising the public about such organizations and their local branches. Support of organizations such as these makes possible continuous cancer research, education and treatment, as well as a variety of services to cancer patients and their families. Films, pamphlets and speakers are available for cancer education for both professional and lay groups.

EXPECTED OUTCOMES

The general public should be able to:
1 State the environmental and life-style factors which predispose to cancer.
2 State seven early symptoms of cancer.
3 Enumerate community resources for information about cancer, cancer prevention and early detection.
4 Utilize services for the detection of cancer.
5 Describe plans to alter life-style to decrease cancer risk factors (e.g. stop smoking).

THE DIAGNOSIS OF CANCER

ASSESSMENT

Assessment of the patient with cancer or at risk of cancer involves the following diagnostic procedures and identification of the physiological and emotional responses related to the diagnosis of cancer.

Diagnostic procedures

X-ray examination. Internal parts of the body may be examined for form and density by x-ray. A radiopaque substance may have to be administered before the examination to provide a contrast medium when soft tissues are to be viewed. For instance, the patient may receive barium by mouth if the oesophagus, stomach or intestine is to be viewed (see p. 495); for kidney and ureteric x-ray a radiopaque dye (an iodide preparation) is given intravenously (see p. 696). Mammography is an x-ray procedure used in examining soft tissue such as the breast. Computerized axial tomography (CAT) produces sharper images than ordinary x-rays and can detect very slight variations in tissue density. It is most useful in confirming a diagnosis of cancer and providing precise estimations of the size, shape and location of the neoplasm.

Radiology has become increasingly useful in the diagnosis and treatment of disease, but it is also potentially harmful unless it is carefully controlled and certain precautions are observed. As is the case with most drugs, an excessive amount can be damaging and may prove fatal. Even an x-ray for diagnostic purposes involves the absorption of a small amount of x-radiation by the patient. Most of the exposed cells recover, but there is a small residual injury which is irreversible—so small that it is insignificant. With many such exposures, however, the irreversible damage is cumulative. For this reason x-rays are to be used judiciously and with precautions.

Ultrasound examination. Sound waves are directed to deep body structures; the reflection or echoes of the waves depicts the condition of the organ or tissues under examination. The procedure is non-invasive and safe for the patient. The picture is examined for different densities of tissue and changes in structure and size.

Thermography. Thermography measures and plots the temperature of skin areas. An elevation of temperature occurs with malignant lesions and inflammation.

Radioactive isotopes. Radioactive isotopes and compounds are also used in diagnosing some cancers. A specific isotope or radioactive tagged compound is given according to the tissue being investigated; some tissues are known to absorb and concentrate a certain chemical. If a radioactive substance is administered, special instruments may then be used to detect and record the localization, distribution and concentration of the substance in the body. This process of detecting radiation within the body is known as *scanning*. The first radioactive isotope used for this purpose was iodine[131] to detect disease of the thyroid. Since then a number of radioactive isotopes have been introduced for both diagnostic and therapeutic purposes. Scanning may be used to detect both primary and secondary cancerous lesions.

Examples of some radioactive chemicals used in diagnosis are iodine[131] (I^{131}) in thyroid disease, rose bengal in liver disease, gold[198] (Au^{198}) in liver disease, radioiodinated serum albumin (RISA) in brain disease and for tracing circulation in the lung, chromium[51] (Cr^{51}) in red blood cell studies, iron[59] (Fe^{59}) in iron absorption and haemoglobin studies, calcium[47] (Ca^{47}) in bone disease, and strontium[85] (Sr^{85}) in bone disease. For a discussion of the nature of radioisotopes and the nursing care of patients who receive a radioactive isotope, please see the section on Internal Radiotherapy in this chapter.

Biopsy and histological examinations. A biopsy is performed to obtain a specimen of tissue to determine whether the cells are cancerous, the type of cancer cells and the degree of differentiation of the cells. Samples of tissue may be obtained by aspiration—a technique which involves removing a small plug of tissue using a needle and syringe—or by open excision of a section of tissue under local or general anaesthesia.

Histological examination of tumour tissue is done periodically to determine the effectiveness of treatment or to monitor progression of the patient's disease.

Clonogenic assay involves the growth of human tumour cells on a special culture medium to predict specific chemotherapy for the individual patient. Culture and sensitivity assays of human tumour cell responsiveness to chemotherapeutic agents provides for more effective drug treatment of cancer.

Exfoliative cytological tests. These tests involve the microscopic examination of smears of secretion or fluid taken from a body cavity. Cells are continuously shed from the epithelial surface tissue of the body cavities; this process is referred to as exfoliation or desquamation. Normally, cell replacement by the basal layer of epithelium parallels the exfoliation. Cancer may attack the epithelial lining of organs or body cavities, and some of the neoplastic cells become separated from the tissue and appear in the secretions found on the internal surface of the cavity. Cancer may be detected through recognition of these malignant cells before there are any other recognizable signs or symptoms, resulting in early successful treatment. Specimens may be taken from the cervix, vagina, respiratory tract, mouth, oesophagus, stomach, urinary tract, prostate and the pleural and peritoneal cavities. The examination generally may be referred to as a Pap smear; 'Pap' is derived from Papanicolaou, the name of the physician who introduced the use of smears for cytological examination. 'Pap smear' in clinical practice refers to a vaginal smear. In the United States, an annual vaginal or cervical Pap smear of all women over 30 years of age is recommended by the National Cancer Society. The increase in this practice has led to early recognition and treatment of cancer of the uterus in many women and may be correlated to the recent decline of deaths due to uterine cancer.

In the United Kingdom, both the Royal College of Nursing and the Royal College of Obstetricians and Gynaecologists recommend that all sexually active women and all women over 30 years of age should have a cervical Pap smear at least once every three years. Other organizations, such as well woman clinics, are now recommending that women should be given an annual cervical smear test.

Endoscopy. This is the introduction of a lighted tube (endoscope) into a body passage or organ for direct inspection of the area. At the same time a biopsy may be obtained by means of a biting forceps passed through the endoscope. This method of examination may be used in the larynx (laryngoscopy), bronchi (bronchoscopy), oesophagus (oesophagoscopy), stomach (gastroscopy), colon (colonoscopy), sigmoid (sigmoidoscopy) and rectum (proctoscopy). These are discussed later in this book in connection with the specific sites.

Haematological and serological tests. Some serological tests are used for certain types of malignant neoplasia. For example, the serum acid phosphatase level is used in investigation for carcinoma of the prostate; it is elevated when the disease is present. Blood and plasma cell evaluations are important in diagnosis and assessment of malignant disease of the bone marrow and reticuloendothelial system.

Physiological responses to cancer
The physiological manifestations and effects of

cancer depend upon the location of the neoplasm, its stage, and whether there are secondary conditions such as ulceration, haemorrhage, infection and metastases. With few exceptions, cancer is a space-occupying lesion. It may obstruct a passageway, compress blood vessels, neighbouring tissue or organs, exert pressure on regional nerves causing pain or even paralysis, or it may interfere with normal function by its invasion and replacement of normal tissue.

Unfortunately, in the early stage of some cancers, signs or symptoms are not evident to the host. The presence of any one of the early disturbances (see p. 146) does not necessarily mean that cancer has developed, but early recognition followed by prompt treatment increases the chances for cure and survival. Frequently at the onset cancer does not cause pain.

As the lesion grows, it outstrips its blood supply and so there are inadequate supplies of oxygen and nutrients for the tumour and the normal tissue. Necrosis of a portion of the tissue results, with subsequent ulceration. Vessels may be eroded, leading to *chronic haemorrhage* and *anaemia*. If the bone marrow is involved, the individual will experience anaemia and also deficient leucocyte and thrombocyte production.

Frequently there is marked *loss of weight and strength* as the rapidly growing cells compete with normal cells for nutrients, and *disturbances develop in the normal metabolic and physiological processes* throughout the body.

Disfigurement and amputations associated with the involvement of superficial tissues and limbs handicap the individual and cause a disturbing change in body image.

Infection also can be a serious problem as a result of decreased efficiency in immunological responses and defence mechanisms and the patient's general debility.

Pain usually develops following the initial stage of the cancer, but may be associated with early development if the neoplasm is close to a sensory nerve or within bone tissue. The pain of cancer generally becomes progressively more severe as the disease infiltrates more and more tissue, causes obstruction, and/or metastasizes.

General debility and malnutrition progressively become severe if the patient's disease is not arrested and nutritional needs are inadequately met. The patient becomes emaciated, extremely weak and has a poor colour. This state may be referred to as *cachexia*.

Emotional responses to diagnosis of cancer
An important effect of malignant disease is the *emotional disturbance* it creates. All ill persons usually experience some psychological as well as physical stress, but this is especially true of those who are advised or even suspect that they have cancer. The individual's anxiety may be concerned with a belief that all cancer is incurable, fear of a prolonged painful illness and death, unfulfilled goals, or the distress that his illness or death will create for the family. The behavioural response will vary from one person to another, depending upon each one's circumstances (e.g. familial experience of cancer) and previous attitude and pattern of responses to stressful situations. Some patients become very depressed and give up; others may withdraw and avoid any discussion or mention of the problem but may show their anxiety in other ways, such as restlessness, inability to sleep and loss of interest in everything and everyone. Certain patients may be resentful that this should happen to them and show anger, and a few become completely disorganized.

Some of the disturbances and discomfort exhibited by the patient with cancer may be due to the effects of the treatment being used (surgery, radiation, and chemotherapy). In some instances, the signs and symptoms of the disease become more severe for a period as a result of the treatment; such effects may be classified as *iatrogenic* (i.e. caused by medical intervention).

IDENTIFICATION OF PATIENT PROBLEMS

Table 9.3 cites three problems common to patients and families at the time of a medical diagnosis of cancer. Identification of factors which influence the patient's and family's responses is important in planning specific intervention. Behavioural responses characteristic of the diagnostic categories are identified. Care is more realistic and patient-centred if the nurse is aware of individual differences and recognizes that fear, anxiety and anticipated grief are normal and useful defence mechanisms for those faced with a diagnosis of cancer and an uncertain future.

Goals during the diagnostic phase
The patient's and family's goals relevant to the diagnostic phase of cancer are to:
1 Reduce the level of anxiety and fear.
2 Communicate feelings and concerns.
3 Minimize the impact of anticipated grief, anxiety and fear on patient participation in diagnostic procedures.
4 Acquire an understanding of the disease, treatment plan and anticipated results.

NURSING INTERVENTION

Planning and implementing nursing intervention for the cancer patient involves the following considerations.

1. Assessment. Prior to planning and initiating nursing intervention for the patient and family faced with a diagnosis of cancer, the nurse should identify:

Table 9.3 Problems likely to be encountered by the patient and family at the time of diagnosis of cancer.

Potential problems	Causes	Signs and symptoms
Anticipatory grieving	Potential threat to life Actual or potential loss of body part Actual and potential disruptions in family stability, roles and life-style	Crying, sobbing and general sadness Verbal expression of distress Denial of diagnosis of cancer and impending treatment Expressions of feeling of guilt Expressions of feeling anger Changes in eating habits Changes in sleeping patterns Changes in activity level Absence of expression of feelings and concerns Withdrawal Avoidance of discussion of diagnosis
Lack of knowledge of the disease, initiation of treatment and implications for self and family	Information not yet provided Lack of readiness for receiving information Anxiety, grief and denial interfering with perception and acceptance	Need for knowledge Does not utilize available resources for information Does not keep appointments for diagnostic tests or treatment Decreased attention span Refusal to accept treatment Does not participate in discussions of diagnosis and treatment
Anxiety	The diagnosis of cancer Future prognosis uncertain Lack of control of events Fear of treatment, pain, mutilation and death	Short attention span Difficulties in making decisions Expressions of anger, denial, fear and anxiety Increased pulse and respiratory rates Increased perspiration Hyperactivity or decreased activity Changes in sleeping pattern Withdrawal from communication with others

- *Patient and family supports and resources.* Are there family members and friends with whom the patient can share feelings and concerns and obtain support? Do these individuals live close to the patient and/or treatment centre? What resources are there in the family unit and community to assist with transport and care? What resources exist in the community to provide support for the family? How have the patient and family dealt with stress in the past and what resources have they found helpful?
- *Pre-existing psychosocial stressors.* What circumstances exist within the family and environment that may influence responses to the current stress? Examples of pre-existing psychosocial stressors might include marriage difficulties, children having problems, unemployment or an unstable work situation, recent experience of cancer within the family or death of a family member as a result of cancer, loneliness caused by the other members of the family living at a distance from the patient.
- *Specific fears and concerns.* What are the major concerns and fears of the patient and family members and how do they think these will affect their present and future relationship and life-style?

What help and support do they require now? Are their fears and anxiety realistic and are they interfering with the diagnostic and treatment plans?
- *Patient and family expectations of the health-care team.* What is their prior experience with illness and medical care? Do they perceive the doctor and/or nurse as sources of information about the disease and treatment plan?
- *Present level of understanding and factors which may influence learning.* Do the patient and family have an understanding of the illness, the type and purpose of the treatment(s) and the need for the procedures and hospitalization? What factors exist that might interfere with learning? For example, cultural belief, language or perceptual problems, or denial of illness may influence their appreciation of the situation and their responses. Are they receptive to explanations and teaching? Do they show confidence in members of the health-care team?

2 Communication. The expression of feelings and concerns by the patient is facilitated when the atmosphere is warm and caring. Excessive cheerfulness or uncomfortable silences hinder the establishment of a trusting relationship. The nurse should spend time with the patient and his family, helping them to express their feelings and encouraging a positive attitude. Privacy is provided for the patient and family to talk together and comfort each other. Members of the care team should give consistent and direct messages to both the patient and his family; conflicting information will only increase their anxiety. Information given to them by the doctor about the patient's disease, treatment and prognosis should be shared with all those caring for the patient. Anxiety and denial may interfere with comprehension; information usually needs to be repeated and misconceptions corrected.

If the nurse can understand and accept the fears and concerns of the patient and his family, she will be better equipped not only to respond to them as people (even if their responses of anger and frustration cause them to behave uncharacteristically) but also to come to terms with her own personal feelings.

3 Planning and initiating patient and family teaching. The patient and his family are told about the treatment plan, procedures and anticipated effects as well as about the disease. Information should be given in short sessions with new information building on previous explanations. Repetition is important. Written material and the use of illustrations help to simplify and reinforce learning. The degree to which the patient and family understand the situation should be assessed continuously and questions encouraged.

EXPECTED OUTCOMES

1 The patient and his family express less anxiety and fear.
2 The patient and his family show increased interest and participation both in the care that is planned and also within the context of the family relationship.
3 The patient adheres to the medical and nursing care plans.
4 The patient and family members participate in discussions and ask pertinent questions about the disease, treatment plan and prognosis.

TREATMENT

Cancer may be treated by surgery, ionizing radiation, drugs, hormones, immunotherapy or a combination of these.

SURGERY

Surgery plays an important role in cancer management. Surgical biopsy may be performed for diagnosis and to evaluate the effectiveness of treatment. Surgical excision is considered the most effective

therapy, provided the disease is still localized. The operation may be simple, as in the case of a basal cell cancer of the skin, or it may be quite radical and probably disfiguring. The lymphatics and lymph nodes which drain the area may also be removed if there is evidence of regional involvement. In some breast cancers, surgery may involve the removal of unaffected glands which secrete hormones that are supportive of the so-called hormone-dependent neoplasm; for example, in breast cancer the ovaries and adrenal glands may be removed.

Palliative surgery may be performed to: decrease symptoms caused by the tumour mass, remove obstructions, reduce the source of hormones (ovaries, testicles or adrenal glands), or to insert equipment for chemotherapy into a body part or organ. Neurosurgical procedures such as a nerve block and cordotomy may be carried out for management of persistent severe pain.

RADIOTHERAPY

Radiation may be used alone or in conjunction with surgery or chemotherapy to treat cancer. It may be derived from an external source, or from a radioactive substance placed within the body or applied to the surface.

Radiation is composed of electromagnetic waves, or streams of nuclear particles from atoms of a radioactive substance. The sources of diagnostic and therapeutic radiation are the x-ray machine and radioactive isotopes.

Units of measurement of radiation
Several units are used in referring to amounts of radiation.[8] The Système Internationale (SI) units are listed, with the former labels in parenthesis as the latter may still be used.[9]

The strength or activity of a radiation source is referred to as the *becquerel* (curie). The absorbed or therapeutic dosage is expressed in *coulombs* (roentgens) which indicate the intensity of the radiation exposure. The gray (rad) is a unit of measurement of the amount of absorbed ionizing radiation (1 gray = 100 rad). The *sievert* (rem) may be defined as the dose equivalent or biological effectiveness of the radiation received (1 sievert = 100 rem).

Types of radiation used
The forms of radiation commonly used for therapy include x-rays, gamma rays, electrons and beta rays. Two or more radiation beams are usually combined in treatment.

X-ray radiation. X-rays are electromagnetic waves which are produced in a special vacuum tube. An

---

[8] Nave & Nave (1985), pp. 370–371.
[9] Hay & Hughes (1983).

electric current of high voltage is passed into an electron source at one end of the tube. Freed electrons rapidly bombard a metal plate (tungsten or molybdenum) at the opposite end of the tube, resulting in the emission of electromagnetic waves (x-rays). Wavelengths can be varied; the higher the voltage of the electrical current applied to the tube, the more penetrating are the x-rays produced. As a result, high or super voltage machines are used in the treatment of cancer in deep-lying structures. Lower voltage machines which produce low-energy rays are used in diagnostic procedures and in the treatment of superficial neoplasms. Heavy dense substances, such as bone tissue, barium, iodides and lead absorb x-rays; soft tissues and less dense elements do not absorb these electromagnetic waves, which is why barium or iodide preparations are used in radiological examination of certain body areas.

Radioactive isotopes. The second source of radiation used in diagnosis and therapy is radioactive isotopes which yield electromagnetic waves (gamma rays) and radiation particles. The latter are fragments of the nuclei of the isotopes. The radiation emitted by these elements is due to instability in their nuclei. Before discussing radioisotope therapy, a brief explanation of the nature of radioactive isotopes may be necessary.

Varying forms of the same element may occur as the result of differences in atomic weights, and are referred to as *isotopes*. The isotopes of an element have a constant number of protons in the nuclei, identical atomic numbers and similar chemical properties, but they differ in the number of neutrons in the nuclei; this results in the variance in atomic weights.[10] To illustrate, there are two isotopes of hydrogen (H)—deuterium (H^2) and tritium (H^3). They each have an atomic number of 1, which is the same as hydrogen. The nucleus of the regular hydrogen atom contains one proton and no neutrons. The deuterium nucleus has one proton and one neutron, making the atomic weight 2; and the atomic weight of tritium is 3 because its atomic nucleus contains one proton and two neutrons.

---

[10] *Atomic structure.* The atom of an element consists of electrons (negatively charged particles), protons (positively charged particles) and neutrons (neutral particles). The protons and neutrons form a dense core, or nucleus, around which the electrons revolve in rings or orbits.

Example: One atom of oxygen consists of eight electrons, eight protons and eight neutrons.

Atomic number. The atomic number of an element is equal to the number of protons or the number of electrons, since both are the same.

Atomic weight or mass. Protons and neutrons are the heavy particles of the atom. The atomic weight, or mass, of an element is equal to the sum of the protons and neutrons in an atom. The mass of an electron is equal to roughly 1/2000 of that of a proton.

Those elements which have an atomic weight greater than 209 tend to be unstable.[11] For example, radium, an unstable element with an atomic weight of 226, has 88 protons and 138 neutrons in its atomic nucleus. The atoms of unstable elements constantly undergo some disintegration or decay until stability is established. This disintegration gives rise to the emission of particles and high-energy electromagnetic waves, and the element or isotope is said to be radioactive. The period of time in which the radioactivity (instability) of an isotope is reduced by half is referred to as the *half-life* of the isotope; this varies from seconds to years with different isotopes.

The particles emitted by the isotope are of two types, alpha (α) and beta (β). The alpha particles are capable of penetrating only a few centimetres of air and a fraction of a millimetre of tissue and are therefore of little therapeutic value. The beta particles are capable of penetrating surface tissue. The waves of energy released in radioactivity are known as gamma (γ) rays, which are similar to x-rays. These are highly penetrating and are capable of passing through concrete several feet thick. A dense metal such as lead is required for shielding from gamma radiation.

Types of radiotherapy

External radiotherapy. This is usually given by a megavoltage x-ray machine which delivers a sharply defined radiation beam with minimal side scatter of rays. It permits penetration without radiation affecting the skin and there is less absorption by bone and the surrounding healthy tissue.

Types of machine include the kilovoltage x-ray machine which produces straight x-rays, the cobalt-60 machine which produces gamma rays, the linear accelerator which produces photon beams, and the electronic linear accelerator which produces photon electron beams.

Equipment that delivers radiation is installed in shielded rooms. While a treatment is in progress, only the patient remains in the room. A means of communication between the patient and the radiographer is provided and a window is available through which the patient may be observed. The size and structure of the machine may be overwhelming to the patient who is left alone during the therapy. An explanation about the machine and its action is necessary to reduce the patient's fears. The patient is positioned prior to treatment and is directed to remain immobile until further instructions are given by the technician.

Internal radiotherapy or brachytherapy. Radioisotopes may be introduced into the body or applied topically to deliver radiation to an affected part. The radioactive element may be encased or sealed within a non-radioactive metal that screens out alpha and beta

---

[11] Flitter (1976).

waves, or the isotope may be unsealed and in liquid form. The radiation may be delivered by administering the radioisotope orally or intravenously, placing it within a body cavity, or implanting it interstitially in the affected area.

The selection of a radioisotope which is to be administered orally or intravenously is based on the affinity of the affected tissue or organ for a particular element. The uptake and concentration of the radioisotope is comparable to that of the non-radioactive form of the element. For instance, radioactive phosphorus (P^{32}) is administered orally or intravenously, and is concentrated in bone tissue from which its radiation readily penetrates to the bone marrow. This accounts for its use in treating polycythaemia (rubra) vera and myelogenous leukaemia. Radioactive iodine (I^{131}) is taken up by the thyroid tissue and is concentrated in the thyroid gland. It may be used in the diagnosis and treatment of thyroid disease.

Colloidal radioactive gold^{198} (Au^{198}), which emits both beta and gamma radiation, is used principally in the treatment of pleural or peritoneal effusion due to cancer of the lung or cancer within the abdomen. The gold suspension is injected into the pleural or peritoneal cavity and the patient is turned every 15 minutes (side, prone, opposite side, back, and sitting positions) for 2 hours, then every half hour for 2 hours and hourly for 3 hours to provide even distribution within the cavity. The gold preparation that is injected is purple; as a result, leakage at the site of injection is readily detected and special precautions are taken in the changing and disposal of the dressing and linens to protect the handler from radiation. A patient who receives radioactive gold is usually very ill; should death occur, the body is conspicuously tagged as having had the radioisotope, and the mortuary is advised as to the necessary precautions.

Radioisotopes sealed in a a metal case are used therapeutically. The encasement containing the radioactive element may be in the form of needles, seeds, tubes, wires or moulds. They are placed within the tissue or a body cavity for a prescribed period of time and then removed, unless the radioisotope used has a short half-life. Seeds which generally contain radon^{222} (Rn^{222}) are frequently permanently implanted; radon is an inert gas that is formed by the disintegration of radium and is radioactive. Its half-life is short (approximately 3.8 days).

Moulds are designed specially for specific areas of the body and may be applied directly to a mucous membrane lining or to the skin.

The implantation of these sealed forms is done under aseptic conditions in an operating theatre. Radioisotopes commonly used in the sealed form in therapy include:

Radium^{226} (Ra^{226})	Half-life	1580 years
Radon^{222} (Rn^{222})	Half-life	3.8 days

Cobalt^{60} (Co^{60})	Half-life	5.3 years
Gold^{198} (Au^{198})	Half-life	2.7 days
Iodine^{131} (I^{131})	Half-life	8.0 days
Phosphorus^{32} (P^{32})	Half-life	14.3 days

Radioisotopes which are not sealed within metal are used in liquid form. They may be given orally or intravenously and are selected on the basis of the specific affinity of the affected tissue for a particular element. The liquid radioisotope may be introduced directly into a body cavity to treat a malignant effusion or may be placed in a non-metal capsule or balloon for irradiation within a body cavity such as the urinary bladder. Examples of radioisotopes used unsealed in therapy include:

Iodine^{131} (I^{131})
Phosphorus^{32} (P^{32})
Gold^{198} (Au^{198})
Bromine^{82} (Br^{82})
Sodium^{20} (Na^{20})

Effects of radiation
In radiation, the rays and particles that are emitted damage or destroy the cells which they enter by the ionizing (molecular dissociation) effect produced. The injury may result in mutations by disrupting chromosomes, or in the inability of the cells to reproduce. If not destroyed, much of the tissue recovers but some permanent residual damage occurs. Subsequent exposures result in increasing accumulations of permanent cellular damage.

The effects of a *prescribed dose* of radiation are influenced by the following:

1 The rate at which the dose is administered. If it is divided and spread over a long period of time, it will produce less damage than if given in one dose.
2 The size of body area being irradiated. The larger the area is, the greater the effects.
3 The depth of penetration of the rays. Low-energy level radiation is absorbed by the skin and superficial structures. Megavoltage or high-energy level therapy minimizes skin destruction and penetrates deeper tissues.
4 The particular tissue cells receiving radiation. Some types of cells are more susceptible to ionizing radiation than others. Haematopoietic cells of the bone marrow, lymphocytes, gonadal cells and those of the mucous membrane of the mouth and gastrointestinal tract are the most sensitive. These are cells which divide and reproduce rapidly. Malignant neoplastic cells which also reproduce rapidly and are poorly differentiated are more susceptible to radiation than normal cells.
5 Individual variability in response. Some individuals have greater reactions than others to similar dosage.

Fortunately, severe reactions are not often seen; increased knowledge and improved therapeutic techniques have reduced radiation side-effects.

Reactions that may occur may be local and/or systemic, and all patients manifest some emotional response. Some patients experience only feelings of tiredness for 2–3 days following each treatment, while others develop disturbances of varying degrees of severity.

Local reactions occur in the area being treated; the therapeutic rays are directed at the cancer but overlying and surrounding healthy tissues also receive some radiation. Usually no reactions are evident for several days or weeks after the treatments are commenced.

Some local skin reaction may be expected with external radiation, since the therapeutic rays are directed through the skin overlying the cancer site. The severity of the skin reaction may be described as mild, moderate or severe. The manifestations of each stage are:

1 Mild reaction. The skin exhibits a slight redness for a brief period, with transitory epilation (loss of hair).
2 Moderate reaction. The skin is erythematous and dry, and some desquamation may occur. A temporary suppression of sweat gland activity develops, as well as some loss of hair.
3 Severe reaction. With larger doses and more sensitive skin, more severe responses are likely to occur. Marked erythema may be followed by purple discoloration, blister formation and moist desquamation. Ulcerated areas may appear and the patient experiences considerable discomfort. Healing is slow and leaves the skin dark, atrophied, thin, and very sensitive to heat, cold and trauma. There is also permanent epilation and destruction of sweat glands in the area.

The reactions of irradiated mucous membrane are similar to those of the skin. Dryness due to suppression of mucus secretion, ulceration and bleeding may follow. If the mouth, throat or gastrointestinal tract is involved, the irritation and damage to the mucous membrane lining frequently interfere with the intake of food and fluids, leading to malnutrition and dehydration; diarrhoea may also contribute to these complications.

If the larynx is treated, the patient is observed for possible oedema and occlusion of the airway which would necessitate prompt intubation or a tracheostomy.

Irradiation of the bladder or neighbouring structures may cause urinary frequency and pain. Radiotherapy of uterine cancer may result in some sloughing of the endometrium and vaginal mucosa. Vaginal discharge or bleeding may be troublesome.

Systemic reactions also occur in varying degrees of severity. Many patients experience anorexia and a sense of fatigue following a treatment. Some are nauseated and vomit, particularly if thoracic or abdominal viscera have been exposed. With large doses, the haematopoietic tissue may be depressed; anaemia,

leucopenia and thrombocytopenia may develop.

Aggressive radiation therapy of large, rapidly dividing tumours which are extremely sensitive to radiation may produce massive necrosis of the tumour cells and the release of potassium, phosphorus and uric acid. This is referred to as *acute tumour lysis*. Life-threatening complications include hyperkalaemia and acute renal failure.

As cited previously, most patients receiving radiation treatments experience some *psychological reaction*, especially when first advised of the need for therapy, and then with the initial treatment. This probably accentuates the nature of the disease, as many lay persons are familiar with the use of 'x-ray treatment' for cancer. Many persons may fear radiotherapy because of knowing or having heard of someone who had severe reactions to treatments before the present improved techniques were introduced. A third factor that causes an emotional reaction is fear of the radiation equipment, which at first appears rather ominous. If internal radiation is used, the patient may react to the precautions that are used to protect those in his environment.

Radiation safety factors
No one would dispute the value of radiation in medicine but, as already indicated, it can be biologically harmful. Like many other things in our environment it has both positive and negative potentials. The negative aspects depend mainly upon whether certain precautions are observed to protect the patient and attendant personnel. When using either external or internal diagnostic or therapeutic radiation, three basic principles regarding protection should be kept in mind and respected in practice. These involve *time, distance,* and *shielding.*

The first principle to be observed is that the shorter the period of time one spends in an area where x-rays or gamma rays are being emitted, the less hazardous is the exposure. When caring for a patient who contains a radioactive substance, necessary treatments and care should be well planned and expedited to minimize the time spent at the bedside. A monitoring badge should be worn so that the amount of exposure can be estimated. If this approaches what is considered the maximum level for safety, a reassignment of personnel is made.

The second basic fact important in radiation protection is that the greater the distance from the source, the less radiation will be received. When the distance is doubled, the intensity decreases by a factor of 4. For instance, at 1.2 m (4 feet) from the source there is only $\frac{1}{16}$ of the exposure that there would be at 0.3 m (1 foot) from the source.

Thirdly, effective shielding materials are available for protection. Ionizing rays lose energy when they come in contact with solid matter. The denser and thicker the matter, the fewer are the rays that will pass through it. Because of its density, lead is used extensively for shielding. Lead 3.12 mm (or ⅛ of an inch), will provide as much protection as several feet of concrete.

Nursing responsibilities in radiotherapy
The nurse caring for the patient whose treatment plan includes radiotherapy requires some understanding of radiation, its sources, how it is administered and its effects on body tissues. This is necessary for the nurse's role in reducing the patient's apprehension, providing the needed psychological support, preparing the patient for therapy and providing adequate postirradiation care. The nurse also requires an appreciation of the radiation hazards that may be experienced by those working in an environment of possible radiation exposure. Protective principles and measures must be familiar to and respected by all personnel working with radiotherapy.

1. Patient teaching. Many lay persons have erroneous ideas of radiation treatment. Some patients have the misconception that this type of treatment means that the disease is advanced, that the surgery that was performed was not successful and that this is a last resort. It is important for the patient to be advised of the purpose of the treatment and of the curative role of radiation in cancer.

Before the initial treatment, an explanation is made to the patient as to what he may expect and what is expected of him; understanding is a defence against fear. If external radiotherapy is to be used, a brief description of the machine, which may appear rather ominous, will help to reduce anxiety. He is advised that although he will be alone in the room he will be under constant observation by the radiotherapist or technician, with whom he may communicate. He is also told that the treatment period will be brief. He should be informed that no pain or sensation will be felt as the rays penetrate, and that it is important for him to maintain the position in which he is placed by the radiotherapist. Time should be taken to talk with the patient and his family, to answer questions, and to reassure them that the treatments are well controlled and adequate protection is used. It should be made clear to all concerned that the patient will not be radioactive following the treatment.

If the patient is to receive internal radiotherapy, it is necessary that the plan of treatment and aftercare be outlined to the patient and family; otherwise, the isolation and protective precautions that may have to be observed for a time are likely to cause great concern. Emphasis is given to the fact that such measures are temporary as well as necessary for the protection of family and friends who might visit, and for hospital staff.

In the case of an outpatient receiving external radiotherapy, possible minor reactions are discussed and the patient and family are advised that any other disorders should be reported promptly. Written instructions concerning skin and mouth care, the need for additional rest, nutritional and fluid intake and the importance of avoiding contact with infection are given. These instructions are reviewed with the patient and a family member, and time should be taken to listen to and answer their questions. They should be given the name of someone to contact if a question or concern arises at home. Emphasis is placed on the importance of keeping the appointment for the next treatment; if the patient is not well enough, the doctor or radiotherapist should be contacted.

2. Physical preparation. The skin of the area to be treated is gently cleansed with water only and dried. It should be intact and free of any lesions or infection. Blood cell counts (erythrocytes, leucocytes and thrombocytes), haemoglobin concentration, and blood urea and uric acid concentrations are usually determined and may be used as a base-line for comparison when assessing radiation reactions later. Special preparation for internal radiotherapy may be necessary, depending upon the site. For example, preparation for internal radiation therapy of uterine cancer may include perineal cleansing and shaving, a cleansing enema and a cleansing antiseptic vaginal douche. The patient will likely receive a general anaesthetic, so food and fluid are withheld as directed (usually for 4–6 hours) preceding the insertion of the applicator with the radioactive isotope.

3. Postexternal radiotherapy care.
(a) *Assessment.* Following the treatment, the skin of the area irradiated is examined daily for reaction; if the mouth was involved, it is checked for dryness and ulceration; the patient is observed for fatigue, weakness and anorexia. Blood studies are repeated and are noted for possible depression of the haematopoietic tissues (anaemia, leucopenia, thrombocytopenia). The temperature is recorded four times daily for 2–3 days for possible elevation, and any observed, or complained of, disturbance or change in body function, such as nausea and vomiting, is reported.

Reactions, their symptoms and severity, and the length of time they last will vary considerably with the site being treated and the amount of tissue irradiated.
(b) *Anxiety.* The occurrence of reactions may alarm the patient; he may interpret them as unfavourable progression of his disease. The nurse should recognize his discouragement, provide the necessary reassurance and explain that the reactions are not unexpected. She should stress their temporary nature and the fact that they are not an indication of a worsening of the cancer.
(c) *Skin integrity.* Some local skin reaction may be expected. The area is cleansed with tepid water and patted dry. Soap is not used and brisk rubbing is avoided. The radiologist usually outlines the area to

which the radiation beam is to be directed; these markings circumscribing the area should remain until the series of treatments is completed. Alcohol, powders, oils, lotions, creams and ointments are not used unless prescribed by the doctor. If the axilla has been irradiated, deodorants must not be applied. The site is kept dry and may be covered lightly with smooth cotton. Adhesive tape is never applied. Pressure is prevented by avoiding any restricting clothing and prolonged periods of lying on the area. No hot or cold applications are used on the site, which must also be protected from exposure to direct sunlight. If the face or neck has received radiation, male patients may be permitted to shave after a few days. If itching and irritation accompany the erythema, the radiotherapist is consulted. Applications of plain calamine lotion (i.e. without phenol) or unscented talcum powder (cornstarch) may be suggested if the area is dry. Later, when the erythema has disappeared, and if the skin is dry and desquamating, a light application of a water-soluble ointment may be permitted.

(d) *Diet and fluids.* Maintaining an adequate nutritional and fluid intake may be a problem because of anorexia and lethargy. A high-protein, high-calorie diet is necessary to promote the patient's resistance, healing and replacement of the tissue destroyed by radiation. An explanation of the importance of food and fluids should be made to the patient. Small amounts of those foods preferred by the patient, offered in small amounts at frequent intervals through the day, may be more acceptable than fewer, larger quantities. An increased fluid intake is encouraged to promote elimination of the products of tissue breakdown (e.g. creatinine).

An antiemetic preparation such as dimenhydrinate (Dramamine, Gravol) may be prescribed for oral or parenteral administration to control nausea.

(e) *Rest.* Extra rest is necessary during the first few days after the treatment, but the patient is encouraged to move about and have some activity. Rest periods are planned with the patient.

4. *Care during internal radiotherapy.* When radioisotopes are implanted or injected for therapeutic purposes, the patient becomes a temporary source of radioactivity. In addition to being concerned with the patient's reactions and psychological and physical needs, the nurse is concerned with the precautions necessary to protect herself and others from radiation that may be emitted from the patient and his body discharges in some instances.

The radioisotope laboratory is consulted as to the precautions to be used with each patient who receives internal radiation; care and precautions vary with different radioisotopes.

(a) *Precautionary measures.* The nurse caring for a patient receiving internal radiotherapy should know the half-life of the radioisotope used and, when it is a liquid, it is also necessary to know how it is excreted from the body. The three safety factors that apply to protection from external radiation sources—time, distance and shielding—must also be kept in mind and respected (see p. 154).

The patient is usually placed in a single room for a period of time equal to the half-life of the radioisotope used. A notice which indicates radioactivity is placed on the door. Preferably the room should have both a window through which the patient can be observed and an intercommunication system, so that the time spent in the room by staff is minimized.

The patient is likely to be apprehensive or resent his isolation unless he understands the plan of treatment, and realizes that it is temporary as well as necessary for the protection of others.

The nurse's time in the room is restricted to a minimum. Those giving care should work quickly and remain only long enough to give the necessary care, having thoughtfully anticipated the patient's needs and planned ahead of time the observations that should be made, as well as the details of care to be carried out. All nurses participating in the patient's care are required to wear a monitoring badge which records the amount of radiation exposure.

Specific directions are necessary regarding the disposal of excreta and contaminated dressings. For instance, radioactive iodine is eliminated in the urine, so it should be collected in a lead-encased container and taken to the laboratory, where it is stored until the radioactivity has decayed. Usually, no special precautions are required for linen or utensils used by the patient.

Any radioactive implant is handled with long forceps, never with the hands. In the event that the implant might become dislodged, a lead storage container is kept at the bedside. If there is a chance of skin contamination during patient contact (as with radioactive iodine), the nurse should wear gloves and carefully wash her hands with soap and running water following each contact with the patient or articles handled by the patient.

The nurse should know the time at which the temporary implant is to be removed. The patient may be returned to the radiotherapy department for this procedure or it may be done in the patient's room. The equipment should be ready in advance and, if necessary, the person responsible for the removal reminded. If the procedure is carried out in the patient's room, the nurse should be familiar with the disposition of the implant.

If the implantations are permanent (e.g. radon seeds), precautions are observed for the half-life of the radioisotope. A permanent type of implant may be used in the treatment of cancer of the urinary bladder. In this case all urine is collected and checked for radioactivity during the half-life of the implant.

The patient is told about the elimination of the isotope so he will not think he is a continuing source of danger to his family and others.

(b) *Anxiety.* The precautionary measures may be

frightening to the patient even if it was explained before the radioisotope was implanted or administered. It is helpful if there is a telephone available during the period of restrictions so he can talk with his family and friends. A radio, television or reading material may also help to relieve the boredom and anxiety. Long periods of total isolation are avoided; brief visits or frequent contact via the communication system will let the patient know he has not been forgotten.

(c) *Assessment*. The patient's temperature is taken every 4 hours; an elevation over 38°C. (100°F) is reported. As with external radiotherapy, any complaint or observed change in body function is reported to the doctor. Blood tests may be done to detect possible changes that might indicate some depression of haematopoietic tissues.

(d) *Physical care*. Nutritional and fluid intake require the same attention as that suggested for the patient who has received external radiation. The usual hygiene care is provided; the nurse works quickly when caring for the patient, keeping the time spent at the patient's bedside to a minimum without making the patient feel at all neglected.

In the case of mouth, lip or tongue therapy specific orders are received as to mouth care. Following a mouthwash, the solution is examined before it is disposed of to make sure no implants have been dislodged.

When the patient has had a uterine implantation, the patient may be required to remain in the dorsal recumbent position. Massage and a small pillow to fill in the space in the 'small of the back' may relieve some discomfort. An indwelling catheter is usually passed at the time the implant is inserted, since the patient is not likely to be able to use the bedpan because of the applicator which protrudes from the vagina. A low-fibre diet may be ordered so that the patient will be less likely to have a bowel movement.

If a liquid isotope has been given, the patient may be ambulatory but is requested to remain in his room during the precautionary period.

C. CHEMOTHERAPY

Drug therapy has assumed increasing importance in recent years in the treatment of some cancers. It may be effective in curing some cancers while in others it produces remissions. Chemotherapy has certainly increased survival and the quality of life for many patients. It may be used alone or in conjunction with surgery or radiation therapy. Unfortunately, the drugs used are non-specific in action, and many are highly toxic and damaging to normal cells as well as to neoplastic cells. As in radiation therapy, the cells that proliferate rapidly are those most susceptible to the toxicity, and patients may experience irritation and ulceration of the mouth and gastrointestinal tract and suppression of the haematopoietic tissues.

The drugs used may be classified as alkylating agents, antimetabolites, plant alkaloids, antibiotics, hormones, steroids, immune agents, or miscellaneous (a few that are used which do not fit into any of the above categories). Chemotherapeutic agents may be used in combinations. Repeated administration of the drugs is more effective in reducing the size of neoplasms than a single course of treatment.

The *alkylating agents*, also known as antimitotic drugs, act within the nucleus of the cell and alter the deoxyribonucleic acid (DNA) molecules, resulting in inhibition of cell growth and reproduction. Their activity is not specific to any one stage of the cell cycle, although reproducing cells are more vulnerable.

The *antimetabolites* resemble substances that are essential to cellular activities, and which are therefore taken up by the cells. These preparations are sufficiently different from normal metabolites as to alter metabolism and inhibit growth and reproduction. They function at a specific phase of the life-cycle of the cell. They include folic acid and purine antagonists and pyrimidine analogues.

The *plant alkaloids* currently in use are derived from periwinkle plants. They block cell reproduction during metaphase (second stage of division of the cell nucleus).

Certain *antibiotics* have been found to be of value in inhibiting some types of neoplastic cells. They act by interfering with DNA and/or RNA synthesis of the cells.

The *hormones* used in the treatment of malignant disease alter the synthesis of RNA and protein in tissues that contain steroid-binding receptors. Adrenal corticosteroids are commonly used because they suppress cell reproduction through inhibition of cellular protein synthesis.

Table 9.4 lists some drugs used in cancer therapy and indicates the method(s) by which they may be administered, the cancer disease in which they may be used, and the possible toxic effects. New drugs are introduced frequently, and the search continues for a drug that will be selective and prove toxic to malignant cells without damaging normal tissue.

Administration of chemotherapeutic agents
The channels by which anticancer drugs are administered are intravenous, oral, intramuscular, intrathecal, intracavity, and intra-arterial.

Intravenous administration of chemotherapeutic drugs requires careful selection of the vein because of the need for repeated administrations. Most chemotherapeutic agents are extremely irritating to tissue and may cause thrombosis of the vein and necrosis of tissue if infiltration occurs. The injection site should be observed closely and frequently for signs of redness or swelling and the patient questioned as to pain, tenderness or burning. Prompt identification and reporting of site infiltration is important to prevent excessive and unnecessary tissue damage. Treatment of drug extravasation includes the admin-

Table 9.4 Drugs used in cancer therapy.*

Chemotherapeutic agent	Methods of administration	Uses in cancer	Toxic effects
Alkylating agents (Act by damaging DNA so cell replication is impaired)			*General* Extravasation (tissue necrosis) Nausea and vomiting Bone marrow suppression Alopecia Non-lymphocytic leukaemia Male sterility, early female menopause
Mustine hydrochloride	Intravenous	Lymphomas (e.g. Hodgkin's disease)	*Specific* As above
Chlorambucil (Leukeran)	Oral	Lymphomas Chronic lymphocytic leukaemia Ovarian carcinoma	Bone marrow suppression Rashes (other side-effects uncommon)
Cyclophosphamide (Endoxana)	Oral Intravenous	Lymphomas Chronic lymphocytic leukaemia Solid tumours	General Haemorrhagic cystitis
Busulphan (Myleran)	Oral	Chronic myeloid leukaemia	General Hyperpigmentation of skin Pulmonary fibrosis (rarely)
Melphalan (Alkeran)	Oral	Myeloma Myelometosis Solid tumours Lymphomas	General Especially bone marrow suppression
Thiotepa	Intravenous Intracavity	Malignant effusions Bladder cancer Breast cancer	General
Antimetabolites (Are incorporated into the nucleus of cells or combine irreversibly with cell enzymes, so preventing normal cell division)			
Mercaptopurine (Puri-Nettol)	Oral	Acute leukaemias	General Interacts with allopurinol
Fluorouracil	Oral Intravenous Topically for malignant skin lesions	Metastatic colon cancer Solid tumours, especially breast cancer	Toxicity rare Bone marrow suppression (occasional) Mucositis—a cerebellar syndrome (rarely)
Cytarabine (Cytosar)	Subcutaneous Intravenous Intrathecal	Acute myeloblastic leukaemia	Bone marrow suppression
Methotrexate	Oral Intravenous Intramuscular Intrathecal	Acute lymphoblastic leukaemia in children Choriocarcinoma Non-Hodgkin's lymphomas Solid tumours	Bone marrow suppression Mucositis Accumulation of drug in renal failure and when serous effusions present Methotrexate interacts with Aspirin, phenylbutazone, probenecid and anti-epileptics

Table 9.4—*continued*

Chemotherapeutic agent	Methods of administration	Uses in cancer	Toxic effects
Thioguanine (Lanvis)	Oral	Acute myeloid leukaemia	General

Azathiaprine (Imuran) is an antimetabolite but is commonly used as an immunosuppressant

Plant alkaloids (Interferes with all division)

Vincristine (Oncovin)	Intravenous	Acute leukaemias Some solid tumours	Peripheral and autonomic nerve toxicity (peripheral paraesthesia, numbness and constipation) Alopecia Bone marrow suppression (rare)
Vinblastine (Velbe)	Intravenous	Lymphomas Some solid tumours (e.g. testicular teratoma)	Bone marrow suppression (less neurotoxicity than vincristine)

Cytotoxic antibiotics

Actinomycin D (Dactinomycin)	Intravenous	Paediatric cancers	Tissue necrosis Nausea and vomiting Bone marrow suppression Alopecia Mucositis
Doxorubicin hydrochloride (Adriamycin)	Intravenous	Acute leukaemias Lymphomas Solid tumours	Tissue necrosis Nausea and vomiting Bone marrow suppression Alopecia Cardiomyopathy
Bleomycin	Intravenous Intracavity	Lymphomas Some solid tumours Malignant effusions	Hyperpigmentation of skin Mucositis Raynaud's phenomenon Progressive pulmonary fibrosis Hypersensitivity—chills and fevers

Hormonal agents

1. *Oestrogens*

Stilboestrol	Oral	Breast and prostate cancer	Nausea Fluid retention Venous arterial thrombosis (in elderly males) Hypercalcaemia Impotence and gynaecomastia in males
Fosfestrol (Honvan)	Oral and intravenous		
Ethinyloestradiol	Oral		

2. *Progestogens*

Norethisterone (Utovlan)	Intramuscular	Possibly of use in breast cancer	Nausea Fluid retention
Gestronol hexanoate (Depostat)	Intramuscular	Endometrial carcinoma Hypernephroma	
Norethisterone	Intramuscular		
Medroxyprogesterone acetate	Oral or intramuscular		

3. *Androgens and anabolic steroids*

Drostanolone propionate (Masteril)	Intramuscular	Second or third line therapy for metastatic breast cancer	Acne Oedema Jaundice Virilism Hypercalcaemia Menstrual irregularities
Nandrolone	Intramuscular		

Table 9.4—*continued*

Chemotherapeutic agent	Methods of administration	Uses in cancer	Toxic effects

4. Hormone antagonists
    Aminoglutethimide
    (Orimeten)
	Oral	Postmenopausal breast cancer	Corticosteroid replacement must be given concurrently
			Drowsiness
			Drug eruption and fever

Tamoxifen (Nolvadex)	Oral	Postmenopausal breast cancer	Bone pain Hypercalcaemia
Other cytotoxic drugs Cisplatin (Neoplatin, Platinex, Platosin)	Intravenous	Ovarian carcinoma and testicular teratoma	Nausea and vomiting Nephrotoxicity Myelotoxicity Bearing loss and tinnitus Peripheral neuropathy
Hydroxyurea (Hydrea)	Oral	Chronic myeloid leukaemia	Bone marrow suppression Nausea Skin reactions
Procarbazine (Natulan)	Oral	Hodgkin's disease and other lymphomas Carcinoma of the bronchus	Bone marrow suppression Nausea Skin reactions (Also a mild monamine oxidase inhibitor so certain foods and alcohol are contraindicated)
Dacarbazine (DTIC-Dome)	Intravenous	Melanoma Second line therapy for Hodgkin's disease	Bone marrow suppression Nausea and vomiting

*This table is not intended to be comprehensive; the reader is referred to the *British National Formulary* (1986).

istration of a prescribed specific antidote (if available) for the drug, or a steroid preparation and the prompt application of ice packs to the site to decrease the spread of the drug.

A peripheral catheter may be inserted into a large vein, or a right atrial catheter may be introduced in patients receiving long-term or repeated courses of chemotherapy. The greater blood volume in the large vein and right atrium dilutes the medication, and thus decreases irritation to the vessel walls. The use of either of these channels reduces the possibility of extravasation of the drug into peripheral tissue and preserves the patient's peripheral veins. A right atrial catheter such as the Hickman catheter allows for greater patient mobility as it is left in and sealed with a cap when not in use. The catheter is flushed at regular intervals with a dilute solution of heparin to prevent blood coagulation in the catheter line.

Intrathecal administration of chemotherapeutic drugs is useful when the neoplasm involves the meninges. Administration is usually done by means of a lumbar puncture.

Intracavity administration of chemotherapeutic agents is usually done following aspiration of fluid from a body compartment such as the intrapleural space or the peritoneal cavity.

Intra-arterial infusion. The drug is introduced directly into the artery that supplies the malignant area. The drug circulates through the affected part in high concentration before it becomes diluted in the general circulation. An arterial catheter is introduced into the appropriate artery under fluoroscopy. For instance, in liver cancer, the organ may be infused with the drug of choice via a small catheter introduced into the hepatic artery. Since it is intra-arterial, pressure is required to overcome the arterial blood pressure. A small mechanical pump may be used which delivers a certain amount of the drug at a prescribed rate.

Intra-arterial perfusion is a more complex procedure, involving extracorporeal circulation, requiring the use of a pump-oxygenator (heart–lung machine). The venous blood from the affected part is diverted into the tube of the pump where the anticancer drug is added. The blood is returned to the artery that supplies the structure to be treated. The isolated circuit is maintained for 30–60 minutes. This method of treatment prevents the circulation of the toxic drug through the total body and maintains a higher concentration in the malignant tissue for a longer period. In some instances, on completion of the perfusion, the blood may be replaced by transfusion blood to prevent the toxic drug from entering the general circulation. Since some blood containing the drug may escape into the systemic circulation, the patient must still be observed for possible toxic reactions.

Preparation of chemotherapeutic agents. Drugs used in the treatment of cancer are very toxic; specific instructions as to the preparation, administration and side-effects of each agent should be carefully identified from the package guidelines, the pharmacy department and guidelines prepared by the hospital or clinic.

In preparing the chemotherapeutic agent, the surface of the preparation area is covered with an absorbent plastic-backed pad and a piece of lint-free paper. The equipment and supplies are placed on this surface. A disposable gown with tight fitting cuffs, two pairs of polyvinyl gloves, and safety splash goggles are worn. The nurse or doctor then prepares the medication using aseptic technique and taking precautions to prevent spillage or splattering. Care is taken to prevent the build-up of pressure in vials by adding small quantities of diluent at a time and withdrawing equal amounts of air. Similar precautions are taken when withdrawing medication from the vial. All the material, including swabs, vials, syringes, needles, disposable gown, mask and gloves are wrapped in the surface covering and placed in a box and plastic rubbish bag which is then tied shut and labelled. The prepared medication is labelled with the name of the drug, the dose, the date and time of preparation, the name of the person preparing it and the name of the patient who is to receive it. It should be noted that rubber or polythene gloves are not worn since some antineoplastic agents may penetrate these materials.

Nursing care of the patient receiving chemotherapy
Anticancer drugs generally cause side-effects that may be quite serious and distressing for some patients. The toxic reactions most commonly associated with the chemotherapeutic agents include bone marrow depression leading to anaemia, leucopenia and thrombocytopenia, stomatitis, nausea and vomiting, diarrhoea or constipation, and fluid retention. Since the side-effects vary with different drugs, it is essential that the nurse knows the chemotherapeutic agent given, the possible toxic reactions of that particular drug, their significance and how they are manifested.

Acute tumour lysis may cause hyperkalaemia, hyperuricaemia, hyperphosphataemia and acute renal failure in patients with large rapidly dividing tumours that are very sensitive to the chemotherapy. This is more likely to occur in patients with Burkitt's lymphoma or acute lymphoblastic leukaemia and is discussed further in Chapter 13.

The routine for administration varies with the drug used and with the patient's reactions to it. In some instances, a course of the anticancer drug is given over several days and then a period of time elapses before it is administered again. Some drugs are given in larger doses for a few days, and then in smaller maintenance doses. The dosage also is a very individual matter, being influenced by the patient's size and weight, whether one anticancer drug or a combination is being used, radiotherapy the patient may also have received, and reactions to the initial dose of the drug.

Patient and family teaching. The patient and family should be informed as to what to expect; otherwise, the side-effects of the drugs may engender alarm and hopelessness. When explaining the treatment plan and drug action, the potential benefits of the drug must be emphasized. The patient and family are advised that persons vary in their reactions to drugs, and the patient should tell the nurse or doctor if he feels different or observes any change in body function after he has received the drug.

The erythrocyte, leucocyte and thrombocyte counts and haemoglobin concentration are determined before the therapeutic regimen is commenced.

Assessment and management of side-effects. When a patient has been given an anticancer drug he is observed closely for manifestations of possible side-effects.

Leucopenia makes the patient very susceptible to infection; the avoidance of contact with persons with infection, frequent antiseptic mouthwash, and good skin care to keep it intact and free of lesions are preventive measures to be observed. The patient's temperature is taken regularly; an elevation above normal may indicate the onset of infection. Antibiotic therapy may be instituted with even a slight elevation of temperature or any other indication of infection. Blood cell counts are usually repeated daily or every other day; a marked decrease in the white blood cells is identified promptly and nursing measures are instituted to protect the patient from infection.

Anaemia may be manifested by weakness, complaints of constant tiredness, pallor and shortness of breath with even slight energy expenditure.

Depression of the bone marrow may also result in a deficiency of thrombocytes and ensuing impairment of the blood clotting process. The patient is observed for signs of haemorrhage, for example ecchymoses, blood in the stool or urine, bleeding into the sclera, or vaginal bleeding. When thrombocytopenia develops parenteral injections are avoided, if possible. Transfusions of whole blood or platelets may be given to support the patient while his bone marrow recovers.

(a) *Nutrition.* Many patients on chemotherapy experience nausea and vomiting which may be relieved by the use of an antiemetic such as dimen-hydrinate (Gravol, Dramamine) or nabilone (Cesamet), a synthetic drug related to tetrahydro-cannabinol. Nabilone may be administered prior to treatment and during the first 2–3 days of treatment. Anorexia is also a problem; every effort is made to encourage the patient to take nourishment and adequate fluids. Small amounts of high-calorie foods which may appeal to him, attractively served at frequent intervals rather than larger amounts served less often, are likely to be more acceptable. If the oral mucosa is irritated and sore, bland non-irritating foods are selected. A mouthwash just before and after each meal may help.

(b) *Bowel elimination*. Diarrhoea may be troublesome with the administration of an antimetabolite or anti-biotic chemotherapeutic agent. An antidiarrhoeic preparation may be prescribed; foods that seem to initiate stools should be identified and eliminated. Bulky foods that absorb fluid (such as bran) may be added to the patient's diet and prove helpful. If the diarrhoea persists dehydration may further compli-cate the patient's condition, and necessitate the administration of parenteral fluids.

(c) *Oral mucosa*. Stomatitis (inflammation of the oral mucosa) is not uncommon in patients receiving some anticancer drugs. The mucosa becomes inflamed and tender and may ulcerate, causing considerable discomfort and interference with the ingestion of food and fluids. The mucosa readily becomes infected.

(d) *Fluid balance*. Retention of fluid commonly occurs in patients receiving steroid drugs. The patient's fluid intake, output and weight should be recorded daily. Observations are made for dependent oedema.

Measures to prevent the development of tumour lysis syndrome include: maintenance of adequate hydration and urinary output to decrease the urinary concentration of uric acid and improve renal excretion of phosphorus; alkalinization of the urine prior to chemotherapy to prevent the precipitation of uric acid in the renal tubules; and the administration of allopurinol to inhibit the formation of uric acid. The serum levels of calcium, phosphate, potassium, uric acid, creatinine and urea nitrogen are monitored closely and the urine output is measured hourly. The patient is assessed for signs of fluid overload and impaired renal functioning.

(e) *Safety*. Sensory and motor innervation may be impaired in a patient receiving one of the plant alka-loid preparations. He may experience some loss of sensation, coordination and reflexes, and severe constipation. Precautions should be taken to prevent possible falls. The patient is encouraged to move and prevent long periods of pressure on any one area.

(f) *Self-image*. Many patients receiving chemotherapy suffer a temporary loss of hair (alopecia). Although the patient was informed of the possibility before receiving his drug, he may have a severe emotional reaction when it occurs. The use of scarves, turbans and wigs is discussed, and the fact that the hair will grow in again when the drug is discontinued is emphasized.

Loss of hair from the head may be reduced by scalp cooling during the intravenous administration of the drug.[12]

(g) *Anxiety*. The patient may become very discou-raged with the discomfort and the illness experi-enced following the administration of an anticancer drug. The patient presents such a distressing picture that his family members may consider 'his suffering is not worth it'. The nurse should indicate that she understands what the patient is experiencing and appreciates the family's reaction, and again empha-sizes that the effects are temporary and stresses the potential benefits. The treatment may mean less suf-fering, a resumption of activities and years of life.

D IMMUNOTHERAPY

Cancer cells produce both specific and non-specific suppression of the patient's immune system. The most common form of immunotherapy is surgical excision of the neoplasm, which eliminates the cause of the immunosuppression and promotes the return of the body's natural immune mechanisms. Stimu-lation of the patient's immune response may be achieved by non-specific immunotherapy or by active or passive immunotherapy.

Non-specific immunotherapy stimulates both cellular and humoral immune mechanisms through the use of interferon (proteins formed by cells invaded by a virus which in turn induce the production of antiviral antibodies by unaffected cells), solutions of bacille Calmette-Guérin (BCG), *Corynebacterium parvum* (a gram-negative anaerobic organism) or levamisole (an antiprotozoan drug). The BCG solution may be administered intradermally, intravenously or directly into the tumour. Side-effects of BCG therapy range from minimal to severe. Local reactions at the side of injection include inflammation, necrosis and scarring. General systemic reactions that may occur are anaphylaxis, fever and tuberculosis.

Active immunotherapy using tumour cell vaccines alone or in combination with BCG, while still experi-mental, has proven to be safe and effective in stimu-lating immune responses and prolonging the remission rate in patients with leukaemia.[13]

Passive or adoptive immunotherapy (serotherapy) involves the administration of antitumour sera or lymphoid cells, or the removal of immunosuppress-ive substances from the patient's plasma by plasma-phaeresis.

---

[12] The Royal Marsden Hospital (1984).
[13] Sabiston (1986), pp. 78 & 79.

A monoclonal antibody is an antibody produced by a single clone of cells and is specific for a specific tumour-associated antigen. Monoclonal antibodies are being used experimentally in cancer treatment. They are attached to 'toxins' or chemotherapeutic agents. The antibody transports the toxic agent to the tumour cells, increasing the destruction of the targeted cancer cells and decreasing the damage to normal cells.

Clinical use of immunotherapy is still limited. It is most useful in combination with surgery, chemotherapy or radiation therapy.

Nursing process

POTENTIAL PATIENT PROBLEMS

The nursing care involved for patients with neoplasms of specific sites is considered in the appropriate following sections. Only patient problems that are common to many cancer patients are discussed here (see Table 9.5).

1. Alterations in oral mucous membrane
Assessment is based on a daily inspection of the patient's mouth and oropharynx using a pentorch. Manifestations of impaired mucosa are:
- Inflammation of the oral mucous membrane (stomatitis)
- Ulceration
- Hyperplasia of gingivae (gums)
- Decreased salivation
- Bleeding of soft tissues
- Difficulty in swallowing (dysphagia)
- Localized pain and soreness
- Swollen, red, dry tongue

Goals are to:
1 Maintain a moist, clean, intact oral mucosa.
2 Relieve localized pain and discomfort of the mouth, oropharynx and tongue.

3 Practise good oral hygiene during the treatment and follow-up phases of cancer management.

Nursing intervention. Prior to cancer therapy, the patient's mouth is assessed for gingivitis, dental caries, plaque, lesions of the mucosa and for the fit of dentures if used. If the mucosa is normal, good oral hygiene is stressed. The patient is advised that the teeth should be brushed four times a day using a soft brush to avoid trauma to soft tissue. The use of dental floss, once or twice daily, to remove plaque from between teeth is recommended. The mouth and throat should be examined daily; the lips, tongue, oral and pharyngeal mucosa are inspected for colour, lesions and moisture. Inflammation, soft puffiness and recession of the gums, and the accumulation of dried secretions are noted. If lesions are present, their location and size are observed.

For the patient with stomatitis, mouth care is carried out every 2–4 hours depending on the severity of the inflammation. A mild mouthwash (e.g. normal saline) is used to rinse the mouth frequently and provide moisture. Commercial mouthwashes are avoided because they contain alcohol which is drying and damaging to the mucosa. A sodium bicarbonate or peroxide solution may be used to remove crusts and dried mucus and is followed by a normal saline rinse. A mouthwash should be provided just prior to meals to reduce interference with the appetite and ingestion and to promote comfort. A very soft toothbrush and unwaxed dental floss are used to clean the teeth. *If the patient's white blood cell and platelet counts are low, cleaning with the toothbrush and dental floss is discontinued to avoid bleeding and trauma* of the soft oral tissue; foam sticks may be used gently to stimulate soft tissue when brushing is contraindicated. The mouth and lips may be moistened by the application of a water-soluble lubricating gel. The secretion of saliva may be increased by the chewing of sugar-free gum or the use of an artificial saliva preparation.

Table 9.5 Common problems of patients with oncological disease.

Problem	Causative factors	Signs and symptoms
Alterations in oral mucous membrane (stomatitis)	Effects of chemotherapy or radiation	Inflammation and ulceration of the oral mucosa Hyperplasia of gingiva Decreased salivation Bleeding of soft tissue Difficulty swallowing (dysphagia) Pain and soreness Tongue, swollen, red and dry
Alteration in nutrition: less than body requirements	Disease process Nausea and vomiting Diarrhoea Loss of appetite Anticipation of effects of therapy Dysphagia (stomatitis)	Weight loss Nausea and vomiting Diarrhoea Inadequate food intake

Table 9.5—*continued*

Problem	Causative factors	Signs and symptoms
Fluid volume deficit	Disease process Nausea and vomiting Diarrhoea Loss of appetite Dysphagia (stomatitis)	Weight loss Nausea and vomiting Diarrhoea Inadequate fluid intake Decreased skin turgor
Disturbance in self-concept: body image	Weight loss Alopecia Loss of body part Skin changes	Expression of actual or perceived changes in body image Alopecia Weight loss Absence of body part Social withdrawal Avoidance of body part Verbalization of feelings of rejection or helplessness

Sexual dysfunction	Biopsychosocial alterations in sexuality related to:
	    altered body structure and function
	    lack of privacy
	    lack of knowledge
	    misinformation
	    communication barriers with partner
	    changes in values
		Discussion of concerns
		Altered family/sex roles
		Altered self-concept
		Physical changes affecting sexual function
		Discussion of difficulties in achieving desired sexual satisfaction

Spiritual distress	Challenged belief and value system:
	    Loss of sense of purpose
	    Remoteness from God
	    Loss of faith
	    Questioning of moral/ethical nature of therapy
	    Sense of guilt/shame
	    Intense mental suffering
	    Unresolved feelings about death
		Discussion of struggles with the meaning of life and death
		Seeking spiritual assistance
		Expressions of anger/guilt
		Crying
		Withdrawal
		Sleep disturbances
		Questioning meaning of suffering
		Discussion of fear of inability to cope
		Consideration of illness as punishment
		Refusal of treatment
		Anger towards God[*]
		Seeking unorthodox therapy

Alteration in family process	Temporary or permanent changes in ability to fulfil family and career roles
	Increased stress on family members
	Role transitions
	Changes in responsibilities
		Family members unable to:
		    Care for children
		    Meet patient's physical care needs
		    Meet patient's emotional needs
		    Meet dietary needs of patient
		    Fulfil work commitments
		    Cope with separation
		    Express feelings and concerns
		    Participate in community activities
		    Seek and utilize resources
		    Talk about the lack of support

Knowledge deficit related to patient care activities, prevention of complications and planning for altered life-style	Lack of information Lack of recall of information Lack of participation in decision-making regarding care Denial of illness situation Patient's expressed desire for no information	Verbal requests for information Non-participation in care activities Inability to perform care activities Expression of anger, denial or disinterest Expressed desire for no information Failure to make use of community resources Discussion of concerns related to ability to cope at home

[*]Kim, McFarland & McLaine (1984), p. 333.

If pain and discomfort are not relieved by the above oral care programme, a topical anaesthetic or analgesic agent may be prescribed.

Infection is a potentially serious problem when mouth lesions exist; a swab is taken for culture to determine the organisms present. The Candida fungus is frequently the cause of lesions and inflammation of the oral mucosa. Nystatin, an antifungal agent, may be prescribed as a mouthwash four times daily to prevent or treat candidiasis.

When the oral mucosa is affected by radiation or an anticancer drug, a bland fluid or soft diet is recommended; irritating food and fluids, alcohol and tobacco are avoided to protect the oral mucosa.

On-going mouth care is necessary since cancer treatment usually is continued on an outpatient basis; also, the effects of radiation may be delayed. The patient should be taught how to inspect the mouth daily, and the necessary oral and teeth hygiene programme should be outlined and its importance stressed. The use of a simple, bland mouthwash and the avoidance of commercial mouthwashes are recommended. If dryness is a problem, the use of an artificial saliva preparation may be suggested. Regular dental care is encouraged but the patient is advised to inform the dentist of the disease and the treatment being used.

Expected outcomes
1 The mucosa of the mouth and oropharynx is normal, clean, pink, moist and intact.
2 Discomfort is reduced allowing the patient to eat and swallow in comfort.
3 The patient performs daily oral inspection and hygiene according to the recommended plan.

2. Alteration in nutritional status and fluid volume deficit
Fluid and nutritional deficits are common to cancer patients. They may be the result of the disease process, side-effects of the treatment such as nausea and vomiting, diarrhoea and loss of appetite, dysphagia and stomatitis or the psychological reaction of the patient when advised of the diagnosis or anticipating the side-effects of therapy.

The *goals* related to fluid and nutritional deficits are to:
1 Maintain weight at or near the normal for the patient.
2 Increase fluid intake.
3 Promote intake of nutrients.

Nursing intervention. The fluid intake for cancer patients may have to be increased by 1000–1500 ml above the normal, particularly if they are receiving radiotherapy or chemotherapy. The products of the rapid cellular breakdown place additional demands on the kidneys. For example, the uric acid concentration increases, and unless it is well diluted and eliminated it may crystallize in the kidney tubules, leading to renal insufficiency or shutdown.

Many of the chemotherapeutic agents are excreted in the urine; adequate hydration is necessary to promote elimination of the drugs and prevent cystitis. Some drugs such as cisplatin (Neoplatin), cause nephrotoxicity if the fluid output is restricted. Creatinine clearance tests are done daily on patients receiving cisplatin.

The patient's cooperation is sought by advising him that plenty of fluids are important, and a supply is kept at the bedside. Assistance should be provided for the person who is weak and finds even taking a drink an effort. If sufficient fluids cannot be taken by mouth, intravenous infusions are administered.

Anorexia, impaired digestion and absorption and severe weight loss are common problems with many cancer patients. Considerable ingenuity may be necessary on the part of the nurse to tempt the patient and to help him maintain a satisfactory nutritional intake. The form of food given will depend on the location of the neoplasm. If the patient is unable to eat, tube feeding or total parenteral nutrition (see Chapter 17) may be necessary. For the patient who can take food in the regular form, preferences and ethnic customs (consistent with his condition) are considered, the family is encouraged to bring in his favourite dishes; protein supplements are used in drinks; and small amounts of high-calorie foods are offered at frequent intervals throughout the day rather than three regular full meals. The patient's surroundings should be clean, tidy and free of odours. Vitamin supplements may be ordered to meet deficiencies and to improve the patient's appetite.

Nausea and vomiting are controlled by administering an antiemetic 30–60 minutes before chemotherapy is initiated and then every 2–4 hours during and immediately following therapy. Non-pharmacological interventions such as relaxation and distraction are important adjuncts to drug management. The goal is to prevent the occurrence of nausea and vomiting and thus avoid the development of anticipatory nausea and vomiting which can occur prior to treatments.

Expected outcomes
1 The patient's fluid intake is sufficiently in excess of 1500 ml to ensure adequate elimination of wastes from tissue destruction and the prescribed chemotherapeutic drug(s).
2 The patient's weight is maintained within 10% of his usual body weight.
3 Nausea and vomiting are absent.

3. Altered body image
Physical changes may result from the cancer itself, surgical removal of a body part or the effects of chemotherapy or radiation treatment. The loss of a limb, a mastectomy, mandibular resection, loss of hair, changes in skin pigmentation, skin rashes and weight loss are examples of visible changes in the

body with which many cancer patients are faced. 'Body image is an adaptive mechanism that maintains equilibrium among the physiologic, psychologic and sociocultural components of the body.'[14]

Assessment. Actual changes in body structure and function can be assessed, but how the individual perceives these changes and how they influence his or her responses is subjective, individual, and difficult to measure. The patient with a disturbance in body image may exhibit: decreased socialization; denial of the changes and avoidance of looking at the affected body part or of looking into a mirror; refusal to touch the affected part; avoidance of physical contact with close family members or friends; expression of fears of rejection; expression of feelings of hopelessness and helplessness; or preoccupation with the change.

Patient *goals* related to altered body image are to:
1 Recognize the physical change and talk about the feelings it provokes.
2 Understand the cause, duration and anticipated long-term implications of the changes.
3 Develop positive feelings about self.
4 Undertake self-care.

Nursing intervention. This includes the establishment of an environment that encourages the patient to discuss feelings and concerns. Grieving for the lost part or previous physical appearance occurs before the patient can adjust to the changes, whether they are temporary, permanent, actual or perceived. During the grieving process, the nurse accepts the patient's responses and acknowledges that his or her feelings and responses are to be expected.

The cause of the physical changes and what may be expected should be explained and suggestions made as to ways of improving the physical appearance. Patients are encouraged to use make-up when skin sensitivity has decreased and to wear a wig or clothing that will cover the defect or scars so long as this is acceptable to them.

Social contact is encouraged and the family is helped to understand and accept the patient's feelings and behaviour. The attitude of those giving care can do much to promote a feeling of self-worth and acceptance of the physical change on the part of the patient. The nurse who is comfortable handling and looking at the patient's colostomy or breast scar, yet aware of the patient's feelings, promotes confidence and encourages the patient gradually to look, touch and talk about the incision and participate in care and future planning. The patient is expected gradually to assume an increasing role in the necessary care.

Expected outcomes
1 The patient openly expresses feelings about physical changes.
2 The patient demonstrates understanding of the

causes and anticipated implications of the physical changes.
3 The patient looks at and touches the body part and/or uses a mirror.
4 Social interactions are increased.
5 Responsibility for self-care is gradually assumed by the patient.

4. Sexual dysfunction
Biopsychosocial alterations in sexuality of the patient with cancer may be influenced by: altered body structure and function resulting from the disease process and/or therapy, lack of privacy in an institutional setting, lack of knowledge or misinformation, and communication barriers between partners.

Human sexuality is a complex phenomenon with individual variations in its meaning and expression.

Assessment. Assessment of sexual health involves the identification of the meaning of sexuality and sexual expression for both the patient and partner. How does each partner view the ways in which the disease and its treatment have altered their relationship and the roles of wife, husband, mother or father? How has the patient's self-concept been altered? Have physical and physiological changes affected sexual functions? What are their usual ways of expressing physical love? What alternative methods of sexual gratification are acceptable to them?

Lamb and Woods point out that 'living' with cancer may enhance some aspects of sexuality as well as impinge on others.[15] Fatigue, pain, decreased physical mobility, sterility, impotence and alterations in body structure resulting from the cancer or therapy may be barriers to sexual expression. Confrontation with a potentially fatal disease encourages some couples to reassess their values and relationship. They may find that sexual expression enhances the feelings of being alive and human, and that it may serve to allay fears and provide comfort to each partner.

Patient and partner *goals* related to sexuality are to:
1 Recognize positive aspects of feelings and expression of sexuality.
2 Understand the actual and potential limitations imposed by the disease and therapy and to correct misconceptions.
3 Explore alternative methods of sexual expression.

Nursing   intervention.   Open   communication regarding sexuality is enhanced when trust and respect are part of the nurse–patient relationship. Discussions on sexuality should begin with the initial nursing assessment to establish its importance and convey a willingness to discuss the topic. Privacy should be provided for the patient and partner.

Discussions with the patient and spouse should identify and correct any misinformation. They are advised in advance of the effects of cancer and its

---

[14] Marino (1981), p. 563.

[15] Lamb and Woods (1981), p. 138.

treatment on sexuality and fertility so that they can make informed choices about treatment and anticipate possible problems.

Patients should be made aware of measures they can take to compensate for the changes resulting from the disease or treatment (e.g. the use of a lubricating gel when vaginal secretions are decreased from hormonal changes).

Alternative ways of expressing physical love may be discussed with the patient and partner. Limitations affecting sexual intercourse may be identified and other possible methods of sexual gratification suggested. When no acceptable alternative is available, the couple will need support and help to cope with their situation. These complex problems may be referred to an appropriate consultant, and counselling should be provided for the patient and spouse.

Expected outcomes.
1 The patient and partner express understanding of the effects of the cancer and therapy on their sexual relationship.
2 Satisfactory alternative methods of sexual expression are identified.

5. Spiritual distress (distress of the human spirit)
Distress of the human spirit can be defined as 'a disruption in the life principle that pervades a person's entire being and that integrates and transcends one's biologic and psychosocial nature.'[16] Spirituality involves the individual's attempt to find meaning and purpose in life and encompasses the concepts of faith, hope and love.

Factors related to the spiritual distress of the patient with cancer may include: challenged belief and value system; loss of sense of purpose; a feeling of remoteness from God; loss of faith; questioning of moral–ethical nature of therapy; a sense of guilt or shame; intense mental suffering; unresolved feelings about death; and anger toward God.[17]

Assessment. Expression of distress of the human spirit is very individualized. Behaviour which may indicate spiritual distress includes: struggles with the meaning of life and death; seeking of spiritual assistance; expressions of anger and/or guilt; crying; withdrawal; sleep disturbances; questioning the meaning of suffering; fear of ability to endure suffering; views of illness as a punishment from God; questioning or refusing therapy; and seeking unorthodox therapy.[17]

Some patients may find the confrontation with their values and religious beliefs to be a rewarding and reassuring experience. The significance of spirituality and religious observances in the patient's life should be assessed.

Patient *goals* related to spiritual distress are to:
1 Explore actual or potential spiritual conflicts.

2 Seek appropriate spiritual guidance.
3 Observe personally meaningful religious practices.

Nursing intervention. The nurse may function as a listener and counsellor in encouraging the patient to express feelings of support or conflict related to spiritual needs. The practice of religious observances can be facilitated by providing privacy for prayers or personal discussions, encouraging attendance at chapel, arranging for bedside religious observances, providing religious articles and reading materials, and by praying with the patient.

Spiritual resources are identified and appropriate referrals made. A religious advisor known and respected by the patient should be sought when possible. Pastoral counsellors or chaplains from within the hospital or from the community are used to provide the relevant services and counselling.

Expected outcomes. The patient:
1 Expresses feelings and discusses spiritual concerns.
2 Receives spiritual consolation.
3 Observes religious practices that are personally meaningful.

6. Alteration in family relationships
The patient's family suffers as a result of temporary or permanent changes in the patient's physical capacity to fulfil family and career roles, the increased stress on family members, role transitions, and changes in responsibilities.

Welch points out that families may have more difficulty coping with the patient's diagnosis and illness than the patient himself.[18] In a study exploring the components of family coping during the cancer experience, Welch identified the following factors as problems in the home settings of the 41 families in the sample: care of children, lack of help with the patient's physical care, having to prepare different meals, being a long distance from the hospital, lack of help with the patient's emotional needs, fear of leaving the patient alone, lack of knowledge about how to care for the patient, and trying to work concurrently.[19]

Family *goals* related to disruption of family life during the experience of cancer in one member are to:
1 Recognize and express feelings and concerns of individuals and the family group.
2 Understand the actual and potential limitations imposed on the patient by the cancer and therapy and correct misconceptions.
3 Find out more about community resources for patient care and social needs.

---

[16] Kim, McFarland & McLaine (1984), p. 57.
[17] Kim & Moritz (1982), p. 333.

[18] Welch (1981), p. 366.
[19] Welch (1981), p. 367.
[20] Welch (1981), p. 368.

4 Identify the personal supports for the family and individual members.

5 Increase participation in decision-making and care-giving activities.

6 Develop effective communication within the family.

7 Develop plans for immediate and long-term changes in roles and responsibilities within the family and explore alternatives.

Nursing intervention. Welch's study identified that the most important nursing measure to help families cope was the provision of excellent, personalized care for the patient.[20] The nurse can further enhance this action by explaining patient care to the family and ensuring that the family understands the plan of care and the reasons behind it. Family members are encouraged to participate in decisions about care and be involved in giving care. The family is informed during the early stages of illness about the disease and the expectations of treatment. Conferences with the family provide the opportunity to advise them of the changes and progress in the patient's condition and enables them to express their needs and concerns. Family members should receive information directly; information delivered second-hand may be incomplete or altered because of differences in perceptions and priorities. The family is advised of available community resources for patient care and social services. Referral to a social worker may be appropriate when the family is facing long-term disruption and when the ability of the family to cope is actually or potentially inadequate.

Family members are encouraged to seek help from those they consider to be helpful and appropriate for them, such as neighbours, vicar, friends and relatives. Immediate and long-term priorities are identified and a readjustment of family roles and responsibilities made. Continuing help and support should be readily available from the nurse, doctor, social worker, pastoral counsellor, hospital chaplain friends and relatives. Continuity in those giving care does much to facilitate communication and long-term planning.

It is important that family members spend time together as well as resume socialization outside the home. In the hospital setting, measures are taken to provide privacy and opportunity for the family to be together as a unit.

Expected outcomes.

1 (a) The patient and family members resume previous family and career goals, *or* (b) when changes in roles and responsibilities cannot be resolved, such problems are discussed and compromises effected.

2 Family members demonstrate an understanding of the limitations on the patient's ability to fulfil family and career roles.

3 The family uses health and social resources in the community.

4 The family uses relevant personal support systems.

5 Family members resume socialization outside the home.

6 Family members maintain employment status.

7 Family members demonstrate healthy patterns of interaction by sharing responsibilities, using touch and physical contact, listening to each other and being together.

7. Lack of knowledge

Advances in cancer treatment are encouraging; patients are living longer and the occurrence and duration of remissions of the disease are increasing. The period of hospitalization for most oncology patients is relatively short in relation to the overall illness experience. Responsibility for day-to-day care of the cancer patient rests to a large extent with the individual and the family, who require knowledge, skills and resources to manage the patient's home care successfully. Understanding of the care plan and reasons for it also facilitate patient and family participation in decision-making regarding treatment and care and provides them with a sense of control and involvement in what is happening to them.

Edstrom and Miller surveyed a group of eight families to identify the needs of families of oncology patients. The needs identified were: (1) skin care—how to prevent and treat skin breakdown; (2) administration of drugs including injections; (3) methods of pain control, including comfort measures and medications; (4) information on maintaining activity and dealing with limitations; and (5) dealing with family changes and problems when living with a member who has a chronic illness.[21]

A teaching plan for health management must take into account the patient's and family's perspectives. What are their major concerns about hospital and home care management? What knowledge and skills do they possess? What resources exist within the family and neighbourhood? What health care and social services are available in the community? How does the patient learn best? What barriers exist to learning?

Patient and family *goals* related to this knowledge deficit are to:

1 Acquire knowledge and skill in management of personal hygiene, diet, activity, medication schedule and special care procedures (including bowel and bladder management, mouth and skin care, pain management and comfort measures, wound care and prevention of infection).

2 Understand the plan for daily patient care.

3 Understand the plan for follow-up care and treatment.

[21] Edstrom & Miller (1981), p. 51.

4 Acquire knowledge of community resources for patient care.
5 Develop realistic plans for patient and family living activities.

Nursing intervention. Teaching sessions should include supervised practice of care as well as information giving. The patient and family can carry out care procedures during the period of hospitalization or with guidance from a visiting nurse in the home. The development of a teaching plan to be achieved within a definite time ensures that necessary content and skills are taught and opportunity is provided for discussion, practice and repetition. Explanations about basic care and treatment should be repeated each time the care is delivered. Dodd and Mood demonstrated that information provided once about chemotherapy to adult oncology patients was not retained. Follow-up information visits by a nurse resulted in increased accuracy and retention of the information.[22]

Written information given to the patient and family enhances learning and facilitates recall. The use of films, slides and pictures helps the patient and family to envisage a technique or problem being discussed. Group sessions are useful to provide basic information and to promote sharing and discussion of experiences. All patients and families require some individualized learning sessions for them to acquire knowledge and skills unique to their particular situation.

A referral may be made to the community nursing services. The community nurse is informed of the patient's and family's progress in developing self-care skills and of specific needs for continuous help and guidance. She can assist with the provision of dressings and drugs (prescribed by the general practitioner) and facilitate access to the home help service, social welfare support and meals-on-wheels. Volunteer workers may be able to assist with transport, social visits and such day-to-day activities as shopping and collecting library books. Visiting nurses can also arrange for the loan of equipment such as hospital beds, wheelchairs and sanitary utensils. These are available in the United Kingdom through the National Health Service.

The teaching programme should include measures to prevent infection, which is a major concern for the immunosuppressed patient during most of the treatment period, and plans to maintain resistance. Contact with persons with any type of infection is to be avoided. Adequate nutrition with increased protein is important as well as hygienic care of the skin and mouth.

The patient and family are taught to be alert for abnormal redness, swelling, warmth and drainage, as well as the occurrence of pain, and are informed of the need for immediate action if these signs and symptoms occur.

Further information relevant to patient and family teaching can be found throughout Chapter 2 and in subsequent chapters of this text.

Expected outcomes. The patient and family:
1 Understand the patient's daily care regimen.
2 Are able to perform specific patient care.
3 State the significance of early recognition of the signs and symptoms of infection and other complications.
4 Understand the follow-up plan of care and keep scheduled appointments.
5 Use community health care and social services.
6 Express a realistic plan for patient and family daily living activities.

POST-TREATMENT PHASE

Following the initial treatment phase, cancer patients may be divided into two groups: those whose disease is cured or in whom a state of remission is achieved, and those whose disease is progressively worsening. The former group usually resumes its accustomed activities and life-style.

Remissions or arrest of the neoplasm

In the post-treatment phase, neoplasia is arrested or there is a remission, i.e. symptoms have subsided. The *goals* related to this phase of cancer are to:
1 Re-establish an appropriate pattern of daily living.
2 Recognize early signs and symptoms of possible disease recurrence.
3 Obtain prompt assessment and treatment when significant signs and symptoms occur.
4 Receive regular medical reassessment and care.

Just as with other patients, those with neoplastic disease are encouraged to resume their normal pattern of life if they are able. Going back to work is good for the patient's and the family's morale; being occupied prevents concentration on his disease. Independence within his physical limitations is encouraged and guidance as to the care required will be necessary. If the patient has a colostomy or tracheostomy or requires a prosthesis, the necessary instruction for care and adaptation for daily life is given. (Specific problems such as these are discussed in the related sections).

Patients whose cancer is arrested or in remission live with the knowledge that their future is uncertain. They are able to function effectively only on a daily basis; long-term planning presents a major problem. They constantly fear recurrence of the disease and are frequently over-anxious about unrelated minor disturbances.

Helping patients to focus on their strengths and the present is a major function of the nurse. During home visits and discussion in clinics, the nurse

---

[22] Dodd & Mood (1981), p. 311.

assists the patient and family to develop positive attitudes and make realistic plans for the present and future.

The patient receives follow-up medical care for at least 5 years following treatment for cancer. Signs and symptoms that might signify recurrence of the disease are identified and investigated promptly. Readmission to hospital or a clinic for follow-up or further treatment immediately arouses fears in the patient and family; the purpose of the test or treatment should be explained and their questions answered.

EXPECTED OUTCOMES

1 The patient resumes daily life and work.
2 The patient's and family's social activities increase.
3 Signs and symptoms of possible disease recurrence are recognized and investigated promptly.
4 Scheduled appointments for follow-up reassessment are observed.
5 Satisfaction with his or her life-style is expressed.

Advanced cancer

Patients with advanced cancer are those with widespread disease. They may have been treated previously but have suffered a recurrence, or the disease was advanced or disseminated before receiving treatment. Management of the patient with advanced cancer involves both *active* treatment and *palliative* care. The latter is directed towards the relief of symptoms and keeping the patient as comfortable as possible, while active treatment is designed to control or cure the disease. Control of advanced cancer is achieved using a multiple modality approach in treatment. Improved methods of treating secondary conditions frequently associated with cancer have made it possible for the doctor to treat the disease aggressively in the advanced stage. For example, infection is controlled by the administration of antibiotics; infusions of blood components counteract the side-effects of chemotherapy.

Patients with advanced cancer undergo long and difficult therapy, general debility and increased psychosocial stress. Physical manifestations vary but may be widespread and severe. The future is uncertain; the patient frequently is faced with progressively severe pain, loss of family and social position, loss of physical abilities and control, and finally death.

IDENTIFICATION OF PATIENT PROBLEMS

Nursing care for the patient with advanced cancer is discussed under the following problems which are common to many patients with advanced cancer:
1 Alterations in comfort: chronic, progressive pain
2 Grieving
3 Alterations in family life related to prolonged dependency and impending death and dying.

Nursing care specific to various treatments and the patient's and family's response to illness and treatment was discussed under the treatment phase of management of the patient with oncological disease.

NURSING INTERVENTION

1. Alteration in comfort: chronic, progressive pain
The patient may be free of pain in the early stages of the disease, but later as the neoplasm invades surrounding tissues it causes pressure, involves bone, blood vessels and sensory nerves, and causes inflammation, infection and necrosis of tissue. It is suggested that moderate to severe pain is experienced by 60–80% of patients with advanced cancer and that the physiological and psychological impact of cancer pain on the patient is usually greater than that of non-malignant chronic pain.[23]

As the disease advances, physical deterioration increases; nutrition may be inadequate, sleep is disturbed and emotional reactions of anxiety and depression become more severe. The patient's pain perception and pain tolerance thresholds are decreased due to depletion of endorphins. The patient's usual coping mechanisms may be inadequate to deal with the pain and the accompanying physical debility and fatigue.

The increasing severity of the pain may be perceived as signifying advance of the cancer. The pain contributes to the physiological and psychological factors that enhance its severity. Loss of sleep and rest due to pain increases the patient's fatigue. Anorexia, nausea and vomiting associated with the pain contribute to nutritional deficiencies and weight loss. Mobility is restricted by the pain, increasing the potential for skin breakdown, constipation, muscle weakness and chest complications. The patient may exhibit anxiety, irritability, anger and withdrawal.

The patient's *goal* in relation to chronic, progressive pain is to gain control of the pain. It has been demonstrated that when chronic, severe pain is relieved, emotional responses decrease.[24] Existing knowledge about pain control is not always fully utilized in clinical practice. Adequate pain control requires the cooperative efforts of the patient, nursing and medical personnel. Assessment of the patient's pain and the effectiveness of interventions must be continuous. The patient is the expert on the pain and only he can determine the effectiveness of treatment. Treatment may include the use of systemic analgesic drugs, nerve blockers, surgical interruption of pain pathways, sensory stimulation and the psychotherapeutic techniques discussed in Chapter 8.

Analgesic medications are given orally when pos-

---

[23] Ajemian & Mount (1980), pp. 113–115.
[24] Ajemian & Mount (1980), p. 115.

sible; this route of administration is easier for the patient and family to manage at home. It may be necessary to increase the dosage and the frequency of administration as the patient's pain becomes more severe. The analgesic is administered prior to the onset of severe pain; maintaining an adequate level of analgesic prevents the patient experiencing overwhelming pain. Frequent observation is necessary for possible side-effects; confusion and drowsiness may be experienced but gradually the patient becomes alert as well as pain-free. Continuous patient assessment is necessary to ensure that the pain is relieved without undue impairment of the patient's ability to function mentally and physically. Addiction is rarely a problem. When an adequate level of analgesia is reached and a preventive approach is used in pain management, dependence on the medication tends to decrease.

It has been suggested that patients in palliative care units such as hospices experience less pain than oncology patients in general hospital wards. The supportive aspects of nursing care in the former situations are considered responsible for the decreased pain perception experienced.

The nurse may decrease the patient's and family's anxiety and fear by providing information and encouraging questions. The patient that knows what to expect and has accurate information about why a situation is occurring is less anxious. Emotional support develops through the relationship established between the patient and nurse. Having the same nursing personnel promotes the development of a trusting nurse–patient relationship. The nurse should provide anticipatory guidance, encourage expression of feelings and questions, listen and respond. Alternative methods of coping are explored and new skills such as relaxation techniques may be taught. Simple nursing measures such as a change of position, turning pillows, massage and the use of pillows to provide support may provide comfort. The day should be planned so that the patient's energy is expended on activities that are most important to him and when the pain is under control.

Expected outcomes.
1 The patient is relatively free of pain.
2 No episodes of severe pain occur.
3 Mental alertness and physical functioning are not decreased by the pain treatment.

2. Grieving
Grieving by the patient with advanced cancer may be due to the loss of a body part, or body function, loss of independence, loss of role in the family and/or society, and the threat to life.

The patient's and family's responses to loss and death may be categorized according to the stages of grieving. Knowledge of these various stages of behaviour help the nurse to understand the patient's responses. It should be remembered that all individ-

uals do not necessarily progress through these phases progressively or within a given space of time. Individuals fluctuate in their reactions, varying in the time spent in any given phase. Labelling of behaviours does not help the patient, but it may be useful to guide the nurse to recognize what is happening to the patient. Hine states that 'perhaps the most useful expectation is that what ought to be happening with the patient and family is what is happening at any given moment'.[25]

The five stages of grieving described by Kübler-Ross are denial, anger, bargaining, depression and acceptance.[26] Behaviour characteristic of the various stages include, shock, disbelief, denial, crying, rage, frustration, anger, sorrow, physical discomfort, detachment, acceptance, calmness and return to realistic functioning and reattachment.

The *goal* for the patient and family related to grieving because of possible, probable or impending loss is to express grief.

Nursing intervention begins with awareness that the patient and family are grieving. The nature and cause of the grief are identified; it cannot be assumed that a patient with advanced cancer is grieving because of the possibility that he will die. The patient may have resolved his imminent death but his grief may be primarily related to loss of independence or the effect his illness and death will have on his family. The nurse may help the grieving patient by acknowledging awareness of what he is experiencing.

The nurse may help the patient to express his feelings of grief, concern, sorrow, anger or frustration by listening and providing opportunities for quiet discussion, and the use of touch. The patient and family are encouraged to share their grief together. Support by the nurse and other health professionals may make it easier for them to express their concerns and grief.

Grieving is a normal process that requires understanding and support but rarely direct intervention. Counselling and help from skilled experienced workers may be necessary when grieving is delayed or one stage is prolonged or the patient is not able to express his feelings. Problems may also arise when the patient and family members are at different stages of the grieving process at a given time. They may require help to understand the responses and feelings of each other and why conflicting emotions are occurring.

Expected outcomes.
1 The patient expresses grief verbally and nonverbally.
2 Family members express their grief and communicate feelings with the patient.

---

[25] Hine (1982), p. 47.
[26] Kübler-Ross (1973), pp. 36–137.

Alterations in family life

The alterations in family life are related to the patient's prolonged illness and dependence and/or his possible or impending death.

The patient with advanced cancer faces progressive debility and pain from the disease process and the many side-effects resulting from therapy. Feelings of helplessness and dependence result from the severity and rapidity of events that seem to be happening to him. The patient may be aware that cure is not possible and that death is imminent, or he may be living with uncertainty about his future. Cure is uncertain and the possibility of severe complications such as infection, haemorrhage and progression of the disease are constantly present. The patient's dependence on others for care and support and the uncertainty about the future cause disruption of family life, role changes, and financial adjustments. Children may feel isolated because one parent is ill and away from home and the other parent is making daily, time-consuming visits to the hospital.

Patient and family *goals* related to alterations in family life are to:
1 Develop skills for patient care.
2 Recognize the realities of what is happening to the patient.
3 Express feelings and concerns.
4 Develop realistic plans for the family and patient during the period of illness.
5 Make realistic plans for reorganization of the structure and function of the family following the period of illness and anticipated death of the patient.
6 Make plans for the patient's death if this is imminent.

Nursing interventions related to the development of health management skills by the patient and family are discussed above under the treatment phase of cancer management (see pp. 168–169). Education related to patient care includes ambulation skills, pain management, comfort measures, diet, bowel functioning and wound and skin care. The family that is disrupted because of the patient's illness and treatment and which has not faced up to the personal crisis of the threatened loss of a member cannot be expected to provide daily patient care or necessary emotional support. The nurse should try to help the family deal with the disruption and resolve their personal crisis. They are taught patient care skills and are helped to make decisions related to home care. Their own personal care (rest, regular meals etc.) is stressed as playing a significant role. Uncertainty about the future may be decreased when the family is kept informed of changes in the patient's status.

Following an assessment of the strengths and deficiencies of the family, the nurse may find that referrals to a social worker and a community nurse are necessary. Home care programmes for the chronically ill and dying, hospice or palliative care units may be available. The family is advised of these resources and is helped to select the services appropriate to their situation and plans. If the decision is that the patient should be at home, the nurse discusses the necessary adjustments to be made by the family so that they can provide adequate care. Home care can have many positive benefits for both the patient and family but consideration must be given to the burden it places on the family. The family's needs should be assessed and they should be helped to set priorities and include significant events in their plans. Although the family may not have the time, energy or resources to indulge in many of their accustomed social events, they can continue to observe a birthday, graduation or special achievement of a child who is feeling isolated or dejected because of the illness and absence of a parent.

Nursing support for the patient's and family's decision regarding care helps them to carry through their plans and provides reassurance that they are doing what is best for them in their situation.

If a patient dies, visits by a community nurse or social worker following the death may help the family to re-establish their daily lives and cope with the loss of a loved one. Follow-up services through national cancer societies or visits by hospital and community personnel can also provide support and guidance for the family during the period of mourning and reorganization.

Expected outcomes.
1 The family provides safe, comfortable care for the patient who is at home.
2 Community and family resources are used for patient care and family support.
3 Sources of financial and social assistance are identified and used as needed.
4 Important family activities are recognized and celebrated to meet the needs of children, spouse and others.
5 The family and/or patient expresses realistic plans for the patient's death, if appropriate.
6 The patient and family share feelings and concerns and discuss them with others if necessary.
7 Realistic plans for reorganization of family structure and function are expressed.

References and Further Reading

BOOKS

Ajemian I & Mount BM (eds) (1980) *The RVH Manual on Palliative and Hospice Care*. New York: Arno Press.
British National Formulary, 11th ed. (1986) London: BMA and Pharmaceutical Society of Great Britain.
Braunwald E et al (eds) (1987) *Harrison's Principles of Internal Medicine*, 11th ed. New York: McGraw-Hill. Chapter 21.

Flitter HH (1976) *An Introduction to Physics in Nursing*, 7th ed. St Louis: CV Mosby.

Fudenberg HH, Stites DP, Caldwell JL & Wells JV (eds) (1980) *Basic and Clinical Immunology*, 3rd ed. Los Altos, CA: Lange. Chapter 23.

Hay GA & Hughes D (1983) *First-Year Physics for Radiographers*. Eastbourne: Baillière Tindall. Chapters 16, 17 & 18.

Hopps HC (1976) *Principles of Pathology*, 2nd ed. New York: Appleton-Century-Crofts.

Kim MJ & Moritz DA (eds) (1982) *Classification of Nursing Diagnosis*. New York: McGraw-Hill.

Kim MJ, McFarland GK & McLaine AM (1984) *Pocket Guide to Nursing Diagnosis*. St Louis: CV Mosby.

Krause MW & Mahon LK (1984) *Food, Nutrition and Diet Therapy*, 7th ed. Philadelphia: WB Saunders. Chapter 36.

Krupp MA & Chatton MJ (1983) *Current Medical Diagnosis and Treatment*. Los Altos, CA: Lange. Chapter 32.

Kübler-Ross E (1973) *On Death and Dying*. New York: Macmillan.

Marino LB (1981) *Cancer Nursing*. St Louis: CV Mosby.

Nave CR & Nave BC (1985) *Physics for the Health Sciences*, 3rd ed. Philadelphia: WB Saunders. Chapter 21.

Office of Population Censuses and Surveys (1983) *Cancer Statistics Registrations; England and Wales 1979*, OPCS series, MBI No. 11. London: HMSO.

Rubin P (ed) (1983) *Clinical Oncology. A Multidisciplinary Approach*, 6th ed. New York: American Cancer Society.

Sabiston DC (1986) *Davis–Christopher Textbook of Surgery*, 13th ed. Philadelphia: WB Saunders. Chapter 21.

Smith LH & Thier SO (1985) *Pathophysiology: The Biological Principles of Disease*, 2nd ed. Philadelphia: WB Saunders. pp. 271–286.

The Canadian Cancer Society (1985) *Cancer Can be Beaten: The Facts*. Toronto. pp. 28 & 29.

The Expert Advisory Committee on the Management of Severe Chronic Pain in Cancer Patients (1984) *Cancer Pain: A Monograph for the Management of Cancer Pain*. Ottawa: Health and Welfare.

The Royal Marsden Hospital Manual of Clinical Nursing Policies and Procedures (1984) London: Harper & Row.

The Royal Marsden Hospital Patient Education Booklets (1985/6) Manchester: Haigh & Hochland.

Twycross RG & Lack S (1983) *Symptom Control in Far Advanced Cancer: Pain Relief*. London: Pitman.

Vredevoe DL, Derdianian A, Sarna LP, Friel M & Shiplacoff JAG (1981) *Concepts of Oncology Nursing*. Englewood Cliffs, NJ: Prentice-Hall.

PERIODICALS

Atwell BM (1984) Sex and the cancer patient, an unspoken concern. *Patient Educ. Couns.*, Vol. 5 No. 3, pp. 123–126.

Bishop MJ (1982) Oncogenes. *Sci. Am.*, Vol. 246 No. 3, pp. 80–92.

Carlson AC (1985) Infection prophylaxis in the patient with cancer. *Oncol. Nurs. Forum*, Vol. 12 No. 3, pp. 56–64.

Cobb SC (1984) Teaching relaxation techniques to cancer patients. *Cancer Nurs.*, Vol. 7 No. 2, pp. 157–161.

Collier RJ & Kaplan DA (1984) Immunotoxins. *Sci. Am.*, Vol. 251 No. 1, pp. 56–64.

Commartin MA (1983) New directions in care: part 1 self help for the cancer patient. *Cancer Nurs.*, Vol. 79 No. 2, pp. 43–44.

Crane LR, Emmer DR & Giguras A (1980) Prevention of infection on the oncology unit. *Nurs. Clin. N. Am.*, Vol. 15 No. 4, pp. 843–856.

Daeffler R (1981) Oral hygiene measures for patients with cancer. III. *Cancer. Nurs.*, Vol. 4 No. 1, pp. 29–35.

Dixon J (1984) Effect of nursing interventions on nutritional and performance status in cancer patients. *Nurs. Res.*, Vol. 33 No. 6, pp. 330–335.

Dodd MJ & Mood DW (1981) Chemotherapy: helping patients to know the drugs they are receiving and their possible side effects. *Cancer Nurs.*, Vol. 4 No. 4, pp. 311–318.

Edstrom S & Miller MW (1981) Preparing the family to care for the cancer patient at home: a home care course. *Cancer Nurs.*, Vol. 4 No. 1, pp. 49–52.

Engelking CH & Steele NE (1984) A model for pretreatment nursing assessment of patients receiving cancer chemotherapy. *Cancer Nurs.*, Vol. 7 No. 3, pp. 203–212.

Epting SP (1981) Coping with stress through peer support. *Top. Clin. Nurs.*, Vol. 2 No. 4, pp. 47–59.

Farrel S, Bubela N & Burlein-Hall S (1985) High volume chemodialysis: a new outpatient program. *Cancer Nurs.*, Vol. 81 No. 2, pp. 44–47.

Faulkenberry JE (1983) Programmed instruction: cancer prevention and detection. Risk assessment: the medical history. *Cancer Nurs.*, Vol. 6 No. 5, pp. 389–401.

Granstrom SL (1985) Spiritual nursing care for oncology patients. *Top. Clin. Nurs.*, Vol. 7 No. 1, pp. 39–45.

Grobe ME, Ilstrup DM & Ahmann DL (1981) Skills needed by family members to maintain the care of the advanced cancer patient. *Cancer Nurs.*, Vol. 4 No. 5, pp. 371–375.

Haughey CW (1981) Understanding ultrasonography. *Nurs. '81.*, Vol. 11 No. 4, pp. 100–104.

Haughey CW (1981) What to say . . . and do . . . when your patient asks about CT scans. *Nurs. '81.*, Vol. 11 No. 12, pp. 72–77.

Hine VH (1982) Holistic dying; the role of the nurse clinician. *Top. Clin. Nurs.*, Vol. 3 No. 4, pp. 45–54.

Hughes CB (1986) Giving cancer drugs IV: some guidelines. *Am. J. Nurs.*, Vol. 86 No. 1, pp. 34–38.

Ignoffo RJ & Freedman MA (1980) Therapy of local toxicities caused by extravasation of cancer therapeutic drugs. *Cancer Treat. Rev.*, Vol. 7 pp. 17–27.

Kelly PP & Tinsley C (1981) Planning care for the patient receiving external radiation. *Am. J. Nurs.*, Vol. 81 No. 2, pp. 338–342.

Lamb MA & Woods NF (1981) Sexuality and the cancer patient. *Cancer Nurs.*, Vol. 4 No. 2, pp. 137–144.

Lane B & Forgay M (1981) Upgrading your oral hygiene protocol for the patient with cancer. *Cancer Nurs.*, Vol. 77, No. 11, pp. 27–29.

Lauer P, Murphy SP & Powers MJ (1982) Learning needs of cancer patients: a comparison of nurse and patient perceptions. *Nurs. Res.*, Vol. 31 No. 1, pp. 11–16.

Leaschenko JM (1981) Assessment and depression in the dying patient. *Top. Clin. Nurs.*, Vol. 2 No. 4, pp. 39–45.

Lev EL (1985) Community support for oncology patient and family. *Top. Clin. Nurs.*, Vol. 7 No. 1, pp. 71–78.

Longman AJ & Rogers BP (1984) Altered cell growth in cancer and the nursing implications. *Cancer Nurs.*, Vol. 7 No. 5, pp. 405–412.

Lum LLQ & Gallagher-Allred CR (1984) Nutrition and the cancer patient: a cooperative effort by nursing and dietetics to overcome problems. *Cancer Nurs.*, Vol. 7 No. 6, pp. 469–474.

Manchester PB (1981) The adolescent with cancer; concerns for care. *Top. Clin. Nurs.*, Vol. 2 No. 4, pp. 31–37.

McNairn N (1981) Helping the patient who wants to die at home. *Nurs. '81.*, Vol. 11 No. 2, p. 66.

Moldawer NP & Murray JL (1985) The clinical uses of monoclonal antibodies in cancer research. *Cancer Nurs.*, Vol. 8 No. 4, pp. 207–213.

Moseley JR (1985) Alterations in comfort. *Nurs. Clin. N. Am.*, Vol. 20 No. 2, pp. 427–438.

Nace CS & Nace GS (1985) Acute tumor lysis syndrome: pathophysiology and nursing management. *Crit. Care Nurs.*, Vol. 5 No. 3, pp. 26–34.

Northhouse LL (1981) Living with cancer. *Am. J. Nurs.*, Vol. 81 No. 5, pp. 961–962.

Nunnally C, Donoghue M & Yasko JM (1982) Nutritional needs of cancer patients. *Nurs. Clin. N. Am.*, Vol. 17 No. 4, pp. 557–578.

Oberst MT & James RH (1985) Going home: patient and spouse adjustment following cancer surgery. *Top. Clin. Nurs.*, Vol. 7 No. 1, pp. 46–57.

O'Donnell L & Papciak B (1981) When all else fails: continuous morphine infusion for controlling intractable pain. *Nurs. '81*, Vol. 11, No. 8, pp 69–72.

Oleske D (1981) Questions about cancer: indicators for patient education. *Top. Clin. Nurs.*, Vol. 2 No. 4, pp. 1–8.

Ostchega Y (1980) Preventing and treating cancer chemotherapy's oral complications. *Nurs. '80*, Vol. 10, No. 8, pp. 47–52.

Rankin M (1980) The progressive pain of cancer. *Top. Clin. Nurs.*, Vol. 2 No. 1, pp. 57–73.

Reich SD (1981) Pharmaceutics: predictive tests of human tumor responsiveness to chemotherapy. *Cancer Nurs.*, Vol. 4 No. 5, pp. 419–421.

Rothwell S (1983) Cancer: advances in prevention, screening and diagnosis. *Cancer Nurs.*, Vol. 79 No. 2, pp. 10–16.

Statland BE (1981) The challenge of cancer testing. *Diagn. Med.*, Vol. 4 No. 4, pp. 12–18. ·

Statland BE (1981) Tumor markers. *Diagn. Med.*, Vol. 4 No. 4, pp. 21–38.

Suppers VJ & McClamrock EA (1985) Biologicals in cancer treatment: future effects on nursing practice. *Oncol. Nurs. Forum*, Vol. 12 No. 3, pp. 27–32.

Tarpy CC (1985) Birth control considerations during chemotherapy. *Oncol. Nurs. Forum*, Vol. 12 No. 2, pp. 75–78.

Trester AK (1982) Nursing management of patients receiving cancer chemotherapy. *Cancer Nurs.*, Vol. 5 No. 3, pp. 201–210.

Varricchio CG (1981) The patient on radiation therapy. *Am. J. Nurs.*, Vol. 81 No. 2, pp. 334–337.

Walter J (1982) Care of the patient receiving antiplastic drugs. *Nurs. Clin. N. Am.*, Vol. 17 No. 4, pp. 607–629.

Watson PM (1982) Patient education: the adult with cancer. *Nurs. Clin. N. Am.*, Vol. 17 No. 4, pp. 739–752.

Welch D (1981) Planning nursing interventions for family members of adult cancer patients. *Cancer Nurs.*, Vol. 4 No. 5, pp. 365–370.

Welch-McCaffrey D (1985) Cancer anxiety and quality of life. *Cancer Nurs.*, Vol. 8 No. 3, pp. 151–158.

Williamson KR (1981) Displatin: delivering a safe infusion. *Am. J. Nurs.*, Vol. 81 No. 4, pp. 320–323.

Woods M & Kowalski J (1982) Assessment of the adult with cancer. *Nurs. Clin. N. Am.*, Vol. 17 No. 4, pp. 539–556.

Wright K & Dyck S (1984) Expressed concern of adult cancer patients' family members. *Cancer Nurs.*, Vol. 7 No. 5, pp. 371–374.

Wroblewski SS & Wroblewski SH (1981) Caring for the patient with chemotherapy-induced thrombocytopenia. *Am. J. Nurs.*, Vol. 81 No. 4, pp. 746–749.

Yasko JM (1982) Care of the patient receiving radiation therapy. *Nurs. Clin. N. Am.*, Vol. 17 No. 4, p. 631–648.

Yasko JM (1985) Holistic management of nausea and vomiting caused by chemotherapy. *Top. Clin. Nurs.*, Vol. 7 No. 1, pp. 26–38.

10

The Patient with an Altered Level of Consciousness

CONSCIOUSNESS

Consciousness may be defined as the complete awareness of self and environment, with appropriate responsiveness to stimuli. It is a dynamic experience involving a series of different elements whose relationship changes incessantly. The precise limits are hard to define as consciousness is inferred from a person's appearance and behaviour.

Two physiological components affect conscious behaviour. These are *content* and *arousal*. Mental activities involve the contents of sensation, perception, attention, memory and volition. Analysis and synthesis of information, along with emotional implications, also occur. The *content* aspects generally refer to those mental functions carried out in the cerebral cortex. The *arousal* aspects are reflected in the person's appearance of wakefulness. Cognitive functions are not possible without some degree of arousal. Arousal can exist without the emotional and thinking components of content.[1]

The system of consciousness is driven by an arousal mechanism. Full consciousness depends upon interaction between the cerebral cortex and the reticular activating system. This is a mesh-like network of undifferentiated neurons located throughout the central portion of the brain stem (see Fig. 10.1). These neurons receive collateral nerve fibres from all sensory pathways that enter the brain via the upper spinal cord or cranial nerves. It has been demonstrated that if the sensory pathways are blocked impulses travel by the collaterals to the reticular activating system then to the thalamus and on to innervate the cortex.[2] This activation of the cortex produces a state of alertness. Further, it has been postulated that impulses are conducted via a feedback loop back to the reticular activating system, which in turn stimulates the cortex.[3] This continuous circuitry of arousal maintains the state of readiness of the cortex to receive and interpret incoming sensory impulses. A further function of the reticular activating system is to screen and modulate incoming messages so that the cortex is able to process significant information.[4]

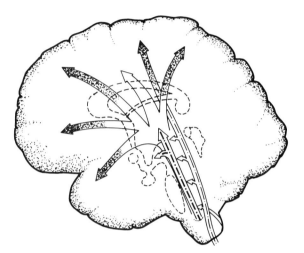

Fig. 10.1 The reticular activating system.

SLEEP

Normal sleep is a periodic depression of the physiological function of the parts of the brain concerned with consciousness from which a person can be aroused to awareness. Sleep occurs in two ways: first, as a result of decreased activity in the reticular activating system, which produces slow-wave or normal sleep.[5] This is a restful type of sleep during which the respiratory and pulse rates and blood pressure fall, the pupils constrict and react more slowly to light, the eyes deviate upwards and tendon reflexes are abolished.

The second way by which sleep occurs results from the abnormal channelling of brain signals and is referred to as paradoxical or desynchronized sleep.[5] Short episodes of paradoxical sleep usually occur about every 90 minutes throughout a night. Heart and respiratory rates and blood pressure alter; cerebral blood flow increases, clonic jerks may occur and rapid eye movements (REM) take place. Most dreams occur during paradoxical sleep.

During normal sleep, activity of the reticular activating system is decreased, while in paradoxical sleep some cerebral areas are active while others are suppressed.

[1] Plum & Posner (1980), p. 3.
[2] Carlson (1977), p. 418.
[3] Guyton (1986), p. 666.
[4] Plum & Posner (1980), p. 13.

[5] Guyton (1986), p. 671.

During sleep a person may be easily aroused to wakefulness or consciousness by cerebral arousal through stimuli such as pain or unaccustomed noise. The return to wakefulness shows that the reticular activating system is still functioning and capable of screening and discrimination.

UNCONSCIOUSNESS

Interruption of impulses from the reticular activating system, or failure of the cerebral cortical neurons to respond to incoming impulses, produces a loss of consciousness. Other than destruction of the cortical or cortical activating cells (reticular formation) by trauma, the basic factors contributing to unconsciousness are considered to be oxygen and glucose deprivation. Neurons require a constant supply of both of these substances for cellular activity. A deficiency of oxygen for even a few seconds decreases neuronal metabolism to a point at which unconsciousness ensues. Fig. 10.2 describes the effects of

alterations in level of consciousness from a state of normal awareness to coma or unconsciousness.

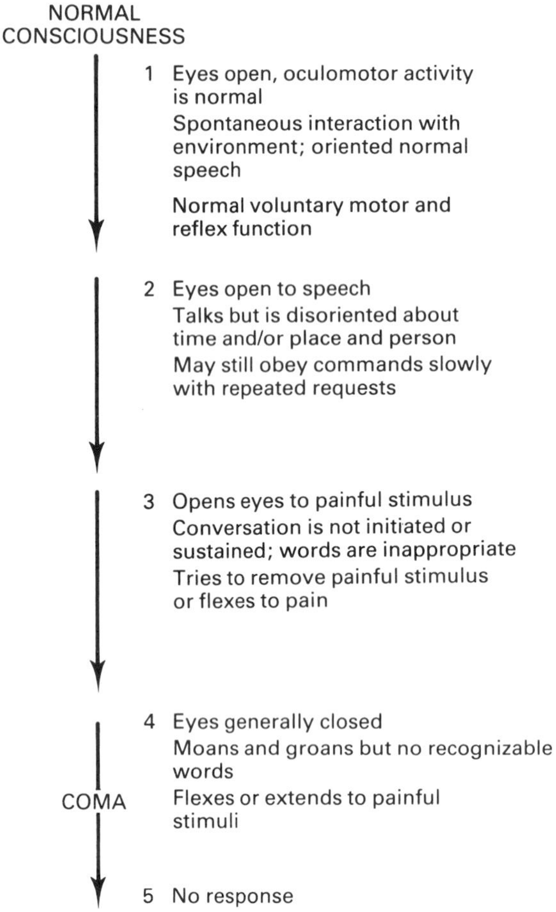

Causes of alterations in consciousness

Causes of an abnormal decrease in the level of consciousness may be classified as (1) abnormal metabolic processes, (2) supratentorial lesions which cause dysfunction of the upper brain stem (see Chapter 22), (3) infratentorial lesions which compress the reticular formation (see Chapter 22) or (4) psychogenic.

1 Processes which may interfere with the metabolism of the brain stem and cerebral cortex include: hypoglycaemia or diabetic ketoacidosis which produces a deficiency of glucose that is essential for cerebral neuronal functioning; cardiac failure, severe blood loss, anaemia, shock and respiratory failure which produce cerebral hypoxia; renal and hepatic failure which cause an accumulation of metabolic wastes; electrolyte imbalance; infections and autoimmune disorders; and drug overdose. Patients' manifestations resulting from altered metabolism show symmetrical changes in motor function. Many warning signals precede hypoglycaemia including nausea, vomiting, pallor, sweating, abdominal pain and light headedness. Overdoses of certain drugs produce varying responses; for example, opiates cause the pupils to constrict, while atropine produces dilation of the pupils. In acute alcoholism the patient will show some reaction to painful stimuli.

2 Supratentorial space-occupying lesions which may alter the level of consciousness include: cerebral haemorrhage from vascular diseases and trauma, tumours, abscess and haematoma from skull injuries. Manifestations are usually unequal on each side and may include hemiplegia and small reactive pupils which later become fixed.

3 Infratentorial lesions that may cause unconsciousness include: cerebral haemorrhage and brain stem infarction, tumours, and abscesses, as well as trauma which produces direct pressure on the reticular formation tissue in the brain stem. Symptoms include loss of reflexes and pupillary reactions. Patients with trauma or metabolic disturbance will show signs of generalized brain dysfunction rather than focal signs; it is important to assess overall brain function and vital signs frequently.

4 Altered consciousness from psychogenic causes may produce lack of responsiveness to environmental stimuli, with physiological responses remaining intact. Patients may manifest episodes of fainting which are sudden and transient and are often precipitated by a stressful event.

(Further discussion on the patient with a head injury and the nursing care of head injured patients is found in Chapter 22.)

NORMAL
CONSCIOUSNESS

1 Eyes open, oculomotor activity is normal
Spontaneous interaction with environment; oriented normal speech

Normal voluntary motor and reflex function

2 Eyes open to speech
Talks but is disoriented about time and/or place and person
May still obey commands slowly with repeated requests

3 Opens eyes to painful stimulus
Conversation is not initiated or sustained; words are inappropriate
Tries to remove painful stimulus or flexes to pain

4 Eyes generally closed
Moans and groans but no recognizable words

COMA   Flexes or extends to painful stimuli

5 No response

Fig. 10.2 Signs of altered consciousness.

Nursing Process

ASSESSMENT OF LEVEL OF CONSCIOUSNESS

HISTORY

The patient with an altered level of consciousness is unable to relate a history. Therefore, information must be obtained from the family members, friends, witnesses, police or rescue workers.

The history should include:

1 A description of the onset of injury. What events, behaviour changes or other unusual factors preceded the incident? When did the injury occur? What type of accident was it and where did it occur? What position was the patient in when found?

2 Whether there is evidence of an infection or a history of a recent infection.

3 History of previous seizures.

4 Information about associated health problems such as diabetes mellitus, cardiovascular or renal disease, respiratory disorder or psychiatric disturbance, which may have affected consciousness or will influence treatment.

5 Recurring headaches, nausea and vomiting, changes in attention span or irritability.[6]

6 The use of prescription and non-prescription drugs. Drug containers in the patient's home, bag or other personal effects or in the area of the incident should be collected and examined in relation to the possible toxic effects of their contents. The nurse should also look for a Medic-Alert bracelet and items such as a diabetic card.

Once information relevant to the initiation of treatment has been obtained and necessary life-support procedures have been instituted, further information is obtained about the patient. This may include identification of the patient and his family or friends who should be notified, past medical history, allergies, sensory deficits and corrective measures (e.g. use of hearing aid, contact lenses, glasses), work experiences, life-style, usual health habits, social and recreational interests, language spoken and relevant cultural and religious beliefs and practices. Knowledge of the patient's daily routine may be useful to the nurse in planning and structuring care that is relevant and meaningful and which may stimulate further awareness on the part of the patient.

PHYSICAL ASSESSMENT

It is difficult to define consciousness and to differentiate between levels or degrees of impairment. Terms such as confusion, drowsiness, stupor, semicomatose and deep coma have obscure meanings and are subject to varying interpretations by different observers. The Glasgow coma scale is a simple assessment tool for consciousness which standardizes observations.[7] It provides for accurate graphical recording of three aspects of behavioural response and the assessor is not required to interpret the observations. Changes in the patient's level of consciousness can be made by comparing current observations with previous results. The scale provides an assessment of overall brain functioning.

Glasgow coma scale
The Glasgow coma scale provides for evaluation of eye opening and the best verbal and motor responses. Within each of these three parameters, there are a variety of responses which are arranged in scales of increasing dysfunction, as outlined in Fig. 10.3. Each aspect is assessed independently of the others.

1 Eye opening.
   (a) *Spontaneous opening* (4). The nurse approaches the patient's bedside and notes whether the eyes are open or closed. Spontaneous opening of the eyes indicates that the arousal mechanism in the reticular activating system of the brain stem is functioning.
   (b) *Opening to speech* (3). If the patient's eyes are closed, the observer speaks to the patient, addressing him by name. If there is no response to a normal speaking voice, the volume should be increased.
   (c) *Opening to pain* (2). Physical stimulation, usually in the form of pressure on the fingernail bed using a pencil or pen is applied. If no response is elicited, pressure may be applied by the thumb over the supraorbital notch. It is important that observers use the same method of applying physical stimulation to ensure consistent, accurate findings.
   (d) *No eye opening* (1). If no response is demonstrated in either eye to increased pain stimuli, there is depression of the arousal system.

The patient may be sufficiently alert to respond by opening his eyes, but is restricted by swelling of the eyelids. If the eyelids are swollen shut, the observer records this as a 'C'.

2 Best verbal response. The patient's ability to speak and to understand the language spoken are determined. If the patient is intubated or has a tracheostomy, verbal response cannot be observed and 'T' is recorded. Speech is first used to stimulate a verbal response by asking the patient simple, direct questions. If there is no response a light touch is used or, if necessary, painful physical stimulation. Patient responses are rated as being: *oriented* (5) if he is able to respond as to who he is, where he is and give the year, month and day; *confused* (4) if not fully oriented to time, place and per-

---

[6] Conway-Rutkowski (1982), p. 202.

[7] Teasdale (1975), pp. 914–917.

				Date						
				Time						
GLASGOW COMA SCALE	Eye Opening	4. Spontaneously								Eyes closed due to swelling = C
		3. To Speech								
		2. To Pain								
		1. None								
	Best Verbal	5. Oriented								Endotracheal tube or Tracheostomy = T
		4. Confused								
		3. Inappropriate								
		2. Incomprehensible								
		1. None								
	Best Motor	6. Obeys commands								Usually record best arm response
		5. Localizes to pain								
		4. Flexion / Withdrawal to pain								
		3. Abnormal flexion								
		2. Abnormal extension								
		1. None								
	Pupils	Right eye	Size							+ = Reacts – = No Reaction C = Eyes Closed
			Reaction							
		Left eye	Size							
			Reaction							
LIMB MOVEMENT	Arms	Normal Power								Record Right (R) and Left (L) separately if there is a difference between the two sides
		Mild Weakness								
		Severe Weakness								
		Spastic Flexion								
		Extension								
		No Response								
	Legs	Normal Power								
		Mild Weakness								
		Severe Weakness								
		Extension								
		No Response								

Pupil Scale mm:
1 ●
2 ●
3 ●
4 ●
5 ●
6 ●
7 ●
8 ●

Blood Pressure
Systolic = V
Diastolic = Λ
Blue = Lying
Red = Sitting
      Standing

Pulse = •
         (Red)

210
200
190
180
170
160
150
140
130
120
110
100
90
80
70
60
50
40

42
41
40
39
38
37
36
35
34
33
32
31
30

°C

Temperature
= •
   (Blue)

Respirations
= •
(Blue)

30
25
20
15
10

30
25
20
15
10

Comments

Fig. 10.3 Assessment: level of consciousness.

son; *inappropriate* (3) if he utters words in a disorganized way, swears or does not engage in meaningful conversation; *incomprehensible* (2) when responses are limited to moaning, groaning or mumbling sounds with no recognizable words; and *no response* (1) when no sounds are made in response to noxious stimuli.

3 Best motor response. The best possible motor response in either arm is usually observed. The patient is asked to raise his arm, or two fingers. Asking the patient to grasp the observer's fingers is unreliable if the grasp reflex is present. In this situation, the patient may be asked to release his grasp. The ratings in order of decreasing levels of function include: *obeys commands* (6) when the patient understands verbal, written instructions or gestures and performs the requested movement, and *localization to pain* (5) occurs when there is no response to command. A painful stimulus is then applied such as pressure on the patient's fingernail bed or stimulation to an area of the head or trunk. The patient moves a limb in an attempt to locate and remove the stimulus.[8] *Flexion withdrawal to pain* (4) occurs when the arm bends at the elbow in response to fingernail bed pressure or other local stimulation. Leg flexion is not a reliable gauge because with brain death, a spinal reflex may be present causing the legs to flex in response to localized pain. *Abnormal flexion* (3) occurs when the arm flexes at the elbow and pronates, making a fist. *Abnormal extension to pain* (2) occurs when the elbow straightens and the arm abducts (usually with internal rotation) in response to localized pain applied to the fingernail bed. If one arm flexes and the other extends, the best response is recorded. *No response* (1) is recorded when no detectable movement or change in the tone of the limbs is observed in response to repeated and varied stimuli.

Assessment of pupil responses and limb movements provides information that assists in localizing lesions; for example, if the pupil starts to dilate, pressure on the third cranial nerve is present, and neighbouring parasympathetic fibres which control pupillary constriction are affected. This may indicate coning or herniation of brain tissue through the tentorial hiatus.

4 Pupils. Each pupil is examined for size and reaction. Normally, the pupils are round in shape, equal in size and constrict in response to direct light. The *size* of each pupil is measured by comparing it with the pupil scale as illustrated in Fig. 10.3. Pupil *reaction* is measured in response to light; the beam of a pentorch is brought in from the patient's side and directed on one eye at a time.

Constriction of the pupil is recorded as '+', or '−' when no reaction is obtained.

The surroundings should be dimly lit and the light beam of adequate intensity to obtain accurate results.

5 Limb movement. Verbal commands are used to elicit movement in each limb. When the patient does not respond to commands, painful stimuli are applied to the nail bed of a finger or great toe. Responses in order of decreasing function are recorded as: *normal power* when the limb movements are appropriate to the normal muscle strength for the patient; *mild weakness* when one limb shows normal strength but its opposite is weaker; *severe weakness* when the difference between two limbs is very much marked; *spastic flexion* when there is slow, stiff movement of the arm with the flexed forearm and hand held against the body; *extension* when the elbow or knee are straightened in response to painful stimulation; and *no response* when painful stimulation produces no movement and the limb remains limp.[9]

It is important to compare each side and to record differences between right and left limbs and changes in the responses of an individual limb.

6 Vital signs. The vital signs (i.e. temperature, pulse, respiration and blood pressure) should be recorded frequently when the patient's level of consciousness is changing or severely impaired. The comatose patient is not able to communicate whether he feels too cold or too warm. With head trauma and certain medical problems, the heat-regulating centre in the hypothalamus is disturbed and the body temperature may fluctuate rapidly. Continuous monitoring of temperature is instituted or individual readings taken every 15–30 minutes. Body temperature may be recorded every 2–4 hours when the patient is in a stable but unconscious condition. Changes in the pulse rate and rhythm and blood pressure provide information about possible increased intracranial pressure, internal bleeding or shock. In addition to observing the rate, rhythm and depth of respirations, the equality of chest movements on both sides and any sounds associated with inspiration or expiration are noted. The chest is auscultated by the doctor for possible retention of secretions and inadequate ventilation of some lung areas.

DIAGNOSTIC TESTS

Investigative procedures used to determine the cause of altered consciousness include the following.

Toxicology screening and *serum drug level* studies are carried out to identify concentration levels of central nervous system depressants and other drugs.

Blood concentrations of arterial gases, electrolytes,

---

[8] *Flexion* and *Extension* are the terms used in this assessment as opposed to *decorticate* and *decerebrate* which involve more subjective interpretation.

[9] Teasdale (1975), pp. 972–973.

creatinine, urea nitrogen and glucose may be determined.

A *computerized axial tomography* (CAT) scan of the skull may be performed to identify fractures, tissue dislocation or changes in the density of cerebral tissues. The location of a haematoma, abscess or tumour may be identified.

A *cerebral angiogram* may be performed to identify changes in the cerebral blood flow or to locate a cerebral aneurysm (a localized outpouching of the wall of a blood vessel).

Electroencephalography (EEG) may be performed to identify changes in neural impulses in the brain. Electrodes are placed on the scalp and electrical impulses produced within the brain are detected and recorded onto a graph. The frequency, amplitude and characteristics of the brain waves recorded are compared to normal expected patterns. Absence of cerebral function for 12 hours or more as identified by EEG is one criterion of brain death.

A lumbar puncture *is not performed* on a patient when increased intracranial pressure is suspected. Removal of cerebrospinal fluid relieves the pressure and may cause coning or herniation of the brain (see Chapter 22).

POTENTIAL PATIENT PROBLEMS

Table 10.1 lists problems relevant to the patient with an altered level of consciousness. These are:

1 Alteration in sensation—visual, auditory, kinaesthetic, gustatory, tactile and olfactory
2 Alteration in thought processes
3 Ineffective airway clearance
4 Impaired physical mobility
5 Potential for injury
6 Potential impairment of skin integrity
7 Alteration in nutrition (less than body requirements)
8 Alteration in patterns of urinary elimination—incontinence
9 Alteration in bowel elimination—incontinence
10 Inability to maintain self-care—feeding, bathing/hygiene, dressing/grooming, and toileting.

Goals for the patient with an altered level of consciousness are to:

1 Identify promptly changes in neurological function
2 Maintain normal body functions and prevent complications
3 Maintain or restore sensation, perception and awareness.

NURSING INTERVENTION

IDENTIFICATION OF CHANGES IN NEUROLOGICAL FUNCTION

Monitoring of the patient's level of consciousness, pupillary responses, limb movements and vital signs is done continuously. If the patient's condition is changing, data are recorded every 15 minutes. When the patient's neurological status stabilizes, recordings are gradually made less often. Early signs of increasing intracranial pressure (see Chapter 22) should be reported promptly to ensure immediate action to prevent cerebral coning. Signs of increasing intracranial pressure include decreasing scores on the coma scale, headache, nausea, altered pupil responses and decreasing limb movement. An intracranial pressure monitor may be used in the intensive care unit.

MAINTENANCE OF BODY FUNCTIONS AND PREVENTION OF COMPLICATIONS

Maintenance of a patent airway. The first priority in caring for an unconscious patient is the establishment of a patent airway. As the patient's level of consciousness decreases, his ability to maintain a clear airway is limited. The cause may be impairment of respiratory regulation by depression of the respiratory centre, obstruction of the airway by the tongue when the jaw and tongue relax, accumulation of secretions and foreign material as a result of depression of the cough reflex and immobility, decreased ventilation from weakness of respiratory muscles, inadequate gas exchange resulting from changes in the rate and depth of respirations or altered metabolic activity.

The unconscious patient is placed in a lateral or semiprone position (unless contraindicated by a chest or spinal injury), with the neck aligned with the spine. Either position facilitates the drainage of mucus and vomit and prevents obstruction of the airway by the relaxed tongue and jaw. If mucus collects in the oropharyngeal cavity, frequent suctioning with a flexible catheter will be necessary. The suction catheter should have several holes at its tip for adequate collection of the mucus during the procedure. The catheter is moistened with water prior to its insertion and is handled gently during insertion and on withdrawal, to avoid trauma to the delicate tracheal mucous membranes (see Chapter 16 for details related to the suctioning procedure).

If the patient is restricted to the dorsal position because of his condition (e.g. a patient who is unconscious due to a motor vehicle accident may also require traction), or his breathing is hindered in the semiprone position, an artificial airway may be needed. An oropharyngeal airway or an endotracheal or tracheostomy tube may be inserted to maintain the airway and facilitate the removal of secretions by suctioning. (See Chapter 16 for a discussion of intubation and tracheostomy.)

Oxygen may be administered by nasal cannulae or mask, or mechanical ventilation may be instituted (see Chapter 16). If the patient is semiconscious or regaining consciousness and is able to follow instruc-

Table 10.1 Potential problems relevant to the patient with an altered level of consciousness.

Problem	Causative factors	Signs and symptoms
Altered sensation: Visual, auditory, kinaesthetic, gustatory, tactile and olfactory	Abnormal metabolic processes Supratentorial lesions Infratentorial lesions Psychogenic	Disoriented in time or place Disoriented with persons Altered abstraction Altered conceptualization[1] Altered problem-solving abilities Altered behaviour or communication patterns Anxiety Irritability Reports auditory or visual hallucinations.
Alterations in thought processes	Abnormal metabolic processes Supratentorial lesions Infratentorial lesions Psychogenic	Disorientation to time, place, person, circumstances and events Altered perception Lack of concentration Memory deficit Hyper/hypovigilance Impaired ability to make decisions Impaired ability to reason[2]
Airway clearance ineffective	Loss of gag reflex Immobility Impaired perception and awareness	Cough ineffective Rapid respirations Râles and rhonchi present on auscultation of lungs Cyanosis Dyspnoea Secretions in oral pharynx
Impaired physical mobility	Neuromuscular impairment Immobilization Impaired perception or awareness	Altered muscle tone Decreased range of joint movement Impaired coordination Decreased muscle strength
Potential for injury	Lack of awareness of environmental hazards Potential for complications from invasive therapeutic measures	Bruises and skin abrasions Altered mobility Impaired coordination Disorientation to circumstances and events
Potential impairment of skin integrity	Immobility Altered muscle tone/spasticity Altered sensation Weight loss Inadequate nutrition Use of restraints, splints, and other devices Urinary incontinence	Redness, oedema, or breaks in skin Immobility Use of restraints, splints or other devices Spasticity Urinary incontinence Decreased sensation
Alterations in nutrition: less than body requirements	Immobility Loss of gag reflex Loss of control of voluntary movement Impaired awareness	Weight loss Decreased daily food/fluid intake Decreased skin thickness Aspiration of food/fluids
Alteration in patterns of urinary elimination: incontinence	Immobility Impaired awareness Sensory motor impairment Neuromuscular impairment	Involuntary voiding
Alteration in bowel elimination: incontinence	Immobility Neuromuscular impairment Impaired awareness Alteration in nutrition	Involuntary passage of stools
Self-care deficit: feeding, bathing/hygiene, dressing/grooming, toileting	Impaired perception and awareness Neuromuscular impairment Decreased strength and endurance	Inability to feed, bathe, dress, groom or toilet self Lack of coordination Inability to follow instructions

[1] Kim (1984), p. 51.
[2] Kim (1984), p. 59.

tions, deep breathing is practised hourly. Hard, sustained coughing is contraindicated as it causes an increase in intracranial pressure. If coughing is necessary to remove secretions and the patient is able to do so, staged coughing is taught. This involves the patient taking a deep breath while relaxing his abdominal muscles, holding the breath, and then exhaling in short, staged intervals involving 4–5 expirations. Postural drainage and chest percussion and vibration are carried out several times a day by the physiotherapist to promote drainage of respiratory secretions.

The patient's position should be changed every two hours. Observations are made following each change of position to determine the effect on respirations. Chest expansion is observed and the rate and rhythm of respirations are noted as well as the patient's colour and general status. The doctor will auscultate the lungs for the presence of wheezes and crackles, which indicate the accumulation of secretions, and for air entry.

Care of the eyes. Loss of the corneal reflex and depression of lacrimal secretion may result in prolonged exposure, drying and injury to the cornea which may lead to ulceration. The eyes should be examined regularly for signs of inflammation or injury. Contact lenses are removed. Ophthalmic solutions may be prescribed to irrigate the eyes three or four times a day. The eyes may be covered with eye patches or closed with butterfly dressings to protect them.

Care of the mouth. Dentures should be removed if the patient is unconscious. The mouth is cleansed several times a day using a solution of bicarbonate of soda to loosen debris and is then cleansed with swabs moistened with a mouthwash solution, e.g. glycothymol, or with water. The teeth are cleaned by brushing when possible. The lips are moistened with a water-soluble ointment or cream. The mouth should be inspected daily for signs of crusting or ulceration of the mucosa.

Positioning. When the patient is placed in the lateral or semiprone position (as cited above), attention is given to good body alignment and to the prevention of contractures, foot and wrist drop, muscle strain, joint injury, and interference with circulation and chest expansion. The head should be positioned so that the neck is aligned with the spine. The arm that is uppermost is flexed at the elbow and rested on a pillow to prevent a drag on the shoulder and wrist drop. The arm that is down is drawn slightly forward, flexed at the elbow, and lies on the bed parallel with the neck and head. The lower limb that is uppermost is flexed at the hip and knee, and supported on a firm, plastic-covered pillow; the other lower limb is slightly flexed. The feet are positioned at a 90° angle to the leg and care is taken that *no* pressure is applied by firm objects placed against the feet.

The patient should be turned at least every 2 hours to promote circulation and to prevent the accumulation of pulmonary secretions and the development of pressure sores. A minimum of two or three persons is necessary to turn the unconscious patient in such a manner that hyperextension and joint and muscle strain are avoided.

Joint movement. The extremities are passively moved through their normal range of motion at least twice daily to preserve joint function and prevent circulatory stasis. Active exercises are initiated as soon as the patient is able to follow instructions.

Protection from injury. The cot-sides of the bed are always maintained in the up position when the patient is unconscious unless someone is in constant attendance on the patient. It may be necessary to pad the sides of the bed if the patient is restless and thrashing about. Placing mittens on the hands may be necessary if the patient is restless, scratches himself, or pulls on the nasogastric or intravenous tube, or the urethral catheter. The mittens are removed at least twice daily; the hands are bathed, the nails are kept clean and short, and the fingers put through their normal range of motion by passive exercise.

The use of restraints is avoided. The patient often becomes more restless if restrained when he is confused or disoriented. The nurse should not attempt to force resisting extremities (such as in spastic flexion or extension) to assume a different position. Forcing a rigid extremity into a different position could result in a fracture of that limb. The use of depressant drugs to control agitation is contraindicated as they may further depress the arousal system.

When the patient is ambulatory but has some impairment of awareness, a safe environment should be provided. Scatter rugs and objects are removed from the patient's path to prevent falling. Sharp objects are removed from the immediate environment.

Fluids and nutrition. The patient is assessed for a gag reflex; as soon as it is present, and the patient is conscious, oral feedings are initiated. Non-milk foods are introduced first. When the patient is unconscious or the gag reflex is absent the patient's nutrition may be sustained by intravenous infusion or feedings given via a nasogastric tube. The liquid feed given by tube contains the essential food elements and the amount is individually calculated to provide adequate caloric intake for the patient's size and metabolic activity. The dietitian should be consulted for advice. Frequency of feeding varies from slow continuous to every 4 hours. If there is any regurgitation (fluid welling up around the tube into the mouth), the volume given at one time is decreased and the frequency of the feedings is increased. If the patient's condition permits, it is helpful to elevate the head of the bed slightly during the feeding and for a brief period following. The tube is rinsed with 30–45 ml of water after each feeding.

The presence of the tube in a nostril tends to irritate the mucous membrane and stimulate mucus secretion. The area is cleansed twice daily with applicators which have been moistened with normal saline, and is then also lubricated lightly. The tube should be secured loosely enough so that it does not continuously press on any one area of the nostril.

When a patient is unconscious for a prolonged period a gastrostomy may be performed. An opening is made into the stomach and a tube is introduced through which food and fluids may be administered. (This technique is rarely used.)

Elimination. The unconscious patient has urinary incontinence. An indwelling catheter is inserted initially only if it is necessary to facilitate accurate monitoring of output or if retention of urine occurs. The catheter is removed as soon as possible to prevent complications and promote the return of normal bladder functioning. Condom drainage is established with the male patient as soon as his condition is stable. While the catheter is in place it is taped to the thigh to prevent undue traction. The complete set of tubes and drainage receptacle constitutes a closed sterile system. The urethral meatus and surrounding area may be cleansed with an antiseptic solution two or three times daily and an antiseptic ointment may be placed around the catheter at the meatus—according to the doctor's instructions.

If a catheter is not used, frequent attention is necessary to protect the skin. Incontinence pads are used to absorb the urine and are changed promptly after voiding. The skin is washed after each voiding and dried thoroughly. A barrier cream may be applied to the skin. The bed linen is changed as necessary.

The patient may be incontinent of faeces, particularly if he is receiving tube feedings. Prompt cleansing and changing of soiled pads and bedding are necessary. If the bowels do not move regularly, the doctor will prescribe an aperient, suppositories or an enema.

Skin care. The unconscious patient is predisposed to the rapid development of pressure sores. Precautions should be taken to keep the skin clean and dry and the bedding free of wrinkles. Pressure areas are bathed and gently dried; talcum powder may also be applied. A resilient, soft material, such as sponge rubber or sheepskin, is placed under the pressure areas, or an alternating air pressure (ripple) mattress may be used. The patient's position is changed at least every 2 hours. If a pressure sore develops it is treated aseptically, just as any wound, and the patient is positioned to avoid pressure on the area.

MAINTENANCE OR RESTORATION OF SENSATION, PERCEPTION AND AWARENESS

Fluctuations in consciousness affect the patient's ability to receive a stimulus, interpret its meaning and respond with appropriate behaviour. The arousal mechanism may be affected so that repeated stimulation may be required to elicit a response. Sensory stimulation is an important aspect of the care of every patient experiencing alterations in the level of consciousness. The type of stimulation, how it is structured and presented and its complexity must be planned for each individual according to his level of consciousness, the cause of the decreased consciousness and the relevance and meaning of the stimulus to this particular individual.

Types of stimuli include the following:[10]

(a) *Auditory* stimulation is provided by the nurse who regularly addresses the patient by name, explains where he is and states the date and time and what is happening to him at any given time. Family members and friends are encouraged to talk to the patient. Radios, tape recordings of music or conversations from friends and family or talking books may also be used to provide auditory stimulation. Environmental noises are interpreted to prevent distortion; bedside curtains and room doors are left open to allow for visualization of the source of sounds.

(b) *Olfactory* stimulation by noxious odours such as sulphur or ammonia may be used to evoke a response. The patient is also exposed to familiar, accustomed pleasant odours; these may include perfumes, coffee, tea, or flowers.

(c) *Visual* stimuli may be provided by a stimulation board placed at the foot or side of the bed; cards, posters and photographs of family members may be pinned to the board. Mobiles can be made to serve the same purpose. Personal possessions, favourite toys and pictures are placed in the patient's line of vision. Television also provides visual stimulation. The human face, especially when it belongs to a friend, is invaluable; visitors are instructed to sit or stand where the patient can see them.

(d) *Tactile* stimulation may be provided by the nurse and family members; the latter are encouraged to use touch and to have the patient touch them in return. Tactile stimuli may take the form of massage, gentle touching or brisk rubbing.

(e) *Kinaesthetic* sensations may be promoted by 'range of motion' exercises of the extremities and by changes in body position. A programme of mat activities may be provided by the physiotherapist.

---

[10] *Stimulation Program for Cognitive Deficits in Traumatic Head Injured Adults.* Unpublished, Hamilton General Hospital, Hamilton, Ontario.

(f) *Vestibular* stimulation may be provided by tilt tables.

(g) *Oral* stimulation may be produced by cotton swabs or flavours may be used on swabs, or ice chips may be given for sucking if the gag reflex is present. Foods of varying textures are provided if the patient is able to swallow, when consciousness returns.

The nurse should always speak to the patient, call him by name and explain what is being done for him. He is told when feeds are being given and that he is being turned. Touch is used as much as possible. Environmental noise is decreased and night orientation is practised to provide rest. Multisensory stimuli sessions may be carried out three or four times a day. Each method of stimulation is introduced one at a time in a form that is meaningful to the patient.

The daily programme for the patient who is able to respond is structured to resemble his usual activities as much as possible. The patient is told what is happening, what is expected of him and what will happen next. Commands are simple, one-step or phase at a time. A variety of sensory procedures are planned and incorporated into the daily care. When the patient is able to follow commands and carry out self-care activities, simple decision-making is included. These may relate to self-care functions or be in the form of games, puzzles, pictures or shapes. Tasks of increasing complexity are introduced when indicated by the responses.

Agitated patients require structure and routine. Extraneous stimuli are eliminated to allow the patient to focus on relevant and meaningful stimuli.

Memory books and diaries are useful tools to help patients recall what they have done and to remind them what is to occur next.

EXPECTED OUTCOMES

1 The patient's level of consciousness as measured by the Glasgow coma scale increases.
2 Complications are prevented as demonstrated by:
 (a) normal vital signs
 (b) absence of corneal injury
 (c) clean, dry and intact skin
 (d) clean and intact oral mucosa
 (e) the range of joint motion within expected limits for the patient
 (f) normal bowel and bladder elimination
 (g) weight within 2.5 kg of usual weight
3 Return of cognitive functioning will vary with each individual.
4 Relearning of self-care skills will vary with each individual and will require a skilled rehabilitation programme.

References and Further Reading

BOOKS

Bannister Sir R (1985) *Brain's Clinical Neurology*, 6th ed. Oxford: Oxford University Press. Chapter 13.

Braunwald E et al (1987) *Harrison's Principles of Internal Medicine*, 11th ed. New York: McGraw-Hill.

Carlson NR (1977) *Physiology of Behavior*. Boston: Allyn & Bacon. Chapter 15.

Conway-Rutkowski BL (1982) *Carini and Owen's Neurological and Neurosurgical Nursing*, 8th ed. St Louis: CV Mosby. Chapter 9.

Guyton AC (1986) *Textbook of Medical Physiology*, 7th ed. Philadelphia: WB Saunders. Chapter 55.

Hart LK, Reese JL & Fearing MO (1981) *Concepts Common to Acute Illness*. St Louis: CV Mosby. Chapter 8.

Kim MJ, McFarland GK & McLane AM (eds) (1984) *Pocket Guide to Nursing Diagnosis*. St Louis: CV Mosby.

Kinney MR, Dear CB, Packa DR & Voorman DMN (eds) (1981) *AACN's Clinical Reference for Critical Care Nursing*. New York: McGraw-Hill. pp. 600–622.

Malasnos L, Barkauskas V, Moss M & Stoltenberg-Allen K (1981) *Health Assessment*, St Louis: CV Mosby. Chapter 8.

Pallett PJ & O'Brien MT (1985) *Textbook of Neurological Nursing*. Boston: Little, Brown. pp. 384–401.

Plum F & Posner JB (1980) *The Diagnosis of Stupor and Coma*, 3rd ed. Philadelphia: FA Davis.

Rudy EB (1984) *Advanced Neurological and Neurosurgical Nursing*. St Louis: CV Mosby. pp. 81–85 & 243–264.

Smith LH & Thier SO (1985) *Pathophysiology: The Biological Principles of Disease*, 2nd ed. Philadelphia: WB Saunders. pp. 1137–1167.

Wilson SF (1979) *Neuronursing*. New York: Springer. Chapter 4.

Wolanin MO & Phillips LRF (1981) *Confusion*. St Louis: CV Mosby.

PERIODICALS

Allen N (1979) Prognostic indicators in coma. *Heart Lung*, Vol. 8 No. 6, pp. 1075–1083.

Anonymous (1980) Head trauma. *Emerg. Med.*, Vol. 12 No. 19, pp. 103–113.

Bowers SA & Marshall LF (1982) Severe head injury: current treatment and research. *J. Neurosurg. Nurs.*, Vol. 14 No. 5, pp. 210–219.

Brigman C, Dickey C & Zegeer LJ (1983) The agitated aggressive patient. *Am. J. Nurs.*, Vol. 83 No. 10, pp. 1409–1412.

Collins VJ (1979) Ethical considerations in therapy for the comatose and dying patient. *Heart Lung*, Vol. 8 No. 6, pp. 1084–1088.

Elliott J & Smith DR (1985) Meeting family needs following severe head injury: a multidisciplinary approach. *J. Neurosurg. Nurs.*, Vol. 17 No. 2, pp. 111–113.

Finklestein S & Ropper A (1979) The diagnosis of coma: its pitfalls and limitations. *Heart Lung*, Vo. 8 No. 6, pp. 1059–1064.

Fritz CP (1981) Concussion. *Nurs. '81*, Vol. 11 No. 9, pp. 13–15.

Gannon EP & Kadezabek E (1980) Giving your patients meticulous mouth care. *Nurs. '80*, Vol. 10 No. 3, pp. 70–75.

Jennett B (1979) If my son had a head injury. *Br. Med. J.*, Vol. 17 No. 6, pp. 1601–1603.

Jones C (1979) Glasgow Coma Scale. *Am. J. Nurs.*, Vol. 79 No. 9, pp. 1551–1553.

Kunkel J & Wiley JK (1979) Acute head injury: what to do when and why. *Nurs. '79*, Vol. 9, No. 3, pp. 22–33.

Mauss-Clum N & Ryan M (1981) Brain injury and the family. *J. Neurosurg. Nurs.*, Vol. 13 No. 4, pp. 165–169.

McGuffin JF (1983) Basic cerebral trauma care. *J. Neurosurg. Nurs.*, Vol. 15 No. 4, pp. 189–193.

Miller M (1981) Emergency management of the unconscious patient. *Nurs. Clin. N. Am.*, Vol. 16 No. 1, pp. 59–73.

Myco F & McGilloway FA (1980) Care of the unconscious patient: a complementary perspective. *J. Adv. Nurs.*, Vol. 5 No. 3, pp. 273–283.

Pemberton L (1979) Assessment and care: nursing an unconscious patient. *Nurs. Mirror*, Vol. 149 No. 11, pp. 41–43.

Rimel RC & Tyson GW (1979) The neurological examination in patients with central nervous system trauma. *J. Neurolog. Nurs.*, Vol. 11 No. 3, pp. 148–155.

Rimel RC, John JA & Edlich RF (1979) An injury severity scale for comprehensive management of central nervous system trauma. *JACEP*, Vol. 8 No. 2, pp. 64–67.

Shpritz DW (1983) Craniocerebral trauma. *Crit. Care Nurs.*, Vol. 3 No. 2, pp. 49, 52, 55–56.

Spielman G (1981) Coma: a clinical review. *Heart Lung*, Vol. 10 No. 4, pp. 700–707.

Teasdale G (1975) Acute impairment of brain function— Part 1, Assessing conscious level. *Nurs. Times*, Vol. 71 No. 24, pp. 914–917.

Teasdale G, Galbraith S & Clarke K (1975) Acute impairment of brain function—Part 2, Observation record chart. *Nurs. Times*, Vol. 71 No. 25, pp. 972–973.

Wong J, Wong S & Dempster IK (1984) Care of the unconscious patient: a problem oriented approach. *J. Neurosurg Nurs.*, Vol. 16 No. 3, pp. 145–150.

Yanko J (1984) Head injuries. *J. Neurosurg. Nurs.*, Vol. 16 No. 4, pp. 173–180.

Young MS (1981) Understanding the signs of intracranial pressure. *Nurs. '81*, Vol. 11 No. 2, pp. 59–62.

11

The Surgical Patient

Surgery is defined as the treatment of disease, injury or deformity by manual or instrumental procedure.[1] This indicates the special feature that categorizes the patient as being surgical, but the care that contributes to the restoration and maintenance of optimum physiological status before and after the operation comprises a large portion of the total surgical treatment and is extremely important in determining the patient's progress and recovery.

Surgical operations may be classified as elective, essential or emergency. An *elective operation* is not necessary for the patient's survival but is expected to improve the patient's comfort and health. *Essential surgery* is considered necessary to remove or to prevent a threat to the patient's life. An *emergency operation* is one which must be done with a minimum of delay in the interest of the patient's survival.

Operative procedures vary greatly. They range from one that is quite simple and uncomplicated, taking only a brief period, to a prolonged, complex, major procedure that has severe traumatic effects. Many necessary considerations and nursing measures are common to the care of all surgical patients, regardless of their particular type of surgery. The basic components of the plan of care may require modification and/or additional specific details according to the particular operation, the individual's psychological or physiological status, and the type of anaesthetic used.

Preparation of the Patient for Surgery

The preoperative period, which begins with the decision that surgery is to be performed, may extend over an hour to several days or weeks. Whenever the patient's condition permits, sufficient time is taken to assess and treat the patient so that he goes to the operation in the best condition possible. Intelligent, conscientious preoperative nursing may contribute much to having the patient achieve an optimum condition that favours a satisfactory postoperative progress and minimizes the possibility of complications. When the surgery is elective or essential, there is usually a period of several days or weeks that the patient is at home awaiting admission to the hospital. A district nurse may contribute to the patient's

---
[1] Miller & Keane (1986), p. 1078.

physical and psychological preparation during this time. Some of the patient's and family's questions may be answered, psychological support provided and advice given on such matters as nutrition and rest. Possible solutions to social and economic problems that are precipitated by the impending surgery may also be suggested by the district nurse.

Psychological preparation

IDENTIFICATION OF PATIENT PROBLEMS

Potential problems common to the patient preoperatively include: (1) anxiety; and (2) lack of knowledge (see Table 11.1).

Preoperative *goals* for nursing intervention are as follows.
1 To decrease anxiety by:
   (a) Identifying the patient's fears and concerns.
   (b) Assessing effectiveness of adaptive responses.
   (c) Supporting effective adaptive responses.
   (d) Answering questions and providing information.
2 Patient teaching. The nurse should:
   (a) Assess the patient's understanding of the operation and events that will occur pre- and postoperatively.
   (b) Inform the patient about the surgical procedure and the pre- and postoperative procedures and activities.
   (c) Teach the patient to perform deep-breathing, coughing and leg exercises, explaining the purpose of each.
   (d) Provide information relating to the expectations of the patient and explain the nurse's pre- and postoperative role.

Anxiety
Few patients face surgery without some degree of anxiety. The concerns and fear vary from one person to another; some may be anxious about the pain and discomfort, others fear possible disfigurement and incapacity, loss of control of self, or death. They may be worried because of absence from work, lack of support for dependants, lack of care for the family or disruption of plans. Many are disturbed because they simply don't know what to expect; the unknown tends to be more threatening than the known.

The patient's emotional state and physical condition should receive equal consideration. Psychologi-

Table 11.1 Potential problems common to the patient preoperatively.

Problem	Causative factors	Goals
Anxiety	Hospitalization Impending surgery Fear of the unknown	To decrease anxiety by: (a) Identifying the patient's fears and concerns (b) Assessing the effectiveness of adaptive responses (c) Supporting effective adaptive responses (d) Answering questions and providing information
Lack of knowledge about preoperative preparation, expectations, the preoperative procedure and postoperative care	Insufficient information given Inexperience Anxiety	To promote patient and family understanding of preoperative care and expectations regarding surgery and postoperative care

cal stress evokes physiological responses (release of adrenaline and noradrenaline) which may have an unfavourable effect, especially if prolonged. The emotionally disturbed patient may experience a greater problem with vomiting, urinary retention, pain and restlessness during the postoperative period.

Assessment. The patient's concerns, perception of the surgery, and usual patterns of dealing with stress should be identified. Understanding the meaning of religion to the patient may help in the selection of appropriate support for the patient and family. Through more prolonged and intimate contact with the patient, the nurse has the opportunity to assess his perception of the situation and identify his attitudes and concerns. Many of his and his family's fears may be unrealistic, based on misinformation and misconceptions about the surgery.

The level of the patient's anxiety may be assessed by observation of behaviours such as hyperactivity, increased talking, repetition of questions, crying, physical withdrawal, decreased social interactions and insomnia. Objective signs of stress include increased heart and respiratory rates, elevated blood pressure, moist palms and restless movements.

Nursing intervention. The patient is encouraged to reveal his fears and concerns, which the nurse should show are accepted, reasonable and to be expected. The problems are explored and, through expressing them and receiving some explanation or available assistance, some of the apprehension may be allayed. The fact that someone expects him to have some qualms and is sufficiently interested to listen to him is in itself a comfort to the patient. Some patients may be reluctant to express their fears because they think of them as a personal weakness, but they may be manifesting their insecurity in other ways such as tenseness, restlessness or withdrawal. The nurse, recognizing the problem, may initiate a discussion by saying, 'I am sure you are concerned about your operation; there may be something I

could clarify for you if you would like to talk about it'. There may be the occasional patient who displays a total lack of concern; this person may have considerable deep underlying concern which for some reason he is denying. Effective adaptive responses and available family and helpful community resources are discussed.

Unrealistic fears based on misinformation and misconceptions can be alleviated by providing factual information. The patient should be kept informed as to the purpose of the operation and what is involved in the investigative and preparatory procedures. What he may expect on the day of operation and in the postoperative period is discussed. Ignorance of what is going to happen usually causes more fear and mental suffering than being advised of the facts.

Any anticipated permanent change in body function or appearance is explored, and the patient is advised as to the available assistance and how he may manage his life; emphasis is placed on the positive aspects. For instance, a woman who is to have a mastectomy may be concerned about her appearance but is relieved when she learns that special prosthetic brassieres are available. A patient who is being prepared for a permanent colostomy may be encouraged to see and talk with a person who has had the same operation and is living a relatively normal, active life. Patients should be referred, where possible, to nurses who have specialized in these particular problems.

It is an established practice in some institutions to have an operating theatre nurse who will be involved with the patient's surgery visit him 2 or 3 days before the day of operation. This has distinct advantages for the patient. It tends to lessen 'the fear of the unknown' for the patient. The visit means that when he is received in the operating theatre, the nurses will not all be complete strangers. It also indicates an interest on the part of the staff, which is reassuring to the patient. The nurse reviews the patient's history, talks with his ward nurse and advises the patient of the purpose of this visit. The discussion includes such matters as transport to the operating theatre, the type of room he will be in, any pre-anaesthetic checks, why staff are gowned and masked, the anaesthetic and the postoperative return to the recovery room or the surgical ward. The patient is encouraged to ask questions. The visit to the ward and patient provides the theatre nurse with information about the patient that enables the theatre staff to be prepared more fully for this particular patient. For example, the patient may have a disability that necessitates preparation for placing him in a different position than that normally used.

Consideration should be given to placement on the ward by selecting a bed that is quiet and nearer to those less likely to increase anxiety in the patient. Long periods in which the patient is entirely alone should be avoided; relatives are encouraged to visit and the nurse should 'drop in' at frequent intervals. Some form of diversion in which he is interested may be provided. The patient may find his local vicar, priest, etc. a source of strength and courage. In some instances help beyond that which the nurse can provide is needed to reduce the patient's fear. It may be necessary to consult the surgeon, anaesthetist or social worker and have one of them talk further with the patient.

Visits with other patients and socializing in the day-room are encouraged. Most patients tend to talk readily to each other about their problems and share their preoperative fears. The fact that many of the same concerns are experienced by others seems to put them in proper perspective and make them less ominous to the patient.

Family members are kept informed, and time is taken to talk with them, answer their questions, and advise them as to how they can offer support to the patient.

Patient teaching

Assessment. The identification of learning needs includes an assessment of the patient's understanding of the surgical procedure and perceptions of the pre- and postoperative experiences. The fact that surgery is scheduled motivates most patients to seek information and their receptiveness to the information provided is increased. In emergency situations, life-threatening needs receive priority over detailed, extensive explanations, but the patient always has the right to some information and to make *informed* decisions. A moderate degree of anxiety enhances learning but when anxiety increases, the attention span and receptiveness decrease.

Nursing intervention. The surgeon will have discussed the operation with the patient and family: why it is necessary, what it involves and the expected results. Frequently the patient and the family are so emotionally overcome at the time that they do not grasp all that has been said. Later, they want clarification of what has been said, and they usually have a number of questions. The nurse determines what information was given to them by the doctor and, in simple, understandable terms, repeats necessary information and answers their questions.

Preoperative procedures and what will be expected of the patient are discussed. Expectations for the postoperative period are outlined. The patient is advised as to where he will be after the operation has taken place; that is, whether he will be taken to a recovery room or the intensive care unit or returned to the present location.

A description of the recovery room and what occurs there is given to the patient, and the family is told that they will be permitted to visit when the patient returns to the ward. The reasons for the *frequent assessment of vital signs*, alertness and responses should also be explained.

Deep breathing is demonstrated and taught; maximal inspirations, which are held for 3–5 seconds and practised several times an hour, increase arterial oxygen saturation and prevent postoperative pulmonary complications. The technique should be demonstrated and the patient given the opportunity to practise it prior to surgery. Use of a spirometer to show the patient how much air is taken into and expelled from the lungs, provides incentive to practise the exercises and provides evidence of the effectiveness of the patient's efforts. The patient is taught to *cough* by supporting the area where the incision will be, taking a deep breath and expelling the air forcefully through the mouth. Coughing is encouraged postoperatively to facilitate the removal of bronchial secretions. Table 11.2 illustrates deep-breathing and coughing techniques. The patient is assured that necessary assistance and support will be provided. Emphasis should be placed on *non-smoking* during the preoperative and postoperative periods; any irritation of the respiratory tract predisposes to pulmonary complications.

Postoperative *lower limb exercises* to prevent circulatory stasis and thrombosis are described and demonstrated. The patient is advised that he will be expected to get out of bed, sit in a chair and walk around the room for brief periods in the early postoperative period; early ambulation promotes normal body functioning and reduces problems such as vomiting, wind pains and urine retention. If the use of drainage tubes (e.g. chest or gastric) or special equipment such as a suction machine is anticipated, preoperative preparation includes an explanation of the purpose and procedure and what will be expected of the patient.

Information is also given about any postoperative pain that may be expected, the cause of the pain and what will be done to control it. The patient is told how he can participate in pain control by asking for medication before the pain becomes severe and by practising relaxation, leg exercises, ambulation and

Table 11.2 Instructions given to patients about breathing and coughing exercises.

Sustained maximal inspiration	Coughing
From a sitting or standing position: 1 Take a deep breath through the mouth, pushing the diaphragm down and distending the abdomen as the chest expands 2 Hold breath for 3–5 seconds 3 Breathe out slowly 4 Repeat several times each hour	From a sitting position: 1 Support incision with hands or pillow 2 Take a deep breath through the mouth pushing the diaphragm down and distending the abdomen as the chest expands 3 Immediately force the air from the lungs out through the mouth 4 Expectorate secretions into a sputum pot 5 Repeat several times every 2–4 hours if secretions are present

other techniques that may have worked previously in relieving pain. Relaxation techniques may be taught if the patient is very anxious, requests it or if severe, prolonged pain is anticipated. Voshall demonstrated that when patients were informed about anticipated pain and given some control over the pain experience, their apprehension was decreased, their pain tolerance increased and they were discharged sooner.[2]

Owens and Hutelmyer showed that cardiac surgical patients who were informed about what to expect and how to deal with experiences such as delirium and decreased ability to concentrate and recognize familiar objects, were better able to cope with the experiences.[3]

Group instruction in deep-breathing, coughing, leg exercises and pain management can be an effective method of teaching. Group instruction saves nursing time and provides opportunity for patients to practise techniques together and share anxieties and fears. Individual instruction is necessary to provide specific information related to the surgical experience of the individual and his family.

Physical preparation

Physical assessment

Common concerns with all surgical patients are cardiac, pulmonary and renal function, blood volume and composition, nutritional status and fluid and electrolyte balance. Basic laboratory tests for all preoperative patients include urinalysis, haematocrit, haemoglobin, white cell count, and bleeding or clotting time. An electrocardiogram is often done, and the chest is examined by auscultation and probably x-ray. Other laboratory tests, functional studies and x-rays may be done, as well as specific investigative procedures relevant to the patient's particular disorder and physiological status. These studies should be understood by the nurse so that the necessary explanation, support for the patient and the

appropriate adaptations in the nursing care plan can be made.

The nurse is constantly alert for signs and symptoms that might indicate a condition or change in the patient which could interfere with the patient's progress and predispose to complications. Such factors as the following are promptly reported to the doctor: a raised temperature; a significant change in pulse, respirations or blood pressure; a rash; a cough, complaint of sore throat or nasal discharge that might point to a respiratory infection; bleeding gums, which may indicate a vitamin C deficiency; onset of menstruation; diarrhoea; nausea and vomiting; and a deficient food or fluid intake.

Patient history

The patient's history includes information that may be significant in the patient's responses to surgery and recovery.

Infants, young children and the elderly are less able to tolerate the stress of surgery. Obesity and nutritional deficiencies interfere with wound healing and predispose to cardiovascular and pulmonary problems. Smoking irritates the respiratory tract and increases secretions, predisposing to respiratory complications; platelet function and blood coagulation are also altered. Existing cardiovascular, renal and liver disorders and diabetes increase the potential for the development of complications postoperatively.

A detailed drug history related to both prescription and non-prescription medications is obtained. Acetylsalicylic acid preparations prolong bleeding. The nurse should be aware of the potential effects of prior drug therapy so that she can identify potential risks and make plans for postoperative observations and interventions for the prevention and prompt identification of problems.

History of any allergic reactions is recorded and an allergy alert bracelet may be placed on the patient's wrist and the chart marked appropriately to alert the surgeon, anaesthetist and nursing personnel.

Nutrition

The patient who is malnourished tolerates surgery less well. Protein deficiency delays healing and decreases the resistance to infection because of a

---

[2] Voshall (1980), pp. 39–43.
[3] Owens & Hutelmyer (1982), p. 61.

slower response in antibody formation. Vitamin C also plays an important role in healing since it is necessary for the laying down of collagen fibres. It also contributes to capillary integrity. Optimum amounts of the vitamin B complex are necessary for normal glucose metabolism and for the maintenance of cellular enzymes. A deficient intake of carbohydrate depletes the liver glycogen, leaving the body without a reserve source of glucose during the period when food intake is decreased, which leads to catabolism of the body tissues.

If the patient is not obese and can tolerate it, he is given a high-calorie (3000–4000 kcal, 12600–16700 kJ) high-carbohydrate diet and vitamin supplements. The patient is more likely to cooperate if he is advised of the significant role nutrition plays in his postoperative progress. Feeding the patient or providing some assistance may be necessary if he is weak or uncomfortable. Frequent small meals may prove more successful than three large meals. When possible, the patient is consulted as to foods that he would prefer.

If the patient's condition is such that the ordinary solid food cannot be taken, fluids containing commercial protein concentrates and glucose may be tolerated. When oral intake is insufficient or not possible, intravenous solutions of glucose, protein preparations, plasma or whole blood may be administered.

There is a considerable increase in the risk in surgery on obese persons. They have a greater tendency to develop cardiovascular, pulmonary and wound complications. The excessive fat tissue frequently makes the operative procedures more difficult. The patient who is overweight is advised of the need to lose weight before his operation and may be given a diet of 800–1200 kcal (3300–5000 kJ).

Fluids and electrolytes
A normal fluid balance is extremely important in the surgical patient; dehydration predisposes to shock, a retention of metabolic wastes and disturbances in electrolyte concentrations. The patient who has been ill for some time, particularly if his disorder is gastrointestinal, frequently has a fluid and electrolyte deficit. A record of the fluid intake and output is kept and the patient is observed for signs of dehydration (see Chapter 6). A minimum intake of 2500–3000 ml is encouraged unless contraindicated. Blood biochemistry studies are done to determine electrolyte concentrations, and any deficiencies are corrected by oral or parenteral preparations.

Rest and exercise
The patient awaiting an operation may find it difficult to rest and sleep because of anxiety and decreased activity. The patient's accustomed presleeping habits are determined and measures which promote relaxation such as massage, warm drinks, reading or soft music are instituted. The physician may be consulted regarding a prescription for a mild sedative to promote relaxation and the necessary rest.

When the patient is well enough, he is usually kept ambulatory and encouraged to get some exercise. This prevents general weakness, contributes to normal fatigue and rest, and diminishes the probability of circulatory complications later.

Specific therapy
Certain treatments to correct secondary physiological disturbances or coexistent disease may comprise a large part of the preoperative preparation. The patient who has developed anaemia because of a loss of blood or nutritional deficiency may receive one or more blood transfusions (see Chapter 13). A course of an antimicrobial drug may be necessary to clear up some infection. A diabetic patient may require dietary and insulin therapy to bring his disease under control, lower the blood sugar, and have the urine free of sugar and ketones. The purpose of any such treatments and their significance to the surgery should be explained to the patient and his family.

INFORMED OPERATIVE CONSENT

Informed consent implies that the patient has been given information by his doctor about the nature of the surgery to be done and that the patient understands that information.[4] It also implies that consent is given freely and that the patient has not been put under undue pressure.

In seeking consent the doctor is required to provide sufficient details and information about what is proposed to enable the patient (or parent or guardian in the case of a minor or a person suffering a disability such as mental illness or subnormality) to form a proper decision and so give an informed consent.

The extent of the explanation given, when seeking consent, will depend on factors such as the patient's age and maturity, physical and mental state and the reason for the operation, and will also be influenced by the questions asked by the patient. Some patients request far more information than others about side-effects, complications, etc.

There is no requirement in English law that every possible complication and side-effect should be explained to the patient.[5] The purpose of informed consent is to protect the hospital, surgeon and anaesthetist against claims of unauthorized anaesthesia and surgery and claims related to possible adverse sequellae to the patient, and to protect the patient against unauthorized procedures.

---

[4] A *consent form* signed by the patient is also necessary for some major and invasive diagnostic procedures.
[5] Palmer (1985).

When asked to sign the consent form the patient must be rational, alert and not under the influence of any drugs or alcohol that might impair comprehension and judgement.

The signing of an operative consent form must be witnessed by a medical practitioner who attests to the fact that in his or her presence the statement has been read by the signatory, who stated that he or she understood and then signed the consent. If the patient is mentally competent, but unable to write, an 'X' indicating a consent is acceptable if witnessed by two signatories.

In England any person of sound mind who has attained the age of 16 years may give a legally valid consent to surgery. A minor's capacity to make his or her own decision depends upon the minor having sufficient understanding and intelligence to make the decision, and is not determined by any fixed age limit. Until the child achieves the capacity to consent, consent must be obtained from a parent or legal guardian.[5]

In the case of a genuine emergency the doctor may safely proceed to do what is reasonably necessary without a formal consent, acting in good faith and in the immediate interests of the patient's health and safety. If the emergency arises in an unconscious patient the doctor should, if time permits, endeavour to obtain the consent of the next of kin.

When the patient is mentally ill or impaired (handicapped), a valid consent can only be given if the matter concerned is within his or her understanding. The patient's relatives or responsible medical officers have no legal power to consent on his behalf though their approval should be obtained.

Immediate preoperative preparation

The following preparatory measures receive consideration the day before and on the day of operation.

Food and fluids
The patient's stomach should be empty when he goes to the operating theatre to prevent the possibility of aspiration of vomit. All food and fluids are withheld for at least 4–6 hours before the scheduled time for surgery and an explanation is given to the patient. Essential oral medication may be given during this time with a small amount of water. If the patient's mouth becomes dry and uncomfortable, he is given a mouthwash. When a patient inadvertently takes food or fluid, the surgeon or anaesthetist should be promptly notified. It will probably necessitate a postponement of the operation or the passing of a gastric tube to evacuate the stomach content.

When the patient is an infant or small child, the doctor may stress the giving of clear sweetened fluids for 24 hours up to 4–6 hours before operation.

This is to promote an optimum glycogen reserve in the liver since it is normally proportionately less than in the adult and will be depleted quickly.

If the patient is to receive a local anaesthetic, a light breakfast may be permitted by the doctor.

Elimination
The doctor's orders may or may not include giving the patient an evacuation enema. If the patient has had a normal bowel movement the day before operation, it may not be considered necessary. Some surgeons prefer all patients having major surgery to have an evacuation enema the evening before surgery to prevent constipation following the operation when diet and activity are restricted.

The bladder should be empty when the patient goes to the operating theatre in order to prevent incontinence during the anaesthetic induction and operation. In the case of low abdominal or pelvic surgery, a full bladder may interfere with the surgical procedure by making the site less accessible, and it may also increase the risk of accidental injury to the bladder wall. The patient is asked to void just before the preoperative medication is administered. If the patient is unable to void, the staff in the operating theatre are informed and, if necessary, catheterization is performed in the operating room prior to the surgery. If an indwelling catheter is needed it is usually inserted in the operating room unless otherwise ordered by the surgeon.

Local site preparation
Although the details of the preparation of the site of the operation vary according to the area and the surgeon's preference, the principles are the same. Preoperative skin care is to have the skin as free as possible of dirt particles, hair, desquamated cells, secretions and organisms. Prior to surgery the patient takes a warm bath or shower, using an antibacterial preparation such as chlorhexidine. The operation site may be further cleansed the morning of surgery using the same solution. Preoperative shaving of the skin may be done when excessive body hair exists over the operative area or when ordered by the surgeon. Care is taken to prevent trauma to the skin; abrasions and lacerations in the skin caused by the razor serve as an entry for microorganisms. When the hair is shaved from the skin, it is recommended that it be done 1–2 hours prior to surgery with a wet-shave. When the skin is to be shaved the surgeon usually specifies the extent of the area to be shaved and the time it is to be done in relation to the surgery. (Some research now indicates that not shaving or using a depilatory cream reduces the risk of postoperative wound infections.[6])

If a patient is discovered to have acne or infected lesions, the operation may be delayed until the con-

---

[6] Cruse & Foord (1980).

dition is corrected. Daily antiseptic baths or the application of an antimicrobial preparation may be prescribed.

Special preparation extending over several days may be ordered by the surgeon for some operations such as skin grafts and orthopaedic procedures. Specific instructions for local preparation are received for any surgery on the head, face and eye.

For rectal and lower bowel surgery, the patient is usually given a bowel clearance preparation such as Picolax, followed by evacuation enemas or rectal washouts until the return fluid is clear. Rectal washouts are given high and slowly, and the patient is allowed to rest following each one. They should also be given early enough to make sure all fluid is expelled before the patient is taken to the operating theatre. The perineum and surrounding area are thoroughly cleansed with water and detergent following the final evacuation.

In the case of operations on the mouth or throat, unless specific preparatory instructions are given, the teeth are cleaned and the mouth rinsed well with an antiseptic mouthwash the night before and the morning of the day of operation.

Personal care
The patient has a bath, shower or bed bath the evening prior to surgery or the morning of surgery using an antibacterial preparation. Prior to surgery the patient is given a clean hospital gown.

The teeth are cleansed and an antiseptic mouthwash may be used the night before and the morning of the day of operation to make sure all food particles are removed. Dentures are removed because they may become displaced and interfere with respiration. They should be placed in an appropriate container, labelled with the patient's name, in the patient's locker. Any prosthesis, such as an artificial eye or limb, is removed and safely stored. If the patient uses a hearing aid, it is usually left in place until he arrives in the anaesthetic room. It is then removed and safely stored.

The hair is combed, neatly arranged back from the face, left free of hairpins, and may be secured under a cap so that it does not become soiled or interfere with the administration of anaesthetic. Coloured nail polish and make-up are removed, since checking of the colour of the lips and nail beds for cyanosis is necessary. All jewellery is removed for safe-keeping. If the patient does not wish to remove a wedding ring, it is securely taped to the hand. The identification wristlet should be checked to make sure it is clearly legible, secure and correct.

Special procedures
Some special procedures may be ordered preceding certain operations. A nasogastric or duodenal tube may have to be passed or an intravenous infusion started. The nurse sees that the necessary equipment is available and that the procedure is completed by the time the patient receives the preoperative medication.

Medication
When the immediate preoperative orders are written, it should be clarified as to whether there are any preceding orders for medications; if so, it should be cleared with the doctor whether these preparations are to be withheld or given. The patient may have been receiving a cardiac drug, insulin or other important drugs and the omission of such could have serious effects.

A sedative is usually given the night before operation to ensure a good night's sleep for the patient. A benzodiazepine such as temazepam (Normison) or a chloral derivative such as dichloralphenazone (Welldorm) or triclofos sodium are commonly used. All patients receiving hypnotic preparations are instructed not to get up after taking the drug but to signal for the nurse if they want something or are unable to sleep. Frequently, simple nursing measures such as a back rub, change of position, turning the pillow or staying with the patient briefly may reduce tension and apprehension and promote sleep.

Approximately 45–90 minutes before operation, the patient usually receives an injection of a drug such as papaveretum (Omnopon) or pethidine to produce relaxation and allay anxiety. The doctor's choice of drugs is based mainly on the patient's condition and age. For example, if the patient is known to develop respiratory problems readily, morphine derivatives are not used because of their depressing effects on the respiratory centre. Milder sedatives such as trimeprazine (Vallergan) or droperidol are used for children.

If a general anaesthetic is to be given, the patient may also receive an anticholinergic preparation such as atropine or hyoscine hydrobromide (scopolamine) to reduce salivary and respiratory secretions and to block vagal impulses that cause bradycardia and hypotension associated with some anaesthetic agents. Scopolamine tends to make the respiratory secretion less tenacious than atropine. It may be administered alone without a sedative to young children since it depresses mental activity as well as secretions.

All preparatory procedures should be completed before the preoperative medication is given. The patient is then left undisturbed and silence is maintained. A relative may remain in the room to provide comfort and security for the patient.

A final check and recording may be made of the pulse, respirations and blood pressure about ½ hour after the preoperative drug has been given.

Patient's chart
Treatments and any pertinent reactions of the patient are recorded, and the complete chart including the nurses' notes, diagnostic reports, progress

notes, patient's history and the operation consent form are put together and taken to the operating theatre with the patient. A sheet on the front of the chart should list any factors that may be considered particularly important for the anaesthetist, surgeon and theatre staff to note. Examples are allergies, drug sensitivity, coexistent disease and limitation of joint movement in a limb. The latter may be significant in relation to positioning the patient on the operating room table. The patient's blood type is also noted.

Patient's family
The family is notified when the operation is to take place and usually one or two members come to the hospital before the operation. They are allowed to visit the patient briefly before the preoperative medication is given. As cited previously, one may remain quietly in the room as long as the patient is not disturbed.

Relatives are normally advised to go home whilst the patient is in theatre and to telephone the ward after the operation has taken place.

Emergency preoperative preparation

Preoperative preparation in emergency surgery is limited to basic essentials. When the patient is in shock or is bleeding, the haemoglobin is checked and the blood typed immediately. An intravenous infusion is started using normal saline or a plasma expander (dextran) until compatible whole blood is available.

If the patient is to have an inhalation anaesthetic and has most likely taken food and fluid within the last 6–8 hours, a gastric tube is passed to evacuate the stomach content. In the case of intestinal obstruction, a nasogastric or duodenal tube is passed and intermittent suction started in order to keep the stomach or duodenum free of fluid and gas.

As soon as possible, the patient is asked to void to obtain a specimen for urinalysis and to have the bladder empty for the surgery. If the patient is unable to void the doctor may ask for the patient to be catheterized, as it is important to know before operation whether the urine contains sugar, or abnormal constituents that might indicate diabetes mellitus or impaired renal function.

The consent form for operation is signed, and preoperative medication is given. Any dentures or prostheses and jewellery are removed, and the hair may be covered with a cap.

If the patient has just been admitted and is not accompanied by a relative, the nurse should make sure she obtains the name and telephone number of a family member and should notify the person as soon as possible.

EXPECTED OUTCOMES

1 The patient identifies concerns related to surgery.

2 The patient's level of anxiety is decreased as evidenced by: blood pressure, pulse rate and respiratory rates within the normal range for the patient; relaxed posture; and ability to sleep the night before surgery.
3 Physical preparation of the patient is completed safely.
4 An understanding of the surgical procedure and the pre- and postoperative events is expressed by the patient.
5 The patient demonstrates the ability to perform deep-breathing, coughing and leg exercises and can state their significance.

Intraoperative Phase

Operating theatre procedures vary greatly from one hospital to another. The information that follows is generally applicable to most situations and may prove helpful to the nurse caring for the patient experiencing surgery. No attempt is made to present the detailed knowledge and techniques essential to nurses who are members of the operating theatre team. Anticipated surgery is a threatening and fearful experience for the patient. Some fear may be allayed if the nurse at the bedside can give the patient some information as to what will take place in the operating room. It is also important that the nurse caring for the patient in the postoperative period has some understanding of what the patient has experienced.

The operating theatre is located, constructed and equipped to promote safety and quiet, prevent infection and facilitate surgical procedures. It is located near the recovery room and surgical intensive care unit. The temperature of the room is readily controlled according to the patient's needs as well as those of the operating personnel. Windows are absent in the operating room; air conditioning is provided by a special ventilation system which filters the air before it enters the room to remove dust and organisms to reduce the risk of infection. It also provides a higher atmospheric pressure within the operating theatre. The higher atmospheric pressure means that when doors into the theatre are opened, air flows out of the theatre rather than in, thereby reducing the risk of airborne infection. Equipment, for example lights and tables, is designed to withstand frequent disinfection and to facilitate aseptic technique and the surgery. Entry to the operating room is controlled to reduce potential transmission of organisms from the wards or outside the hospital.

All operating theatre personnel wear operating room gowns or suits which are laundered by the hospital. Street clothing or ward uniforms are not permitted in the operating theatre. Personnel wear caps to cover their hair, a mask that is impervious to moisture over their nose and mouth and 'covers' over their shoes. If a staff member has an infection (respiratory infection, local skin infection) he is excluded from the operating theatre. The incision and exposure of underlying tissues and viscera place the patient at serious risk of infection, demanding the practice of strict surgical asepsis. Everything that comes in contact with the patient's operative site must be sterile. Table covers, drapes, instruments, sutures, ligaments and sponges are sterilized and are handled only by members of the surgical team who have scrubbed their hands and arms and are dressed in sterile gowns and gloves. Tables, lights and other equipment that does not come in contact with the wound, are kept surgically clean by cleansing with a disinfectant between operations. Floors are similarly cared for.

TRANSFER TO OPERATING THEATRE

At the appropriate time, the patient is taken to the operating theatre, either in his bed or on a trolley.

Before leaving the ward, the personnel responsible for transporting the patient to the operating theatre check the patient's identification bracelet with the ward staff and operating room list to be sure they have the right patient. The patient is lifted on to the stretcher and adequate covers provided to keep the patient warm. Woollen blankets are not allowed within the operating theatre; wool is a potential source of static electricity. Cot-sides are used on the trolley. The patient is disturbed as little as possible; preoperative medication has usually been given to reduce his anxiety and induce drowsiness.

RECEPTION OF PATIENT

The patient is taken to a waiting or holding room or area, where the nurse escorting him from the ward introduces him by name to the operating theatre personnel; it is important not to leave him unattended. An operating theatre nurse introduces herself and proceeds to check the following data:
- The patient's response (drowsy, alert, anxious)
- Name and age. Identification of the patient is made verbally if he is responsive and by the identification bracelet, and his name is also checked with the operating room list
- The operation consent form. Is it correctly signed? The type of anticipated surgery is compared with the operating theatre list and any exceptions are indicated.
- If the surgery to be performed is to be on one of paired organs (e.g. kidneys, lung) or limbs (e.g. leg, arm) or a specific unilateral area (e.g. hernia) is the correct unilateral area clearly identified?
- Special problems (e.g. allergy, rash, joint problem and limited range of motion which may interfere with positioning)

- Laboratory reports; serum electrolytes
  Ca^{2+} (2.2–2.6 mmol/l or 4.5–5.5 mEq/l)
  K^+ (3.5–5.5 mmol/l or 3.5–5.5 mEq/l)
  Na^+ (135–145 mmol/l or 140–145 mEq/l)
  (See Chapter 6 for functions of electrolytes.)
  RBC ($4.5–6.5 \times 10^{12}$ per litre)
  Haematocrit (PCV) (males, 40–50%; females, 37–47%)
  Prothrombin time (PT) 11–15 seconds
  Blood type
- Preoperative medication; what was given and the dose?
  Medication may be given to: allay anxiety; induce drowsiness, which lessens the amount of anaesthetic needed in the induction phase; reduce respiratory secretions; or to diminish undesirable reflex responses during induction (nausea and vomiting)
- Vital signs; these are entered on the operation sheet as base-line data

Any significant observations (e.g. anxiety state; abnormal finding that is recorded, such as allergy, increased prothrombin time; or abnormal vital sign, such as tachycardia) is brought to the anaesthetist's attention before any anaesthetic is administered. A final check is made to make sure the patient has no dentures. The hair is covered with a cap if this has not already been done.

If the patient is sufficiently alert, he is advised of the waiting period; the nurse remains close by and indicates her presence by calmly speaking to the patient or simply by touch if the patient is drowsy. The waiting area should be quiet; loud noises, talking and confusion arouse the patient and heighten his level of anxiety. He may overhear a conversation, misinterpret it because of his drowsiness and preoperative medication and become quite disturbed.

ANAESTHESIA

The type of anaesthesia to be used for each patient is decided by the anaesthetist in consultation with the patient and surgeon. The term anaesthesia implies loss of sensation; that produced may be classified as general or regional. *General anaesthetic* agents produce reversible depression of the cerebral neurons that are responsible for awareness and responses; there is loss of sensation, consciousness, reflex responses and skeletal muscle tone. The muscle relaxation facilitates the surgery. *Regional anaesthesia* temporarily blocks the sensory receptors in the surgical area or the nerve impulses in an area of the sensory impulse conduction pathway. The patient remains conscious but may be drowsy due to preoperative sedation.

Methods of anaesthetic administration
General anaesthesia may be produced by agents administered by inhalation or intravenous infusion

or, alternatively, by hypothermia. Most frequently, the current practice involves rapid induction of anaesthesia by the intravenous injection of an anaesthetic agent such as thiopentone sodium (Intraval), followed by the inhalation administration of one or more anaesthetic agents. Endotracheal intubation is almost routinely done when an inhalation anaesthetic is to be given. Using a laryngoscope, a cuffed tube is introduced by the anaesthetist following the intravenous induction; the chest is observed for rise and fall and is auscultated for air entry to make sure the tube is in the respiratory tract and not the oesophagus. When the tube is in the desirable position, the cuff is inflated with air to maintain an airtight seal. Over-inflation is guarded against; excessive pressure may cause necrosis of the mucosa. The tube is attached to the anaesthetic machine. The inhalation method has the advantage of the control which the anaesthetist can maintain on the amount given. Its disadvantage may be irritation of the respiratory tract and increased secretions. Suction must be readily available. Following the removal of the endotracheal tube, hoarseness or loss of voice due to temporary impairment of the vocal cords, and laryngeal oedema or spasms may occur.

Regional anaesthesia is produced by the following methods.
1 *Local infiltration*. This involves the injection of an anaesthetic agent into the surgical site or into the area to be manipulated. The agent makes the local receptors unresponsive to stimuli. It is used principally on minor superficial surgical procedures.
2 *Peripheral nerve block*. This regional anaesthesia is produced by the injection of an anaesthetic agent into the area of a large nerve trunk or plexus, or into the tissues surrounding the operative site. The conduction of sensory nerve impulses is interrupted. This type of anaesthesia may be used, for example, when a tonsilectomy is done.
3 *Spinal anaesthesia*. This method entails the injection of the anaesthetic agent into the subarachnoid space in the lumbar region of the spine (usually between the second and fourth lumbar vertebrae). The agent blocks impulses at the origin of peripheral nerves. The area anaesthetized is determined by the level to which the drug rises in the spinal canal as well as by the amount of the drug used. This type of anaesthesia may be used in low abdominal and lower limb surgery. Chest and high abdominal surgery would require the agent to be carried to higher levels which would place the patient at risk of respiratory insufficiency as a result of blocking of impulses to the respiratory muscles.
4 *Epidural or caudal anaesthesia*. This regional anaesthesia is induced by the injection of an agent into the extradural space of the lower part of the vertebral canal (the sacrococcygeal region). The drug blocks impulses carried along the fibres of the cauda equina.[7] Epidural anaesthesia may be used in rectal and perineal operative procedures and is commonly used in obstetrics during labour and delivery.
5 *Topical or surface anaesthesia*. This is produced by the application of the agent to the skin or mucous membrane. Absorption of the agent results in a blocking of the sensory receptors. It is used principally in nose and throat procedures.
6 *Hypothermia*. Hypothermia is used rarely as a local anaesthetic in limb surgery. The limb is enclosed in ice or in a hypothermia (cooling) blanket for several hours previous to the surgery. It might be used when the patient's general condition is such that anaesthetic drugs would be hazardous. General hypothermia may be used occasionally in brain or cardiac surgery to slow body metabolism and decrease the body's oxygen requirement. If the surgery places the brain at risk of a decreased blood supply and/or oxygen supply, the body is cooled to reduce cell activity and the oxygen requirement, thus preventing brain damage. (See Chapter 7 for the cooling procedure.)

Anaesthetic agents
A variety of drugs are used as anaesthetic agents. Table 11.3 gives examples of anaesthetic agents used according to the method of administration. The choice depends upon the method of administration to be used, the surgery to be performed, the anticipated time for the procedure, and the physiological and psychological condition of the patient.

The inhalation agents commonly used may be in the form of a gas or a rapidly evaporating (volatile) solution. They are absorbed from the lungs and reach the brain quickly via the circulation. The liquid preparations are vaporized in the anaesthetic machine and usually combined with oxygen for inhalation. For many years, ether and cyclopropane were popular inhalation agents but were extremely hazardous because of their inflammability and explosive potential. They have been entirely replaced with safer agents.

The intravenous anaesthetic agents take effect quickly and recovery is rapid. They are used for induction and for very brief surgical procedures (e.g. incision for drainage of an abscess). A disadvantage of the intravenous method is the greater difficulty in controlling the degree and depth of anaesthesia.

Spinal anaesthetic agents depress motor and autonomic innervation as well as sensory. The patient's blood pressure must be monitored at frequent intervals. A spinal anaesthetic is contraindicated for the patient whose blood pressure is labile or unstable, is in shock or likely to develop it, or has a

___
[7] The *cauda equina* is formed by the spinal nerve roots which extend beyond the terminal portion of the spinal cord in the vertebral canal.

Table 11.3 Examples of commonly used anaesthetic agents.

Types of anaesthesia	Method of administration	Agent

General	Inhalation	Volatile liquids:
		  Halothane (Fluothane)
		  Enflurane (Ethrane)
		  Isoflurane (Forane)
		  Trichloroethylene (Trilene)
		Gas:
		  Nitrous oxide

	Intravenous	Solutions:
		  Thiopentone sodium (Intraval)
		  Methohexitone sodium (Brietal Sodium)
		  Ketamine (Ketalar)
		  Etomidate (Hypnomidate)

Regional	Local infiltration	Solutions:
		  Lignocaine (Xylocaine)
		  Prilocaine (Citanest)

	Spinal	Prilocaine (Citanest) Cinchocaine (Nupercaine) Bupivacaine (Marcain) Lignocaine (Xylocaine)
	Epidural	Lignocaine (Xylocaine) Bupivacaine (Marcain)
	Topical or surface	Cocaine Lignocaine (Xylocaine) Benzocaine Amethocaine (Anethaine)

respiratory problem. Respirations are observed closely for early recognition of the innervation block going to a level that results in impaired function of respiratory muscles. Assisted respiration may be necessary. For administration of a spinal anaesthetic, the patient is placed in a lateral position and the spine arched to increase the intervertebral spaces. He is then turned on to his back and the head of the table lowered.

The agents used in local anaesthesia frequently are combined with adrenaline, which constricts the blood vessels in the area. This reduces the rate at which the anaesthetic agent is absorbed into the bloodstream and the amount of bleeding in the area. The slower absorption maintains anaesthesia in the area for a longer period and prevents undesirable side-effects from rapid absorption. Local and regional anaesthesia are not usually used when there is infection in the area; insertion of the needle tends to spread the infection and breaks down localization.

Epidural anaesthetics may be administered over several hours. A special blunt needle is used to guard against passing through the dura mater into the subarachnoid space.

Muscle relaxants
Muscle relaxation is important in many surgical procedures. Deep anaesthesia, sufficient to produce complete muscle relaxation may place the patient at risk of cardiac and respiratory failure. To facilitate surgery and lessen the amount of anaesthetic required, a muscle relaxant such as suxamethonium (Scoline), pancuronium (Pavulon) or tubocurarine may be given intravenously by the anaesthetist. If given, it is brought to the attention of the nurse in the recovery room; the patient is observed closely for respiratory depression and neurological deficits.

Surgical team
The personnel required for an operation includes the anaesthetist, anaesthetic nurse or operating department assistant (ODA), surgical or 'scrub' nurse(s), circulating nurse, surgeon and surgeon's assistant. The number of personnel required depends upon the surgical procedure being carried out. For example, a radiologist or pathologist may be needed.

The *anaesthetist* assesses the patient's condition, checks the anaesthetic equipment for adequate anaesthetics and oxygen and efficient functioning, induces and maintains anaesthesia and monitors the vital signs throughout the surgery. If special monitoring devices are to be used, the anaesthetist puts them in place before the sterile drapes are applied. He prescribes necessary support during surgery as indicated (e.g. drug to correct cardiac arrhythmia, intravenous solution).

The *scrub nurse* performs the sterile nursing activities. These include the following:
- The setting-up and organization of the necessary tables, drapes, instruments, needles, sutures, ligatures, sponges and special equipment appropriate to the particular surgical procedure.
- Assisting with the application of sterile drapes over the patient.
- During the operation, anticipating the necessary supplies (e.g. sponges, sutures, instruments) and having them readily available for the surgeon.
- On completion of the main surgery and before wound closing, checking sponges, instruments and needles with the circulating nurse to make sure all are accounted for.
- When the wound is closed and area is cleansed of blood, applying the sterile dressing.
- Assisting with the transfer of the patient to the trolley.

The *circulating nurse* carries out non-sterile nursing activities which include:
- Assisting with the preparation and setting-up for the operation.
- Reception of the patient and the checking of the necessary data (see section on Reception of Patient).
- Providing necessary emotional support for the patient.
- Assisting with the transfer of the patient to the operating room table, ensuring a minimum of exposure and securing the wide strap above the knees and placing the arm(s) in the appropriate restraining straps. One arm (the one on the same side as the anaesthetic machine) is usually placed on a padded arm board and a blood pressure cuff applied so it is readily accessible to the anaesthetist.
- Being available to provide necessary equipment, drugs, etc. throughout the operation.
- Positioning of the patient for surgery and exposing the area to be prepared and draped.
- Observing for possible breaks in aseptic technique. This can occur without the awareness of the personnel carrying out the sterile activities.
- Checking of sponges, needles, and other instruments with the scrub nurse.
- Preparing the patient for transfer to the recovery room.
- Accompanying the patient to the recovery room.
- Giving a report of the surgery and patient's condition to the recovery room nurse who takes over the care of the patient.

The *anaesthetic nurse* is available to assist the anaesthetist. Her activities include:
- Assisting the anaesthetist with anaesthesia induction (e.g. intravenous anaesthetic infusion) and the setting-up of monitoring devices to be used.
- Monitoring of the patient's condition throughout the surgery.

- Recording medications and intravenous solutions.

POSITIONS USED IN SURGERY

The patient is positioned to:
1 Provide the necessary accessibility and exposure for the surgery.
2 Provide safety for the patient and prevent injury.
3 Promote normal respiration.
4 Facilitate anaesthesia and efficient monitoring.

The position required will depend on the surgery to be performed. The operating room table is designed so that sections of it may be elevated or lowered when necessary. The positions are shown in Fig. 11.1a–g and include the following.

Supine position (Fig. 11.1a). The patient lies flat on his back with a wide strap over the upper thighs. The arm on the side of the anaesthetic machine is extended on a padded arm board. A blood pressure cuff is applied and the arm secured. In positioning the arm on the board, hyperextension resulting in shoulder injury and discomfort must be avoided. The other arm is placed at the side of the patient, palm down and is secured.

Prone position (Fig. 11.1b). Three or four persons are required to turn the patient on to the anterior body surface. The restraining strap is placed below the knees. The head is turned to one side. One arm is placed at the side, palm up and secured; the other arm is positioned on the arm board, palm up. The feet are elevated off the table by placing a pillow or roll under the ankles. A body roll may have to be placed under each side of the patient to raise the chest off the table and allow for free chest excursion in respiration.

Trendelenburg position (Fig. 11.1c). The patient is placed in the supine position with the knees at a break in the table. The table is adjusted so that the patient is on an incline of about 45°, the head being lower than the hips and knees. The end of the table is lowered so the legs are flexed at the knees. Shoulder supports are in place to hold the patient in the position. This position is used in low abdominal and pelvic surgery; the intestines move into the upper abdomen in the head-down position providing accessibility and greater exposure of the operative organs.

Reverse Trendelenburg position (Fig. 11.1d). In the supine position, the patient is placed on an incline with the feet lower than the shoulders and head. A support is in place at the foot of the table. This position may be used in gallbladder surgery.

Lithotomy position (Fig. 11.1e). The patient is in the

supine position with the buttocks at a break in the table. The thighs and legs are lifted and flexed and the feet placed in stirrups. The arms are supported on the chest or on arm rests. This position is used for perineal, vaginal and rectal surgery. On completion of the surgery, the legs are lowered slowly to prevent a rush of blood into them which could cause a sudden fall in blood pressure.

Lateral position (Fig. 11.1f). The patient is turned on to the unaffected side; sand bags or bed rolls are used to support the patient and maintain the position. A wide strap is placed over the hip region. Precautions are used in positioning the arm and lower limb that are on the 'down' side to prevent hyperextension or prolonged pressure on them. The arms may be folded in front of the patient. This position may be used in chest or kidney surgery. In the latter, the patient is positioned so that the kidney elevator of the table lies between the lower rib and the iliac crest. When the patient is secured in the lateral position the kidney elevator section of the table is raised.

Hyperextension of the head (Fig. 11.1g). This is used for thyroid and neck surgery and may also be necessary for endoscopy (e.g. gastroscopy, bronchoscopy).

POTENTIAL PATIENT PROBLEMS

Table 11.4 lists the potential patient problems common to patients during surgery.
1 Infection. The patient is at risk of infection because of the surgical interruption of the integrity of the skin.
2 Physical injury. The patient's anxiety, drowsiness from preoperative medication and then the loss of sensation and consciousness due to anaesthesia places him at risk of physical injury. The potential causes include:
   (a) Lack of sides on the trolley, or of appropriate restraining straps.
   (b) Leaving the patient unattended which may result in a fall from the trolley or operating table.
   (c) Malpositioning that incurs nerve damage or the occlusion of a blood vessel by prolonged pressure on a part. For example, the ulnar nerve is at risk if the arm is firmly secured to an *unpadded* arm board; the sciatic nerve may be injured if both lower limbs are not flexed together when placing the patient in the lithotomy position. Prolonged pressure on the veins of the calf of the leg may interfere with venous circulation and cause thrombus formation.

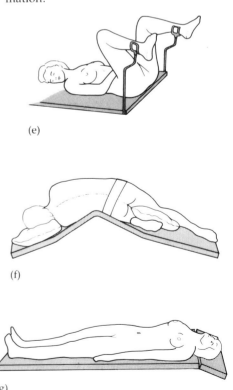

Fig. 11.1 Positions used in surgery: (a) Supine; (b) Prone; (c) Trendelenburg; (d) Reverse Trendelenburg; (e) Lithotomy; (f) Lateral and (g) Hyperextension of the head.

Table 11.4 Potential problems common to the patient during surgery.

Problem	Causative factors	Goals
Potential for infection	Surgical interruption of skin integrity	To prevent infection
Potential for physical injury	Anxiety Altered level of consciousness Loss of sensation Preoperative sedation Anaesthesia Decreased mobility Altered positioning of a body part	To maintain body functioning and prevent injury
Airway clearance ineffective	Endotracheal intubation Inhalation anaesthesia	To maintain a clear airway and adequate respirations
Gas exchange impaired	Altered level of consciousness Increased respiratory secretion Laryngeal oedema or spasm	

(d) Hyperextension in positioning. For example, hyperextension of the arm on the arm board may injure the shoulder, or hyperextension of the head may injure cervical nerves.

(e) Insufficient number of persons to transfer patient from the trolley to the table or vice versa, or to position the patient correctly for surgery.

(f) Omission of a conduction pad under the patient when electric equipment (e.g. cautery) is being used.

3 Airway clearance ineffective and gas exchange impaired. Endotracheal intubation and irritating inhalation anaesthetics place the patient at risk of respiratory dysfunction. The irritation may cause excessive secretions, laryngeal oedema or spasm or temporary impairment of the vocal cords with later hoarseness or loss of voice. Not all patients respond similarly to anaesthetic agents and some agents may depress respirations. If the patient has spinal anaesthesia, there is the risk of the solution going high enough in the subarachnoid space to suppress innervation of the respiratory muscles.

NURSING INTERVENTION

Potential for infection
Measures to prevent infection include the following considerations.
(a) Knowledgeable and conscientious observance of aseptic technique should be shown by all theatre personnel.
(b) Entry of personnel into the operating theatre is restricted.
(c) Regulations regarding the clothing to be worn in the operating room to avoid the possible transmission of organisms by street clothes or ward uniforms should be observed.
(d) Periodic throat and nose cultures are taken from operating theatre personnel and those with pos-

itive results are excluded from the operating theatre—especially for staphylococcus.
(e) Bedding from the ward is not brought into the theatre.
(f) Periodic spot-checking of sterile goods by a bacteriologist should be done to determine sterilization efficiency.
(g) A large skin area (appropriate to the particular surgery) is thoroughly cleaned. The procedure varies with institutions but cleansing with a surgical detergent solution followed by the application of an antiseptic may be the practice. In applying the antiseptic, the pooling of skin preparation solutions between two skin surfaces (e.g. the groin) is avoided because of the risk of irritation and skin damage.
(h) Any break in aseptic technique should be recognized and promptly corrected.
(i) A sterile dressing is securely applied to the wound on completion of the surgery.
(j) In some institutions, a follow-up is made of surgical patients to determine if they remain free of infection. If infection develops, efforts are made to determine its origin. Potential sources include the operating theatre, instruments and materials used at operation, operating theatre staff and the patient's own skin flora.

Potential for physical injury
Some degree of trauma is inevitable with a surgical procedure but nursing measures should aim to minimize that trauma and prevent unnecessary injuries.
(a) The patient should be lifted and positioned very gently; his limbs and head being adequately supported.
(b) The covering sheet is tucked in to support the arms and the cot-sides are also in place on the trolley during transfer to and from the operating theatre.
(c) Similarly, when the patient is on the operating

table, the appropriate restraints are necessary. A wide strap is placed above the knees. A nurse remains with the patient during the induction and early stage of anaesthesia; extra restraint may be necessary because of restlessness. Less of this occurs with the rapid induction that is associated with the commonly used intravenous anaesthetic administration.

(d) When positioning the patient, precautions are observed to avoid hyperextension or exposing vulnerable areas to excessive pressure and interference with blood flow. For example, having the arm board padded, correct positioning of the arm and lower limb that are on the side that the patient is on when in the lateral position and having two persons available to lift and flex the lower limbs together when placing the patient in the lithotomy position are measures that prevent injuries and complications.

(e) In setting-up before surgery, if the use of electric equipment is anticipated such as the electrocautery, placement of a conductive pad under the patient is necessary.

Potential for ineffective airway clearance
The following nursing considerations contribute to the maintenance of respiratory function.

(a) The patient's record is checked for information that indicates his respiratory status (history, vital signs, blood gas analysis report). Auscultation of the chest is done before anaesthetic administration. Anything abnormal or questionable is brought to the anaesthetist's attention.

(b) Anaesthetic equipment is kept in good condition. The anaesthetic machine is tested at frequent intervals by the engineering department; tubes, valves, pressure regulators, flow meters, chemical (soda lime) to absorb carbon dioxide, filters and tubes are checked by engineers as well as by the anaesthetist in preparation for the operation.

(c) Airways, suction equipment, emergency drugs and an Ambu bag are readily available.

(d) The patient is received with a calm reassuring manner and the nurse introduces herself. A quiet, confident patient has a better reaction to anaesthetic than the anxious, fearful and restless patient.

(e) The patient's respirations are monitored throughout the administration of the anaesthesia and surgery. Equipment for taking a specimen for blood gas analysis may be required and should be at hand.

Postoperative Management

All surgery has certain common effects that vary in extent and intensity with each particular individual and each specific operation. It produces tissue trauma, pain, psychological reactions and loss of blood. There is an increased possibility of invasion of body tissues by pathogenic organisms through a break in the continuity of the skin, or by the introduction of foreign objects into the body. In addition, there are disturbances in body functions which are due directly to the surgical procedure or indirectly to the responses of the autonomic nervous system and the adrenal glands to the associated psychological and physical stresses.

The nurse who is caring for a patient following an operation must possess knowledge and understanding of the implications of the particular surgery for the patient, its possible effects on the patient's body functions and the care and support required to assist in his return to normal with a minimum of discomfort and pain. A constant watch of the patient's clinical progress is necessary. Adverse changes and their possible significance must be recognized promptly and the surgeon alerted. If possible, the nurse who is to care for the patient in the postoperative period will have had an opportunity to become acquainted with the patient and learn something of his condition before the operation. The patient may be more confident with a nurse who is not a complete stranger, and the nurse, knowing something of the patient, is better able to evaluate his reactions and condition.

PREPARATION TO RECEIVE THE PATIENT

Most hospitals have a recovery room, either within the operating theatre department or adjacent to it, to which the patient is taken on completion of the surgery. In a few instances, the patient may be returned directly to his ward unit. The recovery room has several distinct advantages; constant surveillance is provided by a staff experienced in immediate postoperative care and whose attention is undivided; proximity to the operating theatre reduces the distance the patient is transported in this critical period; equipment necessary for emergencies is concentrated in the area and is in immediate readiness; and one nurse may care for two or three patients—a situation which would not be possible on the ward, where each patient is in a different location. The patient remains in the recovery room until he fully regains consciousness and his vital signs are stabilized.

Most hospitals have intensive care units apart from the recovery room in which critically ill patients and patients with a special problem, such as respiratory insufficiency, receive care. The patient who has had major surgery or who has developed serious complications may be transferred directly from the operating theatre to the intensive care unit, where the intensive type of care given in the recovery room may be extended for several days. The advantages of such a unit are similar to those of the recovery room, but the latter provides a briefer period of care. In a few situations, the two units may be combined, using the same staff and equipment.

In the surgical unit to which the postoperative patient is to go, certain basic preparations are made to receive the patient. The bed is made up and the top bedding folded to one side to facilitate the transfer of the patient; a draw sheet or transfer sheet may be placed on the bed to facilitate moving and turning of the patient. The bed has cot-sides in place ready for use in the event that the patient becomes restless and confused during recovery from the anaesthesia.

Basic equipment to be assembled at the bedside includes a sphygmomanometer, stethoscope, thermometer, vomit bowl, tissues, face flannel, recording charts and drip stand. Suction apparatus, a portable emergency respirator (Ambu bag with oxygen), and an emergency tray with cardiac and respiratory stimulants, sterile syringes and needles, tourniquet, alcohol swabs, oropharyngeal airway (e.g. a Guedal airway) and endotracheal tubes should be readily available.

Equipment most likely to be needed because of the nature of the surgery should also be assembled in readiness for prompt use. For instance, if the patient is having gastric surgery, equipment for gastric suction or aspiration will be necessary.

The room or bed area is tidied; unnecessary equipment and objects are removed, and daily cleaning is done in order to prevent disturbance of the patient later. The call button is tested to make sure it is in order should assistance be required.

TRANSFER OF THE PATIENT FROM THE OPERATING THEATRE

On completion of the operation, the patient is dried if the skin is moist with perspiration, and a clean gown and sheet are applied. He is then lifted gently and without unnecessary exposure by a mechanical lifting device or by a sufficient number of persons to provide adequate support and prevent strain on any part, particularly the operation site. When the bed is used the patient is placed in the lateral or semiprone position, and the cot-sides are raised. If the transfer is to a trolley, the dorsal recumbent position is more likely to be used and straps may be placed over the patient (one above the elbows, the second just above the knees) and secured for safety. Cot-sides may also be used. Sufficient covers are used to ensure warmth and protection from draughts. The head is extended and an oropharyngeal airway is probably in place to facilitate breathing. If the patient is on his back, the lower jaw must be held up and forward to prevent the tongue from obstructing breathing. The anaesthetist and a nurse accompany the patient to the recovery room. Along with immediate treatment orders, the nurse taking over receives a report on what was done, the patient's condition and anything special for which she should be alert.

IMMEDIATE POSTOPERATIVE CARE

The discussion presented here deals with general postoperative considerations applicable to most surgical patients. Modifications and additional care as related to specific surgery are included in the later respective sections.

The *goals for nursing intervention* in the immediate postoperative period are to:
1 Assess cardiovascular and respiratory functions, level of consciousness, physical activity, emotional responses and level of comfort.
2 Maintain adequate ventilation.
3 Maintain adequate circulation.
4 Identify and evaluate potential or actual complications and initiate emergency treatment promptly if indicated.
5 Protect the patient from injury.

Assessment
When the patient is received in the recovery room, an immediate check is made of the respirations, pulse, blood pressure, colour of the skin and mucous membranes, condition of the skin (warm or cold, dry or moist) and the level of consciousness. The wound area is examined for bleeding and drainage. If there is a catheter or other type of drainage tube, it is checked for patency. These initial observations and the patient's preoperative vital signs serve as a comparative base-line which assists the nurse later in recognizing favourable and unfavourable changes and in making decisions as to actions. Cardiac arrhythmia, weak pulse, a decrease or fluctuations in the systolic blood pressure, abnormal respiratory rate and volume and bleeding in the wound area should be reported promptly to the doctor.

The vital signs are recorded every 15 minutes for 2 hours and observation is made of the patient's colour, skin condition and operative site for any untoward signs, and the patient's responses are noted at frequent intervals.

The fluid intake and output are accurately recorded until normal fluid and food intake and normal urinary elimination have been resumed.

Maintenance of adequate ventilation
Inadequate ventilation (hypoventilation) is a common problem in the immediate postoperative period for the patient who has had a general anaesthetic, and it may lead to serious respiratory complications. Hypoventilation implies that the volume of air being moved in and out of the alveoli (air sacs of the lungs) with each respiration is below normal. It leads to a decrease in the vital capacity and surfactant activity resulting in a decrease in blood oxygen concentration. Pulmonary secretions increase which if retained may obstruct a bronchial tube, resulting in the collapse of a segment of the lung (atelectasis). Bronchitis or pneumonia may develop, since retained secretions provide an excellent medium for

the growth of pathogenic organisms. Postoperative hypoventilation and airway obstruction may result from: (1) central nervous system depression by the anaesthetic agent(s); (2) the depression of respiratory muscle activity by a muscle relaxant; or (3) partial airway obstruction caused by the tongue or lower jaw blocking the pharyngeal area, excessive mucus secretions or laryngeal oedema. Laryngeal oedema may develop if endotracheal intubation was used by the anaesthetist.

Hypoventilation may be recognized by: (1) abnormally slow or shallow respirations; (2) audible, moist, gurgling respirations, indicating excessive secretions; (3) wheezing, or 'crowing' respirations (stridor); (4) râles or non-entry of air into an area detected by auscultation; or (5) restlessness, cyanosis and rapid pulse rate that are characteristic of hypoxaemia.

Measures to promote adequate ventilation include the following:

1 During unconsciousness, unless contraindicated by the nature of the surgery, the patient is placed in a lateral or semiprone position without a pillow under the head. This position lessens the danger of aspiration of mucus and vomit, and of the relaxed tongue and lower jaw 'falling back' to block the pharynx. The head is hyperextended to facilitate free entry of air and expiration. A firm pillow may be placed at the patient's front and back, if necessary, to maintain the desired position. The knees are flexed to reduce strain, and the uppermost limb is flexed to a greater degree than the lower one. The arm that is uppermost is supported on a pillow so that chest expansion is not restricted. If the patient must be kept on his back, an oropharyngeal airway may be necessary during the unconscious period to prevent occlusion of the airway.

2 Excessive secretions may be removed by pharyngeal suction. The suction catheter is directed into the pharyngeal area with the vacuum regulation hole open. When the catheter is in place, the hole is occluded by the thumb and suction established. The catheter is rotated and withdrawn slowly. If the secretions are beyond pharyngeal suction, tracheal suction may have to be undertaken. (See Chapter 16 for details of deep suction.)

3 Oxygen may be administered as a supportive measure and to prevent hypoxaemia. It may be given by nasal cannulae, nasal catheter or mask (see Chapter 16). Oxygen therapy is usually continued until the patient is conscious and able to take deep breaths on command.

4 If hypoventilation persists, the concentration of blood gases is determined. Mechanical ventilatory assistance may be necessary (see Chapter 16 for details).

Aspiration of vomit may occur in the unconscious patient. If vomiting occurs, the head should be kept low, turned to the side and the mouth and pharynx cleared of secretions by suctioning. If aspiration occurs tracheal suctioning is done to remove the secretions.

Maintenance of adequate circulation

The patient's pulse, blood pressure, skin colour and activity are assessed every 5–15 minutes and the surgical area is checked for signs of bleeding. Hypotension, shock, cardiac arrhythmias and haemorrhage are complications that may occur in the immediate postoperative period and during the next few days.

Hypotension results from the anaesthetic agents, reactions to drugs, cardiac arrhythmias, inadequate ventilation and may also result from moving the patient. Following an operation it is common for the patient's blood pressure to be slightly lower than usual. Systolic pressures below 90 mmHg and pulse rates below 60 per minute or above 110 per minute require prompt intervention.

Shock is a circulatory failure that results in an inadequate perfusion of tissues and organs. This failure at the microcirculatory level reduces the delivery of oxygen and other essentials to a level below that required for normal cellular activities. It may develop during or immediately following the surgery, or it may develop more slowly and become evident several hours after operation. It may be secondary to a severe infection or respiratory complication that occurs later.

Early manifestations of shock are a decrease in blood pressure, restlessness, inappropriate anxiety, ashen pallor, cold moist skin, rapid weak pulse and decreased pulse pressure. Shock is serious and immediately life-threatening; prompt recognition and action are necessary to prevent the condition from becoming irreversible. (For details see Chapter 15).

Haemorrhage may occur as a result of a slipped ligature, an increase in blood pressure opening up previously collapsed vessels, or the dislodgement of a clot that plugged a severed vessel.

The haemorrhage may become evident externally at the site of operation, or it may be concealed internally and only manifested and recognized by changes in the vital signs and the patient's general appearance and complaints of weakness. Loss of blood causes a fall in blood pressure, rapid thready pulse, deep rapid respiration (which is referred to as air hunger), pallor, apprehension, restlessness and changes of responses and level of consciousness.

The dressing should be checked frequently for signs of bleeding and the body area checked for swelling or distension. Blood from the incision may run down under the patient and not be apparent on the dressing; it is only discovered by sliding a hand under the patient in the area of the surgery. Any suspicion of haemorrhage must be immediately reported. The dressing should be reinforced and the patient returned to the operating theatre for ligation of the blood vessel(s).

A *cardiac arrhythmia* may develop and is usually caused by the anaesthetic agent or is secondary to cardiac surgery. If the arrhythmia was present pre-operatively, usually no intervention is necessary. Ventricular arrhythmias may lead to cardiac arrest and require continuous monitoring and immediate intervention. Cardiac arrest, although rare, requires rapid, emergency treatment. A cardiac arrest trolley and emergency drugs are always kept available in the recovery room area. External cardiac massage and artificial respirations by the mouth-to-mouth method are initiated immediately. The cardiac arrest is due to failure of the heart muscle to contract, or to ventricular fibrillation. In the latter, the normal synchronized contractions of the ventricular muscle fibres are replaced with rapid, weak, irregular, uncoordinated contractions that result in incomplete filling and emptying of the chambers and insufficient blood being pumped into the systemic circulation. A defibrillator may be used by which one or two electric shocks are delivered to the heart (see Chapter 14). For details of cardiopulmonary resuscitation see Chapter 14.

Protection of the patient from injury
While the patient is emerging from anaesthesia, he may be restless. Cot-sides are used on the bed or trolley to protect the patient. The nurse remains with the patient until he is conscious and ensures that tubes and essential equipment are not dislodged. The patient is addressed by name and given a simple, direct explanation of where he is and what is happening in order to help him orient to the situation as well as reduce fear.

RETURN OF PATIENT TO SURGICAL UNIT

When the patient returns to the surgical unit, the nurse from the recovery room provides an assessment of the patient's condition and information about the surgical procedure and postanaesthetic events.

Assessment
The patient is immediately assessed for level of consciousness, pain and discomfort and status of vital signs. The dressing is checked for signs of bleeding, and drainage and tubes are observed for patency. Equipment is connected, the cot-sides raised and the call-button placed within reach of the patient. If the patient is alert and the vital signs are stable, an assessment is made half hourly and then extended to hourly intervals and then every 2–4 hour intervals over the next 12–24 hours.

Fluid intake and output should be recorded until normal fluid and food intake and normal urinary elimination have been resumed.

The patient is positioned comfortably, maintain-

ing normal body alignment. When a spinal anaesthetic has been given, the bed is kept flat and no pillow is used. This position should be maintained until sensation and motor ability have returned to the lower limbs and the systolic pressure is over 90 mmHg. The family may visit briefly if they wish.

Treatments
The surgeon's orders are noted immediately for specific treatment. For instance, oxygen, intravenous infusion, appropriate drainage system, special positioning and observations, and drug therapy may be indicated by the surgeon's orders.

Any drainage tubes that are to be connected to appropriate bottles or a suction system must receive prompt attention, as they are usually clamped during transit from the operating theatre. If drainage is not quickly established, the tube may become blocked, or sufficient pressure may be built up within the body cavity to cause serious effects. For example, if a gastrointestinal tube remains clamped following gastric or duodenal surgery, distension may cause a leakage of secretions into the peritoneal cavity and may result in peritonitis.

Expected outcomes

1 The patient is conscious, opens eyes spontaneously and in response to speech, makes verbal responses which indicate orientation to time, place and person, and responds appropriately to commands.
2 Blood pressure, pulse and respirations are stable and within the normal range for the patient.
3 There are no complications, or if there were they have abated or are controlled.

CONTINUING POSTOPERATIVE CARE

Table 11.5 lists patient problems which might occur postoperatively.

Goals for nursing intervention during the ensuing postoperative period are to:
1 Promote comfort and control pain.
2 Maintain fluid and electrolyte balance and adequate nutrition.
3 Promote a return to normal patterns of elimination.
4 Promote increasing levels of activity.
5 Promote wound healing.
6 Maintain ventilation.
7 Maintain circulation.
8 Decrease patient anxiety.
9 Prepare patient for discharge and self-management.

Promotion of comfort and control of pain
Discomforts common to many postoperative patients include pain, nausea and vomiting, gas pains and apprehension.

Table 11.5 Potential problems common to the patient postoperatively.

Problem	Causative factors	Goals
Alteration in comfort: pain	Surgical intervention Nausea and vomiting Abdominal distension Anxiety	To control pain
Alteration in fluid and electrolyte balance and nutrition	Decreased oral intake Fluid loss during surgery via drainage tubes Altered gastrointestinal activity	To maintain electrolyte and fluid balance and nutritional status
Alterations in patterns of elimination	Decreased fluid volume Immobility Pain Surgical intervention Altered sensation	To maintain normal patterns of elimination
Reduced mobility	Pain and discomfort Weakness Immobility	To promote early ambulation and physical mobility
Potential for injury	Altered level of consciousness Ineffective airway clearance Decreased sensation Impaired skin integrity Decreased mobility	To maintain body functions To promote healing
Airway clearance ineffective	Respiratory irritation from anaesthesia Pain and discomfort Decreased mobility	To maintain ventilation
Inadequate circulation	Effects of anaesthetic Surgical intervention Increased fluid loss Decreased mobility	To maintain circulation
Anxiety	Fear of unknown Lack of knowledge Pain and discomfort Diagnosis	To reduce anxiety: the patient feels able to talk about his concerns and fears
Insufficient knowledge about health care	Lack of knowledge and skill	To help the patient understand the factors involved in improving his health after discharge

Pain. Pain at the operation site is to be expected because of the unavoidable tissue trauma in surgery. Inadequate control of postoperative pain may cause restlessness and contribute to shock and injury to the operation site.

Assessment of postoperative pain includes data on the nature, duration and location of the pain and the patient's perception of the cause. Pain is not always incisional in origin; it may result from abdominal distension, a full bladder, decreased circulation due to immobility, pressure or muscle spasms. Objective data include observation of the patient's posture and position, facial expression, muscle tension and the respiratory and pulse rates. An elevated temperature may indicate a wound infection which would increase the pain. The surgeon usually orders an analgesic such as papaveretum (Omnopon), pethi-dine or buprenorphine (Temgesic) to be given every 4 hours if required (prn) for the first 24–48 hours. The patient should be kept relatively free of pain by the administration of analgesics before the pain becomes severe. The nurse needs to use her judgement, however, in the administration of analgesics since narcotics tend to depress respirations. When the pain is adequately controlled the patient tends to relax muscles and participate more effectively in deep-breathing and coughing exercises. The use of analgesics is more hazardous with older persons, patients with some respiratory insufficiency (e.g. patients with chronic bronchitis or emphysema) and with young children.

The patient's position is changed, and deep breathing, coughing and necessary treatments are carried out following the drug injection so that the patient may derive maximum benefit. After the first day or two, the dose of the analgesic is usually reduced or a milder drug is substituted.

Prevention of strain on the operation site by good positioning and support with a pillow contributes to the prevention and relief of pain. For instance, a patient with a pendulous abdomen who has had abdominal surgery may suffer less discomfort if the strain on the wound is relieved.

Occasionally, a patient may complain of a backache or pain in a shoulder which may have been caused by prolonged immobilization during surgery. Gentle massage or local application of heat using a heat pad or pack may provide relaxation and relief. If the lower limbs are causing discomfort, the patient is encouraged to do a few simple movements such as flexion of toes, feet and legs. Massage is never used, but a change of position and support under the full length of the limbs may be helpful. Massage of the lower limbs is discouraged because of the danger of dislodging a thrombus that may have formed because of venous stasis. Relaxation techniques, music, sensory stimulation by massage and guided imagery may also be used to lessen the discomfort.

The patient should be encouraged to practise techniques that were taught preoperatively and to inform the nurse about the type and severity of pain and the effectiveness of interventions. The patient who understands the course of his pain and participates in planning and carrying out pain control measures is usually less apprehensive and more tolerant of the discomfort.

Nausea and vomiting. Surgical patients may experience some nausea and vomiting immediately after the operation as a result of the toxic effects of the anaesthetic, pain, anxiety and the handling of viscera in abdominal surgery. Assistance is provided by having a kidney dish available, holding the patient's head, providing a mouthwash and wiping the patient's mouth. If the patient is still under the influence of the anaesthetic or drugs, precautions are taken to prevent aspiration by turning the patient's head to the side and if necessary using suction to make sure the vomit is removed from the mouth and pharynx. Oral fluids are usually withheld, and the patient is kept quiet and is disturbed as little as possible. An antiemetic drug such as metoclopramide (Maxolon) may be administered. Vomit bowls should be emptied promptly and soiled linen changed. Vomiting that persists beyond 24 hours after the operation should be reported, as it may indicate a complication or intolerance to the analgesic being used. (For a fuller discussion of nausea and vomiting see Chapter 17.)

Flatulence and abdominal distension. Patients who have had abdominal surgery may experience some pain and distension which are caused by an accumulation of gas in the gastrointestinal tract. Most of the gas is air that is swallowed during nausea or when the patient is tense and fearful. The depressing effects of anaesthetics and drugs, handling of the intestine during surgery and the lack of food intake in the tract may contribute to a reduction in peristalsis. Distension persists until bowel tone returns and peristalsis resumes. The discomfort may be relieved by the insertion of a rectal tube for a brief period or by an enema. When the distension is high, a nasogastric tube may be passed and suction-decompression used (see Chapter 17). If the distension persists, it may indicate a serious complication such as paralytic ileus, bowel obstruction or peritonitis (see Chapter 17). Frequent turning, early ambulation and normal fluid and food intake are helpful in re-establishing normal peristalsis and preventing distension and gas pains. In some instances, especially gastrointestinal surgery, foods are withheld until bowel sounds are audible on auscultation.

Mechanical intestinal obstruction, paralytic ileus and peritonitis are serious complications which may develop following abdominal surgery. Nursing care of patients with gastrointestinal complications is discussed in Chapter 17.

Apprehension. The postoperative patient may be apprehensive and concerned about his condition; this anxiety is likely to cause restlessness and aggravate discomfort and pain. An explanation of what has taken place and what he may expect may relieve some of his concern. He is also told that the nurse is close by and will be able to help him. Having a family member visit or remain quietly by the bedside may be helpful. It may be necessary for the nurse to spend as much time as possible with the patient and to provide repeated explanations and reassurance until the patient regains sufficient confidence and control. If he is worried about the findings at operation, it may be helpful to have the surgeon advise him as to his condition and the prognosis.

Maintenance of fluid and electrolyte balance and nutrition
A blood transfusion will probably be given during a major operation or immediately after to replace the blood loss or to combat shock if the blood pressure falls below 90 mmHg. Before the transfusion is started, the blood is checked by two persons to be certain that the label bears the patient's name, is the correct blood type and is within the expiry date. The blood bank labels the blood with the patient's name and identification number after making sure it is the right type and is compatible. The blood should be used within 30 minutes of being taken from the fridge. The patient is observed for signs or symptoms of untoward reactions, such as a chill, fever, dyspnoea, pain in the lumbar region or chest, or a fall in blood pressure. Later, the urine may contain haemoglobin because of haemolysis of red blood cells.

The rate of flow is indicated by the doctor; initially, it may be introduced very slowly (2–3 ml per minute). Symptoms of a reaction are usually manifested during the infusion of the first 50–100 ml of each unit of blood. After 100 ml, the rate may be increased to 4–10 ml per minute. The rate of flow will depend on the reduction in the patient's vascular volume, blood pressure and cardiac function. It is usually considerably slower in an elderly person.

If a reaction is manifested, the transfusion is stopped and the doctor is notified immediately. In some situations, the blood and equipment are then returned to the blood bank for examination to determine the cause of the reaction.

Oral fluid and food are restricted during the period of nausea and vomiting and following abdominal operations. Intravenous infusions of electrolyte and glucose solutions are given to meet the patient's daily requirements and maintain normal fluid and electrolyte balance. Frequent rinsing of the mouth and cool, moist compresses laid over the lips will help with the patient's discomfort of thirst.

As soon as fluids are permitted, sips of water are given and gradually increased in amount. The intake is then progressively increased as can be tolerated, through fluids and soft diet to general diet. The resumption of a normal diet as soon as possible promotes normal gastrointestinal functioning, and the patient is less likely to experience abdominal distension, gas pains and constipation. Normal nutrition also favours wound healing, maintenance of strength and a sense of well-being.

In the case of a patient who has had surgery on the alimentary tract (gastric or intestinal), all oral intake is withheld until peristaltic activity is established. Palpation and auscultation of the abdomen will reveal the return of peristaltic movement, as will passage of flatus and bowel sounds usually about the second or third day following gastrointestinal surgery.

Electrolyte balance may be assessed by monitoring serum levels and determining the extent and type of fluid loss. Sodium and potassium depletion occurs with blood loss during surgery and through loss of gastrointestinal secretions in vomiting or nasogastric suctioning. Chloride is also depleted with a loss of gastric secretions. Potassium chloride is often added to intravenous solutions administered to the patient postoperatively.

The postoperative patient may be rather indifferent to food, but he may be encouraged to take more by the offering of small amounts of those foods for which the patient has indicated a preference. Frequently food and fluids are not taken simply because the patient is weak and finds the effort expended in reaching and feeding himself too exhausting. The necessary assistance should be provided until the patient regains sufficient strength. The amounts of food and fluid taken are recorded until a normal diet is resumed.

Promotion of normal elimination
The patient who is adequately hydrated will usually

void within 6–8 hours of surgery. The total urinary output on the operative day will be less than the fluid intake because of fluid loss during surgery and vomiting and fluid retention; fluid retention is due to the increased secretion of ADH which occurs with major surgical trauma and stress. The fluid and electrolyte balance usually returns to normal by 48 hours postsurgery.

The postoperative patient may have a temporary inability to void because of a depression of the bladder sensitivity to distension; the impulses that produce the desire to void and the reflex emptying are not initiated. The inhibition may be due to the anaesthetic, drugs or trauma in the region of the bladder. The recumbent position, nervous tension and fear of pain may also contribute to urinary retention. The patient may have the desire to void but is unable to do so because of spasm of the external sphincter. When the bladder becomes distended, a small amount may be voided frequently, but the bladder is not emptied; this is referred to as retention with overflow. Restlessness, complaints of pain or of a feeling of pressure in the pelvic area, and a palpable fullness above the symphysis pubis are associated with retention.

Distension and stagnation of urine predispose to inflammation and infection of the bladder. If the patient has not voided for 12 hours he is monitored closely; after 24 hours efforts are made to induce voiding. If possible, the patient is assisted out of bed to assume the normal, accustomed position. If the patient is not well enough to be out of bed, a bedpan or a commode by the edge of the bed may be used unless contraindicated. Opening taps to produce the sound of running water or pouring warm water over the vulva of the female patient may be helpful. The male patient may be permitted to stand at the side of the bed to use a urinal. The amount of fluid the patient has had since last voiding should be noted. Catheterization may be ordered if the patient's bladder is distended and retention is prolonged. Strict asepsis and gentleness are necessary in the passing of a catheter to avoid trauma of the mucous membrane and the introduction of infection.

In major abdominal and pelvic surgery, an indwelling catheter may be passed and left in place for 2 or 3 days to avoid repeated catheterization as well as pressure from a full bladder on the internal operation site. An indwelling catheter may also be used to determine hourly secretion of urine if the patient is in shock or has some renal insufficiency due to disease. There is concern if the output is less than 30 ml per hour.

Since the bowel is usually empty at the time of surgery and food intake is restricted for 2 or 3 days, bowel elimination is not an immediate postoperative concern. The patient, probably accustomed to a daily bowel movement, may be worried unless he is advised that the delay is to be expected and will not be harmful.

If a normal diet is quickly re-established, a laxative or enema may not be necessary. Some doctors order a mild laxative, glycerine suppository, or a small enema 2 days after operation. Early ambulation and being allowed to go to the toilet or use a commode help in re-establishing normal bowel elimination.

Increase level of activity
Bed rest and inactivity predispose to problems of flatulence and abdominal distension, retention of urine, loss of strength, joint stiffness, and respiratory and vascular complications. Gastrointestinal peristalsis is sluggish, venous stasis occurs, and respirations are shallow.

To minimize these potential difficulties, some activity and frequent change of position are promoted. Venous stasis and the resultant danger of thrombus formation, particularly in the lower limbs, may be prevented by stimulating the circulation with foot and leg exercises. These are usually commenced 8–10 hours after the operation and done every 2–3 hours until the patient is up and walking. Alternating active flexion and extension of the toes, dorsal and plantar flexion of the feet, and flexion and extension of the legs and thighs are carried out under the direction of the nurse.

If early ambulation is not possible and the surgeon approves, self-care and the following exercises are included as soon as the patient's condition permits: (1) flexion and extension of the head; (2) flexion and extension of the fingers, hands, forearms and arms; (3) abduction, adduction and external rotation of the arms at the shoulders; and (4) contraction of the abdominal muscles. The purpose of self-care and the exercises are explained to the patient; otherwise, he may feel resentful and consider he is not receiving due care. The proposed activities stimulate circulation and respirations and prevent contractures and loss of strength (see Fig. 11.2).

Early ambulation. Within 12–48 hours after surgery, if the vital signs are stable and the general condition satisfactory, the patient is assisted out of bed and encouraged to walk about. At first the patient may take only a few steps, but movement can be progressively increased as the patient feels stronger and more secure. This early ambulation promotes the return of normal physiological activities such as gastrointestinal peristalsis, reduces the incidence of respiratory and circulatory complications, prevents the loss of muscle tone, improves the patient's morale and shortens the period of hospitalization and convalescence.

The patient is likely to be very fearful and helpless the first time he gets out of bed and will need assistance and support. The height of the bed is lowered, and he is turned to a lateral position near the edge of the bed with his legs and thighs flexed. The patient is then slowly assisted to the sitting position and his legs are put over the side of the bed. A change in position from supine to sitting or standing may produce postural hypotension. The patient's pulse rate and rhythm and respirations are determined at this point and a check is made for pallor, feelings of dizziness or light-headedness. The patient remains in the sitting position until his pulse and respirations stabilize. The erect position may then be assumed with the nurse available for support if needed.

Equipment such as an intravenous drip stand and suction machine should not interfere with ambulation. Intravenous bags can be placed on moveable stands and pushed by the nurse or patient. If the patient has a nasogastric tube on suction, the surgeon may indicate that it may be clamped for a brief period of ambulation. When equipment cannot be disconnected, the patient is assisted to walk within the confines of the bed area.

Sitting in a chair may be relaxing and more comfortable for the patient than lying in bed but does not replace ambulation and should not be prolonged. When sitting, patients are encouraged to elevate their legs to prevent venous stasis in the lower limbs and lower abdomen.

The patient is encouraged to use a commode or go to the toilet while up to promote normal bladder and bowel elimination. Precautions against overactivity are necessary when the patient is up more frequently for longer periods because the reparative processes are still going on within the body.

Early ambulation is contraindicated or delayed when there is shock, haemorrhage or cardiac insufficiency.

Wound care
The objectives in wound care are for the wound to remain uninfected and heal firmly with a minimum of scar tissue. When the edges of a wound are in close apposition, healing usually takes place by primary intention (see Chapter 4). A mild inflammatory reaction with fluid and cellular exudate occurs during the first 24 hours. The patient's temperature is usually slightly elevated and the wound edges will be swollen, red and warm. The gap between the incised edges is bridged within 2 or 3 days as epithelial cells migrate across the wound and help to seal it. During the next 10 days, a collagen network forms and regeneration begins. The area will be highly vascular and red in appearance and the edges slightly elevated. The supportive network is usually adequate for the sutures to be removed in 5–10 days. The strength of the wound increases over the next few months and the tissue shrinks and becomes pale. With no complications, the scar will have the appearance of a thin, white line in about 6 months.

On completion of the surgery, the incision is covered with a sterile dressing and the area is inspected frequently during the immediate postoperative period for signs of drainage or bleeding. If the dressing becomes moist with serous drainage, it is reinforced by the application of sterile pads with-

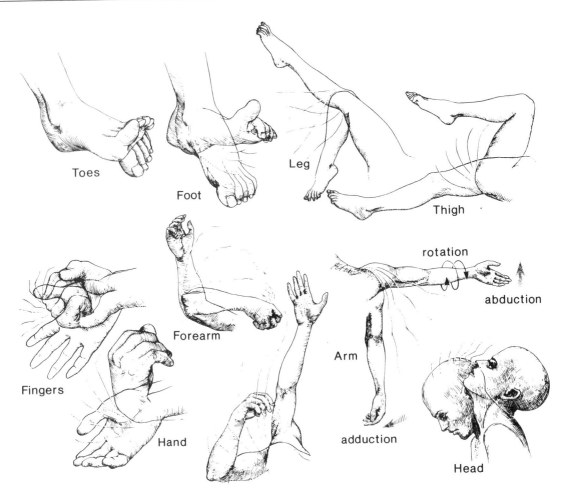

Fig. 11.2 Bed exercises for postoperative patients.

out disturbing the initial dressing. Should bright blood be evident, the doctor is notified promptly. In 2 or 3 days, the surgeon may order the dressing to be removed and the wound left exposed[8,9] or covered with a thin layer of gauze,[10,11]. This is to eliminate warmth and moisture which favour infection and maceration of the wound edges, and the use of adhesive which can be irritating to the skin. Some surgeons prefer to leave the original dressing in place until the sutures are removed. (The rationale for covering the wound is that dehydration retards healing, and a dressing reduces loss of moisture.) The sutures are removed in 5–10 days, depending on the type of suture, rate of healing, etc. If clips or staples have been used to close the wound, these may be removed slightly earlier.

[8] Altemeier (1979).
[9] Hinman & Maibach (1963), p. 377.
[10] Neuberger (1985).
[11] O'Byrne (1979).

A drain may have been inserted at the time of surgery to allow the escape of serum, pus or a body fluid such as bile. The tube may pass through the incision or a separate small stab wound. Specific orders are given as to the required care for this and when the tube is to be removed or shortened. Precautions are necessary when moving or bathing the patient in order to prevent dislodgement of the tube, particularly when it is attached to a drainage system.

Infection. Infection is manifested by fever, increased pulse rate, general malaise and redness, swelling and tenderness of the wound area. Spontaneous purulent drainage occurs unless the infection is deep, in which case the surgeon may remove a suture and probe the area to facilitate drainage. A swab of the first discharge is taken for culture to determine the causative organism. An antimicrobial drug (antibiotic or sulphonamide) is administered and frequent application of hot, moist dressings (e.g. kaolin poultice) may be ordered to increase the blood supply to the area and to promote drainage of the exudate. Even though the wound is infected, strict aseptic dressing technique is used to prevent the introduction of a secondary infection. When the soiled dressings are removed they are immediately placed in a paper bag for disposal, and precautions are taken to avoid contamination of the bedding and other objects in the environment so that the transmission of infection to others is prevented.

Haematoma. A collection of blood, usually clotted, in the surgical wound is usually due to impaired blood clotting. Patients receiving anticoagulant therapy or aspirin for a period of time preoperatively are more at risk of developing a haematoma. The wound edges are elevated and discoloured. If the haematoma is small and causing minimal discomfort, it may be left to be absorbed. If the swelling interferes with vital functions, causes discomfort and/or impairs healing, the surgeon evacuates the clot by needle aspiration or reopening the wound.

Dehiscence. Excessive strain on a wound, such as occurs in prolonged abdominal distension or severe coughing, wound infection, malnutrition, and general debilitation, may cause separation of the edges of the incision; this separation is called *dehiscence*. Resuturing or the application of adhesive strips (Steri-strips) may be used to pull the edges together.

Evisceration. If there is some separation of all the tissue layers (skin, fascia and peritoneum) in an abdominal wound, protrusion of a loop of intestine onto the surface of the abdomen may occur. This is referred to as *evisceration*. It is usually sudden, and the patient experiences 'something giving way' and a warm sensation on the skin surface due to the escape of peritoneal fluid and viscera. The surgeon should be notified and sterile dressings moistened with sterile normal saline are applied to the exposed intestine. If a large portion of the bowel is eviscerated, a sterile towel moistened with the saline will provide better protection. A binder may be applied for support. The patient is requested to lie very still and his head and shoulders and the lower limbs are slightly elevated to reduce the strain on the abdominal wall. Someone remains with the patient to provide reassurance, and a sedative may be ordered to allay fear. Since the patient will most likely be returned to the operating theatre, an anaesthetic and operation consent form is signed after the surgeon has explained what is necessary, and the family is notified. The anaesthetist or surgeon is advised as to when the patient last took food and fluid so that necessary precautions are taken to prevent aspiration. Lavage or induced vomiting are contraindicated since intra-abdominal pressure would be increased and more intestine eviscerated.

Maintenance of ventilation
As soon as the patient regains consciousness, he is encouraged to do the deep-breathing and coughing exercises which were taught preoperatively. Sustained, maximal inspirations are carried out several times each hour. The patient is positioned to allow for maximum chest expansion and is coached by the nurse to take a deep breath, hold it for 3–5 seconds and then breathe out slowly. Coughing exercises are carried out with the incision supported by the patient or nurse. A sitting position is best for both activities. The patient's level of pain is assessed prior to beginning coughing activities and medication given to alleviate the pain if indicated. Pain, fear and lack of understanding of the importance of deep-breathing and coughing activities interfere with patient compliance. Alleviation of pain, provision of support and coaching of the patient in carrying out the exercises are necessary for effectiveness.

The patient is turned from side to side frequently to allow full expansion of both lungs and the drainage of secretions. Early ambulation is essential to promote respiratory functioning and prevent complications caused by hypoventilation and the retention of secretions.

Respiratory complications. The respiratory complications seen most often postoperatively are hypoventilation, atelectasis, pneumonia and pulmonary embolism. Whatever the disorder that develops, the common denominator is hypoxia and hypercapnia. An oxygen deficiency affects the entire body. Hypoxia may be manifested by headache, restlessness and irritability, and then apathy, dullness and clouded consciousness. The pulse rate increases and arrhythmias may develop. The respiratory rate increases as the carbon dioxide level rises.

As noted earlier in this chapter, *hypoventilation* occurs frequently in the immediate postoperative period as a result of respiratory centre depression by drugs or the anaesthetic agent. If the patient does not periodically hyperventilate, atelectasis may develop due to decreased vital capacity and surfactant activity. Suggestions for improving ventilation were presented in the earlier discussion.

Obstruction of a bronchial tube by aspirated material or a plug of mucus results in *atelectasis*, the collapse of the portion of the lung distal to the obstruction. If the collapsed area is large, the patient becomes dyspnoeic and cyanosed; his respirations are rapid and shallow, chest expansion is decreased on the affected side and intercostal retraction may be evident. The pulse rate and temperature are elevated. On examination there is percussion dullness and an absence of breath sounds in the area. Trapped secretions tend to harbour organisms, leading to infection (pneumonia) in the collapsed area.

A chest x-ray may be ordered to determine the extent of the area involved. Frequent deep breathing, coughing and turning are required. Percussion of the chest by a physiotherapist to dislodge the mucus is done several times daily. An increased fluid intake and humidification of the inspired air are used to promote liquefaction of the secretions so they can be raised more easily. Endotracheal (deep) suction may be used, depending upon the location of the collapsed area and the amount of secretions in the tracheobronchial tree. If the mucus plug cannot be dislodged, bronchoscopic aspiration may be necessary. An antimicrobial preparation is prescribed to combat infection.

Pneumonia may develop independently of atelectasis. Any secretions retained in the alveoli and bronchial tubes readily become infected. The patient usually develops a cough and may complain of chest pain. The temperature, pulse and respirations are elevated, and the sputum becomes purulent and streaked with blood. (See Chapter 16 for a detailed discussion of pneumonia.)

Prevention of postoperative respiratory complications begins with the preoperative preparation. Recognition of even a very mild respiratory infection is important and should be reported. Unless the surgery is an emergency, the operation is deferred until the infection is cleared up. A good nutritional status contributes to the patient's resistance to infection, and smoking should be discouraged. It is extremely important that the patient's stomach be empty when receiving an anaesthetic to decrease the danger of aspiration of vomit.

Postoperative nursing measures that contribute to the prevention of respiratory complications include the following: (1) lateral or semiprone positioning of the patient during recovery from general anaesthesia to prevent obstruction of the airway and promote drainage of secretions and vomit; (2) use of suction when necessary to remove secretions from the pharynx and mouth; (3) frequent deep breathing, coughing and change of position; (4) protection of the patient from chilling and exposure to persons with a respiratory infection; (5) early ambulation; and (6) prompt recognition and reporting of adverse signs and symptoms.

Maintenance of circulation

As soon as consciousness is regained and the vital signs are stable, the patient is encouraged to move about in bed, do limb exercises and begin ambulation. Hypotension may result from sudden changes in position during the immediate postoperative period; a change in position should be made slowly and the patient's responses monitored closely. Physical and emotional support are necessary. Leg and arm exercises and ambulation were discussed in an earlier section of this chapter. Circulatory complications including shock, haemorrhage, cardiac arrhythmias and hypotension were also discussed as they related to the postanaesthetic period.

Vascular complications that may develop during the postoperative phase include deep vein thrombosis, thrombophlebitis and embolism.

Deep vein thrombosis (DVT) and thrombophlebitis. Deep vein thrombosis is the formation of a clot in the veins due to a stasis of the blood. It develops most often in the lower limbs. Pressure on the calves of the legs and prolonged flexion of the legs should be avoided. Although the patient may find a pillow under the knees very comfortable, this is hazardous since it promotes venous stasis. Frequent foot and leg exercises play an important role in the prevention of DVT in the bed patient.

The thrombus formation is a 'silent' process; there may be some tenderness in the calf of the leg that is accidentally discovered on pressure, or a positive Homan's sign (pain on stretching of the calf muscle), but there are no evident signs or symptoms. If DVT is suspected or recognized, the patient is placed at rest with the foot of the bed elevated. An anticoagulant (e.g. heparin) is usually prescribed to prevent enlargement of the thrombus. The condition is very dangerous because the clot may be carried along in the bloodstream and eventually may block a vital blood vessel, causing what is called an embolism, which may be fatal. As a precautionary measure the surgeon may order an elastic compression stocking (such as Thrombo-embolic deterrent stockings) or the application of elastic bandages to the lower limbs from the foot to the thigh before surgery. These usually remain in place until just before the patient is discharged or resumes a normal amount of activity. The nurse removes and reapplies them twice daily to give the necessary skin care.

Thrombophlebitis is due to trauma, infection or chemical irritation of the wall of a vein, initiating a local inflammatory reaction and clot formation. In this instance the clot is fairly firmly attached to the wall of the vein. The condition is quickly recognized because the surrounding tissue becomes oedematous, reddened and painful, and there is an elevation of temperature and pulse.

The patient may be kept on bed rest with the affected limb elevated. External heat may help to relieve the pain caused by vasospasm, and an anticoagulant may be ordered to prevent enlargement of the thrombus. The affected limb is handled very gently and is never massaged, in order to avoid dislodging the clot and the possibility of an embolism.

Pulmonary embolism. This is a serious vascular postoperative complication that compromises the individual's gas exchange and the volume of blood returned to the left side of the heart. Embolism involves the transport by the bloodstream of a detached blood clot (thrombus) or mass of 'foreign' material (tissue, fat globules, air) to a site remote from its origin or point of entry into the vascular system. It is most often a thrombus which eventually lodges in a vessel, obstructing the flow of blood and causing an infarction in the area.

A frequent site of embolism is a pulmonary artery,

and the size of the artery occluded determines what happens to the patient. If it is a large pulmonary artery, the patient may experience sudden severe chest pain and respiratory distress and collapse and die immediately. If a smaller pulmonary artery is blocked, the patient experiences chest pain, dyspnoea, coughing and elevation in temperature, pulse rate and respirations. He may expectorate blood-streaked mucus. If it is a relatively large infarction, shock develops rapidly. In a few hours an area of dullness may be detected by percussion, and auscultation may reveal an area in which there are no breath sounds, as the alveoli in the infarct gradually collapse. A chest x-ray is done and the blood pH and gas (oxygen and carbon dioxide) concentrations are determined frequently.

Oxygen is administered by nasal cannulae or a mask, and an analgesic such as morphine sulphate may be ordered to relieve the patient's pain and anxiety. An anticoagulant (heparin) is given by intravenous infusion.

Postoperative embolism occurs more often following pelvic surgery, prolonged bed rest, fractures and orthopaedic surgery. It develops more readily in elderly persons and in those with varicosities or a history of a recent leg injury. It is also suggested that women who have been using an oral contraceptive are predisposed to embolism.[12]

Frequent foot and leg exercises and early mobilization are important measures in the prevention of embolism.

Decreasing patient anxiety
Nursing measures to decrease the patient's anxiety should be specific to the individual patient. What does the surgery mean to the patient? How does the patient perceive the postoperative events and activities? What are the implications for the individual in terms of body image, future life-style changes and social and family functioning?

An opportunity should be provided to discuss the patient's concerns and perception of the surgical experience. Immediate and long-term problems are identified and assistance planned. An explanation of what to expect and what is happening at the present time and correction of misconceptions decreases the patient's anxiety and helps him to develop realistic plans for the future.

When the patient is faced with new and unfamiliar activities including getting out of bed for the first time or walking with complex equipment attached to his body, the nurse should stay with the patient and provide both physical and emotional support.

Preparation for discharge from hospital
Surgical patients remain in the hospital for a much shorter period now than they did a few years ago. Early ambulation, self-care, and early resumption of

a normal diet hasten recovery and help to maintain the patient's strength, making a shorter period of hospitalization possible.

Since the reparative processes continue, the patient and his family receive instructions as to the amount of activity permitted and the necessary rest required. Instructions given will depend on the type of surgery, but in general patients should be encouraged to take some exercise (e.g. walking) daily and will need more rest than usual. The nurse should give explicit advice to each patient, in terms the patient will understand, which should be specific for each patient and his needs. 'Activity' and 'rest' mean different things to different people. If dressings or treatments are required, the patient and a family member are taught how these are carried out, or a referral may be made for a district nurse to visit. The doctor may give the patient some idea of when he may return to work before he leaves the hospital, or it may not be decided until he has his initial follow-up examination.

Expected outcomes

1 The patient is free from pain and discomfort, as shown by verbal expression and participation in physical activities and his ability to rest and sleep.
2 The fluid intake and electrolyte concentrations are normal for the patient.
3 The patient is taking a nutritionally balanced diet.
4 Urinary and bowel elimination are re-established and normal for the patient.
5 The patient is ambulatory, active and participating in his care.
6 The incision is clean, dry and intact.
7 Vital signs are normal for the patient.
8 No manifestations of complications are present.
9 The patient and family demonstrate an understanding of the required care during convalescence and the resources available.

References and Further Reading

BOOKS

Altemeier W (1979) *Manual on Control of Infection in Surgical Patients.* New York: Harper & Row.
Boore J (1978) *Prescription for Recovery.* London: RCN.
British National Formulary, 11th ed. (1986) London: BMA and Pharmaceutical Society of Great Britain.
Dickerson JWT & Booth E (1985) *Clinical Nutrition for Nurses, Dieticians and Health Care Professionals.* Faber and Faber.
Dunphy JE & Way LW (eds) (1981) *Current Surgical Diagnosis and Treatment*, 5th Ed. Los Altos, CA: Lange. Chapters 1, 2, 3, 4, 10 and 14.
Gilman AG, Goodman LS & Gilman A (eds) (1980) *The Pharmacological Basis of Therapeutics*, 6th ed. New York: Macmillan. Chapters 14 and 15.

---

[12] Krupp & Chatton (1981), p. 455.

Gooch J (1984) *The Other Side of Surgery*. London: Macmillan.

Hamilton-Smith S (1972) *Nil by Mouth*. London: RCN.

Hayward J (1975) *Information—A Prescription Against Pain*. London: RCN.

Horsley JA (1981) *Preoperative Sensory Preparation to Promote Recovery*, Michigan Nurses Association; CURN Project. New York: Grune and Stratton.

Krupp MA & Chatton MJ (eds) (1981) *Current Medical Diagnosis and Treatment*. Los Altos, CA: Lange.

LeMaitre GD & Finnegan JA (1980) *The Patient in Surgery: A Guide for Nurses*, 4th ed. Philadelphia: WB Saunders. Part 1.

McCaffrey M (1972) *Nursing the Patient in Pain*. London: Harper & Row.

McFarland J (ed) (1980) *Basic Clinical Surgery*, 2nd ed. London: Butterworths. Chapters 1–6 inclusive.

Miller BF & Keane CR (1986) *Encyclopedia and Dictionary of Medicine, Nursing and Allied Health*, 3rd ed. Philadelphia: WB Saunders.

Palmer RN (1985), *Consent, Confidentiality, Disclosure of Medical Records*. London: Medical Protection Society.

Sabiston DC Jr (ed) (1986) *Davis–Christopher: Textbook of Surgery*, 13th ed. Philadelphia; WB Saunders. Chapters 5, 11 and 13.

Somerville MA (1979) *Consent to Medical Care: Protection of Life Series. A Study Paper Prepared for the Law Commission of Canada*. Ottawa: Ministry of Supply and Services.

Stark DCC (ed) (1985) *Practical Points in Anesthesiology*, 3rd ed. New York: Medical Examination Publishing.

Westaby S (ed) (1985) *Wound Care*. London: Heinemann.

Wilson M (1985) *Surgical Nursing*. London: Baillière Tindall.

PERIODICALS

Preoperative

Brown N (1980) Supreme court judgement; courts may now enforce stricter standards of disclosure on doctors. *Can. Med. Assoc. J.*, Vol. 123 No 11, pp. 1167–1168.

Cruse PJE & Foord R (1980) The epidemiology of wound infection. *Surg. Clin. N. Am.*, Vol. 60 No. 1, pp. 27–40.

Felton G, Huss K, Payne EA & Srsic K (1976) Preoperative nursing intervention with the patient for surgery. *Int. J. Nurs. Stud.*, Vol. 13 No. 2, pp. 83–96.

Ferguson V (1981) Informed consent: given the facts. *Nurs. Mirror*, Vol. 153 No. 1, pp. 35–36.

Fortin F & Kirowac S (1976) A randomised controlled trial of preoperative patient education. *Int. J. Nurs. Stud.*, Vol. 13 No. 1, pp. 11–24.

Metheny N (1981) Preoperative fluid balance assessment. *AORN J.*, Vol. 31 No. 1, pp. 51–56.

Morgan J, Wells N & Robertson E (1985) Effects of preoperative teaching on pain. *Int. J. Nurs. Stud.*, Vol. 23 No. 3, pp. 267–280.

Owens JF & Hutelmyer CM (1982) The effect of preoperative intervention on delirium in cardiac surgical patients. *Nurs. Res.*, Vol. 31 No. 1, pp. 60–62.

Phippen ML (1980) Nursing assessment of preoperative anxiety. *AORN J.*, Vol. 31 No. 6, pp. 1019–1026.

Rice VH & Johnson JE (1984) Preadmission self-instruction booklets; Postadmission exercise programme and teaching time. *Nurs. Res.*, Vol. 33 No. 3, pp. 147–51.

Risser NL (1980) Preoperative and postoperative care to prevent pulmonary complications. *Heart Lung*, Vol. 9 No. 1, pp. 57–67.

Schumann D (1979) Preoperative measures to promote wound healing. *Nurs. Clin. N. Am.*, Vol. 14 No. 4, pp. 683–699.

Seropian R & Reynolds BM (1971) Wound infections after preoperative depilatory vs razor preparation. *Am. J. Surg.*, Vol. 121, p. 251–254.

Stotts N (1982) Nutritional assessment before surgery. *AORN J.*, Vol. 35 No. 2, pp. 207–214.

Tkach JR, Shannon AM & Beastrom R (1979) Pseudofolliculitis due to preoperative shaving. *AORN J.*, Vol. 30 No. 5, pp. 881–884.

Voshall B (1980) The effects of preoperative teaching on postoperative pain. *Top. Clin. Nurs.*, Vol. 2 No. 1, pp. 39–43.

Wang J & Wang S (1985) A randomized controlled trial of a new approach to preoperative teaching and patient compliance. *Int. J. Nurs. Stud.*, Vol. 22 No. 2, pp. 105–115.

Intraoperative

Besst JA & Wallace HL (1979) Wound healing—intraoperative factors. *Nurs. Clin. N. Am.*, Vol. 14 No. 4, pp. 701–712.

Sweeney SS (1981) OR observations: key to postoperative pain. *AORN J.*, Vol. 32 No. 3, pp. 391–400.

Sweetwood HM & Hannelore M (1981) Blood gas analysis in surgery. AORN J., Vol. 34 No. 4, pp. 674–688.

Postoperative

Bauman B (1982) Update your technique for changing dressings; dry to dry. *Nurs. '82*, Vol. 12 No. 1, pp. 64–67.

Bauman B (1982) Update your technique for changing dressings: wet to dry. *Nurs. '82*, Vol. 12 No. 2, pp. 68–71.

Breslin EH (1981) Prevention and treatment of pulmonary complications in patients after surgery of the upper abdomen. *Heart Lung*, Vol. 10 No. 3, pp. 511–519.

Cooper DM & Schumann D (1979) Post-surgical nursing intervention as an adjunct to wound healing. *Nurs. Clin. N. Am.*, Vol. 14 No. 4, pp. 713–726.

deSimone D (1981) Postoperative complications. *Nurs. '81*, Vol. 11 No. 3, pp. 50–53.

Dossey B & Passons JM (1981) Pulmonary embolism: preventing it, treating it. *Nurs. '81*. Vol. 11 No. 3, pp. 26–33.

Ennis CE & Andrassy RJ (1980) Nutritional management of the surgical patient. *AORN J.*, Vol. 31 No. 7, pp. 1217–1224.

Hinman CD & Maibach H (1963) Effects of air exposure and occlusion on experimental human skin wounds. *Nature*, Vol. 200 No. 4904, p. 377.

Lamb K (1979) Effect of positioning of postoperative fractured hip patients as related to comfort. *Nurs. Res.*, Vol. 28 No. 5, pp. 291–294.

Locsin RG (1981) The effect of music on the pain of selected post-operative patients as related to comfort. *Nurs. Res.*, Vol. 6 No. 1, pp. 19–25.

McConnell E (1980) Toward complication-free recoveries for your surgical patients, Part 1. *RN.*, Vol. 43 No. 6, pp. 30–33 & 82–90; Toward complication-free recoveries for your surgical patients, Part 2, *RN*, Vol. 43 No. 7, pp. 34–38 & 70–76.

Marcinek MB (1977) Stress in the surgical patient. *Am. J. Nurs.* Vol. 77 No. 11, pp. 1809–1811.

Nayman J (1981) Management of post-operative pain. *Aust. Fam. Physician*, Vol. 10 No. 4, pp. 276–281.

Neuberger G (1985) A new look at wound care. *Nursing*, Vol. 15 No. 2, pp. 34–42.

O'Byrne CO (1979) Clinical detection and management of postoperative wound sepsis. *Nurs. Clin. N. Am.*, Vol. 14 No. 4, pp. 727–742.

Robusto N (1980) Advising patients on sex after surgery. *AORN J.*, Vol. 32 No. 1, pp. 55–61.

Schumann D (1980) How to help wound healing in your abdominal surgery patient. *Nurs. '80*, Vol. 10 No. 4, pp. 34–40.

Stephenson CA (1977) Stress in the critically ill. *Am. J. Nurs.*, Vol. 77 No. 11, pp. 1806–9.

Weaver TE (1981) New life for lungs . . . through incentive spirometers. *Nurs. '81*, Vol. 11 No. 2, pp. 54–58.

Wong J & Wong S (1981) Surgical care of the aged. *Can. Nurse*, Vol. 77 No. 11, pp. 30–33.

12
Age—Implications for Nursing

Introduction

Significant structural, physiological, intellectual and behavioural differences exist between individuals in different stages of the life cycle. Every nurse should appreciate the growth and developmental processes and the physical and psychological norms characteristic of the various age groups. The chronological and developmental ages of a person greatly influence health care needs, how they are expressed and the ways in which they should be met. It must be recognized that an individual can be an adult chronologically, but may be younger than an adult physically, intellectually and/or behaviourally.

Medical–surgical nursing references generally relate to the mature individual who falls within the physical and psychological norms, but many disorders that are discussed may also occur in children and elderly persons. Adaptations in the care cited are necessary because of existing variants due to age.

Nursing the Younger Patient

Factors in adapting care to children

Nursing a child differs from caring for an adult in several ways. The nurse's responsibilities in assessment, diagnosis and planning of care should include developmental needs. She should consider limitations in the child's ability to understand the illness and its treatment. Adults participate in decisions about their own care; they may be dependent because of physical impairment but if conscious are able to communicate feelings and needs. The young child depends on his parents and the nurse for protection and advocacy of his feelings and needs.

The following paragraphs include some important considerations in the care of the sick child. They are certainly not all-inclusive, but they may serve to indicate that differences do exist and to prompt the reader to refer to paediatric nursing texts for details. Although children may experience many of the illnesses to which adults are subject, infections, dys-

functions associated with congenital defects, nutritional problems and accidents have a much higher incidence. Neoplastic, metabolic and degenerative diseases occur less frequently in the earlier years of life, although neoplasms of the lymphatic and haemopoietic systems are the fifth most common cause of death in children aged 1–14 years.[1]

ILLNESS AND HOSPITALIZATION

Illness and pain are new and frightening experiences to a young child and he has no understanding of them. If hospitalization is necessary, it may impose separation from the parents, strangeness and loneliness, which may have adverse effects on the child. Anything that is strange and unknown is potentially threatening; in addition to physical care he requires attention that will develop a sense of trust and security.

Even young children and toddlers benefit from preparation for hospitalization. Parents can make a simple, truthful explanation of what a hospital is, why boys and girls are there, and why the child must go to the hospital. If the child is not prepared, hospitalization may be interpreted as desertion or punishment. It is helpful if the child receives a general description of his hospital bed, how he will receive his meals, what he will wear, the use of the bedpan, and the personnel who will care for him. The most important assurance however is that he needs to go to hospital to be made better. If his parents are able to be with him, particularly if they are able to sleep in the hospital, this should be emphasized to the child. Not all parents are able to do this however and it is important not to say they will be present if they cannot be. It is comforting if one or two favourite toys are taken along so that he will have something familiar close to him.

A number of picture and story books are available which are useful in preparing the child for admission to hospital. A copy of one of these may be obtained from NAWCH (The National Association for the Welfare of Children in Hospital—see Useful Addresses). Many hospitals now send out their own children's admission leaflet.

---

[1] DHSS (1986).

214

Individual differences in responses to frightening situations occur and depend largely on previous experiences and training. For example, although preparation is still necessary, hospitalization for the child of school age is less difficult. He has had the experience of separation from his mother and home for part of each day and has usually developed some degree of independence.

Usually one or both parents accompany the child and participate in the admission process. When a parent is not available, the young child may fight and resist the nurse or he may withdraw and become listless, possibly because of feelings of being abandoned by his parents. The nurse in understanding and accepting the child's fears, provides attention and care from which the child derives a sense of security and affection.

The mother is usually the most significant support in helping the child to adjust to the new and strange environment. Many paediatric hospitals or units encourage the mother and/or father to consider living-in if this is feasible for them and they are encouraged to participate in care of the child. If the parents are not able to stay, the nurse may need to take over gradually, so that the child, seeing the parents' approval of this, becomes more accepting of the nurse. The child should always be told by the parents when they are leaving and when they will return. The nurse may need to help the parents to say goodbye. She should accept the child's concern and behaviour when the parents have to leave, paying him attention and trying to introduce new interests. Although an occasional child may be inconsolable, the nurse should patiently persist in her efforts to provide comfort and emotional support and establish a relationship that provides security. To give up and leave him alone only adds to his despair and insecurity.

PARENTS

If the child has parents, they are the most important people in his life; his security and source of satisfaction in relation to his physical and emotional needs are vested chiefly in them. They, as well as the child, usually experience considerable emotional disturbance on separation and need the understanding support of the nurse. They may fear the outcome of the illness or be concerned about the child suffering. They may develop feelings of inadequacy and guilt and may attribute the situation to some neglect on their part.

The nurse assesses the parents' reactions and, on recognizing anxiety, makes an effort to avoid giving the impression that she is taking over the child. The mother is encouraged to talk about the child, remain with him as much as possible, especially at first, and to participate in his care. Her participation reassures the child, provides an outlet for the mother and establishes a better nurse–parent relationship in that it acknowledges the normal mother–child relationship. The nurse inquires as to whether there is anything special she should know about the child's accustomed care, such as food likes and dislikes, whether he still has a bottle at bedtime, his special names for urinating and defecation, his sleeping habits (his usual bedtime and whether he has a nap during the day), patterns of play, and what independent behaviour he has developed. As well as providing information to be used in nursing, this manifests an interest in the child and respect for the care he has received from his parents.

Rooming-in and open visiting are usual in paediatric units, and siblings and other visitors are given fairly free access. The mother is usually anxious to spend a good deal of time with her sick child but may require guidance in the interest of the care of other children at home. In participating in the child's care, she should be encouraged to do as much as she feels able to do for her child. The role of the nurse should be one of facilitator and support and back up when the parent is not able to manage. The nurse is still responsible for his total care and must know what takes place. Working with the parents provides an excellent opportunity for teaching and improving health practices which are favourable to the child's health and development. The mother may learn much simply by observing the care given.

GROWTH AND DEVELOPMENT

An important factor that influences the nursing of children is that the patients are in a period of physical growth and psychological and social development. It is necessary for the nurse to be familiar with the norms for the age of the child in her care. She has a responsibility to foster normal growth and developmental processes and recognize abnormalities and regression, as well as to meet the needs incurred by the child's illness. The amount of attention related to this aspect of nursing will vary with the age of the child, the nature and length of his illness, and the parents' understanding of his needs.

Until one has had considerable experience with children and the application of knowledge of growth and development, it may be necessary to refer to texts to determine the norms for the age of the child for whom care is being planned and implemented. It is not the intention to present a review of the characteristics of normal development here since there is an abundance of literature in this field. Several suitable textbooks are included in the references at the end of this chapter.

Illness frequently produces some regression in young children, particularly those in the preschool age group. Earlier patterns of behaviour and greater dependency may be manifested; for example, the child may not indicate a need to go to the toilet and may revert to bedwetting, or he may make no attempt to feed himself. Assessment of the child and information obtained from the parents establish the basis for planning continuing and progressive self-care activities within the limits imposed by his illness. If the need to learn and 'to do for himself' is ignored, overdependence develops, motor skills regress, and the child is less able to cope with the situation.

The child requires opportunities to play, explore, learn, express himself, and achieve in association with his peers if he is to develop. This cannot be left to chance but takes planning, patience and time on the part of the nurse. A variety of toys and amusements are necessary and should be selected according to the child's age, condition, interests and level of development. In many paediatric units there is a playroom which ideally is large enough for bedbound children as well as those who are up and about. Usually a playworker or volunteer is available to organize the activities and they may take play materials to those in cubicles or who have to remain on the ward. It should be remembered that a child has a short attention span and during illness the child will function at a younger age level and have an even shorter attention span. New interests and stimulation are needed. Most paediatric nursing texts include a chapter on play in which specific suggestions are made for play and amusement suitable for the various age groups. Play activities which promote motor coordination and dexterity, perception, and self-expression are also indicated.

A person tends to develop responses that are satisfying to him, but these may not always be acceptable to society. It is important that the child develop patterns of behaviour that are acceptable to those around him. Group play provides opportunities for socialization and the learning of appropriate approved behaviour, particularly 'hospital' play when the children can come to terms with their new experiences.

If the school-child is in the hospital or is confined to bed at home for a prolonged period, his school-work is continued by a visiting teacher provided by the local education authority. The larger children's units have hospital schools or school-rooms which hospitalized children can attend. His diet will probably require periodic adjustment to meet his growth requirements.

SIGNS, SYMPTOMS AND OBSERVATION

Signs and symptoms of illness in an infant and child differ somewhat from those in a mature patient because of the effect of the disorder on immature developing tissues and organs. The onset of an illness is frequently more abrupt and acute. An evident change in behaviour, irritability, refusal of food, vomiting, diarrhoea and fever are common to many conditions in children and do not point to the specific nature or site of the problem. A convulsion is common at the onset of a fever, and the temperature rises to higher levels and is more labile than in an adult. Serious dehydration leading to shock may develop as a result of vomiting, diarrhoea, fever and reduced intake. The child loses weight and becomes debilitated quickly because of the lack of nutritional reserves. The provision of fluids becomes an immediate concern with any sick child, but the fluid requirements are quite different to those of adults and need to be assessed by the paediatrician.

Observation is an important part of all nursing, but it plays an even more significant role in the care of children. The infant and the young child are unable to express and describe their discomforts and needs; the doctor and nurse are dependent on objective signs. Many non-verbal communications in the form of behavioural manifestations have meanings that are just as important as the vital signs. Parents when present can play a vital role in assisting the nurse in the interpretation of the child's behaviour. They are familiar with the child's unique ways of expressing his needs and may quickly recognize changes. The nurse's accurate, objective description of the child's physical, mental and emotional responses are important in the diagnosis and treatment of the child's illness.

Pertinent factors that should be noted and recorded include the following:

1 Crying—whether it is the normal strong vigorous cry or is shrill and piercing, feeble, or a whimper.
2 Body movements and position—whether restless, making purposeless movements, abnormally still and favouring one position, cries and protests when a particular part or area is moved or touched or when he is picked up.
3 Abnormal loss or increase in muscle tension (e.g. rigidity and hyperextension of the neck).
4 Frequent brushing or rubbing of a part (e.g. face or ear).
5 Apathy—passive, withdrawn, indifferent to environment.
6 Increased dependence—appears fearful and bewildered, clings to the nurse or parent.
7 Failure to eat and drink.
8 Change in the number and character of stools.
9 Change in the volume and character of urine.
10 Skin eruptions.
11 Facial expression and colour—drawn, aged appearance, pallor, turgidity of the skin, flaring of the nares, eyes sunken, shadows under the eyes, mottling or cyanosis, dryness of the mouth.
12 Any behaviour that differs from that expected for the age and level of development or from that which was previously exhibited.
13 Excessive sweating is not normal and is brought to the doctor's attention since it may indicate some autonomic nervous system dysfunction.

Continuity of care by the same nurses is important to the child for the development of trust and also facilitates prompt recognition of physical and behavioural changes. Lack of a continuing warm relationship with the parents and siblings or their substitute causes anxiety in the child and can seriously affect his ability to develop trusting relationships in later life.

INFECTION

Children are more susceptible to infection and, the younger the child, the greater the susceptibility. As he becomes older, he develops antibodies and some immunity following repeated infections. The infant is born with a natural passive immunity to some infections through having received antibodies from the mother's blood. Measles, diphtheria, poliomyelitis, and streptococcal and pneumococcal infections are relatively rare in infants up to 6 months of age, especially if they are breast fed. The antibodies which diffused across the placenta from the mother's blood into the fetus gradually diminish over the first 5–6 months of life, and the child begins to manufacture his own antibodies after repeated exposures to invading pathogenic organisms (antigens). The principal defence mechanisms and the reticuloendothelial tissues concerned with antibody formation are immature and slower to respond in the child, contributing to the high incidence of childhood infections.

Parents should be urged to consult their general practitioner or health visitor about the recommended schedule for active immunization for their infant (see Chapter 5). When it is learned that a hospitalized child has had no inoculations, it is brought to the doctor's attention.

Because of their lower resistance, children should be protected from contact with known and suspected sources of infection. The child with an infection requires prompt attention and treatment; his immaturity and lack of antibodies and reserves may lead rapidly to an overwhelming infection.

FLUIDS

There is a proportionately greater volume of water in the body of the child than in the adult; approximately 70–80% of body weight is water, as compared to approximately 60% of the adult's weight. The water in the young is used more rapidly; the increased heat production results in a greater amount being vaporized and the urinary output is proportionately greater since the immature kidneys are less efficient in conserving water and concentrating wastes.

Serious dehydration, acid–base imbalance and shock can develop with startling rapidity when there is a reduced fluid intake or an increased loss of fluid as in vomiting, diarrhoea and fever. Unfortunately all of these latter factors commonly occur together in childhood illnesses. An early assessment of the ill child's state of hydration is necessary. Vomiting, diarrhoea, high fever and failure to take fluids

should be reported promptly so that body fluids may be brought up to the optimal level. Signs of dehydration are dry mouth with thick stringy saliva, loss of tissue turgor, sunken eyes, depressed fontanelles in the infant, apathy and loss of weight. If it is allowed to progress to greater fluid depletion, the reduced intravascular volume causes shock, which is manifested by pallor, cold skin, rapid weak pulse and an abnormally low blood pressure.

Resourcefulness and patience are necessary on the part of the nurse in getting the child to take an adequate amount of fluid by mouth. A pleasant positive approach, assuming the child is going to take the fluid, rather than a demanding, urgent manner is helpful. Overurging may only result in the child's vomiting. Allowing the young child to choose between two or three fluids and to select a coloured straw may capture the child's cooperation. Parents can be of assistance here; they frequently can get the child to drink when others fail. An accurate record of the intake and output is necessary.

When sufficient fluid cannot be given orally, parenteral fluids are administered by intravenous infusion. Sites selected depend on accessibility. In older children any accessible vein may be used. In small infants a scalp vein or a superficial vein in the wrist, hand, foot or arm is usually most convenient. When fluids are urgently needed, they may be given by a central venous line or (more rarely nowadays) a surgical cutdown procedure. Restraints are not permitted so care needs to be taken to secure the intravenous cannula, as the young child does not understand he must keep it there. Mittens and adequate bandaging may be necessary. The parents' presence will be helpful initially.

The volume and rate of flow of the intravenous fluid require careful control to avoid dangerous overload of the cardiovascular system. Modified equipment is used for intravenous infusions in children. Paediatric infusion sets have a special control chamber that holds a limited amount of fluid and is designed to deliver a reduced drop size (60 drops per ml). To facilitate a more precise flow rate, mechanical infusion control pumps are now available and used increasingly for paediatric intravenous fluid administrations.

NUTRITION

Infants and children require more calories in proportion to size and weight than adults in order to support their growth process, higher metabolic rate and physical activity. The daily requirement is approximately 115 kcal/kg (480 kJ/kg) of body weight in the first 2 months, decreasing to 100 kcal/kg (418 kJ/kg) at 4 months and remaining at this figure until the end of the first year of life.[2] The best overall guide

---

[2] DHSS (1979), p. 9.

to food intake is to weigh and measure the height of the child every 3 months. Provided there is satisfactory progress, there is no need to worry about the diet.[3] Malnutrition is manifested quickly in a child with an inadequate caloric intake, as his reserves are very limited.

The sick child frequently presents nutritional problems; food may be refused because of a loss of appetite, the strange environment, despair at being separated from his parents, or because the food is not what he is accustomed to at home. The nurse needs to know the nutritional requirements of the child according to his age, the necessary restrictions because of his disorder, how much he is actually taking and changes in his weight. As with the giving of fluids, resourcefulness and patience are frequently necessary to have the patient receive sufficient nourishment. The following suggestions may be helpful:

1 A positive approach should be used, assuming the child is going to take the food.
2 He should not be hurried or bribed and is commended when he eats what is offered.
3 Milk may be withheld until later if he is inclined to drink it all and then refuse the solid foods.
4 Giving him a choice of food when possible may add some enticement to eat. Self-feeding is permitted and encouraged. The nurse should try to restrict the crisps, sweets etc. that visitors ply children with, until after lunch. When his condition permits, the child usually eats better when at a table with others.

Whenever possible, the parents should be encouraged to visit at mealtime; their presence may provide a situation with which the child is familiar. Home-cooked food may tempt his appetite if food he likes and is accustomed to receiving at home, and which is compatible with his condition, is brought in by his mother.

If the child is obese, fats and starches may be reduced and low calorie drinks offered. In long-term illness, it is important that adjustments be made from time to time in the energy intake and diet according to the child's age and progressive growth requirement.

NAUSEA AND VOMITING

Vomiting commonly occurs with any illness in a child. Nausea may precede the vomiting but the very young cannot draw attention to this. While in the adult vomiting may be anticipated by pallor, increased salivation, restlessness and sweating, the onset is usually quicker in the child.

Regurgitation, which is non-forceful, effortless vomiting that occurs without abdominal muscle contraction, is common in infants because of the incomplete development of the cardiac sphincter. The cause of this type of vomiting is often the swallowing of air or gastric distension due to overfeeding.

The immaturity of the neuromuscular system, which results in less efficient reflexes, increases the possibility of aspiration of vomitus. When a baby tends to regurgitate it is wise either to sit him on a 'baby-sitta' chair or lay him on his front with his hands and arms free so that he can lift his head and neck in case of vomiting. If he aspirates vomitus it is better to hold him head downwards and clear the airway by inserting a finger. It must be remembered, though, that the child lacks the reserve which the adult is likely to have and, in vomiting, will develop serious dehydration and malnutrition more rapidly.

ELIMINATION

The normal infant has a stool frequency of once every 2 days to 7–8 times daily. After the age of 1 year, bowel elimination is usually decreased to one stool per day. Stools are examined for changes in volume, colour, composition and consistency. The characteristics of the stool normally are determined by the food; changes from the normal may indicate a necessary dietary adjustment, particularly in infants.

Elimination which is too frequent or is absent, excessive straining at stool, and abnormality of the stool are reported and recorded. An abnormal stool is saved for the doctor's inspection and for possible laboratory examination. Usually a teaspoon of brown sugar in the bottle will be quite sufficient for the constipated infant. An enema or laxative is only administered when ordered by the doctor since either causes loss of fluid.

REST AND SLEEP

The increased activity, higher metabolic rate and lesser reserve of the young result in their need for more rest and sleep than mature persons. The patient care plan includes plans for regular rest periods and naps during the day as well as a regular early bedtime hour at night. Special bedtime rituals are determined from the parents and followed as much as possible; for example, the child may be accustomed to saying his prayers with someone or to having a certain toy or blanket to cuddle.

VITAL SIGNS

The young child's temperature-regulating mechanism is not fully developed, and as a result fever rises to higher levels than in adolescents or adults. He tolerates exposure to cold less well because his ability to conserve body heat by vascular constriction is less efficient, and his body surface is greater in proportion to his weight than that of an adult.

The temperature is usually taken rectally in infants and by axilla in infants and toddlers to avoid the psy-

---

[3] Passmore & Eastwood (1986), p. 588.

chological trauma of intrusive procedures, and for safety reasons when the glass mercury thermometer is used. The thermometer is held firmly in place and the child supported during the recording to prevent sudden movement and possible breaking of the thermometer. Today electronic recording thermometers are in use and are particularly satisfactory for children. For a fever over 38.8°C (102°F), temperature-reducing measures such as tepid sponging and the administration of antipyretic drugs may be ordered. Paracetamol is the antipyretic drug of choice. The use of aspirin has been discontinued in children because of its association with Reye's syndrome. Tepid sponging is discontinued if cyanosis, weak pulse or a slow respiratory rate is manifested.

The main danger of hyperpyrexia in children is that it can lead to febrile convulsions. Rigorous measures to reduce temperature may therefore be needed, especially as the rise is often very rapid.

The pulse and respirations vary with age, activity, emotions and crying. The volume and rhythm of the pulse are more significant than the rate. More accurate information may be obtained if they are checked when the child is sleeping and before the temperature is taken, since the use of the thermometer may disturb the child and cause variation. The pulse rate gradually decreases, reaching adult levels by adolescence. The average normal range for different age groups is as follows:

Infant	140–120 per minute
1–5 years	120–90 per minute
5–10 years	90–80 per minute
10–16 years	90–74 per minute

The respirations are more rapid and shallow in the infant and preschool-child than in the older child and adult. They vary from 30–50 per minute in infancy and gradually decrease to adult levels of 16–20 per minute by the age of 10–12 years.

The blood pressure is considerably lower in infancy and childhood than in maturity; it gradually increases with weight. The width of the cuff used in determining the blood pressure varies with the size of the child. If the cuff is too narrow, the blood pressure recorded will be higher than it actually is; if it is too wide, a lower reading is obtained. The cuff used should be approximately two-thirds of the length of the upper arm. Cuffs usually appropriate for different ages are as follows:

Infants	cuff of 1–2 inches (5 cm)
2–8 years	cuff of 3 inches (8 cm)
8–12 years	cuff of 4 inches (10 cm)
12–14 years	cuff of 5 inches (13 cm)

The child should be at rest for an accurate recording of blood pressure; fear, restlessness and excitement are likely to produce an erroneously high systolic pressure. The average normal blood pressures according to age are found below.

	Systolic pressure
Infancy	85 mmHg
1–6 years	85–90 mmHg
6–10 years	90–100 mmHg
10–16 years	100–118 mmHg

	Diastolic pressure
Infancy	50 mmHg
1–6 years	50–60 mmHg
6–10 years	60–65 mmHg
10–16 years	65–70 mmHg

Blood pressure recordings for young children are difficult to obtain and consequently are not often requested.

URINARY SYSTEM

The urinary output in infants and young children is proportionately larger than in children over 8–9 years and adults. The immature kidneys have less discriminatory ability; they are unable to conserve water and regulate the output according to the intake and to concentrate wastes to the same extent.

A urinary tract infection caused by *Escherichia coli* is relatively common in young females because of the short urethra. Prevention necessitates prompt changing of soiled nappies or underclothing and thorough cleansing following defecation, always wiping the area from front to back and thus avoiding the possibility of transmitting contamination toward the urethral meatus.

RESPIRATORY SYSTEM

In the early years, on inspiration the chest cavity is enlarged mainly by the contraction and lowering of the diaphragm. The infant's and young child's ribs are horizontal and the intercostal muscles have a lesser role in respiration. As a result, the rise and fall of the chest wall during respiration is less noticeable than in the older child and adult, and movement of the abdomen is more evident.

The lumen of the respiratory tract is smaller and so is more readily occluded in inflammatory conditions and aspiration. The larynx is sensitive, and irritation or inflammation may quickly cause spasmodic contraction, making breathing difficult. The nasal passages, being small, obstruct easily in respiratory infections, making sucking difficult. The cough reflex is absent in the infant and less efficient while developing in the young child; as a result, they do not get rid of secretions or a foreign body as readily as older children and adults. The bronchioles may easily become blocked and 'croup' and infection of the whole respiratory tract can be a paediatric emergency. Because of these several differences, infants and children with respiratory infection require prompt treatment and close observation for respiratory insufficiency. Sternal and intercostal retraction and flaring of the nostrils frequently accompany severe respiratory difficulty and must be reported promptly to the doctor. Prolonged rapid respirations exhaust a young child more rapidly than an older child or adult. Mucus should be wiped away quickly or removed by nasopharyngeal suctioning to prevent aspiration. The patient is kept on his side or in the semiprone position as much as possible to promote drainage of secretions. Cool moist air and increased fluid intake are provided to liquefy the mucus and facilitate its removal.

If oxygen or air is administered directly under pressure into the child's respiratory tract, the pressure must be kept low for a child up to 12 years so that the lungs are not damaged by overdistension. Similarly, caution is also necessary if mouth-to-mouth resuscitation is used.

Middle ear infection (otitis media) is a common complication of respiratory infection in children. The incompletely developed pharyngotympanic tube is straighter and wider, making it a more accessible pathway by which organisms may enter the middle ear from the pharynx.

NERVOUS SYSTEM

The child's developing nervous system is unstable. As a result, convulsions frequently accompany illness in children up to 4–5 years of age, especially if there is a fever. A nurse should remain with the child during the seizure to protect him from injury. Suction is quickly made available to remove excess oral secretions when the child relaxes. The seizure is reported promptly and the following observations recorded:

1 The child's condition and activity immediately preceding the convulsion.
2 The parts of the body involved.
3 Whether the movements are jerky (clonic) or whether the body or involved parts remain contracted and rigid (tonic).
4 The patient's colour, secretions, eye movements and pupillary changes.
5 The length of the convulsion and period of unconsciousness.
6 Incontinence.
7 Temperature, pulse, and respirations, as well as any changes in behaviour and awareness following the seizure. It must be remembered that convulsions may not always be due to the immaturity of the central nervous system; they may be associated with metabolic or central nervous system disorders.

Immature reflexes and lack of complete muscular coordination predispose the developing child to falls and accidents, necessitating greater protective measures on the part of those responsible for him. Blows to the infant's head are more serious because of the open fontanelles and incompletely developed suture lines in the skull.

BLOOD VALUES

Normal blood values for the infant and the child up to 12 years differ from those for adults. Erythrocytes (red blood cells) are more numerous at birth and gradually decrease to a lower level over the first 2–3 months; adult levels are usually reached by the age of 12 years. The leucocyte count is higher in the infant and in the child up to about 12 years with a higher percentage of lymphocytes. In Table 12.1 the normal blood values for various ages are presented.

SAFETY MEASURES

The child's normal curiosity, desire to explore, and lack of experience and understanding necessitate special precautions and constant alertness on the part of the nurse to reduce the possibility of injury from falls, the swallowing or aspiration of foreign bodies, burns, suffocation and poisoning. Essential protective measures include the following: cot-sides must be kept up and securely fastened unless the nurse or a parent is right at the bedside, facing the child. If the nurse must turn from the child to get something during direct care or if the child is on a treatment table, she keeps a hand on the child. The sides should also be kept up on empty cots to discourage ambulant children from climbing. Young children, whether in bed or up, are not left unattended for long periods.

The use of soft pillows and plastic sheeting is avoided; if either is used, it must be secured to the bed to prevent the possibility of the child pulling it over his face and smothering himself. All the windows should have secure locks which cannot be opened by a child. Casement windows must have restricted openings only. Radiators, electrical outlets and fans are covered, and doorways and the entrances to stairways are guarded by gates if children are ambulant. Sharp-edged toys and those with loose or detachable small parts that might be swallowed or aspirated are removed. Safety pins are kept closed and out of reach.

Medications are kept in a locked cupboard and never left at the bedside or within reach of a child. During administration, the nurse must not turn her back on a medicine or a trolley that has medication on it. The term 'sweetie' should not be used as a means of persuasion when giving the child a tablet, as it may lead to his taking an overdose of available tablets at a later date.

A positive identification of the child by checking the necklace or bracelet is necessary before administering a treatment and medication, since the infant or child is not capable of questioning or advising the nurse that he is the wrong patient.

Medications, fluids and foods are not forced because of the possibility of causing aspiration as well as fear and resentment in the child. Infants' feeding bottles must not be propped because of the danger of aspiration.

Table 12.1 Haematological values during infancy and childhood.*

Age	Haemoglobin g/dl %		Haematocrit %		Reticulocytes %	WBC: ×10⁹/l %		Neutrophils %		Lymphocytes % Mean (relatively wide range)	Eosinophils %	Monocytes %
	Mean	Range	Mean	Range	Mean	Mean	Range	Mean	Range		Mean	Mean
Cord blood	16.8	13.7–20.1	55	45–65	5.0	18000	(9.0–30.0)	61	(40–80)	31	2	6
2 weeks	16.5	13.0–20.0	50	42–66	1.0	12000	(5.0–21.0)	40		48	3	9
3 months	12.0	9.5–14.5	36	31–41	1.0	12000	(6.0–18.0)	30		63	2	5
6 months–6 years	12.0	10.5–14.0	37	33–42	1.0	10000	(6.0–15.0)	45		48	2	5
7–12 years	13.0	11.0–16.0	38	34–40	1.0	8000	(4.5–13.5)	55		38	2	5
Adult Female	14	12.0–15.0	42	37–47	1.6	7500	(4.0–11.0)	55	(35–70)	35	3	7
Male	16	13.0–18.0	47	40–50								

*All values represent compromises between a number of standard sources and published reports. Greatest variations in 'normal' are seen in infancy and early childhood. From RE Behrman and VC Vaughan (1983).

Nebulizers are used now and have cold 'steam' rather than the heat steam inhalations of former times which were much more prone to cause accidents.

Sufficient assistance should be available during treatments to provide adequate restraint to ensure safety.

Whenever the opportunity presents, the child who is old enough to understand is taught what is safe and unsafe. The nurse also has a responsibility for educating parents and others about their role in the prevention of accidents.

MEDICATION

Drug dosage for children is based on their weight and age, and must be very accurate. Children and particularly infants are observed closely for the effects of drugs given since their immature enzyme systems, liver and kidneys may not completely metabolize and excrete the drugs. Although the doctor prescribes the dose of the drug to be given, the nurse should be familiar with how a dosage is determined. If not familiar with the drug or if there is reason to question the dosage, the nurse must check before administering the drug. In many instances, the label or brochure accompanying the drug will indicate the dosage or the amount to be given per kilogram of body weight.

When administering drugs to children, a positive, firm approach is used. The nurse's attitude and comment reflect no doubt about the child's cooperation. The child's questions are answered honestly. For infants and children up to 5 or 6 years, medicines are usually given in tablet or syrup form. Medications should not be disguised in food, as this may cause future refusal of that particular food. Many medications are placed in fruit-flavoured syrups which disguise most disagreeable tastes. As

cited under safety measures, special precautions are taken by the nurse to be sure of the right child. Care is taken to avoid force in administering oral medication. The head and shoulders are elevated during the taking of oral medicine to avoid possible aspiration.

Infants and children tolerate opiates differently from adults. Usually children need a higher dose than would be expected for their size and age.

When children are to receive subcutaneous or intramuscular injections, if they are old enough to be frightened and resist, they should receive some preparation. Sufficient assistance should be available to hold the child securely and provide support. Often a parent can hold a young child and thus comfort him. Needles are selected according to the child's size. Afterwards, the child's crying and protestations are accepted; the nurse acknowledges his hurt and tries to comfort the child by picking him up or, in the case of an older child, by staying with him.

The nurse should never wake a child up to give him an injection.

NURSING PROCEDURES

The child's size must always be considered, since it dictates variations in certain procedures. Oversized equipment such as tubes or needles can be traumatizing to the child's tissues and interfere with effectiveness of the treatment.

Procedures are described in simple terms to the child who is old enough to understand even part of what is being said. It is helpful to let the child explore the equipment, see illustrations, or in some instances demonstrate to some extent on the child's doll or toy animal. Resourcefulness is needed to devise approaches and methods. The child is approached with a patient, positive attitude rather than a domineering, demanding manner that threatens him. It is helpful if the child is involved and is asked to do something that contributes. Whenever possible, the same nurse gives the treatment. Sufficient assistance must be available to provide the restraint necessary to make the treatment safe. The temperature of treatment solutions is tested by a thermometer and should not be used if over 40.5°C (105°F) unless specified by the doctor.

When positioning an infant or young child it should be remembered that prolonged pressure from remaining in one position for a long period may alter the shape of young developing bones. It is particularly significant in relation to the skull because of the fontanelles and developing suture lines. Freedom of movement is necessary to promote muscular development and coordination.

When possible, the infant and young child are held during feeding and some nursing care procedures; physical contact is reassuring and tends to make the situation less frightening.

The adolescent

Adolescence is the period of transition from childhood to adulthood and usually is accepted to extend from the thirteenth to the nineteenth year, although physical puberty (which often appears at 10 years or even younger) may be a more accurate guide. It is characterized by marked structural, physiological, emotional and social behavioural changes. The individual is seeking independence and a new set of values and standards, and struggling with identity conflict and developing sexuality.

PHYSIOLOGICAL AND STRUCTURAL FACTORS

There is an increased secretion of the sex and somatotropic (growth) hormones, producing structural and physiological changes which include a spurt in physical growth (an increase in both height and weight), the appearance of secondary sex characteristics, the onset of menstruation in girls and the production of sperm in boys. The physical growth occurs more rapidly than nervous control can be established, resulting in some awkwardness or ungainliness in the young adolescent. The secondary sex characteristics evident in the female are:
1 An enlargement of the breasts and hips.
2 A broadening of the pelvis.
3 The growth of pubic and axillary hair.
4 The onset of menstruation, which indicates increased concentrations of sex hormones, ovulation and the ability to reproduce.

In boys, the secondary sex developments include:
1 Enlargement of the genitals.
2 The growth of hair on the pubis, axillae, chest and face.
3 A general increase in skeletal muscle mass.
4 An increase in the size of the larynx, which produces voice changes.

The activity of the sebaceous and sweat glands is increased in both sexes, giving rise to the common adolescent problem of acne.

PSYCHOSOCIAL FACTORS

Adolescents are faced with the body changes, new feelings and reactions that puberty brings. They become very self-conscious and sensitive and frequently display mood shifts and emotional instability. Their responses to situations are unpredictable; interests, moods and attitudes may vacillate between extreme opposites. For example, teenagers tend to be ambivalent, alternately displaying acceptance and resistance to authority, content and discontent, and independence and dependence. They frequently go through a phase of rebelling against adult opinions and conventional society in general; on the other hand, they place tremendous importance on identification and conformity with their peers. They want to make their own decisions but are generally not sufficiently experienced to sever dependence and parental control entirely. Adults often make the problem more difficult by telling an adolescent he is old enough to know that or to do that and in the next breath tell him he is too young to know or to decide what is best. In this period of life, the decision must also be made as to a vocation or career for the future. Adolescents facing the changes, problems and necessary adjustments characteristic of this period of life require understanding and unobtrusive guidance from adults.

ILLNESS

Illness is disturbing to the adolescent for different reasons than for the child; he resents the interference with his freedom and school and social activities and feels threatened by the imposed dependence. He becomes the focus of his parents' attention at a time when he has been trying to be independent of them. If hospitalization is necessary, the adolescent may feel humiliated if placed in a children's ward, but as adolescent wards are a rarity, a children's ward with its greater freedom may be a more acceptable choice than the general adult wards where they are frequently unwelcome.

In many instances a student nurse may be assigned to care for the patient and, being an adolescent herself, has problems similar to those of the patient. She may find the situation difficult and require the guidance and support of a mature, understanding nurse teacher or staff nurse. The patient's ever-changing moods and attitudes must be accepted, and the nurse's approach adapted to elicit cooperation.

The nurse should be prepared to listen to the adolescent's opinions and concerns, treat them confidentially, and give advice or explanations when the opportunity presents but avoid an authoritarian manner. For example, adolescents usually have great concern about their bodies and welcome assistance in understanding the changes they are experiencing and reassurance that these are normal developments.

Because the adolescent is very sensitive and easily humiliated, it is important that precautions be taken to avoid any unnecessary exposure and to provide adequate privacy. It is helpful to include him as much as possible in planning his care, and procedures are carefully explained. This approach and manifested interest and concern on the part of the nurse mean much to the adolescent; it promotes acceptance and trust. If restrictions on certain activities or foods are necessary, the reason(s) for these are presented in a way that reflects no doubt about the adolescent's cooperation. Being given responsibility for assuming self-discipline and self-care activities, or being asked to assist with other patients or a ward chore, furthers his self-esteem.

The nutritional and energy requirements of the teenager are markedly increased; the daily intake to meet these needs may vary from 2200–3000 kcal (9200–12550 kJ) depending on gender, activities and rate of growth. Protein content should be kept high—80–100 g/day. Emphasis is placed on the inclusion of meat, fish, eggs, cheese, fresh vegetables and fruits, whole grain cereal and milk. When planning the diet during illness, it is important to consider the growth needs of the adolescent as well as the cause of his illness.

Nursing the Elderly (Significant Factors in Nursing the Older Patient)

Ageing and life's stresses result in structural and functional changes which appear throughout the later years of the life span. The changes are degenerative in nature, and the age at which they appear and their rate of progression are individual factors. Chronological age and the degree of change do not necessarily correspond for all persons; stereotyping of the elderly according to their number of years is often erroneous and misleading. It is important for the nurse to know that although there is marked individual variation, there are certain changes which may be expected in the advanced years and that elderly people are structurally and functionally different persons than they were in their youth and maturity. Their needs, the ways in which these are expressed and should be met, and their responses to illness differ.

Care of the elderly focuses on the person as an individual. It is concerned with maintaining health, a satisfying life-style and, following illness, restoring the individual to his normal activities of living as soon as possible.

Illness and hospitalization

Illness is usually more threatening to the older person simply because of his age and his recognition of a difference in his body efficiency. If hospitalization is necessary, he may be very apprehensive and pessimistic in regard to the outcome of his illness, and fear that he may never come out of hospital. In some instances, the older person becomes resentful at being transferred to a hospital or nursing home because it is interpreted by him as an indication that the family does not want to look after him. Adjustment to the hospital is likely to be difficult; the unfamiliar environment and people, and the change in the patient's accustomed routine and way of life produce insecurity. The nurse should be aware that acute illness, the stress of being in hospital, or even constipation may bring about confusion and marked behavioural changes, necessitating special precautions to protect the patient. Frequently, the older person has experienced the loss of his spouse and a number of his contemporaries, and illness and hospitalization seem to further emphasize that he is alone in the world. He is accustomed to having familiar personal possessions around him, and to have all these except a few toilet articles removed suddenly may be very distressing and frequently initiates protests and restlessness.

If the illness necessitates confinement to bed, the enforced inactivity is very hazardous and must be kept to a minimum in the elderly. Circulatory stasis, hypostatic pneumonia, decubitus ulcers and loss of strength become immediate concerns. Arteriosclerosis, which interferes with the circulation to the brain, predisposes to disorientation and confusion. Many older citizens have an income inadequate for the present cost of living. Expenses incurred by fuel bills or special diets during illness may have added to their financial worries.

Repeated orientations to the situation in which the elderly person finds himself are needed because the elderly may forget quickly. Explanations are necessary about such things as to why he is in hospital, how his regular needs (e.g. meals, toilet) will be met, the whereabouts of family members and when they will come, and the location of his personal belongings. A clock and a calendar in the room or ward may help to reduce the confusion that some experience and their possible concern about day and time. The figures on them should be large so they can be seen by the older patient, whose visual acuity may be reduced. Rigid adherence to routines may be very disturbing to the elderly. The individual is encouraged to participate in his care and continue to carry out self-care activities to the extent of his functional ability. Ambulation is very important and the individual is encouraged to dress in his own clothing and to wear good walking shoes for support.

Consideration in regard to the placement of the older person in the hospital ward is necessary; proximity to patients with infections is avoided because of his lowered resistance. The security of being near the bathroom is important for the ambulatory patient. He should not be left unobserved or alone for long periods.

Structural and functional changes—implications for nursing

GENERAL CHANGES

Some basic cellular changes develop gradually as part of the ageing process. The rate of cell division (reproduction), growth and repair becomes slower. In some areas, regeneration becomes less than the rate of cell destruction, resulting in tissue atrophy and, in the case of injury or disease, diminished recovery and healing ability. There is also less specialization in the cells being produced; in many instances, cells are replaced by those of a less specialized order, such as fibrous or fatty tissue cells. These less specialized cells require less oxygen and nutrients but are incapable of the specialized activities of the cells replaced.

There is a reduction in the fluid maintained within the cells and their environment. An inadequate fluid intake or an excessive loss of fluid may quickly lead to serious dehydration. The rate of metabolism decreases with advancing years and reduces the amount of energy and heat produced. The homeostatic mechanisms become less efficient in maintaining the normal constancy of the internal environment (e.g. chemical concentrations, fluid volume, pH, temperature). The reduced efficiency in regulation leaves a decrease in the body's reserves and a lesser margin of safety.

Such general changes obviously influence the functional ability of various organs and systems and must be kept in mind when caring for the elderly.

The elderly person usually adjusts his daily living activities gradually to cope with changes that occur with age. At the same time he may remain a healthy, functioning member of the community. When disease or environmental stress occurs, the body's resources are lessened to an extent that the elderly individual is less able to adapt.

Table 12.2 outlines the physical and functional changes that accompany ageing.

ASSESSMENT

It is important that the nurse identifies an individual's strengths and abilities as well as his weaknesses. It is very easy to concentrate entirely on problems related to the illness, allowing the former to deteriorate while in hospital.

The elderly rarely have one problem alone; assessment can be complicated by a number of deficits as several interrelated body systems degenerate. Although, in the interest of clarity, the rest of the chapter looks at these systems separately, the nurse must regard the elderly person holistically, bearing in mind his particular problems and needs. Further difficulties arise if one problem requires nursing care of a particular kind (e.g. bed rest) when this strategy can lead to complications (e.g. venous stasis or hypostatic pneumonia) which respond better to activity. The holistic approach can therefore help the professional judgement of the nurse to reconcile these otherwise conflicting needs.

CARDIOVASCULAR SYSTEM

The heart is one of the few organs that does not atrophy. More often, it is found to hypertrophy because of the increased demands on it created by vascular changes and hypertension. It no longer has as great a capacity for increasing the rate and strength of contractions to meet increased demands as incurred by physical exercise. The endocardium tends to thicken and patchy sclerosis occurs; the valves become thicker and less pliable, making their closing and opening less efficient. The myocardium gradually becomes slower in recovering irritability and contractility in the cardiac cycle.

The walls of the arteries become less distensible because of a loss of elastic tissue and the development of patchy areas of fatty and calcium deposits in the walls. The intima becomes thicker, and the lumen of the vessels narrows. Resistance is offered to the flow of blood, the blood pressure (both systolic and diastolic) is elevated and there is a diminished blood supply to organs and tissues, lowering their level of function.

The walls of veins are thinner and weaker, predisposing to the slowing of venous drainage and the pooling of blood.

The blood itself has greater constancy than most other tissues in the body. Unless an actual blood dyscrasia develops or dietary deficiencies are experienced, the plasma volume and blood composition show little change. The serum albumin level shows some decrease but the other blood proteins do not usually show any change.

Implications for nursing
Changes in the cardiovascular system necessitate a reduction in the physical demands on the patient. He is cautioned to move more slowly to avoid sudden increases in cardiac demands and output. Physical activity and exercise are important in maintaining and improving health. Activity should be regular and consistent. Physical exercise should be increased gradually; walking at a brisk pace is considered the safest and most beneficial exercise.

If an intravenous infusion is to be administered,

Table 12.2 Physical assessment of the older patient.

	Physical changes	Functional changes
General appearance	Greying of hair Skin wrinkles Loss of stature	Slower, weaker and more easily fatigued
Cardiovascular status	Pulse regular with good volume Resting heart rate slower Systolic blood pressure increased slightly Arteries firmer and more tortuous Serum electrolyte values within normal range	Decreased ability to adapt to sudden change and increased demands Heart rate is slower in returning to resting rate
Respiratory status	Rib cage expanded and more rigid Breaths are shallower Vital capacity decreased Residual volume increased Expiration may be prolonged Discomfort on deep breathing Increased respiratory secretions and cough frequently develop	Increased effort in breathing There is no significant functional impairment unless excessive demands are placed on the respiratory system by physical activity Increased susceptibility to infection
Gastrointestinal status	Increased incidence of constipation and anorexia Weight loss Taste and smell less sensitive	Frequently there is a decreased food and fluid intake due to socioeconomic factors, as well as taste insensitivity and ill-fitting dentures
Genitourinary status	Increased incidence of frequency and incontinence Urine less concentrated with increased odour	Nocturnal frequency Decreased time between the urge to void and the need to void Difficulty initiating and ending the urinary stream in males
Reproductive status	Absence of menstruation Atrophy of breasts and genitalia Mucosa is thinner and paler Vaginal secretions are decreased and thicker	Sexual energy is decreased During sexual intercourse reactions are slower and less intense
Skin, hair and nails	Skin is dry, thin, wrinkled and flabby Dark pigmented areas Total body hair is decreased Hair is grey or white Increased facial hair in females Nails thicken and are brittle	Wound healing is slower Body image is altered
Musculoskeletal status	Bone and muscle mass are decreased Increased stiffness of joints Decreased body weight Decreased muscle strength	Less able to adapt to physical stress and heavy lifting Increased susceptibility to fractures Body movements are slower
Eyes	Eyes appear dry with discolouration of sclera Size of pupil decreased May be loss of some colour in iris Decreased peripheral vision Far-sightedness	Slower adaptation to changes in light Decreased capacity to distinguish colour Increased reaction time for visual stimuli Increased need for corrective glasses especially for reading
Ears	Hearing loss: initially to high frequency tones	Decreased ability to discriminate and localize sounds
Nervous system	Decreased deep tendon reflexes Difficulty remembering recent events Decreased pain and temperature perception	Reaction time is increased and memory for recent events is impaired Shorter attention span

the rate of flow is slower than that used with a younger person. The less elastic arteries and weaker heart may not be capable of accommodating a rapidly increasing intravascular volume.

Immobility and prolonged bed rest are avoided, since they predispose to circulatory stasis and thrombosis. When bed rest is necessary, a change of position every 1–2 hours and passive and active exercises, particularly of the limbs, are important to promote venous drainage and circulation.

RESPIRATORY SYSTEM

In later years, the respiratory system is likely to be less efficient and less resistant to infection. The bronchial walls become thinner. The cough reflex is less responsive and less effective in clearing the tract owing to loss of muscle tone and strength and reduced sensitivity of the tract, resulting in retained secretions which favour infection. The elasticity of the lungs and the compliance of the chest wall are reduced, which results in a reduction in the vital capacity and maximum breathing capacity and an increase in residual air in the alveoli. Underventilation of alveoli, especially in the bases of the lungs, reduces the exchange volumes of carbon dioxide and oxygen between the blood and alveolar air. Oxygen concentration of the blood may be reduced, which encourages degenerative changes throughout the body. When the older patient is at rest, shallow breathing and slower pulmonary circulation predispose to the escape of fluid into the alveoli and ensuing coughing, dyspnoea and hypostatic pneumonia. The cilia are fewer and less efficient in 'sweeping out' mucus and foreign particles as a result of atrophy and dryness of the epithelial lining of the tract.

Implications for nursing
In order to encourage better oxygenation and prevent respiratory complications, it is necessary to have the patient breathe deeply five to ten times, cough and change position every 1–2 hours. One should be sure that the position assumed allows for free chest expansion for better ventilation. Frequent auscultation of the chest will reveal retention of secretions and areas that are not being ventilated. Early ambulation and activity within the limitations imposed by the illness are encouraged. Protection of the elderly patient from exposure to persons with an infection is necessary because of the lowered resistance. Respiratory infection in the older person should receive prompt attention; otherwise, it may become serious very quickly.

DIGESTIVE SYSTEM, NUTRITION AND FLUIDS

The stomach of the elderly person loses muscular strength and tone and takes longer to empty. There is usually some decrease in secretions and acidity; some persons may have a reduced tolerance to certain foods, such as fats. Fewer active taste buds combined with decreased activity contribute to a decrease in appetite. The loss or neglect of teeth may interfere with the taking of essential foods.

Loss of muscular tone in the intestine reduces peristalsis; the content is moved along more slowly, which may cause constipation.

The metabolic rate as well as physical activity is reduced, so that fewer calories are necessary than in previous years. If the person continues the same caloric intake, obesity is likely to develop; this should be avoided since it increases the demands on the cardiovascular system and on the weight-bearing joints.

Implications for nursing
Nutritional deficiencies are frequently found in older persons and may be due to living alone or a reduced interest in and desire for food. In others, the malnutrition may be attributed to an inadequate income, limited cooking facilities and refrigeration, ill health or the lack of dentures.

In order to keep tissue destruction to a minimum, emphasis is placed on high-protein foods, fresh fruits and vegetables in the older person's diet. Vitamin supplements, especially A, B complex and C, may be prescribed to correct deficiencies, improve appetite and the condition and resistance of mucous membranes, correct anaemia and promote a feeling of well-being. A protein concentrate preparation (e.g. dried skim milk) added to liquids may be helpful to make up calories and meet the daily requirements. The nurse may have to combat anorexia with frequent small servings, by determining and respecting the patient's food choices if possible, and by feeding the patient. If he is ambulatory, the meals may be more appealing and pleasant if arrangements are made to have him eat with others. If dentures are posing a problem, the dietary department is advised so that the meat is minced and other foods are appropriately prepared. A referral may be made to a dentist when the patient's condition permits.

As cited previously, the elderly person may develop dehydration very quickly. An explanation of the importance of fluids, the frequent offering of small amounts and giving the patient his choice may be helpful in having him take an adequate amount. The older person will often take twice as much water if it is not ice cold. An accurate record of the intake and output is made until a normal fluid balance is well established. A negative or positive balance is brought promptly to the doctor's attention.

The inadequate fluid intake which is common in illness and the somewhat decreased salivary secretion in the aged readily lead to dryness of the mouth and tongue and an accumulation of tenacious offensive matter (sordes). Frequent care is necessary to keep the mouth moist and clean and to prevent parotitis. Infection and inflammation of a parotid gland is a complication that may occur, in older persons, if good oral hygiene is not maintained.

In preparation for the patient's discharge from the hospital, he should receive counselling as to his nutritional needs and the selection, purchase and preparation of foods in accordance with his circumstances. The reasons for needed dietary changes are explained. Since it is difficult for an older person to remember, written suggestions and pamphlets on recommended dietary allowances should be provided. A referral may be made to the social services department or, if appropriate, the community nursing service so that help and guidance may be provided when he goes home.

BOWEL ELIMINATION

Loss of intestinal muscle tone, inactivity and lack of a well balanced diet and adequate fluids contribute to constipation in an individual in later years. Frequently the older person is overconcerned about daily bowel elimination and resorts too readily to taking non-prescribed laxatives, which may result in excessive fluid and mineral loss.

If constipation is a problem, more bulky foods such as bran, cereals, whole wheat bread, fresh fruits and vegetables, and fluids are gradually introduced into the diet to regulate bowel elimination. If a laxative is needed, the patient receives a bulk-forming laxative such as methylcellulose, an osmotic laxative such as lactulose, or a lubricant such as a liquid paraffin preparation. The latter is used for only a brief period, since it may prevent the absorption of the fat-soluble vitamins. Dependence upon the continuous use of any laxative should be discouraged.

URINARY SYSTEM

Sclerosed areas in the kidneys may develop as a result of a decrease in the renal blood supply. The ability of the kidneys to concentrate wastes may be reduced, and they require solids to be well diluted for elimination. The bladder loses some of its tone and may not be completely emptied during voiding. The residual urine undergoes some decomposition which predisposes to bladder inflammation and infection; the urea releases ammonia which accounts for the ammoniacal odour characteristic of some old persons' urine. Frequency and incontinence are common problems, particularly in illness, and can be embarrassing to the patient and may lead to social withdrawal.

Implications for nursing
The reduced ability of the kidneys to concentrate wastes indicates the need for a minimum of 1500–2000 ml of fluid per day. Because of the urgency and frequency of urination, the ambulatory patient is placed near the bathroom. If incontinence develops, the patient may become very discouraged. Involuntary voiding causes embarrassment, physical discomfort and odour. The individual loses self-esteem, and tends to withdraw and decrease his social interaction.

Every effort must be made to retrain the bladder and correct the incontinence. The patient's fluid intake is increased to 2500–3000 ml daily to improve bladder tone and lessen any irritation that may be contributing to the problem. A variety of fluids is used to make it easier for the patient to take the required amount. The patient goes to the toilet, or is placed on the commode or bedpan, every 2 hours. Fluid intake is discontinued at 8 p.m.; this permits longer uninterrupted periods of rest at night. The schedule and expected outcomes are carefully explained to the patient at the onset.

Understanding and patience are necessary on the part of the nurse with the patient who experiences frequency or incontinence. Manifestations of displeasure and impatience only create more anxiety for the patient, which in turn further aggravates the problem.

The use of an indwelling catheter is discouraged because it provides an entry for bacteria and promotes loss of bladder muscle tone, making re-establishment of normal voluntary control still more difficult. The hazards are emphasized with those caring for the patient who may consider the catheter the procedure of choice. If a retention catheter must be used it should be left in for as short a period as possible. Drainage is by a closed sterile system of tubing and receptacle and the fluid intake is increased to 2500–3000 ml daily, unless contraindicated, to reduce the predisposition to infection and stasis of urine that may lead to the formation of urinary calculi. When the catheter is removed the retraining programme described above is commenced. The intervals between the voiding events are gradually lengthened and, as the patient's general condition improves and he is more secure, the normal conditioned reflex and voluntary control are likely to be resumed.

When the patient is incontinent, the skin should be cleansed and the bedding changed promptly. The skin may be protected by the application of a protective cream or lotion or a moisture-repellant powder following each voiding and cleansing.

REPRODUCTIVE SYSTEM

The earliest changes related to ageing in the female occur in the reproductive organs. Ovulation and menstruation cease and there are changes in the concentrations of sex hormones. The uterus, vagina, genitals and breasts atrophy. The vaginal mucosa becomes thinner, dry and less resistant to infection and irritation.

Reproductive ability persists to a much later age in the male; atrophy of the testicles occurs at a later age than atrophy of the ovaries. There is a decline in sexual energy in both sexes, but some interest and activity in sexual relationships persists for many older persons through the late decades, although reactions are slower and less intense. The need for such intimacy and affection should be accepted and never ridiculed. The older male may experience hypertrophy of the prostate gland which leads to difficulty in voiding and incomplete emptying of the bladder.

Implications for nursing
Careful cleansing and frequent bathing of the female perineal area provides protection against infection. In some countries, patients are encouraged to have a complete physical examination annually.

If the male is a bed patient, he may have difficulty in voiding unless allowed to assume the upright position. If his condition permits, he may be assisted to stand beside the bed or go to the bathroom rather than have to be catheterized.

SKIN

The older person's skin is dry, thin and wrinkled and, as a result, is easily damaged by pressure, chemicals and trauma. Loss of elastic and subcutaneous fatty tissue causes flabbiness and wrinkles. Diminished secretions due to atrophy of the sebaceous and sweat glands contribute to the dryness. Pigmented areas frequently appear on exposed areas. The superficial blood vessels are less efficient in dilating and contracting to regulate body temperature. As a result, in hot weather heat dissipation is poor and, when exposed to cold, the body is not as capable of conserving heat. Local sensation of heat, pressure and painful stimuli may be less acute and are not as reliable in initiating protective reflexes and responses.

Fingernails and toenails tend to thicken and become brittle. The hair loses its colour and tends to become dry, thin and grey.

Implications for nursing
The skin of the elderly patient requires special attention because of the changes associated with the ageing process. Daily bathing may be inadvisable because of the dryness. A mild super-fatted soap is used sparingly, and lanolin or a cold cream is applied after bathing. Bony prominences and pressure areas are examined for any indication of pressure sores or trauma. Frequent changes of position, prompt changing of soiled linen and cleansing of the patient following incontinence, placement of a sheepskin pad under pressure areas, and the use of an alternating air pressure mattress (ripple mattress) contribute to keeping the skin intact and in good condition when the patient is confined to bed.

Soaking of the feet in warm water followed by an application of lanolin or oil will soften and remove much of the hard, dry scaly skin that tends to accumulate. The oil softens the nails, making it easier and safer to cut them.

If local heat applications are used, special precautions are necessary to avoid burns, because of the reduced sensitivity. Exposure to extremes of temperature is avoided. In hot weather, the patient's activity is kept to a minimum, and the room temperature is controlled as much as possible. The older person is more sensitive to cold; he produces less body heat and is less able to conserve body heat. In a room temperature which others find comfortable, he may be chilly. For this reason, the older patient usually requires warm clothing and extra lightweight bedcovers.

Skin wounds heal more slowly and are more easily infected in the aged because of the reduced blood supply to the area and the lower general resistance. Aseptic care of wounds and good nutrition play an important role in preventing infection and promoting healing.

MUSCULOSKELETAL SYSTEM

The bones become more brittle in the later span of life. There is a reduction in the organic material and osteocytes, and some demineralization usually takes place as a result of the changes in the concentration of some endocrine secretions (e.g. oestrogen). These alterations in bone structure increase the incidence of fractures in older people. Joint action may become restricted and painful because of degeneration of the cartilage on the ends of weight-bearing bones. Osteoarthritis, the formation of adhesions, or calcium deposits in the joints interfere with joint function and frequently lead to inactivity and decreased mobility of the patient. The intervertebral discs undergo some atrophy and the vertebrae tend to flatten; as a result the older person loses height.

There is decreased strength and some slowing of response in the muscles. If the person remains active, the muscle tissue shows some atrophy but remains relatively strong. Disuse of the muscles leads to fatty infiltration and marked weakness.

Implications for nursing
Since the elderly tend to fall more readily and their bones fracture easily, their environment and activities are controlled as much as possible to prevent accidents. The patient should be well oriented to his surroundings, which should be well lighted. A light left burning at night so that he can readily find his way to the bathroom if ambulatory or the provision of a commode at the bedside may prevent a fall. Cotsides on the bed may be necessary to lessen the danger of the patient falling out of bed or getting up when his condition does not permit ambulation. Lowering of the bed and removal of the castors also contribute to the prevention of falls. The use of scatter rugs is avoided and footstools or other pieces of furniture over which the patient might trip or stumble are removed. Well-fitting shoes that support the foot, and aids such as walking-sticks and walking-

frames may also be supplied to increase balance and safety.

Overweight in the elderly is to be avoided, as cited previously. In addition to hastening degenerative changes in the joints, it can make mobility and activity practically impossible for the person.

The nurse has to be understanding and patient with the slower responses and movements of the older person and also help the family to accept this change.

Exercise and activity are encouraged within the limitations imposed by the older person's physical condition. The family and friends frequently require guidance in relation to this; with the very best intentions, they may foster inactivity and its undesirable results by waiting on the older person and discouraging self-care and participation in other forms of activity. If left to simply rest in bed or a chair, the person regresses mentally and physically. Complete bed rest is considered one of the most dangerous forms of treatment for the elderly. It predisposes to the complications of thrombosis in the legs, pulmonary embolism, hypostatic pneumonia, loss of calcium from bones, joint stiffness, loss of muscle strength and the breakdown of skin over pressure areas.

Muscle contractures, deformities and restricted joint movement will develop rapidly in the older patient unless emphasis is placed on exercises. Passive movement of the limbs through their normal range by the nurse may be necessary if the patient is too ill or weak to carry out the exercises. It must be remembered that in taking the joints through their range of motion the movement is not forced beyond the range of comfort. Many of these patients may have some permanent joint changes which restrict the range of motion.

When the patient is well enough to be out of bed, it is not sufficient just to have him sitting hour after hour in a chair. He should be encouraged and assisted, if necessary, to walk a few steps and exercise his limbs. If unable to walk, standing up and raising his arms and legs at intervals is encouraged; otherwise blood pools in the lower limbs and pelvis.

SPECIAL SENSES

There is a decline in the older person's special senses, reflected especially by a loss of visual and hearing acuity.

The refractive ability of the eye is reduced owing to changes in the lens which becomes cloudy, allowing less light through to the retina. This cloudiness gradually increases and eventually the lens becomes opaque to light-rays. This change in the lens is referred to as cataract.

The elderly person develops far-sightedness and experiences narrowing of the visual field. Adaptation in dimly lit and darkened rooms is lost and may lead to the person tripping over objects, such as stools or chairs. Similarly, a longer period of time is required for adaptation to a bright light. A white circle may appear at the periphery of the cornea in the very elderly, referred to as the arcus senilis.

Atrophy of the auditory nerve occurs in varying degrees. Acuity for higher pitched tones is lost first. As the ability to communicate is progressively impaired, the older person's interests become limited and he tends to isolate himself socially.

A dulling of temperature perception and a decrease in the speed of the withdrawal reflex may result in burns. For example, an older person may not recognize that a hot water bottle that has been applied is excessively hot. Similarly, pain perception may be decreased; for this reason, lack of the complaint of pain or the severity of pain described is not always dependable, for it may not necessarily correspond to the degree of severity of the causative pathological process. For example, a myocardial infarction may occur in an aged person without any complaint of the chest pain which is considered practically a classical characteristic of such an episode in a middle-aged person.

Implications for nursing

Impaired vision places further emphasis on the need for repeated and thorough orientation of the patient to his surroundings. Good lighting is necessary, particularly for any close work or reading. Glasses and hearing aids should be kept in good repair and kept accessible to the patient. When communicating with an elderly person, the nurse faces him, addresses him by name and speaks slowly and clearly. Adequate time must be allowed for an elderly person to respond since his responses are slower. Teaching strategies relevant to the elderly with altered sensory, motor and memory functions are outlined in Table. 12.3. For further suggestions as to how those with impaired vision or hearing may be helped, please see Chapters 28 and 29.

In relation to the possible decrease in perception of temperature and pain, greater precautions are necessary in the use of heat applications and baths, and it must be kept in mind that the patient's condition may be more serious than is indicated by his complaints.

PSYCHOLOGICAL CHANGES

Some degree of organic cerebral change is associated with the ageing process, but any change in personality or deterioration of cerebral activity varies greatly from one individual to another. Most ageing minds show some loss of memory for recent events, slower comprehension, slower response, and a shorter span of concentration. Learning ability may be sustained to a surprising level if the person's interest and desire to learn are high.

One sees many variants; in addition to the pleasant, alert, elderly persons who adjust readily,

Table 12.3 Teaching the elderly.*

Factors influencing learning	Teaching strategies
Vision Peripheral vision, accommodation to light, colour discrimination, and visual acuity are decreased	1 Ensure that the patient wears corrective glasses that are clean and properly fitted 2 Provide adequate lighting 3 Use visual aids with large bold print and without a lot of detail 4 Check appropriateness of the task; for example, a patient may be unable to discriminate blue–green shades when testing urine for glucose
Hearing Ability to discriminate and localize sounds are decreased Difficulty in discriminating consonants such as s, z, t, f, and g and differentiating phonetically similar words	1 Face the patient 2 Provide a quiet environment 3 Speak clearly, using simple terms 4 Speak slowly–not faster than 140 words per minute 5 Use a one-to-one approach when possible. 6 Check comprehension of material presented in a large group and repeat if necessary
Motor function Body movements are slower and fine movements are decreased	1 Determine appropriateness of task to patient's physical abilities 2 Divide task into sequential parts 3 Increase time for practise
Memory Short term memory is less effective and more susceptible to interference	1 Provide a learning environment free from competing stimuli such as extraneous noise and movement 2 Slow pace of presentation 3 Allow for recall and rehearsal of information
Learning rate Processing of information is slower and it is more difficult for the individual to change his past way of viewing a concept	1 Adjust pace to the individual 2 Avoid large groups where pace must vary for each person 3 Plan teaching over a period of time to allow for assimilation of content (Avoid presenting new information just prior to discharge)
Past and present life experiences Past education, career and accomplishments Adjustment to recent changes such as retirement, loss of support person or change of residence	1 Plan teaching that is realistic to the individual's education, training and work experience 2 Do not underestimate the patient's strengths 3 Consider sociocultural practices and beliefs 4 Identify the individual's motivation to learn
Health/illness status Existing diseases and disabilities Pain Medications	1 Plan teaching sessions when pain or drowsiness and confusion from medication is minimal 2 Plan for constant repetition of information when short-term memory is decreased due to disease 3 Set learning goals that are realistic and achievable 4 Review and revise goals as the patient's situation changes

*Mitchell DM (1981) *Teaching the Elderly*. Hamilton: St Joseph's Hospital. Unpublished.

there are some who are unhappy, irascible, complaining and aggressive. Many of the emotional disturbances and personality differences seen are functional and are not due to organic brain changes. In many instances, they are due to the unfortunate social and economic conditions imposed on the elderly by present-day society. Forced retirement, inadequate income, the current social attitude of society which depreciates the worth of older citizens, and the loss of close family members and friends are factors that contribute to changes in the behaviour of many elderly persons. They may not be consulted or allowed to make decisions in spite of the fact that many older persons have developed greater understanding, foresight and a more balanced sense of values through their experiences in years of living. Occasionally one hears an elderly person say, 'No one cares what I think or how I feel. I am completely ignored and expected to passively accept others' decisions.' Just as in earlier years, these persons have the need for recognition, affection, achievement and some degree of independence. Enforced dependence and loss of self-esteem often lead to introversion; the person withdraws, isolates himself and lives in the past. The individual may experience social deprivation and a lack of sensory input which contribute to a reduced sense of reality, aberrations in behaviour and responses, and confusion. Most older people tend to feel more secure in their established pattern of living and resist new ideas and changes.

Implications for nursing

Any stress in the later years of life, whether physical or psychological, is likely to cause confusion that may last for a varied length of time. Such reactions may be anticipated when an elderly person is ill and hospitalized, which should put the nurses on guard to avoid any possible accident or crisis.

Physical care alone is not adequate for the elderly; they require respect, a voice in matters which concern them and meaningful activity to contribute to an incentive for living. It is important that the nurse understand that many emotional disturbances seen in older persons are due only in part to organic ageing changes.

As with all patients, each aged person is assessed carefully by the nurse; his reactions to the circumstances, interests and mental and physical capacities are noted. The psychological status, obviously, will influence the amount of protective care required and the necessary precautions for safety. An atmosphere of acceptance and respect is reassuring to the patient. When change is necessary, it should be explained, discussed, and when possible introduced gradually. The older person's wishes and pattern of living are given consideration, and unnecessary rigidity in routines should be avoided. By discussing his care with him, respect for the patient's years and individuality is manifested; by showing this respect, the nurse may avoid the reaction of resentment toward the young taking over. Enforced and abrupt change threatens and antagonizes the older patient. Preparation for events and answering questions relating to what is to take place will make the situation less stressful for the patient. Encouraging family members to visit regularly and spend as much time as possible with the older patient will help him to orient to and accept the situation. Close relatives provide ties and identity that are reassuring. If possible, having some familiar personal belongings close by and readily accessible may also help. Use of the proper form of address and using the patient's name indicate respect for his identity.

When his physical condition permits, an effort is made to promote the patient's interests and to encourage activity and socialization with others. Self-care and interest and pride in personal appearance are also encouraged.

Medications and the elderly

Reduced efficiency in metabolism, enzyme systems, renal excretion and circulation in older persons results in a decreased tolerance for many drugs, particularly when they are given in the average adult dosage. Detoxification of drugs by the liver and various enzymes may be incomplete and may occur at a much slower rate. The products may be retained in the blood for a longer period before being eliminated in the urine. A cumulative effect develops more often in the elderly, and may build up a concentration that exceeds the maximum dose. In some instances, a delayed reaction occurs as the result of impaired circulation.

Drug reaction is less predictable than with younger persons. For this reason, these patients are observed closely following the administration of drugs. Sedatives, such as barbiturates, and analgesics, such as opiates, may cause excitement and confusion in some, while others may experience respiratory depression and such sound sleep that the resulting immobility predisposes to circulatory stasis and pressure sores. Usually smaller doses of narcotics and sedatives are used for the aged. The elderly often have multiple complaints and disorders, and one frequently finds several drugs prescribed for the various ailments. The nurse must be alert for the danger of adverse drug interactions.

Older patients are frequently required to continue drug therapy at home following discharge from the hospital. Many studies of elderly patients agree that age is an important factor in medication error and non-compliance.[4] Only 50% of elderly patients accurately take general practitioner-prescribed medications at home; 63% of regular outpatients accurately take medications; and 80% of inpatients in elderly care units that are piloting schemes whereby the patient has responsibility for self-medication take medicines as prescribed. The type of drug regimen may affect this. Only 40% of patients comply with their prescription over a long treatment period, whereas shorter treatment periods are associated with 80% compliance.[5]

Identifying those most at risk of error or non-compliance has to be by individual assessment, as attempts to establish a significant association between error-making and sex, race, marital status, social isolation and educational levels or employment have been unsuccessful.[4]

Instruction and education in taking tablets before discharge from hospital has proved highly effective in reducing errors.[6] If this can be done in association with, or by, the pharmacist then there is also an opportunity to assess the most suitable type of container, packaging and labelling of the drug.

These factors have implications for hospital and community nurses.

Hospital patients who are to continue a medication after discharge should therefore receive a clear,

---

[4] Parish, Doggett & Colleypriest P (1983).
[5] Keet (1976).
[6] Macdonald, Macdonald & Phoenix (1977), p. 618–621.

simple explanation of its purpose, the importance of taking it as prescribed, what may happen if it is omitted and how the supply may be renewed if it is to be continued. Labels and directions for dosage, frequency and method of taking the drug should be clearly written and reviewed with the patient. Some patients responsible for self-administration of drugs require a calendar and time sheet drawn up that will be helpful in reminding them to take the medication. Encouraging the patient to record the taking of his drug immediately may avoid repetition and a toxic dose. If there are family members, one of them should also receive the instructions. In some hospitals there may, perhaps, be opportunities for self-administration of medications with instruction and supervision being provided by the nurse and/or pharmacist. A referral may be made, where appropriate, to the community nursing service so that the patient will receive supervision.

Convalescence and rehabilitation

The convalescent period following an illness is usually longer for the aged than for younger persons. The patient is likely to become discouraged because it takes him longer to regain his strength. In addition to counteracting the undesirable physiological effects of bed rest, early ambulation is promoted to improve the older person's morale. Once he is allowed up he is likely to be more optimistic about his recovery.

Many elderly persons seen by nurses have been socially isolated and emotionally starved prior to their illness. As the patient's physical condition improves, nursing care is planned and implemented to promote activities and mental and physical independence within the limits imposed by ageing and his health status. Interests are determined, and mobility and socialization are encouraged. Suggestions are made to the patient and family as to the activities, interests and sources of assistance that may help to make the older person's life more useful and satisfying and to counteract the apathy, depression and complete dependence so frequently seen. A few simple adjustments such as hand rails on the wall and the side of the bathtub and a seat in the bath may permit self-care.

Most communities now have organized health and social services for senior citizens, but many older persons require information about these services and assistance in making the initial contact with them. Many clubs have been formed to provide certain types of services to older persons; an example is meals-on-wheels. Home visits may be made to those whose health inhibits them from going out; for others, appropriate programmes are planned for entertainment and socialization. Those who are able are encouraged to participate in voluntary services (e.g. baby-sitting, home and hospital visiting); this fosters their self-esteem and sense of usefulness.

Special publications (newspapers, bulletins) are also made available to retired persons free of charge in many localities.

Summary

The elderly compose a large section of our population, and many nursing hours are devoted to the care of elderly persons. Following the mature years of middle life, biological changes are an inevitable component of ageing. The rate and extent of these changes vary with individuals, so that biological age is not characteristic of any particular chronological age. Stereotyping must be avoided. Too often we tend to judge on the basis of age in years and at a glance by skin changes, wrinkles and grey hair. The changes result in a progressive limiting of capacity and compensatory reserve; older persons are more vulnerable to illness and stress. Their immune responses are less efficient, so they require protection from contact with infection and prompt treatment if they become ill. Their physiological changes may cause potentially dangerous reactions to ordinary adult doses and combinations of drugs.

Confusion and behavioural disorders are usually the result of a combination of such factors as strange environment, separation from familiar persons, demands that exceed the individual's capacity, pathological condition (e.g. cerebral circulatory insufficiency), drugs, physical restraints and lengthy periods without sensory input.

In planning nursing care, rehabilitation must be taken into consideration; it is just as important for these patients as for younger persons. They want to be independent and useful. Each person's potential and assets are identified and fostered. The need exists to extend concern beyond physical care; psychological and social needs must not be ignored. These older persons require friendship, understanding, activity and opportunities for communication and social interaction. Otherwise, life lacks meaning, and they withdraw and lose contact with reality. They should not go unnoticed.

References and Further Reading

BOOKS

Nursing children and adolescents
Bee H (1978) *The Developing Child*. London: Harper & Row.
Behrman RE & Vaughan VC (1983) *Nelson Textbook of Pediatrics*, 12th ed. Philadelphia: WB Saunders. p. 1207.
Donaldson M (1978) *Children's Minds*. Glasgow: Fontana.
General Nursing Council (1981) *Aspects of Sick Children's Nursing: A Learning Package*. Newport Pagnell: Learning Materials Design.
Illingworth R (1979) *The Normal Child*, 7th ed. Edinburgh: Churchill Livingstone.

Jolly J (1981) *The Other Side of Paediatrics*. London: Macmillan.

Lewer & Robertson L (1983) *Care of the Child*. London: Macmillan.

Passmore R & Eastwood MA (1986) In: Davidson and Passmore (eds) *Human Nutrition and Dietetics*, 8th ed. Edinburgh: Churchill Livingstone.

Petrillo M & Sanger S (1980) *Emotional Care of Hospitalized Children*, 2nd ed. Philadelphia: JB Lippincott.

Tackett JM & Hunsberger M (1981) *Family-Centred Care of Children and Adolescents: Nursing Concepts in Child Health*. Philadelphia: WB Saunders.

Weller BF (1980) *Helping Sick Children Play*, London: Baillière Tindall.

Nursing elderly people

Brocklehurst JC & Harley T (1981) *Geriatric Medicine for Students*, 2nd ed. Edinburgh: Churchill Livingstone.

Carotenuto R & Bullock J (1980) *Physical Assessment of the Gerontologic Client*. Philadelphia: FA Davis.

Chalmers GL (1980) *Caring for the Elderly Sick*. Tunbridge Wells, Kent: Pitman Medical. Sections A & B.

DHSS (1979) *Recommended Daily Amounts of Food Energy and Nutrients for Groups of People in the United Kingdom*. London: HMSO, p. 9.

DHSS (1986) *On the State of the Public Health for the Year 1984*. London: HMSO.

Hodkinson HM (1981) *An Outline of Geriatrics*, 2nd ed. London: Academic Press.

Hogstel MO (ed) (1981) *Nursing Care of the Older Adult*. New York: John Wiley.

Malasanos L, Barkauskas V, Moss M & Stoltenberg-Allen K (1981) *Health Assessment*, 2nd ed. St Louis: CV Mosby. Chapter 25.

Parish P, Doggett M & Colleypriest P (1983), *The Elderly and Their Use of Medications*. King Edward's Hospital Fund for London.

Schrock MM (1980) *Holistic Assessment of the Healthy Aged*. New York: John Wiley.

Storrs AM (1985) *Geriatric Nursing*, 3rd ed. Eastbourne: Baillière Tindall.

PERIODICALS

Nursing children and adolescents

Caty S, Ellerton ML & Ritchie JA (1984) Coping in hospitalized children: an analysis of published case studies. *Nurs. Res.* Vol. 33 No. 5, pp. 277–282.

Hunsberger H, Love B & Byrne CA (1984) A review of current approaches used to help children and parents cope with health care procedures. *Matern. Child Nurs. J.*, Vo. 13 No. 3, pp. 145–165.

Lattanzi WE & Siegel NJ (1986) A practical guide to fluid and electrolyte therapy, *Curr. Prob. Pediatr.*, Vol. 16 No. 1, pp. 7–43.

Nelms BC (1985) Stress during childhood: long lasting effects: *Pediatr. Nurs.*, Vol. 11 No. 2, pp. 95–98.

Picton JE & Tyack EJ (1986/7) Infancy. *Nurs.: Add-on J. Clin. Nurs.*, Vol. 3 Nos. 12 & 13.

Zurlinden JK (1985) Minimizing the impact of hospitalization for children and their families, *Am. J. Matern. Child Nurs.*, Vol. 10 No. 3, pp. 178–182.

Nursing elderly people

Allen MD (1980) Drug therapy in the elderly. *Am. J. Nurs.*, Vol. 80 No. 8, pp. 1474–1475.

Andrews J & Atkinson L (1981) Home aids and appliances for the elderly handicapped. *Geriatric Medicine*, Vol. 11 No. 7, pp. 17–25.

Atkins John (1981) Care of the scalp and hair, *Geriatric Med.*, Vol. 11 No. 12, pp. 80–85.

Bailey PA (1981) Physical assessment of the elderly. *Top. Clin. Nurs.*, Vol. 3 No. 1, pp. 15–19.

Barrowclough F & Pinel C (1981) The process of ageing. *Adv. Nurs.*, Vol. 6 No. 4, pp. 319–325.

Beaton SR (1980) Reminiscence in old age. *Nurs. Forum*, Vol. 19 No. 3, pp. 270–283.

Beck C (1981) Dining experiences of the institutionalised aged. *J. Gerontol. Nurs.*, Vol. 7 No. 2, pp. 104–107.

Bozian MW & Clark HM (1980) Counteracting sensory changes in the aging. *Am. J. Nurs.*, Vol. 80 No. 3, pp. 473–476.

Brown MM, Cornwell J & Weist JK (1981) Reducing the risks to the institutionalized elderly. Part One: Depersonalisation negative relocation effects and medical care deficiency. Part Two: Fire, food poisoning, decubitus ulcer and drug abuse, *J. Gerontol. Nurs.*, Vol. 7 No. 7, pp. 401–407.

Campbell AJ, Reinken J, Allan BC & Martinez GS (1981) Falls in old age: a study of frequency and related clinical factors. *Age Ageing*, Vol. 10 No. 4, pp. 264–270.

Carpenter GI (1981) The ageing kidney. *Geriatric Med.*, Vol. 11 No. 8, pp. 19–23.

Crooks J & Stevenson IH (1981) Drug response in the elderly—sensitivity and pharmokinetic consideration. *Age Ageing*, Vol. 10 No. 2, pp. 73–80.

Dement WC, Miles LE & Carskadeon MA (1982) White paper on sleep and ageing. *J. Am. Geriatrics Soc.*, Vol. 30 No. 1, pp. 25–50.

Gasek G (1980) How to handle the crotchety elderly patient. *Nurs. '80*, Vol. 10 No. 3, pp. 46–48.

Gault PL (1982) Plan for a patchwork of problems when your patient is elderly, *Nurs. '82*, Vol. 12 No. 1, pp. 50–54.

Hahn K (1980) Using 24-hour reality orientation. *J. Gerontol. Nurs.*, Vol. 6 No. 3, pp. 130–135.

Hayflick L (1980) The cell biology of human aging. *Sci. Am.*, Vol. 242 No. 1, pp. 58–65.

Heller BR & Gaynor EB (1981) Hearing loss and aural rehabilitation of the elderly. *Top. Clin. Nurs.*, Vol. 3 No. 1, pp. 21–29.

Isaacs B (1981) Why do the elderly fall? *Geriatric Med.*, Vol. 11 No. 3, pp. 17–23.

Keet J (1976) Failure of the elderly to take medications as prescribed and ways to improve compliance, *Med. Ann.*, pp. 208–214.

Kieffer JA (1980) A strategy for keeping longer life productive. *Hospitals*, Vol. 54 No. 10, pp. 73–81.

Lancaster J (1981) Maximizing psychological adaptation in an aging population. *Top. Clin. Nurs.*, Vol. 3 No. 1, p. 31–43.

Langstrom NF (1981) Reality orientation and effective reinforcement, *J. Gerontol. Nurs.*, Vol. 7 No. 4, pp. 224–227.

Macdonald ET, Macdonald JB & Phoenix M (1977) *Br. Med. J.*, Vol. 2, pp. 618–621.

Meissner JE (1980) Assessing a geriatric patient's need for institutionalized care. *Nurs. '80*, Vol. 10 No. 3, pp. 86–87.

Miller J (1985) Helping the aged manage bowel function. *J. Gerontol. Nurs.*, Vol. 11 No. 2, pp. 37–41.

Moise JM, Tylko SJ & Dixon HA (1985) The patient who falls . . . and falls again. *J. Gerontol. Nurs.*, Vol. 11 No. 11, pp. 15–18.

Moyer NC (1981) Health promotion and the assessment of health habits in the elderly. *Top. Clin. Nurs.*, Vol. 3 No. 1, pp. 51–58.

Mullen EM & Granholm M (1981) Drugs and the elderly patient *J. Gerontol. Nurs.*, Vol. 7 No. 2, pp. 108–113.

Nordstrom MJ (1980) Criteria leading to quality control in rehabilitation: the elderly patient a team member, *J. Gerontol. Nurs.*, Vol. 6 No. 8, pp. 457–462.

Olsen JK & Cohn BW (1980) Helping families cope with elderly patients. *J. Gerontol. Nurs.*, Vol. 6 No. 3, pp. 151–154.

Price JH & Luther SL (1980) Physical fitness: its role in health for the elderly. *J. Gerontol. Nurs.*, Vol. 6 No. 9, pp. 517–523.

Raab D & Raab N (1985) Nutrition and aging: an overview. *Can. Nurs.*, Vol. 81 No. 3, pp. 24–26.

Rose GK (1981) The geriatric foot. *Geriatric Med.*, Vol. 11 No. 12, pp. 17–23.

Ross M (1981) Nursing the well elderly: the health resource, *Can. Nurs.*, Vol. 77 No. 5, pp. 50–53.

Schwab Sr M, Rader J & Doan J (1985) Relieving the anxiety and fear in dementia. *J. Gerontol. Nurs.*, Vol. 11 No. 5, pp. 8–11, 14 & 15.

Thomas WC (1981) The expectation gap and the stereotype of the stereotype: images of old people. *Gerontologist*, Vol. 21 No. 4, pp. 402–407.

Turnbull EM (1981) The practical problems of footwear hosiery and aids. *Geriatric Med.*, Vol. 11 No. 12, pp. 33–36.

Venglarik JM & Adams M (1985) Which client is a high risk?, *J. Gerontol. Nurs.*, Vol. 11 No. 5, pp. 28–30.

Williams EJ (1980) Food for thought: meeting the nutritional needs of the elderly. *Nurs. '80*, Vol. 10 No. 9, pp. 61–63.

Wolanin MO (1981) Physiologic aspects of confusion. *J. Gerontol. Nurs.*, Vol. 7 No. 4, pp. 236–242.

Yosselle H (1981) Sexuality in the later years. *Top. Clin. Nurs.*, Vol. 3 No. 1, pp. 59–70.

PART II

13

Nursing in Blood Dyscrasias

COMPOSITION AND PHYSIOLOGY OF BLOOD

Blood is a red fluid tissue that is pumped through the vascular system by the heart. It transports cellular requirements and products from one part of the body to another. There is a continuous exchange between the fluid surrounding the cells (interstitial fluid) and the blood; this exchange serves to maintain a suitable cellular environment that varies only within narrow limits.

Blood is opaque and has a viscosity about three to four times that of water. Its colour is dependent on the pigment in the haemoglobin of the red blood cells and varies with the amount of oxygen combined with the haemoglobin. A higher concentration of oxygen produces a brighter red. Blood has a slightly alkaline reaction, with a pH of 7.35–7.45. The average volume in the adult is 5–6 litres, or approximately 70–75 ml per kg of body weight. The volume remains remarkably constant.

Functions of the Blood

The blood performs several important functions:
1 Transportation of oxygen from the lungs to the cells and carbon dioxide from the tissues to the lungs for excretion.
2 Transportation of absorbed nutrients from the alimentary tract to the cells.
3 Conveyance of metabolic wastes from the cells to the organs of excretion (kidneys, lungs, liver and skin).
4 Maintenance of a normal interstitial fluid volume. The interstitial fluid is the medium of exchange between the blood and the cells. Unless its volume is kept relatively constant, the concentration of solutes may be so altered that the passage of substances in and out of the cells is affected.
5 Distribution of hormones and other endogenous chemicals that regulate many body activities.
6 Transference of heat from the site of production to the surface of the body where it can be dissipated.
7 Protection of the individual against excessive loss of blood by coagulation and against injurious agents, such as bacteria and toxins, by its leucocytes and antibodies.

Blood Components

Fifty-five to 60% of the blood is a straw-coloured fluid called plasma, in which the formed elements of the blood (blood cells and platelets) are suspended (Table 13.1).

PLASMA

Composition

The constituents of plasma are water (90–91%) and a wide variety of solutes. The latter include all the substances which cells take in and use as well as many substances produced by the cells. Examples are nutrients (amino acids, glucose and lipids), gases (oxygen and carbon dioxide), electrolytes and salts, and cell products such as hormones, enzymes, urea, uric acid and creatinine. In addition, there are also blood proteins, anticoagulants, clotting factors and antibodies.

The concentration of the solutes remains relatively constant even though water and solutes are continually being added and removed. There are temporary variations, but, under normal conditions, certain complex interactions and mechanisms function quickly to restore the plasma to normal. A good example of a quick readjustment that is made to preserve constancy is the maintenance of the plasma concentration of glucose between 3.9–6.1 mmol/l. Following a meal, the blood sugar becomes elevated, but within 1–2 hours the level returns to normal, owing mainly to liver cells removing excess glucose, converting it to glycogen and storing it. Conversely, much of the plasma glucose may be removed into the cells to be oxidized to produce energy, but a normal concentration in the plasma is maintained by the conversion of glycogen to glucose in the storage depots and its release into the blood.

Blood proteins

Three types of proteins comprise the greater part of the solutes of the plasma. These are referred to as the

Table 13.1 Composition of blood.

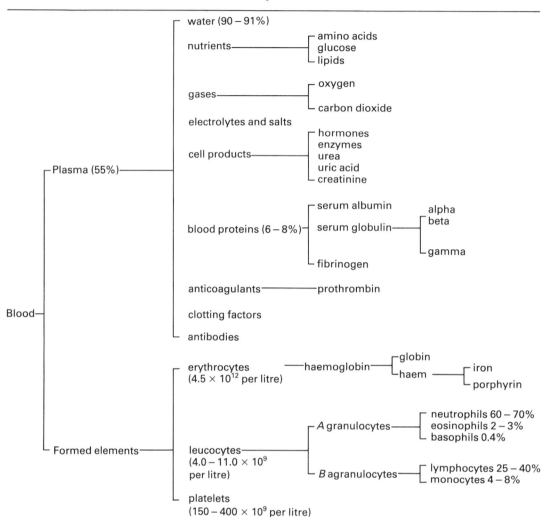

plasma or blood proteins and are *serum albumin, serum globulin,* and *fibrinogen.* The normal concentration of the plasma proteins is about 60–80 g/l. They are large in molecular structure and do not readily diffuse through the capillary walls. The resulting concentration of these non-diffusible substances within the capillaries is responsible for what is referred to as the colloidal osmotic pressure of the plasma. A pressure gradient results between the tissue fluid and the blood that promotes the movement of the fluid from the interstitial spaces back into the capillaries (see Chapter 14). An abnormal decrease in the plasma proteins, especially albumin, reduces the colloidal osmotic pressure, resulting in an accumulation of fluid in the tissues known as oedema. The proteins contribute to the

viscosity of the blood, which influences circulation and blood pressure.

The plasma proteins are formed from the amino acids of ingested foods but in protein starvation they may be synthesized from tissue protein. Serum albumin and fibrinogen are formed by the liver. Albumin, because of its greater molecular weight, functions mainly in producing the colloidal osmotic pressure. Fibrinogen is concerned with the blood clotting process; its role in this is discussed on page 245.

Serum globulin is produced by reticuloendothelial cells (phagocytic cells of the spleen, lymph nodes, liver and bone marrow) and may be separated into three fractions—the alpha, beta, and gamma globulins. The gamma globulin fraction contains antibodies. For this reason it may be administered to provide a temporary immunity against measles or other infections. (See Table 13.2 for normal blood protein values.)

Table 13.2 Normal values of the plasma proteins.

Plasma protein	Concentration (g/l)
Total plasma proteins	60–80
Albumin	40–50
Globulins	20–30
alpha globulin	4.6
beta globulin	8.6
gamma globulin	7.5
Fibrinogen	3.0

In summary, the functions of the plasma proteins are as follows:

1 They exert an intravascular osmotic pressure that influences fluid exchange between the interstitial and intravascular compartments.

2 Fibrinogen plays a role in blood coagulation which protects the individual from an excessive loss of blood.

3 Serum globulin functions in the production of antibodies, protecting the individual against microbial agents and their toxins.

4 At the site of inflammation or injury, fibrinogen forms a medium in which the various tissues can grow and repair themselves (see Reparative Phase p. 43).

5 Plasma proteins provide viscosity to the blood.

6 In starvation, the plasma proteins may be broken down and used as a source of amino acids for the tissues.

7 Plasma proteins will combine with both alkalis and acids and can act as buffers to maintain a normal pH of body fluids. They may accept hydrogen ions from acids or, when necessary, donate hydrogen ions to reduce excessive alkalinity.

8 The proteins bind some substances such as hormones (thyroxine, adrenocorticoids, gonadal secretions), enzymes and essential ions during their transport in the blood. This prevents too rapid escape of these substances by filtration in the renal glomeruli.

FORMED ELEMENTS OF THE BLOOD

The formed elements include the *red blood cells* (erythrocytes), the *white blood cells* (leucocytes) and the *blood platelets* (thrombocytes).

Erythrocytes

The normal red blood cell is an elastic biconcave disc.[1] The approximate number of erythrocytes contained in the blood is $4.5–6.5 \times 10^{12}$ per litre in the adult male and $3.8–5.8 \times 10^{12}$ per litre in the adult

female. The volume percentage of erythrocytes in whole blood is 45–50, and is expressed as the packed cell volume (PCV) or haematocrit.[2] Anaemia is the term applied to a deficiency of red blood cells or to a lack of haemoglobin. An excessive number of red blood cells is referred to as polycythaemia. Each cell has a nucleus when first formed, but the normal mature circulating erythrocyte is devoid of a nucleus.

The *function* of red blood cells, by virtue of their composition, is the transportation of oxygen and carbon dioxide between the tissue cells and the lungs. The major constituent of the cell is *haemoglobin*, which is made up of protein globin and an iron-containing pigment called haem. Haem is formed by the union of iron and the pigment porphyrin; four molecules of haem combine with one molecule of globin to form haemoglobin. Oxygen has an affinity for this compound; four molecules of oxygen combine with one molecule of haemoglobin to form *oxyhaemoglobin*. Approximately 1 g of haemoglobin combines with 1.34–1.36 ml of oxygen. There is a loose combination, so when there is little or no free oxygen in the red cells' environment (plasma), oxygen is freed from the red blood cell and diffuses out of the cell into the plasma, leaving what is known as *reduced oxyhaemoglobin*.

Some of the carbon dioxide in the blood (approximately 27%) is carried by the red blood cells in the form of the compound carbaminohaemoglobin. When the haemoglobin takes on oxygen in the lungs, the carbon dioxide is released into the plasma and then diffuses into the alveoli.

Haemoglobin is produced by the red blood cells themselves before they are released into the circulation from their site of production, the red bone marrow. Because of its pigment content, haemoglobin gives the red colour to the blood. The *normal concentration of haemoglobin* is 14–16 g/dl of blood. It is slightly higher in men than in women, but the mean concentration is 14.8 g/dl.

PRODUCTION OF ERYTHROCYTES (ERYTHROPOIESIS)[3]

After birth, erythrocytes are produced exclusively by the red bone marrow. Prenatally, in the developing organism, they are first produced by the yolk sac and then by the liver, spleen, lymph nodes and thymus from the third month on. During the remaining months the red bone marrow develops and gradually takes over the role. During infancy and childhood most of the bones contain red bone marrow that participates in erythropoiesis. When the

---

[1] Guyton (1986).

[2] The packed cell volume percentage of erythrocytes is determined by centrifuging a blood sample, which separates the cells from the plasma. Erythrocytes normally occupy 45–50% and the plasma 55–60% of the volume of the blood.

[3] *Poiesis* is the Greek word meaning formation or production

growth process is completed, the red blood cells are produced by the red bone marrow of the cancellous (spongy) tissue of the skull bones, vertebrae, ribs, sternum, pelvis and proximal ends of the femora and humeri.

The red blood cells, the white blood cells produced by the marrow, and the platelets (thrombocytes) develop from common primitive stem cells which differentiate to become either red or white blood cells, or platelets. In erythropoiesis, the haemocytoblast forms a proerythroblast which goes through a series of nuclear and cytoplasmic changes, becoming progressively smaller. These changes are outlined in Table 13.3 and compose what is referred to as the maturation process of red blood cells.

REGULATION OF ERYTHROPOIESIS

Under normal conditions the rate of production and maturation of red blood cells approximates the rate of removal of the old cells from the circulation and their destruction. The red blood cell count and the amount of haemoglobin remain relatively constant—sufficient to meet the tissues' oxygen needs but, at the same time, controlled in order to prevent a concentration of cells that would impede the blood flow.

The oxygen concentration of the blood is the essential factor in the regulation of the production of erythrocytes. If the rate of cell destruction is increased or if there is a loss of red blood cells, as in haemorrhage, the concomitant decrease in the oxygen level brings about a prompt increase in erythropoiesis if the bone marrow is normal and the essential substances are available. At high altitudes where the oxygen concentration of the air is low, the body compensates by producing more red blood cells.

The red bone marrow does not respond directly to the hypoxaemia (lowered concentration of oxygen in the blood). The stimulation is brought about by a hormone called *erythropoietin*, or *haemopoietin*, which is produced in response to the hypoxaemia. Most of the erythropoietin is formed by the action of an enzyme (renal erythropoietic factor) produced by the kidneys which acts on one of the plasma proteins. The renal factor (REF) is secreted when the oxygen concentration of the blood falls below normal.[4]

Erythropoietin stimulates the bone marrow to produce haemocytoblasts and hastens the successive nuclear and cytoplasmic maturation changes. As a result of this acceleration, reticulocytes may be released into the bloodstream before complete maturation and the development of a normal amount of haemoglobin.

Protein, iron, vitamin B_{12} (cyanocobalamin), folic acid (pteroylglutamic acid—a member of the vitamin B complex), vitamin C (which is necessary for the maintenance of folic acid reductase—an enzyme necessary to keep folic acid in its active form[5]) and traces of copper must be available to the bone marrow to ensure an adequate production of normal erythrocytes. *Protein* is a necessary element in the structure of the cell and its haemoglobin. *Iron* is essential for the formation of haemoglobin. Only a limited amount of iron is absorbed from the small intestine; it is then loosely combined with transferrin to be transported in the blood plasma. Excess iron is deposited in the liver and other cells where it combines with a protein (apoferritin) to form ferritin, which is referred to as storage iron. Ferritin occurs in

[4] Normal oxygen tension: arterial blood Po_2, 11–13.3 kPa (80–100 mmHg). Normal oxygen content: arterial blood, 7–21 volumes% *venous* blood, 10–16 volumes%.
[5] Williams, Beutler, Erslev & Lichtman (1983), p. 533.

Table 13.3 Production of erythrocytes.*

Stages of development	Description
Stem cell/pronormoblast (earliest differentiated cell) ↓	A nucleated red cell precursor which divides and differentiates to form committed stem cells that are responsive to erythropoietin
Erythroblast/normoblast ↓	A nucleated cell with no haemoglobin that divides into two smaller nucleated cells
Basophilic normoblast (early) ↓	A large nucleated cell with no haemoglobin that divides into two cells. The nucleus is smaller than it was in the previous stages and the cytoplasm is more abundant
Polychromatophilic normoblast (intermediate) ↓	A nucleated cell that divides. The nucleus becomes smaller and more dense and a small amount of haemoglobin appears
Orthochromatic normoblast (late) ↓	A cell in which the nucleus becomes compressed and then is ejected from the cell; the haemoglobin content of the cytoplasm increases. No cell division
Reticulocyte ↓	A non-nucleated cell with an increasing amount of haemoglobin. The cytoplasm has a reticular network. Reticulocytes enter the bloodstream after approximately 24 hours
Erythrocyte	The mature red blood cell from which the nuclear remnants have disappeared. It is almost completely filled with haemoglobin

*Hoffbrand & Pettit (1984), p. 6.

the spleen, bone marrow, kidney, heart, pancreas, intestine and placenta. It is released as iron is needed by the bone marrow. Much of the iron used in the formation of haemoglobin is derived from the breakdown of worn-out erythrocytes. Only a small amount of dietary iron is necessary to maintain that required under normal circumstances. When transferrin and apoferritin are saturated, absorption of iron by the small intestine is inhibited. If erythropoiesis is increased, as it is in haemorrhage, pregnancy or other conditions causing hypoxaemia, more iron is absorbed. In persons who have a normal haemoglobin concentration and a normal amount of iron in storage, extra dietary iron and medicinal iron preparations do not increase the absorption; the excess iron is simply eliminated in the faeces. With increased demands on the bone marrow, the iron stored in the intestinal mucosa and liver is reduced and absorption by the intestine is increased accordingly.

Vitamin B₁₂, which is referred to as the *extrinsic factor*, or *antianaemic factor*, is essential to normal erythropoiesis. It acts as a catalyst, promoting the synthesis of nucleic acids to form normal red blood cells. The extrinsic factor is especially abundant in liver and red meats and is only absorbed in the presence of a factor or enzyme that is secreted by the gastric mucosa. This substance, essential for the absorption of vitamin B₁₂, is known as the intrinsic factor. The vitamin is then stored in the liver and released as it is needed. In the absence of either the extrinsic factor or the intrinsic factor, the number of erythrocytes is reduced, and many that are in circulation are abnormal. Normoblasts do not divide as many times but remain larger and may contain a greater amount of haemoglobin than normal. These large cells are called macrocytes. There may also be large, primitive, nucleated cells in circulation that are known as megaloblasts.

Folic acid (pteroylglutamic acid)[6], acting as a catalyst, also influences the production and maturation of erythroblasts and is sometimes used in the treatment of a deficiency of red blood cells. The richest dietary sources of this vitamin are liver, kidney and fresh green vegetables. Vitamin C is also needed to maintain the active form of folic acid.

Traces of copper are essential to serve as a catalyst for the absorption of iron and its utilization in the formation of haemoglobin.

LIFE SPAN AND NORMAL DESTRUCTION OF
ERYTHROCYTES

The average length of life of the red blood cells is 120 days.[7] As the cell ages, the continuous friction between the blood cells and the vessel walls weakens the cell membrane, and it eventually ruptures. The cell fragments are engulfed by macrophages (large phagocytic cells of the reticuloendothelial tissues) in the liver and spleen. The haemoglobin, which comprises most of the cell substance, is broken down, and the globin and iron fractions are reclaimed for use. The porphyrin molecules are converted to bilirubin and excreted in bile (see Fig. 13.1).

Leucocytes

The white blood cells are less numerous and larger than the erythrocytes, and have nuclei. There are several types, which differ in structure, origin, function and staining reaction. Normally, the blood contains $4.0–11.0 \times 10^9$ per litre (4000–11 000 per μl). The count tends to be lower after a period of rest and increases following a meal or activity. There is a rapid increase to above normal in most infections in defence of the body. The term *leucocytosis* is applied

---

[6] Bouchier, Allan, Hodgson & Keighley (1984), p. 396.
[7] Guyton (1986), p. 48.

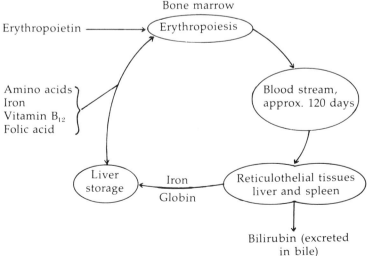

Fig. 13.1 Life-cycle of erythrocytes.

to an increase above the normal number of white blood cells. A decrease in the white blood cells below the normal is called *leucopenia*.

TYPES OF LEUCOCYTES

The leucocytes may be divided into two major groups on the basis of whether their cytoplasm is granular or non-granular—namely, granulocytes or agranulocytes (Table 13.4).

Table 13.4 Types and normal values of leucocytes.*

Type	Percentage of total	Number ($\times 10^9$/l)
Granulocytes		
neutrophils	40–75	2.5–7.5
eosinophils	1–6	0.04–0.44
basophils	<1	0.015–0.1
Agranulocytes		
lymphocytes	20–50	1.5–3.5
monocytes	2–10	0.2–0.8

*The total leucocyte count is normally 4.0–11.0 × 10⁹ per litre.

1 *Polymorphonuclear leucocytes (granulocytes).* The granulocytes are formed in the red bone marrow and have lobulated nuclei. Three types are recognized by the staining quality of their cytoplasm—neutrophils, eosinophils and basophils.
   (a) *Neutrophils* stain with a neutral dye, and their nuclei may have several lobes. The latter characteristic results in the neutrophils also being called *polymorphonuclear* neutrophils. They may comprise 60–70% of the total white blood cells.
   (b) *Eosinophils* stain with eosin, a red acid dye, and normally constitute about 2–3% of the white blood cells.
   (c) *Basophils* stain with basic dyes and comprise about 0.4% of the total leucocytes.
2 *Agranulocytes.* The white blood cells with agranular cytoplasm are of two types—lymphocytes and monocytes.
   (a) The *lymphocytes* are smaller than the granulocytes and have a larger spherical nucleus that fills most of the cell. They are produced in the lymphoid tissue (lymph nodes, spleen, tonsils and thymus) and some are formed in bone marrow. Twenty-five to 40% of the total white blood cells are lymphocytes.
   (b) The *monocytes* are larger than the lymphocytes and have a kidney-shaped nucleus. They are produced in the red bone marrow. Ganong indicates that they circulate in the blood for about 24 hours, and then enter the tissues and become macrophages.[8,9] Monocytes make up about 4–8% of the total number of leucocytes.

---

[8] *Macrophages* are large phagocytic cells—cells that engulf and destroy microorganisms and foreign substances.
[9] Ganong (1985).

LEUCOCYTE COUNT

When a white blood cell count is requested, an estimation is made of the total number of cells per litre. Frequently, a differential white cell count is done, since it is known that certain types of cells are increased in certain disease conditions. For example: in acute infections the neutrophils increase rapidly; in chronic infections, the lymphocytes are increased; the number of monocytes are increased in protozoal infections such as malaria; and the eosinophil count is known to rise in allergic reactions and with parasitic invasion of the body. In a differential count the percentage of the various types of leucocytes is determined.

The various types of white blood cells are produced by the stem cells in the blood cell-forming organs in three primitive forms—the myeloblasts monoblasts and lymphoblasts (Table 13.5). The *myeloblast*, which is produced by stem cells in the red bone marrow, is agranular and the nucleus is not divided into lobules. Successive changes occur and are characterized by the appearance of granules in the cytoplasm; the myeloblasts become promyelocytes, which change to myelocytes. The latter differentiate to form neutrophils, eosinophils and basophils. Following this, nuclear changes develop, resulting in lobulation and the release of the cell into the blood.

The *monoblast* undergoes mitotic division to form the promonocyte. The cell remains large and agranular, but the nucleus changes, becoming oval and then kidney-shaped.

The *lymphoblast*, although produced in lymphoid tissue, goes through developmental phases comparable to the other leucocytes. The lymphoblast divides by mitosis and the cells progressively become condensed to form mature, small lymphocytes.

FACTORS IN LEUCOPOIESIS

Little is known about the physiological stimulus responsible for the production and maturation of leucocytes. It has been observed that the breakdown of white blood cells is followed by the appearance of numerous young white blood cells in the blood. This suggests that a chemical which stimulates leucopoiesis may be released from the disintegrated cells.

Increased leucopoiesis occurs in infection, haemorrhage and tissue destruction. The nutrients, protein and vitamins which are essential to all cells of the body are necessary for the production of leucocytes. Some drugs may depress the production of leucocytes; for example, sulphonamides, gold, thiouracil and cortisone preparations may result in a low white blood cell count.

CHARACTERISTICS AND FUNCTIONS OF LEUCOCYTES

The leucocytes serve as an important body defence.

Table 13.5 Formation of white blood cells (leucopoiesis).

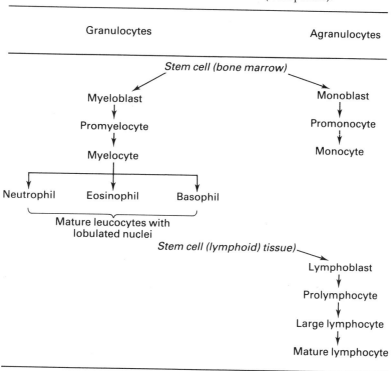

They destroy many injurious substances such as microorganisms and the products of degenerating tissues. This is made possible by certain special properties the cells possess—namely, diapedesis, mobility, chemotaxis and phagocytosis.

Diapedesis is the ability of the leucocytes to squeeze through the capillary walls and escape into the tissues. They are capable of amoeboid movement[10] which takes them through the tissues to the source of irritation. The neutrophils are especially mobile; they are attracted by a chemical substance which is liberated by bacteria or by the irritated tissue cells.

Phagocytosis is the engulfing and digesting of particles and is the most important function of the neutrophils and monocytes in protecting the body against microorganisms.

The lymphocytes play an important role in immunity, discussed in Chapter 4.

LIFE SPAN AND DESTRUCTION OF LEUCOCYTES

The life span of the white blood cells varies greatly with the body's protective needs and with the types of white cells, ranging from a few hours to as long as 200 days. The granulocytes survive for a shorter period than do the agranulocytes. Guyton suggests 12 hours as the average life span for granulocytes, but this may be much shorter if there is infection to combat. Many of the lymphocytes have been found to survive 100–300 days.[11]

It is thought that the white blood cells that are destroyed or die are disposed of by phagocytosis by the macrophages of the reticuloendothelial tissues.

Blood platelets (thrombocytes)

The third and smallest of the formed elements of the blood are the platelets. They are oval, non-nucleated granular structures, numbering $150–400 \times 10^9$ per litre of blood (150 000–400 000 per µl). They are produced in the red bone marrow. The stem cells develop into giant cells called megakaryocytes which may extend parts of their membrane and cytoplasm which separate from the parent cells to form the platelets. The cell contains important substances, including calcium, potassium, several clotting factors, serotonin, adrenaline, adenosine triphosphate (ADP) and enzymes. When an injury occurs to a vessel wall, the platelets clump and adhere to the site. Their membranes are very fragile and readily permit the escape of platelet content. It is suggested

---

[10] *Amoeboid movement* is achieved by the cell protruding a protoplasmic extension into which the remaining cell substance streams.

[11] Guyton (1986), p. 52.

that serotonin and adrenaline are responsible for the vasoconstriction that occurs at the site of injury. The platelets become sticky, resulting in more of them adhering to the original clump and contributing to the formation of a 'haemostatic plug'. The clotting factors released from the thrombocytes promote coagulation.[12]

Platelet production is increased following tissue trauma and destruction and in hypoxaemia. It is suggested that, as well as a reduced oxygen concentration of the blood, chemical substances liberated by degenerating or injured tissue stimulate the bone marrow to increase platelet formation.

FUNCTIONS OF BLOOD PLATELETS

The platelets initiate the blood clotting process through their disintegration and release of thromboplastin (platelet factor) which activates prothrombin (see Blood Coagulation, pp. 244–245). On disintegration, they also liberate serotonin (5-hydroxytryptamine) and adrenaline which causes vasoconstriction that, in turn, contributes to reducing the loss of blood when a vessel is interrupted.

With any slight damage to the inner surface of blood vessels, the platelets clump and stick together at the site, helping to plug leaks and prevent loss of blood.

Blood Groups

Blood may differ from one individual to another according to the presence or absence of specific antigens (agglutinogens) in the red blood cells and the presence or absence of specific antibodies (agglutinins) in the plasma. For this reason, the blood of a person taken at random cannot be used in transfusion since the bloods might be of different types and could cause a serious reaction. The blood groups of greatest clinical significance are the ABO and Rh (Rhesus) types.

ABO BLOOD GROUPS

In the ABO system (see Table 13.6) an individual's blood is typed as A, B, AB, or O, depending on the presence or absence of agglutinogens termed A and B in his erythrocytes. If a person has A or B or both A and B naturally occurring agglutinogens, his plasma will not contain antibodies that will agglutinate his own erythrocytes. Type O is the most common blood type, occurring in 46% of the general population. Type A occurs in 42% of Caucasians. While the incidence of blood group antigens varies from race to race, types B and AB are found less frequently than types O and A.

In blood that is *typed as A*, the erythrocytes contain *agglutinogens A*. The plasma has anti-B agglutinins which only cause clumping of erythrocytes that have agglutinogens B. Blood that is *typed as B* has erythrocytes containing *agglutinogens B* and, in the plasma, *anti-A agglutinins*, which only cause clumping of red blood cells with agglutinogen A. In blood that is *typed as AB*, the erythrocytes bear both *agglutinogens A and AB*. The plasma is free of anti-A and anti-B agglutinins; otherwise, the individual's own red cells would be attacked. In blood that is typed as O, both agglutinogens are absent, but the plasma contains both anti-A and anti-B agglutinins. Antigen A is subdivided into A_1 and A_2. It is suggested that A_2 cells have fewer antigen sites than A_1 cells.[13]

The type of blood is determined by adding specially prepared serum, containing either anti-A and anti-B antibodies. The procedure is as follows:

Anti-A serum is added to a sample of the blood to be typed; if clumping of the red blood cells occurs, the blood is type A.

Anti-B serum is added to a sample of the blood to be typed; if clumping occurs, the blood is type B.

If clumping of the red cells occurs with the addition of anti-A and anti-B sera, the presence of both A and B agglutinogens is indicated, and the blood is type AB.

When there is no agglutination with the addition of either anti-A or anti-B serum, it indicates the absence of both A and B agglutinogens in the erythrocytes. The blood type is O.

The blood type of a person is determined genetically: a gene received from each parent influences the

Table 13.6 ABO System.

Blood type	Agglutinogen in erythrocytes	Agglutinins in plasma	Plasma agglutinates erythrocytes of blood type:
A_1	A_1	anti-B	B, A_1B and A_2B
A_2	A_2	anti-B	B, A_1B and A_2B
B	B	anti-A	A_1, A_2, A_1B and A_2B
A_1B	A_1B	none	none
A_2B	A_2B	none	none
O	none	anti-A_1, anti-A_2 and anti-B	A_1, A_1B, A_2, A_2B and B

---

[12] Ganong (1985).

[13] Smith & Thier (1985), p. 254.

type of blood of the offspring. The genes for A and B agglutinogens are equally dominant. The genotype of an individual of type A may have inherited an A agglutinogen from each parent (AA) or an A agglutinogen from one and none from the other (AO). With type B, it may be BB or BO. In the case of type AB, it is an A and B.

BLOOD TRANSFUSION

When the volume of circulating blood is reduced, the clinical value of the administration of blood donated by another individual is well recognized. The blood used must be of the same type as that of the recipient. If the bloods are not of the same type, the recipient's plasma may contain agglutinins that will clump the red blood cells of the donor's blood. The agglutinated cells may block blood vessels and could prove fatal if the occluded vessels supply vital areas. In a few hours, the clumped cells are destroyed by macrophages (large phagocytic cells) of the reticuloendothelial system, releasing haemoglobin into the plasma. The disintegration of the red cells is referred to as haemolysis. The free haemoglobin in the plasma is treated as foreign protein and is excreted by the kidneys. Backache is one of the prominent symptoms of transfusion reactions because there is intravascular haemolysis, which causes a widespread reaction in the blood vessels including those of the kidney. A urine specimen is collected to detect the presence of free haemoglobin in the urine.

The important precaution to be observed in a blood transfusion is to prevent the donation of red blood cells that will be agglutinated by agglutinins in the recipient's plasma. Since type O has neither A nor B agglutinogens, this blood may be given to a recipient of any one of the four types. For this reason, the person of type O is referred to as a *universal donor*.

Conversely, since an AB type does not have either anti-A or anti-B antibodies in his plasma, the individual is considered to be a *universal recipient*.

The following table indicates possible donors for each blood type in the ABO system.

Recipient	Possible donor
Type A	Types A and O
Type B	Types B and O
Type AB	Types AB, A, B, and O
Type O	Type O

Whenever possible, it is considered safer to use a donor with blood of the same type as that of the person requiring the transfusion. To ensure compatibility of the donor's and recipient's blood, cross matching is done. A small quantity of each of the bloods is centrifuged in separate tubes. Some of the recipient's cells are added to the donor's serum and vice versa. If no agglutination occurs in 15 minutes, the bloods are considered compatible.

RHESUS (Rh) BLOOD GROUPS

This system involves numerous antigens (agglutinogens) having varying degrees of antigenicity. The D factor is the strongest antigen and is of greatest clinical significance. Approximately 85% of Caucasians possess the D factor and are classified as Rh positive. The remaining 15% are said to be Rh negative.

Plasma antibodies (agglutinins) against the D factor do not occur naturally. They only develop in the plasma of Rh(D) negative blood when the D factor is introduced. The anti-D agglutinins will clump erythrocytes containing the D factor. The formation of anti-D antibodies may be evoked within an Rh negative person receiving a transfusion of Rh(D) positive blood, or by the development of an Rh(D) positive fetus within an Rh(D) negative mother. In the case of the blood transfusion, usually no clumping of the Rh positive donor's cells in the Rh negative recipient's blood occurs with the first transfusion, because the anti-D antibodies are developed slowly and may not reach sufficient concentration before the foreign positive cells are terminated. But, if a second transfusion of Rh(D) positive blood is given, a reaction occurs, causing agglutination of the donor's cells.

When an Rh positive fetus develops within an Rh negative mother, some of the fetal red blood cells, or D factors released by worn-out erythrocytes, pass through the placenta into the maternal circulation. The mother then forms anti-D agglutinins which diffuse into the fetal circulation and cause agglutination of the fetal erythrocytes. The clumped cells are ultimately disintegrated, and the haemoglobin is broken down and converted to bilirubin, causing jaundice (yellowness of the skin and conjunctivae). This condition is known as erythroblastosis fetalis. The destruction of red blood cells may prove fatal to the fetus, depending on the concentration of antibodies that reaches the fetal circulation. If the fetus goes to term, at birth the infant will exhibit jaundice, anaemia, oedema and enlargement of the spleen and liver. Prompt treatment by a series of exchange transfusions is necessary. Compatible Rh negative blood is given. The exchange is made by alternate withdrawal and injection of equal amounts of blood.

The first baby sensitizes the Rh negative mother but usually escapes the haemolytic disease. With subsequent pregnancies, the anti-D agglutinins progressively increase if the fetuses are Rh positive. Immunization of Rh negative persons seems to vary; some develop antibodies more readily than others. Sensitization can be prevented by the mother receiving anti-Rh antibodies in the form of Rh immune globulin immediately following the first delivery and in subsequent pregnancies.

The Rh blood group factors are inherited, and the gene for the D agglutinogen is always dominant (Table 13.7). One who is Rh positive may be homozy-

Table 13.7 Rh factor: genetic possibilities for agglutinogen D.*

		Rh negative mother		
		X	X	
Rh positive father (homozygous)	X^D	X^DX	X^DX	Offspring: all heterozygous Rh positive
	Y^D	Y^DX	Y^DX	

		Rh negative mother		
		X	X	
Rh positive father (heterozygous)	X^D	X^DX	X^DX	Offspring: 50% chance of Rh positive; 50% chance of Rh negative
	Y	YX	YX	

		Rh negative mother		
		X	X	
Rh negative father (homozygous)	X	XX	XX	Offspring: all Rh negative (the mother will not form antibodies)
	Y	YX	YX	

* The Rh factor (agglutinogen D) is dominant. If the father is Rh positive and the mother is Rh negative the offspring will be Rh positive and the mother will form antibodies

gous (DD) having inherited a gene for the D factor from each parent, or may be heterozygous (D−), having inherited a gene for D from one parent only. The child of an Rh positive father who is homozygous and an Rh negative mother will always be Rh positive because of the dominance of the D factor. The child of an Rh positive father who is heterozygous and an Rh negative mother has a 50% chance of being Rh positive. If the developing organism in utero is Rh negative, there is no problem.

Haemostatis and Blood Coagulation

Any rupture or severance of a blood vessel is normally followed by certain responses in an effort to reduce the loss of blood. These responses are local vasoconstriction, the formation of a temporary plug, coagulation of the blood and the formation of scar tissue to close the opening in the vessel. These defence responses occur frequently in the body without the individual being aware of them. During normal day-to-day activities and in minor injuries, minute blood vessels are ruptured and the loss of blood is controlled by these mechanisms. If a large vessel, especially an artery, is interrupted, coagulation and vasoconstriction may not be adequate in checking the bleeding. Ligation, pressure or cautery may have to be used.

Vasoconstriction in haemostasis

Local vasoconstriction reduces the blood flow to the injured site and is brought about by direct vascular muscular tissue reaction to the injury and by reflex nerve impulses that occur as a result of the trauma to the vessel. In the latter, sensory impulses arising in the injured vascular wall are transmitted into the central nervous system, causing impulses to be sent to the musculature of the vessels, and stimulating contraction. This vascular spasm is augmented by the release of serotonin (5-hydroxytryptamine) and adrenaline by the disintegrating platelets at the site of injury.

Haemostatic plug

Injury and interruption of a vascular wall results in a clumping of platelets at the site. The aggregation serves as a loose temporary plug in the opening and is the forerunner of blood coagulation and the formation of a clot.

Blood coagulation

Coagulation of the blood is the formation of a jelly-like mass in the blood by the conversion of the soluble plasma protein fibrinogen to an insoluble mass of thin threads called fibrin. Blood cells are enmeshed in the fibrin to form the mass known as a clot. The conversion of fibrinogen to fibrin is dependent upon chain of reactions between several intrinsic factors that are designated by number. Twelve factors are currently indicated; a list of these, their synonyms and their role in the blood clotting process is found in Tables 13.8 and 13.9. Clot formation may be initiated by an extrinsic or intrinsic mechanism. The extrinsic mechanism is initiated by tissue injury. The intrinsic pathway is more complex and may be initiated by Factor XII, the direct action of platelets or by platelet aggregation on blood vessel walls.

The essential major steps in coagulation are:

1 The release and activation of thromboplastin by disintegrating platelets and damaged tissue cells.
2 The conversion of prothrombin to thrombin by thromboplastin (prothrombin activator) in the presence of calcium ions.
3 The conversion of fibrinogen by thrombin to fibrin.

Prothrombin is normally present in the blood and is the inactive form of thrombin. Vitamin K is essential for its production by the liver. The conversion of prothrombin to active thrombin depends upon the presence of calcium ions and thromboplastin. Information concerning the exact role of some factors is incomplete, but the absence of any one produces a bleeding tendency.

NORMAL ANTICOAGULANTS

A remarkable property of blood is its ability to remain fluid in the blood vessels; this is necessary for its circulation. Under normal circumstances, small amounts of thromboplastin are released by the disintegration of some platelets and tissue cells and could initiate coagulation. In order to counteract this, coagulation inhibitors—*heparin* and *antithrombin*—are normally present in the plasma.

Large granular cells in the pericapillary connective tissue that are known as *mast cells* are the principal source of heparin. It inhibits the formation and action of thrombin. If thrombin is produced in relatively small amounts, it is neutralized by antithrombin, an alpha globulin, and the conversion of fibrinogen to fibrin does not take place. The presence of antithrombin and heparin prevents coagulation under normal conditions, but with increased tissue and platelet destruction, the greater concentration of thromboplastin is sufficient to initiate spontaneous coagulation.

Blood that is collected from one person for administration to another is prevented from clotting by the addition of sodium citrate. The citrate combines with the calcium to form insoluble citrate of calcium. Certain blood examinations require that the blood remain fluid; an oxalate which combines with the calcium is usually added.

CLOT RETRACTION AND ORGANIZATION

After a clot forms, the fibrin strands shrink (as a result of Factor XIII) and the plasma that was trapped along with the blood cells is extruded. This fluid is referred to as *serum* and differs from normal plasma because it lacks fibrinogen, clotting Factors II, V and VIII and has a high serotonin content. The fibrin strands of the clot attach to the edges of the injured area of the blood vessel; as they shrink they pull the edges of the opening closer together, helping to check the loss of blood.

The opening in the vessel is repaired by a process called *clot organization*. Fibroblasts proliferate the clot

Table 13.8 Blood clotting factors and their roles in blood coagulation.

Factor Number	Synonym	Role in blood coagulation
I	Fibrinogen	Forms fibrin
II	Prothrombin	Forms thrombin which converts fibrinogen to fibrin
III	Thromboplastin	Converts prothrombin to thrombin
IV	Calcium	Serves as a catalyst in conversion of prothrombin to thrombin
V	Labile factor (accelerator globulin AcG, proaccelerin)	Necessary in the formation of active thromboplastin
VII	Proconvertin (stable factor, serum prothrombin conversion accelerator, SPCA)	Accelerates the action of tissue thromboplastin
VIII	Antihaemophilic factor, AHF (antihaemophilic globulin, AHG)	Promotes the breakdown of thrombocytes and the formation of active platelet thromboplastin
IX	Christmas factor (plasma thromboplastin component, PTC)	Similar to Factor VIII
X	Stuart factor	Promotes the action of thromboplastin
XI	Plasma thromboplastin antecedent (PTA)	Promotes clumping and breakdown of thrombocytes and the release of thromboplastin
XII	Hageman factor	Similar to Factor XI
XIII	Fibrin-stabilizing factor (FSF), Laki-Lorand factor (LLF)	Converts the loose fibrin mesh to a dense tight mass

Table 13.9 Schema of the clotting process.

Stage	Extrinsic pathway	Intrinsic pathway

* A — Activated form.

and, as they mature, the area is filled in by fibrous tissue. Macrophages (large reticuloendothelial phagocytes which develop from monocytes) clear away the trapped blood cells. Endothelial cells of the intima proliferate to replace the vessel lining in the area.

MANAGEMENT OF THE PATIENT WITH A BLOOD DYSCRASIA

The physiological functions of the blood and its components include: internal respiration, cellular nutrition and excretion; defence of the body against infectious organisms and foreign antigens; and protection against the loss of blood from the body.

Blood disorders (dyscrasias) may affect the *erythrocytes, leucocytes* or the *coagulation process*. The problem may be due to a defect originating in the blood-forming organs, the deficiency of an essential element, or the abnormal destruction of cells. The disorders may be primary or secondary to another disease.

Diseases of the blood-forming organs may involve the red bone marrow or reticuloendothelial tissue.

The clinical manifestations of blood dyscrasias are varied and frequently are non-specific. The patient's health history, physical examination, results of diagnostic procedures and knowledge of the haematopoietic system form the data-base on which the nurse and doctor formulate their diagnosis of the patient's problems and develop specific plans for medical and nursing intervention.

DATA COLLECTION

HISTORY

The patient's history includes information about *family history* of any haematological disorders and a *drug history* and exposure to *toxic substances*. Drugs of specific importance are the cytotoxic drugs used in the treatment of some cancers, immunosuppressive drugs including antibiotics, and drugs affecting blood coagulation. An occupational history may provide clues to possible exposure to toxic chemicals.

The most common presenting symptoms are fatigue, lethargy, weakness and weight loss. The history should include details of any fever, night sweats, repeated infections or any indications of unusual bleeding that the patient may have experienced.

PHYSICAL ASSESSMENT

The patient's *general appearance* should be noted for weight loss, pallor and lethargy, and his *skin and mucous membranes* inspected for pallor, petechiae, bruises, dryness and texture.

Blood pressure and pulse rate and rhythm are recorded and compared with normal values for the particular patient. The respiratory rate and rhythm are also assessed; chest expansion and the characteristics of respirations are noted and the anterior and posterior thorax is examined with a stethoscope for breath sounds and possible fluid presence, particularly in the base of the lungs (see Chapter 6).

The patient's *skeletal system* is evaluated for joint movement, deformation and bone tenderness or pain, and his *abdomen* is percussed and palpated to identify any enlargement of the spleen or liver. The *nervous system* is examined for signs of sensory impairment. The person's mental status is evaluated to identify signs of confusion, decreased attention span and disorientation to time, place and person.

Palpable *lymph nodes* in the neck, axillae and groins are examined for enlargement, asymmetry, fixation to surrounding tissue, tenderness and warmth and redness in the surrounding tissue.

INVESTIGATIVE PROCEDURES USED IN BLOOD DISORDERS

Tests used to assess erythrocytes, leucocytes and haemorrhagic disorders are discussed in Table 13.10.

Erythrocyte Disorders

INTRODUCTION

A deficiency or an excess may occur in the number of circulating red blood cells, or the cell composition may be abnormal. Variations in the size, shape and haemoglobin content may be present. Certain descriptive terms are used to denote some of these characteristics.

Erythrocytes that are larger than the normal are referred to as *macrocytes*; if they are smaller than the normal, they are *microcytes*. Cells that possess a normal amount of haemoglobin are said to be *normochromic*, but if it is deficient, they are described as *hypochromic*. Those with a volume of haemoglobin greater than the normal are *hyperchromic*. If the cells present have abnormal shapes, they are described as *poikilocytic*.

Anaemia may sometimes be classified according to the characteristics of the erythrocytes. For example, in anaemia which is due to an iron deficiency, the cells are hypochromic and microcytic; the disease may be referred to as hypochromic-microcytic anaemia.

ERYTHROCYTE AND HAEMOGLOBIN DEFICIENCY (ANAEMIA)

The term anaemia implies a reduction in the oxygen-carrying capacity of the blood as a result of fewer circulating erythrocytes than is normal or a decrease in the concentration of haemoglobin.

CAUSES

The abnormal reduction in the number of erythrocytes may be due to decreased erythropoiesis, excessive red blood cell destruction (haemolysis), or loss of blood. Anaemia may be primary, but frequently is secondary to some other disorder, and because of this the patient may undergo extensive investigation to determine the cause. It may also be classified as acquired or hereditary. Anaemia due to decreased erythropoiesis may be caused by a deficiency of factors essential for normal production or by depressed bone marrow activity. An abnormal rate of destruction of the red blood cells may be associated with intracorpuscular defects or extracorpuscular factors.

Table 13.11 outlines the principal types of anaemia according to cause.

General effects and manifestations of erythrocyte and haemoglobin deficiency

Although there are various causes and types of anaemia, they present a common problem—that of a decrease in the capacity of the blood to transport oxygen. The patient, regardless of the cause or type of anaemia, manifests signs and symptoms attributable to tissue and organ hypoxia and the ensuing reduced metabolism. The occurrence and severity of these manifestations depend on the degree of anaemia present and its rapidity of onset. Table 13.12 lists the manifestations of anaemia.

Table 13.10 Laboratory tests for assessing blood disorders.

Test	Normal values	Description
Assessment of erythrocytes		
Red blood cell count	Males: 4.5–6.5×10^{12} per litre Females: 3.8–5.8×10^{12} per litre	The normal red blood cell count vary with sex, age, altitude and exercise. It will increase with hypovolaemia and decrease with hypervolaemia
Haemoglobin content of erythrocytes	Males: 13–18 g/dl Females: 12–15 g/dl Children (3 months to puberty): 10–14 g/dl	The normal values for haemoglobin vary with age, sex, altitude and exercise. Elevated levels occur with hypovolaemia and decreases are found with excess blood volume
Packed cell volume (haematocrit)	Males: 40–50% Females: 37–47%	The volume of red blood cells in one decilitre of blood (volume percentage of erythrocytes)
Erythrocyte indicies	MCV 76–96 fl (femtolitres) MCH 27–32 pg (picograms) MCHC 30–35 g/dl	Mean corpuscular volume (MCV) is the average size of individual red cells Mean corpuscular haemoglobin (MCH) is the average amount of haemoglobin per red cell Mean corpuscular haemoglobin concentration (MCHC) is the average weight in grams of haemoglobin in one decilitre of red blood cells
Reticulocyte count	0.5–1.5%	The percentage of circulating non-mature, non-nucleated red blood cells. Results are indicative of bone marrow activity

Haemoglobin electro-phoresis
Haemoglobins A_1, A_2, F, C and S
	Adult: $HgbA_1$ 95–98% total Hgb
	          $HgbA_2$ 1.5–3.5%
	          $HgbF_1$ $<2\%$
	          HgbC 0%
	          HgbS 0%
	Newborn: Hgb F 40–70% of total Hgb
	Infant: Hgb F 2–10% total Hgb
	Child (over 6 months): Hgb F 1–2% total Hgb
		The diagnosis of haemolytic anaemias that are resistant to usual therapy requires the separation and identification of the different types of haemoglobin present in the red blood cells. Normal adult haemoglobin and fetal haemoglobin may be identified as well as abnormal haemoglobin. Haemoglobin S is the most common of the abnormal haemoglobins. It is found in sickle cell anaemia, in combination with other variations of haemoglobin or in a symptomatic sickle cell trait

Sickle cell test	Adult: 0 Child: 0	This test demonstrates the presence of haemoglobin S. A reducing agent is used to deoxygenate the erythrocytes and the cells are observed under a microscope for evidence of sickling. Red blood cells containing haemoglobin S become distorted and crescent or sickle shaped when deprived of oxygen
Urinary urobilinogen	0–4 mg in 24 hours	An estimation of the urobilinogen that is excreted in urine. It is increased in excessive red blood cell destruction (haemolytic anaemia) and liver disease
Faecal urobilinogen	50–300 mg in 24 hours	An estimation of the amount of urobilinogen that is excreted in the faeces. It is increased in excessive red blood cell destruction
Schilling test	15–40% of the oral dose	This procedure determines the amount of vitamin B_{12} (cyanocobalamin) absorbed from the gastrointestinal tract. The patient fasts for 8 hours and is then given an oral dose of radioactive vitamin B_{12}. Two hours later, a non-radioactive dose of vitamin B_{12} is given intramuscularly. The urine is collected for the next 24 hours and the amount of radioactive vitamin B_{12} excreted is determined. The administration of the non-radioactive vitamin B_{12} saturates the blood and bone marrow so that the absorbed radioactive vitamin B_{12} is excreted in the urine

Table 13.10—*continued*

Test	Normal values			Description
Bone marrow examination by aspiration or biopsy	Normal values differ with the source used, age of patient and test method. Differential counts are done on each type of cell			Specimens of red bone marrow are obtained by aspiration or percutaneous needle biopsy, usually from the sternum or iliac crest. Smears are made of the marrow specimen and the cells are examined. The number of cells in the various developmental and maturational phases, and the size, shape and characteristics of cell content are noted. The skin is cleansed and a local anaesthetic introduced prior to the test. Discomfort occurs from the pressure needed to pass the needle through the cortex of the bone into the marrow
Osmotic fragility of erythrocytes	Adult	% Haemolysis		Determines the tendency of the red blood cells to haemolyze in increasingly hypotonic solutions. It is used in haemolytic anaemias; the fragility is increased ($>0.46\%$) in some types of haemolytic anaemia (e.g. spherocytosis) and decreased ($<0.30\%$) in others (e.g. sickle cell anaemia)
	% NaCl	Fresh blood	24 hour at blood (37°C)	
	0.30	97–100	85–100	
	0.35	90–98	75–100	
	0.40	50–95	65–100	
	0.45	5–45	55–95	
	0.50	0–5	40–85	
	0.55	0	15–65	
	0.60	0	0–40	

Assessment of leucocytes

Test	Normal values	Description
Leucocyte count	$4.0–11.0 \times 10^9$ per litre	The number of white blood cells in a microlitre of blood
Differential leucocyte count	Neutrophils (polymorphoneuclear leucocytes) 40–75% ($2.5–7.5 \times 10^9$ per litre) Eosinophils 1–6% ($0.04–0.44 \times 10^9$ per litre) Basophils <1% ($0.015–0.1 \times 10^9$ per litre) Monocytes 2–10% ($0.2–0.8 \times 10^9$ per litre) Lymphocytes 20–50% ($1.5–3.5 \times 10^9$ per litre)	
Bone marrow biopsy		See above
Leucocyte alkaline phosphatase (LAP) stain	Quantitative method 15–100 units	Alkaline phosphatase is an enzyme active in neutrophils. The test demonstrates the rate of intracellular metabolism within neutrophils and is useful in diagnosing chronic granulocytic leukaemia

Assessment of haemorrhagic disorders

Test	Normal values	Description
Blood platelet (thrombocyte) count	$150–400 \times 10^9$ per litre	The number of platelets in a microlitre of blood
Bleeding time	2–5 minutes	This is the time it takes bleeding to stop naturally—that is, the period of time blood continues to escape from an 'open' area
Coagulation time	5–12 minutes	This is the time it takes blood to clot after it has been shed
Prothrombin time (PT)	11–15 seconds	This is the time it takes for coagulation following the addition of thromboplastin and calcium to the specimen
Partial thromboplastin time (PTT) to activated partial thromboplastin time (APTT)	PTT 40–100 seconds APTT 30–45 seconds	The partial thromboplastin time is a general test of coagulation used for screening and to monitor anticoagulant therapy. Clotting deficiencies other than Factor VII, XIII and platelets can be detected. The activated partial thromboplastin time (APTT) involves the addition of activators to the regular test reagent to shorten the clotting time

Table 13.10—*continued*

Test	Normal values	Description
Plasma fibrinogen	2–4 g/l	This indicates the fibrinogen concentration
Clot retraction	Adult: complete retraction within 24 hours	Laboratory observation of clot size and retraction characteristics in a test tube provides diagnostic information about platelet deficiencies and dysfunction and the fibrinogen level
Other tests		
Coombs' test	Direct—negative (no agglutination) Indirect—negative	The erythrocytes are examined for the presence of immune bodies (agglutinins) that adhere to the red blood cells and lead to clumping and haemolysis. This is referred to as the direct Coombs' test. An indirect method is done on serum to test for the presence of the antibodies to the erythrocyte antigens. The Coombs' test may be used in identifying haemolytic anaemia or erythroblastosis fetalis
Lymph node biopsy	negative	A tissue specimen of a lymph node that has undergone some change is obtained. The change may be associated with an alteration in the patient's leucocytes, especially the lymphocytes

Table 13.11 Types of anaemia.

A. Anaemia due to decreased erythropoiesis
  1 Deficiency anaemia
    (a) Iron deficiency anaemia
    (b) Vitamin B_{12} deficiency anaemia (pernicious anaemia)
    (c) Folic acid deficiency anaemia
  2 Aplastic anaemia (anaemia due to depressed bone marrow activity)

B. Anaemia due to excessive rate of haemolysis
  1 Haemolytic anaemia due to intracorpuscular defects
    (a) Congenital haemolytic jaundice (hereditary spherocytosis)
    (b) Haemoglobinopathy
        Sickle cell anaemia
        Thalassaemia (Mediterranean anaemia, or Cooley's anaemia)
  2 Haemolytic anaemia due to extracorpuscular factors, such as
    (a) Certain infective agents
    (b) Autoimmune reaction
    (c) Certain drugs and chemicals

C. Anaemia due to blood loss

Table 13.12 Signs and symptoms manifested by a patient with anaemia.

Body structure	Objective and subjective data
Skin	Pallor Brittle nails and dry hair
Mucous membranes	Pale (e.g. conjunctivae)
Respiratory	Shortness of breath on exertion Increased respiratory rate Fluid in base of lungs (with severe anaemia)
Cardiac	Increased pulse rate Cardiac palpitation Cardiac enlargement Angina pectoris (with severe anaemia) Increased stroke volume
Neuromuscular	Headache, dizziness General fatigue Tingling or 'pins and needles' in extremities (vitamin B_{12} deficiency) Fainting Decreased attention span
Gastrointestinal	Anorexia Diarrhoea or constipation Flatulence
Genitourinary	Irregular menstruation Decreased renal function (with severe anaemia)
Metabolism	Increased sensitivity to cold

A. Anaemias due to decreased erythropoiesis

1. DEFICIENCY ANAEMIAS

An essential nutrient for erythrocyte production, such as iron, vitamin B_{12}, folic acid, ascorbic acid or protein, may be lacking in the diet, or there may be defective absorption of an essential factor. In some instances, there may be an increased demand within the person which the normal supply cannot meet. The deficiency anaemias seen most often are those resulting from iron, vitamin B_{12} or folic acid deficiency.

(a) Iron deficiency anaemia

Anaemia due to a deficiency of iron is characterized by small red blood cells with less than the normal content of haemoglobin (microcytic-hypochromic). There is usually some slight reduction in the total number of red blood cells. The deficiency of iron may be due to: (1) an insufficient dietary intake; (2) chronic or acute blood loss; (3) impaired intestinal absorption; or (4) an increased requirement. Iron deficiency is seen frequently in children because of their increased requirements for growth. It is not uncommon in women during their reproductive years because of menstrual blood loss and because of the increased demands during pregnancy and lactation. Anaemia due to an iron deficiency is uncommon in adult males unless there has been a loss of blood or the development of hypochlorhydria secondary to gastric disease or atrophy of the gastric mucosa.

In addition to the general symptoms of anaemia (see Table 13.12), the patient with iron deficiency anaemia may experience soreness and inflammation of the mouth and tongue. The tongue may be very red and may have a smooth, glazed appearance due to atrophy of the papillae. Rarely, the patient with a severe anaemia complains of dysphagia (difficulty in swallowing). The combination of dysphagia, stomatitis (inflammation of the mouth) and atrophic glossitis (inflammation of the tongue with atrophy of papillae) in anaemia may be referred to as the Plummer–Vinson syndrome. Changes in the fingernails are common in prolonged iron deficiency. They become brittle and concave or spoon-shaped.

A well-balanced diet containing an adequate quantity of iron-rich foods is important in the prevention of this type of anaemia. A normal diet contains about 10–18 mg of iron per day, of which only 5–10% is absorbed. It is suggested that absorption is increased as the need for increased production of haemoglobin occurs. It may be necessary to supplement the dietary intake with medicinal iron during periods of increased demands, such as pregnancy and lactation. A supplement may also be necessary for the woman with an excessive menstrual flow.

Unless there is an obvious reason for an iron deficiency anaemia, the patient is investigated to determine the primary cause. For example, malabsorption of iron may be the result of a reduced secretion of hydrochloric acid.

Treatment. Medicinal iron is the principal form of treatment and is usually given orally in the form of a ferrous salt. Examples of preparations commonly used are ferrous sulphate and ferrous gluconate. Oral iron medications may cause gastrointestinal irritation and crampy pain. If the patient complains of distress, the drug is administered with the meal or with a snack. The doctor may recommend that it be given with a glass of orange juice, since it is suggested that vitamin C promotes iron absorption. The patient is advised that his stools will be black and tarry. He may experience some diarrhoea or, with some preparations, may develop constipation, necessitating a mild laxative. Ferrous salt in a syrup or an elixir may be used for children. Any liquid product containing iron should be given well diluted through a drinking tube to prevent staining of the teeth.

For patients who cannot tolerate oral preparations or if oral administration is contraindicated because of some gastrointestinal disturbance or malabsorption, iron may be given parenterally. Injections of iron dextran (Imferon) or iron–sorbitol–citric acid complex (Jectofer) may be given intramuscularly and occasionally dextriferron intravenously, but this is dangerous and rarely done. When giving an iron preparation intramuscularly, the injection is made deeply into the upper outer quadrant of the buttock. The 'Z' track technique[13] is used, since iron is irritating to superficial tissues and may leave a permanent stain. The patient should be observed for toxic reactions which are manifested by headache, dizziness, joint pains and fever. Rarely, an anaphylactic reaction may occur; the patient complains of dyspnoea and chest pain, the pulse is rapid and weak and the blood pressure falls.

The patient with iron deficiency anaemia is encouraged to take an adequate diet that contains iron-rich foods. These are red meats, organ meats (especially liver), eggs, fish, green leafy vegetables, enriched whole grain cereals and bread, and dried fruits.

(b) Vitamin B_{12} deficiency anaemia (pernicious or Addisonian anaemia)

Vitamin B_{12} (cyanocobalamin) is essential for the production of normal red blood cells and may be

---

[13] The 'Z' track technique involves pulling the skin to one side before inserting the needle. After the solution has been introduced, 10 seconds are allowed to elapse before the needle is withdrawn. The purpose of this technique is to prevent the drug leaking into the subcutaneous tissues. The needle used to draw the solution into the syringe is discarded and a new needle is used to prevent tracking of the solution along the insertion path.

referred to as the extrinsic antianaemic factor. When it is not available to the red bone marrow, excessively large cells called megaloblasts are formed. The number of red blood cells produced is less than normal, and they show marked variation in size and shape. The megaloblasts contain a greater than normal amount of haemoglobin, but the deficiency in the total number of erythrocytes results in an inadequate oxygen-carrying capacity of the blood. The condition may be referred to as *megaloblastic anaemia*.

The *cause* of vitamin B_{12} deficiency anaemia is usually non-absorption of the vitamin. Rarely, vitamin B_{12} deficiency occurs because of an inadequate dietary intake (Table 13.13).

Table 13.13 Possible causes of vitamin B_{12} deficiency anaemia.

A. Non-absorption of vitamin B_{12}
  1 Deficiency of intrinsic factor
    (a) Gastric secretory defect
    (b) Gastrectomy (partial or total)
    (c) Autoimmune mechanism
  2 Intestinal resection
  3 Intestinal disease (e.g. regional ileitis, steatorrhoea, intestinal parasites)

B. Malnutrition
  1 Inadequate dietary intake of foods containing vitamin B_{12}
  2 Totally deficient food intake

As cited earlier in this chapter, an intrinsic factor secreted by the gastric mucosa is essential for the absorption of vitamin B_{12}. Non-absorption of the vitamin results from a deficiency of the intrinsic factor, which may be due to a gastric secretory defect, gastrectomy or an autoimmune mechanism. Failure of absorption of the vitamin may also occur as a result of extensive resection of the small intestine or intestinal disease such as ileitis, steatorrhoea and parasitic infestation. Blind or stagnant loops in the small intestine may develop following intestinal surgery or with multiple diverticula (sacs or outpouchings in the walls) and may cause a proliferation of bacteria that use up the available vitamin B_{12} before it can be absorbed.

There appears to be some familial tendency to vitamin B_{12} deficiency anaemia when the deficiency of the intrinsic factor is not secondary to partial or total gastrectomy. It is suggested that a predisposition to the disorder is inherited.[14] An autoimmune mechanism is considered to be active—that is, the individual produces antibodies to the intrinsic factor. This primary form of the disease (that due to a gastric secretory defect or autoimmune mechanism) is known as *pernicious anaemia* or *Addisonian pernicious anaemia*. It is more common in females, has an insidious onset and usually develops between 35 and 65 years of age.

---
[14] Krupp & Chatton (1983), p. 291.

Manifestations. In addition to the general symptoms of anaemia cited previously, the patient may experience gastrointestinal and nervous system changes. The tongue is sore and smooth. There is a loss of appetite and some intolerance for food, but the person does not always show a corresponding loss of weight. The lack of vitamin B_{12} may cause myelin and nerve fibre degeneration in the spinal cord and peripheral nerves. As a result of this degeneration, the patient may develop symmetrical tingling or 'pins and needles' or coldness and numbness in the extremities. Unless the deficiency is corrected, serious motor disturbances may develop in the form of muscular weakness, ataxia (loss of coordination and staggering) and paralysis. In prolonged, severe deficiencies, degeneration of the optic nerves may occur, resulting in serious impairment of vision. When degenerative changes occur in the spinal cord, the condition is referred to as *subacute combined degeneration of the cord*.

In severe pernicious anaemia, the skin may show some jaundice, a result of increased haemolysis. Laboratory examination of the blood reveals a deficiency of erythrocytes. The cells are unusually large with more than the normal amount of haemoglobin (macrocytic-hyperchromic). Gastric analysis demonstrates hypochlorhydria even after stimulation with histamine (see p. 498). Bone marrow aspirated by sternal puncture shows hyperplasia of the bone marrow and failure in normal erythropoiesis. The Schilling test shows that less than the normal amount of vitamin B_{12} is being absorbed.

Treatment. Pernicious anaemia is treated by intramuscular injections of vitamin B_{12}. Since the deficit of vitamin B_{12} is primarily due to malabsorption, intramuscular administration is the method used to achieve adequate blood levels of the vitamin. Oral administration is possible but requires high doses of vitamin B_{12} and careful monitoring of blood levels because the underlying cause is primarily a malabsorption problem. A daily dose may be prescribed for a period of time; then, the interval between injections is gradually increased and the dosage is reduced to a maintenance level according to the patient's response. The patient will require regular maintenance doses of vitamin B_{12} for the rest of his life. The majority of those with pernicious anaemia require 50–1000 mg monthly to maintain normal haemoglobin and erythrocyte levels. Regular red cell counts and haemoglobin estimations are necessary. Initially, the rapid regeneration of erythrocytes in response to treatment may deplete the iron stores, resulting in insufficient haemoglobin production. Ferrous sulphate may be prescribed for a period of time in addition to the vitamin B_{12}.

The recommended diet is light, easily digested, and rich in protein, iron and vitamins. Highly seasoned and coarse foods are avoided if the mouth is sore.

Regular medical examinations are necessary so that early and insidious regressive changes may be recognized before serious degenerative changes develop.

In contrast to pernicious anaemia, the anaemia associated with a dietary deficiency of vitamin B_{12} or intestinal disease does not manifest hypochlorhydria or degenerative changes of the nervous system. The dietary deficiency of vitamin B_{12} (extrinsic factor) usually occurs when the diet lacks animal protein and consists mainly of carbohydrates and vegetables. When the anaemia is secondary to intestinal disease, care of the patient includes treatment of the initial cause as well as parenteral administration of vitamin B_{12}. Oral or parenteral preparations of folic acid may also be prescribed.

(c) Anaemia due to deficiency of folic acid and vitamin C

A lack of folic acid or ascorbic acid may interfere with the production of normal erythrocytes. Either deficiency may result from inadequate intake or a malabsorptive problem. It is also more likely to develop during pregnancy because of the increased demand. Laboratory tests reveal the same haematological changes as appear with vitamin B_{12} deficiency, but the patient does not manifest nervous system involvement, achlorhydria or a decreased vitamin B_{12} absorption.

Folic acid may be given orally or intramuscularly to correct the deficiency. Food sources include dark green leafy vegetables, asparagus, liver and kidney.

Vitamin C enhances the catalytic action of folic acid in erythropoiesis. If the folic acid dietary intake is satisfactory, the administration of vitamin C in anaemia will assist in increasing red cell production.

2. APLASTIC ANAEMIA

This type of anaemia is the result of depressed bone marrow activity. There may be an actual reduction in the amount of blood-forming marrow, or the marrow may have a functional defect. Aplastic anaemia usually results in a deficiency of leucocytes and thrombocytes as well as insufficient red blood cells. The disorder may involve only failure of the bone marrow to produce erythrocytes, causing anaemia alone without leucopenia or thrombocytopenia. When all three formed elements of the blood are reduced, the condition is referred to as *pancytopenia*.

Causes

Depression of bone marrow activity may be the result of the toxic action of certain drugs or industrial chemicals, excessive exposure to radiation, chronic infection or encroachment by tumours or neoplastic tissue. Drugs capable of suppressing bone marrow function include sulphonamides, antineoplastic agents (e.g. nitrogen mustard, busulphan, cyclophosphamide, methotrexate, mercaptopurine), gold salts (sodium aurothiomalate, Myocrisin), chloramphenicol (Chloromycetin) and phenylbutazone

(Butazolidin). Examples of industrial chemicals that may depress erythropoiesis include benzene, aniline dyes, lead, mercury and arsenic. Some insecticides and plant sprays may also be offenders in bone marrow failure. In relation to radiation, drugs and chemicals, there appears to be no direct correlation between the dosage and the development of the anaemia. Sensitivity of the individual seems to be a contributing factor. With some patients their aplastic anaemia may be idiopathic; the cause remains obscure.

Symptoms and treatment

The person with aplastic anaemia is critically ill and, as well as suffering severe hypoxia, he is susceptible to infection because of the deficiency of leucocytes (leucopenia). Spontaneous bleeding is also a problem when the platelet count falls to 20×10^9 per litre or less. With a platelet count of 10×10^9 per litre the tendency to bleed is very high.[15] The onset of the anaemia may be sudden and prostrating, or it may be insidious and gradual. The patient manifests the general symptoms of anaemia (see Table 13.12), oral and throat lesions, fever, infection and haemorrhagic areas.

Treatment includes removal of the cause, frequent transfusions of packed red cells and platelets, oral antibiotic administration to control infection and a corticoid preparation such as prednisone. The latter is thought to have a stimulating effect on the bone marrow. Packed cells are transfused in preference to whole blood to prevent fluid overload. Platelet transfusions are given at the same time or immediately following red cell transfusions to prevent haemorrhage. Platelet counts may be low prior to transfusions and fall during transfusions of red cells either due to a dilutional effect or to immune complex formation.[16]

Bone marrow transplantation is the treatment of choice for patients under 50 years of age with severe aplastic anaemia when a suitable donor is available. Bone marrow transplantation is discussed further on pages 267–269. Immunosuppressive treatment with antilymphocyte globulin (ALG) has been shown to be of benefit to some patients. Treatment with bone marrow transplantation and immunosuppressive therapy provide some hope of a cure or a remission for selected patients. Supportive nursing care is very important. The patient should be observed closely for signs of infection, haemorrhage and increasing hypoxia including dyspnoea, rapid pulse, dizziness, confusion and cyanosis. Precautions are necessary to prevent infection, physical trauma and constipation. The patient is assessed for signs of dizziness and is assisted in walking. His diet is low in roughage and stool softeners are given to prevent gastrointestinal irritation and bleeding. Frequent cleansing of the

---

[15] Brain & Carbone (1985), p. 147.
[16] Brain & Carbone (1985), p. 2.

mouth with an antiseptic solution is important. Subcutaneous and intramuscular injections are avoided as much as possible to keep the skin intact and so prevent infection.

B. Haemolytic anaemias

Excessive haemolysis (disintegration of red blood cells) causes anaemia if the rate of destruction exceeds the erythropoietic ability of the red bone marrow. Premature haemolysis may result from (1) *intracorpuscular (intrinsic) defects* that reduce the ability of the cells to survive the normal life span in circulation, or it may be due to (2) an *extracorpuscular (extrinsic to the erythrocytes) factor or mechanism*.

The patient's symptoms depend on the rate, severity and duration of the cell destruction. As well as the symptoms produced by the reduced oxygen-carrying capacity of the blood, there is an increased concentration of bilirubin in the blood; this may cause jaundice, which is evident first in the sclerae. An increased amount of urobilinogen appears in the urine and faeces and, rarely, free haemoglobin is detected in the plasma and urine. Laboratory examination of the blood reveals an increased number of reticulocytes in circulation (reticulocytosis) because of the constant demand for new cells, as well as a deficiency in the total number of red cells. Examination of a bone marrow specimen demonstrates hyperplasia and hyperactivity of the marrow. Acute haemolytic anaemia may cause a chill followed by a high temperature, prostration, headache and pain in the back and legs.

The haemolytic anaemias caused by a congenital corpuscular defect include hereditary spherocytosis, sickle cell anaemia and thalassaemia. Haemolysis due to extracorpuscular factors may be caused by some infective agents, an autoimmune reaction or certain drugs.

1. HAEMOLYTIC ANAEMIAS DUE TO INTRACORPUSCULAR DEFECT

(a) Hereditary spherocytosis

This type of haemolytic anaemia is also known as congenital haemolytic jaundice, familial haemolytic anaemia and acholuric jaundice. The erythrocyte defect is an abnormal cell membrane that is excessively permeable to sodium. The influx of sodium increases the demand on the 'sodium pump,' adding to the total metabolic work of the cell. The high sodium content of the cells also leads to the entrance of more than the normal amount of water through osmosis, which accounts for the characteristic spherical shape of the cell rather than the normal biconcave disc. This spherical shape predisposes the cells to entrapment in the spleen and their marked fragility results in ready destruction.

The disorder is inherited from an affected parent. The gene with the abnormal trait is dominant; that is,

to have the disorder expressed, one need only receive a gene for the trait from one parent. The age at which the disease is recognized varies, depending on its severity. The patient may have little difficulty and go undiagnosed until adulthood. The enlarged spleen may be discovered during a routine examination. It is usually the jaundice or the symptoms of anaemia that prompt the patient to seek medical assistance. Occasionally, the increased bilirubin leads to the development of gallstones.

Treatment is removal of the spleen, which reduces the excessive destruction of the abnormal red blood cells and relieves the anaemia. The abnormal erythrocytes persist, but the majority survive a normal life span in the absence of the spleen.

(b) Haemoglobinopathy

The complex haemoglobin (Hb) molecule is a combination of globins (protein) and the red pigment haem (porphyrin and ferrous iron). Three forms of haemoglobin occur normally; the type is determined by slight variations in the globin fraction of the compound. The haemoglobin in the erythrocytes of the fetus is type F (Hb-F) and gradually disappears during the first few months of life. About 97% of the haemoglobin that develops after birth is known as type A (Hb-A), and the remainder as type A_2 (Hb-A_2).

The term haemoglobinopathy indicates the presence of red blood cells containing an abnormal type of haemoglobin. The latter is the result of a genetic mutation which causes a disorder in haemoglobin synthesis. The abnormal haemoglobin may cause premature haemolysis of the erythrocytes. The most common haemoglobinopathies are sickle cell disease and thalassaemia. The haemoglobin in the former disease is designated as Hb-S; in the latter various abnormal types may be present.

Sickle cell disease. This recessive, heriditary blood disorder is characterized by erythrocytes that contain Hb-S. It occurs in two forms, sickle cell trait and sickle cell anaemia. *Sickle cell trait* is a heterozygous state; the individual has inherited the Hb-S gene from only one parent. Only a small amount of the individual's haemoglobin is type Hb-S. The person with sickle cell trait usually does not manifest symptoms of sickling except in some very stressful situations, especially those that cause hypoxia. He or she is a carrier, and there is a 50% chance that offspring will inherit the sickle cell trait (see Table 13.14).

Sickle cell anaemia occurs because the individual is homozygous for Hb-S—that is, a gene for the abnormal haemoglobin has been inherited from each parent (see Table 13.14). A large amount of haemoglobin S is present.

The disease affects both males and females and occurs almost exclusively in blacks, the incidence being $1:400–1:500$.

Table 13.14 Possibilities of inheritance in sickle cell disease.

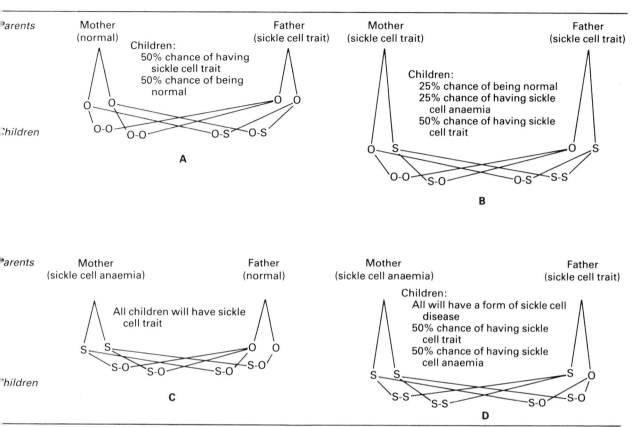

S =gene for sickle cell trait; O = gene for normal erythrocyte

Haemoglobin S is less soluble than normal haemoglobin, especially when it gives up its oxygen to become reduced oxyhaemoglobin, and when the pH is below normal firm crystals form within the cells which are distorted and become crescent-shaped (like a sickle). The blood becomes thicker, heavier and sticky and will not flow as readily through the capillaries. Circulatory stagnation and thrombosis may result, leading to a greater reduction of the oxyhaemoglobin and ensuing local metabolic acidosis (reduced pH). Sickle cells are more fragile and haemolyze readily. Their life span is about 26–35 days, as compared with the 120-day life span of normal erythrocytes. These effects promote more sickling and tend to set up a vicious circle. Sickling and vascular occlusion resulting in an infarcted area may occur in any tissue or organ; the severity and site are not predictable. Frequent sites are the lower limbs, joints, kidneys, mesentery, lungs and brain.

Signs and symptoms. The individual usually has symptom-free periods alternated with exacerbations. There is a continuous premature destruction of red blood cells, resulting in a haemoglobin level of approximately 7–10 g/dl, increased bilirubin in the blood, reticulocytosis, enlargement of the spleen and liver and hyperplasia of the red bone marrow. At intervals, an exacerbation or acute episode, referred to as a sickle cell crisis, occurs. It is frequently precipitated by an infection, stress, dehydration, exposure to cold, acidosis, or any situation in which the individual experiences hypoxia. The acute episode is characterized by sickling, circulatory stagnation and thrombosis. Pain, swelling and impaired function develop in whatever area suffers the interrupted blood supply. The individual is irritable and weak and develops a fever. Jaundice is evident with the increased haemolysis. The symptoms may be quite similar to those of many diseases; for example, if the vascular occlusion occurs in the mesentery, the condition may be mistaken for appendicitis because of the acute abdominal pain and tenderness unless the individual is known to have sickle cell disease. Occlusion of kidney vessels may destroy some nephrons, resulting in renal insufficiency. Obstruction of a cerebral artery may cause some paralysis or reduced mental ability. Growth is retarded and the individual tends to develop a thin short trunk, long extremities, narrow shoulders and hips and increased anterior–posterior diameter of the chest. Symptoms do not usually appear within the first 6 months of life because the individual is protected from sickling during this period by the haemoglobin F that is still present in the erythrocytes.

Thalassaemia. Synonyms that may be used for this type of anaemia are Mediterranean anaemia, homozygous anaemia and heriditary leptocytosis.

This disease occurs in two forms, major and minor, and is seen most frequently in persons of the Mediterranean countries and Southeast Asia. Both forms have the common feature of a genetically determined defect in the cellular synthesis of the globin fraction of the haemoglobin. The red blood cells are smaller than normal, fragile, irregular in shape and deficient in haemoglobin. A large percentage of the haemoglobin is of the fetal type (Hb-F), Haemoglobin A occurs in a greater amount and there is much less Hb-A$_2$ than is found in normal erythrocytes.

Thalassaemia major, also referred to as Cooley's anaemia, is a homozygous state; a gene for the thalassaemia trait has been received from each parent. The disorder is manifested in infancy or early childhood. Fortunately, this form of the disease is of lesser incidence than thalassaemia minor. It produces very severe anaemia and marked hyperplasia of the red bone marrow and may cause pain in the bones. Reticulocytosis occurs and immature nucleated red blood cells may appear in the circulation. The spleen and liver are enlarged as a result of the rapid haemolysis of the abnormal red blood cells, and jaundice may be apparent. The serum bilirubin level is elevated. Growth and development are retarded and the child does not usually survive beyond early childhood. Treatment consists mainly of blood transfusions and splenectomy if the spleen is enlarged.

Thalassaemia minor is a heterozygous state and is less severe. The red blood cells are smaller than normal but are less deficient in haemoglobin than those of the major type and there is less premature haemolysis. The degree of anaemia varies greatly in affected persons; some may be asymptomatic and live a normal life, with their disease only being detected by a blood cell examination. Others may be handicapped to some degree by anaemia.

2. HAEMOLYTIC ANAEMIA DUE TO EXTRACORPUSCULAR FACTORS

Extrinsic mechanisms that may cause haemolysis include (a) some infections, (b) immune bodies, and (c) certain drugs and chemicals.
(a) An increased rate of erythrocyte destruction may be associated with severe infections caused by the haemolytic streptococci, *Staphylococcus aureus*, pneumococcus, *Clostridium perfringens*

(*Bacillus welchii*) and some viruses. Excessive haemolysis may also accompany malaria. The red blood cells may be damaged by the pathogenic organisms or their toxins.
(b) Haemolytic anaemia may be caused by antibodies which may be acquired or may be developed in response to an endogenous or exogenous antigen. Erythroblastosis fetalis (haemolytic disease of the newborn) is an example of haemolytic anaemia occurring as a result of acquired antibodies (see p. 243).

When a person develops antibodies that result in the destruction of his own erythrocytes, the condition is referred to as autoimmune haemolytic anaemia. Frequently, the cause of this condition is not known. In many instances, it is secondary to a collagen disease (e.g. lupus erythematosus) or to a disease involving lymphoid tissue (e.g. Hodgkin's disease). The agglutinins adhere to the red blood cells, predisposing them to entrapment and destruction, especially in the spleen and liver.
(c) Haemolytic jaundice may develop in some persons receiving preparations of quinine, sulphonamide or phenacetin. Its incidence has also been reported in persons exposed to insecticides, arsenic and coal tar products such as aniline dyes and toluene. The mechanism by which certain drugs and chemicals produce haemolysis in some persons is not known.

Treatment of autoimmune haemolytic anaemia includes blood transfusions, splenectomy to reduce the trapping and destruction of the red blood cells, and the administration of a corticoid preparation such as prednisone to decrease sensitivity and antibody formation.

C. Anaemia due to blood loss

The loss of blood removes erythrocytes from the circulation, reducing the oxygen-carrying capacity of the blood. A blood count taken immediately after a haemorrhage does not reflect the degree of anaemia since the total intravascular volume is reduced. Over a period of 24–48 hours, the intravascular volume is restored by the entrance of extracellular fluid into the vascular compartment and probably by intravenous infusion. The red blood cells at this time are those that remained after the blood loss and are now dispersed in a greater volume of plasma. The count (per litre) now gives a more accurate indication of the severity of the anaemia.

Normally, the bone marrow responds quickly to the tissue hypoxia, and the erythrocyte count returns to normal over a period of 4–5 weeks. At first, more than the normal number of reticulocytes are in circulation and some immature nucleated normoblasts may also be released. Since a considerable amount of iron is lost from the body in haemorrhage, haemoglobin production may lag behind red blood cell production. The administration of an iron preparation may be necessary to bring the haemoglobin concentration back to normal.

If the blood loss is 20% or more of the total blood volume, rapid replacement by means of a blood transfusion is necessary to prevent renal failure and endocrine and sympathetic nervous system responses which can lead to cardiac, renal, respiratory and gastrointestinal problems (see Signs and Symptoms of Shock, Chapter 15). This quickly increases the total circulating volume as well as the number of erythrocytes to carry oxygen.

In cases of chronic blood loss in which there is a continuous loss of a relatively small amount over a long period, the bone marrow may keep the erythrocyte count close to normal. The continuous loss of iron, however, creates a deficiency of that essential element, and the erythrocytes in circulation are small and lack a full complement of haemoglobin. The anaemia may be described as microcytic-hypochromic. Treatment includes correction of the cause of the bleeding and the administration of an iron preparation such as ferrous sulphate.

Nursing process

The care required by the anaemia patient varies with the severity and cause of his disease. The anaemia may not be severe enough to necessitate bed rest or hospitalization. It may be chronic, as in pernicious and sickle cell anaemia, resulting in the patient's need for continuous treatment and supervision and modification in his way of life. With some, their anaemia may be entirely cured by correction of the cause. Depending on the causative factor, there may be symptoms and problems in addition to those attributable to anaemia. For example, in haemolytic anaemia there may be the problem of jaundice; in the sickle cell type there is the serious problem of vascular obstruction. Regardless of the type of anaemia, the patients have one common difficulty: namely, a decreased capacity of their blood to transport oxygen.

ASSESSMENT

The patient with pernicious anaemia is observed for signs of degenerative changes in the nervous system. Any complaint of tingling, numbness and sensations of 'pins and needles' in distal portions of the extremities, loss of finer movements, difficulty in holding small objects, weakness of limbs, ataxia and impaired vision are immediately recorded and brought to the doctor's attention. The patient's tolerance for activity is noted.

The colour of the patient's sclerae and skin is noted daily for pallor and, in the case of haemolytic anaemia, for initial or increasing jaundice.

If the patient has sickle cell anaemia, frequent close observation is made for swollen, tender and painful

areas, and changes in body functions or the patient's mental and physical abilities that may indicate areas of thrombotic disease.

Reports of laboratory studies are followed and nursing measures adapted to indicated changes. For example, a decrease in the haemoglobin, packed cell volume or erythrocyte count may be such that the patient's activity should be further reduced.

POTENTIAL PATIENT PROBLEMS

1 Alteration in nutrition: less than body requirements related to a deficient dietary intake of iron, folic acid or vitamin B_{12}, or to the inability to digest and absorb the essential nutrient.
2 Activity intolerance related to inadequate tissue oxygenation.
3 Potential for injury related to impaired cellular function as a result of erythrocyte and haemoglobin deficiency and tissue oxygenation.
4 Alteration in thought processes related to decreased cerebral oxygenation.
5 Knowledge deficit related to the cause, manifestations, prevention and management of the anaemia and of measures to promote health and maintain daily functioning.

NURSING INTERVENTION

Goals for the patient with erythrocyte and/or haemoglobin deficiency are to:
1 Maintain adequate nutrition.
2 Achieve and maintain an acceptable level of activity.
3 Maintain body functioning and prevent the development of complications. Prevent infection.
4 Maintain adequate oxygenation of cerebral tissue.
5 Acquire knowledge of the anaemia and the therapeutic plan of care, and achieve an acceptable daily life-style when the anaemia is chronic.

1. Maintenance of adequate nutrition
Diet has an important role in erythropoiesis. It should be light, easily digestible and selected to provide the protein, iron, vitamins, folic acid and vitamin B_{12} necessary for the production of red blood cells and haemoglobin. Dietary sources of iron include red meats, liver, eggs, fish, green leafy vegetables, enriched whole grain cereals and bread and dried fruits. Meat is an excellent source of protein. Sources of vitamin B_{12} include red meats, liver, eggs and dairy products. Folic acid is present in meats (especially liver), whole grain cereals, leafy vegetables, beans, brewer's yeast and dairy products. Citrus fruits and other fruits and vegetables are good sources of vitamin C.

The nurse and dietitian should discuss with the patient and family the importance of food in increasing the red blood cells and haemoglobin. Food preferences are identified and help is given to plan menus that will provide the necessary nutrients in a form that is acceptable to the patient.

Anorexia frequently poses a problem; if the patient's mouth, tongue and oesophagus are sore, roughage and hot spicy foods should be avoided. Small, frequent meals may be more acceptable to the patient than the usual three meals a day. Giving mouth care just before the food is served, remaining with the patient, providing the necessary assistance if weakness is a problem, and a well ventilated, clean and tidy environment that is free of commotion and disturbing sights are conducive to having the patient take his food.

Extra fluids are important for the patient with haemolytic anaemia, especially sickle cell, to counteract the increased blood viscosity and circulatory stagnation. The daily fluid intake should be recorded. If an adequate oral intake is not tolerated, an intravenous infusion is given.

Iron preparations, folic acid and vitamin C may be prescribed to supplement the patient's dietary intake. Vitamin B_{12} injections are administered when the patient has a deficiency of the intrinsic factor and is not able to absorb the vitamin.

2. Attainment and maintenance of acceptable level of activity
The anaemic patient fatigues quickly and may complain of light-headedness or may faint on exertion. Energy expenditure is reduced in order to decrease the demand for oxygen. Nursing care is planned to conserve the patient's energy in order to decrease the demand for oxygen. When the anaemia is severe, the patient is assisted in turning and transferring from the bed to a chair. Uninterrupted rest periods should be scheduled to follow periods of activity.

An explanation of the basis of the fatigue and weakness and the importance of rest and activity may help the patient to understand what is happening and to accept limitations. If the patient is still active or employed it may be necessary for him to lighten the activity load and to rest at intervals throughout the day. The nurse helps the patient and family evaluate the usual daily routine and to identify activities that are important to him. Together, a plan is developed that permits gradual increased activity and participation in recreational interests. The importance of resting before fatigue and breathlessness develop, avoiding sudden strenuous activity, scheduling rest periods before and after planned activities is stressed. The patient's performance of specific daily activities is reviewed and, if necessary, changes in body movements and/or the environment are suggested in the interest of less energy expenditure.

3. Maintenance of body functioning and the prevention of complications
Alterations in body functioning results from decreased cellular oxygenation and ensuing cellular dysfunction. Medical and nursing intervention vary according to the cause and the severity of the anaemia.

(a) *Nutrition and fluids.* Adequate intake of iron, vitamins and protein is provided in the patient's diet and supplemented with iron and vitamin preparations administered orally or parenterally. Blood transfusions are given when the anaemia is severe and acute.

(b) *Rest and activity.* Activity is encouraged but the importance of resting before the patient becomes fatigued and breathless should be stressed. Scheduled rest periods are provided and the patient is helped to perform essential activities with the minimum expenditure of energy.

(c) *Respiratory support.* Severe anaemia may cause shortness of breath or dyspnoea. The patient may be more comfortable with the head of the bed elevated and the room well ventilated. If the dyspnoea is present with the patient at rest, oxygen administration may be necessary. Sufficient assistance should be given to the patient to avoid unnecessary expenditure of energy and increased oxygen demand. A blood transfusion of packed cells may be given to increase the oxygen-carrying capacity.

(d) *Mouth care.* In pernicious and iron deficiency anaemias, a common problem is ulcerative lesions of the oral mucosa and a sore 'raw' tongue. Frequent cool, mildly alkaline mouthwashes are necessary. A soft-bristled toothbrush or an absorbent applicator is used to clean the teeth. The mouth is cleansed before and after taking nourishment. As cited above, roughage and hot spicy foods are avoided.

(e) *Skin care.* The skin is more susceptible to pressure and breaks down readily because of the reduced oxygen supply in the tissues. If the patient is confined to bed, his position is changed every 1–2 hours and his pressure areas are protected by the use of sponge rubber, sheepskin or a ripple (alternating air pressure) mattress.

If the anaemia is haemolytic, there may be jaundice and pruritis (itching of the skin). Slightly warm or tepid water is used for bathing. Sodium bicarbonate added to the bath water, or oatmeal that is tied in a gauze bag and squeezed through the water, may help to relieve the irritation. The use of soap is avoided. Calamine lotion or caladryl may be applied for relief. The patient's fingernails are kept short and clean to prevent excoriation and infection of the skin should the patient scratch the irritated areas.

(f) *Warmth.* As a result of the reduced amount of oxygen available for metabolism, the anaemic patient produces less body heat. He may require extra clothing and bedding and a warm, ventilated room. Local heat applications are rarely used, especially with the pernicious anaemia patient, since he may have some sensory loss.

(g) *Pain and headache.* Patients with anaemia frequently experience severe headache as a result of the cerebral hypoxia. Symtomatic relief measures are used: the patient is encouraged to remain quiet and inactive; environmental stimuli such as bright light and noise are reduced to a minimum. Cold compresses may be helpful and an analgesic such as paracetamol is prescribed.

Hyperplasia of the red bone marrow is associated with anaemia; the increased production of marrow cells in response to the concomitant hypoxia results in pressure from the volume of tissue, which causes pain. A cradle is used to protect the site from the weight of the bedclothes. Local heat application may provide some relief and an analgesic is prescribed.

(h) *Prevention of infection.* The patient with severe anaemia is more susceptible to infections. Consideration is given to his placement in the hospital ward to avoid contact with a patient with infection. Visitors and personnel with any infection, such as a cold or sore throat, should not be permitted contact with the patient. The person with aplastic anaemia may be placed in reverse isolation or a single room, since he is lacking leucocytes to provide him ordinary protection.

(i) *Cerebral function.* Observe the patient for signs of confusion and slow intellectual responses.

4. *Knowledge of the anaemia and of the health management plan*

Knowledge of the anaemia. An explanation of the nature of the disorder is made to the patient and family; the symptoms such as weakness, fatigue, and shortness of breath are related to his anaemia and the resulting deficiency of oxygen.

The type and degree of activity which precipitate signs of fatigue should be identified to help the patient recognize changes which may indicate recurrence of the disorder and the need for further medical assessment.

In the case of sickle cell anaemia, the parents receive an explanation of the disease and factors that predispose to crises.

Individuals with an hereditary anaemia or a family history of anaemia are encouraged to seek genetic counselling. Decisions on whether to have children or not should be based on factual information about the potential risk of future offspring inheriting the disease or trait and the implications of this. The patient and family are advised of available genetic counselling resources.

Knowledge of the health management plan. The instruction programme includes the following: information about the prescribed plan of care; evaluation of the patient's understanding of the plan; having the patient carry out the prescribed procedures, such as administration of medications and the planning and preparation of the required diet; and information about available community resources and the importance of regular medical check-ups.

(a) *Medications.* Various medications are used in the treatment of anaemia. The drug used depends on the cause and type of the anaemia. These drugs have been cited in the preceding discussion of the various types of anaemia. The principal antianaemic drugs are preparations of iron, vitamin B_{12} and folic acid. Explanations are provided about the action, method of administration and possible adverse effects of the drugs. The necessity of maintenance doses of vitamin B_{12} should be explained to the pernicious anaemia patient; even though he feels well he must not omit the prescribed dose of vitamin B_{12}. If the disease is severe and a weekly injection is prescribed, a referral may be made to the district nurse so the patient may receive the drug at home rather than having to go to the clinic so frequently.

(b) *Nutrition.* The patient and family are taught the importance of obtaining a daily diet containing adequate iron, vitamins and protein as described previously.

(c) *Activity and rest.* Patients are taught the importance of obtaining adequate rest and of maintaining daily activity. Adjustments to the daily routine may be planned to incorporate rest periods. The patient learns to perform essential activities with the minimum energy expenditure.

5. *Long-term alterations in life-style*

Individuals with chronic anaemia requiring on-going therapy and supervision include those with pernicious anaemia or a hereditary form of anaemia (e.g. sickle cell). Those at high risk include persons with chronic disease such as renal failure. Care is directed towards relief of symptoms and the prevention of complications.

Children with sickle cell anaemia and their parents are taught the importance of prophylactic care during remission and the factors that may precipitate a crisis. The affected person is encouraged to live as normal a life as possible, but to avoid chilling, contact with infected persons, high altitude, overfatigue and stressful situations. A well-balanced, nutritious diet, adequate fluids and plenty of regular rest are important. Proper dental hygiene and immunization against infectious diseases are stressed. Regular visits to the clinic or the doctor are necessary for physical and blood examinations. In the case of the school-child, the parents are encouraged to inform the teacher and the school nurse of the child's problem. Identification indicating that the individual has sickle cell disease should be carried or worn at all times; as cited previously, presenting symptoms are similar to those of many other disorders. Membership of a specific support group or association (for example the Sickle Cell Society) may be useful.

Care during a crisis includes bed rest, analgesics for the relief of pain and increased fluid intake. Clear fluids are given orally but, if they are not tolerated, intravenous infusions are used. A close check is kept on the vital signs and urinary output, and for the appearance of 'new' signs and symptoms. If the anaemia is severe, the patient may receive blood transfusions and oxygen. Oxygen is used only during the acute emergency period, since prolonged use and the ensuing high oxygen concentration in the blood may cause suppression of erythropoiesis.

The adult with chronic anaemia is taught to modify his life-style to accommodate the disease. A well-balanced diet is stressed as well as curtailment of activity before fatigue and dyspnoea develop. Work schedules should be organized to allow for rest periods. The individual is given help in setting priorities and determining what activities are preferable. The prevention of infection, recognition of early symptoms and the need for prompt treatment are explained. Soaps and abrasive substances are avoided because the skin and hair may be thin and dry due to oxygen deprivation. The patient is encouraged to use skin creams and make-up and to take an interest in his appearance.

EXPECTED OUTCOMES

The patient:
1 Devise a plan to maintain the necessary dietary intake of iron, vitamins and protein.
2 States a plan to continue a medication regimen following discharge from hospital.
3 States a plan to maintain essential activities and to obtain adequate rest.
4 Describes signs and symptoms of complications of anaemia.
5 States action to take when complications arise.
6 States the cause and manifestations of the anaemia.
7 Describes a plan to implement the therapeutic plan of care.
8 Outlines a plan to adjust life-style to promote health and maintain daily activities.

POLYCYTHAEMIA (ERYTHROCYTE EXCESS)

An excessive number of erythrocytes and a corresponding increase in the concentration of haemoglobin is referred to as polycythaemia. The red blood cell count may be 7–10 × 10^{12} per litre (7–10 million per μl) with a haemoglobin concentration of 18–25 g/dl. The condition may be primary or secondary.

Secondary polycythaemia is a physiological compensatory increase in the number of erythrocytes by the red bone marrow in response to a low concentration of oxygen in the blood. It occurs normally at high altitudes where the atmospheric oxygen tension is low, and in pathologic conditions in which there is inadequate oxygenation of the blood. Examples of the latter are congenital malformations of the heart which lead to blood bypassing the pulmonary–circulatory system and pulmonary conditions that interfere with normal gas exchange (e.g. emphysema).

Primary polycythaemia is known as *polycythaemia vera*; it is a rare proliferative disorder of the red bone marrow in which there is an uncontrolled production of an excessive number of red blood cells and haemoglobin. It may be accompanied by some overproduction of myelocytes (leucocytes produced by the marrow) and platelets. The cause is unknown. The onset is usually in middle-aged persons, with a higher incidence in males and Jewish persons.

Signs and symptoms

Polycythaemia vera increases the total volume and viscosity of the blood. The blood pressure is elevated and the work load of the heart is increased. The rate of flow through the vessels is reduced and, with the increased number of thrombocytes and blood viscosity, predisposes to the development of thrombi. Occlusion of a vessel may occur, causing a cerebral vascular accident, coronary thrombosis, pulmonary infarction or gangrene of a limb. Heart failure may develop insidiously as a result of the increased cardiac demands. The spleen enlarges because of the increased number of red blood cells to be destroyed.

Symptoms vary greatly with patients; the individual may not experience any discomfort and be totally unaware of any problem until the excessive number of erythrocytes are discovered during the course of a regular physical examination. Symptoms may include headache, dizziness, a full feeling in the head, weakness and ready fatigue. The patient may complain of pruritis, especially after a hot bath, and pain in the bones as a result of hyperplasia of the red bone marrow. A high colour (deep dusky red) is manifested in the lips, nose, cheeks, ears and neck. The distal parts of the limbs (especially lower) may be cyanotic at times, owing to the sluggish circulation incurred by the increased viscosity of the blood. These patients also have a tendency to develop a peptic ulcer which is attributed to an associated increase in gastric secretions.

Treatment and care

Treatment and care of patients with polycythaemia vera are aimed at decreasing the activity of the red bone marrow and at reducing the volume and viscosity of the blood. Radioactive phosphorus (P^{32}), which is taken up by the bone marrow cells, may be administered to suppress the bone marrow. Irradiation of the long bones by x-rays may be used. Drugs such as chlorambucil, busulphan (Myleran) or cyclophosphamide (Endoxana) may also be given to inhibit erythropoiesis. A phlebotomy (venesection) may be done at regular intervals to provide a temporary reduction in the blood volume. Five hundred to 1000 ml may be withdrawn each time. The normal blood donor equipment for the collection of blood is used. Red and glandular meats and iron-containing foods are restricted in the patient's diet. Allopurinol is administered daily to lower the excessive serum uric acid level and relieve the inflammation and pain in the joints of the extremities.

These people are not usually treated as inpatients until a complication such as thrombosis, peptic ulcer or cardiac insufficiency develops. A reasonable amount of activity is encouraged to prevent circulatory stasis. They are advised of the need for regular, frequent visits to their general practitioner or the haematology clinic for close supervision. The family and patient are alerted to early indications of impending complications and advised of the importance of promptly contacting their general practitioner.

Leucocyte Disorders

Alterations in the number of leucocytes may involve an increased or decreased production of the cells.

LEUCOCYTOSIS

The number of leucocytes in circulation normally increases to a level in excess of the normal $4.0–11.0 \times 10^9/l$ in defence of the body in most infections and in response to necrotic tissue. This increase is referred to as leucocytosis and is usually predominant in one type of white cell. Information as to which type of leucocytes are in excess of the normal provides significant information for the doctor, since some leucocytoses are known to be associated with certain pathological conditions. For instance: neutrophil leucocytosis normally develops quickly in response to most infections (e.g. appendicitis, pneumonia) and tissue destruction (e.g. myocardial infarction); lymphocytosis is characteristic of certain infections such as measles, mumps, pertussis, and infectious hepatitis; and an increase in eosinophils (eosinophilia) accompanies many allergic conditions. The white blood cell count returns to normal when the infection is controlled, the necrotic tissue is disposed of, or the initiating factor, such as an allergen, is removed.

Leukaemia

Normal leucocytes progress from differentiated, proliferating blast cells (myeloblasts, lymphoblasts, monoblasts) to mature, non-proliferating, functioning white blood cells. Leukaemia is a disease in which there is an excessive uncontrolled production of leucocytes in blast form. They continue to prolifer-

ate and remain immature, and consequently are unable to perform their normal functions. The cell production is comparable to the uncontrolled production of cells in malignant neoplastic disease. For this reason leukaemia is sometimes referred to as cancer of the blood.

There usually is a marked increase in the number of leucocytes in circulation, and many of these are immature and abnormal. Their inability to perform their normal role in body defence makes the individual very susceptible to infection. Hyperplasia of the haemopoietic tissue, the accumulation of leucoblasts within it and disturbance of the normal regulatory mechanisms hamper the formation and maturation of erythrocytes and thrombocytes, leading to anaemia and thrombocytopenia. The circulating leukaemic cells infiltrate organs and tissues and cause dysfunction in these areas. The liver, spleen and lymph nodes enlarge. The enlargement of viscera, in addition to hyperplasia of the bone marrow, causes discomfort, pain and interference with neighbouring structures.

The marked overproduction of leucocytes and the rapid rate of their destruction result in an increase in the body's metabolic rate. The use of certain substances in the proliferation of these cells deprives other cells of essential metabolic elements, and the increased amount of cell destruction increases the concentration of metabolic wastes.

TYPES OF LEUKAEMIA

The leukaemias are divided into two basic types, each of which may be acute or chronic. Lymphoblastic leukaemia (LL) begins in the lymphocytic precursors of the lymph nodes or other lymphogenous tissue. Non-lymphoblastic leukaemia (NLL) or myelogenous leukaemia (ML) begins in the myelogenous cells of the bone marrow and then spreads to other areas of the body.

The French–American–British (FAB) Cooperative Group has subdivided the two types of acute leukaemias as follows:

1 *Acute lymphoblastic leukaemias* (ALL)
    (a) L_1—small usually homogeneous cells (child type)
    (b) L_2—larger more heterogeneous cells (adult type)
    (c) L_3—large, homogeneous cells (lymphoma-like leukaemia)

The L_1 type of leukaemia has a more favourable prognosis than does the L_2 type. The presence of lymphocytes which lack B and T cell markers (null cells) also indicates a more positive prognosis. T cell (cellular immunity) markers are present in 15–20% of patients with acute lymphoblastic leukaemia while B cell (humoral immunity) markers occur rarely.[16] The

---

[16] Bennet, Catovsky, Daniel et al (1981), p. 553.

level of the enzyme terminal deoxynucleotidyl transferase (TDT) is elevated at diagnosis and during relapse with both the T and null cell types.[17] Determination of levels of this enzyme aid in diagnosis and in identifying remissions of the disease.

2 *Acute myeloid leukaemia* (AML) or *acute non-lymphoblastic leukaemia* (ANLL) is subdivided as follows[18]:

  (a) Classification M_1 to M_3 designates myeloblastic leukaemia which differs in the extent of maturation of the white blood cells. Type M_1 cells are immature while M_2 cells are predominantly myeloblasts and promyeloblasts. Type M_3 cells are mostly abnormal promyeloblasts with extensive granulation
  (b) M_4—myelomonocytic leukaemia
  (c) M_5—monocytic leukaemia with monoblasts predominating
  (d) M_6—erythroleukaemia

The presence of Auer's bodies (rod-shaped granules) in the cytoplasm of M_1 to M_4 types of myelogenous leukaemia aids in the diagnosis and indicates a more favourable prognosis.[19]

Incidence

Leukaemia occurs in all age groups and approximately 50% of the diagnosed cases are acute and the remainder chronic. About half of those with acute leukaemia are under the age of 20 years. The incidence of ALL and AML is equal but ALL comprises 80% of the childhood leukaemias. Chronic lymphocytic leukaemia (CLL) accounts for 25% of leukaemias seen in clinical practice and chronic myeloid leukaemia (CML) accounts for 20%.[20] While extensive research continues to search for the cause of leukaemia and for a means of preventing and curing the disorder, chemotherapeutic agents used in recent years have produced remissions and prolonged the life of those with acute leukaemia. The therapeutic regimen is directed toward reducing the production of leukaemic cells and preventing associated complications, such as infection, anaemia and haemorrhage. The chronic forms of the disease progress slowly, are less malignant and manifest more normal mature leucocytes in the blood.

Aetiology

Leukaemia is considered to be a fatal disease of unknown aetiology in most instances. Factors within the patient that predispose to leukaemia include: chromosomal abnormality (e.g. Down's syndrome), chronic marrow dysfunction (e.g. aplastic anaemia),

immunodeficiency and heredity. Environmental factors contributing to the development of leukaemia include: radiation, chemicals and viruses.[21] There is significant evidence that overexposure to ionizing radiation is the causative factor in some cases. This is substantiated by the high incidence of leukaemia found in the survivors of the Hiroshima and Nagasaki atomic bombing, radiologists and patients with ankylosing spondylitis (arthritis of the spine) who were treated by x-ray radiation. Absorption of the chemicals benzol, pyridine and aniline dyes have been strongly suspected of being leukaemogenic. Viruses have been identified as an aetiological factor for some leukaemias in animals.[21] Guyton states that regardless of the initial cause, the uncontrolled production of leucocytes is the result of a cancerous mutation of a myelogenous or a lymphogenous cell.[22] Studies have shown that chromosomal abnormalities are present in the leucocytes involved.

Manifestations

Acute leukaemia usually has an abrupt onset that is frequently accompanied by weakness, general malaise and non-specific complaints. Fever, excessive perspiration, lowered heat tolerance, tachycardia and weight loss develop because of the increased metabolic rate. Bone marrow dysfunction and the resulting anaemia are manifested by pallor, shortness of breath, extreme fatigue, weakness and palpitation. External and internal bleeding may occur due to the reduced production of thrombocytes. Bleeding of the gums, nose and gastrointestinal tract is common. Petechiae or ecchymoses may appear as further evidence of the reduced ability of the blood to coagulate. The patient with myelogenous leukaemia will most likely complain of tenderness and pain in the long bones and sternum from the hyperplasia and crowding in the bone marrow.

Although there is an excessive number of leucocytes, they are immature and do not provide the normal defence against infection; the patient may complain of a sore mouth and throat which exhibit infected necrotic ulcers. An acute infection such as pneumonia, septicaemia or perirectal abscess may develop. The spleen and liver enlarge and, in the later stages, infiltration of the leukaemic cells into the kidneys may cause renal insufficiency. Renal dysfunction also occurs as a result of the excessive blood concentration of uric acid produced by the rapid destruction of the leucocytes. Urate crystals may form and obstruct renal tubules. Sensory and motor disturbances, severe headache, convulsions or disorientation may occur, indicating central nervous system involvement. Lymph nodes enlarge and are tender, owing to infiltration by the leukaemic cells.

[17] Hoffbrand, Ma & Webster (1982), pp. 719–741.
[18] Eastham (1984), p. 202.
[19] Eastham (1984), p. 230.
[20] Hoffbrand & Pettit (1984).

[21] Truman (1981), p. 313.
[22] Guyton (1981), p. 73.

This may be readily detected in the axillary, cervical and inguinal lymph nodes.

The leucocyte count varies greatly but is usually above normal and may exceed 100×10^9 per litre. In some instances, the count is within normal levels or may even be below normal. This is attributed to the bone marrow retaining the leucocytes because of their immature state; normally, they are not released until mature. The erythrocyte and thrombocyte counts are abnormally low. A specimen of aspirated bone marrow demonstrates the proliferation of leukaemic cells.

The *chronic forms of leukaemia* have an insidious onset, but are slowly progressive. They may go unrecognized for a lengthy period. The discovery is often made when the individual undergoes a regular physical checkup or is being investigated for some unrelated condition.

Chronic myelocytic (granulocytic) leukaemia is manifested by a progressive development of weakness, loss of weight, anaemia and thrombocytopenia. The granulocytes are in excess and upon examination reveal a deficiency of alkaline phosphatase and glycogen and an increased histamine content. An abnormality (Philadelphia chromosome) of the cells, detectable in 90% of patients, is produced by the bone marrow of patients with this chronic form of leukaemia.[23] In the advanced stage of the disorder, the enlarged spleen may cause considerable discomfort; an infarction within it may precipitate acute, severe pain in the upper left abdomen. Large ecchymoses and other signs of bleeding appear. The temperature is elevated and the patient becomes progressively weaker because of the increased anaemia. In this later stage the number of immature granulocytes (myeloblasts) in circulation shows a marked increase. Pain is experienced in the sternum and long bones owing to marrow hyperplasia. Within 3–6 years following diagnosis the disease may evolve into acute leukaemia (acute blastic crisis).[24]

The rate at which *chronic lymphocytic leukaemia* progressively develops varies with patients. Some remain free of symptoms and in relatively good health with only mild anaemia and a moderate increase in lymphocytes for several years. In others the leukaemic process slowly but steadily increases in severity. The blood picture is one of an increased leucocyte count, with small atypical lymphocytes predominating. There is a decrease below normal in erythrocytes and thrombocytes. The patient experiences recurring infections because the immune and defence mechanisms are impaired; antibodies are not formed in antigenic response to organisms. The spleen, liver and lymph nodes enlarge; pressure on neighbouring structures may cause impaired function, discomfort and pain. In the advanced stage

many more immature lymphocytes (lymphoblasts) appear in the circulation and the anaemia and deficiency of thrombocytes become severe.

Treatment of the patient with leukaemia

The treatment and care of the patient with leukaemia are directed toward suppressing the abnormal cell production, the prevention of complications (infection and haemorrhage), and supporting the patient physiologically and psychologically.

DRUG THERAPY

The chemotherapeutic programme for the patient with acute leukaemia involves a variety of drugs which are given in combinations or singly. Selection of the drugs depends on accurate identification of the type of leukaemia. Administration usually extends over a period of 3 years. Antileukaemic agents act by interfering with cell mitosis and the synthesis of the leucocyte cellular substance, and by depressing the red bone marrow. Unfortunately they affect normal cells, especially those which reproduce rapidly (e.g. mucous membrane, erythrocytes), in addition to leukaemic cells, and produce serious side-effects with which the nurse must be familiar as they necessitate physiological and psychological supportive measures. Table 13.15 lists common antileukaemic agents. The most common side-effects associated with these chemotherapeutic agents are nausea, vomiting, stomatitis and ulceration, alopecia (loss of hair), change in bowel habit (diarrhoea or constipation) and bone marrow suppression that predisposes the individual to infection and haemorrhage.

An example of a therapeutic regimen that may be prescribed for adults with ALL follows. Diagnostic studies and classification are completed. The patient is given extra fluids orally and/or intravenously to provide adequate hydration, and allopurinol is administered daily to lower the uric acid level. If the uric acid level remains high, the urine is made alkaline through administration of sodium bicarbonate. Treatment is divided into phases. The patient is advised of the possible side-effects. A signed consent form is usually required. Initially the patient receives vincristine, prednisone, daunorubicin and L-asparaginase for 4 weeks to induce a remission, evidenced by a marked reduction or total absence of leukaemic cells in the blood and bone marrow. Vincristine is given intravenously weekly, usually through a right atrial catheter, and the patient is observed for possible side-effects which include alopecia, abdominal cramps, constipation and neurological disturbances. Signs and symptoms of neurological disturbances are an abnormal gait, stumbling, a decrease in reflex responses, loss of coordination, paralysis and paralytic ileus. Prednisone, an adrenocorticosteroid, is given by mouth daily. Its serious side-effect is the individual's increased susceptibility to infection.

---

[23] Smith & Thier (1985), p. 276.
[24] Truman (1981), p. 321.

Table 13.15 Antileukaemic agents.

Agent	Classification	Administration	Potential side-effects
Vincristine (Oncovin)	Plant alkaloid Inhibits mitosis of leukaemic cells	Intravenous	Alopecia Abdominal cramps Constipation Nervous system disturbances: hyporeflexia, abnormal gait, loss of coordination, stumbling, paralysis, paralytic ileus Stomatitis
Prednisone	Hormone—an adrenocorticosteroid Retards leukaemic cell reproduction	Oral	Gastric distress and ulceration Decreased immune responses and increased susceptibility to infection Retention of fluid
L-Asparaginase	Enzyme Deprives leukaemic cells of amino acid, L-asparagine	Intravenous	Anaphylactic shock Allergic reactions Impaired liver and pancreatic functions (hyperglycaemia) Depression (psychological)
Methotrexate	Folic acid analogue Deprives leukaemic cells of folic acid	Oral Intravenous Intrathecal	Bone marrow depression Oral and gastrointestinal ulceration and bleeding Nausea, vomiting, diarrhoea Dermatitis Impaired liver function and renal failure Alopecia
6-Mercaptopurine	Purine analogue Deprives leukaemic cells of essential purine	Oral	Bone marrow depression Nausea and vomiting Intestinal ulceration Dermatitis
Cyclophosphamide (Endoxana)	Alkylating agent Suppresses leukaemic cell reproduction	Oral Intravenous	Bone marrow depression Haemorrhagic cystitis Alopecia and sterility
Daunorubicin (daunomycin, rubidomycin)	Antibiotic Inhibits synthesis of normal cellular substance (DNA)	Intravenous	Nausea and vomiting Stomatitis Alopecia Bone marrow depression Cardiac arrhythmia
Doxorubicin (Adriamycin)	Antibiotic Inhibits DNA synthesis and DNA-dependent RNA synthesis	Intravenous	Nausea, vomiting Fever Bone marrow depression Anaemia Stomatitis Alopecia Liver and cardiac toxicity
Cytarabine (cystosine arabinoside ara-C, Cytosar)	Pyrimidine analogue	Intravenous Intrathecal Subcutaneous	Nausea and vomiting Bone marrow depression Stomatitis and ulceration Neurotoxicity with intrathecal use
Thioguanine (6TG)	Purine analogue	Oral	Bone marrow depression Stomatitis and diarrhoea Hepatitis

Table 13.15—*continued*

Agent	Classification	Administration	Potential side-effects
Busulphan (Myleran)	Alkylating agent Interferes with mitosis	Oral	Bone marrow depression Alopecia Nausea, vomiting, diarrhoea Stomatitis Pulmonary fibrosis Hyperpigmentation of the skin
Chlorambucil (Leukeran)	Alkylating agent Antimetabolic action	Oral	Nausea and vomiting Bone marrow depression
Hydroxyurea	Antimetabolic	Oral	Nausea and vomiting Bone marrow depression Skin changes Stomatitis Alopecia
5-Azactidine	Pyrimidine analogue	Intravenous	Bone marrow depression Liver toxicity Neuromuscular disturbances: myalgia, lethargy and confusion Nausea, vomiting, diarrhoea Hypotension
Amsacrine (Amsidine)	Inhibits DNA synthesis	Intravenous	Bone marrow depression Mucositis Nausea and vomiting Headache, dizziness Alopecia, skin rash Liver and cardiac toxicity
Vinblastine (Velbe)	Plant alkaloid Inhibits mitosis of leukaemic cell	Intravenous	Nausea, vomiting Headache, neuropathy Alopecia Cellulitis
Vindesine (Eldisine)	Plant alkaloid Inhibits mitosis of leukaemic cell	Intravenous	Neurotoxicity Alopecia Constipation, abdominal pain Nausea, vomiting Depression

Gastric distress and ulceration may develop but may be prevented if the drug is given with milk or an antacid preparation such as Maalox. Daunorubicin is given intravenously weekly. It produces side-effects of nausea, vomiting, stomatitis, bone marrow depression and alopecia. L-Asparaginase is administered intravenously from day 15–28. Side-effects include allergic reactions, psychological depression and liver and pancreatic impairment. Initial treatment brings about a remission of the disease and a return to a normal haematological state in 70–80% of the patients with ALL.

Infiltration of the central nervous system by leukaemic cells may be referred to as 'central nervous system leukaemia'. It usually develops late in the disease and may be manifested by headache, nausea, vomiting, exaggerated reflex responses, irritability, disorientation, papilloedema[25] and head retraction with rigidity of the neck. The drugs cited above (vincristine, prednisone and L-asparaginase) are ineffective in destroying the leukaemic cells which infiltrate into the brain and cervical area of the cord. This ineffectiveness is attributed to the limited amount of those drugs that crosses the blood–brain barrier, which is readily traversed by the leukaemic cells. The therapeutic regimen usually includes prophylactic measures before central nervous system leukaemia becomes evident. As soon as the bone marrow is in remission, intrathecal administration of methotrexate, a folic acid antagonist, is commenced.

---

[25] *Papilloedema*, also referred to as choked disc, is hyperaemia and oedema of the optic disc and is usually associated with increased intracranial pressure.

A series of cranial radiation sessions or intravenous administrations of high doses of methotrexate follow.

The patient receiving methotrexate should be observed for anaemia, haemorrhage and infection because of the potential bone marrow and antibody suppression. He may also develop oral and gastrointestinal ulceration. The latter may be manifested by abdominal discomfort and pain, vomiting, haematemesis, diarrhoea and blood in the stool. Liver function may be impaired. The 8 week period of induction therapy is reinforced by 6 weeks of consolidation therapy to further eradicate the leukaemic cells and improve remission quality. Repeated cycles of alternating drug combinations are used, e.g. a combination of prednisone, vincristine and adriamycin or cyclophosphamide, cytosine arabinoside and thioguanine. Maintenance chemotherapy continues for 2–3 years for most patients and consists of combinations of methotrexate, mercaptopurine, L-asparaginase and cyclophosphamide with periodic doses of vincristine and prednisone. Mercaptopurine may cause bone marrow depression and intestinal ulceration. Cyclophosphamide may depress the bone marrow and also causes alopecia. It is eliminated in the urine and may result in severe haemorrhagic cystitis unless well diluted by an adequate daily fluid intake (a minimum of 3000 ml). In order to provide an adequate fluid intake, an antiemetic preparation, such as metoclopramide hydrochloride 10 mg (Maxolon) or prochlorperazine maleate 5 mg (Stemetil), is administered.

The treatment of chronic lymphocytic leukaemia consists of symptomatic care and the administration of an alkylating agent such as chlorambucil or cyclophosphamide. Prednisone may also be used, as well as radiation of the lymph nodes and spleen.[26]

The treatment of chronic myelocytic leukaemia is symptomatic rather than curative. Busulphan is given to decrease the size of the cell mass. Hydroxyurea and mercaptopurine or radiation therapy may be used to control the disease.[27]

Nursing responsibilities associated with drug therapy include the following. It is important that the nurse be familiar with the expected action, route of administration used and the potential side-effects of the antileukaemic agents. The patient is advised of the possible effects, that support will be provided and that those drugs now available do bring about a remission and permit the individual to leave the hospital and resume many former activities. Opportunities should be provided for the patient to ask questions and discuss his feelings about his therapy and reactions to it. If the patient's need for information and assurance are not met he becomes resentful, frustrated and depressed.

A frequent assessment is made of the patient for

changes and manifestations of reactions to the drug(s). Nursing measures are instituted promptly to provide necessary support and relief. For example, nausea may be prevented by administering an antiemetic before the antileukaemic drug is given and throughout the course of the infusion, relaxation techniques, reducing external stimuli by dimming the light, and leaving him undisturbed.

Since most patients receive repeated courses of intravenous chemotherapy and also require many laboratory tests necessitating withdrawal of blood samples, care must be taken to preserve the integrity of the patient's veins. The need for tests should be reviewed and if necessary withdrawal of blood specimens should be done when the intravenous line is being started to decrease the number of venepunctures. A right atrial catheter such as the Hickman catheter may be left in place for 9 months to a year and can be used for both drug administration and the withdrawal of blood samples. (A Portocath may be left in place for several years.) Right atrial catheters (see Fig. 13.2) may have a single lumen, or may have double, triple or quadruple lumens. Each lumen runs the length of the catheter and varies in diameter. Multiple lumens in the catheter facilitate the administration of several infusions at one time. Patients may be receiving total parenteral nutrition, antibiotics, antiemetics, platelets and chemotherapeutic agents intravenously. The larger lumen of the catheter is reserved for the withdrawal of blood and the administration of blood and blood products and total parenteral nutrition. Precautions include the use of Luer lock connections on all intravenous tubing and the taping of all connections. Tuff link adaptors are used when Luer lock connections are not available. Each line of the catheter has a coloured marker to facilitate identification. Care must be taken not to confuse the lines of the catheter and intravenous solution and the tubing connected to each line. The catheter is capped when not in use allowing the patient to participate in most daily activities. Each lumen of the catheter is flushed regularly with a solution of heparin to keep it patent when it is not being used. The patient or a family member is taught to irrigate the catheter lines regularly with a solution of heparin or a referral is made to the district nurse. Table 13.16 lists the content for a programme to teach patients and families to care for the right atrial catheter, to prevent complications and what to do if problems occur. Table 13.16 also lists expected outcomes for the patient-teaching programme.

Supportive therapy during periods of bone marrow depression may consist of the administration of red blood cells to combat the associated anaemia, platelets to control bleeding and transfusions of granulocytes to control infection. Packed red blood cells are administered if the patient's haemoglobin is less than 10 g/dl. Platelets are administered to prevent bleeding as well as to treat active bleeding. Dur-

[26] Truman (1981), p. 318.
[27] Truman (1981), p. 322.

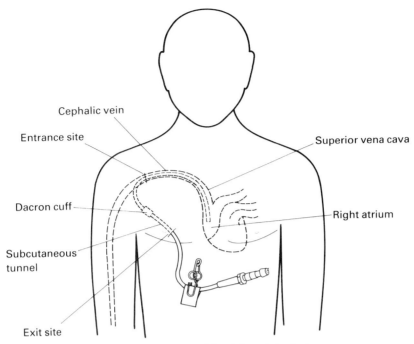

Fig. 13.2 Placement of the right atrial catheter.

Check that....

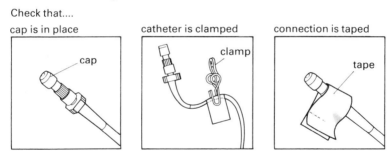

Fig. 13.3 Safety precautions: right atrial catheter.

ing periods of severe bone marrow depression from the induction chemotherapy, platelet transfusions may be given daily to maintain a platelet count greater than 20×10^9 per litre. During and immediately following a transfusion of red blood cells, platelets or granulocytes, the patient is observed closely for adverse reactions which may be manifested by a chill, fever, urticaria, severe headache, lumbar pain, dyspnoea, oliguria and discoloration of the urine due to haemoglobin released by haemolysis. If a reaction occurs, the transfusion is discontinued. Granulocyte transfusions are administered slowly and the patient may receive corticosteroids, paracetamol (Panadol), pethidine or diphenhydramine (Benadryl) prior to the transfusion to reduce the possibility of reaction.[28]

A combination of antibiotics, including an aminoglycoside (tobramycin or gentamycin) and a semisynthetic penicillin (tecarcillin or carbenicillin), are administered promptly when signs of infection appear. The neutropenic patient with an altered immune system is very susceptible to infection, which can be life-threatening. Antibiotic therapy is continued until the patient's white blood cell count rises following chemotherapy. Granulocyte transfusions may also be prescribed.

Total parenteral nutrition may be administered if the patient has severe stomatitis and is unable to swallow or retain nutrients. Care of the patient receiving total parenteral nutrition is discussed in Chapter 17.

BONE MARROW TRANSPLANTATION

A bone marrow transplant consists of the intrave-

---

[28] Graham & Rubal (1980), p. 99.

Table 13.16 Patient teaching programme: right atrial catheters.*

1 Information about the right atrial catheter
- *What is a right atrial (Hickman) catheter?* The right atrial (Hickman) catheter is a narrow, silicone rubber tube which is inserted through the skin and into a vein on the upper chest or shoulder. The tip of the catheter is situated in the right atrium of the heart. The outer end is tunnelled a few inches along the chest wall just under the skin and then comes out to the surface. This is the section you can see. The end of the catheter has a cap, taped in place, and is clamped with a metal clamp to ensure that the catheter is closed off when it is not being used.
- *The purpose and use of right atrial catheters:* The right atrial catheter provides a ready access to the circulation. It can be used to administer medications, blood transfusions or blood products, for nutritional therapy or as an access to the circulation for plasma phoresis.
- *Three essential safety points:* When the catheter is not being used you will check it on arising in the morning, before and after bathing, when dressing and before going to bed to ensure that:
  (a) the catheter cap is in place
  (b) the catheter is clamped
  (c) all catheter connections are taped
- *Maintaining patency of the catheter:* Each catheter lumen is heparinized to prevent blood from clotting in the line and to keep the line patent when not in use. The catheter is heparinized twice daily. There is no standard for the frequency of heparinization of each catheter line. Daily heparinization appears to be adequate. Frequency of heparinization may also vary according to the concentration of heparin solution used. The volume of heparin solution may also vary in different centres but should exceed the 3.5 ml capacity of the larger lumen. This is usually done on arising in the morning and before going to bed at night. On occasion, you may adjust your schedule. Be sure there is an interval of 9–14 hours between heparinization times.

2 Heparinization of the catheter
Filling a syringe with heparin solution
(a) assemble equipment
(b) wash hands thoroughly
(c) check the label on the bottle: heparin solution 10 units/ml
(d) vigorously wipe the top of the heparin bottle with an alcohol swab
(e) open package containing syringe and needle
(f) pull back on the plunger of the syringe to the 6 ml mark
(g) remove the cap from the needle, being careful not to touch the needle
(h) holding the bottle on a firm surface, insert the needle of the syringe into the rubber cap of the bottle
(i) push the plunger down to inject the air into the bottle
(j) invert the bottle and syringe. Be sure the tip of the needle is in the solution
(k) pull back on the plunger and fill the syringe to the 6 ml mark with the heparin solution
(l) check that there are no air bubbles in the syringe. If there are, tap the syringe to force the bubbles to rise to the needle hub. Push the plunger to rid syringe of air bubbles. Re-fill the syringe to the 6 ml mark with solution
(m) withdraw the needle from the bottle

(n) replace the cap on the needle and return the heparin solution to the refrigerator

Flushing the catheter with heparin solution
(a) remove the tape from the catheter cap
(b) vigorously clean the end of the cap with an alcohol swab
(c) insert the needle of the syringe prepared with 6 ml of heparin solution into the cap
(d) release the clamp from the catheter
(e) draw back on the plunger to make sure there is no air in the catheter
(f) inject the heparin solution slowly up to 5.5 ml
(g) replace the clamp
(h) gently press on the plunger of the syringe to check that no more solution goes in
(i) remove the needle from the cap
(j) tape the cap connection

3 Safety precautions
If you follow the instructions to check your catheter several times a day and to heparinize it twice a day, you should not encounter any problems. Problems that might occur are that air enters the catheter, the cap loosens, the catheter is punctured, the catheter becomes blocked, or the exit site becomes infected. The handling of these problems is quite simple, but it is important that you take immediate action if any of these situations develop.
- *Air in the catheter.* The catheter is always checked for the presence of air prior to heparinization by pulling back on the plunger of the syringe. If air comes back into the syringe:
  (a) continue to pull back on the plunger until blood enters the syringe
  (b) with the needle and syringe still in place, clamp the catheter
  (c) remove the needle from the cap
  (d) expel the air from the syringe
  (e) repeat the procedure. If no further air is present, inject the heparin
  (f) if the tubing cannot be cleared of air, call the district nurse or go to the emergency or outpatient department of the hospital where the catheter was inserted
- *If the cap comes off.* If the catheter cap loosens or comes off:
  (a) check that the clamp is in place and replace it immediately if it is off
  (b) vigorously clean the end of the catheter with an alcohol swab
  (c) put a new sterile cap on the catheter. An extra sterile cap should be kept with you at home
  (d) retape the cap in place
- *Preventing puncture of the catheter.* The catheter is made of silicone rubber and can be easily punctured by a needle, pin or other sharp objects. To prevent puncture of the catheter:
  (a) take care when heparinizing the catheter. Hold the catheter straight and insert the needle into the centre of the cap and tubing
  (b) avoid wearing jewellery, pins or other sharp objects on clothing over the area of the catheter
- *If the catheter is punctured.* If the catheter should be punctured, clamp the catheter between the puncture and the exit site on the chest and go to the emergency department of the hospital where the catheter was inserted. If living outside the city, contact the community nurse.
- *If the catheter is blocked.* If heparin solution cannot be injected into the catheter, first check that the catheter is

not kinked and that the clamp is released. Take a deep breath, raise both arms above your head and change your body position. If these actions are not successful and the heparin solution still cannot be injected, contact the visiting nurse or go to the emergency department of the hospital where the catheter was inserted.

- *Signs of infection at the catheter exit site.* The exit site of the catheter should be checked daily through the transparent dressing for any signs of infection. Changes that might indicate an infection at the exit site are: redness, tenderness, swelling and drainage. An elevation of body temperature may also indicate infection at the exit site or elsewhere in the body.
- *If signs of infection are present.* Any signs of infection should be reported immediately to the doctor and to the community nurse.
- *Medic Alert identification.* The presence of a right atrial catheter is not apparent under your clothing. The general public and some health care professionals may not be familiar with the catheter and may not initiate appropriate action promptly in emergency situations. It is therefore important that you wear a Medic Alert bracelet or necklace and carry a card describing the catheter.

4 Use of community resources

- *Plans for dressing changes at home.* The transparent adhesive dressing over the exit site is changed once each week. With the assistance of a family member or friend, you may learn to change the dressing. Arrangements may also be made to have the dressing changed at the time of a weekly visit to an outpatient clinic. Home care nursing services are available to change the dressing for you or to teach you or a family member to change the dressing if you did not learn this prior to discharge from hospital.
- *Patient and family plans for home care services.* Home care services are provided by the district or community nurses and health visitors. You and your family will participate in planning what services you will require and be told of the referrals that are made for follow-up care at home. The names of individuals to contact in the hospital and community and the phone number will be given to you so you can contact these resource persons at any time.

5 Expected patient outcomes: self-care and management of right atrial catheters

- *Information.* The patient and/or family members will be able to:
  (a) state the purpose and use of right atrial catheters
  (b) state three essential safety points that should be checked several times daily
  (c) state the purpose of heparinizing the catheter
  (d) state the frequency of performing the heparinization procedure
- *Practice.* The patient and/or family members will be able to:
  (a) demonstrate ability to safely fill a syringe with heparin solution
  (b) demonstrate ability to safely heparinize the right atrial catheter
- *Safety precautions.* The patient and/or family members will be able to:
  (a) state actions to take if air is present in the catheter
  (b) state actions to take if the catheter cap comes off
  (c) state action to take to prevent puncture of the catheter
  (d) state actions to take if the catheter is punctured
  (e) state actions to take if the catheter becomes blocked
  (f) describe signs which may indicate infection at the catheter site
  (g) state actions to take if signs of infection are present
  (h) state plans to obtain a Medic Alert identification
- *Use of community resources.* The patient and/or family members will be able to:
  (a) describe plans for changing the dressing at the catheter site
  (b) describe plans for community nursing services

*Royle & Green (1985).

nous administration of marrow cells from a compatible donor; it is used in the treatment of some leukaemias, especially acute myelogenous leukaemia. The patient receives total body irradiation and large doses of cyclophosphamide prior to the bone marrow transplant. This not only destroys leukaemic cells but also suppresses his immune system and so he must be cared for in a controlled germ-free environment. Long-term survival of patients receiving bone marrow transplants is greatest in patients who achieved a complete remission of the disease following induction therapy. When making a decision related to bone marrow transplantation, the patient should be aware of alternative treatment and consideration should be given to the patient's age and personal wishes.

Nursing care of the patient receiving a bone marrow transplant focuses on the prevention of infection, maintaining nutritional status, prevention and control of bleeding.

Graft-versus-host disease, in which the donor T lymphocytes immunologically attack host tissue, is a major complication. All blood products administered to the patient, with the exception of the donor marrow, are irradiated prior to use. Treatment of the syndrome includes the administration of corticosteroids, cyclosporine or methotrexate.

Nursing process

The patient with leukaemia experiences fear and uncertainty about hospitalization, prolonged treatment, possible death from the disease and/or complications of the treatment. The course of the disease varies with the type and acuteness of the leukaemia and the patient's responses to treatment. Most patients achieve a remission in response to the initial treatment; the duration of the remission may be very short or last several years. Patient care, as always, must be individualized and includes both

Table 13.17 Patient care plan: the patient with leukaemia.

Problem	Patient goals	Nursing intervention	Expected outcomes
1 Anxiety related to the diagnosis of leukaemia, fear of the unknown, lack of control over events and uncertainty about the future	**a** To identify the causes of the anxiety **b** To decrease the level of anxiety	**a** Observe non-verbal and verbal behaviour that may indicate anxiety and fear, such as crying, hyperactivity or withdrawal **b** Assess the patient's prior experience of illness and hospitalization **c** Assess the patient's understanding of leukaemia, diagnostic tests, treatment plan and prognosis **d** Assess the family members' responses to patient's illness and hospitalization and how this affects the patient **e** Listen to the patient **f** Express awareness and acceptance of concerns and anxiety **g** Provide privacy and time for expression of feelings and asking of questions **h** Provide information about the leukaemia, hospitalization, diagnostic tests, treatments and anticipated outcomes to the patient and family **i** Allow the patient time to prepare for tests and treatments following the explanations **j** Allow opportunity for the patient to state preferences and make choices about care and hospital routines whenever possible **k** Ensure that the patient's decisions and preferences are communicated to all staff and incorporated in the individual plan of care **l** Create opportunities for the patient to socialize with family and friends **m** Provide opportunities for family members to participate in patient care activities **n** Support family for participating in care activities and provide instruction and guidance as needed	The patient: 1 Expresses decreased feelings of anxiety 2 Participates in decision-making regarding care 3 Increases social interaction with others
2 Lack of knowledge concerning the leukaemia, hospitalization, treatment plan, effects of treatment and prognosis	To understand leukaemia, need for hospitalization, diagnostic tests, treatment plan, short-term prognosis and anticipated long-term outcome	**a** Assess the patient and family's understanding of the leukaemia, diagnostic tests, treatment plan and expected prognosis **b** Discuss with other health professionals the information that has been communicated to the patient and family **c** Assess the patient's and family's response to the diagnosis **d** Assess the patient's previous experience with illness and hospitalization **e** Identify barriers to learning, such as language, cultural and religious beliefs, level of education, intelligence, sensory losses, anxiety and denial **f** Identify factors influencing learning such as: readiness to learn, asking of questions, acceptance of diagnosis, family support **g** Plan a teaching programme: there should be short sessions and repetition of information, building on previous content, opportunities	1 The patient expresses understanding of: (a) How leukaemia affects the body (b) The components of the blood and their functions (c) The reasons for diagnostic tests (d) Expectations for the patient before, during and following tests and treatments (e) The treatment plan (f) Effects of treatment on the blood components and the body (g) What can be done to relieve the effects of the disease and drugs (h) Anticipated course of initial

Table 13.17—*continued*

Problem	Patient goals	Nursing intervention	Expected outcomes
2 Lack of knowledge (continued)		to ask questions, opportunities for family involvement, and written information to reinforce verbal explanations **h** Provide the following information: • Definition of leukaemia • Identification and functions of components of the blood, especially white blood cells, red blood cells and platelets • Reasons for diagnostic tests: bone marrow examination and blood studies • Preparation for tests and expectations for the patient before, during and after the test • The treatment plan, including the actions and side-effects of drugs • Measures to alleviate side-effects of disease and chemotherapy • Plans for continuing treatment as an outpatient • Duration of expected treatment • Anticipated results of treatment, especially over a 3 year period **i** Assess effectiveness of teaching on an on-going basis by having the patient review information and by identifying when the patient applies information to self-care	treatment and hospitalization and follow-up treatment
3 Increased potential for infection related to the leukaemia process and chemotherapeutic-induced immunosuppression	**a** To minimize contact with infectious agents in the environment **b** To decrease potential for endogenous infections **c** To promptly identify and treat infections	**a** Observe the skin and mucous membranes for signs of redness, swelling, drainage or open lesions **b** Assess and record the patient's temperature every 4 hours and report any elevation **c** Instruct the patient to promptly report the occurrence of tenderness or pain and signs of redness, warmth, swelling, drainage or open lesions on skin or mucous membranes **d** Monitor the patient's white blood cell count and institute *all protective measures* when levels fall below 5.0×10^9 per litre **e** Place the patient in a single room **f** Limit visitors to significant family members and select friends **g** Prevent all contact with individuals with known or potential infections **h** Implement the practice of good hand-washing techniques by all staff and visitors **i** Take the patient's temperature orally or axillary—never rectally **j** Avoid, if possible, parenteral administration of medications **k** Provide regular oral hygiene **l** Give a daily bath using a mild antiseptic soap to reduce the skin flora **m** Keep the patient's nails short and clean	The patient: **1** is free from infection as evidenced by: temperature within normal range, absence of pain, tenderness, swelling, redness, warmth or drainage on skin or mucous membranes **2** has clean, intact skin and mucous membranes **3** promptly reports changes in temperature, the occurrence of pain or tenderness, skin or mucosal swelling, redness, drainage or open lesions

Table 13.17—*continued*

Problem	Patient goals	Nursing intervention	Expected outcomes
3 Increased potential for infection (continued)		n Provide fruit and plenty of fluids in the patient's diet and administer a stool softener such as dioctyl sodium sulpho-succinate (Dioctyl) to prevent constipation o If a local infected area is identified, a swab for culture and sensitivity is taken immediately and an antibiotic is administered as prescribed p Teach the patient protective measures to institute following discharge including avoidance of crowds and individuals with infections. Advise of the need to report his condition to the dentist and others prior to receiving care q Report signs of possible infections promptly to ensure immediate treatment	
4 Increased potential for bleeding (injury) related to the leukaemia process and chemotherapy-induced bone marrow suppression	a To promptly identify signs of bleeding b To prevent bleeding due to trauma	a Observe the patient for signs of bleeding which may be petechiae, bruises, joint swelling, mucous membrane oozing, pain, abdominal discomfort, restlessness or observable bleeding b Monitor the patient's platelet count and test stools for occult blood c When the platelet count is below 50×10^9 per litre institute preventive measures: • Avoid unnecessary invasive procedures including injections • Do not take the temperatures rectally • Use only electric razors for shaving male patients • Use a soft toothbrush or swabs for mouth care. (Do not use dental floss or hard toothbrushes.) • Do not administer medications affecting blood coagulation such as acetylsalicylic acid (aspirin). • Prevent constipation by dietary measures and stool softeners • Prevent trauma by assisting patient when unsteady on feet, eliminating environmental hazards d Administer platelets as ordered e Observe the patient frequently for signs of bleeding following any invasive procedure f Instruct the patient about preventive measures to be carried out in the hospital and home g Teach the patient to observe for signs of bleeding and to report them promptly if they appear	1 Signs of bleeding are identified immediately 2 Bleeding due to tissue trauma does not occur 3 The patient demonstrates an understanding of precautionary measures 4 The patient complies with precautionary measures

Table 13.17—*continued*

Problem	Patient goals	Nursing intervention	Expected outcomes
4 Increased potential for bleeding (continued)		**h** Institute measures to control bleeding. When bleeding occurs: apply pressure, elevate the part, notify the doctor, administer platelets as ordered	
5 Impairment of oropharyngeal mucosa due to the leukaemia process and the effects of chemotherapy	**a** To prevent complications and trauma to the oropharyngeal mucosa **b** To promote comfort **c** To treat complications of oropharyngeal mucosa promptly	**a** Inspect (and record any changes) the mouth, tongue and oropharynx daily for appearance of mucosa, location, size and appearance of lesions and bleeding **b** Record changes in mucosa of mouth, tongue and oropharynx **c** Teach the patient to inspect his mouth daily and report any changes **d** Teach patient to carry out regular oral hygiene during periods of remission when platelet count is close to normal range: • Brush teeth after each meal with soft brush • Use dental floss to remove plaque from teeth • Use mild, diluted mouth-wash **e** When stomatitis is present and/or platelet count is decreased, give mouth care every 2 hours: • Cleanse mouth with hydrogen peroxide solution diluted with normal saline • Use toothettes, foam swabs or soft toothbrush for cleaning • Irrigate mouth with normal saline • Remove dentures • Rinse mouth with mycostatin solution to prevent or treat fungal infections • Apply a water-soluble lubricating ointment to lips **f** Instruct the patient how to carry out prescribed mouth care **g** Apply analgesic solutions to mouth and throat as prescribed **h** Administer systemic analgesics on a regular basis when needed **i** Suction oral cavity gently using a soft, rubber catheter to control excess salivation **j** Instruct patient to obtain regular dental care and to inform the dentist of disease, treatment and problems of stomatitis, thrombocytopenia and leucopenia	**1** The mucosa of the mouth, tongue and oropharynx is clean, pink, moist and intact **2** When stomatitis is present oral hygiene is provided every 2 hours **3** Complications due to trauma do not occur **4** Changes in the status of the oral mucosa are identified promptly **5** There is an absence of pain from oral lesions **6** The patient inspects his mouth and performs the prescribed oral hygiene
6 Alteration in nutrition: less than body requirements related to the increased metabolic rate associated with leucocyte overproduction and rapid destruction; and stomatitis, nausea, vomiting, anorexia and	**a** To maintain an adequate intake of essential nutrients **b** To prevent or minimize weight loss	**a** Identify the patient's usual eating habits, food preferences and dislikes, cultural influences and weight patterns **b** Note the patient's height, weight, body build and skin folds	**1** Weight loss is less than 10% **2** The essential nutrients are obtained from the daily food intake **3** The patient and

Table 13.17—*continued*

Problem	Patient goals	Nursing intervention	Expected outcomes
diarrhoea resulting from the leukaemic process and chemotherapy		c Provide small appetizing meals that are high in calories and vitamins, non-spicy, bland, and include food preferences of the patient d Administer antiemetics as prescribed to control nausea and vomiting resulting from chemotherapy e When stomatitis is present, rinse the patient's mouth with water or a mild antiseptic mouthwash before each meal f Rinse the mouth with an analgesic agent before meals g Instruct the patient and family on the contents and preparation of nutritious meals h Assist the patient and family to develop a plan for meeting nutritional needs following discharge i Record the patient's weight on a regular schedule	family discuss plans for meeting nutritional and fluid needs following discharge
7 Fluid volume deficit related to the increased fluid requirements needed to eliminate waste products and the decreased fluid intake resulting from stomatitis, nausea, vomiting and diarrhoea	a To maintain an adequate fluid intake b To maintain adequate elimination	a Provide a minimal fluid intake of 2500–3000 ml per day by mouth and supplement with intravenous fluids as necessary b Include fluids that are cool, non-irritating and soothing to the mouth, concentrated for increased caloric value and contain supplemental vitamins c Keep fluids available within reach of the patient d Offer fluid frequently and assist with taking it when the patient is weak e Provide frequent mouth care and oral analgesics when stomatitis is present f Instruct the patient and family about the need for adequate daily fluid intake g Record daily fluid intake and output	1 Fluid intake is 2500–3000 ml per day 2 Urine output is over 1500 ml per day 3 Patient expresses an awareness of the need to maintain adequate daily fluid intake
8 Health management deficit related to lack of knowledge and skills in implementing a long-term treatment plan and measures to prevent complications	a To develop plan to continue prescribed treatment programme b To develop plans for self-care and prevention of complications during periods of remission of the disease c To be able to identify early symptoms of exacerbation of leukaemia and complications d To develop plans to resume daily activities and modified life-style during remission of disease	a Identify the patient's and family's needs and resources for on-going care b Inform the patient and family of community resources for transportation, meals, home care and nursing services c Instruct the patient and family about the diet, oral hygiene, prevention of infection and prevention and control of bleeding d Teach the patient or family members to perform special care procedures such as care of the central venous catheter line or arrange for care by a community nurse e Teach the patient and family to identify changes that might indicate infection, bleeding and exacerbation of disease f Advise the patient who to call or the clinic to contact	The patient: 1 Demonstrates understanding of the treatment plan 2 States plans for continuing treatment on an outpatient basis, transportation and assistance at home 3 Demonstrates knowledge of and skill in preventive measures and special procedures: diet, oral hygiene, prevention of infection, prevention of bleeding, care of central venous catheter 4 Expresses awareness of actions to take when complications develop

Table 13.17—*continued*

Problem	Patient goals	Nursing intervention	Expected outcomes
8 Health management deficit (continued)		when a complication develops **g** Assist the patient and family to develop realistic plans for a return to school or work and resumption of usual daily activities **h** Identify factors interfering with increased socialization and activity and help the patient and family in dealing with, or adjusting to, these: for example, the purchase of a wig when hair loss occurs; wearing clothing that covers bruises; supporting decision-making activities when dependency results from illness and hospitalization **i** Make referrals to appropriate health-care workers or community resources to assist the patient and family with home care and management, financial assistance, spiritual guidance and individual and family coping	5 Is aware of relevant health care resources 6 Resumes activities of daily living
9 Family disruption related to diagnosis, hospitalization, prolonged treatment and resulting changes in role performance and relationships	**a** To maintain functioning of the individual and family as a unit **b** To promote continued growth and development of patient (child)	**a** Assess the impact of illness and hospitalization on the roles and functions of the patient and other members of his family **b** Assist the family to identify resources, such as neighbours, friends and community family services **c** Encourage the participation of the family in care activities and planning meetings **d** Provide privacy for family meetings and interactions **e** Assist the patient and family to develop plans to maintain family functioning and to support individual members by celebrating birthdays, graduations, and encouraging sports and other activities of children **f** Assess the level of growth and development of the child patient **g** Implement play and learning activities that are appropriate for the child's level of development **h** Assist the family to make plans for the child to have contact with other children and return to school as soon as possible **i** Encourage the adult patient to return to work and to resume the parenting role when appropriate **j** Identify communication, sexual, financial or other problems which may arise in the family as a result of the patient's illness and make appropriate referrals for assistance	1 Pre-illness roles by the patient and other members of the family are resumed 2 Plans for an altered role of functioning during periods of illness and treatment are developed 3 There is progression through the normal stages of growth and development for the child

immediate and long-term planning. In Chapter 9, nursing measures for the patient with cancer were discussed for the diagnostic, therapeutic and post-treatment phases of malignant diseases. Table 13.17 identifies patient's problems, goals of nursing, nursing intervention and expected outcomes relevant to patients with leukaemia.

LEUCOPENIA

Leucopenia may be defined as a reduction in the number of leucocytes below the normal lower limit of 5.0×10^9 per litre. It may be due to a decreased production or excessive destruction of leucocytes. The deficiency occurs most often in the granulocytes, especially in neutrophils. Lymphopenia, a deficiency of lymphocytes, occurs rarely but is seen occasionally in patients receiving an adrenocorticoid preparation or adrenocorticotropic hormone (ACTH) and in those with uraemia.

AGRANULOCYTOSIS (NEUTROPENIA)

Agranulocytosis is characterized by a marked reduction in neutrophils.

Causes

In most instances, this blood disorder is the result of the toxic effects of certain drugs in persons with a sensitivity or idiosyncrasy. The drugs found most frequently to be offenders include gold salts, sulphonamides, amidopyrine, phenylbutazone (Butazolidin), chlorpromazine (Largactil) and thiouracil preparations. The condition may also be associated with typhoid fever, malaria, miliary (widespread throughout the body) tuberculosis or any severe, overwhelming infection (e.g. septicaemia).

Neutropenia may be an integral part of the aplastic anaemia that may develop with radiation and anticancer drug therapy, or it may be due to an excessive destruction of the neutrophils by the spleen (hypersplenism). The disease has a higher incidence in females than in males.

Manifestations

Neutrophils play an important role in defending the body against infection because of their ability to ingest and destroy organisms. Neutropenia lowers the normal resistance to infection, resulting in prompt invasion of the mucous membranes and skin by pathogenic organisms. The source of the infecting organisms may be the individual's own body flora.

The disease usually has a sudden onset and is manifested by chills, fever and prostration. The patient complains of a very sore throat and has difficulty in swallowing. Infected, ulcerated areas appear on the mucous membranes in the mouth, throat, rectum and vagina. Skin and respiratory infections may develop. Some patients complain of severe joint pain (arthralgia). The white cell count may be less than 1.5×10^9 per litre of blood.

Treatment and nursing care

Goals for the patient with neutropenia are to: (1) prevent infection, and (2) identify and treat infections promptly when they occur.

Treatment of neutropenia includes prompt elimination of any suspected cause. Antibiotic therapy in large doses is commenced promptly to prevent infection and check that which may be established. If the neutropenia is a part of pancytopenia, a blood transfusion may be given to relieve the anaemia. Granulocyte transfusions may be given in conjunction with antibiotic therapy or alone to patients who fail to respond to antibiotics. If the infection can be controlled and supportive care provided, a gradual increase in the number of neutrophils and improvement in the patient's condition may be expected in 1–2 weeks.

Nursing intervention for the patient with neutropenia is directed toward controlling the patient's environment in order to decrease contact with infectious agents and prompt identification and treatment of infections. The assessment, goals, identification of problems, nursing intervention and expected outcomes for the patient with an increased potential for infection are presented in Chapter 5.

The patient should be cared for in a single room. When the neutropenia is severe, reverse isolation may be used or the patient may be placed in a room with a laminar air-flow system. People contacting or caring for the patient are screened for possible infection and are required to wash their hands thoroughly before attending to the patient. Protective isolation is considered of questionable value by many since infection is usually caused by the patient's own flora. Visitors are restricted to one or two immediate family members who are free of infection, and who are instructed to wash their hands on entering the patient's room or prior to contact.

The prevention of tissue trauma is necessary in the prevention of infection. Care of the mouth is extremely important. It is rinsed or irrigated every 1–2 hours with normal saline or a mild, antiseptic mouthwash. The patient should receive 2000–2500 ml of fluids per day and a high-protein, high-vitamin diet. Because of the oral lesions, the patient may have difficulty taking adequate food. Nutritious fluids, soft bland foods, protein concentrates and vitamin supplements may be used. Raw fruits and vegetables and tap water may be eliminated in the patient's diet and replaced with cooked foods and bottled or boiled water.

Constipation is avoided; the hard stool may injure the intestinal mucosa, making it more vulnerable to infection.

Expected outcomes

The patient:
1 Understands measures to prevent infection.
2 Describes signs of infection and action to take.
3 Demonstrates understanding of the need to maintain optimum general health through good nutrition, personal hygiene, exercise and rest.

Prevention of neutropenia

In some instances, neutropenia might have been prevented if the affected person had understood the danger inherent in self-medication. Whenever the opportunity presents, the nurse has the responsibility of informing lay persons that drugs should only be taken under medical supervision and according to the specific directions of the doctor. It is not uncommon to learn of someone who has been taking a potentially dangerous drug on his own over an abnormally long period of time. Equally dangerous is the situation in which a family member, neighbour or friend shares a drug or suggests one that has been prescribed for him and has proved helpful. They do not appreciate that a drug may affect one person quite differently from another and that it is prescribed by the doctor on an individual basis following a careful study of the patient's condition. Reactions and side-effects are unpredictable; some supervision is necessary to recognize early toxic manifestations.

Disorders of the Plasma Cells

MULTIPLE MYELOMA (MYELOMATOSIS)

Multiple myeloma is a malignant disease characterized by a proliferation of abnormal plasma cells in the bone marrow. Plasma cells are involved in the synthesis of the immunoglobulins that function as antibodies. In multiple myeloma the malignant plasma cells proliferate in the bone marrow, forming diffuse, multiple solid tumours. It occurs in middle to late age and affects both sexes.

Effects and manifestations

Diffuse areas of bone destruction develop; these areas may coalesce and leave large 'punched out lesions'. The breakdown in bone structure frequently results in pathological fractures, especially in weight-bearing bones such as the vertebrae. The patient experiences pain in the areas of the bone lesions, which worsens with movement, jarring and pressure. The vertebrae are a common site of involvement, and pressure on nerve roots by the tumours and/or collapsing vertebrae causes severe back and/or lower limb pain; interruption of nerve

impulses may give rise to paraplegia. Changes in posture and stature become evident. The ribs and skull bones are frequently affected. As tumours and areas of bone destruction develop in the skull, soft subcutaneous masses may be palpated. As the disease progresses, the patient has more and more pain and becomes increasingly incapacitated and deformed. Skeletal x-rays show areas of bone destruction.

The excessive production of abnormal plasma cells results in a decrease in the synthesis of normal immunoglobulins. This decrease in normal antibodies predisposes the patient to infection. The patient experiences recurring infections which are usually respiratory, but bladder infection and skin lesions are not uncommon.

The production of leucocytes, erythrocytes and thrombocytes diminishes as the bone marrow is crowded and replaced by the myeloma. The reduction in white blood cells further predisposes the individual to infection. Symptoms of anaemia (shortness of breath on exertion, pallor, chilliness, weakness) and a bleeding tendency (bleeding gums, petechiae, ecchymoses, melaena) may be manifested.

The breakdown of bone tissue gives rise to the release of calcium and hypercalcaemia develops (normal calcium: 2.2–2.6 mmol/l). The excretion of the serum calcium by the kidneys entails an increased loss of water. If the fluid intake is not correspondingly increased, the patient manifests dehydration, the serum calcium is retained and the urinary output falls. Nausea, loss of appetite, impaired cardiac function and disorientation may occur with hypercalcaemia.

An abnormal protein, referred to as Bence-Jones protein, is excreted by the kidneys. In high concentration this protein may be precipitated in the renal tubules, forming casts and damaging the tubules and possibly resulting in renal insufficiency. The high serum urate (normal: 250 μmol/l or 3–7 mg/dl) incurred by the rapid destruction of cells further contributes to impaired renal function; precipitation of the uric acid in renal tubules can obstruct and destroy them. Another factor that contributes to impaired renal function is the hypercalcaemia cited above.

Laboratory blood tests reveal an elevation in erythrocyte sedimentation rate, erythrocyte, leucocyte and platelet counts below normal, and elevated serum calcium and uric acid levels. Urinalysis may record the presence of Bence-Jones protein. Examination of a bone marrow specimen shows the presence of abnormal plasma cells. Serum electrophoresis demonstrates the presence of abnormal globulin.

Treatment

Care of the patient with multiple myeloma involves the administration of chemotherapeutic agents, radiation therapy and supportive care.

DRUG THERAPY

The chemotherapeutic agents used in the treatment of multiple myeloma are melphalan (Alkeran), cyclophosphamide (Endoxana), prednisone and vincristine (Oncovin). Melphalan is given daily orally in combination with prednisone; it may cause nausea and bone marrow depression. Cyclophosphamide is given daily orally and may cause nausea and vomiting, bone marrow depression, alopecia and haemorrhagic cystitis. The bone marrow depression results in a decreased production of erythrocytes, platelets and leucocytes, in addition to destruction of the plasma cells. This contributes to the anaemia, haemorrhagic tendency and leucopenia that are also caused by bone marrow crowding and replacement by the abnormal plasma cells. The blood cell counts are followed closely; the dosage or protocol for the drug administration may have to be readjusted.

Allopurinol is prescribed to decrease uric acid production and prevent impaired renal function.

RADIATION THERAPY

A series of x-ray treatments to the local areas of involvement may be used to reduce the tumour mass and lessen the pain caused by pressure.

SUPPORTIVE CARE

The patient's anaemia and thrombocytopenia may necessitate blood transfusions. If the fluid balance is negative, whole blood is used. If the oral intake has been adequate, packed red blood cells and platelets are transfused to prevent overtaxing the heart by overload. The patient is observed closely for reactions during and following the transfusion (see pp. 291–293).

Nursing process

ASSESSMENT

Frequent assessments are necessary, as significant changes may occur in a very short period of time. Laboratory data are noted so that the nurse may make the necessary modifications in the care plan according to the findings. For example, it is important to know if the patient's anaemia is worsening or improving, to be aware of the leucocyte count in order to judge susceptibility to infection, and to ascertain whether the platelet count is such that there is a predisposition to haemorrhage. The specific gravity of the urine is noted; if it is high, it may indicate an increase in serum calcium and/or urate and the need to increase the fluid intake.

The fluid intake and output are recorded and the balance noted.

The patient should be observed frequently for signs of infection; the temperature is taken, respirations noted and the skin and mouth checked for lesions.

Posture, the degree of freedom or difficulty with which the patient moves and the amount of incapacity are evaluated constantly. Any numbness or loss of movement is promptly reported to the doctor. Observations are also made for the possible toxic effects of the chemotherapeutic agent(s) that the patient is receiving.

POTENTIAL PATIENT PROBLEMS

The problems likely to be encountered by the patient with plasma cell disorders (multiple myeloma) are as follows:
1 Anxiety related to diagnosis of a potentially fatal disease, impending treatment and discomfort.
2 Impaired physical mobility related to the disease process and complications, particularly bone and spinal cord involvement and pain.
3 Alterations in comfort (chronic, progressive pain) related to bone lesions.
4 Fluid volume deficit related to decreased fluid intake due to oral lesions and increased fluid requirements for adequate elimination of calcium and urates.
5 Potential for infection related to altered immune system and decreased white blood cell production.
6 Lack of knowledge related to alterations in mobility, safety, fluid intake, prevention of infection, comfort, treatment plan and health care resources.

Goals for the patient with multiple myeloma are to:
1 Decrease the level of anxiety
2 (a) Promote and attain realistic mobility and functioning
   (b) Prevent injury and complications
3 Minimize pain and promote comfort
4 Maintain an adequate fluid intake
5 (a) Prevent infection
   (b) Identify and treat infections promptly when they occur
6 Understand the health management plan

NURSING INTERVENTION

1. *Decrease anxiety*
The nature of the disease, therapeutic programme and potential side-effects of the chemotherapeutic agents should be outlined to the patient and his family by the doctor. It is important for the nurse to know if they have been told. Obviously it is a blow to learn that the disorder is malignant. The nurse should provide opportunities and time for the patient and family to ask questions and she should be willing and prepared to listen to them and discuss the situation. The patient may be fearful of the pain becoming more severe; assurance is given that measures will be used to effectively control the pain.

2. Mobility and positioning

Ambulation and activity are promoted within the limits of the individual's capacity. Inactivity, bed rest and immobilization cause decalcification of osseous tissue, adding to the demineralization of bone tissue by the disease process and contributing to the hypercalcaemia. The patient moves slowly and precautions are taken to prevent the possibility of falls.

As the disease advances and the patient becomes more incapacitated, walking with assistance and limb exercises are encouraged as long as possible. Activities that are important to the patient are planned; rest periods are scheduled to prevent exhaustion. If pathological fractures occur, bed rest and casts are used only if absolutely necessary. When the spine is involved, a brace or corset may be helpful when the patient is out of bed. Whenever assistance is provided, the nurse 'handles' the patient with gentle, slow movements; support is provided for limbs and joints. Quick, jarring movements may cause a fracture or muscle spasm with severe pain.

A fracture board (or a firm-based bed) and firm mattress are necessary. Moving and bumping against the bed should be avoided since even very slight jarring of the patient may cause muscle spasm and pain. Frequently the patient finds it difficult to find a comfortable position. The nurse must be patient as well as resourceful; soft and firm pillows of various sizes are used to provide support, and a cradle is used to take the weight of the bedding. In the advanced stages of the disease it may be easier for the patient if he is cared for on a Stryker frame.

3. Pain control

Gentle supportive movement and positioning are important in reducing discomfort and providing relief of pain. If the patient is experiencing considerable muscle spasm, a muscle relaxant may be prescribed. Analgesics are used; initially, a mild preparation such as paracetamol (Panadol), dextropropoxylene hydrochloride (Distalgesic) may provide relief. Later a stronger preparation is required. It may be helpful to give the patient an analgesic 15–30 minutes before bathing, getting him up or carrying out an exercise schedule.

4. Fluids

A daily fluid intake of at least 3000 ml is necessary to replace the increased loss incurred by the hypercalcaemia and to promote elimination of urate. The patient's preferences are determined and the fluids must be placed within easy reach since movement is painful. If the oral intake is inadequate, intravenous infusion is used to meet the requirement.

Because of oliguria or other renal symptoms, renal function tests or an intravenous pyelogram may be done. Fluids must not be withheld for any of these since dehydration could cause acute renal failure.

5. Protection from infection

The patient's susceptibility to infection necessitates special precautions. Measures to protect the patient from infection are discussed in detail in Chapter 5.

6. Patient teaching

When the initial chemotherapeutic course is completed the patient is usually permitted to go home. He and his family are advised about the following:

(a) The need to keep active/moving and the importance of setting priorities. Activities that the patient will enjoy are planned provided that they will not make excessive demands on his energy. The plan includes frequent rest periods.

(b) Precautions against falling. Suggestions are made to remove scatter rugs, footstools and anything that might trip him. Waxed and highly polished floors should be avoided.

(c) The importance of an adequate fluid intake to prevent kidney complications.

(d) The need for a fracture board (or firm-based bed) and firm mattress.

(e) Protection against infection. Such measures as avoiding contact with those with an infection, disinfecting the infected person's dishes in the case of a respiratory infection, avoiding chilling, and using good mouth and skin hygienic measures are emphasized.

(f) Early recognition of respiratory infection, mouth and skin lesions, and impaired renal function, and the need for prompt contact with the clinic or the doctor if these appear.

(g) The need to promptly report change in posture or the contour of a limb (which might indicate a fracture), any numbness, marked weakness or loss of movement, inability to void and increased severity in pain.

(h) Medications. Following the initial course of chemotherapy, the patient is continued on maintenance doses. He will also require an analgesic preparation. Allopurinol may also be continued. The purpose of these drugs, the administration schedule and early signs of toxic reactions are reviewed. Pertinent information (dosage, frequency time and reactions that should prompt contacting the doctor) should be given to the family in writing.

(i) Sources of assistance. A referral should be made to the district or community liaison nurse. The patient and family are usually reassured by the nurse's visits. They provide frequent assessment of the patient's progress and the family situation and suggestions and guidance are provided as new problems arise.

(j) The importance of keeping the frequent appointments with the clinic or doctor. Frequent reassessment of the patient and blood studies are necessary. The patient's capacity is evaluated; he may be forcing himself to 'keep going' to protect the family.

EXPECTED OUTCOMES

The patient:
1 Expresses decreased feelings of anxiety.
2 Receives prompt identification and treatment of infections when they occur.
3 Takes fluids in excess of 2500 ml per day.
4 Continues activities within the limits of his ability.
5 Does not acquire complications from immobility such as contractures, renal impairment or decubitus ulcers.
6 Bone fractures from trauma do not occur.
7 Does not experience pain of moderate or severe intensity.
8 Demonstrates understanding of the health management plan and community resources.

Disorders of the Lymphatic System

INFECTIOUS MONONUCLEOSIS

This is a benign infectious disease involving the lymphatic system and is seen most commonly in adolescents and young adults. The causative organism is the Epstein-Barr virus (EBV). The disease is not highly infectious, but may be transmitted by close personal contact.

Manifestations

The symptoms vary from one patient to another. Common complaints are sore throat, gingivitis, headache, tiredness, anorexia and general malaise. The patient has a fever which may be intermittent, and there is enlargement and tenderness of the superficial lymph nodes (cervical, axillary and inguinal). The spleen is usually enlarged and tender, and palpation may also reveal abdominal tenderness due to involvement of the mesenteric lymph nodes. Some patients develop an erythematous or maculopapular rash. Some patients are jaundiced as a result of the development of hepatitis.

The total leucocyte count is elevated and may range from $10.0–20.0 \times 10^9$ per litre. A differential count reveals an increase in lymphocytes and monocytes, and many of the lymphocytes are atypical. The percentage of granulocytes may be below normal. The patient may experience anaemia due to increased haemolysis. Diagnosis may be confirmed by a positive Paul–Bunnell test. Heterophile antibodies appear in the serum of patients with infectious mononucleosis; these antibodies cause the agglutination of sheep blood cells, which is the basis of the Paul–Bunnell test. The Paul–Bunnell reaction does not usually become positive until after the first week of infection. Recently a mononucleosis spot test (Monospot test) has been used; it is easier to carry out and is considered to be more specific.

Treatment and nursing care

Goals for the patient with infectious mononucleosis are to:
1 Obtain adequate rest until the temperature returns to normal
2 Relieve discomfort
3 Prevent spread of the infection to others
4 Prevent secondary infections

The disease usually runs a self-limited course of 2–4 weeks. The treatment is symptomatic and supportive. The patient is in bed until the temperature is normal. Aspirin or aspirin compound (e.g. aspirin, caffeine and codeine) or Distalgesic is usually prescribed to relieve the headache, general body discomfort and sore throat. Warm saline throat irrigations may also help to relieve the sore throat. A high-calorie, high-protein diet is recommended to support the patient's resistance. The patient may become discouraged and depressed as the illness continues for weeks; he may even be fearful of the outcome. The nurse should convey understanding to the patient, accept his reactions and provide reassurance that although improvement appears slow he will return to normal activities. Convalescence is usually prolonged; an effort is made to find an interest for the patient (e.g. reading, radio, television): the occupational therapy department may provide assistance. He is warned that fatigue and having less than his accustomed strength and tolerance may be expected for several weeks. His previous activities should be resumed gradually and the need for extra rest is stressed.

The patient may develop a secondary throat infection; frequently it is due to ß-haemolytic streptococci and is treated with an antibiotic.

Expected outcomes

The patient with infectious mononucleosis:
1 Demonstrates an understanding of the disease, method of transmission and the need to avoid fatigue.
2 Describes a plan to obtain rest and prevent fatigue.
3 Describes measures to promote comfort.
4 Understands the measures required to prevent spread of the infection.
5 Promptly recognizes the occurrence of secondary infections and seeks treatment.

Malignant Lymphomas

This is a term that may be applied to a group of neoplastic diseases that primarily affect lymphoid tissue (nodes and spleen). They are characterized by painless, progressive enlargement of lymph nodes and spleen. In some the proliferating cells invade extralymphatic tissues and organs. These diseases include Hodgkin's disease (lymphadenoma), lymphocytic lymphoma (lymphosarcoma), histiocytic lymphoma (reticulum cell sarcoma) and Burkitt's lymphoma (stem cell lymphoma). They are classified according to the cells identified with lymph node biopsy. Histologically they show marked differences, but the signs and symptoms are similar for all types. The painless enlargement of one or more lymph nodes is usually the initial presenting disturbance. The patient gradually develops general malaise, fatigue, weight loss, fever, sweating and splenic enlargement. Investigation and assessment of the extent of the disease is similar for the various types of lymphomas.

HODGKIN'S DISEASE (LYMPHADENOMA)

Hodgkin's disease is a disease of unknown aetiology that involves lymphoid tissue. It may develop at any age but usually occurs in adolescents and young adults. There is a higher incidence of the disorder in males. Until recently Hodgkin's disease was always considered a fatal condition. Impressive advances have been made in assessing the extent of the lymph node involvement and treating the affected areas with radiation and chemotherapeutic agents.

Signs and symptoms

The disease has an insidious onset and is manifested by painless enlargement of one group of lymph nodes (usually cervical at the beginning). The disease spreads progressively to other lymphoid tissues throughout the body and a variety of symptoms develop, depending upon the lymphoid tissue involved. The enlarging lymph nodes may cause pressure on nerves, resulting in pain, or may impose on neighbouring organs, causing dysfunction. Axillary and inguinal nodes frequently interfere with venous and lymph drainage, leading to oedema in the arms and legs. Enlarged mediastinal nodes may produce a distressing cough, dyspnoea or difficulty in swallowing (dysphagia). The spleen becomes enlarged, causing abdominal discomfort.

Constitutional symptoms are not prominent until the later stages. The patient gradually develops fatigue, weakness, fever, anorexia, loss of weight and pruritis. These are likely to be seriously aggravated by the treatments used (radiation, chemotherapy). Fluctuations in the symptoms and size of the nodes may occur.

The leucocyte count varies with patients; it may be increased or it may be normal or below normal. The differential count indicates a deficiency in the lymphocytes. Diagnosis is established by biopsy of an affected lymph node. Large atypical cells known as Reed–Sternberg giant cells are characteristic of Hodgkin's disease.

Assessment of extent of disease (staging)

When the diagnosis of Hodgkin's disease has been confirmed, a series of investigative procedures are carried out to determine the extent of lymphoid tissue involvement. The treatment and prognosis depend upon the findings. A classification into four stages has been made according to the degree of involvement (Table 13.18). The classifying process may be referred to as 'staging'.

Table 13.18 Classification of extent of involvement in Hodgkin's disease (staging).*

Stage	Degree of involvement
I	Disease confined to one anatomic site or two contiguous anatomic sites on the same side of the diaphragm
II	Disease in more than two anatomic sites or in two non-contiguous sites and confined to one side of the diaphragm
III	Disease on both sides of the diaphragm but confined to lymph nodes, spleen and Waldeyer's ring
IV	Involvement of extranodal sites other than by direct invasion from affected node

For each stage of the classification:
A = Asymptomatic
B = Presence of typical symptoms (fever, night sweats and weight loss)

*Smith & Thier (1985), p. 279.

The assessment made to determine the stage of the disease may include chest x-rays, computerized axial tomography (CAT), lymphangiography, inferior venacavography, liver, spleen and bone scans, liver function tests and laparoscopy or exploratory laparotomy.

A *lymphangiogram* involves the introduction of a radiopaque preparation into a lymphatic vessel in each foot. The 'dye' is injected over 1–2 hours and x-rays are then taken of the lower limbs, abdomen and chest. Enlarged and diseased lymph nodes may be visualized on the films. Follow-up x-rays may be taken over a period of time to assess the effect of the treatment without further injection of the dye, since the initial dose remains in the lymphatic nodes for many weeks.

A *venacavogram* requires the injection of a radiopaque preparation through a catheter into a femoral vein. Abdominal x-ray films are then made.

A *laparoscopy* may be done to determine extralymphatic involvement. The exploratory laparotomy provides more thorough evaluation of the extent of abdominal visceral and mesenteric lymphatic node involvement. Biopsies may be done and the spleen may be removed.

An explanation of the purpose(s) of each investigational procedure is made to the patient and what he may expect is outlined. A signed consent is required. No special preparations are required for the angiography. Laparoscopy and laparotomy may require preoperative shaving and cleansing of the abdomen. A sedative is usually given ½–1 hour before the scheduled time, and food and fluid are withheld for the preceding 8 hours. Following the laparoscopy, the patient is observed closely for the possible complications of haemorrhage and shock. Abdominal pain, distension or rigidity is reported promptly to the doctor. Laparotomy involves complete postoperative care (see p. 201).

The scans that may be done on the liver, spleen and bones require the administration of a radioisotope for which each of these structures has an affinity. A graph of the rays emitted by the radioactive substance is made, which indicates its concentration in the particular organ or structure being evaluated. *Computerized axial tomography (CAT scan)* is a non-invasive radiological technique which provides a cross-sectional view of a body area and information about the density and size of body organs and tissues.

Treatment and nursing care

Treatment may consist of radiation therapy, chemotherapy or a combination of both. The patient requires psychological and physiological supportive care.

RADIATION THERAPY

This is used when the Hodgkin's disease is regionally localized. The patients in stages I and II receive a series of irradiation to all involved sites. Depending upon the extralymphatic involvement, patients in stages III and IV may also receive radiation therapy. The series of treatments, what may be expected during the x-ray treatment, the necessary care and possible reactions should be discussed with the patient and family (see p. 155). When the location of the lymph nodes being irradiated is the neck, chest or abdomen, the patient is observed for coughing, dyspnoea, sore throat, dysphagia, nausea and vomiting. Haemoglobin concentration and blood cell counts are determined frequently, since bone marrow depression may occur. Nausea and persisting fatigue are the most common problems. The patient is advised to plan for rest periods during the day and to retire early. Antiemetics and small, frequent, selective meals may be necessary to relieve the nausea. The patient is reassured that these problems will be temporary.

CHEMOTHERAPY

This may be used to treat patients of stage III disease. The drugs used include mustine hydrochloride (nitrogen mustard), vincristine (Oncovin), prednisone, procarbazine (Natulan), vinblastine and cyclophosphamide (Cytoxan). A combination of three or four drugs may be given over 14 days followed by 2 weeks rest without treatment. Three to six series of treatment, each followed by 2 weeks rest, are usually given.

Toxic reactions to the drugs include nausea, vomiting, diarrhoea, stomatitis, bone marrow depression, alopecia and dermatitis. Vincristine and vinblastine are administered intravenously and precautions must be observed to avoid extravasation of the solution into the tissues because of the necrosis that may follow. These two drugs may also have some side-effects on the central nervous system. The patient is observed for loss of reflexes, coordination, sensation and ability to move (see Table 13.15).

NURSING INTERVENTION

The potential patient problems, goals and nursing interventions for the patient with Hodgkin's disease are similar to those for the patient with leukaemia. (See patient care plan for the patient with leukaemia p. 270). Following the investigational procedures and initial therapy, the patient—especially one with stage I, II or III disease—returns home and is encouraged to resume, as much as possible, his former pattern of life. The patient's care is fully discussed with him and the family; such factors as prevention of infection, the importance of regular visits to the doctor or clinic for reassessment, the need for extra rest, medications and coping with therapy reactions are emphasized.

LYMPHOCYTIC LYMPHOMA (LYMPHOMA SARCOMA)

This is a neoplastic disease of lymphoid tissue characterized by a proliferation of lymphocytes. Unlike leukaemia, the cells are confined within the lymphoid tissues until the later stages of the disease. It occurs more often in males and in those over 40 years of age.

The disease progresses similarly to Hodgkin's disease; usually only one area of lymphoid tissue is affected at first, but there is a gradual dissemination to other regions. The symptoms are largely dependent upon the location of the tumours. They reflect the pressure and interference imposed on neighbouring structures by the enlarging lymphoid tissues. Fever and progressive debilitation accompany the extension and increasing severity of the disease. The treatment employed is the same as that used for Hodgkin's disease.

CUTANEOUS T CELL LYMPHOMA (MYCOSIS FUNGOIDES AND SÉZARY'S SYNDROME)

These two disorders are characterized by T cell infiltrations in the skin. Mycosis fungoides, a chronic malignant lymphoreticular skin disease, begins with round or oval, superficial scaling areas of the skin resembling eczema or psoriasis. The lesions are itchy and may spontaneously disappear and then reappear. The premycotic stage may last up to 6 years. The second stage is characterized by irregular thickening of the skin, with raised plaques and red–brown or red–yellow hues. The third stage is characterized by mushroom-like growths, painful fissures, scalp involvement with alopecia and enlarged lymph nodes. Infiltration of other organs can occur in the second and third stages.

Sézary's syndrome is characterized by a generalized pruritus and erythroderma with thick scaly plaques on the palms and soles, alopecia, nail dystrophy, enlarged lymph nodes (due to the infiltration of lymphocytes) and the presence of circulating abnormal 'Sezary cells' and increased leucocytes.

Treatment consists of total body electron beam radiation of approximately 12 treatments over 3 weeks. If a skin biopsy performed 3 months later is positive, topical nitrogen mustard therapy is initiated.[29] Chemotherapy is initiated if the disease fails to respond and in the late stages. A combination drug regimen from doxorubicin (Adriamycin), methotrexate, vincristine, bleomycin, cyclosphosphamide and prednisone is prescribed and may be accompanied by electron beam therapy. Other treatment forms may include the use of ultraviolet radiation with an oral photosensitizing drug (PUVA) or leucapheresis which removes circulating leucocytes or anti-T cell antibodies.

In the early stages, patients are able to continue their usual daily activities. As the disease progresses, the patient requires instruction about keeping the skin clean and moist and preventing infection. Also in the later stages, the patient's physical appearance changes, and lesions become painful with large amounts of drainage.

Haemorrhagic Disorders

An abnormal tendency to bleed may be due to a disorder of the clotting mechanism, an excess of anticoagulant or a vascular defect. A haemorrhagic disorder is characterized by: prolonged bleeding following tissue damage; spontaneous bleeding into mucous membrane, skin and organs; and bleeding in more than one area of the body.

Failure of the clotting mechanism may result from a deficiency of any of the essential factors in the coagulation process (see p. 245). These disorders include haemophilia, hypoprothrombinaemia and thrombocytopenia.

When a haemorrhagic disorder is suspected it is important to note the form in which the bleeding presents; purpural areas, haematoma, ecchymoses, oozing or free flow from wound, and whether from single or multiple sites. Wallerstein states that

'Purpuric spots suggest a capillary or platelet defect; they are not characteristic of haemophilia. Hematomas, hemarthroses, or large ecchymoses at the site of trauma suggest hemophilia. Sudden, severe bleeding from multiple sites after prolonged surgery or during obstetric procedures suggests acquired fibrinogen deficiency. Massive bleeding from a single site without a history of purpura or previous bleeding suggests a surgical or anatomic defect rather than a coagulation defect.'[30]

It is important to determine:
1 If the individual has a history of bleeding—that is, has this type of response been occurring since early childhood, or is this the initial incidence?
2 How long the bleeding has been taking place.
3 If there is anyone in the family with a history of a similar problem.
4 What precipitated this bleeding (e.g. trauma, visit to the dentist).

THROMBOCYTOPENIA (THROMBOCYTOPENIC PURPURA)

Failure of the coagulation process may be due to a deficiency of circulating thrombocytes (blood platelets), known as thrombocytopenia. Thrombocyte deficiency may be due to failure in the production of thrombocytes, pooling of platelets in splenomegaly, dilutional loss resulting from excessive blood transfusions within a short period or increased destruction of thrombocytes.

Insufficient thrombocyte production may be associated with leukaemia or lupus erythematosus or may be caused by bone marrow suppression resulting from drugs or radiation. Destruction of thrombocytes may result from excessive intravascular coagulation, damage to thrombocytes from abnormal blood vessel walls or from an antigen–antibody reaction in which the person develops antibodies (agglutins) which destroy the thrombocytes. The latter is referred to as immune thrombocytopenia which may be idiopathic (cause unknown) or caused by drugs, transfusions of platelets carrying PLA–1 antigen, or transfer of maternal antibodies across the placenta to the neonate. The normal life span for platelets is approximately 8–10 days; in idiopathic thrombocytopenia their survival rate is only 1–3 days. The cause of the antibody production

[29] Brain & Carbone (1985), pp. 92–93.

[30] Krupp & Chatton (1983), p. 324.

is not known, but in most cases of idiopathic thrombocytopenia antibodies can be detected.

Manifestations

The disorder is manifested by bleeding in any site. Petechiae and purpuric areas may appear in the skin or mucous membranes and bleeding from the nose or from the gastrointestinal or urinary tract may occur. Children and young adults, especially females, are more often affected. The severity of the disease varies, and alternating remissions and relapses may occur.

Treatment

Treatment is directed toward removing the cause of the thrombocytopenia (e.g. withdrawal of drugs that suppress the bone marrow) to protect the patient from trauma and ensuing bleeding.

The patient is kept at rest and is treated with an adrenocorticoid preparation (e.g. prednisone) and transfusions of fresh blood or platelets. If the patient does not respond favourably to these measures, splenectomy may be performed. Although the spleen does not become enlarged, it appears to be active in thrombocytopenia. It separates out and harbours the platelets and is suspected of producing some antibody.

BLOOD CLOTTING FACTOR DEFICIENCY

Failure of the coagulation process may result from a decrease in the quantity or abnormal function of any one of the factors which promote the blood clotting process. A deficiency of some factors occurs rarely and symptoms of factor deficiencies vary from mild to severe. The disorders include haemophilia (A and B), Factor VIII and Factor IX deficiencies.

Haemophilia is a coagulation disorder that occurs in males as a result of a deficiency of the Factor VIII (the antihaemophilic factor) or Factor IX (the Christmas factor). If the bleeding tendency is the result of a deficiency of Factor VIII, the disease is referred to as *haemophilia A*; if it is the result of a deficiency of Factor IX, it is known as *haemophilia B* or *Christmas disease*. It is inherited as a sex-linked recessive trait. The defective gene is carried on an X chromosome and is transmitted from mother to son.

The female has two X sex chromosomes, and the male has one X and one Y. If a female inherits an X chromosome bearing the haemophilic gene from her father, she becomes a carrier. The disorder is not manifested in her because the X chromosome with the abnormal gene is dominated by the normal X chromosome. If the carrier marries a non-haemophiliac, there is a 50% chance her daughters will be carriers. Her male progeny have a 50% chance of being haemophilic (see Table 13.19). The sons of a haemophilic father receive only a Y chromosome

from him, so the disorder is not passed on to them or their descendants. All daughters of a haemophilic male carry the trait since the father's genetic contribution to each is an X chromosome, which in his case bears the defective gene (see Table 13.19).

Manifestations

Haemophilia is usually recognized within the first year or two of life. Excessive bleeding from the umbilical cord does not occur because of the transplacental transfer of the mother's clotting factors to the fetus. Occasionally, persistent bleeding when the infant is circumcised leads to early diagnosis of the disorder.

The severity varies in individuals; some bleed excessively with very slight trauma and others bleed only with a more severe injury or during incidents such as tooth extraction or surgery. The important characteristic feature of the bleeding is its persistence rather than the amount. Most children experience some bleeding into joints, especially the knees, ankles and elbows. With some, this may be so severe that, as well as causing pain, it produces crippling deformities. As the blood clot organizes, fibrous adhesions may cause ankylosis. Haematomas and haematuria may be manifested. Early death may occur as a result of the pressure of a haematoma (collection of blood within tissue) on a vital structure, or from the loss of blood. The latter is rarely fatal since blood and plasma have become so readily available.

Laboratory blood studies indicate a prolonged whole blood clotting time (normal: 5–11 minutes when glass tubes are used); the bleeding time (normal: 2–9 minutes), blood platelet count (normal: 150–400 × 10^9 per litre) and prothrombin time (normal 11–15 seconds) are normal. The activated partial thromboplastin time is prolonged (normal: 30–45 seconds). Quantitative assays of Factors VIII and IX are performed.

Treatment and care

The patient (if old enough) and the family are alerted to the need for continuous on-going care.

A. TREATMENT OF EPISODES OF BLEEDING

Control of bleeding will depend on the level of the clotting factors in the blood. If Factor VIII is low, it can be replaced by Factor VIII infusion, fresh frozen plasma or cryoprecipitate (children). Fibrinogen can also be used. Factor VIII concentrate is heat-treated. If the patient is Factor IX deficient it can be replaced, although it is only available as a commercial product. If Factor VIII levels are below 2%, synthetic vasopressin may also be used.

Cryoprecipitate of the antihaemophilic factor (prepared from frozen fresh plasma) may be used when treating the patient with haemophilia A.

Table 13.19 Genetic possibilities in haemophilia.

		Normal male		
		X	Y	
Female carrier	X	XX	XY	XX Normal female
	X^h	X^hX	X^hY	XY Normal male
				X^hX Female carrier
				X^hY Male with haemophilia

		Male with haemophilia		
		X^h	Y	
Normal female	X	XX^h	XY	XX^h Female carrier
	X	XX^h	XY	XY Normal male

The advantage of the commercial concentrates and cryoprecipitate is that either can be infused in a small volume; this prevents overloading of the individual's cardiovascular system.

During an episode of bleeding the patient is confined to bed. If there is bleeding into a joint, the joint is immobilized and attention is given to positioning with good alignment to reduce possible deformity. The patient may be fearful of using the joint after the bleeding has been arrested in case of further haemorrhage; he must be encouraged to resume activity as soon as possible to prevent ankylosis. Full range-of-motion exercises are started 48 hours after the bleeding has been controlled

B. PROPHYLACTIC AND SUPPORTIVE MEASURES

Nursing responsibilities include planning and implementing instruction for the patient and family about the nature of the disorder, safe activities, necessary precautions, recognition of the need for factor replacement, and appropriate action when bleeding occurs. In some instances one or two members of the family may be taught the administration of the prescribed concentrate.

Patients are urged to seek prompt treatment following trauma and on the earliest symptoms of bleeding; for example, replacement of the deficient factor is recommended as soon as the patient experiences slight tightness or pressure in a joint, especially if he knows it has received a bump.

It should be emphasized that the person with haemophilia should always carry some form of identification indicating the disorder and blood type.

The patient and family are advised to carry on as normal a life as possible. The severity of the disease determines the restrictions placed on the individual's activities; they must be consistent with safety but there are non-traumatic sports, occupations and

forms of recreation in which he may and should be encouraged to participate. Parents and siblings are warned against overprotection and promoting dependency. If of school age, the patient is usually able to attend a normal school. The teachers should be informed of the individual's condition, the necessary restrictions and precautions and what to do if he receives an injury or bleeding commences. For the child whose disease is severe, arrangements may be made for him to pursue his education at home or to attend special classes. The problem must be kept in mind when selecting toys and sport equipment.

During the teaching sessions the patient and family are informed that patients with haemophilia must not be given aspirin because of its tendency to promote bleeding. Parenteral administrations must also be kept to a minimum; usually the introduction of a needle is restricted to the administration of the antihaemophilic factor.

Good dental hygiene is stressed so that extractions may be avoided. A very soft brush to clean the teeth is recommended to prevent trauma and bleeding of the gums. The patient's dentist is advised of the disorder on the initial visit so that the necessary precautions can be taken.

A referral may be given to the district nurse and health visitor so that home visits may be made to provide necessary assistance and supervision. The patient and family are acquainted with the resources of a local haemophilia society.

The genetic possibilities in offspring are reviewed with parents and young adults in the family. A referral may be made to the appropriate clinic for genetic counselling.

C. COMPLICATIONS

Some patients, after receiving several doses of a factor concentrate, develop antibodies to the factor.

Precautions and activity restrictions have to be reassessed and are usually made more rigid. If a bleeding episode occurs, a much larger dose of the antihaemophilic preparation may be prescribed in an effort to counteract the antibody activity.

Repeated haemarthroses (bleeding into joints) may lead to ankylosis and crippling.

WILLEBRAND'S DISEASE

This disorder resembles haemophilia but occurs in both sexes. It is characterized by prolonged bleeding, bruising and nose-bleeds.

This is an autosomally transmitted disorder caused by a deficiency of a protein, the von Willebrand factor. This factor is necessary for normal platelet function and interacts with another protein involved in Factor VIII production. The patient therefore has a deficiency of Factor VIII and defective platelet adhesion resulting in a prolonged bleeding time. The platelet count is normal. Bleeding is controlled by the administration of cryoprecipitate.

PROTHROMBIN, FACTOR VII, FACTOR IX AND FACTOR X DEFICIENCIES (VITAMIN K DEFICIENCY)

Vitamin K is essential in the production of prothrombin and Factors VII, IX and X by the liver. A deficiency may result from a deficient supply, impaired absorption or defective utilization of vitamin K. If the diet does not supply an adequate amount, it is synthesized by the bacteria which normally inhabit the intestinal tract. The bleeding tendency in the newborn is attributed to the lack of bacterial synthesis of vitamin K during the first 2–3 days of life when the tract is free of organisms. Sterilization of the bowel by the oral administration of sulphonamides or antibiotics may produce a vitamin K deficiency.

Bile salts are essential in the intestine for the absorption of vitamin K. A frequent cause of a deficiency of prothrombin and Factors VII, IX and X is obstruction to the flow of bile into the small intestine. An insufficient production of prothrombin may also occur in liver disease, such as chronic cirrhosis.

Vitamin K deficiency due to impaired synthesis or absorption is treated with a synthetic preparation of vitamin K [phytomenadione, (Konakion)] which may be administered parenterally or orally. When the deficiency is due to liver disease, the patient may receive blood transfusions to supply prothrombin and the deficient factors.

EXCESS OF ANTICOAGULANT (COUMARIN/HEPARIN TOXICITY)

Haemorrhage may be a complication of excessive anticoagulant drug therapy. The products commonly used are heparin and preparations of coumarins (e.g. warfarin) and phenindione (Dindevan). Heparin inhibits the conversion of prothrombin to thrombin. Coumarin preparations prevent the utilization of vitamin K to form prothrombin. If bleeding occurs, administration of the drug is stopped. Whole blood transfusion may be necessary and, in the case of heparin, protamine sulphate is used as an antidote. If the bleeding is due to the other two anticoagulants cited above, parenteral injections of vitamin K are administered as well as blood transfusions.

Prolonged administration of aspirin may cause bleeding in some patients; it causes reduced platelet stickiness. High doses reduce amounts of Factors V, VII and X and prothrombin.[30b]

VASCULAR PURPURA

In some instances, bleeding into tissues and organs occurs because of damage to or a defect in the small blood vessels. The result may be increased permeability or inadequate vasoconstriction, predisposing to blood loss. This type of disorder may be associated with an allergic reaction, septicaemia or a vitamin C deficiency (scurvy).

A rare hereditary bleeding disorder known as hereditary haemorrhagic telangiectasia is characterized by dilated, thin-walled vessels (especially veins) that lack the normal amount of muscular tissue. Angiomas (tumours composed of blood vessels) appear on the skin and mucous membrane surfaces, and normal vasoconstriction does not take place in the affected vessels.

DISSEMINATED INTRAVASCULAR COAGULATION (DIC) (DEFIBRINATION SYNDROME)

Disseminated intravascular coagulation (DIC) is a potentially fatal condition that is a secondary development in a serious primary illness. It is characterized by two phases. In the first phase multiple diffuse microthrombi develop within the vascular system. This widespread coagulation depletes the blood of thrombocytes and several clotting factors to the extent that haemorrhage occurs. This is the second phase of the disorder. Contributing to the haemorrhagic phase is the fibrinolysis that occurs.

DIC may be seen as a complication in many disorders which include any condition associated with extensive tissue damage, shock, severe infections (especially those associated with gram-negative organisms), severe trauma, burns, extensive metastatic disease, surgery involving extracorporeal shunts, and obstetrical complications (toxaemia and abruptio placentae).

Factors involved with the onset of DIC include hypotension, usually associated with shock acidaemia, and stasis of capillary blood.[31] The process

[30b] Richards, Linch & Goldstone (1984).
[31] Voegelpohl (1981), p. 38.

involves diffuse traumatization of tissue cells and/or blood platelets by the primary disorder; thromboplastin is released which triggers the clotting process. The blood clots may seriously interfere with the blood supply to some tissues and organs, resulting in impaired function. Respiratory insufficiency and renal failure are common ensuing problems.

Plasminogen is activated during the pathological clotting and forms the enzyme plasmin, which breaks down the fibrin of clots and fibrinogen. The degradation products of this dissolution process inhibit the thrombin–fibrinogen reaction which yields fibrin. They cause a prolonged thrombin time and retard the production of thromboplastin. Obviously, these reactions inhibit coagulation and cause haemorrhage.

Disseminated intravascular coagulation differs from normal clotting in that: (1) it is diffuse rather than localized; (2) it damages, rather than fulfils, the normal protective role; and (3) it consumes prothrombin, fibrinogen, platelets, Factor V and Factor VIII faster than they can be produced and so bleeding occurs.[32]

Manifestations

There are indications in the patient's general condition of regression. Diffuse bleeding occurs in various areas and may be evident by petechiae, ecchymoses, haematuria, gastrointestinal bleeding, vaginal bleeding, epistaxis, or persistent oozing from a surgical wound or needle puncture. The patient may complain of pain as a result of bleeding into tissues. Oliguria and respiratory distress may develop.

Laboratory blood studies indicate a marked decrease in the number of blood platelets, decreased levels of fibrinogen and Factors V and VIII, and prolonged prothrombin, thrombin and partial thromboplastin times.

Treatment and nursing care

Treatment is directed toward reversing the primary disorder and arresting the diffuse coagulation process.

Heparin may be given intravenously to interrupt the formation of thrombi; this allows the level of blood platelets and fibrinogen to rise. Cryoprecipitate may be administered to increase other blood clotting factors. A transfusion of whole blood is given to compensate for the loss incurred, and platelets may be given for thrombocytopenia.

The patient is critically ill and the nurse is concerned with the primary condition as well as the blood disorder. Care includes: (1) maintaining blood pressure and volume, (2) preventing trauma that could initiate further bleeding, and (3) preventing stasis and correcting hypoxaemia and acidosis.[33] Close observation is made for bleeding, and frequent assessment of the patient's vital signs and general condition is necessary. The hourly urinary output is noted. Continuous cardiac monitoring may be set up and, if respiratory insufficiency occurs, the patient may be put on a mechanical ventilator (see p. 448).

Nursing patients with a tendency to bleed

Specific nursing needs of patients with haemorrhagic disorders vary with each individual and with the cause, associated symptoms, and severity of the disease, but there are some common problems and general considerations applicable to all. These are presented in the patient care plan in Table 13.20.

Blood Transfusion

An infusion of blood or blood components may be given to: (1) replace blood lost during surgery or in haemorrhage; (2) replace a deficiency of specific blood components, such as erythrocytes, platelets and clotting factors; (3) increase the oxygen-carrying capacity of the blood, as in anaemia; and (4) to increase the intravascular volume in shock.

When blood is taken from the donor, it is received in a special sterile container that contains anticoagulant. The anticoagulant most frequently used is a mixture of sodium citrate, citric acid and dextrose (acid citrate dextrose). The sodium citrate prevents clotting, the citric acid serves as a preservative and the dextrose prolongs the life of the erythrocytes. Heparin is used as an anticoagulant in blood that is to be transfused within 24 hours of procurement. Heparinized blood is necessary for extracorporeal shunts (as in open heart surgery). The heparin is less damaging to platelets and to the enzyme 2.3–diphosphoglycerate (DPG) which promotes the release of oxygen from oxyhaemoglobin.

The blood is labelled clearly to indicate donor number, blood type, whether Rh negative or positive, anticoagulant used, and expiration date. The blood may be given as whole blood or some of the components may be separated out for administration. Blood is stored at a temperature of 2–4°C and may be used up to 21 days of having been obtained, except that which is heparinized.

Preparations used in transfusions (Table 13.21)

1 *Whole blood*. Whole blood is administered to

---

[32] Eastham (1984), pp. 361–364.

[33] Voegelpohl (1981), p. 41.

Table 13.20 Patient care plan: the patient with a haemorrhagic disorder.

Problem	Patient goals	Nursing intervention	Expected outcomes
1 Potential for injury: bleeding related to a disorder of the clotting mechanism, excess of anticoagulant or a vascular deficit	a To promptly identify bleeding and to prevent blood loss	a Inspect the skin and mouth for the appearance of petechiae and purple patches (purpura) b Record the size, location and colour of petechiae and areas or purpura c Examine joints for oedema, limitation of movement or tenderness d Observe open lesions, incisions, intravenous and intramuscular injection sites for bleeding, oozing or haematomas e Examine and test excreta (urine, stools and vomit) for blood f Assess for symptoms of internal bleeding such as pallor, weakness, air hunger (rapid deep respirations), rapid weak pulse, fall in blood pressure g Observe for signs of cerebral dysfunction, such as confusion, disorientation and restlessness due to bleeding into the brain h Inform the patient about the causes, signs, and symptoms of bleeding i Teach the patient to recognize signs of bleeding	1 Signs of bleeding are identified immediately 2 The patient describes signs of bleeding
	b To prevent further bleeding by avoidance of tissue trauma	a Handle the patient gently. Avoid the use of restraints b Decrease the amount and duration of pressure on tissues by: Turning the patient every 1–2 hours Using foam pads, alternating pressure mattresses or sheepskin under the patient in bed Placing a 4 inch foam pad on the chair Padding the cot-sides of the bed c Instruct the patient to avoid falls, bumps, scratches, cuts and pressure d Remove furniture or other obstacles that may lead to bumps or falls in ambulatory patients e Have the patient: • Clean the teeth with a soft toothbrush or toothettes • Rinse the mouth frequently with a mild, cool mouthwash f Instruct the patient to avoid very hot, rough and highly seasoned foods to prevent damage of the oral and oesophageal mucosa g Avoid invasive procedures when possible: no intramuscular injections; coordinate all laboratory work to minimize the number of venepunctures h Apply direct pressure to venepuncture sites for 10 minutes i Take the blood pressure only when needed and rotate sites used to avoid unnecessary pressure to the arms j Instruct the patient to avoid constrictive clothing k Instruct male patients to use only electric razors l Keep the patient's nails clean and short	1 Bleeding due to tissue trauma does not occur 2 The patient describes measures to prevent bleeding

Table 13.20—*continued*

Problem	Patient goals	Nursing intervention	Expected outcomes
1 Potential for injury (continued)		**m** Instruct the paient to prevent constipation and injury to the rectal mucosa by maintaining adequate fluid intake and using a stool softener if necessary **n** Warn the patient against taking any non-prescribed medication, especially acetylsalicylic acid (aspirin), any product containing aspirin, and alcohol **o** Teach the patient to avoid forceful sneezing and coughing and to maintain an adequate fluid intake to keep the nasal and bronchial mucosa moist	
	c To control bleeding when it occurs	**a** Keep the patient at rest in bed **b** Administer blood products and medications as prescribed **c** Assess the patient during and following transfusions for signs of possible reaction (chills, fever, skin rashes, itching, headache, nausea, backache and restlessness) **d** Measure and record fluid intake and output **e** Estimate and record blood loss in vomit, nasogastric drainage, stools and on dressings or sanitary pads as accurately as possible **f** Institute measures listed about how to prevent further trauma and bleeding **g** Immobilize limbs or joints if bleeding is present in the area. Position in good alignment **h** Instruct patient to obtain medical care immediately when bleeding occurs	**1** Bleeding is controlled as evidenced by absence of overt bleeding; stabilization of areas of purpura and swelling in joints; return of blood pressure, pulse and respiratory rates to normal range; absence of restlessness; increase in serum platelet count and fibrinogen level and decrease in prothrombin time to the normal range
2 Anxiety related to: fear of bleeding, injury and pain; lack of understanding of the disease process and treatment plan; and lack of control over events	**a** To minimize anxiety and fear	**a** Assess the patient for behaviour indicative of anxiety and fear (restlessness, hyperactivity, withdrawal, crying, sobbing, expression of fear or anger) **b** Acknowledge awareness of the patient's fear **c** Repeatedly explain procedures and activities before and during the experiences **d** Explain to the patient what is happening and what is expected of him **e** Inform the patient that the doctor is aware of his problem, that he is being kept informed and everything possible is being done **f** Stay with the patient **g** If the patient is left alone be sure that his call-button is within reach and that he knows when you will return **h** Listen to the patient and encourage him to ask questions **i** Encourage family members to stay with the patient and to participate when possible in care activities **j** Inform the patient and family that they will receive help and instructions on how to prevent and control bleeding episodes **k** When possible, inform the patient of the anticipated duration and outcomes of the problem	**1** The patient expresses decreased anxiety and fear **2** The patient's behaviour indicates that his anxiety and fear are less frequent and intense **3** The patient cooperates with the treatment plan **4** The patient is able to rest and sleep

Table 13.20—*continued*

Problem	Patient goals	Nursing intervention	Expected outcomes
3 Impaired physical mobility related to pain, decreased joint movement and immobilization due to treatment	To prevent complications and deformities resulting from immobility	**a** If there is bleeding into joints, immobilize the limbs in optimum alignment **b** Use a bed-cradle to keep the weight of bedding off the affected part **c** Begin range-of-motion exercises 48 hours after the bleeding has been controlled **d** Preventive measures as cited above are used to prevent pressure sores and maintain the integrity of the skin mucous membranes	**1** Joint movement returns to pre-bleeding functional level **2** Complications such as decubitus ulcers and skin lesions do not occur
4 Lack of knowledge about the disease process, necessary management and resulting adaptations in daily living	**a** To understand the disease process and health management plan **b** To develop a realistic plan for continuing care and resumption of daily living activities	**a** Instruct the patient and family regarding the nature of the disease and signs of bleeding **b** Outline the limitations imposed by the disorder on daily activities and life-style **c** Instruct the patient regarding measures that can be taken to prevent bleeding **d** Provide information about prescribed medications and plans for follow-up medical care **e** Instruct the patient to avoid contact sports and occupations that present the risk of trauma to the body **f** Identify daily activities, recreational activities, hobbies and interests that are safe for the patient **g** Encourage the patient and family in planning to participate in appropriate recreation and other activities **h** Assist the child and family to develop realistic plans that promote growth, development and education **i** Provide information about health care and social community resources **j** Provide an application form for a Medic Alert bracelet and information about the importance of always wearing an identification bracelet or pendant and carrying a card with the necessary information about the person's condition **k** Inform the family of resources for genetic counselling if the disorder is hereditary	**1** The patient demonstrates understanding of: (a) Nature of the disease (b) Signs of bleeding (c) Medication regimen (d) Plans for follow-up medical care (e) Measures to prevent bleeding (f) Actions to take should bleeding occur (g) Community resources **2** The patient and family describe plans for resuming daily activities and modifying their life-style to accommodate limitations **3** Plans to obtain Medic Alert identification are stated

replace blood loss or to increase the intravascular volume in shock. *Fresh* whole blood is needed for the patient who is on extracorporeal shunt (e.g. as in open heart surgery) or receiving an exchange transfusion or a massive transfusion (ten or more units in 24 hours). Fresh blood may also be required for patients with bone marrow depression who require platelets in addition to erythrocytes.

2 *Packed red cells*. A large portion of the plasma is removed from whole blood by centrifuging. The remaining cells are given to increase the oxygen-carrying capacity of the recipient's blood. The advantage of packed cells is that a lesser volume is added to the patient's intravascular volume, thus preventing the risk of overload. The cells may be administered in a small volume of normal saline or plasma.

3 *Plasma*. Fresh frozen plasma may be stored for several months. It contains all the clotting factors except platelets, so it may be used to control bleeding in some patients.

4 *Thrombocytes*. Platelets may be concentrated and given in a small volume to avoid the administration of a large volume of fluid. This avoids the risk of overtaxing the recipient's heart and overloading the circulatory system. The platelets must be given while fresh (within 12–24 hours). The administration time is ½–1 hour. Transfusion of platelets is used to con-

Table 13.21 The administration of blood and blood products.

Blood/blood product and composition	Administration	Common complications

Whole blood
Red blood cells, leucocytes, plasma, platelets, clotting factors, (500 ml/unit)
	1 Warm blood 20–30 minutes at room temperature before administering
	2 Check label carefully with the patient's identification number
	3 Use a parenteral administration set with a blood filter inside the drip chamber
	4 Use only normal saline (0.9% NaCl) solution for intravenous infusion
	5 Fill the drip chamber to cover the filter with the blood
	6 Agitate the blood bag gently before and during administration
	7 Begin the transfusion at a flow rate of 20–30 drops per minute and observe patient constantly for the first 15 minutes. Adjust rate if there are no adverse reactions
	8 Complete transfusion in 1.5–2 hours
	9 Discard any blood not transfused within 4 hours
		Transfusion reactions include:
		  fever
		  chills
		  headache
		  restlessness
		  back pain
		  dyspnoea
		  tachycardia
		  palpitation
		  hypotension
		  cold clammy skin
		  thready pulse
		  altered level of consciousness
		  risk of circulatory overload

Packed red cells Fresh—red blood cells, 20% plasma, some leucocytes and platelets (300 ml per unit) Frozen—red blood cells, no plasma and few leucocytes or platelets (200–300 ml/unit)	1 Use a Y-connector set with normal saline solution to improve infusion rate. 2 Use blood administration set with blood filter 3 Fill drip chamber to cover filter 4 Agitate bag before and every 20–30 minutes during administration 5 Administer over 1–2 hours	Transfusion reactions are the same as with blood but are less frequent
Plasma Fresh, frozen or dried—all plasma proteins and clotting factors (no RBC, WBC or platelets) (200 ml/unit)	1 Use a standard intravenous administration set 2 Administer as rapidly as necessary and tolerated for volume replacement 3 Administer fresh, frozen plasma promptly after thawing to prevent deterioration of clotting factors	Greater risk of allergic reactions and viral hepatitis than with whole blood because of multiple donors Risk of fluid overload with rapid infusions
Platelets Platelets, lymphocytes and some plasma (40–50 ml/unit)	1 Use standard blood filter infusion set or a special filter 2 Administer as rapidly as tolerated (½–1 hour) 3 Use Y-set with normal saline	Chills, fever Alloimmunization producing rapid destruction of transfused platelets Risk of hepatitis or AIDS because of multiple donors
Granulocytes White blood cells and plasma with some red blood cells, platelets and other white blood cells (200–300 ml per suspension)	1 Use a standard blood filter infusion set 2 Use a Y-connector set with normal saline solution only 3 Administer first 50–75 ml slowly and observe for transfusion reaction 4 Administer over 2–4 hours	Chills, fever Allergic reactions (urticaria, wheezing) Hypotension, shock Respiratory distress
Albumin Albumin with plasma and normal saline (5% in 250–300 ml units, 25% in 25–50 ml units)	1 The rate of administration should not exceed: 2–4 ml/min for 5% albumin and 1 ml/min for 25% albumin 2 Use administration set with filtered air inlet	Fluid volume overload
Clotting factors Cryoprecipitated antihaemolytic factor Factor VIII plus 50 mg fibrinogen in each 20 ml unit	1 Administer by standard intravenous drip set 2 Administer promptly on thawing 3 Multiple units are usually administered	Chills and fever Risk of hepatitis Bleeding if infusions are not repeated because of short half-life of product
Factor IV—prothrombin (complex concentrates)	1 Administer by standard straight-line intravenous set	Chills and fever Allergic reactions Risk of hepatitis

trol bleeding in patients with thrombocytopenia. The development of alloimmunization or sensitivity to the ABO antigens and Rh factor found on platelets is a common complication of platelet transfusions. The rate of platelet destruction is increased in the sensitized individual.

5 *Granulocytes*. White blood cells from a compatible donor are prepared by differential centrifugation leucapheresis (cell separation) or filtration leucapheresis. For both methods, the donor is connected to the leucapheresis machine and blood is drawn from one vein into the machine and returned to the donor by another vein. Concentrated granulocytes are administered to neutrogenic patients within 24–48 hours of their collection. Administration is over a 2–4 hour period, with the first 50–75 ml being transfused very slowly and the patient observed for reactions.

6 Albumin is prepared from plasma and is available in 5% and 25% solutions. It is used to rapidly expand plasma volume in severe hypovolaemia.

7 *Clotting factors*. Concentrates of certain clotting factors (e.g. VIII, IX) are prepared from fresh frozen plasma to control bleeding in haemophilia A and B or in fibrinogen deficiency. The preparation is known as cryoprecipitate.

Patient care

1 The patient is advised that he is to receive a transfusion; the purpose and what is involved are explained. He will probably have questions which should be answered.

2 The patient is made as comfortable as possible, as he may be less free to turn and move while the transfusion is being administered.

3 The patient's blood type has been determined and his blood crossmatched with donor blood for compatibility. Before the matched blood is given, a check is made by two persons to ensure that the blood that has been received is for this particular patient, and is of the correct type. The expiration date on the blood label should also be checked and contents examined for abnormal cloudiness and particles.

4 The rate of administration depends upon the patient's condition; if the blood volume has been markedly depleted by haemorrhage or if the patient is in severe shock, it may be delivered at a faster rate than is used if the intravascular volume is normal. A rate commonly used is 30 drops per minute or the delivery of a unit (500 ml) over 4 hours. If the blood volume has not been depleted or if there is a risk of overtaxing the patient's heart, the rate should be reduced to 15–20 drops per minute. Blood should be administered within a 4-hour period because of the potential for bacterial contamination. If the transfusion has not been completed within 4 hours it is discontinued and a new unit set up. The patient should be observed closely throughout the administration for signs of overloading (dyspnoea, coughing, pink frothy sputum, weak pulse).

5 Precautionary measures are used. The blood is infused through a filter and is *gently* mixed at intervals to keep cells suspended throughout the plasma. A normal saline infusion is started so that the tube can be flushed before and after the blood is administered.

No medication should be given into the blood that is being administered; if a drug must be given, the blood is temporarily stopped and the normal saline infusion restarted.

The nurse remains with the patient for a period of 15–20 minutes following the beginning of the blood transfusion, or until at least 100 ml has been delivered; the patient may be very apprehensive at first and most reactions usually develop within that period. The patient is assessed frequently for possible reactions and the rate of flow is checked. Observations should continue for at least one hour after stopping the infusion.

Reactions

The transfer of blood or any component of it carries a risk of a reaction. The blood or its components may act as a foreign protein or antigen that prompts an immune response or tissue reaction.

Unfavourable responses to transfusions include the following:

1. HAEMOLYTIC REACTION

This is agglutination of the donor's red blood cells followed by their haemolysis, which occurs as a result of incompatibility. Antibodies within the recipient's blood attack the donor's erythrocytes. Haemoglobin and other products of the haemolysis are circulated throughout the body.

Early manifestations of incompatibility include chill, headache or full feeling in the head, anxiety, restlessness, pain in the kidney area (backache), and/or chest, dyspnoea, tachycardia and palpitation. Anaphylactic shock may develop; the patient's blood pressure falls, the skin becomes cold and clammy, respiratory distress is increasingly more severe, the pulse weakens and consciousness is clouded.

After several hours, even though the patient's general condition has improved markedly, haemoglobinuria and/or oliguria may appear. The haemoglobin released by the haemolyzed cells is excreted in the urine, colouring it red. The haemoglobin may be precipitated in the renal tubules by the acidity of the urine. The tubules become blocked and are damaged, reducing the urinary output. Acute renal failure and anuria may develop if the haemolysis is extensive as a result of the patient receiving approximately 100 ml or more of the incompatible blood.

A complication associated with a haemolytic reaction is hyperkalaemia. The haemolysis of the donor's red blood cells releases potassium. The impaired renal function results in retention of the potassium, and its serum concentration exceeds the normal level. Hyperkalaemia may develop when the whole blood that is being given has been stored for 5 days or more. Some red cells are broken down and the serum potassium concentration of the donor blood is increased.

Treatment

The administration of the blood or blood component is stopped promptly with the initial manifestation(s) of reaction. The normal saline is started again slowly to maintain an open intravenous line in case medications may have to be administered intravenously. A urine specimen is obtained and sent to the laboratory.

If the patient complains of shortness of breath and 'tightness' in the chest, adrenaline 1:1000 (0.5–1 ml) subcutaneously or intramuscularly may be prescribed. A marked fall in blood pressure (hypotension) may be treated by increasing the intravascular volume with intravenous plasma or dextran.

Treatment is instituted to promote urinary output and reduce impairment of renal function by the haemoglobin released through haemolysis. The fluid intake and output must be accurately measured and recorded. An indwelling catheter may be passed so the urinary output may be measured hourly. Fluids containing potassium must be avoided. Manitol (25 g), an osmotic diuretic, may be slowly infused intravenously. If the urinary output progressively decreases, the fluid intake is limited to insensible fluid loss and losses by other channels (vomiting, bowel elimination). Anuria and renal failure may develop, necessitating haemodialysis.

2. FEBRILE REACTION

A fairly common reaction to a transfusion is fever preceded by a chill. It is attributed to the recipient's sensitivity to the donor's leucocytes, thrombocytes or plasma proteins. It may also develop as a result of a pyrogenic material in the equipment or solution used. Pethidine may be administered and the transfusion is slowed to relieve the discomfort of the febrile reaction and chills in the patient receiving a granulocyte transfusion.[34]

3. ALLERGIC REACTION

A component of the donor's blood may act as an antigen and initiate an allergic response. It is also suggested that the cause of an allergic reaction may be the response of antibodies in the donor's blood to an antigen within the recipient. The most common manifestations are urticaria and asthma. Severe bronchospasm and anaphylaxis occur less frequently. An antihistamine preparation, such as diphenhydramine hydrochloride (Benadryl), may provide relief. If the bronchospasm is severe or anaphylaxis develops, adrenaline 1:1000 may be administered parenterally as well as a corticosteroid preparation.

4. CIRCULATORY OVERLOAD

The giving of a transfusion too rapidly, or the administration of whole blood or plasma to someone with a normal intravascular volume or who has or is predisposed to cardiac or renal insufficiency, is dangerous. The resulting increased intravascular volume places too great a demand on the heart. Heart failure and pulmonary oedema ensue. The patient develops severe dyspnoea, coughing, anxiety, weak pulse and cyanosis. A pink frothy sputum is expectorated.

Circulatory overload may be prevented by the slow administration of packed red cells while the central venous pressure is monitored carefully. (See p. 321 for central venous pressure monitoring).

5. INFECTION

Hepatitis is the most common infectious problem associated with transfusions. Donors' blood is tested in blood banks for the hepatitis B antigen, but the transmission of hepatitis is still a possibility. The onset of manifestations of the infection may occur many weeks after the transfusion.

Syphilis, malaria, AIDS and hepatitis B, non-A and non-B may be transmitted by transfusion, but the possibility is minimal because of the screening of donors and the tests that are performed on all donor blood.

If a transfusion reaction occurs

1 The transfusion should be stopped promptly: slow infusion of normal saline is resumed to maintain an open line, and the doctor is notified.
2 The remaining blood or blood component is returned in the container with the tubing to the blood bank for analysis and determination of the cause of the reaction.
3 The blood bank is notified of the nature of the reaction.
4 Blood specimens are taken from a vein other than the one that was used to administer the blood. They are sent to the laboratory for retyping, culture and estimation of free plasma haemoglobin.
5 A nurse remains with the patient; vital signs are monitored frequently and continuous assessment of the patient's condition is necessary. The patient is likely to be very apprehensive and fearful. He

---

[34] Patterson (1980), p. 103.

requires some information about what is happening and reassurance that everything possible is being done.

6 A urine specimen is collected from the patient as soon as possible and sent to the laboratory for haemoglobin determination.

References and Further Reading

BOOKS

Alspach JG & Williams S (1985) *Core Curriculum for Critical Care Nursing*. Philadelphia: WB Saunders.

Aronstam A (1985) *Haemophilic Bleeding—Early Management at Home*. London: Baillière Tindall.

Beck WS (ed) (1981) *Hematology*, 3rd ed. Cambridge, MA: MIT Press.

Brain MC & Carbone PP (1985) *Current Therapy in Hematology–Oncology*. St Louis: CV Mosby.

Bouchier IAD, Allan RN, Hodgson HJF & Keighley MRB (1984) *Textbook of Gastroenterology*. Eastbourne: Baillière Tindall.

Byrne CJ, Saxton DF, Pelikan PK & Nugent PM (1981) *Laboratory Tests*. Menlo Park, CA: Addison Wesley. Chapters 2, 3 & 9.

Chanarin I, Brozovic M, Tidmarsh E & Waters DAW (1984) *Blood and Its Diseases*. Edinburgh: Churchill Livingstone.

Eastham R (1984) *Clinical Haematology*, 6th ed. Bristol: Wright.

Ganong WF (1985) *Review of Medical Physiology*, 11th ed. San Francisco: Lange. Chapters 240 & 242.

Goldman JM & Preisler HD (eds) (1984) *Haematology 1: Leukaemias*. London: Butterworths.

Guyton AC (1986) *Textbook of Medical Physiology*, 7th ed. WB Saunders. Philadelphia: Part 2.

Hoffbrand AV & Pettit JE (1984) *Essential Haematology*, 2nd ed. Oxford: Blackwell.

Howe PS (1981) *Basic Nutrition in Health and Disease*, 7th ed. Philadelphia: WB Saunders. Chapter 25.

Hughes-Jones NC (1984) *Lecture Notes in Haematology*. Oxford: Blackwell Scientific.

Krause MV & Mahan LK (1984) *Food, Nutrition and Diet Therapy*, 7th ed. Philadelphia: WB Saunders. Chapter 29.

Krupp MA & Chatton MJ (1983) *Current Medical Diagnosis and Treatment*. Los Altos, CA: Lange. Chapter 9.

Richards JDM, Linch DL & Goldstone AH (1984) *A Synopsis of Haematology*. Bristol; Wright.

Smith LH & Thier SO (1985) *Pathophysiology*, 2nd ed. Philadelphia: WB Saunders. Chapter 5.

Theml H (1985) *Pocket Atlas of Haematology—Morphological Diagnosis for the Clinician*. New York: Georg Thieme Verlag.

Truman JT (1981) The leukemias. In: WS Beck (ed), *Hematology*, 3rd ed. Cambridge, MA: MIT Press.

Williams WJ, Beutler EEAJ, Erslev AJ & Lichtman MA (1983) *Hematology*, 3rd ed. New York: McGraw-Hill.

Woodliff HJ & Herrman RP (1979) *Concise Haematology*, London: Edward Arnold.

PERIODICALS

Arkel YS (1981) Shedding light on platelet dysfunction. *Diagn. Med.*, Vol. 5, No. 1, pp. 27–35.

Bennet JM, Catovsky D, Daniel MT et al (1981) Classification of acute lymphoblastic leukaemias. *Br. J. Haematol.*, Vol. 47 No. 4, p. 553–561.

Brandt B (1984) A nursing protocol for the client with neutropenia, *Oncol. Nurs. Forum*, Vol. 11 No. 2, pp. 24–28.

Brown MH & Kiss ME (1979) Nursing patient-care outcome audit: acute non-lymphoblastic leukaemia, Part 2. *Cancer Nurs.*, Vol. 2 No. 2, pp. 139–147.

Caza B & Ross CA (1981) Living with leukaemia. *Can. Nurs.*, Vol. 77 No. 9, pp. 32–35.

Darden ML (1981) Blood loss determination, *AORN J.*, Vol. 33 No. 7, pp. 1368–1380.

de la Montaigne M, de Mao J, Nuscher R & Stutzer CA (1981) Standards of Care for the patient with 'graft–versus host disease' post-bone marrow transplant. *Cancer Nurs.*, Vol. 4 No. 3, pp. 191–198.

Dressler D (1980) Understanding and treating haemophilia, *Nurs. '80*, Vol. 10 No. 8, pp. 72–73.

Dwyer JE & Held DM (1982) Home management of the adult patient with leukaemia. *Nurs. Clin. N. Am.*, Vol. 17 No. 4, pp. 665–675.

Eddy JL, Selgas-Cordes R & Curran M (1984) Cutaneous T-cell lymphoma. *Am. J. Nurs.*, Vol. 84 No. 2, pp. 202–206.

Ern M (1981) Programmed instruction: cancer care. Leukaemia. *Cancer Nurs.*, Vol. 4 No. 6, pp. 493–497.

Feeley AM & Houlihan NG (1981) Programmed instruction: cancer care. Leukaemia: the treatment of leukaemia. *Cancer Nurs.*, Vol. 4 No. 3, pp. 233–245.

Fergusson JH (1981) Cognitive late effects of treatment for acute lymphocytic leukaemia in childhood. *Top. Clin. Nurs.*, Vol. 2 No. 4, pp. 21–29.

Fox LS (1981) Granulocytopenia in the adult cancer patient. *Cancer Nurs.*, Vol. 4 No. 6, pp. 459–466.

Fuller BF (1981) Haemostasis: a balanced system. *AORN J.*, Vol. 34 No. 2, pp. 225–230.

Graham V & Rubal BJ (1980) Recipient and donor response to granulocyte transfusion and leukapheresis. *Cancer Nurs.*, Vol. 3 No. 2, pp. 97–100.

Hays K & Rafferty DC (1982) Care of the patient with malignant lymphoma. *Nurs. Clin. N. Am.*, Vol. 17 No. 4, pp. 677–695.

Heller PH (1981) Bleeding disorders in the ER. *Emerg. Med.*, Vol. 13 No. 11, pp. 100–110.

Hoffbrand AV, Ma DDF & Webster ADB (1982) Enzyme patterns in normal lymphocyte subpopulation lymphoid leukemias and immunodeficiency syndrome. *Clin Haematol.*, Vol. 11 No. 3, pp. 719–741.

Houlihan NG (1981) Programmed instruction: cancer care. Leukaemia: a haematology review. *Cancer Nurs.*, Vol. 4 No. 2, pp. 149–160.

Houlihan NG & Feeley AM (1981a) Programmed instruction: cancer care. Leukaemia: the acute and chronic leukaemias. *Cancer Nurs.*, Vol. 4 No. 4, pp. 323–338.

Houlihan NG & Feeley AM (1981b) Programmed instruction: cancer care: Leukaemia. *Cancer Nurs.*, Vol. 4 No. 5, pp. 397–405.

Hutchinson MM & Itoh K (1982) Nursing care of the patient undergoing bone marrow transplantation for acute leukaemia. *Nurs. Clin. N. Am.*, Vol. 17 No. 4, pp. 697–711.

Kelly JO (1983) Standards of clinical nursing practice for leukaemia: neutropenia and thrombocytopenia. *Cancer Nurs.*, Vol. 6 no. 6, pp. 487–494.

Lane B & Forgay M (1981) Upgrading your oral hygiene protocol for the patient with cancer. *Cancer Nurs.*, Vol. 77 No. 11, pp. 27–29.

Layton PB, Gallucci BB & Aker SN (1981) Nutritional assessment of allogenic bone marrow recipients, *Cancer Nurs.*, Vol. 4 No. 2, pp. 127–134.

Leser DR (1982) Synthetic blood: a future alternative. *Am. J. of Nurs.*, Vol. 82 No. 3, pp. 452–455.

Markus S (1981) Taking the fear out of bone marrow examination. *Nurs. '81*, Vol. 11 No. 4, pp. 64–67.

Megliola B (1980) Multiple myeloma. *Cancer Nurs.*, Vol. 3 No. 3, pp. 209–218.

Nace CS & Nace SG (1985) Acute tumor lysis syndrome: pathophysiology and nursing management. *Crit. Care Nurs.*, Vol. 5 No. 3, pp. 26–34.

Nuscher R, Baltzer L, Repinec DA et al (1984) Bone marrow transplantation. *Am. J. Nurs.*, Vol. 84 No. 6, pp. 764–772.

Ostechega Y (1980) Preventing and treating cancer chemotherapy's oral complications. *Nurs. '80.*, Vol. 10 No. 8, pp. 47–52.

Owen H, Klove C & Cotanch PH (1981) Bone marrow harvesting and high dose BCNU therapy: nursing implications. *Cancer Nurs.*, Vol. 4 No. 3, pp. 199–205.

Parker JW (1981) A new look at malignant lymphomas. *Diagn. Med.*, Vol. 4 No. 4, pp. 77–113.

Patterson P (1980) Granulocyte transfusion: nursing considerations. *Cancer Nurs.*, Vol. 3 No. 2, pp. 101–104.

Querin JJ & Stahl LD (1983) 12 Simple, sensible steps for successful blood transfusions. *Nurs. '83.*, Vol. 13 No. 11, pp. 34–43.

Reheis CE (1985) Neutropenia: causes, complications, treatment and resulting nursing care. *Nurs. Clin. N. Am.*, Vol. 20 No. 1, pp. 219–225.

Rice L & Jackson D (1981) Can heparin cause clotting? *Heart Lung*, Vol. 10 No. 2, pp. 331–335.

Rooks Y & Pack B (1983) A profile of sickle cell disease.

Nurs. Clin. N. Am., Vol. 18 No. 1, pp. 131–138.

Rooney A & Haviley C (1985) Nursing management of disseminated intravascular coagulation. *Oncol. Nurs. Forum*, Vol. 12 No. 1, pp. 15–22.

Royle J & Green E (1985) Right atrial catheters: a patient and family education program. *Can. Nurs.*, Vol. 81 No. 3, pp. 51–54.

Schmidt PJ (1981) Transfusion mortality: with special reference to surgical and intensive care facilities, *AORN J.* Vol. 34 No. 6, pp. 1114–1122.

Smith LG (1984) Reactions to blood transfusion. *Am. J. Nurs.*, Vol. 84 No. 9, pp. 1096–1101.

Stream P, Harrington E & Clark M (1980) Bone marrow transplantation: an option for children with acute leukaemia, *Cancer Nurs.*, Vol. 3 No. 3, pp. 195–199.

Tishler CL (1981) The psychological aspects of genetic counselling. *Am. J. Nurs.*, Vol. 81 No. 4, pp. 733–734.

Voegelpohl RA (1981) Disseminated intravascular coagulation. *Crit. Care Nurs.*, Vol. 1 No. 4, pp. 38–43.

Walters I, Baysinger M, Buchanan I, et al (1983) Complications of sickle cell disease. *Nurs. Clin. N. Am.*, Vol. 18 No. 1, pp. 139–184.

Wessler RM (1982) Care of the hospitalized adult patient with leukaemia. *Nurs. Clin. N. Am.*, Vol. 17 No. 4, pp. 649–663.

Williams I, Earles AN & Pack B (1983) Psychological considerations in sickle cell disease. *Nurs. Clin. N. Am.*, Vol. 18 No. 1, pp. 215–229.

Woods ME & Mazza I (1980) Blood and component therapy. *Nurs. Clin. N. Am.*, Vol. 15 No. 3, pp. 629–646.

Wroblewski SS & Wroblewski SH (1981) Caring for the patient with chemotherapy-induced thrombocytopenia. *Am. J. Nurs.*, Vol. 81 No. 4, pp. 746–749.

14

Nursing in Cardiovascular Disease

Circulation

Normal cellular activity is dependent upon a constant supply of oxygen, nutrients, and certain chemicals, as well as the removal of metabolic waste products. The unicellular organism is in direct contact with the outside environmental source of its essentials, but in complex multicellular organisms cell needs are not as simply met. Specialized organs are necessary for the processes of oxygenation, nutrition and excretion, as well as a transportation system between these organs and the cells throughout the body. This transportation of materials to and from tissue cells by the propulsion of blood through a closed system of tubes is the process referred to as circulation.

CIRCULATORY STRUCTURES

The circulatory system consists of the heart and the vascular system.

HEART

The heart is a hollow, cone-shaped, muscular organ lying obliquely in the thoracic cavity. Approximately two-thirds of it is situated to the left of the midline. The upper border (or base) lies just below the second rib; the apex, which is directed downward, forward and to the left, lies on the diaphragm at the level of the fifth intercostal space in the left midclavicular line. *These boundary locations are significant in determining any abnormal enlargement and in counting the apex beat.* The structural organization of the heart includes the pericardium, heart walls, chambers, orifices, valves and coronary system.

Pericardium
The pericardium is a strong, non distensible sac which loosely encloses the heart and attaches to the large blood vessels at the base of the heart and to the diaphragm at the apex. It consists of two layers. The outer one forms the fibrous pericardium, and the inner one, the serous pericardium, is also divided into two layers; one layer lines the sac, and the other is reflected over the surface of the heart as the epicardium, or visceral pericardium. The space formed between the sac and the heart is normally only a potential space. The surfaces are in close contact, and sufficient serum is secreted to keep them moist so that adhesion and friction

between the heart and the sac are prevented. The fibrous pericardium, because of its inextensible nature, prevents over-distension of the heart. It also supports the heart, preventing change of its position during postural changes. Although the pericardial sac is firm and considered non-extensible, it does extend in response to the gradual, sustained stretching imposed by enlargement of the heart (hypertrophy).

Heart walls and chambers
From shortly after birth, the human heart is divided longitudinally by a partition into two halves between which there is no direct communication. The cavity of each side is divided horizontally by an incomplete partition which results in two upper chambers, called the right and left atria, and two lower ones, which are the right and left ventricles (see Fig. 14.1).

The walls of the heart consist of three layers—the epicardium, myocardium and endocardium. The myocardium (heart muscle) comprises the main functional part of the heart wall; its rhythmic contractions provide the pumping force which maintains circulation. It is formed of involuntary striated muscle fibres which interlace, branch, anastomose and coalesce. This arrangement produces a very firm, closely related mass of tissue through which an excitatory impulse for contraction spreads very quickly. The muscle fibres of the atria are continuous and behave as a single mass. Similarly, those of the ventricles are also continuous and act as a single mass. Atrial muscle fibres are completely separated from those of the ventricles by fibrous tissue.

The atrial myocardium is much thinner than that of the ventricles and the left ventricular wall is thicker than that of the right. This difference can be correlated with the force that must be given to the contained blood. The atria are receiving chambers and are only required to deliver the blood to the ventricles, which discharge blood from the heart. The right ventricle pumps blood through the lungs to the left atrium, forming the circuit referred to as the pulmonary circulatory system. The left ventricle must provide sufficient pressure to carry blood through all parts of the body and return it to the right atrium. This latter circuit is referred to as the systemic circulatory system.

Special structures
Two small masses of specialized tissue lie within the atrial myocardium—the sino-atrial (SA) node and

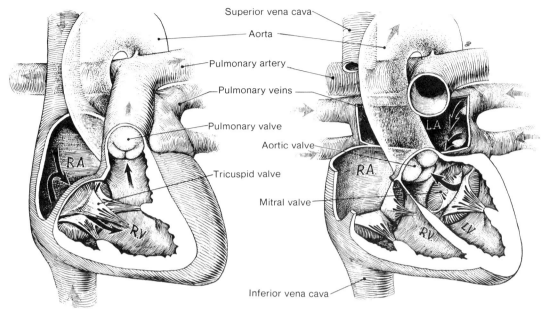

Superior vena cava
Aorta
Pulmonary artery
Pulmonary veins
Pulmonary valve
Aortic valve
Tricuspid valve
Mitral valve
Inferior vena cava

Fig. 14.1 The heart.

the atrioventricular (AV) node. The SA node is located in the upper part of the right atrium near the superior vena cava and is responsible for initiating the impulses for the rhythmic heart beats.

The AV node lies in the lower part of the interatrial septum and is a part of the system that conducts impulses from the atria to the ventricles. A bundle of fibres called the bundle of His proceeds from junctional tissue at the AV node into the ventricular septum where it divides into two, forming the left and right bundle branches. The left bundle branch further divides into the anterior (superior) and posterior (inferior) divisions (Fig. 14.2). As it descends, each bundle branch gives rise to a network of fine fibres which are known as the Purkinje fibres. They are distributed to the ventricular myocardial cells.

Orifices in the chambers

The right atrium has three inlets and one outlet. Blood is received from two large veins, the superior and inferior venae cavae, and the coronary sinus. The outlet channels the blood into the right ventricle. The right ventricle has two openings—the inlet from the right atrium and an outlet into the pulmonary artery.

The left atrium has four inlets, which are the terminations of the four pulmonary veins, and one outlet into the left ventricle. The blood received from the left atrium is discharged by the left ventricle into the aorta.

Endocardium

The endocardium is the smooth endothelial lining of the heart chambers. It covers the valves and is conti-

nuous with the lining of the blood vessels entering and leaving the heart. Its smooth surface reduces friction between the blood and the vessel.

Cardiac valves

Normal circulation requires the flow of the blood in one direction only. This is maintained in the heart by a set of four valves—two atrioventricular and two semilunar.

The atrioventricular valves are formed of fibrous cusps, or leaflets, which derive from the fibrous ring that encircles each atrioventricular opening. They are covered with endothelial tissue which is continuous with the endocardium. The right atrioventricular valve has three cusps and is referred to as the tricuspid valve; the left one has two cusps and is called the mitral valve. These valves open into the ventricles but are prevented from opening into the atria by fine tendinous cords (chordae tendineae) which insert on the free border of the leaflets and originate in small pillars of muscle projecting from the ventricular walls (papillary muscles). When the ventricles fill, the valve cusps are forced up in the direction of the atrioventricular opening. They meet, closing off the opening and, with the contraction of the papillary muscles, sufficient tension is exerted by the chordae tendineae to prevent the valves from opening into the atria (see Fig. 14.1).

The semilunar valves guard the openings from the ventricles into the pulmonary artery and aorta. Each consists of three pocket-like pouches arranged around the origin of the artery, with the free borders being distal to the ventricle (see Fig. 14.1). During the contraction of the ventricles and ejection of blood

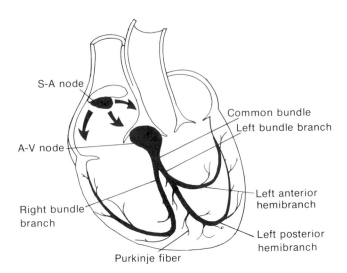

Fig. 14.2 The impulse conduction system.

under considerable pressure into the aorta and pulmonary artery, the valve cusps lie free in the stream, offering no resistance to the flow of the blood. When the ventricles relax and there is a reversal in the direction of pressure, blood fills out the semilunar pouches, bringing their surfaces together. This closes off the aperture into each ventricle, preventing a backflow.

Cardiac blood supply (coronary system) (See Fig. 14.3)
The myocardium receives its blood supply from the right or left coronary arteries, which arise from the sinuses of Valsalva in the root of the aorta. The left coronary artery divides into the anterior descending artery and the circumflex artery. The anterior descending branch is distributed to the anterior part of the left ventricle and portions of the right ventricle. In addition to the anterior wall of the left ventricle, the anterior descending artery supplies the anterior papillary muscle of the left ventricle, the anterior two-thirds of the interventricular septum, and distal parts of the conduction system. The circumflex artery carries blood to the lateral and lower posterior, left ventricular walls and to the left atrium. Branches of the right coronary artery supply the remaining portions of the myocardium. The right coronary artery nourishes the sinoatrial (SA) node in approximately 55% of people and the atrioventricular (AV) node in 90% of people. At other times, the blood supply to these structures is provided by the left circumflex artery. The large arteries divide and subdivide to form a network of smaller arteries and capillaries throughout the heart muscle. The blood is returned to the right atrium through a system of progressively enlarging veins which terminate in the coronary sinus.

The myocardium requires a large blood supply since it must work continuously and adapt its activity to the varying needs of tissues throughout the body.

The coronary vessels dilate to increase the supply when demands are increased. They also dilate when there is an increase in the carbon dioxide concentration of the blood and a decrease in the pH.

The flow of blood through the coronary system is dependent upon the pressure of the blood in the aorta; a reduction in blood pressure will result in a lesser volume entering the coronary arteries. The coronary volume is greater during myocardial relaxation. In systole, with the myocardium contracted, the vessels are compressed and their volume is reduced. When a person is at rest, the blood entering the coronary system is approximately 4% of the total cardiac output. The coronary blood supply can be increased, but to a lesser degree than the cardiac output. That is, the work of the myocardium can be increased to a greater extent than its blood supply.

VASCULAR SYSTEM

The blood travels from the heart successively through arteries, arterioles, capillaries and veins back to the heart (see Fig. 14.4). The structure of each type of vessel is modified according to its function and location. One common structural characteristic of all the vessels is the smooth endothelial lining, known as the intima. The arteries and arterioles form a high-pressure distributing system; the capillaries are structured and organized for exchanging substances between the blood and interstitial fluid; the venules and veins serve as a low-pressure collecting system which returns the blood to the heart.

Arteries
The large arteries carry blood away from the heart and branch and subdivide many times. Their structure varies with their size, the larger ones being more elastic and less muscular. Elasticity is an important property of these vessels; with the ejection of blood

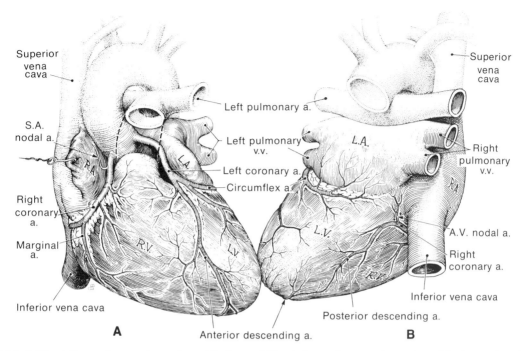

Fig. 14.3 *A*, Circulation to the anterior surface of the heart. *B* Circulation to the posterior surface of the heart, showing the AV nodal artery as a branch of the right coronary artery.

from the heart, the vessel distends and on recoil exerts a slight pressure on the contained fluid, helping to force it forward. If resistance is offered to the flow of the blood, normally the arteries can stretch to accommodate the increased volume of blood, and the pressure of the blood remains within the normal range. Reduced elasticity and a thickening of the arterial walls with a narrowing of the lumen, as seen in arteriosclerosis and atherosclerosis, result in a rise in the arterial blood pressure.

Arterioles

The smallest arteries emerge as arterioles which have walls composed mainly of a well developed muscular coat over the endothelium. The muscle tissue may contract or relax to decrease or increase the amount of blood through the arterioles. This feature of the arterioles gives them an important role in determining arterial blood pressure and in controlling the blood supply to tissues.

Capillaries

Each arteriole channels its content into microscopic endothelial tubes, the capillaries, which anastomose with each other to form a capillary bed. These vessels are the principal functional unit of the cardiovascular system. The functions of the other structures (heart, arteries and veins) are contributory to that of the capillaries. The exchange of substances to maintain and regulate cell activity takes place as the blood

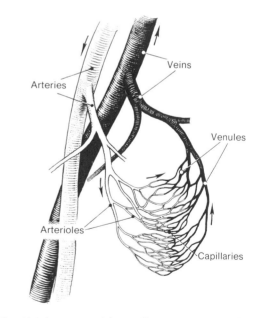

Fig. 14.4 Artery–arteriole–capillary–vein sequence in circulation.

passes through these minute, semipermeable vessels.

Not all the capillaries are open at all times. There are wide variations in the amount of activity in some tissues (e.g. skeletal muscle), while in others a more constant blood supply is necessary, as in brain tissue. Similarly, when an area is irritated, more blood is brought to that part in its defence (e.g. inflammation). The number of capillaries through which blood is passing at any given time is adjusted locally to meet the needs of the tissues in the area. Guyton indicates that a small proportion of the blood is located in the capillaries in resting states; the volume increases as tissue activity increases.[1] This adjustment is made possible by the fact that some capillaries have at their origin a ring of plain muscular tissue which forms a precapillary sphincter.

Venules and veins

The collecting part of the vascular system originates in venules which drain the capillaries and progressively unite and enlarge to form the veins. They differ from arteries in several ways: (1) they carry blood toward the heart; (2) their walls are much thinner and less elastic with the result that they collapse when empty; (3) the contained blood is under a much lower pressure; and (4) many of the veins have valves.

The structure of veins changes as they increase in size; more muscle and fibrous tissue appear in the walls but, in comparison with arteries, the muscle fibres are sparse. Most of the pressure of the blood created by the heart is dissipated in the arterioles and capillaries and, in order to maintain the flow in one direction, valves similar in structure to the semilunar valves of the heart occur at intervals in many of the veins. They are particularly numerous in the lower extremities where the blood is flowing against gravity. The thinner walls of the veins are readily compressed by skeletal muscle contraction; this assists the blood along its course toward the heart, since backflow toward the capillaries is prevented by the valves.

PHYSIOLOGY OF CIRCULATION

Normal circulation through the cardiovascular system is dependent upon an appropriate pressure gradient throughout the system, an adequate volume of blood, a closed system of unobstructed tubes and a set of valves to ensure flow in one direction only.

PRINCIPLES APPLICABLE TO THE FLOW OF FLUIDS THROUGH TUBES

Since circulation is the continuous flow of blood in a pressure system composed of a pump and a series of tubes filled with the blood, it might be well at this point to consider some physical factors which govern the flow of any liquid through tubes. The rate at which a fluid moves through a tube depends upon the pressure gradient and the resistance to flow.

Pressure gradient

Fluids flow from an area of high pressure to one of lower pressure. The pressure of fluid at any given point in the system must be greater than that in the succeeding area into which it is to flow. This difference is referred to as the pressure gradient, or driving force. If the pressure should become the same throughout the system, no movement of fluid takes place.

The pressure gradient which maintains the normal flow of blood through the vessels is the difference between the pressure of the blood in the arterial system and that of the venous system. The main source of the driving force is the pumping action of the heart which produces a relatively high pressure in the arteries.

Resistance to flow

The amount of resistance offered to the flow of fluid is determined by the dimensions of the tube and the viscosity of the fluid.

The pressure of a fluid progressively decreases as it flows through a tube because of the friction between the fluid and the walls of the tube. This friction, which is referred to as peripheral resistance, causes a loss of energy. Fluid flows more slowly through a tube of smaller diameter since more friction is created between the walls and the fluid, resulting in an increase in resistance. As the blood flows through blood vessels having a lesser radius (arterioles and capillaries) resistance is increased, causing a decrease in the rate of flow and blood pressure.

Similarly, resistance is increased as the length of the tube increases, since the greater amount of surface provides more friction.

If the volume of fluid remains the same in a system of tubes, the rate of flow decreases as the tubular space (capacity) increases. This factor contributes to the marked decrease in the velocity of the blood in the capillaries. Although the radius of the capillaries is extremely small, the total cross-sectional area of the vast number of these minute tubes exceeds the total area of all the other vessels combined.

The viscosity of a fluid is an internal resistance to flow created by the friction between the molecules of fluid and their tendency to cohere. Obviously, a greater concentration of particles in a fluid produces an increased internal resistance. For example, an excessive number of blood cells, particularly erythrocytes, increases the viscosity of the blood and retards its rate of flow.

In summary, resistance to flow is inversely proportional to the diameter of the tube, directly proportional to the length of the tube, and directly proportional to the viscosity of the fluid. If the volume of fluid remains the same, the rate of flow decreases as the diameter of the tube increases.

[1] Guyton (1984), p. 284.

The preceding principles are based on the flow of fluids through rigid tubes. Some modification is necessary in applying them to circulation. The blood vessels are not rigid tubes and their diameters are variable. Branches, division and curves occur at frequent intervals in the blood vessels. Blood is viscous and its flow is pulsatile, rather than steady, in a large part of the circulatory system.

THE ROLE OF THE HEART IN CIRCULATION

The pressure that keeps the blood in continuous movement through the circulatory system originates in the heart and is augmented slightly by the elastic recoil of the large arteries. A continuous succession of alternate myocardial contractions and relaxations, occurring rhythmically on an average of 60–70 times per minute, pumps the blood through the body.

IMPULSE ORIGIN AND CONDUCTION IN HEART CONTRACTION

The cells of the myocardium are of two types—those which contract when stimulated and those which originate and conduct impulses. The ability to originate and conduct impulses is referred to as the electrical activity of the heart. The heart has three electrical properties: (1) automaticity, or the ability to initiate an electrical impulse; (2) excitability, or the ability to respond to an electrical impulse; and (3) conductivity, or the ability to transmit an impulse from one cell to another. The muscle fibres have an absolute and a relative refractory period. The fibres are unresponsive to any stimulus during the absolute refractory period which immediately follows a contraction. The relative refractory period is the interval in which the muscle fibres gradually recover their excitability (ability to respond to a stimulus) but will respond to a stimulus if it is stronger than the usual. The refractory period in cardiac muscle is longer than in other muscle tissue. Excitability is more slowly regained, giving the heart chambers time to fill effectively.

Contraction of the myocardium is dependent upon impulses which arise within the myocardium itself. The structures capable of generating and conducting impulses within the myocardium form the conduction system. They are the SA node, tracts of conducting fibres originating with the SA node, the AV node, the bundle of His, bundle branches and the Purkinje fibres. Several areas of the conduction system are capable of the spontaneous generation of impulses—namely, the SA node, the junctional tissue where the conducting fibres join the AV node, the bundle of His and the Purkinje fibres. The rate at which impulses are normally fired varies in the different areas: the SA node originates approximately 60–80 impulses per minute; the junctional tissue, 50–60 impulses per minute; the bundle of His, 40–50 impulses per minute; and the Purkinje fibres,

30–40 per minute. Since the region which is producing the highest rate of impulses sets the heart rhythm (number of contractions per minute), the SA node is referred to as the normal pacemaker.

Impulses arising in the SA node are quickly conducted through the atria, initiating their contraction. At the same time, impulses are transmitted to the AV node where they are delayed; this delay allows for completion of atrial emptying and ventricular filling. From the AV node and junctional tissue they travel through the bundle of His and along the right and left bundle branches and the widely distributed Purkinje fibres to the ventricular contractile fibres.

ELECTROPHYSIOLOGY

Electrical currents in cardiac cells are produced by ion movement across the cell membrane. There is a marked difference in the intracellular and extracellular concentrations of ions, the most important of which are sodium and potassium. The potassium concentration is approximately 30 times greater inside the cell than outside, and the sodium concentration is approximately 30 times less within the cell than outside.

During the resting state the inside of the cardiac cell is negatively charged while the outside is positively charged, and the membrane is referred to as polarized. By inserting microelectrodes inside the cardiac cell, researchers have been able to measure the potential difference in voltage across the membrane. In the resting state, the potential is −90 millivolts, as shown in Fig. 14.5 and is called the resting membrane potential. At this time the cell membrane is impermeable to the movement of ions through it.

During depolarization, the cell membrane becomes permeable to sodium, which rapidly shifts inside the cell. This sudden influx of sodium reverses the transmembrane potential and potassium moves out of the cell.

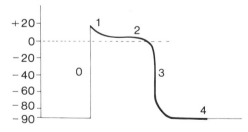

Fig. 14.5 The electrophysiology of the cell.

In Fig. 14.5 the resting or polarized phase is shown as the straight line at −90 millivolts. The change in transmembrane potential is represented by the upstroke, phase 0. After excitation the action potential rapidly declines and then levels off for a short period, as represented by phases 1 and 2. This time is referred to as the absolute refractory period and further stimulation produces no response.

Repolarization, or return to the normal resting potential, occurs during phase 3—the relative refractory period. The inside of the cell gradually resumes its negative electrical charge. During this time a stimulus of greater than normal intensity could reactivate the cell. Phase 4 shows a period of stable resting potential which remains until the next wave of excitation.

During depolarization ions move into and out of the cell because of differences in concentration gradients on either side of the cell membrane. During repolarization, however, an active transport system is required to pump out the sodium which has entered the cell and to pump in an equivalent amount of potassium. This mechanism is known as the 'sodium pump' and requires energy.

THE CARDIAC CYCLE

The succession of events which occurs with each heart-beat is called the cardiac cycle. It consists of the relaxation and contraction of the atria and ventricles and the opening and closing of the cardiac valves in a sequence that permits the filling and emptying of the heart chambers. Contraction of the atria or ventricles is called systole; their relaxation is known as diastole. In referring to contraction or relaxation of the atria or ventricles, the terms used are atrial or ventricular systole or atrial or ventricular diastole respectively. If systole or diastole is used alone, it refers to ventricular performance only.

The sequence of events of the cardiac cycle is as follows. The atria in diastole fill with blood received from their inlet vessels. In the early part of the relaxation period, the AV valves are closed but, as pressure builds up in the atria, it becomes greater than that in the ventricles, forcing the AV valves open, and the blood starts to flow through into the ventricles. Atrial diastole is followed in a fraction of a second by contraction, to complete the emptying of the two upper chambers, and the atria again enter their diastole.

During the filling and contraction of the ventricles the blood floats the AV valve cusps up, closing off the AV openings and preventing a regurgitation of blood into the atria. In order to receive the blood from the atria, the ventricles must be in diastole and, at this time, the semilunar valves are closed. With ventricular filling the intraventricular pressure builds up until it exceeds that in the aorta and pulmonary artery, with the result that the semilunar valves open, allowing blood to flow into the arteries. The ventricular muscle contracts, and the ventricles are emptied.

During ventricular systole, the papillary muscles also contract, exerting tension on the fine tendons (chordae tendineae) inserted on the AV valve cusps. This prevents the cusps from opening into the atria.

If this control was not placed on the AV valves, there would be a backflow into the atria, especially with the ventricular contraction. The ventricles relax following their systole and emptying. This results in the pressure being greater in the arteries than in the ventricles, thus favouring the backflow of blood into the ventricles. But flow in the direction of the heart brings about the closure of the semilunar valves by the filling of the semilunar pouches; their free borders are brought together, preventing the blood from re-entering the ventricles from the arteries. The cardiac cycle is now completed.

The cycle in a heart beating approximately 70 times per minute is completed in 0.7–0.8 of a second. The length of each phase of the cycle varies; atrial diastole lasts approximately 0.7 second, while its systole is approximately 0.1 second. Ventricular diastole is about 0.4–0.5 second, and its systole takes about 0.3 second. Following the ventricular contraction there is a brief period, approximately 0.4 second, in which the entire myocardium is relaxed. The ventricular diastole overlaps the atrial diastole.[2]

HEART SOUNDS

Two sounds are produced in quick succession in each cardiac cycle. These are followed by a brief pause before being repeated in the next cycle. Through a stethoscope the heart sounds will be heard as a lub-dub and are produced by closure of the heart valves.

The first heart sound, S_1, is a prolonged low-pitched sound (lub). It is produced by the closing of both atrioventricular valves, the mitral and the tricuspid, just before ventricular systole. Although closure of the two valves occurs almost simultaneously, the mitral valve closes slightly before the tricuspid valve. Therefore, the mitral component is heard slightly before the tricuspid and is the main component of the first heart sound.

The second sound, S_2, is briefer and higher pitched (dub). It is produced by the closing of both semilunar valves, the aortic and the pulmonary, just before diastole. Since the aortic valve closes slightly before the pulmonary valve, the aortic component of S_2 will be heard slightly before the pulmonary. The components of the second sound are normally affected by respiration. During inspiration, closure of the pulmonary valve is delayed because of the increased venous return to the right heart. The difference in the two components of S_2 is therefore more apparent. This is referred to as physiological splitting and disappears during expiration.

The heart sounds will differ as one listens at different locations on the chest (Fig. 14.6). The mitral component of S_1 (M_1) is best heard over the apex of the heart (the patient's fifth left intercostal space near

[2] Ganong (1985), p. 460.

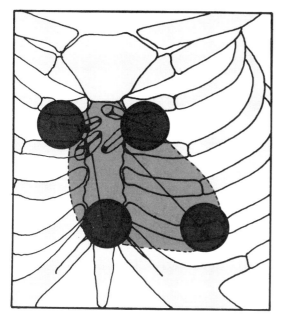

Fig. 14.6 Auscultatory areas on the chest.

the left midclavicular line). The tricuspid component (T_1) is softer than the mitral component and may be best heard over the patient's lower left sternal border.

The aortic component of the second heart sound (A_2) is louder than the pulmonary component and is best heard in the patient's second right intercostal space. The pulmonary valve closure (P_2) is best heard in the patient's second left intercostal space.

A third and fourth heart sound may also be heard. S_3 is a low-pitched sound produced in the ventricle by rapid filling. It may indicate ventricular decompensation and is heard in patients with congestive heart failure. An audible fourth sound (S_4), also called presystolic, is low-pitched and generated by forceful contractions of the atria. It may be present in healthy individuals but is frequently heard in patients with systemic hypertension.

Other unusual or abnormal sounds may also be heard, such as rubs, clicks, splits and murmurs, and usually indicate some pathology in the heart.

CARDIAC OUTPUT

The volume of blood ejected from each ventricle in a minute is known as the cardiac output. The output of each ventricle with each contraction is called the stroke volume. In an adult, the cardiac output varies from 3000–5000 ml per minute, and the stroke volume is about 60–70 ml. If it were 60 ml in a person with a heart rate of 60, the cardiac output would be 3600 ml. (Stroke volume × heart rate = cardiac output per minute.)

The volume of blood that the normal heart pumps out each minute is increased in any situation that increases the body demands and activity. This is readily seen in physical exercise. In strenuous exertion the cardiac output may increase to a volume 13 times greater than the output during rest. This is achieved by an increase in the heart rate and the stroke volume. An increase in the cardiac output also occurs in high environmental temperature, emotional responses such as fear, anger or other excitement, after a heavy meal and in the later months of pregnancy.

Physiologically, the cardiac output is dependent upon preload, afterload, the contractile state of the myocardium and heart rate. In order to eject blood during systole, the ventricle must overcome the pressure of the blood it contains and the back pressure in the vessels into which it is ejecting the blood. The work performed by the ventricle in overcoming these pressures is called the ventricular load. Preload looks at pressures to be overcome at the end of diastole: that is, the pressure of the blood contained in the ventricle just before contraction. Another term to describe this pressure is left ventricular end-diastolic pressure which is related to the volume of blood in the ventricle at the end of diastole.

Afterload describes the force against which the ventricle is working, or the resistance to the ejection of blood. This resistance is also called impedance and is reflected in the tension which ventricular muscle develops during systole.

The contractile state of the myocardium is the ability of the heart to contract. Normal heart structures, absence of disease and an adequate supply of nutrients and oxygen are important factors in the heart's ability to produce the necessary force to eject the contained blood.

Preload
Preload is determined by venous return, ejection fraction and residual volume.

Ejection fraction. The percentage of the total volume of blood in the ventricle which is ejected with each contraction is called the ejection fraction. Normally, this represents 56–72% of the total volume.

Residual volume. Residual volume is the amount of blood left in the ventricle after systole. Normally, it is approximately 28–44% of the total volume in the ventricle.

Venous return. Venous return is affected by total blood volume, and by exercise and respirations which influence the distribution of that volume within the circulatory system.

Blood volume and blood pressure
A decrease in the volume or pressure of the blood in the systemic circulation causes a decrease in the

venous return. This is seen in haemorrhage in which the volume is reduced, and in shock, which is characterized by a fall in blood pressure. Certain areas of the body normally contain a relatively large volume of blood which may be moved out when the normal circulating volume is threatened. These areas are referred to as blood reservoirs and are the liver, spleen, large abdominal veins and venous plexuses of the skin. When necessary, the liver will increase its output into the hepatic vein, and the spleen will contract to empty as much as three-quarters of its contained blood into the circulation. Similarly, when the total circulating volume is reduced, the large abdominal veins constrict to increase their outflow. The venous plexuses of the skin, which normally contain a considerable volume of blood, will also constrict when necessary to provide a greater flow to the heart.

Resistance to blood flow
Increased resistance to the blood flow anywhere in the circulatory system may reduce venous return to the heart and cause a corresponding decrease in cardiac output.

Exercise
Muscular exercise is one of the most significant factors in promoting venous return. When skeletal muscles contract, veins are compressed, and more blood is forced out of them. It must move toward the heart since the valves prevent a backward flow. Also, the increased metabolism in the muscles during exercise increases their need for oxygen and nutrients, resulting in local vasodilation of the arterioles and capillaries which reduces resistance to the flow of blood in the muscles. Since exercise usually involves a large number of muscles, this causes an appreciable decrease in the total resistance in the systemic circulation, favouring an increased venous return and cardiac output.

Respiration
The rate and depth of respirations also have a marked effect on venous return; increased respirations increase the volume of blood entering the right atrium. On inspiration, the diaphragm descends, compressing the abdominal cavity and increasing the pressure on the veins in that area. At the same time the thoracic cavity enlarges and the pressure on regional veins is reduced. This increases the pressure gradient between the blood in the abdominal veins and that in the thoracic veins so that a greater volume flows from the abdominal veins into the thoracic vena cava and on into the heart.

The foregoing explanation of the effects of exercise and respirations on the venous return and cardiac output explains the importance of having inactive and bed patients breathe deeply at frequent intervals and do some physical exercises. These activities promote circulation and help to prevent complications that may occur with circulatory stasis.

Sympathetic (nervous) innervation may augment the volume of blood in circulation, and thus the venous return, by causing organs such as the liver and spleen to reduce their intrinsic volume.

The ability of the heart to increase its output commensurate with increased tissue activity and needs is referred to as cardiac reserve. The normal heart is capable of forwarding the volume of blood delivered to it and of responding to an increased demand without difficulty. It does this without causing breathlessness, tachycardia or palpitation beyond 5–10 minutes. It can do approximately 13 times what it does at rest if its reserve is normal.

Afterload
Afterload is affected by the level of aortic pressure and peripheral vascular resistance and the size of the heart.

Contractile state of heart
If the heart is undamaged and is in a condition to respond, the strength of the heart-beat is determined mainly by the length of the muscle fibres when contraction begins. Stretching of muscle fibres, within limits, increases the strength of their contraction. The length or stretching of the myocardial fibres is dependent upon the volume of blood entering the heart. This principle is known as Starling's law of the heart and may be expressed in this manner: 'the energy of contraction is proportional to the initial length of the cardiac muscle fibres.'[3]

The inotropic state of the heart is also affected by local and circulating catecholamines, the rate and rhythm of ventricular contractions, physiological depressants such as acidosis or myocardial hypoxia, the amount of ventricular substance and certain drugs such as digoxin and/or caffeine.

HEART RATE

The number of heart-beats per minute varies in different people and under different conditions. The average normal rate for an adult is 70 beats per minute, but it may range from 60–90. Several factors influence the heart rate. In the infant a rate of 110–130 is normal. It becomes progressively slower as the child grows older; by the early teens it is usually about 80. Muscular exertion will produce a marked increase, especially if one is unaccustomed to physical exercise. The rate usually increases during emotional reactions, with fever, and in the lower atmospheric pressures found at high altitudes.

REGULATION OF CARDIAC ACTIVITY

Certain nervous, chemical and mechanical factors play an important role in the action of the heart.

---

[3] Ganong (1985), p. 418.

Nervous influence

The heart muscle is capable of generating its own impulses for contraction, but nerve impulses from the parasympathetic and sympathetic divisions of the autonomic nervous system may modify the rate and strength of the contractions. Nervous regulation is mediated by impulses which arise in the medulla oblongata in a group of neurons known as the cardiac centre. Parasympathetic impulses reach the heart by way of branches of the vagus nerve (10th cranial nerve) and are delivered to the SA and AV nodes and to the atrial muscle. Vagal or parasympathetic innervation has an inhibitory effect on cardiac activity; it slows the heart rate and decreases the force of the atrial contraction by reducing the excitability of the pacemaker (SA node) and the conductivity of the AV node and conducting system.

Sympathetic impulses enter the heart by the cardiac accelerator nerves, originating in a cervical ganglion. These impulses are transmitted to the SA node, the conducting system, and the atrial and ventricular muscle. Sympathetic stimulation increases the heart rate and the strength of the heart contractions.

Parasympathetic innervation predominates in heart action. Normally, it exerts a fairly constant check on the heart rate, thus conserving the heart's strength.

The cardiac centre may be stimulated by impulses originating in higher levels of the brain or in some part of the body which is outside the central nervous system (brain and spinal cord). One need only recall the change experienced in one's own heart action during fear, anger or other excitement. The response of increased or decreased heart activity is due to impulses being discharged by the cerebral cortical level to the cardiac centre.

Sensory impulses from outside the central nervous system enter the cord or brain and may be relayed to the cardiac centre, resulting in innervation of the heart. The response of the heart to peripheral sensory impulses may be referred to as a cardiac reflex. The most significant of these are the vasosensory impulses originating in the baroreceptors and chemoreceptors. A group of sensory nerve endings in the aortic arch and in the carotid arteries at their bifurcation are sensitive to changes in the blood pressure and are called baroreceptors. In the same areas are nerve endings that are sensitive to changes in the carbon dioxide and oxygen concentration and the pH (hydrogen ion concentration) of the blood. These are known as the chemoreceptors. Impulses initiated in these receptors enter the brain or cord and are relayed to the cardiac centre.

An increase in blood pressure produces a response in the cardio-inhibitory centre. Vagal stimulation of the heart is increased and the heart rate decreases.[4] A decrease in the oxygen concentration, an increase in carbon dioxide concentration and a decrease in the pH of the blood result in stimulation of the cardio-accelerator centre and in elevation of the heart rate.

Chemical influence

Normal, rhythmic heart contractions are greatly dependent upon an optimal concentration of potassium, sodium and calcium in the extracellular fluid.[5] These minerals play an important role in the excitability of the cardiac muscle cells and their contraction.

If the potassium level is greater than its normal concentration in the extracellular fluid, an impairment in conduction and contraction occurs. It causes a prolonged relaxation of the heart with abnormal dilation of the chambers. The pulse becomes slow. A decrease below the normal concentration of sodium results in weaker contractions. The pulse is rapid and weak, and there is a fall in blood pressure. An excess sodium concentration does not directly affect cardiac action. An excess of calcium produces a stronger and prolonged systole. Conversely, a lack of calcium prolongs the diastole.

Other chemicals of significance in heart action are oxygen and carbon dioxide. Any deficiency of oxygen is quickly reflected in a weakening of heart action. The myocardium is much more sensitive to oxygen lack than skeletal muscle; it will stand only one-fifth as much oxygen deficiency as skeletal muscle. The pulse becomes rapid, weak and irregular. With an excess of carbon dioxide in the blood, as may occur in respiratory insufficiency, heart action is impaired. Conduction is slowed, the relaxation period is prolonged and the contraction is briefer than normal.

Mechanical influence

The principal mechanical influence on cardiac activity is the stretching of the myocardial fibres by the volume of blood entering the chambers. As previously stated, stretching of muscle fibres increases the strength of their contraction (Starling's law of the heart, p. 304). An increase in arterial blood pressure also demands a greater force of contraction; the heart muscle must release a greater amount of energy to perform its function because of meeting greater resistance.

BLOOD PRESSURE AND PULSE

Blood pressure

Blood pressure may be defined as the pressure exerted laterally on the walls of the blood vessels. It varies in different parts of the circulatory system, being greatest in the large arteries, with a progressive decrease as the blood continues on through the

---

[4] Marey's Law. The pulse rate is inversely related to the arterial blood pressure.

[5] Optimal serum concentrations: K^+, 3.5–5.5 mmol/l; Na^+, 135–145 mmol/l; and Ca^{2+}, 2.2–2.6 mmol/l.

smaller arteries, arterioles, capillaries and veins. The pressure is highest in the aorta and lowest in the large caval veins which enter the heart. Blood pressure at any point in the vascular system is dependent upon the force with which the heart pumps the blood out of the ventricles, the volume of blood in the system, the elasticity of the arteries and the amount of resistance to the flow of the blood from one portion of the circulatory system to the next.

ARTERIAL BLOOD PRESSURE

The blood pressure of greatest clinical interest is that in the arteries. The pulsatile nature of heart activity causes fluctuations in the pressure. With each contraction of the left ventricle a volume of blood is pumped into the aorta, which is already filled with blood. This causes an appreciable increase in the pressure of the blood and stretches the aortic walls. If the aorta were not elastic, the rise in pressure would be much higher and sharper. During the ventricular diastole, the elastic walls of the aorta recoil, exerting a pressure on the contained blood. If the aorta were a rigid tube which did not recoil, the pressure of the blood would fall more rapidly and to a much lower level than it does normally. The higher pressure produced by the ventricular systole is referred to as the *systolic blood pressure*. The lower pressure that occurs during the ventricular diastole is dependent upon the recoil of the large arteries and is known as the *diastolic blood pressure*. The difference between these two pressures is called the *pulse pressure*. Pulse pressure varies inversely with the elasticity of the arteries. Rigid vessels with a loss of ability to distend and recoil produce a higher systolic pressure and a lower diastolic pressure, resulting in an increased pulse pressure.

Measurement
Arterial blood pressure is most frequently measured in millimeters of mercury (mmHg) by means of a sphygmomanometer and a stethoscope, using the brachial artery. The rubber cuff of the blood pressure apparatus is applied to the upper arm just above the elbow and is inflated with air, which compresses the brachial artery. The pressure in the cuff is transmitted to the column of mercury of the manometer. The stethoscope is applied over the brachial artery just below the cuff.

When the cuff pressure becomes greater than the blood pressure, no pulse is heard. The air in the cuff is slowly released and the height of the mercury on the manometer is noted when the pulse is first heard. This corresponds to the systolic blood pressure.

With further slow deflation of the cuff, the pulse gradually becomes softer. The level of the mercury is again noted just before the pulse becomes inaudible; this represents the diastolic blood pressure. If the blood pressure is recorded as 100 mmHg, it simply means that the pressure of the blood on the walls of the vessel is sufficient to raise a column of mercury to a height of 100 mm. The normal systolic pressure in a healthy young adult in a sitting position is 100–135 mmHg; the normal diastolic pressure is 60–80 mmHg. Blood pressure may also be determined by a more direct method. A needle or a cannula is placed in an artery and connected to a mercury manometer on which the blood pressure is indicated. For continuous monitoring of blood pressure, the needle may be connected to a transducer for electronic recording.

Factors which determine arterial blood pressure
Arterial blood pressure is influenced by the strength of the heart-beat, volume of blood, elasticity of the vessels and the resistance offered to the flow of blood.

Strength of the heart-beat. If the myocardial strength is weakened by disease, lack of essential materials or a deficiency in stimulation, it follows that the pressure under which the blood is ejected into the arteries would be reduced, as well as the volume of blood emitted. The arterial pressure is directly proportional to the cardiac output.

Blood volume. Any reduction in the intravascular volume will reduce the head of pressure and the stretch and recoil of the arteries, resulting in an appreciable decrease in the pressure of the blood. Small decreases in the volume are compensated for by the contraction of vessels but, in some conditions (e.g. haemorrhage, severe dehydration, burns), the loss may be beyond compensation. In some instances, vasodilation may occur (e.g. shock, anaphylaxis), increasing the capacity of the system beyond that of the contained volume, and the blood pressure falls. A disproportion between the volume of blood and the capacity of the vascular system due to widespread vasodilation or a diminished blood volume, as in haemorrhage, reduces the venous return to the heart. This is an important factor in determining the cardiac output, the strength of the heart-beat and the blood pressure.

Aldosterone, a hormone secreted by the adrenal cortex, produces an increase in the intravascular volume and a corresponding increase in blood pressure by its effect on kidney activity. It promotes absorption of sodium by the kidney tubules. The increased sodium concentration of the blood in turn causes more water to be absorbed by the renal tubules, increasing the total vascular volume and, as a result, the blood pressure. Conversely, a reduction in aldosterone secretion will reduce the intravascular volume, and the blood pressure falls. The mechanism that regulates the amount of aldosterone secreted by the adrenal cortices is not yet established.

Elasticity of the vessels. The elastic quality of the large arteries has an important role in determining blood pressure. It allows for an increase in the capacity of the arteries when the blood is ejected by each heartbeat. The stretch factor reduces the resistance offered to the flow of blood from the heart, thus reducing somewhat the demand on that organ. With ventricular diastole and the run-off of blood into succeeding vessels, the elastic arterial wall recoils. This provides some pressure on the contained blood to augment its forward movement, and helps to maintain a continuous flow of blood between ventricular contractions. The pressure of the blood at this time (i.e. during arterial recoil and between ventricular contractions) represents the diastolic blood pressure. If the elasticity of the arteries is reduced, as in arteriosclerosis, the blood is pumped into rigid, nondistensible tubes; the systolic pressure is increased because of the lack of vascular stretching and the diastolic pressure is reduced because of the reduced force of recoil.

Resistance to blood flow. The amount of resistance with which the blood is met as it flows through the vascular system depends mainly on the calibre of the arterioles and the viscosity of the blood.

1 *Calibre of the arterioles.* The relatively large lumen of the arteries offers little peripheral resistance to the flow of blood, but their subsequent branching into numerous arterioles introduces more surface contact for the blood, which increases friction and resistance to the flow. This resistance determines the rate at which blood can flow from the arteries into the arterioles, which in turn influences the volume of blood confined in the arteries and, hence, the arterial blood pressure.

Normally the arterioles are in a constant state of partial contraction, referred to as the basic level of tone, but the calibre of the vessels may be modified by contraction or relaxation of the well developed, circular, smooth muscle in the walls in response to various factors. Obviously, with relaxation, the increased diameter of the arterioles will offer less resistance, more blood will pass from the arteries through the arterioles to the capillaries and the arterial blood pressure will tend to be normal or below normal. Conversely, with contraction of the arterioles, the decreased diameter increases the resistance to the blood flow, less blood escapes from the arteries and arterial blood pressure is maintained at a normal or above normal level. The calibre of the arterioles is controlled by nerve impulses delivered to the musculature of the arterioles and by certain chemical changes in the extracellular fluids. The latter may exercise their influence directly on the vessels or indirectly through the autonomic nervous system.

Neural control of vascular tone is exerted by the autonomic nervous system. The vessels are supplied by two types of nerve fibres: those whose impulses cause contraction of the muscle tissue of the vessel are the excitatory or vasoconstrictor nerves, and those which cause relaxation are the inhibitory or vasodilator nerves. All vasoconstrictor nerves derive from the sympathetic division of the autonomic nervous system and are thought to act on the alpha (α) receptor sites of smooth muscle. Sympathetic vasoconstrictors are located in the kidneys, skin, gut and spleen. Vasodilation may be initiated by a decrease in sympathetic innervation which allows a relaxation of the smooth muscle of the vessel or, in some instances, dilation results from impulses delivered by nerves to the vessel walls. The vasodilator, or inhibitory, nerves in some areas of the body belong to the parasympathetic division; in others the vasodilator as well as the vasoconstrictor nerves originate in the sympathetic nervous system. Sympathetic vasodilators are distributed to the vessels of skeletal muscles, the intestines, the coronary system and some areas of the skin. Parasympathetic vasodilators supply the vessels in the tongue, sweat and salivary glands, external genitalia and possibly the bladder and rectum.

The principal source of the impulses that regulate the calibre of the blood vessels is the vasomotor centre in the medulla. Some impulses may arise from spinal cord neurons in the thoracolumbar areas. These areas may be influenced by impulses received from the blood vessels themselves, the baroreceptors and chemoreceptors of the carotid sinus and aortic arch, the cerebral cortex, the hypothalamus and various other regions of the body, such as the skin, muscles and viscera.

Chemical influence of the smooth muscle in the vessels may be direct or may be indirect through the nervous system. Certain chemical changes in the composition of the extracellular fluid may result in the initiation of nerve impulses which influence the blood vessels. Increased carbon dioxide or decreased oxygen tension results in vasoconstriction and a corresponding increase in resistance. Similarly, an increase in the hydrogen ion concentration (decreased pH) causes vasoconstriction.

A direct effect on the arterioles may be produced by metabolites and hormones. Metabolites produce the opposite effect locally to that caused indirectly through the nervous system. An increase in the concentration of hydrogen ions and carbon dioxide and a diminished oxygen tension in an area cause dilatation of the arterioles in that area. The indirect action of the nervous system produces a more general vasoconstriction and a rise in blood pressure, increasing the rate of flow through the locally dilated arterioles, when there is an increased need for more oxygen and nutrients, and for the removal of more metabolites.

When tissue cells are irritated or injured, chemical substances are released which produce relaxation in the local arterioles and capillaries, resulting in more blood in the area. One of these substances is identified as histamine, a strong vasodilator.

Still another chemical substance, renin, stimulates vasoconstriction and increases arterial blood pressure. It is produced by kidney tissue in response to a diminished blood supply (renal ischaemia). Renin is a proteolytic enzyme which, when released into the bloodstream, acts upon a globulin fraction, producing the vasoconstrictor angiotensin (hypertensin) that acts directly on the arterioles. It would appear that angiotensin has no significant role in the maintenance of normal blood pressure, since it is quickly destroyed in the healthy person. It remains active for a longer period in persons with a blood pressure higher than normal and is receiving some attention in relation to the disease of hypertension.

The hormones associated with vasomotor activity are adrenaline and antidiuretic hormone (ADH). Adrenaline, secreted by the adrenal medulla or administered parenterally, has a direct vasoconstricting effect on the arterioles in the skin, mucous membranes and the splanchnic area. At the same time, it inhibits the tone in the arterioles of the skeletal muscles and the coronary system. Guyton suggests that the effect of adrenaline on the coronaries may be indirect, since the hormone stimulates metabolism which causes the local metabolic regulatory system to increase blood flow.[6]

The secretion of the neurohypophysis or posterior lobe of the pituitary gland contains ADH. It excites the smooth muscle of most blood vessels, but its effect is slower than that of adrenaline.

It may be seen from the foregoing discussion of vasomotor regulation that peripheral resistance is a complex affair. Resistance is directly proportional to the length of vessels and inversely proportional to the diameter, and many factors may influence the diameter. A moderate degree of vasoconstriction is essential; most of the arterioles must be in a partial state of constriction at all times. If too many vessels relax at one time blood pressure falls to dangerously low levels, and circulation becomes seriously impaired.

Frequent and quick readjustments in the calibre of the arterioles are necessary to maintain a relatively constant level of blood pressure and to meet the changing needs of tissue cells. Increased activity of structures or areas demands more blood in those parts and vasodilation occurs. To compensate for the increased volume in one area, vasoconstriction must occur in other parts of the body to maintain a forward movement of the blood and a normal cardiac output and blood pressure. For example, when a person moves from the recumbent to the upright position, the blood tends to collect in the lower part of the body because of gravity. This causes a decrease in the blood pressure in the aorta and carotid arteries, and the baroreceptors then initiate the reflex response of vasoconstriction in the arterioles. This response maintains an adequate circulation throughout the upper parts of the body.

2 *Blood viscosity.* The second factor on which the resistance to the flow of blood depends is the viscosity of the blood. It is a much less significant factor than the calibre of the arterioles. Viscosity is the resistance to flow created within the fluid itself by the friction and cohesiveness between its molecules. Resistance of a fluid is directly proportional to its viscosity.

Blood viscosity is mainly dependent on the concentration of the red blood cells and blood proteins. It is approximately 2.5–5 times the viscosity of water. An increase above the normal number of red blood cells (polycythaemia) impedes the flow of blood and may cause an appreciable increase above normal in the arterial blood pressure. The calibre of the arterioles is subject to frequent fluctuations, but usually viscosity only changes when blood is diluted or when there is an increase or decrease in the number of red blood cells.

Normal variations in arterial blood pressure
Age, exercise, emotions and weight influence blood pressure.

Blood pressure changes with age. During infancy and childhood, blood pressure is lower than later in life. In the newborn infant systolic pressure is approximately 55–90 mmHg; the diastolic is approximately 40–55 mmHg. This gradually increases throughout childhood, reaching adult level about puberty. Usually in the fifties, the systolic pressure begins to show a slight increase which progresses with age, corresponding to the loss of elasticity and to the thickening of the walls of the arteries characteristic of the ageing process.

Physical exertion is accompanied by a rise in the arterial blood pressure due to the increased venous return and the increased production of metabolites such as carbon dioxide and lactic acid. The systolic pressure may increase as much as 60–70 mmHg in strenuous exercise.

Emotions may also cause an elevation in blood pressure; the more excited, anxious, angry or fearful a person becomes, the higher the blood pressure goes. Vasoconstriction is increased due to sympathetic innervation and the release of adrenaline into the bloodstream.

Blood pressure increases with increased body weight, especially after middle age. This is of significance in our present-day society in which overweight and hypertension have a high incidence.

CAPILLARY BLOOD PRESSURE

The pressure of the blood on entry to the capillaries is approximately 20–35 mmHg. This varies with the constriction and dilation of the arterioles. It is this pressure that is responsible for the movement of fluid and dissolved particles through the semipermeable capillary walls into the interstitial spaces, making them available to cells. The volume of fluid

---

[6] Guyton (1984), p. 289.

that moves out into the interstitial spaces is dependent upon the capillary blood pressure and the opposing pressure exerted by the interstitial fluid. The capillary blood pressure is quickly reduced by this loss of fluid and to some extent by the resistance of the minute vessels. As a result, by the time the blood leaves the capillaries, the pressure is reduced to approximately 10–20 mmHg. The movement of fluid across the capillary walls is more fully discussed under Fluids and Electrolyte Balance, pp. 80–82.

VENOUS BLOOD PRESSURE

The pressure of the blood is reduced slowly but progressively from the time it leaves the capillaries until it reaches the right atrium.

Venous blood pressure is influenced by cardiac strength, blood volume, respirations and posture. Venous pressure is actually the force that remains of that created by the left ventricular contraction. The blood enters the venous system under a pressure of approximately 10 mmHg. The walls of the veins continue to offer some resistance and the blood, particularly in the lower parts of the body, must travel a considerable distance before reaching the heart.[7] As a result, the pressure is dissipated progressively, and by the time it reaches the right atrium is very low—0–10 cmH$_2$O (0–1 mmHg). Obviously, if the left ventricular systole is weak and the blood starts out at a lower than normal arterial pressure, it will tend to move more slowly in the veins toward the heart.

Cardiac strength
Maintenance of normal pressure and flow of the venous blood are influenced by the ability of the right heart chambers to empty sufficiently to receive the volume of blood being forwarded by the large veins. If the heart cannot pass on the blood it receives, the normal volume cannot enter and there is a damming back in the veins. The resulting increased volume causes an increase in the blood pressure. Normal emptying of the right atrium actually promotes venous flow; in diastole, the empty right atrium tends to produce an aspirating effect on the large veins.

Blood volume
The greater the volume of blood flowing into the veins from the arterioles and capillaries, the greater will be the venous pressure. If the arterioles are constricted, the pressure in the veins will be lower. If the arterioles are dilated, as in muscular exercise, the greater volume escaping into the veins will increase the venous pressure. Normally, marked changes do not occur since the veins have the ability to adjust by

either vasoconstriction or dilation to the volume of blood being received. This is accomplished mainly in the smaller veins.

Respiration
On inspiration there is a decrease in intrathoracic pressure and an increase in intra-abdominal pressure. Abdominal venous pressure increases while that in the thoracic veins is lowered, causing a larger volume of blood to move into the thoracic veins. On expiration, intrathoracic pressure increases, compressing the veins and raising the pressure within them, thus helping to move the blood into the atria.

Posture
Due to gravity, the upright position favours an increase in venous pressure in the lower parts of the body, but continuous venous return is preserved by compensatory mechanisms. The baroreceptors initiate reflex vascular constriction which usually preserves an adequate blood pressure. In spite of the compensatory vasoconstriction, a greater volume of blood is likely to accumulate in the lower veins during long periods of standing. This may be seen in persons who faint when required to stand for a relatively long period.

For measurement of venous blood pressure see p. 321.

Pulse

Each ventricular contraction ejects a volume of blood into the aorta, producing an increase in the blood pressure which causes an expansion of the artery. During ventricular diastole, the elastic recoil of the aorta moves the blood into the next portion of the artery, which stretches and then recoils. This alternating expansion and recoil spreads along the whole arterial system, producing a pulse wave. Each pulsation corresponds to a heart-beat and is the result of the impact of the ejected volume of blood on the arterial wall. The pulsations occur in the arteries of the pulmonary circulatory system as well as in the systemic circulation.

A pulse may be felt in arteries near the surface of the body, and is a valuable source of information about the heart and vessels. The radial artery at the wrist is the most convenient site for feeling the pulse, but it may also be felt in the temporal, carotid, brachial, external submaxillary, abdominal aorta, femoral, popliteal and dorsalis pedis arteries. When palpating a pulse, the observer notes the following:
1 The frequency per minute, which represents the number of left ventricular contractions that are strong enough to produce pulse waves that will reach the peripheral artery being used.
2 The volume, which indicates the strength of the heart contraction.

---

[7] Pressure is inversely proportional to frictional resistance and the length of the tube.

3 The rhythm, or regularity, of the intervals between pulsations.
4 The tension and thickness of the arterial wall, which gives some indication of the resistance.

The loss of pressure of the blood in arterioles and capillaries results in the absence of a venous pulse. There is one exception—a feeble venous pulse may be palpated in the internal jugular veins while the subject is in a recumbent position. It is caused by the atrial systole. Since no valves guard the openings of the vena caval veins into the right atrium, a small amount of blood is regurgitated into the large veins with atrial contraction, producing a weak pulse.

FETAL CIRCULATION

The circulatory pathway in the fetus differs from that established at birth (Fig. 14.7). This is a necessity, since the developing organism is dependent upon the maternal blood for its oxygen and nutrients, as well as for the elimination of its metabolic wastes.

SPECIAL CIRCULATORY STRUCTURES

Several special structures are developed in the fetal circulatory system, and they function to support the developing organism during intrauterine life. Two umbilical arteries arise from the fetal hypogastric or internal iliac arteries and deliver fetal blood from the aorta to the placenta. One umbilical vein originates in the placenta. The blood which is transported has taken on oxygen and nutrients in the placenta in exchange for carbon dioxide and other metabolic wastes. The placenta is a mass of finger-like projections (chorionic villi) which penetrate deeply into the thick endometrium early in pregnancy. The villi become highly vascularized and lie in close contact with the maternal blood in the wall of the uterus to allow for an exchange of substances. The ductus venosus is a vein formed by a continuation of the umbilical vein along the undersurface of the liver. It receives blood from the portal vein and gives rise to a few small vessels which enter the liver. The ductus venosus terminates in the inferior vena cava. The

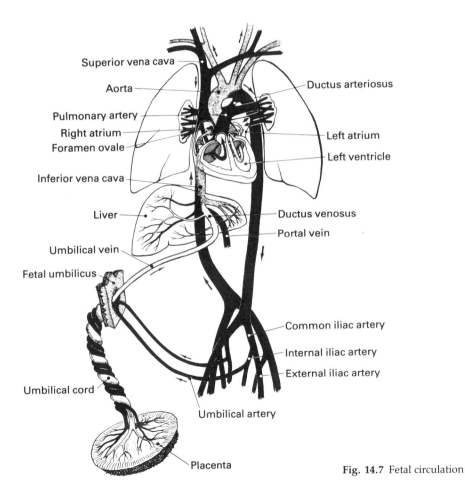

Fig. 14.7 Fetal circulation

ductus arteriosus is a short vessel between the pulmonary artery and the descending thoracic aorta. Blood flowing through this vessel bypasses the pulmonary system. The foramen ovale is an opening between the right and left atria. A valve permits blood to flow from the right atrium into the left atrium, thus bypassing the pulmonary system.

THE CIRCULATORY PATHWAY IN THE FETUS

With these special structures in mind, the course which fetal blood takes may be outlined (Table 14.1).

Starting with the left ventricle of the fetal heart, the blood is received into the aorta and continues on the usual route. A supply is distributed through aortic branches to structures in the thoracic and abdominal regions. Some of the blood continues on to the lower limbs via the external iliac arteries, but the greater volume of it is delivered to the placenta by the two umbilical arteries which derive from the hypogastric arteries (internal iliac arteries). The umbilical arteries leave the fetus in the umbilical cord and pass to the placenta, where they divide and subdivide into thin-walled capillaries contained in the villi of the placenta. The semipermeable walls of the capillaries permit the movement of oxygen, nutrients and other substances into fetal blood from maternal blood and movement of wastes from fetal blood to maternal blood. Since this exchange is through capillary walls, there is no direct mixing of the fetal and maternal bloods.

The fetal blood is collected in the placenta into the umbilical vein and passes via the umbilical cord to the fetus. Within the fetal body, the umbilical vein proceeds toward the liver where it becomes the ductus venosus. Most of the blood bypasses the liver, continuing on into the right inferior vena cava by which it enters the right atrium.

A volume of the blood in the right atrium passes through the foramen ovale into the left atrium because the pressure of the blood in the right atrium is greater than that in the left atrium. The remainder of the blood flows into the right ventricle and out into the pulmonary artery. Only a small portion of this blood continues on through the lungs, and is eventually delivered to the left atrium by the four pulmonary veins. The larger portion is shunted through the ductus arteriosus into the aorta, thus bypassing the lungs.

The shunting of the blood through the foramen ovale and the ductus arteriosus into the aorta greatly reduces the volume of blood in the pulmonary circulation. This particular pathway would seem to be so designed because the lungs of the fetus are not functioning, and no purpose would be served by having all the blood pass through the pulmonary system.

The blood in the left atrium passes into the left ventricle and out into the aorta to join that received from the ductus arteriosus. The circuit is now complete.

CHANGES IN FETAL CIRCULATION AT BIRTH

After birth, the baby must function independently, so the special structures are no longer useful. With the cutting of the umbilical cord, no blood enters

Table 14.1 Schematic outline of fetal circulation.

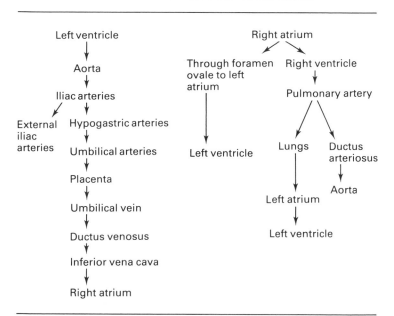

either the umbilical vein or arteries. The portion of these vessels within the body cavity contract, thrombose and eventually become fibrous cords. The ductus venosus, now non-functional, also becomes fibrous. All the blood in the portal vein is now directed into the liver.

When the lungs expand and become functional, a greater volume of blood enters the pulmonary circulation and flows into the left atrium. The pressure of the blood in the left atrium is now higher than that in the right atrium and the foramen ovale in the atrial septum is closed. A gradual constriction and atrophy of the ductus arteriosus takes place, and its closure is usually complete within a few weeks of birth.

Nursing in Impaired Cardiac Function

Heart disease is a national health problem of considerable proportions. It is a leading cause of death in the United Kingdom, Canada and the United States. Many nursing hours in hospitals, homes and clinics are devoted to patients with heart disease.

NURSE'S ROLE IN PREVENTION OF HEART DISEASE

The nurse has many opportunities to contribute to the prevention of cardiac insufficiency. Whether the work is in the hospital, clinic, home, industry or school, the role may be participation in health screening, education or provision of care. In order to recognize and fulfil the responsibilities in the preventive programme, the nurse must be informed and must make a personal effort to keep abreast of new knowledge. In addition to an understanding of the role of the heart in supplying all the cells throughout the body with materials essential to their survival and activities, a knowledge of how this function may be impaired by various pathological processes is necessary. This information serves as the basis for the recognition of excessive demands on the heart, significant signs and symptoms and the need for medical attention. It also provides the basis for explanations and appropriate health education as well as for the planning and giving of safe and effective care.

People are urged to secure an early diagnosis and treatment of illnesses which may damage the heart. Examples of such conditions are rheumatic fever, hypertension, syphilis and hyperthyroidism. The promotion of immunization for diphtheria contributes to the prevention of heart disease because the toxin produced by the causative organisms may have a serious effect on the heart muscle.

Opportunities often arise for the nurse to discuss the hazards of obesity and its possible effects on the heart. Similarly, the advantages of such factors as moderate exercise, annual physical examinations and the reduction of animal fat in the diet are stressed. Avoidance of unaccustomed strenuous physical activities and overexcitement, particularly by older people, are stressed in health education in relation to the prevention of heart disease. All too often one reads of sudden deaths due to a heart attack suffered while shovelling snow or while participating in competitive sports. The nurse has an important role in helping both adults and children to develop good health habits and to live a balanced life of physical activity, rest, work and recreation.

Studies have indicated a higher incidence of coronary heart disease among cigarette smokers. Established smokers are encouraged to stop or at least reduce the number of cigarettes smoked per day. Every effort should be made to discourage young people from starting the smoking habit.

The nurse should be ever alert to the possible significance of shortness of breath, cyanosis, oedema and chest pain on exertion. Recognition leading to an early diagnosis and treatment may prevent irreparable damage which can eventually incapacitate the person.

It must be understood that much heart disease can be and is cured. Many people with a heart condition or reduced cardiac efficiency live useful, satisfactory lives by readjusting their activities. The nurse must appreciate these facts to develop an optimistic, encouraging attitude with cardiac patients. Any pessimism on her part may readily be conveyed to a patient or family who, generally, tends to be overpessimistic about heart disease. Motivation, instruction and planning to have the heart patient live within the functional ability of his heart may prevent progression of the heart disease and possible heart failure. Follow-up of patients to provide guidance in following the doctor's suggestions may prevent problems and relapses. For example, visits to the child who has had rheumatic fever may ensure the continuation of prescribed prophylactic doses of penicillin.

ASSESSMENT OF IMPAIRED HEART FUNCTION

At the present time the nurse often assumes more responsibility than formerly for assessing the clinical status of patients. Assessment includes taking a nursing history, monitoring and recording physical signs and symptoms, and observing emotional and psychological reactions. The nurse may also participate in the administration of invasive and non-invasive diagnostic tests.

The responsibility of the nurse in patient assessment varies with the practice setting. In all instances the nurse is responsible for observing, recording and reporting specific physical signs and symptoms, understanding their implications and preparing and supporting the patient for various diagnostic procedures. In some situations certain physical assessments or diagnostic measures may be delegated to the nurse by the doctor—for example, electrocardiographic monitoring. In assessing the person with heart disease the nurse should collect subjective and objective information. A list of the patient's problems or needs can then be formulated and the goals set. This forms the basis for planning and implementing the nursing care of the patient.

MANIFESTATIONS OF IMPAIRED HEART FUNCTION

Any impairment in circulation due to an abnormal heart condition is reflected in signs and symptoms which are produced by various factors: (1) a reduced blood supply to the heart and tissues throughout the body, causing a reduced nutrient and oxygen supply and an accumulation of metabolic wastes; (2) malfunctioning of the conduction system; and (3) the inability of the heart to eject the blood it receives. The latter results in an excessive volume in the venous system, creating congestion and increased pressure that interfere with the function of tissues and organs.

The signs and symptoms of cardiac conditions vary with the degree to which circulation is impaired and with the form and location of the heart condition. All those which are discussed here do not necessarily occur in every patient, nor are they all inclusive but are the more common problems presented by cardiac patients.

Abnormal pulse
The pulse rate may be abnormally fast or slow and the intervals between the heart-beat may be unequal. The volume may vary. Some specific abnormalities of the arterial pulse are as follows:

Pulsus alternans. With pulsus alternans, the heart-beats are regular but vary in amplitude. This condition is produced by changes in the left ventricular contractile force and is often precipitated by a premature ventricular beat. It is frequently associated with left ventricular failure resulting from hypertension, cardiomyopathy or aortic valve disease.

Pulsus bigeminus. Premature contractions occurring after every other heart-beat result in variation in the strength of the heart-beats. This alteration in pulse volume from beat to beat is called bigeminal pulse. It differs from pulsus alternans in that the weaker beat occurs regularly after a stronger, normally conducted beat.

Pulsus paradoxus. Normally, the strength of the arterial pulse falls during inspiration because of pooling of blood in the pulmonary vascular system. This occurs because of the more negative intrathoracic pressure and expansion of the lungs causing a reduced left ventricular stroke volume. If the blood pressure falls more than 10 mmHg (the normal fall during inspiration), the pulse is called pulsus para-

doxus. Causes include cardiac tamponade, chronic constrictive pericarditis, emphysema and bronchial asthma.

Abnormal venous pulse
The time and amplitude of jugular venous pulses are observed with the trunk of the patient elevated to the degree at which maximum venous pulsation occurs. The degree of elevation required will vary from person to person, from less than 45° for the normal person to 90° in some patients with heart disease. A beam of light is shone tangentially across the skin over the vein and the character of the venous wave and the level of venous pressure are observed. Elevation of jugular venous pressure indicates an increase in right atrial pressure. Causes include tricuspid stenosis, decreased right ventricular compliance, cardiac tamponade and acute and chronic cor pulmonale.

Blood pressure
Arterial blood pressure is an important indicator of the patient's circulatory status. The systolic pressure depends on the cardiac output and, obviously, will fall with a reduced output by the left side of the heart. Venous pressure is frequently used to assess the ability of the heart to accept the inflow into the right side of the heart. A venous pressure in excess of the normal may indicate cardiac insufficiency or failure or an excessive intravascular volume.

Dyspnoea
The patient may experience shortness of breath or laboured breathing only on exertion, or it may be present even at rest. This is due to pulmonary congestion. The left side of the heart may not be forwarding all the blood it receives, and the blood is dammed back in the pulmonary veins. The pulmonary congestion and hypertension resist alveolar expansion, increasing the work of breathing and decreasing the vital capacity. If the congestion is long standing, alveolar tissue changes occur; the elastic tissue is replaced with fibrous tissue, and normal gas exchange is disturbed.

Dyspnoea that occurs when the patient is recumbent is referred to as orthopnoea. It may be relieved when the patient sits upright.

Cough
Fluid escapes into the alveoli from the capillaries in the congested pulmonary system and acts as a cough stimulus. This collection of transudate in the alveoli may be referred to as pulmonary oedema. The fluid may be expectorated as a frothy sputum and in severe heart failure may contain blood.

Hypoxia
Any impairment in circulation will create an oxygen deficiency in tissues. The cardiac output may be reduced, or a disturbance in pulmonary circulation

may reduce the exchange of gases in the lung. Symptoms of an oxygen deficiency are many and varied, since the function of all structures is affected. The brain quickly reflects oxygen deprivation and reduced mental efficiency, apathy and disorientation are manifested. If the deficiency is severe, consciousness is lost and, unless the supply to the brain is promptly re-established, there is likely to be permanent tissue damage.

Severe pain occurs when muscle tissue, such as the myocardium, is deprived of adequate oxygen. Hypoxia may also cause cyanosis, a bluish colour, which is usually seen first in the lips and nail beds.

Oedema (see p. 92)
Excess fluid accumulates in the interstitial spaces of the tissues in cardiac disease when the heart cannot forward the blood it receives. The blood backs up in the veins and venules, raising the venous blood pressure. Normally, at the venous end of the capillaries, the colloidal osmotic pressure exceeds the hydrostatic pressure of the blood, and interstitial fluid moves into the capillary. However, if the hydrostatic pressure of the blood in the distal portion of the capillaries exceeds the blood protein osmotic pressure, interstitial fluid will not be moved into the capillaries.

The retention of sodium ions also contributes to the formation of oedema in the cardiac patient. The decreased sodium excretion is promoted by the reduced blood flow through the kidneys which results from the impaired circulation. It is also suggested that some mechanism may exist which causes an increased secretion of aldosterone by the adrenal cortices. This hormone promotes reabsorption of sodium in the kidney tubules.

Oedema is a very characteristic sign of some weakening in heart function. Considerable fluid accumulates before the oedema becomes apparent; a person may retain 4.5–7.0 kg (10–15 lb) of excess fluid before the oedema becomes evident. It appears first in the dependent parts of the body where the venous and capillary blood pressures always tend to be greater. If the patient is ambulant, it becomes evident first in the ankles and feet but, if he is in bed, it appears initially in the sacral region.

Pain
Chest pain may result from a variety of conditions. Non-cardiac causes include: musculoskeletal disorders such as cervical arthritis, gastrointestinal disorders such as reflux oesophagitis and gallbladder disease, pulmonary conditions such as pulmonary embolus, and psychological states such as severe anxiety.

The discomfort may mimic in both severity and description that of cardiac origin. For example, the pain of oesophageal spasm is usually burning in nature, located substernally and may be relieved by nitroglycerine. Non-cardiac disease is ruled out by a careful history, physical examination and specific diagnostic tests such as gastric or gallbladder investigations. The chest pain which cardiac patients experience is usually due to the deficiency of oxygen in the myocardium. It is important to determine the location, nature and precipitating or contributing factors of chest pain in order to distinguish the specific cause. The pain may be described as sharp, aching, squeezing, a feeling of heaviness or weight on the chest or a sensation of pressure within the chest. It may be mild or excruciating. It may be localized to one area or may spread across the chest, and into the back, neck, jaw, shoulders and/or arms. It may be precipitated or aggravated by activity, breathing cold air, or certain bodily positions, and may be relieved by resting or a change of position. Table 14.2 describes some cardiac problems and the pain often associated with them.

Palpitation
Change in heart function may cause the person to be conscious of his heart-beats. Palpitation may be due to the apex of the enlarged heart striking the chest wall with each contraction, or it may occur with an increased stroke volume in extrasystole, or ectopic beats (see Arrhythmias. p. 339).

General debilitation, loss of strength and decreased mental and physical efficiency
Weakness, loss of appetite and weight, general apathy and reduced efficiency occur as the result of the reduced nutrient and oxygen supply, venous congestion and the accumulation of metabolic wastes. In a child, growth and development may be retarded.

Abnormal heart sounds
Cardiac murmurs are abnormal sounds caused by small jets of blood which create eddies in the bloodstream. Movements of these currents produce audible vibrations which are referred to as murmurs. The most frequent causes of heart murmurs are stenosed and incompetent valves and openings between the right and left sides of the heart. Murmurs may also occur in an aneurysm, a localized saccular dilation of an artery.

The doctor, in determining the significance of a murmur, considers when it occurs in the cardiac cycle, its intensity, quality of sound, duration, factors which alter the sound (such as respiration and change of position) and the patient's history. Murmurs in some persons may have no great significance.

Occasionally, in tachycardia, a third heart sound becomes audible, producing then a quick sequence of three sounds during each cardiac cycle. This phenomenon is referred to as gallop rhythm and is an unfavourable sign since it indicates a weakening and dilatation of the heart and often precedes heart failure.

Table 14.2 Differentiating characteristics of chest pain.

Medical condition	Characteristics of pain	Location
Angina	Pressing; squeezing Precipitated by cold, physical activity, large meals, emotional upsets Usually relieved within a few minutes by rest and/or glyceryl trinitrate	Retrosternal May start in midchest and may radiate to jaw, shoulders, arms or fingers (often the left arm) May only be present in the neck, jaw, shoulders or arm(s)
Myocardial infarction	Similar pain to angina but longer-lasting and usually more severe Not relieved by rest or glyceryl trinitrate	Same locations as angina
Pericarditis	More stabbing or burning than pain of myocardial infarction Usually aggravated by deep inspiration or twisting the thorax May be relieved by high Fowler's position or bending forward	Substernal May radiate to the precordium trapezius muscle area or upper part of abdomen
Pulmonary embolus	Small pulmonary emboli may produce no pain, but with larger emboli pain is sharp and often sudden May be aggravated by deep breathing Accompanied by cyanosis, dyspnoea, cough, haemoptysis	Often located laterally but may be central
Dissecting aneurysm	Often sudden and excruciating Described as burning or tearing	May originate in anterior chest but often shifts to intrascapular region

Friction rub is a sound produced by the contact between the two pericardial surfaces with each heart-beat. Because of disease the surfaces are rough, causing audible vibrations.

DIAGNOSTIC PROCEDURES

The nurse requires some understanding of the diagnostic procedures in order to meet the associated nursing needs.

Blood tests
Various blood tests are used in investigating heart disease. Those used depend on the presenting signs and symptoms.

Leucocyte count. The number of white blood cells may be of significance, since these will be increased if there is an inflammatory process as occurs in bacterial endocarditis and rheumatic fever. Leucocytosis also occurs following a myocardial infarction as a result of the necrotic tissue.
Normal: $4.0–11.0 \times 10^9$ per litre.

Erythrocyte count and haemoglobin concentration. These are observed to determine the oxygen-carrying capacity of the patient's blood. In congenital cardiac defects which establish an abnormal blood pathway, the red blood cells and haemoglobin may be increased as a compensatory mechanism, since areas of the body are deficient in oxygen.

An increase in erythrocytes increases the viscosity of the blood, adding to the work of the heart and predisposing to thrombus formation.
In those with rheumatic fever or bacterial endocarditis, there may be fewer erythrocytes and less haemoglobin than normal.
Normal:
Erythrocytes, men, $4.5–6.5 \times 10^{12}$ per litre; women, $3.8–5.8 \times 10^{12}$ per litre.
Haemoglobin, men, 13–18 g/dl; women, 12–15 g/dl.
Haematocrit, men, 40–50%; women, 0.37–0.47%.

Erythrocyte sedimentation rate. The rate at which erythrocytes settle in a blood sample is increased in inflammatory conditions and in myocardial infarction. Periodic checking of the sedimentation rate gives information as to the progress of the disease; as the inflammatory process subsides or as the infarcted area heals, the rate decreases.
Normal:
Westergren method: male, 0–15 mm in 1 hour; female, 0–20 mm in 1 hour.
Wintrobe method: male, 0–9 mm in 1 hour; female, 0–15 mm in 1 hour.

Blood culture. Studies may be made to determine the causative organism in bacterial endocarditis.

Prothrombin time. This test indicates the amount of prothrombin in the blood. Some heart patients receive anticoagulant therapy and a frequent check must be made of the concentration of prothrombin, which serves as a guide to the dosage of the drugs. From 1½–2½ times the normal level is considered a therapeutic range.

Normal: 11–15 seconds.

Partial thromboplastin time (PTT). This test assesses the intrinsic clotting system. It defines abnormalities of certain factors usually present in the coagulation pathway. It is also used as a guide for the administration of heparin which is given parenterally, either subcutaneously or intravenously. A therapeutic level is 1½–2 times the normal range.

Normal range: 50–80 seconds.

Clotting time. This test measures the total time for fibrin formation. In some institutions it is used to monitor the administration of heparin, but it is less reliable than partial thromboplastin time.

Normal range: 5–10 minutes.

Serum enzymes. Certain intracellular enzymes known to be present in myocardial cells are released into the blood when the cells are damaged or destroyed. Determination of the serum concentration of these enzymes provides information that assists in confirming myocardial infarction and the extent of the damage. Changes may also occur with shock and cardiac surgery. In addition, these enzymes are present in other tissues and may therefore be elevated in other than myocardial conditions (e.g. pulmonary embolus).

The enzyme tests include serum aspartate aminotransferase (AST) (formerly referred to as serum glutamic oxaloacetic transaminase–SGOT) and estimation of the concentration in the serum of lactic dehydrogenase (LDH), creatine phosphokinase (CPK) and alpha-hydroxybutyrate dehydrogenase (HBD) (see Table 14.3).

The concentration of AST rises within 6–8 hours after a myocardial infarction, reaching a peak in 24–48 hours and usually returning to normal within 4–8 days. AST may also be elevated in liver cell

necrosis, in acute pancreatitis and with severe skeletal muscle damage.

Normal range: 8–40 units/l.

Following an infarction, the LDH level becomes elevated in 24–48 hours, reaching a peak in 48–72 hours. The increase persists for 5–10 days and then gradually returns to normal. The LDH level may also increase in patients with megaloblastic and haemolytic anaemias, pulmonary infarctions and haemolysis of red blood cells. LDH may be separated into five main fractions (isoenzymes) for greater specificity. Cardiac necrosis would show an elevation of LDH-1 and LDH-2 (using standard international nomenclature). LDH-1 and 2 may rise in patients with myocardial infarction even though there is no change in total LDH.

Normal range: 150–300 units/l.

HBD is associated with the cardiospecific isoenzymes of LDH. It is elevated within 12 hours after a myocardial infarction, peaks in 48–72 hours and remains elevated for up to 3 weeks. Slight elevations may also appear in liver disease, muscular dystrophy and megaloblastic anaemia.

Normal range: 50–250 units/l.

CPK has a more limited distribution than the other enzymes; it is found only in skeletal muscle, brain tissue and cardiac muscle. Therefore it is considered by some to be more cardiospecific than the other enzymes. CPK begins to show a postinfarction increase in approximately 2–5 hours, reaching its peak within 12–24 hours. It usually returns to normal within 2–3 days. Conditions other than myocardial infarction that may result in elevated total CPK include pericarditis, myocarditis, electrical cardioversion and severe congestive heart failure. CPK is often elevated following intramuscular injections.

CPK may also be fractionated to isoenzymes, with MBCPK being the isoenzyme found only in the myocardium. Studies have shown that CK-MB (or MBCPK) was 100% sensitive and specific for the diagnosis of acute myocardial infarction, provided that it was determined between 6–36 hours after the

Table 14.3 Serum enzymes following myocardial infarction.*

Enzymes	Normal values per litre (units)†	Begins to rise (hours)	Peaks (hours)	Returns to normal
AST	8–40	6–8	24–48	4–8 days
LDH	150–300	24–48	48–72	5–10 days
HBD	50–250	12	48–72	1–3 weeks
CPK	0–4	2–5	12–24	2–3 days
MBCPK	0–2	6	8–16	36 hours

*AST: serum aspartate aminotransferase (formerly SGOT)
LDH: serum lactic dehydrogenase
HBD: serum alpha-hydroxybutyrate dehydrogenase
CPK: serum creatine phosphokinase
MBCPK: cardiospecific creatine phosphokinase
†Hurst et al (1986).

onset.[8] Although total CPK may be influenced by intramuscular injections, MBCPK seems to be unaffected.[9]

Normal range: 0–4 units/l.

Some doctors suggest that, because of its lack of specificity for myocardial infarction, AST should not be included as one of the diagnostic tests. They support the use of total LDH and CPK and their isoenzymes.[9]

Normal values of serum enzymes may vary slightly from one laboratory to another depending upon the techniques and sampling methods used.

Blood gases. The circulatory status of a patient is reflected in the blood concentrations of oxygen and carbon dioxide. The volumes differ in arterial and venous blood for obvious reasons. The amount of oxygen is usually expressed as tension or pressure in mmHg. Rarely, the volumes per cent are recorded.

Normal:

Po_2, arterial, 11–13.3 kPa (80–100 mmHg).

O_2, arterial, 15–23 volumes%.

Po_2, venous, 4.8–6.0 kPa (35–45 mmHg).

O_2, venous, 10–16 volumes %.

The partial pressure of carbon dioxide in the blood provides information about the pH of the body fluids and is usually given in mmHg. The carbon dioxide combining power indicates the available alkali and reflects the amount of carbon dioxide in the blood available to form carbonic acid.

Normal:

Pco_2, arterial, 4.8–6.0 kPa (35–45 mmHg).

Pco_2 venous, 6.0–7.2 kPa (45–54 mmHg).

CO_2 combining power, 50–58 volumes %.

Hydrogen carbonate (alkali), 22–28 mmol/l (22–28 mEq/l).

pH is an indicator of the hydrogen ion concentration of the blood. When within the normal range, the body is said to be in a state of acid–base balance.

Normal range: 7.35–7.45 (pH arterial)

A pH below 7.35 signifies an increased hydrogen ion concentration, or acidosis, while a pH above 7.45 indicates a decreased hydrogen ion concentration, or alkalosis.

Electrocardiography

Electrocardiography is the study of the electrical activity associated with heart contractions. The electrocardiogram (ECG), which produces a visible record of heart activity, provides one of the most dependable aids in assessing heart function and in diagnosing heart disease.

Each heart contraction results from electrical currents which spread from the heart and can be monitored from the surface of the body. These currents, which reflect the electrical activity of the heart, are detected when electrodes are placed on the external surface of the body. An application of contact jelly is made to the skin beneath the electrodes in order to facilitate conduction. The ebb and flow of the electrical forces result in a specific pattern, called a complex or cardiac cycle. Each part of the complex represents the electrical pathway of a specific part of the heart and normally occurs over a specific period of time.

The waves for each cycle are identified as P, Q, R, S and T, as shown in Fig. 14.8, and are recorded on special graph paper. The base line of the graph represents zero electrical potential. Three of the waves (P, R, and T) appear above the base line and two (Q and S) appear below.

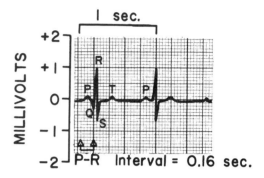

Fig. 14.8 A normal electrocardiogram.

The P wave, or first rounded contour, represents atrial depolarization. Although depolarization of the S-A node precedes depolarization of the atria, it cannot be picked up by body surface leads.

The P-R interval indicates the time from the beginning of the P wave to the beginning of the QRS complex. The QRS complex represents conduction through the ventricles. The Q wave is the initial downward (negative) deflection following the P wave, the R wave is the initial upward (positive) deflection following the Q wave, and the S wave is the downward deflection following the R wave. The ST segment is an interval of zero potential, the period between completion of depolarization and the beginning of repolarization (recovery) of the ventricles. The T wave represents the recovery phase after contraction or return of the ventricular muscular fibres to their resting state.

The horizontal axis of the graph paper represents time. Each small square indicates 0.04 second. Each large square is composed of five small squares and is therefore equal to 0.20 second.

The vertical axis of the graph indicates voltage. Each small vertical square represents 0.1 millivolt, while a large square composed of five small squares equals 0.5 millivolt.

The P wave should not be longer than 0.10 second duration, or 2 or 3 mm in height. Normally the P-R interval is between 0.12 and 0.20 second. The QRS

[8] Blomberg et al (1975), pp. 464–469.
[9] Roberts (1981), pp. 486–506.

complex should not exceed 0.10 second in duration, or 5 to 20 or 25 mm in height. The T wave is of 0.20 second duration and normally not above 5–10 mm in height, depending upon the lead.[10]

The tracing is studied for deviations by comparing it to a tracing made by a normal heart; the direction, contour and timing of the waves and segments are noted. Information is obtained that is related to impulse formation and conduction and to the condition and response of the myocardium.

A nursing responsibility associated with this diagnostic procedure is to give the patient a brief explanation of the test. Some patients are fearful that they will receive a shock from the electrodes. The patient is advised that he should relax and that he will not feel anything as the instrument records his heart's action. If digitalis or quinidine has been prescribed for the patient, it must be noted on the requisition form as well as on a conspicuous place on the patient's chart, as either drug may influence the interpretation of the tracing.

If the patient is very ill the nurse remains with him during the test. In some instances the nurse is responsible for obtaining the electrocardiogram.

Ambulatory electrocardiography

The Halter technique of electrocardiography is a means of studying, over a prolonged period of time, the electrical activity of the heart during a person's normal daily activities. By this method, intermittent arrhythmias can be detected and when applicable, can be related to specific activities and to any symptoms the patient is experiencing.

Electrodes are applied to the chest and a light, portable tape recorder is carried by the patient at all times. A description of activities and symptoms as well as the time they occur are documented in a diary. The continuous ECG is analysed in relation to the contents of the diary.

This technique is particularly helpful in studying patients who have periodic symptoms such as dizziness or palpitations but in whom normal, single ECGs have been obtained. It may also be used to study the presence of ST-T changes during normal activities. Alternatively a telemetry monitoring system can be used. This method incorporates a transmitter (a small battery-powered unit), which can fit into a pyjama jacket pocket, and a receiver and monitor, which are commonly housed in the coronary care unit. The patient, attached to the transmitter by means of chest electrodes, can be in a ward in another part of the hospital as long as he is within the working radius of the transmitter and receiver. The cardiac rhythm can thus be monitored in the coronary care unit by nurses who are able to recognize cardiac arrhythmias.

---
[10] Marriott (1983).

Exercise electrocardiograms

This test is done to assist in the diagnosis of myocardial ischaemia in a patient with atypical symptoms. Many patients with angina pectoris have normal ECGs at rest but changes may occur during exercise. The exercise ECG is also used to assess the effect of specific treatments for angina and in rehabilitation following a myocardial infarction or cardiac surgery.

Electrodes are attached to the body and recordings taken while the patient exercises. One of the earliest stress tests was the 'Master's two-step stress test', in which a person climbed two 9-inch steps a selected number of times at a specific speed. The test was considered positive if the recordings showed an ST depression of at least 0.5 mm.

Graded exercise testing has been developed in which the patient exercises on a treadmill or rides a bicycle at gradually increasing speeds against a regulated amount of resistance. Of these, the graduated treadmill provides the best form of exercise for this test. The exercise continues until the patient reaches a predetermined maximal heart rate (according to age and sex). The test is discontinued earlier if the patient develops chest pain, hypotension, signs of cerebral insufficiency or undue dyspnoea. The test is considered positive if the electrocardiogram shows an ST segment displacement of 1 mm or more.

Chest radiographs

An x-ray of the chest may be made to note the size and shape of the heart. Visualization of the lungs may show a density that may indicate an increased volume of blood in the pulmonary circulation and fluid in the alveoli. The size and shape of the pulmonary artery and aorta may also be noted.

Fluoroscopic examination allows the doctor to observe the heart in action. The functioning of different chambers and large vessels may be noted.

A brief explanation of the patient's role may be necessary if he is apprehensive and completely unfamiliar with the x-ray procedure.

Cardiac angiogram

In this test, also known as a cardiopulmonary angiogram, visualization of the heart and vessels is made possible by the injection of a radiopaque dye into a vein or artery or directly into a heart chamber. The site depends on the type of abnormality suspected. A series of x-ray pictures is taken, or a fluoroscopic study is made, as the blood flows through the heart and pulmonary system. The pathway of the blood is followed, and the size, shape and filling and emptying of the various structures are noted. This examination is of particular importance in identifying congenital defects of the heart and large vessels.

Preparation of the patient includes an explanation of the test so that he will have some idea of what to expect. This may be given by the doctor but, if it is not, the nurse must have sufficient understanding of the procedure to be able to prepare the patient and reduce his fear.

Depending upon hospital policy, it is likely that informed written consent will be required from the patient undergoing cardiac angiography. Food and fluids are withheld for 6–8 hours previous to the hour of the test, and a sedative may be ordered ½–1 hour before the patient is taken to the x-ray or cardiology department.

An iodine patch test is performed. Alternatively the radiologist administers a test dose of the radiopaque dye before proceeding with the angiocardiogram in case of a hypersensitivity to such substances. This examination is not done on a person with a history of asthma or allergic reaction. A reaction to the dye might be manifested in respiratory distress, fall in blood pressure, shock, urticaria, and nausea and vomiting. Antihistamines, steroids, adrenaline and oxygen should be quickly available in the event of a reaction. Postexamination care involves close observation for signs of delayed reaction. The site of injection should be examined for a few days for signs of irritation or thrombosis.

Cardiac catheterization

Cardiac catheterization is a useful diagnostic procedure for certain patients. It is undertaken to evaluate the severity of known cardiac lesions, such as acquired valvular heart disease, congenital defects and coronary artery disease, when these conditions might be amenable to surgical treatment. It is also used for diagnosing heart disease and for the evaluation of the long-term effects of cardiac surgery.

Under local anaesthesia a long radiopaque catheter is passed into the right and left side of the heart. Pressures within the chambers of the heart and oxygen concentrations in certain chambers are determined (see Table 14.4 for normal values.) An example of an abnormal finding is an atrial septal defect which results in an oxygen tension higher than normal in the right side of the heart.

A contrast material or radiopaque dye is usually introduced into the heart through the catheter. The pathway of this dye is filmed, and obstructions in the coronary arteries may be evaluated. The cardiac output is also measured.

Right heart catheterization provides information about the right side of the heart and the pulmonary circulation. The catheter is introduced through a cutdown in the femoral vein of the right leg or the basilic vein of the right arm and, under a fluoroscope, is passed through the inferior or superior vena cava into the right atrium. It may then be guided through the tricuspid valve into the right ventricle and on into the pulmonary artery. An x-ray may be taken with the catheter in various positions for future studies.

Left heart catheterization generally involves the retrograde passage of the catheter into a femoral artery up through the aorta and aortic valve to the left ventricle; it may then be advanced through the mitral valve into the left atrium. It may also be directed from the aorta into the right and left coronary arteries. Alternatively, an approach using the right brachial artery is adopted.

Preparation of the patient for a cardiac catheterization includes an explanation of the procedure and obtaining a written consent. Although the doctor usually talks with the patient and family, the nurse should be conversant with the procedure. It is understandable that the patient and relatives are apprehensive. The nurse encourages them to express their fears and is prepared to answer questions. The patient is informed of the equipment he may see during the procedure, the sterile precautions that will be taken, and some of the physical sensations that he will experience, such as a feeling of pressure when the catheter is introduced and the warm flush which immediately follows the injection

Table 14.4 Range of normal resting haemodynamic values.*

	a wave	*v* wave	Mean	Systolic	End Diastolic	Mean
Pressures						
Right atrium	2–10	2–10	0–8			
Right ventricle				15–30	0–8	
Pulmonary artery				15–30	3–12	9–16
Pulmonary artery wedge and left atrium	3–15	3–12	1–10			
Left ventricle				100–140	3–12	
Systemic arteries				100–140	60–90	70–105
Oxygen consumption index (ml·min^{-1}·m^{-2}) (ml/min/m^2)	110–150					
Arteriovenous oxygen difference (ml/1)	30–50					
Cardiac output index (l·min^{-1}·m^{-2})	2.5–4.2					
Resistances (units)						
Pulmonary vascular	<2.5					
Systemic vascular	10–20					

*Braunwald (1985).

of the dye. Although each step is usually explained during the procedure, the patient's anxiety is often decreased when given this information beforehand. Some institutions may provide leaflets describing the experience.

Food and fluid are withheld for a stated number of hours preceding the catheterization. A sedative may be ordered.

The patient's reaction must be observed closely during the procedure. Heart action is constantly observed on the oscilloscope, an instrument which visibly registers and traces the electrical activity of the heart. Irritation of the myocardium by the catheter may precipitate ventricular fibrillation, so a defibrillator is close at hand. The patient experiences little discomfort but may complain of a fluttering or irritation in the chest, especially during movement of the catheter. He is advised that this is a temporary sensation.

Following the catheterization, which may have taken 2 or 3 hours, the patient is given fluids and nourishment and is allowed to rest. The pulse is checked at frequent intervals—every 15 minutes for the first hour and then at gradually increased intervals if it remains normal. An irregular, rapid or weak pulse is promptly reported to the doctor. If the catheter was passed through a femoral artery the patient remains in bed for 12–24 hours, and the site where the catheter was inserted is examined frequently for possible bleeding. A pressure dressing is applied. The wound is observed for redness and tenderness which may indicate irritation or phlebitis.

Patients frequently wish to discuss their feelings following the procedure. Although one probable reaction is relief that the procedure is completed, anxiety about the findings and their implications is often evident.

Vital capacity
Vital capacity represents the maximum volume of air that a person can exhale after inhaling to the maximum. The normal is approximately 2500–5000 ml. Usually it is higher in males than females, and will be greater in those accustomed to regular and fairly strenuous activity.

In the procedure, the patient is required to take a maximum breath and then exhale into the mouthpiece of a spirometer which makes a graphic record of the volume of air exhaled. The nurse advises the patient as to the value of the test and what will be required of him.

Lung capacity may be reduced in heart conditions by an excessive volume and pressure of blood in the pulmonary circulatory system. Expansion of the lungs meets with resistance and fluid escapes into the alveoli, reducing respiratory efficiency.

Phonocardiography
Heart sounds may be picked up, amplified and recorded by a microphone placed on the chest. A study of the phonocardiogram is helpful in cases in which the doctor has difficulty in distinguishing heart sounds and murmurs by the usual auscultation.

Echocardiography
This is a non-invasive test used to detect valvular abnormalities, intracardiac tumours, pericardial effusion, ventricular dysfunctions and some congenital defects. Through a transducer placed against the chest wall, ultrasound waves at a level of approximately 2–3 million cycles/sec or 2–3 MHz (mega hertz) are aimed at the heart and a recording is made of the echo. In adults, lower frequency ultrasonic beams are used as high frequency beams are unable to penetrate a thick chest wall.

As the sound waves hit various structures while passing through the heart, some of them are bounced back, producing patterns characteristic of each structure. Ultrasound is poorly transmitted through bony or air-containing material (bony thorax and lungs). The transducer must, therefore, be placed in a position to avoid these structures.

A conductive jelly is applied to the chest to provide a stable interface between the patient and the transducer and to minimize the loss of sound waves in the air. Views may be taken with the patient in the left lateral or supine position, depending upon the part of the heart to be examined.

There are two echocardiographic techniques: the M-mode (M standing for motion) and the two-dimensional (2-D) mode. With the M-mode technique, a beam of sound is aimed at one position on the chest wall. A detailed one-dimensional view of the heart is produced and continuously recorded in a strip chart. M-mode echocardiography is especially useful in diagnosing pericardial effusion and mitral valve disease. However, this technique does not visualize the spatial orientation of intracardiac structures.

With 2-D echocardiography, an ultrasonic beam scans the heart in an arc from 30°–80°, showing cardiac shape and lateral motion. It can reliably evaluate left ventricular aneurysm, wall motion abnormalities and ventricular dysfunction in patients with coronary artery disease as well as visualizing intracardiac tumours.

Doppler echocardiography is a new application of ultrasound. By assessing blood velocity at a specific area of the heart, information is provided on blood flow patterns.

Although the test is painless it does require the patient to remain motionless for 10–30 minutes. An explanation of the purpose, procedure and equipment is given to the patient prior to the test.

Nuclear cardiology
Nuclear cardiology includes a group of diagnostic tests in which tracer substances called radionuclides are injected into the bloodstream and their distribu-

tion in cardiac chambers is measured using a computer and a gamma camera. Tracer substances are composed of two components: the radionuclide and the substance to be tagged. The measurement to be made determines the choice of nuclide and substance to be tagged.

Tracers are characterized by their chemical behaviour, their physiological and biological half-life and by the type, number and energy of radiations emitted. For example, tracers that emit gamma radiations are used to make most of the measurements in nuclear cardiology. Gamma photons can usually be detected externally and have the greatest chance of penetrating tissues.

The heat, excitation or ionization which occurs when gamma photons interact with matter, can be detected by special gamma radiation detectors. Development in detectors has progressed from simple, rudimentary scanners to the scintillation gamma camera which allows for more precise and comprehensive examinations. Other equipment such as analyzers, recorders and computers are also utilized.

Nuclear cardiology techniques are non-invasive except for a peripheral intravenous injection and are considered safer and are more easily repeated than invasive techniques. Some measures are carried out while the patient is at rest and others during exercise.

Information provided varies with the test performed. Some tests estimate myocardial blood flow: others, cardiac haemodynamics such as cardiac output, stroke volume or ventricular performance. Radionuclide techniques may be divided into two general types: (1) first-pass techniques, in which only the first transit of a radionuclide bolus through the circulation is analyzed and (2) equilibrium studies in which serial studies can be obtained over time.

Multigated blood-pool imaging (Muga scan)

The radiopharmaceutical used in this test is technetium–99m pertechnetate, which is tagged to the patient's red blood cells. The physical half-life of this radionuclide is 6 hours. In Muga scanning, images are collected at various times during cardiac contractions. The mechanical activity of the heart usually has a fixed relation to the electrical activity. By triggering the computer to record from a specific phase of the electrical cycle, information can be obtained about cardiac mechanical function. The electrocardiographic trigger with which the scanner is synchronized is the R wave of the patient's ECG. Information is obtained from one R wave to the next. Each R–R interval, is subdivided into frames, usually 16–24 equal divisions. Each frame is arranged in the computer image according to its time relationship to the beginning of the R wave.

When the R–R intervals are equal, each sequential frame will have the same data. Images are taken over several heart-beats so that several cardiac cycles can

be recorded. Measurements of ejection fraction and left ventricular wall motion can also be obtained. A left ventricular time–activity curve can be generated by the computer and the ejection fraction can be estimated by measuring this curve.

Left ventricular wall motion can be examined by observing if the left ventricle contracts symmetrically or has areas contracting dyskinetically. Imaging is performed in the anterior and left anterior oblique positions for complete analysis.

To obtain reliable information, the heart rate must be regular during the test and the time period must be long enough to provide an adequate count density.

Thallium myocardial scintography

Thallium-201 is an element with properties similar to potassium and is the radiopharmaceutical of choice for myocardial perfusion scintography. Clearance from the blood is rapid and extraction by the myocardium is high.

Thallium-201 scanning provides an assessment of regional myocardial blood flow and the amount of viable myocardium. Normally, the coronary blood flow is equal throughout the myocardium, and thallium-201 would be distributed evenly through the coronary arteries. It is extracted from the blood by viable myocardium. In normal tissue the concentration of thallium should show a similar intensity in each portion of the myocardium.

In coronary artery stenosis, thallium-201 would be distributed unevenly and the camera would detect less thallium activity in the portion of the myocardium nourished by the diseased artery. In some patients, blood flow may be normal at rest, even with severe coronary disease. With exercise, however, the blood supply will differ in the area supplied by the diseased vessels to that supplied by normal vessels.

Measurement of venous blood pressure

Venous blood pressure is an important parameter in the care of seriously ill patients. It reflects the intravascular volume and the ability of the heart to forward the blood it receives. Measurement of the venous pressure may be made in a peripheral vein, such as the medial basilic, or in a large central vein, such as the superior vena cava.

Central venous pressure. Central venous pressure (CVP) is more reliable than the peripheral, and is being used clinically more often in assessing the patient's condition. It may be used as a guide for fluid replacement for the dehydrated or postoperative patient, or for a critically ill patient.

An intravenous catheter is passed into the superior vena cava via the subclavian or internal jugular veins, or occasionally into the inferior vena cava via a femoral vein. The catheter is attached to a three-way stopcock which is also connected to a water manometer and intravenous infusion. In setting up the CVP line the zero level of the manometer is positioned at the level of the right atrium, which is approximately in line with the mid-axillary and suprasternal notch. The most important factor is that the equipment is at the same level for each recording, so the initial level is usually marked on the patient's skin. In most instances the changes in the venous pressure are more significant than the actual level. The patient must be in the same position for each reading. The pressure is generally recorded hourly. When the catheter is introduced, the stopcock is adjusted to allow fluid to flow to the patient. Then, to determine the venous pressure, the stopcock is turned to direct the fluid up into the manometer to a level of 30–35 cm. The valve is then adjusted to close off the flow from the intravenous bag and to establish a flow line between the manometer and the catheter. When the fluid reaches the level of the venous pressure it remains at a relatively stationary level, rhythmically rising and falling 1–2 cm with respirations. Following the recording the stopcock is readjusted to allow the intravenous solution to flow to the patient.

The normal central venous pressure is approximately 5–10 cm of water. This varies with the patient's size, position and state of hydration. The significance of the pressure is determined in conjunction with the arterial blood pressure, the hourly output of urine, pulse rate and volume, and ECG. The nurse needs to know the levels at which the doctor is to be informed, and the type, volume and rate of flow of the infusion must be prescribed.

Other nursing responsibilities include observation for complications such as inflammation at the insertion site. This may be prevented by the use of aseptic technique during catheter insertion and during the application of dressings. Interference with flow may be minimized by periodic flushing with a solution of heparinized saline to prevent clotting and loosely coiling the tubing to prevent it from kinking.

Measurement of pulmonary artery pressure (wedge pressure)

To obtain more specific information about the functioning of the left side of the heart, pulmonary artery and pulmonary capillary pressures are measured. This procedure is used for critically ill patients in whom early detection of left ventricular dysfunction is important.

A flow-directed (Swan–Ganz) catheter is inserted into a peripheral vein. A balloon at the tip of the catheter is partially inflated and the catheter floats into the right atrium, right ventricle and pulmonary artery at which time the pulmonary artery pressure may be measured. The catheter is then advanced into a branch of the pulmonary artery until it becomes wedged in a pulmonary capillary. Pressure measurements are obtained which reflect pressures

in the left atrium. The balloon is then deflated until the next pressure reading.

- The nurse is responsible for monitoring pressures, reporting abnormalities and preventing complications. The normal pulmonary artery pressure is 25/10 mmHg, and the normal pulmonary capillary wedge pressure is 4–12 mmHg.

CLASSIFICATION OF PATIENTS WITH A CARDIAC CONDITION (see Table 14.5)

The required care is not the same for all patients with a cardiac condition, since there are varying degrees of heart impairment and reduced efficiency, in addition to different pathological conditions.

There are those individuals who have a slight abnormality or who have had a condition which has been cured. The heart may carry some structural change or scar, but the cardiac efficiency and reserve are such that no restrictions on activities are necessary. Some of these people have unwarranted fears and restrict their activities unnecessarily, even though they have been advised by their doctors to live a normal, active life. The role of the nurse with these patients is to try to dispel their unsound fears and encourage them to be active. In some instances, overprotection by the family may be a problem.

A second group of people whom the nurse may help are those who are not ill but who have a reduced cardiac reserve. The heart condition has resulted in adaptive changes (dilatation, hypertrophy and/or acceleration) to compensate for the defect in order to maintain circulation. Energy expenditure must be restricted to correspond to the functional capacity of the heart in order to avoid failure. Obviously, the limitations vary with the extent of pathology and physiological changes in the heart and its resulting

Table 14.5 The functional classification of patients with diseases of the heart.*

Class I	*No limitation:* Ordinary physical activity does not cause undue fatigue, dyspnoea or palpitation
Class II	*Slight limitation of physical activity:* Such patients are comfortable at rest. Ordinary physical activity results in fatigue, palpitation, dyspnoea or angina
Class III	*Marked limitation of physical activity:* Although patients are comfortable at rest, less than ordinary activity will lead to symptoms
Class IV	*Inability to carry on any physical activity without discomfort:* Symptoms of congestive failure are present even at rest. With any physical activity, increased discomfort is experienced. The accuracy and reproducibility of this classification are limited

*Braunwald (1985), p. 496.

capacity. For some it may mean only giving up strenuous competitive sports; for others, greater restrictions are necessary. The aim of the care of these people is to have each one live within his compensatory limits and, at the same time, live as useful and satisfying a life as possible. Continuous treatment may be necessary for some to remain asymptomatic. The doctor assesses each patient's capacity, and the nurse helps the patient and family accept and adjust to the necessary restrictions. Positive emphasis is placed upon certain activities; suggestions are made as to what the patient can do, remembering that appropriate amounts of work, recreation and rest are more satisfying and beneficial.

The functional capacity of some cardiac patients may be so limited that they cannot participate in any physical activity without experiencing symptoms of cardiac insufficiency. They may be restricted to self-care activities or may be confined to a chair or bed, completely dependent upon others. The nurse's role with these patients is to provide the prescribed treatment and necessary care.

The doctor may use the functional and therapeutic classifications developed by the New York Heart Association and published by the American Heart Association. This serves as a general guide to the type of care required and may influence the choice of suitable employment for the patient (see p. 322).

CAUSES AND TYPES OF HEART DISORDERS

Heart disorders may be classified as congenital or acquired. Various subclassifications may be used in acquired heart disease. Some authors concentrate on structure, such as pericardium, myocardium and endocardium. Others highlight the causes of heart disease, such as trauma, infections, degenerative processes, and hyper- and hypometabolic processes. This text classifies heart disorders as:
1 Congenital cardiovascular defects
2 Inflammatory diseases which may result in structural changes within the heart
3 Deficiency in the blood supply to the myocardium
4 Disturbances in conduction
5 Decompensation, or heart failure

Congenital cardiovascular defects

Congenital cardiovascular defect implies a structural abnormality that was present at birth in the heart or the large proximal blood vessels. It has only been within the last two to three decades that many of the congenital cardiovascular defects have been identified and successfully treated by surgery. Many are recognized shortly after birth if the infant survives. Others may go undiscovered for months or years because the heart maintains an adequate circulation by compensation. As in so many congenital deformities, the cause remains obscure. In some instances it is thought that a viral infection, such as German measles, occurring in the mother in the first trimester of pregnancy, may cause the defect. Frequently, cardiovascular malformations accompany other congenital defects such as cataract, mental retardation and deaf–mutism.

Many types of heart malformations occur. They may be classified into three main groups: (1) those which produce a left-to-right shunt of blood; (2) those which offer resistance to the blood flow; and (3) those which cause a right-to-left shunt (Fig. 14.9).

ANOMALIES WHICH CAUSE A LEFT-TO-RIGHT SHUNT

Several malformations occur which produce an abnormal pathway that permits a direct flow of blood from the left side of the heart or aorta to the right heart or pulmonary artery, creating a bypass of the systemic circulation and an overloading of the pulmonary circulation. These anomalies include patent ductus arteriosus and septal defects.

Atrial septal defect

An opening between the two atria may be due to failure of the foramen ovale to close after birth or to a gap in the septum, either above or below the foramen ovale. Blood in the left atrium will flow through the opening into the right atrium, increasing the volume of blood in the pulmonary system. The right atrium, right ventricle and pulmonary artery enlarge. Pulmonary hypertension develops and causes dyspnoea, particularly on exertion. The reduced systemic circulatory volume retards physical and mental development and efficiency. The size of the opening may be so small that it goes undiscovered, and the patient may not experience any respiratory or circulatory difficulty.

Surgical repair of an atrial septal defect is usually accomplished by open heart surgery. Some defects may be closed simply by suturing while others may require a patch of Teflon, an inert material to which tissues do not react.

Ventricular septal defect

An opening in the ventricular septum results in a left-to-right shunt and produces problems similar to those cited in atrial septal defect—pulmonary hypertension, enlargement of the right ventricle and pulmonary arteries, and a deficient systemic circulation. If the defect is small and the patient is asymptomatic, surgery is not indicated. Moderate to severe defects may be closed by patching with either pericardial tissue or Teflon. Occasionally the defect closes spontaneously in the young child.

Patent ductus arteriosus

Normally, after birth, a gradual spontaneous con-

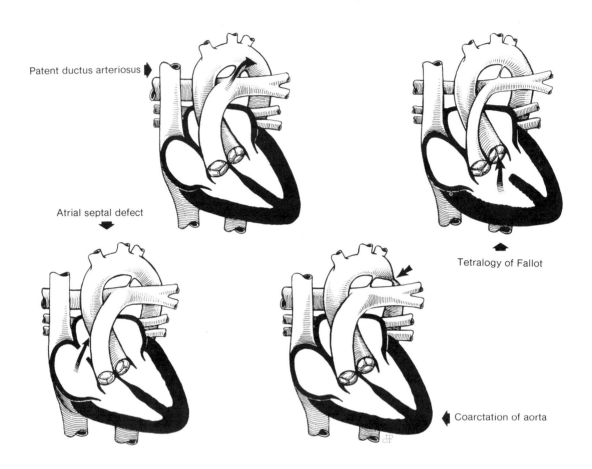

Fig. 14.9 Congenital cardiac defects.

striction and atrophy of the ductus takes place. If it remains open the blood in the aorta, under a pressure approximately five–six times that in the pulmonary artery, is shunted into the pulmonary artery. This increases the volume of blood entering the lungs, resulting in a high pulmonary blood pressure and dilatation of the pulmonary vessels. The patient experiences dyspnoea, particularly on exertion. There is a corresponding increase in the venous flow into the left atrium and left ventricle, causing dilatation and hypertrophy of the left side of the heart. The volume of blood in the systemic circulatory system is less than normal, and the resulting oxygen and nutritional deficiencies retard normal mental and physical development.

The patent ductus arteriosus is corrected by surgical division and suturing of the two ends of the vessel.

ANOMALIES WHICH CAUSE RESISTANCE TO BLOOD FLOW WITHIN THE CIRCULATION

The seriousness of the resistance is determined by the degree of constriction or stenosis which may be found in the pulmonary artery or the aorta.

Pulmonary stenosis
A stenosis of the pulmonary valve or artery offers resistance to the outflow of blood from the right side of the heart. The right ventricle enlarges and the pressure in both the right ventricle and atrium is above normal. Blood may be backed up in the venous system, while the blood volume entering the pulmonary system is below normal. The latter creates an oxygen deficiency throughout the body which is manifested by fatigue, shortness of breath and, less

frequently, cyanosis. Symptoms may not be present for several years.

This malformation may be treated surgically by incision of the constricted ring.

Aortic stenosis

A defect comparable to pulmonary stenosis may occur in the aorta and offer resistance to left ventricular outflow. The left side of the heart enlarges and the pressure in both left chambers is above normal: this may be reflected in an increased pulmonary pressure if the restriction is severe. The cardiac output is lower and reduces arterial blood pressure and the systemic circulation as well as the blood supply into the coronary arteries. The defect may be treated by surgery, using an extracorporeal pump-oxygenator (cardio-pulmonary bypass) during the procedure.

Coarctation of the thoracic aorta

Coarctation is a stricture in a segment of the aorta. Postductal coarctation occurs just beyond the obliterated ductus arteriosus and distal to the origin of the left subclavian artery. The second type, preductal coarctation, develops in the segment of aorta before the entrance of the ductus arteriosus. With this latter type the ductus usually remains patent.

Blood volume and pressure are increased behind the stricture, and the work of the left side of the heart is increased greatly. The blood volume and pressure are high in the upper extremities and head, but are abnormally low in the body parts which derive their blood supply from below the stricture. A difference in growth and development may be seen between the areas supplied from behind the stricture and those supplied from the aortic flow distal to the stricture. The patient may experience headaches, epistaxis, dyspnoea on exertion, leg cramps and fatigue.

Surgical treatment of the condition involves resection of the constricted area and an end-to-end anastomosis or, in some instances, the area is excised and a graft of inert material introduced.

ANOMALIES WHICH CAUSE A RIGHT-TO-LEFT SHUNT

A shunting of blood from the right side of the heart to the left involves a combination of two or more anomalies. Normally, the pressure is much higher in the left side of the heart than in the right side. A stenosis which offers resistance to flow from the right ventricle may increase the pressure in the right side to a level exceeding that in the left side. If a septal defect coexists with this increased pressure, blood is shunted from the right to the left side of the heart.

One of the most frequently seen combinations of anomalies which produces a right-to-left shunt is the tetralogy of Fallot. Tetralogy denotes a set of four conditions: pulmonary stenosis, ventricular septal defect, dextraposition of the aorta which causes it to over-ride the septal defect, and right ventricular hypertrophy. The pulmonic stenosis produces an increased pressure in the right ventricle, causing a right-to-left shunt. The volume of blood flowing through the pulmonary system for oxygenation is reduced. Unoxygenated blood escapes into the aorta and a general systemic hypoxia occurs, manifested by cyanosis and dyspnoea, especially on physical exertion, and by clubbing of the fingers. Compensatory responses to the oxygen deficiency develop in the form of polycythaemia, high haemoglobin level and increased pulse and respiratory rates.

Correction of these defects is possible by means of open heart surgery and the use of the pump-oxygenator. The septal opening is patched, and the pulmonary stenosis is relieved. Occasionally the surgeon may decide not to perform corrective surgery but will proceed with a palliative surgical procedure, referred to as a 'shunt'. This consists of an anastomosis between the subclavian and pulmonary arteries (Blalock's operation) or between the aorta and pulmonary artery (Potts' operation). The purpose of the anastomosis is to divert a larger volume of blood through the lungs for oxygenation.

MISCELLANEOUS CONGENITAL CARDIAC ANOMALIES

Only the more common anomalies that are recognized and treated have been presented here. A wide variety of anomalies can occur, many are not yet amenable to treatment, and others may be so severe that the infant cannot survive. Transposition of the great vessels is relatively common and may be treated surgically. In this anomaly, the pulmonary artery originates from the left side of the heart and conducts the oxygenated blood back to the lungs, and the aorta rises from the right ventricle, carrying unoxygenated blood into the systemic circulation.

Rarely, transposition of the pulmonary veins to the right of the heart is seen, and transplantation of the veins to the left atrium may be attempted.

Valvular atresia (absence of an opening) is another form of anomaly which occurs most frequently with the tricuspid valve but may also develop with the aortic valve. Tricuspid atresia raises the pressure within the right atrium to a level exceeding that in the left atrium, and blood flows through the foramen ovale. This anomaly frequently is accompanied by a ventricular septal defect which permits some blood to enter the right ventricle and pass into the pulmonary artery. Either the Blalock or Potts operation (see above), or an anastomosis between the superior vena cava and the pulmonary artery may be done to increase the volume of blood through the lungs.

Inflammatory disease involving heart structures

In any tissue, the inflammatory process may result in destruction of normal functional tissue followed by its replacement with scar tissue, which is fibrous in nature and less specialized.

Diseases which produce inflammatory heart lesions and impaired function include rheumatic fever, bacterial endocarditis, syphilis and pericarditis.

RHEUMATIC FEVER

This is the most common cause of inflammation in the heart structures. Although any or all parts may be affected by rheumatic fever, the valves and the myocardium are the most frequent sites and tend to sustain greater permanent damage. The disease is a complication of a group A streptococcal infection which is usually respiratory. A period of 1–5 weeks may lapse between the infection and the onset of the rheumatic fever, during which time the patient may have recovered completely from the infection.

The inflammatory response, which may occur in the joints as well as in the heart, is thought to be due to a sensitivity of the affected individuals to the antibodies that were formed in response to the invading bacteria. The antistreptococcal lysin titre is found to be high in these people at the onset of rheumatic fever. This sensitivity is only present in certain individuals, since not all those with streptococcal infection develop rheumatic fever. The symptoms of the acute stage vary in intensity and may be so mild that they go unrecognized. In some, joint involvement and fever may be predominant with no evident symptoms referable to the heart, and it is not until much later that it becomes known that cardiac tissue was involved and received permanent damage.

Rheumatic fever may cause acute myocarditis with subsequent scarred areas that reduce myocardial efficiency and impair the conduction system.

The valves are the most common area of the heart to be affected, and the mitral and aortic valves are the most susceptible. They frequently become scarred, distorted and functionally impaired. Both the valve ring at the opening and the valve cusps may be affected. Following the acute inflammation scarring occurs, the orifice is diminished and the edges of the cusps may fuse. These changes result in resistance to the forward movement of the blood, thus increasing the work of the heart chamber behind the obstruction. Damage of this type is referred to as a stenosis. Normally, the mitral opening in an adult is large enough to admit three fingers; in severe stenosis it can become so restricted that only one finger may be introduced.

In some instances, the scarring of the valvular cusps produces a thickening and loss of tissue that prevents them from coming together to close off the opening completely. This incomplete closure allows a regurgitation or backflow of blood through the valve, and is called valvular incompetence or regurgitation. An added strain is placed on the heart chamber behind the incompetent valve. Many patients with rheumatic heart disease have a combined stenosis and incompetence in the affected valve. If the mitral valve is involved, the left atrium develops dilatation and hypertrophy to compensate for the resistance of stenosis and the backflow of valvular incompetence (i.e. the leaking of the blood back through the valve). In the case of aortic valvular damage, the left ventricle dilates and hypertrophies. Prolonged strain created by a damaged valve, increased demands on the already weakened heart, or further progress of the initial rheumatic disease process may result in decompensation or heart failure.

Treatment of rheumatic fever includes drug therapy (antimicrobial preparations, salicylates, corticosteroids), rest and possible surgery.

In the acute stage of rheumatic heart disease the patient may receive large doses of *penicillin* to destroy any haemolytic streptococci which may still be active in the body. Reactivation of the disease occurs very readily with any subsequent streptococcal infection. Patients with rheumatic fever, particularly children, continue on prophylactic doses of oral penicillin or on a monthly intramuscular injection of a large dose which is slowly absorbed. For better absorption, the oral penicillin is given before food is taken in the morning and again at bedtime when the stomach is empty. Very occasionally, sulphadiazine may be used for prophylactic therapy instead of penicillin. The patient is advised to drink a minimum of six to eight glasses of fluid each day to prevent precipitation of this drug in the renal tubules.

With the initial administration of penicillin the nurse is alert for symptoms of allergic reactions. If the patient has had the drug previously, a test dose may be given. Any information of previous reactions or of asthma or hay fever should be passed on to the doctor before the drug is given.

Aspirin is commonly used in rheumatic fever. It relieves symptoms by suppressing tissue reaction. It is given orally and may produce gastric distress, so should be given with meals or with a snack or a large volume of fluid. If the patient complains of dizziness, headache, tinnitus or dullness of hearing, the doctor is informed. Enteric-coated aspirin tablets can be used to prevent gastric irritation

Julian[11a] suggests that although controversy continues as to the relative merits of salicylates and steroids in the treatment of rheumatic heart disease, it is now common practice to use salicylates in rheumatic fever in the absence of carditis but that corticosteroids are added, or substituted, where there is definite evidence of cardiac involvement.

Activity restrictions may vary from bed rest in the

[11a] Julian (1983).

acute stage to gradually increasing periods out of bed as symptoms abate.

Therapy for valvular damage includes restriction of activity to within tolerated limits, treatment of complications such as heart failure and, in some instances, surgical replacement of valves.

BACTERIAL ENDOCARDITIS

Inflammation of the endocardium, including the valves, may be caused by many different pathogenic organisms, but the viridans streptococcus causes the greatest number of cases. Bacterial endocarditis has a higher incidence in those who have some valvular abnormality, either acquired or congenital in origin, or who have a history of rheumatic fever. Special precautions should be taken with such people when they experience minor infections, tooth extraction, and surgery, all of which predispose to the entrance of organisms into the blood.

Bacterial endocarditis may be further defined as acute or subacute. The differentiation is based upon the causative organism and the rapidity of onset. Subacute bacterial endocarditis is most commonly caused by the viridans streptococcus and the onset of symptoms may be insidious. The acute form is caused by more virulent organisms such as *Staphylococcus aureus*, pneumococcus, group A streptococcus and gonococcus. This form of the disease progresses more rapidly and more often attacks the normal heart.

Symptoms include fever, weakness, fatigue, anorexia, chills and petechial lesions in the mucous membranes of the mouth, pharynx or conjunctiva. Cardiac auscultation usually reveals the presence of a heart murmur. In bacterial endocarditis the organisms, transient in the blood, implant on areas of the endocardium and clusters of vegetative structures form which consist of inflammatory exudate, fibrin, platelets and bacteria. These are quite friable and may break off to form an embolus which may then lodge in an artery, interrupting the blood supply to an area of tissue. Should the embolus derive from the right side of the heart, it is likely to obstruct a pulmonary artery, causing a pulmonary infarct.[11b] If the embolus originates in the left side of the heart, it may enter any systemic artery, resulting in an infarction. For example, it may lodge in a cerebral artery, leading to a stroke, or in a femoral artery, interrupting the blood supply to the limb.

Treatment for bacterial endocarditis includes antibiotic therapy, the choice of drug being determined by the organism isolated in blood cultures. Antibiotics are administered in large doses, usually intravenously for at least 2 weeks, and treatment is continued for at least 4 weeks. Nursing care includes the usual nursing measures for a patient with an inflammatory condition.

[11b] An *infarct* is an area of tissue which undergoes necrosis because it is deprived of its blood supply.

As the infection subsides in endocarditis, the affected areas become scarred; if a valve was involved incompetence is likely to develop, and the patient then has the same problems as mentioned in relation to the patient with rheumatic fever.

SYPHILIS

Another type of infection that may produce a valvular lesion is syphilis. Most frequently it is the aortic valve that is affected, and incompetence develops.

PERICARDITIS

Pericarditis may occur as the result of an infectious or noninfectious process, or may be due to an autoimmune reaction (see p. 338 for a discussion of hypersensitivity reaction following a myocardial infarction). Fluid accumulates in the pericardium as part of the inflammatory response. The pressure exerted on the heart by this fluid may prevent its normal filling, creating a condition referred to as cardiac tamponade. In some instances extensive scarring of the visceral pericardium may prevent normal stretching and filling of the heart chambers.

Pericarditis is characterized by chest pain, which is often pleuritic in nature. There may be electrocardiographic changes (elevation of ST segments followed several days later by T wave inversions) and a pericardial friction rub on auscultation. A paradoxical pulse may be present if cardiac tamponade has occurred.

Treatment includes salicylates, indomethacin and occasionally corticosteroids to combat the inflammatory response. The patient must be observed carefully for complications such as cardiac tamponade.

In the inflammatory conditions discussed in the preceding paragraphs, it can be seen that permanent heart damage can occur from the formation of scar tissue. The patient may remain active as long as his heart compensates, but may have limitations due to reduced cardiac efficiency.

Deficiency in the blood supply to the myocardium (ischaemic heart disease)

CORONARY ATHEROSCLEROSIS

A narrowing or obstruction in the coronary arteries reduces the blood supply to the myocardium, and causes what is called ischaemic heart disease. It results in a deficiency of oxygen and nutrients to the muscle. The reduced oxygen supply is most significant and is quickly reflected in reduced myocardial efficiency. The heart muscle can withstand only a very small oxygen debt, as it is much more susceptible to a reduced oxygen supply than skeletal muscle. In most instances the decreased blood supply to the myocardium is due to degenerative changes in the arteries that produce a narrowing of the lumen of the vessels. Fatty substances, which include cholesterol, are deposited within the intima of the arteries to cause *atherosclerosis*. These fatty plaques interfere with the nutrition of the cells in the intima, leading to necrosis, scarring and calcification, which leave the surface rough and the lumen reduced. These roughened constricted areas allow less blood through and predispose to thrombus formation and occlusion of the vessel.

Atherosclerosis usually develops gradually. While the blood supply through the artery is being reduced, a collateral circulation develops in an effort to increase the supply to the myocardium, but this supplementary circulation is rarely sufficient to provide enough oxygen to the heart muscle during strenuous physical exertion.

Coronary atherosclerosis is a disease having many causes. Its development seems to result from the interaction of personal and environmental factors; the incidence increases with age and shows a strong familial tendency. It is less common in women of childbearing age than men of the same age but after this period gradually becomes as frequent in women. A number of surveys have shown a greater incidence of coronary atherosclerosis among populations whose diet regularly contains high amounts of calories, total fats, saturated fats, cholesterol and refined sugars.

The major risk factors associated with the development of coronary atherosclerosis are hyperlipoproteinaemia (especially hypercholesteraemia), hypertension, cigarette smoking and diabetes mellitus. These factors may usually be controlled—hyperlipoproteinaemia by diet and/or medications, and hypertension by medications. Cigarette smoking should be discontinued, although for some individuals this represents considerable difficulty. Other suggested risk factors include lack of exercise and psychosocial tensions. Obese individuals may develop atherosclerosis through a predisposition to hypertension, diabetes mellitus, hyperlipidaemia and possibly the association with lack of physical activity.[12]

Although control of risk factors does not guarantee elimination of atherosclerotic heart disease, evidence suggests that modifying dietary, smoking and exercise habits and reducing emotional stress may decrease its incidence.

Hyperlipoproteinaemia
Blood lipids include cholesterol, triglycerides, phospholipids and free fatty acids. Cholesterol and triglycerides are of clinical significance and are transported in plasma as lipoproteins. There are four major classes of lipoproteins, which are chylomicrons and prebeta, beta, and alpha lipoproteins; each contains varying proportions of protein and the three blood lipids. The lipoproteins may be separated by the process of electrophoresis.

Chylomicrons are mainly of dietary origin. Prebeta lipoproteins contain a large amount of triglycerides, primarily of hepatic origin, synthesized from fatty acids and carbohydrate. Beta lipoproteins carry one-half to two-thirds of the total plasma cholesterol. Alpha lipoproteins carry little triglycerides but larger amounts of protein and an appreciable amount of cholesterol. Certain studies have suggested that high levels of high density lipoproteins (HDL) may protect against the development of coronary atherosclerosis, although it is uncertain how this occurs.[13]

Hyperlipoproteinaemia may be classified as Type I, II, III, IV or V. Types I and V hyperlipidaemia are rare. Types II, III and IV are associated with an increased incidence of coronary heart disease. Hyperlipoproteinaemia may be secondary to another disease such as obstructive liver disease, due to an excessive intake of saturated fats and cholesterol in the diet, or may result from a primary or familial disorder. Determination of serum cholesterol and triglyceride levels will detect hyperlipoproteinaemia in most cases and is less costly than other laboratory procedures. However, in some instances, further studies may be warranted. Control of hypercholesteraemia is directed toward lowering the serum cholesterol levels by diet and in some instances by medications.

Studies suggest that by modifying the dietary intake of fats, carbohydrate and calories, the blood lipid levels of most patients with primary hyperlipidaemia can be lowered. The contribution of diet to the prevention of coronary atherosclerosis is not clear but evidence suggests that this approach might be worthwhile.

The purpose of the diet is to reduce body weight when required and to lower the intake of total fat, saturated fatty acids and cholesterol, while increasing the intake of unsaturated fatty acids. Saturated fat and cholesterol are found in high-fat meats and dairy products and in some commercially baked goods. Polyunsaturated fats are contained in vegetable and fish oils.

The modified diet emphasizes substitution of lean meat (veal, lean beef), poultry and fish for fattier meats (pork, organ meats, visible meat fat). It also includes non-fat products such as corn oil, margarine, skimmed milk and low fat cheese, whole grain or enriched flour products, fruits, vegetables and polyunsaturated vegetable oils.

The degree of dietary restriction depends upon the type of hyperlipidaemia and the age and condition of the patient. Dietary teaching is a combined function of the doctor, nurse and dietitian. The dietitian is the

---

[12] Wenger & Schlant (1986), p. 824.

[13] Castelli, Hjortland, Kannel & Dowberm (1977), p. 707.

primary person involved if the diet is complex, but the nurse also needs to be informed so that she can reinforce the teaching. Some patients may require much support and understanding to continue on their diets, especially if drastic changes in eating habits are needed. Compliance will probably be greater if the diet is adjusted as much as possible to individual tastes.

Lipid-lowering drugs may be ordered for selected patients who do not respond to diet therapy alone. These include:

Clofibrate (Atromid-S). This drug interferes with cholesterol synthesis. It reduces cholesterol and triglyceride levels in patients with Types III, IV and V hyperlipidaemia and, to a small degree, may alter the cholesterol levels of patients with Type II. Its side-effects include weight gain, gastrointestinal upsets, gallstones and increased levels of the enzymes AST and ALT. It also prolongs the prothrombin time of patients on warfarin so that anticoagulant dosage of the drug may need to be adjusted.

Nicotinic acid. This drug inhibits cholesterol synthesis and the release of free fatty acids from adipose tissue. Almost all types of hyperlipidaemia, including Type II, respond to it. Marked flushing, pruritis, nausea and vomiting are among its side-effects. Liver function may be abnormally altered but this situation is reversible if the drug is discontinued. Gradual increases in dosage may prevent the side-effects.

Cholestyramine. This drug acts by binding bile acids and preventing their reabsorption in the intestine. Increased breakdown of cholesterol results. It is used for patients with familial Type II hyperlipidaemia. Cholestyramine is administered with meals. Side-effects include gastrointestinal disturbances.

The development of coronary atherosclerosis produces the ischaemic heart diseases known as angina pectoris and myocardial infarction.

ANGINA PECTORIS

The term angina pectoris describes a clinical syndrome characterized by chest pain. 'Pectoris' indicates the general location (chest) and 'angina' refers to the choking, suffocating nature of the pain. This condition arises because of a discrepancy between the oxygen being supplied to the myocardium and the energy expenditure. The pain, arising from heart muscle fibres which are deficient in oxygen, is usually precipitated by physical exertion or emotional stress which increases the work load of the heart. There is a need for a greater blood supply than is being delivered by the coronary circulation. The patient suddenly develops chest pain retrosternally which may radiate to the left or both shoulders and arms and occasionally up the neck to the jaws. The pain may, however, be atypical and

arise only in the arms, jaw or neck and not in the chest. It is usually relieved within a few minutes by resting and/or by glyceryl trinitrate (GTN) but may last as long as 30 minutes. The patient may become short of breath.

Angina may remain a stable condition brought about by predictable precipitating factors with no change in the severity or frequency of the attacks. It is then controlled by limiting those activities or situations known to cause pain, and by medication. The pain may progress in frequency and intensity if the atherosclerosis process in the coronary arteries proceeds more rapidly than the development of collateral circulation. Activities may then need to be curtailed greatly and the patient may even experience pain at rest.

Unstable angina is distinguished from stable angina by four characteristics:
1 The syndrome has developed within the previous month, brought on by minimal exertion.
2 A pattern of stable exertion-related angina pain becomes less predictable, more prolonged, frequent or severe and may have a different radiation.
3 The syndrome occurs at rest as well as with minimal exertion.
4 The pain is not relieved as promptly with glyceryl trinitrate as it is with stable angina.

Unstable angina frequently precedes myocardial infarction and may be referred to as pre-infarction syndrome or crescendo angina.

Prinzmetal angina refers to a type of unstable angina in which the pain occurs at rest and at the same time each day. It is not precipitated by exertion. The underlying cause is spasm of the coronary arteries and obstructive coronary artery disease may or may not be present.

Management of angina pectoris
Immediate care in an anginal episode involves the following: The patient stops whatever activity he may be engaged in and the prescribed medication is administered [e.g. glyceryl trinitrate (GTN)]. The pulse, respirations and blood pressure are checked during the episode. The doctor may want an ECG taken while the patient is experiencing pain.

The patient is advised that strenuous physical exertion and emotional outbursts should be avoided. In many instances normal functioning can be maintained by modifying aspects of his occupation, recreation and social life. Risk factors such as smoking and obesity are eliminated in an effort to prevent progression of the disease. Smoking favours vasoconstriction and obesity increases the demand on the heart.

Moderate exercise below the point of producing pain is encouraged. Walking is excellent exercise and should be done on a regular basis. The individual should begin with short walks on level ground, gradually increasing the distance over a period of weeks. Regular, medically supervised exercise programmes are recommended for some patients. Regular exercise improves muscle tone and general well-being and stimulates the development of collateral circulation in the myocardium. Normal weight is more easily maintained. The psychological benefit of exercise to the patient cannot be overestimated.

Drugs used in angina pectoris include the following (Table 14.6):

Nitrates. Nitrates act by relaxing vascular smooth muscle. This results in decreased peripheral vascular resistance and venous return, with a subsequent decrease in heart size, stroke volume and cardiac output. The net effect is a decrease in the oxygen consumption of the heart.

Glyceryl trinitrate (GTN) is a short-acting vasodilator administered in tablet form. The tablet is placed under the tongue where it is absorbed very quickly.

The patient will experience a tingling feeling on the tongue when first taken and should obtain relief in 1–2 minutes. Patients should not take multiple doses to get quick relief of pain. If relief is not apparent after 3 tablets taken at 5 minute intervals a doctor should be called. Initial dosage should be 0.3 mg. This reduces the likelihood of severe headaches, which often occur in the initial stage of treatment. People who suffer attacks of angina are advised to carry the drug at all times. It should be replaced periodically so that a fresh supply is available when required. Tablets should be kept in a dark glass container and those not being carried should be stored in a cool, dark place, since GTN is affected by both light and heat. The patient is advised that he may experience mild fullness, warmth or throbbing in the head, but fortunately with continued use side-effects usually diminish. GTN may also be used prophylactically 2–3 minutes prior to activities which are known to precipitate anginal attacks.

Table 14.6 Drugs used in patients with angina pectoris.

Drug	Action	Side-effects
Nitrates 　Short-acting 　　Glyceryl trinitrate	Relaxes vascular smooth muscle, thus decreasing peripheral vascular resistance	Headache or sense of fullness in the head
Long-acting 　　Isosorbide dinitrate 　　(Isordil)		Headache Postural hypotension
Pentaerythritol 　　　tetranitrate (Peritrate)	As above	As above
Beta-blockers 　Propranolol (Inderal)	Decreases myocardial oxygen requirements by decreasing heart rate, depressing myocardial contractility and decreasing left ventricular tension development	Excessive bradycardia Congestive heart failure Bronchospasm AV block May worsen diabetes
Metoprolol 　(Lopresor, Betaloc) Timolol 　(Blocadren) Oxprenolol 　(Trasicor) Atenolol 　(Tenormin) Pindolol 　(Visken) Nadolol 　(Corgard)	As above, but depresses B_1 receptors (heart) to a greater degree than B_2 receptors (bronchioles, peripheral vessels)	
Calcium channel-blockers Nifedipine 　(Adalat)	Dilates coronary and peripheral vessels	Nausea, headache, flushing, peripheral oedema, constipation, dizziness, fatigue
Verapamil 　(Cordilox)	Same as above Also prolongs the refractory period of the AV node	

GTN ointment (e.g. Percutol) is used prophylactically to prevent attacks of angina but is not used for treating them. The doctor will prescribe the amount of glyceryl trinitrate ointment to be applied and the nurse must be aware of the correct manner of application. The ointment is measured out in 1–5 cm lengths according to the order. It is then spread over the application paper, providing an application area of approximately 5–8 cm. The paper is then applied to the skin of the patient and may be covered with any commercial plastic covering to facilitate maximum absorption.

GTN ointment may be applied to skin on the arms, legs, chest or abdomen. Sites should be rotated. It is best to keep the size of the application site constant, to prevent the side-effects which may occur when it is enlarged. Side-effects are the same as those of GTN tablets.

Transdermal GTN patches[14] have now been developed which deliver glyceryl trinitrate into the bloodstream at a constant rate for 24 hours. They are less messy and difficult to use than ointment and may enhance patient compliance.

In certain emergency situations, it is preferable to administer GTN intravenously. It may be added to either 5% dextrose in water or normal saline. The concentration of the solution and the rate of flow will vary with the patient. Although intravenous GTN does not have to be protected from light, certain other precautions should be taken.[15] Because it is absorbed by plastic and therefore rapidly lost to the solution, it is recommended that the drug only be added to intravenous solution in glass bottles. Some institutions suggest flushing the intravenous tubing with 30–35 ml of the solution, which then binds tubing sides and prevents the absorption of the rest of the solution.

Isosorbide dinitrate (Isordil) is a slower- and longer-acting nitrate given sublingually in small doses or orally in larger doses. It is ordered for patients experiencing regular attacks of angina. Since it reduces vascular tone, some patients may experience hypotension on standing, especially when taking larger doses. The patient is usually started on small doses, which are gradually increased as the drug becomes tolerated. Isordil is frequently prescribed in combination with propranolol. The effects of both drugs may be complimentary; the increase in heart rate and contractility induced by nitrates is offset by propranolol.

Pentaerythritol tetranitrate (Peritrate) is also a slower-acting vasodilator and is effective for a longer period. It is given orally in doses of 80–320 mg daily. Some patients may require doses of oral Peritrate and Isordil much greater than those generally recommended.

Beta-adrenergic blockers. These drugs block sympathetic stimulation of the beta receptors.

Propranolol (Inderal) relieves anginal symptoms by decreasing myocardial oxygen requirements. It does this by depressing myocardial contractility and decreasing heart rate and left ventricular tension development. It significantly reduces pulse rate, sometimes to as low as 40 beats per minute.

Another property of beta-adrenergic blockers is that of 'intrinsic sympathomimetic activity (ISA)' which means that they weakly stimulate the beta-adrenergic receptors. Drugs with ISA usually do not slow the resting heart rate. However, the effect of these drugs during adrenergic stimulation (e.g. exercise) is equivalent to beta blockers that do not have this property.

The patient is usually started on a low dose (e.g. 10–20 mg) every 6 hours, which is gradually increased until relief is obtained. However, in some patients, this goal may not be achieved because of significant bradycardia or the occurrence of side-effects. Because of variability in metabolism, the individual therapeutic dose of propranolol may vary from 80–1000 mg per day. Patients with congestive heart failure or a history of bronchial asthma are not given the drug because it will increase the failure and its beta-blocking properties will prevent dilatation of the bronchioles. Mild cardiac failure is not an absolute contraindication to the use of propranolol. The benefit–risk ratio is considered by the doctor in deciding whether or not to start propranolol in these patients. There are however several beta-blockers that block B_1 receptors (heart) to a greater degree than B_2 receptors (bronchioles, peripheral vessels). This is referred to as cardioselectivity and allows the use of these agents when a non-selective beta-blocker would be less desirable, for example, for patients with asthma, diabetes, or peripheral vascular disease.

Calcium channel blockers. Certain drugs act by decreasing the cellular uptake of calcium, which is required for the contraction of vascular smooth muscle. This results in coronary vasodilatation. Although the effect of these drugs is similar to nitrates, the mechanism of action differs. These drugs are particularly effective in coronary artery spasm. Examples are nifedipine and verapamil. Verapamil may also be administered for acute tachyarrhythmias; it is then given intravenously. The usual oral dose for angina is 80–120 mg three times daily. Nifedipine is administered orally in divided doses to a total dose of 40–120 mg daily.

For those patients who do not obtain adequate relief with medications, surgery may be indicated (see p. 364).

Percutaneous transluminal coronary angioplasty (PTCA)
PTCA provides an alternative for some patients who might otherwise require coronary artery bypass

---

[14] Dasta & Geraets (1982), pp. 23–32.
[15] Baaske, Yacoui & Amann (1982), p. 36–39.

surgery. PTCA is a non-surgical method of relieving stenotic or occlusive lesions in the coronary arterial system. However, since emergency aortocoronary bypass surgery may be required if complications occur, the preparation of the patient includes that required for surgery.

Criteria for selection of patients include: (1) recent onset of angina pectoris, (2) angina refractory to medical treatment, (3) angina symptoms of sufficient severity to compromise the quality of life of the patient, (4) single vessel disease with the lesion situated high in the vessel so that it is easily accessible to the catheter and (5) the patient is an acceptable candidate for bypass surgery.

Diagnostic testing prior to this procedure is similar to that for coronary bypass surgery. Nursing care includes giving both physical and emotional support to the patient, as the procedure is relatively new and often frightening. Educational responsibilities include an explanation of coronary artery disease if this has not been given and of all the tests carried out prior to the procedure. The doctor will explain the procedure, the risks involved, the possible need for bypass surgery and the expected results of this treatment. The nurse reinforces and gives further information as required.

After a local anaesthetic is administered, a guide catheter is introduced into the right or left femoral or brachial artery. This catheter is advanced under fluoroscopy to the affected coronary artery. Once through the stenotic narrowing in the coronary artery, a dilating catheter is slipped through the guide catheter. When positioned within the atherosclerotic lesion, the dilating balloon is inflated with a mixture of saline and contrast media. The resultant stretching of the coronary arterial muscle wall widens the lumen of the artery, allowing blood to flow more freely. In addition, work is being carried out into the application of laser energy in this treatment of atheromatous disease.

Possible complications include bleeding or thrombosis of the affected artery due to injury of the vascular endothelium, coronary artery spasm and rupture of the artery, causing cardiac tamponade. These complications may result in acute myocardial infarction.

Medications such as nifedipine and beta-blockers are given either prior to or during the procedure to prevent coronary artery spasm. They also include intravenous glyceryl trinitrate to promote vasodilation. Antithrombotic medications such as aspirin and persantin may be given. Generally patients receive an anticoagulant such as heparin, which may be followed by treatment with warfarin.

Following the procedure, ECG monitoring is maintained continuously and the patient is observed closely for signs or symptoms indicating bleeding, myocardial ischaemia, impaired left ventricular function or electrolyte imbalance.

Bed rest is maintained for 24 hours and the patient is gradually mobilized and usually discharged within 2–4 days. Prior to discharge, instruction is given on all the aspects of the medication regimen which the patient must follow. The name, purpose, dosage, and times to take the drugs are reviewed. The importance of avoiding activities, food or over-the-counter medications which might interfere with or enhance the effect of the medication should also be stressed. Activities allowed and to be avoided are discussed, as well as the importance of medical follow-up.

Intra-aortic balloon pump
Occasionally counter-pulsation with the intra-aortic balloon pump is utilized for the patient with unstable angina prior to coronary artery surgery. The intra-aortic balloon is inserted into the aorta from one of the femoral arteries; it is inflated during diastole and is deflated as the heart ejects its contents during systole. In this way it reduces afterload and myocardial oxygen demand, increases myocardial ischaemia and relieves angina. The intra-aortic balloon pump is an invasive method of treatment; consequently, the patient and his family require a great deal of support from nursing and medical staff.

ACUTE MYOCARDIAL INFARCTION

Acute myocardial infarction (also known as coronary occlusion or thrombosis) is the most serious and acute form of ischaemic heart disease. A coronary artery becomes blocked and the myocardial area which it supplies suffers oxygen deficiency and necrosis. It occurs suddenly, and compensation through collateral channels is inadequate to maintain the myocardial cells. The resulting area of necrotic tissue is referred to as an infarction.

The extent of the infarction varies from patches of 1 or 2 cm in diameter to widespread areas of necrosis. One or more layers of the heart may be involved. The area of infarction becomes soft and then eventually fills in with firm, fibrous scar tissue. Survival and the extent of subsequent restrictions depend upon the amount of myocardial damage and the area of the heart affected. Death may occur immediately or within a few hours. Obviously, the remaining viable heart tissue must compensate for the loss of functional tissue.

Occlusion may be preceded by some manifestations of coronary insufficiency such as angina, or it may occur suddenly without any previous warning.

Types of myocardial infarction
It is difficult to delineate the precise area of the myocardium which is affected, but general areas can be identified. Although other areas of the heart may be involved, most infarctions occur in the left ventricle.

Anterior wall infarction. The anterior wall of the left ventricle is infarcted due to an occlusion of the left anterior descending artery. The papillary muscles of the left ventricle and the intraventricular septum may also be involved. In the latter instances, the infarction would be referred to as anteroseptal.

Lateral wall infarction. An infarction in the lateral wall of the left ventricle is associated with an occlusion of the lateral branch of the left circumflex artery. Occasionally both the anterior descending and the left circumflex branches are obstructed, and the infarction is designated anterolateral.

Inferior wall infarction. This term implies an infarction of the part of the left ventricle which rests on the diaphragm. It is usually due to occlusion of the right coronary artery. Occasionally it is called a diaphragmatic infarction.

Posterior wall infarction. This type is usually due to occlusion of the posterior branch of either the right coronary or left circumflex artery. It is sometimes called a true posterior infarction to distinguish it from an inferior infarction.

Nursing process
In most instances of myocardial infarction the patient suddenly becomes seriously ill, and prompt action is necessary. The doctor is called immediately. The patient is kept at rest in a position that is most comfortable and facilitates breathing—usually semi-recumbent. Tight clothing (collars, belts, etc.) is loosened and the patient covered sufficiently to prevent chilling. Food and fluids may be withheld initially.

The patient may be transported to a hospital and admitted to a coronary care unit. (Since the work of Mather et al.[16] there has been a debate as to whether this is the most appropriate place for such a patient. Some will therefore remain at home or be cared for in a hospital ward.) When his condition has stabilized, he is transferred to a general care ward. Hospitalization for patients without complications varies from a few days to 3 weeks. Total convalescence ranges from 8–12 weeks.

The objective of care of the patient with myocardial infarction is to restore the ability of the heart to maintain adequate circulation, and to prevent deterioration.

Assessment. Constant observations of the patient are necessary in the acute stage. The nurse must be alert to significant changes and must make decisions about the need for prompt reporting, the seeking of assistance and the use of emergency measures.
- *Pulse.* The pulse becomes rapid and weak and may be imperceptible at the time of the attack. Initially, a few patients may exhibit bradycardia, followed by tachycardia. The monitor gives more specific information about the type of disorder in

rate and rhythm during the acute stage. The patient's pulse is checked every 2–4 hours during the acute stage and more frequently if it is showing great variability. Once the heart rate and rhythm have stabilized, the pulse is taken four times daily. Changes in rate or rhythm are reported. Pulse rate is noted in response to activity.
- *Blood pressure.* Due to the decreased pumping efficiency of the heart, the blood pressure falls but may be elevated in the first few hours following an attack due to an augmented sympathetic response. It is taken every 2–4 hours during the acute stage, and more often if there is variation or abnormality. It is also checked following the administration of medications such as diamorphine, and if the patient is experiencing signs or symptoms such as pain, faintness or cyanosis. When the acute episode is over and the patient's condition has stabilized, the blood pressure is taken four times daily. Blood pressure may be checked when the patient is lying down and after assuming the upright position to detect postural hypotension. Either a fall in blood pressure or continuous hypertension is reported immediately.
- *Pain.* The most common presenting complaint of patients with myocardial infarction is severe chest pain. The nurse must ascertain the exact location and character of the chest discomfort (see p. 314 for a description of various types of chest pain), whether it is aggravated by any particular movement or change of position, and how it is relieved. The pain may last for several hours or until relieved by analgesics. It should not persist for days; prolonged pain may be an indication of pericarditis or an extending infarction.
- *Dyspnoea.* Dyspnoea may be due to pulmonary congestion or pain. It may also occur as activity is increased. Relief of pain and congestion may relieve the dyspnoea. It is important to note whether shortness of breath is present at all times or, if intermittent, how it is precipitated and what measures relieve it. In the acute stage, respirations are checked at least every 2–4 hours, or more often as changes occur. During the convalescent stage, they are observed and recorded four times daily and in relationship to various activities.
- *Skin.* The skin may be cool, moist and a greyish colour in response to the decreased cardiac output. The colour, temperature and moistness of the skin are observed frequently and any changes noted.
- *Nausea and vomiting.* Nausea and vomiting may be experienced at the time of the attack, lasting from several hours to 2 or 3 days. Occasionally, nausea and vomiting occur in response to the opiates being administered. The nurse notes the presence of nausea and vomiting and any possible precipitating factors.
- *Temperature.* Myocardial necrosis causes an elevation of body temperature ranging from 37.7–39°C

---

[16] Mather et al (1976), pp. 925–929.

(100–102°F). The temperature usually rises within 24–48 hours and returns to normal by the sixth or seventh day. If the temperature persists longer, it may be due to complications. The patient's temperature is taken four times daily until it has been normal for several days. It may then be taken once or twice daily. Rectal temperatures are avoided to prevent rectal stimulation which may lead to straining at stool.

- *Weakness and tiredness.* Extreme weakness may be experienced and may persist for many days. Many patients complain of tiredness for weeks after their infarction. The exact cause of this is not clearly defined. Some suggest it results from decreased oxygen perfusion of the tissues due to a lowered cardiac output. It has also been attributed to weakened skeletal muscles as a result of even a brief period of immobilization. The patient may have been in a state of physical exhaustion prior to his attack or he may be emotionally exhausted from the experience.

  The nurse observes the extent to which the patient tolerates any activity (such as walking). She also notes how much he sleeps during the day and how quickly he falls asleep following activities.

- *Psychological reactions.* A heart attack carries the threat of death or invalidism for the patient. The sudden change in his well-being leaves feelings of vulnerability and helplessness. The patient is required to make very rapid adjustments to both his illness and change in environment.

  Anxiety is the most common psychological response. It is manifested by various overt and covert behaviours, such as tenseness, restlessness, short attention span, inability to concentrate, crying, constant talking and expression of feelings of anxiety. The patient may appear generally relaxed but may exhibit more subtle manifestations of anxiety such as darting eye movements. Patients may also show denial, and may be angry and/or depressed. These emotional responses may appear in varying degrees and at any time during hospitalization or may not become evident until after discharge from the hospital. The individual's interpretation of his experience and his personal coping pattern influence his responses. Continuing restlessness and apprehension are noted and reported.

- *Electrocardiographic monitoring.* In the coronary care unit a constant monitoring of heart action is established for continuous assessment of cardiac activity. Electrodes are applied to the chest wall and are connected to an electrocardiograph with an oscilloscope. The purpose of the monitor is explained to the patient and his family. The patient is advised that he need not lie immobile because of the electrodes. The nurse responsible for the patient must become sufficiently familiar with the monitoring system and ECG so that she is able to recognize changes and arrhythmias that demand prompt action. The basic rhythm of the patient's heart is observed and recorded each shift. Any changes in the rhythm are immediately observed and decisions made as to further action required.

- *Diagnostic tests.* The nurse must be aware of the results of diagnostic tests and their significance following a myocardial infarction. Assessment includes: (1) noting on-going changes in the ECG; (2) serum enzymes; and (3) leucocyte count and erythrocyte sedimentation rate.

1 Changes in the electrocardiogram. Theoretically, three types of changes are present in the myocardium when an infarction develops. These define three areas, referred to clinically as the area of infarction, the area of injury and the zone of ischaemia, resulting in a distinctive electrocardiographic pattern. In the infarcted area, irreversible structural changes occur with resulting necrosis of the tissue. Since electrical impulses cannot be conducted through this tissue, electrical energy is lost, causing a relative gain of electromotive forces directed away from the necrotic area. These developments produce a negative deflection (Q wave) in electrodes facing the infarcted area, indicating that electrical forces are not being directed toward it but away from it. An increased positive deflection (R wave) will be seen in leads facing the opposite surface of the heart, indicating forces moving toward the leads and away from the infarcted area.

Surrounding the zone of infarction is an area of injury which suffers a decreased blood supply, but the damage is not permanent. Although specific abnormal electrocardiographic changes are produced, these may revert to normal if the blood supply is restored. Electrodes placed over the injured area will record an ST segment elevation.

The zone of ischaemia surrounds the area of injury and may also return to normal once the blood supply is restored. Inverted T waves indicate ischaemia.

ST elevations appear within several hours following an infarction and disappear in a few days. In the early stages T waves become taller and appear as an extension of the elevated ST segment. They later become inverted. Q waves appear within 1–2 days and persist (see Fig. 14.10). The area of infarction will be reflected in leads which view that portion of the heart. Thus, inferior infarctions can be identified in leads II, III and AVF, anterior infarctions can be identified in the anterior leads V_1 to V_4 and lateral wall infarction in leads I, AVL, V_5 and V_6. Since under normal conditions no leads face the posterior wall of the heart, diagnosis is based upon reciprocal changes in leads facing the

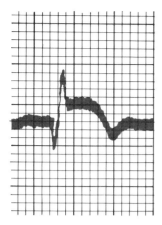

Fig. 14.10 Electrocardiographic changes indicating acute myocardial infarction: Q wave, ST elevation, and T wave inversion.

opposite wall—that is, increased R waves in leads V_1 and V_2.

2 Serum enzymes. Diagnosis of a myocardial infarction is confirmed by the elevation of specific intracellular serum enzymes and by a characteristic electrocardiographic pattern (see pp. 316–317 for a description of enzymes). Table 14.7 demonstrates enzyme elevations in one patient with an acute myocardial infarction. CPK and aspartate aminotransferase (AST) (SGOT) levels increased early and peaked within 48 hours. The LDH level increased more gradually and remained elevated after 7 days.

3 Leucocyte count and erythrocyte sedimentation rate. Leucocytosis and an increased erythrocyte sedimentation rate occur in response to necrosis but are non-specific diagnostic measures. The white blood count rises a few hours after the infarction and returns to normal within 7 days. The sedimentation rate becomes elevated by the third or fourth day and may remain so for weeks.

Table 14.7 The elevation of serum enzyme levels in one patient following a myocardial infarction (units/litre).

Enzyme	Day of admission	Day 2	Day 3	Day 7
CPK	6	162	5	5
AST	14	177	201	23
LDH	151	513	789	419

Identification of patient problems. During her assessment of the patient, the nurse may identify the following actual and potential problems.

1 Alteration in comfort (both physical and psychological).
 (a) The patient is likely to experience pain in the chest (on account of the decreased oxygen perfusion)
 (b) The patient is likely to suffer from hypoxia and dyspnoea related to the stiffness of his lungs secondary to heart failure
 (c) Nausea and vomiting are also likely
 (d) The patient may become extremely anxious, as may his family.

2 Problems associated with immobility and the reduction of energy demands
 (a) The patient may find the necessity to rest and restrict his activity very difficult to cope with.
 (b) He may become bored.
 (c) He may become constipated.

3 Lack of knowledge about the illness and its implications for his life-style.

4 Inability of the patient to recognize complications and lack of knowledge about what to do.

5 Problems in adjusting to transfer from the coronary care unit.

Nursing intervention.

1 Relief of discomfort (physical and psychological).
 (a) *Pain.* An analgesic such as diamorphine is usually given to relieve the severe pain associated with myocardial infarction. The drug is administered intravenously in small doses in the accident and emergency department and in the coronary care unit. Intramuscular injections elevate CPK readings, as this enzyme is also present in skeletal muscle and diagnosis of a myocardial infarction may be obscured. The effect of the drug on the respirations should be noted, since depression of the respiratory centre may occur.
 (b) *Hypoxia and dyspnoea.* Oxygen is usually administered by mask or nasal cannulae in order to increase arterial oxygen tension, which may help to relieve the myocardial pain caused by hypoxia and prevent extension of the infarction. Mechanical respiration using intermittent positive pressure ventilation may be necessary in cases of severe insufficiency.

  The nurse briefly explains the procedure to the patient and remains with him until he is accustomed to the mask or nasal cannulae. Observations are made of the patient's response to the oxygen. Its effectiveness will be indicated by reduced pulse rate, less dyspnoea, improvement in colour and less restlessness. (For details of administration of oxygen, see p. 445).

Some degree of dyspnoea may be prevented by helping the patient avoid exertion. Explanations are given concerning the easiest way to move in bed, the importance of avoiding straining and the Valsalva manoeuvre. The patient is positioned in a low semi-Fowler's position. This allows for greater expansion of the lungs and reduces the venous return to the heart, thus reducing the stress on it.

(c) *Nausea and vomiting.* Metoclopramide 10 mg intravenously or intramuscularly, cyclizine 50 mg intramuscularly or orally, or prochlorperazine (Stemetil) intramuscularly should be given as an antiemetic. Nursing measures cited in Chapter 17 are observed.

(d) *Anxiety.* Mental rest is a considerable part of therapy for the heart patient. Anxiety may be somewhat reduced by the relief of physical symptoms. In the coronary care unit, brief and precise explanations of all equipment, routines, tests and procedures prove very helpful. Patients are also reassured by prompt attention to their needs and constant monitoring. Competent, quiet performance without apparent concern and hurry provides some reassurance for the patient. Anticipation of needs and preparedness for treatments contribute to more effective care. Articles likely to be wanted are left within reach so that the patient is neither tempted to get up nor reach for something rather than ask.

Patients may pose direct questions about their condition, such as 'Is it serious?' or 'Will I recover?' Answers should be honest and supportive. Klein and Garrity suggest a relationship between long-term survival and emotional responses as well as severity of infarction, and state that each patient must be helped to find a coping strategy appropriate to his personal situation and his own strengths and weaknesses.[17] This is done through effective communication with the patient; it is the only means by which he may influence his environment and be assisted in working out appropriate coping strategies.[18] Effective communication includes listening to the patient and responding to his cues, introducing statements to which the patient might respond and allowing the patient to discuss his

feelings. Considerable help and peace of mind may be derived from a vicar, priest or other religious leader.

If the patient is very upset the nurse remains with the patient until he becomes less apprehensive, and then assures him that someone is close by and will be in and out frequently. The presence of a close member of the family who will not disturb the patient may provide additional comfort. Occasionally, diazepam (Valium) or another anti-anxiety drug may be prescribed.

Members of the patient's family also experience shock and anxiety in response to the patient's illness. Seeing someone close to us in pain and seriously ill is a very frightening experience. Relatives of patients have described their initial reaction as 'feeling numbed and dazed'. As reality sets in, anxiety about the patient's survival and future increases.

The doctor and nurse speak to a member of the family shortly after the patient's admission to the hospital, explaining the suspected diagnosis and the treatment to be given during the next few hours. The nurse then attempts to speak to close family members whenever they visit to answer any questions and to show some understanding of the anxiety they are experiencing. Relatives as well as patients are reassured by simple explanations of equipment, procedures and routines. In talking to the family, the nurse may elicit information about the patient's habits, likes and dislikes and emotional reactions, which may be helpful in planning care.

Alleviating the anxieties of relatives and/or close family friends allows them to be more supportive of the patient. As with the patient, concern may prevent the member of the family from absorbing all that he or she is told. Explanations and instructions may have to be repeated. The family should be included in teaching programmes provided for the patient or in programmes specifically designed for them.

2 Reduction of energy demands

(a) *Rest and restriction of activity.* This is of the utmost importance in the treatment and care of the patient with an acute myocardial infarction. The patient is placed on complete bed rest until symptoms such as pain and shortness of breath have abated; this means that he remains in bed and all care is provided for him. This necessary dependence should be discussed with the patient as to its purpose and importance, its temporary nature and what it involves. Previously, the patient remained at this level of activity for several days to several weeks. In recent years the trend has been to mobilize the patients early once pain and severe shortness of breath are no longer present; research has shown that fewer complications occur. Also, the psychological effect of early ambulation is worth a great deal.

By the second day, strict inactivity is

---

[17] Garrity & Klein (1975), pp. 730–737.
[18] Garrity & Klein (1975), p. 734.

modified. The patient is allowed mild activities such as cleaning his teeth, washing his face and hands and feeding himself, as long as reaching is avoided. Exercising of the lower limbs to prevent venous stasis is commenced. By the second day, most patients are permitted to use a bedside commode, since this demands less energy than using a bedpan; indeed, many patients are able to use a commode, rather than a bedpan, from the time of admission. Undisturbed rest periods are provided following short periods of activity—for instance, after eating and after bathing.

Activities and ambulation are gradually increased. The days of long-term bedrest for a patient following acute myocardial infarction are over. Having begun gentle limb exercises in bed about 24 hours following admission, he may sit out in a chair when pain-free. The patient is advised to sit up gradually to prevent feelings of dizziness or faintness. Continual cardiac monitoring immediately identifies any arrhythmias accompanying changes in activity. Blood pressure is recorded in the lying and sitting positions and the patient is observed closely for reactions such as weakness, fatigue, shortness of breath and chest pain.

The degree to which activities and exertion are restricted varies with the patient's response, the size and location of the infarction, the presence of complications and the doctor's philosophy. The body temperature, enzyme concentrations, leucocyte count, sedimentation rate and electrocardiographic changes are used as guides. An important determining principle is that activities should be increased gradually, that rest periods are alternated with activities and that certain activities such as pushing, pulling, lifting or straining are avoided. By the time the patient leaves the coronary care unit, he may be sitting in a chair three times a day for 30–45 minutes, using a bedside commode, feeding and bathing himself and taking short walks around his bed.

The progression in activities continues after the patient is transferred from the coronary care unit and in the weeks after he leaves the hospital. He will begin walking short distances on the ward, progressing in most cases to the length of the ward hallway by discharge, and he may have climbed stairs. Limitations are applied to those activities which precipitate dyspnoea and pain.

Once the patient is free of pain and other early symptoms, he feels quite well but must still be restricted. Time hangs heavy on his hands, so some effort is made to provide suitable diversions in which the patient is inter-ested. Reading and radio and television programmes may occupy the patient. He may have some hobby he can pursue without overtaxing his heart. Visitors are restricted at first, but later they help relieve the patient's boredom. Visitor selection should be made by the family to avoid those who might excite or distress the patient. Visitors should be made aware of time limitations as it may be difficult for the patient to ask them to leave if he becomes tired.

(b) *Nutrition.* Liquids are given in small amounts at first following a myocardial infarction. The diet is increased gradually to easily digested, non-gas-forming solids as tolerated. Large meals are avoided. If necessary, the caloric intake is decreased. Salt is usually restricted. Fluids may be restricted if the patient has heart failure (see p. 359).

(c) *Elimination.* Constipation should be prevented and the patient cautioned against straining at stool because of the stress it places on the heart. A mild laxative or stool softener may be given as necessary.

3 Assisting the patient to understand his illness and to adjust to the imposed limitations.

(a) *Patient teaching.* In order to make the best possible adjustment to his illness and recovery, the patient must have some understanding of the illness and how he can assist in recovery. Providing this information helps give the patient some control over his situation. Teaching programmes are adjusted to specific patient needs and capabilities, since learning capacity varies among individuals. Patients experiencing myocardial infarctions often have many misconceptions of their condition and how it will affect their future. It is useful for the nurse to find out what the patient already knows and to obtain information about his life-style. The nurse has many opportunities to reinforce and elaborate on explanations given by the doctor and to respond to further questions.

During the acute stage, the patient is often too anxious to absorb much information. *Simple* explanations of equipment being used and procedures common to coronary care units are usually adequate. Following transfer to the general ward, the patient is usually better able to participate in a planned programme. Written as well as verbal instruction can be provided. Visual aids such as heart models or diagrams help to enhance learning. Suggested topics include basic information on how the heart functions, what happens to the heart with a myocardial infarction, how the heart heals and the purpose of treatment. For 6–10 weeks the patient is advised to avoid heavy lifting, pushing, mental and physical fatigue and driving. Sex should be discussed with the patient. Intercourse is probably best avoided for one month only following myocardial infarction but can be resumed when the person feels able. Travel abroad should be discouraged for about two months. Activity and ambulation is increased gradually, interspersed regularly with rest periods. Some explanation is given of risk factors, how these factors relate to the patients, and how they may be reduced. Any prescribed special diet or medication is reviewed. In some instances the dietitian or clinical pharmacologist as well as the doctor and nurse may be involved in teaching the patient.

Short teaching sessions are necessary, as many patients with myocardial infarction tire easily. It is helpful if one of the family can be present in the teaching session. Acknowledgement is made of the feelings that the patient has in response to his illness. He may wish to express verbally the feelings that he is experiencing, such as discouragement, fear, anger and/or depression; the nurse should provide opportunities for free expression and should be a willing listener.

4 Recognition of complications. Complications following myocardial infarction include arrhythmias, congestive heart failure, pericarditis, mitral regurgitation, myocardial rupture, aneurysm and systemic or pulmonary emboli.
  (a) *Arrhythmias.* Arrhythmias usually occur early following a myocardial infarction (see p. 339) for a discussion of arrhythmias). The most serious arrhythmia that may be seen is ventricular fibrillation: this is treated by cardiac defibrillation. Bradyarrhythmias, such as sinus bradycardia, first degree atrioventricular block and Wenckebach heart block are most often associated with inferior wall infarctions. Since the SA node and the AV junctional tissue are most often supplied by the right coronary artery, occlusion of this vessel will lead to their decreased functioning. Anterior myocardial infarctions are more prone to heart failure and arrhythmias that accompany it, such as sinus tachycardia and rapid atrial arrhythmias, and to intraventricular conduction disturbances, such as Mobitz Type II block. Complete AV block (third degree or complete heart block) can follow either inferior or anterior wall infarction and may necessitate a temporary pacemaker.
  (b) *Heart failure.* Mild congestive heart failure occurs in many patients due to the decreased efficiency with which the heart contracts. Gross left ventricular failure is more common following an anterior infarction. Heart failure is diagnosed by the presence of râles on chest auscultation, complaints of shortness of breath and a chest x-ray. (See p. 355 for management).
  (c) *Pericarditis.* Pericarditis following a myocardial infarction is thought to be due to an autoimmune reaction in which antigens originate from the injured myocardial tissue, initiating inflammation of the pericardium. It may occur as early as 24 hours after the infarction. The pain which accompanies pericarditis is similar to that of a myocardial infarction but is sometimes more excruciating. It is alarming to the patient, who may think that he is having another heart attack. A distinction may be made if the pain is increased by deep breathing or twisting the trunk, or if it is relieved by leaning forward, lying on the right side or sitting in an upright position with the trunk straight. A friction rub may be heard on auscultation but is not always present in the early stages. The patient's temperature may remain elevated for more than one week. Treatment is usually with non-steroidal antiinflammatory drugs such as indomethacin or soluble aspirin. A corticosteroid preparation may be employed.
  (d) *Mitral regurgitation.* This complication may occur when a papillary muscle dysfunctions or ruptures, causing the valve to become incompetent. This is a grave complication which may be corrected by surgery. Less severe mitral insufficiency may be due to infarction of the papillary muscle.
  (e) *Myocardial rupture.* Myocardial rupture, when present, usually occurs within 7 days. It is more often seen in patients with transmural infarctions. Rupture of the interventricular septum usually occurs within the first 2 weeks and is a very grave prognostic sign. Instead of flowing normally from the left ventricle into the aorta, blood is re-routed to the right ventricle, increasing the demands on it and flooding the lungs. Surgery is the only effective treatment.
  (f) *Aneurysm.* An aneurysm is a ballooning out of the infarcted myocardial tissue, causing the heart to contract in a disruptive fashion. If large, it seriously impedes the maintenance of normal cardiac output. The extent of the aneurysm may be determined by a myocardial scan and in some instances may be corrected by surgery.
  (g) *Emboli.* Emboli occur because clots formed in the healing area of the myocardium break loose and escape into the circulation. Pulmonary emboli may arise in the leg veins due to circulatory stasis, and may be prevented by exercising the limbs. The treatment for emboli includes anticoagulant drugs.
  (h) *Shoulder–hand syndrome.* In the weeks following a myocardial infarction a few patients may develop a stiffness or tenderness in the left arm and shoulder. Immobility during the early period of recovery has been suggested as a cause.

5 Transfer from the coronary care unit.

Transfer out of the coronary care unit is often a difficult period of adjustment for patients.

Although interpreting transfer as a sign of progress, patients often miss the security of constant observation by the staff as well as their continual contact. Concern may also be related to the increased independence expected, particularly in relation to physical care and decision making. This transition is much less difficult if the patient is prepared for it and if the change to independence is not abrupt. When explanations are given as to why the patient no longer needs to be monitored and what schedules and routines he might expect on the ward, adjustment is much easier. A gradual reduction in the amount of physical care provided and a gradual increase in the amount of responsibility assumed by the patient helps him to feel more secure. Specific information about the patient's regimen, likes and dislikes and problems should be communicated by the coronary care staff to the nurses assuming responsibility for the patient. This helps to facilitate continuity of care.

Arrhythmias and conduction disturbances

Normally, the rate and rhythm of the heart contractions are established by impulses generated in the SA node at a rate between 60 and 100 beats per minute (Fig. 14.11A). A disorder of rate or rhythm is referred to as a cardiac arrhythmia, and is due to some disturbance in the formation or conduction of impulses. The arrhythmia may be of short duration or persistent and may be functional in origin, result from organic heart disease or be associated with an electrolyte imbalance, such as hypokalaemia.

An arrhythmia may have significant haemodynamic consequences. For example, an excessively slow or fast heart rate may decrease the cardiac output and blood pressure, thus compromising the perfusion of vital organs such as the brain, kidneys, liver and heart itself. Arrhythmias may also predispose the patient to thrombus formation.

Common irregularities include tachycardia, bradycardia, ectopic beats (extrasystoles), flutter, fibrillation and heart block. The arrhythmia is further defined by the site of its origin; sinus arrhythmia originates in the SA node, atrial originates in an atrium, nodal or junctional originates in the AV node, and ventricular originates in the ventricle.

TACHYCARDIAS

Sinus tachycardia

In this rhythm the heart rate is greater than 100 beats per minute, and the impulse originates in the SA node. It is not always an abnormal rhythm, since it occurs during and after exercise and in response to emotional stress. It may be due to an abnormal state such as fever, anaemia, infection, hyperthyroidism, myocardial infarction and heart failure. It also may result from medications—for example, atropine, adrenaline, isoprenaline hydrochloride and thyroid extract, or other drugs such as alcohol and nicotine (see Fig. 14.11B).

Tachycardia is significant for two reasons: coronary blood flow occurs predominantly during diastole. With tachycardia, the diastolic time is shortened, reducing the time for perfusion of the myocardium. Also, an increased heart rate increases the need of the myocardium for oxygen. In someone with narrowed coronary arteries, tachycardia may precipitate myocardial ischaemia.

Treatment may be directed at correcting the underlying cause or it may be necessary to reduce the rate by giving a drug such as a digitalis preparation or propranolol (Inderal).

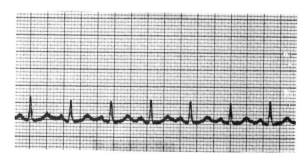

Fig. 14.11B Sinus tachycardia: rate over 100 per minute; P wave and QRS are normal in 1:1 relationship.

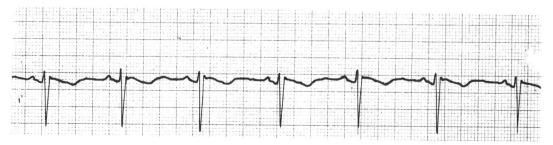

Fig. 14.11A Normal sinus rhythm.

Paroxysmal atrial tachycardia (PAT)
This is an abrupt onset of a very rapid heart rate, usually 150–250 beats per minute, initiated in the atria. It may last a few seconds or longer. Such attacks cannot be explained in some persons; in others they may be related to organic heart disease (Fig. 14.11C).

A rapid heart rate of this type is serious if imposed on a diseased heart. When this arrhythmia occurs, the patient is advised to rest and the doctor is notified. If the patient is subject to recurring attacks, he is encouraged to recognize and avoid possible precipitating factors such as fatigue, emotional stress, reaching, or excessive smoking or coffee drinking. In some instances an attack may be relieved by measures that increase parasympathetic (vagal) innervation to the heart. Among those suggested is pressure on the carotid sinus or eyeballs. *Caution must be used in relation to both these manoeuvres.* Carotid sinus massage applied injudiciously may result in asystole; too frequent and too heavy pressure on the eyeballs may predispose to retinal detachment in the eye. These manoeuvres are not performed by nurses.

Some people who experience paroxysmal tachycardia find that it may be checked by assuming a certain position, such as flexion of the trunk or holding the arms over the head. The Valsalva manoeuvre, which involves an inspiration followed by voluntary closure of the glottis and an effort to exhale, may prove helpful. This reduces the venous return from the extremities and head, thus reducing the volume of blood entering the heart which in turn decreases the cardiac output and the arterial blood pressure. An antiarrhythmic agent such as verapamil a beta-blocker or digoxin may be used. Disopyramide or amiodarone may be useful. Long acting quinidine preparations are sometimes still prescribed.

Ventricular tachycardia
Usually the term ventricular tachycardia refers to a run of rapidly repeated ventricular beats, essentially regular in rhythm, at a rate of 100–210 per minute. Any rate above 60 per minute which is initiated in the ventricles might be considered tachycardia, because the ventricles normally do not initiate impulses at more than 25–40 beats per minute. However, rates between 60 and 100 per minute are usually distinguished from the faster rates. Marriott refers to them as 'accelerated idioventricular rhythms'[19] but they are also called 'slow ventricular tachycardia' or 'nonparoxysmal ventricular tachycardia' (see Fig. 14.11D).

Ventricular tachycardia is a more serious arrhythmia than atrial tachycardia, as there is always the danger it will lead to ventricular fibrillation. It is usually due to ischaemic heart disease and is frequently present following a myocardial infarction.

Treatment includes electrical defibrillation (DC shock), and/or antiarrhythmic drugs such as intravenous lignocaine. Other drugs that may be used

---

[19] Marriott (1983), p. 107

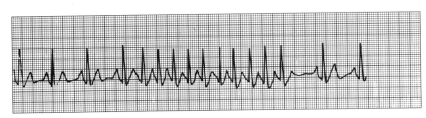

Fig. 14.11C Paroxysmal atrial tachycardia.

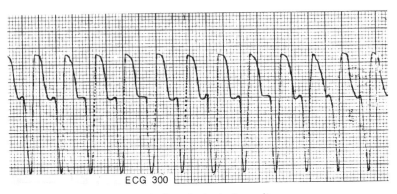

Fig. 14.11D Ventricular tachycardia.

include intravenous disopyramide or ajmaline or mexiletine, tocainide or a beta-blocking agent. In the sick patient with ventricular tachycardia, bretylium tosylate may be administered.

BRADYCARDIAS

Sinus bradycardia

This is the term used for an abnormally slow pulse rate. It is applied when the pulse rate is below 59 per minute in an adult, less than 80 per minute in a child and less than 100 per minute in an infant. (See Fig. 14.11E).

Circulation may be adequately maintained by an increased stroke volume in a person with brady-cardia. With fewer contractions more blood collects in the heart chambers to produce greater stretching of the myocardial fibres, resulting in a stronger con-traction and increased output. Obviously this can only occur if the myocardium is in good condition. If the heart rate is less than 30–40 per minute circula-tory insufficiency is likely to occur, especially with physical activity.

The most common causes of bradycardia are a decreased blood supply to the SA node, increased vagal tone, old age, head injury, amyloidosis and obstructive jaundice. Circulatory reflexes may ini-tiate a compensatory increase in the heart rate but, if the cause persists and becomes progressively severe, the heart muscle will gradually become weaker and less responsive, producing fewer contractions. Any disturbance which initiates an increase in vagal nerve impulses to the heart will produce a decrease in the heart rate. An example of this would be brady-cardia produced by carotid sinus massage or, in some people, by vomiting. Other examples of condi-tions in which slowing of the heart rate may be secondary are increased intracranial pressure and myxoedema (a deficiency of thyroid secretion).

The pulse rate may normally be slower in those with well developed cardiac reserve, such as well trained athletes. In such people, the venous return is of greater strength, producing an increased stroke volume with each contraction.

ECTOPIC BEATS

When impulses which influence the heart rate and rhythm are generated elsewhere than in the SA node, the contractions are called *ectopic* or *premature beats* or *extrasystoles*. The ectopic or premature beat occurs when the myocardial fibres are in the relative refractory period following a normal contraction. The impulse from the SA node for the succeeding normal contraction is ineffective, since it arrives when the muscle fibres are in the absolute refractory period following the premature beat, and no contrac-tion takes place. This causes a longer than normal pause before the next normal contraction and the heart 'misses' a beat. The next normal contraction may be stronger because of the prolonged filling period. The time between the normal heart contrac-tion which precedes the extrasystole and the one that follows is equal to two normal cardiac cycles. The subject usually describes the experience as his heart 'missing a beat and then a thud'.

Extrasystoles, or premature beats, may be due to ischaemic areas or to inflammation in the heart muscle. The fibres may also become irritated and hypersensitive as a result of certain toxic conditions, such as may occur with the excessive use of tobacco, coffee, tea or alcohol. The extrasystoles may occur irregularly, with varying lengths of time between them. The incidence may be so rare as to have no clinical significance but they should be investigated if persistent, even though they occur irregularly and at relatively long intervals. Premature beats may arise regularly and at a rate in excess of that of the normal SA pacemaker, resulting in paroxysmal tachycardia.

Atrial premature beats

The ectopic focus is in the atria and the complex occurs earlier than expected. Atrial premature beats are significant because, if they occur during the vul-nerable period of the atria, they may precipitate more serious atrial arrhythmias, such as atrial flutter or atrial fibrillation. They may or may not be conducted to the ventricles, depending upon the state of con-duction through the AV node and the refractory period at which they occur. Treatment is usually not

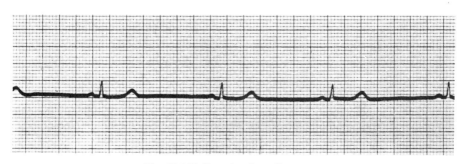

Fig. 14.11E Sinus bradycardia.

required unless they occur with great frequency or unless progression to more serious arrhythmias is feared, as may occur following a myocardial infarction. If a precipitating cause is recognized, it should be eliminated. (See Fig. 14.11F.)

Ventricular premature beats (VPBs)

The ectopic focus is in the ventricle, and therefore there will be no related P wave on the electrocardiogram. Occasional ventricular premature beats may be innocuous but they may also precipitate ventricular tachycardia and/or fibrillation. If they occur in a diseased heart, in groups of two, three or more, more frequently than five per minute, arise from more than one focus (multifocal) or are on the T wave of the preceding complex, they are considered serious and require treatment. The usual immediate treatment is lignocaine (Xylocard) given by bolus intravenous injection followed by a continuous intravenous drip. An oral drug such as 'disopyramide might be given when the lignocaine infusion is gradually tapered off; however, many patients do not require this. (See Fig. 14.11G.)

FLUTTER

Atrial flutter

As with atrial tachycardia, atrial flutter is due to a rapidly firing ectopic focus in the atria. There is some dispute as to whether atrial flutter should be differentiated from atrial tachycardia; some cardiologists describe both as supraventricular tachycardia, while others differentiate on the basis of rate and pattern. The rate usually falls between 250 and 350 beats per minute and a characteristic sawtooth pattern is seen on the ECG. AV block is usually present, so that the ventricular response may vary from 150–175 beats per minute (see Fig. 14.11H). Atrial flutter may occur with mitral stenosis, ischaemic heart disease and chronic obstructive pulmonary disease. The usual treatment is a DC shock with 25–50 joules in emergency situations, or the administration of digoxin, which blocks impulses at the AV node and may produce atrial fibrillation which is easier to manage. Alternatively amiodarone may be given. This drug, unlike digoxin, will not increase myocardial oxygen demand.

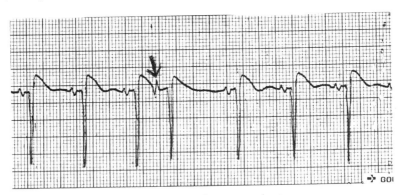

Fig. 14.11F Atrial premature beat.

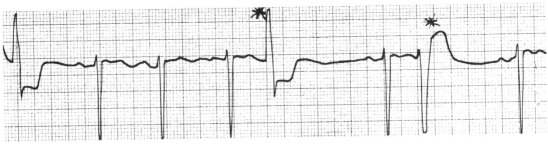

Fig. 14.11G Ventricular premature beat.

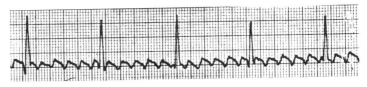

Fig. 14.11H Atrial flutter.

FIBRILLATION

This is an arrhythmia in which the normal rhythmic contractions of the myocardium of either the atria or ventricles are replaced by extremely rapid (250–500 per minute), ineffective contractions, irregular in force and rhythm. Some area of the heart gives rise to very rapid and irregular impulses, and the myocardial contractile fibres do not achieve the contraction and relaxation that permit normal emptying and filling of the chambers.

Atrial fibrillation
Atrial fibrillation is a fairly common arrhythmia in which electrical activity in the atria is totally disorganized. It is due to some myocardial weakness or disease which may be the result of coronary insufficiency, rheumatic heart disease, thyrotoxicosis or acute infection. The atria are never completely empty, and normal filling cannot occur. Since little pressure is created by the atrial contractions, the flow of blood into the ventricles is due mainly to the pressure created by the volume of blood. Circulation may become seriously impaired. Only a proportion of the impulses arising in the atria are conducted through the AV node to the ventricles, but those that do pass through may far exceed the normal in frequency, and are irregular (see Fig. 14.11I). Normal filling and emptying of the ventricles do not take place, cardiac output is reduced, arterial blood pressure falls and the blood is backed up in the large veins.

The pulse is very rapid, weak and irregular. With some ventricular contractions, the stroke volume may be so reduced that radial pulsation does not occur. This sets up an *apex-radial deficit*, defined as the difference between the apical and radial pulses. To determine a pulse deficit accurately, the ventricular rate is counted for a full minute, using a stethoscope placed over the apical region of the heart. At the same time, a second person counts the radial pulse for a full minute. If two people are not available, one may count one pulse and then the other, each for a full minute.

Established atrial fibrillation may be treated with digoxin. Digoxin slows the heart rate by depressing the impulse conduction through the AV node and by increasing the vagal nerve stimulation. The myocardial contractions are strengthened, resulting in more efficient emptying of the heart chambers. Beta-blockers may also be used. Alternatively, if left ventricular function is poor, verapamil may be selected.

When the atrial fibrillation is paroxysmal, amiodarone, disopyramide or quinidine can be employed.

Cardioversion (synchronized DC shock) is sometimes used for treatment of a first attack or if the patient is an emergency. Should cardioversion be selected for the person with established atrial fibrillation, then a minimum of 3 days anticoagulation with heparin, or preferably a week of oral agents, is prescribed. This is to reduce the risk of emboli arising from the atria entering the circulation following restoration of sinus rhythm. Furthermore if the person has been receiving digoxin this should be withheld for 24 hours prior to cardioversion.

A complication that may follow atrial fibrillation is embolism. The blood that was not forwarded into the ventricles during fibrillation may have formed a thrombus in an atrial chamber and then, when normal heart action is re-established, the thrombus may be moved out into the circulation.

Ventricular fibrillation
In ventricular fibrillation very rapid, asynchronous contractions arise in the ventricular myocardium because the electrical activity occurs in a totally disorganized sequence (see Fig. 14.11J). The contractions are so ineffective in pumping that the condition may very quickly prove fatal. The pulse and blood pressure become unobtainable in a few seconds, the patient quickly loses consciousness, his pupils dilate, his reflexes are lost and cyanosis is likely to develop. Prompt emergency treatment may re-establish circulation. If the patient is being monitored in a coronary care unit, the arrhythmia may be identified immediately at onset and treatment would

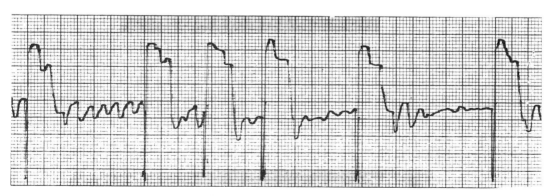

Fig. 14.11I Atrial fibrillation with varying ventricular responses.

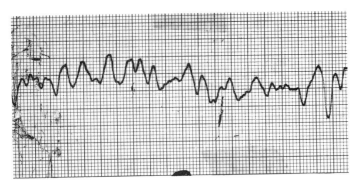

Fig. 14.11J Ventricular fibrillation: chaotic ventricular activity.

consist of immediate DC shock. In many coronary care units nurses who are taught this procedure implement it. *Hospital policy will dictate who may defibrillate a patient, as it constitutes part of the nurse's extended role.* An important guideline is that it must be initiated within minutes.

Although an electrical shock may cause fibrillation, it may also be used to stop it. In defibrillation two electrodes ('paddles') are placed on the chest wall, one on each side of the heart or one on the ventral wall with a second on the dorsal wall. A strong current (approximately 200–400 j) is passed through the electrodes for a brief period. All the muscle fibres of the myocardium are thrown into contraction together and then enter a refractory period simultaneously. This quiescent period may give the normal pacemaker, the SA node, an opportunity to take over. It is important to make sure that no one is touching the bed or the patient during the electrical discharge to prevent their receiving a severe shock. When a defibrillator is not available, cardiac massage accompanied by artificial respiration may sustain life and restore circulation (see Cardiac Arrest, p. 352).

Ventricular fibrillation may occur with irritation of the heart during heart catheterization because of coronary occlusion by the catheter, myocardial infarction, hypothermia, hypoxia, hypokalaemia and electrical shock. Very frequently ventricular fibrillation is preceded by ventricular premature beats. Prompt administration of an antiarrhythmic drug such as lignocaine (Xylocard) may prevent serious ventricular tachycardia and fibrillation.

HEART BLOCK

This is a condition in which impulse formation is depressed or impulse conduction is blocked. Although conduction may be interrupted between the SA node and the atria, the term 'heart block' usually refers to a disorder of conduction at the junctional tisues, which are the atrioventricular node and the common bundle (bundle of His). The SA node or the conduction pathway may be damaged by inflammatory disease such as rheumatic fever, coronary insufficiency, pressure from scarred or calcified tissue, or surgical trauma.

Sinoatrial block

In sinoatrial block, impulses either are not formed in the SA node, fail to be conducted from it or emerge very slowly. If sinoatrial impulses are not received by the atria, occasional beats may be dropped, cardiac standstill may occur, or the ventricles may respond to impulses arising from a lower pacemaker, such as the junctional tissue. In the latter instance a junctional rhythm will result (see Fig. 14.11K).

The seriousness of an SA block depends on the extent to which the heart rate is slowed and cardiac output is decreased. A slow rate may precipitate other arrhythmias. Specific precipitating causes include drugs such as digoxin and some antiarrhythmic drugs, salicylates, coronary artery disease, myocardial infarction and increased vagal tone.

Treatment is directed at removing the cause, when possible, and improving conduction between the SA

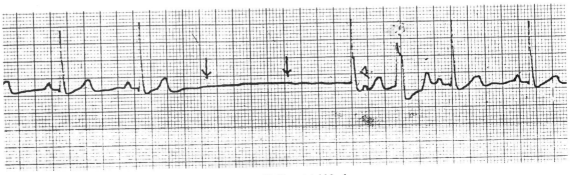

Fig. 14.11K Sinoatrial block.

node and the atria by drugs such as atropine and iso-prenaline. If drug therapy is not effective, artificial pacing may be required.

Heart block at junctional tissues occurs in varying degrees of severity and may be categorized as first degree, second degree—Type I and Type II—and third degree, or complete heart block. Conduction may be impaired in the bundle branches, referred to as right or left bundle branch block.

First degree heart block

First degree heart block is usually due to delayed conduction through the AV node, and the interval between atrial and ventricular contractions is lengthened. This is exhibited on the ECG by a prolonged P-R interval (greater than 0.20 sec). Fig.14.11L). It may be caused by increased vagal tone in the normal person, fatigue in the conduction system because of prolonged tachycardia, digoxin toxicity, inflammatory heart disease, or coronary artery disease. Although the patient often has no characteristic physical symptoms, auscultation may reveal a decline in the intensity of the first heart sound. First degree heart block may progress to second and third degree heart block but in the absence of evidence of disease requires no treatment. Digoxin may be discontinued or the dosage reduced.

Second degree heart block

Second degree or partial heart block refers to a more advanced disturbance in which some of the sinus impulses fail to get through and activate the ven-tricles. It may be divided into Mobitz Type I or Wenckebach and Mobitz Type II.

In Wenckebach block the period of time between atrial and ventricular conduction becomes progressively longer, until finally an atrial impulse is completely blocked. The ECG shows progressively longer P-R intervals, until finally a P-wave is not followed by a QRS complex. The P-R interval following this dropped ventricular beat is close to the normal range, but with each successive beat it lengthens and the cycle repeats itself. The patient may be conscious of a decreased ventricular rate if the change occurs suddenly but may exhibit no physical symptoms. On examination, the intensity of the first heart sound may be weak or may decrease over several beats (see Fig. 14.11M).

Type II, second degree block, is usually more serious than Type I. At definite intervals impulses are blocked at the AV node and an atrial beat fails to be followed by a ventricular beat. The ratio of atrial to ventricular beats may vary—for example 2:1, 3:1, 4:3, 3:2. The P-R interval is fixed and unvarying and there may be evidence of right bundle branch block on the ECG. The patient may experience syncopal (fainting) attacks. (See Fig. 14.11N.)

Both second degree blocks may be due to inflammatory or fibrotic processes, coronary artery disease, infarction, or drugs such as digoxin, beta-blockers or verapamil.

Third degree heart block

In this block, conduction is so disturbed that no impulses reach the ventricles and the atria and ven-

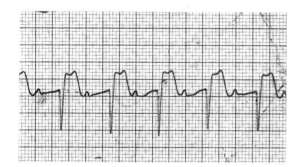

Fig. 14.11L First degree heart block.

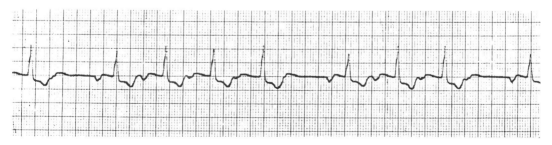

Fig. 14.11M Wenckebach block.

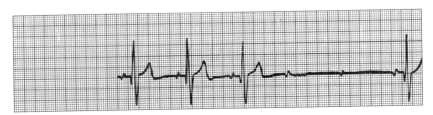

Fig. 14.11N Type II second degree block.

tricles beat independently at their own inherent rhythms. The block may occur at the AV node, or the main part of the bundle of His. It is a more advanced block and may be caused by any of the disorders responsible for Type II partial blocks. Since atrial impulses are unable to penetrate the AV node, a lower pacemaker takes over and controls the ventricles. If this 'rescuing' pacemaker is initiated in the junctional tissue, the ECG will show a QRS complex which is normal in appearance and not wide unless there is an associated bundle branch block. If the pacemaker is in the ventricles, the QRS complexes will be wide and abnormal in shape (see Fig. 14.11O).

Palpation of the pulse will usually reveal a rate of 45 or less because the rhythm is ventricular. On physical examination, the first heart sound varies markedly from beat to beat and may occasionally be quite loud (bruit de canon) when the ventricular contractions happen to follow very quickly after the atrial. The prognosis for complete heart block is uncertain but, in the event that Stokes–Adams syndrome occurs, it is poor without immediate treatment.

Heart block may be a temporary or permanent condition. If it is permanent, the independent ventricular rhythm may become firmly established and, with some restrictions of activities, the patient may live a fairly normal life. In some instances the ventricular rhythm may be irregular and episodes of cardiac arrest may threaten the patient. Cardiac asystole lasting 10 seconds or longer may occur, reducing the cardiac output to a level that causes cerebral ischaemia. The patient becomes dizzy and may faint or convulse, or sudden death may occur. This type of episode is referred to as a Stokes–Adams attack or syndrome.

TREATMENT

Treatment of heart arrhythmias includes the use of a pacemaker and/or drugs.

Artificial cardiac pacemakers

In serious conduction defects, and sometimes in the treatment of tachyarrhythmias, electrical stimulation may be provided by an electronic battery-operated pacemaker to stimulate or control cardiac contractions. The pacemaker consists of a power unit which generates electrical impulses and two fine insulated wires, each terminating in an electrode (one positive and the other negative, to complete the electrical circuit). Previously, the pulse-generating system of most pacemakers consisted of small mercury or transistor batteries which lasted approximately 18–30 months. The primary source of power in the immediate future will probably be lithium. Lithium cells have several advantages over existing sources and have an operating life span of 5 years and longer. Nuclear power batteries are another generating source available, lasting a great deal longer. The much greater cost limits their availability and use.

The strength (milliamperes) of the power impulses and the rate at which they are discharged by the artificial pacemaker are adjustable and are preset on an individual basis. The electrodes of the early pacemakers were applied externally to the chest wall over the heart. More recent models deliver the charges by an electrode placed in direct contact with the heart.

If the conduction defect is transient, a temporary pacemaker is used. A pacing electrode is introduced through the external jugular, subclavian, antecubital

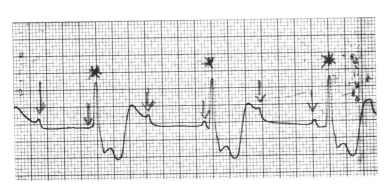

Fig. 14.11O Third degree heart block.

or femoral vein and advanced into the right ventricle under fluoroscopy. The electrode wire is connected to an external battery-operated pacemaker. The site of insertion of the electrode is secured with a sterile dressing (Fig. 14.12A).

When the conduction defect is irreversible, a permanent pacemaker is implanted within the body. The electrode is introduced transvenously, usually through the right cephalic or the right external jugular vein, and the battery unit is implanted subcutaneously in a supermammary pouch on the chest wall. Alternatively, it is implanted beneath the muscle of the upper abdominal wall. This requires a small incision (Fig. 14.12B). To simplify the categorization of pulse generators, a code has been developed, identified as the Intersociety Commission for Heart Disease Resource Code (ICHD). Using the ICHD identification code, pacemakers are described according to: (1) the chamber in which the pacing electrode is located; (2) the chamber in which the heart's intrinsic electrical impulse is sensed; and (3) the mode of response of the pacemaker (see Fig. 14.12C). Additional codes are likely to develop in order to cope with facilities on newer programmable units and with 'telemetric' capabilities.

There are several types of pacemakers, categorized according to their pattern of activity. The pacemaker may be preset to discharge at a fixed rate, by demand or at a rate that corresponds to cardiac activity.

In asynchronous pacing, which may also be referred to as fixed-rate pacing (AOO, VOO, DOO), the pacemaker delivers a predetermined fixed number of electrical impulses irrespective of the impulses generated by the heart itself. In other words, fixed-rate pacing is not synchronized with generic cardiac activity. There is a risk of causing tachycardia or ventricular fibrillation due to additional spontaneous impulse formation as the condition of the heart improves. A second disadvantage of fixed-rate pacing is that it will not increase or decrease heart activity to correspond with body activity and demands.

The ventricular and atrial inhibited (VVI and AAI) pacemaker, also called demand or standby pacemaker, is preset to discharge impulses only when the patient's heart rhythm falls below a preset rate. A device in the power unit of the demand pacemaker is sensitive to the electrical currents generated by spontaneous heart impulses. These electrical stimuli are conveyed via the electrode wire to the sensor and inhibit the release of impulses by the power unit. If no stimulation of the sensory device is generated by spontaneous heart impulses, the pacemaker is activated to discharge at a constant preset rate. The advantage of demand (standby) pacing is the elimination of the risk of intrinsic impulses in addition to pacemaker impulses, resulting in an arrhythmia.

Atrial synchronous pacemakers (VAT) are capable of varying the rate of impulses discharged producing synchronous pacing. A device sensitive to the atrial contraction is placed in the right atrium. The stimulus is conveyed to the power unit of the pacemaker and an impulse is initiated and conveyed to an electrode in the right ventricle, resulting in a ventricular contraction (see Fig. 14.12D). This arrangement produces a delay in the delivery of the impulse to the ventricle similar to that normally occurring in the AV conduction system. It also provides a means by which ventricular contractions correspond with the impulses initiated by the SA node and atrial contractions. Normally the SA node responds to increased physiological needs, as in exercise and fever, by discharging more impulses; this is evidenced by an increase in the pulse rate. Conversely, the rate of discharge by the SA node becomes slower with a decrease in physiological demands (e.g. during rest). Thus, the synchronous type of pacemaker has the distinct advantage of varying the rate according to the patient's physiological needs, and synchronizes ventricular contractions with the intrinsic atrial impulses and contractions.

Ventricular- and atrial-triggered (VVT and AAT) pacemakers pace the heart synchronously in response to the natural impulse of the chamber paced and asynchronously in the absence of the normal impulse. One electrode is placed in either the ventricle (VVT) or the atrium (AAT) and acts as both a sensor and a pacer. Since normal electrical activity in the heart is sensed and an impulse generated during the early refractory periods of the QRS and P waves, the ventricular- and atrial-triggered pulse generators do not compete with the heart's own rhythm; however, the spontaneous ECG complexes are distorted.

Nursing care of the patient with a pacemaker. Nursing care involves assisting in the preparation of the patient for implantation. He may be apprehensive because of the symptoms he is experiencing, such as dizziness and fainting, and may also be fearful of the procedure and his dependence on a mechanical device. When explaining the need for a pacemaker the doctor reviews the procedure with the patient. The nurse reinforces this explanation and answers any further questions before the patient signs the consent form. Explanations are also given to the family.

The patient receives a sedative before the implantation. Temporary pacemakers are usually implanted under local anaesthetic in the angiography department, in the radiology department or occasionally, in an emergency, at the bedside. Permanent pacemakers are inserted in the operating theatre or the angiography department.

Following the implantation of a permanent pacemaker, the patient is monitored continuously until it has been established that the pacemaker is functioning properly. Bed rest is indicated for the remainder of the day. If a temporary pacemaker has

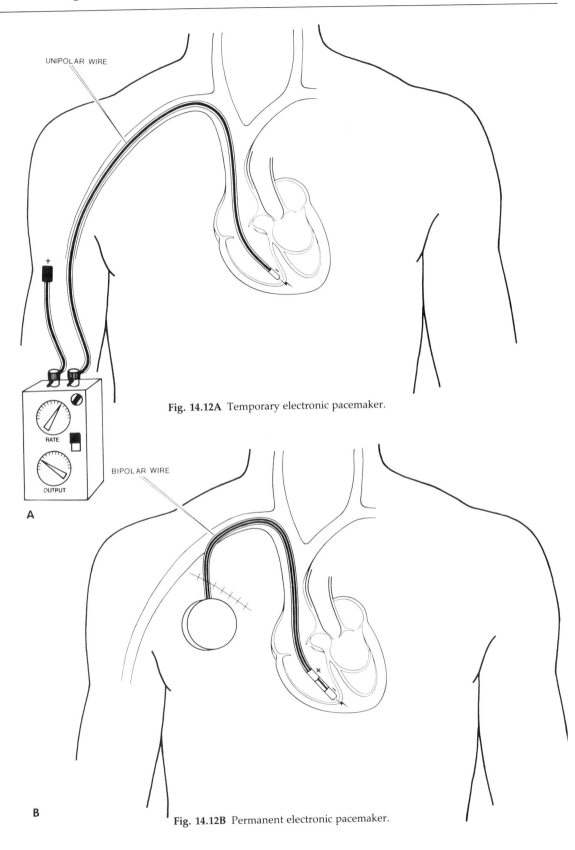

UNIPOLAR WIRE

RATE

OUTPUT

A

Fig. 14.12A Temporary electronic pacemaker.

BIPOLAR WIRE

B

Fig. 14.12B Permanent electronic pacemaker.

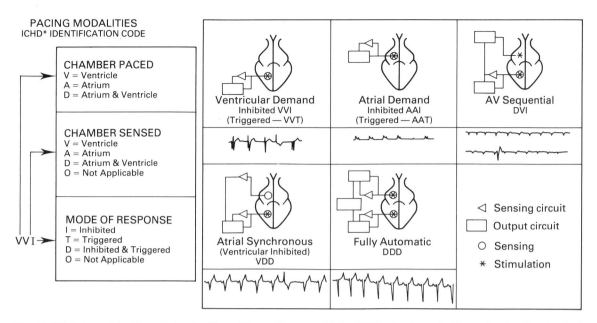

PACING MODALITIES
ICHD* IDENTIFICATION CODE

CHAMBER PACED
V = Ventricle
A = Atrium
D = Atrium & Ventricle

CHAMBER SENSED
V = Ventricle
A = Atrium
D = Atrium & Ventricle
O = Not Applicable

MODE OF RESPONSE
I = Inhibited
T = Triggered
D = Inhibited & Triggered
O = Not Applicable

V V I →

Ventricular Demand
Inhibited VVI
(Triggered — VVT)

Atrial Demand
Inhibited AAI
(Triggered — AAT)

AV Sequential
DVI

Atrial Synchronous
(Ventricular Inhibited)
VDD

Fully Automatic
DDD

◁ Sensing circuit
▢ Output circuit
○ Sensing
* Stimulation

Fig. 14.12C Intersociety Commission for Heart Disease Resource Code. (1) The first letter indicates the chamber in which the pacing electrode is located. (2) The second letter indicates the chamber in which the heart's own impulse is sensed. (3) The third letter indicates the mode of response.

For example, VVI indicates that the pacing electrode is in the ventricle, the sensing electrode is also in the ventricle and that the pulse generator is the 'inhibited' type. The letter D (for Double) indicates that the sensing or pacing device is in both chambers or that the mode of response is both triggered and inhibited.

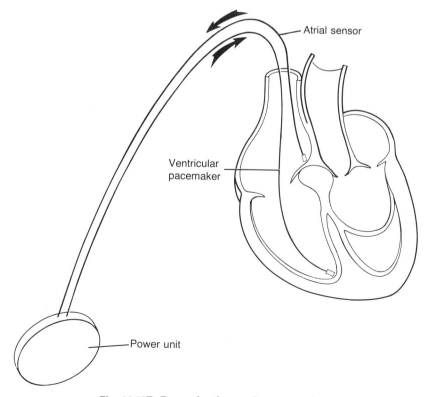

Atrial sensor

Ventricular
pacemaker

Power unit

Fig. 14.12D Pacemaker for synchronous pacing.

been inserted mobility is restricted, depending upon the site of insertion as well as the patient's general condition. Cardiac monitoring may be continued as long as the temporary pacemaker is being used.

The nurse is responsible for monitoring and reporting the patient's rhythm, for checking the operation site and cleansing the wound as necessary, for assessing and reporting any complications and for supporting the patient and providing him with information as needed.

Complications which could occur include mechanical malfunction of the pacemaker, perforation of the myocardial wall by an electrode, breakage or dislodgement of the electrodes, thrombus formation, and infection, such as phlebitis, endocarditis or septicaemia. Mechanical malfunctions may occur because the pacemaker fails to fire, fires too rapidly or fires erratically. Malfunctioning may be detected by cardiac monitoring or by an ECG, as well as by the presence of certain physical signs and symptoms, such as decreased pulse rate, dizziness and/or fainting.

Following perforation of the myocardium blood seeps into the pericardium, causing cardiac tamponade. The resulting compression of the heart causes low blood pressure, tachycardia, increased central venous pressure and distended neck veins. The electrode may also stimulate innervation to the upper abdominal or lower chest muscles, resulting in spasm. Breakage or dislodgement of the electrode will result in a change in the shape of the QRS complex and in the heart rate.

The nurse is also alert to electrical hazards in the environment. Electrical equipment in the patient's environment must be properly earthed and the external pulse generator of temporary pacemakers must be kept dry.

Caution regarding electrical hazards includes avoiding close contact with large electrical motors; for example, in a machine shop the patient may develop arrhythmias as a result of the electrical interference. Microwave ovens may cause similar interference with some pacemakers if the oven is faulty with an inadequate door seal. Small home appliances, if properly earthed, produce no untoward effects. Contact sports should be avoided, although other sports might be allowed on the doctor's advice. The patient's dentist should be advised that he is wearing a pacemaker before any electrical equipment is used.

The amount of information given to the patient depends upon his interest and capacity for learning. Certain points are reviewed with him and a member of his family. Basic information is given on the functioning of the heart, the way in which the pacemaker works, activities allowed, battery changes, and precautions regarding electrical hazards. A follow-up appointment is made for the patient to visit the pacemaker clinic or the outpatient department and it is stressed to the patient that

regular checks are necessary.

The patient should carry an identification card indicating the type of pacemaker he is wearing and the doctor to be notified in case of difficulty. Before travelling he should obtain the name of a local doctor or hospital in case of an emergency.

Drugs used in cardiac arrhythmias
Drugs commonly used (Table 14.8) include:

Digoxin. This drug is used to strengthen and slow the myocardial contraction without increasing oxygen utilization by the myocardium, thereby increasing cardiac output.

It slows the pulse rate by depressing the AV conduction and by increasing vagal nerve stimulation. The resulting fewer contractions give the heart muscle time to rest and recover.

A secondary action is diuresis; as circulation is improved, the urinary output increases which helps to reduce oedema, if present.

There are many cardiac glycosides; however, digoxin is the most commonly used. There are preparations for intravenous and oral administration. A large dose may be prescribed for the first 2–3 days in order to achieve a therapeutic concentration of the drug in the blood; this is referred to as digitalization. The dosage is then reduced to a smaller maintenance dose.

Nursing responsibilities in administering digoxin include assessing and reporting changes in physical signs and symptoms, such as less dyspnoea and decreased fatigue. Observations are also made for signs of toxicity such as anorexia, nausea and vomiting, diarrhoea, abdominal discomfort and visual disturbances. The cardiovascular signs of toxicity are extreme slowing of the pulse and/or a sudden change in rhythm. Patients with hypokalaemia are predisposed to cardiac arrhythmias when receiving digoxin.

The radial pulse is taken before each dose is given. If it has slowed considerably the apex beat is checked. If the apical pulse is also very slow the doctor should be consulted before administering the drug. A rate below 60 is usually given as the point at which to notify the doctor, but some patients may have a rate as low as 50 without toxicity. Specific arrhythmias cannot be determined without an ECG and one should be obtained if there is concern.

Digoxin should be given at the same time every day. Occasionally, serum digoxin levels are determined for patients who become toxic or who do not show a therapeutic response with normal dosage. In these situations the serum digoxin level helps the doctor to decide whether to increase or decrease the dosage.

Digoxin should not be given intramuscularly because it causes intense local pain and because of unpredictable and erratic absorption from this site. Parenteral preparations should not be added to intravenous fluids other than normal saline (small

Table 14.8 Drugs used in cardiac arrhythmias and failure.

Drug	Action	Clinical uses	Toxic effects
Cardiac glycosides			
Digoxin	Increases force of contraction without significantly increasing oxygen utilization; decreases conduction through the AV node; increases vagal stimulation	Congestive heart failure Atrial arrhythmias (e.g. fibrillation)	Anorexia Nausea and/or vomiting Diarrhoea Blurred or coloured vision Arrhythmias (e.g. junctional rhythms and blocks)
Ouabain	As above		
Antiarrhythmic drugs			
Disopyramide (Rythmodan)	Similar to quinidine	Ventricular arrhythmias	Dry mouth Urinary hesitancy Constipation Blurred vision
Amiodarone (Cordarone X)	Increases the duration of the action potential	Wolff–Parkinson– White syndrome Atrial flutter Atrial fibrillation Ventricular tachycardia Recurrent ventricular fibrillation	Corneal micro-deposits Peripheral neuropathy Headache Phototoxicity Skin rash Skin discoloration (rare) Tremor Hypo- and hyperthyroidism Diffuse pulmonary alveolitis Hepatitis
Mexiletine (Mexitil)	Similar to lignocaine	Ventricular arrhythmias, especially following myocardial infarction	Bradycardia Hypotension Confusion Dysarthria Nystagmus Tremor
Lignocaine (Xylocard)	Depresses ventricular ectopic foci	Premature ventricular contractions	Central nervous system disturbances (e.g. convulsions)
Verapamil (Cordilox)	Prolongs refractory period of the AV node	Paroxysmal supraventricular tachycardia Atrial flutter Atrial fibrillation	Constipation Nausea Hypotension Fatigue Dizziness Headache Atrioventricular block Asystole (with intravenous injection)
Quinidine sulphate	Decreases automaticity; slows conduction; acts as a vasodilator; decreases contractility	Paroxysmal atrial tachycardia Atrial flutter and fibrillation Premature ventricular contractions	Nausea and/or vomiting Diarrhoea Visual disturbances Arrhythmias, e.g. ventricular tachyarrhythmias and AV block
Procainamide hydrochloride (Pronestyl)	Similar to quinidine	More useful in ventricular than atrial arrhythmias	Gastrointestinal symptoms Lupus erythematosus syndrome

volumes up to 50 ml). Patients are instructed to take their drug every day at the same time and not to miss doses.

Disopyramide (Rythmodan). This agent has no chemical similarities to other existing antiarrhythmic agents but it resembles quinidine in its activity. It is as effective as quinidine and procainamide in controlling certain arrhythmias and is generally better tolerated. The most common side-effects of disopyramide are primarily related to its anticholinergic action, which limits its use in people with glaucoma or urinary retention. The side-effects include dry mouth, urinary hesitancy, constipation and blurred vision. Because it has a negative inotropic effect it may cause or worsen congestive heart failure. The usual dose is 100–200 mg every 6 hours.

Amiodarone (Cordarone X). This is used in the treatment of Wolff–Parkinson–White syndrome and may be used for the treatment of other arrhythmias when other drugs cannot be used. These include supraventricular tachycardias, atrial flutter and fibrillation and recurrent ventricular fibrillation. It is given once daily at the lowest effective dose. Patients may develop small deposits in the cornea which only occasionally interfere with vision. Other side-effects include phototoxic reactions, and both hypothyroidism and hyperthyroidism. The oral dose is 200 mg three times daily for 1 week; 200 mg twice daily for another week and then 200 mg daily.

Mexiletine (Mexitil). This drug has an action similar to lignocaine and is used to treat ventricular arrhythmias. It can be given as a slow intravenous injection followed by an infusion; however, nausea and vomiting may prevent an effective dose being given. The usual oral dose is 400 mg initially followed in 2 hours by 200–250 mg three to four times daily.

Lignocaine (Xylocard). This preparation is commonly used to decrease premature ventricular contractions and ventricular tachycardia which may precede ventricular fibrillation. It depresses the rate of impulse discharge and conduction. Lignocaine is administered intravenously. An initial dose of 50–100 mg by direct intravenous injection may be given followed by an intravenous infusion at the rate of 1–4 mg per minute.

The drug acts rapidly within a matter of 2–4 minutes. The patient is observed closely for possible hypotension, and the heart action is checked by monitor. This drug should be kept readily available for use following a myocardial infarction, during a cardiac catheterization and following cardiac surgery.

Verapamil (Cordilox). Verapamil is given for acute tachyarrhythmias as well as angina (see page 330).

Quinidine sulphate. This drug may be prescribed in the treatment of atrial flutter or fibrillation, recurrent paroxysmal atrial tachycardia and ventricular ectopic beats. It slows the rate by decreasing automaticity and conduction at the SA node and ectopic pacemakers. It also depresses the excitability of both atrial and ventricular myocardium and has

vasodilator effects, which may result in hypotension.

The drug is administered by mouth, and radial and apical pulses are taken before each dose. The blood pressure should also be checked. Reactions to the drug may include nausea, vomiting, diarrhoea, tinnitus, headache, visual disturbances and fever. Cardiovascular abnormalities include heart block and ventricular rhythm disorders (e.g. ventricular fibrillation). A patient may have an idiosyncrasy to the drug and the nurse is required to observe him closely for any toxic effects. Oral membranes are inspected frequently for signs of petechial haemorrhages which may indicate thrombocytopenic purpura.

Procainamide hydrochloride (Pronestyl). This drug has a similar action to quinidine. It was originally used for both atrial and ventricular arrhythmias but is more useful for ventricular disorders. It may be given intravenously, intramuscularly or orally. Because of the short half-life of the drug it is usually given at frequent intervals (e.g. every 3–4 hours). The blood pressure is checked during intravenous administration and the patient is observed closely for any indication of hypersensitivity. This may be manifested by a chill, joint pain, itching, weakness, dizziness or gastrointestinal disturbances. Noradrenaline and adrenaline should be readily available in the event of an adverse reaction.

Cardiac arrest

Cardiac standstill or arrest means the sudden cessation of effective ventricular contraction. It includes ventricular fibrillation and ventricular asystole. Possible causes are myocardial ischaemia, respiratory insufficiency, heart block, electric shock, metabolic acidosis and adverse reactions to an anaesthetic or a drug.

The condition must be recognized as an emergency. It is urgent that circulation be sufficiently re-established to deliver oxygen to the brain within 4 minutes to prevent permanent cerebral damage. Cardiac arrest may be manifested by sudden collapse and loss of consciousness, an absence of pulse in the radial, carotid and femoral arteries, apnoea and dilatation of the pupils.

Cardiopulmonary resuscitation (CPR) must be commenced at once. This comprises external cardiac massage (chest massage) and artificial respiration (see Fig. 14.13 and Table 14.9).

ARTIFICIAL RESPIRATIONS (MOUTH-TO-MOUTH)

A. Airway
Since cardiac arrest causes respiratory failure, artificial respirations must accompany external cardiac massage, otherwise the persisting oxygen deficiency

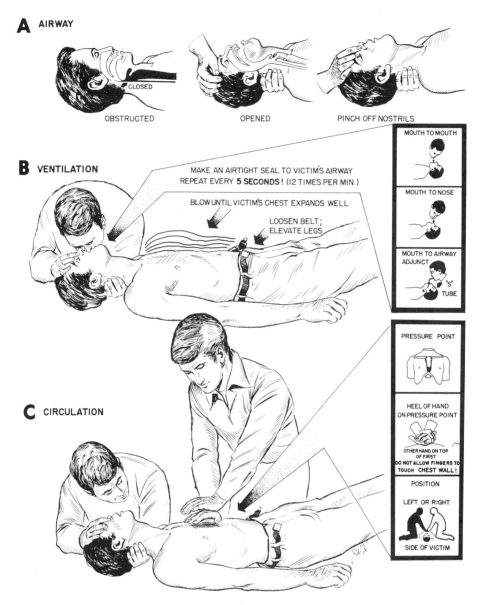

A AIRWAY

OBSTRUCTED

CLOSED

OPENED

PINCH OFF NOSTRILS

B VENTILATION

MAKE AN AIRTIGHT SEAL TO VICTIM'S AIRWAY
REPEAT EVERY **5 SECONDS**! (12 TIMES PER MIN.)

BLOW UNTIL VICTIM'S CHEST EXPANDS WELL

LOOSEN BELT;
ELEVATE LEGS

MOUTH TO MOUTH

MOUTH TO NOSE

MOUTH TO AIRWAY
ADJUNCT

"S"
TUBE

C CIRCULATION

PRESSURE POINT

HEEL OF HAND
ON PRESSURE POINT

OTHER HAND ON TOP
OF FIRST
DO NOT ALLOW FINGERS TO
TOUCH CHEST WALL!

POSITION

LEFT OR RIGHT

SIDE OF VICTIM

Fig. 14.13 Resuscitation in cardiac arrest.

to the cardiac muscle will prevent its response and increase the possibility of cerebral damage.

The most important factor for successful resuscitation is immediate opening of the airway. This can be accomplished easily and quickly by tilting the victim's head backwards as far as possible.

B. Breathing
The mouth-to-mouth method of artificial respiration is the one of choice unless the victim is in a situation where a self-inflating (Ambu) bag is available. After establishing breathlessness, the rescuer gives four initial quick and full breaths. If required, cardiac

compressions are then commenced. If a second person is not available to perform the respiratory resuscitation efforts, external cardiac massage is interrupted every 15 pressure strokes to ventilate the victim's lungs twice. In a hospital, mouth-to-mouth respirations may be replaced by an intermittent positive pressure ventilator which will deliver a higher concentration of oxygen.

EXTERNAL CARDIAC MASSAGE

C. Circulation
External cardiac massage consists of the intermittent

Table 14.9 Cardiopulmonary resuscitation.*

Cardiopulmonary resuscitation is an emergency first aid measure, and must proceed in an organized manner. It includes assessing the need for both artificial ventilation and artificial circulation. The steps which should be started and the order in which they should be performed are:
1 Establishing an open airway
2 Initiating artificial ventilation
3 Initiating external cardiac massage

Steps in artificial ventilation

1 The mouth is cleared of any foreign matter
2 One hand is placed under the victim's neck to lift and support it.
3 The heel of the other hand is placed on victim's forehead so that the head may be tilted back as far as possible.
4 With the thumb and forefinger of the hand that is on the forehead, the operator gently pinches the nostrils closed.
5 The operator takes a large breath, places his mouth tightly over the patient's mouth and blows out his breath to inflate the patient's lungs. In the case of a small child, the operator's mouth is placed over the mouth and nose. If effective, the chest will rise with each blowing.
6 The operator removes his mouth. Air should be heard escaping from the patient's lungs, and the chest should fall.
7 The procedure is repeated approximately 12 times per minute.
8 If the patient's chest does not rise with the first respiration, the position of the head, neck and lower jaw are checked again to ensure an open airway. If air still does not enter the patient's lungs, check the mouth for mucus and turn him to one side. Several sharp blows with the heel of the hand are then struck between the shoulder blades to dislodge a mucus plug or foreign substance which may be blocking the airway.
9 The artificial respirations and the pressure strokes of the external cardiac massage must be coordinated. About one respiration to five pressure strokes is given, and the

blowing in of air must occur during the release of sternal pressure. When there is only one rescuer, two respirations are given after every 15 pressure strokes.

Steps in external cardiac massage

1 Someone is dispatched for the necessary medical assistance and equipment.
2 The victim is placed on his back on a firm surface, such as the floor or ground. In the case of a bed patient, a board is placed under the patient. Each hospital ward is usually equipped with an 'emergency board' that is easily handled and may be quickly placed under the upper half of the patient's trunk.
3 The operator places the heel of one hand over the lower one-half of the sternum and the heel of the other hand over the first hand. The hands should not be placed over the lower tip of the sternum (the xiphoid process). Pressure is applied vertically downward, depressing the sternum 1–2 inches about once each second. The pressure should be sufficient to produce a carotid and femoral pulse, which may be checked by a second person. Less pressure is required in cardiac massage for children up to 10–12 years, since the thoracic cage is very flexible. The pressure delivered by the heel of one hand is sufficient. In infants, the pressure is exerted by the fingers of one hand.
4 At the end of each pressure stroke, the hands are completely relaxed but kept in position.
5 Mouth-to-mouth respirations are started as soon as possible if assistance is at hand. If the person doing the cardiac massage is alone he initially gives four quick ventilations and then interrupts the massage approximately every 15 pressure strokes (every 15 seconds) to give two artificial respirations.
6 The massage is continued until heart action resumes and is producing a strong peripheral pulse or until some other form of treatment is instituted. As circulation is restored, spontaneous respirations and constriction of the pupils should occur.

*Canadian Heart Foundation. *Cardiopulmonary Resuscitation (CPR), Part I.* Recommended Standards for Basic Life Support.

application of vertical pressure over the lower third of the sternum. The pressure stroke compresses the heart between the sternum and the spine and empties the ventricles. To be effective, the compression must force a volume of blood into the arteries sufficient to produce pulsation in the carotid and femoral arteries. The pressure should depress the sternum 1–2 inches and is exerted about once a second. The thoracic cage is quite flexible in an unconscious person and thus the possibility of injury to the ribs is reduced. Relief of pressure allows the heart to refill. This technique of resuscitation is simple, requires no special equipment and may be done anywhere.

Once cardiopulmonary resuscitation has begun, diagnosis and definitive therapy are attempted. One member of the team attaches electrodes to the patient and continuous cardiac monitoring is begun to determine the underlying cardiac rhythm. Another member of the team inserts an intravenous line for

the infusion of medications. If ventricular fibrillation has caused the arrest, an electric defibrillator is used whereby an electric current is delivered through electrodes into the chest wall.

Since metabolic acidosis rapidly develops, Hurst advises that 'an immediate injection of 44 mEq/l of sodium bicarbonate (HCO_3^-) is given and repeated at 10-minute intervals as long as resuscitation efforts are continued.'[20] Arterial blood is withdrawn for blood gas analysis; the carbon dioxide level serves as a guide for the sodium bicarbonate administration. Other emergency drugs are given as required.

Every institution has written policies governing the responsibilities of medical and nursing personnel and members of the cardiac arrest team. The nurse should review and be aware of which responsibilities and procedures she is expected to assume, and those for which she is not legally responsible.

[20] McCall (1978).

The patient who has been resuscitated requires constant observation of the vital signs. If possible, he is transferred to an intensive care unit and continuous monitoring of heart action is established. A pacemaker may be applied which will deliver a stimulus to the heart in the event of recurring asystole. Peripheral pulses are checked for volume, rhythm and rate.

Respirations and blood pressure are noted and recorded at frequent intervals (every 15 minutes); the temperature is checked hourly. The defibrillator and mechanical ventilator are kept nearby and ready for immediate use.

The patient will be very apprehensive. He is advised of improvement in his condition and of the importance of rest and minimal emotional stress, and is assured that someone will either be with him or close by so that treatment may be quickly instituted should he need it.

Heart failure or decompensation

The ability of the heart to dilate and hypertrophy to compensate for an abnormal condition is limited. Excessive dilatation overstretches the muscle fibres to the point of injury; increasing hypertrophy creates a need for a corresponding increase in oxygen and nutrients, but there is no proportional increase in the coronary blood supply.

Prolonged strain, progressive disease and demands exceeding the individual's cardiac compensation are likely to lead to a reduced cardiac output that will not meet the needs of the body. The heart is then said to be *decompensated* or *in failure*. Heart failure may be designated as left-sided or right-sided heart failure, acute or chronic failure, or congestive heart failure.

Failure of the heart to forward the volume of blood it receives is usually confined to one side of the heart, although the other side may later fail as a result of the primary failure. The side affected is determined by the site of the causative lesion. If the *left side of the heart* cannot forward the blood offered to it, blood is backed up in the pulmonary circulatory system. The vessels become engorged and fluid escapes into the alveoli, producing acute pulmonary oedema manifested by dyspnoea and cough. In severe failure of the left side of the heart, more blood is pumped into the pulmonary system than the left side of the heart can receive and forward. The vessels become congested, and the alveoli gradually fill with serous fluid and blood. Unless this is checked, the respiratory exchange is cut off and the patient literally drowns in his own secretions.

This may be referred to as acute pulmonary oedema. Acute pulmonary oedema is an emergency which demands prompt action. Efforts are made to reduce preload and afterload and, at the same time, strengthen the contractility of the heart in order to increase the output from the left side.

Right-sided failure may be secondary to that of the left side, or it may occur independently. If the right heart chambers cannot forward the blood being returned to the heart by the venae cavae, the system becomes congested and oedema develops in the tissues and organs.

Acute cardiac failure occurs suddenly and is considered a more serious threat to the patient's life. Chronic heart failure develops gradually and may only appear when the patient increases his activities and energy expenditure.

The term congestive is applied to cardiac failure to describe the condition in the circulatory system behind the failure. It implies an excessive accumulation of blood in the system because the heart cannot accept and forward it.

Specific precipitating causes of heart failure include myocardial infarction, systemic hypertension, pulmonary emboli, cardiac arrhythmias, anaemia, chronic obstructive pulmonary disease, thyrotoxicosis and pregnancy with underlying heart disease.

NURSING PROCESS

Assessment

- *Respirations.* Dyspnoea is the most common symptom of heart failure. Pulmonary oedema impairs gas exchange and may induce hypoxia. In mild or early failure, dyspnoea may only be experienced with exertion. With severe heart failure, it is present at rest. With acute pulmonary oedema, it is severe. The respirations are checked every ½–1 hour in acute failure and every 4 hours in moderate or mild failure. With breathlessness related to activity, the degree of exertion is noted. The lungs are auscultated by the doctor for the presence of râles or rhonchi.
- *Pulse.* The pulse may be rapid, weak and irregular, as tachycardia frequently accompanies severe heart failure. The strength, rate and rhythm of the pulse are noted frequently and in relation to activities.
- *Cough.* Due to congestion and fluid in the alveoli and bronchial tubes, cough may be present. The frequency, characteristics and amount of sputum are noted. Frothy, colourless sputum occurs in pulmonary oedema, and blood may appear from the rupture of capillaries and arterioles in severe congestion.
- *Colour.* The colour of the lips, nail beds and skin is observed, and any changes noted. There may be cyanosis of lips and nail beds. The skin may show pallor due to generalized vasoconstriction.
- *Blood pressure.* The blood pressure is checked frequently since it reflects the cardiac output.
- *Body temperature.* Many patients with cardiac insufficiency register a subnormal temperature,

since their heat production is reduced because of inadequate circulation, deficiency in oxygen and resulting decrease in metabolism.

- *Generalized oedema.* Failure of the right side of the heart causes fluid to accumulate in the systemic venous circulation. The reduced venous return to the heart leads to a reduction in left ventricular output and compensatory mechanisms occur in an attempt to maintain adequate perfusion of vital organs. This causes further retention of fluid. Systemic venous and capillary pressures are raised due to the inability of the heart to receive the blood. Fluid escapes from the vascular system into the interstitial tissues, resulting in oedema.

One looks for oedema in the dependent areas of the body. If the person is mobile, swelling first appears in the feet and ankles, but, if he is confined to bed, oedema may first become apparent in the back and sacral region. As it becomes more severe all body tissues become affected, and even ascites and hydrothorax may develop. The latter further embarrass the patient's breathing.

The most accurate method of observing the patient for oedema is by weighing him daily if his condition makes this possible. He should be weighed at the same time each day with the same weight of clothes. Before oedema becomes apparent, 4.5–7.0 kg (10–15 lb) of water may be retained.

- *Fluid balance.* An accurate record is kept of the patient's fluid intake and output. A positive balance is brought to the attention of the doctor, particularly if the urinary output is decreased to 20–25 ml per hour. The amount of sweating is noted, as a large amount of fluid may be lost in this manner.
- *Fatigue.* The degree of fatigue is noted at rest as well as in relationship to specific activities.
- *Orientation and level of consciousness.* When circulation and/or the oxygen content of the blood perfusing the brain is inadequate, the patient's cerebral functioning may decrease. Observations are made as to the patient's level of consciousness, his orientation to person, time and surroundings, and his response to stimuli such as questioning.
- *Anxiety.* It is very important to observe the patient for fear and apprehension. Anxiety may initiate the release of adrenaline, which increases the demands on the heart. The patient's apprehension may indicate a need for information, explanations or sedation.
- *Anorexia.* The patient may not eat because of lack of strength to feed himself or because of dietary restrictions which make meals unpalatable. Congestion of internal organs due to oedema may contribute to loss of appetite. Anorexia may also result from drug toxicity (e.g. digoxin). The amount and type of food the patient eats should be observed at every meal.
- *Chest or abdominal pain.* Chest pain and any

apparent precipitating causes are observed and reported immediately. Abdominal pain may be due to the congestion and poor perfusion of internal organs. Abdominal distension may be associated with reduced peristalsis as a result of congestion and reduced blood supply.

Identification of patient problems
The following problems are examples that might be identified for the patient with congestive heart failure. The list must be individualized to meet the problems of the specific patient.

1 Alteration in cardiac output: the decrease is related to change in preload, afterload, heart rate, contractility or conduction disturbance.
2 Ineffective breathing patterns (dyspnoea) related to impaired gas exchange.
3 Activity intolerance due to an imbalance between oxygen supply and demand.
4 Lack of self-care related to decreased strength and endurance.
5 Alteration in fluid volume: excess related to compromised regulatory mechanisms.
6 Possible sensory–perceptual alteration related to oxygen deficit, electrolyte imbalance, inappropriate environmental stimuli or psychological stress.
7 Possible disturbance in self-concept related to changes in body image and role performance.
8 Potential alteration in sleep pattern: lack of sleep may be related to anxiety, physical discomfort and unfamiliar environment.
9 Potential alteration in bowel function (constipation, diarrhoea) related to immobilization.
10 Anxiety of patient/family related to the threat of the illness.
11 Lack of knowledge regarding the illness and recovery.

Nursing intervention
The nursing goals for the patient with heart failure are to:

1 Improve cardiac contractility by administering medications as ordered.
2 Improve oxygenation of the tissues.
3 Reduce the work load of the heart by the administration of medications as ordered (vasodilator therapy).
4 Reduce excess fluid accumulation by the administration of diuretics and other treatments as ordered.
5 Reduce energy demands on the heart.
6 Help the patient/family understand the illness so that he/she may live within cardiac capacity.
7 Promote the patient's safety by preventing complications.

1. Improving cardiac contractility. Heart contractility is improved by pharmacological agents ordered by the doctor. The nurse is responsible for administering them and observing their effects and possible side-effects. Drugs commonly used to improve cardiac contractility are inotropic agents such as cardiac glycosides (see p. 351), dopamine hydrochloride and dobutamine.

(a) *Dopamine hydrochloride (Intropin)*. This drug acts directly on beta receptors in the myocardium to stimulate myocardial contractility. It acts indirectly by releasing noradrenaline from sympathetic nerve terminals which also stimulate beta receptors in the heart. Its effect is dose-related. In small amounts it causes renal vasodilatation with a resultant increase in renal perfusion, glomerular filtration rate and sodium excretion. With large doses, however, it causes renal vasoconstriction.

Toxic effects include cardiac arrhythmias, nausea and vomiting, anginal pain and headache. It is administered intravenously. Extravasation of the tissues should be avoided by observing closely for any signs that the intravenous infusion is interstitial. If it does occur, it is recommended that phentolamine is injected into the area.

(b) *Dobutamine*. Dobutamine is a synthetic sympathomimetic amine which improves cardiac contractile force. It stimulates beta receptors in the myocardium. In addition, it stimulates beta$_2$- and alpha-adrenergic receptors but with less effect. In contrast to dopamine, it does not alter renal blood flow but does increase blood flow to the coronary and skeletal beds over mesenteric and renal vascular beds. Side-effects are similar to those of dopamine hydrochloride.

2. Oxygenation of the tissues. Oxygen may be administered by mask or nasal cannulae to increase arterial oxygen concentration. It will only be effective if delivery to the tissues is improved.

The nurse should explain the procedure to the patient briefly and remain with him until he is accustomed to the mask or nasal cannulae. Observations are made of the patient's response to the oxygen. Its effectiveness will be indicated by reduced pulse rate, less dyspnoea, improvement in colour and less restlessness. (For details of administration see p. 446).

In severe pulmonary oedema, the doctor may administer oxygen under positive pressure to counteract the movement of fluid from the capillaries into the alveoli.

3. Reducing work load of the heart by vasodilator therapy.
(a) *Arterial vasodilators*. Arterial vasodilators reduce afterload by reducing peripheral vascular resistance.

Hydralazine (Apresoline) acts directly on vascular smooth muscle to cause vasodilation.

Phentolamine is a secondary choice of treatment and acts by blocking adrenergic stimulation of the arterioles. It is occasionally given

intravenously and begins to act immediately. Since its action stops within minutes after being discontinued, it has a quickly reversible effect. It also improves myocardial contractility. Side-effects include nausea, vomiting, abdominal pain and tachycardia. The initial dose is 0.1 mg/min and may be increased in steps of 0.1 mg/min every 5 minutes up to a maximum of 2.0 mg/min.

(b) *Venous vasodilators*. Venous vasodilators reduce preload. By reducing the venous return to the heart, these drugs alleviate heart failure. Drugs commonly used are glyceryl trinitrate tablets or ointment and isosorbide dinitrate.

(c) *Dual acting vasodilators*. This group of vasodilators affect both arterial and venous muscle tone. Included are sodium nitroprusside and prazosin and captopril.

Captopril is a vasodilator which acts by inhibiting the enzyme necessary for converting angiotensin I to angiotensin II, thus preventing the formation of a powerful vasoconstrictor. It also interferes with the breakdown of the vasodilator bradykinin. Side-effects include rash, fever, proteinuria and rarely agranulocytosis.

4. Reducing excess fluid accumulation. Measures directed towards reducing the oedema associated with cardiac failure include (a) drugs, (b) dietary measures and (c) occasionally phlebotomy or (d) tourniquets (see below). The selection of measures is dictated by the severity and location of the oedema. In the case of sudden left-sided cardiac failure, acute pulmonary oedema develops quickly. Prompt treatment is necessary to save the patient's life. The nurse, when advised that such a patient is to be admitted, quickly assembles the necessary equipment and medications for treatment so that there will be no delay.

The patient with severe pulmonary oedema is naturally very fearful, which further aggravates the primary condition. The doctor will probably administer diamorphine intravenously to reduce pulmonary artery pressure and to provide sedation, an inotropic drug to strengthen myocardial contractions and a diuretic intravenously to decrease circulating blood volume further. Additional efforts to reduce venous return may be made by the application of tourniquets and a phlebotomy.

Generalized oedema generally develops gradually and is usually associated with right-sided heart failure.

(a) *Drugs to produce diuresis:* There are various groups of diuretics which act directly on the kidneys and are administered orally and/or parenterally. They increase the rate of urine formation and indirectly cause the removal of fluid from the tissues. Commonly used diuretics include the following (see Table 14.10).

Table 14.10 Diuretics.

Name	Action	Onset of action	Length of action	Possible side-effects
Frusemide (Lasix)	Inhibits sodium and chloride reabsorption; acts primarily at ascending loop of Henle	½–1 hour	6–8 hours	Hypokalaemia Hyponatraemia Hypovolaemia
Ethacrynic acid (Edecrin)	As above	1 hour	6–8 hours	Hypokalaemia Hyponatraemia Hypovolaemia Skin rash Granulocytopenia
Spironolactone (Aldactone)	Aldosterone antagonist in distal renal tubule	24–48 hours	2–3 days	Hyperkalaemia; Gastrointestinal upsets Gynaecomastia Drowsiness
Amiloride	A potassium-sparing diuretic Influences renal tubular transport of electrolytes	2 hours	24 hours	Gastrointestinal disturbances, e.g. nausea, vomiting, anorexia Dry mouth and thirst Dizziness Weakness Paraesthesia Rash
Bendrofluazide	Direct effect on arteriolar smooth muscle Inhibits sodium and chloride and therefore water reabsorption by the distal renal tubules	1 hour	12–18 hours	Hypokalaemia Hypochloraemic alkalosis Mild hyperglycaemia Incontinence in the elderly

Thiazides. The thiazide diuretics are used because of their effectiveness and the fact that they may be administered orally and are well tolerated. This group of drugs inhibits the reabsorption of sodium and chloride ions, and therefore water, by the distal renal tubules. Potassium depletion also occurs and potassium supplements are usually given. Hypokalaemia is particularly important in patients taking digoxin because a low potassium level can predispose a patient to digitalis toxicity. Other complications associated with thiazide therapy include hyperglycaemia, hyperuricaemia and rarely cholistatic hepatitis and hypersensitivity. Bendrofluazide is an example of this type of diuretic. It is appropriate for use in mild or moderate cardiac failure when the patient is not desperately ill and does not have severe pulmonary oedema.

Frusemide. This loop diuretic inhibits sodium reabsorption especially in the ascending loop of Henle. It acts quickly, producing diuresis in ½–1 hour following oral administration; it is widely used.

For patients with acute pulmonary oedema frusemide is administered intravenously. The rate of intravenous administration should not exceed 5 mg/min, since rapid intravenous administration may result in deafness. A close check is kept on serum electrolyte levels. Frusemide is often prescribed for patients with severe heart failure who might be refractory to the thiazide diuretics.

Ethacrynic acid (Edecrin). This is a very potent diuretic which inhibits sodium reabsorption at the ascending loop of Henle. It is well absorbed when administered orally and may also be given intravenously. With the intravenous route extravasation should be avoided, as it is very irritating to the superficial tissues. It should not be given intramuscularly. Serum electrolyte levels are monitored closely as chloride, potassium and hydrogen ions are also excreted. Because of its powerful effect the patient may become hypovolaemic. Ethacrynic acid and frusemide are the agents of choice for patients with severe heart failure refractory to thiazides.

Mercurial diuretics. The potency and effectiveness of frusemide when given orally and its relatively low incidence of side-effects has resulted in the virtual abandonment of the use of the mercurial preparations.

They act quickly within 1–2 hours, but excretion of the drug begins in 3 hours.

Spironolactone (Aldactone). This diuretic acts by inhibiting the action of aldosterone which is secreted by the cortex of the adrenal glands and promotes the absorption of sodium ions and water by the kidney tubules and the excretion of potassium. By inhibiting the action of aldosterone, spironolactone promotes the excretion of sodium and water and the retention of potassium. Hyperkalaemia may result if spironolactone is administered concomitantly with potassium supplements, or it may occur in patients with uraemia. Occasionally gynaecomastia (enlargement of the mammary glands in the male) may develop. Spironolactone is most effective when administered with thiazide diuretics. It is contraindicated (unless administered with other diuretics) for patients with hyperkalaemia. It has a slow onset of action and does not reach peak effectiveness for 2–3 days.

Spironolactone is a weak diuretic which potentiates thiazide and loop diuretics, and helps to prevent hypokalaemia.

Amiloride (Midamor) is another weak diuretic which causes retention of potassium. This diuretic is useful in patients with oedema, but should not be given if hyperkalaemia or renal failure are present.

(b) *Nutrition and fluids.* Modifications in the diet for patients with heart failure are based first on their retention of an excess of sodium which causes the formation of oedema, and secondly on the knowledge that overeating and overweight increase the work load of the heart.

Low-sodium diets are prescribed to reduce oedema and to prevent further accumulation of fluid in the tissues. The sodium restriction varies with patients, depending upon their heart efficiency and amount of oedema. Normally the average daily salt intake is 10–12 g. If no salt is added to food either at the table or in cooking and no salted foods are used, the intake may be reduced to approximately 3 g. In congestive heart failure more stringent restrictions are sometimes necessary, and foods are selected that will provide still less sodium. Diets that contain as low as 0.25 g can be prepared.

Low-sodium diets are unpalatable, and the patient finds it difficult to adhere to the prescribed restriction. Frequently the result is that he does not take sufficient food to meet his nutritional needs. The nurse should explain the purpose of the diet and relate it to symptoms the patient is experiencing. There are many spices and foods allowable that help to make a low-sodium diet more palatable. In prolonged, severe restriction of sodium, the patient may develop a sodium deficiency. The doctor is informed of any complaints of muscular cramps and weakness.

Braunwald suggests that with the advent of the newer and more potent diuretic drugs, severe dietary sodium restriction is not as mandatory as it was previously for the average patient with heart failure.[22] Obviously salty foods, however, should be avoided, as well as extra salt at the table.

The normal daily salt intake may be reduced by half by eliminating salt-rich foods and salt added at the table. This reduction would be required for the patient with mild or moderate heart failure. Omitting all salt from cooking reduces salt intake to one quarter of the normal. Even further reductions to between 500 and 1000 mg may be obtained for the patient in severe heart failure by eliminating milk, cheese, bread, cereals, canned vegetables and soups, some salted cuts of meat and fresh vegetables such as spinach, celery and beets that have a high sodium content.

If the patient with heart failure is overweight, the caloric intake is reduced in an effort to reduce the weight to normal. A maintenance diet is then prescribed. The lower-calorie diet should contain less fat but enough of the other foods to meet nutritional requirements.

In addition, curtailing the fluid intake to about 1500 ml daily can be advantageous. It is unusual, however, to find that a more rigorous restriction is warranted.

(c) *Phlebotomy.* A measure that may be used to reduce venous return and total blood volume is phlebotomy. The doctor withdraws 250–700 ml of blood from a vein. A blood donor set is quickly made available for this procedure and the blood may be donated to the blood bank.

(d) *Tourniquets.* A reduction in venous return to the heart may be achieved by rotating the application of tourniquets; however, the technique is only very rarely employed. Three tourniquets are necessary; one is applied to the upper part of three extremities with just enough pressure to interfere with superficial venous circulation. One tourniquet is moved to the free limb every 10–15 minutes and a definite pattern, either clockwise or counterclockwise is established (see Fig. 14.14). The doctor will indicate the period between moves and how long the tourniquet procedure is to be used. Too long a period of venous compression may produce the risk of phlebothrombosis and embolism.

5. Reducing energy demands on the heart.

(a) *Rest.* Rest is important in the treatment of the patient with heart failure since it reduces the demand on the heart by reducing body requirements for oxygen. For the patient in failure, rest in bed is necessary until the oedema is decreased. The doctor's order may read 'complete (or absolute) bed rest' or simply 'bed rest'. These usually mean something different, and the nurse must

---

[22] Braunwald (1985).

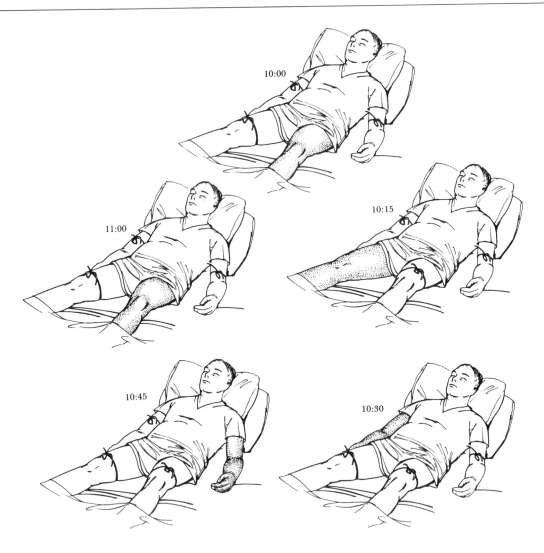

Fig. 14.14 Rotation of tourniquets at 15-minute intervals.

determine exactly what is meant by each in the particular situation. Generally, 'complete bed rest' is interpreted as absolute minimal activity on the patient's part, with the nurse doing everything possible for him. He is fed, bathed, turned, and assisted on and off the commode or bedpan; his teeth are cleaned and his hair combed. 'Bed rest' usually means that the patient may participate to some degree in his personal care, and the nurse observes the effects of such activities on the patient. If they produce shortness of breath, an increase in pulse rate and excessive fatigue, his activities are reduced.

Once the acute episode has passed, the patient is allowed out of bed for gradually increasing intervals. Intermittent rest periods during the day and following activities are arranged, and the patient rests before and after meals and between procedures.

(b) *Psychological support.* Mental rest is as important as physical rest, but is often difficult to promote. The common knowledge that the heart is a most vital organ and that heart disease is a frequent cause of death produces a greater emotional reaction in the person advised of a diagnosis of a heart failure. He becomes fearful and apprehensive; his life, his job, his family's security and his whole future are threatened. Rarely does any other condition, even though it may be an equally severe threat, engender as much fear and concern. Frequently the anxiety reaction may be completely out of proportion to the actual threat. Emotional reactions increase respirations and the work load of the heart. A patient may appear to be at rest but is actually in mental turmoil. The sensitive, observant nurse who understands the possible implications that illness has for this patient is likely to detect his mental unrest and endeavours to promote the peace of mind essential to optimum rest.

The nurse who understands the patient's condition, knows what to look for and what to do, usually displays calm and composure which contribute to the patient's confidence and security. A quiet, controlled atmosphere does more toward allaying fear than verbal reassurance.

It is helpful to have someone remain with the anxious patient; alone, he may panic, thinking he is cut off from help. If a nurse is not available, the presence of an auxiliary nurse or a member of the family will provide some reassurance. Emotionally disturbed relatives should not be permitted to visit or remain with the patient unless they can conceal their feelings and control their reactions.

There may be a problem at home that contributes to the patient's unrest. Some solution may be suggested or arrangements made for assistance from the social services or primary health-care team. The nurse encourages the patient to express his anxieties and tries to identify his feelings and his problems as he sees them. Frequently, verbal expression of concerns may reduce their proportions: having shared them, he now has the support of someone who knows his problems. It may be necessary with some patients to seek the assistance of the doctor or the patient's religious adviser to deal with questions or expressions of fear.

In the interest of providing optimum rest for the patient, consideration is given to his location on the ward. He is not placed next to people who might disturb him, and will most likely feel more secure if he is close to the nursing station. A light left on at night may contribute to a feeling of security, as well as make it easier for the nurse to make frequent, reassuring visits and the necessary observations. If his degree of activity permits, reading or listening to the radio may provide diversion and relaxation.

There is no specific formula for dealing with the cardiac patient's anxiety in order to provide the much needed rest. The nurse must be alert to the problem and work at it: that which proves successful with one patient will not be the answer for all.

Physical comfort will contribute to the patient's rest and may be promoted by change of position, bathing, warmth, etc. Anticipation of need and the planning and provision of undisturbed rest periods are important. Cooperation is sought from the laboratory, dietary and housekeeping staffs to control the interruptions. A sedative may be prescribed to reduce anxiety and restlessness, and the nurse provides the necessary attention to ensure maximum benefits from the drug.

(c) *Activity.* Rest has been emphasized as an important phase of the treatment of cardiac patients, but it is well known that there are certain disadvantages inherent in bed rest. The limbs should be put through passive movements to promote venous drainage and prevent phlebothrombosis. Gentle massage will also be helpful. If the patient's condition permits, it may be suggested that he gradually commences foot, leg and arm exercises. The patient is also encouraged to take five to ten deep breaths every 1–2 hours. As soon as possible he is allowed to get out of bed to use a commode, since the use of a bedpan for defecation places considerable strain on the patient.

Observations are made of reactions to any activity so that undue stress on the heart may be avoided. These will also assist the doctor in defining the patient's future activities and the amount of rest and restriction that will be necessary.

(d) *Positioning.* The position the patient with heart failure finds most comfortable in bed is determined by his breathing. The patient who is experiencing dyspnoea will be more comfortable with the head of the bed elevated, but the height of elevation should only be that at which the dyspnoea is minimal.

Patients with congestive failure manifest orthopnoea—that is, less difficulty in breathing with the trunk in the upright position. Semi- or high Fowler's position increases the vital capacity and tends to reduce the volume of blood returned to the heart and to the pulmonary system. Pressure of abdominal viscera on the diaphragm is reduced. Some patients may be still more comfortable in a true sitting position—that is, with the lower limbs down. A special cardiac bed on which the foot of the bed can be lowered to provide a chair-like support is available. Alternatively the patient may find comfort from sitting in a chair. The sitting position promotes the formation of peripheral oedema in the dependent parts but relieves the pulmonary congestion to some extent; peripheral oedema is much less serious than pulmonary oedema.

In the sitting position a pillow placed longitudinally at the patient's back may help provide some comfort. Pillows should be used at the sides to support the arms and relieve the fatiguing pull on the shoulders. A change may be effected by arranging a table and pillow over the bed in front of him, upon which he may rest his head and arms. Cot-sides may be kept up on the bed to safeguard the patient when he is in the upright position, since he may become drowsy and fall to the side, or may experience cerebral hypoxia which causes disorientation. The sides are also useful when a change of position is made since they may be grasped by the patient and used for added support. Patients in the upright position are encouraged to assume the recumbent position for brief periods to help reduce circulatory stasis and oedema in the lower parts of the body. However, patients should not be forced to do this if they are suffering from severe dyspnoea.

In patients with heart conditions, as with all patients, the general principles of positioning apply. Good body alignment is respected to prevent contractures, hyperextension and circulatory stasis. *Even a slight change in position* every 1–2 hours is helpful. A footboard is used to prevent foot drop.

(e) *Elimination.* Constipation and straining at defecation are to be avoided because of the undue strain placed on the heart. A mild laxative may have to be given to keep the stool soft. If constipation does occur, a micro-enema, for example Microlax or an oil enema, may be given. Abdominal distension is also to be avoided, since it raises the diaphragm and further embarrasses the patient's breathing. It has been shown that the use of the bedpan requires more energy than getting out of bed and using a commode. Therefore the doctor may prefer to have the patient use a bedside commode for defecation.

When a patient receives a diuretic it will mean frequent use of the urinal, bedpan or commode, which can be very exhausting. The nurse provides the necessary assistance, and the patient is allowed to rest undisturbed between voidings.

(f) *Care of the mouth and skin.* The dyspnoea and retention of sodium experienced by the cardiac patient cause a decrease in normal salivary secretions. The tongue is rough and dry, and a thick mucus accumulates and adheres to the teeth and mucous membrane, providing a medium for organisms. Under such conditions, older patients are especially predisposed to parotitis. The mouth should be cleansed every 2–3 hours and kept moist.

The poor circulation, oedema, bed rest and restricted activity necessitate special skin care to prevent pressure sores. Bony prominences and pressure areas are kept clean and dry. The alternating air pressure mattress is useful in protecting pressure areas but, if not available, a sponge rubber mattress may be used, or a piece of sponge rubber or sheepskin may be placed under pressure areas such as the sacrum, buttocks and heels.

6. *Rehabilitation of the patient with cardiac dysfunction.* The philosophy and principles of rehabilitation are applicable to heart patients just as they are to patients with other conditions in which there is some residual damage or progressive disease. These people may require help to learn to live within the limits of their cardiac capacity and, at the same time, achieve personal satisfaction and be able to function as productive members of society.

When a patient learns that he has a heart condition or recovers from an acute cardiac illness, he is advised as to whether he may resume his former activities or if it will be necessary for him to curtail some activities. The amount of activity and necessary restrictions are defined by the doctor on the basis of the functional capacity of the heart (see Table 14.5). Many of these people consider themselves doomed to complete invalidism and an early death. They may have an unjustified fear of another attack or of participating in any activity and may become helpless and dependent, creating unnecessary problems and hardships for themselves and their families.

Heart disease does not differ from many other diseases in that the patient may recover and take up his life where he left off. Some may find that a few simple adjustments in their pattern of living are necessary, while others are more restricted.

The doctor has several ways of assessing the patient's capacity for activity and his limitations. He may observe the patient's responses to a gradual increase in energy expenditure. This will probably begin with self-care activities which are progressively extended to include more strenuous efforts. The assessment programme may go on over several weeks or months, and the patient may require considerable encouragement to persevere.

An evaluation by standardized tests may be made in a heart clinic. In some situations, work evaluation clinics are established and serve to determine how much activity the patient's heart will permit. Following an assessment, a functional and therapeutic classification may be made. This is particularly useful in placing the patient in employment.

The nurse may assist in the assessment of the patient by observing and recording his responses to various activities. Any complaint of shortness of breath, palpitation, fatigue or an undue increase in the pulse rate are reported, and the effort is discontinued until the patient is checked by the doctor.

It is sometimes helpful to have the patient list his accustomed pattern of activities. The doctor may then indicate what changes, if any, are necessary. This is useful in getting the patient to think and talk about how much he will be able to do. It encourages him to plan independently and to reach a compromise between activity and restrictions.

The patient should realize that he has some responsibility for his future. The length of time he will live, and with what degree of satisfaction, depends largely on his own efforts. Each person reacts differently to illness and to restrictions. One may refuse to take advice or accept limitations and decide to 'live it up'. Another may become depressed or may display hostility, and still others become overdependent. It is usually more difficult for the adult patient to accept and adjust to restrictions. Heart disease so often occurs just when the patient has reached a high position in his job and when life has become easier. The adult required to change to a less strenuous occupation finds it difficult to face a retraining programme. Often his age makes it difficult for him to get another job.

With emphasis on the positive aspects, the nurse helps the patient and family understand and accept the decision of the doctor and to plan for the necessary adjustments. In the following paragraphs, consideration is given to the planning for assistance and guidance for these patients, remembering that every programme must be planned in relation to each individual.

The nurse should have a copy of the many useful pamphlets and booklets available from the British Heart Foundation. Many of these deal with rehabilitation, and appropriate copies may be given to the patient to read with the doctor's approval.

Progressively increased activity is encouraged and directed by the nurse to condition the patient to the level of activity that corresponds to his heart's ability.

Changes may be necessary in the patient's home if he is not allowed to use stairs. It may be helpful to have a member of the primary health-care team or an occupational therapist or social worker assess the home situation before the patient returns to it. Suggestions may be made in the interest of the patient and those who will be caring for him. For example, a bedroom and bathroom may have to be provided on the ground floor. Distance from public transportation and work may be factors that require consideration for some patients.

It should be pointed out to the patient and his family that moderation in everything is a good rule for persons who have had a heart illness. Some work, exercise, rest and recreation are important for everyone. Situations that are likely to add undue strain should be anticipated and avoided. Enough time should be allowed to prevent rushing. For example, rather than run the risk of running for a bus, the patient should plan to leave earlier. Climbing, walking against a strong wind, lifting, pushing and fatigue are to be avoided. Constipation, infections and emotional upsets also tend to increase the demands on the heart. The patient should strive for equanimity and develop the philosophy that what cannot be changed must be accepted. Suitable recreational activities, which meet both his interests and his cardiac functional capacity, may be suggested. Some exercise is beneficial and appropriate forms are discussed. Walking is considered a good exercise. Regular hours of rest at night and, if necessary, a rest period during the day are recommended.

The doctor, a social worker or the nurse may discuss necessary adjustments in the persons's work situation with his employer or the industrial nurse. Assistance might be given to find suitable employ-

ment or to obtain retraining if a change in occupation is indicated.

Since smoking, particularly cigarettes, is found to be vasoconstricting, the patient is advised to discontinue smoking.

Shortness of breath, palpitation, faintness, persisting fatigue, pain and oedema are indications for the person to slow up and report to the clinic or his doctor.

Clarification of the prescribed diet is made. Many patients are advised to continue with a low sodium intake and a limited number of calories. Foods allowed, those restricted and meal planning are discussed. The importance of keeping the weight normal and avoiding large meals is explained. Preferably, the discussion of the diet should be with the family as well as the patient. Directions and suggestions are given to the patient in writing, and an appropriate diet booklet can be obtained from the British Heart Foundation or the Health Education Council.

The medications that are to be continued are discussed, and written instructions are provided. Early signs of untoward reactions are cited, and included with these are directions about what to do if they develop. For example, if an anticoagulant such as warfarin is to be continued, the patient and a family member are advised of the action of the drug and the necessary observations to recognize bleeding. They are told that bleeding from body orifices, discoloured areas of the skin (bruises and petechiae), bleeding gums, and persistent bleeding from minor cuts or injuries are to be reported immediately to the doctor or clinic. If he is to have dental work done, the patient should advise his dentist that he is receiving warfarin. He is given an identification card to carry which states that he is receiving warfarin. A weekly visit to clinic for prothrombin time evaluation is usually requested by the doctor.

Many patients with heart conditions are required to take digoxin continuously and should understand that loss of appetite, nausea or diarrhoea may indicate the need for some adjustment in the dosage of the drug. If the patient is an elderly person who lives alone, he is advised to keep a calendar available with the days that he is to take a medication clearly marked. It is stressed that he adopt the habit of marking off the medication as soon as he takes it.

Some follow-up service is important. The patient and family are advised of the resources outside the hospital, and a referral may be made to the general practitioner and district nurse. Home visits by a nurse can be very helpful; they provide an opportunity for the patient and family to ask questions and receive counselling on the various aspects of care. At the same time the patient's condition and progress are noted.

If the patient's heart condition demands fairly stringent restrictions on his activities, it may be necessary to assist the family in planning how they will provide the required care. Some patients need provision made for their ordinary personal care. The family is advised about the amount of care needed, how to provide it and how to protect their own health. They are encouraged not to overprotect the patient or foster an overdependent role. The family should plan together and all share in the necessary care. The nurse may recognize that the care of the patient will impose too heavy a burden on the family and help them to seek some other solution. A referral may be made for home nursing or the patient may be transferred to a nursing home. Circumstances might necessitate the family receiving supplementary benefit. The nurse may have to help the patient accept this situation.

The importance of regular medical supervision is stressed. The severely handicapped person may have difficulty getting to the outpatient clinic or doctor's surgery. Transport may be requested of a voluntary organization such as the Red Cross Society, the ambulance service or hospital car service.

The housewife with a cardiac condition is given assistance in learning to continue her home functions within her heart capacity. Again, the reader is referred to the appropriate publications available through the British Heart Foundation. Much work has been done on work simplification in the home, and there are many simple and inexpensive ways of making it possible to achieve more with less effort. Some physical changes, a reorganization in the placement of equipment, elimination of unnecessary chores by provision of a home help, and the management of many tasks to economize on time and motion may be suggested and demonstrated. The success of rehabilitating the housewife is largely dependent on how willing she is to change her way of doing things. Members of the caring team may find that much time will have to be devoted to persuasion.

The patient's health and degree of satisfaction in living will depend to a large extent on his recognition and acceptance of the limitations imposed.

NURSING THE CARDIAC SURGICAL PATIENT

Significant advances have been made in the field of cardiac surgery, in correcting both congenital and acquired heart defects. Correction of acquired heart disease includes surgery for coronary artery disease and for stenosed or incompetent cardiac valves. The fact that the heart must function immediately after the surgery presents a problem different from that in many areas of the body. It must heal while continuing to maintain adequate circulation. This creates the need for greater support and for minimizing physiological demands.

Progress in this area of surgery was delayed until the introduction of the pump-oxygenator. This machine permits extracorporeal oxygenation of the blood and maintenance of circulation while the heart is arrested and opened to provide a direct approach to defects within the heart. Circulation bypasses the heart and lungs. The venae cavae are cannulated, and the blood passes from them into tubes leading to the mechanical oxygenator, which takes the place of the lungs. It is then pumped through a heat exchanger and filtered back into the arterial system, generally via the aorta. Sufficient blood enters the coronary system to sustain the myocardial cells. The blood is heparinized in order to prevent coagulation and thrombus formation. On completion of the cardiopulmonary bypass, the heparin is neutralized by the administration of protamine sulphate.

Hypothermia may be used to reduce the metabolic activity of the heart so the cells can survive interruption of the coronary circulation. Reducing the body temperature to within a range of 20–30°C (hypothermia) may be used in heart surgery either alone or as an adjunct to the extracorporeal circulation. It reduces the metabolic activity of cells throughout the body and therefore their oxygen and nutritional needs. Hypothermia prevents damage to the brain and other vital organs when an interruption of circulation or a reduction in oxygenated blood to a dangerously low level is anticipated (see section on hypothermia, p. 121).

SURGERY FOR CORONARY ARTERY DISEASE

Both direct and indirect methods are used to revascularize the myocardium. The indirect method, or Vineberg procedure, involves implanting the internal mammary artery into the myocardium and is rarely used. Collateral circulation develops over a period of months; revascularization is not immediate. Consequently, infarction and mortality rates are higher during this period than with direct revascularization procedures.

The most popular procedure is the aortocoronary bypass surgery, in which one end of a resected saphenous vein is anastomosed to the aorta and the other to the coronary artery beyond the point of obstruction. The blood supply to the myocardium is immediately improved.

Angioplasty may also be used in coronary artery disease (see p. 331).

SURGERY FOR DISEASED VALVES

The surgeon can significantly enlarge the size of the orifice of stenosed valves in some individuals by dilating the valve, either manually or instrumentally. Others, however, may require valve replacement.

Certain patients with regurgitation of the aortic, mitral and/or tricuspid valves, who no longer respond to medical treatment, require total replacement. This is accomplished with an artificial valve prosthesis or the use of tissue homografts.

The preoperative preparation for cardiac surgery may extend through days to weeks, while the patient is thoroughly investigated and his physical and mental conditions are improved.

Psychological preparation

In most instances, heart surgery carries more than the ordinary risk. The incision may be midsternal, which avoids entrance into the left pleural cavity and collapse of the left lung, or it may be through the left chest and may result in collapse of the left lung. Because of the tremendous emphasis placed on the heart by the average person, it is understandable that the patient and his family will be very apprehensive. The surgeon describes the patient's condition to the patient and his family, and the likely prognosis if he continues untreated. An explanation is then made of what can be done surgically and the inherent risk.

It takes courage to face heart surgery; the patient, or (in the case of a child) the parents, may find it difficult to arrive at a decision. They require a great deal of emotional support. The nurse assesses the patient's anxiety and fears, and efforts are directed towards minimizing them, since they will affect the patient's reaction to surgery and his postoperative progress. He is encouraged to talk about his concerns and to ask questions. Worries may become less significant through talking about them and being able to share them. Socioeconomic problems may come to light which should be referred to the social worker. The patient may fear death and may wish to talk about this. A visit from the patient's spiritual adviser may provide considerable support.

Acquainting the patient with what to expect when he goes to the operating theatre and after the surgery will reduce some of his fear of the future. As the patient talks more and more about the whole major event, he will begin to accept it with less stress. Nursing research has demonstrated that when appropriate information is given to patients preoperatively, postoperative pain and stress are reduced.[23,24] In all discussions with the patient and family, what is said should be informative, in understandable terms, and judiciously selected to prevent inducing unnecessary anxiety. Sincere interest and understanding of their problems are frequently better expressed by feeling tones than by words.

To prevent unnecessary concern, the patient is advised of the multiple and complex equipment that will surround him after his operation. It may be helpful with some patients to actually let them see some of the equipment in this preoperative period. The patient is told that he will have a tube in his throat (endotracheal) so that he may receive oxygen by a ventilator which will reduce the work of breathing,

that his blood pressure and pulse will be taken at very frequent intervals to reveal information about his condition, and that there will be a tube in the chest as well as an intravenous tube and an indwelling catheter. The nurses will be making frequent checks of these tubes and the drainage. He is advised that he will likely experience a sensation of heaviness and tightness as well as some pain in the chest, and is reassured that the staff will do everything possible to provide relief. In many hospitals, the patient is visited the day before surgery by the nurse who will be caring for him in the intensive care unit. This preoperative visit establishes a contact for the patient as well as helping the nurse to know him better.

Observations

During the preoperative period, vital signs, fluid intake and output, daily weight and reactions to any exertion are noted. The patient is also observed closely for indications of any condition, such as a cold or skin infection, which could cause serious postoperative complications. A detailed knowledge of the patient and his vital signs serves as a basis for comparison postoperatively.

Operative consent

The patient, if responsible and of age, will sign his consent form for operation. The patient should have had a description of the operation and its expected outcome before being asked to sign the operation consent form. In the case of a minor, a parent is required to give permission.

Functional tests (see p. 315)

Cardiac and respiratory functional tests, as well as complete blood studies, are done to further assess the patient's condition. The blood work will include typing and crossmatching so that compatible blood will be available at the time of operation. Serum electrolytes, cardiac enzymes, serum creatinine and blood urea determinations are also performed, and blood clotting tests such as prothrombin time and partial thromboplastin time are done. A preoperative urinalysis is carried out.

The nurse explains the tests to the patient and provides the required preparation and aftercare applicable to each one. For several hours following the more complex cardiac tests, such as heart catheterization, close observation is necessary for manifestations of reactions or complications. Bleeding or irritation at the site of entrance into the blood vessel, reaction to the radiopaque substance, fibrillation and cardiac arrest occur rarely.

For some patients, tests such as cardiac catheterization may be done several weeks preoperatively, and the patient may re-enter the hospital 1–3 days prior to surgery.

Physical preparation

Optimum nutritional status is important; attention is

[23] Hayward J (1975).
[24] Boore JRP (1978).

directed to having the patient take adequate meals. Protein and vitamin C are particularly important, for they contribute to tissue repair. If the patient has been having a low-sodium diet previously, this will be continued. Optimum hydration is desirable; a daily intake of 2000–2500 ml is encouraged as long as his output is adequate and the patient is not in cardiac failure.

The patient is advised that he will be required to cough, take five to ten deep respirations, change position and do some simple leg and foot exercises frequently, for several days after the operation. Arm and shoulder exercises will also be necessary later. The purposes of these activities should be explained. Instructions are given on how to cough and do the exercises, and the patient is encouraged to practise. To cough, he is instructed to take a deep breath, contract the abdominal muscles and then cough with the mouth and throat open. Postoperative coughing and deep breathing promote expansion of the lungs, the removal of secretions from the respiratory tract and the removal of air and fluid from the thoracic cavity. The foot and leg exercises are to prevent phlebothrombosis. The arm exercises promote a return to the full range of motion of the arms, since the patient will tend to favour them following the operation.

Particular attention is paid to skin and oral hygiene during this period. Daily bathing with a mild antiseptic solution or soap minimizes the possibility of staphylococcal wound infection. This will be done 1–2 days prior to surgery. Antiseptic mouthwash will help to prevent mouth and respiratory infection.

Immediate preoperative care
Extra precautions are taken with these patients in preparing the skin. Infection superimposed on their surgery could prove fatal. The day before operation almost the whole trunk is shaved and cleansed, including the axillae. The pubic area and upper thighs are also prepared. The surgeon will indicate what antiseptic, if any, is to be applied; following the shave, the patient may be given an antiseptic bath and placed in fresh bed linen. Care is taken during the shave to keep the skin intact. It is important that the fingernails are free of nail polish so that their true colour may be detected.

Solid food is withheld for 10–12 hours previous to operation and the meal preceding this period should be light. Water may be given up to 4–6 hours prior to operation.

The doctor may or may not want the patient to have a small cleansing enema the afternoon before operation. A sedative is prescribed to ensure the patient a good sleep the night before operation. The nurse makes a final check to see that the urinalysis report and vital signs are satisfactory, that the operative consent has been signed, and that the patient is wearing an identification bracelet. This may be on his ankle for convenience.

The morning of operation the patient may be required to take an antiseptic bath, and he empties his bladder just before the sedative is given. All procedures are completed before the patient receives his preoperative medication so that he may be left undisturbed to derive the maximum benefit from the drug. A nurse accompanies the patient to the operating theatre and remains with him until the anaesthetist or theatre staff take over.

In the operating theatre, a Foley catheter is inserted into the patient's bladder and attached to a drainage tube and bag, a venous catheter is forwarded into the right heart for measurement of central venous pressure, and an arterial catheter is inserted to be used postoperatively to obtain samples of arterial blood for measurement of blood gases and to monitor blood pressure. Some patients may require a Swan–Ganz catheter for assessment of pulmonary artery and pulmonary capillary pressures.

Family
Consideration is given to the relatives during this stressful situation. A spouse, parent or someone close whom the patient wishes to have may be allowed to visit before the preoperative medication is administered. The family may wish to remain at the hospital during the operation, or may decide to return home to await word by telephone. If they remain, they are shown to a sitting room and are given emotional support during the long wait. The nurse should take a few moments at intervals to go and speak with them and to see that they have refreshments. Recognition on the part of the nurse or others that this is a difficult time will help. Many surgeons, knowing the family's stress, may forward a message from time to time to reassure them.

POSTOPERATIVE NURSING CARE

The patient who has had cardiac surgery is cared for in an intensive care unit where the necessary special equipment is assembled. Continuous observation and constant, expert nursing care are required. The patient becomes very anxious and fearful if left alone for even a very brief period the first day or two.

The care must be adapted to the patient's particular needs and the surgeon's directives. The following points of care may not be applicable nor complete in all situations, but may serve as a guide to the nurse who is planning and providing care for the surgical cardiac patient.

Preparation to receive the patient
During the operation the necessary equipment is assembled at the patient's bedside. In many intensive care units, much of the monitoring equipment is attached to the wall beside the patient's bed.

Reception of the patient
The closed chest drainage, urinary drainage, intravenous infusion, arterial line, and central venous

and pulmonary arterial pressure lines are checked for function. The endotracheal tube is attached to the mechanical ventilator and respiratory support and the administration of oxygen are continued as ordered. Limbs with infusions are secured and continuous cardiac monitoring is started.

Positioning
The patient is kept flat until the systolic blood pressure is 100 mmHg or more. He is raised gradually and his responses noted. Unless otherwise directed, his position is changed every 2 hours from back to left side to back and to right side, etc. Precautions are necessary to avoid dislodging any tubes when turning the patient.

Observations
A constant monitoring of the heart action is used so that cardiac arrhythmias and change of rate may be quickly detected. Blood pressure, radial pulse and apex beat, respirations and colour are checked and recorded every 15 minutes at first and every hour once the vital signs become stabilized.

Venous pressure readings are taken as an indication of intravascular volume and right heart function. Pulmonary artery and pulmonary capillary wedge pressures, when ordered, are measured as an indication of left heart functioning. These measurements are continued for at least 48 hours following surgery.

Initially the patient is supported by mechanical ventilation, either pressure- or volume-controlled. The adequacy of this ventilation is assessed by measurement of arterial blood gases as well as by observation of the patient's responses which include colour, blood pressure, restlessness and pulse rate. Arterial blood specimens are collected from the inter-arterial line by the doctor when the patient is first admitted to the intensive care unit and periodically thereafter. Observations related to the ventilator are discussed in Chapter 16. The arterial line is flushed with normal saline hourly.

Movement of both sides of the chest is noted; unequal expansion of the two sides, audible moist sounds and dyspnoea should be reported.

Continuous recording of the rectal and peripheral temperature by an electric thermometer may be used for the first day or two. The wounds are observed at frequent intervals for possible bleeding.

Orientation, level of consciousness, restlessness and anxiety are significant and should be noted. Stasis of circulation during surgery may have resulted in the formation of a thrombus which later may move out as an embolus. Also, a small amount of air left in the heart on closing may cause an air embolism. For these reasons the patient's ability to move his limbs and his speech are tested every 1–2 hours. Any weakness or loss of function is promptly reported. Peripheral pulses in the limbs, as well as the radial pulse, are checked (dorsalis pedis, femoral and posterior tibial). The absence of one of these may point to a thrombosis or embolism.

Fluid intake and output are recorded. When his condition permits, the patient is weighed daily to detect possible retention of fluid.

Respiratory tests may be required at frequent intervals; the expiratory volume per minute may be estimated by the use of a spirometer. Blood specimens are collected for determination of blood gases, electrolyte concentrations, haemoglobin, and haematocrit.

Assisting respiratory function
As mentioned, the patient's endotracheal tube is attached to a mechanical ventilator. While the endotracheal tube is in place the patient is given suction every hour, or more often if necessary. The secretions are assessed for amount, colour and consistency. Suction can be a very frightening experience for the patient, so the procedure is explained before it is carried out. Careful aseptic technique is observed and each suction should not exceed 10 seconds.

After approximately 12–24 hours the patient is assessed to see if he can breathe spontaneously and adequately. If lung expansion is adequate and arterial blood gases are within acceptable limits, the endotracheal tube is removed. The patient then receives warm, humidified oxygen. If the patient is unable to be weaned from the ventilator, intermittent positive pressure ventilation is maintained. Should this situation persist, a tracheostomy may be performed.

Coughing every 1–2 hours is started as soon as the blood pressure is stabilized. The nurse assists the patient by elevating him to a sitting position and supporting the chest, back and front. If the coughing is not productive, and it is evident that secretions are present, suction is used.

Intermittent positive pressure ventilation may be used prior to chest physiotherapy to help loosen and moisten secretions and to help in lung expansion. When the patient is not being ventilated, he is encouraged to take five to ten deep breaths every 1–2 hours.

Deep breathing, coughing, turning and skin care are done at one time in order to provide a longer, undisturbed period for the patient.

Management of fluid loss
Drainage tubes are inserted into the thoracic cavity at the end of surgery to promote the drainage of blood and secretions. These tubes are connected to a tube which extends into the fluid in a drainage bottle. Keeping the end of the tube submerged in the water allows fluid and air to escape from the chest cavity but prevents air from entering the chest. (For details of closed, water-sealed drainage in chest surgery, see Chapter 16.) The system is observed at frequent intervals for functioning; the level of the fluid should

fluctuate in the tube in the bottle, with respirations and with coughing. To prevent blockage by a clot the tubes are 'milked' at least hourly for the first 24 hours. If the tubes are not draining it is reported promptly, since an accumulation of fluid in the thoracic cavity could cause serious cardiac embarrassment. The drainage is examined for possible bleeding, and the volume is measured. The tube must be clamped with two clamps close to the chest wall in the event of any disruption of the system.

The urine drainage is checked hourly for the first 24–36 hours, particularly if the blood pressure is low. An hourly output of 30 ml or less is brought to the doctor's attention since it may indicate the onset of a renal shutdown.

The total 12-hour or 24-hour output is recorded and the fluid balance determined.

Nutrition and fluids

For the first 24–48 hours the patient is maintained with intravenous fluids. The maximum amount to be given in an hour is specified and the rate of flow carefully controlled to prevent overloading the circulatory system and increasing the demand on the heart. The intravenous fluid is usually glucose 5% rather than saline.

Sips of water may be permitted to relieve the thirst sensation once the endotracheal tube is removed and the patient is able to swallow. Frequent mouth care also helps and is necessary to prevent infection. All fluid intake is measured and recorded. A positive balance may necessitate restricting the fluid intake to a prescribed volume.

The diet progresses from fluids to soft foods and then to light solid foods as tolerated. Frequent small amounts are more acceptable than larger amounts less often. Gas-forming foods are to be avoided, and sodium restriction may be indicated.

Rest

Uninterrupted periods of rest are important to reduce the demands on the heart. The various observations that must be made and the treatments, tests and doctors' visits sometimes make it difficult for the patient to get sufficient rest. The nurse should be alert to the problem and, if necessary, consult the doctor.

Psychological care

The patient who has had considerable preparation for what will follow the operation tends to accept the postoperative situation with less anxiety than patients who have not had a similar preparation. It is important that his questions are answered and that he receive some information as to his progress. Brief explanations of what is going to be done are appreciated by the patient and a visit from a family member is also reassuring.

It is not uncommon for the patient's spirits to fluctuate; he may have brief periods of depression and may become very irritable. Patience and understanding on the part of the nurse are important. An expression that indicates to the patient that she knows how he feels may provide some support.

Medications

Analgesics and sedatives are used sparingly with the cardiac surgical patient since they tend to depress respirations and the cough reflex.

A small dose of papaveretum (Omnopon) may be prescribed for the relief of pain. Close observation of the patient's response to the drug is necessary; respirations are checked before the administration and during the period following. Very judicious use of these drugs is necessary; to withhold the drug unnecessarily may be harmful, since pain and the patient's response to it may increase the demands on the respiratory system and the heart. The narcotic ordered by the doctor should be used only for pain—not for restlessness. The latter condition indicates the need for increased observation to determine its cause; it may be due to hypoxia or haemorrhage and should be reported.

A prophylactic antibiotic may be administered for a period of 5–10 days. The number of days will depend on the patient's history; if he has had rheumatic fever and rheumatic heart disease he will probably receive the antibiotic for a longer period to prevent reactivation of the rheumatic disease.

Digoxin may be prescribed to strengthen the heart. Quinidine sulphate or another antiarrhythmic drug may be necessary to treat fibrillation. If the patient experiences cardiac arrhythmias cautious use of antiarrhythmic drugs may be advised.

Exercises and mobility

To prevent circulatory stasis and thrombus formation some activity is desirable. Passive movements of the limbs are initiated first and are followed by active foot and leg exercises when indicated by the doctor. Later, active exercises are extended to include the arms and shoulders. A pull cord by which the patient may pull himself up may be attached to the foot of the bed. His next move will be to the side of the bed, then to a chair, and finally to self-care activities and walking.

The patient tends to immobilize the shoulders and arms and may develop 'frozen shoulders'. Gentle passive movement is all he may tolerate at first, but as soon as possible he is encouraged to use his arms and put them through a full range of motion as he was instructed preoperatively.

The starting of exercises and the rate of progression and degree of mobility will be decided for each patient. For example, the patient who has had surgical correction of a coarctation of the aorta must remain inactive for a much longer period than many other patients. The patient's responses will also be a factor in determining the amount of activity and when it should be started.

The family

When the operation has been performed, the family will be seen. They will be informed about what was done and advised about the patient's condition. It is then helpful if they may see the patient without disturbing him. Before taking them to the patient's room, a brief description of some of the equipment in use may reduce their concern when they enter the room. A close family member may wish to remain in the hospital for most of the day and may be allowed to look in on the patient briefly at intervals. The nurse who stops to speak briefly with the family and inform them of the patient's condition conveys to them an understanding of their anxiety.

Transfer from the intensive care unit

When patients are moved to various wards as their condition changes, the problem arises in the patient's adjustment to different environments and variations in the nursing care provided. Patients experience discomfort and anxiety upon leaving the intensive care unit where they receive more frequent observation and attention. The adjustment required may seem abrupt to the patient. Although requiring less monitoring and technical support, patients still need measures for relief of pain and fatigue, assistance with personal hygiene, teaching and guidance regarding activity, medications and diet, and opportunities to express emotional reactions to the experience of heart surgery. To make the transition as smooth as possible, communication is required between the staff of the units involved as to the patient's progress, individual reactions and needs.

Convalescence and rehabilitation

While the patient's physical activity is increased, his tolerance is noted. Any shortness of breath, cardiac pain, significant increase in heart rate or oedema is promptly reported and activity is stopped until the doctor has seen the patient.

Prescribed exercises are continued throughout convalescence and rehabilitation. A member of the family and the patient are given instructions about his care after discharge. How long he must curtail his activities and to what extent will depend on the patient's condition before and after the operation and on his responses to activity.

Planning for his return home and his rehabilitation should include consideration of the factors suggested on page 362 under Rehabilitation, recognizing of course that every programme must be determined on an individual basis.

SYSTEMIC DISEASE

Cardiac disease may be a secondary development in a disease in an area other than the heart. The primary disease may have placed an added strain on the circulation, or may have produced toxins or deficiencies in essential materials. Examples of these are diphtheria, hyperthyroidism, anaemia, septicaemia and pneumonia. Diphtheria produces a toxin that may cause myocarditis or may damage the conduction system. Diseases in which there is a prolonged and marked increase in the metabolic rate, as in hyperthyroidism, place an increased demand on the circulatory system to keep the overactive body cells supplied. Pulmonary conditions, such as pneumonia and emphysema, may produce a respiratory insufficiency that results in an inadequate oxygen supply to the heart muscle and a consequent cardiac inefficiency. They may also increase pulmonary pressures, putting an added strain on the heart.

HEART DISEASE IN PREGNANCY

The woman with a heart disease who contemplates having a child should consult a cardiologist. Many such women are quite able to bear a child and come through safely if they are closely supervised throughout pregnancy and follow the doctor's instructions. For others, pregnancy may carry considerable risk, since it creates increased demands on the heart.

During pregnancy, the total blood volume is increased as much as 25% by the seventh or eighth month. This increases the work load of the heart and persists 24 hours of the day, not just with physical activity. Some enlargement of the heart usually occurs in the normal pregnant woman. The changes in the concentration of certain hormones in pregnancy cause some retention of sodium. This varies in different women but does produce a hazard for the patient with a heart condition who, because of some cardiac insufficiency, may already be retaining an excess of sodium. The pregnant woman also experiences some shortness of breath as the enlarging uterus rises in the abdominal cavity, causing pressure on the diaphragm.

The nurse may be asked by the woman with a heart condition whether it is safe for her to become pregnant. She is advised to consult her doctor. If the woman confides in the nurse that she thinks she is already pregnant, she is urged to see her doctor at once. A thorough history is taken, and her heart's functional capacity is assessed. The doctor may tell her he believes it would be safe for her to have a child, but that it will be necessary for her to follow his instructions closely. The fact that pregnancy imposes an increased work load on the heart and that she has a reduced cardiac reserve should be explained to her and to her husband. Pregnancy for her will necessitate reduced activity, longer and more frequent rest periods, avoidance of infection and emotional stresses, weight control and restricted salt intake.

The patient and her husband will be instructed to get in touch promptly with the doctor if she experiences shortness of breath, palpitation, vomiting, any infection or gain in weight in excess of that suggested by the doctor. Frequent visits to the obstetrician and cardiologist are necessary. Weekly visits alternating between these two doctors may be requested.

If the woman develops any signs of cardiac failure she is put to bed and digoxin and a diuretic are prescribed. More stringent restrictions of sodium will be used. The midwife can give this patient a great deal of help and support and should know that the strain on the heart reaches a peak in the seventh and eighth months. During these later months of pregnancy, closer observation of the patient and a strict regimen are very important.

The patient may be allowed to go to full term, or the doctor may think it advisable to induce labour a few weeks before term. In caring for the patient during labour, the midwife is alert for early signs of cardiac failure. The pulse, blood pressure and respirations are noted at frequent intervals. Every effort is made to prevent unnecessary exertion and to provide the patient with as much rest as possible. Fluid intake and output are measured and recorded. The equipment and supplies used in the treatment of any heart patient are kept at hand.

Following delivery, close observation for manifestations of cardiac insufficiency and precautions to reduce the work load of the heart are continued.

THE SURGICAL PATIENT WITH IMPAIRED CARDIAC FUNCTION

The person with some cardiac insufficiency may require an operation. Unless it is an emergency, time is taken to assess carefully the functional capacity of the heart. Several tests are likely to be done which bear nursing responsibilities as discussed on page 315. The patient is closely observed during the period of preparation for any signs of failure; the recognition of such signs may influence his treatment and the risk which the surgery may carry.

This patient, knowing he has a heart condition, is likely to be more fearful than other surgical patients. The nurse encourages him to talk about his concerns and takes time to help him work through them. He should be advised that there will be a nurse with him constantly until he is conscious, that when he regains consciousness one will remain close by and visit him at frequent intervals, and that a doctor will be notified promptly of any change in his condition.

Surgery carries less risk for these patients than it did formerly; recent knowledge and new and improved techniques, equipment and anaesthetics have made surgery safer and provide more physiological support.

Postoperatively, the nurse provides even closer attention for this patient, since his condition could change suddenly. Frequent checking of vital signs, colour, level of consciousness and accurate recording of the fluid intake and output are necessary for several days longer than for most surgical patients. Any dyspnoea, cyanosis, abnormal pulse rate, rhythm or volume, positive fluid balance, apathy

and loss of consciousness are reported to the doctor promptly since they may indicate reduced cardiac function. If the patient is to receive intravenous fluids, the rate of flow and volume must be carefully controlled to avoid a sudden increase in the intravascular volume and an overloading of the impaired heart. Any surgical complications, such as infection and phlebitis, are extremely hazardous because they may precipitate failure.

Nursing in Vascular Diseases

Disturbance of circulation within the vascular system may originate in the arterial system (arteries and arterioles) or in the veins. In the case of the former, a partial or complete occlusion reduces the volume of blood into the part which the vessel supplies, and the tissues suffer oxygen and nutritional deficiency. If the site of the vascular problem is the veins, there is interference with the normal outflow of venous blood, causing congestion and oedema within the tissues. Vascular conditions may be chronic, developing slowly over a considerable period of time, or they may be sudden and acute.

ARTERIAL DISORDERS

AORTIC ANEURYSM

An aneurysm is a saccular dilatation of the wall of an artery and develops as a result of weakness in the wall of the vessel in that area. The weakness in the majority of cases is due to atherosclerosis but may also be caused by an infectious disease (e.g. syphilis), congenital defect or trauma. The aorta and cerebral arteries are the most common sites of aneurysms.

The aneurysm that does not extend completely around the artery is referred to as a *saccular aneurysm*. If it involves the complete circumference, it is classified as a *fusiform aneurysm*.

Separation of the layers of the aorta is referred to as a *dissecting aortic aneurysm*, even though no dilatation may be present. The tear is often in the intima and may be due to bleeding in the medial layer from the vasa vasorum. The dissection may extend lengthwise for a considerable distance and may involve branches of the aorta. The aortic aneurysm may also be classified according to the section of the artery in which the defect is located; for example, it may be designated as a thoracic or abdominal aortic aneurysm. The former may be further categorized as an ascending thoracic aortic aneurysm, a transverse thoracic aneurysm or a descending thoracic aortic aneurysm.

A serious threat to any patient with an aneurysm is

rupture of the weakened vascular area; the rapid loss of blood almost always proves fatal.

Manifestations

Signs and symptoms may be absent until the aneurysm is large enough to compress adjacent structures. The patient with a thoracic aneurysm may experience chest pain, dyspnoea, hoarseness due to vocal cord paralysis and/or congestion of the veins in the neck because of pressure on the superior vena cava. With an abdominal aneurysm, the patient may complain of midabdominal, lumbar or pelvic pain, often severe. Physical examination may reveal an expansile, abdominal mass. Femoral pulses may be reduced. Careful physical examination, x-rays, echocardiograms and/or aortography are means of confirming the diagnosis.

Symptoms of a dissecting aortic aneurysm include pain, often described as ripping or tearing in nature, and may involve the chest, back and/or abdomen. Blood pressure drops and there may be a discrepancy in pulses in various locations in the body.

Treatment

In recent years, encouraging advances have been made in the surgical treatment of aneurysms. If a small blood vessel is affected, it may be tied off and the flow of blood is diverted to another artery. In treating an aortic aneurysm, the area is resected and replaced with a graft of inert synthetic material such as Teflon or Dacron which does not cause tissue reaction.

Nursing management of the patient is similar to that for the patient having heart surgery see (p. 365).

ACUTE ARTERIAL OCCLUSION

Acute occlusion occurs suddenly as a result of external compression, thrombosis or embolism. It is serious because there is a lack of collateral circulation to the tissues supplied by this artery.

Arterial thrombosis occurs with the formation of an abnormal blood clot (thrombus) within an artery, usually as the result of narrowing of the lumen of the artery by atherosclerotic changes. The stasis in the blood flow predisposes to the formation of the clot, partially or completely blocking the vessel. If the vessel is not completely blocked, treatment is directed toward preventing the clot from enlarging to occlude the vessel and toward keeping it at the site of formation to prevent an embolism.

Arterial embolism is the blocking of an artery by a foreign mass that has been carried by the bloodstream until it reaches an artery too small for it to pass through. The foreign mass is referred to as an embolus.

Most frequently it is a thrombus that breaks loose from its site of origin, but it may consist of air, fragments of vegetations from diseased cardiac valves, fat, atherosclerotic plaques or small masses of tissue or cancerous cells. The effects of an embolism are determined by the localization of the embolus. The vessel which the embolus obstructs depends upon the size of the embolus, its origin, and whether the artery blocked is an end-artery or one that anastomoses above the block with smaller vessels in the part supplied. Obviously, if it is an end-artery, the tissue entirely dependent upon it becomes necrotic. An embolus originating in a vein or the right side of the heart is likely to cause a pulmonary embolism (see Chapter 16). One arising from the left side of the heart or a large systemic artery may produce a cerebral embolism or may plug a smaller artery. The site of arterial occlusion by an embolus may also be a lower extremity.

CHRONIC ARTERIAL OCCLUSION

This most frequently develops as a result of gradual changes in the walls of the vessels, causing narrowing of the lumen. It may also be of functional origin due to a hyperactivity of the sympathetic nervous system, causing an excessive vasoconstriction. Gradual occlusion of the vessels allows for collateral circulation to be established, lessening the problem of deprivation in the tissues distal to the occlusion.

The most common causes of chronic occlusion are atherosclerosis and arteriosclerosis. The arteries in any area of the body may be affected, but the coronary, cerebral and renal arteries are frequent sites. The problems caused by their insufficiency are discussed under disorders of the relative structures. When the abdominal aorta and/or medium- and large-sized arteries are involved, the condition may be referred to as *arteriosclerosis obliterans*. The arteries of the extremities are also a relatively frequent site of chronic occlusion that may be referred to as *peripheral vascular disease*. Two common forms of peripheral vascular disease are Raynaud's disease and thromboangiitis obliterans.

Raynaud's disease is a condition in which episodes of excessive vasoconstriction occur in the digits of the hands and/or feet. The cause is obscure, but the episodes are most frequently precipitated by cold or emotional stress. The disease is more common in females, usually develops before the age of 40–45 years and is bilateral.

Thromboangiitis obliterans (Buerger's disease) is a chronic occlusive disease in which there is an inflammation and thickening of the walls of limb arteries, predisposing to thrombosis. It has a higher incidence in young males and in Jewish people. The parts are very tender and painful, and necrotic areas develop in the distal portions of the digits. The condition is seriously aggravated if the person smokes. The cause of this disease is unknown.

Manifestations of arterial insufficiency in the extremities
These manifestations are due to the deficiencies in oxygen and nutrients to the tissues resulting from

the decreased blood supply into the limb. If there is a complete deprivation, the tissue cells die, and necrosis occurs in the form of ulceration or gangrene.

Pain. The patient may experience intermittent claudication. This is pain that occurs on exercise and is relieved by rest. The blood supply is sufficient to meet the tissue needs only when the part is at rest; on exercise, oxygen demands cannot be met. The pain may be constant even with the part at rest, indicating a decreased blood flow into the tissues or a complete obstruction. The pain may be described as aching or cramp-like and is often severe. The patient may complain of a numbness or tingling in the extremity.

Pulse. A weakness or absence of peripheral pulses may be evident. In the arm, the radial, ulnar, brachial or axillary artery may be palpated with the fingertips, and in the leg the dorsalis pedis, popliteal or femoral artery may be felt. An oscillometer or Doppler flowmeter may be used to palpate the pulsation of arteries in an area where the vessels are deeper and cannot be palpated by the fingers. A comparison is made of the pulse in the different arteries and would reveal a partial block if one were present. Complete occlusion would be indicated by an absence of the pulse.

Colour. A difference in the colour of the two extremities or an abnormal change in both extremities, if both are involved, will most likely be present. The skin may become white and blanched, or it may become a dusky red or cyanosed, depending on the amount of blood in the capillaries and the amount of reduced haemoglobin in the blood. On being raised, the limb becomes even paler as the venous drainage increases but, on being lowered, it fails to increase its colour as the normal limb would do quickly with the rush of arterial blood into it. The superficial veins are slow in filling when the limb is lowered; normally, they fill in approximately 5 seconds.

Skin temperature. The skin temperature and moisture may be different in the two limbs. The affected one exhibits a coldness to the touch and may be unusually moist. The warmth of the skin is dependent on the heat brought to the part by the blood. The moisture may point to excessive sympathetic stimulation, causing vasospasm.

Atrophy of tissues. Limb tissues may atrophy, causing the affected limb to become smaller than the other. The skin becomes dry and shiny and loses its hair. Nails thicken and become brittle and ridged.

Necrosis. Ulcerated or gangrenous areas may develop, denoting areas of tissue completely deprived of a blood supply. Ulceration is a superficial area of devitalized tissue; gangrene is a more massive area of dead tissue.

Diagnostic procedures
'In most instances, a thorough history and an adequate vascular physical examination result in an accurate diagnosis of occlusive arterial disease. Non-invasive instrumentation is helpful in confirming the diagnosis . . .'[25]
Various tests may be used by the doctor in diagnosing and assessing vascular disease.

Exercise tolerance. The patient is required to walk or perform some form of exercise until intermittent claudication occurs. The length of time from the start of activity until the occurrence of pain is noted.

Angiography. The method frequently used to locate the site of occlusion precisely is angiography, either aortography or selective arteriography. A radiopaque dye is introduced into the arteries, and x-rays are made of the vessels. The site of narrowing or obstruction may be located in this way, and some information as to the amount of collateral circulation present may also be obtained.

Ultrasonic arteriography. Images of arteries, which are comparable to x-ray angiography, are produced by ultrasonic technique. By this non-invasive method, the dimensions and configurations of arteries are mapped.

Reactive hyperaemia. In this test, the flow of blood into the limb is reduced by the application of a tourniquet or blood pressure cuff for 2–3 minutes. On release, vasodilation normally follows, and blood flows in very quickly to produce warmth and flushing of the skin. In arterial insufficiency the flow of blood into the part is delayed.

Radiography. If the problem is arteriosclerosis, calcified deposits may show up in x-ray pictures but this does not necessarily indicate an obstruction to blood flow.

Treatment and nursing care of the patient with arterial occlusive disease
The aims in the care of the patient are:
1 To prevent further progress of the condition causing the ischaemia in the limbs.
2 To prevent complications, such as dryness and cracking of the skin, infection and ulceration, since the resistance of the tissues is lower.
3 To increase the blood supply to the extremities.
4 To keep the demands of the tissues within the limits of the existing blood supply into the limb.

Arterial occlusive disease (peripheral vascular disease) is a chronic condition, and the patient will most likely have to continue with the prescribed care and precautions indefinitely. It may create consider-

---

[25] Young & de Wolfe (1982), p. 1459.

able hardship for the patient and his family, depending on the severity of the disease and the limitations it imposes. Adjustments may have to be made in his occupational and social life; he may become partially or completely dependent financially and for his personal care. The patient will certainly find it difficult to accept the situation and will react accordingly. The nurse must be alert to the possible implications for the patient and family and should provide the necessary assistance and guidance.

The patient and a member of his family are instructed in the necessary care. They should understand that adherence to the doctor's suggestions and regular supervision are all important in preventing serious complications.

Diet. Obesity should be avoided, since excess tissue always increases the demands on the circulatory system. Overweight people tend to be less active, which does not favour circulation. Protein and vitamin C are usually increased to provide maximum maintenance and support of the tissues suffering a degree of ischaemia. An increase in B vitamins may be recommended, especially if there is peripheral nerve involvement and the patient is experiencing peripheral neuritis. The saturated fat and cholesterol content of the diet will probably be reduced and vegetable fat substituted for most of the animal fat if the arterial insufficiency is due to atherosclerosis.

An optimum fluid intake is important in maintaining a normal vascular volume and in preventing possible haemoconcentration predisposing to thrombus formation.

Smoking. The use of tobacco is discontinued, since it promotes vasoconstriction and aggravates the disease. The close relationship between thromboangiitis obliterans and cigarette smoking suggests that tobacco is a causative agent in this condition.

Protection from cold. Exposure to cold with lowering of normal body temperature produces undesirable responses—namely, peripheral vasoconstriction and increased metabolism. Special precautions are necessary in cold weather. Extra, warm clothing should be worn, and a change of residence to a warmer climate may be helpful. If exposure to cold precipitates an episode, the patient is advised to take a warm drink and seek a warm environment. A warm bath or a heating pad to the abdomen may be used to produce reflex vasodilation in the limbs. Local heat applications to the affected parts are discouraged because the tissue resistance is lowered and, frequently, there is a reduced nerve sensitivity. The patient is advised to wear warm socks or to wrap his feet in a warm blanket rather than applying a hot water bottle.

Protection of the affected limbs. Extra precautions are necessary to protect the affected limbs from trauma and infection. Daily bathing in comfortably warm (not hot) water using a mild soap is recommended. Gentle and thorough drying is important, and special attention is given to the areas between the digits. If the skin is dry, the limbs may be gently massaged with lanolin or some light emollient. Nails are cut straight across but not right down to the soft tissue. A pumice stone may be used on calluses, but corns should be removed by a chiropodist; the patient should not undertake to 'pare' them with sharp instruments. The extremities, especially the terminal portions, are examined daily for changes: any discoloration, blister, broken area of skin, tenderness and swelling are to be promptly seen by the doctor.

The patient is advised of the importance of well-fitting shoes and socks or stockings. Socks should be loose and are changed daily. The patient is instructed to avoid walking about in bare feet; a cut, abrasion, sliver or infection could be quite serious, since the tissue resistance is lowered and healing is poor. If injury does occur, even of a minor nature, it should receive prompt medical attention. Anything tight or restricting, such as round garters, must not be worn. The pressure of bedclothes can be prevented by using a footboard or bed-cradle at the foot of the bed.

Positioning. The horizontal position is used when the patient rests unless the doctor suggests otherwise. Occasionally, raising the head of the bed may be used to encourage the flow of blood into the lower limbs by gravity. Position should be changed at frequent intervals throughout the day, and long periods of standing must be avoided. The patient is advised not to cross his legs and, when sitting, pressure on the popliteal region is avoided. If ambulatory, he sits or lies down every 2–3 hours and elevates his feet for 10–15 minutes.

Measures to increase the blood supply to the extremities

Activity. Many authorities indicate the most effective treatment for intermittent claudication is physical exercise, especially walking. It is suggested that the patient should exercise 20–30 minutes daily. He may do this by walking to the point of distress, stopping until the discomfort disappears, and then continuing to walk until the distress develops again. The patient repeats this exercise for the prescribed period. The underlying theory is that exercise increases collateral circulation.

Exercises. Buerger–Allen exercises may be used for arterial insufficiency in the lower limbs. The leg is raised to approximately 45° above the horizontal and held until it blanches (1–2 minutes). It is then lowered to below the horizontal (over the side of the bed) until it becomes pink and then returned to the horizontal level for 1–2 minutes. This is repeated five to ten times every 6 or 8 hours. A padded support at the required height is provided for the elevation part of the cycle. The timing is determined by how long it takes for venous drainage and for refilling of the vessels, so the colour must be observed closely and timed at first.

Passive and active exercises may also be prescribed; flexion and extension of the legs, feet and toes may be used for lower limbs, and similar exercises may be employed for the arms and fingers if these are the sites of the arterial insufficiency. Exercises promote emptying and filling of the vessels and stimulate the development of collateral circulation.

Reflex dilatation. Warm baths or increasing general body warmth by a higher environmental temperature may produce a reflex vasodilatation.

Oscillating bed. Alternate raising and lowering of the limbs to promote more efficient emptying and filling of the blood vessels may be achieved passively by placing the patient on an electric oscillating bed. A rocking motion is produced by a motor that can be set to tilt the bed longitudinally at a definite rate. The length of the period for operation may gradually be increased as the patient adjusts to the repeated tilting. It may be operated day and night and is helpful in relieving and preventing the pain which is associated with immobility. The patient is taught how to operate the motor, since the switch is readily available to him.

Drugs. Vasodilating and anticoagulant drugs have been used to treat patients with arterial occlusive disease.

Although many drugs are promoted as agents capable of increasing peripheral blood flow, many are universally ineffective.[26] Any alpha-adrenergic blocking drug will increase the flow through the skin but no drug can increase flow to muscles when the underlying disease is atherosclerosis of a major artery.

Anticoagulant drugs may be prescribed to prevent and treat thrombosis. The most widely used anticoagulants are heparin and warfarin. Aspirin or sulphinpyrazone (Anturan) may be used. Heparin is given parenterally since it has no effect orally. It is thought to block the effect of thrombin on fibrinogen, thereby preventing clot formation. Heparin begins to be effective within minutes after administration and is prolonged for 3–4 hours. It may be given in a continuous intravenous drip or at regularly spaced intervals. Heparin therapy is usually extended over several days and then gradually replaced by a warfarin preparation given orally. Warfarin takes effect in approximately 48 hours, so it is started before the heparin is withdrawn.

---

[26] Bailey, Hampton, Jones et al (1983), pp. 164–185.

The dosage and frequency of warfarin administration is dependent each day upon the prothrombin time of that day. The dosage of heparin is decided by the partial thromboplastin time (PTT). A therapeutic level is generally considered to be one and one-half times to twice the normal values for the PTT. A clotting time is done when partial thromboplastin time cannot be measured.

These drugs produce the risk of bleeding but their therapeutic value may be considered to outweigh this risk.

The nurse's responsibilities include close observation for signs of haemorrhage. Profuse bleeding from minor cuts, bleeding gums, haematuria, haematemesis, blood in the stool, petechiae and abnormal vaginal bleeding are reported promptly. In the event of bleeding the drug is discontinued, and vitamin K and a blood transfusion may be given to counteract the reduced coagulation. Protamine sulphate, a heparin antagonist, is given if severe bleeding occurs as a result of heparin administration.

The prothrombin or partial thromboplastin time is determined by the doctor before the anticoagulant drug is administered. Patients outside the hospital taking anticoagulants are usually required to report to the clinic weekly for a prothrombin time check. More recently, drugs which prevent platelet aggregation, such as aspirin and sulphinpyrazone (Anturan), are being used to prevent arterial thrombosis.

Surgical treatment and care. If there is evidence of a decrease in vasomotor tone and improved circulation in the limbs in a diagnostic sympathetic block, a lumbar sympathectomy (removal of the second, third and fourth ganglia) may be performed.

A direct surgical approach may be employed in which the surgeon chooses to do an endarteriectomy, a bypass or a graft. An endarteriectomy is the removal of the thickened intima and atheromatous plaques from the artery and is used when the disease is localized to a relatively small area. The establishment of a bypass channel in order to reduce the arterial insufficiency may be achieved by transplanting one end of another artery into the occluded artery below the site of obstruction or by an autogenous venous graft. The latter consists of the removal of a section of a vein (usually the saphenous), reversing it (because of the valves) to ensure flow in the right direction and attaching it to the affected artery above and below the occlusion. The surgeon often elects to resect the affected segment of the artery and replace it with an inert synthetic (Teflon or Dacron) graft. This type of graft is relatively porous and is eventually incorporated into host tissues. An intima develops within it fairly quickly as cells proliferate through the interstices and from the host intima of the artery at each end of the graft. A layer of fibrous tissue also develops on the exterior surface, reinforcing the tube.

The most frequent site of major vascular surgery

for occlusive disease is the aorta and the iliac and femoral arteries.

Nursing responsibilities in the care of a patient having major vascular surgery include those applicable to most surgical patients, as cited in Chapter 11, as well as the following considerations.

1 *Preoperative preparation.* Local preparation involves the shaving and cleansing of the skin from the nipple line to the knees. The patient's blood is typed and crossmatched in readiness for transfusions during and after the operation.

The patient and family are advised that he may be taken to the intensive care unit following surgery. To avoid unnecessary concern later, they are given some information about the nasogastric tube and the suction decompression, intravenous infusion, urinary catheter drainage, cardiac monitoring and frequent checking of pulse and blood pressure that will follow surgery.

2 *Postoperative care.* It is very important that the nurse understands the patient's disease process and the corrective surgical procedure used.

(a) Observations. The nurse is alerted to the possible complications of thrombosis in the graft, haemorrhage and embolism. Heart action is constantly monitored so that any adverse change is quickly detected. Arterial pressures are recorded at frequent intervals.

Peripheral pulses in the lower limbs are checked frequently. Those in the feet may not be detectable after surgery but, if they cannot be felt, it is brought to the surgeon's attention. The pulses used are the femoral, popliteal, dorsalis pedis and posterior tibial. The femoral pulse may be felt in the middle of the groin, and the popliteal is located behind the knee. The dorsalis pedis pulse is found in the central region of the dorsum of the foot, and the posterior tibial behind the medial malleolus. With the latter two, it is helpful to mark the location on the skin so they can be readily checked. When only one limb has been affected, a comparison of the distal pulse is made with that of the unaffected limb.

Skin temperature and colour are assessed and, where applicable, a comparison is made between the affected and unaffected limbs. Blanching or cyanosis and a lowering of the temperature in areas distal to the operative site must be reported quickly.

Restlessness, general pallor, a rapid pulse of decreased volume, increased respirations and a fall in arterial blood pressures associated with bleeding necessitate prompt medical attention.

The patient's level of consciousness, speech, strength of hand grip and ability to move his limbs are checked frequently. A disturbance in any one area may indicate a cerebral embolism.

(b) Positioning. The revascularized area is usually elevated to a level above that of the heart to promote venous and lymphatic drainage and to prevent oedema. The sudden increase in the blood supply may exceed the drainage capacity unless it is assisted by gravity.

(c) Care of affected limb. The skin breaks down very easily, necessitating special protective measures against pressure and trauma. A bed-cradle is used to relieve the limb of the weight of bedclothes, and the foot rests on sheepskin. The toes are separated by loose absorbent cotton to prevent maceration. The skin is bathed and handled gently. A light application of lanolin may be used to relieve dryness and scaling.

(d) Coughing and exercises. The patient is required to breath deeply and cough hourly to improve pulmonary ventilation. The ankles and toes are flexed 10 times hourly to prevent venous stasis. These flexion exercises may have to be passive until the patient is sufficiently responsive to carry them out himself.

(e) Fluids and nutrition. The patient is sustained by intravenous infusions of 5% glucose. Saline solutions are avoided with most patients with circulatory problems because of their tendency to retain the sodium.

Aspiration of the nasogastric tube is discontinued and the tube removed 2 or 3 days after surgery if there is no nausea or abdominal distension. The patient receives clear fluids at first and, if these are tolerated, the diet is gradually increased. High protein and vitamin C content contribute to the healing and resistance of affected tissues.

(f) Instruction. In preparation for the patient's discharge from hospital, he is advised of his need to avoid sitting with his hips and knees flexed for long periods. If necessary, continued abstinence from smoking is stressed. He is made aware of ominous changes (pain, discoloration, cold, abrasions, oedema) in his limbs that would necessitate prompt medical attention. The doctor gives him some idea of when he may expect to resume former activities and makes an appointment for a follow-up visit to him or the clinic.

VENOUS DISORDERS

As stated earlier, interference with the flow of blood through the veins reduces venous return from the part, inducing congestion and oedema, which interfere with normal cell function and eventually prevent a normal arterial volume from reaching the tissue cells. Common venous conditions are varicose veins, thrombophlebitis and phlebothrombosis.

VARICOSE VEINS

When venous blood meets with increased resistance

to its forward flow, the walls of the veins become dilated and tortuous, the valves become damaged and incompetent and the blood tends to pool and stagnate. The condition may be referred to as varicosities, or as varicose veins. The superficial veins of the lower extremities are most susceptible. Because of our upright position, the venous pressure in the lower limbs is increased by gravity. Other common sites of varicosities are the veins of the anal canal (haemorrhoids), spermatic veins (varicocele), oesophageal veins (oesophageal varices), and the vulvar veins in pregnant women due to pressure from the enlarging uterus. Although resistance to the flow of blood is the main cause of varicosities, an inherited weakness of the valves of the veins is said to be a factor. Long periods of standing also predispose to the development of varicose veins in the lower extremities.

The overfull veins result in local oedema of the tissues, crampy pains or aching, and a full, heavy feeling in the affected area. The congestion and oedema in the tissues interfere with the normal supply of oxygen and nutrients reaching the cells, leading to fibrosing of subcutaneous tissues and, in some instances, necrosis of superficial tissue, producing what is referred to as a varicose ulcer. The affected area appears swollen and discoloured, and the veins are seen as tortuous, bulbous protrusions. These veins readily develop phlebitis, and occasionally the vessel wall ruptures, causing haemorrhage.

The test most frequently done for varicosities in the lower limbs is the Trendelenburg test. While the patient is in the horizontal position, the leg is elevated above the level of the pelvis until the superficial veins appear to be empty. The patient then stands, and the veins are observed as they fill. Normally they fill relatively slowly from below; in varicosities, the incompetent valves allow them to fill from above as well.

Treatment and nursing care of a patient with varicose veins
Treatment may be conservative. The patient is instructed to avoid situations and factors that tend to increase the resistance to venous flow, to provide support to the veins and tissues by bandages or elastic compression stockings, and to assist drainage by elevation of the limb at intervals.

If the varicosity is not extensive, the doctor may inject a sclerosing agent (e.g. sodium tetradecyl sulphate or ethanolamine oleate) into the veins. The varicosed segment becomes inflamed, scarred and thrombosed by the sclerosing agent. Antihistamines and the emergency drug tray are kept readily available in the event of a reaction.

With more severe varicosities in the lower limbs, surgical treatment in the form of ligation and stripping of the veins may be employed, usually under general anaesthesia. The affected vein is ligated above the varicosity, its connecting branches

are severed and tied, and the vein removed. The venous blood then returns via the deep veins. The great saphenous vein is the one most frequently ligated and removed from the groin to the ankle. This necessitates several small horizontal incisions along the course of the vein. Elastic bandages are applied from the foot to the groin after the operation, and the foot of the bed is elevated. Beginning soon after operation, usually the day following surgery, the patient will be required to get up at regular intervals and walk about to prevent thrombosis. He may experience stiffness and some pain on movement and is given the necessary assistance and support. Early regular activity is very important and is explained to the patient in order to gain his cooperation.

In the postoperative period, the nurse observes the limb at regular, frequent intervals. The wound areas are checked for bleeding, and the feet and toes are examined for colour, warmth and sensation, so that any disturbance in the circulation will receive early recognition. If there is bleeding, if the distal parts are cold or cyanosed, or the patient experiences numbness, pain or 'pins and needles,' the bandage should be removed and the surgeon informed promptly.

The patient is usually only hospitalized for a brief period of 2–3 days. He is advised as to how long to continue the alternating periods of rest and walking and the bandaging and elevation of the limbs. He is taught how to apply and care for the elastic bandages or stockings and is told when to return to the doctor or clinic. Since the superficial tissue continues to be tender and has less resistance, he is instructed to use precautions against injuries and abrasions. Long periods of standing are still be be avoided.

All patients with leg varicosities should avoid constricting clothing, such as round garters and tight girdles. They are also advised not to sit with their legs crossed. As with all circulatory conditions, obesity is to be avoided.

Varicose ulcers develop very easily with the circulatory stasis but are very slow to heal. The patient may have to rest in bed with the affected leg elevated or, if he remains active, an elastic bandage or stocking is applied in an effort to reduce the oedema and congestion.

There are a variety of methods for treating varicose ulcers, commonly involving aseptic cleansing, a dressing and the application of pressure on the whole limb by means of a variety of bandages or elastic compression stockings. Antiseptic solutions are often used. Leaper argues that evidence is beginning to suggest that this may not always be appropriate, particularly since the introduction of the 'moist environment for healing', offered by the occlusive and semipermeable dressings.[27] Normal saline is

---

[27] Leaper (1986) pp. 45 & 47.

sometimes the agent used and, if healing does not occur, grafts with porcine dermis have been employed.

THROMBOPHLEBITIS AND PHLEBOTHROMBOSIS

Phlebitis is an inflammation of the walls of a vein and may be caused by injury, prolonged pressure or infection. The endothelial lining is damaged and a thrombus develops at the site of inflammation, producing a secondary condition known as thrombophlebitis.

Phlebothrombosis is the formation of a blood clot within a vein with no associated inflammation and for this reason may be referred to as a bland or silent thrombosis. It is nearly always due to slowness or stasis of the circulation, such as occurs with prolonged bed rest, inactivity or pressure causing resistance to the venous blood flow. The serious factor in both phlebothrombosis and thrombophlebitis is the blood clot, which becomes a potential embolus. The silent thrombus or that associated with inflammation may be carried along in the bloodstream and may eventually lodge in an artery to cause an embolism. Phlebitis and venous thrombosis may occur in any vein, but the most frequent site is the saphenous veins of the legs.

Manifestations

Thrombophlebitis in superficial veins produces local pain, tenderness and swelling. The pain may vary from moderate discomfort on touching the limb to severe cramping. If the leg is involved, there may be calf pain during dorsiflexion of the foot (Homans' sign). Systemic symptoms such as fever, headache, and general malaise develop. If the vein is superficial, the overlying skin becomes red and hot. It may be taut and shiny.

With deep vein thrombosis, the process may be silent. No symptoms may be present until the thrombus is swept along and causes an embolism. In either phlebothrombosis or thrombophlebitis, the thrombus may become large enough to block the vein, causing severe congestion, oedema and pain.

Prevention

Circulatory stasis in the lower limbs is the principal cause of phlebothrombosis, so efforts are directed toward avoiding prolonged inactivity and positions which favour its development. Passive movement and active exercises, especially of the lower limbs, and frequent change of position are used for patients who are inactive or confined to bed. Early ambulation is always to be encouraged when the condition permits. A dorsal recumbent position with the knees flexed and supported by a pillow is always contraindicated, since it promotes a venous stasis in the legs. Sitting for hours is discouraged because the legs are dependent and there is a risk of pressure on the veins in the popliteal region. Sitting should be alternated with periods of walking around or lying down. The patient is instructed not to sit with his legs crossed, but to extend his legs, rotate his feet at the ankles, and flex and extend his toes five to ten times hourly when sitting for an extended period. People with leg varicosities are predisposed to phlebothrombosis and thrombophlebitis. Bandaging their lower limbs up to the groin with elastic bandages or stockings provides support to the veins and promotes venous return when they are not mobile.

Treatment and nursing care of a patient with thrombophlebitis

When thrombophlebitis develops, care is directed toward preventing an embolism and relieving the congestion and oedema of the tissues. The patient is confined to bed, and the affected limb immobilized in an elevated position to promote venous and lymphatic drainage. Active exercise and massage of the limb are contraindicated to avoid possible dislodging of the thrombus and ensuing embolism, but are applied to unaffected extremities. All strenuous activity, straining at stool, coughing and deep breathing are discouraged. The circulation of the affected extremity is checked frequently.

Local heat applications, moist or dry, may be prescribed. Precautions are taken to avoid burns since the skin is very susceptible to injury. A footboard or cradle is used to keep the weight of the bedclothes off the limbs.

Anticoagulant therapy is started as soon as the thrombosis is recognized (see p. 374). Rarely, if the patient is experiencing severe pain from vascular spasm, a sympathetic ganglionic block may be done to relax the veins. Analgesics are ordered for the relief of pain.

If the clot is dislodged, it will be carried along by the venous blood through the right side of the heart into the pulmonary circulation, where it is likely to cause a pulmonary embolism. Pain in the chest, dyspnoea, coughing, haemoptysis, rapid weak pulse and pallor are reported promptly. A lung scan (see Chapter 16) may be done to confirm the diagnosis.

After 7–10 days, if the symptoms have subsided, mobility is permitted. An elastic bandage or antiembolic stocking is applied before the patient gets out of bed. Activity is alternated with periods of rest. During the rest period the limb is elevated to the horizontal position or higher. The leg is examined for swelling and discoloration following ambulation and following a period of sitting. The patient may have to wear an elastic support indefinitely and must plan to avoid prolonged periods in which the limb is in the dependent position. The doctor may suggest that it is important that the limb be elevated above heart level for several brief periods through the day. This is more often necessary following a thrombosis of the larger deep veins. Before going home, the nurse teaches the patient the application and care of the bandages or elastic stockings. He is helped to understand the importance of the prescribed periods of elevation of the limbs and that he must be in the dorsal recumbent position to do this. The patient is also advised not to stand for long periods of time, to alternately flex and extend the legs frequently when sitting, to avoid constricting clothing, not to smoke and to report any further symptoms to his doctor immediately. If discharged on anticoagulant medication, the purpose, dosage, times of administration and side-effects are reviewed with the patient and, if possible, a member of his family or other significant person. The patient is followed closely in the clinic or the doctor's office for some time following the phlebothrombosis.

Nursing in Hypertension

Hypertension is a condition in which there is a sustained elevation of the arterial blood pressure. The level at which the normal blood pressure becomes abnormally high is not firmly established, but Dustan states that borderline hypertension is used for those readings consistently between 140/90 and 160/95 mmHg. Readings above 160/95 are termed definite hypertension.[28] These readings may be further classified as mild, moderate and severe: the diastolic pressures being 95–104, mmHg, 105–114 mmHg and 115 mmHg or greater.[28] The diastolic pressure is the more significant since it reflects the degree of peripheral resistance.

Hypertension is a serious condition. It is a common cause of heart failure and cerebral vascular haemorrhage. The sustained elevation in the arterial blood pressure seriously increases the work load of the heart and causes organic changes in the arteries. The myocardium hypertrophies in response to the increased demands, but there is not an adequate increase in the coronary blood supply and eventually some failure develops. The changes in the arterial walls involve thickening and sclerosis which alter the blood supply to tissues and ultimately may reduce their functional ability. The arteries may develop necrotic areas that weaken and tend to rupture under the high pressure of the blood, or they may thicken and narrow the lumen, predisposing to thrombosis. The areas of most serious damage are the heart, kidneys, brain and eyes, and these most often account for the symptoms seen in hypertensive patients. Cerebral vascular accident (stroke) is a common sequela. Kidney function becomes impaired as the result of sclerosing haemorrhage or thrombosis of the renal arteries which destroys functional tissue. Retinal haemorrhages and oedema of the optic disc occur frequently, resulting in degenerative changes in the eyes. Thickening and sclerosis of the coronary

arteries may cause ischaemic heart disease; the patient may experience angina pectoris or suffer a coronary occlusion in addition to developing the myocardial hypertrophy previously mentioned.

TYPES OF HYPERTENSION

Hypertension may be classified as primary (essential) or secondary. Approximately 90% of people with hypertensive disease are said to have essential hypertension; the remaining 10% have secondary hypertension.[29]

PRIMARY OR IDIOPATHIC HYPERTENSION

Primary hypertension is most frequently referred to as essential or idiopathic hypertension. The cause of this type of hypertensive disease is not known; no initial disturbance in the areas commonly associated with secondary hypertension has been established. It may cause cardiac or kidney disease but is not preceded by either. Heredity is thought to be a factor, since most persons with the condition have a history of a parent or grandparent having had it. There is a higher incidence in females, and the majority of hypertensive women are overweight.

Essential hypertension may be referred to as benign or malignant. The term benign, rarely used, is applied to essential hypertension that persists over 10–20 years without causing serious problems. Malignant indicates a rapidly progressive and serious condition. The patient develops kidney and heart complications and other sequelae very quickly and survives only a few months to 1 or 2 years at the most.

Essential hypertension may be classified according to the degree of severity of the disease. The numerical grading is based on changes in the ocular fundi, the response to treatment, the amount of cardiac hypertrophy and the effect on kidney function. Grades 3 and 4 are considered serious, and the patient with a Grade 4 hypertension as well as papilloedema may be said to have a malignant hypertension.

SECONDARY HYPERTENSION

Causes of secondary hypertension include the following:

Coarctation of the aorta
Obviously, a congenital stricture of an area of the aorta increases the resistance to the flow of blood through the vessel, causing an increase in the arterial pressure behind the coarctation. This may be corrected by surgery.

---

[28] Dustan (1986), p. 1042.

[29] Guyton (1984), p. 284.

Disturbances within the central nervous system
Interference with the vasomotor centre or with pathways from the centre may result in an increased vasoconstriction and peripheral resistance. Space-occupying lesions, such as a brain tumour, increased intracranial pressure, a cerebral thrombosis or poliomyelitis are examples of conditions which may lead to the malfunctioning of the vasomotor centre or pathway.

Endocrine disturbance
A phaeochromocytoma is a tumour of the adrenal medulla. Tumours may be single or multiple. The tumour cells secrete adrenaline in the same way as normal medullary cells, which produces vasoconstriction and an increased cardiac output with a corresponding elevation in arterial blood pressure. Removal of the tumour restores a normal blood pressure.

An increased output of aldosterone by the cortex of the adrenal glands may also be responsible for hypertension. The increased secretion may be idiopathic or may be due to a tumour. Aldosterone increases the reabsorption of sodium by the kidney, leading to water retention and an expansion of the intravascular volume, increasing the arterial blood pressure. It is suggested that aldosterone may also have a direct vasoconstricting effect. A general increase in the secretion of all of the adrenocorticoids causes Cushing's disease, which is also accompanied by hypertension.

Oral contraceptives
Some women taking oral contraceptives may develop hypertension. It is thought that the oestrogen component of the pills may be responsible by stimulating hepatic synthesis of angiotensinogen which leads to increased amounts of angiotensin.[30] The contraceptive agents are discontinued for 6 months and the blood pressure usually returns to normal.

Kidney disturbance
Any condition which reduces the blood flow through the kidneys or destroys renal functional tissue causes hypertension. Examples of such conditions are sclerotic changes or stenosis of a renal artery, nephritis and polycystic disease. The ischaemic kidney reacts by secreting a proteolytic enzyme called renin (see Fig. 14.15). In the bloodstream, renin acts upon a plasma protein to produce angiotensin I which is then converted to angiotensin II by another enzyme. This angiotensin II causes widespread vasoconstriction of the arterioles and increased peripheral resistance, leading to an elevation of arterial blood pressure. Angiotensin II is also alleged to increase

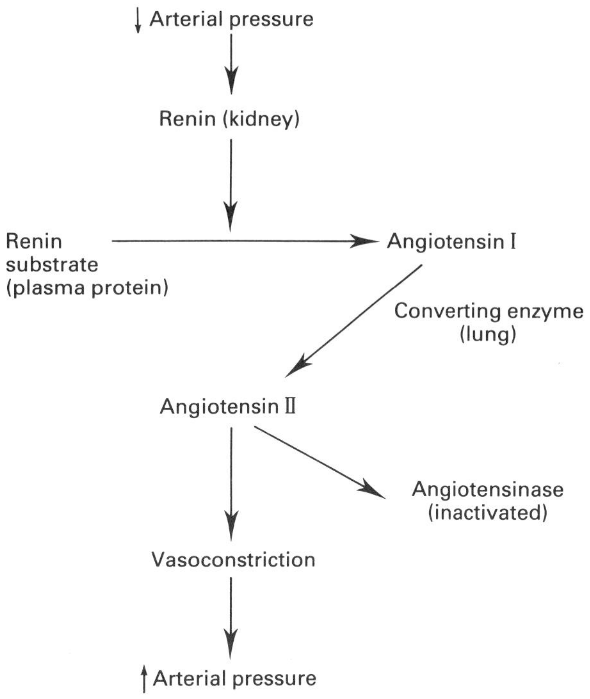

Fig. 14.15 Renin–angiotensin vasoconstriction mechanism for arterial pressure control.

the secretion of aldosterone by the adrenal glands[31] which, as previously cited, increases the blood pressure through its influence on sodium and water retention.

Toxaemia of pregnancy
Hypertension is a feature of toxaemia in pregnancy in which there is renal involvement.

MANIFESTATIONS OF HYPERTENSION

A person may have an abnormally high arterial blood pressure for a long period without symptoms. The condition is often discovered on a routine physical examination. Some people may exhibit a higher than average normal blood pressure and, on investigation, may produce a higher than average response to stimuli that normally elicit an increase in blood pressure. The stimuli under which people are observed are generally cold and exertion. Those who manifest an excessively high response are said to have vascular hyperactivity and are most likely headed for hypertension.

Those who do experience symptoms may complain of a throbbing occipital headache, especially on wakening in the morning, dizziness, visual disturbance, fatigue, irritability and restlessness,

---

[30] Hurst (1986), p. 1564.

[31] Guyton (1984).

vomiting, emotional instability or epistaxis. Patients with phaeochromocytoma often have pounding headaches, excessive sweating and flushing of the face, and are often under the age of 30. Later, more serious manifestations appear as the heart, kidneys, brain or eyes become damaged by the persisting hypertension. The person who manifests even a slight elevation above the normal in both systolic and diastolic blood pressures undergoes careful investigation to determine a possible primary cause.

DIAGNOSTIC PROCEDURES

Several systems may be investigated in an attempt to identify the cause of the hypertension. The renal and endocrine systems are the more important of these.

RENAL SYSTEM

Blood levels of creatinine and urea are determined. Twenty-four-hour urine collections may be ordered and examined for proteins, creatinine and electrolytes. When the renal system is damaged, proteins not normally present may leak into the urine. An intravenous pyelogram may be ordered in which serial 1-minute films are taken. The differential secretion rates of the two kidneys are studied. Minor differences may be apparent in rapid films that might go unrecognized in the standard 5-, 10- and 20-minute films. A renal scan and renal arteriograms are occasionally done.

ENDOCRINE SYSTEM

Adrenal secretions
A 24-hour urine collection is tested for levels of 17-ketosteroids and 17-hydroxycorticosteroids. The former is the excreted form of the androgen hormone and the latter is the product of the breakdown of the hormones cortisone and hydrocortisone. A more precise screening test for Cushing's syndrome is the dexamethasone suppression test. When dexamethasone 0.5 mg is given every 6 hours for 48 hours to people with normally functioning adrenal glands, adrenal corticoid production is suppressed, as evidenced by decreased amounts of cortisol in the urine. This does not occur in persons with bilateral adrenal hyperplasia.

The 24-hour urine collection is also tested for electrolytes. With increased mineralocorticoid production, sodium excretion is decreased while potassium excretion is increased. Tests for sugar, serum cortisol and serum electrolytes are also done. With Cushing's disease, the blood sugar and cortisol levels are elevated. Serum potassium will be below normal.

Test for phaeochromocytoma
The urine is collected over 24 hours and examined for the presence of vanillylmandelic acid (VMA). The latter is a metabolite of catecholamines which is secreted in the urine. In some institutions, the patient is put on a special diet for 3 days before the test and foods such as bananas, coffee, tea, chocolate and vanilla are excluded. The urine is collected in a bottle containing hydrochloric acid as a preservative and is refrigerated during the collection period. When a tumour of an adrenal gland is present the level of vanillylmandelic acid in the urine is elevated above normal.

Very occasionally, a Rogitine (phentolamine) test is ordered. The arterial blood pressure is recorded before the test. Phentolamine (Rogitine) 5 mg, an adrenergic blocking drug, is given intravenously. The blood pressure is then checked every 30 seconds for 5–10 minutes. The test is considered positive for phaeochromocytoma if the fall in systolic pressure is greater than 35 mmHg and the diastolic pressure falls more than 25 mmHg, and if they remain decreased for more than 3–4 minutes.

TREATMENT AND NURSING CARE OF HYPERTENSION

If the hypertension is secondary, treatment is directed toward correcting the primary condition. In essential hypertension, treatment is directed at: (1) lowering the blood pressure in an effort to prevent serious complications; and (2) having the patient adjust his life to reduce the demands on the cardiovascular system and kidneys. The treatment depends on the height and constancy of the blood pressure and the signs and symptoms of impaired function in vulnerable organs. The patient with mild hypertension may simply be advised to reduce his weight to normal, avoid overwork and overexcitement, and decrease his salt intake to a prescribed level in order to prevent the development of hypertension.

People with more severe hypertension may receive a drug to lower the blood pressure and are likely to be more restricted in activities and diet. The patients seen in the hospital are usually those with Grade 3 or Grade 4 hypertension and those with cardiac, cerebral or renal complications.

Observations
The blood pressure is determined at regular intervals with the patient in the same position each time. The doctor may request several casual readings at times when the patient is not anticipating the recording. A record of the pressure each morning before the patient moves about may also be necessary and, in some instances, there may be a request to obtain a reading while the patient is asleep. The nurse should know the patient's activities or experiences for the period preceding any reading. If frequent recordings cause anxiety, this is brought to the doctor's attention. Fluid balance is noted, as a positive balance may point to either renal or cardiac failure. The patient's

weight is recorded daily, either to indicate progress to his normal weight level or to indicate possible sodium and water retention. The pulse rate and volume are recorded at least twice daily, and the respirations are observed for any signs of dyspnoea, particularly on exertion. Any complaint of headache or pain is reported.

Rest and activity
The amount of rest needed, and whether it must be bed rest or not, will depend on the severity of the hypertension. Moderately severe hypertensive patients may require a period of bed rest. When activity is permitted, it is graduated and the patient's blood pressure response noted. Moderate exercise, such as walking and golfing, is encouraged once the blood pressure has been somewhat lowered, and as long as there is no dyspnoea nor undue fatigue.

Diet
The caloric intake is reduced to 1000–1200 calories daily until the weight is normal: then a maintenance diet is established. The sodium intake is usually reduced, and the degree of restriction depends upon the severity of the patient's disease. If the salt restriction is prolonged, one should be alert for sodium deficiency, which is manifested by muscular cramps, weakness, nausea and vomiting. The amount of coffee, tea and alcohol is usually limited with most hypertensive persons.

Elimination
Constipation is to be avoided since straining raises the blood pressure and could cause the rupture of a damaged sclerosed artery.

Medications
When therapeutic measures such as weight reduction, cessation of smoking, reduced salt intake and regular isotonic exercise have not proved successful in lowering blood pressure to the desired level, antihypertensive medications are added to the regimen. An individual or stepped-care approach is used in selecting appropriate drug therapy.

Therapy usually begins with a diuretic but may commence with a beta-blocking agent. If the desired blood pressure is not reached after a trial period, other drugs may be added. These will include a beta-blocker, and if blood pressure control is still not achieved, a vasodilator is included. If further therapy is required, a centrally acting drug or a sympathetic neuron blocker is administered or there is a change to captopril and frusemide.[32]

Diuretics. Diuretics decrease blood pressure by increasing sodium excretion and reducing both plasma volume and extracellular fluid. A thiazide

diuretic is the first diuretic of choice. It may be given in conjunction with a sodium-restricted diet and a hypotensive drug. If administration is prolonged, the patient is observed for possible potassium deficiency and skin rash. As with the administration of any diuretic, the urinary output is measured and the patient is weighed daily during hospitalization.

Vasodilators
- *Hydralazine (Apresoline)*. This drug may be used in the emergency treatment of high blood pressure as well as in the management of less urgent instances of hypertension. It acts primarily on the arterioles, rather than on the nervous system, causing smooth muscle relaxation. Peripheral vascular resistance is lowered and arterial pressure falls. It may cause sodium and water retention and is much more effective when combined with a diuretic. In addition, it can cause reflex tachycardia and therefore is used cautiously for patients with angina. This reflex increase in sympathetic discharge may be offset by combining it with a drug which blocks the sympathetic nervous system, such as propranolol. Toxic reactions are manifested by headache, dizziness, rapid pulse, palpitation, precordial pain and shortness of breath. Large doses, in excess of 200 mg daily, have been associated with a lupus erythematosus-like syndrome.

  Diazoxide (Eudemine). This is a fast-acting vasodilator used for the emergency treatment of hypertensive crisis. It is usually given as a 300 mg bolus within 15–30 seconds and the effect lasts approximately 5–8 hours. The typical response is an immediate and precipitous fall in blood pressure, which may compromise the blood flow to the heart and brain in patients with atherosclerotic coronary and cerebral disease, diazoxide may be given by slow infusion over 10–30 minutes or smaller boluses (75–100 mg intravenously) may be given every 5–10 minutes. Diazoxide also causes sodium and water retention and is usually given with frusemide (intravenously) to counteract these effects. Reflex tachycardia similar to that observed with hydralazine can be controlled with the use of parenteral propranolol (Inderal). It is used with caution for patients with angina. Extravasation must be avoided. This infusion should not be added to intravenous fluids; it should be given undiluted in a calibrated drip chamber.
- *Sodium nitroprusside*. This drug is also used to treat hypertensive crisis. The hypotensive response to this potent vasodilator occurs within seconds, so blood pressure must be monitored very frequently. Fifty to 100 mg is added to 1 litre of 5% dextrose. The drug is started as a continuous drip at the rate of 10 drops per minute. The concentration and rate of administration are then adjusted to maintain the desired level of blood pressure.

[32] Fentem, Tunstall-Pedoe & Wilcox (1983).

Adverse effects include nausea, vomiting, muscle twitching, apprehension and sweating. Since sodium nitroprusside is air- and light-sensitive, the infusion bottle should be protected from light during administration. A fresh solution should be prepared after 12 hours.

- *Minoxidil (Loniten).* This drug markedly reduces peripheral vascular resistance, causing more pronounced vasodilation than hydralazine. Reflex sympathetic action and sodium retention also occur and so minoxidil is often combined with a beta-blocker and a potent diuretic. A relatively common side-effect is excess hair on the face, chest and brow.
- *Captopril.* Captopril is a powerful vasodilator, with a different mechanism of action from the above medications (see p. 357).

Peripheral adrenergic blockers
- *Guanethidine (Ismelin).* This agent has generally been reserved for severe or resistant hypertension, although it may be useful in selected patients with less severe disease. It acts by inhibiting the release of noradrenaline at sympathetic neuro-effector junctions and by depleting tissue stores of catecholamines. The patient should be warned against activities that cause vasodilation, such as taking hot showers, drinking alcohol and long exposure to the sun, as they may result in severe postural hypotension. Patients are advised to avoid sudden changes in posture. Guanethidine has a long period of onset of action (1 week) and a long duration of action. When the patient is being changed from this to another antihypertensive drug, a few days without guanethidine are advisable before he is started on the new drug.

    Side-effects are dose-related and include diarrhoea (often severe) and sexual problems in men, such as inhibition of ejaculation or retrograde ejaculation, as well as postural hypotension. Like other antihypertensive agents, it is more effective when combined with a diuretic.
- *Bethanidine.* This drug acts similarly to guanethidine and has comparable potency and produces similar side-effects, except that it causes less diarrhoea. The main difference is its shorter duration of action, 8–12 hours, so that alteration of dosage is easier.
- *Prazosin (Hypovase).* Although originally considered to be a vasodilator, prazosin also acts as an alpha-adrenergic blocker. It is moderately effective in lowering blood pressure in hypertensive patients. The drug seems equivalent to alpha-methyldopa in antihypertensive potency and side-effects. Prazosin is frequently combined with beta-blockers and diuretics. To prevent profound hypotension and collapse, the initial dose should not exceed 0.5 mg, preferably taken at bedtime. Other side-effects include lassitude, oedema, anti-

cholinergic effects and CNS symptoms (headache, drowsiness and nervousness).

Centrally acting adreneregic blockers
- *Alpha-methyldopa.* It is currently believed that this drug lowers blood pressure primarily by acting on vasomotor centres in the brain, resulting in decreased sympathetic outflow. Peripheral sympathetic inhibition may add to the cardiovascular effect of the drug. It is used in the treatment of patients with mild to moderate hypertension. The most common side-effects are drowsiness and fatigue. In approximately 20% of patients it causes a positive reaction to the direct Coombs' test. Occasionally patients develop haemolytic anaemia and hepatitis. The hepatic damage seen with alpha-methyldopa is generally preceded by a flu-like syndrome characterized by chills, fever and muscle aches. If these occur, the drug should be discontinued immediately. Some patients may experience an inability to concentrate and a marked slowing of mental performance.

- *Clonidine (Catapres).* Clonidine is a centrally acting antihypertensive agent. It reduces blood pressure by inhibiting the outflow of adrenergic impulses, resulting in decreased sympathetic stimulation of the heart, kidney and peripheral vasculature. It is effective in moderate to severe hypertension. The onset of action is usually within 30 minutes and maximum effect occurs within 2–4 hours. The most frequent side-effects associated with clonidine are sedation and dry mouth. These usually disappear as the patient develops a tolerance for the drug. An unusual reaction attributed to clonidine is rebound hypertension following abrupt discontinuance of the drug. Patients should be warned against sudden withdrawal of the drug. Dosage reduction is gradual over a period of a week.

Beta-adrenergic blocking agents
- *Propranolol (Inderal).* Propranolol works directly on the heart to slow the rate and force of contraction. It is also thought to interfere with renin release from the kidney and to have a central mechanism of action. It may be combined with other agents in the treatment of hypertensive patients (see p. 381).
- *Metoprolol, timolol, pindolol, atenolol.* These drugs are beta-blockers which block B_1 receptors to a greater degree than B_2 receptors (see p. 330).

Sedatives. Frequent small doses of a tranquillizing drug may be ordered for the hypertensive patient to promote relaxation and rest.

Precautions. When a patient is receiving a hypotensive drug, he must be observed for the particular side-effects that are associated with the drug he is receiving. If they occur, the doctor is informed promptly. Most of these drugs can cause postural hypotension—a sudden fall of blood pressure to below the normal when a patient assumes the upright position. The nurse instructs the patient to move slowly and to assume the recumbent position on the first feeling of faintness. When getting up, he should sit on the side of the bed for a few minutes before standing.

The blood pressure is recorded at frequent intervals as indicated by the doctor. The nurse may be requested to take the blood pressure with the patient standing, especially if the patient is having ganglionic blocking drugs. It may be necessary to take the blood pressure before each dose of the drug. The level frequently determines whether the drug should be given and in what dosage. The antihypertensive drug and the dosage are prescribed individually; one drug may be more effective than another with one patient, and the effective dosage will often vary from one patient to another.

If the patient develops a fever or a spell of hot weather occurs, the dosage of the antihypertensive drug may have to be reduced, since a higher temperature seems to intensify the effect of the drug.

HYPERTENSIVE CRISIS

Hypertensive crisis is a syndrome characterized by a sudden elevation of the blood pressure accompanied by severe headache, nausea, vomiting, visual disturbances, transient neurological disturbances, disorientation and drowsiness which may progress to coma. The retinopathy seen in malignant hypertension is often present. The blood pressure is extremely high, often as great as 250/150 mmHg. Rarely, hypertensive encephalopathy occurs. This is associated with cerebrovascular spasm and ensuing ischaemia, oedema and possibly thrombosis. It constitutes a medical emergency requiring prompt treatment.

Immediate treatment for the patient in a hypertensive crisis includes the intravenous administration of hydralazine or sodium nitroprusside and frusemide. Because of the potency of the medications being used, the patient is observed for sudden hypotension. The blood pressure is monitored every 5–10 minutes or more often. Anticonvulsant medications or sedatives may be required. The patient is maintained on bed rest. The pulse, respirations and neurological signs are checked every 5–10 minutes and the intake and output of fluids measured. It is important to maintain a calm, quiet environment.

References and Further Reading

BOOKS

Andreoli KG et al (1983) *Comprehensive Cardiac Care*, 5th ed. St Louis: CV Mosby.

Ashworth PM (1980) *Care to Communicate*. London: RCN.

Boore JRP (1978) *Prescription for Recovery*. London: RCN.

Bailey JS, Hampton JR, Jones JSP et al (1983) Arterial disease. In: JR Hampton (ed) *Cardiovascular Disease* (Integrated Clinical Science Series). London: Heinemann Medical, Chapter 8.

Berne RM & Levy MN (1981) *Cardiovascular Physiology*, 4th ed. St Louis: CV Mosby.

Braunwald E (ed.) (1985) *Heart Disease: A Texbook of Cardiovascular Medicine*, 2nd ed. Philadelphia: WB Saunders.

Cornett SJ & Watson JE (1984) *Cardiac Rehabilitation: An Interdisciplinary Team Approach*. New York: Wiley & Sons.

Doenges ME, Jeffries MF & Moorhouse MF (1984) *Nursing Care Plans: Nursing Diagnoses in Planning Patient Care*, Philadelphia: FA Davis.

Dustan HP (1986) Pathophysiology of hypertension. In: JW Hurst et al (eds), *The Heart*, 6th ed. New York: McGraw-Hill.

Fentem PH, Tunstall-Pedoe H & Wilcox RG (1983) The blood pressure. In: JR Hampton (ed), *Cardiovascular Disease* (Integrated Clinical Science Series). London: Heinemann Medical.

Ganong WF (1985) *Review of Medical Physiology*, 12th ed. San Francisco: Lange.

Guyton AC (1984) *Physiology of the Human Body*, 6th ed. Philadelphia: WB Saunders.

Guzzetta CE & Dossey BM (1984) *Cardiovascular Nursing: Bodymind tapestry*. St Louis: CV Mosby.

Hayward J (1975) *Information—A Prescription Against Pain*. London: RCN.

Hurst JW et al (1986) *The Heart*, 6th ed. New York: McGraw-Hill.

Julian DG (1983) *Cardiology*, 4th ed. London: Baillière Tindall.

Kim MJ, McFarland GK & McLane AM (1984) *Pocket Guide to Nursing Diagnosis*. St Louis: CV Mosby.

McCall MM, III (1978) Cardiopulmonary resuscitation. In: JW Hurst et al, (eds) *The Heart*, 3rd ed. New York: McGraw–Hill.

Marriott HJ (1983) *Practical Electrocardiography*, 7th ed. Baltimore: Williams & Wilkins.

Schamroth L (1984) *The Electrocardiology of Coronary Artery Disease*, 2nd ed. Boston: Blackwell Scientific.

Underhill SL et al (1982) *Cardiac Nursing*. Philadelphia: JB Lippincott.

Weissler A (1982) *Non-invasive Cardiology*. New York: Grune & Stratton.

Wenger N & Schlant R (1986) Prevention of coronary atherosclerosis. In: JW Hurst et al (eds), *The Heart*, 6th ed. New York: McGraw-Hill.

Wyngaardin JB & Smith LH (1985) *Cecil Textbook of Medicine*. Philadelphia: WB Saunders.

Young JR & de Wolfe VG (1982) Diseases of the peripheral arteries. In: JW Hurst et al (eds), *The Heart*, 5th ed. New York: McGraw-Hill.

PERIODICALS

Ashworth PM (1984) Staff–patient communication in coronary care units. *J. A. Nurs.*, Vol. 9, pp. 35–42.

Baaste DM, Yacoui C & Amann AH (1982) Intravenous nitroglycerin. A review. *Am. Pharm.* Vol. 22 No. 2, pp. 36–39.

Berger HJ & Zaret BL (1981) Nuclear cardiology: Part I. *New Eng. J. Med.*, Vol. 305 No. 14, pp. 799–807.

Berger HJ & Zaret BL (1981) Nuclear cardiology: Part II. *New Eng. J. Med.*, Vol. 305 No. 15, pp. 855–865.

Berkovits BV (1980) A–V sequential demand pacemakers for treatment of cardiac arrhythmias. *CVP*, Vol. 8, pp. 29–35.

Blomberg DJ et al (1975) Creatinine kinase isoenzymes: predictive value in the early diagnosis of acute myocardial infarction. *Am. J. Med.*, Vol. 59 No. 4.

Castelli GWP, Hjortland M, Kannel WB & Dowberm (1977) High density lipoprotein as a protective factor against coronary artery disease. The Framingham study. *Am. J. Med.*, Vol. 62, p. 707.

Cooper T et al (1981) Coronary prone behaviour and coronary heart disease: a critical review, *Circulation*, Vol. 63 No. 6, pp. 1199–1215.

Donaldson R (1981) Sounding out the heart. *Nurs. Mirr.*, Vol. 152 No. 8, pp. 40–41.

Dosta J & Geraets DR (1982) Topical nitroglycerin: a new twist to an old stand-by. *Am. Pharm.* Vol. 22 No. 2, pp. 23–32.

Fletcher GF & Murphy P (1981) Cardiac procedures in acute care situations. *Med. Clin. N. Am.*, Vol. 65 No. 1, pp. 67–81.

Fox J (1980) Keeping pace with pacemaker design. *CVP*, Vol. 8, pp. 25–27.

Friedenreich K (1981) Pacemakers today: the beat goes on. *CVP*, Vol. 9, pp. 33–37, 59.

Garrity TF & Klein RF (1975) Emotional responses and clinical severity as early determinants of six-month mortality after myocardial infarction. *Heart Lung*, Vol. 4 No. 5.

Gentry W, Doyle O-W Jan Deterd Musch F & Hall RP (1981) Differences in types A and B behaviour in response to acute myocardial infarction. *Heart Lung*, Vol. 10 No. 6, pp. 1101–1105.

Iskandrian A, Wasserman L & Segal B (1980) Thallium-201 myocardial scintography: advantages and limitations. *Arch. Int. Med.*, Vol. 140, pp. 320–327.

Katler MN, Mintz G, S Segal, Bernard L & Parry WR (May 1980) Clinical uses of two dimensional echocardiography. *Am. J. Med.*, Vol. 45 No. 5, pp. 1061–1082.

Leaper D (1986) Antiseptics and their effect on healing tissues. *Nurs. Times*, Vol. 82 No. 22, pp. 45 & 47.

McLane M, Krop H & Mehta J (1980) Psychosexual adjustment and counselling after myocardial infarction. *Ann. Int. Med.* Vol. 92 No. 4, pp. 514–519.

McNeal GJ (1978) Twenty-four hour ambulatory monitoring. *Nurs. Clin. N. Am.*, Vol. 13 No. 3, pp.437–448.

Mather HG, Morgan DC, Pearson NG et al (1976) Myocardial infarction: a comparison between home and hospital care for patients. *Br. Med. J.*, Vol. 1, pp. 925–929.

Mechner F & Brown GE (1976) Examination of the heart and great vessels—Part I., *Am. J. Nurs.* Vol. 76 No. 11, pp. 1–23.

Mechner F & Brown GE (1977) Patient assessment: auscultation of the heart—Part II, *Am. J. Nurs.*, Vol. 77 No. 2, pp. 1–79.

Owen PM (1984) Defibrillating pacemaker patients. *Am. J. Nurs.*, Vol. 84 No. 9, pp. 1129–1132.

Perry S & Viederman M (1981) Management of emotional reactions to acute medical illness. *Med. Clin. N. A.*, Vol. 65 No. 1, pp. 3–14.

Purcell JA & Giffen PA (1981) Percutaneous transluminal coronary angioplasty. *Am. J. Nurs.*, Vol. 81 No. 9, pp. 1620–1626.

Purcell JA & Haynes L (1984) Using the ECG to detect MI *Am. J. Nurs.*, Vol. 84 No. 5, pp. 627–642.

Purcell JA & Burrows SG (1985) A pacemaker primer. *Am. J. Nurs.*, Vol. 85 No. 5, pp. 552–568.

Quint RA (1981) Percutaneous transluminal coronary angioplasty: pre- and postprocedural care *C.V.P.*, Vol. 41, pp. 35–42.

Rahimtoola SH (1980) Coronary arteriography in asymptomatic patients after myocardial infarction. *Chest*, Vol. 77 No. 1, pp. 53–57.

Raines J & Traad E (1980) Non-invasive evaluation of peripheral vascular disease. *Med. Clin. N. Am.*, Vol. 64 No. 2, pp. 283–299.

Roberts R (1981) Diagnostic assessment of myocardial infarction based on lactic dehydrogenase and creatine kinase enzymes. *Heart Lung*, Vol. 10 No. 3, pp. 486–506.

Schneider GN (1980) Programmable pacemaker: wave of the future. *C.V.P.*, Vol. 8, pp. 18–20.

Schneider RR & Seckler SG (1981) Evaluation of acute chest pain. *Med. Clin. N. Am.*, Vol. 65 No. 1, pp. 53–66.

Swanson–Kauffman K (1981) Echocardiography: an access route to the heart. *Crit. Care Nurs.*, pp. 20–26.

Tannenbaum RP, Sohn CA, Cantwell R, Rogers M & Hollis R (1981) Pain—angina pectoris: how to recognize it; how to manage it. *Nurs.*, '81, Vol. 11 No. 9, pp. 44–51.

Tinker JH (1976) Understanding chest x-rays. *Am. J. Nurs.*, Vol. 76 No. 1, pp. 54–58.

Wenger NK (1980) Rehabilitation of the patient with symptomatic coronary atherosclerotic heart disease: part I. *Cardiol. Series Inc.*, Vol. 3 No. 2, pp. 6–27.

Wilson-Barnett J (1979) A review of the research into the experience of patients suffering from coronary thrombosis. *Int. J. Nurs. Stud.* Vol. 16; pp. 183–198.

15
Nursing in Shock

Introduction

Shock is a pathophysiological condition, characterized by inadequate tissue and organ perfusion, which seriously reduces the delivery of oxygen and other essential substances to a level below that required for normal cellular activities. Cellular injury or destruction may occur, and tissue and organ functions deteriorate.

CAUSES OF SHOCK

The basic pathophysiological mechanisms involved in the production of shock are:

1 Widespread vasoconstriction or vasodilation which alters the peripheral vascular tone and resistance.
2 Reduction in the intravascular volume (hypovolaemia).
3 Inadequate cardiac output.

The disturbance or initiating event may occur in any part of the cardiovascular system but will inevitably be reflected in a reduction in the microcirculatory or capillary flow throughout the body.

Shock may be associated with any trauma or stress, regardless of its clinical orientation. The causative factor in alteration of the peripheral vascular tone and resistance may be anaphylaxis, neurogenic trauma, or sepsis. In the case of hypovolaemia the cause may be haemorrhage, plasma loss as in burns and peritonitis, or dehydration. Inadequate cardiac output may be the result of myocardial infarction, congestive heart failure, cardiac arrhythmia, obstruction of a major arterial pathway as in pulmonary embolism, cardiac tamponade or tension pneumothorax.[1]

TYPES OF SHOCK

Table 15.1 lists the various types of shock according to their causative factors.

Hypovolaemic shock implies a deficiency in the intravascular volume which may be due to haemor-

rhage or dehydration as a result of vomiting, diarrhoea, loss of plasma in burns or into the peritoneal cavity in peritonitis, inadequate fluid intake, or excessive urinary output caused by adrenal crisis or overdosage of a diuretic.

When the intravascular volume drops, the mean systolic blood pressure is reduced, which causes a decrease in venous return to the heart; the atrial pressure during diastole is decreased because of the drop in venous return, the ventricular volume decreases and the stroke volume and cardiac output diminish. The arterial blood pressure is lowered and

Table 15.1 Classification of shock according to cause.

Type of shock	Causative factors
1 Hypovolaemic	Fluid volume deficit
Haemorrhagic	Blood loss related to minor or major trauma; gastrointestinal bleeding; blood coagulation deficits; or surgery
Dehydration	Fluid volume loss related to prolonged vomiting and/or diarrhoea; fluid-shift into peritoneal cavity in peritonitis, intestinal obstruction; inadequate fluid intake; excessive urinary output with diuretic therapy, uncontrolled diabetes mellitus, adrenal insufficiency
Burn	Plasma loss through damaged body surface
2 Cardiogenic	Decreased tissue perfusion from inadequate cardiac output related to congestive heart failure, cardiac arrhythmia, myocardial infarction, pulmonary embolism, pericardial tamponade, or pneumothorax
3 Vascular	Inadequate circulatory blood volume as a result of decreased peripheral resistance and increased vascular capacity
4 Neurogenic	Loss of sympathetic nervous system control with spinal cord trauma, spinal anaesthesia
5 Septic	Infection with the release of endotoxins
6 Toxic shock syndrome	Localized *Staphylococcus aureus* infection with release of toxins
7 Anaphylactic	Antigen-antibody reaction with release of histamine

---

[1] *Tension pneumothorax* is caused by the escape of air from the lung into the pleural cavity where it progressively accumulates, increasing the intrapleural pressure and compressing the heart as well as the lung.

blood flow through the tissues becomes inadequate. The degree of shock produced depends on the volume of blood lost and the rate of the loss. Compensatory mechanisms are more effective when the loss occurs slowly.

Cardiogenic shock indicates an inadequate cardiac output and may be associated with congestive heart failure, cardiac arrhythmia, myocardial infarction, pulmonary embolism, pericardial tamponade or pneumothorax.

The ability of the heart to pump blood is impaired; this results in an increase in the ventricular filling pressures but a decrease in the stroke volume and cardiac output. Tissue perfusion is inadequate, but pulmonary pressures increase, resulting in pulmonary oedema.

Vascular shock (vasomotor, distributive or low-resistance shock) results from decreased peripheral resistance and increased vascular capacity. The blood volume is unchanged but is inadequate because of the expansion of the vascular system. Disorders leading to vascular shock include neurogenic, toxic and *anaphylactic reactions*.

Neurogenic shock is produced by autonomic nervous system activity in response to the primary trauma or stress, resulting in reflex vasodilation and loss of arteriolar tone with consequent pooling of blood and a reduction in the venous return to the heart. This type of shock may be caused by spinal cord injury, spinal anaesthesia, severe pain (e.g. renal colic), accidental injury, or extreme fright.

Septic or *bacteraemic shock* is caused by an overwhelming infection. The offending organisms are most often gram-negative (e.g. intestinal bacilli) and their endotoxin causes an initial brief vasoconstriction followed by vasodilation and pooling of blood. The toxaemia also has a direct depressant effect on the heart.

Toxic shock syndrome results from a process which resembles septic shock. Toxic shock syndrome is believed to be caused by a toxin produced by *Staphylococcus aureus*. The incidence is greatest in women during a menstrual period (when it is associated with the use of tampons) but it has occurred in all age groups and both sexes. A focal infection with penicillin-resistant *Staphylococcus aureus* appears to be the common factor.[2] Manifestations of the disorder include a temperature greater than 38.9°C, diarrhoea, vomiting and a diffuse rash which progresses to exfoliation in addition to the hypovolaemia, hypotension, and respiratory, renal, liver, coagulation and cardiac impairments found in patients with other types of shock.

Anaphylactic shock is the result of an antigen–antibody reaction that causes the release into the bloodstream of toxic substances (e.g. histamine) that produce vasodilation and pooling of blood (see Chapter 4).

CONCEPT OF PATHOPHYSIOLOGICAL RESPONSES IN SHOCK

Whatever the primary cause or type of shock, the body responses follow a similar pattern. Guyton identifies three stages of shock which form a useful framework for examining the pathophysiological responses which occur. The stages are: (1) non-progressive or compensated, (2) progressive, and (3) irreversible.[3] Table 15.2 outlines the signs and symptoms of these stages of shock.

1 *Non-progressive or compensated stage*. This stage is characterized by neurogenic, hormonal and chemical responses.[4] In Fig. 15.1, the *neurogenic compensation* in response to a decrease in blood pressure is outlined. The baroreceptors in the aorta and carotid arteries respond immediately to the fall in blood pressure and signal the vasomotor centre in the medulla, resulting in stimulation of the sympathetic nervous system. The sympathetic nervous system activation initiates an increase in the rate and force of the cardiac contractions, resulting in increased cardiac output and a rise in blood pressure. Selective vasoconstriction occurs in the skin, lungs, gastrointestinal tract and kidneys, ensuring a greater volume of blood in the coronary and cerebral vascular systems. This maintains the blood flow to the heart and brain. The cerebral blood vessels lack sympathetic innervation and do not respond to the vasoconstrictor response. Smith states that control of coronary vascular resistance is dominated by local metabolism, which prevents coronary vasoconstriction.[5] The skeletal muscles show some immediate reduction in blood flow due to vasoconstriction.[5] The net effect is an increase in the cardiac output and improved perfusion of the most vital areas—the heart and brain. The respirations increase in rate and depth. The skin becomes moist and clammy as the sweat glands respond to the sympathetic innervation, and the pupils dilate.

Hormonal responses in the compensatory phase of shock include the release of catecholamines (adrenaline and noradrenaline) through stimulation of the sympathetic nervous system (see Fig. 15.2). The fall in renal blood volume and pressure stimulates the juxtaglomerular apparatus to release renin which reacts with angiotensinogen to form angiotensin I; this is then converted to angiotensin II which causes vasoconstriction. The blood pressure rises and venous return to the heart increases. The adrenal cortex responds to angiotensin II by releasing aldosterone, which functions

---

[2] Heimburger (1981), p. 34.

[3] Guyton (1981), p. 322.
[4] Rice (1981), p. 4.
[5] Smith & Thier (1985), p. 1000.

Table 15.2 Assessment of the patient in shock.

	Non-progressive or compensated stage	Progressive stage	Irreversible or refractory stage
Subjective data	Restlessness, apprehension and anxiety Nausea Thirst	Listlessness or apathy Anorexia Confusion	Non-responsive
Objective data			
Skin and mucous membrane	Ashen, pale, cold, moist and clammy Mouth dry	Cyanotic, moist and clammy Mouth dry	Cyanotic, cold and clammy Jaundice, petechiae and bleeding from mucous membranes and lesions
Cardiovascular	Pulse rapid and thready ↑ Heart rate Blood pressure normal	Pulse weak, rapid and thready ↑ Heart rate Cardiac arrhythmias ↓ Blood pressure ↑ Pulse pressure	Pulse slow, irregular or imperceptible Cardiac arrhythmias ↓ Blood pressure–diastolic may be difficult to obtain
Respiratory	↑ Respiratory rate and depth	↑ Respiratory rate Shallow respirations	Respirations slow, shallow and irregular Crackles and wheezes heard
Temperature	↓ Body temperature or ↑ Body temperature (septic and toxic shock)	↓ Body temperature	↓ Body temperature
Urinary	↓ Urinary output	↓ Urinary output	↓ Urinary output or no urine output
Gastrointestinal	↓ Bowel sounds	↓ Bowel sounds or absent Haematemesis, melaena	Bowel sounds decreased or absent Abdominal distension Haematemesis, melaena
Level of consciousness	Confused as to time, place and person Judgement impaired	Confused or inappropriate verbal responses Flexion, extension or no response to painful stimuli	Absence of verbal and motor responses to noxious stimuli

with the antidiuretic hormone (ADH) to increase the reabsorption of sodium and water by the renal tubules.

Adrenocorticotrophic hormone (ACTH), released by the anterior pituitary gland, stimulates the adrenal cortex to release glucocorticoids which increase gluconeogenesis in the liver and raise the serum glucose level.

When the pulmonary blood flow and pressure are decreased, a ventilation–perfusion imbalance occurs. Gas exchange between the air in the alveoli and pulmonary capillaries is decreased primarily as a result of inadequate pulmonary perfusion. Carbon dioxide is retained in the blood and the oxygen concentration decreases. These changes in blood gases lead to *chemical compensatory responses* (see Fig. 15.3). Chemoreceptors in the aorta and carotid arteries respond to the decreased oxygen tension by increasing the rate and depth of respi-

rations. The carbon dioxide concentration drops as the respiratory rate increases and the amount of carbon dioxide exhaled increases, thus producing respiratory alkalosis. Cerebral blood vessels constrict in response to the lowered carbon dioxide tension and the alkalosis which leads to cerebral hypoxia. Stimulation of the chemoreceptors also activates the vasomotor centre of the medulla producing the sympathetic responses illustrated in Fig. 15.1.

2 *Progressive stage.* This stage of shock occurs when the compensatory mechanisms fail to maintain an adequate cardiac output.[6] If tissue perfusion is reduced sufficiently, ischaemic hypoxia results. Under these conditions anaerobic metabolism takes place and metabolites such as pyruvate, lac-

---

[6] Rice (1981), p. 6.

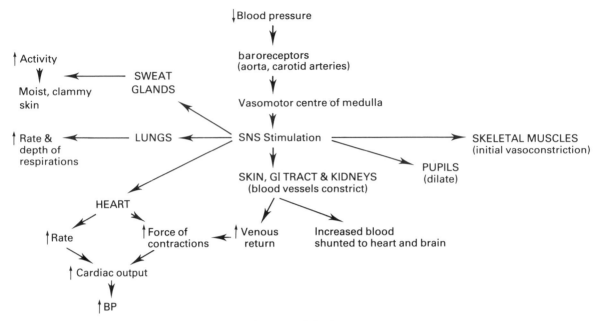

Fig. 15.1 Non-progressive stage of shock (nervous compensation).

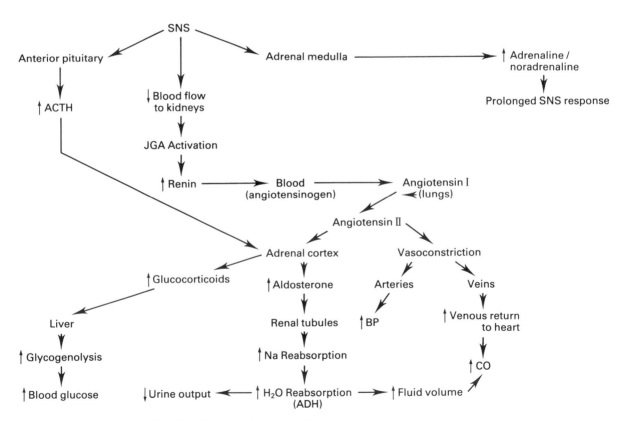

Fig. 15.2 Compensatory stage of shock (hormonal compensation).

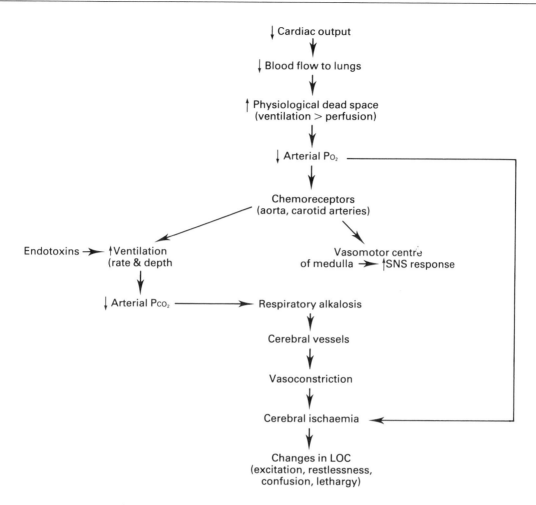

Fig. 15.3 Compensatory stage of shock (chemical compensation).

tic acid, carbon dioxide, and hydrogen ions accumulate. The pH of the blood decreases and metabolic acidosis develops. The presence of excessive metabolites and the lowered pH cause vasodilation of the arterioles, while the venule constriction continues. Pooling of the blood ensues, and stagnant hypoxia results. Cellular metabolic disturbances result in failure of the active (energy-requiring) transport system of cell membranes. Enzymes, potassium and other cellular components move out. Oedema occurs as a result of a fluid shift from the dilated capillaries to the interstitial spaces. Protein also leaks through the enlarged capillary pores, resulting in a lowered serum osmotic pressure which further promotes the fluid shift. Interstitial fluid moves into the cells causing cellular oedema and worsening their dysfunction.[7]

Capillary blood flow is impaired by the decreased intravascular volume, increased blood viscosity and the resulting clumping together of erythrocytes and platelets. Cardiac contractility is impaired by the depressing effect of a myocardial toxic factor (MTF) that is released by the ischaemic pancreas. These responses contribute to the progression of the shock, resulting in further impairment of circulation and cardiac output.

3 *Irreversible stage of shock*. This stage develops when the process cannot be reversed. Cardiac output decreases and the force of contractions weaken as a result of the decreased coronary blood supply and the presence of acidosis and toxins; cardiac failure occurs.

Figure 15.4 depicts the cycle of acidosis which is perpetuated during the irreversible stage. Respiratory failure, decreased ventilation and carbon dioxide retention lead to respiratory acidosis which adds to the metabolic acidosis already present. Cellular function is further impaired and

---

[7] Rice (1981), p. 7.

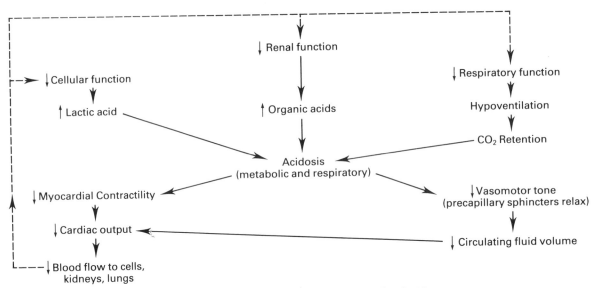

Fig. 15.4 Irreversible stage of shock (cycle of acidosis).

renal failure causes the retention of metabolic products.

Tissue and organ perfusion is further compromised by disseminated intravascular coagulation (DIC) (see Chapter 13) which develops with the stagnation of capillary blood and the ensuing clumping of erythrocytes and platelets. Eventually the blood-clotting factors are consumed by the widespread microcoagulation; the fibrin clots break down and diffuse bleeding occurs.

Cerebral ischaemia increases the sympathetic response which perpetuates the ischaemia. Cardiac and respiratory failure lead to further depression of vital cerebral centres. The irreversible stage of shock progresses to failure of all body systems and, ultimately, to death. Guyton indicates that with modern therapy it is deterioration of the heart that is usually the final factor that leads to the irreversibility of shock.[8]

MANIFESTATIONS OF SHOCK

The degree of shock is not always the same for all persons following stress and injuries of equal intensity. There is considerable variation in the response and also in the rapidity with which some patients progress to the irreversible stage. Those who are elderly or very young, have chronic disease or infection or are emotionally fragile are more susceptible to shock. Signs of shock reflect failure in the perfusion of vital organs and the responsive mechanisms set in operation.

[8] Guyton (1986), p. 336 & 389.

It is important that the nurse be constantly alert for early changes in patients' conditions that may indicate shock, especially in those with conditions in which it is more likely to develop (e.g. burns, trauma, haemorrhage, dehydration and severe infection). Early recognition and treatment substantially increase the patient's chance for survival.

Altered level of consciousness. Unless the shock is very severe and develops very quickly, early signs are restlessness, apprehension and anxiety. Later, the restlessness and apprehension may be replaced by listlessness, apathy and confusion. Verbal responses may be inappropriate as cerebral hypoxia increases. Painful stimulation may elicit withdrawal, flexion, extension or no response. In the irreversible stage of shock the patient is unconscious and shows no response to painful stimulation.

Skin. Initially, the skin is ashen pale and cold due to increased peripheral vascular resistance and decreased perfusion of the superficial tissues. Cyanosis develops, reflecting a reduction in the cardiac output (as in cardiogenic and progressive shock) and decreased oxygen saturation. The latter occurs due to the pooling of blood and the diminished flow of blood through the lungs. If the skin vessels are blanched by pressure, they refill slowly.

The skin may be moist (clammy) due to sympathetic activity to the sweat glands. In the early stages of septic shock, the skin is warm, dry and less pale.

Cardiovascular signs. The pulse is rapid and thready. Tachycardia is a compensatory response to the decreased cardiac output. During the progressive or irreversible stages, the pulse progressively weakens, becoming slower and irregular and eventually imperceptible.

Initially the blood pressure may be normal, as adaptive mechanisms function to maintain cardiac output. As shock progresses, the blood pressure falls as the cardiac output decreases. Familiarity with the patient's previous blood pressure helps to determine the significance of readings. Serial readings of blood pressure are essential in providing information about trends or changes. The pulse pressure (the difference between the diastolic and systolic pressures) decreases. This decrease is due to the rise in the diastolic pressure as a result of the vasoconstriction and a decrease in the systolic pressure as a result of the decreased stroke volume.[9]

Respiratory changes. Respirations increase in rate and depth in response to hypoxia. If the initial cause is a loss of intravascular volume (e.g. haemorrhage) the patient may show signs of air hunger. In severe and progressive shock, depression of the respiratory centre causes slower, shallow and possibly irregular respirations. Many patients in shock develop serious pulmonary dysfunction characterized by pathophysiological changes in the lungs. These changes are usually not manifested until 3–6 days after the event which initiated the shock. Changes include a decrease in the secretion of surfactant with a concomitant increase in surface tension which results in areas of atelectasis, interstitial oedema, congestion, disseminated intravascular coagulation, thromboses and pulmonary emboli. Pulmonary capillary perfusion is greatly reduced and oxygen and carbon dioxide transport across the alveolar membrane progressively decreases; severe hypoxaemia and hypercarbia develop. The complication may be referred to as adult respiratory distress syndrome (ARDS), 'shock lung' and, rarely, as 'wet lung' (see Chapter 16).

Temperature. The body temperature is usually subnormal; cellular metabolism and heat production are reduced by hypoxia. The exception to this occurs with a patient in whom the primary cause of the shock is infection. This type of shock may be referred to as hyperdynamic or warm septic shock in the early stages.

Urinary output. Renal output is diminished as a result of decreased renal perfusion. The output may become less than 30 ml per hour; urea, nitrogen and creatinine are retained, as indicated by increasing blood levels.

Thirst. This is very distressing, especially in hypovolaemic shock. The mouth becomes parched as a result of the increased withdrawal of fluid from the interstitial spaces into the intravascular compartment.

Gastrointestinal symptoms. Gastric motility decreases because of the sympathetic innervation and vasoconstriction. Decreased bowel sounds indicate reduced peristalsis and, if shock progresses, the sounds are absent. Haematemesis and melaena may occur because of the diffuse bleeding associated with disseminated intravascular coagulation.

Diffuse intravascular clotting (coagulation). Prolonged and severe shock, especially that of septic origin, is frequently complicated by diffuse intravascular clotting. The coagulation and formation of thromboses block small vessels and may cause serious tissue necrosis. Clotting elements may become depleted and then diffuse bleeding occurs. The condition is suspected with the appearance of petechiae and ecchymoses or bleeding from the nasal or oral mucous membrane. It may go unrecognized until there is evident haemorrhage (e.g. epistaxis, gastric, rectal, bladder). Blood studies reveal a prolonged prothrombin time, reduced number of platelets, and deficiency of fibrinogen. Multiple coagulation factors may be involved.

Acidosis. Changes that occur in the patient's responses and vital functions are worsened by the rapid development of acidosis associated with shock. As mentioned previously, the impairment of tissue perfusion and the resulting hypoxia incur anaerobic metabolism; metabolic acids accumulate and interfere with normal cell functioning. Cardiac arrhythmia and myocardial failure are likely to develop if acidosis persists.

Nursing Process

ASSESSMENT

Shock is an unstable, dynamic state in which the patient's condition either improves or worsens. Continuous monitoring is essential to identify changes which dictate necessary therapeutic and care measures.

The blood pressure, pulse, respiratory status, colour and hourly urinary output are noted immediately when taking over a patient's care. It is important to have a base-line in order to determine whether changes indicate improvement or further deterioration. Changes are frequently of greater significance than absolute values.

The nurse requires an understanding of the importance of the data obtained in assessment procedures and monitoring in order to take appropriate action.

---

[9] Rice (1981), p. 11.

Various parameters and observations are used to assess the cardiovascular status, respiratory functions and certain biochemical levels.

CARDIOVASCULAR ASSESSMENT

Assessment of the patient's cardiovascular status includes the following procedures.

Blood pressure and pulse
These are recorded at 15-minute intervals, and the intervals are lengthened only as the patient's condition improves. They reflect cardiac functioning and cardiac output.

The arterial blood pressure may be monitored by the sphygmomanometer but is likely to be lower than that obtained by intra-arterial measurement because of the peripheral vasoconstriction. An ultrasound flowmeter (Doppler) may be placed over a major artery to obtain a more accurate measure of blood pressure. Direct measurement by means of an intra-arterial catheter is more reliable. A catheter is passed via the radial or brachial artery into the subclavian artery. It is attached to a transducer which converts the mechanical pressure exerted by the blood to electrical impulses that appear on the monitor.

The pulse is counted and evaluated for a full minute. The radial artery may be used but, if it is inaccessible, the carotid, femoral or pedal pulses may be used. A stethoscope may be used to determine cardiac rhythm and apical rate.

Electrocardiograph
Continuous electrocardiographic monitoring is employed for early detection of arrhythmias and arrest.

Pulse pressure
The pulse pressure, which is the difference between the systolic and diastolic blood pressures, is noted. It decreases with a decrease in cardiac output. There is cause for concern when it becomes less than 30 mmHg.

Jugular veins
The jugular veins are observed for distension, pulsation or reflux, which would indicate cardiac insufficiency in receiving and forwarding the venous return.

Central venous pressure
A line may be established by which central venous pressure (CVP) is determined. A catheter is passed into the superior vena cava and attached to a giving set and a manometer using a three-way stopcock or may be connected to a transducer and monitor. The pressure indicated on the manometer or monitor screen reflects the intravascular volume and the venous return to the right side of the heart. The normal value is 10–12 cmH$_2$O or 0–4 mmHg; an increase above normal may indicate weakening or failure of the right side of the heart, or may be due to an excessive intravascular volume that may be the result of too rapid fluid infusion. A pressure below 5–6 cmH$_2$O usually reflects an intravascular volume deficit.

Pulmonary artery pressure (PAP)
This determination provides information about the pressure within the pulmonary vascular system and the functional ability of the heart. A floating balloon-tipped (Swan–Ganz) catheter with two, three or four lumens is passed into the superior vena cava. The balloon is then inflated, and the catheter is carried by the bloodstream through the right side of the heart into the pulmonary artery. The non-balloon lumen of the catheter is filled with water or saline which recedes in a monitoring tube until the pressure of the blood that it meets is equal to its pressure. The normal range of the PAP is 15–30 mmHg during systole and 5–15 mmHg during diastole, with a mean value of 10–20 mmHg, and in shock it is monitored continuously.

Pulmonary artery wedge pressure (PAWP; pulmonary capillary pressure)
This is obtained to provide information about the functional ability of the left side of the heart. A balloon-tipped flow-directed catheter (Swan–Ganz) is introduced into the pulmonary artery and advanced until the inflated balloon wedges in a branch of the artery. The tip of the open lumen is closed off from the pressure in the proximal pulmonary artery which is that created by the right side of the heart. The use of the Swan–Ganz catheter permits frequent determinations at short intervals.

The PAWP is the back pressure of the blood being delivered to the left side of the heart and reflects the ability of the left atrium and left ventricle to receive and forward the blood. The normal is approximately 10–12 mmHg.

Urine output
The hourly urinary output serves as a useful parameter in assessing a patient's cardiovascular status. An indwelling catheter is passed, and the urine excreted per hour is measured. The output reflects renal perfusion.

Normal ranges are:

Age	ml/h
Infant	8–20
1–4 years	20–25
4–7 years	25–30
7–10 years	25–30
Adult	30–60

Temperature
Body temperature is monitored continuously or by

means of rectal, skin or oesophageal probes, or may be recorded every 1–2 hours. The temperature may be elevated in the early stages of septic or toxic shock: in other types of shock, it is usually subnormal as shock progresses.

Skin
The colour and temperature of the skin are noted frequently. Lessening of the pallor, warming, and quick refilling of the capillaries and veins following compression are favourable signs. In severe shock, and that associated with sepsis, the nurse should be alert for petechiae or other signs of subcutaneous bleeding that may indicate disseminated intravascular coagulation.

Level of consciousness
Eye movement, the best verbal and best motor responses to verbal and painful stimulation are determined at regular intervals since they reflect cerebral perfusion and the oxygen supply. (See discussion of Glasgow Coma Scale p. 178).

RESPIRATORY ASSESSMENT

This should be carried out at frequent intervals.

Rate and volume of respirations
The rate and volume of respirations are recorded every 15–30 minutes. Hyperventilation may develop in the early stages of shock in response to the decrease in the pulmonary blood flow and the stimulation of the respiratory centre by the decreased oxygen tension; this greatly increases the work of breathing. As cited previously, respirations may become slow, irregular and shallow as a result of ischaemia of the respiratory centre and weakness of the respiratory muscles.

When assessing the patient the nurse should be aware of the serious changes that may develop in the lung in shock. Alternate intercostal ballooning and retraction, asymmetry in chest movement and dyspnoea are events to be reported. Auscultation of the anterior and posterior chests is used by the doctor, or trained intensive care nurse, to assess air entry and to listen for sounds of moisture in the airways. The presence of secretions and non-ventilated areas require prompt attention.

If ventilatory dysfunction occurs, the tidal volume is measured by means of a spirometer (see Chapter 16).

Arterial blood tests
Arterial blood specimens are collected every 2–3 hours for blood gases and hydrogen ion concentrations or pH determinations. The nurse should be able to understand the significance of the results; unfavourable changes may occur quickly and should be brought to the doctor's attention promptly so that appropriate therapeutic measures may be instituted. The Pao_2 content is elevated when compensation by hyperventilation is present, but falls as shock progresses (see Table 15.3). A Pao_2 of 11 kPa (80 mmHg) or less necessitates the administration of oxygen and, if it falls to 8 kPa (60 mmHg) or less, mechanical ventilatory assistance may be indicated (see Chapter 16). The pH is likely to be elevated, due to the respiratory alkalosis which occurs in response to the compensatory hyperventilation, but falls as shock progresses and metabolic and respiratory acidosis occur. The $Paco_2$ may fall due to hyperventilation, but is elevated in the progressive stage as respirations become depressed. The serum hydrogen carbonate level will likely be below normal as the shock progresses since it is being used for buffering the increased carbonic acid. If the $Paco_2$ rises and the serum hydrogen carbonate and pH remain low, respiratory compensation is inadequate and the doctor is notified. Ventilatory assistance may be necessary to remove the excess carbon dioxide.

BIOCHEMICAL LEVELS

The levels of certain biochemical factors provide necessary information about the patient's progress, as well as serving as a basis for some therapeutic measures (see Table 15.3). A considerable number of laboratory blood tests are performed. Blood specimens are collected for determination of lactic acid, hydrogen carbonate, potassium, chloride, sodium and calcium levels. These levels indicate the degree of anaerobic metabolism, acidosis and the disturbances or breakdown in cells. Determinations of blood urea and creatinine are also carried out for evaluation of tissue damage, kidney function and nitrogenous waste retention. Serum enzyme levels may be requested, since they reflect the amount of tissue damage and are especially significant in cardiogenic shock (see p. 335). Serum glucose levels are elevated in non-progressive shock and fall as shock progresses due to liver dysfunction and depletion of glycogen stores. Haematology studies provide information about the body's response to blood loss or sepsis. Platelet counts and coagulation tests determine clotting disturbances which occur with progressive and irreversible shock.

Urine tests provide information about renal function. With non-progressive shock the urine specific gravity will be elevated, the sodium content decreased and urine osmolality increased due to the retention of sodium and water. As shock progresses and renal failure develops creatinine clearance and urine osmolality decrease.

Treatment

Therapy is directed toward improving tissue perfusion and oxygenation and correcting the specific cause. The treatment and care presented here relate to shock and do not deal in detail with the specific initiating factor, although one is determined by the other.

Table 15.3 Summary of laboratory data in shock.

Laboratory test	Normal values	Changes in shock	Causative factors
Arterial blood gases			
pH	7.35–7.45	Elevated (compensatory) Decreased (progressive shock)	Respiratory alkalosis with hyperventilation Depressed respirations Metabolic acidosis
Pao_2	11–13 kPa (80–100 mmHg)	Elevated (compensatory) Decreased (progressive shock)	Hyperventilation Hypoventilation Ventilation–perfusion imbalance
$Paco_2$	4.8–6.0 kPa (35–40 mmHg)	Decreased (compensatory) Elevated (progressive shock)	Hyperventilation Hypoventilation
Biochemical levels			
Hydrogen carbonate	24–28 mmol/l	Decreased (progressive shock)	Acidosis
Serum lactate	0.5–2.0 mmol/l	Elevated (progressive shock)	Tissue hypoxia, acidosis
Sodium	135–145 mmol/l	Elevated (compensatory) Elevated or decreased (progressive shock)	Decreased renal excretion Altered renal perfusion
Chloride	100–106 mmol/l	Decreased (compensatory) Elevated (progressive shock)	Alkalosis Acidosis
Potassium	3.5–5.5 mmol/l	Decreased (compensatory) Elevated (progressive shock)	Increased renal excretion Acidosis Decreased renal excretion
Calcium	2.2–2.6 mmol/l	Decreased (progressive shock)	Renal failure
Phosphate	0.8–1.5 mmol/l	Elevated (progressive shock)	Renal failure
Magnesium	0.8–1.3 mmol/l	Decreased (progressive shock) or elevated (progressive shock)	Prolonged gastric suctioning and malnutrition Renal failure
Glucose	3.9–6.1 mmol/l	Elevated (compensatory) Decreased (progressive shock)	Sympathetic activity Depletion of glycogen stores Impaired liver function
Total serum protein albumin globulin	60–80 g/l 40–50 g/l 20–30 g/l	Decreased (progressive shock)	Leakage through capillaries
Blood urea	2.9–8.9 mmol/l	Elevated (progressive shock)	Decreased renal excretion
Creatinine	60–120 μmol/l	Elevated (progressive shock)	Decreased renal excretion
Haematology			
Haemoglobin	Males: 13–18 g/dl Females: 12–15 g/dl	Decreased	Blood loss
Haematocrit	Males: 40–50% Females: 37–47%	Increased	Fluid volume (loss) Plasma loss (burns)
Red blood cell count	Males: $4.5–6.5 \times 10^{12}$ per litre Females: $3.8–5.8 \times 10^{12}$ per litre	Decreased	Blood loss
White blood cell count	$4.0–11.0 \times 10^9$ per litre	Increased	Infection
Platelet count	$150–400 \times 10^9$ per litre	Decreased (progressive and irreversible shock)	Clotting disturbances
Prothrombin time (PT)	11–15 s	Prolonged (progressive and irreversible shock)	Clotting disturbances
Partial thromboplastin	60–70 s	Prolonged (progressive and irreversible shock)	Clotting disturbances

OBJECTIVES OF TREATMENT

In cardiogenic shock, the treatment focuses on strengthening the heart to increase the cardiac output and preventing arrhythmias by the use of certain drugs. Surgical revascularization of the heart muscle may be done in the case of myocardial infarction to improve coronary circulation. Immediate attention is also given to the correction of acidosis.

In hypovolaemic shock, the objective is expansion of the intravascular volume. For example, if the cause of the shock is haemorrhage, the treatment is directed toward arresting the bleeding and replacing the blood lost so that blood pressure is increased and tissue perfusion restored. The intravenous infusion solution of choice initially is a crystalloid solution, usually Ringer's lactate solution (an isotonic electrolyte solution) or normal saline. Colloid solutions of whole blood or fresh frozen plasma may be given in conjunction with the crystalloid solutions (see Table 6.5).

Septic shock is treated by an appropriate antibiotic to combat infection, possible drainage and excision of the source of infection in conjunction with attempts to improve tissue perfusion and oxygenation. A corticosteroid preparation (e.g. methylprednisolone) may be administered in large doses in the early stages. This drug enhances susceptibility to infection, increasing the need for close observation for signs of infection.

Neurogenic shock is usually associated with a spinal cord injury or may be incurred by spinal anaesthesia. Since there is a widespread loss of vasomotor tone and a disproportion between intravascular capacity and intravascular volume, an intravenous infusion is given to increase intravascular volume, and a vasoconstrictor drug such as methoxamine hydrochloride (Vasoxine) may be administered slowly, at a rate specified by the doctor, by intravenous infusion or intramuscular injection.

A vasoconstrictor preparation such as methoxamine hydrochloride is sometimes used in an emergency and in shock due to general or spinal anaesthesia, but inotropic agents which strengthen the force of muscular contractions are thought to be more effective. Examples of these drugs include dobutamine hydrochloride (Dobutrex) and dopamine hydrochloride (Intropin). Dobutamine acts on sympathetic receptors in cardiac muscle, increasing contractility. It is frequently used in septic and cardiogenic shock. Methoxamine hydrochloride raises the blood pressure but often at the expense of perfusion of vital organs such as the kidneys. Since the aim is to prevent this, the use of methoxamine in shock is usually deprecated.

IDENTIFICATION OF PATIENT PROBLEMS

Because of the complexity and diverse mani-

festations of shock, many nursing diagnoses are relevant. The major problem is alteration in tissue perfusion. Nursing interventions for the other problems contribute to the improvement of tissue perfusion. The patient's problems include:
1 Alteration in tissue perfusion
2 Fluid volume deficit
3 Alteration in cardiac output: decreased
4 Impaired oxygen and carbon dioxide exchange
5 Alteration in nutrition: less than body requirements
6 Anxiety
7 Alteration in comfort
8 Impaired mobility
9 Alteration in patterns of urinary output

NURSING INTERVENTION

PREVENTION OF SHOCK

Anticipation of shock by identification of patients at risk of developing it and identification and recording of early signs and symptoms by the nurse are essential if prompt treatment is to be initiated. High risk patients include those with acute myocardial infarction, spinal cord injury, burns, and altered immune systems and those who have had major surgery. Significant nursing assessments in the early identification and prevention of shock include: cardiac monitoring for prompt identification of arrhythmias, monitoring of fluid balance for haemodynamic changes, recognition of early signs of infection and documentation and communication of allergies and previous allergic reactions.

The nurse is responsible for the prevention of sepsis through consistent application of the principles of asepsis and the avoidance of non-essential invasive procedures.

1. Alteration in tissue perfusion

Cerebral, cardiopulmonary, renal, gastrointestinal, and peripheral perfusion are reduced due to hypovolaemia, altered cardiac output, increased peripheral vasoconstriction, decreased gas exchange and increased energy expenditure.

The goals are to:
1 Promote tissue perfusion
2 Decrease the metabolic needs of the cells

PROMOTION OF TISSUE PERFUSION

Measures to promote cellular perfusion include: replacing circulating blood volume, increasing cardiac output by treating arrhythmia, improving cardiac contractility, altering peripheral vascular resistance and improving gas exchange.

Acid–base imbalance. The measures which promote tissue perfusion also contribute to the correction of the acid–base imbalance. When the metabolic acidosis is severe, sodium bicarbonate may be administered intravenously.

Administration of corticosteroids. High doses of corticosteroids may be prescribed in the early stages of shock. It is believed that corticosteroid preparations stabilize the lysosomal membrane in cells and prevent the release of lysosomal enzymes into the cell cytoplasm. Corticosteroids also may improve tissue perfusion by decreasing interstitial oedema and enhancing cardiovascular response to catecholamines.

MEASURES TO DECREASE ENERGY DEMANDS

Planning of care. Monitoring, therapy and nursing care are organized to permit uninterrupted rest periods. The patient's energy expenditure is kept to a minimum by anticipating his needs, reducing discomfort and apprehension and providing adequate assistance when turning or lifting. Environmental stimuli (e.g. conversation, visitors, noise) are controlled to reduce disturbances. The usual 24-hour cycles of day and night should be respected (consistent with essential monitoring and treatment); lights should be dimmed and noise kept to a minimum at night to promote rest.

Body temperature. The patient is kept comfortably warm by the use of light covers and control of room temperature. Heat applications are not used because they increase peripheral vasodilation and body fluid loss. It is important to avoid overheating and chilling; extremes of temperature involve increased metabolism and, as a result, a greater demand for oxygen and increased carbon dioxide production. If hyperpyrexia develops the patient is given tepid sponges and is exposed to cool air. Conversely, a warming or hypothermia blanket may be used in cases of hypothermia, but careful checks should be made of the patient's temperature and the blanket removed before he becomes overheated.

Decrease anxiety and fear. Shock is a critical and life-threatening condition and creates fear and anxiety in the patient. In the critical care environment, the patient experiences loss of privacy and independence, strange sights and sounds, the absence of familiar persons and meaningful stimuli and a sense of aloneness. What it means to the patient and the effect of his fear and concerns on his condition should not be underestimated. Anxiety created by the situation and environment in which the patient finds himself aggravates respiratory distress and increases catecholamine secretion and metabolic demands. The nurse should identify the patient's concerns and fears and provide explanations relating to all nursing care activities. The patient's right to be treated with dignity and respect for his privacy are considered at all times. The intensive care environment is made as quiet and supportive as possible.

2. Fluid volume deficit

There is a reduced fluid volume because of blood loss, inadequate cardiac output or altered peripheral vascular tone and resistance.

The goal is to promote tissue perfusion by restoring the circulating blood volume.

FLUID REPLACEMENT

An intravenous line is established immediately so that fluids may be administered to expand the intravascular volume, blood loss may be replaced, and a readily accessible channel is provided for the administration of medications. Usually, an infusion of sodium chloride 0.9% is used while the patient is being assessed. The doctor then prescribes the appropriate solution, volume, and rate of administration according to the cause of shock, clinical manifestations and laboratory reports of the haematocrit, electrolytes, blood gases and pH levels. Solutions that may be used include crystalloid solutions such as Ringer's lactate solution and normal saline to replace electrolytes, and colloid solutions of whole blood, dextran, plasma or albumin. The volume and rate of administration of fluids are based on the blood pressure, central venous pressure, pulmonary artery pressure and pulmonary artery wedge pressure. Urinary output is also a useful parameter in this context. Frequent monitoring of the patient's reactions and the flow of these solutions is a primary responsibility of the nurse; adjustments in the rate of flow may be made when necessary to improve tissue perfusion, correct hypovolaemia and prevent fluid overload. The initial infusion is usually administered rapidly to arrest the progression of shock, but precautions against overloading the vascular system are necessary.

Oral fluids are not given to patients in shock because of impaired gastrointestinal absorption.

REDISTRIBUTION OF BLOOD FLOW

The patient should be in the supine position to promote venous return. Until recently the practice was to elevate the lower limbs or place the patient in the Trendelenberg position. The supine position promotes venous return without interfering with the descent of the diaphragm during inspiration. This position also reduces the possibility of aortic and carotid sinus baroreceptor reflexes which result in vasoconstriction of the cerebral vessels.

External devices such as medical anti-shock trousers (MAST) may be used to redistribute blood from the legs into the central circulation. The trousers have three chambers, one for each leg and one which covers the abdomen. Each chamber can be inflated separately to a prescribed pressure to compress underlying peripheral vessels. The compression returns 20–30% of the blood immediately to the central circulation. The use of this device is contraindicated in cardiogenic shock because of the rapid fluid shift that is created. Pressure should not be maintained for more than 2 hours and should be reduced gradually. During and following the decompression, close monitoring of infusions is necessary to prevent sudden intravascular overload.

3. Alteration in cardiac output

Cardiac output may be decreased due to cardiac disease, decreased blood volume, altered peripheral resistance, or altered cardiac contractility from the effects of shock and the presence of cardiac depressant factors.

The goals are to:
1 Increase cardiac output
2 Promote tissue perfusion

Cardiac support measures include maintaining the circulating fluid volume (fluid replacement) and decreasing the work load of the heart by placing the patient at rest in a supine position. Measures which decrease the body's demands for oxygen facilitate cardiac functioning.

The patient is monitored continuously for the development of cardiac arrhythmias; antiarrhythmic medication is administered if indicated. Medications may also be ordered to increase cardiac contractility and to alter peripheral resistance. The choice of drugs used in shock depends upon the cause and severity of hypotension, and they are given intravenously. Examples of drugs which may be prescribed include dopamine (Intropin), vasoactive preparations such as adrenaline, metaraminol (Aramine) and isoprenaline hydrochloride.

Dopamine may be used to improve the strength and rate of cardiac contractions. It increases the cardiac output and blood pressure and has the added advantage of increasing renal perfusion when given in small doses. Prolonged administration may produce ventricular arrhythmia and peripheral vasoconstriction.

A digitalis glycoside preparation may be given to increase the strength of the heart muscle and decrease the frequency of its contractions.

The role of vasoactive drugs in shock therapy is controversial except where anaphylactic shock occurs; adrenaline is the drug of choice in anaphylaxis because it produces vasoconstriction and also stimulates the heart. Isoprenaline hydrochloride causes vasodilation and an increased heart rate and output. A close check is kept on the pulse. If tachycardia or an arrhythmia develops, infusion of the drug is discontinued and the response reported. As well as increasing the cardiac output and blood flow, isoprenaline hydrochloride also accelerates the metabolic rate, increasing the oxygen demands.

Nursing responsibilities in drug therapy in shock include: being aware of the action and possible side-effects of the drugs; close monitoring for cardiac arrhythmias; monitoring the blood pressure every 5 minutes until the patient's condition is stable following the administration of a vasoactive drug; hourly measurement of the urinary output; observation of the infusion site for signs of infiltration or inflammation of the surrounding tissue; and the prompt reporting and recording of the patient's responses.

Intra-aortic balloon counter-pulsation may be instituted when cardiogenic shock occurs or when heart failure develops in the late stage of other types of shock. A balloon-tipped catheter (Swan–Ganz) is inserted through the femoral artery and aorta to the mid-thoracic level. Diastolic pressure is increased when the balloon is inflated and blood flow to the coronary arteries and peripheral blood vessels is increased. Deflation of the balloon prior to systole decreases peripheral resistance and promotes ventricular ejection of blood at a lower pressure, reducing the stress on the left ventricle. The coronary circulation is enhanced, the work load of the heart is decreased and the cardiac output is increased.

4. Impaired oxygen and carbon dioxide exchange

The impaired oxygen and carbon dioxide exchange are related to ventilation–perfusion imbalance, altered ventilation rate, decreased cardiac output and impaired circulation.

The goal is to promote gas exchange by supporting ventilation.

VENTILATION

Immediate attention is given to establishing and maintaining a patent airway. Oxygen is given by nasal cannulae or mask unless the blood gas determinations indicate the need for the delivery of a higher and more controlled concentration of oxygen by means of an endotracheal tube and mechanical ventilator (see Chapter 16). The aim is to restore and maintain a Pao_2 tension of at least 8 kPa (60 mmHg). High concentrations of oxygen cause alveolar damage so the lowest concentration necessary to maintain this level is administered. If intubation and ventilatory assistance are still necessary after a prolonged period, a tracheostomy may be performed to replace the endotracheal tube (see Chapter 16). Intubation by either means and the use of mechanical ventilation have several distinct advantages: they provide better control of ventilatory volume and oxygen concentration, decrease the work of breathing, provide a means by which the elimination of carbon dioxide can be regulated, and permit more effective deep suctioning and clearance of the airway.

If the patient is able, he is encouraged to perform deep-breathing and coughing exercises at frequent intervals with the necessary support. Maximum inspirations are carried out several times each hour. A change of position half-hourly or hourly is recommended to improve oxygenation.[10] Changing the patient's position alters the dependent areas of the lung, which decreases the possibility of consolidation developing and ventilation–perfusion inequality, promoting better gas exchange.

5. Alteration in nutrition: less than body requirements

The patient's nutritional status is altered due to inadequate gastrointestinal perfusion and increased needs.

The goals are to:
1 Avoid increased circulatory demands
2 Prevent excessive weight loss
3 Prevent a negative nitrogen balance

Food and fluids are not given orally to patients in shock because of the presence of paralytic ileus and the resulting increased need for blood flow to the gastrointestinal tract. A nasogastric tube is inserted to drain the stomach contents and prevent abdominal distension. Nutrition and hydration are maintained primarily by intravenous infusions. If the shock state is prolonged, total parenteral nutrition may be used to provide adequate nutrition (see Chapter 17). Oral feeding is resumed only after bowel sounds return.

6. Anxiety

The patient's anxiety may be related to his health and life expectancy, loss of control of events, unfamiliar hospital environment and separation from his family and friends.

The goals are to:
1 Identify the patient's concerns
2 Decrease his anxiety

As discussed earlier, anxiety increases the metabolic demands of the body and thus contributes to the shock.

A positive nurse–patient relationship provides a basis for establishing trust and confidence. The patient who is advised of his progress and receives simple explanations of tests and therapeutic measures, so he knows why they are necessary and what to expect, is generally less apprehensive. The constant presence of a nurse and the provision of opportunities to talk will help to allay the patient's anxiety. When communication is impaired because of intubation, the nurse should still speak to the patient and encourage written or hand signals from the patient. Anticipation of the patient's needs and awareness of preferences does much to relieve anxiety.

Family or friends are encouraged to visit; the duration of the visits should be adjusted to the patient's physical condition and his response to the visitors. It may be helpful to have a reliable, composed relative or friend remain quietly in the room. This familiar person's presence may provide reassurance and alleviate the patient's feelings of aloneness.

Non-essential noise and conversations with co-workers within hearing of the patient should be minimized. Unnecessary concern may arise if the patient misinterprets something he has heard, or applies it erroneously to himself.

Family. The family members also need consideration and support. Illness of a family member is a stressful, threatening event which represents a crisis for the family. Fear and concern for their loved one, the disruption of their accustomed life-style and additional burdens may disorganize their resources. They may suddenly be unable to cope and may need help.

The nurse should convey understanding and acceptance of their concern and reactions. They are kept informed about the patient's treatment and progress. Time is taken to listen to and answer their questions.

The family is advised where they may wait, of the location of a telephone they may use and where they may get a meal if they plan to remain in the hospital. They should not be left for long periods without contact with someone who can talk to them about the patient. Brief visits to the patient will mean much to them as well as indicate the nurse's appreciation of their feelings. They should receive assistance to mobilize their own resources. Guidance is provided, but they should be involved in solving their own problems if possible.

7. Alteration in comfort

The patient's alteration in comfort may be related to immobility, invasive procedures, fever and causative factors of shock, for example trauma.

The goals are to:
1 Promote comfort
2 Control pain

Bathing promotes relaxation and rest but should be planned to coincide with other activities of turning and assessment procedures. Frequent mouth care is important in contributing to comfort and in preventing sores, ulcers and infection.

Pain also increases anxiety, restlessness and metabolic demands, and so every effort should be made to provide prompt relief. Analgesics are usually administered intravenously; the patient is then observed for any respiratory depression that may result from the analgesic preparation used.

---

[10] Shafer (1981), p. 40.

8. Impaired mobility

Injury, decreased energy, fatigue, altered level of consciousness and/or treatment may all decrease the patient's mobility.

The goal is to prevent musculoskeletal and skin complications, which can be caused by decreased mobility.

Immobility predisposes the patient to serious complications such as circulatory stasis, thrombosis, accumulation of pulmonary secretions, atelectasis, decubitus ulcer and flexion contractures. Although rest and immobilization are necessary to decrease the patient's energy demands, it is essential that nursing measures are taken to prevent complications.

(a) Measures to prevent sores include: frequent inspection of the skin for areas of redness; turning the patient every ½–1 hour to relieve pressure as well as promoting drainage of pulmonary secretions; relieving pressure on the buttocks and shoulders by lifting every 1–2 hours; and by placing the patient on an alternating pressure (ripple) mattress.

(b) Measures to prevent contractures and foot drop include: positioning the patient in good body alignment; frequent change of position; positioning the feet at 90° to the ankles; passive movement of the limbs (especially the lower limbs); and active limb exercises when the patient's condition permits. The feet should not touch a firm surface or board as this could initiate a reflex spasm of muscles and lead to contracture. A bed-cradle to prevent pressure from the weight of the bedclothes is also useful.

9. Alteration in patterns of urinary elimination

Inadequate renal perfusion reduces urinary elimination. The goal is to maintain adequate urinary output.

An indwelling catheter is introduced using aseptic technique in order to determine the hourly urinary output, as renal failure or shutdown is a possible complication in shock. If renal insufficiency develops, peritoneal dialysis or haemodialysis may be necessary to remove urea, creatinine, water and other nitrogenous wastes (see Chapter 21).

Measures to replace fluid volume and increase cardiac output and tissue perfusion also promote increased urinary output.

EXPECTED OUTCOMES

1 The circulating fluid volume returns to normal as indicated by the following:
  (a) The arterial blood pressure is within 20 mmHg of preshock level.
  (b) The central venous pressure is between 10–12 cmH$_2$O (0–4 mmHg).
  (c) The pulmonary artery pressure is 10–20 mmHg.
  (d) The pulmonary artery wedge pressure is 10–12 mmHg.
2 The urinary output is greater than 30 ml/h.
3 The serum electrolytes are within the normal range:

Sodium	135–145 mmol
Chloride	100–106 mmol/l
Potassium	3.5–5.5 mmol/l
Calcium	2.2–2.6 mmol/l
Phosphate	0.8–1.5 mmol/l
Magnesium	0.8–1.3 mmol/l
Glucose	3.9–6.1 mmol/l (fasting: 2.5–5.6 mmol/l)

4 The cardiac output returns to preshock level:
  (a) The heart rate is ± 10 of the preshock rate.
  (b) The heart rhythm is regular.
5 The blood gases are within the normal range: Pao_2, 11–13 kPa; $Paco_2$; 4.8–6.0 kPa (35–40 mmHg).
6 Respiratory function returns to normal:
  (a) The respiratory rate is 16–22 per minute and regular
  (b) The lungs are free of crackles or wheezes on auscultation
7 Metabolic needs are decreased as evidenced by:
  (a) The patient is able to rest and sleep.
  (b) The body temperature is normal (37°C).
  (c) The patient is comfortable and free of pain.
  (d) The patient is less anxious.
8 Acid–base balance is restored:
  pH 7.35–7.45
  [H$^+$] 35–45 nmol/l
  HCO$_3^-$ 24–28 mmol/l
  serum lactate 0.5–2.0 mmol/l
9 Blood urea and creatinine levels are normal: Blood urea, 2.9–8.9 mmol/l; creatinine, 100–120 mmol/l.
10 The patient is alert and conscious:
  (a) Eyes open spontaneously.
  (b) Verbal responses show orientation to time, place and person.
  (c) Motor responses are coordinated and appropriate to command.
11 The skin is warm, dry and normal in colour.
12 Complications from immobility are absent:
  (a) The skin is dry and intact.
  (b) The limbs are free of contractures.

Transfer and Rehabilitation

With reversal of the shock state, the patient is transferred from the intensive care unit to a general ward. This usually engenders considerable apprehension and concern even though it indicates favourable progress. The patient has been under constant observation and care. In this new situation he will likely be left to himself for lengthy periods.

The move should be discussed with him in the intensive care unit. The staff in the general ward should have some knowledge and appreciation of what the patient and family have experienced during the acute shock state, and should be aware of any residual problems.

Preparation for discharge includes a discussion of the resumption of activities and the necessary care. There may be a tendency following such a severe illness for the patient to be fearful of doing some things and for the family to be overprotective.

References and Further Reading

BOOKS

Bordicks KJ (1980) *Patterns of Shock: Implications for Nursing Care*. 2nd ed. New York: Macmillan.

Guyton AC (1986) *Textbook of Medical Physiology*, 7th ed. Philadelphia: WB Saunders. pp. 386 & 390.

Hart LK, Reese JL & Fearing MO (eds), (1981) *Concepts Common to Acute Illness*. St Louis: CV Mosby. Chapter 15.

Holloway NM (1984) *Nursing the Critically Ill Adult*, 2nd ed. Menlo Park, CA: Addison–Wesley. pp. 223–238.

Kinney MR, Dear CB, Packa DR & Voorman DMN (eds) (1981) *AACN's Clinical Reference for Critical Care Nursing*. New York: McGraw-Hill. pp. 309–311 & 697–701.

Krupp MA & Chatton MJ (1983) *Current Medical Diagnosis and Treatment*. Los Altos, CA: Lange. pp. 9–13.

Niedringhaus L, Smith-Collins A & Myers JL (1983), In: Perry AG & Potter PA (eds), *Shock: Comprehensive Nursing Management*, St Louis: CV Mosby.

Sabiston DC Jr (ed) (1981) *Davis–Christopher: Textbook of Surgery*, 12th ed. Philadelphia: WB Saunders. Chapter 3.

Smith LH & Thier SO (1985) *Pathophysiology*, 2nd ed. Philadelphia; WB Saunders. pp. 999–1003.

PERIODICALS

Barrows JJ (1982) Shock demands drugs—but which one is best for your patient. *Nurs. '82*, Vol. 12 No. 2, pp. 34–41.

Beyer A (1979) Shock lung. *Br. J. Hosp. Med.*, pp. 248–257.

Bihari DJ & Tinker J (1982) Steroids in intensive care. *Br. J. Hosp. Med.*, pp. 323–330.

Bourbonnais F (1980) Adult respiratory distress syndrome. *Can. Nurs.*, Vol. 76 No. 10, pp. 51–54.

Brown LK (1981) Toxic shock syndrome. *Am. J. Mat. Child Nurs.*, Vol. 6 No. 1, pp. 57–59.

Bull S (1981) Vascular pressures and critical care management. *Nurs. Clin. N. Am.*, Vol. 16 No. 2, pp. 225–239.

Cohen S (1982) Nursing care of patients in shock—Part 3. Evaluating the patient: programmed instruction. *Am. J. Nurs.*, Vol. 82 No. 11, pp. 1723–1746.

Cooper TJ & Tinker J (1984) The adult respiratory distress syndrome. *Hosp. Update*, pp. 849–859.

Crumlish CM (1981) Cardiogenic shock—catch it early. *Nurs. '81*. Vol. 11 No. 8, pp. 34–41.

Davis JM (1982) Cardiovascular problems (1). *Hosp. Update*, pp. 1359–1369.

Davis JM (1982) Cardiovascular problems (2). *Hosp. Update*, pp. 1521–1534.

Ewertz M & Shpritz D (1980) Your best strategy when 'shock lung' strikes, *R.N.* Vol. 43 No. 10, pp. 43–45.

Geddes JS, Adgey AAJ & Partridge JF (1980) Prevention of cardiogenic shock. *Am. Heart J.*, Vol. 99 No. 2, pp. 243–254.

George RJD, Banks RA (1983) Bedside measurement of pulmonary capillary wedge pressure, *Br. J. Hosp. Med.*, pp. 286–291.

Hall KV (1981) Detecting septic shock before it's too late. *R.N.*, Vol. 44 No. 9, pp. 28–32.

Harmon AL & Harmon DC (1980) Anaphylaxis—sudden death anytime. *Nurs. '80*, Vol. 10 No. 10, pp. 40–43.

Heimburger DC (1984) Toxic shock syndrome. *Crit. Care Nurs.*, Vol. 1 No. 4, pp. 32–36.

Huestes DW (1984) Platelet transfusion: some general considerations. *J. Med. Tech,*. Vol. 1 No. 9, pp. 703–707.

Lamb LS (1982) Think you know septic shock? Read this. *Nurs. '82.*, Vol. 12 No. 1, pp. 34–43.

Ledingham IMcA & Routh GS (1979) The pathophysiology of shock. *Br. J. Hosp. Med.*, pp. 472–482.

Ledingham IMcA, Cowan BN, Burns HJG (1982) Prognosis in severe shock. *Br. Med. J.*, Vol. 284, pp. 443–444.

Nagel RL, Fabry ME & Paul DK (1984) New insights on sickle cell anaemia. *Diagn. Med.*, Vol. 7 No. 5, pp. 26–33.

Preston FE (1982) Disseminated intravascular coagulation. *Br. J. Hosp. Med.*, pp. 129–137.

Pursley PM (1981) Arterial catheters: nursing management to decrease complication. *Crit. Care Nurs.*, Vol. 1 No. 5, pp. 16–21.

Rice V (1981) Shock, a clinical syndrome part 1. Definition, etiology and pathophysiology. *Crit. Care Nurs.*, Vol. 1 No. 3, pp. 44–50.

Rice V (1981) Shock, a clinical syndrome part II. The stages of shock. *Crit. Care Nurs.*, Vol. 1 No. 4, pp. 4–14.

Rice V (1981) Shock, a clinical syndrome part III. The nursing care: prevention and patient assessment., *Crit. Care Nurs.*, Vol. 1 No. 5, pp. 36–47.

Rice V (1981) Shock, a clinical syndrome part IV. Nursing Intervention. *Crit. Care Nurs.*, Vol. 1 No. 6, pp. 34–43.

Rice V (1984) The clinical continuum of septic shock. *Crit. Care Nurs.*, Vol. 4 No. 5, pp. 84–109.

Rice V (1984) Shock management part 1: fluid volume replacement. *Crit. Care Nurs.*, Vol. 4 No. 6, pp. 69–82.

Shafer T (1981) Nursing care of the patient with ARDS. *Crit. Care Nurs.*, Vol. 1 No. 3, pp. 34–43.

Shine KI, Kuhn M, Young LS & Tillisch JH (1980) Aspects of management of shock. *Ann. Int. Med.*, Vol. 93 No. 5, pp. 723–734.

Sumner SM & Grau PA (1981) To defeat hypovolemic shock anticipate and act swiftly. *Nurs. '81.*, Vol. 11 No. 10, pp. 47–51.

Tinker J (1979) A pharmacological approach to the treatment of shock. *Br. J. Hosp. Med.*, pp. 261–268.

Wallace PGM & Spence AA (1983) Adult respiratory distress syndrome. *Br. Med. J.*, Vol. 286, pp. 1167–1168.

Wardle N (1979) Bacteraemic and endotoxic shock. *Br. J. Hosp. Med.*, pp. 223–245.

Wroblewski SS (1980) Shock. *Emerg. Med.*, Vol. 12 No. 19, pp. 47–53 & 58–62.

Wroblewski SS (1981) Toxic shock syndrome, *Am. J. Nurs.*, Vol. 81 No. 1, pp. 82–85.

Wroblewski SS (1981) Cardiogenic shock needn't spell death. *Emerg. Med.*, Vol. 13 No. 4, pp. 124–128.

Wroblewski SS (1984) Caring for the patient in hypovolemic shock. *Nurs. '84*, Vol. 14 No. 3, pp. 24–27.

16
Nursing in Respiratory Disorders

Respiration

A constant exchange of oxygen and carbon dioxide between the living organism and its environment is essential for survival. Respiration is the process which performs this function. The exchange takes place between the total organism and the external environment and between the tissue cells and the blood. The former involves pulmonary ventilation and diffusion of the gases through the alveolar membrane of the lungs. The exchange between the cells and the blood (sometimes called internal or tissue respiration) requires transportation of the gases by the blood and an exchange of oxygen and carbon dioxide between the capillaries and tissue cells.

Pulmonary ventilation or breathing consists of the movement of air into and out of the lungs (inspiration and expiration). Diffusion involves the movement of gases between the air in the pulmonary air sacs (alveoli) and the blood in the pulmonary capillaries in the direction of the lower pressure or concentration.

In addition to providing oxygen for cellular metabolism and removing the cellular metabolite carbon dioxide, the respiratory system also plays an important role in voice production, regulation of the pH of body fluids and the elimination of heat and water. Ventilation enhances venous return to the right side of the heart by alternating positive and negative intrathoracic pressure, and also contributes to compression of the abdominal viscera to aid in parturition and defecation.

Metabolic functions of the lungs include synthesis of phospholipids (surfactant) and protein, carbohydrate metabolism and chemical changes of some vasoactive substances (e.g. conversion of angiotensin I to angiotensin II. The lung also secretes immunoglobulins which contribute to pulmonary defence against infection.[1]

RESPIRATORY STRUCTURES

The structures concerned with ventilation are the upper and lower respiratory tracts, respiratory muscles, thorax and portions of the nervous system. (Fig. 16.1).

[1] Cherniak & Cherniak (1983), p. 145.

The upper airway is formed by the nose, mouth, pharynx and larynx. It serves as a passageway for air being inspired and expired, filters, warms and moistens the inhaled air, and provides the protective reflexes of sneezing and the closing off of the larynx to prevent aspiration of fluid and solids. Irritation of the pharynx and larynx may also initiate the cough reflex.

Nose
The nose has a highly vascularized and ciliated mucous membrane lining which serves to moisten, warm and filter inhaled air. The nasal cavities and their connecting sinuses act as resonating chambers in sound production. The posterior portion of the cavities contains olfactory receptors concerned with the sense of smell (olfactory sense). The external orifices are called the nostrils, or anterior nares.

Pharynx
The pharynx, a muscular tube lined with mucous membrane, provides a common passageway for air entering the larynx and food entering the oesophagus. Air reaching the pharynx passes readily into the larynx, but the presence of food or fluid stimulates a reflex contraction of the pharyngeal tube. The posterior nares (openings into the nasal cavities) are then blocked off and the larynx is closed off by a lowering of the leaf-shaped structure, the *epiglottis*. These closures prevent the entrance of food or fluid into the nose and lower respiratory tract. As a result of the contraction, the pharyngeal content is directed into the oesophagus.

Larynx
The larynx is composed of muscle tissue and cartilage and is lined with mucous membrane. It functions as an air passage and contains the *vocal cords*, which are responsible for sound production. The laryngeal passageway is narrowed in one area by membranous folds reflected over the vocal cords. The slit-like space between these two folds is referred to as the *glottis* and is varied in size to produce the different levels of pitch in voice production. In normal quiet inspiration and expiration the vocal cords are relaxed and the glottis is open.

LOWER RESPIRATORY TRACT

The lower tract consists of the trachea, bronchi and two lungs.

401

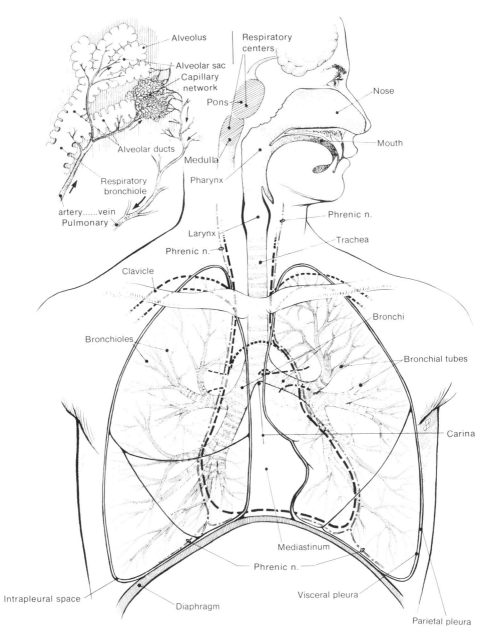

Fig. 16.1 The respiratory system.

Trachea
The trachea is a continuation of the inferior end of the larynx and divides into two tubes—the right and left bronchi. The right bronchus is shorter and more vertical than the left; this accounts for aspirated foreign particles entering the right bronchus more often than the left. The tracheal walls are composed of fibroelastic tissue in which incomplete cartilaginous rings are imbedded to prevent collapse of the tube. The trachea simply serves as an air passageway.

Bronchi, bronchial tubes and bronchioles
Each bronchus enters a lung where it branches like a tree to form the bronchial tubes and, eventually, the very small tubes, the bronchioles. As the branches become more distal, the lumen of the tubes narrows and the walls change structure. The bronchi and bronchial tubes are similar in structure to the trachea except for the addition of plain muscle tissue in their walls. In the bronchioles, the cartilaginous tissue disappears and the smooth muscle tissue becomes more abundant.

The trachea and bronchial air passages are lined by a ciliated mucous membrane continuous with that of the upper air passages. The cilia are hair-like projections of protoplasm which alternately bend in one direction and straighten, providing a sweeping motion to remove the mucus secreted and any foreign particles that may have been inhaled. Excessive secretions may initiate the cough reflex, which is a defence mechanism to rid the tract of such substances (see p. 427). The bronchi conduct air between the external environment and terminal structures where gas exchange takes place, as well as serving in the clearance of secretions. Some bronchioles function only as air conductors, others participate in gas exchange as well as conduction of air.[2]

Terminal respiratory units

The bronchioles divide and subdivide, progressively becoming smaller. Each bronchiole eventually gives rise to a spray of microscopic tubes known as *alveolar ducts*. Microscopic sacs called *alveoli* (singular—alveolus) increase in number along the terminal bronchioles and completely line the alveolar ducts and terminate in alveolar sacs containing alveolar projections. Collectively, these structures are referred to as the *terminal respiratory units* or parenchyma. Their function is gas exchange. The walls of the alveoli consist of thin epithelial cells, elastic connective tissue and a network of capillaries. The air in each alveolus is separated from the blood in the capillaries by a very thin semipermeable tissue which permits diffusion of the oxygen and carbon dioxide through it. The surface area of the alveolar surface is very great and is estimated to be approximately 30–40 times that of the skin surface.

Lungs

Each lung is made up of conducting airways comprising: the bronchial tubes, with their successive branches; the terminal respiratory units, composed of respiratory bronchioles; alveolar ducts and alveoli; and the many blood vessels of the pulmonary circulatory system. The right lung is divided into three lobes, and the left is divided into two lobes only. The portion of lung derived from each main bronchial tube is referred to as a *bronchopulmonary segment* (see Fig. 16.2). Each lung is enclosed in an adherent serous membrane called the visceral pleura, which is continuous from the hilum of the lung with a similar layer that lines the thoracic wall—the *parietal pleura*.

Blood supply to the lungs

Blood from two sources enters the lungs. The bronchial arteries convey blood from the aorta to nourish the conducting airways (from the main bronchi to the terminal bronchioles). The pulmonary artery delivers the blood from the right side of the heart to the terminal respiratory units to be oxygenated. Blood from both sources is then collected from the capillaries around the alveoli and other structures into veins and is returned to the left side of the heart by the four pulmonary veins. Some blood from the bronchial arteries, around the area of the hilum, enters bronchial veins which empty into larger veins to be transported to the right atrium.

Lymphatic drainage

Two pulmonary lymphatic systems exist: the superficial network located within the connective layer of the visceral pleura, and the deep or parenchymal system which surrounds the airways, arteries, veins and terminal respiratory units.[3] Lymphocytes and plasma cells are found throughout the tracheobronchial structures. Small lymph nodes are also found in the lungs. Smith indicates that the lymphatic system of the lungs plays a vital role in defence against infection; lymphoid tissue in the mucous membrane of the tracheobronchial tree provides antibody- and cell-mediated immune responses. Pulmonary lymphatic dysfunction causes pulmonary oedema and infection.[4]

Thorax

The lungs are well protected by the bony thoracic cage which is formed by the sternum, ribs and thoracic vertebrae. The apices of the lungs extend about 2.5 cm above the clavicles. The thorax acts as an airtight box in which the lungs are suspended and in which pressure can be varied by contraction of respiratory muscles, altering the thoracic cavity dimensions.

SECRETIONS

The respiratory tract produces two secretions: *mucus* and *surfactant*. The inner surfaces of the alveoli and alveolar ducts are covered with a film of fluid called *surfactant* (or surface active substance), a phospholipid compound synthesized by special epithelial cells in the walls of the alveoli. The composition of this solution is such that it reduces the surface tension, facilitating inflation and preventing collapse of the alveoli on expiration. Surfactant also prevents the movement of fluid from the capillaries into the alveoli (pulmonary oedema) by reducing the surface tension.

Inactivation of surfactant or a deficiency in the amount secreted increases the surface tension, resulting in resistance to the inflow of air and reduced lung expansion. The condition may be congenital, and is referred to as hyaline membrane disease or respiratory distress syndrome of the newborn. Inactivation of the secretion or a deficiency may also be associated with hypoxia, excessively

---

[2] Smith & Thier (1985), p. 754.

[3] Smith & Thier (1985), pp. 765–766.
[4] Smith & Thier (1985), p. 833.

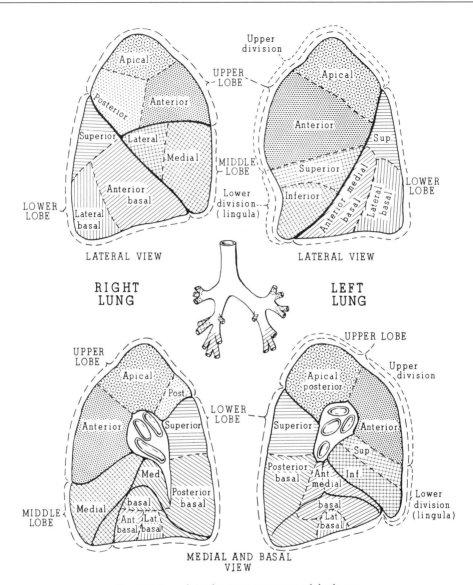

Fig. 16.2 Bronchopulmonary segments of the lungs.

high concentrations of oxygen, acidosis, inadequate perfusion (flow of blood through the capillaries) or severe stress (trauma).

The *mucus* which is secreted by the glandular (goblet) cells of the mucous membrane lining of the respiratory tract serves to protect the organism in several ways. It provides a protective barrier against inhaled irritants and traps foreign particles, facilitating their removal by the cilia. It also waterproofs the surface, thus diminishing the loss of body water as well as setting up a barrier to inhaled organisms. Insufficient secretion of mucus or the production of a thick tenacious mucoid such as occurs in the congenital disorder mucoviscidosis (fibrocystic disease of the new-born) prevents the action of the cilia, predisposing to infection and partial or complete obstruction of bronchial tubes and bronchioles.

CHEST CAVITIES AND THEIR PRESSURES

The spaces between the visceral and parietal pleurae form the intrapleural or *pleural cavities*. (Each lung has its own closed pleural cavity.) Each pleural cavity is only a potential space, since the visceral and parietal pleurae are separated normally by just a thin film of fluid that moistens the surfaces. The surfaces of the lungs are in close apposition with the chest walls. The pressure within the pleural cavities is approximately 5 mmHg less than atmospheric pressure, which is 760 mmHg at sea level. It may also be expressed as a negative pressure equal to that exerted by a column of water 10 cm in depth.

The *intrapulmonary cavity* is the space within the lungs and, since it communicates with atmosphere, the intrapulmonary pressure varies above and below atmospheric pressure during expiration and inspiration, respectively. Between expiration and inspiration, when there is no movement of air, the intrapulmonary pressure is the same as that of the atmosphere. Normally, alveolar pressure falls and then inspiration occurs.

The space in between the two lungs and their pleurae is known as the *mediastinum*. It contains the large blood vessels, heart, oesophagus, trachea, bronchi, and lymphatic ducts and nodes.

RESPIRATORY MUSCLES

The muscles used in normal breathing are principally the diaphragm and the intercostal muscles. The *diaphragm* is a dome-shaped muscular partition between the thoracic and abdominal cavities and is the most important respiratory muscle. When the diaphragm is relaxed, its thoracic surface is convex. On contraction, the convexity is reduced and the thoracic cavity is lengthened. The diaphragm also functions in coughing and sneezing and, in conjunction with the abdominal muscles, is used in defecation, vomiting and parturition.

The *external intercostal muscles* increase the lateral and anteroposterior diameters of the thoracic cavity by elevating the sternum and moving the ribs into a more horizontal position.

Accessory muscles may be used to facilitate breathing. In laboured and forced inspiration, the sternocleidomastoid muscles elevate the sternum, and the scalene and pectoralis muscles contract to raise the upper ribs. At the same time the nostrils dilate and the glottis widens. Forced or difficult expiration involves the abdominal and internal intercostal muscles. The abdominal muscles contract to raise the relaxed diaphragm higher in order to compress the lungs and facilitate expiration.

RESPIRATORY FUNCTIONS

MECHANICS OF PULMONARY VENTILATION

Each respiration involves inspiration and expiration. Inspiration is an active phase during which air moves into the lungs. Expiration, in normal breathing, is a passive phase during which air moves out of the lungs. Pulmonary ventilation is made possible by rhythmic variations in the dimensions of the thoracic and intrapulmonary spaces brought about by the alternating contraction and relaxation of the respiratory muscles.

Gases possess certain physical properties which explain the movement and exchange of respiratory gases. They differ from fluids in that their molecules spread out to fill the space available to them. The molecules of a gas are in a ceaseless movement and strike the walls of the container, creating a pressure. Within a given space, the greater the number of molecules of gas, the higher is the pressure produced. *The pressure of a gas varies inversely with the space in which it is contained if the temperature remains constant* (Boyle's law). If the space in which the volume of gas is confined is reduced, more gas molecules strike a smaller area of the container, increasing the pressure. Conversely, if the space is increased, the pressure of the gas is decreased. *Gas molecules move from an area of higher pressure to one of lower pressure.*

According to Dalton's law of partial pressure, *each gas in a mixture of gases exerts the same pressure that it would exert if it were not in a mixture, and that pressure is proportional to its concentration.* The pressure of the mixture is the sum of the pressures of the constituent gases. The pressure of each gas in the mixture is termed the partial pressure of that gas, and is indicated by a '*P*' preceding the gas symbol. For example, the pressure of oxygen in a mixture of gases is recorded as Po_2.

The amount of a gas absorbed by a fluid (i.e. its solubility) *is directly proportional to the partial pressure of the gas.* The fluid will absorb the gas until the pressure of the gas is the same as that at the surface. This is referred to as Henry's law of the solution of gases.

Inspiration

The diaphragm and external intercostal muscles contract, increasing the closed, airtight thoracic space and resulting in a pressure decrease of approximately 4–5 mmHg within the cavity. The moist visceral and parietal pleurae are apposed and resist separation in the same way that two pieces of plastic or glass whose surfaces are wet are difficult to separate but slide readily on each other. As the adherent moist parietal pleura moves out with the thoracic walls, the visceral pleura follows because of the cohesion between the two moist serous surfaces. The pressure in the intrapulmonary space is atmospheric and is greater than that of the expanded thoracic cavity. This pressure differential, combined with the cohesion of the pleurae, promotes a stretching of the elastic alveoli, resulting in the expansion of the lungs. The intrapulmonary space is now increased and the pressure of the contained air is reduced. A pressure gradient is produced between the atmospheric air and that in the lungs, so air moves into the respiratory tract, producing an inspiration.

Expiration

Relaxation of the respiratory muscles reverses the above process. As the intrathoracic space decreases with the muscular relaxation, the pressure within the cavity increases. The elastic alveoli which were stretched now recoil also, diminishing the intrapulmonary space. The pressure of the air within the lungs is increased then to a level above that of the atmospheric air. This causes air to move out until the intrapulmonary pressure is equal to that of the atmosphere, thus producing an expiration. Normally, this cycle of inspiration and expiration is completed 14–18 times per minute in the adult.

The work of breathing

The inspiratory phase of breathing requires energy to overcome the elastic forces in the lungs (compliance work), the flow-resistant forces within the air passages (airway resistance work) and the viscosity of the lungs and thoracic cage (tissue resistance work). Owing to their elastic property, the lungs and chest wall constantly tend to maintain the position they occupy at the end of a normal expiration. When the respiratory muscles contract to expand the intrathoracic and intrapulmonary spaces to provide inhalation, they must overcome this elastic resistance. *Compliance* is the term used to indicate the distensibility of the lungs and the thorax, or the ease with which they are stretched. Pulmonary disease may produce changes in the lung tissue that make it 'stiffer' and less elastic, causing a reduction in compliance. Similarly, the compliance of the thorax may be decreased by disorders affecting the chest wall.

Some energy is also necessary to overcome the frictional and viscous resistance offered by the surface tissues in the air passages. Any condition which reduces the calibre of the passages, causes an excessive production of mucus, or increases the surface tension increases the flow-resistant forces. These changes create a demand for greater energy to move air in and out in ventilation.

Control of ventilation

The control of ventilation is complex, and knowledge of this control is incomplete and unclear. Respirations are regulated by both nervous and chemical mechanisms.

Neural regulation. Inspiration and expiration are dependent upon alternate contraction and relaxation of muscles which are subordinate to impulses initiated by groups of neurons in the medulla and pons of the brain stem. These groups of neurons make up the *respiratory centres* (see Fig. 16.1).

The *medullary centre* is considered responsible for spontaneous, rhythmic respiration. Some neurons in this centre discharge impulses that result in contraction of the respiratory muscles and inspiration; others discharge impulses that cause relaxation of the muscles and expiration. The rhythmic discharge of the neurons in the medulla may be modified by impulses generated by groups of neurons (centres) in the pons (*pontine centre*) and by impulses transmitted to the medullary centres by afferent (sensory) nerve fibres of the vagus nerves. These nerve fibres transmit impulses from receptors in the lungs that are sensitive to stretching (pulmonary stretch receptors), irritation (irritant receptors), possibly capillary distension and increased interstitial fluid volume (juxtacapillary receptors). Stretching of the lungs by inflation produces impulses that have an inhibitory effect on the neurons that generate inspiratory impulses. The pulmonary stretch stimulus and ensuing inhibitory response is known as the *Hering–Breuer reflex*. It is more active in infants and young children and is quite weak in adults. Stimulation of the irritant receptors causes bronchoconstriction and hyperpnoea while the juxtacapillary receptors are believed to play a role in the sensation of dyspnoea and in producing rapid, shallow breathing.

Impulses from the respiratory centre descend into the spinal cord. Those carried to the diaphragm are transmitted by the phrenic nerves, which originate with the third, fourth and fifth cervical spinal nerves. The impulses to the intercostal muscles are delivered by the intercostal nerves that arise from the spinal cord with the third, fourth, fifth and sixth thoracic spinal nerves. The activity of the respiratory centre is influenced by the level of activity of the reticular formation. Mental alertness and wakefulness normally have a stimulating effect on breathing, but sleep, sedatives and anaesthesia tend to reduce the rate and volume of ventilation.

Respiratory muscle activities may be modified by impulses originating in the cerebral cortex that are delivered to the respiratory centres. For example, breathing may be controlled voluntarily for a limited period, as in breath-holding or the taking of large deep breaths. Voluntary control and a high level of central nervous system coordination and integration are needed in speaking and singing. Changes in the rhythm, rate and depth of respirations are frequently associated with emotional states (e.g. excitement, laughing, crying, depression, fear).

Certain sensory impulses may influence respirations. Severe pain produces faster and deeper respirations. Muscle activity increases respirations; this is attributed both to an increase in carbon dioxide production and to impulses originating in the stretch and pressure receptors of muscles, tendons and joints. A sudden cold application to the body produces a brief reflex apnoea (cessation of breathing) followed by increased ventilation.

Chemical regulation. The major chemical factors that exert a control on ventilation are the P_{CO_2}, pH or [H+] and P_{O_2} of the blood.

The *arterial carbon dioxide* tension plays an important role in the regulation of breathing. An increase above the normal P_{CO_2} results in an increase in the activity of the respiratory centres and a corresponding increase in the volume and frequency of respirations. A decrease below the normal slows the respiratory rate. An increase in the *hydrogen ion concentration* (decrease in the pH) produces a similar response as that to an increase above normal in the P_{CO_2}. The *arterial oxygen tension* influences respirations to a lesser extent than the carbon dioxide content. The cells which are sensitive to changes in these chemicals are not highly sensitive to slight variations in P_{O_2}; the oxygen content may fall below 14 volumes % before there is a noticeable increase in respiratory activity.

Changes in the pH (or hydrogen ion concentration) and tensions of carbon dioxide and oxygen in the blood bring about respiratory changes through *respiratory chemoreceptors*. These are groups of cells that are sensitive to certain changes in the chemistry of the blood. According to their location in relation to the nervous system the chemoreceptors are of two types, peripheral and central.

Central chemoreceptors are located in the medulla and respond to changes in the hydrogen ion concentration in the extracellular fluid surrounding the receptors. An increase in the P_{CO_2} in the blood results in carbon dioxide diffusing into the cerebrospinal fluid from the cerebral blood vessels. Hydrogen ions are then liberated and stimulate the chemoreceptors; the resulting increase in the rate and volume of respirations reduces the P_{CO_2} in the blood and in the cerebral spinal fluid.[5] A decrease in the hydrogen ion concentration in the surrounding extracellular fluid inhibits the central receptors.

The peripheral chemoreceptors are located in the carotid and aortic bodies[6] and are sensitive to decreases in the arterial P_{O_2} and to a lesser extent to increases in P_{CO_2}. The carotid bodies also respond to decreases in the pH or increases in the hydrogen ion concentrations. Impulses are initiated in these receptors and are then transmitted to the respiratory neurons via the glossopharyngeal and vagus nerves, resulting in changes in the rate and volume of respirations.

When body metabolism increases, more oxygen is used by the tissues and more carbon dioxide and acid metabolites are produced. Normally, this decreases the P_{O_2} and increases the P_{CO_2} and hydrogen ion concentration in the blood, and a corresponding increase in the rate and volume of respirations occurs.

Other factors influencing respiration. Other factors which influence ventilatory activity include blood pressure changes, changes in body temperature, drugs, and age.

Pressoreceptors in the aortic and carotid bodies are sensitive to changes in blood pressure. When they are stimulated, impulses are delivered to the respiratory centres which produce the appropriate response. A fall in blood pressure produces increased ventilation and, conversely, an elevated blood pressure generates impulses that give rise to a slower respiratory rate.

A high fever produces a noticeable increase in respiration which may be attributed principally to the increased oxygen consumption and carbon dioxide production by the accelerated cell metabolism. A decrease in temperature well below the normal, such as is produced in hypothermia, results in shallow, slow respirations.

Some drugs are known to depress the respiratory centre, and overdosage may prove fatal for this reason. Narcotics such as morphine, barbiturates, anaesthetics, alcohol and some tranquillizers are examples of drugs that reduce respiratory activity. Certain drugs, such as prostaglandin inhibitors, have the reverse effect and in excess may cause hyperpnoea (increased rate and volume of respiration). This could lead to exhaustion and respiratory alkalosis because of the excessive elimination of carbon dioxide. Salicylate preparations and other anti-inflammatory drugs, such as phenylbutazone (Butazolidin) used in the treatment of rheumatoid arthritis, are the most common offenders in this area.

Rate of respiration

Respiratory rate varies with age; it is more rapid in the young, decreasing with age. The rate at birth may be 40–70 respirations per minute, at 5 years of age it is approximately 25–30 per minute, at 10 years it is 20–22 per minute, and at 15 years of age and older it is 16–20 per minute.

COMPOSITION OF INSPIRED, EXPIRED AND ALVEOLAR AIR

Inspired air

Dry, inspired or atmospheric air at sea level is composed of nitrogen, oxygen and carbon dioxide in the following proportions:

oxygen	21 volumes %
carbon dioxide	0.04 volume %
nitrogen	79 volumes %

Various quantities of water vapour, dust particles, and insignificant amounts of rare gases such as argon, neon and ozone may be present. Oxygen and carbon dioxide are the respiratory gases; nitrogen is not of concern since it is inert in the body. Some nitrogen does diffuse in and out of the blood, but under normal atmospheric pressures it has no physiological significance.

Expired air

This shows a reduction in oxygen and an increase in the carbon dioxide as compared with atmospheric air. It is a mixture of alveolar and atmospheric air from the passages above the alveoli. No exchange of gases is made in the air passages above the terminal respiratory units. This non-respiratory area is called

---

[5] West (1979), p. 117.
[6] The *carotid bodies* lie in the bifurcations of the carotid arteries; the *aortic bodies* are located on the wall of the aortic arch.

the *anatomical dead space*. If any alveoli are not perfused by capillary blood flow, those alveolar spaces combined with the anatomical dead space compose the *physiological dead space*. If a person breathes through a tube, the dead space is increased; less of the inspired air reaches the alveoli.

Alveolar air
Since it is at the level of the terminal respiratory units that an exchange of the respiratory gases takes place with the capillary blood, the volume of oxygen in the contained air is reduced and that of carbon dioxide increases. Air that moves into the alveoli with each inspiration is a mixture of newly inspired air and air that moved into the dead space from the air sacs on previous expirations. In other words, as inspiration begins, alveolar air which had moved into the dead space on expiration is drawn back into the alveoli mixed with a portion of newly inspired air. Thus air entering the alveoli does not have exactly the same composition as inspired atmosphere air.

A comparison of the approximate volumes of respiratory gases in inspired, expired and alveolar air may be made from Table 16.1.

Table 16.1 Tension of respiratory gases in inspired, expired and alveolar air.

	Volumes %		Partial pressure (kPa)	
	Oxygen	Carbon dioxide	Oxygen	Carbon dioxide
Inspired (atmospheric) air	20.95	0.04	21	0.04
Expired air	16.3	4.5	15.4	3.7
Alveolar air	14.0	·5.6	13.3	5.3

Alveolar ventilation may be increased by increasing the inspiratory volume and the frequency of respirations per minute. The latter will only be effective if the inspiratory volume is increased at the same time. Rapid shallow respirations simply ventilate the dead space and expend considerable muscular energy to no avail. In exercise, when more oxygen is being used and more carbon dioxide is being produced, both the frequency of respirations and the inspired volume are automatically increased. These factors have a practical application in caring for inactive patients and emphasize the importance of having them take several deep breaths at regular intervals in order to ventilate the alveoli adequately.

DIFFUSION AND TRANSPORTATION OF RESPIRATORY GASES

Diffusion
The diffusion component of pulmonary respiration is the interchange of oxygen and carbon dioxide across the alveolar and capillary membranes. Gases move rapidly from areas of higher to lower pressure. The rate of transfer of gases across the alveolar membrane is 'proportional to the tissue area and the difference in gas partial pressure between the two sides and inversely proportional to the tissue thickness (Fick's law)'.[7] The alveolar area is very large and thin and the tissue characteristics are ideal to promote the transfer of gas. Gas characteristics relevant to diffusion include solubility and molecular weight; carbon dioxide diffuses more rapidly than oxygen because it is more soluble, even though the molecular weights of the two gases are similar. A pressure differential occurs between the oxygen in the alveolar air and that in the blood in the pulmonary capillaries and, as a result, oxygen moves from the alveoli into the blood. Carbon dioxide moves in the opposite direction for the same reason.

Blood enters the vast number of pulmonary capillaries with the Po_2 at about 5.3 kPa (40 mmHg) and the Pco_2 at approximately 6.0 kPa (46 mmHg). Alveolar air has a Po_2 of approximately 13.0 kPa (100 mmHg) and a Pco_2 of about 5.3 kPa (40 mmHg). As a result of the diffusion exchange that quickly takes place as the blood flows through the pulmonary capillaries, blood enters the pulmonary veins with a Po_2 of 12.6–13.0 kPa (95–100 mmHg) and a Pco_2 of approximately 5.3 kPa (40 mmHg) (see Table 16.2 and Fig. 16.3).

Table 16.2 Partial pressures of respiratory gases.*

	Po_2 (kPa)	Pco_2 (kPa)
Alveolar air	13.0 (100)	5.3 (40)
Venous blood	5.3 (40)	6.0 (46)
Arterial blood	12.6 (95)	5.3 (40)

*Figures given in brackets are values for mmHg.

Transportation of respiratory gases by the blood
Oxygen is transported by the blood in solution in plasma and as a chemical compound in the red blood cells. The amount of gas that can be carried in solution is very limited; in order to carry sufficient oxygen through the body to meet the needs of the cells, most of the gas that enters the blood in the alveoli diffuses from the plasma into the red blood cells where it combines loosely with the haemoglobin to form the compound oxyhaemoglobin. If the haemoglobin has its normal complement of iron, each gram can carry 1.34 ml of oxygen and is about 97% saturated. The chemical process that produces oxyhaemoglobin is reversible so that as the oxygen in solution is used up by the tissues, more is made available by the dissociation of the unstable oxyhaemoglobin (Hb + $O_2 \leftrightarrows HbO_2$). Of the 20 volumes %

---

[7] West (1979), p. 23.

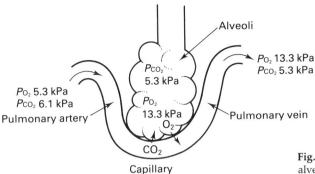

Fig. 16.3 Oxygen and carbon dioxide exchange through alveolar–capillary membranes.

of oxygen in the arterial blood, only about 0.5 volumes % remains in solution in plasma; the remaining 19.5 volumes % are carried as oxyhaemoglobin.

The rate at which haemoglobin combines with oxygen and the rate of dissociation of oxyhaemoglobin is influenced by the Po_2 and Pco_2 of the plasma (Fig. 16.4). An increase in the Po_2 and a decrease in the Pco_2 hasten the formation of oxyhaemoglobin. Conversely, a decrease in the Po_2, and an increase in the Pco_2, as occurs in the systemic capillaries, promote the release of oxygen from haemoglobin; the saturation of haemoglobin declines. The pH of the blood has a significant effect on the dissociation of oxygen and haemoglobin. A decrease in the alkalinity below the normal (i.e. a decrease in the pH) promotes release of oxygen from the haemoglobin molecule. Body temperature also influences oxygen–haemoglobin dissociation; an elevated temperature also promotes the release of oxygen from oxyhaemoglobin.

Carbon dioxide is produced within the body by cellular metabolism and diffuses out of the cells through the tissue fluid into the blood, where it is carried in several forms. Only a very limited amount remains in solution in plasma; the larger proportion is carried in the form of hydrogen carbonate (HCO_3^-) and in combination with haemoglobin and plasma proteins (carbamino compounds). About two-thirds (70%) of the total blood carbon dioxide is carried as sodium bicarbonate ($NaHCO_3$) in the plasma and serves to maintain the normal blood alkalinity (pH 7.4). Carbon dioxide diffuses from the tissues into the plasma and on into the red blood cells where the enzyme carbonic anhydrase rapidly promotes a reaction with water to form carbonic acid.

$$CO_2 + H_2O \xrightarrow{\text{carbonic anhydrase}} H_2CO_3$$

This is a very unstable acid and readily ionizes to hydrogen and hydrogen carbonate ions.

$$H_2CO_3 \rightarrow H^+ + HCO_3^-$$

The hydrogen ions are buffered by haemoglobin while the hydrogen carbonate ions diffuse from the red blood cells into the plasma in exchange for chloride ions. This is referred to as the *chloride shift*. A small, essential amount of potassium bicarbonate ($KHCO_3$) is found in the erythrocytes.

The chemical compounds are unstable and tend to dissociate with changes in the pressures of the gases in the blood. As the blood is circulated through the tissues, the increasing Pco_2 and decreasing Po_2 promote the formation of the compounds. A reverse of the pressure of these gases promotes dissociation of the compounds. In the pulmonary capillaries, where the Po_2 increases and Pco_2 decreases, a rapid dissociation takes place to release some of the carbon dioxide.

Tissue respiration

The exchange of carbon dioxide and oxygen which takes place between the cells and the blood in the systemic capillaries throughout the body comprises tissue or internal respiration. The basis of the gaseous exchange is the pressure gradient of each of the respiratory gases between the cells and the tissue fluid, and between the tissue fluid and the blood. The Po_2 of the arterial blood when it enters the systemic capillaries is approximately 12.6 kPa (95 mmHg) (20 volumes %) and is much higher than that of the interstitial fluid, so oxygen diffuses from the plasma into the tissue fluid. Continuous cell activity uses

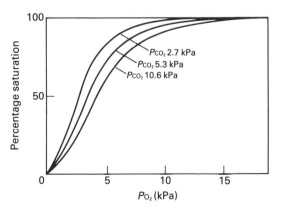

Fig. 16.4 Oxyhaemoglobin dissociation curve.

oxygen, so the higher Po_2 of the tissue fluid results in a movement of the oxygen into the cells. As the oxygen tension is reduced in the plasma, the loosely combined oxyhaemoglobin dissociates to free oxygen. By the time the blood again reaches the pulmonary capillaries the oxyhaemoglobin has given up considerable oxygen.

The chemical activities of the cells (metabolism) produce carbon dioxide. Its concentration in the cell produces a pressure gradient that results in its movement into the tissue fluid. From here, because of the pressure difference, it moves into the capillary blood and gradually accumulates a higher concentration in the venous blood than that of alveolar air. This promotes the diffusion of carbon dioxide from the pulmonary capillary blood into alveolar air.

The amount of gas exchanged in tissue respiration varies in different tissues and organs and with a decrease or increase in activity. The brain tissue, myocardium and skeletal muscles require a constant supply of oxygen. Any deficiency is quickly reflected in impaired function of these structures.

ACID–BASE REGULATION

The transport of carbon dioxide alters the acid–base balance of the blood. Arterial blood normally has a pH of 7.4. As the blood acquires carbon dioxide in the tissue capillaries, the pH falls to approximately 7.36 in the venous circulation. The reverse occurs in the lungs.[8] Carbonic acid (an unstable acid) is formed when carbon dioxide enters the bloodstream in the tissues. In the lungs the carbonic acid readily dissociates, releasing carbon dioxide which diffuses into the alveoli because of the pressure gradient; the pH of the blood rises. Since 70% of the carbon dioxide is transported as carbonic acid, respiratory elimination of carbon dioxide has a profound effect on acid–base balance. The buffers in the blood function to control an elevation in the hydrogen ion concentration by producing the weak unstable carbonic acid. Hydrogen ions combine with hydrogen carbonate to form carbonic acid which in turn forms carbon dioxide and water:
$$H^+ + HCO_3^- \rightarrow H_2CO_3 \rightarrow H_2O + CO_2$$
The increase in carbon dioxide and H^+ ions stimulates the respiratory centre, increasing the rate and depth of respirations which facilitates the elimination of carbon dioxide.

A decrease below the normal concentration of carbon dioxide causes respiratory alkalosis and an increase in the pH. This may be due to hyperventilation. Respiratory acidosis is seen with hypoventilation; less than normal amounts of carbon dioxide are removed in ventilation. A rise in Pco_2 and a decrease in pH occurs. Renal compensatory mechanisms function to correct the imbalance (see Chapter 6).

Factors which influence pulmonary diffusion
The volumes of oxygen and carbon dioxide which diffuse across the pulmonary membrane depend upon the pressure gradient of each gas between the alveolar air and capillary blood. Alveolar ventilation must be adequate to maintain an effective Po_2 to drive oxygen into the blood. Sufficient elimination of carbon dioxide in expiration to reduce the Pco_2 in the alveolar air is necessary to promote the movement of carbon dioxide out of the blood into the alveoli. Increased respiratory rate alone does not necessarily provide alveolar ventilation. If the respirations are shallow, it is mainly the dead space that is being ventilated. Shunting of blood through non-ventilated areas of the lung lowers the Po_2.

Diffusion is greatly influenced by the ventilation–perfusion ratio. Normally, ventilation of the alveoli and perfusion (flow of blood) are relatively uniform. Any disparity that incurs underperfusion or underventilation results in reduced diffusion, which results in decreased blood Po_2 and possibly an increased Pco_2.[9] A disturbance in the ventilation–perfusion ratio may be referred to as the mismatching or imbalance of ventilation and blood flow. Mismatching may be caused by such conditions as pulmonary embolism, which causes underperfusion, and emphysema, bronchial constriction or pneumonia, which result in a number of alveoli being underventilated.

Diffusion may be decreased by the presence of increased fluid in the alveoli, collapse of the alveoli or, rarely, by alveolar tissue changes resulting from chronic pulmonary disease (e.g. pulmonary fibrosis).

Any reduction in the alveolar surface area, such as occurs with lobectomy, pneumonectomy or emphysema diminishes the diffusion volume of respiratory gases.

RESPIRATION AND HIGH ALTITUDE

Atmospheric pressure decreases as the distance above sea level increases. The corresponding decreases in the partial pressure of oxygen at high altitudes reduces the pressure of oxygen in alveolar air and less oxygen diffuses into the blood, causing a deficiency throughout the body. The height at which symptoms of hypoxia (deficiency of oxygen) are first experienced varies somewhat with different individuals and according to the speed with which they ascend. A rapid ascent to 10 000 feet (3050 m) where atmospheric pressure is approximately 523 mmHg and the Po_2 in alveolar air is 9.0 kPa (67 mmHg) produces symptoms of oxygen deficiency in the brain. The person manifests reduced mental effeciency and

---

[8] Guyton (1986) p. 442.

[9] Carbon dioxide is much more soluble than oxygen, so it diffuses more rapidly. Impaired diffusion is likely to cause hypoxia before hypercapnia.

a decrease in visual and auditory acuity. Greater heights produce further deterioration, and at 20 000–25 000 feet (6100–7600 m) the person lapses into coma.

In a gradual ascent to a high altitude the person's physiology makes some adjustments to acclimatize. Respirations increase in rate and volume and the heart rate and output are increased. The number of red blood cells and the amount of haemoglobin are increased when one is exposed to a higher altitude for a period of 1 or more weeks. Since more carbon dioxide is lost at these heights, owing to the lower carbon dioxide pressure in the air and the increased respirations, blood alkalinity is increased. More base ions are excreted by the kidneys in an effort to maintain a normal pH of the body fluids.

In aviation, the low atmospheric pressure of high altitudes is overcome by breathing pure oxygen to increase the oxygen concentration in the alveolar air or by pressurizing the cabin of the plane.

RESPIRATION AND HIGH ATMOSPHERIC PRESSURE

Atmospheric pressure increases as the distance below sea level increases. A depth of 33 feet (10 m) below sea level doubles the atmospheric pressure. An abnormally high atmospheric pressure is experienced by deep-sea divers and by workers in chambers or tunnels which are filled with compressed air to prevent cave-ins that might result from the increased pressure from without. The high pressure of the air causes greater amounts of oxygen and nitrogen to diffuse into the blood.

Excessive amounts of these gases are carried in solution in the body fluids. The high oxygen concentration may interfere with normal cellular activity; impaired brain function may be manifested by twitching, convulsions, confusion, stupor and coma. The excessive volume of nitrogen may also affect behaviour. Most frequently, it has a depressing or anaesthetizing effect on the central nervous system and the person becomes very drowsy and inefficient. Nitrogen frequently causes more problems when the person ascends to normal atmospheric pressure. While exposed to the greater pressure the nitrogen remains in solution, but when the individual ascends to the surface the decreased pressure on the body causes the nitrogen to expand and form bubbles in the tissues or fluids. These may cause an embolism and tissue damage in any area of the body; severe pain, brain damage, paralysis or severe gastrointestinal distension may occur. To prevent bubble formation, the person is brought to sea level very slowly or is confined within a chamber in which the pressure is very gradually decreased while the excess nitrogen escapes.

Deep-sea divers prevent the entry of excess gases into their blood by reducing the amount of oxygen in the gas they breathe, and in some instances they add helium. Disturbances due to extremely high atmospheric pressure may be referred to as *caisson disease, decompression sickness or the bends*.

Nursing Process

ASSESSMENT

Assessment of the patient with respiratory dysfunction begins with: (1) an overview of the patient's general appearance; (2) the history of the problem as experienced by the patient; (3) the psychosocial history to identify the unique qualities of the individual, his perception of the illness and coping skills and resources for adapting to the potential limitations; (4) physical examination of the chest; (5) measurement of respiratory functioning; (6) other diagnostic procedures; and (7) a knowledge of manifestations of the respiratory disorder and treatment plan. The nurse analyses the data obtained from the assessment and, with the essential knowledge base, formulates the nursing diagnoses and develops a patient-centred, goal-directed plan of care.

Patient's general appearance

In order to determine nursing needs, the nurse begins with an overview of the patient's general appearance.

Factors that are noted include:
1 *Facial expression*. Does the patient appear alert, anxious, dull, exhausted, depressed or forbidding? Grimaces, distortions or biting of the lips are noted as these may indicate pain. The colour may be significant; for example, the face may be flushed because of a fever, or cyanosis may be observed.
2 *Posture*. The observer notes the patient's position; does he appear comfortable and relaxed, or tense and apprehensive? Does he assume an erect, slouched or crouched-forward position?

History of the problem

1 *Symptoms of respiratory impairment*. The initial history of the patient manifesting signs of acute respiratory distress should be limited to enquiries about precipitating factors and the nature and severity of the presenting symptoms. When the individual is not in obvious distress, more detailed information may be obtained, which should include:
   • The symptoms which prompted the patient to seek health care
   • A description of the precipitating events
   • Duration of the symptoms
   • The patient's perception of the causes and implications of the symptoms

The symptoms manifested by the patient may include:

(a) *Cough.* The presence, frequency and depth of the cough are noted as well as the nature and sound of the cough. It may be hard and racking, croupy, hacking, shallow, deep and rattling or may have a whooping sound. The cough may be worse at certain times of the day and the patient should be asked if pain accompanies the cough. It is noted if the cough is productive or non-productive. Finally, it is important to assess the effect of the cough on the patient; does the exertion exhaust the patient, create anxiety or disrupt sleep or daily activities?

(b) *Sputum.* It is necessary to determine the consistency (mucus, watery, purulent, tenacious, frothy, caseous or blood-streaked), colour, amount and if the amount has increased recently.

(c) *Breathlessness.* The patient may complain of breathlessness and the assessment should reveal if it occurs with usual activity, increased effort or when at rest, and whether it interferes with daily activities and sleep pattern. It should be noted if the patient's speech is audible, clear and effortless, or if the responses are weak, short and jerky phrases with apparent effort. The patient is questioned as to what was done to prevent or modify the breathlessness and if the suggested actions were effective in preventing or alleviating the breathlessness.

(d) *Fever.* The patient may have a fever and give a history of having night sweats.

(e) *Pain and discomfort* may be associated with the chest, breathing activities or coughing; the nature, severity, duration and precipitating factors are noted.

2 *Causative and risk factors.* Assessment involves learning if the patient: has been exposed to infectious agents; smokes (what, how much and how long he has smoked); has any known allergy (and if so, what the antigen is and the nature of the reaction when exposed to it). Are there risk factors or irritants to which the patient is exposed at work, home or in the community?

3 *Past history related to respiratory disorders.* The patient is questioned as to whether he has had any recent trauma or surgery to chest or respiratory passages, respiratory infections (and their frequency); and any history of tuberculosis.

4 *General health status.* The history should include: any associated acute or chronic illnesses, the quality of the patient's diet, and his usual daily routine and exercise pattern. What is an acceptable level of daily activities to the patient?

5 *Medications.* It is important to know what prescription and non-prescription drugs the patient has been taking regularly or intermittently. The dosage, frequency, purpose and effectiveness of each drug should be noted.

Psychosocial history

1 Individual characteristics. Significant facts are age, education, life experiences, religious beliefs and general socioeconomic status.

2 Occupational history. Health hazards in the patient's place of work are identified. For example, chemicals or dust exposure may be a predisposing factor in the person's respiratory disorder.

3 Home history. The home environment and conditions are reviewed. Some knowledge of the people in the home, physical characteristics of the home and problems disclosed during the discussion may prove relevant. What are the implications of the patient's illness for the family? Who are the significant people in the patient's life who care for him and can be depended upon for support?

4 Patient's perception of the illness and ability to cope. How does the patient perceive his present illness? Efforts are made to assess his understanding of the disorder and treatment; for example, is the meaning of 'chronic' clear if such is the case? It is important to discern what implications of the illness are perceived by the patient.

In discussing previous illnesses and crises, the patient's methods of coping are identified and their success determined. The nurse asks questions to help her discover what coping mechanisms are currently being employed by the patient.

Physical examination of the chest

Assessment involves physical examination of the chest by inspection, palpation, percussion and auscultation. Physical examination is normally carried out by a doctor or specialist nurse only.

Inspection

Thorax. Normally, the thorax is symmetrical. It is important to note any difference on either side and any apparent abnormality in the shape or bony framework of the thorax. Scoliosis or kyphosis may interfere with normal breathing. If the chest is barrel-shaped (slight kyphosis with the ribs in a horizontal position, the sternal angle prominent and the anterior posterior diameter enlarged) it may indicate chronic airflow limitation. A funnel-shaped chest is characterized by depression of the sternum while a 'pigeon' chest involves an outward location of the sternum and inward depression of the first few ribs with minimal impairment of breathing.

Chest movements associated with respirations. The frequency, rhythm and depth of respirations are noted by observing the chest. If the individual's breathing is laboured, the intercostal spaces are observed for any 'ballooning out' during exhalation or retraction during inspiration. Either indicates a serious respiratory problem. Normally, on inspiration, the diaphragm descends, the lower rib cage moves slightly upward and outward and there is slight expansion of the upper chest. Expiration is passive, and of slightly longer duration than inspiration. A short pause occurs prior to the next inspiration.

Accessory muscles. Rhythmic movement of the diaphragm is observed with normal respiration. Use of the accessory muscles indicates some degree of respiratory distress and is characterized by retraction of the supraclavicular and suprasternal areas and elevation of the shoulders during inspiration. Enlargement of the accessory muscles, particularly the sternocleidomastoid muscles occurs with chronic airflow limitation.

Palpation

This method of examination is used to assess chest excursion, symmetry, vocal fremitus, structural abnormalities and tenderness.

Chest excursion and symmetry. The chest excursion on inspiration reflects the extent of expansion and depth of respiration. It may be assessed by placing the hands on the chest with the fingers slightly outspread and the thumbs just meeting at the midline (Fig. 16.5). As the patient breathes in, the hands are normally separated by the chest expansion. Whether the range of the chest excursion is the same on both sides is also noted; if it is equal, the thumbs will be moved an equal distance from the midline on each side. Normally the movements of the two sides are symmetrical.

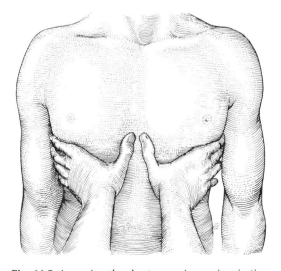

Fig. 16.5 Assessing the chest excursion on inspiration.

Vocal fremitus. Palpation is used to detect the presence and intensity of vibrations produced in the chest wall by voice sounds. The vibrations are conducted throughout the air passages to the chest wall and are referred to as *vocal fremitus*. They may be felt by the examiner's hand (tactile fremitus) or may be heard through a stethoscope (auditory vocal fremitus).

In the tactile method of chest palpation, the examiner places a hand on the chest and, beginning in the apical region and working down, moves from one side of the chest to the other (see Fig. 16.6). The patient is asked to repeat 'ninety-nine' during the examination. Auditory fremitus simply requires the use of a stethoscope in place of the hand.

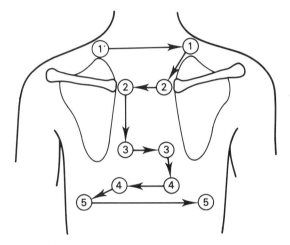

Fig. 16.6 Chest palpation (The numbers and arrows show the sequence of examination).

The vibrations are more intense in the areas of the larger bronchial tubes and are weakest in the areas of the lung bases. They are more prominent when conducted through solid matter and are not conducted as well through air and fluid. Decreased fremitus may be due to trapped air, as in emphysema or asthma, or to pleural effusion or pneumothorax. Increased fremitus occurs when underlying tissues become more dense, as in atelectasis, pneumonia or a neoplasm.

Tracheal deviation. The trachea is observed for position, movement and evidence of shortening. Normally the space between the trachea and the sternal notch is the width of 2–4 fingers. Shortening and deviation to one side occurs when airflow obstruction is present.

Tenderness. Palpation may also detect sensitive areas or a mass in the chest wall.

Percussion

This procedure involves tapping the chest with the

fingertips to elicit sounds that reflect the density of underlying structures. The chest is examined anteriorly and posteriorly, going from apex to base over each side. The percussion sounds are compared with those produced on the contralateral side. Those structures that contain air result in low-pitched, resonant percussion sounds. Solid tissue and inflammatory exudate produce higher-pitched, flat or dull sound. Percussion helps to determine the location, size and density of underlying organs.

Percussion may be performed by placing the palmar surface of the middle finger over an intercostal space. Then, with the index or middle finger of the other hand, a sharp tap is delivered to the finger on the chest, and the sound noted. This method is called mediate or indirect percussion. A more direct method may be used by tapping the chest directly (immediate percussion).

Auscultation
Normal respirations present characteristic sounds as air enters and leaves the lower respiratory tract. Listening to the breath sounds is done through a stethoscope and the process is known as auscultation.[10] The diaphragm of the stethoscope is placed firmly against the chest wall and the patient is asked to breathe deeply and slowly through the mouth. The examiner begins at the upper lobes of the lungs and progresses in a symmetrical manner to the lung bases. Comparisons are made with the corresponding point on the opposite hemithorax, assessing equality of air entry and any abnormal sounds or absence of sounds (see Fig. 16.5). The environment should be as quiet as possible and the patient protected from unnecessary exposure and chilling. The diaphragm of the stethoscope is warmed before being placed on the patient.

The sounds heard in normal respirations are called *vesicular breath sounds*. They produce a soft, low pitched sound and are heard over all the lung areas except over the apex of the right lung. This is because of the proximity of the large bronchial tubes to the chest wall. The inspiratory phase of a vesicular sound is longer and louder than the expiratory phase. The differences may be attributed to the movement of inspiratory air into progressively smaller air passages (and vice versa in the case of the air being exhaled).

Bronchial breath sounds are associated with a short inspiratory phase and a longer expiratory phase. The sounds are higher-pitched and equally loud in both phases. They are abnormal, and indicate some disease process such as pneumonia in the lung.

Bronchovesicular breath sounds are characterized by inspiratory and expiratory phases of equal duration. The sounds are moderate in pitch and intensity, being more muffled than bronchial breath sounds. Bronchovesicular sounds are heard normally along the sides of the sternum and between the scapulae where the major bronchi are situated.

Adventitious sounds are abnormal sounds superimposed on breath sounds as a result of a disease process within the tracheobronchial tree and/or lungs. These include crackles, wheezes and pleural friction rub.

Crackles may be described as fizzing or popping sounds created by the equalization of airway pressures during the explosive reopening of previously closed terminal respiratory units. They vary in frequency, pitch, loudness and time of occurrence within the breathing cycle. Harper states that crackles occurring during the early inspiration phase are found in the larger airways and are usually 'few in number, low-pitched, varying in loudness, and not abolished by coughing'[11]. They occur with airway obstruction. Late inspiratory crackles result from the late opening of deflated alveoli with disease of the peripheral airways (e.g. pneumonia, pulmonary oedema and pulmonary fibrosis) and are usually numerous. They are found in the peripheral airways and are heard over various regions of the lungs and are gravity dependent, as they are abolished with changes in position.[12]

Wheezes (rhonchi) are whistling, musical sounds and are divided into two types: monophonic and polyphonic. They are attributed to spasm of the bronchial walls. Monophonic wheezes are characterized by single notes which originate and end at different times during the breathing cycle.[13] There are numerous types of monophonic wheezes and they vary in pitch. They are usually heard in asthma.[14] Polyphonic wheezes or rhonchi are coarse, wheezing sounds that are predominant during expiration. They are associated with a narrowing of a portion of the tracheobronchial tree in patients with chronic lung disease.

Pleural friction rub is a characteristic rough, grating sound produced when inflamed roughened pleurae rub against each other on inspiration. It becomes audible during the latter part of the inspiratory phase.

Measurements of respiratory function

Respiratory function tests reveal the individual's ability to move air in and out of the lungs and indicate the status of gas exchange across the alveolar–capillary membrane. Impaired function may be

---

[10] Auscultation is defined as the listening to sounds produced by an organ within the body. The procedure is used most frequently in the assessment of cardiac and pulmonary function but it may also be used to evaluate gastrointestinal activity.

[11] Harper (1981), p. 181.
[12] Harper (1981), p. 181 & 183.
[13] Harper (1981), p. 183.
[14] Rokosky (1981), p. 208.

detected and information obtained concerning the nature and extent of the defect. Diffusion and exchange of the respiratory gases are reflected in the arterial oxygen and carbon dioxide tensions, hydrogen ion concentration (pH) and oxyhaemoglobin saturation.

Several objective measurements of respiratory function are used routinely to diagnose respiratory problems, monitor the patient's progress and to determine changes in the status of patients with chronic respiratory disease.

Laboratory measurements of pulmonary function

Measurements of lung volumes (see Table 16.3). Lung volumes may be determined by spirometry[15] at the bedside, in the clinic, doctor's surgery or patient's home. Changes in lung volumes provide the best objective measurement of airflow limitation. Lung volume determinations are used to identify potential risks of respiratory complications in preoperative patients and to monitor changes in the postoperative

period. Vital capacity and timed forced expiratory volume are used most frequently at the bedside.

The normal values for the different lung volumes have been established from studies made on normal subjects. They vary with height, age and sex; tables of normal values are available.

Vital capacity (VC) is represented by the maximal volume of air exhaled following a maximal inspiration. To determine the VC, the individual breathes through a mouthpiece which is connected to a tube leading to a spirometer. The normal VC ranges from 3500–5000 ml.

The VC provides information about the compliance, since the person made an effort to expand his lungs fully when taking the maximal inspiration.

Vital capacity is below normal in obstructive lung disease (e.g. emphysema and chronic bronchitis) because the airways reduce the volume of air exhaled. It is below normal in restrictive lung disease (e.g. fibrosis or limited chest expansion due to neuromuscular defects or weakness) because of the limited expansion of the lungs which reduces the volume of air inspired and exhaled.

Tidal volume (V_T) is the volume of air exhaled following a normal breath. It is determined by using the

---

[15] Spirometry is the measurement of air taken into and expelled from the lungs.

Table 16.3 Summary of pulmonary function measurement.

Test	Symbol	Description	Comments
Vital capacity	VC	The maximal volume of air exhaled following a maximal inspiration (Normal: 3500–5000 ml)	Reduced in restrictive airway disease because of limited lung expansion. In obstructive airway disease, the total lung capacity is increased but vital capacity may be reduced due to decreased volume of air exhaled (air trapping)
Tidal volume	V_T	The volume of air exhaled following a normal breath (Normal: 450–500 ml)	
Forced vital capacity	FVC	The maximal volume of air that can be forcibly and rapidly exhaled following a maximal inspiration	Reduced in obstructive airway disease due to air trapping
Timed vital capacity	FEV_T	The percentage of vital capacity that can be expelled in 1 second (FEV_1), 2 seconds (FEV_2) and 3 seconds (FEV_3) (Normal ranges: FEV_1, 80%; FEV_2, 90%; FEV_3, 95%)	Reduced in obstructive airway disease because of increased airway resistance: usually normal in restrictive airway disease
Maximal voluntary ventilation	MVV	The maximal volume of air that can be breathed in a given time interval (Normal: about 40–70 breaths per minute breathing half of the vital capacity with each breath)	The least accurate of timed breathing tests. Useful indication of exercise tolerance
Residual volume	RV	The volume of gas remaining in the lungs at the end of a maximal expiration (Normal: 25–40% of total lung capacity, e.g. 1500 ml)	Increased in obstructive airway disease
Functional residual capacity	FRC	The volume of air remaining in the lung after a passive exhalation in normal breathing (Normal: about 3000 ml)	Increased in obstructive airway disease

same method as cited above, except that the individual breathes quietly and is *not* asked to take a maximal inspiration and force out as much air as possible. The normal is usually stated as being 450–500 ml with the individual at rest, but varies with individuals and their activities. *Minute ventilation* (or minute respiratory volume) is determined by multiplying the tidal volume by the number of respirations per minute.

Forced vital capacity (FVC) is the maximal volume of air that can be forcibly and rapidly exhaled following a maximal inspiration. The patient's nasal passages are closed off and he is asked to take a maximum inspiration through his mouth, and then rapidly and forcibly to exhale as much air as possible into the spirometer.

Timed forced expiratory volume (FEV_T) records the percentage of vital capacity that can be expelled in 1 second (FEV_1), 2 seconds (FEV_2) and 3 seconds (FEV_3). The individual inhales as deeply as he can and then exhales as quickly and as much as possible into the spirometer; the volume is noted for the indicated time interval. A calculation is then made to determine what percentage the volume is of the individual's vital capacity. Normally about 80% of the vital capacity is expired in 1 second, 90% in 2 seconds and 95% within 3 seconds.

Timed forced expiratory volumes provide information about the resistance to expiratory airflow. In obstructive airway disease such as chronic bronchitis the FEV_1 and FEV_T volumes are reduced. In restrictive airway disease such as pulmonary fibrosis in which the compliance is reduced, with a resulting decrease in vital capacity, the expiratory airflow is usually normal.

Residual volume (RV) is the volume of gas remaining in the lungs at the end of a maximal expiration.

Functional residual capacity (FRC) is the air remaining in the lung after passive exhalation in normal breathing; no forceful or increased effort is used.

Patient care in pulmonary function tests. If the patient is in the hospital he is advised of the purpose of the tests and what to expect before he is taken for pulmonary assessment. Bronchodilators are withheld for 8 hours prior to the test except when the patient has severe airflow limitation. Before each test, the physiotherapist or technician exlains what is to occur and gives the patient instructions how to carry out his role. The patient should not be rushed. The use of the mouthpiece produces anxiety in some patients. Fear can affect the results obtained. The patient is told that the tests may be repeated following the inhalation of a bronchodilator.

The tests can be very exhausting for the patient; the repeated maximal inspirations and rapid forceful exhalations are energy-demanding. Observations are made of the patient's reactions to the various tests; he may require assistance to move from one place to another. A rest period is provided following such a series of tests. The patient should be advised of the results.

Blood gas analysis. Determinations of the partial pressures of oxygen and carbon dioxide, the hydrogen ion concentration (pH) and the oxygen–haemoglobin saturation of the arterial blood are useful in diagnosis and in on-going assessment of patients with respiratory insufficiency.

Normal values are:

Pao_2	11–13.3 kPa (80–100 mmHg)
$Paco_2$	4.8–6.0 kPa (35–45 mmHg)
pH	7.35–7.45
$[H^+]$	35–45 nmol/l
Plasma CO_2	(20–32 mmol/l) (20–32 mEq/l)
Arterial oxyhaemoglobin saturation	95–97%

A blood specimen for gas analysis is withdrawn from an artery with a syringe that has been rinsed with heparin or is received in a heparinized vacuum tube. If frequent analyses are necessary, an indwelling arterial cannula may be introduced to avoid repeated arterial punctures. The site used for the withdrawal of blood may be a femoral, radial or brachial artery.

It is very important that the specimen does not become exposed to air in order to obtain an accurate gas measurement. This is ensured with the use of the vacuum tube. If a syringe is used, all air must be excluded before withdrawal of the specimen and, when the needle is withdrawn, it must be capped *immediately* or plunged into a rubber stopper.

The tube or syringe is placed on ice in a special, labelled container and delivered promptly to the laboratory.

Firm pressure is applied to the arterial puncture site for at least 5 minutes; it is then protected with a sterile dressing. Frequent observation is made of the site for bleeding. If the patient has been receiving an anticoagulant preparation, it is necessary to apply pressure to the site for 15–20 minutes, or longer if necessary. The arm or lower limb in which the arterial puncture was made is checked for adequate blood supply in the distal part in case of arterial occlusion.

If an arterial cannula is used, it is closed off following the blood withdrawal. It is kept patent by periodic flushing with a heparin solution.

As cited previously, an important function of the respiratory system is the provision of *oxygen* which is essential to all cells for normal metabolism. If the oxygen tension is inadequate, cellular metabolism becomes abnormal and anaerobic; lactic acid is produced and accumulates, decreasing the blood pH and causing metabolic acidosis. In assessing the arterial oxygen tension, the *oxyhaemoglobin saturation* is also determined. Only a small amount of oxygen is in solution in plasma; the remainder is combined with haemoglobin. If the plasma concentration is lowered, oxygen is dissociated from the haemoglobin and moves out into the plasma. The haemoglobin is no longer saturated and the total amount of oxygen is less.

A second important function of respiration is the removal of *carbon dioxide* from the blood, keeping the $Paco_2$ within a very narrow range. Impaired ventilation or gas exchange that causes an increase above or a decrease below the normal $Paco_2$ produces an acid–base imbalance which is reflected in the pH. If ventilation or diffusion is decreased, less carbon dioxide is removed from the blood; the hydrogen ion concentration is increased (the pH is below normal), and respiratory acidosis develops.

Hyperventilation removes carbon dioxide in excess of the normal. The $Paco_2$ and plasma CO_2 concentration fall below normal, the pH is above normal and respiratory alkalosis develops.

Electrolyte concentrations. Determination of electrolyte values, particularly hydrogen carbonate ions (24–28 mmol/l) is necessary to interpret changes in acid–base balance. Table 16.4 provides a useful framework for analysing arterial blood gases.

Other diagnostic procedures

Other assessment procedures used to detect respiratory disease may include radiological examinations, examination by direct visualization (e.g. bronchoscopy), blood and sputum studies and skin tests.

Radiological examinations

X-ray of the chest. Radiological studies of the chest may reveal a lesion in the respiratory tract or thoracic cavity, its location, the size of the area involved and something of the nature of the lesion. They also provide information about the mediastinum, the structure of the thorax, the size of the heart and aorta and the level of the diaphragm. The initial films requested are usually postero–anterior (PA) and lateral (L) views. If certain chest or lung areas are suspected of being diseased, films may be requested that provide views from special positions. For example, right and left anterior oblique films will visualize the mediastinum and some areas of the lung that are not seen in PA and L films.

The procedure is explained to the patient if it is unfamiliar to him so he will know what to expect. His clothing is removed to the waist to prevent the possibility of objects such as buttons restricting the entrance of x-rays. If the patient is wearing an identification tag or a necklace, it is also removed. The patient is given a cotton gown to prevent exposure. He is advised to take a deep breath and hold it while the x-ray is being taken, and then to breathe normally.

Table 16.4 Analysis of arterial blood gases.*

Look at pH. For this manoeuvre, only a pH of 7.4 is considered to be normal, even though the range of normal is actually 7.35–7.45
   A pH under 7.4 indicates acidaemia
   A pH over 7.4 indicates alkalaemia

Look at $Paco_2$ (normal: 4.8–6.0 kPa [35–45 mmHg]). If $Paco_2$ is normal, there is no primary respiratory problem and no respiratory compensation for a metabolic problem.
Abnormal $Paco_2$ values are interpreted in relation to pH:

Increased $Paco_2$ plus decreased pH:	acidosis of respiratory origin
Increased $Paco_2$ plus increased pH:	respiratory retention of CO_2 to compensate for metabolic alkalosis
Decreased $Paco_2$ plus increased pH:	alkalosis of respiratory origin
Decreased $Paco_2$ plus decreased pH:	respiratory elimination of CO_2 to compensate for metabolic acidosis

Look at hydrogen carbonate (HCO_3^-) (range of normal: 24–28 mmol/l). If HCO_3^- is normal, there is no primary metabolic problem and no metabolic compensation for a respiratory problem.
Abnormal HCO_3^- values are interpreted in relation to pH:

Decreased HCO_3^- plus decreased pH:	acidosis of metabolic origin
Decreased HCO_3^- plus increased pH:	renal retention of H^+ or elimination of HCO_3^- to compensate for respiratory alkalosis
Increased HCO_3^- plus increased pH:	alkalosis of metabolic origin
Increased HCO_3^- plus decreased pH:	renal retention of HCO_3^- or elimination of H^+ to compensate for respiratory acidosis

Use above findings to diagnose acid–base status. Possible disorders include compensated or uncompensated respiratory acidosis (synonym 'hypoventilation'), compensated or uncompensated respiratory alkalosis (synonym 'hyperventilation'), compensated or uncompensated metabolic acidosis, and compensated or uncompensated metabolic alkalosis. Simultaneous respiratory and metabolic disorders are also possible. If $Paco_2$, HCO_3^-, and pH are *all* within their normal ranges, acid–base status is normal

Look at Pao_2 (normal: 11 kPa (80 mmHg) for elderly adults at sea level; 13.3 kPa (100 mmHg) for young adults at sea level). A Pao_2 below normal for age indicates hypoxaemia

---

*Rokosky (1981), p. 198.

Radiological investigation may include making a series of films of the lungs at different planes. This type of radiology is referred to as *tomography*. In these films the lung tissue is visualized at different depths. They provide details that are not revealed in ordinary x-rays because of overlying structures. Tomographs are helpful in recognizing solid or calcified lesions and cavitations.

Computerized axial tomography (CAT) *scan* provides a cross-sectional depiction of a section of lung tissue and is particularly useful in identifying small nodules, calcification and invasion of lesions into adjoining structures that may not be detected by other techniques.

A *stereoscopic* (three-dimensional) x-ray picture may be used (although it is not common) to delineate or confirm the presence and location of a lesion.

Fluoroscopic examination (direct viewing by x-ray) of the chest may be done to view lung expansion and the respiratory excursion of the diaphragm.

The patient may be too ill to be moved to the x-ray department to be x-rayed. A portable x-ray machine is brought to the bedside and a film of the chest is made. Staff members leave the room while the x-ray is taken to avoid unnecessary radiation exposure.

Pulmonary and bronchial angiography. A film of the pulmonary vessels may be made to confirm the presence of thrombi or an embolism, detect abnormalities in the pulmonary vasculature or assess perfusion in pulmonary disease. A radiopaque liquid is injected rapidly through a catheter into a large systemic vein, the right heart chambers or pulmonary artery. A film is then made to show the distribution of the opaque material throughout the pulmonary vasculature.

The site through which the catheter was introduced into the body is observed for any local reaction and signs of inflammation.

Bronchial angiography may be used to identify bleeding sites in the lungs. A catheter is inserted into the bronchial arteries and a radiopaque dye injected.

Bronchography. This involves the introduction of a radiopaque liquid into the tracheobronchial tree through a catheter passed through the pharynx and larynx. The patient is then placed in various positions to distribute the fluid, and x-rays are taken in which the trachea and bronchial tubes are outlined.

The procedure may be combined with a bronchoscopy. With the fibreoptic bronchoscope, the dye may be confined to a particular lobe or segment of a lung. The bronchogram is used to confirm bronchiectasis or locate obstruction, constriction or malformation of the air passages.

The procedure is explained to the patient beforehand and a signed consent form is required. No food or fluid is given for 6–8 hours preceding the broncho-gram. Postural drainage (see p. 429) may be necessary before the procedure to clear the smaller distal tubes so the fluid can enter them. Dentures are removed, a mouthwash is given, and a sedative may be ordered.

Following the bronchogram, postural drainage is used to promote drainage of the fluid from the bronchial tree. Food and fluid are withheld until the swallowing reflex returns, as a local anaesthetic is used during the procedure and the same precautions are used for aftercare following a laryngoscopy (see p. 419).

Lung scan (pulmonary scintigram). A lung scan may involve the administration of a radioisotope by inhalation or intravenous injection (e.g. Xenon[133], radioiodinated albumin). A scintiscanner[16] is then used to make a graphic record of the concentration of the isotope in the lungs. The scan provides information about the equality of ventilation throughout the lung if the radioisotope is inhaled.

Perfusion scanning is performed by intravenous injection of a solution of albumin which is tagged with radioactive particles. The particles are small enough to pass readily through the circulation until they reach the capillary beds of the lung where they are trapped, providing a picture of pulmonary circulation. Abnormalities of pulmonary blood flow, particularly if due to pulmonary emboli, can be detected.

Ventilation scanning involves inhaling a gas mixture containing a small amount of radioactive gas (Xenon[133]). Following a single deep inhalation, the patient holds his breath and a scan is made of the distribution of the gas throughout the bronchi and alveoli. Poorly ventilated areas of the lung are identified.

Examination by direct visualization
This involves endoscopic investigation. An endoscope is a hollow instrument which is equipped with a light and is used for direct examination of an area within the body. Each one is constructed for use in specific body areas; examples are the laryngoscope, bronchoscope, gastroscope, cystoscope, and colonoscope. These instruments have been improved markedly in recent years; they are made of flexible fibreoptic material and are smaller in diameter, which makes possible their direction into areas that could not be examined with the original rigid metal endoscopes. Their flexibility and size make them less traumatizing than the previous models and the procedure less painful and uncomfortable for the patients.

The fibreoptic endoscope contains two fibreoptic bundles; one transmits light from a remote source

---

[16] A *scintiscanner* is a machine that is sensitive to gamma rays and records the concentration of the radioisotope emitting the rays.

into the field being viewed. The second bundle, which has a lens at each end, transmits the image to the proximal lens which focuses and magnifies the image, resulting in clearer viewing of the area.

In addition to permitting direct examination of a part, endoscopy may also include an aspiration or excision biopsy; specially constructed instruments are available that may be introduced through the endoscope to obtain the specimen for biopsy. Investigation of a patient with a respiratory disorder may include a laryngoscopy or a bronchoscopy.

Laryngoscopy. Direct examination of the larynx may be done with a flexible fibreoptic bronchoscope or rarely with the traditional short, hollow metal laryngoscope which has a light at the distal end.

Preparation of a patient for a laryngoscopy includes an explanation of the procedure and the signing of a consent form. He is advised of the purpose of the procedure, that he will be on his back with his head hyperextended and that he will remain conscious throughout, since only topical anaesthesia is used to introduce the instrument. The patient should know that the room will be darkened and his eyes covered.

Food and fluids are withheld for the 6–8 hours previous to the scheduled examination time to avoid vomiting and aspiration. Dentures are removed and atropine is generally prescribed to reduce secretions. Some sedation may also be ordered to promote relaxation and reduce the patient's anxiety.

Following the examination the head of the bed is elevated, and the patient is encouraged to breathe deeply. The swallowing and gag reflexes are usually absent for a few hours because of the local anaesthesia used; fluids and food are withheld until these reflexes return. The patient is usually able to take a soft diet in 8 hours and his regular diet by the end of 24 hours. He is encouraged to rest quietly and not attempt to talk, cough or clear his throat.

Trauma of the larynx may produce hoarseness or loss of the voice; the patient needs reassurance that either is only temporary, and he is given a pencil and paper by which he can communicate.

The sputum may be streaked with blood if a biopsy was done but should clear in 24–48 hours. Any excessive amount of blood is reported promptly as it may manifest haemorrhage from the biopsy site.

A tracheostomy tray is kept close at hand following a laryngoscopy because, occasionally, laryngeal spasm or oedema and difficulty in breathing develop. The patient is kept under close observation for several hours. Any indication of respiratory distress is brought to the doctor's attention immediately.

Bronchoscopy. The bronchoscope used most commonly is a flexible fibreoptic tube that permits direct visual examination of the trachea, the left and right bronchi, the lobar and segmental bronchi and the bifurcations of their smaller subdivisions.

A topical anaesthetic (e.g. lignocaine spray or Xylocaine spray 2%) is applied to the nostrils and throat and the bronchoscope is introduced through the nose. In some instances the tube is introduced through an endotracheal tube such as when a culture specimen is required.

The purpose of the bronchoscopy is to inspect accessible parts of the respiratory tract, aspirate secretions and exudate that are obstructing air passages, remove a foreign body or obtain a biopsy specimen.

The care of the patient before and after the bronchoscopic examination is similar to that cited above for the patient having a laryngoscopy.

Bacteriological and cytological studies
Specimens of sputum, throat secretions, pleural fluid or tissue may be examined for pathogenic organisms and malignant cells.

Sputum is examined microscopically in a smear or by culture for disease organisms, bronchial casts, eosinophils and cancer cells. Tests are also done to identify the antimicrobial drug(s) (usually antibiotics) to which the infecting organisms present in the sputum are sensitive. This denotes the drug that will be effective for the patient.

The sputum specimen should be collected first thing in the morning, since the secretions that accumulate during the night may have a higher concentration of organisms. The mouth should be clean and free of residual food particles. The patient is given a small sputum container and is instructed to cough deeply to raise the sputum from the lungs. When the specimen is obtained, the container is labelled and delivered to the laboratory. Sputum specimens may be collected during or following postural drainage. They may also be obtained by tracheal aspiration if the patient is unconscious or too weak to cough. The sputum specimen container is attached to the suction catheter, which allows the sputum to flow directly into the container.

If the patient is unable to expectorate a satisfactory amount of sputum, a specimen of the gastric content may be requested, since some sputum may have been swallowed while sleeping. A gastric aspiration is done in the morning before anything is taken by mouth. A sterile gastric tube is passed and a syringe is used to withdraw a specimen. The fluid is placed in a sterile container.

Bacteriological studies may also be made of secretions from the *throat* and *pleura*. Pleural fluid is obtained by thoracentesis which involves the introduction of a needle into a pleural cavity. Aseptic technique is used in withdrawing the fluid. The patient is informed of what is to be done and the purpose, and is placed in a sitting position, leaning forward with his head and arms resting on a table over the bed or on several pillows. Following the cleansing of the skin and sterile draping, the doctor uses a local anaesthetic before introducing the needle. Nursing responsibilities in caring for the patient having a thoracentesis are discussed in Table 16.8.

The amount and characteristics of the aspirate are noted and a sterile specimen is labelled and sent to the laboratory for examination. When the needle is withdrawn, the puncture wound is covered with a sterile dressing and tightly sealed. The patient's pulse and respirations are checked frequently for at least 2 hours. Any unfavourable changes in respiration and colour, rapid pulse rate, excessive coughing or blood-tinged sputum are promptly noted.

Cytological examination of a sputum specimen, pleural fluid and tissues obtained by biopsy may be carried out to identify malignant cells.

Skin tests for tuberculosis. A tuberculin skin test is used in the diagnosis of tuberculosis and to identify those who have been exposed. The test involves an intradermal injection of tuberculin bacillus extract using a syringe and needle (Mantoux test) or a multiple puncture apparatus (Heaf, Tine or Mono-Vac). Tuberculin extract preparations include purified protein derivative (PPD) and old tuberculin (OT) which are available in several strengths. The forearm is the usual site of innoculation. Results are interpreted in 48–72 hours. A positive reaction is characterized by an area of induration of 10 mm or greater.

Blood studies
The following blood analyses may be made in investigating the patient with respiratory disturbances.

Leucocyte count. A total and differential count of the white blood cells may be ordered since this information may be useful in confirming infection and distinguishing between an acute disease, such as pneumonia, and a chronic one, such as tuberculosis. A leucocytosis, with the increase being mainly in the polymorphonuclear granulocytes is generally associated with an acute infection. In chronic infection there is usually only a slight increase above the normal in the total number of leucocytes, and it is usually the lymphocytes that account for any increase. The eosinophils are increased in allergic asthma. The normal leucocyte count value is 4.0–11.0 $\times 10^9$ per litre.

Erythrocyte count and haemoglobin and haematocrit determination. It is important to know if the erythrocyte count is normal since erythrocytes contain the haemoglobin which carries the oxygen (normal: men, 4.5–6.5 $\times 10^{12}$ per litre; women, 3.8–5.8 $\times 10^{12}$ per litre). Similarly, an assessment of the patient includes a determination of the haemoglobin concentration (normal: men, 13–18 g/dl; women, 12–15 g/dl). Obviously, a deficiency of red blood cells or haemoglobin may produce an oxygen deficiency. The haematocrit represents the volume percentage of erythrocytes (normal: men, 40–50%: women, 37–47%).

Histological examination

Bronchial biopsy. Bronchial tissue can be visually examined through a bronchoscope and samples of tissue and cells obtained by brushing or aspirating secretions from the involved areas.

Lung biopsy. A lung biopsy may be necessary to confirm a diagnosis when radiological studies reveal pulmonary infiltration or lesions. Lung tissue can be obtained for examination by open thoracotomy, bronchoscopy or percutaneous needle biopsy. Transbronchial biopsy involves the introduction of a bronchoscope, using fluoroscopy, and the insertion of long flexible forceps into the involved area. Small samples of tissue may be obtained in this manner. Percutaneous needle biopsy involves the insertion of a needle into the diseased area to obtain a small sample of tissue. The procedure is useful when the lesion is localized but other diseased areas may be missed.

Lymph node biopsy. The scalene lymph nodes, which are situated in a pad of fat anterior to the scalenus anterior muscle in the neck, drain the lungs and mediastinum. The nodes are examined histologically to help determine the spread of a bronchogenic carcinoma and the indications for surgical resection or the prognosis in diseases such as sarcoidosis, tuberculosis or lymphomas such as Hodgkin's disease.

Pleural biopsy. Pleural fluid and tissue may be obtained during open thoracotomy but is usually obtained by thoracentesis. A specially designed needle is inserted into the pleura and samples are taken. Tissue from several sites may be required to confirm a diagnosis of tuberculosis or a malignancy.

Manifestations of respiratory disorders

Irritation of the airway or an accumulation of secretions initiates the need for *airway clearance*, which may be manifested by cough, expectoration of secretions or moist breathing sounds.

COUGH

A cough is a sudden, expulsive expiration for the purpose of removing an irritant from the air passages. It is a protective reflex that indicates the presence of some irritation in the tract.

Mechanism. The cough mechanism involves stimulation of receptors in the mucous membrane of the bronchial tubes, trachea, larynx or pharynx or stimulation at a point along the vagus nerve. The impulses travel via afferent fibres of the vagus nerve or the glossopharyngeal nerve to the cough centre, formed by a group of neurons in the medulla of the brain. Responsive impulses are initiated in the centre and travel to the respiratory muscles and the larynx, producing, in succession, a quick inhalation, closure of the glottis, relaxation of the diaphragm and contraction of the abdominal and internal intercostal muscles to increase the intrathoracic and intrapulmonary pressures. The latter is exerted against the closed glottis which opens suddenly, releasing a forceful gust-like expiration. A review of the sequence of activities shows three phases—namely, the inspiratory, compressive and expulsive phases. During the compressive phase, pressure is placed on the alveoli and their secretions are moved into the small bronchial tubes. The increased velocity of the airflow in the expiratory phase results in secretions being expelled from the air passages.

The cough is generally an involuntary response, although some voluntary control may be exerted to inhibit it or produce it. If a cough is unproductive, it may be helpful to instruct the patient to make an effort to inhibit the cough in order to conserve his energy and prevent exhaustion. In other instances, the patient may be required to initiate a series of coughs at regular intervals to prevent the accumulation of secretions in the air passages. The strength or vigor of a cough is determined by the volume of the precough inspiration, the strength of the compression and the rate of expulsion of air.

Causes. The origin of the cough stimulus may be within the respiratory tract or may be extrinsic to it. *Intrinsic stimuli* include inflammation, secretions, fluid, scar tissue which causes traction on the nerve endings, bronchial hyperreactivity, newgrowths, inhaled or aspirated particles of dust, irritating gases and foreign bodies and very cold or very hot air. *Extrinsic stimuli* are abnormal conditions in neighbouring structures which exert pressure on some area of the tracheobronchial tree. Pleurisy, neoplasms of the oesophagus, enlarged lymph nodes in the mediastinum and aortic aneurysm are examples of extrinsic causes. Rarely, a cough is psychogenic. Emotional tension may result in a failure of the epiglottis to close in swallowing, allowing saliva, fluid or food to enter the respiratory tract. Occasionally, a cough is used as an attention-seeking device or as a release of nervous tension.

Implications for nursing. A persistent cough should always be considered as an indication of something abnormal that requires investigation. It is not unusual to find persons ignoring a cough until some more distressing sign or symptom appears, at which time the cause may have progressed to a serious or advanced stage.

SECRETIONS

Normally, the adult produces about 100 ml of mucus daily. This is increased when there is some irritation in the air passages and may change in colour and consistency. The expectoration of blood occurs in many respiratory disorders and in varying degrees of severity. There may be only a slight streaking of the mucus with blood or there may be expectoration of frank blood. The latter is referred to as *haemoptysis*. Blood in the sputum is commonly associated with inflammatory conditions and lesions which cause erosion and necrosis of the tissues and blood vessels, such as bronchitis, pneumonia, tuberculosis, carcinoma and pulmonary infarction.

ABNORMAL BREATHING PATTERN

Normal involuntary respirations are regular, effortless and quiet. Irregularities in breathing may relate to rate, volume, rhythm or the ease with which the person breathes. The following terms are used to indicate characteristic breathing patterns.

Eupnoea is quiet normal breathing at the rate of about 16–20 times per minute in the adult. Respirations are more rapid and shallow in the infant and preschool child; they vary from 30–50 per minute in infancy, gradually decreasing to adult levels by the age of 10–12 years.

Tachypnoea is rapid breathing with the volume of the respirations usually below normal.

Bradypnoea is an abnormally slow rate of respirations.

Hyperpnoea is an increase in the volume of air breathed per minute due to either an increase in the rate or depth of respirations or to both.

Dyspnoea refers to a subjective awareness of a disturbance in breathing. The patient experiences discomfort and/or the need for increased effort or work in ventilation. The individual's perception of difficult breathing or shortness of breath may be due to physiological or psychological stress. The experience is anxiety provoking, since the person knows that breathing is essential to life; the emotional reaction tends to aggravate and perpetuate the problem further. The individual may describe it as 'tightness in the chest', 'shortness of breath', 'unable to get enough air', or 'suffocating'. The dyspnoeic patient frequently has a distressed appearance, is restless and may be perspiring. The difficulty may only be present on exertion and may be episodic. The frequency of the episodes and whether their occurrence is related to a particular time of day, activity or certain situations or factors are noted.

Orthopnoea is dyspnoea which is present in the recumbent position but is relieved to some extent by elevation of the trunk.

Cheyne–Stokes respirations are characterized by a few seconds of apnoea followed by respirations that gradually increase in frequency and volume to a peak intensity and then gradually subside to a period of apnoea. This pattern is cyclic.

Biot's pattern of breathing is characterized by a few respirations varying in volume, followed by a prolonged period of apnoea.

Kussmaul's respirations are rapid and very deep.[17]

ABNORMAL BREATH SOUNDS

Normal respirations present characteristic sounds as air enters and leaves the lower respiratory tract. Absence of such sounds or the accompaniment of other sounds may indicate excessive secretions of fluid in an area or constriction or blockage of a section of the system (see Chest Examination, p. 412).

CHEST PAIN

Pain associated with respiratory disorders originates mainly in the upper air passages or in the pleurae. Inflammation of the trachea or bronchial tubes causes a burning 'raw' type of pain which is not affected by respirations but becomes worse on coughing. Pleural pain tends to be localized to one side of the chest and is due to the stretching of the affected pleura. It is sharp and stabbing on inspiration, causing the patient to take shallow breaths.

ABNORMAL CHEST MOVEMENTS

Unequal participation of the two sides of the chest in respiratory movements may be evident, or unusual retraction or ballooning of the intercostal spaces may occur. For example, in atelectasis or pneumothorax, in which a part or all of the lung is not being inflated, there is diminished movement of the chest wall on the affected side. Similarly, this may occur if a large section of alveoli is consolidated with fluid or secretions. Excessive retraction or ballooning is associated with extreme difficulty in getting air in or out of the air passages.

ABNORMAL BLOOD GAS LEVELS

Manifestations of disturbances in respiratory ventilation and/or gas exchange may be reflected in changes in the arterial Po_2, Pco_2 and pH. For normal values see p. 408. Blood gas levels provide objective measurements of respiratory functioning. Table 16.4 provides guidelines for the nurse in interpreting blood gas levels and analysing their significance in relation to the blood pH and hydrogen carbonate concentration.

HYPOXIA

This means that the supply of oxygen available to the

---

[17] Kussmaul's respirations are usually associated with metabolic acidosis.

tissues is insufficient to meet cellular needs for normal metabolism.

Causes of hypoxia
The causes of hypoxia may be inadequate oxygenation of the blood, impaired delivery of oxygen to the tissues, increased oxygen demand by the body cells or inability of the cells to use the oxygen.

Inadequate oxygenation of the blood. This may be the result of:
- *Hypoventilation.* If less than the normal volume of air enters the alveoli, then obviously the exchange of gases is decreased. This may occur as a result of weak shallow respirations which may be due to a disorder of the nervous system that depresses the respiratory centres or gives rise to paralysis of the respiratory muscles. Hypoventilation may also develop because of a reduction in functional alveoli due to atelectasis (collapse of alveoli) or a collection of exudate in the air sacs, as in pneumonia and pulmonary fibrosis which restricts lung expansion and ventilation.
- *Low atmospheric tension.* A decline in the oxygen tension in the atmosphere, as at high altitudes, is a cause of inadequate oxygenation of the blood. Haemoglobin saturation decreases gradually after an altitude of about 5000 feet (1500 m) above sea level is reached.
- *Ventilation–perfusion mismatching.* Some alveolar capillaries may not be perfused; the alveoli are ventilated but inadequate blood perfusion results in a reduction in the oxygenation of the blood. This condition may be referred to as mismatching or inequality of perfusion and ventilation.
- *Diffusion defect.* Fibrosing changes or oedema of the alveolar walls produces a decrease in the amount of oxygen that diffuses from the alveolar air into the blood. Oxygen is less soluble than carbon dioxide, and is 20 times slower in its transfer to the blood than is carbon dioxide in its diffusion from the blood into the alveoli.
- *Venoarterial shunts.* A shunt within the circulatory system that causes a mixing of arterial (oxygenated) and venous (reduced oxygen) bloods reduces the oxygen tension of the blood delivered to the tissues. The blood that is shunted bypasses the lungs or ventilated areas of the lungs and therefore is not oxygenated. The Po_2 decreases but the Pco_2 is usually normal. Administration of oxygen does not raise the Po_2 level because the shunted blood which bypasses ventilated alveoli is not exposed to the increased alveolar oxygen concentration. The cause is usually a congenital cardiac condition which causes blood to move directly from the right to left side, or the blockage of a large pulmonary vessel by a large pulmonary embolus.

Impaired transportation of oxygen to the tissues. This may be due to:

- *Anaemia.* Fewer than the normal number of erythrocytes or less than a normal complement of haemoglobin reduces the amount of oxygen uptake by the blood.
- *Abnormal haemoglobin.* Hypoxia may be caused by a chemical alteration of the haemoglobin to a form that reduces its oxygen-carrying capacity (e.g. as seen in carbon monoxide poisoning). The offending gas unites with haemoglobin even more readily than oxygen to form a compound (carboxy-haemoglobin) that is more stable than oxyhae-moglobin).

  Certain drugs may also alter haemoglobin and prevent its combination with oxygen. Examples of these drugs are sulfathiazole and phenacetin.
- *Cardiac failure.* Failure of the heart to pump blood throughout body tissues results in stagnation. The oxygen becomes depleted and is not being replaced.

  Inadequate transportation of oxygenated blood may be limited to a certain area of the body (ischaemia) as a result of thrombosis or embolism, and the tissues in that area experience hypoxia.

Increased oxygen requirement. This may develop in:

- *Severe hyperthyroidism.* The utilization of oxygen is increased in severe hyperthyroidism by the rapid rate of metabolism. Similarly, hypoxia may also develop in the person with a high fever; an excessive amount of oxygen is used by the cells in accelerated metabolism and the production of increased body heat.

Tissue cell impairment. This may result in the cells being unable to use the oxygen that is in the blood. The cellular defect is usually in the enzyme system, and is such that the normal oxidative processes are inhibited. This may occur in narcotic or cyanide poisoning.

Tissue oedema contributes to hypoxia by increasing the distances that gases must diffuse to reach the cells.

Classification of hypoxia
Hypoxia may be classified according to the above causes as:

Arterial hypoxia, which indicates inadequate oxygenation of the blood.

Anaemic hypoxia, which is an oxygen deficiency in the blood due to a reduction in its oxygen-carrying power.

Circulatory hypoxia, which is characterized by a decline in the delivery of an adequate volume of oxygenated blood to the tissues.

Metabolic hypoxia, which is an imbalance between the oxygen demands of the tissue cells and the quantity of oxygen available.

Histotoxic hypoxia, which occurs when the cells become defective due to a toxic substance and, as a result, are unable to utilize oxygen.

Effects and symptoms of hypoxia
The effects and symptoms of hypoxia depend upon the severity of the hypoxia and the causative condition, and whether the oxygen deficiency is acute or chronic. If it is chronic, physiological adaptation by increasing the number of red blood cells (polycythaemia) may occur, such as when a person resides at a high altitude or has chronic airflow limitation.

General hypoxia produces some impairment of cellular activities throughout the body. The brain, heart, kidneys and liver are the most sensitive structures, and may suffer permanent damage due to the restricted oxygen supply. Metabolic processes are incomplete; the anaerobic situation results in an accumulation of lactic acid, producing tissue acidosis.

Initially an acute deficiency of oxygen in the blood (hypoxaemia) induces an increased cardiac output and dilates the peripheral vessels. The pulse rate and blood pressure increase; then the pulse weakens as the myocardium suffers hypoxia. The patient may experience nausea and vomiting and complain of precordial pain.

The cerebral hypoxia and a consequent general reduction in metabolism produce a large range of symptoms. Early manifestations may be headache, restlessness, weakness, muscle incoordination, and loss of visual acuity. If the oxygen deficit continues, reduced cerebral efficiency may progress through confusion and stupor to coma. Respirations may be increased, especially if there is a concomitant increase in the carbon dioxide content of the blood. They may be interspersed with sighing and yawning, and the patient may complain of dyspnoea. If the hypoxia persists, respirations gradually fail as the respiratory centres become depressed.

Cyanosis (bluish colour of mucous membranes and skin) is seen due to an excessive reduction of oxyhaemoglobin. Since it is dependent upon the presence of reduced haemoglobin, cyanosis is not present in individuals whose haemoglobin is reduced to 5–6 g/dl or less.

HYPERCAPNIA

Hypercapnia or hypercarbia is the retention of carbon dioxide in excess of the normal range (normal $Paco_2$, 4.8–6.0 kPa (35–45 mmHg)). It develops more slowly than hypoxia because it is more soluble and diffuses more readily than oxygen.

Causes of hypercapnia
Normally, the individual eliminates excess carbon dioxide by increasing the volume and rate of respirations. The respiratory centres and chemoreceptors are sensitive to the blood tension of carbon dioxide,

which provides what may be referred to as the 'respiratory drive'.

The causes of retention of carbon dioxide are hypoventilation, mismatching of alveolar ventilation and perfusion, circulatory failure and, rarely, increased metabolic production of carbon dioxide.

Effects and manifestations of hypercapnia
Initially the retention of an excess of carbon dioxide increases the respiratory drive and the respiratory rate and volume show a notable increase. If prolonged, the associated effort and energy expenditure cause the patient to experience dyspnoea and exhaustion. If the hypercapnia is severe the person becomes lethargic and the level of consciousness decreases.

If the hypercapnia becomes chronic there is a decreased respiratory response as the respiratory centres and chemoreceptors become accustomed to the higher Pco_2 of the blood. Breathing becomes more dependent upon the hypoxic drive.

The retained carbon dioxide is hydrated to form carbonic acid ($H_2O + CO_2 \rightarrow H_2CO_3$), the pH is decreased and the patient develops respiratory acidosis. The normal hydrogen carbonate–carbonic acid ratio of 20:1 is altered. The kidneys adjust to compensate for the decreased alkalinity by eliminating more chloride and hydrogen ions and by forming more hydrogen carbonate ions. Renal compensation takes several days. Serum hydrogen carbonate levels rise (normal: 24–28 mmol/l) and the urine becomes more acidic.

Circulatory changes include dilation of peripheral and cerebral vessels. The skin is warm and flushed; the patient complains of headache and manifests apathy, reduced mental ability which may progress to confusion, and loss of muscle coordination. The cerebral vascular dilation causes increased intracranial pressure, cerebral oedema and papilloedema.

Acidaemia impairs myocardial function; the cardiac output is decreased, arrhythmias may develop and, unless cardiac dysfunction is reversed, circulatory failure occurs. The pulse becomes weak and the blood pressure falls. This promotes hypoxia, which reduces metabolism and leads to metabolic acidosis; the pH decreases even further.

CYANOSIS

A dusky bluish colour of the mucous membranes (central cyanosis) or of the skin and nail beds (peripheral cyanosis) may be associated with respiratory disease due to excessive deoxygenation of the haemoglobin.

The absence of cyanosis is not always a reassuring sign unless the haemoglobin level is known. In a person with 50% or less of the normal complement, the reduced haemoglobin may not be sufficiently concentrated to reflected through superficial tissues.

HYPOCAPNIA

Hypocapnia or hypocarbia occurs when the carbon dioxide content of the blood falls below the normal range.

Causes of hypocapnia
The excessive loss of carbon dioxide is due to hyperventilation resulting from overstimulation of the respiratory centre. The latter may be caused by an intracranial disorder (e.g. cerebrovascular accident), salicylate poisoning, hypermetabolism (as in thyrotoxicosis), extreme apprehension or emotional disturbance or a severe asthmatic attack.

Effects and manifestations of hypocapnia
The ventilating off of too much carbon dioxide alters the normal hydrogen carbonate–carbonic acid ratio 20:1. The base ions are increased in proportion to the acid ions, the pH increases to above normal and respiratory alkalosis develops. The kidneys excrete more base ions and conserve hydrogen and chloride ions, but the ratio of hydrogen carbonate to carbonic acid still remains too high. The patient complains of vertigo, blurred vision and palpitation. The cerebral disturbance causes neuromuscular irritability, reflexes are exaggerated, skeletal muscles manifest twitching and tetany may develop.

CONSTITUTIONAL SYMPTOMS IN RESPIRATORY DISORDERS

If the respiratory disturbance is due to infection or trauma, or if there is degeneration of tissue as in pulmonary infarction, the patient usually develops a fever and a corresponding increase in pulse rate. General debilitation occurs quickly in most respiratory diseases; the patient complains of anorexia, weakness and fatigue and loses weight.

CLUBBING OF THE FINGERS AND TOES

This unusual sign develops in some patients with primary pulmonary malignancies and occasionally in chronic respiratory disease and, although its cause is not known, it is thought to be due to increased vascularity in response to hypoxia.

IDENTIFICATION OF PATIENT PROBLEMS

Analysis of the information gathered during assessment reveals the potential for a number of problems related to the patient's respiratory function, emotional responses, alterations in life-style and self-care (see Table 16.5). The problems are:
1 Ineffective airway clearance
2 Ineffective breathing pattern
3 Impaired gas exchange

4 Anxiety
5 Disturbance in self-image
6 Alteration in family relationships
7 Lack of knowledge of the disease and treatment plan and activity intolerance

NURSING INTERVENTION

1 Ineffective airway clearance

The *goals* are to:
1 promote mechanisms in airway clearance
2 prevent impairment of airway function
3 maintain a patent airway

PROMOTION OF AIRWAY CLEARANCE

Education related to respiratory functioning and airway clearance begins with an understanding of the lung mechanisms that function in the healthy individual to clear particles from the airways. These are the cough reflex, the production of mucus to which particles adhere, cilia (hair-like projections) on the lining of the air passages which move the mucus towards the oropharynx, and macrophages in the alveoli which engulf and destroy particles.[18]

Factors which increase the demands on normal lung defence mechanisms include: cigarette smoking, repeated respiratory infections, atmospheric pollutants, and irritation of the respiratory mucosa by over use of prescription and non-prescription nasal drops and sprays.

Prolonged irritation of the respiratory mucosa, regardless of the irritant, results in a breakdown of the lung's defences. Cigarette smoke and polluted environments contain a large number of irritants. Although much is known about the actions of certain chemicals, there is still much to learn about their collective actions when mixed in cigarette smoke, or the work, home or community environments.

Knowledge of the effects of irritants on the respiratory mucosa is necessary for children and adolescents to develop healthy life-styles and to motivate adults to eliminate health hazards and establish positive health practices.

Smoking affects respiratory functions in the following ways:
(a) It produces an allergic response. Tobacco glycoprotein is a specific antigen that produces an antigen–antibody reaction similar to asthma.
(b) Movement of particles and mucus from the airways is impaired as a result of inhibition of the cilia. Mucus and particles from deeper portions of the lungs accumulate and are retained, providing a medium for infective organisms.
(c) The production of mucus is increased in response to the irritation.

(d) The airways narrow. Mucus-secreting glands increase in number and/or size, increasing the space they occupy in the airway. The walls of the smaller airways thicken and the muscle tissue in the walls contracts, adding to the constriction of the airways.
(e) Destruction of the structures of the terminal respiratory units develops due to the release of enzymes from the macrophages when they are destroyed by the constituents in the smoke. Destruction of the macrophages also eliminates their protective action in engulfing and destroying particles in the alveoli.[19]

Promotion of non-smoking should be directed to younger individuals before they begin to smoke. The hazards are well documented and extensively publicized. Public education about health-promoting activities such as exercise should be included to encourage the development of positive life-styles and health habits. Changing the behaviour of smokers is difficult to achieve but documentation does show that giving up smoking does influence the incidence of disorders of airflow limitation as well as the mortality rate.[20]

Control of atmospheric pollution requires the collective efforts of governments, industries, communities and individuals. Consumers should exert pressure for improved emission controls on all motor vehicles. Employers and employees should be requested to meet high standards of pollutant control.

The development of industrial health programmes which include frequent routine medical and radiological examinations and employee education should be encouraged, and every effort made to prevent inhalation of hazardous dust. Protection is achieved by damping systems, improved exhaust and ventilation systems and the use of masks and respirators by employees.

PREVENTION OF IMPAIRMENT OF AIRWAY FUNCTION

- Stop-smoking programmes are available in most communities to assist individuals to stop smoking.
- Early detection of respiratory disorders may be achieved through industrial health programmes, regular physical examinations by general practitioners and screening clinics in the community.
- Public education on the possible effects of prolonged use of non-prescription nasal sprays, drops and inhalers is needed to discourage the abuse of these preparations.
- Individuals prone to repeated respiratory tract infection should be taught to recognize early signs

---

[18] Jones (1981), p. 388.

[19] Jones (1981), pp. 388–390.
[20] Jones (1981), p. 390.

Table 16.5 Potential problems of patients with respiratory disease.

Problem	Causative factors	Signs and symptoms
Problems related to respiratory function		
1 Ineffective airway clearance	1 Increased respiratory secretions 2 Increased obstruction of airflow 3 Increased bronchial reactivity 4 Neuromuscular and skeletal impairment 5 Decreased energy/fatigue 6 Altered level of consciousness 7 Ineffective breathing pattern 8 Ineffective cough mechanisms	1 Change in rate and depth of respirations 2 Presence of crackles and wheezes 3 Normal breath sound diminished or absent 4 Increased heart rate 5 Cough 6 Increased sputum (decreased sputum in some patients) 7 Dyspnoea 8 Cyanosis 9 Altered arterial blood gases, pH and electrolytes 10 Increased length of expiration (FET) 11 Decreased vital capacity and forced expiratory time 12 Increased anteroposterior chest diameter
2 Ineffective breathing pattern	1 Neuromuscular impairment 2 Skeletal impairment 3 Pain 4 Altered level of consciousness 5 Trauma 6 Anxiety 7 Decreased energy or fatigue	1 Altered rate and depth of respirations 2 Dyspnoea 3 Use of accessory muscles 4 Pursed-lip breathing—increased duration of expiration 5 Altered arterial blood gases, pH and electrolytes 6 Increased anteroposterior chest diameter
3 Impaired gas exchange	1 Altered ventilation 2 Decreased perfusion 3 Ventilation–perfusion imbalance 4 Shunting of blood 5 Impaired transportation of gas 6 Increased oxygen requirements 7 Inability of cells to utilize oxygen or exchange gases	1 Confusion and irritability 2 Lethargy and fatigue 3 Altered respiratory rate 4 Increased heart rate 5 Increased respiratory secretions 6 Altered arterial blood, gases, pH and electrolytes (hypoxia, or hypercapnoea or hypocapnoea) 7 Cyanosis 8 Headaches and tremors 9 Altered sleep patterns
Problems related to emotional responses of the patient		
4 Anxiety	1 Feelings of breathlessness 2 Loss of control of events 3 Lack of understanding of respiratory disorder, health-management plan, and expected outcomes 4 Change in health status	1 Expression of fears of suffocation, feelings of helplessness 2 Fatigue 3 Apprehension 4 Worried, anxious facial expression 5 Focus on self and illness
5 Disturbances in self-image, body image and role performance	1 Increased production of sputum of a different colour and odour 2 Altered body posture 3 Fatigue 4 Decreased level of awareness 5 Inability to fulfil usual roles and functions	1 Non-compliance with treatment regimen 2 Discussion about changes in chest structure, posture, fatigue and/or confusion 3 Withdrawal from usual social activities 4 Decreased or absent touching or physical contact with others 5 Withdrawal from verbal communication
6 Alteration in family relationships	1 Disruption of family roles and functions related to patient's illness, hospitalization and treatment	1 Willingness to talk about difficulties in meeting physical and health care needs of patient

Table 16.5—*continued*

Problem	Causative factors	Signs and symptoms
6 Alteration in family relationships (continued)	**2** Lack of knowledge of disease process, health-management plan and expectations for patient and family **3** Altered sexual function **4** Ineffective coping	**2** Decreased family involvement in social and community activities **3** Failure to participate in usual family celebrations and activities **4** Lack of participation of family in decision-making about patient care
Problems related to alterations in life-style and self-care		
7 Lack of knowledge about the disease process, health-management plan and need to alter daily routine and life-style	**1** Lack of knowledge **2** Lack of recall of teaching	**1** Non-compliance with health-management plan **2** Lack of use of community resources **3** Inability to perform prescribed breathing exercises **4** Requests for information
8 Exercise/effort intolerance	**1** Decreased physical tolerance as a result of increased effort required to breathe and decreased oxygen to tissues **2** Lack of knowledge	**1** Decreased energy **2** Fatigue **3** Dyspnoea on exertion **4** Inactivity **5** Dependence on others for basic needs

of infection and to seek medical treatment promptly.

- Prevention of aspiration of foreign objects may be achieved through education of the public on the hazards of toys with small, detachable parts, ingestion of large mouthfuls of food and fluid, and the taking of food containing small bones.

MAINTENANCE OF A PATENT AIRWAY

The maintenance of a patent airway so that air can reach the lungs requires passages free of foreign objects and secretions. When mechanical obstruction occurs, an artificial airway must be established.

Removal of a foreign object
Obstruction of the airway by an aspirated foreign body presents an acute emergency. The patient should be slapped vigorously between the scapulae. Alternatively, someone standing behind the individual places his arms around the victim's trunk just below the diaphragm, clasping the hands in front. Pressure is applied with the arms and hands (Fig. 16.7). The compression (Heimlich hug or manoeuvre) forces air under pressure through the airway and may dislodge the aspirated mass.

Removal of secretions
The methods used to promote the removal of secretions include (1) coughing, (2) suction, (3) chest physiotherapy, (4) postural drainage and (5) humidification.
1 *Coughing*. Coughing is necessary to remove secretions from the trachea and bronchial tree. The retention of pulmonary secretions predisposes to infection, atelectasis and reduced alveolar venti-

lation and gas exchange. Harper emphasized that coughing 'is an expiratory manoeuvre that produces alveolar deflation, a reduction in lung volume and increased pleural pressure which reduces venous return to the heart'.[21] The purpose of the cough manoeuvre should be explained to the patient and instruction is given as to how to cough effectively. The patient assumes the sitting position, if possible, and a deep breath is taken through the mouth. The patient is instructed to hold his breath to the count of three, contract his abdominal muscles and forcibly exhale. Effectiveness of the cough depends on the volume of air and the force of the expiration. Repetition of the cough procedure helps the patient to expel the secretions that were mobilized by the initial cough.

Staged coughing is taught to patients with cardiovascular disorders who cannot tolerate the increases in vascular pressure from forceful coughs. It involves a slow deep inspiration and then the patient is asked to cough in three short 'bursts'. Short coughs use less energy and are less likely to cause wheezing or airway collapse.

Liquefaction and raising of the secretions are facilitated by a generous fluid intake as well as by humidification of the air. A fluid intake of 3000–4000 ml is recommended unless contraindicated by cardiac or renal insufficiency.

If the patient has difficulty in producing a cough, stimulation of the pharynx with the tip of a suction catheter may precipitate the desired response. Coughing by the surgical patient may be facilitated by the application of firm support over the incision to lessen the pain. 'Huff' coughing is another technique that is believed to facilitate

---

[21] Harper (1981), p. 272.

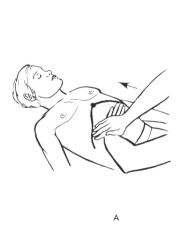

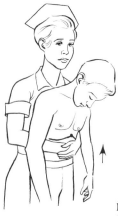

A   B

Fig. 16.7 The Heimlich method of dislodging a foreign body from larynx or trachea.

mobilization of secretions while stabilizing the airways and preventing airway collapse.[22] The patient is instructed to breathe in as much air as possible and to exhale sharply and rapidly while whispering the word 'huff' two to three times. The glottis remains open during this manoeuvre and explosive forces are avoided. This procedure is contraindicated during acute asthmatic attacks.

During coughing the patient is observed for signs of fatigue and allowed to rest when indicated.

The doctor is advised if symptoms and chest auscultation indicate the presence of secretions that the patient is unable to raise. Deep suction may be necessary.

2 *Suction.* This is a very important procedure used to remove secretions from the oropharynx, trachea and bronchi. A sterile disposable catheter, connected to a wall source of negative pressure, or to a suction machine, may be gently passed directly into the oropharynx or trachea or through an endotracheal or tracheostomy tube into the trachea or proximal portion of either bronchus.

(a) *Suction of the oropharynx.* This involves the use of a sterile catheter with a whistle tip which is connected to a tube leading to the source of negative pressure. A suction catheter has a 'built in' vent (thumb valve) that is normally open until a finger or thumb is placed over the opening. The patient is advised of what is to be done and its purpose. The catheter may be passed through the mouth or a nostril to the pharyngeal region. When the tip of the catheter is in position, a finger or thumb is placed over the vent to establish suction. The catheter is gently rotated and withdrawn.

The introduction of the catheter frequently initiates the cough reflex, resulting in the

removal of deeper secretions in addition to those in the pharynx.

(b) *Intratracheal suction.* Deeper suction is used to remove pulmonary secretions or aspirated material (food or vomitus). The procedure and its purpose are explained to the patient and any dentures are removed. An emergency trolley should be close at hand in case of complications. Before and after suctioning the patient may be given oxygen.

The nurse wears gloves and introduces a sterile suction catheter moistened with sterile normal saline through a nostril. The diameter of the catheter must not exceed one-third that of the trachea. When it reaches the nasopharynx (which can be noted by looking through the mouth), the tongue is grasped and drawn forward, using a square of gauze. The patient is then asked to take several deep breaths and the catheter is advanced; force should not be used when inserting the catheter. When it enters the larynx, coughing is initiated and, as the glottis opens widely, the catheter is readily moved into the trachea. The vent on the catheter is left open during the passing of the catheter, and is occluded to establish suction.

The catheter is gently rotated and suction is applied intermittently while it is being withdrawn. The aspiration must be brief since it removes air as well as secretions and may deplete the patient's oxygen supply. Suction is not applied for longer than 5–10 consecutive seconds. Intermittent application of suction also minimizes damage to the mucosa. If the aspiration was not sufficiently effective, allow ventilation for a few minutes before reapplying the negative pressure.

The pulse is monitored during and following suctioning; cardiac arrhythmia may develop, especially if the patient's Pao_2, was below normal before starting. The pulse is observed

[22] Harper (1981), p. 273.

for an increase in rate and irregularity that may occur as a result of hypoxaemia and vagal nerve disturbance. Tachycardia may develop, followed by premature ventricular contractions due to the hypoxia and ensuing acidosis. The disturbance may progress to bradycardia and asystole. To increase the patient's Pao_2 before and after each suctioning 100% oxygen may be prescribed and is administered for up to 5 minutes for some patients. Intratracheal suctioning is contraindicated, unless absolutely necessary, in patients with cardiac arrhythmia or failure, hypotension or acidosis. The patient's respirations are observed and the lungs auscultated for adventitious sounds to assess the effect of the suctioning. Frequency of endotracheal suctioning is determined by patient assessment. Mobilization of secretions by other means is encouraged in order to decrease the need for suctioning.

3 *Chest Physiotherapy* is used to loosen secretions so that they can be coughed up. Percussion or clapping and vibration of the chest are the manual procedures used. The physiotherapist determines which affected lung segments require drainage. This information may be obtained by auscultation or may be indicated by the doctor. Chest percussion may be used routinely over the lung bases or the complete chest during the postoperative period, or if the patient is immobilized over a long period, especially when there is a history of obstructive pulmonary disease or repeated chest infections.

Chest percussion is applied by clapping the chest with cupped hands over the area to be drained. The chest wall is struck rhythmically using both hands rapidly and alternately with uniform force for 1 or 2 minutes. The therapist's shoulders are relaxed, the wrists are flexed and extended in rhythmical movements producing a hollow sound. Obviously, surgical or injured areas are avoided, as are bony prominences, kidney areas and female breasts. It is also contraindicated in patients with a pulmonary embolism. Percussion is not performed below the lower ribs.

Chest vibration may be used after 30–40 seconds of percussion or as an alternative in the patient's pulmonary physical therapy. The procedure is performed by placing one hand flat over the other on the chest area to be vibrated and, while exerting moderate pressure, uniform vibratory movements are made to dislodge and mobilize secretions. The vibration is done to coincide with an exhalation, and pressure is relieved during inhalation. It is repeated three or four times.

Chest physiotherapy is usually used in conjunction with deep breathing and coughing. Postural drainage may also be used as an adjunct.

4 *Postural drainage* requires placing the patient in certain positions to promote the elimination of pulmonary secretions. The position assumed initiates gravitational movement of fluid and mucus to a level of the tracheobronchial tree that favours its removal by coughing or suctioning. As cited above, postural drainage may be accompanied by percussion and/or vibration to dislodge the secretions in the lung segment requiring drainage.

The position assumed depends upon the lung segment or particular area to be drained. To promote the movement of secretions out of *upper lobes*, the patient is placed in a sitting position and alternately leans forward and to each side to drain different segments. For drainage of the *middle lobe*, *lower lobes* and *lingula*,[23] various side-lying, prone and supine positions are used. The patient may be horizontal or, to remove accumulations in lower segments, he may be tilted so that his head and chest are lower (see Table 16.6). An ambulatory patient may be positioned prone and crosswise on the bed so that his head and thorax are leaning over one side. This position especially facilitates drainage of larger bronchial tubes and, if used, precautions are necessary to ensure safety and to prevent a fall and possible injury; it is contraindicated for patients with cerebral disorders, severe pain, unstable vital signs and severe dyspnoea. The nurse remains with the patient each time until assured that he can safely handle the situation.

An explanation is made to the patient before commencing chest physiotherapy and/or postural drainage so that he will know what to expect. He is advised that he will be required to cough. The patient's condition and the treatments being used (e.g. intravenous infusion) may necessitate modification of some positions, but the nurse should be familiar with the one appropriate to the drainage of various lung segments. The patient is made as comfortable as possible in whatever position is used; for example, in the lateral positions at a 45° angle a pillow is placed in front of the patient to provide support.

Each position is maintained for 20–30 minutes, if possible. The patient is then encouraged to cough, and suction may also be necessary to assist in elimination of the dislodged secretions.

5 *Humidification.* An important consideration in the care of a patient with a respiratory disorder is the need for supplemental humidification of inspired air or oxygen.

Normally the inspired air is adequately moistened within the respiratory tract by moisture evaporated from the mucosal surface and the cilia. In a disorder the process is impaired and the mucosa is irritated and depleted of water, the mucus becomes viscous and crusted, and ciliary activity is depressed. The ensuing retention of the

---

[23] The *lingula* is the small projection from the lower portion of the upper lobe of the left lung.

Table 16.6 Postural drainage positions.

Areas to be drained	Posture
Apical lobes	
Apical segment	Sitting position; patient alternately leans forward and to each side
Anterior segment	Supine position
Posterior segment	Right/left lateral, about 45° angle
Lingula	
Superior and inferior segments	Foot of bed elevated 35–40 cm; turned slightly to right
Middle lobe	
Medial and lateral segments	Foot of bed elevated 35–40 cm; turned slightly to left
Lower lobes	
Superior segment	Prone position with hips elevated on a pillow
Medial basal segment	Right lateral with hips elevated or foot of bed elevated 40 cm
Anterior basal segment	Supine position with hips elevated or foot of bed elevated 40cm
Lateral basal segment	Lateral right/left with hips elevated or foot of bed elevated 40 cm
Posterior basal segment	Prone position with hips elevated or foot of bed elevated 40 cm

tenacious secretions increases airway resistance and promotes infection.

Various methods are used to humidify the air or gas to be inspired. The method used depends mainly upon: (1) whether or not the upper airway is bypassed: (2) the degree of dehydration of the mucosa and secretions: (3) the equipment available, and (4) the flow rate of oxygen administration. Humidification is not required when oxygen is administered at low flow rates (e.g. 3 or 4 l/min) at 24% oxygen. A steam kettle, vapourizer or room humidifier is probably the simplest means of increasing the moisture in the inspired air.

A method commonly used to humidify inspired gas is to bubble it through water (or a prescribed diluent) to increase the water vapour content of the inhaled gas. Water vapour molecules are absorbed into the gas bubbles. The amount absorbed may be increased by heating the water. The water vapour in inspired gas also may be increased by passing the gas slowly over a large surface of water.

A more efficient method of humidification is to deliver the water in an aerosol or nebulized form. The more sophisticated humidifiers include electrically operated jet nebulizers, ultrasonic nebulizers and centrifugal aerosol generators.

The jet-type nebulizer produces a coarse spray of fluid which is directed into a stream of rapidly moving gas. Before the gas with the fluid leaves the nebulizer, it may be directed onto a baffle or the walls of the container to reduce the size of the water particles carried into the respiratory tract.

In ultrasonic nebulization, ultrahigh frequency sound waves are transmitted into water, resulting in a very fine particulate spray. The gas to be inspired is directed across the surface of the water so that the fine spray is carried with it into the respiratory tract. This humidifying technique is considered one of the most efficient means of delivering an aerosol of high density.

The centrifugal aerosol generator has a rapidly spinning disc that throws the water against a baffle or container wall breaking it into small aerosol particles.

The cascade humidifier, in which the inspired gas is bubbled through heated water, is used frequently for humidification of the inspired gas during continuous mechanical ventilation.

The diluent used in humidifiers may be sterile distilled water, normal (0.9%) saline, half-strength normal (0.45%) saline or hypertonic saline.

Unless specified by the doctor, water is used. It must be remembered that it is hypotonic and, with prolonged humidification, may cause mucosal oedema in high density delivery. Half-strength saline is usually the choice for prolonged administration and when the ultrasonic or heated aerosol methods are used. Hypertonic saline promotes liquefaction and elimination of secretions.

Medications, principally bronchodilators, may be administered by metered-dose aerosol inhalers. This method is frequently used for patients with chronic airway limitation. The advantage is that it avoids systemic administration and the possible associated side-effects, and ensures that the desired amount of medication is administered. The patient directs the mouthpiece of the inhaler towards the back of the mouth and slowly inhales while pressing the canister down to release the drug. After inhaling fully, the breath is held for 5–10 seconds before exhaling. The frequency and number of puffs the patient takes each time are prescribed by the doctor.

Artificial airways

Endotracheal intubation. This procedure involves the

passage of a tube through the mouth or nose and larynx into the trachea. Intubation is used to establish an airway to improve ventilation or facilitate ventilatory assistance and to aspirate secretions. The passing of an endotracheal tube is a rapid means of establishing an airway in an emergency as compared with the surgical procedure of tracheotomy.

If the patient is sufficiently alert he is advised of what the procedure involves, its purpose and the ensuing interference with communication and swallowing. He is told that he will be under constant surveillance, the treatment is of a temporary nature, and a slate and pencil will be available by which he can communicate, and his fluid and nutritional needs will be met by parenteral solutions. The family receives a similar explanation of the purpose, procedure and interference with communication.

If the patient has dentures they are removed, and he is then positioned on his back with the head extended and supported on a 5–10 cm firm pad to align the mouth, pharynx and larynx.

Using the laryngoscope, the doctor introduces the endotracheal tube, and the proximal portion of the tube is secured to the patient's face. The tube, made of soft plastic, is more pliable and less traumatizing to tissue than a rubber tube (Fig. 16.8). The tube is equipped with an inflatable cuff a short distance above the distal end. The cuff, when inflated, remains soft, which reduces the pressure on the tissue and the possibility of ischaemia and trauma, When inflated it prevents the aspiration of vomitus and oral secretions. It also permits more effective ventilation by preventing the escape of gases being delivered under pressure.

When the tube is in position the cuff is inflated with air if the patient is to receive mechanical ventilatory assistance. A slight leak around the cuff is advisable to prevent pressure necrosis of the tracheal wall by the cuff. The air leak is detected by a stethoscope placed over the lateral surface of the trachea just above the area of the cuff. Near the proximal end of the fine tube leading to the cuff, and through which the air is introduced, there is a small balloon-like dilation which remains inflated when the tube is clamped. It is observed frequently and as long as it remains inflated the cuff is also inflated. A pharyngeal airway or bite block is inserted into the patient's mouth.

Immediately following insertion of the tube, and then at regular intervals, the chest is auscultated to determine if air is entering both lungs. If the tube is too low, the inflated cuff could completely block off a bronchus and cause atelectasis of the respective lung. An x-ray may be made to check the position of the tube; if the end rests against the carina, the terminal opening will be blocked and air entry into the bronchi will be cut off.

The endotracheal tube is distressing and a source of discomfort to the conscious patient. Prolonged use may cause damage to the vocal cords and ulceration in the trachea. If an artificial airway is necessary for a prolonged period, a tracheostomy is done and the endotracheal tube removed.

Periodic deflation of the cuff should not be necessary if a large-volume, low-pressure cuff is used. The

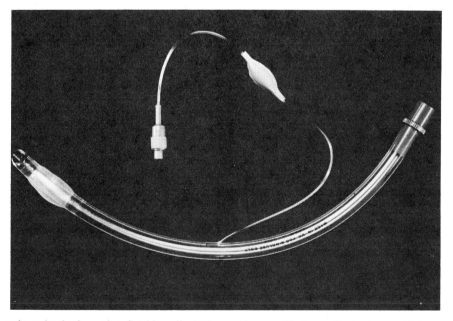

Fig. 16.8 An endotracheal tube with inflatable cuff which provides a seal between the trachea and tube. After the tube is inserted, the cuff is inflated by the introduction of a specified volume of air through the fine, attached tube, which is then clamped.

inspired gas is humidified before entering the endotracheal tube to liquefy secretions and prevent
encrusting within the tract and tube. Frequent deep
suction through the endotracheal tube is necessary.
The procedure involves hyperoxygenation, oropharyngeal suction, tracheal suction, and hyperoxygenation.

Suctioning may deplete the amount of oxygen
reaching the alveoli. The patient may be given
oxygen prior to suction, and again following suction.
The patient's pulse is monitored for possible cardiac
dysfunction and arrhythmias (due to hypoxia)
during and after the suctioning. If any irregularity
occurs, suctioning is immediately discontinued and
oxygen is administered with the self-inflating bag
and mask.

Using sterile gloves, the nurse passes a sterile
catheter, moistened in sterile water or normal saline,
through the tube into the trachea. Suction is not
applied while the catheter is being introduced. When
in position, suction is applied intermittently and the
catheter is rotated and withdrawn. If the airway is
not clear of secretions, the catheter is not allowed to
become contaminated and may be reintroduced into
the trachea. It will likely be necessary to ventilate the
patient with the self-inflating bag before passing the
catheter again. If the secretions are tenacious,
5–10 ml of a sterile saline solution may be introduced
into the tube, followed by immediate suction. Following suction the patient is hyperoxygenated.

Frequent mouth care is necessary, and suctioning
of the oropharyngeal area at frequent intervals is
done to remove the secretions that may be a response
to the presence of the tube.

When the patient is to be *extubated*, the emergency
(resuscitation) trolley should be accessible so the
patient can be quickly reintubated if necessary.

Before the cuff is deflated and the doctor removes
the tube, secretions are suctioned from the oropharynx to prevent aspiration. Following the removal of
the tube, the patient is observed for respiratory distress and insufficiency. A nurse remains in attendance, constantly monitoring the patient's respirations, pulse and colour. The patient is usually
apprehensive and needs the nurse's presence and
reassurance.

Tracheostomy. This is a surgical procedure in which an
incision is made in the anterior wall of the trachea
and a special tube is inserted. An airway is established which bypasses the larynx and air passages
above.

Indications for a tracheostomy include:

1 An upper airway obstruction (e.g. laryngeal newgrowth).
2 Prolonged, mechanically assisted ventilation
where a seal is necessary to prevent loss of ventilatory gas that is under pressure.
3 The need for more efficient access to retained pulmonary secretions which, unless removed, may

cause serious respiratory problems such as atelectasis and pneumonia.
4 The prevention of recurrent aspiration of oral
secretions and vomitus.

A tracheostomy may be done in primary respiratory
disorders, but it is frequently necessary with patients
whose respiratory difficulty or insufficiency is
secondary to disease elsewhere or to trauma. For
example, it may be necessary following cerebral
injury or cardiac surgery or for the patient with
myasthenia gravis who has developed dysfunction
of the respiratory muscles. A tracheostomy reduces
the work of breathing by eliminating the resistance
offered by the upper airway. It also reduces the dead
space by almost 50% (the normal is approximately
150 ml).

Since endotracheal intubation has been more
commonly used and can be performed very quickly,
tracheostomy is rarely used in an emergency
situation. The current procedure is generally
elective, and is performed with an endotracheal tube
in position and under aseptic conditions in an operating room. It may be necessary as an emergency
measure if the patient cannot be intubated because of
facial injuries or burns, laryngeal oedema or severe
upper airway infection. If the tracheostomy is associated with laryngectomy, it becomes permanent.

The *operative procedure* is undertaken with the
patient in the dorsal position, head and neck hyperextended. A pillow or folded sheet is placed under the
shoulders. A vertical or horizontal incision is made
about 2 cm above the suprasternal notch to expose
the upper part of the trachea. This is then opened,
usually at the level of the second and third cartilaginous rings, and a tracheostomy tube is introduced.
The tube is held in position by laterally attached
tapes which are tied securely around the patient's
neck.

Tracheostomy tubes are available in various sizes.[24]
The diameter and length of the tube selected
depends upon the size of the trachea, and is slightly
smaller in diameter than the trachea. This necessitates having several sizes sterile and available at the
time of the tracheostomy.

The tracheostomy tubes may be made of plastic
(plastic and polyethylene) and may be single or consist of two parts, an inner and outer cannula (see
Fig. 16.9). A silver double cannulated tube is also
available and may be used. The plastic tubes tend to
become more pliable as they approach body temperature and are less subject to accumulating
secretion encrustations. When the metal tube is
used, the outer cannula is fitted with an obturator
that extends beyond the distal end of the tube. Its

---

[24] The size of the tubes may be indicated in the Jackson
scale of sizes, which goes from No. 00 to 10, the external
diameter scale, which goes from 4.5 mm to 14 mm, or the
French gauge, which goes from 13 to 42.

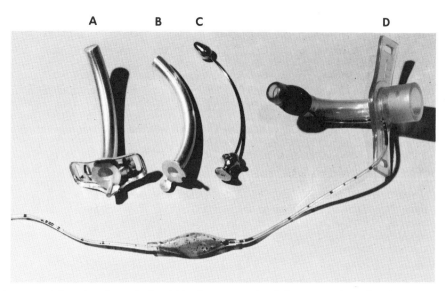

Fig. 16.9 Tracheostomy tubes, *A*, outer part of metal tracheostomy tube. *B*, Inner part of metal tracheostomy tube. *C*, Obturator used during insertion of the outer metal tube. *D*, Polyethylene cuffed tube.

end is blunt and smooth which facilitates the introduction of the tube. As soon as the tube is in position, the obturator is removed and the inner tube is inserted and secured.

The tube with an inner cannula provides a more efficient means of clearing the airway of secretions, since the inner tube can be removed and readily cleansed without the risk of compromising the patient's airway. The single tube (without an inner cannula) must be changed about every 3 days or more often if secretions accumulate within the tube. The tube with an inner cannula may be left for a longer period.

Most synthetic tubes now in use have a high-volume, low-pressure cuff which encircles the lower part of the outer tubes (Fig. 16.10). After the tube is in position, the cuff is inflated by introducing a small amount of air via a fine tube that leads into it. The cuff creates a seal between the trachea and the tube and prevents air from entering or escaping around the tube, in addition to preventing the aspiration of

secretions or fluid into the tract below. This type of tube is used most frequently in patients who require mechanical assistance in breathing. A disadvantage of the cuff is possible ulceration of the tracheal mucosa due to pressure at the site. The cuff must be deflated at frequent, regular intervals and must remain deflated for a stated period of time.

The amount of air required to produce a seal without unnecessary pressure on tracheal tissue varies from 2–10 ml. While introducing the air, the nurse listens and tests for the escape of air from around the tube. The tracheostomy tube may be blocked off momentarily while testing for leakage around the tube. A slight leak is desirable to prevent pressure ischaemia of the tracheal mucosa. When the inflation is completed, the end of the fine tube is clamped. The amount of air used in inflating the cuff is recorded each time; any significant change observed from one time to another is reported. A decreased amount of air used may indicate swelling and oedema in the 'air passage' tissues.

Near the proximal end of the fine inflating tube is a small balloon-like dilation. This is inflated and, since it is visible, may be checked frequently to determine if the tube and the cuff below remain inflated. Obviously, if the small pilot balloon becomes deflated, a leak in the system is indicated and the cuff will be deflated, thus losing the intratracheal seal.

A variety of tubes are available which facilitate upper respiratory breathing or speaking and are used when weaning patients from mechanical ventilation.

Tracheostomy care is very important. The nurse should appreciate that the patient is dependent upon the patency of the tracheostomy tube for getting air in

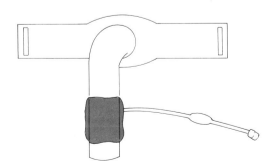

Fig. 16.10 A cuffed tracheostomy tube.

and out. Constant attention and meticulous care are necessary to prevent serious complications and to reduce the patient's fear of 'choking'. Sensitivity to the patient's fears and needs is important, since he cannot communicate verbally.

- *Preparation for the tracheostomy*. If the patient is sufficiently alert, and if the delay does not invoke any risk, he is advised about the need for a tracheostomy and what it involves. An explanation is made of his breathing and removal of secretions through the tube and of his temporary loss of voice. He is then reassured that someone will be in constant, close attendance and that provision will be made for him to communicate by writing if he wishes. A similar explanation is given to the family. Opportunities are provided for the patient and family members to ask questions and to receive further clarification.

- *Preparation to receive the patient*. This includes assembling sterile suction equipment, respirator if indicated, adapter to fit tracheostomy tube, oxygen, sterile tracheostomy tray with various sizes of tracheostomy tubes in case the one inserted becomes dislodged, sterile tape for securing the tube in place, gauze squares, tracheal dilator and artery forceps, sterile syringe to inflate the cuff, humidifier (the type will depend upon whether or not the patient is to receive mechanical ventilatory assistance; if not, a nebulizer may be available which fits over the opening of the tube), equipment for frequent mouth cleansing, and a pencil and slate or pad.

- *Position*. The head of the bed is usually elevated to appoximately a 45° angle if the patient is conscious and the blood pressure and pulse are stable.

- *Assessment*. Frequent monitoring of the patient's blood pressure, respiratory rate and sounds, pulse and colour is necessary. An increase in the respiratory rate, crackles and wheezes and an increased pulse rate may indicate the need for suction. The patient may still experience respiratory insufficiency due to obstruction in the tract below the tracheostomy. This could be evidenced by marked respiratory effort, unequal movement of the sides of the chest and retraction of the soft tissues in the intercostal and supraclavicular spaces. Cyanosis and distress not relieved by suctioning are reported promptly. Increasing restlessness, especially if accompanied by a rapid pulse rate, may indicate hypoxia or bleeding.

   The neck and area around the incision are inspected for possible interstitial emphysema due to air leaking into the subcutaneous tissue. The wound is observed for bleeding in the immediate postoperative period and then checked daily for signs of infection and sloughing.

   The tube is checked frequently for patency and the characteristics (consistency, colour, amount) of the tracheobronchial secretions are noted. Increased secretion occurs in response to the tracheal trauma and is usually coloured by blood at first, but the blood content should gradually diminish and disappear. A daily specimen of the secretions for staining and culture may be requested.

   If the patient is receiving mechanical ventilatory assistance, both sides of the chest are observed for movement or are auscultated for air entry. The tidal volume and minute volume are recorded hourly.

- *Suction*. The patient's cough is less effective in clearing the airway, so suction is necessary. Frequency of suction is determined by assessment of the patient's breathing and auscultation of the chest for wheezes and crackles. The frequency is decreased as the secretions become less. One has to be sure they are less and not thick and tenacious and retained because of lack of fluids and humidification. Sterile saline may be instilled into the tube and followed immediately by suction.

   If the patient is receiving mechanical ventilatory assistance or oxygen, he is hyperoxygenated before suction (O_2, 100% for 3–5 minutes). Suction removes air and oxygen from the respiratory tract, as well as removing secretions, and may cause hypoxaemia and ensuing cardiac arrhythmia.

   The trachea is suctioned using a sterile glove and a sterile suction catheter moistened in sterile water or normal saline. The negative pressure is not applied during the insertion of the catheter but is applied when it is in position and intermittently during withdrawal. Suction must be brief, not longer than 10–15 seconds. If it must be repeated, the patient is allowed several breaths or is given oxygen again.

   Secretions and suction may initiate coughing. Secretions escaping from the tracheostomy tube are gently wiped away with sterile unfrayed gauze (free of lint and absorbent). The mucus and exudate must be cleaned away quickly before being drawn back into the tube with a breath.

- *Tube and wound care*. The wound and surrounding skin are kept as dry and free of secretions as possible; moisture predisposes to infection and maceration of the tissues. Hydrogen peroxide 3% is frequently the solution of choice for cleansing the area around the tracheostomy tube. The wound and area under the tube are protected with sterile dry gauze to fit around the tube. The gauze should be unfrayed and free of lint and absorbent to prevent possible aspiration of a loose thread or particle. If the tapes securing the tube become soiled they are replaced with fresh sterile tapes.

   The inner cannula of the tracheostomy tube is carefully removed and cleansed every 3–6 hours, or as often as necessary (perhaps even hourly). The cannula is cleansed thoroughly using a small tube brush or applicator and hydrogen peroxide. It is then rinsed in water and sterilized. The outer cannula is suctioned if necessary before the inner cannula is reinserted. Any delay is avoided to prevent the drying and adherence of secretions in the lumen of the outer tube. It may be necessary to suction the outer tube to remove secretions before replacing the inner cannula. Precautions must be taken not to displace the outer tube; the tapes which secure it are checked frequently.

Single tubes are usually changed by the surgeon every 3 days; the tube with an inner cannula may be changed weekly. A tray with sterile replacement tubes and the necessary equipment is kept at the bedside.

If a mechanical ventilator is being used, the tube leading to the tracheostomy tube should be supported so it does not pull on the tracheostomy tube and cause pressure on the wound. A flexible swivel connector is used to attach the ventilatory tube of the machine to the tracheostomy tube. This permits movement and turning of the patient with minimal risk of moving or dislodging the tracheostomy tube.

Should the tube come out of the trachea because of vigorous coughing or carelessly tied tapes, the tracheal opening closes and the patient is threatened with asphyxia. Prompt action is necessary. The tracheal wound is quickly reopened with the sterile tracheal dilator or artery forceps which are always kept at the bedside in the event of such an emergency. The opening is held open until the doctor (or specialist nurse) arrives and inserts the sterile tracheostomy tube.

- *Humidification*. Adequate humidification of the inspired gas is very important to prevent encrustations forming within the trachea and the tube, which increase airway resistance. As cited above, the method used will depend upon whether or not mechanical ventilation is necessary. Equipment which provides a nebulized solution is more efficient (see p. 430).

- *Fluids and nutrition*. A minimum fluid intake of 3000 ml is recommended to help liquefy pulmonary secretions, unless contraindicated by cardiac insufficiency and oedema. An accurate record is kept of the intake and output. The patient is not usually permitted any fluids or food by mouth; they are administered intravenously. Some patients receive feedings via a nasogastric tube (see Chapter 17).

If the tracheostomy is going to be permanent, or if the patient is not on a respirator, oral fluids are introduced gradually; if tolerated, a soft diet is given and increased gradually to a regular diet. The patient is at first fed by the nurse, and then he is encouraged to feed himself as he overcomes his apprehension about choking. The nurse remains with him until he gains sufficient confidence.

- *Mouth care*. Oral hygiene is important for the patient's comfort and to reduce the possibility of infection. The mouth is cleansed and rinsed every 2 hours until the patient is taking normal meals, at which time regular cleansing of the teeth and rinsing of the mouth after each meal and at bedtime suffice.

- *Psychological support*. The patient is likely to be fearful of choking and concerned about his inability to cough up the secretions and to communicate. When the nurse leaves the bedside the patient is advised of the errand and how long it will take. A call-bell is given to the patient; he will be more secure if he knows he can call someone if necessary.

The nurse talks to the patient, advises him of his progress and what is going to be done, and endeavours to anticipate information the patient might want to have but cannot ask for verbally. He especially wants information about how long he is likely to be unable to breathe and communicate normally. A slate or pad and pencil are kept readily within his reach, and he is encouraged to communicate his feelings and needs. Hand signals are developed to enable the patient to communicate 'yes' or 'no' or make routine requests by raising one or more fingers. Family members are encouraged to talk to him.

A mild sedative or tranquillizer may be prescribed if the patient is fearful and emotionally disturbed. Analgesics and sedatives that may depress the respiratory centre and the cough reflex are avoided.

- *Extubation*. If the patient has been receiving mechanical ventilatory assistance, removal of the tracheostomy tube is not considered until he is successfully weaned from the ventilator. When the tracheostomy is a temporary measure, the patient is gradually returned to breathing through the upper tract. In order to lessen tracheal injury and scarring the tube is removed as soon as possible, but without compromising adequate ventilation. The protective reflexes should be responsive; the epiglottis and glottis should close to prevent aspiration, the gag reflex should be present and the patient should be able to swallow fluids and food without risk of aspiration.

If a cuffed tube has been used, the cuff is deflated for 24–48 hours before the tube is removed and the patient's ability to keep upper tract secretions out of the lower tract is observed. An alternative method is by replacing the single tube with a tube that enables upper respiratory breathing. It may be fenestrated or have a one-way attachment for only inspiration; expiration occurs through the mouth. Until the protective reflexes have been demonstrated the cuff is reinflated during and for 20 minutes after meals. A methylene blue test may be done to determine the effectiveness of the reflexes. The test involves giving the patient about 100 ml–120 ml of water containing 1 ml of methylene blue. The trachea is then suctioned every 15 minutes for 1 hour. If the suctioned secretions do not show the presence of the methylene blue solution, the protective reflexes are considered effective.

A sterile tracheostomy tray with tubes of several sizes is kept at the bedside in case a tube may have to be reinserted after extubation. Sterile suction equipment should also be available.

When the tracheostomy tube is removed, the wound is cleansed, the wound edges are approximated and taped and a firm dressing is applied. Healing occurs spontaneously; sutures are not considered necessary. The patient is advised to place his hand over the area and exert some pressure when he coughs. He may be fearful of not being able to breathe when the tube is removed, so he is assured beforehand that his breathing is adequate via the normal route. A nurse remains with him following removal to be certain that he experiences no difficulty. Blood specimens may be taken for a day or two to determine the Pao_2 and $Paco_2$ levels. Following discharge, the doctor or clinic keeps track of the patient who has had a tracheostomy for at least a year. He is checked for possible scarring and tracheal stricture resulting from irritation and trauma.

- *Home tracheostomy care.* If the tracheostomy is permanent, the patient is instructed about the care of the tube and the stoma (an artificial opening to the surface). This is done as soon as he is well enough to undertake the care in the hospital so he will develop confidence. A member of the family also receives instructions about the necessary care and precautions.

  The patient and family are referred to the district nurse who is able to obtain the necessary suction equipment and dressing supplies, and also give instruction in the use and care of the equipment.

  The patient and family are advised how to conceal the site of the tracheostomy. The shirt will cover the stoma in a man; a woman may wear a scarf or high-necked blouse or dress. Small 'bibs' can be made or may be available from the district nurse.

  An explanation is made of the danger of aspirating water through the tracheostomy tube; this precludes swimming or immersion in water to a high level. Precautions must also be used when taking a shower.

  The patient is advised to return to the outpatient department or to his general practitioner at regular intervals, as directed, for changing the tube and examination of the stoma. Eventually, when the stoma is firmly healed and the tracheal opening remains patent, the patient or a member of the family may be taught to change the outer cannula, or the tube may be removed permanently. Precautions should be used to avoid close contact with those in the environment with respiratory infection.

Drugs to improve function of the airways
1 *Bronchodilators* are administered to prevent or correct bronchoconstriction. Examples of these are:
 (a) *Salbutamol (Ventolin).* This drug is available in aerosol form in a small cartridge-type dispenser for inhalation. The valve is metered to deliver a specific amount of the drug each time it is released by pressure. The dosage usually prescribed is two puffs three or four times daily. The inhalation is not repeated within 3–4 hours of the last dose.

     Salbutamol may also be administered orally or nebulized. If given by this route the patient may experience palpitation and muscle tremor.
 (b) *Terbutaline (Bricanyl).* This drug is a potent, long-acting bronchodilator which is administered orally or by inhalation. Aerosol dosage is one to two puffs three or four times a day, or as necessary.
 (c) *Fenoterol (Berotec).* This is a newer drug which is similar to salbutamol and terbutaline acting specifically on beta$_2$ (β_2) receptors to relax bronchial smooth muscle.
 (d) *Ipratropium (Atrovent).* This is usually inhaled in aerosol or nebulized form. It is useful in preventing and controlling attacks and is often used with salbutamol. It may cause dryness of the mouth and (rarely) constipation.
 (e) *Aminophylline.* This is an effective bronchodilator which may be administered orally or intravenously, or by rectal suppository. It is used in combination with salbutamol. It may cause headache, cardiac arrhythmia or palpitation and hypotension, and tachycardia.
 (f) *Adrenaline.* This drug is usually given subcutaneously but a preparation is also available for inhalation. It is a powerful and quick-acting bronchodilator, but its adverse cardiac side-effects limit its use. If it is given the patient is observed closely for a rapid, irregular, weak pulse. Tremors, anxiety and restlessness are commonly manifested.
2 *Corticosteroids.* A corticoid preparation may be prescribed in conjunction with another bronchodilator to enhance the effect of the latter and to reduce bronchial reactivity. It may be administered intravenously or orally if the patient has severe respiratory insufficiency, but is gradually tapered off and terminated as the condition improves. The preparation beclomethasone dipropionate (Becloforte or Becotide) for inhalation is available in nebulized form in a small pressurized dispenser. Applied locally, it reduces the bronchial response of spasm without producing the side-effects characteristic of long-term general administration of corticosteroids.
3 *Antibiotics.* A broad-spectrum antibiotic [e.g. tetracycline, amoxycillin (Amoxil)] is given when

the earliest signs of infection appear. These may be purulent sputum, general malaise, fever, decreased effort tolerance and increased shortness of breath. A sputum specimen may first be collected so that the organism may be identified and sensitivity tests made in order for a specific antimicrobial drug to be prescribed and administered.

Rarely, an antibiotic is administered by aerosol. If the infection is unresponsive to antibiotics which may be given safely by the oral or parenteral routes, or the required antimicrobial drug is toxic, the administration may be by inhalation.

EXPECTED OUTCOMES

The patient:
1 States the effects of smoking and atmospheric pollutants on airway clearance.
2 Describes measures which may be initiated by the individual, industry and community to prevent the development of airway dysfunction.
3 Demonstrates signs and symptoms of improved or stable airway clearance:
   (a) The respiratory rate and depth are normal for the individual.
   (b) The vesicular breath sounds are audible on auscultation.
   (c) The heart rate is within the patient's usual range.
   (d) Respirations are rhythmical and effortless.
   (e) There is an absence of crackles and wheezes in the lungs.
   (f) Arterial blood gases are within the normal range for the individual.
   (g) Forced expiratory time (FET) and vital capacity (VC) are within the normal range for the individual.
4 Demonstrates improved physical tolerance in carrying out daily living activities.

2 Ineffective breathing pattern

The *goal* is to increase the effectiveness of breathing.

Normally, increased activity leads to increases in ventilation and cardiac output, and more effective oxygen uptake by tissues. Respiration is regular and more effective. Increased activity on the part of individuals with respiratory disease usually causes ventilation–perfusion mismatching and air-trapping. The alveoli may be adequately perfused but unevenly ventilated and/or uniform ventilation may exist with unequal blood flow. When the respiratory rate increases in response to hypoxia and hypercapnia the irregularity of respirations is increased.[25] Shallow respirations frequently associated with neuromuscular and skeletal impairment, pain or anxiety also decrease the effectiveness of respirations.

When disease or injury affects one area of the lung or chest wall the chest excursion may be unequal. Efforts to improve the effectiveness of respirations include localized breathing exercises and diaphragmatic and pursed-lip breathing.

Localized breathing exercises. These techniques are used to promote equal and symmetrical chest expansion when disease or injury are confined to one area of the lung or chest wall. The patient is assisted to a sitting position in bed or sitting on the side of the bed with legs dangling and arms supported. The physiotherapist or specialist nurse places hands over the base of the ribs with thumbs extended along the costal margins (see Fig. 16.5) and instructs the patient to breathe slowly and deeply; this should expand the chest and push the physiotherapist's hands outward. Expansion of the upper chest is encouraged using the same technique of making the patient aware of the limitation in chest expansion and having him consciously expand the area. Observing and feeling the movement of the hands as the ribs expand outward, reinforces the effectiveness of the breathing exercise. As the patient exhales through his mouth, slight pressure is applied against his chest. The patient is taught to carry out the exercise by himself. Incisional pain may be minimized for the surgical patient by supporting the area with the hands or a pillow.

Diaphragmatic breathing. Harper states that by increasing diaphragmatic excursions and reducing the use of accessory muscles the following objectives are achieved: ventilation of the lung bases is improved by improving breathing efficiency and reducing upper alveolar overinflation; the work of breathing is reduced; uncoordinated breathing patterns are eliminated; activity tolerance improves; and the patient learns to control his breathing when dyspnoeic, reducing the anxious feelings and panic.[26]

Diaphragmatic breathing involves:
1 Placing the patient's or instructor's hands on the patient's abdomen below the ribs
2 Relaxation of the shoulders
3 Taking a deep breath through the nose while pushing the abdomen outward against the hands
4 Holding the breath for 1 or 2 seconds to keep the alveoli open
5 and breathing out slowly through the mouth while applying gentle pressure to the abdomen with the hands.[27]

The exercise is repeated several times and the patient is encouraged to concentrate on the abdominal movement.

Pursed-lip breathing. Pursed-lip breathing involves taking a deep breath and exhaling slowly and fully

---

[25] Blegis (1981), pp. 10.

[26] Harper (1981), p. 275.
[27] Harper (1981), p. 275.

through pursed lips. The aim of this technique is to prolong expiration and slow the respiratory rate.

The patient is taught to practise diaphragmatic and pursed-lip breathing together. The patient relaxes his shoulders and takes a slow deep breath while relaxing and 'protruding' the abdomen; he then leans forward slightly, and exhales slowly through pursed lips while contracting the abdominal muscles. This controlled breathing pattern is used by the patient with chronic airflow limitation when carrying out the activities of daily living and during episodes of stress and anxiety.

MAINTENANCE OF INTRATHORACIC PRESSURE

The intrathoracic space is that between the visceral and parietal pleurae; the membranes are normally only separated by a thin film of fluid. Disruption of the pleura by disease, trauma or chest surgery results in air or fluid entering this space; the normal negative intrapleural pressure is lost. The increased pressure restricts lung expansion on inspiration and may cause collapse of the lung. Closed chest drainage is usually established. A thoracentesis (pleural aspiration) may be performed to remove fluid from the pleural cavity as well as for diagnostic tests (see Table 16.8.

Closed chest drainage
A closed or water-seal drainage system is established to allow the escape of air and fluid from the pleural cavity and re-establish the normal negative pressure, while preventing any reflux. Two tubes are generally placed in the affected area of the chest and are secured by a suture to the chest wall. One tube is placed in the anterior upper part of the area and mainly serves in the escape of air; the second tube is usually placed in the posterior base of the cavity for fluid drainage. A single tube placed high in the anterior or lateral chest is used for a pneumothorax when air, not fluid, is present in the pleural space.

Methods. Various methods are used to achieve closed drainage, but the principle is the same with all—that is, to allow air and fluid to pass in one direction only. The difference in the methods is generally in the number of bottles or bags used, whether or not suction is applied and whether or not a flutter valve is introduced into the system.

Water-seal drainage may be established with one bottle fitted with a two-holed stopper through which two glass or plastic tubes pass (Fig. 16.11). The chest tubes are connected to a fairly long tube leading to the drainage bottle, where it is connected to a glass or plastic tube which has its distal end submerged at all times in sterile water or sterile normal saline to a designated depth (usually 3–5 cm). The depth of tube submersion determines the pressure exerted by the water—hence the term 'water-seal drainage'. A small, short tube, serving as an air vent, passes through the second hole of the tight-fitting, two-holed stopper. The water level must be marked clearly on the bottle so that the amount of drainage can be determined accurately. When preparing the set-up, a strip of adhesive may be placed lengthwise on the drainage bottle and marked off at calibrations of 100 ml, 200 ml, 300 ml, etc. if the container is not already calibrated.

With each expiration, the respiratory muscles relax, the intrapleural space is diminished and the pressure within the space is increased; this pressure exceeds that exerted by the water at the end of the tube, so fluid and air are forced from the cavity into the water in the bottle. The air may be seen bubbling through the water, from which it passes, escaping from the bottle through the vent. With inspiration the pleural space enlarges and the pressure within it decreases, causing water to rise several centimetres in the distal end of the tube. The evacuation of fluid and air from the intrapleural space results in greater space and less pressure. As a result, lung expansion is increased.

The alternating changes in pressure in the pleural cavity result in repeated fluctuations in the water level in the distal end of the drainage tube; these fluctuations correspond to the patient's breathing in and out and indicate a patent system, serving as a guide to the nurse. If the water level does not oscillate, it may be suspected that the tube is blocked by a blood clot or fibrin. If this occurs, the tube is 'milked' toward the drainage bottle in an effort to relieve the blockage and, if this is not successful, the doctor is notified at once. In order to prevent blocking, the tube may be 'milked' or stripped' at stated intervals. This practice is controversial as stripping a chest tube may create excessive negative pressures. It is recommended that stripping of the tubing be done only when necessary to prevent blocking by clots when there is intrapleural bleeding.[28] Fluctuation of the fluid level in the tube ceases when the lung has fully re-expanded. The doctor confirms this by an x-ray of the chest before removing the drainage tube.

Coughing and deep abdominal breathing alter the intrapleural space and pressure to a greater degree than normal respirations and, as a result, are important in promoting drainage of the cavity, removal of air and fluid and the re-expansaion of remaining lung tissue.

To prevent water from being sucked into the chest, the drainage bottle must be kept well below the level of the patient (2–3 feet below the patient's chest). The negative chest pressure is equivalent to 10–20 cm of water and sucks the water up into the tube only to that level. If the bottle must be lifted or moved, caution is observed to prevent traction on the tube, which might result in its dislodgement.

A safer method for preventing the possibility of water accidentally entering the chest cavity, and

---

[28] Erickson (1981), p. 40.

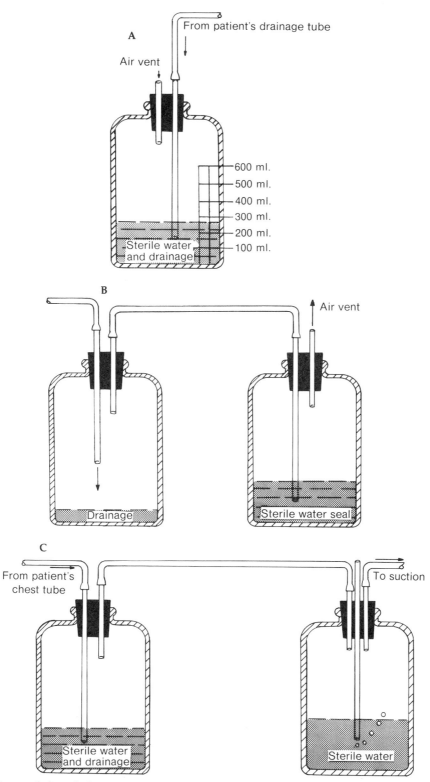

Fig. 16.11 *A,* Water-seal chest drainage system using one bottle. *B,* Water-seal chest drainage system using two bottles. *C,* Water-seal chest drainage system using two bottles and suction.

Table 16.7 Nursing intervention in the management of the patient with water-seal chest drainage.

Goals	Nursing intervention	Rationale/discussion	Expected outcomes
1 To increase the effectiveness of breathing 2 To remove secretions and gas from the pleural space 3 To promote safety and prevent injury	*Connection of the closed drainage system* Wash hands thoroughly and use sterile technique when opening the disposable or bottle drainage unit	To prevent contamination of the unit and spread of microorganisms to the pleural space	1 The drainage system is patent as evidenced by fluctuations in the fluid level in the drainage bottle 2 The patient's respiratory rate, depth and pattern are within normal limits 3 Deep breathing and coughing are performed at regular intervals 4 Chest x-ray demonstrates expansion of the lung prior to removal of the chest tube
	Place the bottles, a stand and disposable unit on a designated rack away from where it can be knocked over and below the level of the patient	To decrease the potential for accidental breakage or disconnection of the system, and to prevent fluid from being sucked into the pleural cavity	
	Add sterile normal saline to the bottle or disposable system and adjust the tube in the bottle to designated depth (3–5 cm) of submersion	The depth of the tube determines the pressure exerted	
	Check that the air vent tube or opening is open	To permit escape of air from the system	
	Mark the fluid level on a strip of adhesive tape placed lengthwise on the bottle or indicate the calibration level on the disposable system	To provide a double check that the water level is adequate, and to enable measurement of the amount of drainage in single-bottle system	
	Connect extension tube to suction if ordered	To promote drainage with low level suction	
	Connect drainage tubing to the submerged tube in the bottle and attach the tube and connector to the chest tube	To connect the system	
	Tape all connections	To make certain the system is airtight and to prevent accidental disconnection	
	Arrange tubing, coiling it loosely to prevent kinks and fasten it to the bedside	To prevent kinks and obstruction of tubing and to prevent tubing from interfering with patient movement	
	Place two clamps at the patient's bedside where they are readily visible and attainable	To clamp the system in case of accidental disconnection and thus prevent air entry into the pleural cavity	
	Assessment Patency of the system as evidenced by fluctuations in the water level in the drainage bottle; air bubbling through the water	To determine patency of the closed drainage system Fluctuation in the water level will not occur when continuous suction is used	
	Safety: all connections are intact and taped; the bottles/disposable system are below the level of the patient; the tubing is not kinked	To ensure that all safety precautions are observed	

Table 16.7—*continued*

Goals	Nursing intervention	Rationale/discussion	Expected outcomes
(see p. 440 opposite)	The drainage is observed for volume, colour and consistency, especially during the first 24–48 hours	To determine the effectiveness of the drainage system and to promptly identify complications such as bleeding	(see p. 440 opposite)
	The patient is assessed for: rate, depth, pattern and frequency of respirations; signs of dyspnoea and cyanosis; and chest pain and rapid pulse. Lungs are auscultated for air entry and the presence of wheezes and râles	Accumulation of air in the pleural cavity can cause collapse of the lung on the affected side	
	Maintenance of the closed drainage system If blockage of the tubing is suspected, check for kinking and inspect tubing for clots. 'Milk' or strip the tubing in the direction of the drainage bottle	'Milking' of the tubing clears the tubing of clots. Since it creates excessive negative pressures it should be done only when necessary	
	Encourage the patient to deep breathe and cough at frequent, regular intervals	Coughing and deep abdominal breathing increase the intrapulmonary and intrapleural pressures promoting drainage and preventing tension pneumothorax	
	Changing of the drainage bottle is done by an experienced person. Clamp each drainage tube close to the chest with two clamps and quickly disconnect the drainage bottle and connect the new sterile, calibrated container	To prevent air being sucked into the pleural cavity and to prevent contamination with microorganisms	
	Accidental interruption of the drainage system. Immediately clamp the tubing close to the chest wall with two clamps. A new sterile drainage system and tubing are connected	To prevent air from entering the pleural cavity and collapse of the lung	
	Discontinuation of the closed drainage system The patient is instructed to take a large breath and hold it as the doctor clamps the tube and removes it. A sterile petroleum gauze dressing is simultaneously applied to the exit site and sealed with tape or a transparent adhesive dressing	To prevent air from entering the pleural cavity To protect the wound from microorganisms	

which also keeps the drainage separated from the water, is to use *two* bottles. The second one contains the water, leaving the drainage bottle dry (Fig. 16.11). When only one bottle is used, fluid drainage from the chest raises the level of the fluid, increasing the pressure at the distal end of the tube. More pressure is then required to force the fluid down on expiration and allow the escape of air and fluid. Blood and serum are more likely to collect and clot in the tube. In the two-bottle system, the first bottle is sealed and does not contain water; the shorter of the tubes is connected to the second bottle, which also has two tubes. The first (drainage) bottle is connected to the longer tube in the second bottle. The distal end of this tube is submerged in sterile water to a designated depth (3–5 cm). The second tube in bottle 2 is short and acts as an air vent.

If there is a considerable amount of air leaking into the pleural cavity from the intrapulmonary space, or if the patient's cough and respirations are not sufficiently strong to facilitate the clearance of fluid and air from the chest cavity, *continuous gentle suction* may be applied. This necessitates a two-bottle system; the first bottle serves as a drainage bottle and *water-seal*. The short air-vent tube in bottle 1 is connected to the second bottle which has a three-holed stopper through which two short tubes and one longer tube pass (see Fig. 16.11). The lower end of the longer tube is submerged in water to a designated depth. The upper end is open to the air. This tube controls the degree of suction applied to the pleural cavity. One short tube is connected to bottle 1; the second short tube is connected to a suction apparatus. The usual suction machine creates too strong a negative pressure to be applied directly to the pleural cavity. This may be reduced by a valve and meter (such as is used in 'wall suction') inserted between the suction and the water-seal bottle. If the portable suction machine is used, the negative pressure is controlled by the depth of submersion of the lower end of the open glass tube in bottle 2. A continuous bubbling in the control bottle (bottle 2) indicates that the suction is being maintained.

Disposable closed drainage receptacles with two compartments comparable to the two-bottle system are available. The receptacle is attached to suction and is suspended from the side of the bed, eliminating the danger of bottles being knocked over and broken.

The water-seal system is cumbersome and also restricts patients' mobility. The nurse and patient are continuously apprehensive of such things as tubes becoming disconnected and bottles being broken. As a safety measure and to permit greater freedom in turning and earlier ambulation, some surgeons prefer to introduce a plastic flutter valve into the system. It is placed between the chest drainage tube and the drainage bottle. Suction may still be applied. The system may be placed on a small cart or pole with wheels to allow the patient to move around the unit.

Responsibilities and precautions (see Table 16.7). When any method of water-seal drainage is used, nursing responsibilities include the following considerations.

It is important that the nurse understands the purpose and operating principles of the system, as well as the precautions to be observed to prevent air and fluid from entering the chest cavity, which could cause a pneumothorax (collapse of the lung) and life-threatening respiratory insufficiency.

If the bottle system is used, a directive should be received from the doctor as to the depth to which the underwater tube should be submerged. The bottle should be calibrated so that the volume of water used is known and the drainage may be measured.

The system must be checked at frequent intervals for patency. This is determined by noting the oscillating water level in the submerged tube; this rises with inspiration and falls with expiration. When suction is employed, fluctuations of the water level do not occur because the continuous suction holds the water level in the tube at a fixed level. The suction may be interrupted briefly and the column of water observed for fluctuations. If the water level does not fluctuate in a closed system, the tube should be examined for possible kinks or compression caused by the patient lying on it. A clot may be obstructing the tube and may be dislodged by 'milking' or 'stripping' the tube toward the drainage bottle. If the system remains non-functional, the doctor is informed at once.

As a precaution, all connections are taped with adhesive to prevent their separation and to keep air from entering the system. The bottles are placed in a rack or taped to the floor to prevent accidental moving or knocking over. Visitors and ward personnel are warned not to disturb them, and a warning sign placed by the bottles is helpful.

The drainage tube is supported and lies free in a fold in the sheet, to which it is secured by a clip or tape. It should not be looped but should be long enough to avoid marked restriction of the patient's moving and turning.

The characteristics and volume of the drainage are noted and recorded frequently, especially during the first 24–48 hours. The drainage may be coloured by blood at first, but gradually clears and decreases in amount.

Changing the drainage bottle is done by someone who fully understands closed drainage. Each drainage tube is clamped close to the chest wall with two chest drain clamps, and the bottle is quickly replaced by a clean, calibrated sterile bottle.

If an interruption or break in the closed system should occur as a result of the disconnection of a tube or a broken bottle, the drainage tube(s) should be clamped off close to the chest wall immediately to prevent air from entering the chest cavity. An accumulation of air in the pleural cavity could cause a collapse of the lung on the affected side and produce compression of the unaffected lung, heart and large blood vessels. Associated symptoms are a complaint by the patient of tightness or pressure in the chest, dyspnoea, cyanosis and a rapid pulse. The doctor is notified promptly and the clamps remain in place until the integrity of the system is re-established. As a precaution, an extra set of sterile bottles and connections should always be available.

Regular frequent staged coughing and deep breathing are important since they increase the intrapulmonary and intrapleural pressures, forcing air and fluid out of the cavity and promoting lung expansion. The patient should be ambulatory as soon as possible.

When turning the patient, or when giving any care, precautions are taken not to dislodge or disconnect the drainage tubes. A final check is made to make sure the patient is not lying on a portion of the tube and that there are no loops or kinks present to interfere with drainage.

Even if the system appears to be functioning satisfactorily, any patient complaint of pressure or pain in the chest, dyspnoea, cyanosis or a rapid, weak pulse is reported promptly.

When the lung is fully expanded and no fluid remains in the pleural cavity, the tubes are removed. The water in the closed drainage bottle will have stopped fluctuating, and the lung expansion is confirmed by the doctor by percussion, auscultation and a chest x-ray.

When the tube is withdrawn from the chest cavity, the wound is covered with a dry, secure dressing. In some cases a purse-string suture has been inserted around the tube and this is tightened off when the tube is removed and covered with a dry, secure dressing. The patient is observed closely for the next 24 hours for possible leakage of air into the chest and ensuing pneumothorax.

Thoracentesis (pleural aspiration) (see Table 16.8)
A thoracentesis is the withdrawal of fluid or air from the pleural cavity. Normally pleural fluid serves to lubricate the pleura. Excessive fluid and air interfere with lung expansion. Chest expansion will be asymmetrical with distension and decreased movement present on the affected side. A thoracentesis is performed to remove excessive pleural fluid to facilitate lung expansion, for diagnostic purposes or to instil medication into the pleural cavity. Following preparation of the skin and injection of a local anaesthetic, the doctor inserts a needle through an intercostal space into the pleural cavity. A three-way adaptor (stop-cock) is attached to the needle to enable withdrawal of fluid through attached tubing or a syringe and closing of the system when fluid is not being aspirated. Care must be taken to maintain a closed system and to prevent air from entering the pleural space.

EXPECTED OUTCOMES

The patient:
1 Uses controlled breathing techniques during activities of daily living.
2 Demonstrates slow and deep respirations.
3 Expands his chest symmetrically during inspiration.
4 Relaxes his abdominal muscles during inspiration and contracts them during expiration.
5 Experiences fewer, shorter and milder episodes of dyspnoea.

3 Impairment of gas exchange

The *goals* are to:
1 Promote pulmonary ventilation
2 Maintain adequate pulmonary ventilation
3 Maintain adequate transportation of oxygen to the tissues
4 Decrease tissue demands for oxygen

PROMOTION OF PULMONARY VENTILATION

Exercise. Immobility and lack of exercise have adverse effects on the respiratory system. Secretions tend to accumulate and stagnate in the airways. Regular exercise should be part of everyone's lifestyle. Benefits of regular exercise to the respiratory system include increased rate and depth of ventilation, increased pulmonary perfusion and increased rate of diffusion of oxygen and carbon dioxide.[29]

Exercise is equally beneficial to the person with respiratory impairment. Patients who increase their physical activities gradually and consistently show improvement in tolerance levels and a decrease in the effects of the disease.

Incentive spirometer. This device gives visual feedback to patients; it is used to promote maximum ventilation of the lungs. The patient sits comfortably, breathes through the mouthpiece of the spirometer, takes a deep breath, holds it for 3 seconds and then exhales. The visual cues provided by the spirometer (e.g. ball rising to a certain level, staying there for 3 seconds, and falling, and the number of deep breaths performed) encourage patients to increase their respiratory effort and their tidal volumes.

MAINTENANCE OF PULMONARY VENTILATION

Nursing interventions directed towards promoting airway clearance and establishing effective breathing patterns contribute to pulmonary ventilation. Additional measures include: (1) changes of position, and (2) administration of oxygen.

Changes of position
Changes in body position affect ventilation and perfusion in healthy individuals and in patients with

---

[29] Halfman & Hojnacki (1981), p. 5.

Table 16.8 Nursing intervention in the management of the patient having a thoracentesis.

Goals	Nursing intervention	Rationale/discussion	Expected outcomes
1 To increase the effectiveness of breathing 2 To remove pleural fluid and tissue for diagnostic studies 3 To instil medication into the pleural cavity	The patient is informed of the procedure, and what to expect during the procedure	Knowledge of what to expect can reduce anxiety and opportunity is provided to answer the patient's concerns	1 The patient understands the procedure and what to expect during the procedure 2 The patient's breathing is regular, rhythmical and not laboured 3 Chest expansion is symmetrical, with a usual degree of excursion
	The nurse checks that the consent form has been signed following the doctor's explanation to the patient of the purpose of the test and expected and other possible outcomes, and that chest x-rays have been carried out	X-rays provide information as to the exact anatomical location of the fluid and air in the pleural cavity	
	The prescribed sedation is administered prior to the start of the procedure	Sedation may be required to promote relaxation and decrease discomfort and anticipatory pain	
	The patient is placed in a sitting position, leaning forward, with head and arms resting on a table or several pillows	Fluid is dependent and therefore accumulates in the lower portions of the pleural cavity when the patient is upright, making it easier to remove	
	During the procedure the nurse provides physical support for the patient and instructs him to remain still while the needle is being inserted and while it is in place	To prevent spontaneous movement by the patient which may result in trauma to the pleura and lung	
	During the procedure the nurse provides on-going explanations as to what is occurring. As the antiseptic solution is applied, the patient is told to expect a feeling of cold; injection of the local anaesthetic will be felt and a pressure will be experienced as the thoracentesis needle is inserted	Patient cooperation increases and anxiety is decreased when he is aware of what is happening	
	A sterile transparent dressing or a gauze dressing sealed with tape is applied as the doctor withdraws the thoracentesis needle	To prevent air from entering the pleural cavity To protect the site from microorganisms	
	The patient is assisted to a comfortable position in bed and assessed at least every 15 minutes for the first 2 hours. Observations include respiratory rate, depth and rhythm, pulse rate, presence of blood, frothy sputum, uncontrolled cough, dyspnoea, cyanosis, chest pain or tightness and feelings of dizziness or faintness. The site is inspected and the surrounding tissue palpated for puffiness or crackling	If a large amount of fluid is removed, lung expansion occurs suddenly and pulmonary and cardiac distress may occur Spontaneous pneumothorax and subcutaneous emphysema may occur following thoracentesis A portable chest x-ray is usually ordered to verify that a pneumothorax is not present	

Table 16.8—*continued*

Goals	Nursing intervention	Rationale/discussion	Expected outcomes
	The volume, colour and consistency of the pleural fluid is determined and recorded. The specimen containers are labelled and sent promptly to the laboratory	Accurate, prompt documentation is a legal requirement. Prompt labelling and discharge of specimens ensures identification of the specimen and that contamination of the specimen does not occur	

lung diseases. West demonstrated that in the upright position the base of the lung is better ventilated and perfusion is greater than in the apex, producing regional differences in gas exchange.[30] In the supine, prone and lateral positions ventilation and perfusion are more uniform. Changes in body position significantly affect the rate of ventilation, the amount of lung capacity and the amount of physiological dead space.[31]

Knowledge of the effects of position changes on pulmonary ventilation and perfusion in healthy subjects illustrates the need for nurses to assess the effects of various positions on patients with altered lung ventilation and perfusion. Ng and McCormick point out that studies have shown that in patients with chronic airflow limitation, differences in ventilation–perfusion ratios and gas exchange do not occur in the sitting position.[32] Turning the patient with acute respiratory failure from the supine to prone position enhances gas exchange. Patients with disease predominantly affecting one lung showed improvement when turned from the supine position to a lateral position with the diseased lung uppermost. This illustrated that the patient should be turned on to the side of the affected lung.[33] Measurements of lung volumes, blood gases and oxygen saturation by ear oximeter provide objective measures of ventilation and perfusion when evaluating a patient's response to changes in position. The nurse can also use the following parameters: observation of respiratory rate and depth; breath sounds; use of accessory muscles; pulse rate; skin colour; and the patient's general state of relaxation or tension.

Position changes for a patient with respiratory impairment are individualized and based on the assessment of the patient's responses to various positions.

Administration of oxygen
Oxygen administration is used to increase the arterial oxygen tension in conjunction with treatment directed toward the cause of the hypoxia.

Oxygen is not usually prescribed for patients unless their Pao_2 is reduced to 15–30% below normal (normal Pao_2 is 11.0–13.3 kPa or 80–100 mmHg) or the oxygen saturation is less than 85%. As with any medication, it should not be used indiscriminately. For instance, the administration of oxygen, except in a very low concentration, could be fatal to patients with hypoxia associated with chronic pulmonary disease. This is because these patients may have some retention of carbon dioxide (chronic hypercapnia). Normally, increased carbon dioxide tension stimulates the respiratory centres and elicits a ventilatory response that increases carbon dioxide elimination. The sensitivity of the chemoreceptors to hypercarbia is diminished in chronic hypercapnia and the patient becomes dependent upon hypoxia as a respiratory stimulus. If oxygen is given to correct the hypoxaemia, the patient's 'respiratory drive' is removed, hypoventilation develops and carbon dioxide retention is increased.

The concentration of oxygen administered to raise the oxygen level depends upon the patient's Pao_2, the effectiveness of the transportation of blood gases to the tissues, and on the tissue needs for oxygen and ability to utilize oxygen. Commonly, the flow rate per minute is set to deliver an oxygen concentration of about 30–40%. A frequent policy observed is to commence therapy with a low concentration (the flow rate will depend on the method used to deliver the oxygen); after 30 minutes the arterial blood gas concentrations and pH are determined. The flow rate is then adjusted on the basis of the findings. The arterial blood gases, pH, and the patient's responses are monitored at frequent intervals throughout oxygen therapy to indicate progress and any adjustment to be made in the concentration of oxygen administered or the method of delivery.

When using oxygen, it should be remembered that it is colourless, odourless, tasteless and heavier than air, and that it is hazardous because it supports combustion. Certain *precautions* must constantly be observed to avoid possible fire: (1) smoking is prohibited in the area, and signs indicating the restriction are posted; (2) cigarettes, pipe and matches are removed from the patient's bedside; (3) electrical devices such as electric razors are kept at least 5 feet from the primary source of oxygen; (4) the use of oil and alcohol-based lotion for skin care is avoided; (5) portable oxygen systems should be stored in a cool,

---

[30] West (1979), pp. 62 & 63.
[31] Ng & McCormick (1982), p. 18.
[32] Ng & McCormick (1982), p. 22.
[33] Ng & McCormick (1982), p. 23.

dry, well-ventilated area;[34] and (6) patients should receive instructions about safety precautions.

Methods of administering oxygen. The oxygen therapy device that is selected should be capable of delivering a consistent concentration of oxygen and be comfortable for the patient.

Oxygen delivery systems may be classified as *low flow* or *high flow*. Low-flow systems let the patient inhale room air which mixes freely with the oxygen. As the patient's ventilatory pattern changes so does the concentration of oxygen he receives. Low-flow systems are economical and comfortable but they do not provide a fixed concentration of oxygen. High-flow systems deliver a precise concentration of oxygen regardless of the patient's ventilatory pattern. Most of these systems use a Venturi mask which controls the amount of room air entering the system. The orifice size regulates the ratio of room air to oxygen, controls the velocity and directly affects the oxygen concentration being administered. Changes in the patient's respiration do not affect the inspired oxygen concentration as long as the correct litre flow is used and the mask fits snugly.

1 *Low-flow oxygen therapy devices.* Low-flow devices include the nasal cannulae, nasal catheter (rare), and the simple face mask.

   (a) *Nasal cannulae.* These are two fine, plastic tubes that stem from a common tube that connects with the oxygen source (Fig. 16.12). The cannulae are inserted just inside the anterior nares and oxygen is directed into the nasal sinuses which form a reservoir for the oxygen.

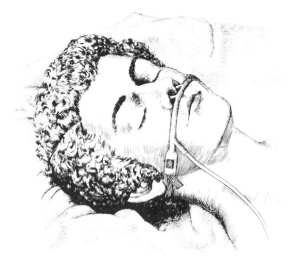

Fig. 16.12 Plastic cannulae or prongs inserted into the nostrils to deliver oxygen.

On inspiration, room air is drawn in and mixes with the oxygen in the reservoir. A flow rate of 1–6 l/min can deliver a concentration of 25–35% inspired oxygen. Cannulae are usually run at low flow rates. Flow rates in excess of 6 l/min may produce headache and discomfort for the patient. Inspired oxygen concentrations vary widely in relation to the patient's ventilatory pattern. The cannulae do not deliver the required concentration if the patient is a mouth breather. Advantages of using the nasal cannulae are comfort for the patient, fewer problems with prolonged use and lack of interference with daily activities and verbal communication. Occasionally, the patient complains of soreness around the nares or ears with long-term use which may be relieved by the application of a water-based lubricant around the nares and padding behind the ears.

   (b) *Nasal catheter.* The catheter used for the administration of oxygen is flexible and has a rounded tip and several holes in the distal 2–5 cm. The tube is moistened and passed through a nostril into the nasopharynx. The tip of the catheter should be visible just below the soft palate.

The catheter is secured and the patient advised to breathe through his nose. The catheter is changed every 8–10 hours; the nostrils are used alternately to minimize irritation of the mucous membrane. Oxygen is directed into the oropharynx. Room air is drawn in with each inspiration and mixes with the oxygen. The nasal catheter is rarely used because studies have shown that the nasal cannulae provide similar inspired oxygen concentration with less discomfort to the patient.[35] This method of administration interferes less with treatments and nursing care, and patients are usually more tolerant of it than of the mask. This is not a common method in British hospitals though it is used more often for infants.

   (c) *Simple oxygen mask.* This plastic mask fits over the nose and mouth and with the nasal sinuses forms reservoirs for oxygen. Room air is drawn in around the edges of the mask and through holes in the sides of the mask on inspiration and mixes with oxygen in the reservoirs. The patient's respiratory pattern influences the concentration of inspired oxygen. Flow rates of 5–8 l/min can produce inspired oxygen concentrations of 40–80%. A minimum flow rate of 5 l/min will flush exhaled gas out of the mask and prevent rebreathing of expired carbon dioxide. Flow rates in excess of 8 l/min do not increase inspired oxygen concentrations because the reservoirs are filled.

Masks interfere with patient activities, especially talking and eating. They are less comfortable than the nasal cannulae but can deliver higher concentrations of oxygen.

Oxygen supplied from wall or tank systems lacks humidity and may cause drying of the mucosa. At low flow rates (e.g. 3–4 l/min) humidification of the oxygen is not needed and if supplied may cause 'feelings of suffocation'. At higher flow rates, humidification of the inspired oxygen may be supplied by humidifiers such as the bubble humidifiers. The oxygen is bubbled through sterile water allowing the oxygen to pick up water vapour.

2 *High-flow oxygen therapy devices/controlled oxygen therapy.* These devices include Venturi masks and non-rebreathing masks.

(a) *Venturi mask (entrainment mask).* This mask can deliver 28–35% oxygen which is fairly precisely controlled. When oxygen enters the mask, it passes through a narrow jet opening which increases the velocity of the flow. Room air is drawn through the entrainment ports into the stream of oxygen. Oxygen concentration is varied by changing the size of the jet or the size of the entrainment ports (see Fig. 16.13). The jets are calibrated which allows control of the ratio of oxygen to air. The larger the jet, the more room air inhaled. These masks are recommended for use by patients with chronic airflow limitation because oxygen concentrations can be controlled. However, like other masks, it interferes with patient activities. Humidifiers are not recommended with Venturi masks as the humidity may clog the jet openings and cause changes in the concentration of the oxygen delivered. Usually, enough room air is entrained to maintain sufficient humidity of the inspired gas. If more humidification is required, the room air may be

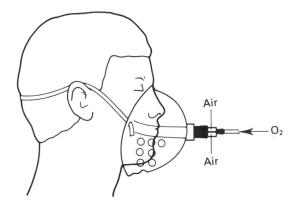

Fig. 16.13 Venturi mask (entrainment mask).

humidified by use of a vaporizer. A head tent has been developed using the Venturi principle. It is equally suitable for giving controlled oxygen therapy.

(b) *Non-rebreathing mask.* A bag is attached to the base of this mask to serve as a large reservoir for the oxygen (see Fig. 16.14). On inspiration, a one-way flap valve between the bag and the mask opens so that oxygen can be inhaled and one-way flap valves over the exhalation ports close to prevent entrainment of room air. If the mask fits securely, the patient breathes only the oxygen from the bag, permitting delivery of 90–100% oxygen concentrations. Exhaled air is directed through the exhalation ports and cannot enter the bag as the flap valve between the bag and the mask closes.

The flow rate of the oxygen should be high enough to keep the reservoir bag partially full at all times. Collapse of the bag on inspiration would mean that the only air the patient can obtain is room air entrained from around the edges of the mask.

Humidifiers are not recommended for use with non-rebreathing masks as the water vapour condenses in the reservoir bag and interferes with the opening and closing of the flap valves. Generally these masks are used for only short periods of time.

(c) *Partial rebreathing mask.* This mask also contains a reservoir bag but has no valve, therefore the patient's expired gas flows back into the bag. The first third of the patient's exhaled breath enters the bag with the remainder going out the exhalation ports of the mask. The portion of exhaled gas entering the bag is primarily from the anatomical dead spaces of the respiratory tract. The concentrations of carbon dioxide and oxygen in this gas are the same as in the inhaled gas. The concentration of oxygen administered is fairly consistent.

The inspired oxygen concentration is slightly lower than that delivered by a non-rebreathing mask ranging from 60–90%. As with other masks, the fit of the mask affects the entry of room air and the inspired oxygen concentration.

(d) *Manual resuscitation bag (Ambu bag).* This is part of the standard equipment on any ward emergency or resuscitation trolley. It is a portable ventilator that is operated manually (Fig. 16.14). It consists of a self-inflating bag which connects with a source of 100% oxygen and has a short tube to which a mask is attached. A connecting adapter replaces the mask when the bag is used for a patient with an endotracheal or tracheostomy tube.

After applying the mask so that there is as tight a seal as possible, or after connecting the tube to the patient's artificial airway, the bag is

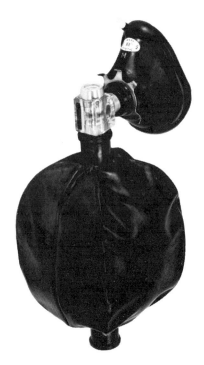

Fig. 16.14 An Ambu resuscitator, a self-inflating hand-compressible breathing bag with mask.

squeezed with both hands. Collapse of the bag delivers an adequate tidal volume of oxygen into the patient's airway.

The self-inflating hand ventilator is useful for resuscitation in an emergency. It is kept at the bedside of a patient who is receiving mechanical ventilatory assistance so it is readily available to ventilate the patient in case of malfunction of the respirator.

Oxygen toxicity. The nurse must be aware of additional precautions when administering oxygen. High concentrations of oxygen over prolonged periods can cause oxygen toxicity. Concentrations greater than 60% oxygen over 24 hours can cause pathological changes in the lungs and central nervous system. The alveolar–capillary membrane is damaged, resulting in increased permeability and ensuing oedema of the interstitial tissues and alveoli. Oxygen and carbon dioxide diffusion is impaired. Some alveoli collapse. The Pao_2 falls and causes what is referred to as 'refractory hypoxaemia'. Retention of carbon dioxide and acidosis develop.

Neurological manifestations include muscular irritability that may progress to convulsions and impaired vision. Premature infants exposed to a high oxygen concentration develop vascular changes in their eyes that lead to blindness.

Mechanical ventilators

When a patient is unable to ventilate his lungs effectively and maintain adequate alveolar–blood gas exchange, a mechanical ventilator (respirator) may be used to inflate the lungs and assist the individual's inspiratory effort. The ventilator introduces air or a mixture of air and oxygen intermittently into the patient's airway by producing a positive pressure.[36] Expiration is passive when the inflow-regulating valve closes. The indications for ventilator use are ventilatory insufficiency, hypovolaemia and hypercapnia.

An artificial airway is necessary when a respirator is being used so that a seal is produced by a cuffed tube to prevent escape of the inspiratory gas. Initially, an endotracheal tube is generally used, but if mechanical respiratory support is necessary for a prolonged period, a tracheostomy is done and the ventilator is connected to a cuffed tracheostomy tube.

Types of ventilators

Three basic types of positive-pressure ventilators are available: (1) pressure-cycled; (2) volume-cycled; and (3) time-cycled.

The classification reflects the mechanism that terminates the inspiratory phase. With *volume-cycled ventilators*, the inspiratory phase ends after a preset tidal volume has been delivered. *Pressure-cycled ventilators* deliver the inspiratory gas until a preset pressure is reached which then terminates inspiration.

Volume-cycled ventilators are the most widely used and accepted as they permit greater control of patient ventilation. The time and pressure required to deliver the set volume change in relation to changes in the patient's airway resistance and pulmonary compliance.[37] The volume of gas is delivered regardless of the patient's pulmonary status. Changes in pulmonary resistance and compliance affect the volume of gas delivered by pressure or time-cycle ventilators. The alterations in total ventilation affect gas exchange and necessitate frequent adjusting of the ventilator to ensure that the rate and volume of respirations are adequate and consistent.

The use of pressure- and time-cycled ventilators is limited to intensive care settings, where nurses and doctors are skilled in adjusting the ventilator and where constant patient observation is assured.

Operational factors. The ventilator is selected and regulated to meet the specific needs of the individual patient. The mode of administration is chosen and then the volume of gas is set, the respiratory rate determined and the oxygen concentration prescribed. Respirators may be used to provide con-

---

[36] *Positive pressure* implies a gas pressure greater than that of the atmosphere.

[37] Brooks (1981a), p. 15.

trolled ventilation or assisted ventilation. In *controlled ventilation* the machine is set for automatic operation and for producing a set number of cycles per minute at a predetermined flow rate. This mode can be used only when the patient cannot make any respiratory effort at all.[38] This may necessitate administration of drugs to maintain respiratory paralysis in the patient.

In *assisted ventilation* the inspiratory phase of the respirator's cycle is triggered by the patient's spontaneous inspiration; it may either complement the patient's ventilatory volume or augment his respiratory efforts with a preset rate of ventilation. Most respirators that can be set for assisted ventilation are equipped with a safety control, so that if the patient's respiratory function fails to trigger the ventilator by a preset interval of time, controlled ventilation automatically takes over.

The tidal volume is determined by the patient's pulmonary and cardiac status. Tidal volumes greater than normal are usually selected to improve compliance, decrease the incidence of microatelectasis and improve gas exchange.[38]

The volume of air left in the lung at the end of expiration may be increased to prevent airway collapse in patients where a deficit of surfactant is suspected (e.g. adult respiratory distress syndrome). This is referred to as positive end-expiratory pressure (PEEP).

The respiratory rate is adjusted in relation to the tidal volume; slow respiratory rates are used with larger tidal volumes.

The oxygen concentration of the inspired gas will be prescribed on the basis of the patient's Pao_2. It does not usually exceed 40–50%, but can occasionally go up to 100% for a short period. The concentration is kept as low as possible without the patient experiencing hypoxia so as to prevent oxygen toxicity (see p. 448).

Nursing responsibilities. The nursing care plan for the patient who requires mechanical ventilatory assistance will vary according to the cause of the respiratory insufficiency and general condition.

The nurse, who is constantly at the patient's bedside, should have an understanding of the underlying principles of mechanical ventilation. She should be familiar with the operation of the particular machine being used and the prescribed inspiratory gas composition (percentage of air and oxygen). It is also necessary to know whether the ventilation is controlled or assisted and volume- or pressure-cycled, the prescribed volume or pressure setting for the delivery of the inspiratory gas and the flow rate and cycles per minute. A very important nursing responsibility is the immediate recognition of the indications of ventilator malfunction and untoward

reactions in the patient, as well as the initiation of prompt appropriate action.

It is essential that any nurse assuming responsibility for the care of a patient requiring mechanical ventilatory assistance has received adequate instruction and supervision in order to provide safe and effective care.

The patient who is receiving mechanical ventilation requires constant supervision. Visual and auditory alarm systems alert the nurse to ventilator malfunction and if the system fails to deliver the preset volume. If malfunction of the respirator or unfavourable changes in the patient are not immediately recognized and prompt action taken, the patient's life is threatened.

- *Assessment.* When mechanical ventilation is first established, it is necessary to note the patient's blood pressure, pulse rate and volume, colour, level of consciousness, and blood pH, gases ($Paco_2$, Pao_2) and electrolyte levels to establish base-lines for ongoing assessment. A chest x-ray may have been done and the findings are reviewed.

  Arterial blood samples are collected at frequent intervals for pH, blood gas and electrolyte (especially hydrogen carbonate, sodium, and potassium) determinations. These assessment parameters are monitored frequently and usually recorded as necessary, while the patient is in an acute setting because of the physiological effects of the positive pressure on the thoracic structures. In the intensive care unit, monitoring of *pulmonary capillary wedge pressure* (PCWP) will provide information about pulmonary congestion and cardiac function. A balloon-tipped (Swan–Ganz) catheter (see Chapter 14) is inserted so that the balloon obstructs a branch of the pulmonary artery and recordings of the pulmonary capillary wedge pressure and the pulmonary artery pressure can be made. The normal PCWP is 4–12 mmHg. Decreases in PCWP values are seen in hypovolaemia and increases are seen with pulmonary congestion and fluid overload. PCWP readings also provide indirect measurement of left ventricular function. Additional considerations in patient care include: (1) maintenance of a patent airway by suctioning; (2) positioning of the patient to promote effective ventilation, (3) range-of-motion exercises to prevent complications of immobility; and (4) maintenance of adequate hydration.

- *Emotional support.* The patient who requires mechanical ventilation, if sufficiently alert, finds the situation very frightening and threatening. A brief explanation of the ventilator and what it is expected to achieve will allay some fear. Reassurance that someone will always be close to the bedside also helps.

  The nurse must guard against becoming so preoccupied with the machine and technical procedures that she forgets that the patient is a

---

[38] Brooks (1981a), p. 16.

person. It is important to address the patient by name. Being unable to communicate verbally, the patient is dependent upon signs and facial and eye expressions to convey his feelings and needs, unless he is able to write, and provision should be made for this. Recognizing the nature of the situation and its implications for the patient, the nurse acknowledges the individual's fears and concerns, talks to the patient and provides information. Touching the patient (laying one's hands on the patient's shoulder, arm or hand) also conveys empathy.

- *Family.* It is only natural that the family will be very concerned about the patient who is ill enough to require ventilatory assistance. The care and treatments that the patient is receiving are likely to restrict the amount of time a relative may spend with the patient. Frequently, family members remain for hours in the hospital visiting room hoping for some information and to be told that they may see the patient. The nurse may become so involved with the responsibility of patient care that thought for the family's concern is neglected. Part of total patient care is ensuring some consideration for the family; members should be informed at intervals about what is being done for the patient and what his progress is. They are told that someone will talk with them periodically and will let them know when they may see the patient.

  A family member is permitted to visit briefly at frequent intervals. Such visits are important to the family and are also supportive and reassuring to the patient. In some instances a relative may be of assistance in turning the patient or in performing some similar comfort measure. This participation in care is helpful to the worried person who is probably thinking 'if I could only help or do something'.

  Family members remaining close by are advised of the location of a telephone, washroom and restaurant.

- *Emergency care.* If there is a disturbance in the mechanical ventilation, it may be due to an obstruction in the airway or to malfunctioning of the ventilator. It may be that the latter can be immediately recognized and corrected; if not, help is summoned and the respirator is disconnected from the patient's airway. The patient is ventilated with a self-inflating resuscitation bag. If the problem is in the patient's airway and is not relieved by suctioning, it may be necessary to call the doctor to change the tube. It is possible that air may enter the patient's airway but exhalation may be blocked by a mucus plug being drawn against the end of the tube. Air is trapped and the lung becomes overdistended.

- *Weaning.* The weaning process is the process by which the patient is encouraged to breathe independently. It begins as soon as it is established that the patient is physiologically capable of maintaining respirations. If prolonged mechanical ventilation is necessary, the patient may become very dependent upon the respirator and is fearful of its use being discontinued. He is advised that he will be observed closely and that his respirations and blood gases will be monitored frequently. Gradual weaning from the machine is introduced as soon as the patient can do his own work of breathing and when gas exchange and transportation are adequate.

  The first stage is to introduce synchronized, intermittent mandatory ventilation. The patient may breathe spontaneously from a reservoir bag within the ventilator circuit while the ventilator will deliver a specified number of respirations (usually 4–6 per minute). *It is important that the use of the respiratory muscles is re-established as soon as possible to prevent loss of tone and slowness of response.* Specific physiological responses are observed to determine the patient's readiness for weaning— that is blood gas analyses, vital capacity, minute volume and tidal volume, blood pressure, and whether there is sweating. It is also important to evaluate how tired the patient is.

  The patient requires considerable emotional support since he may be anxious and fearful, even though many patients are anxious to get off the ventilator.

MAINTENANCE OF OXYGEN TRANSPORTATION

Transportation of oxygen from the lungs to the tissues requires adequate ventilation in the alveoli, diffusion of gases in the alveoli, an adequate cardiac output and peripheral circulation to perfuse body tissues. Measures to maintain and support pulmonary ventilation and perfusion have been discussed above.

Maintenance of cardiac output and peripheral circulation involves: (1) ensuring an adequate fluid volume by replacing lost fluids; (2) maintaining blood pressure by correction of fluid deficits and administration of vasopressor drugs; and (3) improvement and support of cardiac function by the administration of drugs to strengthen myocardial contractions and increase cardiac output, and by decreasing the work load of the heart.

The oxygen-carrying capacity of the blood depends on the number of red blood cells and the haemoglobin available for oxygen transport. Measures to replace blood loss and stimulate the production of red blood cells and haemoglobin should be initiated if this is the cause of inadequate tissue perfusion. Such measures include increasing the amount of iron, folic acid, vitamins and protein in the diet and the parenteral administration of vitamin B_{12} and iron.

DECREASE TISSUE DEMANDS FOR OXYGEN

Patients with respiratory limitations experience

fatigue as a result of the hypoxia and ensuing decrease in cellular metabolism. Efficient planning of nursing interventions can help to decrease oxygen requirements. Nursing care should be organized to permit uninterrupted rest periods; the patient's needs are anticipated and objects that may be required are left within easy reach. Assistance is provided in turning and moving to minimize the patient's energy expenditure. Exercises can be performed passively by the nurse. Pain and discomfort are controlled before they become severe. Anxiety and apprehension are decreased by providing explanations of what is happening, communicating expectations for patient participation and reassuring the patient of his progress. Environmental stimuli, including noise and lighting are controlled.

If the patient is in an intensive care unit, where possible the usual day–night cycle is maintained. Lights are dimmed and noise and disruptions are kept to a minimum at night to promote sleep. The patient's usual pre-sleep habits are incorporated into his care if possible to reinforce familiar routines which promote relaxation and sleep.

Patients with chronic respiratory impairment are taught to organize their daily activities to allow for periods of rest and to carry out activities in ways that expend the least amount of energy.

If the patient experiences increased breathlessness following meals, he may find it easier to have smaller and more frequent meals, with rest periods before and after. Gas-forming foods should be avoided.

EXPECTED OUTCOMES

1 Exercise is a regular component of the individual's life-style.
2 The patient is alert and oriented.
3 The patient is able to perform activities of daily living.
4 Cardiac and respiratory rates are within the patient's normal limits.
5 Arterial blood oxygen and carbon dioxide levels are adequate and within the patient's usual range.
6 Serum electrolytes and pH are within normal ranges.
7 The patient is able to sleep and rest.
8 Cyanosis is absent.

4 Anxiety

The *goals* are to:
1 Decrease anxiety
2 Acquire a realistic perspective of the implications of the disease process and treatment plan.

DECREASING ANXIETY

Shortness of breath is a frightening experience for any individual. Fears of suffocation and death are enhanced by feelings of helplessness and the inability to control what is happening. Fatigue from the hypoxia and the extra work involved in breathing further decrease the patient's ability to cope with the situation. Cerebral manifestations of hypoxia, including headache, confusion and disorientation, interfere with the individual's ability to perceive the situation realistically, and increase anxiety. Lack of understanding of the disease process and management plan contributes to the individual's fear and loss of control. Medications to relieve anxiety, restlessness and sleeplessness (hypnotics and analgesics) depress respirations and further complicate the situation.

Nursing measures to decrease fear and anxiety include the following:

(a) Assessment of the individual's level of understanding of the disease process and plan of care.
(b) Provision of information about the disease and its management.
(c) Explaining to the patient: what is happening to him now; what is being done to alleviate his distress; what is expected of him in relation to the procedure and activities; and what additional resources are available.
(d) Maintaining a consistent nurse–patient relationship to develop the patient's confidence. The nurse also assures the patient that his needs and the agreed-upon plan of care will be communicated to other staff members.
(e) Provision of time and privacy for the patient to discuss his feelings and concerns.
(f) Helping the patient to recognise which breathing techniques work for him when breathlessness occurs and assisting him to develop the skill to implement them.
(g) The patient is consulted about all aspects of his care. He knows what works best for him and what activities or measures are ineffective or detrimental.
(h) Helping the patient to recognize the causes of his fears and anxiety and factors that precipitate these responses. Awareness of the causes of anxiety is necessary before realistic long-term plans can be developed to control them.
(i) Explaining relaxation techniques, which may be useful in breaking the cycle of anxiety and fear. Physical and emotional relaxation decrease oxygen requirements and alleviate tension. Abdominal and pursed-lip breathing may be used to slow the respiratory rate and increase the depth of respirations. As the breathing pattern improves, guided imagery and total body relaxation can be incorporated. By diverting the patient's attention to pleasant things, the nurse helps break the overwhelming focus on breathing.

The patient:
1 Expresses decreased anxiety.
2 Uses breathing and relaxation techniques to control anxiety.
3 Is able to rest and sleep.

5 Disturbance in self-image

The *goal* is to re-establish a positive self-image.

Changes in body image and self-concept may be precipitated by: physical changes in chest structure and posture, fatigue, confusion and decreased ability to carry out significant social roles. Frequent coughing and expectoration of sputum create a distasteful image for the patient and probably for others. Family members may consciously or unconsciously limit the usual amount of touching and increase the space between themselves and the patient. The patient may also decrease the use of touch and physical closeness to others as a result of his self-image or because of the response of others to him. Frequently commercials on television exaggerating the horrors of 'bad breath' reinforce the view that respiratory secretions and coughing are socially unacceptable.

Shortness of breath also interferes with speaking. Speech requires control of exhaled air; this makes an extra demand on the patient with airway limitation. He may speak in short phrases and have to stop for breath frequently. This difficulty limits the patient's ability to communicate; it may be perceived by others as rudeness or lack of consideration.

The nurse should instruct the patient on the acceptable use and disposal of tissues and the use of a covered sputum cup. Frequent mouth care is recommended, which the patient probably finds refreshing. Self-image is enhanced when one is clean, well groomed and neatly dressed.

The patient, family and friends are assisted in understanding that establishing the recommended breathing pattern requires time and energy and that speaking and appearance become secondary when dyspnoea is severe. Awareness of the patient's feelings and needs helps friends to adjust to the imposed changes and accept the person as he is. Family members can provide support and encouragement and show their understanding by waiting until the patient is able to continue speaking, assisting him with physical activities and acknowledging their awareness of the efforts made by the patient when he socializes and does things for others.

The patient:
1 Presents a neat, clean, well-groomed appearance.
2 Is able to talk about his self-image and the perceptions of others.
3 Disposes of respiratory secretions safely.

6 Alteration in family relationships

The *goal* is to help the family adapt to changes in daily routines, roles and functions.

The patient's illness, treatment and hospitalization disrupt usual family routines and increase the demands on all members. The family may have to adjust their daily patterns of living to accommodate the patient's treatment programme and decreased ability to fulfil his previous roles and responsibilities. Fatigue and physical limitations resulting from chronic respiratory impairment usually develop gradually as the patient's disease progresses, and the family is required to adjust. Acute respiratory problems present sudden crises for the family but are usually resolved in a limited time period.

Family members should become familiar with the patient's disease management and rehabilitation programme. They require support and reassurance that by encouraging increased patient activity, they are helping the patient toward the long-term goals of an acceptable and satisfactory life-style.

The physiotherapist will teach the patient's relatives how to assist him with his care programme, which may include breathing exercises, postural drainage, coughing and suctioning.

The nurse helps the family to look at their strengths and resources and advises them of appropriate available community resources. The family structure, age and development of children and roles and functions of the patient within the family, influence their ability to adjust to crises and illness within the family. Members require continuous support as the patient and family situation changes throughout the course of chronic respiratory disease.

The family:
1 Expresses feelings of support and understanding of the situation and indicates knowledge of available resources.
2 Participates in the patient's treatment and rehabilitation programme.

7 Alterations in life-style and self-care

The two main problems related to alterations in life-style and self-care are: (a) the patient's lack of knowledge about the disease process, health management plan and need to alter his daily routine and life-style, and (b) activity intolerance.

The patient's *goals* are to:
1 Understand the disease process and health management plan
2 Recognize his present level of psychosocial and physical functioning
3 Develop and implement a plan to assimilate the disease process and management plan into his daily life
4 Develop and/or maintain an exercise tolerance that

is compatible with an acceptable level of daily activity

IMPLICATIONS OF DISEASE AND MANAGEMENT

Chronic respiratory limitations present many implications for the patient's present and future functioning and life-style. Before he can realistically assess the meaning of these limitations he must acquire an understanding of the disease process, learn techniques to control the manifestations, and accept the fact that permanent limitations exist. The nurse assists in this process by providing information, discussing his disorder and the limitations and changes in life-style which are necessary to lessen the energy demands, providing instruction in breathing techniques and about the prescribed medications, and advising the patient about available community resources. The patient is encouraged to discuss his life-style, roles and relationships and to identify what is an acceptable level of health and functioning. Short-term and long-term goals are set, and the patient, family and health-team members plan together how best to achieve these goals and set realistic priorities. The patient may need help in setting realistic limits. Control of breathing and ability to manage self-care activities should be achieved before attempting larger steps such as returning to work.

KNOWLEDGE OF DISEASE PROCESS

Information about the disease process is presented to the patient and family using simple terms and charts or models of the chest and lung. The amount of detail presented at each session is adapted to the patient's level of understanding, readiness to learn and duration of concentration. An assessment of the patient's understanding is made at each session and wrong information is corrected.

Factors which precipitate or intensify disease manifestations and relief measures are explored. The patient learns to assess his usual pattern of breathing and to identify changes when they occur. Monitoring changes in the amount, consistency and colour of sputum is emphasized, as well as early signs of infection and indications of the need for prompt medical attention. How the disease process affects the individual's attitudes and functioning is discussed in detail.

PSYCHOSOCIAL AND FUNCTIONAL ASSESSMENT

A detailed *psychosocial history* (see p. 412) provides information which assists in determining the patient's needs and existing resources. The assessment includes the following:
1 Identification of the individual's usual health habits, including diet, rest and sleep patterns. Habits that support health are identified, as well as actions such as smoking which are detrimental to health.

2 How has the patient dealt with stress in the past and how does he adapt to change?
  (a) What coping skills are conducive to change in the present situation?
  (b) How does the patient cope with breathlessness?
3 How does the patient's disease and health management affect the patient and the patient's family?
  (a) How do the patient and family perceive the dysfunction?
  (b) What role changes have occurred within the family structure?
  (c) What problems or potential problems exist (e.g. altered finances, meeting developmental needs of children or altered sexual function)?
4 What social support exists?
  (a) Who are the significant people in the patient's life who love and care about him and can provide support and assistance?
5 What factors in the patient's home such as 'support' people and physical environment promote or hinder his rehabilitation?
  (a) What factors in the work environment support his continued functioning or hinder his return?
Functional assessment and investigations of the patient's effort tolerance are carried out to determine how he can reduce his energy expenditure in performing various activities and how his environment can be modified to facilitate his functioning:
1 What is the patient's usual level of daily activity?
  (a) Is he eating?
  (b) Can he dress himself, shave or shower without assistance?
  (c) Can he climb stairs?
  (d) What household activities can be performed, for example, vacuuming, making beds, preparing food?
  (e) What occupational activities is the patient capable of performing (e.g. sedentary or physical)?[39]
2 When does breathlessness occur? Is it:
  (a) With simple daily tasks such as shaving, dressing, tying shoe-laces?
  (b) With extra effort such as climbing stairs?
  (c) During the night?
  (d) On getting up in the morning?
3 Can the breathlessness be prevented by modifying the breathing pattern or by taking a bronchodilator before the activity?[40]
4 *Effort–tolerance* may be assessed by the 12-minute walk which is carried out in a level, enclosed corridor of a specific length. The patient is requested to walk as many lengths as possible in 12 minutes. A chair should be available if the patient should have

---

[39] Roberts L (1982) Assessment of Effort Tolerance—Exercise and Functional. Hamilton, Ontario: St Joseph's Hospital. Unpublished.
[40] Robinson & Pugsley (1981), p. 182.

to stop and rest. The resting heart rate is recorded as well as the pulse rate on completion of the test. An ear oximeter is used to determine the changes in the arterial oxygen saturation associated with the exercise. The test estimates the patient's horizontal walking capacity.

This information about the patient's energy assists in planning an acceptable daily routine and an exercise programme to increase the effort tolerance.

5 Further data are obtained to identify how the patient perceives his respiratory dysfunction.
   (a) What does it mean to him?
   (b) What losses in functioning are most relevant to him?
   (c) What losses is he able to accept?
   (d) How does he feel about it?
   (e) Is his attitude one of hopeless resignation or unrealistic denial?
   (f) Is he motivated to pursue a self-care programme?

DEVELOPMENT AND IMPLEMENTATION OF THE
SELF-CARE PLAN

Development of plan
The rehabilitation plan is patient-centred and goal-directed. If the patient is to achieve the goals of self-management and self-monitoring of his disease and is to adapt his care regimen into his daily life, he must be an active participant in planning and implementing the programme. It is the patient who decides what level of health or functioning is acceptable to him. Once goals are established, strengths and assets are identified that support achievement of the goal. Lack of knowledge, skills and support, and activities and habits which need to be altered, are identified. Priorities are then set based on the patient's desires and goals, his disease management needs and the realities of his present functional capabilities. Goals are reviewed on an on-going basis in relation to changes in the patient's respiratory status and how realistic and achievable they are for the individual patient. Functional expectations may then be increased when the patient achieves the minimal level agreed to, or they can be decreased when it is recognized and accepted that they cannot be achieved.

Factors affecting learning are identified as well as the patient's specific learning needs.

Factors influencing learning include the patient's past education and experience, level of alertness, duration of attention span, effort tolerance, communication impairment, visual or hearing deficits, manual dexterity, language, cultural beliefs, usual learning styles, readiness to change, and availability of supports.

Learning needs are identified based on: the patient's level of understanding and existence of misinformation; skill in performing care functions;

the existence and meaning of unhealthy habits, such as smoking, which need to be changed; and the nature of the actual potential alterations in daily life required.

Assimilation of respiratory disease and its management into one's life-style begins with the acquisition of knowledge and skills, but also involves a process of change that necessitates continuous re-evaluation and adaptation.

Self-care plan
Components of a self-management programme include:
1 Maintaining a clear airway.
   (a) *Coughing techniques.* The patient is taught to inhale slowly and deeply, hold the breath, lean forward, contract his abdominal muscles, exhale forcefully, and to repeat the procedure.
   (b) *Postural drainage.* The patient should be able to identify the time of day secretions are increased, (e.g. on arising in the morning, following activity or exposure to atmospheric irritants) and to establish a daily schedule that allows adequate time to carry out this procedure. The hospital schedule should conform as closely as possible to the proposed home programme.
   (c) *Chest percussion and vibration.* Family members or others in the patient's home are taught to perform chest percussion and vibration. Supervised practice is provided in the hospital, in an outpatient setting or the home to be sure that it is carried out safely and effectively.
   (d) *Avoidance of irritants.* Identification of irritants in the home and work environments is made. The patient is helped to recognize how these affect him and measures are recommended to make the necessary modifications in these environments. If necessary, a programme is established to assist the patient to stop smoking and the patient and family work together to make plans to eliminate tobacco smoke from the patient's environment at home.
      Aerosol spray and perfumes should not be used. The home environment should be as free of dust as possible; the temperature should be warm but fluctuations avoided. The humidity of the home should be maintained at 40–50%.
   (e) *Signs and symptoms of airflow limitation.* Patients are taught to observe their usual patterns of respiration, to identify changes and recognize factors which precipitate the changes. Respiratory infection is the most frequent cause of increased airflow obstruction. Alterations of the amount, colour and consistency of sputum should be recognized and acted on quickly. The doctor may give the patient a prescription for a broad-spectrum antibiotic to be obtained

at the first indication of an infection. The 7–10 day course of treatment should be completed. If the sputum has not cleared and the symptoms persist after 2 or 3 days, medical evaluation should be sought.

2 *Maintenance of effective breathing patterns.* Patients are taught techniques to improve the effectiveness of their breathing pattern by slowing the rate, prolonging the duration and increasing the depth of inspirations. Pursed-lip and diaphragmatic breathing can be carried out during daily activities which require extra effort, such as climbing stairs, bathing, shaving or dressing. The patient relaxes his shoulders and abdominal muscles, takes a deep, slow inspiration pushing the abdomen out, holds his breath for 1–2 seconds, and expels the air slowly through pursed-lips by contracting his abdominal muscles.

The patient should be constantly aware of his breathing pattern and the effectiveness of it.

3 *Maintaining adequate gas exchange.* Ventilation may be improved by keeping the airway cleared and controlling breathing patterns as discussed above. The patient is also taught measures to decrease oxygen requirements by:

(a) Pacing his activities, and moving slowly and purposefully
(b) Planning rest periods before and after activities requiring extra effort
(c) Obtaining adequate rest and sleep
(d) Stopping to rest when dyspnoea occurs
(e) The use of breath control during all activity and exhalation with the strenuous part of an activity
(f) Sitting while doing things, when possible
(g) Organizing work and living space so that everything needed is within easy reach
(h) Pushing or sliding objects rather than carrying or lifting them.

The patient is helped to pre-plan activities for each day, to space activities and provide time to rest. Activities requiring extra effort should be planned for the time of day when the patient feels best.

The patient also needs help in implementing these measures in socially appropriate ways, as he may have to stop and rest when walking down a street or while at work or a social gathering.

Additional measures that facilitate ventilation include eating smaller and more frequent meals and avoiding gas-forming foods which increase abdominal distension and oppose movement of the diaphragm.

Supplementary oxygen will be required by some patients throughout the day or during the night. The number of hours of oxygen therapy depends on the patient's degree of hypoxia and presence of pulmonary hypertension. The patient is taught safe handling and storage of oxygen equipment. Resources for obtaining equipment are identified and the patient is helped to choose the type of equipment most appropriate for his needs and resources. Portable oxygen cylinders are available and can be replaced.

The patient is also taught to recognize the signs and symptoms of hypoxia and hypercapnia. If a headache increases, or fatigue, lethargy, emotional irritability, confusion, tachycardia, cyanosis or tremors develop, immediate action should be taken to improve ventilation.

4 *Administration of medications.*

(a) The patient is taught the action, duration of effect, method of administration and side-effects of prescribed medications (especially bronchodilators and corticosteroids).
(b) The patient is instructed in the proper use of metered dose inhalers for optimal delivery of the medication into the bronchial tree (shake inhaler; open mouth; close mouth and lips over inhaler mouthpiece; trigger the inhaler once at the beginning of a full slow inhalation; hold breath for several seconds).
(c) The patient's medication schedule is developed to meet his particular needs. The duration of action of bronchodilators is approximately 4 hours; therefore, these drugs are usually administered four to six times per day. Administration may be planned to coincide with the beginning of specific activities to promote optimal functioning. The dose of corticosteroid preparations is adjusted so that the smallest dose necessary to maintain improvement in airflow is administered. Inhalation preparations are used because there are no systemic effects when the drug is inhaled. Also, a smaller dose is effective.

5 *Exercise programme* to increase and maintain tolerance. Participation in graded exercise programmes produces improved exercise tolerance and facilitates performance of daily activities. Patients have been able to achieve activities in a supervised programme that they would not otherwise attempt because of fear of dyspnoea. Both physiological and psychological benefits result. Selection of an exercise modality should be based on its relevance to the patient's life-style. Does the patient need to climb stairs at home or walk long distances on his job? The exercise programme should be integrated into the total rehabilitation plan. Abdominal and pursed-lip breathing are used by the patient while walking, climbing stairs, riding a stationary bicycle or on a treadmill. Controlled breathing helps increase the tidal volume and arterial oxygen concentration and reduces the respiratory rate.[41]

The administration of bronchodilators prior to exercise has been found to be beneficial for some individuals. Other studies have evaluated the effects of oxygen administration during exercise

---

[41] Casciari (1981), pp. 393–398.

and found it produced an increased exercise tolerance with less effort for some patients.[42]

Exercise should be regular and graded to produce increases in activity. It usually starts with less demanding exercises such as walking on the level for 5–10 minutes twice a day and gradually increases to 30 minutes. Walking on a slope, and jogging may be introduced as increased tolerance develops. In cold, damp weather, patients are advised to exercise indoors and use a treadmill or stationary bicycle, if available. The patient is reminded to think about his breathing technique throughout the activity. Lack of activity and exercise leads to increased shortness of breath and decreased tolerance; therefore, it is important for the patient to maintain his exercise routine, and the duration and intensity of the programme should be adapted to reflect the patient's level of functioning.

6 *Knowledge of community resources.* The patient requires a knowledge of the available resources for equipment and services. These include:
(a) Sources where equipment can be purchased, rented or borrowed.
(b) Community nursing services, home help services and meals on wheels.
(c) Transportation available to and from the clinic.
(d) Who to contact when problems occur.
(e) Services provided by the health centre, general practitioner or hospital.
(f) 'Stop smoking' support groups.

Achievement of self-monitoring and care by the patient requires time and continuous guidance. Health professionals should reinforce behaviour at each opportunity, pointing out the patient's progress and what he should be alert to.

EXPECTED OUTCOMES:

The patient:
1 Is able to talk with understanding about:
(a) The disease process
(b) Measures to maintain airway clearance
(c) Measures to maintain effective breathing patterns
(d) Measures to maintain gas exchange
(e) Actions and side-effects of medications
(f) Techniques for administration of medications
(g) Signs and symptoms of impaired airflow
(h) Early signs of infection
(i) Signs of altered breathing patterns
(j) Signs and symptoms of hypoxia and hypercapnia
(k) Resources available in the community.

2 Describes a plan for home management and a schedule for daily and weekly activities.
3 Demonstrates evidence of assimilation of the disease management plan in his daily life. He:
(a) Carries out coughing, postural drainage and chest therapy techniques as prescribed.
(b) Takes medications regularly according to his individualized schedule.
(c) Identifies early signs of infection and takes the recommended action.
(d) Practises breathing control measures while performing daily activities.
(e) Maintains an optimal exercise programme.
(f) Performs the usual activities of daily living to the extent of his functional capabilities.
(g) Recognizes alterations in respiratory functioning and adjusts his management plan and daily activities accordingly.
(h) Arranges home and work environments to conserve energy expenditure.
(i) Uses community resources as needed.

Respiratory Disorders and Treatment

There are many different disorders which may adversely affect the movement of a normal volume of air in and out of the alveoli or interfere with the diffusion of the respiratory gases across the alveolar capillary membrane. Respiratory failure occurs when the individual is unable to maintain adequate gas exchange. Respiratory disorders may be acute or chronic; they both have a very high incidence and account for a large part of absenteeism at work and school as well as for permanent disability and dependence. Pulmonary disorders may be classified as:
1 Obstructive disorders affecting the airways
2 Restrictive disorders affecting ventilation by a reduction in lung volume
3 Vascular lung diseases affecting pulmonary circulation and gas exchange
4 Infection
5 Trauma

Because it is impossible to discuss all disorders of respiration, a brief overview of the pathophysiological principles that are relevant to each disease pattern will be presented, with reference being made to the most common diseases which are encountered.

OBSTRUCTIVE DISORDERS OF THE AIRWAY

Obstructive diseases of the lung and their complications affect a large number of individuals. With adequate care and treatment these patients can lead useful, enjoyable lives with minimal hospitalization.

---

[42] Stein & Bradley (1982), p. 6.

CAUSES

The cause of narrowing or obstruction of the airway may be within the lumen or walls or may be extramural. Either or both the central and peripheral airways may be affected.

1 Lumenal causes include: excess mucus as occurs in bronchitis, asthma and bronchiolitis; aspiration of fluid or a foreign body; tumours; and retention of secretions postoperatively.

2 Intramural causes include: constriction of the smooth muscle as in asthma; hypertrophy of the mucus glands which takes place in chronic bronchitis; inflammation or oedema of the wall, which may occur in the larynx; development of scar tissue and thickening of the wall; benign or malignant tumours; and tracheo- or bronchomalacia which is a softening of the cartilaginous structure.

3 Extramural causes include: compression of the trachea, bronchi or bronchioles by enlarged lymph nodes or tumours; destruction of the lung parenchyma as occurs in emphysema; a loss of radial traction on the terminal bronchioles and subsequent narrowing.[43] Narrowing of the airways results in: expiratory air flow limitation, maldistribution of ventilation resulting in underventilation of the area of lung beyond the narrowing, and overinflation as a result of the increase in the volume of air trapped in the lungs.[44]

Chronic Obstructive Airways Disease (COAD)

Chronic obstructive airways disease is a term used to describe the airflow limitation in the bronchial tree when it is greater than expected for the person's age, height and sex.[45] Other terms used to describe this problem include chronic airflow obstruction (CAO) and chronic obstructive lung disease (COLD). Causative factors are chronic bronchitis, emphysema, bronchiectasis and asthma.

Chronic bronchitis

This disease is characterized by hyperactivity of the mucus-secreting glands of the bronchial mucosa in response to prolonged or frequently recurring irritation. The common irritants are tobacco smoke, infection and atmospheric pollutants such as dust, industrial fumes and smoke. The most frequent offender is tobacco smoke. The patient experiences frequent, productive coughing. A higher incidence is seen in older persons and in persons of poor socioeconomic circumstances. Dampness, wind and winter cold are considered to be aggravating factors.

The bronchial mucosa undergoes a chronic inflammatory process, along with hypertrophy and an increase in the number of mucus-secreting glands. The mucus predisposes to infection. Destruction of the normal epithelial lining and the cilia occurs. The mucosa becomes oedematous, thickened and scarred, leading to distortion and narrowing of the lumina of the air passages. The excessive mucus is retained, blocking bronchioles and reducing ventilation further. Some bronchospasm may be present. The obstruction to the flow of air is greater during expiration, resulting in air being trapped in the bronchioles and alveoli. Eventually the air sacs become permanently overdistended. Pulmonary circulation may be affected; the underventilated areas produce a deficiency of oxygen that may initiate a vasoconstrictive response in the local pulmonary vessels. If this persists, the individual is likely to develop pulmonary hypertension, resulting in resistance to the output of the right side of the heart into the pulmonary artery, and the patient may develop right-sided heart failure.

The disease has an insidious onset and, unless reversed, the disease process is gradually progressive. Ventilation is impaired by progressive airway obstruction, the work of breathing is increased, and hypoxaemia and hypercapnia may develop.

Pulmonary emphysema[46]

This chronic disorder is characterized by overdistension of the terminal respiratory units or pulmonary lobules by entrapped air. This leads to increased lung capacity, loss of elasticity of the lungs and destruction of intra-alveolar septal tissue and the capillary bed. The damage is not uniform. It may affect only the central portion of the pulmonary lobules (centralobular emphysema) or it may result in destruction of most of the structures within a terminal unit, including the alveolar ducts and alveoli (panlobular emphysema).

The onset is insidious but, once initiated, is progressive and non-reversible. The lung damage cannot be repaired but the patient can be helped to breathe more effectively and live with less disability. Both emphysema and chronic bronchitis are frequently present in the same patient. There is usually a long history of chronic bronchitis in which the blocking of the small terminal bronchioles with mucoid secretions leads to the entrapping of air in the alveoli and the eventual emphysema. Rarely, emphysema is primary. Heredity is suspected to play a role in some cases, since a deficiency of an enzyme is present in some individuals with panlobular emphysema. The incidence of emphysema is higher in middle-aged and older males.

---

[43] Tisi (1980), p. 41.
[44] Tisi (1980), p. 42 & 43.
[45] Robinson & Pugsley (1981), p. 177.

[46] Emphysema is the Greek word meaning inflation. In medicine, it implies a swelling or distension due to an accumulation of air. It may occur in any tissue. Pulmonary emphysema indicates overdistension of air sacs in the lungs.

Bronchiectasis

This disorder is a chronic dilatation of bronchial tubes resulting from destruction of elastic and muscular tissue of the walls. It may involve any part of the lung, but the lower dependent segments are the areas affected most often.

The cause of bronchiectasis is repeated or prolonged pulmonary infection, bronchial obstruction by extrinsic pressure, a mucus plug or an aspirated foreign body. The dilatation occurs above the obstruction.

Dilatation of the tubes results in the retention and pooling of secretions which readily become infected. The infection is perpetuated and extends, causing further tissue damage. The degree of impairment of pulmonary ventilation and oxygen uptake depends upon the amount of chronic infection and lung damage. Retention of secretions causes bronchial obstruction and inadequate aeration of the bronchioles and alveoli distal to the bronchiectatic area, altering pulmonary ventilation and perfusion.

The onset of bronchiectasis has a higher incidence in childhood. A congenital malformation of the affected bronchial tubes and debilitation are considered to be predisposing factors in the development of the disease. The incidence of bronchiectasis has decreased with the prevention and antibiotic treatment of bronchopneumonia. The decrease in childhood communicable diseases which predispose to respiratory infections has been an important contributory factor to the lesser incidence.

Asthma

An accepted British definition of asthma has been made by Scadding. He defines asthma, in terms of pathophysiology, as 'a disease characterized by wide variations over short periods of time in resistance to flow in intrapulmonary airways'. He goes on to say that this should be followed by a brief statement of the ways of defining disorder of function. 'The use of the term "asthma" without further specification should imply no more than clinically important variability in airflow resistance.'[47]

More recently, a committee of the American Thoracic Society defined asthma as 'a disease characterized by an increased responsiveness of the trachea and bronchi to various stimuli and manifested by widespread narrowing of the airways that changes in severity either spontaneously or as a result of treatment.'[48] The reaction of the over-responsive airway to stimuli is oedema and thickening of the mucosa, hypersecretion by the mucus glands and contraction of bronchial and bronchiolar muscle tissue. This causes diffuse narrowing of the tracheobronchial tree and obstruction to airflow. The bronchoconstriction is attributed to: (1) the action of chemical mediators such as histamine, and other

slow-reacting substances of anaphylaxis, and prostaglandins released in response to an antigen. They act on receptor sites on the membrane of smooth muscle cells, producing contraction of the smooth muscle or (2) an abnormality in the neural regulation of the smooth muscle tissue of the airway.[49] It is considered possible that both mechanisms may play a role in causing bronchoconstriction. Narrowing of the airway in asthma also results from the changes that take place in the mucosa of the airways.

Stimuli which may precipitate the asthmatic response include allergens, infection, irritating inhalants (chemicals, air pollutants), cold air, acetylsalicylic acid (aspirin), emotional stress, physical exercise and laughing. Frequently, there is a personal and/or family history of one or more allergies. Asthma usually begins in childhood but may develop at any age. Warning signs of increasing bronchial reactivity include frequent awakening at night, decreased physical effort tolerance, shortness of breath on getting up in the morning and cough.

During an acute asthmatic attack the patient experiences tightness in the chest, wheezing and dyspnoea. The accessory muscles of respiration are used and expiration is prolonged. The patient appears distraught and assumes an upright sitting position. The sputum is scant and thick and the pulse is rapid.

SIGNS AND SYMPTOMS OF COAD

COAD has physical, psychological, social and functional implications for the patient. The major symptom is shortness of breath, which varies on a daily basis with usual activity, increased effort and during sleep. Physical signs and objective measures of respiratory function which occur with COAD are listed in Table 16.9.

MANAGEMENT OF THE PATIENT WITH COAD

Although COAD is irreversible, management of the patients has improved over the past few decades to enable them to live useful and satisfying lives. Nursing intervention is directed toward increasing airflow by clearing the airway, improving the patient's breathing pattern and eliminating possible irritants from the environment. Bronchodilators and corticosteroids are the medications most often administered to these patients. Self-monitoring and self-care are essential components of the management programme. The patient must learn to cope with the limitations imposed by the disease, prevent complications and comply with the treatment plan if a satisfactory life-style is to be achieved. As with any chronic disorder, the individual must learn to live with the disease process and to manage his daily

[47] Scadding (1977).
[48] Smith and Thier (1985), p. 819.

[49] Smith & Thier (1985), pp. 819–820.

Table 16.9 Signs and symptoms of chronic obstructive airways disease.*

Physical signs
  Clavicles are prominent (sculpturing)
  Hypertrophy of accessory muscles of respiration
  Tracheal shortening
  Tracheal descent on inspiration
  Costal margins of the rib cage move inward on respiration
  Diminished breath sounds
  Sputum production increased in many but not all patients

Symptoms
  Breathlessness
  Weakness

Measurements
1 Lung volumes:
  Forced expiratory time (FET)—increased (greater than 4 seconds)
  Forced expiratory volume (FEV)—decreased
  Vital capacity—normal or slightly reduced
  Ratio of FEV/VC—decreased

2 Blood gases:
  Pao_2—less than 8.0 kPa (60 mmHg)
  $Paco_2$—greater than 6.0 kPa (45 mmHg)

---

*Robinson & Pugsley (1981), pp. 177–179.

living. Discussions of specific measures to achieve these goals are included under nursing intervention earlier in this chapter.

Localized airway obstruction

Localized obstruction of airflow is less common than chronic airflow limitation and causes less residual impairment.

Obstruction of the nasal passages
The narrow nasal passages are particularly susceptible to obstruction. Obstruction may be the result of: trauma causing deviation of the septum and nasal fractures; foreign bodies in the nose, which are common in childhood; growths and polyps; and inflammation of the nasal mucosa as a result of irritation from pollution, allergies, smoking or infection. Signs and symptoms include assymetry of the nose from trauma, bleeding, and thin clear to thick purulent drainage. The patient breathes through one nostril or the mouth when obstruction is present.

Obstruction of the pharynx
Inflammation and enlargement of the adenoids in the nasopharynx and the palatine tonsils in the oropharynx interfere with breathing and swallowing. Foreign bodies that are of sufficient size to lodge in the oropharynx are usually relatively easy to remove. Smaller objects that pass on to the larynx and bronchi pose a greater hazard.

Obstruction of the larynx
Oedema, laryngeal spasm, or aspiration of a foreign body may cause obstruction in the larynx. Any constriction or obstruction in the larynx is manifested quickly by hoarseness, dyspnoea, stridor (high-pitched crowing breath sound), cyanosis and increased but ineffective inspiratory effort, evidenced by the retraction of the intercostal spaces. Prompt emergency measures are necessary or death may ensue as a result of asphyxia.

Obstruction of the trachea
Aspiration of a foreign body, scarring following trauma or surgery, or pressure from an aortic aneurysm or neoplasm of a neighbouring structure may narrow the trachea and offer resistance to the flow of air. Inspiratory and expiratory stridor result and hypoventilation leads to hypercapnoea and hypoxaemia.

Removal of a foreign body from the trachea may be achieved by the Heimlich procedure (see p. 427). If this procedure does not dislodge the object, a laryngoscope may be quickly introduced by the doctor through whch the offending object may be retrieved. If the patient's breathing is completely obstructed, an emergency tracheostomy may have to be performed to establish an airway before the foreign body can be removed (see p. 432).

For *oedema* or *spasm*, intubation may be performed in which a tube is passed beyond the obstruction into the trachea to establish an airway, or the doctor may do a tracheostomy (see p. 431). If oedema of the larynx is due to an allergic response, the patient is given adrenaline 1:1000 subcutaneously. An adrenal corticosteroid preparation such as prednisone may be prescribed for a brief period to reduce tissue sensitivity. Local applications of ice to the neck may also be suggested.

When laryngeal muscle spasm is the cause of the obstruction, intravenous calcium chloride or calcium gluconate may be prescribed.

Obstruction of a bronchus
If a foreign body is inhaled, it may pass into either bronchus but most often it is the right one that is blocked. Localized obstruction may also be caused by enlarged lymph nodes surrounding the bronchus. Complete obstruction leads to atelectasis (collapse of the lung) beyond the obstruction.

Restrictive disorders of ventilation

In restrictive disorders of ventilation, there is limited lung expansion resulting in a reduction in lung volumes, particularly vital capacity (VC) and total lung capacity (TLC). Manifestations include (1) reduced lung volumes, (2) decreased maximal expiratory flow, (3) increased work of breathing and (4) maldistribution of ventilation.[50]

---

[50] Tisi (1980), p. 46.

CAUSES

1 Changes in the chest wall. Ventilation may be restricted if the bony structure is abnormal or if there is rigidity of the wall. *Scoliosis* (a deformity in which the spine is S-shaped with one shoulder higher than the other) causes stiffness of the chest wall, as well as limiting the size. Surgical removal of ribs (*thoracoplasty*) results primarily in a reduction in the size of the thoracic cavity. Restriction to thoracic expansion may also occur following chest surgery when the patient tends to immobilize the chest and take shallow respirations to minimize the pain.

2 Respiratory muscle dysfunction. Restricted lung expansion may be the result of impaired innervation to the respiratory muscles as occurs in the Guillain–Barré syndrome, poliomyelitis and amyotrophic lateral sclerosis, or it may be due to muscular weakness incurred by a chemical deficit at the myoneural junction (myasthenia gravis). The impaired muscle contraction causes dyspnoea and, if severe enough, respiratory failure. Involvement of the diaphragm increases symptoms and assisted ventilation is usually necessary. Severe obesity may also cause restricted lung expansion by compression on the diaphragm.

3 Disorders of the pleurae. These include effusion and pneumothorax. Pleural effusion is an accumulation of an abnormal quantity of fluid in the interpleural space and is a symptom associated with a variety of conditions. The fluid may be a transudate or an exudate. A *transudate* may collect in the pleural space as a result of increased venous pressure incurred by congestive heart failure or an intrathoracic tumour which interferes with venous drainage in the area. Cirrhosis of the liver may cause a pleural effusion, as well as ascites. An accumulation of exudate in the pleural space indicates irritation and inflammation of the pleura associated with infection.

The patient with an effusion may experience some pleuritic pain, which is stabbing and is worse on inspiration before the excess fluid collects. The condition may develop insidiously and may go unrecognized until the increasing volume of fluid commences to compress the lung, causing dyspnoea and impaired pulmonary ventilation.

A chest aspiration (thoracentesis) is done to relieve the pressure on the lung and to obtain a specimen of fluid for examination. Treatment is directed toward the disease causing the effusion. A culture is made of the aspirated fluid for identification of the causative organisms and their antibiotic sensitivity. The patient receives antibiotics parenterally or orally, and the drug may also be injected into the thoracic cavity following aspiration. Surgical drainage may be necessary, especially if the pus is thick. Early breathing exercises to promote re-expansion of the lung are important,

since the visceral pleura tends to become thick, fibrous and resistant to stretching, reducing lung compliance and the vital capacity.

Pneumothorax occurs when air is introduced into the pleural space. It may enter from the lung or through an injury to the chest wall and causes collapse of the lung, outward expansion of the chest wall, and depression of the diaphragm on the affected side. The vital capacity and forced expiratory volumes are reduced. Air in the pleural space is gradually reabsorbed but if the patient is experiencing dyspnoea and pain, a tube may be inserted through the chest wall and connected to an underwater seal allowing the air to escape from the pleural cavity (see p. 438).

4 Disorders of the lung parenchyma. Restriction of ventilation may be caused by a decrease in the lung tissue as seen with the surgical removal of a lung (pneumonectomy) or by increased stiffness of lung tissue due to fibrosis.

Diffuse interstitial pulmonary fibrosis is frequently seen and is characterized by scattered areas of thickening of the interstitium of the alveolar walls. The respiratory bronchioles dilate and the alveoli coalesce forming larger air sacs. The cause is unknown in some patients. It may be associated with collagen–vascular diseases, prolonged occupational exposure to irritants or lung injuries.[51] It has a higher incidence in older adults and results in dyspnoea and rapid shallow breathing on exertion. The larger airways, chest cage and respiratory muscles remain normal. Distensibility of the lung is reduced, causing increased effort on inspiration and decreased lung volumes. Gas exchange is impaired and both the arterial Po_2 and Pco_2 are reduced.

Treatment usually includes corticosteroid therapy and breathing exercises to improve the patient's pattern of breathing and to establish more effective respirations.

Pulmonary vascular disorders

CAUSES

The causes of pulmonary vascular disease may be hypertension, oedema or embolism.

Pulmonary hypertension

This condition may develop as a result of: (1) a decrease in the pulmonary intravascular space due to vasoconstriction or structural changes in the vessels, or a combination of these; (2) poor ventilation of lung areas which causes low alveolar oxygen tension, initiating the pulmonary vascular response of constriction. If acidosis develops, this vasoconstriction response is enhanced; and (3) left-sided heart failure or a congenital heart defect (e.g. interatrial septal defect).

---

[51] Smith and Thier (1985), p. 814.

Sustained pulmonary arterial hypertension causes secondary changes in the walls of the pulmonary arteries and ventricular hypertrophy which may lead to heart failure. The latter, when secondary to respiratory disease may be referred to as *cor pulmonale*.

Pulmonary Oedema

This is an abnormal accumulation of fluid within the lungs. The rate of development of the oedema varies, but when acute becomes a life-threatening emergency.

Pulmonary oedema may be caused by:

1 Left-sided heart failure. The heart cannot take the blood being carried to it by the pulmonary veins; as a result the back-flow raises the pulmonary capillary pressure and fluid escapes into the alveoli. Vascular overload may incur the same problem.

2 Irritation of the alveoli may result in capillary dilation and the increased diffusion of fluid into the alveoli. Causes of irritation may be the inhalation of toxic gases, exudate from pneumonia, oxygen toxicity or adult respiratory distress syndrome.

3 Lymphatic drainage from the lungs may be obstructed by tumours or as a result of fibrosis, as occurs in silicosis.

4 Rapid removal of pleural effusion or pneumothorax and the concomitant decrease in pressure on capillary walls, resulting in the escape of fluid.

5 A decrease in the intravascular osmotic pressure due to hypoproteinaemia, or to overloading with intravenous saline infusion, which also promotes the escape of fluid into the alveoli.

6 Other factors which may precipitate pulmonary oedema, include very high altitudes, heroin overdose and trauma of the central nervous system.[52]

The patient with pulmonary oedema is dyspnoeic, cyanosed and fearful. Sputum is copious, frothy and usually blood-streaked. The respirations are rapid and shallow. As the oedema increases musical rhonchi are heard on auscultation of the lung bases. In non-cardiogenic pulmonary oedema infusions of albumin may be given to decrease intravascular fluid volume and pressure. High concentrations of oxygen are administered usually by mechanical ventilation, using PEEP (see p. 449) to improve the hypoxaemia.[53]

Pulmonary embolism

This involves sudden obstruction of a pulmonary vessel and its branches by an embolus which is usually a blood clot from the peripheral circulation. Pulmonary emboli frequently are preventable by instituting measures which promote venous return to prevent venous stasis which develops with immobility. Early detection of peripheral thrombi by means of a scan may be used as a preventive measure. Obstruction of a pulmonary vessel produces sudden dyspnoea, chest pain, blood-streaked sputum and extreme apprehension. Massive emboli produce shock, chest pain, rapid thready pulse, hypotension and unconsciousness. They can also cause cardiac arrest and/or sudden death.

Treatment consists of oxygen administration and, when necessary, vasopressor drugs to maintain blood pressure. Anticoagulant therapy is initiated to prevent recurrence. Surgical removal of the clot(s) from the pulmonary circulation is rarely done.

INFECTIOUS DISEASES

Rhinitis

Rhinitis is an acute or chronic inflammation of the nasal mucous membrane caused by infection or an allergic reaction. It may also result from nasal polyps or a deviated nasal septum. Symptoms are those of the common cold. The nasal mucosa is red and oedematous and there is a clear nasal discharge which becomes purulent with some infections. The individual breathes through the mouth. (See below for treatment).

Sinusitis

Sinusitis is an acute or chronic inflammation of the sinus cavities resulting from infection or allergies. It is accompanied by rhinitis because the mucous membranes of the sinuses are continuous with those of the nose. As secretions accumulate in the sinuses feelings of heaviness, discomfort and headache develop. General malaise and fever accompany the local symptoms when infection is present.

Treatment of rhinitis and sinusitis is usually symptomatic. Aspirin may be taken by adults to decrease inflammation and promote comfort. Fluid intake is increased, a balanced diet eaten and adequate rest obtained. If the problem persists or becomes severe, a general practitioner's advice should be sought.

Pharyngitis (sore throat)

Pharyngitis is a common respiratory inflammatory disorder caused by allergies, viral or bacterial infections. Symptoms include dryness, soreness of the throat, difficulty swallowing, fever and general malaise. Sore throats of bacterial origin are treated with antibiotic therapy. Other measures include rest, increased fluid intake, warm saline gargles and mild analgesics such as aspirin.

Tonsillitis

Tonsillitis is usually of bacterial origin and is most common in children and adolescents. Swabs are taken of the throat to identify the causative agent and antibiotic therapy is prescribed for acute tonsillitis.

---

[52] West (1982), p. 117.
[53] Harper et al (1981), p. 116.

Symptoms include a sore throat, difficulty swallowing, chills, fever and malaise. The white blood cell count will be elevated. Complications include acute otitis media, acute rhinitis and sinusitis and peritonsillar abscess. Tonsillitis usually resolves spontaneously in 5–7 days. Acute peritonsillar abscess (quinsy) requires treatment with antibiotics, and incision and drainage of the abscess may be necessary. Adequate analgesia (e.g. pethidine or papaveretum for adults) should be administered. Airway obstruction can be life-threatening if treatment is not instituted promptly.

Surgical removal of tonsils and adenoids is usually indicated only when the individual experiences recurrent, incapacitating infections.

Pneumonia

Pneumonia is the term generally used to indicate infection and inflammation of lung tissue. Pneumonitis is a synonymous term but is used less frequently than pneumonia. Guyton defines pneumonia as 'any inflammatory condition of the lung in which the alveoli are usually filled with fluid and blood cells'.[54]

Pneumonia caused by pneumococci is a common type of pneumonia, but other bacteria or viruses may be the cause. Non-bacterial and non-viral causes include: aspiration of gastric secretions, food, fluids or lipoids (aspiration pneumonia), and retention of secretions, which occurs frequently in the immobilized elderly or debilitated individual (hypostatic pneumonia).

Manifestations. The onset, symptoms and course of disease vary with different types of pneumonia. Infection of the alveoli results in their filling with inflammatory exudate (plasma, blood cells, pathological organisms and cellular debris) that readily overflows into other alveoli, extending the infection. A whole lobe of lung tissue may become consolidated or the consolidation may be patchy; pulmonary ventilation and diffusion are impaired, and the oxygen tension of the blood is reduced to below normal. The Pco_2 level generally remains normal; the increased respiratory rate caused by the initial increase in the Pco_2 results in increased amounts of carbon dioxide being excreted by the normal areas of the lung. In a few days the exudate becomes more liquid and may be gradually eliminated from the alveoli by expectoration and absorption. This process is referred to as *resolution*. The disease may clear up with dramatic rapidity when specific antibacterial drugs are administered. It may run a course of 5–10 days; untreated, it may rapidly prove terminal.

The onset of some infective pneumonias may be very sudden; they frequently begin with a chill, followed by fever (e.g. pneumococcal and Friedlaender's). Hypostatic, staphylococcal and atypical (viral) pneumonias have a gradual onset (less abrupt than the pneumococcal type). The latter two may be associated at the onset with upper respiratory infection.

The pulse rate and respirations increase. The latter may be shallow and accompanied by an audible grunt characteristic of pleuritic pain. The nostrils flare on inspiration and the face may be flushed. Cyanosis of the lips, tongue and nail beds may develop. The patient's cough may be hacking, painful and unproductive at first; later, it becomes less painful and is productive. In bronchopneumonia the sputum is tenacious, blood-streaked and mucopurulent. In pneumococcal pneumonia, the sputum is usually rust-coloured and becomes purulent as resolution takes place. In Friedlaender's pneumonia the pulmonary secretions are dark, reddish-brown and very tenacious.

The patient experiences general malaise, weakness, headache and aching pains. The leucocyte count is elevated in some types (e.g. pneumococcal, staphylococcal) and normal or below normal in others (e.g. atypical). Sputum examination and culture and blood culture are used to identify the causative organism. Specific antimicrobial therapy is determined by culture and sensitivity tests.

Pulmonary tuberculosis

Tuberculosis is an infectious disease that is caused by the tubercle bacillus. The organism may attack other tissues in the body, but in Europe and North America the lungs are most frequently the primary site of invasion.

Infection is usually by inhalation of droplets bearing tubercle bacilli. The droplets have been expelled into the air by the sneezing or coughing of a person with active disease.

Disease process. Small, rounded nodules, with a tendency toward central necrosis, develop at the site of tissue invasion by the bacilli. These are referred to as *tubercles* and are composed of lung tissue cells, leucocytes, other phagocytic cells, fibroblasts and tubercle bacilli. If the body defences are strong enough to destroy the organisms the lesion heals and may calcify.

In some instances, the reproduction of the tubercle bacilli may be minimal; a few continue to survive within the tubercle but remain confined and dormant. This person, having been infected and still harbouring live bacilli, will show a positive tuberculin test in approximately 2–10 weeks after the initial infection; defensive cells have become sensitized and tend to inhibit or slow up the growth of tubercle bacilli. At a later date, if his resistance is lowered, the reproduction of the tubercle bacilli may be accelerated and he develops active disease. When the bacilli continue to multiply, the tubercle necroses centrally, producing soft, caseous material that may

---

[54] Guyton (1986), p. 520.

eventually be discharged from the tubercle, leaving a cavity. This caseous discharge is highly infective.

The initial infection does not affect pulmonary function. The later stages of tuberculosis, which are becoming again more common in Britain and Europe, produce systemic and local symptoms. The constitutional symptoms are vague and non-specific; they include lassitude, fatigue, malaise, loss of appetite and weight, fever (usually low grade) in the latter part of the day, tachycardia and night sweats. Symptoms produced by the local disease process at the site of the lesion in the lungs are cough, sputum, haemoptysis, dyspnoea and chest pain if the pleura is involved.

Diagnostic investigation. The investigation of a patient for pulmonary tuberculosis involves tuberculin testing, chest x-ray and bacteriological examination of sputum (see p. 420).

Treatment. The treatment and care of tuberculosis has undergone dynamic changes in recent years. Patients are no longer isolated in special hospitals for months and years. They remain at home and continue to work and live a normal, useful life without endangering others. The principal factors in the plan of patient care are prolonged chemotherapy, rest, and patient and family education.

The administration of specific antimicrobial drugs over a long period of time has proved very successful in the treatment of tuberculous patients. Drugs currently in use include the following:

- *Isoniazid.* This is taken orally in one or two prescribed doses daily. This drug is usually well tolerated; sensitivity or toxic reaction is uncommon. Rarely, the patient may develop general malaise, anorexia, nausea, vomiting, fever or a rash. Polyneuritis, apathy and anaemia may occur.
- *Ethambutol.* This is given orally in a single daily dose in combination with another antibacterial drug. It inhibits the synthesis of RNA and cellular phosphate, and so destroys and arrests the reproduction of the tubercle bacilli. A side-effect that may occur is reduced visual acuity.
- *Rifampicin.* This is given orally with one or two other antitubercular agents (usually ethambutol and/or isoniazid). The patient is observed for possible hepatitis.
- *Streptomycin.* This antibiotic may be administered intramuscularly for a shorter period than the other antitubercular preparations—usually not longer than 4 or 6 months. Serious side-effects of this drug are damage of the auditory nerves and consequent loss of hearing.
- *Para-aminosalicylic acid* (PAS). This drug was one of the earliest antitubercular preparations used but is poorly tolerated for prolonged administration. Side-effects include anorexia, nausea, vomiting, diarrhoea, chills and fever and skin rash.

Initially the patient may receive a combination of two or three of the drugs for a period of time. Later a change to one or two may be made. Isoniazid is the only preparation used singly. An example regimen is isoniazid and rifampicin daily for 4–6 months, and then isoniazid and ethambutol; eventually, isoniazid only may be prescribed.

Drug therapy is continued for 9 months to 2 years. It is important for the nurse to be familiar with the possible toxic and side-effects of the drugs so that early reactions may be recognized. For example, the patient's visual acuity is determined before ethanbutol is administered. An assessment of the patient's vision is made every month as long as the patient is receiving the drug.

CHEST INJURIES

The commonest form of chest injury is a *fracture of the ribs* but, unless the fragments penetrate or injure the pleura and lung, it is not considered serious. However, the pain interferes with normal respiratory function, since the patient tends to immobilize the chest and take shallow respirations to minimize the pain. The hypoventilation predisposes to retention of secretions, atelectasis and pulmonary infection.

An analgesic is prescribed to relieve the pain and the patient is encouraged to breathe deeply during the period in which the analgesic is effective. If the pain cannot be controlled by analgesics, an intercostal nerve block may be done to provide relief. The patient is usually more comfortable in an elevated position. Sudden, sharp chest pain, dyspnoea and blood-streaked sputum are promptly brought to the doctor's attention.

A *crushing injury* of the chest is frequently sustained by an automobile driver in an accident. His chest is crushed by the steering wheel and several ribs may receive multiple fractures. A portion of the rib cage is detached and displaced inward, producing a *flail chest*, which is serious (see Fig. 16.15). On inspiration, the flail section of the chest wall is pulled in, and on expiration it moves out. This is referred to as *paradoxical respiration*. Obviously, the patient suffers respiratory insufficiency, leading to hypoxia and retention of carbon dioxide, which further stimulate respirations. Secretions are also retained, predisposing to infection.

Emergency treatment is the application of a rigid dressing to the chest wall to reduce the paradoxical movement. When hospitalized, mechanical ventilation is used to inflate the chest by positive pressure, and immobilization of the chest by external application is usually not necessary. Currently, only patients with severe chest instability are intubated and mechanically ventilated.[55]

---

[55] Henshaw & Murray (1980), p. 782.

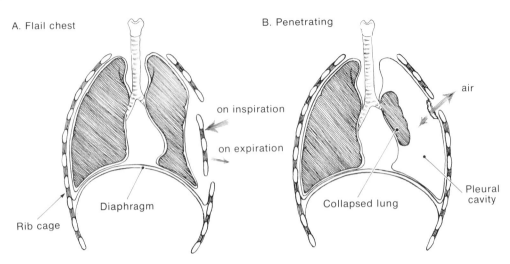

A. Flail chest

B. Penetrating

on inspiration

on expiration

air

Diaphragm

Rib cage

Collapsed lung

Pleural cavity

Fig. 16.15 A flail chest caused by a crushing injury and multiple rib fractures. *B*, A penetrating chest injury which produces a sucking wound.

Injury to the pleura or lung frequently complicates the condition, causing pneumothorax (collapse of the lung) or haemothorax (collection of blood in the thoracic cavity). Chest aspiration will probably be necessary to remove serum and blood, and a catheter may be left in the pleural cavity to allow for a continuous escape of air and fluid. An effort may be made to reduce the patient's pain with an intercostal nerve block. Narcotics are used sparingly, since they depress respirations and the cough reflex. The condition is usually complicated by severe shock and probably by other injuries.

Penetrating chest wounds produce what is commonly referred to as a *sucking wound*. Air passes freely in and out of the pleural cavity, and the lung of the affected side collapses. The air may accumulate to displace the mediastinum to the unaffected side, interfering with the normal respiratory capacity of the lung on that side by compression.

An immediate effort to seal off the opening into the chest wall is mandatory. In the emergency situation, a towel, handkerchief or any clean material at hand should be used until surgical treatment is available. A thoracotomy may be done to control the bleeding and repair damaged tissues. The intrapleural cavity has been entered and the nursing care of the patient following the surgery is similar to that of any patient who has chest surgery.

ACUTE RESPIRATORY FAILURE

Respiratory failure is a disorder of respiratory function that is present when a person is unable to maintain adequate arterial blood levels of oxygen and carbon dioxide. A Pao_2 of less than 8.0 kPa (60 mmHg) or a $Paco_2$ of more than 6.2 kPa (50 mmHg) are parameters used to define respiratory failure.

CAUSE

Respiratory failure may be encountered in any clinical area and may be associated with a variety of disorders, including: (1) trauma and surgery that incur shock; (2) intrapulmonary disorders, such as acute and chronic airway obstruction, resistive disorders and pulmonary vascular disorders; (3) central nervous system disorders, such as drug overdose, brain tumour, cerebral injury or haemorrhage; (4) neuromuscular disease that involves respiratory muscle innervation (e.g. myasthenia gravis and Guillain-Barré syndrome); (5) sepsis, especially if the organisms are gram-negative; and (6) obstructive and central sleep apnoea.

Patients with a history of chronic obstructive pulmonary disease (asthma, chronic bronchitis) and cardiac or kidney disease, and those who are obese or debilitated are predisposed to develop acute respiratory failure when illness occurs.

Respiratory failure may be the result of alveolar hypoventilation, inadequate oxygenation of the blood (as occurs in ventilation–perfusion imbalance) or right-to-left shunt. In some instances more than one problem is present. Ventilation–perfusion inequality is the most frequent cause and is largely responsible for the low Po_2 in respiratory failure resulting as a complication of obstructive and restrictive diseases and adult respiratory distress syndrome. Hypoventilation is characterized by the retention of an excessive volume of carbon dioxide (hypercarbia), accompanied by hypoxaemia. The patient develops respiratory acidosis because of the elevated $Paco_2$. It is frequently associated with general hypoventilation due to neuromuscular disturbances and chest wall injury. When diffusion is impaired the carbon dioxide retention is initially slight and hypoxia is usually minimal.

Failure to oxygenate the blood adequately may be due to abnormal distribution of the inspired gas, ventilation–perfusion inequality or shunting of the blood through unventilated areas of the lung. The alveoli may be filled with fluid, or the alveoli are not ventilated because of an airway obstruction or atelectasis. As a result, the blood may flow through the capillaries around the alveoli without gas exchange taking place. When blood enters the arterial system without going through ventilated areas of the lung, it is referred to as a shunt, such as occurs with a heart defect when the blood moves directly from the right side of the heart to the left. In other instances the alveoli may be ventilated but the respective capillaries do not receive an adequate blood supply or are occluded (ventilation–perfusion mismatching).

When respiratory failure is severe pulmonary capillary epithelium is damaged, which leads to haemorrhage and interstitial oedema. The oedema decreases diffusion because fluid lies between the alveoli and capillaries. Fluid infiltrates the alveoli; surfactant is destroyed by proteins which leak through the permeable capillaries, and functional terminal respiratory units collapse. The capillaries dilate, the alveolar walls hypertrophy and the lungs become fibrotic. Defective gas diffusion becomes extensive and very serious. This severe form of respiratory failure may be referred to as *adult respiratory distress syndrome* (ARDS) or *shock lung*. There is increased resistance to air entry in the airways and alveoli.[56]

MANIFESTATIONS

The patient may manifest the effects of hypoxaemia or hypercarbia, or both. Dyspnoea or tachypnoea may be present, or in ventilatory failure respirations may be depressed and are slow, irregular and shallow. Cyanosis may not be present at the onset. The pulse rate increases and arrhythmias may develop. The patient may be restless and complain of headache or dizziness. Disorientation, apathy and slow responses develop as a result of the cerebral hypoxia, and may progress to unconsciousness. Periodic sustained contraction of a group of skeletal muscles (asterixis), slurred speech and mood fluctuations may occur if there is marked retention of carbon dioxide. The tidal and minute volumes are usually reduced.

Auscultation and an x-ray of the chest reveal patchy consolidated areas (no air entry). Measurement of the arterial blood gases may show levels as: Pao_2, 6.5 kPa or less (50 mmHg); and $Paco_2$, 6.5–8.0 kPa or more (50–60 mmHg). The pH is always checked to determine the presence and degree of acidosis or alkalosis.

Respiratory failure may develop quickly in a few hours after the initial insult, or the onset may be insidious over a few days or weeks. Serial monitoring of the patient's blood gases and tidal volume, and close observation of the characteristics of the respirations in circumstances where respiratory insufficiency may occur are important in early recognition of the problem.

TREATMENT

The underlying disorder which initiated the respiratory failure is treated and therapy is immediately directed toward improving ventilation and oxygenation of the blood. Airway obstruction is alleviated by removing retained secretions, coughing, postural drainage and suctioning. A bronchodilator (e.g. salbutamol) is administered and respiratory stimulants may be given. Respiratory depressants are avoided.

Infections are treated promptly as they may produce respiratory failure in patients with chronic airflow limitation.

Oxygen may be administered by nasal cannulae or mask, or by means of mechanical ventilation. Tracheal intubation may be necessary (see p. 431).

When respiratory failure is acute and severe, intensive nursing care and constant monitoring are required. Specific nursing measures to improve respiratory function are discussed under Nursing Intervention on pages 425–456.

Surgery of the Respiratory Tract

SURGERY OF THE UPPER RESPIRATORY TRACT

Major surgery of the upper respiratory tract usually is done because of benign or malignant tumours of the larynx and local tissues in the neck. A benign papilloma or polyp may develop within the larynx, the most frequent source being the vocal cords. Hoarseness and coughing are generally the initial symptoms, but gradually, as the tumour enlarges, breathing may become difficult. The tumour may be removed through the laryngoscope or by open surgery. Rarely is there any permanent voice impairment with this type of neoplasm.

Symptoms of laryngeal tumours include hoarseness, dyspnoea, cough, expectoration of blood, pain, enlargement of cervical lymph nodes and possibily dysphagia (difficulty in swallowing) as the mass encroaches on the oesophagus.

Early recognition by laryngoscopy and biopsy is important. A few cases may be treated by radiation alone, but the majority of patients undergo surgical treatment. A partial laryngectomy may be done if the newgrowth appears localized. Some residual impair-

[56] Shafer (1981), p. 35.

ment of voice is likely, necessitating speech therapy following recovery from the surgery.

Many patients have a total laryngectomy, which means they will be left voiceless and with a permanent tracheostomy through which they will breathe (see Table 16.10). The tracheostomy tube used for this type of operation is shorter than the tube used when the opening is temporary to facilitate ventilation and suction (i.e. it does not extend as far into the trachea). The tube remains until the tissues have healed and the stoma is well established. Following recovery from surgery, the patient is helped to develop oesophageal speech or to use an artificial larynx (Fig. 16.16).

Surgical reconstruction may also be done following laryngectomy to provide communication of pulmonary air with the pharyngo-oesophagus.

Radical neck dissection often accompanies total laryngectomy. This radical procedure involves the excision of a large portion of the neck tissue because of metastases to the cervical lymph nodes. The surgery removes the lymph network and the sternocleidomastoid muscles, the omohyoid muscle, the internal jugular vein and often the spinal accessory nerve. Modified procedures attempt to preserve the sternocleidomastoid muscle, jugular vein and spinal accessory nerve, thus producing less structural deformity.

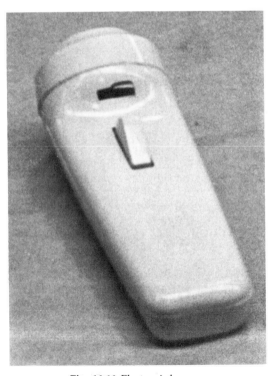

Fig. 16.16 Electronic larynx.

NURSING THE THORACIC SURGICAL PATIENT

In pulmonary disorders, the thoracic operative procedures performed include pneumonectomy, lobectomy, segmental resection and decortication.

Pneumonectomy, in which an entire lung is removed, involves the ligation of a large pulmonary artery, two large pulmonary veins and a bronchus. The phrenic nerve on the operative side is crushed or severed to permit the diaphragm to rise to reduce the size of the cavity that remains. Pneumonectomy is used in cancer of the lung or for widespread unilateral bronchiectasis, tuberculosis or abscesses.

A *lobectomy* is the removal of a lobe of a lung and is used when the disease is confined to that particular lobe.

Segmental resection is used when the person's disease is localized to a segment of a lung, making it possible to conserve functional tissue and lessen the degree of overdistension in the other lung by removing only the affected segment.

Wedge resection is used when the disease is localized and small. Only a part of a lung segment is removed.

Decortication is a surgical procedure in which a thick fibrous membrane that has replaced the visceral pleura is removed. The membrane, which causes restrictive respiratory insufficiency, may develop with empyema (a collection of pus in the pleural cavity), pleural effusion or prolonged haemothorax (blood in the pleural cavity).

PREOPERATIVE NURSING CARE

The patient who is to have chest surgery usually undergoes a period in which evaluation studies are made and care is given to improve his general condition (see Table 16.11a).

POSTOPERATIVE NURSING CARE (see Table 16.11b)

During the operation certain pieces of equipment are assembled in the patient's unit and are checked for functioning. These include the following, as well as those prepared for all patients having major surgery (see Chapter 11).

1 Respiratory suction equipment
2 Equipment for closed chest (water-seal) drainage
3 Two large artery forceps or clamps
4 Equipment for oxygen administration; mask, catheter or cannulae, tubing and bottle for humidification
5 Equipment for measuring central venous pressure
6 Thoracentesis (chest aspiration) tray

Patient assessment

The arterial blood pressure, pulse and respirations are noted every 15 minutes for the first 2–3 hours and then the interval is increased to ½–1 hour for the succeeding 8–10 hours if the vital signs are stabilized.

Table 16.10a Care of the patient undergoing laryngectomy: preoperative patient care plan.

Potential patient problems	Goals	Nursing intervention	Expected outcomes
1 Increased anxiety related to surgical procedure, possible diagnosis of cancer, threat to breathing and communication and disfigurement	a To alleviate anxiety	a Provide the patient and family with information about the surgical procedure, the reason for the surgery, and what to expect preoperatively and in the immediate postoperative period b Listen to the patient, provide privacy and encourage expression of feelings regarding the surgical procedure, loss of speech and disfigurement, and the opening into the trachea c Arrange for a visit by someone who has undergone similar surgery and achieved communication by oesophageal speech. The person may be located through the local cancer society	1 Patient expresses decreased anxiety 2 Patient and family are able to talk about impending surgery and its implications for future life-style
2 Lack of knowledge about preoperative care, surgical procedure and implications of the surgery for future life-style and functioning	a To acquire understanding of the operative procedure and expectations for preoperative and postoperative periods b To acquire understanding of the implications of the surgery on future life-style	a Explain the procedures to be followed preoperatively: • Instruction and practice in deep-breathing techniques • Preparation of the operative area as prescribed • Preoperative medications • Laboratory tests • Practise exercises for head support if neck muscles are to be removed b Explain what to expect on arrival in the operating theatre. Arrange for a nurse from the operating theatre to visit the patient c Explain postoperative routines and procedures. If the patient is to be transferred to the intensive care or a special head and neck surgical unit, arrange for the patient and family to visit the unit and meet the nursing staff Teach patient hand signs for communicating basic needs postoperatively and explain that someone will be close by at all times Demonstrate the use of the tracheostomy tube Explain suctioning procedures and the insertion of a nasogastric tube for feeding Arrange for a speech therapist to meet the patient and to explain the rehabilitation programme that will be instituted preoperatively d Allow the patient and family an opportunity to ask questions Provide repeated explanations as indicated e Show family members where the waiting rooms and facilities for food are located and advise them of arrangements for obtaining information about the patient's progress during and following surgery	1 Patient and family express understanding of preoperative routines, the surgical procedure, immediate postoperative care 2 Patient and family express awareness of effects of surgery on life-style and functioning

Table 16.10b Care of the patient undergoing laryngectomy: postoperative patient care plan.

Potential patient problems	Goals	Nursing intervention	Expected outcomes
1 Ineffective airway clearance related to: tracheostomy, absence of cough reflex, oedema of neck, and effects of anaesthesia	**a** To maintain a patent airway **b** To prevent respiratory complications	**a** Assess rate and depth of respirations and chest expansion; auscultate lungs for presence of crackles and wheezes Observe tracheostomy tube for presence of secretions **b** Monitor pulse and blood pressure **c** Suction tracheostomy tube and trachea as often as indicated by assessment for presence of secretions **d** Remove and cleanse the inner cannula of the tracheostomy tube every 3–6 hours, or more frequently if needed **e** Check the tracheostomy tube to make sure it is secure—see that the tapes are securely tied and the inner cannula is locked in place **f** Assist the patient to take deep, prolonged breaths while providing support for the head and neck Provide humidification with oxygen administration or by humidification of room air **g** If Haemovac drainage is used in the wound, it is checked frequently to be sure suction is maintained Observe and record the amount and type of drainage Empty Haemovac container as required	**1** No crackles or wheezes are heard on auscultation of lung **2** Pao_2 and $Paco_2$ levels are within normal range **3** The respiratory rate is within normal range **4** Breathing pattern rhythmical with symmetrical chest expansion **5** Tracheostomy clean and patent
2 Altered nutrition and fluid intake due to inability to swallow, and potential for wound contamination	**a** To maintain adequate fluid and nutritional intake	**a** Intravenous fluids are administered until fluids are permitted orally **b** A nasogastric tube is inserted preoperatively or following surgery to allow feedings and prevent wound contamination The nasogastric feedings are given slowly with the patient's head and shoulders elevated. Small amounts are given initially and the patient is observed for signs of regurgitation; the volume is increased as the patient is able to tolerate it **c** When the nasogastric tube is removed, the patient's ability to swallow is tested by administering small sips of water. If there is no difficulty, clear fluids are given by mouth, progressing to soft foods and gradually resuming a normal diet when tolerated	**1** Fluid intake exceeds 1500 ml daily **2** Weight loss is less than 2 kg
3 Wound healing incomplete, due to surgical incision	**a** To promote wound healing **b** To prevent wound infection	**a** Observe the incision frequently for redness, swelling, drainage and for signs of fluids when oral feedings are commenced **b** Monitor the patency of the Haemovac drainage	**1** The incision is clean and dry **2** Wound drainage is maintained

Table 16.10b—*continued*

Potential patient problems	Goals	Nursing intervention	Expected outcomes
3 Wound healing incomplete (continued)		**c** Cleanse the incision with antiseptic solution and apply sterile dressings as indicated **d** Cleanse the area proximal to the tracheostomy tube with hydrogen peroxide solution, removing encrustations	
4 Potential for impairment of oral mucosa increased due to inability to take fluids orally and to decreased saliva following oral surgery	**a** To maintain integrity of oral mucosa **b** To prevent discomfort	**a** Frequent mouth care is necessary. As soon as possible, re-establish brushing of teeth and stimulation of gums **b** Inspect the mouth daily for redness and ulcerations **c** If oral surgery was also performed, special mouth care is carried out frequently and artificial saliva is supplied to maintain moisture	**1** The oral mucosa is clean, moist and intact
5 Mobility impaired due to anaesthesia and surgery and possibly to excision of muscles of neck	**a** To prevent complications of immobility **b** To support head and initiate exercise programme to develop head support and arm functioning on the affected side	**a** Assist patient to carry out leg exercises as soon as possible and repeat every few hours **b** Ambulation usually begins within the first postoperative day. Assist the patient to a chair and then to walk around the room **c** When radical neck dissection is performed, teach the patient to place his hands behind his head to lift it An exercise programme is established by the physiotherapist to strengthen the remaining muscle groups to take over the function of the excised muscles	**1** The patient is ambulatory as soon as possible **2** The patient supports his head with both hands when moving (following radical neck surgery) **3** An exercise programme is started to facilitate head support and shoulder movement
6 Communication deficit related to removal of larynx	**a** To establish alternate patterns of communication for immediate use **b** To provide oesophageal speech training	**a** In the immediate postoperative period teach the patient to use hand signals to communicate needs **b** Paper, slate or communication board and pencils are kept at the bedside **c** Take time to read and respond to the patient's messages Advise the patient as to what is happening and what is expected of him **d** The call-button is kept within reach at all times **e** Encourage the patient and family to use touch and forms of communication other than speech **f** An intra-oral electrolarynx may be used during the immediate postoperative period to enable the patients to articulate sounds without putting stress on the wound **g** A speech therapy programme is commenced as soon as possible—usually when the patient is able to take food orally. The speech therapist teaches oesophageal speech and provides instruction for nurses and family on how to assist the patient.	**1** Patient begins speech programme **2** Patient indicates plans for continuing speech development programme

Table 16.10b—*continued*

Potential patient problem	Goals	Nursing intervention	Expected outcomes
Communication deficit (continued)		Oesophageal voice is produced when residual intra-oral air descends and is immediately raised from the upper oesophagus to vibrate at the level of the pharyngo-oesophageal segment. When residual air has passed down from the oral and pharyngeal cavities, it is immediately redirected upward through the pharynx, and vibrates to create sound **h** The patient requires support and encouragement for each small step taken as this is a long difficult process **i** For the patient who is unable to learn oesophageal speech or for whom speech is not relevant to a meaningful life, devices such as the artificial larynx in Fig. 16.16 are available. Electrolaryngeal devices may also be used until the patient learns oesophageal speech. They may be introduced when the wound is healed and tolerant of light internal pressure Talking machines are also useful for some patients. They provide sounds, words and phrases which can be retrieved, or picture symbols or printed words	
7 Body image altered due to physical deformities and loss of speech	**a** To recognize feelings about physical changes and loss of speech **b** To begin speech training **c** To learn techniques which maximize positive attributes and minimize deficits	**a** Provide time and privacy for the patient to share his feelings, using an electrolarynx device or pencil and pad **b** Face the patient and indicate understanding of his messages **c** Encourage the patient and family to participate in the care programme **d** Compliment the patient for achievement in caring for the tracheostomy and in oesophageal speech learning **e** Arrange opportunities for the patient to have contact with other patients and to participate in activities with others **f** Assist the patient to develop a plan for re-establishing social contacts following discharge **g** Give advice about wearing a scarf or high collar over the tracheostomy to provide a light covering **h** If the patient has had a radical neck dissection, use of erect posture, normal shoulder position and the exercise programme are emphasized **i** Advise the patient about non-allergic make-up to cover scars once healing takes place	1 Patient expresses feelings about appearance and loss of speech 2 Patient explores implications for daily functioning 3 Patient begins speech training 4 Patient shows an interest in appearance and uses suggestions to minimize deformities
8 Lack of knowledge about health management and skill in performing self-care	**a** To understand self-care needs **b** To develop and implement a plan for	**a** Instruct the patient in self-care measures Reinforce teaching each time care is provided	1 Patient and family indicate understanding of self-care procedures and safety measures

Table **16.10b**—*continued*

Potential patient problems	Goals	Nursing intervention	Expected outcomes
8 Lack of knowledge about health management and skill in performing self-care (continued)	post-hospital management and rehabilitation	**b** Provide opportunities for the patient and family to practise skills with supervision **c** Assist patient and family in developing care that will be compatible with the patient's usual daily activities and life-style **d** *Instructions include:* • Care of tracheostomy tube and stoma: When the stoma is healed and the opening remains patent, the tube is removed • Removal of secretions: Suctioning techniques are practised with supervision. If the patient requires suction equipment, he is advised of community resources for loan or purchase of home equipment. (e.g. a cancer society or the Red Cross) The need for a minimum of 2000 ml of fluid daily, unless contraindicated, to liquefy respiratory secretions is stressed • Safety precautions include: The use of smooth light-weight, lint-free material over the stoma to prevent foreign particles being inhaled and for aesthetic purposes Precautions when taking a shower to avoid aspiration of water. Shields are available that may be used and the shower spray is directed below neck level Swimming or immersion in water must be avoided • Speech therapy: Arrangements are made with the speech therapist to continue speech therapy as an outpatient • The prescribed exercise programme for head, neck and shoulders is taught and arrangements are made for continuation of the programme following discharge • Continuing medical supervision: Arrangements are made for follow-up medical care. Referrals are made to appropriate community services such as district or community nurses • Vocational retraining: Assessment is initiated if the patient is unable to return to his former occupation	**2** Patient and family express plans for implementing health-management plan **3** Patient and family begin to participate in care activities

Since venous return to the right atrium is influenced by respiratory movements, and intrathoracic pressure changes, hourly recording of the central venous pressure may be required. This pressure also reflects the ability of the right side of the heart to forward the blood. The reduction in the pulmonary vascular bed following lung resection may offer resistance to the outflow of the right side of the heart, causing an elevation of venous blood pressure. The pressure is obtained by the installation of a fine venous catheter threaded through an antecubital vein (basilic or cephalic vein) into the superior vena cava (see Chapter 14). The surgeon usually indicates the level of elevation of venous pressure at which he is to be notified and at which the fluid intake is restricted.

Table 16.11a Preoperative care plan for a patient undergoing thoracic surgery.

Problem	Goals	Nursing intervention	Expected outcomes
1 Anxiety increased due to operative procedure and outcome	1 To alleviate anxiety	1 To provide patient and family with information about his condition, the proposed surgery and expectations for the patient and family during the preoperative, intraoperative and postoperative periods 2 Answer questions raised by patient and family and reinforce information provided by the doctor 3 Provide opportunities for the expression of fears and concerns 4 Identify actual and potential home problems and make referrals to social workers or others who may provide the necessary assistance	1 The patient expresses feelings of decreased anxiety 2 The patient and family state that their questions have been answered
2 Lack of knowledge about surgical procedure, preoperative preparation and postoperative expectations	1 To acquire an understanding of the operative procedure and expectations for preoperative and postoperative periods	1 Explain the procedures and routines to be followed preoperatively 2 Explain the procedure on the patient's arrival in operating theatre and arrangements for the family to wait during surgery Arrange for a nurse to come from the operating theatre to talk with the patient, if possible 3 Explain postoperative expectations and care Advise the patient if he will be transferred to intensive care from the operating theatre Describe chest tubes that will be in place Describe the expected routines for coughing, deep breathing, changing position and explain what will be done to relieve pain and discomfort Explain the probable need for the administration of oxygen	1 Patient and family demonstrate an understanding of the surgical procedure, preoperative routine, what will happen on arrival in the operating theatre and the postoperative routine and expectations 2 Patient demonstrates an ability to perform deep-breathing and coughing techniques and to use the respiratory equipment
3 Airway clearance ineffective due to pulmonary disease and potential effects of anaesthesia and surgical procedure	1 To promote airflow prior to surgery	1 If necessary, promote clearance of secretions by postural drainage and chest percussion. Secretions are observed for volume, colour and consistency and cultures are taken Antibiotics are administered as prescribed Frequent mouth care is provided	1 The patient's airways are as clear of secretions as possible preoperatively as evidenced by: absence of crackles and wheezes 2 Temperature is within normal range

Table 16.11b Postoperative care plan for a patient undergoing thoracic surgery.

Problem	Goals	Nursing intervention	Expected outcomes
1 Airway clearance ineffective due to anaesthesia, surgical procedure and incisional pain	To promote and maintain airway clearance	**a** As soon as the blood pressure is stabilized, the patient is asked to cough every 1–2 hours, or more often if there is evidence of retained secretions. It is important that the patient is wakened to cough at regular intervals throughout the night. Even with preoperative instruction and practice, the patient is usually fearful and may find the procedure difficult **b** Suctioning is used to clear the pharyngeal part of the tract and will also precipitate coughing. The latter loosens secretions in the lower tracheobronchial passages and raises them to the upper tract from which the patient may cough them up, or they may be reached by suction **c** The nurse assists the patient to a sitting position for coughing and, standing at the side of the bed which is opposite to the patient's incision, supports the operative side of the chest, back and front, with her hands. The patient is asked to take several deep breaths and to cough with each expiration. If the cough and suctioning are not productive, listen to the chest for evidence of crackles and wheezes. A nebulized solution may be prescribed to liquefy the secretions, making them easier to raise **d** Physical therapy (vibration and percussion) may be used to dislodge secretions from peripheral bronchial tubes and bronchioles. A humidifier in the room may also be helpful. Endotracheal suctioning may have to be done if the secretions continue	1 The patient deep breathes and coughs as instructed 2 There is an absence of crackles and wheezes 3 The respiratory rate is normal for the patient 4 Respirations are deep, regular and symmetrical 5 The temperature is within the normal postoperative range
2 Breathing patterns altered due to anaesthesia, surgical procedure, pain and presence of fluid and/or air in the intrapleural space	To promote effective patterns of respirations	**a** *Deep breathing*. The patient is encouraged to take five to ten deep breaths hourly and is given an explanation of the need to promote full expansion of the remaining lung tissue and the drainage of air and fluid from the thoracic cavity. As the lung expands to occupy more space, the pressure increases within the pleural cavity, forcing air and fluid through the drainage tube. Incentive spirometry may be used to encourage maximum inspirations	1 Respirations are deep, regular and symmetrical (except with pneumonectomy) 2 Inspiratory volume increases progressively 3 Chest tubes are patent and drainage equipment is functioning

Table 16.11b—*continued*

Problem	Goals	Nursing intervention	Expected outcomes
2 Breathing patterns altered (continued)		**b** *Positioning.* With the return of consciousness and stabilization of the blood pressure and pulse, the head of the bed is raised gradually to a 30–45° angle. This facilitates the patient's breathing by lowering the diaphragm. The patient is turned every 1–2 hours and the doctor usually specifies whether he may be turned on either side or to one side only. In the case of a pneumonectomy, turning is from the back to the affected side only so that there is no restriction placed on the remaining lung, which is carrying the full respiratory load. With partial resection, the patient usually may be turned from his back to left side, to back to right side, and so on. If a sternum-splitting incision is used, the patient is generally most comfortable on his back, but is encouraged to assume a lateral position for at least brief periods. During any moving or turning of the patient, precautions are necessary to prevent dislodging the chest drainage tubes **c** *Chest tubes and drainage.* All connections should be checked to make sure they are taped and airtight. Drainage receptacles are placed below the level of the patient. The system is checked regularly for functioning (see p. 438). The colour, volume and consistency of drainage is observed and recorded every hour, initially and then every 2–4 hours	
3 Impaired gas exchange, related to anaesthesia, surgery and pain	To promote and maintain pulmonary ventilation	**a** *Oxygen administration.* The patient usually receives oxygen by mask, cathether or nasal cannulae for at least the first 24–36 hours. The administration is not prolonged unless the patient is experiencing some respiratory insufficiency	1 Pulse and respiratory rates are normal for the patient 2 The patient's colour is good 3 Arterial blood gases are within the normal range 4 The patient is rational, oriented and does not complain of a headache
4 Fluid volume deficit due to loss during surgery and decreased fluid intake	To maintain adequate hydration and ventilation	**a** The blood loss at operation is replaced by a blood transfusion, and fluids are usually given intravenously for the first 24–48 hours. The rate at which the fluid is given must be carefully controlled to prevent too rapid filling of the reduced vascular compartment and subsequent pulmonary oedema, which is manifested by dyspnoea, bubbling sounds and frothy sputum. The doctor may indicate	1 The central venous pressure is within the normal range 2 The blood pressure is within the normal range for the patient 3 Urinary output exceeds 50 ml/h 4 The patient's skin tone is maintained

Table 16.11b—*continued*

Problem	Goals	Nursing intervention	Expected outcomes
4 Fluid volume deficit (continued)		the rate at which the intravenous fluid may be administered, which usually does not exceed 40 drops per minute. The rate of flow is also regulated according to the central venous pressure **b** Clear fluids may be given as soon as there is no nausea and vomiting, and gradually are increased in volume as tolerated. The patient may have a soft diet the first postoperative day, if he can take it, and a regular diet the following day. Extra fluids are provided, unless contraindicated by increased venous pressure, to reduce the tenaciousness of the respiratory secretions	
5 Alterations in comfort—pain related to thoracic incision and chest tubes	To promote comfort	**a** Narcotic drugs are used sparingly since they generally depress respirations and the cough reflex. A small dose of morphine or pethidine hydrochloride may be prescribed for pain, but judgement must be used in administering it. The patient should not be allowed to suffer unnecessarily, but it is also important for him to cough to remove secretions and to breathe deeply to ventilate the remaining lung tissue adequately Administer medications regularly and before pain is severe. Plan breathing and coughing exercises to follow administration of medications	**1** The patient expresses absence of severe pain experiences **2** The patient indicates that measures to decrease pain are effective **3** The patient performs breathing and turning activities as directed
6 Mobility impaired due to surgery and decreased energy and effort tolerance	**a** To prevent complications of immobility **b** To promote a full range of motion of arm on the affected side	**a** Passive extension and flexion movements of the lower limbs are carried out every 3–4 hours **b** During the first day postoperatively, assist the patient to a sitting position over the side of the bed and then into a chair Monitor respiratory responses, pulse and blood pressure. Observe patient for signs of dizziness **c** When the patient's condition is stable, assist him in walking around the room. Increase walking distance daily from the second postoperative day to include the ward corridor **d** Carry out passive range-of-motion exercises on affected arm and shoulder four times a day Begin physical therapy and active arm and shoulder exercises by the third day Encourage the patient to use affected arm in self-care activities	**1** Leg exercises are performed as directed **2** Arm exercises are carried out four times a day **3** The patient uses affected arm to perform self-care activities **4** The patient is up on the first postoperative day **5** The distance and duration of walking activity increases each day

Table 16.11b—*continued*

Problem	Goals	Nursing intervention	Expected outcomes
7 Wound healing incomplete, related to surgery and chest tube sites	a To promote wound healing b To prevent wound infection	a Observe dressing for signs of drainage or bleeding when the patient returns to the unit and every 4 hours during the first day b Observe incision and chest tube sites for signs of redness, tenderness, drainage and oedema during each dressing change and every 8 hours after the removal of the dressing The dressing is usually removed within 48 hours Cleanse the incision with antiseptic (e.g. providone-iodine) daily c Take a swab for culture and sensitivity if signs of infection are present d When chest tubes are removed cover the areas with occlusive dressings of petroleum jelly gauze and seal tightly for about 48 hours	1 The incision and chest tube sites are clean, dry and intact
8 Lack of knowledge about post-hospital care and rehabilitation	a To understand expectations for post-hospital period and on-going rehabilitation b To be aware of resources for continued physiotherapy and medical supervision	a The convalescence and rehabilitation must be adapted to each individual patient. Generally, the patient requires a fairly long period of convalescence during which he is encouraged to continue his exercises and deep breathing. Activity is gradually increased, and the patient's reaction to it is noted. The body has to adjust to a reduced respiratory capacity, and the patient who has had a pneumonectomy will require a greater period of adjustment. The patient may not be able to resume his former occupation and may need help to find lighter work within his respiratory capacity b In preparation for going home, the patient receives instructions about the exercises, deep breathing and coughing which are to be continued. The recommended amounts of rest and activity are explained. If distance and travel do not present too great a problem, the patient may be requested to return to the physiotherapy department for exercise supervision once or twice weekly, or arrangements may be made to have a physiotherapist or a nurse visit him at home to counsel and assess his progress. He may experience some numbness, pain, or heaviness in the operative area due to interruption of the intercostal nerves but may be reassured that this is generally temporary	1 Patient and family demonstrate understanding of post-discharge care related to deep breathing and coughing, mobility exercises, rest, self-care activities, diet and fluids 2 Plans for continued physiotherapy and on-going medical supervision are understood

The rise and fall of both sides of the chest in respiration should be noted. Dyspnoea, decreased movement of one side of the chest on inspiration (except in pneumonectomy), cyanosis or chest pain may manifest a pneumothorax and should be reported promptly to the doctor. This may develop as a result of air or fluid collecting in the pleural cavity and compressing the lung. It must be treated quickly by chest aspiration (thoracentesis), or the patient may die of respiratory insufficiency. Respirations are also observed for audible moist sounds. A portable chest x-ray may be done daily for 2–3 days to determine lung expansion and detect the presence of fluid and air in the pleural cavity.

The wound area and chest drainage are examined frequently for any indications of bleeding. The sealed drainage system is checked frequently for functioning (see p. 438), and the tubing connections are examined for security. The volume of drainage is measured at regular 8-hour intervals. The intake and output are recorded, and the fluid balance is estimated.

The nurse measures the patient's tidal and minute volumes. Arterial blood specimens may be necessary for blood gas determinations which indicate possible respiratory insufficiency and the need for mechanical assistance and/or increased oxygen inhalation.

LUNG AND HEART TRANSPLANTATION

Several successful heart–lung transplantations have taken place. Difficulties arise because the transplanted lungs are continually exposed to air and infection. Disruption of the cough mechanism also predisposes to complications. The use of cyclosporin to suppress the recipient's immune responses has led to improved success because the bone marrow suppression is less than with other immunosuppressive agents. The length of survival, and the quality of life, for transplantation patients is progressively improving as new techniques evolve.

References and Further Reading

BOOKS

Anderson SVD & Bauwens EE (1981) *Chronic Health Problems*. St Louis: CV Mosby. Chapter 11.

Bates B (1983) *A Guide to Physical Examination*, 3rd ed. Philadelphia: JB Lippincott. Chapter 6.

Braunwald E et al (1987) *Harrison's Principles of Internal Medicine*, 11th ed. New York: McGraw–Hill. Part 4.

Byrne CJ, Saxton DF, Pelikon PK & Nugent PM (1981) *Laboratory Tests*. Menlo Park, CA: Addison-Wesley. pp. 193–202 & 252–256.

Cherniack RM & Cherniack L (1983) *Respiration in Health and Disease*, 3rd ed. Philadelphia: WB Saunders.

Ganong WF (1985) *Review of Medical Physiology*. 12th ed. San Francisco: Lange.

Guyton AC (1986) *Textbook of Medical Physiology*, 7th ed. Philadelphia: WB Saunders. Parts VII & VIII.

Harper HA, Rodwell VW & Mayes PA (eds) (1979) *Review of Physiological Chemistry*. Los Altos, CA: Lange Medical. Chapter 15.

Harper RW (1981) *A Guide to Respiratory Care*. Philadelphia: JB Lippincott.

Hart LK, Reese JL & Fearing MO (eds) (1981) *Concepts Common to Acute Illness*. St Louis: CV Mosby. Chapter 18.

Henshaw HC & Murray JF (1980) *Diseases of the Chest*, 4th ed. Philadelphia: WB Saunders.

Keers RY (1978) *Pulmonary Tuberculosis*. A Journey Down the Centuries. London: Ballière Tindall.

Kinney MR, Dear CB, Parka DR & Voorman DMN (eds) (1981) *A.A.C.N.'s Reference for Critical Care Nursing*. New York: McGraw-Hill. Chapters 3, 19, 23 & 38.

Jones E (1981) *Essential Intensive Care*. Lancaster, England: MTP Press.

Malasanos L, Barkauskas V, Moss M, & Soltenberg-Allen K (1981) *Health Assessment*. St Louis: CV Mosby. Chapter 15.

Miller S, Simpson LK, Soukup M & Weinburg SL (eds) (1980) *Methods in Critical Care: The A.C.C.N. Manual*. Philadelphia: WB Saunders. pp. 189–255.

Robinson LA & Pugsley SO (1981) Dealing with chronic airflow obstruction. In: SVD Anderson & EE Bauwens (eds), *Chronic Health Problems*. St Louis: CV Mosby.

Sabiston DC Jr (ed) (1985) *Davis–Christopher Textbook of Surgery*, 13th ed. Philadelphia: WB Saunders. Chapter 54.

Scadding JG (1977) *Definition and Clinical Categories in Asthma*. London: Chapman & Hall.

Sexton DL (1981) *Chronic Obstructive Pulmonary Disease*. St Louis: CV Mosby.

Smith LH & Thier SO (1985) *Pathophysiology*, 2nd ed. Philadelphia: WB Saunders. Section 11.

Tisi GM (1980) *Pulmonary Physiology in Clinical Medicine*. Baltimore: Williams & Wilkins.

West JB (1979) *Respiratory Physiology—The Essentials*, 2nd ed. Baltimore: Williams & Wilkins.

West JB (1982) *Respiratory Pathophysiology—The Essentials*, 2nd ed. Baltimore: Williams & Wilkins.

PERIODICALS

Belitz J (1983) Minimizing the psychological complications of patients who require mechanical ventilation. *Crit. Care Nurs.*, Vol. 3 No. 3, pp. 42–46.

Blegis MA (1981) Controlled breathing patterns in COPD. *Rehab. Nurs.*, Vol. 6 No. 2, pp. 10–14.

Bourbonnais F (1980) Adult respiratory distress syndrome. *Can. Nurs.*, Vol. 76 No. 10, pp. 51–54.

Boyd G (1984) Drugs and respiratory system. *Nursing* (Oxford), No. 27, pp. 805–806.

Brooks CG Jr (1981a) Artificial mechanical ventilation of the adult. Part I: getting it started. *Crit. Care Nurs.*, Vol. 1 No. 4, pp. 15–18.

Brooks CG Jr (1981b) Artificial mechanical ventilation of the adult. Part II: fine tuning. *Crit. Care Nurs.*, Vol. 1 No. 5, pp. 8–15.

Brooks CG Jr (1983) The adult way to wean from mechanical ventilation. *Crit. Care Nurs.*, Vol. 3 No. 6, pp. 64–65 & 78.

Brooks CG Jr (1984) Respiratory mathematics: adjusting the Pao_2. *Crit. Care Nurs.*, Vol. 4 No. 6, pp. 20–24.

Brown I (1982) Trach care? Take care—infections on the prowl. *Nurs. '82*, Vol. 12 No. 5, pp. 45–49.

Bull S (1981) Vascular pressures and critical care management. *Nurs. Clin. N. Am.*, Vol. 16 No. 2, pp. 225–239.

Callahan M (1982) C.O.P.D. makes a bad first impression, but you'll find wonderful people underneath. *Nurs. '82*, Vol. 12 No. 5, pp. 67–72.

Casciari RJ, Fairshter RD, Morrison JT & Wilson AF (1981) Effects of breathing retraining in patients with chronic obstructive pulmonary disease. *Chest*, Vol. 79 No. 4, pp. 393–398.

Chalmers KL (1984) A closer look at how people cope with chronic airflow obstruction. *Can. Nurs.*, Vol. 80 No. 2, pp. 35–38.

Cimprich B (1981) Quality assurance: a program for nursing care for patients with lung cancer. *Cancer Nurs.*, Vol. 4 No. 5, pp. 409–418.

Cline BA & Fisher ML (1982) A.R.D.S. means emergency. *Nurs. '82*, Vol. 12 No. 2, pp. 62–67.

Creighton H (1985) Organ transplantation. Part I: law for the nurse manager. *Nurs. Management*, Vol. 16 No. 9, pp. 16–17.

Curran FJ (1981) Night ventilation by body respirators for patients in chronic respiratory failure due to late stage Duchenne muscular dystrophy. *Arch. Phys. Med. Rehab.*, Vol. 62 No. 6, pp. 270–274.

Darovic GO (1983) Ten perils of mechanical ventilation and how to hold them in check. *RN*, Vol. 46 No. 5, pp. 37–42.

Davido J (1981) Pulmonary rehabilitation. *Nurs. Clin. N. Am.*, Vol. 16 No. 2, pp. 275–283.

Dossey B & Passons JM (1981) Pulmonary embolism: preventing it, treating it. *Nurs. '81*, Vol. 11 No. 3, pp. 26–33.

Dropkin MJ (1981) Development of a self-care teaching program for postoperative head and neck surgery patients. *Cancer Nurs.*, Vol. 4 No. 2, pp. 103–106.

Durie M (1984) Respiratory problems and nursing interventions. *Nursing* (Oxford), No. 28, pp. 826–828.

Edlund BJ & Wheeler EC (1980) Adaption to breathlessness. *Top. Clin. Nurs.*, Vol. 2 No. 3, pp. 11–25.

Ellmyer P & Thomas NJ (1982) Ambulatory nursing: A guide to your patient's safe home use of oxygen. *Nurs. '82*, Vol. 12 No. 1, pp. 56–57.

Erickson R (1981) Chest tubes—they're really not that complicated. *Nurs. '81*, Vol. 11 No. 5, pp. 34–43.

Erickson R (1981) Solving chest tube problems. *Nurs. '81*, Vol. 11 No. 6, pp. 62–68.

Fuchs PL (1980) Getting the best out of oxygen delivery systems. *Nurs. '81*, Vol. 10 No. 12, pp. 34–43.

Fuchs PL (1984) Streamlining your suction techniques. Part I: nasotracheal suctioning. *Nurs. '84*, Vol. 14 No. 5, pp. 55–61.

Glass LB (1981) Exercise therapy for the patient with pulmonary dysfunction. *Top. Clin. Nurs.*, Vol. 3 No. 2, pp. 87–93.

Grossbach-Landis I (1980) Successful weaning of ventilator dependent patients. *Top. Clin. Nurs.*, Vol. 2 No. 3, pp. 45–68.

Halfman MA & Hojnacki LH (1981) Exercise and the maintenance of health. *Top. Clin. Nurs.*, Vol. 3 No. 2, pp. 1–10.

Hall JP & Jackson VD (1981) Adult respiratory medical emergencies. *Nurs. Clin. N. Am.*, Vol. 16 No. 1, pp. 75–84.

Heimbecker RO, McKenzie N, Stiller C, Kostuk WJ & Silver MD (1984) Heart and heart–lung transplantation. *Heart Lung*, Vol. 13 No. 1, pp. 1–4.

Hudson LO (1984) Management of C.O.P.D.: state of the art. *Chest*, Vol. 85 No. 6, pp.765–815.

Humbrecht B & Van Parys E (1982) From assessment to intervention: how to use heart and breath sounds as part of your nursing care plan. *Nurs. '82*, Vol. 12 No. 4, pp. 34–41.

Hunter PM (1981) Bedside monitoring of respiratory function. *Nurs. Clin. N. Am.*, Vol. 16 No. 2, pp. 211–224.

Jones NL (1981) The pathophysiological consequences of smoking on the respiratory system. *Can. J. Public Health*, Vol. 72 No. 6, pp. 388–390.

Laschinger HK (1984) Demystifying arterial blood gases. *Can. Nurs.*, Vol. 80 No. 10, pp. 45–47.

Luce JM (1980) Respiratory complications of obesity. *Chest*, Vol. 78 No. 4, pp. 626–637.

Mathewson M (1983) Nursing rules—Fact or myth? A nasal cannula guarantees a low oxygen concentration to the patient. *Crit. Care Nurs.*, Vol. 3 No. 5, p. 30.

McCormick GP, White MJ, Simotoski FJ, Stanley LH & McGuiness K (1982) Artificial speech devices. *Am. J. Nurs.*, Vol. 82 No. 1, pp. 121–122.

McDonald GJ (1981) A home care program for patients with chronic lung disease. *Nurs. Clin. N. Am.*, Vol. 16 No. 2, pp. 259–274.

McGavin CR, Gupta SP & McHardy GJR (1976) Twelve-minute walking test for assessing disability in chronic bronchitis. *Br. Med. J.*, Vol. 3 No. 1, pp. 822–823.

McMillan E (1984) Oxygen therapy. *Nursing* (Oxford), Vol. 2 No. 28, pp. 822–825.

Murphy PA & Schare BL (1981) Timely techniques in caring for the patient with an endotracheal tube: Part I. *Nurs. '81*, Vol. 11 No. 9, pp. 70–73.

Nielsen L (1980) Mechanical ventilation: patient assessment and nursing care. *Am. J. Nurs.*, Vol. 80 No. 12, pp. 2191–2217.

Ng L & McCormick KA (1982) Position changes and their physiological consequences. *Adv. Nurs. Sci.*, Vol. 4 No. 4, pp. 12–25.

O'Malley P & Zankofski MA (1979) Disposable suction catheters: a nursing '79 product survey. *Nurs. '79*, Vol. 9 No. 5, pp. 7–75.

Peterson GM (1981) Application and assessment of oxygen therapy devices. *Nurs. Clin. N. Am.*, Vol. 16 No. 2, pp. 241–257.

Petty TL (1979) Clinical evaluation of patients with chronic respiratory insufficiency. *Semin. Resp. Med.*, Vol. 1 No. 1, pp. 1–17.

Petty TL (1979) Management of chronic airflow obstruction. *Semin. Resp. Med.*, Vol. 1 No. 1, pp. 29–46.

Petty TL & Scoggen CV (1979) Diseases with chronic airflow limitation. *Semin. Resp. Med.*, Vol. 1 No. 1, pp. 18–29.

Pfister S (1982) Manual resuscitation bags: uses, features and troubleshooting. *Crit. Care Nurs.*, Vol. 2 No. 2, pp. 27–35.

Pfister S & Bullas J (1984) Caring for a patient with an endotracheal tube. *Crit. Care Nurs.*, Vol. 4 No. 1, pp. 29 & 56–61.

Pfister S & Bullas J (1985) Caring for a patient with a chest tube connected to the emersion pump. *Crit. Care Nurs.*, Vol. 5 No. 2, pp. 26, 27, 30–32.

Promisloff RA (1980) Administering oxygen safely: when, why and how. *Nurs. '80*, Vol. 10 No. 10, pp. 54–56.

Rathley MC (1982) Teaching families to give tracheal care at home. *Nurs. '82*, Vol. 12 No. 6, pp. 70–71.

Rich W & Reichenberger M (1981) Managing flail chest: a

matter of monitoring breathing. *Nurs. '81*, Vol. 11 No. 12, pp. 26–31.

Richard E & Shepard AC (1981) Giving up smoking: a lesson in loss theory. *Am. J. Nurs.*, Vol. 81 No. 4, pp. 755–757.

Riegel B et al (1985) A review and critique of the literature on preoxygenation for endotracheal suctioning. *Heart Lung*, Vol. 14 No. 5, pp. 507–518.

Rogers TR (1981) Clinical problems in the adult with asthma. *Nurs. Clin. N. Am.*, Vol. 16 No. 2, pp. 293–297.

Rokosky JS (1981) Assessment of the individual with altered respiratory function. *Nurs. Clin. N. Am.*, Vol. 16 No. 2, pp. 195–209.

Shafer T (1981) Nursing care of the patient with ARDS. *Crit. Care Nurs.*, Vol. 1 No. 3, p. 35.

Shell G (1980) Upper and lower respiratory tract infection. *Nurs. Clin. N. Am.*, Vol. 15 No. 4, pp. 715–727.

Snider GL (1985) Distinguishing among asthma, chronic bronchitis and emphysema. *Chest*, Vol. 87 No. 1, pp. 355–395.

Sumner SM & Lewandowski V (1983) Guidelines for using artificial breathing devices. *Nurs. '83*, Vol. 13 No. 10, pp. 54–57.

Stein DA & Bradley BL (1982) Mechanisms of oxygen effects on exercise in patients with chronic obstructive pulmonary disease. *Chest*, Vol. 81 No. 1, pp. 6–10.

Talabere LR (1980) The child with a tracheostomy: a holistic approach to home care. *Top. Clin. Nurs.*, Vol. 2 No. 3, pp. 27–44.

Thompson MC (1984) Physiotherapy—essentials of chest care. *Nursing* (Oxford), Vol. 2 No. 27, pp. 796–800.

Twohig RG (1984) Respiratory function tests. *Nursing* (Oxford), Vol. 2 No. 27, pp. 807–810.

Weber BA (1981) Living to the limit: exercise for the chronic breathless patient. *Physiotherapy*, Vol. 67 No. 5, pp. 128–130.

Westra B (1984) Assessment under pressure: when your patient says 'I can't breath'. *Nurs. '84*, Vol. 14 No. 5, pp. 34–40.

White HA & Briggs AM (1980) Home care of persons with respiratory problems: optimization of breathing and life potential. *Top. Clin. Nurs.*, Vol. 2 No. 3, pp. 69–77.

Woodin LM (1980) Rehabilitating the COPD Patient. *Rehab. Brief*, Vol. 3 No. 7.

Woodin LM (1982) Your patient with pneumothorax: a patient in distress. *Nurs. '82*, Vol. 12 No. 11, pp. 50–56.

Woodin LM (1982) Fight the frustration of status asthmaticus. *Nurs. '82*, Vol. 12 No. 3, pp. 58–62.

Woodin LM (1982) Guidelines for nursing care of patients with altered ventilation. *Oncology Nurs. Forum*, Vol. 10 No. 2, pp. 113–116.

17

Nursing in Disorders of the Alimentary Canal

The Alimentary Canal

The alimentary canal, or what is frequently referred to as the gastrointestinal tract, consists of a long hollow tube extending from the lips to the anus. It provides a non-sterile pathway for nutrients in the body and it is divided into the mouth, pharynx, oesophagus, stomach (Greek, *gaster*) and intestines (Greek, *enteron*). Modifications in structure occur in different parts of the tract, and are correlated with the particular functions featured in the respective area and the likely condition of the content when it reaches that part. The primary function of the gastrointestinal tract is to provide the body cells with a continual supply of nutrients, electrolytes and water in a form that is acceptable to the system. To do so it performs the functions of ingestion, digestion and absorption of food and fluid into the blood and elimination of residue and waste products. These functions are regulated by autonomic innervation, endocrine secretions and important local intrinsic controls. The latter promote activities without any extrinsic direction; that is, cells may secrete chemicals and the smooth muscle in the walls of the tract contracts rhythmically in response to specific local environmental conditions without extrinsic stimulation and controls.

Food sustains life and determines an individual's nutritional status, as reflected in his state of health, activities, levels of achievement and resistance to and ability to handle disease. It supplies the body with the energy required for all its activities (e.g. respiration, circulation of the blood, muscular activity and work). Food provides the materials for tissue growth and repair and those essential for the production of substances by the body cells (e.g. hormones and enzymes). Essential regulatory substances such as vitamins are also obtained from foods. Most foods are complex compounds; chemical and mechanical processes occur in the gastrointestinal tract to break them down into absorbable forms.

If food is withheld or a disorder within the tract interrupts the essential processing of the nutrients, the individual's survival is threatened.

Structural divisions of the gastrointestinal tract (see Fig. 17.1)

MOUTH

The mouth, or oral cavity, the initial part of the tract, is lined by a mucous membrane which secretes mucus to mix with the food, facilitating its movement through the pharynx and oesophagus. Although the mouth is primarily concerned with the ingestion of food, it also plays an important role in speech.

The tongue, teeth and salivary glands are contained within the mouth. The *tongue* is comprised of muscular tissue enclosed in mucous membrane. The upper surface is studded with numerous papillae and contains taste buds. The tongue functions in swallowing and speech as well as in taste.

Early in life, the human organism develops 20 primary deciduous *teeth*—10 upper and 10 lower. Beginning in the fifth or sixth year and continuing over a period of several years, the deciduous teeth are replaced by a permanent set of 16 in the upper jaw and 16 in the lower jaw. The front teeth are shaped for biting and tearing, and the remainder for grinding and masticating food. Hence, loss of teeth, or defects in them, can lead to indigestion or malnutrition.

Each tooth consists of a crown and root (see Fig. 17.8). The crown is the exposed portion which has a hard external covering of enamel and an internal substance called dentine. The root is the part buried in the jaw bone and has a covering of cementum, a substance softer and less smooth than the enamel. A central cavity running the length of the tooth contains nerves and blood vessels.

There are three pairs of *salivary glands* whose ducts open onto the surface of the mouth. The parotid glands lie in front of and just below the ear and produce a thin, watery secretion that includes an important digestive enzyme, ptyalin. The submaxillary and sublingual glands are located in the floor of the mouth. The sublingual glands secrete only mucus; the submaxillary glands produce both a watery and mucous secretion. The secretions of the salivary glands and the oral mucosa collectively form the saliva. For the composition and functions of saliva see p. 485).

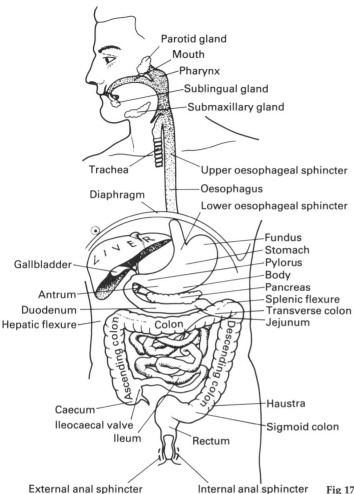

Fig 17.1 Structural divisions of the alimentary canal.

PHARYNX

The second segment of the tract is the pharynx, which is a funnel-shaped muscular tube lined with mucous membrane that is continuous with that of the mouth, respiratory tract and oesophagus. It serves as a common pathway for food and air. When its muscular tissue contracts, the band of striated muscle known as the cricopharyngeal or upper oeso-phageal sphincter relaxes; food and fluid are directed into the oesophagus and the entrances to the larynx and the oral and nasal cavities are closed simul-taneously.

OESOPHAGUS

The oesophagus is a narrow muscular tube, approxi-mately 10 inches long, that passes down behind the trachea and heart, through the mediastinum and diaphragm to the stomach. The upper third is striated muscle, the middle third is mixed striated and smooth muscle and the lower third smooth muscle. A thickened band of smooth muscle forms the lower oesophageal or gastrointestinal sphincter which opens when food is swallowed. It is lined with mucous membrane and has an outer protective coat of fibrous tissue.

STOMACH

The stomach and the intestines, the remaining portions of the digestive tract, lie within the abdomi-nal cavity. The stomach is located just below the dia-phragm and is the widest part of the alimentary canal which makes possible its retention of a considerable amount of food while it undergoes certain changes. The stomach is divided into three segments: the fun-dus, body and pylorus (see Fig. 17.1).

The gastric walls have three layers of muscle tissue; one in which the fibres run longitudinally, a second one in which they are circular, and a third in which they run obliquely to the others (Fig. 17.2). The circular muscle layer is thickened at the opening

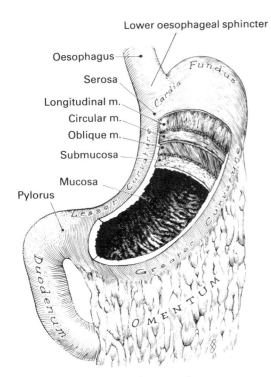

Fig 17.2 The stomach.

of the oesophagus into the stomach to form the *cardiac* or *lower oesophageal sphincter*. Similarly, the opening into the small intestine is guarded by the *pyloric sphincter*.

The mucous membrane lining is thick and lies in folds to allow for distensibility as the stomach fills. It contains numerous minute glands made up of three types of secreting cells: the chief, or zymogen cells secrete the gastric enzymes, the parietal cells produce hydrochloric acid, and mucous glands provide mucus. The glandular secretions are poured out into the stomach to form collectively the gastric juice.

SMALL INTESTINE

The small intestine is the longest portion of the alimentary canal, being approximately 18–20 feet, and is divided into the *duodenum, jejunum* and *ileum*. The duodenum is the short, proximal portion which originates with the gastric pylorus. It receives the bile and the pancreatic enzymes through a sphincter (sphincter of Oddi) at the junction of the common bile duct and the duodenum. The long jejunum and ileum lie in loops and fill the greater part of the abdominal cavity.

The mucosal surface of the small intestine is covered with many finger-like processes called villi, (see Fig. 17.3), each of which contains a central lymph channel called a lacteal and a network of capillaries. Each villus is covered with a single layer of specialized epithelial cells, the luminal surface of which is covered with small projections called micro-villi (brush border) (see Fig. 17.4). Most digestion and absorption takes place in the small intestine where circular folds increase the surface area and somewhat retard the passage of the food, thus favouring absorption. The villi with their microvilli serve to greatly increase the absorptive area. The molecules of digested food are picked up by the blood in the capillaries and the lymph in the lacteals.

The small intestine contains many glands which secrete digestive enzymes (see p. 487) and hormones onto a sticky layer called the glycolax which covers the microvilli. Lymph nodes appear in clusters throughout the small intestine and are referred to as Peyer's patches. Other lymphoid cells located in the intestinal mucosa and between the epithelial cells lining the villi, play an important role in the immunological defence of the body.[1]

LARGE INTESTINE

The large intestine has a greater diameter than that of the small intestine and is divided into the *caecum, colon, rectum* and *anal canal*. The ileum opens into a pouch-like structure, the caecum, in the right lower abdominal quadrant. The *appendix*, a slender blind tube, is attached to the caecum and is a frequent site of inflammation and infection (appendicitis). At the junction of the ileum and caecum, an *ileocaecal valve* functions to allow contents to pass in one direction only—from the ileum to the caecum.

The large intestine ascends the right side of the abdominal cavity from the caecum as the ascending colon and flexes at the undersurface of the liver to form the transverse colon. The descending colon passes down the left side of the abdomen and, since it takes an S-shaped course through the pelvis, becomes the sigmoid colon.

The mucosa of the large intestine has no villi but has many goblet cells which secrete mucus. The longitudinal muscle tissue is arranged in three strips that are shorter than the other tissues. This muscular arrangement along with the contraction of segments of circular muscle, especially the transverse colon, form small sacs along the tube which are referred to as *haustra* (see Fig. 17.1).

The rectum is a continuation of the sigmoid along the anterior surface of the sacrum and coccyx. It is about 6–7 inches long and contains vertical folds referred to as rectal columns. Each column contains an artery and vein. The veins frequently become varicosed, forming haemorrhoids.

The short terminal portion of the alimentary tube, the anal canal, opens onto the body surface at the anus. The opening between the rectum and the anal canal is controlled by the *internal anal sphincter*, which is not under the control of the will. The anus is con-

---

[1] Smith & Thier (1985), pp. 1212–1214.

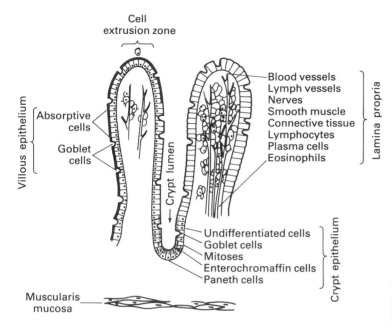

Cell
extrusion zone

Villous epithelium

Absorptive
cells

Goblet
cells

Crypt lumen

Blood vessels
Lymph vessels
Nerves
Smooth muscle
Connective tissue
Lymphocytes
Plasma cells
Eosinophils

Lamina propria

Undifferentiated cells
Goblet cells
Mitoses
Enterochromaffin cells
Paneth cells

Crypt epithelium

Muscularis
mucosa

Fig. 17.3 Schematic diagram of two sectioned villi and a crypt to illustrate the histological organization of the small intestinal mucosa.

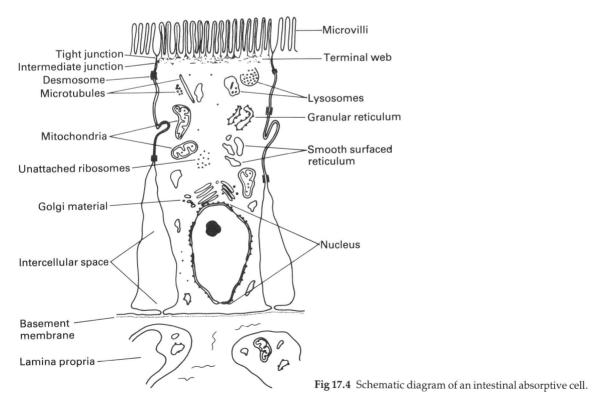

Microvilli

Tight junction
Intermediate junction
Desmosome
Microtubules

Terminal web

Lysosomes

Granular reticulum

Mitochondria

Smooth surfaced
reticulum

Unattached ribosomes

Golgi material

Nucleus

Intercellular space

Basement
membrane

Lamina propria

Fig 17.4 Schematic diagram of an intestinal absorptive cell.

trolled by the *external anal sphincter* which, after infancy, is under voluntary control.

PERITONEUM

The outer protective coat of the stomach and intestines is serous membrane and is known as the *visceral peritoneum*. The abdominal cavity is lined with serous membrane called the *parietal peritoneum*. A fan-like expanse is reflected off the posterior abdominal wall and extends to the intestine where it becomes continuous with the visceral peritoneum. This portion of serous membrane is known as the *mesentery*; it supports the intestine and transmits blood vessels, lymphatics and nerves. A sheet of peritoneum, the *great omentum*, is reflected off the stomach to lie like an apron in front of the intestines. The great omentum protects the intestines and, when infection or inflammation of the peritoneum (peritonitis) occurs, it makes an effort to wall off the affected area by surrounding it to prevent a spread of the infection. The *lesser omentum* is a fold of peritoneum extending from the liver to the stomach.

BLOOD SUPPLY TO THE ALIMENTARY CANAL

The mouth, tongue and pharynx derive their blood supply from the external carotid arteries via the lingual and external maxillary arteries. The oesophageal artery arises from the thoracic aorta. Three main arteries supply the stomach, the left, right and short gastric arteries. The left gastric is a branch of the coeliac which is a large, shorter artery arising from the abdominal aorta. The other two gastric arteries originate from the other main branches of the coeliac, the hepatic and splenic arteries.

The remainder of the tract is nourished by the superior and inferior mesenteric arteries, direct branches of the abdominal aorta.

The blood into which the digested food products are absorbed is carried by the superior and inferior mesenteric veins into the portal vein, which transmits it to the liver. This makes the food products immediately available to the liver for its functions.

Accessory structures of digestion

THE BILE SYSTEM AND PANCREAS

The biliary system and exocrine pancreas are important contributory structures in digestion and absorption (see Chapter 18).

DIGESTION

Digestion consists of mechanical and chemical processes. The mechanical processes involve the neuromuscular tissues of the alimentary tract and have as their purposes the movement of food through the tract, the mixing of it with digestive secretions, and the repeated breaking up of the food mass to bring more of it in contact with the absorptive surface. These processes include mastication, deglutition (swallowing), movements of the stomach and intestines, and defecation. The chemical processes are chemical reactions catalyzed by enzymes to reduce the food to simpler compounds.

The digestive enzymes are substances secreted by mucosal cells of the alimentary tract and by the associated digestive organs (pancreas and liver). Like all enzymes in the body they act as catalysts (i.e. they promote and speed up chemical reactions without becoming a part of them). All enzymes are specific and, in the case of the digestive enzymes, each is secreted only by cells in a certain area of the digestive system. They are classified according to the food they act upon. An enzyme which promotes the breakdown of protein is called a *proteolytic enzyme* or *peptidase*; one that acts upon starches is an *amylase*; and a fat-splitting enzyme is known as a *lipase*.

Digestion takes place within the lumen of the alimentary canal or the cells lining the tract. The principal reaction in chemical digestion is hydrolysis, which is the breaking up of a large molecule of a substance into smaller molecules by combining it with water. For example, in the digestion of cane sugar, one molecule of sugar and one molecule of water yields two molecules of simple diffusible glucose that can be absorbed:

$$C_{12}H_{22}O_{11} + H_2O \xrightarrow{\text{enzyme}} 2(C_6H_{12}O_6)$$

Most food undergoes several chemical reactions before it is reduced to a form that can be absorbed. The steps in the digestive breakdown of protein, carbohydrate and fat follow.

Protein → proteoses → peptones → polypeptides → amino acids

Seventy to 80% of protein digestion is intracellular therefore, only about 10–12% is broken down into amino acids within the intestinal lumen.[2]

Carbohydrate
    Starch (polysaccharide) → maltose → glucose
    Disaccharides
        maltose → glucose
        sucrose → glucose and fructose
        lactose → glucose and galactose
Fat → glycerol and fatty acids

The motility and secretions vary from one area of the digestive tract to another. In the following section, digestion is discussed as it occurs in each of the different parts of the alimentary tract.

---

[2] Davenport (1982), p. 205.

Motility, secretion and digestion in the mouth, pharynx and oesophagus

MOTILITY IN THE MOUTH, PHARYNX AND OESOPHAGUS

The mouth performs mastication and the initial part of swallowing. The pharynx and oesophagus are concerned only with swallowing.

Mastication

Most of the food entering the mouth undergoes biting and grinding by the teeth to reduce its size for swallowing and mixing with the saliva to produce a moist pulpy mass, called a bolus. Mastication is achieved by the contractions of the muscles of the lower jaw, lips, cheeks, and tongue. Movement of the lower jaw is responsible for the biting and grinding done by the teeth.

Deglutition

Deglutition is the term applied to the transmission of food and fluid from the mouth to the stomach and is commonly referred to as swallowing. When mastication is completed, the food is moved to the posterior oral cavity by the tongue and cheeks and is then forced into the pharynx. Certain reflexes then occur in rapid succession. Muscles in the walls of the pharynx contract, drawing the soft palate up and back and closing off the entrance to the nasal cavities. The larynx is raised, bringing its opening against the epiglottis and the base of the tongue, thus preventing the food from entering the respiratory tract. The upper oesophageal sphincter relaxes and food cannot re-enter the mouth, for the back of the tongue is raised to block the opening. The pressure exerted on the bolus by the tongue and pharyngeal constriction forces the food into the only open route, the oesophagus.

The reflex responses of the pharynx to the entrance of food or fluid may be depressed by local anaesthetic. To prevent aspiration following anaesthetization of the pharynx, food and fluid are withheld until the swallowing reflexes have returned. This also applies following laryngoscopy, bronchoscopy, oesophagoscopy, gastroscopy and surgery on the mouth or throat.

When the bolus enters the oesophagus, it stimulates the circular muscle of the section it is in and inhibits that of the portion immediately ahead. Thus, the food is squeezed out of the first section into the relaxed portion. A complex series of reflexes coordinated in the medulla of the brain are brought into play, producing a wave of alternating contractions and relaxations along the oesophagus. The wave of inhibition which precedes the bolus reaches the cardiac sphincter, causing it to open, and the bolus enters the stomach.

The more liquid the bolus, the more rapidly it travels through the oesophagus. The passage of food through the oesophagus may be aided by gravity unless the person is in an antigravitational position.

SECRETION AND DIGESTION IN THE MOUTH, PHARYNX AND OESOPHAGUS

Saliva is secreted by the salivary glands; added to it is a small amount of mucus produced by the mucous membrane of the oral cavity. The amount of saliva secreted varies from approximately 1–1.5 litres per day, depending on the quantity and quality of food taken. A greater volume of food requires an increased output of saliva, and appetizing foods also stimulate the output. The saliva is swallowed and much of the fluid is reclaimed by absorption. Any interference with swallowing or any condition that provokes loss of saliva from the mouth results in a considerable loss of body fluid, contributing to dehydration.

Saliva is usually slightly acidic with a pH of 6.6–6.9 and consists of:

Water (97–99%)
Mucin
Sodium, potassium, bicarbonate and chloride.
(The bicarbonate salts of saliva are responsible for the formation of most of the tartar on the teeth. The salts, when exposed to air, release carbon dioxide and the bicarbonate is transformed to an insoluble carbonate.)
Enzyme ptyalin
Organisms
Epithelial cells from the mucosa
Antibacterial agents

Functions of saliva

One of the functions of saliva is to moisten the food and lubricate the oral cavity in order to facilitate swallowing. Dry food is put into solution by saliva, making possible the taste sensation, since only food in solution reaches the taste buds which are recessed in small pits in the tongue. Speech is made more articulate when the oral structures are moist.

The enzyme ptyalin acts on starches, reducing them to maltose. This is the only chemical digestive function performed by the saliva. The action of ptyalin may be continued for a brief period in the stomach, as the saliva is swallowed with the food. Ptyalin is only effective in an alkaline or very mild acid medium; in the stomach it is inactivated by the presence of the hydrochloric acid.

Saliva has a cleansing effect; it washes away food particles and other debris. If these are allowed to accumulate, they could act as a culture medium for organisms. Patients who are not secreting the normal amount of saliva require frequent cleansing mouth care. Disorders and a lack of the natural antibacterial agents may lead to ulcers and tooth decay.

The salivary glands excrete certain substances from the blood into the saliva. Lead, sulphur and potassium iodide may be transferred to the saliva. Similarly, urea may be noticeable in the saliva of persons whose kidneys fail to excrete the normal amount of urea.

Finally, saliva has a role in relation to the water balance. The moisture of the mouth largely determines the sense of thirst. A reduction in salivary output occurs with dehydration and a sense of thirst accompanies the dry mouth. When the fluids are replenished, the mouth again becomes moistened by saliva and the sense of thirst is alleviated.

Regulation of salivary secretion. Control of the salivary glands is by the autonomic nervous system; each gland has both a parasympathetic and sympathetic nerve supply which deliver impulses from a salivary centre in the medulla of the brain stem. Sensory nerves conduct impulses from the mouth to the salivary centre to influence its action. The sensory impulses arise from taste and from pressure created by the presence of food or some instrument in the mouth. One is familiar with the experience of increased salivation when the dentist is working in the mouth.

Until recently, an increased output of saliva may have been considered a conditioned response to the sight, smell or thought of food. Current studies do not always support this notion.[3,4]

Parasympathetic innervation results in an increased volume of a watery secretion containing the enzyme ptyalin; sympathetic innervation causes a scanty flow of a thick, viscous saliva. The generalized sympathetic innervation associated with fright or nervousness and stress frequently produces a dry, 'sticky' mouth. Release of vasoactive intestinal polypeptide seems to complement the action of parasympathetic nerve stimulation in increasing salivation.[5]

No enzymes are secreted by the pharynx and oesophagus; therefore, no chemical digestion is attributed to these areas. The mucous membrane produces mucus that facilitates the movement of food in swallowing. The mucus also protects the mucosa from any abrasive effect the food might have upon it and from tissue digestion by gastric juice that might escape into the oesophagus.

There is an oesophagosalivary reflex that increases salivation. A mass of bolus pressing on the walls of the oesophagus for any length of time gives rise to sensory impulses, resulting in stimulation of the salivary glands. The increased volume of saliva which is swallowed is an effort to 'wash down' the mass. One sees this in the patient with cancer of the oesophagus who experiences the problem of excessive salivation. Intense salivation is also associated with nausea and vomiting and may act to lubricate the vomitus and facilitate the emesis.

Motility, secretion and digestion in the stomach

GASTRIC MOTILITY

The stomach retains the food and churns it about for a period of time until it undergoes certain chemical and physical changes. Each section of the stomach performs its own function. The fundus acts as a storage vessel by receptively relaxing with the entry of the food into the stomach. The body or corpus of the stomach contracts rhythmically about three times per minute to mix the food with enzymes, producing a mixture referred to as chyme. The antrum acts as a pump where waves intensify and circular peristaltic contractions propel the chyme toward the pylorus. The pylorus is narrow, therefore only a small portion of the contents is ejected into the duodenum with each peristaltic wave. The remainder of the pyloric content passes back into the body of the stomach.

Approximately 3–5 hours after the last meal, strong contractions which originate in the lower oesophagus and stomach, sweep the entire length of the small intestine at about 90 minute intervals. These waves of contractions are known as the interdigestive myoelectric complex. They expel undigested residue and seem to sweep debris along through the small intestines to the colon.

Gastric motility and emptying are regulated by gastric and duodenal factors and hormonal and nervous controls. The presence of food in the stomach stimulates volume-sensitive nerve receptors as well as chemical receptors. Volume stretches the stomach wall which increases contractility force. The presence of proteins stimulates the release of gastrin and other polypeptide hormones which increase motility and enhance the activity of the pyloric pump, promoting gastric emptying. At the same time, acid and enzyme secretion is stimulated. As the gastric content is liquefied, more chyme is forced into the duodenum.

The duodenum acts to brake the gastric motility and secretion, preventing overloading. Distension of the duodenum and the presence of increased acid or high fat content induces neural inhibition of gastric emptying and stimulates the release of duodenal hormones and secretions. These include cholecystokinin, vasoactive intestinal polypeptide and gastric inhibitory polypeptide which act in various ways to inhibit both gastric motility and secretion.

To summarize, gastric emptying is controlled by the volume and consistency of the stomach content, the effects of gastrin in stimulating motor functions, and by neural and hormonal feedback from the duodenum.

GASTRIC SECRETION AND DIGESTION

The gastric glands secrete a clear, colourless, slimy fluid of high acidity (pH 0.9–1.5) that contributes to chemical digestion and changes the food to a more fluid consistency.

[3] Davenport (1982), p. 110.
[4] Liang & Cascieri (1981), p. 1133.
[5] Lundberg, Anggard & Fahrenkrug (1981), p. 329.

The constituents of gastric juice are:
Water (97–99%)
Hydrochloric acid (0.2–0.5%)
Enzymes:
    pepsinogen (inactive pepsin)
    rennin
    gastric lipase
Inorganic salts of sodium, potassium and magnesium.
Haematopoietic or intrinsic factor (promotes absorption of Vitamin B_{12})
Mucus

The hydrochloric acid and enzymes are the substances concerned with chemical digestion. Pepsinogen is activated to pepsin by the hydrochloric acid and the initial breakdown of proteins occurs. Pepsin reduces proteins to proteoses and peptones. Rennin is a specific proteolytic enzyme that converts the soluble caseinogen of milk to insoluble paracasein. The paracasein, with the calcium of the milk, produces a curd, a more solid form that results in its retention in the stomach while it is digested by pepsin. Gastric lipase is produced in small amounts. Emulsified fats may undergo some reduction but fat digestion in the stomach is relatively insignificant.

The hydrochloric acid secreted by the parietal cells destroys many bacteria which are ingested with food. The acidity of chyme, due to the hydrochloric acid secretion, stimulates the secretion of the hormone secretin (prosecretin) by the duodenal mucosa. Secretin influences the pancreatic cells to release a fluid high in sodium bicarbonate.

Regulation of gastric secretion

The amount of gastric juice produced varies somewhat with the types of food taken, but with average meals, it is about 2 litres per day. With fasting, and during the night, the volume is reduced.

Secretion is influenced by mechanical, nervous and hormonal factors, and it is customary to describe gastric secretion as occurring in certain phases—the cephalic, gastric and intestinal phases. The *cephalic (psychic) phase* of gastric secretion occurs before the food reaches the stomach. When food is anticipated, tasted and chewed, sensory impulses from the mouth enter the central nervous system and result in parasympathetic innervation via vagus nerve fibres, stimulating the gastric glands to pour out their secretions. The more appetizing the food is, the greater will be the vagal innervation and the response of the gastric glands. Psychic stimulation by the thought, smell or sight of appetizing food may produce the same effect. Conversely, excessive sympathetic innervation depresses the gastric glands and secretion is reduced. Emotional disturbances such as worry, fear and grief result in a decrease in gastric secretion.

Food reaching the stomach further stimulates its secretion, producing what is known as the *gastric phase*. The food causes a direct mechanical stimu-

lation of the gastric glands and initiates sensory nerve impulses that are delivered via vagus nerve fibres to the medulla, resulting in return impulses, via vagal motor fibres that increase the activity of the gastric glands. Chemical stimulation is by a hormone, gastrin, that is released by the gastric mucosa into the blood. Distension of the stomach, particularly in the pyloric region, and certain foods, referred to as secretogogues, evoke the release of gastrin. Proteins, particularly meats, are high in secretogogues, which are soluble in water. Meat soups and broths increase gastric secretion and therefore are often used at the beginning of a meal in preparation for the food to follow.

The question has always arisen as to why the pepsinogen activated by the hydrochloric acid (pepsin) does not digest the gastric tissue. A natural mucosal resistance and the mucus secreted by the mucosal glands are thought to play an important role in protecting the surface. The gastric mucosal barrier may be broken down by some substances, such as ethyl alcohol, acetylsalicylic acid and bile acids. The mucosa repairs itself when the agent breaking the barrier is removed.[6]

Histamine which is produced, stored and released by enterochromaffin cells in the gastric mucosa, has been found to stimulate the parietal cells of the gastric glands, resulting in an increased output of hydrochloric acid. The gastric mucosal cells have a high histamine content. It is suggested that two types of histamine receptors, H_1 and H_2 are present, and the H_2 receptors initiate the release of histamine which stimulates the secretion of hydrochloric acid. The recent preparation of H_2 antagonists (e.g. cimetidine) aids in the treatment of ulcerative gastric disease by inhibiting histamine-stimulated acid secretion.[7] If the doctor finds it necessary to determine if the patient's cells are producing acid, or if he is lacking hydrochloric acid (achlorhydric), a histamine-like substance is injected and the gastric juice aspirated for analysis.

The *intestinal phase* of gastric secretion involves an increase in the concentration of various hormones which are associated with the passage of chyme from the stomach into the duodenum. The increased concentration of these stimulates pepsinogen and hydrochloric acid secretion.

Motility, secretions and digestion in the small intestine

MOTILITY OF THE SMALL INTESTINE

Food moves slowly through the small intestine so that digestion may be completed and the simpler molecules absorbed. The motor activities perform

[6] Davenport (1982), p. 138.
[7] Davenport (1982), p. 122.

three functions: food is mixed with bile and with pancreatic and intestinal secretions, the mass is broken up to bring it into contact with the absorptive surfaces, and the unabsorbed content is moved into the large intestine.

Rhythmicity and automaticity are two notable features of the muscle tissue of this division of the alimentary canal; waves of contractions move down the tract at an orderly rate, appropriate to the stage of digestion and absorption. Approximately 16 rhythmic contractions per minute occur in the duodenum and about 11 per minute in the ileum. Contractions of the longitudinal and circular layers of muscle tissue produce two major types of movement, namely, *segmentation* and *mixing*. Segmentation occurs with areas of the circular muscle contracting and dividing the intestine into a series of alternating constricted and relaxed areas, giving the tube the appearance of a string of sausages. The mass of food stimulates the circular muscle of the section it is in, while those areas behind and ahead remain relaxed. The content in the contracted area is divided into two segments; one is squeezed into the relaxed portion of the intestine ahead and the other is forced back into the relaxed area behind the constriction. The area of contracted circular muscle relaxes and contraction occurs in the previously relaxed areas. Segmentation serves to break up the mass of content so it is mixed with the digestive juice and so more of it is brought into contact with the absorptive surfaces.

Mixing of the chyme and intestinal juice and absorption are facilitated by oscillations of the villi of the mucosa. The slow mixing and segmentation movements push the food along the tract. Any residue of a meal is cleared by the first wave of the interdigestive myoelectric complex as it moves along the tract.

Peristalsis is a wave-like muscular activity consisting of a wave of inhibition followed by a wave of contraction. The advancing portion of the wave involves relaxation of an area of the circular muscle and contraction of the longitudinal muscle, producing a sac-like dilatation. The posterior part of the wave consists of contraction of the circular muscle, producing a constricted area in the tube. The peristaltic waves vary in intensity and in the distance they travel. Some go only a short distance while others pass over a long section, pushing the content much further along the tract. Those that traverse a considerable length of the tract may be referred to as peristaltic rushes.

The small intestine terminates with the ileocaecal valve, which guards the opening into the caecum. The pressure in the small intestine forces open the valve and the fluid passes through into the large bowel.

Muscular and villi activity of the small intestine is regulated by both an intrinsic and extrinsic mechanism. The intrinsic control is by two neural plexuses (networks). One, the myenteric or Auerbach's plexus, is located between the longitudinal and circular layers of muscle tissue. The second intrinsic plexus lies between the circular muscular tissue and the submucosa. The receptors associated with the plexuses are sensitive to stretch or irritation of the mucosa. The reflex response is contraction of the muscle tissues which initiates segmentation, peristalsis and movements of the villi.

The extrinsic mechanism concerned with the motility of the small intestine is parasympathetic innervation via vagal nerve fibres and sympathetic innervation through splanchnic nerves. Parasympathetic impulses stimulate the muscle tissue and conversely sympathetic innervation tends to slow motility. Autonomic nerve impulses are not essential to intestinal motility but do influence it. The recent finding of multiple types of peptidergic nerves in both the myenteric and submucosal plexus has led to intense study of their involvement in the control of motility, blood flow and secretion in health and disease.[8]

SECRETION IN THE SMALL INTESTINE

The digestive juice in the small intestine includes external pancreatic secretions and bile as well as the secretions of the intestinal mucosal glands.

Pancreatic juice and bile
Approximately 700–1200 ml of pancreatic secretions enter the duodenum daily and consist of:
Water (97–98%)
Enzymes:
amylase (amylolytic)
amylopsin
proteinases (proteolytic)
trypsinogen (inactive trypsin)
chymotrypsinogen (inactive chymotrypsin)
procarboxypeptidase (inactive carboxypeptidase)
lipase (lipolytic)
steapsin
Salts: principal ones are sodium and potassium bicarbonate and sodium alkaline phosphate.

Because of the salts, the pancreatic secretion is alkaline, with a pH of 7.5–8.4, and neutralizes the acid chyme.

For the secretion and composition of bile, see p. 586. Bile does not contain a digestive enzyme, but the bile salts do facilitate the digestion of fat by the pancreatic lipase.

Regulation of pancreatic enzyme and bile secretion. Pancreatic secretion into the intestine is regulated mainly by hormones secreted by the intestinal mucosa. The entrance of the acid solution chyme into the duodenum causes the release of secretin (prosecretin) into

---

[8] Polak & Bloom (1980), p. 46.

the blood. When secretin reaches the pancreas, it activates the cells to secrete a fluid high in sodium bicarbonate. Failure to produce this alkaline solution may result in damage to the duodenum by the chyme, which is strongly acid and contains pepsin. The duodenal mucosa is not as well protected by mucus as the gastric mucosa.

A second hormone, cholecystokinin-pancreo-zymin (CCK), is also produced by the duodenal mucosa when food enters from the stomach. It is carried to the pancreas where it causes the cells to produce a thicker solution rich in enzymes. CCK also produces contractions of the gallbladder and enhances the action of secretin stimulating the alkaline pancreatic fluid. Secretion of CCK by the duodenal mucosa is stimulated by the presence of fatty acids and amino acids in the chyme.

Some control of pancreatic secretion is also exerted via the vagus nerve and local peptidergic nerves. It is suggested that this is part of the gastric reflex. Sensory impulses are initiated by food in the stomach and result in vagal stimulation of the pancreatic cells to produce enzymes.

The liver cells secrete bile continuously, but the amount is increased when food is taken, especially fat and protein. It is thought that the hormone secretin, which excites the pancreas, may also cause an increased output of bile. Probably the most effective mechanism is stimulation of the liver cells by bile salts. The bile salts are absorbed from the intestine and activate the liver cells to form bile. As noted above, CCK causes the gallbladder to contract and bile flows into the common bile duct. It also causes relaxation of the sphincter of Oddi, and bile that has been stored in the gallbladder enters the intestine. Bile salts are then available to be absorbed in the ileum and recirculated to stimulate the liver cells. In a fasting state, bile does not enter the duodenum and the secretion of bile is decreased.

Intestinal juice (succus entericus)
The mucosa of the small intestine produces 2–3 litres of fluid per day. The solution, called succus entericus, is rich in bicarbonate, and the pH varies from 7.0–9.0, depending on the region of the intestine. The composition of succus entericus is:
  Water
  Salts
  Mucin
  Epithelial cells
  Enzymes:
    enterokinase, which activates the trypsinogen
      and probably procarboxypeptidase
    erepsin
    lipase
    sucrase
    maltase
    lactase
These enzymes act mainly on the glycocalyx (the sticky covering of the microvilli) and are shed into the intestinal lumen due to sloughing of the cells of the villi tips.

Regulation of secretion in the small intestine. The volume of fluid in the lumen of the small intestine is the net result of fluid between the mucosa and the serosa to maintain an isotonic state. Water moves passively with the active movement of material in either direction. The chyme entering the intestine from the stomach is hypertonic. Water diffuses from the serosa to the mucosa and into the hypertonic solution in the lumen. The presence of non-absorbable material in the lumen also moves water by osmosis. For example, mannitol, a non-absorbable sugar produces diarrhoea by holding water in the lumen of the intestine. Active absorption of nutrients and salts increases the net mucosal flow to the serosa, decreasing the fluid volume in the lumen.

Toxins such as those produced by a salmonella infection or cholera greatly increase water movement from the intestinal wall into the lumen as well as the active secretions of ions, producing diarrhoea, dehydration and metabolic acidosis.

Most of the polypeptide hormones located in the mucosa of the small intestine influence either secretion or absorption. Of note is the secretory action of a vasoactive intestinal polypeptide which is produced in excessive amounts by certain tumours and results in diarrhoea. The opioid peptide enkephalin has an absorptive action which is a powerful antidiarrhoea mechanism. This is probably the mechanism by which opiate drugs act to control diarrhoea.

DIGESTION IN THE SMALL INTESTINE

Most chemical digestion takes place in the small intestine.

Any polysaccharides which have not been reduced by ptyalin to maltase are acted upon by the pancreatic enzyme amylase (amylopsin). Disaccharidases (enzymes) reduce disaccharides to monosaccharides by hydrolysis, producing the simple absorbable sugars glucose, galactose and fructose. The intestinal enzyme maltase hydrolyzes maltose, lactase splits lactose, and sucrase breaks down sucrose. These enzymes are secreted by the absorptive cells and are an integral part of the sticky layer, the glycocalyx. The final splitting of the disaccharides takes place at the microvillus level.

Protein digestion initiated in the stomach by pepsin is completed by several pancreatic and intestinal enzymes. Trypsinogen is activated in the intestine by enterokinase and is then known as trypsin. Chymotrypsinogen is converted to the active form chymotrypsin by trypsin, and procarboxypeptidase becomes active carboxypeptidase. The proteolytic enzymes trypsin, chymotrypsin, carboxypeptidase and intestinal erepsin reduce proteins (polypeptides) to simpler forms of peptides. A considerable amount of ingested protein may be absorbed in the form of di- and tripeptides rather than amino acids.[9] The latter are more slowly absorbed than the peptides.

The breakdown of fats into glycerol and fatty acids is done mainly by the pancreatic lipase, steapsin. The intestinal lipase is less effective. Fat digestion is greatly facilitated by bile, which emulsifies the fat.

Fats are absorbed in a multistep process; the fat globules are emulsified by bile which allows the triglycerides to be reduced to monoglycerides and fatty acids. These soluble products form micelles, or small polymolecular colloidal particles, which move toward the microvilli where the fats move through the membrane and then are transferred to the systemic circulation via the lacteals of the lymphatic system.

Motility, secretion and digestion in the large intestine

MOTILITY OF THE LARGE INTESTINE

Contractions of the muscular tissue in the large intestine mix and knead the content as well as move it through the large intestine toward the terminal portion. The mixing and kneading movements are performed in the ascending and transverse colons and facilitate the absorption of water.

Propulsion in the colon occurs as a mass movement three or four times a day, moving the content toward the rectum. When the content reaches the distal portion of the colon, it is then moved into the rectum. As the food proceeds through the mouth, stomach and small intestine, a large amount of water is added to it. Much of this water is reclaimed by absorption in the colon which changes the consistency of the remaining content. The latter becomes a soft, solid mass referred to as faeces.[10]

Peristaltic movements in the large intestine are reflexly stimulated by the entrance of food into the stomach. This gastrocolic reflex, as it is termed, is usually most evident after breakfast when the stomach has been empty for a longer period of time. It results in the faeces being moved into the rectum, giving rise to the desire to defecate. Reflex stimulation originating with emotion, and distension or irritation of the colon, will also initiate movement.

Defecation is the term applied to the expulsion of faeces from the rectum and has both an involuntary and voluntary phase. Normally, the rectum remains empty until just before defecation. When faeces enter the rectum, the local distension and pressure give rise to sensory impulses that initiate reflex impulses to the internal anal sphincter and to the muscle tissue of the sigmoid colon and the rectum. The internal smooth muscle sphincter relaxes and the muscle tissue contracts, moving the faeces into the anal canal. The external anal sphincter is under voluntary control and must relax for evacuation of the rectum. Defecation may be assisted voluntarily by contracting the abdominal muscles and by forceful expiration with the glottis closed to increase the intra-abdominal pressure.

If the defecation reflex is ignored and the external sphincter is kept closed, the defecation desire soon wanes. Eventually, with repeated ignoring of the defecation reflex, local stimulation by distension and pressure is lost. Faeces accumulate in the rectum and lower colon, causing constipation.

Normally 8–10 hours are required for the chyme to pass through the small intestine and to reach the distal portion of the colon, where it accumulates until defecation. The content of the alimentary canal that is not absorbed may take 24 hours or longer to pass through the entire canal. Excessive mixing and local contractile motility of the colon lead to greater exposure of the material to the absorptive surface. This leads to dehydration of the contents and constipation. Material such as fibre holds water in the faeces and facilitates the mass movements. Lack of mixing contractions and diminished absorption combined with strong frequent propulsive contractile activity result in diarrhoea.

Faecal matter consists of unabsorbed food residue, mucus, digestive secretions (gastric, intestinal, pancreatic and liver), water and microorganisms. The water content is progressively reduced by absorption as the faeces move through the large intestine so that, normally, on elimination the stool is a formed mass. If the faeces are moved rapidly through the large intestine, less water is absorbed and the stool is unformed and liquid. If movement of the faeces and elimination are delayed, an excessive amount of water is absorbed and the stool becomes hard and dry.

SECRETION AND DIGESTION IN THE LARGE INTESTINE

The large intestine has no role in digestion. It secretes a large amount of viscous alkaline mucus that lubricates the faeces, facilitating their movement through the large bowel. The mucus also protects the mucosa from mechanical and chemical injury, and its alkalinity neutralizes acids formed by bacterial action, which is considerable in the colon.

Irritation of an area of the large intestine results in an increased output of mucus as well as an outpouring by the mucosa of large amounts of water and electrolytes in an effort to dilute and wash away the irritant. This causes the condition known as diarrhoea (frequent liquid stools). The loss of fluid and electrolytes may cause dehydration and an electrolyte imbalance.

INTESTINAL MICROORGANISMS

Many microorganisms inhabit the intestine, and

---

[9] Mathews (1977), p. 277.
[10] *Faeces* is the Latin word for dregs.

colon bacilli are present in large numbers. The tract is sterile at birth, but in a short time organisms which have been ingested with food are present in the intestine. These organisms are useful in that they synthesize vitamin K, which is essential to the production of prothrombin. A deficiency of vitamin K can result in uncontrollable haemorrhage. Intestinal bacteria also synthesize thiamine, riboflavin, and folic acid. The organisms normally found in the intestine are non-pathogenic to the tract but may cause disease if they are carried into other tissues.

Bacteria cause some fermentation and putrefaction of the intestinal content. The fermentation process breaks the content down into still simpler components and at the same time produces gas. The organisms may cause a breakdown of unabsorbed amino acids which may release poisonous substances such as histamine, indole, choline, ammonia, skatole and hydrogen sulphide. However, since this usually takes place in the large bowel, little of these toxic products are absorbed. If they are absorbed, the normal liver detoxifies them.

Absorption

Absorption is the movement of food, water, or drugs from the alimentary canal into the blood to make them available to the cells throughout the body. It is performed passively by the physicochemical processes of diffusion, osmosis and by active transport by the cells.

There are two channels by which food may be absorbed—the capillaries of the mucosa and the lacteals. That absorbed into the capillaries is carried via the portal vein to the liver. That absorbed into the lacteals is transported by the lymph to the thoracic lymphatic duct which empties into the junction of the subclavian and internal jugular veins. Water, salts, glucose, amino acids and some fatty acids and glycerol are absorbed into the capillaries. The larger proportion of the products of fat digestion is absorbed into the lacteals.

Like digestion, most absorption takes place in the small intestine. Its surface is especially adapted by the many circular folds in the mucous membrane to increase the surface area. The whole surface is also studded with millions of villi which contain epithelial mucosal cells that are specially adapted for both absorption and secretion. The network of capillaries and the central lymph channel of each villus take up much of the digested food.

ABSORPTION IN THE MOUTH

No food is absorbed from the mouth, but a few drugs may be taken into the blood through the buccal mucosa. Examples of these are glyceryl trinitrate and adrenaline.

ABSORPTION IN THE STOMACH

Absorption in the stomach is relatively negligible. The gastric mucosa does not actively transport food molecules across it but, if the concentration is high in the stomach (creating a considerable gradient between the blood and the stomach), glucose, water and electrolytes may be absorbed. Alcohol and some drugs are also absorbed from the stomach.

ABSORPTION IN THE SMALL INTESTINE

Minerals, vitamins, water, drugs, amino acids, simple sugars, fatty acids and glycerol are freely absorbed from the small intestine. Most absorption takes place in the upper part of the small intestine.

ABSORPTION IN THE COLON

Large amounts of water are absorbed in the colon. Approximately 500 ml of fluid pass from the small intestine into the colon daily. About 400 ml of water are absorbed from this, leaving 100 ml to be excreted in the faeces. Small amounts of glucose and salts are also absorbed by the large intestine, and a number of drugs may be administered by this channel. The absorptive capacity of the colon is seldom reached but water toxicity can be induced by excessive fluid introduced into the colon, especially in infants.

ABSORPTION OF VITAMINS

The water-soluble vitamins B complex and C are generally readily absorbed from the small intestine. The exception is vitamin B_{12}. For absorption of B_{12}, a substance called the intrinsic factor is necessary and is secreted by the mucosa of the stomach. A deficiency of the intrinsic factor or of vitamin B_{12} causes a deficiency in the production of mature red blood cells.

The fat-soluble vitamins A, D, E and K are absorbed from the small intestine if bile salts and pancreatic lipase are present.

PROTECTIVE AND IMMUNOLOGICAL FUNCTIONS OF THE GASTROINTESTINAL TRACT

The gastrointestinal tract is a continuity of the skin and is formed by special endothelial cells. The material it receives does not have to be sterile. Bacteria are found in most foods ingested, yet rarely do these bacteria invade the system. This is in part due to the pH in the stomach and to enzymatic degradation of the bacteria themselves.

It has been shown that the gastrointestinal tract has its own immune system and the immunoglobulins produced in these areas differ from those produced elsewhere. These lymphoid cells are formed from precursor cells located in the Peyer's patches in the small intestine, and produce an immunity against antigens which enter the gastrointestinal tract.[11] Oral poliomyelitis vaccine uses the immunological system of the gastrointestinal tract to produce local and systemic immunity to the poliomyelitis virus. Many persons with poliomyelitis exhibit systemic symptoms of poliomyelitis; others only manifest disturbances in the gastrointestinal tract.

Smith indicates that it is likely that the IgA antibodies found in breast milk are present through movement of the immunologically competent plasma cells of the intestine to the mammary glands.[11] These antibodies protect the infant who is unable to produce antibodies immediately after birth. As with the systemic immune system, allergic reactions can occur in the gastrointestinal tract of sensitized individuals. For example, certain seafoods may be the offender.

Nursing Process

Disorders and abnormal functioning of the gastrointestinal tract may be manifested by a wide variety of symptoms. Disturbances may occur in one or more functions of the tract (ingestion, digestion, absorption and elimination). The disorder may be of organic or psychological origin or may be secondary to dysfunction in another body system (e.g. vomiting in renal failure; diarrhoea in hyperthyroidism). Organic disorders may be neoplastic, inflammatory, vascular or traumatic. Stress or emotional disturbances (e.g. anxiety, grief) may cause dysfunction within the tract. Impaired function of a component part of the tract may be reflected in secondary problems, because all body systems are dependent on the nutritional supply and elimination of waste provided by the functions of the gastrointestinal tract.

ASSESSMENT

History

A patient history relevant to the functioning of the gastrointestinal tract includes: (1) eating pattern—food intake, eating habits, factors affecting eating and responses to food; (2) past history of disorders of the gastrointestinal tract and the treatment (prescribed or non-prescribed); and (3) bowel elimination pattern.

Eating pattern

Food intake. If the patient is well enough and responsible enough, his food intake may be determined by his own verbal description of what is taken or by having the patient list the food taken in the last 24 hours. This method of assessment is subject to error as the patient may list what he thinks he ought to have consumed rather than stating what he actually ate. Recording a patient's history is usually undertaken by a dietitian, or (increasingly) a nurse. It includes breakfast, lunch, dinner, snacks and nonessential foods such as alcohol and coffee. If more specific information is required, the outpatient may be asked to record his total food intake for a 3–7 day period while carrying out usual daily activities.

The analysis of the food intake includes an estimate of the total calories consumed; this is considered in relation to the patient's activities, and whether the diet includes the required amounts of the various essential foods. For example: Does the patient consume adequate milk or milk products to meet the requirements for his age? Does the patient receive four servings of fruit and vegetables daily and are at least one green and one yellow vegetable included? Is one serving of citrus fruit included? Are two or more servings of protein foods (meat, poultry, fish or eggs) taken? Are four servings of bread or cereal incorporated into the daily diet?

Eating habits. The significance of food is not the same for everyone. Having an understanding of what food means to the patient and his accustomed eating habits and rituals helps the nurse to plan care that is patient-centred as well as therapeutic. Data include usual meal-times, the social milieu in which eating occurs, rituals or lack of rituals that accompany eating, and if meals are considered pleasant social events or if the patient eats alone.

Who prepares the food and does the shopping are also determined. The patient is questioned as to whether changes in eating habits have occurred.

Factors influencing nutrition. Important determining factors in the patient's food intake are economic status and the living and cooking arrangements. Social, ethnic and religious customs also greatly influence diet and eating habits. The history should record likes and dislikes, and the patient may be asked to list dislikes and the foods that 'disagree with him'. Known food allergies are also recorded.

Physical and emotional stress produce various gastrointestinal changes. An effort is made to learn how the patient usually responds to stress and whether it affects his eating pattern.

Responses to food. The patient is questioned about his experience with and feelings about taking food. Some significant adverse responses to be noted include: no appetite; disagreeable taste; difficulty in chewing or swallowing; nausea, vomiting or regurgitation of food; heartburn; excessive gas after eating; a bloated and distended feeling; pain or discomfort before, during or after eating; and fear

---

[11] Smith & Thier (1985), p. 213.

of eating. It is important to know if the patient's weight has changed and, if so, the loss or gain. If any of these symptoms occur, detailed data are collected as to the severity, frequency, duration and pattern of occurrence (i.e. Do certain foods or circumstances precipitate them?) Information is elicited as to what action was taken to relieve the symptoms.

Past history
The data include information about: previous surgery; in particular, abdominal and dental procedures.
- Previous significant acute or chronic illnesses, which include peptic ulcer, gallbladder disorder, jaundice, recurring diarrhoea, cancer or anaemia
- Any family history of gastrointestinal disorders
- Any psychiatric- or stress-related disorders and how these were manifested
- Prescribed special diet and medications which the patient has been receiving and the responses to them.
  Self-prescribed drugs and diet
  Ingestion of alcohol and acetylsalicylic acid (aspirin)

Bowel elimination pattern
The patient's usual pattern of bowel elimination is identified: the frequency, usual time and general characteristics (consistency, colour, volume and odour) of the stools are indicated. Questions are raised as to whether pain, discomfort or unusual effort is experienced with bowel elimination and if mucus or blood has ever been present. If blood has been noted, the patient is asked whether it was bright red, dark red, superficial or mixed. The practice of dietary adjustment, the use of stool softeners, laxatives, enemas or digital stimulation are recorded in the history.

An important aspect related to elimination is the patient's perception of normal and abnormal bowel elimination and his interpretation of the changes that have occurred.

Physical examination

Assessment of the patient with a disorder of the alimentary canal is usually carried out by the doctor, although the nurse will assist in certain aspects of the examination. The assessment includes:
1 Noting the patient's height, weight, skin-fold thickness and mid upper-arm circumference measurement.
2 Examination of the oral cavity and lips, skin condition, abdomen, anus and rectum; this involves inspection, palpation, auscultation and/or percussion.

Height and weight
The patient's height and weight are measured, using reliable, calibrated instruments, and are compared with the normal range for his age and sex.

Skinfold thickness
A general assessment of subcutaneous body fat may be made on obese or undernourished patients. Calibrated callipers (such as Harpenden callipers) may be used to measure skinfold thickness. The skin is pinched up, being careful to avoid muscle tissue, and the callipers are applied. Measurements are usually taken over the triceps, sub-scapular region and the upper abdomen.

For further information about methods of nutritional assessment, see Grant et al (1981).[12] Results are compared with the normal value according to age and sex.[13]

Measurements of circumferences
Mid-arm circumferences provide information about the individual's musculature and aid in an indirect estimate of protein and caloric deficiencies. The measurements are usually made with a tape-measure over the mid-point of the upper arm. Compression of the muscle tissue is avoided. Tables of normal values are available and serve as gross comparisons of patient circumferences.[14] When using these tables allowances must always be made for individual differences.[15]

Oral cavity and lips
A tongue depressor and light are needed to examine the oral cavity and tongue for lesions, sordes, dehydration, bleeding and discoloured areas (e.g. leucoplakia). Whether or not the tongue is coated or is abnormally smooth is noted. The condition of the teeth and gums (gingivae) are also checked. The former are inspected for jaggedness and caries, and the gums for excessive redness, soft puffiness, recession and bleeding. The odour of the breath is noted to determine if it is offensive or is characteristic of that associated with a specific condition. For example, the odour of acetone may be associated with acidosis or starvation, that of urea with renal insufficiency and that of alcohol with alcoholism. Observation of the mouth may elicit significant information as to the patient's state of hydration and nutrition as well as manifestations of systemic disease and local disorders. The tongue and mouth are the first sites to reflect dehydration; the mouth and tongue become dry and the latter may be furred. Dryness in some instances may be a side-effect of a drug that is being administered. Bleeding of the gums may indicate a deficiency of vitamin C or an infection. Excessive salivation (sialorrhoea) may be associated with a vitamin B deficiency or certain medications or a neoplasm in the mouth or neighbouring structure.

The lips are scrutinized for lesions (e.g. lumps,

---

[12] Grant, Coster & Thurlow (1981), p. 437–463.
[13] Malasanos et al (1981), p. 104–105.
[14] Malasanos et al (1981), pp. 106 & 107.
[15] Jelliffe (1966).

cracks, blisters, ulcers), dryness and abnormal colour and palpated if necessary to determine the presence and extent of a mass.

Abdomen
The doctor performing the examination requires the patient to lie on his back with arms at his sides, a pillow under his head and knees flexed. The latter promote relaxation of the abdominal muscles. The patient is protected from unnecessary exposure and chilling and is advised of what is to take place.

Observation of the abdomen will yield information regarding contour, distension, discoloured areas, unusual pigmentation, masses, symmetry and movement with respirations. Scars may indicate the site of previous surgery or trauma. Hernias may also be detected.

The patient is also assessed to determine whether he is suffering from any abdominal pain or tenderness. The nature of any discomfort is a guide to the diagnosis. Prominent dilated veins which may indicate obstruction of the portal circulation as a result of liver disease and pulsation of an artery are recorded. The latter might be due to an aortic aneurysm. Rarely, an excessive amount of hair may be encountered and is usually associated with an adrenocortical disturbance.

Auscultation of the abdomen is carried out by the doctor and is used to assess peristalsis by listening for bowel sounds. It should precede percussion and palpation as these activities may increase bowel motility. The diaphragm of the stethoscope is used. Normal bowel sounds are high pitched, gurgling sounds. One should listen for a period of 5 minutes, since normal peristaltic activity occurs at intervals of 5–15 seconds in the small intestine. An absence of bowel sounds occurs in peritonitis and paralytic ileus. Excessive activity may occur in an area in an effort to overcome an obstruction. Palpation or movement of a part may produce a splashing sound (succussion), indicating fluid and air within.

Abnormal vascular sounds (bruits) may also be detected by abdominal auscultation using the bell-shaped end on the stethoscope. For example, an aortic aneurysm or a tortuous vessel compressed by a tumour or enlarged viscus produces a bruit.

Percussion is most often used to determine the presence of gas or air in the intestine, detect urinary bladder distension or identify the location and size of solid viscera. The fingers of one hand are placed on the abdomen while the fingers of the other hand are used to tap the second finger. A hollow resonant sound (tympany) is heard if there is gas; a dull, flat sound reflects density or solid tissue such as liver, spleen or neoplasm.

In palpation of the abdomen, a very light pressure is applied at first, using the palmar surfaces of the fingers which are extended and together. The examiner proceeds systematically over the four quadrants of the abdomen. A superficial mass, which may be distended viscera, areas of tenderness and resistance offered by abdominal muscles may be detected. If tenderness is elicted by gentle palpation over McBurney's point,[16] appendicitis is suspected (see Fig. 17.5). Rebound tenderness following the abrupt release of palpation pressure on the abdominal wall is associated with peritoneal inflammation.

When the entire abdomen has been palpated superficially, deep palpation may be used to identify deeper-lying tenderness and to obtain information as to the size and mobility of a mass and the enlargement or position of an organ (e.g. locating the lower border of the liver and determining if the spleen is enlarged). Normally, the lower edge of the liver lies just above the lower right costal margin. If it extends below, it is enlarged. Normally, only the lower tip of the spleen is palpable on deep inspiration but if it is enlarged it is readily identified by deep palpation.

Anus and rectum
The patient is placed in the left lateral position with the knees flexed for examination of the anus and rectum. The knee position may be used; the patient is prone with the shoulders and head resting on the bed or examining table and the knees flexed raising the hips at a 75–80 degree angle.

The buttocks are spread with both hands to permit inspection of the exterior anal surface. Skin pigmentation, moisture, rashes, lesions, scars, external haemorrhoids or fistula are noted and described. The presence of external haemorrhoids, polyps, fissures or rectal prolapse may be identified by asking the patient to take a deep breath and bear down or strain as for a bowel movement. The skin of the pilonidal area is inspected for dimples, inflammation or sinus opening.

Examination of the anus and rectum permits assessment of the anorectal area, the male prostate gland, inguinal area and some lower pelvic structures. A gloved index finger is lubricated and inserted slowly and gently through the anal sphincter as the patient strains down relaxing the sphincter. The finger is rotated to feel the external sphincter and muscle ring and the wall of the lower rectum. The sphincter tone, any tenderness and the presence of nodules are noted. The male prostate gland lies anterior to the rectum and can be palpated through the mucosal wall, as can the female cervix.

Diagnostic tests

Except for the mouth, which is readily accessible to viewing and palpation, diagnosis of disorders of the

---

[16] *McBurney's point* lies in the lower right quadrant approximately two inches from the right anterior spine of the ileum and corresponds to the area in which the appendix is usually located.

digestive system are rarely made without the assistance of various investigative procedures. These include: (1) blood studies; (2) x-ray examinations and scans; (3) endoscopy; (4) oesophageal function studies; (5) gastric secretory tests; (6) exfoliative cytotocrit, 40–50% (males), and 37–47% (females).

BLOOD STUDIES

Leucocyte count
An increase in the number of white blood cells (leucocytosis), particularly neutrophils, may indicate infection and an acute inflammatory process. This test is of significance in conditions such as appendicitis, acute enteritis, colitis and acute gallbladder disease (cholecystitis). Normal: leucocyte count: $4–11 \times 10^9$ per litre µl)

Erythrocyte count, haemoglobin concentration and haematocrit
A deficiency in the number of red blood cells and in the amount of haemoglobin may indicate the loss of blood or nutritional deficiency and provide information as to the patient's condition. Normal: erythrocytes $4.5–6.5 \times 10^{12}$ litres (males) and $3.8–5.8 \times 10^{12}$ litres (females); haemoglobin, 13–18 g/dl (males) and 12–15 g/dl (females).
The haematocrit may be determined to indicate the volume percentage of erythrocytes. Normal: haematocrit, 40–50% (males), and 37–47% (females).

Bleeding time and prothrombin time
Although bleeding time is not routinely carried out, both bleeding time and prothrombin time can be important if there are indications of haemorrhage. An increase in either predisposes the individual to a greater loss of blood. Normal: bleeding time, 2–5 minutes; prothrombin time, 11–15 seconds (usually recorded as a ratio–normal 1:1).

DIAGNOSTIC X-RAY TECHNIQUES AND FLUOROSCOPY

Radiological examination is a very valuable procedure in diagnosing disorders of the digestive system, particularly those of the alimentary canal. A radiopaque substance, barium sulphate, may be given by mouth ('barium swallow or barium meal'), and fluoroscopic studies are made and x-ray pictures taken as it passes through the oesophagus, stomach and intestines. The rate at which it moves through the tract, and outlines of the various parts are studied. When the barium is followed by a series of x-rays taken at intervals of several hours the procedure may be referred to as a gastrointestinal x-ray series.
The patient who is to have a barium swallow usually has a light evening meal and then nothing but sips of water until several hours after he has received the barium the next morning. As soon as the radiologist indicates that the patient may have a meal, it should be served promptly. The patient may

be very tired and may be experiencing weakness and discomfort because of the lack of food.
Following the taking of the barium, and when the first studies of the series are completed, the patient is offered a mouthwash, since the barium is chalky and clings to the oral mucosa. When the series is completed, which may be the day after the barium was administered, the patient is instructed to increase his fluid intake to promote the elimination of the barium. A mild laxative or a cleansing enema may be needed to relieve constipation and prevent faecal impaction and considerable discomfort.
X-ray examination of the large intestine and rectum is done by giving an enema of the barium solution. In some instances, an air contrast barium enema study may be done; this involves the introduction of air as well as barium to increase visualization of the mucosal surface of the colon. The lower bowel has been emptied previously by the administration of a laxative and a cleansing enema. Specific directions as to which laxative and enema solution are to be used and the time they are to be administered should be received from the x-ray department or the attending doctor. Food may be restricted to some extent for 18–24 hours preceding the barium enema. A low residue diet may be given the day before the enema. On the day of examination only clear fluids are allowed. If the patient is thought to have an intestinal obstruction, he will be fasted prior to the examination.
The patient receives an explanation as to why the food is withheld. Also, he is advised as to what will happen when he goes to the x-ray department and the importance of his retaining the barium until the necessary studies and films are made.
The barium enema is given in the x-ray room, and its progress through the rectum and colon are observed by fluoroscopy. X-ray films are also made to be studied later. Provision is made for the expelling of the enema, and then more films are made. The fluid intake is increased following the procedure and a mild laxative may be prescribed to ensure complete elimination of residual barium.

Computerized axial tomography (CAT) scan
This non-invasive examination of the abdomen is useful to locate neoplasms (benign, primary and metastatic), abscesses and cysts by providing more specific information about changes in tissue density than is available with the standard x-ray procedures. A timed series of x-rays are passed through the body at different angles as the x-ray machine revolves in a half circle over the abdomen or part being examined. The images produced are recorded immediately on a detector and passed to a computer. The amount of x-rays absorbed by different tissues and fluid is then computed.
Since the amount of radiation passing through to the detector is influenced by the density of the substance through which it passes, the image reflects

varying density in areas of tissue or body fluids. The dark, shaded and light areas on the image reflect the density gradients and are compared with the normal. The computer print-out can be transferred to a film as a permanent record.

Preparation of the patient for the scan includes an explanation of what will take place. The person will be required to lie still during the scan. The investigation is not painful and normal activities may be resumed immediately after the test. It may be done on an outpatient basis. An abdominal or *total body* scan requires an empty gastrointestinal tract. Food and fluids are withheld for 6–8 hours preceding the test. A laxative or enema may also be prescribed.

ENDOSCOPY

The introduction of the fibreoptic endoscopes has made it possible to view the oesophagus, stomach, duodenum, colon and rectum more thoroughly. Their flexibility facilitates passage of the endoscope and more efficient examination, with much less trauma and discomfort for the patient. Two bundles of flexible, very fine glass fibres are carried in the shaft. One bundle transmits light which illuminates the organ being viewed, and the second transmits an image back to the operator. A tube in the shaft makes it possible to inflate the area being viewed, eradicating folds so that the complete surface may be seen. A camera may be attached for taking pictures of a lesion or of an area that requires further study. Instruments may also be passed through the shaft to obtain specimens for biopsy or to coagulate a site of gastrointestinal bleeding. Specimens and pressure recording from the pancreatic and bile ducts can also be obtained. Radiopaque dyes may be injected for x-ray visualisation of the pancreatic and biliary ducts.

Oesophagoscopy and gastroscopy

The oesophagus may be examined and a biopsy specimen obtained by *oesophagoscopy* if the patient has complained of dysphagia, gastric reflux or regurgitation, or haematemesis. Oesophagoscopy is useful in localizing bleeding and is also used to remove a foreign body or a bolus that has lodged in the oesophagus.

Gastroscopy is usually used to obtain more detailed information about a lesion (e.g. ulcer) that has been identified as being present by previous barium x-ray. A biopsy is taken and pictures may be made of the lesion. It may also be used to assess the healing of an ulcer.

The improvement in endoscopic instruments has made it possible in some instances to arrest haemorrhage by the direct application of electrocautery or a haemostatic preparation to the bleeding site.

The gastroscope may be passed through the pylorus to examine the duodenum. The ampulla of Vater may be cannulated and viewed, and a radiopaque dye injected to demonstrate the pancreatic and common bile ducts (cholangiopancreatograph). Endoscopic examination may also be extended into the jejunum.

Nursing care in oesophagoscopy and gastroscopy. Preparation for either of these diagnostic procedures should begin with an explanation to the patient of what to expect. The doctor may have described the examination and its values, but the patient will most likely still have questions. The nurse should have sufficient understanding of the procedure to be able to answer the patient's questions judiciously.

The patient is advised that he will be taken to the endoscopy unit or to the operating theatre for the examination. A written consent for the procedure is obtained. The oesophagus and the stomach must be completely empty. No food or fluid is given for 6–8 hours before the procedure. In gastroscopy, the doctor may request a gastric lavage to be done several hours before the examination in patients in whom some pyloric obstruction is suspected. The teeth are cleaned and a mouthwash provided before the procedure; dentures and jewellery are removed and kept safe.

A sedative such as pethidine may be administered 30–60 minutes before the scheduled time or an analgesic may be administered intravenously during the procedure. The patient empties his bladder before leaving his room to avoid such need during the procedure.

The pharyngeal area is sprayed with a local anaesthetic before the gastroscope or oesophagoscope is introduced. A general anaesthetic may be given in the case of a child or, rarely, it may be used for a nervous adult in order to get better relaxation. A nurse remains beside the patient to give reassurance and support during the procedure and to assist with positioning. The patient is unable to speak when the endoscope is in position. In oesophagoscopy, the patient's head and shoulders are extended over the head of the table. In gastroscopy, a lateral position may be used.

Following the examination, the patient is allowed to rest. All food and fluids are withheld until the effect of the local anaesthetic has worn off and the gag reflex returns (usually 4–6 hours). Before giving any fluid, the reflex may be tested by gently touching the back of the throat with an applicator or spoon. The patient may complain of a sore throat or soreness in midchest. Warm fluids may be soothing and may provide some relief. Any expectoration or vomiting of blood or severe pain should be reported promptly to the doctor.

Colonoscopy

The flexible fibreoptic colonoscope has made possible the visualization of the complete colon, the taking of a biopsy and pictures of a lesion and the removal of polyps. Insufflation of air is used during the procedure to distend the bowel, permitting better visualization.

Nursing care in colonoscopy. The patient is advised of the purpose of the examination and what to expect and is asked to sign a statement giving consent. The bowel must be absolutely clean. The patient is usually admitted 1 or 2 days before the colonoscopy and given a low residue or clear-fluids only diet. On the day of the examination only a cup of black tea is allowed. Laxatives are given for 2 days prior to the colonoscopy to ensure that the bowel is empty. The regimen is modified if the patient is suffering from acute colitis or rectal bleeding. The patient is expected to stay overnight in the hospital after the examination.

The patient is told that it will be helpful during the examination to take deep breaths with his mouth slightly open and to relax the abdominal muscles. Sedation (pethidine or diazepam) may be given 30 minutes–1 hour before the scheduled colonoscopy, or an intravenous infusion may be started and diazepam (Valium) or pethidine administered intravenously during the procedure. A general anaesthetic is not given because the patient is requested to indicate pain during the examination. The patient is usually placed in the recumbent position on his left side and the nurse remains at the patient's head, providing necessary support.

Following the colonoscopy, the patient is allowed to rest and receives food and fluids. The patient is observed for signs of bleeding, pain and abdominal tenderness and rigidity. If polyps were removed, a specific directive is received from the doctor as to the patient's diet. The intake may be restricted to fluids for a period of time, and then a low-residue diet is gradually introduced.

Sigmoidoscopy and proctoscopy
A direct examination of the anal canal, the rectum and the sigmoid colon may be made by means of a sigmoidoscope. Proctoscopy is direct viewing of the rectum and anal canal by means of a proctoscope.

Nursing care in sigmoidoscopy and proctoscopy. These examinations may be performed in the doctor's surgery or in the ward treatment room of the hospital. A tissue specimen (biopsy) may also be obtained at the same time.

An explanation of the procedure is given to the patient in which he is advised of the position that he will be required to assume. The knee-chest and the left lateral are the positions commonly used. The lower bowel should be empty; cleansing enemas are usually given 2–3 hours before the scheduled time. A low-residue diet may be prescribed for the preceding day. The patient is required to sign a consent form.

A nurse remains with the patient to assist with the positioning and provide support. Unnecessary exposure should be avoided by adequate drapes. In the knee-chest position the patient lies face down and draws his knees up so that his weight is borne by the chest and knees. The feet are extended over the end of the table, arms at the sides or at sides of the head, and the head is turned to one side. In the left lateral or Sims' position the lower limbs are flexed, with the right one being drawn up further than the left. Suction is made available to remove any secretion or fluid faeces that interfere with visualization of the bowel mucosa.

After the examination, the anal region is cleansed and the patient is allowed to rest. The nurse may be responsible for seeing that the tissue specimen is placed in the appropriate container, correctly labelled and delivered to the pathology laboratory.

OESOPHAGEAL FUNCTION STUDIES

These studies include the determining of lower oesophageal sphincter pressure, oesophageal swallowing waves, the presence of gastric reflux, oesophageal acid clearance and simulation of gastro-oesophageal reflux.

The patient fasts prior to the tests which are performed in a specially equipped room. Three tubes, the ends of which are 5 cm apart, are swallowed by the patient and passed into the stomach. The tubes are slowly pulled back and the lower oesophageal sphincter pressure is recorded (normal 10–20 mmHg). The patient is asked to swallow and the pattern of the peristaltic waves is recorded on a graph. Normal swallowing produces synchronized and propulsive peristaltic waves in the oesophagus. When spasm is present strong, asynchronized, non-propulsive waves are demonstrated.

The tubes are returned to the stomach and hydrochloric acid (HCl) is instilled through them. The oesophageal pH is measured through a fourth tube inserted into the oesophagus. Acid reflux is identified by a drop in the pH in the oesophagus. The tubes are then raised into the oesophagus and HCl is instilled. The number of swallows required to clear the acid are determined.

The Bernstein test is then performed. HCl and saline are alternately instilled into the oesophagus in an attempt to reproduce the symptoms of gastro-oesophageal reflux. Complaints of heartburn during instillation of the acid indicate a positive test.

The procedure is explained to the patient before the tests and during each step of the studies. Sedation is not administered as it may alter the lower oesophageal sphincter pressures and patient responses.

GASTRIC SECRETORY TESTS

Common gastric function tests used in the investigation of patients with symptoms of gastrointestinal disease include the measurement of the volume of secretions over a stated period and the determination of HCl secretion under basal conditions and then in response to a gastric stimulant. Gastric analysis in which a quantitative estimation is required involves the use of a nasogastric tube to aspirate the gastric contents. If the test is done only to determine whether HCl is being secreted or not, aspiration of the gastric contents is unnecessary.

Analysis of gastric contents
A fasting period of 8–10 hours precedes the test and the patient is instructed not to smoke, as smoking stimulates gastric secretion. Anticholinergic drugs (e.g. propantheline bromide) are also withheld for 24 hours prior to the test as they inhibit the histamine stimulation of gastric acid secretion. A tube is passed into the stomach and the gastric content is aspirated by a syringe. The volume of this aspirate is noted, recorded and labelled for determination of the acid concentration.

Following this initial specimen, the directions may be to aspirate the gastric secretion at intervals of 15 minutes for 1 hour. Each specimen is placed in a separate tube and numbered according to the order in which it is collected. These specimens provide information about the *basal secretory activity*[17] of the stomach.

Occasionally, this fractional analysis procedure to evaluate secretory function includes the parenteral administration of a secretory stimulant such as pentagastrin, given intramuscularly, or (less frequently) insulin, given subcutaneously. The drug is administered after the initial aspiration. Aspiration specimens are then collected at intervals of 15 minutes for one hour.

If insulin is used as a secretory stimulant, the patient is observed closely for signs of hypoglycaemia (insulin shock). Complaints of nervousness, hunger pains, weakness or faintness or signs of cold, clammy perspiration should be reported promptly. The doctor may start an intravenous infusion of normal saline before the insulin is given so that 50% glucose may be given without delay if hypoglycaemia develops.

The normal basal gastric secretion is 30–70 ml/h and the HCl production (basal acid output, BAO) is 2–5 mmol/h during the resting state. The normal maximum acid output (MAO) in response to a secretory stimulant is 10–20 mmol/h.[18]

Achlorhydria indicates a deficiency in the gastric secretion of HCl. The term is applied when the pH of the gastric content is more than 6 following the administration of a secretory stimulant. Achlorhydria may be associated with cancer of the stomach, chronic gastritis, gastric ulcer or pernicious anaemia.

Hyperchlorhydria is a term used to describe an excessive secretion of HCl. An increase in acid secretion is seen in duodenal ulcer and the Zollinger–Ellison syndrome.

Serum gastrin level
Gastrin is a polypeptide hormone secreted by cells in the pylorus which stimulates the secretion of gastric acid and pepsin. An excessive release of gastrin may be associated with tumours of non-beta cell/islets in the pancreas (see Zollinger–Ellison syndrome p. 539). Normal serum gastrin levels are 40–150 ng/l.

Nightly gastric aspiration
When the patient has partial pyloric obstruction, the doctor may order a nightly aspiration. The patient receives his prescribed diet during the day; then, at about 10 p.m. his stomach content is aspirated and measured. The amount of food residue and secretions in the stomach at this time gives the doctor information as to the severity of the obstruction. It also relieves the patient of the sense of fullness, pain and discomfort resulting from the overdistended stomach and prevents vomiting.

Analysis of gastric content or vomitus
Examination of a specimen of vomitus or aspirated gastric content may be made to detect the presence of blood, bile or organisms (e.g. tubercle bacillus).

STOOL EXAMINATION

A stool specimen may be examined in the investigation of disorders of the digestive system for blood, urobilinogen, parasites, organisms or specific food residue such as fat. A small amount of stool is removed on a tongue depressor to the appropriate container (a waxed cardboard container with a lid). If the examination is for parasites, the specimen is kept warm and must be delivered to the laboratory promptly. If an enema is necessary to obtain a stool specimen, the solution used is clear water or normal saline.

When anything unusual is noted about a patient's stool, such as the presence of blood, excessive mucus or parasites, a specimen of the stool should be sent to the laboratory; a detailed description is recorded and the doctor notified.

LAPAROSCOPY

Rarely, an endoscope is introduced into the peritoneal cavity to examine its contents. A small area of the abdominal wall is surgically prepared as for any surgery, a local anaesthetic is introduced into the abdominal tissue and a small incision is then made through which the laparoscope is passed. The procedure is performed under strict surgical asepsis. A biopsy or a specimen of fluid may be obtained.

Following the examination, the wound is surgically dressed and the patient is observed for signs of bleeding or visceral trauma.

---

[17] *Basal secretion* is the secretion produced during a fasting period and in which the patient has received no secretory stimulant.
[18] Pagana & Pagana (1982), p. 41.

EXFOLIATIVE CYTOLOGY

In this test cells shed from the gastric mucosa are examined to determine if they are normal or manifest malignant changes. The cells are obtained by lavaging the stomach through a gastric tube (e.g. Levin tube) with normal saline. The patient is required to fast for the 6–8 hours preceding the lavage. The volume of lavage solution is indicated by the doctor or laboratory. All the aspirate is sent for analysis.

Manifestations of disorders of the alimentary canal

The signs and symptoms depend largely on the location of the disorder in the gastrointestinal tract as well as the nature of the aetiological factor. In some instances, some disorders cause similar disturbances in function—that is, several manifestations that develop are non-specific (e.g. nausea and vomiting, abdominal pain). Frequently a disturbance of function in the alimentary tract is secondary to a disorder in another part of the body. For example, some disorders of the brain may be manifested by vomiting or difficulty in swallowing; diarrhoea may be due to some medications. Some persons readily experience some malfunctioning of the gastrointestinal system coincidental with some form of stress. The patient may worry about the symptoms, creating stress which contributes to perpetuation of the dysfunction.

The patient whose medical investigation rules out organic and structural disease still requires the nurse's understanding support and must be observed for emotional stress that may be the basis of his problem.

PAIN

Pain caused by a digestive disorder may be due to strong contractions of muscle tissue, stretching of a viscus, chemical or mechanical irritation of the mucosa, inflammation of the peritoneum, or direct irritation or pressure on associated nerves. It may occur in any part of the abdomen or in some instances is referred to a site remote from its origin. For example, pain arising from a peptic ulcer or from the biliary tract may be referred to an upper area of the back.

Heartburn is a form of pain that is described as a burning sensation felt behind the sternum. It is usually attributed to irritation of the oesophageal mucosa by reflux of gastric acid fluid into the oesophagus and may be accompanied by regurgitation of some stomach content into the mouth.

A patient may complain of a sense of fullness, especially after eating. Normally, the stomach relaxes and distends to accommodate food without increasing the intragastric pressure. This accommodation may not occur if there is a disease, such as carcinoma, or if the patient is in an anxious state.

Significant characteristics of the pain must be noted and recorded. Meaningful clues include the duration, location (see Fig. 17.5), and the nature and onset of the pain as described by the patient. Aggravating factors such as activity, the taking of food or medicine, or some specific experience or emotional stress may exist. Nausea, vomiting, flatulence and defecation associated with the pain are pertinent observations. The effect of pain on each individual varies and also varies with the cause and nature of the pain. For example, the patient experiencing gallstone or kidney stone colic writhes in agony while the patient with peritonitis or paralytic ileus tends to remain immobile. The patient is observed for such changes as restlessness, pallor, perspiration, weakness and changes in the vital signs.

For a general and more detailed discussion of pain, the reader is referred to Chapter 8.

ANOREXIA

Anorexia is a loss of appetite for food and is a common complaint of patients with a digestive disorder but is also associated with disorders in practically all parts of the body. The individual may even express a revulsion to the odours of food. It may be functional in origin, resulting from an emotional upset. Persistent refusal of food due to psychological disturbance is referred to as *anorexia nervosa*. It leads to emaciation and, occasionally, to death (see Chapter 19).

NAUSEA AND VOMITING

Nausea is an unpleasant sensation in which one has a feeling of discomfort in the region of the stomach and the inclination to vomit.

Vomiting is the ejection of the gastric contents through the mouth and is usually preceded by nausea and hypersalivation. There may be nausea without vomiting, and vomiting may occasionally occur without being preceded by nausea. The involuntary muscular activity that precedes or accompanies vomiting is referred to as *retching*.

Nausea and vomiting are very common symptoms and are seen in a great variety of conditions. They can be manifestations of a digestive dysfunction, may represent hormonal changes such as occur in early pregnancy, or they may accompany practically any acute illness or stress situation. The nurse is frequently called upon to comfort and support a patient who is vomiting and to make pertinent observations which may prove significant to the doctor in making a diagnosis and planning treatment.

The vomiting process is initiated by a vomiting or emetic centre in the medulla oblongata. This centre may be excited by sensory impulses originating in the stomach or intestines, by impulses of psychic origin when fright, unpleasant sights, odours or severe pain are experienced, or by impulses from a group of

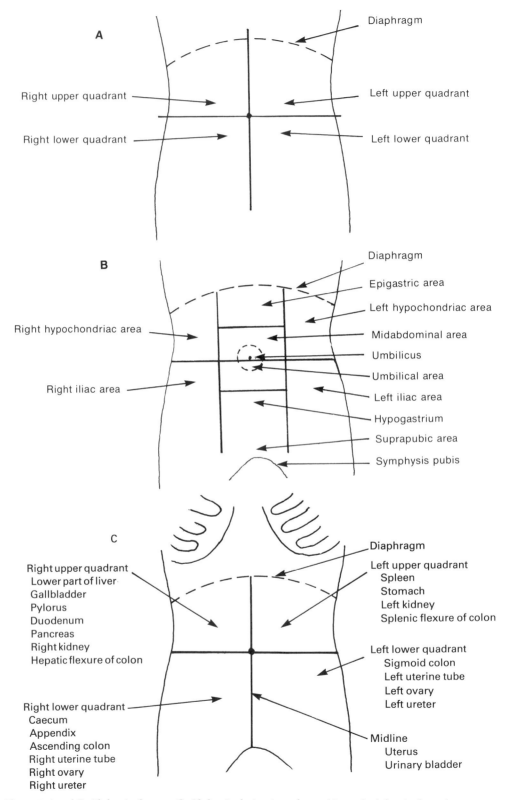

Fig 17.5 *A* and *B*, Abdominal areas. *C*, Abdominal structures located in each abdominal quadrant.

neurons referred to as the chemoreceptor trigger zone in the floor of the fourth ventricle. The cells in the trigger zone are sensitive to certain chemicals in the blood and to impulses from the portion of the internal ear concerned with equilibrium. Vomiting in motion sickness, radiation therapy, toxaemia and with the taking of certain drugs such as digoxin results from impulses that arise from the chemoreceptor trigger zone. The sensitivity of the vomiting centre varies in different individuals; some vomit very readily and with little effort while others are not affected even though the stimulus may be similar and of equal intensity.

The impulses discharged by the vomiting centre result in excessive salivation, a quick, deep inspiration followed by closure of the glottis and epiglottis, closure of the nasopharynx by elevation of the soft palate, and relaxation of the oesophagus, cardiac sphincter and stomach. Vigorous contraction of the diaphragm and abdominal muscles increases intragastric pressure and simultaneously, strong reverse peristalsis begins in the stomach. The gastric contents are forced up through the relaxed oesophagus into the mouth. The retching or heaving that is experienced before and after vomiting results from the back-and-forth movement of the stomach contents between the negative pressure in the thorax and the positive pressure in the abdomen. The vomiting is accompanied by pallor, cold, clammy skin, increased heart rate and increased salivation and swallowing.[19]

One should be alert to the possible effects of vomiting, regardless of its cause. Considerable muscular energy can be expended in frequent vomiting and may result in exhaustion.

Obviously, nausea and vomiting interfere with normal nutrition and, if prolonged, malnutrition and loss of weight and strength occur. The reduced intake and loss of fluid may rapidly lead to dehydration. Loss of gastric secretion may deplete the body electrolytes and cause acid–base imbalance. Acidosis may develop as the patient becomes dependent on his body fat as a source of energy. The patient may complain of abdominal soreness from the retching and muscular effort and may become extremely worried about his condition, which may further aggravate the disturbance.

REGURGITATION

Ejection of small amounts of chyme or gastric secretion through the oesophagus into the mouth without the vomiting mechanism being employed is referred to as regurgitation. It may occur owing to some incompetency of the oesophageal–gastric (cardiac) sphincter, as seen in infants or those with hiatus hernia, or it may be a symptom of organic disease.

---

[19] Yasko (1985), p. 29.

DYSPHAGIA

Dysphagia is defined as difficulty in swallowing. The patient may be able to swallow soft foods and liquids but may be unable to take firmer, more solid foods. Others may be able to swallow but complain of pain on doing so.

Dysphagia may be due to mechanical obstruction, dysfunction in the neuromuscular structures involved in swallowing or to diseases of the mouth, pharynx or larynx. Pain associated with swallowing frequently indicates an organic lesion such as an ulcer due to acid reflux from the stomach.

LOSS OF WEIGHT AND STRENGTH

Obviously, if food cannot be taken, digested or absorbed, body tissue cells are deprived of their requirements for normal functioning. Body stores and actual tissues are mobilized to meet the needs, but eventually these may be depleted. The patient manifests loss of weight, strength and efficiency.

If the problem is related to a specific food, symptoms characteristic of a lack of that particular food will appear. For example, effects of a protein deficiency include muscle wasting, weakness, hypoalbuminaemia, oedema, anaemia and, in the child, retarded growth and development. If there is a disturbance in the absorption of vitamin K due to a lack of bile salts in the intestine, the deficiency may be manifested by bleeding, since prothrombin, necessary for blood coagulation, will not be produced by the liver.

CHANGES IN THE MOUTH

Changes in the mouth may be of local origin or may be associated with digestive or general disorders. Disturbances may take the form of a coated or furry tongue, dryness, soreness, small ulcers (aphthous ulcers) and halitosis. Changes due to local conditions may be caused by inflammation, infection, neoplastic disease or injury of the tongue, buccal mucosa or lips. Any sore that does not heal in 2 weeks should be investigated.

HICCUP (HICCOUGH, SINGULTUS)

Persisting hiccups or frequent attacks of hiccups may be associated with organic disease of the digestive system. They are caused by intermittent spasms of the diaphragm due to gastric distension, irritation of the phrenic nerve or a metabolic disorder such as uraemia or toxaemia which affects the central nervous system. The frequency of the attacks and the effect of the hiccups on the patient should be noted. Dehydration, acid–base imbalance and malnutrition may develop, since hiccups may interfere with the taking of fluids and food. Disturbed rest and the expenditure of muscular energy may cause exhaustion. In many instances, the patient becomes fearful because of the persistence of the condition.

A simple nursing measure is to have the patient breathe into a paper bag held closely over the mouth and nose. Rebreathing the air in the bag gradually increases the carbon dioxide content of the air in the lungs and eventually the blood. The respiratory centres stimulate the diaphragm to contract normally in an effort to eliminate the carbon dioxide. The inhalation of a prescribed mixture of oxygen and carbon dioxide may be ordered. A sedative or tranquillizer may also be prescribed if the hiccups persist. Rarely, if they persist and are having serious effects on the patient (exhaustion, dehydration, etc.) a phrenic nerve block or crush is done.

FLATULENCE

Flatulence is an excessive amount of gas in the gastrointestinal tract. The patient may complain of a 'full, bloated feeling,' pressure or actual pain. The abdomen may be distended and the patient may eructate gas from the stomach through the mouth or may expel gas (flatus) from the bowel. Excessive gas in the stomach or bowel is frequently due to swallowed air. Aerophagia, or the unconscious swallowing of air, may be seen in nervous persons and in patients who are nauseated or experiencing some digestive stress. It is sometimes helpful to advise patients to make a conscious effort to avoid the swallowing or to hold something such as a wooden or plastic applicator between their teeth.

Excessive gas in the intestine may result from the ingestion of excessive amounts of gas-forming foods (cabbage, turnips, onions, etc.) or from abnormal fermentation of the food due to bacterial action. Flatulence and distension occur with any obstruction in the tract and with paralysis of peristalsis. Another frequent cause is ingestion of milk in individuals who as adults do not possess the enzyme lactose. This can also occur in individuals who increase milk intake when they have been accustomed to very little.

Borborygmi (singular, borborygmus) is a term applied to the sounds made by the movement of a gas and fluid mixture in the intestines that are loud enough to be heard by the patient and others close by. The sound can be a significant observation, especially where there is some question of obstruction. The sounds do occur in the normal alimentary tract on occasion.

ABDOMINAL RIGIDITY

Rigidity of any area of the abdominal wall due to excessively tense muscle tone may be evident in patients with disease of the gastrointestinal tract. The muscle contraction is usually a response to irritation of an underlying structure. This symptom is usually noted by palpation of the abdomen when examining the patient.

CHANGE IN THE NORMAL PATTERN OF BOWEL ELIMINATION

A disorder of the intestine may cause a retarded or an accelerated movement of contents through the intestine. Delayed movement may cause *constipation* characterized by infrequent, hard, dry stools or may result in a complete failure of the passage of faeces. Acceleration of the content causes *diarrhoea*, which is frequent liquid or unformed stools. The person who experiences any persistent change in his normal pattern of bowel elimination should consult a doctor.

For a discussion on constipation and diarrhoea (see pp. 513–521).

FAECAL INCONTINENCE

Involuntary defecation is referred to as faecal incontinence. Elderly individuals who are immobilized become constipated and may develop incontinence; the patient is constantly soiled with semiformed stools. This form of incontinence is usually preventable. Involuntary defecation may also be caused by underlying bowel disease or neurogenic impairment.

BLEEDING FROM THE GASTROINTESTINAL TRACT

Bleeding in the alimentary canal may be manifested by the vomiting of blood (haematemesis), by melaena (the passage of a black, tarry stool containing blood pigments), or by the passage of frank blood from the bowel. Haematemesis and melaena occur as a result of bleeding in the upper digestive tract. The characteristic black tarry appearance of the stool is due to the effect of the digestive enzymes on the blood. Frank blood in the stool usually originates with bleeding in the colon, rectum or anal canal.

It may be necessary in some instances to examine the blood that has been ejected through the mouth to determine whether it has been coughed up (haemoptysis) or vomited. Blood from the respiratory tract is a brighter red and frothy because of the contained air; that from the stomach is usually darker and may contain small clots and food particles. Melaena may be so slight that it goes unrecognized unless a stool specimen is submitted for laboratory examination for *occult blood*.

The most frequent cause of haematemesis and melaena is peptic ulcer, but oesophageal varices, carcinoma, injuries or a blood dyscrasia may account for the bleeding. Any evidence of bleeding should be promptly reported to the doctor. The patient who has haematemesis or tarry stool is put at rest and his blood pressure, pulse, respirations, colour and general state (e.g. strength and consciousness) are checked frequently.

Frank bleeding from the lower part of the tract may be due to erosion of the mucosa, a congenital malformation of arterioles, a neoplasm, ulcerative colitis, haemorrhoids or an anorectal fissure. The patient is advised to see a doctor immediately for early diagnosis and treatment.

Gastric or intestinal intubation

The investigation, treatment and feeding of many medical and surgical patients may include the passage of a tube into the stomach or small intestine via the nose or mouth and the oesophagus. The purpose may be to withdraw fluid from the stomach or intestine for analysis, to remove fluid and gas (decompression of the stomach or intestine), to wash out the stomach (gastric lavage), to apply cold or pressure to the walls of the oesophagus, stomach or small intestine, or to administer feedings or drugs.

TYPES OF TUBES

Many different tubes are encountered and the type used varies with the purpose. The composition varies and the tube may have one or two lumens and may have a small inflatable bag attached at the distal end. Longer tubes are necessary for intestinal intubation. The following are commonly used (see Fig. 17.6).

Levin tube. This tube has a single lumen with several openings at the distal end and is used for gastric intubation.

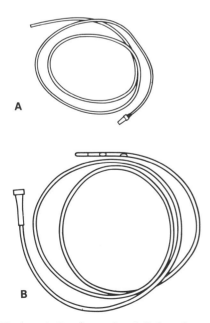

Fig 17.6 *A*, Fine-bore tube. *B*, Ryles tube.

Miller–Abbott tube. The Miller–Abbott tube used for intestinal intubation is quite long and has two lumens. One lumen serves to aspirate intestinal fluid and gas, and the other opens into a small rubber bag which is inflated after the tube is passed. The balloon causes pressure which stimulates intestinal motility. In some instances, mercury is used in the balloon instead of air; its weight facilitates the movement of the tube through the pylorus and along the intestine.

The inlets at the proximal end must be clearly marked to indicate which lumen is for drainage and which is kept clamped off to maintain the inflation of the balloon. The tube is marked off in centimetres so the distance it has passed may be determined.

Cantor tube. The Cantor tube is used for intestinal aspiration. It has a small rubber bag at its distal end which contains 5–10 mm of mercury. The lumen of the tube is sealed off at its junction with the bag, and the openings that permit aspiration are above the bag.

Harris tube. This tube is smaller than the Cantor tube but resembles it in that it has a single lumen and a bag containing mercury attached below the holes. In both the Cantor and Harris tubes the mercury is introduced into the balloons before intubation. The mercury will not escape through the fine needle hole.

The tubes which are most frequently used are nasogastric tubes:

Ryle's tube. This is a plastic, single lumen, fairly rigid nasogastric tube. There is a hole at the gastric end and a cuff at the nasal end to allow syringes or connection tubing to be fitted. There are a variety of diameters of tube available to be used according to the size of the patient. The tube is used for intermittent or continuous aspiration of gastric contents. If a bag is attached to the tube with a length of connection tubing and placed below stomach level, free continuous drainage of gastric contents will occur. Alternatively contents can be withdrawn using a syringe at prescribed intervals. The tube can also be used to give fluid or medication to the patient who is unable to swallow.

Fine bore tube. Fine bore tubes such as the Clinifeed tube have a 1 mm internal diameter, and are made of soft-flexible plastic. They are designed for long-term use for patients requiring enteral feeding. They are introduced into the patient with a guide wire inside them, which is removed once the tube has been placed into the stomach via the nose and oesophagus. The position of the tube is confirmed by an x-ray.

NURSING RESPONSIBILITIES

Suction may be applied intermittently or continuously

for aspiration of gastric or intestinal contents. The suction may be provided by a syringe for the purpose of collecting specimens or for occasional aspiration of a small amount. More frequent or continuous suction may be provided by a suction machine. The electric suction apparatus may be set for intermittent or continuous suctioning. Piped suction from a central source may be available through a wall outlet with a valve and gauge by which the amount of suction is controlled.

Gastrointestinal suctioning must be gentle; the amount of suction or pull exerted is kept low to avoid drawing the soft tissue structures to the openings which would obstruct drainage and possibly damage the tissues.

Following gastric surgery, aspiration may be achieved by applying suction to a gastrostomy tube. A catheter with several side openings is inserted into the stomach through an abdominal incision and secured by sutures. This method of aspiration eliminates the discomfort and irritation associated with a nasogastric tube that is necessary for several days.

Assisting with the insertion of the nasogastric tube

An explanation of the treatment is made to the patient. This includes the purpose and what may be expected both during and following the insertion of the tube. He is advised that the insertion will be easier and quicker if he relaxes, breathes deeply through his mouth and swallows when instructed to do so to advance the tube.

The tube is usually made of plastic and can be placed in the refrigerator prior to use so that it is stiffer and less likely to curl up; it is lubricated with water or a water-soluble jelly. If the tube is too stiff it is immersed in warm water.

The distance from the patient's ear lobe to the bridge of his nose and from this point to the xiphoid process provides a fairly close estimate of the length of tube required to reach the stomach.

The head of the bed is elevated, and the patient's head is hyperextended during the initial introduction of the tube through a naris. When the patient is asked to swallow, the head is slightly flexed to the more natural position for swallowing. The tube is gently passed downward as the patient swallows, but it should not be advanced faster than the swallowing or it will curl up in the pharynx and cause gagging. The patient may be allowed sips of water to make the swallowing easier. If resistance is met, the tube is rotated slowly and directed back and down.

To make sure the tube is in the oesophagus and not in the trachea, the proximal end may be submerged in water; bubbles will appear as the patient exhales if the tube is in the trachea. Or the patient may be asked to speak or hum, which is not possible if the tube is in the larynx. The tube is withdrawn immediately if any change in the patient's respiratory status is observed during insertion.

To make sure the tube is in the stomach, a syringe is attached to aspirate a small amount of gastric content; alternatively, 5–15 ml of air may be injected into the tube while listening over the stomach with a stethoscope for the entry of the air into the stomach.

In intestinal intubation, when the tube reaches the stomach the patient is required to assume various positions to promote its passage through the pylorus and the duodenum. The usual procedure is to place the patient on his right side for 1–2 hours, and then on his back with the head of the bed elevated for 1–2 hours. Advancement of the tube may be followed by radiography and suggestions are made as to the desirable positioning of the patient. When the Miller–Abbott tube is used, the doctor may inflate the balloon when it reaches the stomach on the basis that it simulates a food mass and stimulates motility to carry it through the pylorus. In other instances, the balloon may not be inflated until the tube has passed into the duodenum.

Securing the tube

The tube is secured to the face with narrow strips of non-allergenic adhesive when it has been advanced to the desired position if it is to be left in place for several hours or days. It must be checked several times daily for security, and the skin is examined for possible irritation from the adhesive.

If the tube is attached to a drainage bottle, it should be supported in a 'trough' made in the bottom sheet or by a tape or towel pinned to the bedding to prevent tension on the nasogastric tube. The connecting tube should be long enough to prevent displacement of the gastrointestinal tube and to permit free movement of the patient in bed.

Mouth and nose care

The patient usually experiences considerable discomfort from the tube being in the nose and throat and from the dryness due to mouth breathing and restricted oral intake. The mouth should be cleansed and rinsed frequently. Normal cleansing of the teeth is encouraged and need not interfere with the nasogastric tube. A water-soluble ointment, face cream or oil may be applied to the lips. In some instances, small sips of water may be allowed to stimulate salivary secretion.

The nostril may become irritated and secretions accumulate and encrust. It should be gently cleansed with a swab moistened in water or normal saline and a light application of water-soluble jelly or mineral oil made.

Turning the patient hourly helps to shift the tube sufficiently to relieve constant pressure on one area of the throat. Throat lozenges may be ordered to lessen throat irritation.

Maintenance of drainage

After the tube is in place and connected to the suction apparatus, it is necessary to check the system at frequent intervals for functioning. Mechanical failure of the apparatus might occur, or drainage may be interrupted by a blocking of the tube by mucus or a blood clot and could result in pain, vomiting, or serious distension of the stomach or intestine. The surgeon may order the tube to be irrigated by syringe at regular intervals or only if it is blocked. The solution and volume to be used for irrigating are specifically stated. Normal saline is usually used to irrigate gastric tubes since water promotes electrolyte loss from the gastric mucosa. After injection of the solution, some of the fluid may be aspirated using the syringe to determine if the tube is clear. The amounts of solution injected and aspirated are accurately measured and recorded on the fluid balance sheet.

The characteristics of the drainage fluid are noted and the total volume is recorded every 8–12 hours. The volume is an important factor in determining the fluid and electrolyte replacement needed. Loss of gastric secretions incurs a loss of hydrogen ions (H^+) and chloride ions (Cl^-) that may result in alkalosis. Loss of intestinal fluid may result in a severe loss of hydrogen carbonate (HCO_3^-) and potassium and cause acidosis. The bottle is washed each time it is emptied as well as the connecting tubing.

Removal of the tube
Before removal, the tube may be clamped and left in place while oral fluid is introduced. If the fluid is tolerated, an order may then be given to remove the tube. The gastric tube is withdrawn gently and quickly. The patient is instructed to hold his breath to avoid possible aspiration of fluid or mucus that may escape from the tube into the oropharynx during removal.

The intestinal tube is removed slowly, a few inches at a time. The lumen into the air-inflated balloon is opened, and the air is allowed to escape. When slight resistance is encountered owing to the intestinal peristalsis, the tube is left for a few minutes and then withdrawal is resumed. The doctor should be notified if resistance to removal persists; force should not be used. If the tube has a mercury-filled bag at its distal end, the latter is brought out through the mouth and the bag removed. The remainder of the tube may then be pulled through the nostril. As with the removal of the gastric tube, the patient is asked to hold his breath as the terminal portion of the tube is drawn from the oesophagus.

The mouth should be cleansed and rinsed immediately following the removal of the tube. The patient may complain of some soreness in the throat and nose which usually subsides in a day or two.

POTENTIAL PATIENT PROBLEMS (GASTROINTESTINAL DISORDERS OR DYSFUNCTION)

1 Nutritional intake of less than body requirements
The problem of a nutritional intake of less than body requirements is related to inefficiency in ingestion, digestion or absorption.

Causative factors and *defining* characteristics for the assessment of the patient with nutritional deficiencies are identified in Table 17.1. Nutritional intake of more than body requirements, and excessive food intake in relation to energy output are discussed in Chapter 19. Inadequate nutrition resulting from insufficient intake of food due to non-physiological factors is also discussed in Chapter 19.

The *goals* are to:
1 Promote oral hygiene
2 Maintain the ability to masticate food
3 Maintain the integrity of the oral mucosa
4 Relieve dysphagia
5 Alleviate discomfort, dehydration, malnutrition and acid–base imbalance associated with nausea and vomiting
6 Maintain adequate nutritional intake when ingestion, digestion and/or absorption are impaired

Table 17.1 Patient problem: (1) nutritional intake of less than body requirements.*

Causative factors	Signs and symptoms
Inability to ingest, digest or absorb nutrients due to pathological disorders	Weight loss with adequate food intake
	Lack of body fat
	Oral mucosal inflammation
	Absence of teeth
	Difficulty swallowing
	Heartburn
	Abdominal pain, cramping or tenderness
	Abdominal distension and bloating
	Altered bowel sounds
	Abnormal loose, bulky, odorous stools
	Flatulence
	Weakness and fatigue
	Altered muscle tone
	Peripheral oedema

*Kim & Moritz (1982), p. 300.

1. PROMOTION OF ORAL HYGIENE

Assessment
The teeth, gums and oral mucosa should be inspected to identify abnormalities. In a normal, healthy mouth:
• The lips are moist and intact.
• Breath is free from odour.
• Teeth are white, intact, firm and free from caries, jaggedness and plaque.
• The gums are moist, pink, intact and adhere to the teeth.
• The mucosa is moist, pink, soft and intact.
• The tongue is pink and moist with minute papillae on the superior surface.

Nursing intervention
The patient is taught oral hygiene to prevent the development of disorders of the teeth and oral mucosa. The teeth are brushed after each meal or snack by placing the side of a soft toothbrush along the gum-line and moving the brush gently down along the surface of the teeth. Vibratory motions are used, directing the brush across the tooth surface. Teeth on the lower jaw are brushed from the gum upwards along the surface of the teeth. Plaque is removed from the teeth by passing dental floss between the teeth. Gentle pressure is applied to the floss as it is moved up and down against the side surface of each tooth. If it is not possible to use a toothbrush, oral hygiene packs containing soft sponges with attached handles are available and can be used to help clean a patient's mouth. The sponges are immersed in an appropriate mouthwash solution such as sodium bicarbonate or glycerol of thymol, and then used to clean the teeth, gums, oral mucosa and tongue. The packs are designed to be used once and then discarded. The importance of dental care by a dentist twice yearly is stressed as well as the importance of maintaining adequate nutrition and fluid intake.

Expected outcomes
1 The teeth are white, intact and firm.
2 The gums and oral mucosa are pink, moist and intact.
3 The tongue is pink and moist with minute papillae on the superior surface.
4 The patient understands the need for:
  (a) Daily oral hygiene
  (b) A dental check by a dentist every 6 months
  (c) Maintaining nutritional and fluid needs.

2. MAINTENANCE OF ABILITY TO MASTICATE

Assessment
The patient's history and inspection of the patient's teeth and oral mucosa may reveal:
● Absence of some teeth.
● Dentures that are ill-fitting as evidenced by movement on mastication; redness or swelling of the mucosa under or around dentures or jagged teeth; discomfort on chewing; a tendency to eat only soft and liquid foods.
● Dental caries.
● Pain and tenderness in response to hot, cold or sweet foods.

Nursing intervention
● Refer the patient for dental assessment and care.
● Remove dentures (if removable) and clean with a brush and denture cream or other mild cleansing agent.
● Teach the patient to inspect the tissue under and around the dentures for redness and lesions.
● Instruct the patient to eat a balanced diet that includes foods that are easily chewed and swallowed.
● Alleviate pain of dental caries with oral analgesics and instruct the patient to avoid hot and cold foods until dental care is received.
● Teach the patient oral hygiene as outlined above.
● Teach the patient to inspect the oral mucosa and teeth for signs of irritation and breaks or discoloration in enamel of the teeth.

Expected outcomes
1 Dental care is evidenced by dentures that fit snugly and occlude with the opposing teeth, and dental caries are repaired.
2 The oral mucosa under or around the dentures or adjacent to previously irregular teeth, is pink, moist, firm and intact.
3 The patient understands the need for:
  (a) Carrying out daily oral hygiene
  (b) Maintaining nutritional and fluid needs
  (c) Obtaining regular dental care.
4 The patient inspects his mouth regularly for signs of irritation and breaks or discoloration in the enamel of the teeth.

3. MAINTENANCE OF INTEGRITY OF THE ORAL MUCOSA

Assessment
Inspection of the lips and oral cavity may reveal:
● Dryness, roughness, cracks, crusts or ulcerations of the lips.
● Periodontal disease, as evidenced by gums that are red, oedematous and receded from the teeth. Bleeding and tenderness may be present on brushing. Some teeth may be loose and plaque is present.
● Stomatitis, which is recognized when the oral mucosa is shiny, red, oedematous and tender. Ulcerative areas may be present.
● Oral infection symptoms, which include areas of localized redness, oedema, pearly appearance, vesicles, ulceration, necrosis, bleeding, tenderness and offensive odour of breath.

Nursing intervention
● The lips are cleansed with normal saline and gauze, and patted dry. Moisture is provided by applying a water-soluble ointment every 2–4 hours.
● Periodontal disease requires a referral to a dentist for treatment. The patient is taught oral hygiene and to inspect his gums to identify early signs and symptoms of periodontal disease. Supervision of the patient in carrying out brushing techniques, gum stimulation and removal of plaque may be necessary. The diet appropriate to the disorder and treatment are discussed; nutritious, bland, soft, vitamin C-containing foods are recommended. Hot and spicy food and fluids should be avoided.

- Stomatitis is inflammation of the oral mucosa. The patient's mouth is rinsed every 2–4 hours with a normal saline solution. Debris is removed from the mouth by cleansing with gauze applicators and a 3% solution of hydrogen peroxide followed by thorough rinsing to avoid further irritation.

  The patient's diet is evaluated for adequate intake of fluids, vitamins and protein. It should be bland and soft or liquid. Spicy and hot foods are avoided as well as tobacco and alcohol.

Oral infections. A swab for culture is taken of infected lesions prior to initiation of any therapeutic measures. Mouth care includes cleansing every 2–4 hours with normal saline. If the tongue is coated and the mucus is thick, the mouth is cleaned with a sodium bicarbonate solution followed by a normal saline rinse. Debris is removed from the mouth with a 3% solution of hydrogen peroxide followed by rinsing or irrigation with normal saline.

If the patient is malnourished, vitamin supplements such as vitamin B complex and vitamin C may be prescribed. Analgesic lozenges are given to alleviate pain and discomfort. Antibiotics may be prescribed for some infections. Fungal infections such as candidiasis is treated with an oral suspension of nystatin; the patient is instructed to swish the fluid around in the mouth.

The diet should be bland and soft or liquid. Irritants such as spices, hot foods, alcohol and tobacco are avoided. Nutritious foods and fluids are encouraged to promote the healing of lesions, resistance and normal salivary secretion. Transfer of the infection to others is prevented by personal mouth care equipment and careful handling of dishes and cutlery and other objects which have been in contact with the patient's mouth and oral secretions. The patient and family are instructed to avoid direct oral contact while the infection is present and to thoroughly wash their hands under running water following mouth care and any contact between hands and the mouth or oral secretions. Nursing personnel should wash their hands following each contact with the patient.

Expected outcomes
1 The lips are soft, moist and intact.
2 The patient receives dental care and treatment for periodontal disease.
3 The patient understands the plan for daily oral hygiene.
4 The patient inspects the mouth regularly for oral irritation, gum disease or infection.
5 The diet is adjusted to maintain adequate nutrition and fluid intake.
6 Mucosal lesions have healed, tenderness abated and the oral mucosa is clean, moist, pink and intact.
7 The patient carries out measures to prevent transfer of infection to others.

4. ALLEVIATION OF DYSPHAGIA

Assessment
The patient's history and physical examination may reveal:
- Decreased production of saliva as evidenced by dryness of the mouth and difficulty in chewing and swallowing. Salivary glands may be enlarged and tender on palpation
- Inflammation of the mouth and pharynx producing pain and discomfort during the initial stage of swallowing
- Avoidance of solid, spicy and very hot foods
- Frequent episodes of aspiration of food into the trachea and posterior nasal passages
- The patient experiences the feeling that food is lodged in the throat or chest and complains of heartburn, pain and discomfort. The pain may radiate to the back or shoulder
- Regurgitation of the bolus of food.

Nursing intervention
A lack of salivary secretion may be associated with a disease of the mouth, the salivary glands or with a condition in which the mouth is kept open and the individual continuously breathes through his mouth. It frequently occurs when the patient has had radiation treatment for cancer of the mouth. The fluid intake is increased unless contraindicated. Frequent oral irrigation or mouthwashes with a bland non-irritating solution followed by the application of mineral oil or glycerin and lemon juice are usually helpful. The sucking of fruit (lemon) lozenges which are sufficiently tart to stimulate salivary secretion may also provide some relief. Artificial saliva may also be administered to moisten the mouth and lubricate foods.

When oesophagitis is chronic, the head of the patient's bed is elevated at night to reduce the reflux of gastric secretions during sleep. At home, the patient can place a wedge under the upper portion of the mattress, place the head of the bed on blocks or he may use several pillows for sleeping.

Antacid medications such as magnesium trisilicate mixture may be administered orally at regular intervals during the day. Cimetidine (Tagamet) or ranitidine (Zantac) may be prescribed to inhibit the secretion of gastric acid if the cause of the dysphagia is acid reflux.

The patient with dysphagia of oesophageal origin is taught to swallow twice in rapid succession when symptoms occur. Fox has demonstrated that this simple manoeuvre of the double swallow may convert the painful oesophageal contractions into contractions of normal amplitude and duration and thus relieve the symptoms.[20]

The patient records the food taken and assists in identifying foods which exacerbate the problem.

---

[20] Fox & Monna (1980), p. 209.

Citrus fruits, tomatoes and alcoholic beverages are likely to cause pain and discomfort in patients during swallowing. The patient should be in a sitting position when eating to facilitate ingestion by gravity. Stress has also been identified as a precipitating factor. The nurse provides reassurance and remains with the patient when discomfort occurs. These techniques are carried out before and after eating to produce muscular and emotional relaxation.

Since the pain of dysphagia is not constant, long pain-free periods are common. It is important to work with the patient to identify foods and stresses which exacerbate the symptoms and to help adjust eating habits and daily routines to avoid these factors.

Expected outcomes
1 Factors in the diet, lack of saliva and stressful events contributing to dysphagia are identified.
2 Episodes of dysphagia are decreased in frequency, severity and duration.

5. ALLEVIATION OF NAUSEA AND VOMITING

Assessment
Assessment of the patient who is nauseated and is vomiting involves noting the following factors:
• Was the vomiting preceded by nausea?
• Was there retching or was the vomitus regurgitated without effort?
• Was pain associated with the vomiting?
• Was there any association with the ingestion of food or drugs?
• Do the nausea and vomiting occur at any time or are they more severe at a particular time of day?
• How frequent is the emesis?
• What is the quantity, consistency, colour and content of the vomitus?
• What are the effects—physical and emotional—on the patient?

Nursing intervention
The care must be individualized; what may prove helpful with one person may not be tolerated by another. It is also influenced by the cause of the vomiting.

Supportive measures. Sympathetic attention and understanding can mean a great deal to the patient. Since worry and fear can perpetuate nausea and vomiting, the patient is encouraged to express his concerns. Problems may come to light which may be explained or solved. The plan of care and any diagnostic and therapeutic measures should be explained to the patient; knowing that something is being done or going to be done provides reassurance.

Support is also provided by remaining with the patient, supporting the head or painful site (e.g. incision), holding the basin, cleansing the mouth and lips and making sincere efforts to relieve the discomfort.

Fluid and food. Oral intake is usually withheld for a period of time and is resumed gradually in small amounts. If the vomiting is due to local irritation, it may be helpful to have the patient take a whole glass of water to 'wash out' the stomach. If vomiting is prolonged, an intravenous infusion of fluids may be necessary to prevent or correct dehydration and replace electrolytes. An accurate record is made of the fluid intake and output. The skin and oral mucous membrane are observed for dryness, and skin turgor is assessed to identify dehydration. Laboratory reports of the concentration of plasma electrolytes (sodium, potassium, chloride) are followed closely so that imbalances may be corrected by appropriate intravenous fluids. The patient's weight is recorded daily or every second day.

Hygienic and comfort measures. The mouth is rinsed after each emesis and the basin emptied and disposed of promptly. Soiled bedding and clothing are changed and the room ventilated. The odour or sight of vomitus may contribute to the patient's discomfort and may cause repetitive vomiting. The patient may be reassured by having tissues and a clean basin always within reach, but it is less suggestive if covered with a clean towel.

Rest, quiet and a minimum of disturbance may reduce the incidence of vomiting. Encouraging the patient to take several deep breaths may help to lessen nausea and offset vomiting. Nausea tends to increase with motion; any change of position should be made slowly. Positioning should facilitate drainage of the vomitus from the mouth to prevent possible aspiration. Subdued lighting may reduce external stimuli and be conducive to rest.

Medication. An antiemetic or a sedative may be prescribed. Diazepam (Valium) may be administered orally or parenterally for sedation. Prochlorperazine or metaclopramide are examples of antiemetics which may be used.

The use of antiemetics or other drugs is restricted if there is any question of pregnancy to prevent any effects on fetal development. Anticipatory nausea and vomiting are also controlled by preventative and regular doses of antiemetics. Nausea and vomiting due to chemotherapy is prevented or controlled by the administration of antiemetics ½–1 hour prior to the chemotherapeutic drugs and throughout the infusion. Relaxation techniques are also useful in the control and management of nausea and vomiting.

If the vomiting continues, gastric drainage by means of a nasogastric tube may be established (see p. 503).

Expected outcomes
1 Nausea and vomiting are relieved.
2 The urinary output is within the normal range, the oral mucosa is moist and skin turgor is normal.

6. MAINTENANCE OF ADEQUATE NUTRITIONAL INTAKE

When impairment of ingestion, digestion or absorption of nutrients exists, the nutritional intake is maintained by decreasing stimulation of certain secretions, adapting the patient's diet to relieve the problem or by using alternative routes to administer nutrients.

Dietary measures
Measures to decrease stimulation of gastric secretions include withholding food for 24–48 hours to allow the stomach to rest. Fluids are given intravenously as even water taken by mouth will stimulate gastric acid secretion. Gastric intubation with suctioning may be used to remove gastric secretions to promote healing (see p. 503).

Recommended dietary modifications for the patient with *increased gastric secretions* include the following principles:
- The patient receives a nutritionally adequate diet.
- Substances which stimulate gastric secretion (e.g. coffee, strong tea, highly seasoned foods, especially those with pepper, citrus fruit and alcohol) are avoided.
- Meals are taken regularly at frequent intervals of about 3 hours to maintain the buffering action of food in the stomach.
- Meals should be small to avoid gastric distension which stimulates gastric acid secretion.
- Foods which the patient recognizes as actually precipitating symptoms are avoided.
- The patient should not smoke.
- Drugs such as acetylsalicylic acid (aspirin) which are known to damage the gastrointestinal mucosa are avoided.
- Meals are taken in a pleasant, relaxed atmosphere.[21]

The diet for patients with *deficiencies of digestive enzymes* avoids foods that are not digested by the individual and provides nutrients in simpler forms than those found in normal diets to promote absorption. The patient with lactase deficiency avoids milk and other foods containing lactose.

Prepared formula feeds (elemental food) contain carbohydrates in the form of glucose and dextrans, and protein as amino acids and peptides. The fat content of prepared formula feeds is usually minimal.[22] Formula preparations are taken orally when possible but can be administered through a nasogastric or gastrostomy tube. Foods that the individual can digest and absorb should be included in an individualized diet with the formula preparation to ensure the taking of all essential nutrients.

Dietary measures for the individual with a *malabsorption syndrome* include elimination of the specific inabsorbable nutrient from the diet and administration of unabsorbed nutrients through other routes if necessary; for example, a gluten-free diet for the patient with gluten-sensitive enteropathy eliminates wheat, rye, barley and oats from the diet and substitutes cornmeal and potato, rice and soy bean flour. Vitamins B_{12} and K are administered parenterally when a deficiency exists.

Alternative routes for the administration of nutrients
Oral intake of food is preferred, but when this is not possible nutrients can be administered intravenously or by nasogastric or gastric routes.

Nasogastric tube feeding. When a patient is unable to take fluid and foods by mouth, a nasogastric tube may be passed, through which a specially prepared solution of essential nutrients is introduced directly into the stomach. This method of feeding a patient is known as enteral feeding. The nurse assists with the intubation as described on p. 504. The tube may be left in place, but should be removed every 5–6 days, and a clean tube reinserted through the other nostril. With infants and young children the tube is inserted prior to each feeding. When a Ryle's tube is to be left in place, it is secured to the patient's face with narrow strips of adhesive.

The medical, dietetic and nursing staff are involved in enteral nutrition of patients. The doctor decides if a particular therapeutic diet is required, the dietitian plans the regimen and the nurse administers the diet. Various feeds are used. The foods of a normal diet may be liquefied in a blender and then given to the patient via the tube, or a protein supplement and vitamins may be added to a mixture of eggs, milk and orange juice.

Most commonly, commercial preparations are used. These feeds are ready mixed in a can and therefore require less time to prepare them, are less likely to become infected because once opened the can is emptied into a sterile feed container and administered to the patient via a giving set attached to the nasogastric tube, and are advantageous as the constituents of the feed care are known. Such feeds are given continuously via the giving set and the regimen is determined according to the requirements of the patient for fluid and nutrients. For example, a regimen of 500 ml of feed per 5 hours may be given for 20 hours of the day, and the patient rested for the remaining 4 hours. The cycle of feeds may then be resumed or may be slightly modified if the patient's needs have altered.

When evaluating a formula, consideration is given to its osmolality, caloric value and protein, carbohydrate, fat, vitamin and mineral composition.[23] Nutrients are present in simple forms, are easily digested and absorbed and leave minimal residue in

---

[21] Krause & Mahan (1984) p. 428.
[22] Krause & Mahan (1984), p. 724.

[23] Krause & Mahan (1984), p. 716.

the bowel. Patients with some malabsorption disorders may not tolerate some of the prepared formulae. Functioning of the patient's digestive tract and hydrational status are assessed before the preparation is selected.

The prescribed amount of solution is administered at room temperature or may be given cold from the refrigerator if preferred by the patient. If this is the initial feeding, an explanation of the procedure is given to the patient. The head of the bed is elevated. Using a syringe, a small amount of gastric content is aspirated to make sure the tube is in the stomach. The aspirate is returned through the tube. In some instances, 5–10 ml of air may be introduced into the tube; the nurse listens for the entry of air through a stethoscope placed over the stomach. A continuous infusion of the feed is given via a giving set attached to the nasogastric tube. The container with the liquid feed is hung on an intravenous stand. The fluid feed is given slowly, for example 500 ml over 6 hour, and the speed is regulated by a pressure regulator on the tubing.

The feed is administered slowly and allowed to flow into the stomach by gravity. To avoid air entering the stomach, the feeding container is not allowed to empty completely until all the fluid is given. When the feed is completed, the tube is cleansed by rinsing it with 30–40 ml of water and is then clamped. If regurgitation or vomiting occurs, it may be that the prescribed volume is too great. A smaller amount given more frequently may be tolerated.

Frequent mouth care is necessary and the nostril through which the tube passes requires attention.

For removal of the tube see p. 505.

Gastrostomy. This is the surgical establishment of an opening into the stomach through the abdominal wall and the insertion of a tube through which fluids and liquefied food may be introduced directly into the stomach. This procedure is rarely used nowadays.

Before the gastrostomy, the procedure is discussed with the patient so he understands the purpose of the surgery and what is entailed postoperatively. The patient's written consent and the usual preoperative preparation for abdominal surgery are necessary. General or local anaesthesia is used and a small incision made in the abdominal wall and stomach. A large catheter (No. 20 or 22F) is inserted into the stomach and secured by sutures put through the tissues and the tube. In some instances, a Foley catheter is used and a purse string suture used around it. The layers of tissue are then closed around the tube.

A gastrostomy may be a temporary procedure during a period of corrective surgery or it may be permanent when an oesophageal obstruction is considered inoperable or there has been an oesophagectomy.

The patient generally finds it difficult to accept a gastrostomy. He is denied the natural process of eating and its associated pleasures such as taste and sociability. Personnel caring for the patient, the family and friends should acknowledge to the patient that they understand his concern and tendency to withdraw. An effort is made to find interests for the patient and to treat him as normally as possible.

For the first day or two postoperatively, water or a glucose solution in prescribed amounts is given through the tube; then, regular feeds are given according to the doctor's orders. The food preparations used in gastrostomy are similar to those cited above for gastric tube feedings or are regular foods put through a blender. The required amount of feeds is given through a funnel or the barrel of a syringe attached to the gastric tube. The patient's head and shoulders are elevated and he remains in this position for ½ hour after the feeding to prevent regurgitation into the oesophagus and leakage around the tube. The tube is cleansed following the feeding by rinsing it with 30–40 ml of water and is then clamped.

A gauze or transparent (Op Site) dressing is applied to the wound following inspection of the skin for excoriation. The escape of even a small amount of gastric juice from around the tube may irritate the skin because of its acid-pepsin content. The gauze dressing is changed whenever there is drainage, and the skin is cleansed thoroughly with soap and water and dried. A protective coating of petroleum jelly or a prescribed ointment or powder is then applied. A transparent sheet such as Op Site may be applied; it provides protection for the skin and permits visualization of the area. It may be left in place for as long as 1 week.

The feeds may have to be adjusted from time to time. Too much fat or carbohydrate may cause diarrhoea. Complaints of a full feeling or abdominal discomfort may necessitate a decrease in the amount of feeds given. A record of the patient's weight is made which also serves as a guide in adjusting the caloric value of the feeds formula.

The tube is removed in approximately 1–2 weeks when the opening (stoma) and the channel through the layers of tissue are well established and healing has sealed off the peritoneal cavity. The tube is reinserted for each feed and the stoma covered with a small dressing pad between feedings. A shorter tube with a flange that holds the tube in place is available for a permanent stoma. The tube also has a screw cap that seals the tube off between feedings.

Since the feeds correspond to the patient's meals, meticulous care should be used in relation to the equipment and to the preparation and administration. Such consideration as a clean, fresh towel covering the tray and clean equipment free of stains may lessen the patient's aversion to this unnatural method of taking his meal. When the patient receives blender feeds he may feel more hopeful and 'less different' if advised he is receiving foods included in a normal diet. Strict privacy should be provided during the feed as the patient is sensitive.

The patient's mouth will require special attention. Frequent cleansing and rinsing are essential. Some satisfaction may be derived from the taking of various fluids (e.g. fruit juice), retaining them in the mouth for a brief period and then expectorating them. The doctor may encourage the patient to take foods which he desires, masticate them and then expectorate the bolus. These measures help to keep the mouth in better condition, stimulate gastric secretion and may provide some satisfaction through taste for the patient.

If the patient is to be fed by gastrostomy over a long period while various stages of treatment are carried out or if the gastrostomy is permanent, he is taught to feed himself. Instruction is given to the patient and a member of the family in the preparation of the feeding and the care of the stoma. Financial assistance may be necessary to provide a blender or prescribed commercial feeding preparations. The nurse may direct the family to the appropriate community resources for the necessary assistance or make the contact for them.

Total parenteral nutrition (TPN). Parenteral nutrition is the infusion, into a large central vein or right atrium, of solutions of protein, glucose, electrolytes, trace amounts of essential minerals, vitamins, and lipids (fat emulsions) in sufficient concentrations to meet individual requirements for normal metabolism, tissue maintenance, repair and energy demands.[24] It may also be used to supplement nutrition received orally.

Parenteral nutrition may be used with patients who; (1) are unable or unwilling to take nutrition orally or receive it by nasogastric tube; (2) are unconscious for a prolonged period; (3) have a condition such as Crohn's disease or a bowel fistula that requires that the intestinal tract be given a rest; (4) have had a massive intestinal resection which may have been necessitated by a mesenteric thrombosis or a volvulus; (5) are in a hypercatabolic state, in which body tissue is broken down and a negative nitrogen balance results (e.g. burns) or (6) have cancer and cannot tolerate oral food because of chemotherapy reactions. In the case of an intestinal resection, if only a part of the small intestine is removed, parenteral nutrition is used while the remaining small bowel adapts and increases its

absorption of food to compensate for the section removed. If there is insufficient absorptive area left (total intestinal resection), the parenteral nutrition procedure becomes the permanent means by which the individual receives nutrition.

The *procedure* is carried out by an experienced team, who start and supervise these complex intravenous infusions. The team is usually composed of the nurse, clinical pharmacist, dietitian and the patient's (consultant or registrar) doctor. Their responsibility includes teaching the patient and family to manage the feeds at home.

Strict surgical asepsis is mandatory throughout the insertion of the catheter, when handling the solutions and tubes, and when caring for the 'wound' (site of insertion). Infection causes a serious problem; the parenteral line serves as an excellent culture medium and, since it leads directly into the blood, bacterial invasion will cause septicaemia.

It is important to *prepare the patient*. If the patient is conscious, and especially if total parenteral nutrition is to be prolonged or permanent, he and his family receive a detailed explanation of the procedure, its purpose and subsequent care. They are encouraged to ask questions and time is taken to answer them. They may require assurance that the patient will be able to eat normally after a period of being fed this way.

The site of insertion is shaved and cleansed first with alcohol to remove fatty secretion and then with a strong antiseptic (e.g. povidone-iodine).

Care is taken on *insertion of the catheter.* The alimentation solution is infused into a large, valveless intrathoracic vein; a plastic vascular catheter is usually passed via an internal jugular vein or subclavian vein into the superior vena cava. It is necessary to use a large vein since highly concentrated (hyperosmolar) solutions are likely to cause severe phlebitis in smaller peripheral veins. When the solution is dripped into a large vein it is rapidly diluted in the large volume of blood and osmolality of the plasma is therefore not notably increased.

If the condition permits, the patient is positioned for a brief period with the head lower than the rest of his body; this distends the neck and upper intrathoracic vessels which facilitates the passage of the catheter.

A sterile field around the site of insertion is provided by the application of sterile drapes and the doctor and assistants wear sterile gloves. They, as well as the patient, wear masks to prevent airborne contamination by mouth and nose organisms. A local anaesthetic is used in the area to be punctured and a large needle is passed into the subclavian or internal jugular vein. Entry into the subclavian vein is made just below the clavicle (subclavicular) which provides greater freedom of movement for the patient's neck and arms. A small intravascular catheter is threaded through the needle and advanced

---

[24] The *electrolytes* included in the solutions are sodium, potassium, chlorine, calcium, magnesium, phosphate and acetate. The *minerals* essential in trace amounts are iron, copper, cobalt, zinc, iodine, manganese, chromium, and selenium. The recommended daily allowance of multiple vitamins is added to the solutions. In addition, folic acid is added daily, vitamin K daily or weekly and vitamin B_{12} is given once a month.

into the superior vena cava. The patient is instructed to perform the Valsalva manoeuvre as the catheter is threaded into the superior vena cava.[25] The needle is withdrawn and an isotonic solution is attached for infusion. The doctor may suture the catheter to the skin at the site of insertion to prevent dislodgement or movement of the tube in and out. The site is cleansed of any blood and dried, and a temporary dressing is applied until after the placement is verified. An air-occlusive dressing is then applied.

A chest x-ray is taken before infusion of the parenteral nutrition solution to determine the position of the catheter.

Insertion of a right atrial catheter is usually done under radiographic control to ensure it is in place. The catheter is threaded through the subclavian vein and may also be tunnelled a few inches under the skin to permit anchoring it in position with two dacron cuffs that are attached. The separate entrance and exit sites decrease the potential for infection. The right atrial catheter has a wider bore than the peripheral catheters and can be flushed with a dilute heparin solution and capped when not in use. It is best suited for patients undergoing long-term parenteral nutrition at home. A double lumen catheter is usually used for parenteral nutrition, but a single or triple lumen catheter may be used.

The *solutions* used to provide total parenteral nutrition are very concentrated and are prescribed individually. They are contained in collapsible plastic bags to avoid possible air embolism.

The infusion tube which is attached to the catheter when not connected to a solution flask is sealed with a sterile cap. The frequency with which the intravenous tubing and/or filter(s) are changed is indicated by hospital policy. If contamination occurs or is even suspected, a doctor or nurse is notified and the tubing is changed. All tubing changes are made quickly while the catheter is clamped to prevent air entry and the risk of embolism. If the catheter cannot be clamped, the patient is instructed to bear down and hold his breath before the tubing is disconnected and to breathe again once the connection is made (Valsalva manoeuvre). The infusion line may contain one or two micropore filters. Tubing connections are always reinforced with adhesive to ensure maintenance of an intact line. Total parenteral nutrition solutions consist of an amino acid/dextrose solution and a fat emulsion solution which are infused at the same time. Replacement fluids for gastric losses may also be infused simultaneously.

A specific directive is received from the doctor as to the rate of flow of the solution. *The rate must be kept constant* for maximum benefit. If the infusion is too

rapid, glucose is not metabolized rapidly enough to maintain a normal blood sugar level. The latter is likely to exceed the glucose renal threshold and glucose is excreted in the urine, taking with it essential water and electrolytes. The rate of flow (drops per minute) is checked frequently, since the rate of a gravity drip may vary with changes in the patient's position. A volume-control pump may be used to provide better regulation of the rate of flow.

Only the prescribed parenteral nutrition solutions are administered through the catheter into the superior vena cava. *No medications* (e.g. antibiotic, digoxin), *plasma*, or *other solutions* are given via the parenteral line. Also, the parenteral nutrition line must not be used for drawing blood for specimens into the tube following the administration of the solutions. Right atrial catheters may be used for withdrawing blood or administering medications but should be used only when necessary because of the danger of contamination.

On *dressing* the site strict aseptic technique similar to that cited for the insertion of the catheter is observed and a mask is worn. Caution is necessary to avoid dislodging the catheter. The catheter site is inspected for redness, swelling or drainage; a swab is taken for culture if any irritation is observed. The skin is cleansed with alcohol followed by an application of povidone-iodine which is left for 2–3 minutes to dry. A small amount of povidone-iodine ointment is applied to the skin around the catheter and the dressing applied. The dressing of choice is a transparent, elastic, self-adhesive film (e.g. Op Site) that is water and bacteria proof but permeable to air and water vapour. The transparency permits frequent visualization of the area without disturbing the dressing which can be left in place for as long as a week.

Frequent *mouth care* is essential. Regular, frequent cleaning of the teeth followed by a mouthwash is very important. The lack of oral food and fluid intake causes discomfort and favours the growth of organisms present in the mouth, producing sordes, inflammation and tooth cavities. If the parenteral nutrition is prolonged or permanent, the patient may be permitted hard candy or sugarless gum, or a small amount of food which he chews and then expectorates. Some patients may be able to take small amounts of clear fluids or specified nutrients if their gastrointestinal tract is intact.

When *assessing* the patient the following observations are very important.

The patient's blood pressure, pulse, respirations and colour are recorded frequently following the insertion of the catheter.

Any complaint of pain or tightness in the chest or change in level of consciousness is reported promptly. It may be associated with an air embolism or a pneumothorax or haemothorax.

The temperature, pulse and respirations are recorded one to four times daily. An elevation of

---

[25] The *Valsalva* manoeuvre involves a forcible expiratory effort against a closed glottis. This increases intrathoracic pressure and reduces the possibility of air entering the circulatory system.

temperature and increased pulse rate may indicate infection.

A urine specimen is examined every 6 hours for sugar and acetone. Blood specimens are submitted at stated intervals for determination of glucose, urea and serum electrolyte levels. Hyperglycaemia may develop, necessitating the administration of regular insulin.

Blood cultures are done and checked for fungi as well as bacteria.

The patient's weight is recorded daily. The intake and output are recorded and the fluid balance noted.

The site of insertion is examined carefully each time the dressing is changed and is inspected daily through the transparent dressing for inflammation, oedema, sloughing or purulent discharge.

Psychological support is necessary for the patient receiving total parenteral nutrition for a prolonged period as he feels 'very different'. Repeated explanations of the purpose and value of the feedings are necessary. As he gradually acquires an understanding of the procedure, it becomes more acceptable. Active and passive exercises and ambulation are encouraged. Exercise promotes protein synthesis as well as improving the patient's psychological well-being. The patient is encouraged when advised of his weight gain.

Bowel *elimination* decreases and the patient may worry about this. He is advised that nothing enters the tract.

When TPN is *discontinued* the solutions are reduced gradually over 48 hours to prevent a sudden fall in blood glucose. When the parenteral nutrition solutions are withdrawn, a solution of glucose 5% is infused over several hours before the doctor removes the catheter. Oral intake is gradually increased. The catheter tip is sent to the laboratory for culture.

Instruction must be given to the patient who requires long-term parenteral nutrition. Appetite decreases during parenteral feedings. This is attributed to the caloric intake, decreased gastric motility and underlying disease. Appetite remains suppressed when parenteral feedings are discontinued. Martyn, Hansen and Jen (1984) demonstrated that suppression of appetite following parenteral nutrition was self-limiting but lasted for 1–2 weeks in healthy rhesus monkeys.[26] Patients are assessed for feelings of satiety when parenteral nutrition is discontinued and their dietary intake is closely monitored for 1–2 weeks.

If this method of receiving nutrition is to be permanent or prolonged, the family and patient are prepared for his discharge from the hospital. They are taught how to put up the solutions, the maintenance of asepsis, indications of problems (e.g. symptoms of infection), care of the site of catheter insertion, and how often the tube is changed and by whom. They are advised of the necessary supplies

and how they are obtained. The patient is also taught to test his urine for glucose and acetone and to make a daily record of his weight.

The patient is not discharged until he has demonstrated efficient self-care. A referral for nursing supervision at home is made. The district nurse usually makes weekly visits to change the dressing, assess the patient's progress and identify any signs of infection or other untoward reactions.

Expected outcomes
The patient:
1 Demonstrates awareness of the causes and effects of his nutritional deficiencies.
2 Describes dietary and other therapeutic measures to meet his specific nutritional needs.
3 Is able to plan and maintain adequate nutrition on a daily basis.
4 Is able to perform prescribed feeding techniques (e.g. tube feeding or total parenteral nutrition) safely.
5 Shows progressive increases in body weight towards normal.
6 Demonstrates a decrease in signs and symptoms of disturbance in ingestion, digestion and absorption. This is shown by: an increased feeling of well-being; fewer episodes of steatorrhoea or diarrhoea; and an absence of bloating, flatulence, abdominal distension, abdominal cramps and peripheral oedema.

2 Alteration in bowel elimination

Causative factors and defining characteristics for the assessment of problems *relevant to elimination* are listed in Table 17.2.

1. DIARRHOEA

The term diarrhoea implies an accelerated movement of content through the intestine with a decrease in mixing and absorptive processes resulting in frequent liquid or unformed stools. The faeces pass through the colon before the normal amount of water is absorbed.

Diarrhoea is a symptom of many different disorders which may be within the bowel or may be extrinsic to the intestine. Changes characteristic of organic disease may occur in the intestine and result in diarrhoea, or the bowel may be structurally normal with the hypermotility being functional. The more common causes of diarrhoea are presented here as intrinsic or extrinsic, although there are many different aetiologic classifications in medical literature.

Intrinsic causes
Normally the stimulus for peristalsis arises within the intestine. It may cause direct stimulation of the muscle tissue, or it may initiate sensory nerve

---

[26] Martyn, Hansen & Jen (1984), p. 336.

Table 17.2 Patient problems: (2) alteration in bowel elimination.*

Problem	Causative factors	Signs and symptoms
Alteration in bowel elimination 1 Diarrhoea	Bacterial organisms and enterotoxins Intestinal neoplasms Diet high in roughage or spicy foods Allergy to ingested foods Malabsorption syndrome Diverticulitis Laxatives Antibiotics Inflammatory disorders of the intestinal tract Emotional stress Systemic diseases causing toxaemia (e.g. hyperthyroidism, uraemia)	Loose, watery stools Several bowel movements per day Dehydration: loss of skin turgor, weight loss, dry mouth Abdominal cramping and pain Weakness Increased bowel sounds
2 Constipation	Disease of the bowel Decreased intestinal motility Altered innervation to bowel and anal sphincter Megacolon Inadequate fluid intake Lack of fibre or cellulose in diet Physical inactivity Medication (e.g. opiates) Weakness of abdominal muscles and diaphragm Irregular habits of defecation Loss of bowel tone from excessive use of laxatives Haemorrhoids	Abdominal pain Abdominal distension Sensation of fullness and pressure in rectum Loss of appetite Headache Dry, hard, formed stools Infrequent bowel movements (less than three times per week) Straining on defecation
3 Impaction	Altered tone, motility and sensation in bowel as a result of ageing process Immobility Central nervous system disorders	Cramping pain Oozing liquid stools Headache Loss of appetite Abdominal distension Dry, hard formed stools Palpable hard rectal mass Straining at defecation No bowel movement for over three days
4 Incontinence	Constipation Faecal impaction Excessive use of laxatives and enemas Drugs (e.g. iron, methyldopa) Diabetes Diverticulitis Proctitis Carcinoma Rectal prolapse Regional enteritis (Crohn's disease) Malabsorption syndrome Ischaemic colitis Neurogenic disorders	Involuntary defecation Constant soiling of clothing Faeces soft and semiformed or loose Absence of sensation or urge to defecate Diminished propulsive contractions on rectogram

*Brochlehurst & Hanley (1981), p. 85.

impulses that are transmitted into the central nervous system, resulting in parasympathetic nerve impulses being carried out to the intestine that then stimulate its motility. Disease or irritations within the bowel which may increase either direct stimulation or reflex hypermotility include the following:

Malabsorption. Impaired absorption of foods may be due to incomplete digestion or to a defect in the absorptive process of the small intestine. Obviously, with reduced digestion and absorption, an increase in the bulk of the colon content results and is a stimulus to intestinal motility. The stools are bulky, have an offensive odour and usually contain large amounts of fats which are irritating to the bowel mucosa and initiate reflex peristalsis. The presence of unabsorbed osmotically active substances such as glucose or a disaccharide that cannot be split, causes osmotic diarrhoea. The increased intraluminal osmotic pressure causes water to move into the intestine, producing diarrhoea. General malnutrition is also evident.

Diverticulitis.   A pouch or sac may occur in the wall of the intestine and is known as a diverticulum (Fig. 17.7). It may be congenital or may develop as a result of a weakening of an area of the muscle tissue in the wall. There may be several diverticula, or the defect may occur singly.

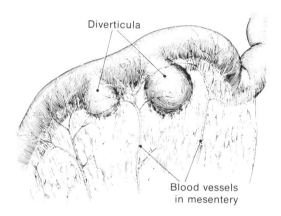

Diverticula

Blood vessels
in mesentery

Fig 17.7 Intestinal diverticulum.

Diverticula of the large intestine are more likely to give rise to trouble, as the more solid faecal content tends to collect and be retained in the sac, setting up an inflammation that causes increased reflex peristalsis and diarrhoea.

Laxatives.   Many laxatives act by direct irritation of the intestinal mucosa, resulting in the content being hurried through the colon before the normal amount of water is absorbed.

Infection.   Food or fluid contaminated by salmonella, shigella or staphylococcal organisms is the most common cause of intestinal infection and may be referred to as bacterial food poisoning.
The shigella bacilli cause bacillary dysentery, and the primary source is usually the excreta of an infected person. This disease is rare, except under crowded and poor sanitary conditions.
The salmonella bacilli may inhabit the intestine of man, fowl and animals and may be the source of infection to others. It may be transmitted by the meat of infected animals and by food or water contaminated by the excreta of infected humans or animals.

Sporadic outbreaks occur and may be due to a human carrier employed in the handling of food. Ingested salmonella or shigella organisms multiply, causing irritation and inflammation of the intestine, resulting in diarrhoea accompanied by crampy abdominal pain, fever, nausea and vomiting.
Hypersecretory bacterial diarrhoea may be caused by toxin-producing organisms such as staphylococci, salmonella, shigella and Vibrio cholera. The enterotoxins stimulate the release of excessive amounts of fluid and electrolytes by the small intestine.

Neoplasms.   Diarrhoea may be a symptom of a malignant neoplasm of the colon and may be alternated with periods of constipation.

Dietary Factors.   An excessive amount of coarse foods or highly seasoned irritating foods may produce hypermotility of the bowel. Occasionally, allergy to a certain food may account for diarrhoea; if the intestinal mucosa is sensitive to the food, it becomes hyperaemic and oedematous and causes increased reflex hypermotility.

Antibiotics.   Diarrhoea sometimes accompanies the oral administration of antibiotics. They may irritate the mucosa or alter the normal bacterial flora of the intestinal tract. The most frequent offenders are the tetracycline preparations.

Idiopathic inflammation.   Patients with ulcerative colitis or regional enteritis experience severe diarrhoea. No specific cause has been recognized for either condition.

Extrinsic causes
Diarrhoea accompanies a variety of disorders in which the stimulus that results in increased parasympathetic innervation to the bowel originates outside the intestine.

Emotional stress.   Anxiety or underlying tension is frequently the basis of diarrhoea, producing a condition which may be referred to as the irritable bowel or colon syndrome. On investigation, disturbances may be revealed that are secondary to the diarrhoea, but there is no organic disease in the intestine or elsewhere. The intestinal hypermotility is entirely functional and is considered psychogenic. The patient is usually sensitive and has a nervous temperament; a study of the patient's total life situation may reveal a specific emotional conflict that will probably account for his diarrhoea.

General or systemic disorders.   Frequently, diarrhoea is associated with general diseases, particularly if they cause toxaemia. Examples of such conditions are acute infectious disease, hyperthyroidism and uraemia.

Assessment

It is important to obtain the following information:
- The patient's previous bowel habits
- The number of bowel movements each day
- The volume and consistency of the stools
- Whether the stools contain abnormal components, such as blood and excessive mucus
- Whether the patient experiences abdominal pain
- Whether there is exacerbation with certain foods or activities, and
- Whether the diarrhoea is worse during the day or the night. Functional diarrhoea tends to occur during the day, while that associated with organic disease is generally as disturbing at night as during the day.
- The systemic effects on the patient:
    (a) What is the hydrational status?
    (b) What are the electrolyte, pH, and haematocrit levels?
    (c) Is the temperature elevated?
    (d) Is the patient exhausted because of loss of sleep?
    (e) Is the patient losing weight?
- Whether or not there are increased bowel sounds
- The patient's perception of and reaction to the diarrhoea
- The condition of the skin around the anus and over pressure areas
- Fluid and electrolyte balances. The fluid balance is monitored and the serum haematocrit and electrolyte levels are determined at regular intervals if diarrhoea is prolonged.

Nursing intervention

Measures to decrease peristalsis. Peristalsis of the small and large intestines may be slowed by the following measures:

1 Removal of the cause of the diarrhoea. This may involve the administration of prescribed antibiotics for intestinal infection, avoidance of specific foods for the patient with a malabsorption disorder or an intestinal allergy, and avoidance of laxatives and treatment for systemic diseases such as hyperthyroidism or uraemia.
2 Changing the diet to eliminate spicy foods, fruit juices, raw fruits and vegetables and gas-forming foods
3 Use of drugs. Various medications may be used in the treatment of diarrhoea:
    (a) Drugs to reduce intestinal spasm and motility may be ordered. Examples are diphenoxylate hydrochloride (Lomotil) and loperamide hydrochloride (Imodium).
    (b) Opiates such as codeine phosphate are believed to increase absorption by acting on the opiate receptors, e.g. kaolin and morphine mixture.
    (c) Drugs to provide a protective coating on the intestinal mucosa or to provide an adsorbent,

which condenses and holds irritating substances, are used. Examples are kaolin, aluminium hydroxide gel and bismuth subcarbonate.
    (d) An anti-infective drug may be ordered if the diarrhoea is of microbial origin. Sulphonamide preparations that are poorly absorbed, have a local effect but are less frequently used orally; examples are calcium sulphaloxate, phthalyl-sulphathiazole and sulphaguanidine. Sulphasalazine (Salazopyrin) is indicated for the maintenance of remission in ulcerative colitis and Crohn's disease.

Rest. The patient with diarrhoea feels weak and fatigued. Rest periods are provided and the patient is encouraged to relax and pursue sedentary activities such as reading or watching television. If necessary, the patient is assisted to the bathroom or a commode chair may be used at the bedside. The call-button should be answered promptly to avoid unnecessary effort or anxiety for the patient in attempting to reach the bathroom in time. Some patients are unable to relax and rest because of a constant fear of not receiving the bedpan in time; in such instances it may be helpful to make an exception and leave a clean covered bedpan at the bedside within the patient's reach.

Fluids and nutrition. Fluids and electrolytes are replaced by intravenous infusions. If oral fluids are tolerated, water, sweetened clear tea, fat-free broth and gruel may be given. Carbonated drinks, whole milk, fruit juice and iced fluids are usually avoided.

The diet is expanded as soon as possible to reduce the possibility of nutritional deficiencies. A high-calorie, high-vitamin and high-protein bland diet is gradually introduced, and the patient is observed as to the intestinal response. Roughage and gas-producing foods are restricted at first; whole grain bread and cereals, raw fruits and vegetables and highly seasoned and fried foods are not used. Concentrated sweets and fats are likely to be poorly tolerated. Fibre-containing foods and roughage are gradually introduced as tolerated. A prolonged bland diet is likely to become unpalatable, resulting in an inadequate nutritional intake. If the diarrhoea is due to malabsorption, a gluten-free diet may be ordered in which foods are avoided that contain any wheat, rye, and barley grains or flour.

The first few mouthfuls of a meal may initiate a mass peristaltic wave, and the meal is interrupted. The patient's tray should be removed from the room and the hot foods kept warm. Following the necessary postdefecation care, the tray is returned. The patient may require some persuasion to complete his meal, as he is discouraged and is afraid that if he eats it will just precipitate another stool.

Aesthetic and hygienic factors. Placement of the patient

on the ward receives consideration. If ambulatory, he should be near toilet facilities; if confined to bed, privacy should be provided so the patient is less embarrassed by his frequent use of the bedpan.

The anal region should be left clean after each defecation and, if the skin around the anus is irritated, it is washed and a protective cream applied. Soiled bedding or clothing is changed promptly. Provision is made for thorough washing of the patient's hands after each defecation and the room is ventilated to avoid embarassment for him.

Diversion. Something to occupy the patient and divert his attention may prove beneficial. If the diarrhoea is a reaction to stress, efforts are directed toward identifying the source of the emotional disturbance. The patient is encouraged to express his feelings and is reassured that there is no serious disease. New interests and activity in hobbies or sports may be suggested. Sedatives or tranquillizers may be ordered to relieve the emotional tension.

Medical asepsis. Cases of acute diarrhoea are considered potentially infectious until otherwise indicated. Precautions are used to prevent the possible spread of infection to others. A gown is worn by all personnel when giving care, and the hands are scrubbed with soap and running water after each contact. Contaminated waste such as soiled dressings or swabs are put into bags which are sealed and labelled with a biohazard warning. Linen is put into a linen skip which is lined with a plastic bag, tied, and labelled appropriately. Used equipment such as syringes, needles, giving sets and lancets are placed directly into suitable containers such as Burn Bins. These are sealed when only three-quarters full and labelled with a biohazard warning. All waste is then sent for incineration. Excreta and vomit are put directly into the sluice disposal machine and, after being disposed of, the cycle is repeated to ensure the machine is flushed through.

When performing any nursing care procedures requiring contact with the patient's faeces, disposable gloves are worn. Visitors are restricted to members of the family who may be asked to wear a gown and to avoid contact with the patient and his bed.

Acute infectious diarrhoea may readily spread throughout a family, school or neighbourhood because of a common source of infected food or water or by the spread from an infected person. The nurse may play an important role in the prevention of diarrhoea by alerting people to the hazards of exposed and unrefrigerated foods, particularly meat and those with cream filling or topping. Opportunities may arise to emphasize the hygienic handling of food and the importance of thorough hand washing after going to the toilet and the handling of soiled clothing.

The family in which a member develops acute diarrhoea should be advised of the necessary precautions in caring for him to prevent the spread to others. If several members of a family become ill at one time, questions should be raised as to recently ingested food and its source.

If a large number of cases are found in a school or community, the local health authorities should be notified so that a systematic investigation as to the possible source may be instituted. Occasionally, acute diarrhoea may spread through the patients on one ward of a hospital. The primary source of such an outbreak should be sought. Ward personnel are urged to practise rigid medical asepsis, for infection may be carried from one patient to another or from a ward worker to patients through failure to thoroughly wash the hands between patients, after handling bedpans or linen, or after going to the toilet.

Expected outcomes
1 The patient's stools are formed.
2 The frequency of defecation approximates the patient's usual pattern.
3 The patient's skin turgor is adequate, urinary output is normal and serum haematocrit and serum electrolyte levels are within the normal range.

2. CONSTIPATION

The majority of persons normally defecate once every 24 hours but there is considerable variance in the frequency among healthy persons. Some persons have more than one bowel movement daily, while others may have an evacuation of a normally moist stool once every 2 or 3 days. Such variances in frequency of bowel elimination may be compatible with health. An individual is considered to be constipated if bowel elimination is unexplainably delayed for several days or if the stool is so hard and dry that it is difficult to expel.

Constipation may be a delay in the passage of faeces through the colon, referred to as colonic constipation, or it may be a prolonged retention of the faeces in the rectum, designated as *rectal constipation* or *dyschezia*.

Causes
The causes of constipation are many and varied. It may be associated with organic disease, or it may be a functional disturbance.

Disease within the colon or rectum may narrow the lumen of the bowel and offer resistance to the forward movement of content. Common examples are: neoplasms of the intestine; inflammation, which causes spasm, scarring and adhesions; and partial volvulus (twisting of the bowel). Severe ascites (accumulation of fluid in the peritoneal cavity) or a tumour, such as an ovarian cyst or uterine fibroid, may compress the colon and delay the movement of intestinal content.

Failure of the normal propulsive movement may occur due to some disturbance or imbalance in the innervation of the intestine. The derangement may result in excessive tone and spasm in a segment of the bowel that retards the movement of the content. The spasm may be induced by a hypersensitivity of the colon or by anxiety. Constipation may be associated with injury or degeneration of the spinal cord or cauda equina, which affects the nerve supply to the colon and rectum.

Megacolon (large colon) may account for constipation in infants. It is a congenital anomaly in which there is an absence of certain nerve structures (parasympathetic ganglia) in a segment of the colon, resulting in failure of peristalsis in the affected portion of the bowel. The most frequent site is the sigmoid and it is seen more often in males. The affected segment is constricted and does not participate in normal peristaltic activity. Faecal content accumulates in the adjacent preceding colon and dilation occurs. The condition is also known as *Hirschsprung's disease*. Surgical resection of the colon may be considered necessary and is done in two stages: a colostomy is done first, and then resection of the affected area and anastomosis are performed.

Constipation may be associated with any illness in which there is diminished intake of food and fluid or in cases in which the diet is modified and lacks fibre, resulting in less residue. The lesser amount of food does not provide sufficient bulk to stimulate peristalsis. Dehydration causes a small, dry, hard stool that may irritate the colon, causing spasm, or may fail to stimulate normal colon motility.

Constipation is frequently secondary to physical inactivity or prolonged bed rest. It is a common complaint among persons with sedentary occupations who probably ride to and from work and do not participate in any type of physical exercise.

Occasionally, drugs used in treatment may decrease intestinal motility and delay excretion. This increases mixing of the faeces and exposure to the absorptive surface, which dries out the faeces and produces constipation. Common examples of such drugs are opiates (e.g. codeine) and anticholinergic drugs [e.g. propantheline bromide (Pro-Banthine)].

Expulsion of the faeces is aided by increasing the intra-abdominal pressure to compress the colon and rectum. This involves contraction of the muscles of the abdominal wall and of the diaphragm. Weakness of these muscles due to disease, senility, malnutrition or inactivity may contribute to constipation. Similarly, lack of tone in the intestinal musculature or weakness of the levator ani muscles may impair peristalsis and the expulsive power.

Frequent causes of constipation in persons who are not ill are faulty defecation habits, faulty diet and the habitual use of laxatives. If the urge to defecate is ignored and evacuation delayed, the reflex becomes weak as the rectal mucosa adapts to the pressure of the content. Repeated failure to respond to defecation reflex may eventually result in the rectum's becoming insensitive to the presence of a faecal mass and the reflex is not initiated. The person may delay response to the defecation urge because he does not find it convenient to interrupt what he is doing or because toilet facilities may not be available.

A deficiency of foods with cellulose and fibrous content in the diet may be the cause of constipation. Refined foods and those that leave little residue after absorption fail to produce sufficient bulk to stimulate colonic motility.

Many persons have an inordinate concern about bowel elimination and think they must have a daily bowel movement or a frequent purge and resort to unnecessary, repeated use of a laxative. Loss of intestinal tone and reduced peristaltic response to normal food residue follow the use of a laxative, and then too often the laxative is repeated. The colon is not allowed to regain its natural rhythmic response to the normal faecal mass.

Constipation may cause considerable discomfort; the person may experience abdominal pain, a full feeling and abdominal distension. There is a loss of appetite accompanied by headache and eventually nausea and vomiting. The hard dry masses of faecal matter may damage the intestinal mucosa and lead to a fissure. Haemorrhoids are frequently the result of chronic constipation.

The *goals* are to:

1 Relieve the constipation
2 Develop regular bowel elimination

Assessment

The nursing history includes information about:

- The patient's usual bowel elimination habits
  (a) The time of day defecation usually occurs
  (b) The usual frequency of defecation
  (c) Any unusual effort or stimulation used to promote defecation
  (d) The use of laxatives or enemas
- The patient's perceptions of what is normal bowel elimination for him
- The patient's eating habits: types of foods taken and the volume of fluid taken daily
- The patient's usual activities
- The patient's level of awareness of his surroundings and bodily functions
- The patient's problem of constipation and potentially related factors:
  (a) The duration and severity of the problem
  (b) Recent changes in usual eating habits, fluid intake and physical activity
  (c) The patient's perceptions of the problem
  (d) Measures the patient has used to relieve the constipation and the effectiveness of these.
  (e) Pain, abdominal cramps, passing of gas associated with constipation
  (f) History of disorders or medication therapy

that may have altered food intake, digestion or absorption of foods or bowel motility or sensation

- The patient's living arrangements and availability of toilet facilities
- The patient and family's knowledge of: foods that contain fibre and the function of fibre in promoting bowel function; the need to maintain an adequate fluid intake; the benefits of exercise and activity; and the action and untoward effects of various types of laxatives.

The patient may be observed over 2–4 days to determine the frequency and time of bowel elimination, the volume and characteristics of the faeces as well as the patient's reactions. Any warning signs of constipation experienced by the patient, such as abdominal cramps, passing of gas, restlessness, rubbing of the abdomen, moaning or other verbal responses, should be noted.

Nursing intervention
Table 17.3 lists the steps to be implemented in formulating a plan to develop regular bowel elimination habits for a patient.

Table 17.3 Steps to establish regular bowel elimination habits.

---

1 Identify factors contributing to constipation
2 Discontinue the use of laxatives and enemas
3 Develop a diet plan to increase fibre and fluid intake
4 Develop a plan to increase daily physical activity
5 Establish a schedule for daily bowel elimination
6 Implement diet, exercise plans and elimination schedule daily
7 Evaluate effectiveness of plan each day
8 Modify plan as necessary

Establishing a regular schedule. It is helpful to explain to the person in simple terms the physiological mechanism of defecation so he may grasp the significance of responding to the initial urge for defecation. The importance of establishing a regular time for bowel elimination is stressed, for most individuals about one half hour after breakfast is the usual time for defecation; the ingestion of food stimulates the necessary wave of intestinal peristalsis. The frequency of bowel elimination varies with individuals. It should be stressed to the patient that daily bowel elimination is not essential to health; defecation every 2–3 days may be normal for some persons.

Dietary modifications. The nurse and/or dietitian works with the patient and family to evaluate current dietary habits and then helps them to plan a diet that provides a liberal amount of fibre-containing foods, taking into consideration the person's food preferences, financial resources and daily routine. Emphasis is placed on whole grain cereals and bread,

fresh fruits and vegetables and fruit juices. A daily fluid intake of 2000–2500 ml is recommended unless contraindicated by a cardiovascular condition.

Peristalsis may be promoted by the drinking of a cup of hot water on rising in the morning (approximately one half hour before breakfast).

Techniques to promote defecation. Table 17.4 lists various measures the patient may use to promote regular bowel elimination: a scheduled time for defecation is stressed as is the importance of prompt response to the urge to defecate. Peristalsis may be stimulated by the taking of a cup of warm liquid or eating a meal about one half hour before attempting to defecate. Ensuring comfort and privacy during the defecation attempt, contracting abdominal muscles, leaning forward and bearing down to increase abdominal pressure and application of manual pressure to the abdomen may be helpful.

The patient is instructed to implement these techniques daily until defecation occurs. If no bowel movement occurs in 2–3 days glycerine suppositories may be used. If this is still not effective, a stool softener or a bulk laxative may be administered. Once the patient establishes a regular schedule, other laxatives or enemas should not be necessary.

Table 17.4 Techniques to promote bowel elimination.

---

1 Increase the amount of fibre in the diet
2 Increase daily fluid intake
3 Increase daily physical activity
4 Respond promptly to the urge for a bowel movement
5 Drink a cup of warm liquid ½ hour before usual time of defecation
6 Go to the bathroom at usual time of defecation
7 Sit comfortably on the toilet in an environment that provides privacy, quiet and warmth
8 Use the following techniques to stimulate peristalsis:
  (a) contract abdominal muscles, lean forward and bear down
  (b) exert manual pressure downward on the abdomen
9 If the above techniques are not successful in producing a bowel movement consider use of the following in this order:
  (a) glycerine suppository
  (b) emollient laxative or stool softener
  (c) bulk-forming laxative
  (d) enema

Physical exercise. Some physical exercise is essential; walking is especially good. Good tone in the abdominal muscles is important; exercises to increase the strength of the abdominal muscles may be suggested. Examples of prescribed exercises are as follows: The patient lies on his back on the floor or bed with his arms folded across his chest and raises himself to the sitting position, keeping his heels on the floor. From the supine position, the patient raises his lower limbs without bending his knees. These exercises are done two or three times daily, and the patient is also encouraged to contract his abdominal muscles several times at frequent intervals through the day.

Laxatives and enemas. Laxatives, enemas and suppositories that the patient may be accustomed to using are discontinued. If increased dietary fibre, fluids and exercise are not sufficient at the beginning to establish normal bowel elimination, mild laxatives may be employed until the defecation reflex is restored and bowel irritability and spasm are reduced. Glycerine suppositories placed high against the wall of the anus may be used one half hour before the usual time of defecation to stimulate peristalsis. The suppository may be repeated daily for several days. If this is not effective a stool softener may be ordered to prevent severe straining at stool and injury to the rectal and anal tissues. The stool softeners in use are mineral oil and preparations of dioctyl sodium sulphosuccinate (Dioctyl). These latter preparations act as wetting agents, allowing water to penetrate and mix with the faecal mass. Mineral oil should not be used for prolonged periods because it may prevent normal intestinal absorption, especially of fat-soluble vitamins. Prolonged use also predisposes to lipoid pneumonia.

Bulk-forming laxatives may also be recommended. These preparations swell when combined with fluid in the gastrointestinal tract and have a stimulating effect. Examples of bulk-forming laxatives are bran and Fybogel. Use of these laxatives should be assessed carefully in the elderly if dehydration is present. Osmotic laxatives such as lactulose syrup are disaccharides that are not absorbed in the small intestine. It is broken down by bacteria in the colon and acidifies the colonic contents, which then stimulates peristalsis and serves as an effective laxative for the elderly. Magnesium hydroxide (Milk of Magnesia) is a cathartic which is not completely absorbed in the small intestine and causes retention of water in the intestinal lumen stimulating peristalsis. It is contraindicated for those with any renal insufficiency.

Expected outcomes
The patient:
1 Gains an understanding of the role of dietary fibre and fluid intake in stool formation and defecation.
2 Indicates appreciation of physical activity in normal bowel elimination.
3 Develops a satisfactory plan to increase dietary fibre, fluid intake and physical activity.
4 Plans a regular schedule for defecation and applies techniques to promote regular bowel elimination.
5 Experiences regular bowel elimination.
6 Does not use laxatives and enemas.

3. FAECAL IMPACTION

Occasionally, faeces accumulate in the rectum, producing a hard dry mass that forms a partial or complete obstruction. It occurs most often in older persons and in those with central nervous system disorders. These patients frequently suffer a loss of intestinal musculature motility and sensation. It may be associated with dehydration, lack of dietary fibre and volume, immobilization or narcotics. Manifestations include crampy pain, the passage of liquid stools without expulsion of the hard palpable faecal mass. The patient may complain of headache, fatigue, loss of appetite and pressure and discomfort in the rectal and anal regions.
The *goals* are to:
1 Relieve the impaction
2 Develop regular bowel elimination.

Assessment
● Faecal impaction is identified by the presence of a palpable hard mass in the rectum, the oozing of liquid stools without passing the faecal mass and the absence of a bowel movement for over 3 days.
● The patient's usual bowel habits, dietary intake of fibre and fluids and daily activity are assessed as outlined for the patient with constipation.

Nursing intervention

Relief of impaction. The faecal impaction is treated by the administration of an oil-retention enema to soften the impacted stool and by oral administration of an emollient laxative such as dioctyl sodium sulphosuccinate which also softens the stools. The enema is followed in a few hours by digital breaking up and removal of the faecal mass. The nurse lubricates a gloved finger and gently inserts it into the patient's rectum to loosen the impacted faeces. A cleansing enema of saline or tap water is then given. This process is usually very exhausting; following the enema the patient is made comfortable and allowed to rest.

Development of regular bowel elimination habits. The patient experiencing faecal impaction is helped to develop a regular bowel elimination programme which includes dietary management, increased activity, a regular schedule, and the use of techniques to stimulate peristalsis. Glycerine suppositories, stool softeners or bulk laxatives may be required initially. Impaction occurs most often in the elderly who do not eat adequate fibre and who have problems with mobility and experience difficulties in getting to the bathroom. The patient's living environment is assessed and the accessibility of the toilet is taken into consideration. Assistance may be required from the district nurse, neighbours and friends to ensure the aged or incapacitated individual receives an adequate diet and necessary physical assistance. If the patient is in a hospital or a nursing home, a plan for bowel elimination is an integral part of the patient care plan. The nurse assumes responsibility for guiding the patient's compliance with the plan. Excessive bed rest is avoided and physical activity encouraged.

Expected outcomes
The patient:
1 Experiences regular bowel elimination.
2 Indicates understanding of the function of dietary fibre and fluid intake in stool formation and defecation.
3 Indicates knowledge of the role of physical activity in normal bowel elimination.
4 Makes a plan to increase dietary fibre, fluid intake and physical activity.
5 Develops a schedule and applies techniques to promote regular bowel elimination.

4. INCONTINENCE (FAECAL)

The *goal*: to re-establish regular bowel evacuation.

Assessment
The nursing history is reviewed to determine the patient's usual bowel elimination habits. The problem of incontinence is assessed by observing and recording the frequency of defecation, the consistency of the stools, and warning signs experienced or expressed by the patient related to defecation. It is important to note if the patient experiences an urge to defecate and if he manifests abdominal discomfort, massages his abdomen, or provides verbal clues that defecation is occurring. The abdominal muscles are observed for tone, strength and voluntary control and the anus is digitally palpated to determine muscle control and sensation. Mental alertness is evaluated to determine the patient's ability to respond to the urge to defecate and to follow a bowel elimination schedule.

Nursing intervention

Establishment of a regular bowel routine. Faecal continence can be established by developing regular bowel elimination habits as discussed for the patient experiencing constipation or by establishing a programme for regular bowel evacuation.

Programme to stimulate peristalsis. When the cause of the incontinence is constipation or faecal impaction, as commonly occurs in the elderly, a programme to adjust the diet and activity, maintain regularity and stimulate peristaltic activity is usually effective.

Prevention of reflex bowel emptying. When neuromuscular control is impaired, management of incontinence is directed to preventing reflex emptying of the bowel in response to rectal distension by faeces. If the patient has a predictable pattern of defecation such as after breakfast each morning, a schedule can be developed to ensure that the patient is assisted to the bathroom or to a commode each morning following breakfast. If the patient's pattern of defecation is irregular, attempts are made to establish a regular time for bowel evacuation. A daily routine is established similar to that described for the patient who is constipated. The techniques described in Table 17.4 to stimulate peristalsis are employed. If no bowel movement occurs, the routine is repeated the next day. A glycerine suppository may be used on the second or third day to further stimulate defecation. If the patient usually defecates every two days, this measure would be introduced on the second day prior to the expected involuntary defecation. A stool softener may also be used. Patients with spinal cord injury or neurological disease are usually able to establish a regular defecation pattern and avoid episodes of incontinence. Routine enemas and laxatives are avoided. Patient participation in developing and implementing a bowel retraining programme is important if long-term results are to be achieved. When the patient cannot take an active part, the plan is documented and followed by all staff (see Chapter 3).

Personal hygiene. Until regular bowel evacuation is established, the incontinent patient is kept clean and dry, and skin irritation is avoided. Following faecal incontinence the skin is washed with soap, rinsed well and patted dry. Protective ointment may be applied to provide a coating over the skin. The clothing and bedding are changed as often as necessary to keep the patient clean. The nurse reduces the patient's embarrassment and concern by reassuring the patient that it is understood that the patient cannot control the bowel movements but that control can be achieved with the bowel-retraining programme. Episodes of incontinence may still occur if the patient develops diarrhoea or if his routine is changed, but most patients can achieve acceptable control if the programme is followed.

Expected outcomes
1 The patient's bowel evacuation is regular.
2 Episodes of incontinence do not occur or occur only sporadically when the patient's routine is disrupted.

Disorders of the Digestive System

Disorders of the digestive system are many and varied; they may interfere with the ingestion, digestion, absorption of food and fluids, elimination of residue and/or with the immunological defence mechanism of the body. Any dysfunction threatens the well-being, functional capacity, and perhaps the survival of the person. The manifestations depend largely on the location of the disorder in the system as well as the nature of the aetiological factor. Different diseases may cause similar disorders of function—that is, several manifestations that develop are non-specific.

Modern health education places much emphasis on nutrition, and any interference with the ability to take and retain food creates anxiety in the individual. The common knowledge of the high incidence of malignant disease in the gastrointestinal tract may cause considerable concern in anyone with any digestive upset. Fortunately, the digestive system has considerable reserve; parts of it may be removed and the patient, with some necessary adjustments in diet and living habits, may continue to live a useful life.

Frequently a disturbance of function in the alimentary tract is secondary to disease in another part of the body. For example, some disorders of the brain may be manifested first by vomiting or difficulty in swallowing. It may be a complaint of indigestion that brings the patient with primary anaemia to the doctor. Fatigue or emotional stress may be the basis of malfunctioning of the gastrointestinal tract and most of us at some time have experienced functional disturbance in the stomach or bowel during a period of anxiety or grief. The patient whose medical investigation rules out organic and structural disease still requires the nurse's understanding sympathy; efforts are made to identify problems that are causing emotional stress which may be the basis of the illness.

DISORDERS OF MOTILITY, SECRETION AND DIGESTION IN MOUTH, PHARYNX AND OESOPHAGUS

Disorders of the mouth and contained structures are numerous and, as cited previously, may be of local origin or may be secondary to disease elsewhere in the digestive system or in some other system. Primary lesions may be due to bacterial, viral or fungal infection, chemical irritation, congenital malformation, injury or neoplastic disease. General diseases frequently accompanied by a mouth disorder include vitamin B complex or vitamin C deficiency, blood dyscrasias, metallic medication intoxication, infectious disease and any condition that interferes with the normal fluid and food intake or salivary secretion.

Predisposing factors in mouth lesions are debilitation, poor dietary habits, poor oral and dental hygiene, dehydration, emotional stress and mouth breathing.

Disorders of the mouth

Manifestations of mouth disorders include discomfort or toothache, especially when taking food, and as a result the patient rejects adequate nutrition. There may be a palpable mass or a swollen area evident within the oral cavity or on the external surface. Bleeding of the gums or from a lesion may be present. An offensive breath may indicate sordes or infection. Excessive salivation or dryness and/or disagreeable taste may be present. The individual may experience difficulty with clear speech or with swallowing.

MASTICATION DISORDERS

Food is taken into the mouth where it is broken up, mixed with saliva, lubricated and then swallowed. The act of chewing is partly voluntary and partly reflex. The teeth serve to break up the food and jaw and tongue movements shift the bolus of food around in the mouth.

A healthy oral mucosa is moist, intact and of a dark pink colour. Healthy gums (gingivae) are a lighter pink and firm and fit closely to the teeth, forming papillae to fill the interdental spaces. The tongue, a light pink, is moist and has minute papillae on the superior surface. A slight white 'fur' may be present, particularly in the morning.

DENTAL CARIES

Tooth decay is a major health problem caused by the action of organisms on ingested refined carbohydrates; acids are produced which eventually destroy the enamel surface of the teeth. Tooth decay, cavity formation, inflammation and eventual loss of teeth result if measures are not instituted to prevent progression of the process. Prevention, particularly during childhood, includes: regular brushing of the teeth following eating; restriction of refined carbohydrate foods; and the use of fluoride in topical applications, toothpaste and drinking water. Fig. 17.8 illustrates the normal structure of a tooth and adjoining gum and the effects of build-up of debris on the tooth and gums.

PERIODONTAL DISEASE

This disorder affects the tissues that support the teeth. Development of periodontal disease is influenced by the build-up of plaque on the teeth, poor nutrition, poor oral hygiene, malocclusion of the teeth and by some metabolic disorders. Symptoms include inflammation, bleeding and tenderness of the gums and loosening of the teeth. Formation of plaque is prevented by regular use of dental floss and regular examination and care by a dentist.

ACUTE TOOTH INFECTION

Infection of the dental pulp or development of an abscess at the 'root' of a tooth is very painful and may cause an elevated temperature and general malaise. The person is advised to seek prompt treatment by a dentist. An opening or canal is made to provide drainage and an antibiotic preparation may be pre-

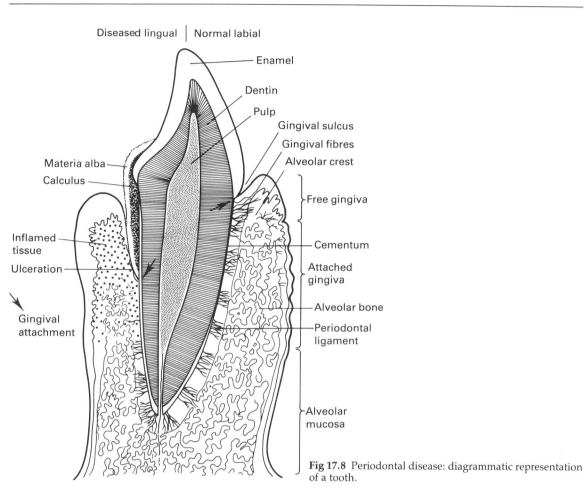

Fig 17.8 Periodontal disease: diagrammatic representation of a tooth.

scribed. In some instances, the tooth may be extracted. Frequent antiseptic or saline mouth-washes are recommended.

STOMATITIS

This is a term applied to inflammation of the oral mucosa. In some instances, it may involve the gums and the lips.

The *causes* are numerous, and include excessive smoking, dental sepsis, dehydration, vitamin deficiency, blood dyscrasia such as primary anaemia and leukaemia, local or systemic infection and a sensitivity to certain foods or drugs. The mucosa is very red and tender and ulcerative areas may develop.

Herpetic stomatitis. The lesion may occur singly or in crops on the mucosa of the mouth or on the tongue. It is commonly referred to as a mouth ulcer and appears first as a small, sore inflamed area, followed by vesicle formation. The vesicle ruptures, leaving an ulcer which usually heals in a few days. The condition is painful and the patient complains of a burning sensation.

Frequent attacks of multiple lesions can be very distressing to the patient and may interfere with food intake. Treatment is usually on an empirical basis; what may be effective for one patient may not be so with another. Since herpetic stomatitis is usually secondary to some other disorder (e.g. inflammatory intestinal disease, vitamin B_{12} deficiency), it tends to be recurrent. Various diagnostic procedures may be necessary before the primary cause is identified.

Local therapeutic measures are mainly palliative and are aimed at relief of the discomfort, prevention of infection and promotion of healing of the ulcers. Caustic agents such as silver nitrate should not be applied to the lesions as they only increase the erosion of tissue. A mild mouthwash such as sodium bicarbonate is used. Vitamin B complex and vitamin C may be prescribed. The doctor may also suggest some form of analgesic lozenge to relieve the discomfort. Bland foods and fluids, not too hot, are taken.

THRUSH (MONILIASIS)

Thrush is caused by the fungus *Candida albicans* and may also be referred to as *candidiasis*. It may develop in the vagina as well as in the mouth. It occurs most frequently in infants and children and in the very old, but may also appear in debilitated persons. Occasionally, it follows prolonged use of certain antibacterial drugs such as tetracycline (Achromycin) and chloramphenicol (Chloromycetin). Areas of superficial ulceration occur in the oral mucosa or gums, and the membrane over the lesion becomes white and is easily detached. The lesions respond to the local application of 1% gentian violet or to an antifungal antibiotic solution such as nystatin. Attention is also directed to the patient's diet in an effort to improve his resistance and general condition.

GINGIVITIS (VINCENT'S ANGINA, TRENCH MOUTH)

This is an inflammation of the gums (gingivae) followed by ulceration and necrosis. It is thought to be caused by proliferation of specific fusiform bacilli and spirochetes which are present in only small numbers in normal mouths.

The gums are swollen and painful and bleed readily. Excessive salivary secretion and an offensive breath are usually present. There is a loss of marginal gum tissue and of the interdental papillae by the ulceration and necrosis. Lesions may develop on the buccal and pharyngeal mucosa. A smear may be made from the affected area to confirm the diagnosis. Predisposing factors are poor oral and dental hygiene, malnutrition and debilitation. It may be associated with dietary deficiencies, infections, mononucleosis, alcoholism or a blood dyscrasia.

Mouthwashes are given frequently: a solution of hydrogen peroxide, saline or sodium perborate may be used. An antibiotic by parenteral administration is prescribed and may be supplemented by topical application. The person is advised not to smoke, and a soft, nutritious diet of non-irritating foods is recommended. The patient will require instrumentative treatment by a dentist as soon as the acute stage is over.

The condition is infectious and can be transmitted to other persons unless precautions are taken.

LEUCOPLAKIA

This condition is characterized by patchy, yellowish-white, firm, thickened areas of the oral mucous membrane or of the tongue. The lesion results from hyperplasia of surface epithelial tissue and keratinization.

The lesions are painless and are considered serious since they may be precancerous. They occur most frequently in men after the fourth decade of life. The lessions usually develop in response to chronic irritation that may be mechanical, chemical, thermal or infective in origin. The lesions may disappear with elimination of the irritation. In many instances, the cause is unknown.

Teeth are checked and defects corrected that may be causing irritation. Smoking should be discontinued and a high-vitamin diet is prescribed. If the area is fissured or ulcerated, a biopsy is done to determine if cancer has developed. If malignant changes have taken place, surgical excision and radiation therapy are used.

CANCER OF THE MOUTH

Carcinoma may develop on the tongue, floor of the mouth, oropharynx or buccal mucosa, but the most frequent site is the lower lip. It has a much higher incidence in males between the ages of 50 and 60 years.

The most common malignant lesion occurring in the mouth is squamous cell carcinoma. Smoking (especially pipe smoking in the case of lip cancer), excessive exposure to the sun, prolonged irritation by a jagged tooth or poorly fitting denture and chronic infection are considered to be predisposing factors. It usually appears first on the lip or mucosa as leucoplakia, as a roughened area or as a persisting ulcer.

The lesion in cancer of the tongue or buccal mucosa usually appears as a small firm lump. Later the area breaks down, leaving a painful ulcer. If the condition goes untreated, swallowing and speech become difficult, hypersalivation develops, the mucosa becomes infected and the malignant growth metastasizes to the jaw and to the lymph nodes in the neck.

As with all malignant disease, early recognition and treatment are extremely important; *any sore that resists treatment and persists for 3 weeks should receive prompt medical attention.*

Treatment involves surgical excision of the cancerous tissue and radiation therapy. Irradiation may be by interstitial implantation of needles, seeds or moulds containing radium (see Chapter 9). When metastasis to lymph nodes is suspected, more radical surgery may be performed to include dissection of the cervical lymphatics and chemotherapy may be employed (see Chapter 9). Extension of the malignant disease into the jaw may necessitate extirpation of the jaw (see Tables 17.5 and 17.6).

Table 17.5 Oral surgical procedures.

Lip resection is the excision of a portion of a lip. It is usually done to remove a benign or malignant tumour.
Glossectomy is the removal of the tongue for the treatment of carcinoma
Hemiglossectomy is the excision of a part of the tongue
Mandibulectomy is the removal of the lower jaw bone; it may be partial or complete
Buccal resection is the excision of a section of a cheek (bucca)
Radical neck dissection (eu bloc dissection) involves the extensive excision of cervical lymph nodes and non-vital tissues on the side of a primary malignant neoplasm of the salivary gland, tongue or mouth

Table 17.6 Plan of care for the patient undergoing oral surgery.

Identification of problems	Goals	Nursing intervention	Expected outcomes
Preoperative preparation			
1 Anxiety, related to lack of knowledge of the disease process, impending surgical intervention, concern for potential deformity and disfigurement and loss of the ability to ingest food and communicate	**a** To alleviate anxiety **b** To acquire knowledge of the disease, the surgical procedure and expectations for the postoperative period	**a** Provide opportunity and privacy for the patient to express his fears and concerns **b** Evaluate the patient's and family's understanding of the disease process, hospitalization, surgery and expectations for the postoperative period **c** Provide information about the disorder, surgery, hospital routines, pre- and postoperative care to be provided and expected patient participation **d** Correct any misconceptions the patient and family may have about the disorder and treatment **e** Excisions of the lip and tongue may interfere with speech and communication. Discuss communication measures that may be used such as writing with pad and pencil, hand signals or communication boards **f** If a hemiglossectomy is to be performed discuss alternative feeding methods that will be used, such as nasogastric tube feedings or total parenteral nutrition **g** If possible introduce the patient and family to other members of the care team and personnel from the operating room **h** Inform the family of services available to them while they wait for the patient to return from surgery	1 The patient's anxiety is decreased, as evidenced by normal pulse and respiratory rates and rhythm and minimal agitation when discussing surgery 2 The patient indicates understanding of the reasons for the surgery, the surgical procedures and what may be expected in the postoperative period regarding his fluid and nutritional needs, pain management, communication, mouth and wound care and visits from his family 3 Patient participates in preoperative routines and care
2 Alteration in nutrition: less than body requirements, related to inadequate food intake due to the discomfort incurred by the oral lesions	To alleviate fluid and nutritional deficiencies prior to surgery	**a** Assess the patient's hydration and nutritional status **b** Provide oral fluids and nutrients as tolerated **c** Provide supplementary fluids and nutrients as prescribed by intravenous route, nasogastric feedings or parenteral nutrition through a central venous catheter **d** Record fluid intake and output	1 Further weight loss does not occur 2 Fluid balance is adequate, as measured by normal volume of urine output, normal serum haematocrit level and skin turgor 3 Serum electrolytes and pH are within the normal range
3 Alteration in oral mucous membrane related to interruption of normal defences of the mouth from the disease and impending surgery	To decrease potential for infection of the mouth	**a** Provide oral hygiene every 4 hours. Debris is removed with hydrogen peroxide solution followed by an irrigation of normal saline. Teeth are cleaned with a soft toothbrush or sponge swabs. Sodium bicarbonate solutions may be used to rinse the mouth if saliva is thick. This is followed by rinsing with normal saline **b** Oral and/or topical antibiotics may be prescribed	1 The lips, oral mucosa and tongue are clean, moist and free of debris and crusts

Table 17.6—*continued*

Identification of problems	Goals	Nursing intervention	Expected outcomes
Postoperative care **1** Ineffective airway clearance, related to: oedema of the mouth, tongue and throat; impaired swallowing; and accumulation of secretions in the mouth and throat	To maintain a patent airway	**a** Extensive resection of the tongue and larynx may necessitate a tracheostomy (see care of patient with a tracheostomy pp. 433–436) **b** Assess the respiratory status of the patient (constantly at first). Note: the respiratory rate, rhythm and pattern; pulse rate and volume; accumulation of oral secretions; and difficulty in swallowing. Tissue of the face and neck are observed for swelling **c** Place the patient in a semi-prone or lateral position to facilitate drainage of secretions and prevent aspiration. As soon as the vital signs are stable, elevate the head of the bed **d** If secretions are excessive, place a gauze wick in the corner of the mouth to facilitate drainage. Avoid suctioning if a hemiglossectomy was performed, as the tongue is very vascular and haemorrhage may occur	**1** Respiratory rate and rhythm are within the normal range for the patient **2** Chest expansion is symmetrical and abdominal movements are observed **3** Pulse rate and volume are normal for patient **4** Wheezes and crackles are absent on auscultation of the lungs
2 Altered nutrition: less than body requirements, related to altered ability to ingest food and fluids	To maintain adequate nutritional intake	The method of supplying fluids and nutrition will depend on the nature and extent of the surgery: **a** Supply intravenously for the first few days **b** Nasogastric tube feedings are usually administered to allow healing of the mouth **c** If the patient has prolonged difficulty with swallowing or if reconstructive plastic surgery is undertaken, total parenteral nutrition is instituted (see text). **d** When oral fluids and foods are permitted, begin with a small amount of clear fluid to evaluate the patient's ability to swallow and to minimize the possibility of aspiration and regurgitation. Fluids are gradually increased as tolerated, and soft, puréed foods are introduced. Fluids and food should be at room temperature. There should be gradual progression to a soft then regular diet as tolerated	**1** Weight loss is less than 2 kg in the postoperative period **2** Urine output is maintained within a normal range **3** Serum electrolytes and pH are within the normal range
3 Impaired verbal communication, related to the surgical procedure, oedema and pain	To be able to communicate needs to others	**a** A pencil and paper, and/or a communication board are kept within the patient's reach while speech is impaired **b** Teach the patient hand signals so that he can convey his needs and respond to questions	**1** The patient communicates by writing, hand signals or touch **2** Difficulties with swallowing and speaking are minimized by control of pain, maintenance of

Table 17.6—*continued*

Identification of problems	Goals	Nursing intervention	Expected outcomes
3 Impaired verbal communication (continued)		**c** Administer analgesics regularly to control pain **d** The mouth is irrigated with sterile normal saline and artificial saliva is provided if indicated to lubricate the mouth to facilitate speaking and swallowing. Precautions are observed to prevent aspiration **e** Place the patient's call-button within reach and advise him of the nurse's leaving and expected time of return **f** Encourage family members to sit with the patient and to use and encourage use of touch and other forms of communication in order to decrease the effort required by the patient in speaking **g** Use statements requiring 'yes', 'no' or short answers when conversing with the patient **h** Arrange for speech retraining if extensive resection of the tongue has been performed	moisture of mouth and limiting the need for conversation
4 Alteration in oral mucous membrane, related to surgical intervention and interruption of normal defences of the mouth and oral mucosa	To restore integrity of the oral mucosa and prevent infection	**a** Perform oral hygiene every 2–4 hours initially and following food intake when the patient begins oral feeding. Debris may be removed from uninvolved areas of the mouth with cotton swabs moistened with hydrogen peroxide. Teeth are cleaned with sponge swabs. Brushing is usually contraindicated because of trauma to tissues. The mouth may be irrigated with sterile normal saline using a small catheter. With the patient's head tilted to the side, the fluid drains into a basin. Precautions are taken to avoid soiling the dressing by the return flow **b** Administer antibiotics as prescribed **c** Inspect the mouth for healing of the surgical area and signs of redness, oedema, crusting and fluid accumulation	**1** The mouth is clean and moist **2** The surgical area is clean and intact **3** Areas of the mouth unaffected by the surgery are clean, moist, soft and intact
5 Disturbance in body image related to physical changes resulting from the surgical excision and reconstruction of tissues, and difficulty in speaking and swallowing	To express feelings and concern about his physical appearance	**a** Encourage the patient to express his feelings and concerns **b** Provide information about the healing process and help the patient to set realistic expectations about how he will look when healing has taken place and the swelling has gone **c** Difficulty with swallowing and speaking may be temporary but if permanent changes are anticipated the patient is told what can and will be done to help him	**1** The patient expresses concerns and feelings about his appearance **2** Social contact with family, friends, and other patients increases

Table 17.6—*continued*

Identification of problems	Goals	Nursing intervention	Expected outcomes
5 Disturbance in body image (continued)		**d** Facilitate social interaction by encouraging family visits and placing the patient in a room with a compatible patient **e** If reconstructive surgery is done, introduce the patient to someone who has had a similar experience **f** Provide assistance and faciulities for the patient to care for hair and personal appearance. Encourage the patient to dress in his own clothing as soon as he is ambulatory	
6 Lack of knowledge about health care needs, skills in performing care, and awareness of available resources	To develop skills in self-management of nutritional needs, oral hygiene and continuing care that may be required	**a** As soon as the patient is alert and able, encourage him to participate in his feeding and oral hygiene **b** Provide oral and written instructions for feeding and oral hygiene before discharge **c** If tube feedings or parenteral nutrition are to be continued, teach the patient and family the specific procedure and give them opportunities to practise with supervision. Referral is made to the community health nursing organization if necessary **d** Provide instructions regarding on-going care. Radiation therapy may be necessary and continuing speech therapy should be arranged **e** A referral to a dentist for a dental prosthesis is made as indicated	1 The patient and family indicate a plan to meet nutritional needs and perform oral hygienic measures following discharge 2 The patient and family communicate a plan to carry out recommended care (e.g. speech therapy, dental prosthesis etc.) following discharge

INFLAMMATION OF THE PAROTID GLAND

Inflammation of a parotid gland is the most common disturbance of the salivary glands and may be due to infection by the specific virus that causes mumps, or it may develop as a result of any non-specific bacterial invasion of the gland. Non-specific parotitis may occur as a complication in febrile diseases or when dehydration is present and there is a lack of attention to oral hygiene. It tends to develop more readily in older and debilitated persons. The onset is sudden, the gland becomes swollen and painful and the patient develops a fever.

Preventive measures include frequent mouth care and keeping the mouth moist by ample fluid intake, sucking sour sweets (lemon) and chewing gum. The disorder is treated by the parenteral administration of antibiotics. If suppuration develops, surgical drainage is necessary. The fluid intake is increased and frequent mouth care is necessary. The local application of an ice bag to the area may be prescribed if pus has not formed.

OBSTRUCTION TO THE FLOW OF SALIVA

Obstruction of any one of the salivary glands may be due to *intrinsic* or *extrinsic* causes. Disease *within* the gland or duct may be infection, newgrowth or a calculus. In conditions that cause inflammation, the duct may be occluded by swelling and oedema or later by the resulting scar tissue. *Extrinsic* causes such as a tumour or infection in neighbouring structures may compress the duct, or scar tissue resulting from stomatitis may close off the duct orifice.

The obstruction is manifested by swelling of the affected gland. The swelling is most pronounced during meals because of the salivary stimulation and may subside between meals. Pain and tenderness may be due to the pressure or to the condition causing the obstruction. Fever and general malaise may accompany infection.

Constriction of the duct is treated by probing and dilatation. A calculus may be removed via the duct or, if this approach should fail, surgical removal may have to be undertaken.

A *tumour in a salivary gland* causes a more gradual swelling unrelated to salivary stimulation. It is treated by prompt surgical excision of the gland. The parotid gland is the most frequent site of salivary tumours; the submaxillary gland is next in order of incidence. If the doctor suspects the tumour is malignant because of its firmness, fixation and involvement of the facial nerve, a biopsy may be done to confirm the diagnosis. Surgery is the therapy of choice since malignant neoplasms of the salivary glands are radiation resistant. Carcinoma involves radical surgery. In the case of cancer of a parotid gland, removal of the mandible and dissection of the cervical lymphatics may be necessary. Surgical excision of the submaxillary gland for malignancy includes dissection of the cervical lymphatics and possibly resection of the mandible. Following such disfiguring surgery as the extirpation of the lower jaw, a prosthesis may be constructed of a synthetic material which is physically and chemically inert and is implanted in the area to restore a normal appearance.

Following any surgery on the parotid gland, the patient is observed for signs of facial paralysis because of the close proximity of the facial nerve to the operative site. In some instances the facial nerve may be involved by a malignant tumour and is removed with the gland, leaving the patient with some permanent facial paralysis.

FRACTURE OF THE JAW

Fracture of the jaw is a relatively common injury in motor accidents, some sports and violent disagreements. Diagnosis may be made on crepitus, apparent deformity, and abnormal, painful movement of the mandible, and is confirmed by x-ray.

Treatment and nursing intervention for fracture of the jaw. If the fragments are displaced, they are approximated and the lower jaw is immobilized. The latter may be achieved by wiring the lower jaw to the upper jaw or by attaching soft metal bars to the upper and lower teeth. These bars have hooks from which rubber bands extend between the upper and lower jaws, applying traction and fixation.

Following immobilization of the lower jaw, the patient is placed in a semiprone or lateral position to promote oral drainage and prevent aspiration of secretions during recovery from anaesthesia. A wire cutter is kept at the bedside; if the patient vomits, the wire or bands that immobilize the lower jaw must be released immediately so the mouth can be opened to prevent aspiration. A nasogastric tube may be passed and attached to low suction to remove gastric contents and reduce the risk of aspiration. Pharyngeal and oral suctioning with a small catheter may be necessary to remove secretions; trauma and resulting oedema of pharyngeal tissues may interfere with swallowing.

The patient receives a high-calorie fluid diet. It may be given for a brief period via the nasogastric tube but as soon as possible it is taken orally through a straw.

The mouth is thoroughly cleansed every 2 hours after each feeding. Normal saline or a mild antiseptic mouthwash may be used. The buccal mucosa and exposed areas of the gums are examined twice daily for lesions and sordes.

Early ambulation is encouraged and the patient may be discharged from the hospital as soon as he can care for himself. The nurse will be responsible for teaching the patient and/or a family member the importance of good oral hygiene and how to carry out the necessary cleansing and inspection. The diet, with suggestions for variation, and its preparation and digestion are discussed in detail. When the wires are removed the patient is urged to see a dentist.

NURSING INTERVENTION

When caring for a patient with an oral disorder, it should be remembered that the mouth and associated structures are concerned with the ingestion, mastication and swallowing of food, the sense of taste, speech and physical appearance. Some disorders of the mouth may also cause respiratory difficulty.

Factors to be considered when planning patient care will depend upon the nature and severity of the disorder, whether surgery is involved and the degree to which there is impairment of functions and disfigurement.

ORAL SURGERY

The major surgical procedures are most frequently done for carcinoma. They include resection of the buccal mucosa, glossectomy, hemiglossectomy, mandibulectomy and radical neck dissection (Table 17.5). For *nursing management* of the patient requiring intra-oral or radical neck dissection, see Table 17.6. The reader is also referred to Chapter 11 for consideration of the care of the patient prior to surgery, and during the intraoperative and postoperative periods.

Rehabilitation exercises are used after a radical neck dissection: These exercises are started when the wounds are firmly healed. The type of exercises prescribed varies for each individual. The frequency of exercise is limited to start with and gradually increased as the patient's tolerance improves. They are commenced slowly and gently; quick, jerky movements are avoided.

Head exercises. The patient: (1) turns the head to each side, (2) alternately flexes it laterally and forward, and (3) then extends it.

Shoulder exercises. The patient assumes the sitting position with arms and hands placed in front of the trunk. The arms and shoulders are drawn back, elevated and then rotated.

Further shoulder exercises are prescribed for the individual patient according to the extent of the surgery and the degree of wound healing that has occurred.

Disorders of the oesophagus

Manifestations of oesophageal disorders include dysphagia (difficulty in swallowing), regurgitation, pyrosis (heartburn), substernal pain and bleeding.

CAUSES

Interference with the transmission of food and fluid from the mouth to the stomach may be due to an abnormal condition within the oesophagus or to an extrinsic disorder. Swallowing may be impaired by a disturbance in innervation to the oesophageal muscle tissue, a decrease in or an obstruction of the lumen or the tube or by mucosal irritation and inflammation.

Disease of neighbouring structures
Since the mouth, tongue and pharynx are involved in directing food and fluid into the oesophagus, it is obvious that disease in any one of these structures may interefere with the initial phase of swallowing. This may be seen in severe stomatitis, pharyngitis, tonsillitis, cleft palate and neoplastic disease of the mouth or tongue. The condition may actually interfere with the swallowing process or cause so much pain that the patient avoids swallowing.

Compression of the oesophagus by enlargement or neoplasms of neighbouring structures occurs rarely. Examples are goitre (enlargement of the thyroid), aortic aneurysm and enlargement of the mediastinal lymph glands.

Neurological disorder
Dysphagia may result from a nervous system disorder that affects innervation to the central striated muscle tissue of the oesophagus. Damage to the swallowing centre in the medulla or to nerve fibres of the tenth cranial (vagus) nerve concerned with the swallowing mechanism may cause a partial or complete paralysis. Paralysis may occur in the pharyngeal area owing to interference with normal innervation via the ninth (glossopharyngeal) cranial nerve. Failure of the normal pharyngeal phase of swallowing may result in food passing into the trachea and the nasal cavities. The sphincter at the oesophageal opening may remain relaxed, allowing air to be drawn into the oesophagus during inspiration.

Conditions in which paralysis of swallowing is commonly seen include myasthenia gravis (failure of nerve impulse transmission at the neuromuscular junction), poliomyelitis that involves the motor neurons in the swallowing centre, and cerebrovascular accident (stroke).

Congenital abnormalities
A congenital abnormality may occasionally be the cause of impaired swallowing in the newborn infant. The commonest malformations of the oesophagus include atresia, stenosis and tracheo-oesophageal fistula. In atresia, the oesophagus is interrupted, ending in a blind pouch. Stenosis is a constriction of the tube at one point that prevents the passage of food to the stomach. In a tracheo-oesophageal fistula there is an opening between the trachea and the oesophagus. This may be combined with atresia, in which case the oesophagus opens into and ends in the trachea. In other instances, the oesophagus may be complete, but a short tube exists between it and the trachea.

Manifestations of an oesophageal malformation in the newborn may be continuous drooling (since the normal amount of saliva cannot be swallowed), regurgitation of the feeding, choking and cyanosis. Prompt recognition and reporting of any indication of difficulty in swallowing may save the infant's life. Early diagnosis and surgical treatment are necessary in the first few days of life if the infant is to survive. The infant's need for fluids and nourishment is paramount. A gastrostomy may be done in which an opening is made into the stomach through which a tube may be passed. Food is then introduced directly into the stomach. Later, surgery is undertaken to correct the anomaly.

Reflux oesophagitis
The most common cause of oesophageal mucosal irritation is regurgitation of gastric content. Bacterial, viral or fungal infection may be imposed on the inflammation. Diagnosis is usually made on the basis of the patient's complaint of dysphagia, intolerance to hot, spicy foods and substernal pain and heartburn. X-ray and endoscopy may be performed to confirm the diagnosis.

In the case of chronic regurgitation of acid gastric content into the oesophagus, function studies are made (see p. 497). The Bernstein test evaluates the patient's responses to acid in the oesophagus. Oesophageal motility is recorded and manometry is used to assess the competency of the lower oesophageal sphincter. The sphincter may be incompetent; it is relaxed permitting passage of gastric content into the oesophagus. The patient complains of a burning sensation in the oesophagus. The lower oesophageal sphincter is positioned within the abdomen (just below the diaphragm). When it is displaced into the thorax, as in a hiatus hernia, the lower oesophageal sphincter pressure is less than the intra-abdominal pressure, and reflux occurs.[27] Sphincter incomp-

---

[27] Davenport (1982) p. 48.

etency also occurs in degenerative disorders of smooth muscle.

Treatment of chronic oesophagitis may include: elevation of the head of the bed to reduce the reflux of acid gastric content during sleep; administration of an antacid orally or by a continuous drip; and inhibition of gastric secretion by a histamine H_2 receptor antagonist such as cimetidine (Tagamet). Regular meals of equal quantity and low fat are recommended as well as the avoidance of coffee, alcohol and smoking. The person is advised to remain upright for at least 2 hours following a meal. If the cause of persistent oesophagitis is an incompetent lower oesophageal sphincter, surgical repair to prevent reflux may be necessary. The operative procedure frequently used is a fundoplication, in which the fundus of the stomach is wrapped around the lower end of the oesophagus and sutured to it, or a modified form of this may be performed.

Chronic oesophagitis may incur progressive formation of scar tissue leading to stricture. This may be treated by intralumenal dilation by the insertion of bougies at intervals over a period of time, or may necessitate surgical correction.

Oesophageal achalasia

This is the term used to describe the inability of the lower oesophageal sphincter to open in response to swallowing, accompanied by a lack of tone in the musculature above the sphincter and loss of peristalsis in that area. In the northern hemisphere the cause of achalasia is unknown. In South America it can be due to Chagas disease, caused by the parasite *Trypanosoma cruzi* which causes denervation of the gastrointestinal tract probably by an autoimmune mechanism. The oesophagus gradually dilates above the denervated sphincter. The result is an accumulation and stagnation of food and fluids in the dilated segment.

The symptoms of the disorder are: a full, uncomfortable feeling in substernal region, pyrosis, dysphagia and regurgitation. The patient may also experience coughing and dyspnoea due to pressure on the trachea by the distended oesophagus; a disturbance in normal cardiac functioning may even be manifested.

Achalasia may be treated by the surgical procedure oesophagomyotomy which involves the division of the muscle fibres at the lower end of the oesophagus. The patient tends then to develop reflux oesophagitis. In some instances, the sphincter and lower end of the oesophagus may be dilated by the introduction of an inflatable bag under x-ray control.

If dysphagia is accompanied by severe chest pain, the patient may experience many cardiovascular examinations. A diagnosis of an oesophageal origin of the pain may reduce the anxiety and the dysphagia since emotional stress and anxiety tend to aggravate the disorder. When the innervation of the oesophagus is intact and the dysphagia is myogenic

in origin, multiple swallows in rapid succession may relieve the muscular hypercontractility of the sphincter and thus the pain.

Trauma of the oesophagus

Dysphagia or aphagia may occur as a result of the ingestion of a caustic substance, foreign objects or too large a mass of food.

When a *caustic substance* such as a strong acid (e.g. sulphuric or nitric acid) or base (e.g. household bleach) is swallowed, serious corrosive burning occurs in the oesophagus. The larynx may also be affected as well as the lips, mouth and pharynx. The mucosa manifests acute inflammation, blisters, oedema and possible ulceration. If the chemical is not removed or neutralized promptly, burning and corrosion of deeper layers of tissue occurs. Later with healing, scar tissue forms and the lumen of the oesophagus is constricted. Dysphagia progressively becomes more serious over several weeks as scar tissue is laid down.

There will be evident corrosive burns on the lips and in the mouth; the voice may be hoarse and the patient experiences dysphagia and probably dyspnoea and difficulty with speech due to laryngeal irritation and oedema. Shock may develop quickly.

Management of the person who has swallowed a caustic substance includes the following.

1 The chemical swallowed is immediately identified: The lips, mouth and clothing are examined if necessary for evidence. If a container of the chemical that was taken is available, the label is checked for suggestions as to an effective antidote. Milk may serve as a neutralizing agent.

2 Vital signs are assessed and treatment for respiratory insufficiency and shock promptly commenced.

3 An oesophagoscopy is done as soon as possible (within 12–24 hours) to determine the extent and depth of the burns.

4 An analgesic is prescribed for relief of pain.

5 Oropharyngeal suctioning may be necessary to prevent aspiration of secretions.

6 Sips of water may be permitted to satisfy the patient. Gastric lavage and induced vomiting are contraindicated to prevent further damage to the oesophageal wall. An intravenous infusion is given to provide fluid and electrolytes.

7 A tracheostomy may be necessary if laryngeal oedema is indicated by respiratory distress and stridor (see p. 432). Blood gases are monitored.

8 A corticosteroid preparation is prescribed to reduce the inflammatory response and to lessen scar tissue formation and ensuing stricture. An antibiotic preparation is usually given to prevent serious infection.

9 A gastrostomy may be necessary in severe constriction in order to provide adequate food and fluids.

10 Stricture of the oesophagus is treated by bougie-

nage; as soon as sufficient healing has taken place, bougies are passed into the oesophagus every day or two to dilate the lumen. The interval between treatment is gradually lengthened, but the bougienage may extend for over a period of a year or more. If a gastrostomy is necessary, it may serve for retrograde bougienage as well as for feedings. A very fine bougie is passed into the oesophagus and remains in place between treatments, one end protruding from the nose, the other from the gastrostomy opening. The two ends are then tied together. During dilatations, the larger bougie is attached to the lower end of the finer bougie and is then pulled up through the oesophagus.

11 If bougie therapy is not successful, surgical resection of the constricted area with end-to-end anastomosis may be performed. When the area is extensive, surgical reconstruction of the oesophagus may be undertaken. A plastic tube or a section of intestine may be implanted to provide a patent passageway.

Nursing intervention for the patient requiring surgery on the oesophagus is described in the plan of nursing care in Table 17.7.

The oesophagus may be injured by a rough or sharp foreign body (e.g. pen, nail, meat or fish bone, small toy). The object may cause dysphagia or aphagia. The patient experiences choking and becomes frightened and agitated. An oesophagoscopy is done and the foreign body located and removed. The patient may complain of soreness and dysphagia for a few days.

Occasionally a large mass of food may lodge in the oesophagus (meat is the most common offender) causing obstruction of the lumen and respiratory distress by pressure on the trachea. Prompt emergency care is necessary; an airway is established. Oesophagoscopy may be done to locate and remove the mass and assess the injury to the oesophagus.

Neoplasms of the oesophagus

Benign neoplasms. These occur rarely in the oesophagus. The most common of these are leiomyomas which are tumours of non-striated muscle tissue. Those encountered less frequently are polyps, cysts, fibromas, adenomas and fibrolipomas. As the tumour imposes itself on the lumen of the oesophagus or interferes with normal muscle activity, dysphagia occurs. The patient first experiences difficulty in swallowing the more solid foods, such as meat and bread. The tumour is excised and whether the approach is transoesophageal, cervical or thoracic will depend on the location and the nature of the tumour.

Carcinoma. Cancer of the oesophagus tends to develop more often in the older age group. Its incidence is mainly in males between 50 and 70 years of age, and the lower third of the oesophagus is the most common site. The majority of malignant tumours of the oesophagus are squamous cell cancer (epidermoid cancer). Adenocarcinoma may occur but is most frequently secondary to gastric carcinoma.

The patient complains first of dysphagia with solid foods which gradually progresses to difficulty with liquids. Substernal discomfort and pain, regurgitation and loss of weight and strength are experienced with steadily increasing severity. In advanced stages, bleeding may occur. Structures adjacent to the primary lesion may become involved: the disease may spread to the trachea, bronchi, stomach, diaphragm or associated lymph nodes, depending upon its location in the oesophagus.

Diagnosis is made by x-ray examination and an oesophagoscopy. A biopsy is obtained and a smear from the lesion is probably taken for cytologic study during the endoscopic examination.

Treatment may be by surgical resection and/or irradiation. Various surgical procedures are employed. The affected part of the oesophagus is resected with a wide margin of normal tissue as well as the regional lymph nodes. If the lesion is in the lower part, the upper portion of the stomach is also removed (oesophagogastrectomy). The remaining proximal portion of the oesophagus is anastomosed to the stomach which is drawn up into the thoracic cavity (oesophagogastrostomy). A nasogastric tube is passed and remains until the anastomosis is fairly well healed and peristalsis is established.

If the cancer is located in the middle or upper portions of the oesophagus, or if a large area is involved, it is more difficult to treat the patient surgically. A segment of the patient's intestine (jejunum or colon) may be implanted to replace the resected oesophagus. More recently, a plastic tube has been used to re-establish a passageway between the remaining oesophagus and the stomach.

Following diagnosis and investigation of the patient's general condition, the surgeon may conclude that radical surgery is inadvisable. Radiation therapy may be used with some benefit. A plastic nasogastric tube may be inserted through the constricted area and left in place so the patient can be given fluids and nourishment. Complications of ulceration and bleeding may develop with this latter palliative procedure. More often, a gastrostomy is employed by which nutrition is maintained for the remainder of the patient's life (see p. 510).

Oesophageal varices

This serious condition is associated with cirrhosis of the liver and is discussed in Chapter 18.

HIATUS HERNIA (DIAPHRAGMATIC HERNIA)

The openings in the diaphragm which accommodate

Table 17.7 Plan of care for the patient requiring surgery of the oesophagus.

Potential problem	Goals	Nursing intervention	Expected outcomes
Preoperative preparation **1** Anxiety due to lack of knowledge of the disease process and surgical intervention, inability to swallow, and potential deformity	**a** To alleviate anxiety **b** To acquire some understanding of the disorder, surgical procedure and expectations for the postoperative period	**a** Acknowledge the patient's and family's feelings of apprehension and concern for the future **b** Identify specific fears, misconceptions and learning needs regarding the disorder, hospital routines, surgery, postoperative expectations and implications for future functioning **c** Explain what may be expected in the postoperative period and answer the patient's and family's questions willingly. An explanation is given of the numerous pieces of equipment that will be necessary at his bedside after the operation and of the need for the nasogastric, chest and intravenous tubes and frequent suctioning. Stress the importance of deep breathing, frequent turning and the simple foot and leg exercises and instruct the patient how to breathe deeply, cough and do the exercises. The discussion of the postoperative period is extended over several periods and, as the patient talks about it and asks questions, his apprehension of the situation may be reduced	**1** The patient experiences decreased anxiety **2** Pulse and respiratory rates are within the normal range for the patient **3** Posturing, excessive verbalization, crying or other indications of anxiety decrease **4** The patient states the purpose and expectations of the surgical procedure and postoperative routines **5** The patient practises deep-breathing exercises and coughing
2 Alteration in nutrition: less than body requirements, related to inadequate food and fluid intake as a result of dysphagia	To correct fluid and nutritional deficiencies prior to surgery	**a** Assess the patient's nutritional status by obtaining a recent diet history and recording weight and body fat. His hydrational status is also assessed **b** Encourage the patient to take as much food and fluids as he can manage orally. High-calorie, high-protein liquids or semiliquid foods may be given, but if the condition limits the oral intake and the patient is emaciated and dehydrated, tube feedings and parenteral fluids may be ordered, or a gastrostomy may even be considered necessary. Blood transfusions may be necessary to correct anaemia that has resulted from nutritional deficiency	**1** Fluid balance is adequate. The serum haematocrit level and skin turgor are normal **2** Serum electrolytes and pH are within the normal range
3 Potential for injury: infection related to surgical intervention and abnormal nutritional state	To decrease the potential for infection	**a** Perform oral hygiene regularly using an antiseptic mouthwash to decrease organisms and accumulated secretions in the mouth **b** If reconstructive surgery is anticipated which may involve the use of a segment of the patient's intestine (jejunum or colon) to replace the resected	**1** Oral mucosa is clean, moist, soft and intact **2** Preparation of the gastrointestinal tract for surgery is carried out as ordered

Table 17.7—*continued*

Potential problem	Goals	Nursing intervention	Expected outcomes
3 Potential for injury (continued)		oesophagus, an oral antibiotic or sulphonamide may be ordered for several days prior to the resection to reduce the intestinal bacteria. If the patient is being tube-fed, the preparation is put into solution and given through the nasogastric or gastrostomy tube.	
Postoperative care **1** Ineffective breathing pattern, related to the chest incision and the presence of chest drainage tubes	To maintain effective respiratory functioning	**a** Care of the patient following chest surgery is discussed in Chapter 16 **b** Maximum inspirations are performed several times each hour. The nurse assists the patient to a sitting position and supports the incision **c** Staged coughing is performed to mobilize secretions; forced coughing is avoided because the increased pressure created presents a hazard to the oesophageal sutures	**1** The patient's respirations are regular, rhythmic and deep **2** Chest expansion is symmetrical **3** Wheezes and crackles are absent on auscultation of lungs **4** Arterial blood gas concentrations are within the normal range
2 Potential for injury, related to surgical intervention and incomplete healing process	To promote healing	**a** If a nasogastric tube has been introduced in the operating room, it is usually attached to a suction apparatus for continuous removal of gastric secretions. The drainage may be coloured with blood for the first few hours but should gradually assume the characteristics of normal secretions. Directions will be given when the suction is to be discontinued and when nasogastric fluids and feedings are to be given **b** A temporary gastrostomy may be used for drainage and feedings; a nasogastric tube may simply be kept in position to maintain a patent oesophagus. (See care of the patient requiring gastric surgery, Table 17.8) **c** A frequent check is made of the patient's temperature and white blood cell count for any indication of infection. If either is increased to levels above the normal, parenteral administration of an antibiotic is ordered. In some instances the surgeon may prefer to start the antibiotic administration after the operation as a prophylactic measure against infection **d** Perform oral hygiene several times a day to promote comfort and prevent possible infection of the oral mucosa which could spread to the oesophagus	**1** The patient is able to swallow clear fluids without regurgitation when the nasogastric tube is removed in 4–7 days **2** Body temperature and white blood cell count are within the normal range 1 week postoperatively

Table 17.7—*continued*

Potential problem	Goals	Nursing intervention	Expected outcomes
3 Alteration in nutrition: less than body requirements, related to inability to swallow, surgical intervention and nasogastric intubation	To maintain adequate nutritional intake	**a** The nasogastric tube may be removed in 4–7 days, and small amounts of water may then be given. Any difficulty in swallowing or regurgitation is promptly reported. The patient will find swallowing easier if he is sitting up. If he has no difficulty with water, the fluids are gradually varied and increased in volume. The diet gradually progresses through semiliquids, blended or soft foods and a normal diet. Parenteral fluids and gastrostomy feedings are continued until the patient is able to swallow adequate amounts of fluids and food. If the surgical procedure entailed an oesophagogastric anastomosis with the stomach being drawn up into the thoracic cavity, the patient may not be able to take the ordinary amount of food or fluid at one time without experiencing pressure in his chest and some dyspnoea. In this event, the patient is fed smaller amounts at more frequent intervals and should remain upright in the sitting position for 1–2 hours after eating **b** A record is kept of the patient's fluid intake and output and the balance is noted until a normal intake by mouth is well established **c** Serum electrolytes are closely monitored because of the loss of gastric secretions through the nasogastric tube. Electrolytes, especially potassium and chloride, may be needed in the intravenous infusions	**1** Weight loss is less than 2 kg over the postoperative period **2** Fluid intake is adequate and the urinary output is maintained within the normal range **3** Serum electrolytes and pH are within normal ranges **4** Oral fluids and soft foods are taken and tolerated
4 Alteration in comfort: pain, related to surgical intervention	To control pain and discomfort	**a** Simple nursing measures such as change of position, rubbing the back and remaining with the patient for brief periods may help **b** An analgesic may be necessary to provide relief but is used sparingly to avoid depression of respirations	**1** The patient expresses relief, relaxes and sleeps
5 Mobility is impaired as a result of surgery, decreased energy and the presence of tubes and suction equipment	To prevent complications of immobility	**a** Assist the patient to perform deep breathing every 2–4 hours postoperatively **b** Change the patient's position every 2–4 hours. An alternating pressure mattress is placed on the bed if the patient is emaciated and malnourished to reduce the risk of developing pressure sores. A sheepskin is placed under pressure areas	**1** The patient's skin is intact with no areas of redness or oedema **2** Patient moves about freely. Ambulation progressively increases over the first few days postoperatively

Table 17.7—*continued*

Potential problem	Goals	Nursing intervention	Expected outcomes
5 Impaired mobility (continued)		**c** Assist the patient to sit on the side of the bed and to move around the bed as soon as possible after the surgery. Ambulation is increased each day	
6 Inadequate knowledge about dietary modifications and post-hospital health management	To develop: **a** A plan for post-hospital health management **b** Skills needed for self-care at home	**a** Inform the patient that the convalescent period is usually long **b** Explain necessary dietary modifications and meal pattern to the patient and family. Instruct the patient not to swallow large amounts at one time. A brief rest period should follow each feeding or meal **c** Refer the patient to the district nurse or a social agency if necessary. The patient and family may require social and financial counselling if the patient is not able to return to work for a prolonged period of time	The patient and family: **1** Indicate a satisfactory plan to meet nutritional and other health needs at home **2** Exhibit an awareness of community resources for nursing care and social services

the oesophagus and aorta are potential sites for the herniation of abdominal viscera into the thoracic cavity. The hiatus through which the oesophagus passes is the most vulnerable area; normally, when oesophageal content passes into the stomach it does not return to the oesophagus. If it does, it is referred to as reflux (a return flow).

Cause

The chief causes of the defect in the diaphragm are considered to be a congenital weakness and the ageing process. The former probably results from a defect in the fusion of tissues around the opening. The incidence of hiatal hernia is much greater in middle-aged and elderly persons, and is probably due to weakening of the diaphragmatic muscle. The weakness or gap that occurs results in imperfect closure of the hiatus around the oesophagus. Rarely, the hernia may be caused by trauma such as a fractured rib or perforating foreign object (e.g. bullet) or prolonged, extreme intra-abdominal pressure as occurs in ascites or pregnancy.

Classification

The hernia may be classified as sliding (oesophago-gastric) or rolling (paroesophageal) (see Fig. 17.9). A *sliding hiatal hernia* is one in which the oesophago-gastric junction and a portion of the fundus of the stomach ride up into the thoracic cavity. In a sliding hernia, the lower oesophageal sphincter at the oeso-phagogastric opening (cardia) loses competency, resulting in reflux of the gastric contents into the oesophagus. In a *rolling* or *paraoesophageal hernia*, a sac-like portion of the peritoneum and stomach her-niates through into the thorax alongside the oesoph-agus. A section of omentum may also be extruded. The cardiac sphincter usually remains competent but the displaced portion of the stomach occupies space within the mediastinum and may cause respiratory distress or impaired cardiac function by direct pressure on the heart. Distension of the herniated segment or strangulation may develop, which demands emergency surgery.

Manifestations

The symptoms depend upon the size of the hernia and the amount of displaced viscus. Intermittent mild digestive disturbances only may be experi-enced. The patient may complain of substernal burn-ing pain or discomfort (heartburn), regurgitation of acid fluid, belching, a feeling of fullness and shortness of breath. The symptoms are frequently precipitated by stooping over, straining associated with increased intra-abdominal pressure or a large meal. It may also be brought on when the patient is recumbent and may be relieved when he sits up.

Frequent reflux may cause oesophagitis, ulcer-ation and bleeding. Scarring may develop that causes some constriction and probably dysphagia. Rarely, the herniated portion is so large that it becomes incarcerated and even strangulated. Respi-rations and cardiac function are likely to be com-promised.

Diagnosis

This is made by the patient's history and by a barium meal or barium swallow. The pain of reflux oesopha-gitis associated with hiatal hernia is frequently simi-

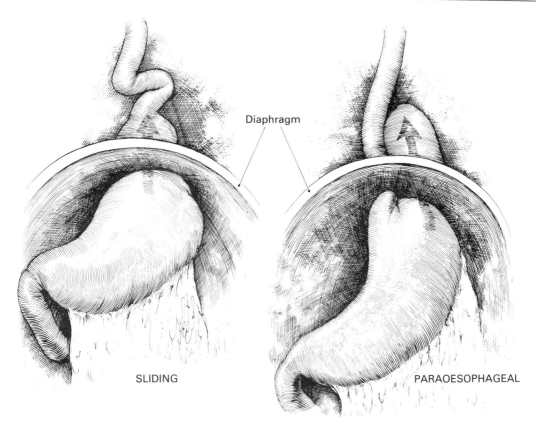

Diaphragm

SLIDING

PARAOESOPHAGEAL

Fig 17.9 *A*, Sliding hiatus hernia. *B*, Paraoesophageal hernia.

lar to that associated with angina pectoris and myocardial infarction. It may radiate up into the neck and down the left arm. As a result, when the patient initially presents with an acute episode, the doctor has an electrocardiograph made to differentiate.

Therapeutic management
A slight hernia may be controlled and the patient kept relatively asymptomatic by loss of weight (if he is obese), the avoidance of heavy lifting, and frequent, small, bland meals. Gas-forming foods, coffee and alcohol are avoided. An antacid such as an aluminium hydroxide preparation is usually prescribed to be taken after meals and at bedtime. The patient is advised to remain in an upright position for at least 2 hours after a meal. The head of his bed is elevated.

If a loop of the intestine or a portion of the stomach becomes confined in the thoracic cavity, surgical treatment is essential to return the viscus to the abdominal cavity. The surgical approach is usually made through the chest but occasionally may be made via the abdominal cavity. Following replacement of the viscus, the hiatus hernia is repaired. A nasogastric tube is likely to be introduced, and mild suction is applied to prevent vomiting and intestinal distension. Fluids are

administered by intravenous infusion for the first day or two, and then gradually introduced by mouth when the gastric suction is discontinued. For nursing care when a thoracotomy is used, see Chapter 16. For nursing care when the abdominal approach is used see Chapter 11.

NURSING INTERVENTION

Nursing intervention to alleviate dysphagia and maintain adequate nutrition and fluid intake were discussed earlier in the chapter. The care plan for the patient with oesophageal disorders adapts these measures to the specific needs of the individual.

Care of the patient requiring surgery
Surgical intervention in oesophageal disorders involves entering the thoracic cavity in most instances. In planning care, the factors cited in the section on care in chest surgery are considered. Since surgery on the lower oesophageal sphincter also involves gastric surgery and the lower end of the oesophagus, the principles which apply to nursing in gastric surgery also apply (see Table 17.8).

A pre- and postoperative care plan for the patient requiring surgery of the oesophagus is outlined in

Table 17.7. In clinical practice, the plan is adjusted to meet the needs of the individual patient.

DISORDERS OF SECRETION, DIGESTION AND MOTILITY IN THE STOMACH AND DUODENUM

The gastric and duodenal disorders most frequently seen include gastritis, peptic ulcer and carcinoma.

GASTRITIS

The term gastritis implies inflammation of the stomach. The condition may be acute or chronic and the pathological process is usually limited to the mucosa.

The causes of *acute inflammation* may be the ingestion of large quantities of alcohol, contaminated foods, or foods to which the person is sensitive or allergic, such as seafood, mushrooms or salicylates (e.g. aspirin). Infective gastritis is most frequently due to the ingestion of foods bearing staphylococci or salmonella organisms.

The patient with acute gastritis becomes ill suddenly and suffers severe epigastric pain, nausea, vomiting and fever. The attack may last a few hours to a few days. Dehydration develops rapidly and the patient becomes prostrate. The treatment includes nothing by mouth, bed rest and parenteral fluids. Clear fluids are given when the symptoms subside and, if tolerated, a bland diet of soft foods is introduced and progressively increased until a normal diet is resumed.

Chronic gastritis occurs with prolonged and repeated irritation of the mucosa and results in atrophic changes in the mucosa and glands. The cause may be evasive, since the condition may be associated with other diseases such as pernicious anaemia, and with the degenerative changes of ageing. It may result from constant subjection of the stomach to an ingested irritant, such as alcohol, and frequently accompanies a gastric ulcer or gastric carcinoma.

The symptoms of chronic gastritis are usually ill-defined but may include anorexia, discomfort and a full feeling after meals, flatulence, heartburn, nausea and occasionally haematemesis. A bland diet is recommended with abstinence from foods and fluids that seem to aggravate the condition. Spicy and raw foods, fats and very hot foods are poorly tolerated. Alcohol, coffee and salicylates should be avoided. The patient may lose considerable weight as he tends to restrict his food intake to avoid the distress it may precipitate. Attention is directed toward improving his general nutritional status by encouraging a well-balanced diet of non-irritating foods. Milk, buttermilk and egg-nogs between meals may be tolerated and are nutritious.

PEPTIC ULCER

A peptic ulcer is the erosion of a circumscribed area of tissue in the wall of the gastrointestinal tract that is accessible to gastric secretions. The actual erosion is caused by the digestive action of hydrochloric acid and pepsin. The most frequent sites of an ulcer are the stomach (*gastric ulcer*) and the proximal portion of the duodenum (*duodenal ulcer*) but the oesophagus or jejunum or any other part of the gastrointestinal mucosa may be susceptible if the surface comes in contact with gastric secretions.

The ulcer penetrates the mucosa and may invade the underlying submucosal and muscular tissues. Ulcers tend to recur; some heal promptly while others become chronic.

Causes

There is no conclusion as to the initiating cause of peptic ulcer. Normally, hydrochloric acid and pepsin are secreted but ulceration does not occur. This is attributed to the following defensive factors. The mucosa secretes sufficient mucus to dilute the secretions and provides a protective coating that prevents mucosal digestion by the acid–pepsin action. The duodenum has the additional protection of the strong alkalinity of the bile and pancreatic and intestinal secretions which neutralize the acidic chyme. Still another defence is a healthy resistant mucosa which has a good blood supply and is capable of continuous rapid regeneration of the mucosal epithelial cells.

A peptic ulcer may develop when the secretory output of hydrochloric acid and pepsin is in excess of the normal or when the protective mechanisms are inadequate in relation to the amount of acid and pepsin produced. Guyton states, 'The usual cause of peptic ulceration is an imbalance between the rate of secretion of gastric juice and the degree of protection afforded by the gastroduodenal mucosal barrier and the neutralization of the gastric acid by duodenal juices.'[28]

An increased acid level is not usually present in gastric ulcer while duodenal ulcer is associated with a high acid level. The problem is: what causes a hypersecretion of acid and pepsin or lowers mucosal resistance? Factors that are suspect include individual physiological differences such as greater parietal cell mass, greater sensitivity of the cells to the stimulating hormone gastrin, excessive production of gastrin and more rapid passage of gastric contents into the duodenum, resulting in more free acid and pepsin being delivered to the duodenum. A disturbance in the autonomic nervous control of gastric secretion that results in increased vagal (parasympathetic) innervation causes prolonged secretion of hydrochloric acid and pepsin.

The following are considered to be potential contributing factors in the development of an imbalance between the secretion of hydrochloric acid and pepsin and the defensive mechanisms of the mucosa.

---

[28] Guyton (1986), p. 799.

- *Emotional factors.* Emotional tension, anxiety, frustration and stress may cause an imbalance in the autonomic nervous system, resulting in increased vagal stimulation of gastric secretion.
- *Inflammation.*   Gastritis and trauma of the mucosa reduces the resistance of the membrane to digestion. Cell destruction is accelerated and cell reproduction, which normally renews the superficial layers quickly, may be retarded.
- *Heredity.*   Genetic factors appear to have a role, since studies on incidence show there is a tendency for peptic disease to occur in families and in persons of certain blood types. There is correlation between duodenal ulcer and the blood type O while gastric ulcer patients are more often of the blood group A.
- *Trauma and serious illness.* The patient with severe tissue injury such as that produced by extensive burns may develop severe peptic ulceration. It has been recognized as a complication frequently associated with any serious illness, especially if it is characterized by hypotension or respiratory insufficiency. These ulcers may be referred to as *stress ulcers*.
- *Certain drugs.* Some drugs, e.g. acetylsalicylic acid (aspirin), adrenal steroids (cortisone), indomethacin (Indocid) and phenylbutazone (Butazolidin), are ulcerogenic in some persons.
- *Bile reflux.* The reflux of bile and pancreatic enzymes into the stomach due to an incompetent pyloric sphincter may lead to a gastric ulcer. The bile salts damage the gastric mucosa, predisposing it to ulceration.
- *Endocrine secretions.* Rarely, severe peptic ulceration is caused by marked gastric hypersecretion that occurs in response to an excessive gastrin concentration in the blood. The gastrin is produced by a tumour of the islets of the pancreas or the submucosa of the duodenum and stomach or regional lymph nodes (Zollinger–Ellison syndrome).
   Peptic ulceration also develops in hyperparathyroidism. The disturbance is attributed to the altered serum calcium level.
- *Histamine.* Histamine promotes stimulation of acid secretion; H_2-receptor antagonists which inhibit histamine action have been found in gastric parietal cells.
- *Sex.* Peptic ulcer has a much higher incidence in men than in women. It has been suggested that oestrogenic hormones in the female may account for this.
- *Other factors.* Poor dietary habits, particularly irregular meals, are thought to be an aggravating factor. Abnormally long periods between meals in persons with a prolonged hypersecretion of acid and pepsin leave the mucosa vulnerable. The protective mechanisms cannot withstand the acid–pepsin action without the diluting and neutralizing assistance of food. Smoking and excessive amounts of alcohol or coffee increase gastric secretion.

Incidence
Peptic ulcer is a common disease and has a higher incidence in males between the ages of 40 and 55 years. Duodenal ulcer is much more common than gastric ulcer, and the incidence of gastric ulcer (not associated with cancer) is higher in females than in males. The patients frequently experience seasonal exacerbations in the spring and autumn.

Manifestations
The prominent symptom of peptic ulcer is epigastric *pain* with definite characteristics. It may radiate to the back. The pain is usually described by the patient as gnawing or burning and of being rhythmic in its development and relief in relation to the ingestion of food. The onset of pain may be immediately or up to 4 hours after a meal, depending upon the location of the ulcer, and is relieved by taking food or an antacid. In the case of an *oesophageal ulcer*, the pain develops within a few minutes after the meal. It may be intermittent and the patient usually complains of heartburn and regurgitation. Pain associated with a *gastric ulcer* usually occurs ½–1 hour after the ingestion of food; that of *duodenal ulcer* is delayed for approximately 2–4 hours. The patient's rest is frequently disturbed by nocturnal pain, especially with a duodenal ulcer. Although the ingestion of food generally provides relief, in a few instances it may be the initiating factor of the ulcer pain, particularly if the food is coarse or highly seasoned.
   Vomiting is not a common incident in peptic ulcer but may occur if the ulcer pain is very severe or if the ulcer is in the pyloric region. In the case of the latter, inflammation and oedema of the surrounding tissues, pyloric spasm or contracted scar tissue resulting from ulceration may narrow the lumen of the pylorus. This may delay the emptying of the stomach and may cause vomiting.
   The ulcer patient usually maintains his *weight*, since he eats frequently to relieve his pain unless his condition is complicated by vomiting.

Diagnosis
Investigation of the patient for peptic ulcer may include endoscopy, x-rays with a barium meal, gastric analysis to determine the hydrochloric acid secretion, gastroscopy, serum gastrin assays, exfoliative cytology and stool examination for occult blood. (See earlier in this chapter.)

Management
Treatment of the peptic ulcer patient is directed toward the relief of symptoms, healing of the ulcer and the prevention of complications and recurrence. A regimen of rest, non-irritating diet and various medications is designed to reduce gastric secretory and motor activity, dilute the gastric juice and neutralize much of the hydrochloric acid that is secreted in order to promote healing.
   Hospitalization is not always necessary. It may be

that the patient's home situation and his understanding and acceptance of the treatment are such that he may progress satisfactorily at home. A period in the hospital may be beneficial if the patient's usual environment is the source of incompatibilities, anxiety and frustration that aggravate his disease. Treatment and care should be individualized for all patients, but it is extremely important with the ulcer patient. This means that those concerned with his care must get to know the patient and his pattern of living.

Diet. Considerable controversy has arisen in recent years regarding the value and effectiveness of restrictive bland diets. Strict dietary control is not considered necessary. A regular well-balanced diet, free of foods which are upsetting to the individual, is recommended. Foods that patients usually find difficult to tolerate include coffee, tea, alcohol, highly seasoned foods and gas-forming foods. In the acute phase, small frequents meals will be more tolerable to the patient. These are gradually modified to the more customary three larger meals per day. In some instances five or six smaller meals may have to be continued.

Medications. The drugs used in the treatment of the patient with a gastric or duodenal ulcer include antacids, H_2 receptor antagonists, anticholinergic preparations, sedatives and tranquillizers.

1 *Antacids.* An antacid is given to raise the pH of gastric contents. To be effective, it must be taken frequently throughout the day and night. It is administered 1 hour after each meal and at night as prescribed. The dose is individualized on the basis of that required to reduce the patient's pain. For this reason it is important for the nurse to note the patient's response. Initially, the antacid may be indicated in hourly doses; then, as the pain diminishes, it is taken less frequently (probably four doses a day).

The antacids commonly used singly or in combination are aluminum hydroxide, magnesium oxide and calcium carbonate. The preparations of aluminium hydroxide and calcium carbonate (especially the latter) tend to cause constipation, whereas magnesium oxide has a laxative effect. Calcium carbonate is contraindicated for patients with fluid or electrolyte imbalance or a history of renal disease or calculi; it may cause hypercalcaemia and hypercalcuria. These drugs are non-absorbable; *absorbable antacids such as sodium bicarbonate are not used*, since they would produce alkalosis.

2 *H_2 receptor antagonists.* Cimetidine and ranitidine are H_2 receptor antagonists. They block the H_2 receptors in the parietal cells, inhibiting the secretion of acid. They can only be used in confirmed ulceration and are not prescribed for non-specific dyspepsia.

Abrupt withdrawal of these drugs is avoided as it leads to increased risks of complications. Side-effects such as diarrhoea, dizziness, skin rashes and mental confusion are rare. Cimetidine also potentiates the actions of certain drugs such as oral anticoagulants and phenytoin.

Cimetidine and ranitidine should only be given in single short courses of 4–6 weeks as they carry an increased risk of producing gastric cancer. Patients with resistant ulcers may have their period of treatment extended for 2–5 months.

Eighty to 90% of duodenal ulcers will recur within a year of stopping the drug and long-term use of the drug should be weighed against the benefit of surgery.[29]

3 *Anti-cholinergic drugs.* These drugs depress gastric secretion and motility. However, side-effects such as dry mouth, blurred vision, tachycardia, and urinary retention are fairly common and these drugs, with the exception of propantheline and dicyclomine, are rarely used.

4 *Sedatives and tranquillizers.* Tension and emotional stress are capable of increasing gastric secretion and motility. For this reason, sedatives are frequently a part of the treatment regimen of the ulcer patient. Small doses may be ordered throughout the day, with a larger dose being given at bedtime. Small doses of phenobarbital may be used, or amylobarbitone (Amytal), diazepam (Valium) or flurazepam (Dalmane) may be the drug of choice.

5 *Parasympathetic stimulant.* If the patient's ulcer is located in the oesophagus, a parasympathetic stimulant may be prescribed in addition to an antacid. The purpose is to tighten up the cardiac sphincter at the junction of the oesophagus and stomach and reduce reflux. An example of a parasympathetic stimulant used is metoclopramide (Maxolon). The patient is observed for side-effects, which may be disturbances in vision, crampy abdominal pain or dyspnoea.

6 *Contraindicated drugs.* Salicylate medications such as acetylsalicylic acid (aspirin) are contraindicated for the patient with a peptic or reflux ulcer or with a history of one. They are considered ulcerogenic and predispose the individual to gastrointestinal bleeding. If a mild analgesic is needed, as for a headache, paracetamol may be ordered.

Corticosteroid preparations, phenylbutazone and indomethacin (Indocin) are also considered ulcerogenic to some people.

Smoking. Ulcer patients are advised to abstain from smoking, particularly cigarettes. It is considered to increase gastric motility and secretion and delay healing of the ulcer.

Continuing assessment. The patient's understanding of and willingness to cooperate in the prescribed dietary modifications, the adherence to regular medication and abstinence of smoking, alcohol and irritating foods are assessed. Observations are made

---

[29] British National Formulary (1986).

for evidence of mental conflicts and emotional factors that may be influencing the patient's disorder. The response to the prescribed medications is noted. Prompt recognition and reporting of early symptoms of complications which may develop are an important responsibility (see below).

Education in modification of life style. It is important that the patient has some understanding of the nature of his disorder and the prescribed therapeutic measures. With adequate knowledge, he is more likely to cooperate. The person is advised that ulcers are prone to recur and that respect or lack of it for the suggested regimen plays an important role in whether he remains symptom-free or has a recurrence.

Assessment of the patient may reveal concerns or situations which are a source of anxiety and stress that predispose to peptic ulceration. The patient is encouraged to express these and is given assistance to resolve the problems(s).

The following factors in the recommended therapeutic regimen are discussed and clarified for the patient: diet, medications, the important role of regularly relaxing and resting, the avoidance of extremes and excesses, eating, abstinence from alcohol and smoking and the avoidance of taking aspirin and any medication that is not prescribed.

It is also important for the person with a peptic ulcer to know that any persisting pain, vomiting, haematemesis or abdominal distension should be reported promptly to a doctor so early treatment can be instituted.

Surgical treatment. If the symptoms persist and the ulcer becomes intractable, or if there has been bleeding or the ulcer has resulted in some obstruction in the gastric outlet, surgical treatment may be considered necessary. Various operative procedures are used in the surgical treatment of an uncomplicated ulcer in order to reduce the potential gastric acid secretion. Current operative approaches include the following procedures:

Gastric resection (subtotal gastrectomy) is the removal of a portion of the stomach, including the ulcer-bearing area and part of the parietal cell mass. An anastomosis is then made between the gastric stump and the duodenum (*gastroduodenostomy; Billroth I*) or jejunum (*gastrojejunostomy; Billroth II*) to restore gastrointestinal continuity.

Gastric resection plus vagotomy may be done. Vagotomy is a resection of the vagus nerve to reduce the stimulation of gastric secretion. It also reduces the motility of the stomach and may interfere with gastric emptying. For this reason it is rarely performed alone but is combined with a gastric resection or with a gastroenterostomy to provide effective gastric emptying.

A combined vagotomy and resection of the antrum of the stomach (antrectomy) may be performed. The vagotomy reduces the innervation that increases the gastric secretion; removal of the antrum removes the source of the chemical stimulus, gastrin.

Vagotomy with pyloroplasty involves plastic surgery of the pylorus to relieve pyloric stricture as well as interruption of the vagus nerve fibres. In some instances a *gastroenterostomy* may be done instead of the pyloroplasty.

For nursing management of the patient who requires gastric surgery, see Table 17.8.

Complications of peptic ulceration
The complications that commonly occur with peptic ulcer are serious and usually account for the deaths attributed to peptic ulcer. They are haemorrhage, perforation, and pyloric obstruction.

1. Haemorrhage. Peptic ulceration is the commonest cause of haematemesis and melaena. The loss of blood is due to erosion of a blood vessel at the ulcer site. Most of the patients who have a haemorrhage are known to have or to have had an ulcer but, in a few, it may be the first symptom that prompts them to seek treatment.

Vomiting of blood and the passing of black tarry stools are the prominent indications of serious ulcer bleeding. The patient experiences weakness, apprehension, dizziness and faintness which may progress rapidly to prostration and loss of consciousness. The skin becomes pale, cold and clammy. The pulse is rapid and thready and the blood pressure is abnormally low. Rapid respirations indicate air hunger and hypoxaemia. If a large vessel is eroded, the signs and symptoms appear rapidly and collapse occurs quickly.

Management of the patient with haemorrhage may be conservative or require surgery. The complication of haemorrhage is serious and demands prompt treatment by absolute rest, blood and fluid replacement, oxygen if necessary and treatment of the site of the bleeding.

If bleeding cannot be brought under control by conservative measures, emergency surgery may be undertaken. The ulcer area is resected and the vessels leading to it are ligated.

In *assessing* the patient with a haemorrhage, the blood pressure, pulse and respirations are monitored frequently and the level of consciousness, colour and body temperature are noted.

Blood typing and cross-matching are done immediately. The haematocrit and haemoglobin levels are determined, initially to determine the extent of the blood loss then later, at intervals, to assess the patient's response to treatment.

Accurate recording of the volume and characteristics of the emesis and drainage via the nasogastric tube is important. (Is the blood bright? Does the emesis contain clots?) An indwelling catheter may be passed so that urinary output per hour can be monitored.

It is important to assess the person's reaction to the situation, since fear and anxiety aggravate his condition.

Nursing intervention for a patient with haemorrhage includes the following:
- Normal saline or plasma is given intravenously according to medical direction until compatible whole blood is available. The rate of flow is usually slowed as the patient's blood pressure increases; too rapid an increase in the blood pressure has the risk of increasing the bleeding. The blood pressure is measured every 15–30 minutes.

  The patient is kept at absolute rest with a minimum of disturbance. A sedative may be prescribed to promote rest and relaxation.
- Precautions are taken by those around the patient against exhibiting apprehension. The patient may be less fearful if he is told something about his condition and is advised that treatment is well under control. Someone should remain with the patient. Relatives are asked to control their emotions when in the patient's immediate environment.
- A nasogastric tube may be passed into the stomach and *gentle* suction may be applied to remove the blood and gastric secretions (see pp. 503–504). Removal of the latter removes the acid and pepsin which could cause further irritation and erosion of the ulcer.

  A gastroscopy may be done to locate the bleeding site and electrocautery or a topical application of a haemostatic preparation applied to control the bleeding. If the gastroscopy indicates that the patient is still bleeding he is prepared for urgent surgical intervention. If the bleeding has stopped the patient remains fasting, and close observation is continued until the patient's condition is stable. Alternatively, the patient is fasted and taken to theatre for surgery.
- The patient is treated conservatively and when the bleeding has ceased, and he is no longer shocked, he is allowed to take small amounts of water orally. If this is tolerated, his intake is gradually increased to include clear fluids, fluid diet, soft food, and eventually an ordinary diet. Being able to take food and fluid again improves the patient's morale and lessens his anxiety. A preparation of iron may be ordered to promote development of haemoglobin.
- Frequent mouth care is necessary because of the haematemesis, dehydration and the discomfort of extreme thirst. A sedative may be necessary to relieve the pain caused by the ulcer.

2. Perforation. A peptic ulcer may progressively erode the submucosal, muscular and serous layers of the gastrointestinal wall. When the serous membranous layer is penetrated, some of the stomach or duodenal content escapes into the peritoneal cavity and causes a generalized peritonitis by chemical irritation and infection.

When perforation takes place, the patient immediately experiences sudden, incapacitating abdominal pain that begins in the epigastric region but spreads through the abdomen as more of the peritoneum becomes irritated by the intragastrointestinal content. The patient exhibits pallor, a cold clammy skin, rapid pulse, shallow grunting respirations and probably nausea and vomiting. The abdomen becomes rigid and board-like.

Perforation demands immediate treatment; emergency surgery may be performed to close the perforation or resect the affected area, or the patient's condition and history may be such that the perforation is treated by non-surgical conservative methods. The surgical procedure may consist of gastric resection or simple closure of the perforation by suturing the serous layer and reinforcing the area with a patch of omentum. The peritoneal cavity is cleared of the intragastrointestinal fluid that seeped through the perforation. In addition to the usual preoperative procedures for emergency surgery, preparation will include the insertion of a nasogastric tube and an intravenous infusion of electrolytes and fluids. An explanation of the need for surgery and what it entails will be made by the surgeon, and the nurse briefly explains the necessary preparatory procedures as she proceeds with them. For postoperative nursing care, see Table 17.8.

Non-operative treatment usually includes an analgesic such as morphine by parenteral administration, aspiration of the stomach content using a large tube followed by the insertion of a nasogastric tube and continuous gastric suctioning, intravenous electrolytes and fluids (fluids may include whole blood) and antibiotic therapy. If the patient's condition is satisfactory, continuous gastric suctioning is replaced by intermittent aspiration after 30–48 hours.

3. Pyloric obstruction. This may be caused by inflammation, oedema and spasm when the ulcer is in the acute stage or by scar tissue which is formed as the ulcer heals. The ulcer may be gastric in the region of the pylorus, or it may be in the duodenum. The constriction causes gastric retention and dilatation.

The *symptoms* which the patient complains of include a 'full feeling' which causes greater discomfort toward the end of the day. Pain may be experienced following eating as gastric contractions increase in intensity in an effort to overcome the obstruction. The contractions gradually decline and the stomach becomes atonic and dilates. Severe anorexia develops and the patient vomits large amounts irregularly. The loss of nutrients, water and electrolytes leads to loss of weight, weakness, dehydration and acid–base imbalance (alkalosis).

If the obstruction is due to the active ulceration process, it is treated medically by gastric aspiration and intravenous fluids.

Obstruction due to contraction of fibrous scar tissue is treated by surgery. A gastric resection with a gastroenterostomy or pyloroplasty may be performed. For a nursing care plan see Table 17.8.

CANCER OF THE STOMACH

Although cancer of the stomach still accounts for a large number of deaths each year, there has been a significant decline over the last three decades. The incidence is higher in males and in those 60 years of age and over.

The cause is unknown but certain factors are considered predisposing. Familial or hereditary tendency is thought to play a role. There is a higher incidence in persons belonging to blood group A and in persons with atrophy of the gastric mucosa, achlorhydria and chronic gastric ulceration.

Any region of the stomach may be involved, but the most frequent sites are the pylorus and antrum.

Symptoms
The manifestations are vague and insidious. At first, the patient may complain of some mild discomfort after he eats but, as the disease advances, belching, regurgitation, nausea and vomiting may be experienced, and there is a progressive loss of appetite, weight and strength. Blood may appear in the vomitus and stool when there is ulceration at the cancer site. Pain is usually a late symptom. Unfortunately, because the early symptoms are mild and vague, the person tends to delay seeing a doctor, and the disease becomes well advanced before there is medical intervention. Nurses should be aware of this problem and, on learning that a patient is experiencing even mild 'digestive' disturbances, should urge him to seek medical advice.

Diagnosis
Investigation of the patient includes x-ray examinations, analysis of gastric content for acidity, cytological studies of gastric fluid, gastroscopy and biopsy, examination of the stool for blood, haemoglobin estimation and blood cell counts.

The gastric analysis is done to determine if there is a decrease in the secretion of hydrochloric acid as the majority of patients with cancer of the stomach demonstrate a hypochlorhydria or an achlorhydria. The blood examinations will probably show some deficiency of haemoglobin and red blood cells, as anaemia is a characteristic of gastric cancer due to the chronic bleeding, reduced production of the intrinsic factor by the gastric mucosa, reduced absorption of iron because of the hypochlorhydria and nutritional deficits.

Metastases
Gastric carcinoma develops and metastasizes rapidly; all too often there has been a spread to some other structure(s) by the time of diagnosis. There may be direct extension to neighbouring organs (e.g. oesophagus, duodenum) or an indirect spread via the lymph and venous blood. The spleen, abdominal lymph nodes, peritoneum, liver, pancreas and lungs are frequent sites of metastases from gastric carcinoma. The left supraclavicular and axillary nodes may also be affected.

Treatment
At present, surgery is considered to be the only therapeutic approach to gastric cancer. The surgical procedure used will depend on the site of the cancer and its extension or possible course of extension. A subtotal gastrectomy or, rarely, a total gastrectomy is performed and may include resection of the duodenum, excision of the areas of lymphatic spread (omentum, spleen), resection of the pancreas or resection of the lower oesophagus. In subtotal gastrectomy, the stomach is anastomosed to the jejunum (gastrojejunostomy) if it has been the lower part of the stomach that has been removed. In the case of removal of the proximal portion of the stomach the operation is completed by anastomosis of the oesophagus to the remaining stomach (oesophagoantrostomy). Total gastrectomy and a resection of the oesophagus necessitate entrance into the thoracic cavity. Continuity of the alimentary tract is restored by an oesophagojejunostomy.

The preoperative and postoperative nursing care of the gastric surgical patient is presented in Table 17.8. Care of the patient following a complete gastrectomy will include the care necessary for any patient who has had chest surgery (Chapter 16). The patient who has had his stomach or a large part of it removed will require small frequent meals of easily digested bland foods and vitamin B_{12} injections throughout the remainder of his life.

CARE OF THE PATIENT REQUIRING GASTRIC SURGERY

Gastric surgery may be performed: when a peptic ulcer perforates the wall of the stomach or erodes a blood vessel causing haemorrhage; to remove a malignant tumour; or to treat pyloric obstruction. Gastric perforation and haemorrhage necessitate emergency surgery.

Care of the patient requiring surgery is discussed in Chapter 11. The same general principles apply for the patient undergoing gastric surgery. Special considerations applicable to the patient experiencing gastric surgery are outlined in Table 17.8. The amount of gastric drainage obtained postoperatively and the extent of the nutritional deficit resulting from the surgical intervention vary according to the type and extent of gastric tissue excised during the surgical procedure. In clinical practice, the care plan is modified to meet the specific needs of the individual.

Dumping syndrome (see Table 17.8)
Normally, the gastric content is delivered in small amounts into the intestine by the pylorus. Following a gastric resection, vagotomy or gastroenterostomy,

Table 17.8 Plan of care for the patient requiring gastric surgery.

Potential problems	Goals	Nursing intervention	Expected outcomes
Preoperative preparation			
1 Anxiety, related to being in hospital and the prospect of surgery, fear of cancer and concern about the possible loss of the stomach and the implications of this for survival	a To alleviate anxiety b To acquire understanding of the operative procedure, its purpose and implications for future functioning	a Assess the patient's and family's level of understanding of the surgery, its purpose and implications b Reinforce the surgeon's explanation of the type of surgical procedure to be done and the reason for it c Discuss the long-term implications of the surgery: what it will mean to the patient's future activities (including dietary adjustments, relief of symptoms, weight control) and quality of life. Encourage the patient to share his fears and concerns d Reassure the patient that the continuity of the gastrointestinal tract will be re-established, that he will be able to take food in the normal way, and that only a few dietary modifications may be necessary because of diminished gastric capacity e If the patient is acutely ill or in shock, provide short, simple and reassuring explanations. Check with the patient and family to be sure that urgent concerns are dealt with. Plan to deal with other concerns postoperatively when the patient's condition permits	1 The patient and his family show a decrease in anxiety 2 Pulse and respiratory rates decrease towards normal; physical posturing decreases and crying ceases 3 Patient and family demonstrate an understanding of the surgery and implications for the patient
2 Lack of knowledge about hospital routines and pre- and postoperative care and expectations for the patient	To acquire understanding of hospital routines, pre- and postoperative care and the expected patient role	a Orient the patient and family to hospital routines and procedures. If possible, introduce a member of the nursing staff in the operating room to advise the patient what to expect on arrival in the operating room. The anticipated postoperative care is discussed so that the patient may have some idea as to what to expect and will not be alarmed by the frequent checking of his pulse and blood pressure, gastric suction and intravenous administration b Family members are advised of the services available to them while they wait during the surgery and when and how information about the patient's progress will be conveyed to them c Postoperatively, the patient who has had gastric surgery tends to take very shallow breaths. The normal movement of the diaphragm and chest walls may cause pain in the operative area so the patient restricts respiratory movements. Shallow respirations decrease the respiratory exchange of oxygen and carbon dioxide and	1 The patient and family convey a general understanding of hospital policies, preoperative care and postoperative management of the patient 2 The patient demonstrates deep breathing and staged coughing techniques

Table 17.8—*continued*

Potential problems	Goals	Nursing intervention	Expected outcomes
2 Lack of knowledge about hospital routines and pre- and postoperative care and expectations for the patient (continued)		promote the accumulation of respiratory secretions in the alveoli and bronchioles predisposing to serious pulmonary complications. The importance of deep breathing, coughing, and early ambulation, which will be part of his postoperative care, is discussed. Demonstrations of these activities by the nurse and physiotherapist, and practise by the patient accompany the explanation to make it easier for him after the operation and to ensure greater cooperation on his part. The patient is asked to stop smoking and is given the reasons for this	
3 Alteration in nutrition: less than body requirements, related to the gastric disorder	To improve fluid and nutritional status prior to surgery	**a** Assess the patient's recent nutritional history, hydrational status and serum electrolyte levels **b** If solid food is permitted, total calories and protein and vitamin content are increased and given in frequent small feedings. Foods that are normally contraindicated for patients with peptic ulcer are avoided (fried and raw foods, spices, etc.) Fluids are provided between meals; if diluted citrus fruit juices are tolerated, they are encouraged, since they provide vitamin C, potassium and calories. If solid food cannot be taken, semifluids, blender feeds or liquids containing commercial protein preparations may be given. Various intravenous solutions (glucose, electrolytes, amino acids) may be necessary to improve the patient's fluid and nutritional status. Supplementary parenteral preparations of vitamin B complex, C and K may also be given. If the patient has been receiving oral feedings, these may be reduced to clear fluids the day before operation; nothing is given in the immediate 8–12 hours preceding the operation, and suction may be used to empty the stomach of secretions and any food residue. The tube is left in place when the patient goes to the operating room	**1** Fluid balance is normal; the serum haematocrit and skin turgor are normal **2** Serum electrolytes and pH are within the normal range
Postoperative care **1** Potential for injury related to surgical intervention, altered level of consciousness, and incomplete healing	**a** To maintain body functioning **b** To promote healing	**a** Equipment and supplies to be assembled in the patient's room include equipment for gastric suctioning, intravenous infusion and a sphygmomanometer and stethoscope	**1** The patient's vital signs are stable **2** Blood in the gastric drainage decreases and disappears over the first 12 hours **3** Bright red blood and large

Table 17.8—*continued*

Potential problems	Goals	Nursing intervention	Expected outcomes
1 Potential for injury (continued)		**b** When the patient is transferred from the operating room, the nasogastric or gastrostomy tube is connected to the suction as ordered, and the intravenous infusion is checked to make sure the transfer has not displaced the needle **c** Close observation is made of the patient for the first 24–48 hours for early signs of shock, haemorrhage and interference with the gastric drainage system. Check the blood pressure, pulse, respirations, colour, temperature and moisture of the skin, gastric drainage, wound site and the patient's level of consciousness frequently and record them **d** An accurate record is made of the fluid intake and output. The latter will include any emesis and gastric drainage as well as the urinary output **e** Gastric drainage (see pp. 503–504). Gentle gastric suctioning and 'nothing by mouth' are continued for the first few days to prevent the escape of gastric secretions and fluid through the stomach suture line into the peritoneal cavity, and to minimize vomiting and distension Drainage may be via a nasogastric or gastrostomy tube that is positioned in the stomach through a stab wound. The characteristics and exact volume of the drainage are noted; it will probably be coloured by blood at first but usually clears in a few hours. The doctor is notified if large amounts of blood appear or if the drainage continues to be blood-coloured. The tube may become obstructed by mucus or a small blood clot. An order may be received to clear it with a syringe and a small amount of normal saline or water (25–30 ml). The order may be for continuous low suction or, the drainage tube may be attached to a pump which automatically applies intermittent suction. After 24–36 hours, the tube may be connected to the suction apparatus only for stated periods at intervals; the volume which is aspirated is recorded each time. The number of days the nasogastric tube is left in and oral fluids are withheld varies with each surgeon and will also depend on the patient's progress.	amounts of blood do not occur **4** The nasogastric tube is patent **5** Blood in drainage decreases and disappears in about 12 hours **6** The patient's temperature shows minimal elevation in response to the inflammation associated with surgery and decreases over a few days to normal **7** The incision is clean, dry and healed

Table 17.8—*continued*

Potential problems	Goals	Nursing intervention	Expected outcomes
1 Potential for injury (continued)		The nasogastric tube is usually removed when normal bowel sounds return. **f** Take and record the patient's temperature every 4 hours for the first few days and then daily **g** Inspect the dressing for signs of bleeding and drainage; when changed, inspect the incision for redness, swelling or drainage	
2 Alteration in nutrition: less than body requirements, related to inability to ingest foods and fluids	To maintain nutritional and fluid status	**a** Parenteral fluids are used to sustain the patient over the first few days. Different procedures are used to introduce the first fluids into the gastrointestinal tract; the surgeon may have the nasogastric tube removed and small stated amounts of water given every half hour or every hour. The amount is gradually increased if tolerated. The directive may be to introduce a specific amount of water at intervals through the nasogastric tube, which is then clamped **b** If the patient tolerates the increased amounts of water without experiencing vomiting, pain or distension, feedings of clear sweetened tea, equal parts of milk and water, whole milk, creamed soups, gruel and blender preparations are progressively added over 2–3 days but only when normal bowel sounds are heard on auscultation **c** With normal progress, the patient is usually receiving a soft bland diet by the fifth to seventh day. The volume given at any one time remains small because of the reduced capacity of the stomach. Foods high in calories are selected and served frequently. The patient's weight is recorded regularly, and the doctor is advised if there is a loss or a failure to gain. Inability of the patient to take the prescribed diet, any regurgitation, vomiting, abdominal distension or complaint of pain is reported **d** By the time the patient is ready to leave the hospital, a light bland diet of high-calorie foods divided into six meals is usually tolerated. Fluids may be omitted from the meals and taken in between so their volume will not prevent the patient from taking sufficient solid food. The patient is advised that he may gradually increase the amount taken at regular meals and, if no discomfort is	**1** Total weight loss is less than 2 kg **2** Urinary output is maintained within the normal range **3** Serum electrolytes and pH are within normal ranges **4** Oral fluids and soft foods are taken and tolerated in small, frequent amounts

Table 17.8—*continued*

Potential problems	Goals	Nursing intervention	Expected outcomes
2 Alteration in nutrition (continued)		experienced, he may eventually resume three or four meals with milk and other fluids taken between them **e** Vitamins B complex and vitamin C and iron may be ordered, since the natural food sources of these will be restricted in the diet for a period of time	
3 Breathing pattern ineffective, related to thoracic and/or high abdominal incision, pain and decreased mobility	To maintain respiratory functioning	**a** If a total gastrectomy was performed the incision may involve the thorax, and chest drainage tubes will have been established (see care of the patient requiring thoracic surgery p. 466) **b** Remind the patient hourly to take five to ten deep breaths and to cough several times using the staged coughing technique to prevent undue tension on the suture line. Provide necessary encouragement and support by holding a small pillow lightly over the operative site and placing a hand on the patient's back during the coughing. Acknowledge the patient's distress but at the same time emphasize the importance of deep breathing and coughing in the prevention of other problems **c** When vital signs are stable, the head of the bed may be gradually elevated to promote deeper breathing and gastric drainage **d** Change the patient's position at regular frequent intervals: side to side to back to side	**1** The patient's respirations are regular, rhythmic and deep **2** Chest expansion is symmetrical **3** Wheezes and crackles are absent on auscultation of the lungs **4** Arterial blood gas concentrations are within the normal range
4 Mobility impaired related to surgical procedure, decreased energy, pain and therapeutic equipment	To prevent complications of immobility	**a** Limb exercises are started the evening of surgery and continued every 2–4 hours during the day until the patient is ambulatory **b** Assist the patient to sit on the side of the bed (usually on the evening of surgery) **c** Ambulation usually starts on the first postoperative day **d** Self-care activities are encouraged	**1** Ambulation increases over the first few days following surgery **2** Patient participates in self-care
5 Potential impairment of skin integrity related to immobility, malnutrition and dehydration	To maintain skin integrity	If the patient is emaciated, place an alternating pressure mattress on the bed. Pressure areas are protected by the use of sheepskin pads. The patient is turned every 2–4 hours, until ambulatory and able to turn by himself	**1** The patient's skin is free of pressure sores and areas of redness or oedema
6 Alteration in comfort: pain related to surgery and irritation from nasogastric tube	To control pain and discomfort	**a** Considerable pain is experienced by the patient who has had gastric surgery. An analgesic, such as pethidine, given intramuscularly, is usually ordered to relieve the patient's discomfort. The analgesic is	**1** The patient indicates comfort

Table 17.8—*continued*

Potential problems	Goals	Nursing intervention	Expected outcomes
6 Alteration in comfort (continued)		administered regularly for the first few days and should be given prior to the onset of severe pain. The patient is assessed for indications of respiratory depression and encouraged to breathe deeply and cough to expectorate respiratory secretions **b** Frequent regular change of position helps to relieve pain and discomfort **c** Frequent cleansing and moistening of the mouth are necessary to lessen the patient's discomfort while the nasogastric tube is in place and oral fluids are restricted. The tube may cause irritation that results in mucus secretion which, if allowed to collect, might be aspirated. The nostril through which the tube is passed is cleansed and moistened and receives a very light application of mineral oil or water soluble lubricant to prevent the accumulation and crusting of secretions	
7 Inadequate nutrition, related to the surgical disruption or bypass of the pyloric sphincter or from gastric resection or gastrectomy	To maintain adequate nutritional status on a long-term basis	**a** Dumping syndrome (see p. 543) • The patient is observed for signs of the 'dumping syndrome', which is precipitated by eating. These include: nausea, crampy abdominal pains, distension, diarrhoea, muscular weakness, dizziness, fainting, palpitation, sweating, rapid pulse and paleness • Explain to the patient and family that these symptoms occur when gastric surgery results in disruption or bypass of the pyloric sphincter • Assess the patient for emotional factors which may contribute to the development of the dumping syndrome • Measures to relieve the dumping syndrome include the avoidance of large meals and a reduced intake of salty and sweet foods; no fluids are given with meals. Six small, dry meals consisting mainly of proteins and fats are planned to meet the patient's caloric requirement. Liquids are taken between meals to maintain normal hydration but should be limited during the half hour preceding and following a meal. The patient is advised to eat slowly and to lie down for a half hour following each meal. The symptoms cause considerable emotional reaction	**1** The patient and family state the symptoms of nutritional alterations that require follow-up (nausea, vomiting, abdominal distension, diarrhoea, weakness, fatigue) **2** The patient describes a plan for continuing health care

Table 17.8—*continued*

Potential problems	Goals	Nursing intervention	Expected outcomes
7 Inadequate nutrition (continued)		in the patient. He requires encouragement to persevere with the suggested dietary regimen and reassurance that the condition will gradually subside as the gastrointestinal tract adapts to the structural changes. To avoid the distressing symptoms, the patient may tend to reduce his food intake to dangerously low amounts that result in weight loss and nutritional deficiencies. Anticholinergic drugs may be prescribed to decrease gastrointestinal motility **b** Nutritional deficiency ● Assess the patient for signs and symptoms of nutritional deficiencies, which include: the inability to maintain normal weight; insufficient food intake; feelings of satiety and overfullness following a small amount of food ● Assist the patient in developing a dietary plan that includes frequent high-caloric feedings (small amounts at first and gradually increased as tolerated) ● Assess the patient's perception and responses to the necessary continuing dietary modifications following surgery. The need for a period of time for the digestive system to adjust to the changes is discussed **c** Anaemia ● Monitoring of the patient's red blood cell count and haemoglobin is done regularly following gastric resection and information is elicited as to energy, fatigue and food elements in the diet. The patient may develop an iron deficiency as a result of decreased iron absorption. Normal absorption is facilitated by gastric acidity which is reduced if a gastrectomy is done. The bypassing of the duodenum by a gastrojejunostomy may also reduce the amount of iron absorption The deficiency may in some instances be due to a poor dietary intake of foods that provide iron (red meat, liver, leafy vegetables, whole milk, eggs and certain cereals) A supplemental preparation of iron is prescribed and the diet corrected to contain the necessary sources	

Table 17.8—*continued*

Potential problems	Goals	Nursing intervention	Expected outcomes
7 Inadequate nutrition (continued)		Anaemia frequently develops as a result of a deficiency in the secretion of the intrinsic factor (due to the loss of gastric mucosa by the gastric resection) which promotes the absorption of vitamin B_{12}. It may develop within a few months or not until 2–3 years after the gastrectomy. The patient may be given weekly vitamin B_{12} by subcutaneous or intramuscular injections until a normal erythrocyte count is established A maintenance dose is then given monthly throughout the remainder of the patient's life **d** Postprandial hypoglycaemia • The patient who has extensive gastric surgery may develop hypoglycaemia 2–3 hours after taking a meal. Symptoms include: weakness, tremulousness, faintness, sweating and palpitation. The blood sugar level may fall to 2.7–3.3 mmol/l • The hypoglycaemia is attributed to an abnormally rapid absorption of glucose from the intestine, causing a sudden hyperglycaemia. This stimulates a release of excessive insulin which rapidly lowers the blood sugar concentration to an abnormally low level A high protein, low carbohydrate diet is recommended to eliminate the problem. Frequent small meals are helpful Some forms of sugar (candy, honey, lump sugar or orange juice) should be quickly available and taken when the early symptoms of hypoglycaemia are experienced **e** Osteomalacia, which is characterized by decalcification of the bones and weakening of their structure, is a rare complication following gastrectomy. This is attributed to decreased absorption of vitamin D and calcium. Associated symptoms include diarrhoea and steatorrhoea. Treatment involves vitamin D and calcium supplements	
8 Lack of knowledge about dietary modifications and treatment regimen	**a** To acquire knowledge of necessary dietary modifications and treatment regimen **b** To develop a plan for continuing care	**a** The patient and family are helped to develop a plan to modify the diet and activity to accommodate temporary and long-term limitations imposed by the surgery. The importance of frequent small meals of	**1** The patient describes a plan to implement the necessary dietary modifications following discharge **2** The patient describes a plan for rest after meals **3** The patient indicates an

Table 17.8—*continued*

Potential problems	Goals	Nursing intervention	Expected outcomes
8 Lack of knowledge about dietary modifications and treatment regimen (continued)		non-irritating foods high in calories is explained. The size of the meals may be gradually increased when comfortably tolerated, as the remaining portion of the stomach progressively adapts to larger quantities. After several months, the person may find that he can manage three regular meals. Suggestions are made as to food selection and preparation. Written dietary instructions and outlines may be necessary for some patients The patient is advised to weigh himself regularly and to report to the clinic or doctor on scheduled dates. If pain, vomiting, progressive loss of weight or other distressing symptoms occur the doctor is contacted promptly Considerable rest will be necessary for some time and he should lie down for at least ½ hour after each meal. Normal activities are resumed gradually and should not interfere with regularity of meals **b** If a total gastrectomy has been done or a large section of the stomach removed, the patient will require regular parenteral administration of a maintenance dose of cyanocobalamin (vitamin B_{12}). The importance of receiving this is stressed and arrangements are made for the vitamin B_{12} administration at the scheduled times; it may be given at the clinic or in the doctor's office or by a visiting nurse or a family member who is taught to give the drug subcutaneously **c** The patient and family are informed of the assistance available to them from the community nurse. Economic problems may be a concern because of the prolonged illness and convalescence, and it may be difficult to provide the diet and care suggested for the patient. A social worker may be asked to see them to arrange for the necessary assistance, or the nurse may refer the problem to an appropriate source	awareness of symptoms of digestive disorders requiring prompt medical attention **4** The patient and family know the available relevant community resources

the normal pyloric control of the volume moving from the stomach into the small intestine is absent. The dumping syndrome is caused by the precipitous passage into the small intestine of a relatively large amount of gastric content that has not undergone the usual dilution by gastric secretions and digestive changes. The exact mechanism by which the characteristic responses are initiated is not entirely clear; it is suggested that the following factors are implicated.

First, the sudden distension of the proximal portion of the small intestine initiates sympathetic reflexes. Second, the fluid that moved quickly out of the stomach is hypertonic, having a high concentration of sugar and/or electrolytes. The resulting hyperosmolarity on the intestine results in the movement of fluid from the intravascular spaces into the jejunum. Only a small percentage of patients develop the problem; patients who are emotionally unstable are more likely to develop it.

DISORDERS OF MOTILITY, SECRETION AND ABSORPTION IN THE INTESTINES

Disorders of the *small intestine* may cause disturbances in: the movement of the content along the alimentary canal; secretion, which may incur a problem in digestion or absorption; or absorption alone. A prolonged or serious dysfunction threatens the patient's nutritional status.

A disturbance in the function of the *large intestine* interferes with the excretion of bowel waste and, if the right half of the colon is involved, the normal absorption of water and salts may be reduced and cause dehydration.

A disorder in motility, secretion or absorption rarely occurs independently; a disturbance in one is usually accompanied by dysfunction in one or both of the other intestinal functions. For example, increased secretion may accelerate motility, decreased absorption causes dysfunction in motility and elimination, and inflammation usually causes a disturbance in all three functions.

Disorders of secretion of the small intestine

SECRETORY DIARRHOEA

This condition occurs when the intestine secretes excessive fluid and electrolytes because of increased hydrostatic and tissue pressure, or because of increased secretion by the mucosal cells. Increased hydrostatic and tissue pressure occurs with intestinal obstruction and inflammatory and ischaemic diseases of the bowel. Increased secretion occurs with gastrinomas, secretory tumours of the pancreas and thyroid gland, dysentery (*Shigella*), cholera and malabsorption. Other causes include excessive use of laxatives, and drugs such as anti-

biotics, theophylline, caffeine and alcohol.[30] Excessive amounts of fluid and electrolytes move from the serosa to the mucosa of the intestine and into the lumen, producing dehydration and diarrhoea; this may also lead to metabolic acidosis.

Disorders of digestion and absorption of the small intestine

MALABSORPTION SYNDROME

Malabsorption involves failure to transport nutrients from the intestinal lumen to the body fluids and loss of nutrients in the stool. It results from impairment of either the digestive or the absorptive process. Digestion involves the break down or hydrolysis of nutrients to smaller molecules which can be transported across the intestinal cells; it depends on the secretion of gastric acid and pepsin and on the actions of pancreatic enzymes and bile in the small intestine. Transportation mechanisms include facilitated active transport, which involves a carrier mechanism and energy to move substances across the cell membrane, and diffusion.

Nutrients are absorbed: (1) into the capillaries and from there are carried through the portal vein into the liver and then into the systemic circulation; or (2) through the lacteals into the thoracic lymphatic system and on into the systemic circulation. The absorptive cells of the intestinal villi are especially adapted for both absorption and secretion.

The causes of malabsorption may be: (1) a lack of normal intralumenal digestion, (2) dysfunction of the absorptive cells of the intestinal mucosa, or (3) impairment in the intestinal circulation or lymphatic system.

Manifestations. The signs and symptoms of the malabsorption syndrome vary from severe to very mild; with the latter the disorder may go undetected for years. The major manifestations are: weight loss; abnormal stools which are bulky, soft, light yellow to grey in colour and have a rancid odour; abdominal distension; anorexia; muscle wasting; peripheral oedema; weakness and skeletal disorders. Table 17.9 lists the signs and symptoms of malabsorption with their aetiological factors.

Digestive disturbances
Malabsorption due to *digestive disturbances* occurs with liver and biliary tract disease, following a gastrectomy and with bacterial overgrowth in the small bowel. With liver and biliary tract disease the primary symptom of inadequate digestion and absorption is the presence of steatorrhoea or undigested fat in the stool. Decreased synthesis or excretion of bile salts results in impaired digestion of

---

[30] Smith & Thier (1985), pp. 1211–1212.

Table 17.9 Assessment of the patient with systemic manifestations of malabsorption.*

Problem	Signs and symptoms	Causative factors
1 Altered body image	Muscle wasting, weight loss and oedema	Malabsorption of fat, carbohydrate or protein; calorie loss; and protein loss (albumin)
2 Altered bowel elimination	Diarrhoea, abdominal distension and flatulence Pale, bulky, odorous stools	Impaired absorption or increased secretion of water and electrolytes; increased secretion of water and electrolytes with unabsorbed bile and fatty acids; fluid and electrolyte load in excess of absorptive capacity of colon; impaired carbohydrate absorption Impaired fat absorption and increased loss of fat
3 Altered urinary elimination	Nocturia and dehydration	Delayed absorption of water; hypokalaemia
4 Weakness and fatigue	Anaemia, and weakness	Impaired absorption of iron, vitamin B_{12}, folate; loss of electrolytes (potassium)
5 Increased potential for bleeding	Ecchymoses and haematuria	Impaired vitamin K absorption; increased prothrombin time
6 Altered muscle tone and sensation	Muscle cramps, tetany and prickling and burning sensations Muscle flaccidity, weakness, decreased tendon reflexes and cardiac arrhythmia	Impaired calcium and magnesium absorption Impaired potassium absorption
7 Increased potential for injury	Skeletal deformities and bone fractures	Impaired absorption of calcium and protein; demineralization of bone
8 Altered sexual function	Amenorrhoea Decreased libido	Impaired protein absorption; loss of calories
9 Altered integrity of skin and oral mucosa	Dermatitis, glossitis and dry fissures of the lips	Impaired absorption of iron, vitamin B_{12}, folate and other vitamins
10 Altered visual acuity	Night blindness	Impaired absorption of vitamin A

* Smith & Thier (1985), p. 1206; Braunwald et al (1987), p. 1268.

fat and interferes with the absorption of vitamin D and calcium. Following a gastric resection, emptying of the stomach occurs more rapidly; the duodenum may be bypassed, decreasing the stimulation of pancreatic enzymes; mixing of bile salts may be inadequate; stasis of intestinal contents may occur and protein intake may be decreased.

Management includes the administration of pancreatic enzymes. Bacterial growth in the small bowel is controlled by normal peristalsis. When intestinal motility is impaired, bacterial proliferation occurs, resulting in changes in the action of the bile salts. Fat absorption is impaired and steatorrhoea is present. Vitamin B_{12} absorption is also decreased due to its utilization by the microorganisms. Treatment involves antibiotic therapy.

Dysfunction of absorbing cells
Malabsorption due to *dysfunction or destruction of the absorbing cells* may be due to an inadequate absorptive surface resulting from extensive resection of the small bowel, intestinal bypass or extensive inflammatory disease. The extent and site of the area involved determines which nutrients are most affected. Iron, calcium, water-soluble vitamins and

fats (monoglycerides and fatty acids) are absorbed in the proximal intestine. Sugars are absorbed in the proximal and mid-intestine. Amino acids are mostly absorbed in the mid-intestine and jejunum while bile salts and vitamin B_{12} are mostly absorbed in the distal portion of the small intestine. Water and electrolyte absorption occurs in the colon.[31] Patient management includes a high caloric diet—high in carbohydrates and protein and low in fat. Vitamin and mineral supplements are administered. Drugs such as belladonna alkaloids and codeine may be given to decrease intestinal motility. Cimetidine (Tagamet) may be given to decrease gastric acid secretion. Long-term parenteral nutrition may be required in very extensive resection or total removal of the intestine.

Enzyme deficiencies
The malabsorption syndrome may be due to *enzyme deficiencies* in the intestinal mucosal cells. Adult lactase deficiency is a common disorder which causes an intolerance to lactose, the sugar found in milk.

---

[31] Braunwald et al (1987), p. 1263.

Hydrolysis of disaccharides takes place on the glycocalyx of the microvilli of the intestinal cells. When lactase is deficient, lactose is not hydrolyzed to galactose, and glucose and is not absorbed; it remains in the intestinal lumen and draws water by osmosis into the lumen. Symptoms include abdominal cramps, distension, flatulence and diarrhoea following ingestion of milk. The diagnosis is made by taking a history and by a lactose tolerance test. The disorder is more common in negroid, oriental and South American people than in Caucasians. Treatment consists of a milk-free diet; cheese contains a minimal amount of lactose and is tolerated by most patients.

Gluten-sensitive enteropathy
Gluten-sensitive enteropathy (coeliac disease) is an immunological disorder characterized by a reaction of the intestinal mucosa, particularly in the jejunum, to gliadin, (a component of the gluten of wheat).[32] The mucosa is damaged, the villi atrophy and absorptive cells are infiltrated by lymphocytes and plasma cells. Other enzyme alterations may occur. Mucosal damage results in decreased stimulation of pancreatic hormones, impaired absorption of water and electrolytes and the excretion of unabsorbed fats. Symptoms include weight loss, distension, diarrhoea and steatorrhoea.

A gluten-free diet is recommended; wheat, rye, barley and oats are avoided. Rice, corn, soy bean and potato flours are used as substitutes in the diet.

Lymphatic obstruction
Lymphatic obstruction as a cause of malabsorption occurs rarely and is associated with Whipple's disease (intestinal lipodystrophy). It is due to the invasion of the intestinal mucosa by an unidentified organism and impaired cell-mediated immunity. Characteristics of the disease include arthralgia, skin pigmentation, abdominal pain, diarrhoea, weight loss and impaired absorption. The patient receives antibiotic therapy.

Drugs
Certain drugs may also interfere with intestinal absorption. Examples of drugs which affect the absorption in the intestine include: antacids and phosphorus; anticonvulsants and folates; biguanides and glucose, amino acids and vitamin B_{12}; xylose and folic acid and tetracycline and ferrous ions.[33]

Inflammatory disorders of the intestines

Inflammation may develop in any area of the small and large intestines and alter motility, secretion and/or absorption. The most prevalent inflammatory intestinal diseases include appendicitis, gastroenteritis, diverticulitis, Crohn's disease and ulcerative colitis.

APPENDICITIS

The appendix, a narrow blind tube extending from the inferior part of the caecum, is a common site of inflammation which may necessitate its surgical removal. The appendix has no essential function in the human and there is no change in body function when it has been removed.

The commonest cause of appendicitis is obstruction of the lumen by a faecalith (a small, hard mass of accumulated faeces) or a solid foreign body, or by disease or scar tissue in the walls of the appendix. Secretion collects in the tube, causing distension that results in pressure on the intramural blood vessels. The mucosa becomes inflamed, ulcerates and readily becomes infected; the walls may become gangrenous because of the interference with the blood supply, and perforation is likely to occur. A ruptured appendix is serious; it allows the escape of organisms into the peritoneal cavity and may cause an abscess in the appendiceal region or a generalized peritonitis.

The disease may occur at any age but is more common in children over 4 years of age, adolescents and young adults. Early diagnosis and treatment of appendicitis is important to prevent serious complications.

Manifestations of appendicitis are abdominal pain, nausea and vomiting, a moderate elevation in temperature and a leucocytosis with the increase being in the polymorphonuclear cells. At the onset, the pain may be diffuse or referred to the central portion of the abdomen or the lower epigastric region, and is described as crampy. As the inflammation involves the walls of the appendix, the pain becomes localized to the lower right quadrant or McBurney's point.[34] The area is tender on palpation, and rigidity gradually develops in the muscles (muscle guarding). Rebound tenderness may be present which is determined by palpation of the left lower quadrant. With the sudden release of the pressure, the patient experiences pain or discomfort in the appendix region. The patient moves slowly and carefully to avoid jolting and movement that increase the pain, and tends to keep his right thigh flexed.

The omentum and adjacent bowel may become adherent to the inflamed appendix, walling off the area. If the appendix ruptures, an abscess will most likely form in the walled-off cavity. But, if perforation occurs before the area is walled off, a generalized peritonitis develops; the patient complains

[32] Smith & Thier (1985), p. 216.
[33] Braunwald et al (1987), pp. 1264–1265.

[34] *McBurney's point* refers to the area about 2 inches from the anterior superior iliac spine on a line with the umbilicus. It corresponds with the normal position of the appendix.

of pain and tenderness over the whole abdomen which becomes rigid (board-like) and distended. The distension is due to inhibited bowel motility, which may be referred to as paralytic or adynamic ileus.

Examination of the patient includes palpation of the abdomen and a differential leucocyte determination. The doctor may also do a rectal examination, and a vaginal pelvic examination may be done on the female.

The *treatment* of appendicitis depends on the stage to which the disease has advanced. If it is still localized to the appendix, an appendectomy is done as soon as the diagnosis is established. If the appendix has ruptured and there is an abscess or peritonitis, the patient may be treated conservatively with antibiotics and parenteral fluids and given very little or nothing by mouth to reduce the gastrointestinal activity. Gastrointestinal decompression is used if there are generalized peritonitis and a paralytic ileus. Surgery may be undertaken later to remove the appendix.

Nursing intervention

The person with abdominal pain is urged to seek medical advice and self-treatment is discouraged, particularly the taking of a laxative or an enema which could be serious, since either could cause perforation of the appendix through stimulation of peristalsis. The patient is also advised not to take food or fluid until seen by the doctor. This is in case immediate surgery is necessary. In most instances, surgery is performed as soon as the diagnosis is established unless perforation is suspected. If the appendix was intact at the time of removal, the patient usually makes a rapid, uneventful recovery with a short period of hospitalization (5–7 days). For postoperative nursing care, see Table 17.11.

If an abscess is present, a drainage tube is placed in the abscess cavity at the time of operation. This necessitates cleansing of the wound and changing of the dressing at intervals. Alternatively, a drainage bag can be put over the end of the drain to collect wound drainage, thus avoiding the need to continually change dressings. The bag also allows observation of the discharge and accurate measurement of the volume of fluid draining. Large doses of an antibiotic are ordered, and the patient should receive plenty of fluids. An accurate record of the intake should be kept and, if the patient cannot take sufficient quantities by mouth, parenteral supplements may be ordered. Close observations are made for possible extension of the infection and generalized peritonitis. Abdominal distension, nausea and vomiting, lack of bowel sounds, an elevated temperature and rapid pulse are brought promptly to the surgeon's attention.

PERITONITIS

Peritonitis is a localized or generalized inflammation of the peritoneum and is most often a secondary condition. It is usually acute but may be chronic. The inflammatory response may be due to bacterial invasion or chemical irritation caused by bile, pancreatic, gastric or intestinal secretions, urine or blood escaping into the peritoneal cavity. A common infectious agent is *Escherichia coli* which has escaped from the intestinal lumen.

Intestinal motility is depressed and the intestine becomes distended with gas and fluid. The peritoneal serous membrane becomes hyperaemic and oedematous and there is an outpouring of fluid into the cavity that incurs serious fluid, electrolyte and protein imbalances.

The patient experiences abdominal pain, nausea, vomiting and distension. The abdomen becomes rigid (muscle guarding) and progressively more distended. A leucocytosis and fever may develop. The pulse becomes rapid and there is a decrease in blood volume due to loss of intravascular volume. The respirations may be shallow and rapid as a result of ventilatory interference by extreme abdominal distension. Unless quickly reversed, the patient shows signs of shock. He is pale and prostrate; the skin is cool and moist. Bowel sounds are absent as peristalsis is arrested.

Treatment is directed toward the primary condition (e.g. surgery to close a perforated ulcer), relieving the distension and re-establishing peristalsis, combating infection and shock, and replacing fluids and electrolytes.

Gastric and intestinal intubation and continuous suctioning are established. Nothing is given orally. An intravenous infusion is administered and the solutions used may be based upon laboratory determinations of serum electrolyte levels. A blood transfusion may be given to counteract shock and replace protein lost in the inflammatory exudate. An antibiotic is administered if organisms are the causative factor of the peritonitis.

The patient is very ill and requires constant supportive nursing care. He is nursed in the position in which he is most comfortable (e.g. a medium Fowler's position), with regular changes to avoid the development of pressure sores.

GASTROENTERITIS

This is an acute inflammation of the stomach and intestines. Causes include microorganisms (e.g. salmonella bacillus, staphylococcus), parasites (e.g. roundworm) and chemical irritants (e.g. excessive alcohol). Rarely, the condition may be attributed to an allergic reaction to a certain food or drug.

The patient experiences vomiting, diarrhoea, diffuse abdominal tenderness and pain, fever and leucocytosis.

Management

The patient is advised to rest in bed. Food and oral

fluids are withheld until vomiting has ceased. An intravenous infusion may be necessary to prevent severe dehydration. Strict medical asepsis is observed to prevent the spread of the disorder if due to infection. The nursing care of the patient who is experiencing vomiting or diarrhoea has been discussed elsewhere.

The patient may be very fearful during the acute stage about the outcome of the disorder; reassurance is given that the disorder runs a definitive course with complete recovery.

When the nausea and vomiting are controlled the patient receives clear fluids and jelly. The volume is gradually increased as tolerated and then bland solid food is introduced.

CROHN'S DISEASE (REGIONAL ENTERITIS, GRANULOMATOUS ILEOCOLITIS)

Crohn's disease is a chronic inflammatory disease which may affect any part of the gastrointestinal tract but has a predilection for the terminal portion of the ileum. Patches of granulomatous inflammation and ulceration develop in segments of the intestine and involve all layers of the wall. The bowel may perforate and form an internal or external fistula (an abnormal passage) into another loop of intestine or onto the skin. As the inflammation subsides, there is scarring and some stenosis which may lead to a partial obstruction. During investigation of the disorder, the patient receives a barium meal and radiological studies are made of the intestine. In Crohn's disease the ileum presents a string-like appearance. The cause is unknown but the disorder is thought to be related to an autoimmune reaction.

Manifestations

The patient experiences abdominal pain and tenderness, a low-grade fever and frequent watery stools that may contain mucus and particles of undigested food. Some abdominal rigidity due to peritoneal irritation may be seen, and there is usually a slight leucocytosis. As the disease progresses, malnutrition, loss of weight and strength, dehydration, and anaemia develop because of loss of appetite and interference with normal intestinal absorption. The condition may persist, or there may be remissions and exacerbations. The course is very unpredictable, varying considerably with the individual. Some patients develop serious complications such as fistula, obstruction and perforation. In others the disease may become progressively less severe over a lengthy period.

Treatment and nursing intervention

Care of the patient with Crohn's disease is principally supportive and symptomatic. Efforts are directed toward relief of pain, control of diarrhoea, correction of fluid, electrolyte and nutritional defi-ciencies, treatment of secondary infection, and reduction of the patient's emotional distress. The physical condition and emotional state of the patient have important roles in the progress of the disease and in preventing an exacerbation.

Supportive care. The amount of assistance and the extent of modification in life pattern required by the patient depends upon the severity of the disease and his strength and nutritional status. Much of the nursing care discussed in the section on diarrhoea is applicable to the patient with Crohn's disease.

● *Rest and psychological support.* Physical and mental rest are important for the person with regional enteritis. In severe attacks, bed rest is recommended. A reduction in energy expenditure and extra hours of rest during the day may be suggested for less debilitated patients whose disease is less active. In addition to advising the patient that he can contribute to favourable progress by getting adequate rest, the avoidance of emotional disturbance is stressed. This is difficult, since the patient has been advised of the nature of his disease and the limited success of current treatment. He should know that the course and severity vary, and that many patients do lead relatively normal lives. The nurse may help by being a willing listener when the patient and family express their concerns and despair. Acceptance of their feelings, working through problems and providing realistic encouragement contribute to support. Realization that his problems are recognized and that his reactions are understood and accepted assists the patient to cope with circumstances and reality. Some type of diversion should be provided; constant worry about the condition may increase intestinal motility.

● *Fluids and nutrition.* An excessive loss of fluid in diarrhoea and a probable reduced intake by the patient because of abdominal pain and 'feeling sick' may lead to dehydration. The daily intake and output are recorded and the fluid balance is noted. The patient is encouraged and, if necessary, given assistance to take adequate amounts of fluid. Intravenous infusion may be necessary to correct dehydration and maintain sufficient intake.

Serum electrolyte levels, especially potassium and sodium, are determined, as an abnormal amount may be lost in the stools or through fistula drainage. Replacement is made by intravenous fluids. A blood transfusion may be necessary to correct anaemia that has resulted from nutritional deficiencies. These develop due to insufficient food intake and/or impaired intestinal absorption. The patient is encouraged to take a well-balanced, nutritious diet. He is advised to eliminate only those foods which he cannot tolerate or digest. These vary among patients, but usually raw vegetables, raw fruits and fats are common problems. Fat intolerance is attributed to the loss of bile salts (failure of the intestine to reabsorb the salts). Some patients may find that they have to keep the roughage content low and that vitamin supplements may be necessary.

As part of the treatment of an acute attack, the doctor may have the patient sustained by total parenteral nutrition. Nothing is given orally and the intestine is 'placed at rest.' If a patient is not taking or absorbing enough to support even limited body activity, his dietary intake may be supplemented by intravenous nutrition (see p. 511 for total parenteral nutrition).

Medications.   Several types of drugs are used in the treatment of regional enteritis. Those commonly administered include:

1 *Corticosteroid preparations.*   These (e.g. prednisone) are prescribed for their antiinflammatory action. The patient receives large doses for 1–2 weeks and the dose is then progressively decreased to a maintenance level. Observations are necessary for side-effects such as retention of sodium and water, hypokalaemia and hypertension.

2 *Azathioprine (Imuran).*   This is antiinflammatory and immunosuppressive. Although the prescribed dosage in regional enteritis is smaller (1.5–3 mg per kg body weight) than that used for the prevention of transplant rejection (1.5–5 mg per kg body weight), the patient's resistance to infection is lowered. The nurse and patient observe the necessary measures to prevent infection.

3 *Sulphasalazine.*   This is an anti-infective drug. When prescribed, it is important that the patient take a minimum of 2500 ml of fluid daily, as with any sulphonamide preparation. This is to prevent possible crystallization of the sulphonamide in the renal tubules.

4 *Antibiotics.*   A fistula complicated by infection or a stagnant area or loop of intestine in which there is an overgrowth of bacteria may be treated with an antimicrobial agent (e.g. tetracycline).

5 *Codeine.*   This may be prescribed in small doses to relieve abdominal pain and help control the diarrhoea.

6 *Mild sedatives.*   One of these, such as diazepam (Valium), in small doses may be ordered to reduce the patient's anxiety and emotional stress.

7 *Nutritional supplements.*   Due to malabsorption the patient may require various supplements such as iron, cyanacobalamin (vitamin B_{12}), folic acid and multiple vitamins. Fat-soluble vitamins may have to be given parenterally because of malabsorption.

Complications.   These are common in regional enteritis. The ensuing scar tissue of the inflammatory process narrows the lumen of the intestine and may cause partial or complete bowel obstruction. Damaged areas of intestine result in impaired absorption which may lead to various nutritional abnormalities.

An abscess may develop at the site of active disease; inflamed loops of intestine may be bound together to form blind loops. The inflammation involves all layers of the intestinal wall which predisposes to perforation, leading to generalized peritonitis or the development of a fistula. The latter may form between the intestine and another abdominal organ or may form a passage to the skin surface.

Surgical intervention.   This is usually reserved for the patient with complications or where the disease is intractable and incapacitating. The surgical procedures used may be a resection and end-to-end anastomosis, resection and ileostomy, bypass of the diseased area by anastomosis, or bypass with closure of the proximal end of the bypassed portion. Unfortunately, following surgery, the disease tends to recur. If an extensive resection is done, the absorptive surface is so diminished that malnutrition is a very serious problem. Massive resection may necessitate permanent total parenteral nutrition.

ULCERATIVE COLITIS

Ulcerative colitis is characterized by severe inflammation and ulceration of the mucosa of the rectum and of a part or all of the colon. The process usually begins in the rectosigmoid area and spreads up the descending colon. There is marked inflammation and oedema in the affected area, followed by ulceration. The denuded areas result in infection, abscesses and a loss of fluid, electrolytes and blood.

Cause

The cause of this disease remains obscure. There is at present support for the theory that it is due to an autoimmune reaction in which the body forms antibodies that destroy the normal protective mucus which coats the bowel. A genetic factor is thought to be involved because of the familial incidence of the disease. Infection, hypersensitivity to a particular food, insecurity and emotional stress have been considered to be implicated in the development of colitis but none has been proven conclusively to be an aetiological factor. The personality characteristics of excessive dependence, immaturity, hostility and depression frequently manifested by the patient with colitis are probably the result of the disorder rather than the cause; they are common to persons with any chronic disease characterized by exacerbations and remissions. Frequently arthritis, skin lesions or iritis is associated with ulcerative colitis and is considered to be a response to the same causative factor responsible for the disease in the colon.

Ulcerative colitis affects both sexes equally and, although it may occur at any age, the onset occurs most frequently during the second and third decades.

Manifestations and course.

The onset is usually insidious; rarely it may develop suddenly with intense severity. The patient has frequent diarrhoeal stools containing blood, mucus and pus, accompanied by colicky abdominal pain. There is abdominal tenderness, especially on the left side, and rectal involvement causes tenesmus (painful, ineffective straining). Dehydration, anaemia and loss of weight and strength develop, and the patient may have a low-grade fever. The prolonged and distressing symptoms and incapacitation cause emotional stress, and the patient may become very discouraged and depressed.

Diagnostic investigation includes a sigmoidoscopy or colonoscopy (see p. 496). The examination reveals a friable mucosa that bleeds readily, ulcers and sloughing areas and probably loss of haustra, which are the normal pouch-like structures of the colon. A biopsy is carried out during the endoscopic examination. A barium enema may be used with an x-ray examination but is not given in severe, acute colitis because of the danger of perforation of the bowel. Laboratory tests include determinations of haemoglobin, haematocrit, leucocyte count and sedimentation rate. The latter two are elevated with colitis. Electrolyte level and blood protein determinations are necessary, since there may be dysfunction in absorption in the proximal portion of the colon and excessive losses in the frequent, diarrhoeal stools.

The course of ulcerative colitis is unpredictable. The patient may have a complete recovery but, more often, there are relapses in subsequent months or years. An acute exacerbation may be precipitated by nervous or physical strain. The patient's history may reveal a recent bereavement, a home or job conflict, an acute infection or probably dietary indiscretions or bowel irritation by laxatives.

Persisting and frequent recurrences are likely to cause serious *complications*. Severe haemorrhage may occur if a large vessel is eroded, necessitating emergency surgical treatment in which a colectomy is usually done. Perforation of an ulcerated area of the bowel, leading to generalized peritonitis, is a less common complication but very serious. Perforation of the rectum frequently causes an abscess and fistula in the perirectal or perianal regions. When the disease is prolonged, the affected colon tends to become a smooth, narrow, inflexible tube. The mucosa becomes thin and the walls are infiltrated by scar tissue that causes a stenosis that may result in obstruction. Occasionally, polyps develop in the ulcerated colon and may give rise to bleeding. The incidence of cancer of the colon is higher in persons who have had ulcerative colitis for several years than in the general population.

Treatment and nursing intervention.
The patient is usually hospitalized during an acute attack of ulcerative colitis so that a more intensive therapeutic and supportive programme may be provided. Also, hospitalization may remove the patient from an environment that has stress factors which aggravate his disease. Treatment and care are directed toward reducing colonic activity, combating secondary infection, improving the patient's general condition by correcting the malnutrition and anaemia, and alleviating emotional stress.

Emotional support. It should be understood by all those caring for the ulcerative colitis patient that sensitivity, dependence and insecurity are common characteristics of these patients and that they tend to have inner tensions and bottled-up feelings which are not expressed. Every appropriate means possible should be considered to make the patient mentally and physically comfortable. It is important that the nurse convey to the patient by thoughtful attention and words that she knows and cares about what he is experiencing and how he feels about his total situation.

Understanding sympathetic care is extremely important in gradually establishing confidence and a relationship that is conducive to more effective treatment. The patient is encouraged to talk about himself and his life activities while the nurse listens carefully for problems that may be responsible for aggravating his disorder. He may feel better after talking to the nurse because someone has been interested enough to listen.

Orientation to the environment and an explanation of care and treatments are necessary. The best timing for certain activities and the beneficial effects of such may be discussed; for example, it may be advisable to leave the patient undisturbed following a meal and to delay the bath or other care procedures to avoid movement and activities that may stimulate bowel activity. If the sensitive patient is not advised of the purpose of the delay, he may feel neglected.

Some form of appropriate diversion should be provided to reduce the patient's preoccupation with his disease. Mild sedation may be necessary to promote rest and reduce his level of anxiety.

Assessment. The number, volume, consistency and content of the stools are noted and recorded. A close check is made of the patient's hydration and nutritional status from day to day. His weight is recorded daily unless it proves a source of concern to the patient, in which case it is discontinued and only noted once or twice weekly.

The nurse is alert to the possibility of perforation and haemorrhage and should promptly report any changes in the patient that might be early indications of these complications.

The foods taken by the patient are noted and observations made as to whether the patient's diarrhoea increases after any one particular food is taken.

Rest. Bed rest, quiet and relaxation tend to reduce intestinal motility and are recommended during the acute phase. Activity is gradually resumed as the severe diarrhoea and fever subside. Nursing care is planned to permit undisturbed periods of rest.

Assistance is given the weak and debilitated patient in turning and in getting on and off the bedpan or getting in and out of bed to go to the bathroom, which can be exhausting to him.

Positioning and skin care.   The patient with ulcerative colitis may become emaciated, which necessitates special attention to the bony prominences to prevent decubitis ulcers. The areas are kept clean and dry. Pressure on the bony prominences may be relieved by using a ripple (alternating air pressure mattress. The anal region is washed after each defecation, and a protective ointment or cream such as petroleum jelly or zinc oxide is applied. If severe tenesmus is experienced, warm compresses or an ointment such as lignocaine (Xylocaine) may be applied to the anus for relief.

The patient tends to lie curled up in one position with the legs and thighs continuously flexed, which predisposes to contractures. There is a reluctance to move about in bed or turn for fear of stimulating peristalsis and another bowel movement. He must be encouraged to turn and change his position every 1–2 hours. Full extension of the lower limbs should be required at frequent intervals and, if possible, the prone position should be assumed for a few minutes two or three times daily.

Nutrition and hydration.   In serious acute attacks, oral food and fluids may be withdrawn for a brief period in an effort to reduce intestinal activity to a minimum while the patient is maintained on parenteral fluids or total parenteral nutrition.

When food is permitted, a high-calorie, high-protein, non-irritating low-residue diet is given. Milk is usually poorly tolerated. Iced fluids, carbonated drinks, raw fruits and vegetables and all foods suspected of stimulating bowel activity are avoided. Recently, a more liberal diet with elimination of only those foods that the patient recognizes as increasing the diarrhoea has been recommended.

Nutrition of the patient requires a great deal of attention. The patient may develop serious nutritional deficiencies. Anorexia presents a problem, and there are serious losses of essential nutrients, fluid and electrolytes in the frequent stools. In many instances, the nurse must work at getting the patient to take sufficient nourishment; it may be necessary to provide frequent small meals. An effort is made to serve foods the patient likes, to provide variety, and to have the tray attractively arranged. A discouraging factor commonly encountered is that, as soon as the patient starts to eat, peristalsis is stimulated and he must have the bedpan. When this happens the tray should be removed from the room and returned after the patient has used the pan and received the necessary hygienic care. Hot foods should be kept warm or reheated. Encouragement and praise are given as the patient manages to take larger amounts of food.

Even though a fair amount may be taken orally, fluid and electrolyte losses may have to be replaced by intravenous infusions. Blood transfusions may be given to correct anaemia and to restore a normal blood volume. Impaired absorption of the foods and vitamins, as well as restriction of certain foods, contributes to the need for vitamin supplements, particularly ascorbic acid and the vitamin B complex.

Environment.   Preferably, the ulcerative colitis patient should be in a room by himself so he will be less embarrassed by his frequent use of the bedpan and the odour involved. If this is not possible, he should be placed in an area that can be screened to provide privacy and can be readily ventilated. If he is permitted to walk to the bathroom, his bed should be positioned as near as possible.

It may be necessary to keep a clean, covered bedpan at the bedside because of the patient's urgency and to prevent concern about getting it in time. The bed linen is kept clean and fresh. Extra covers may be needed for the patient for warmth; chilling should be avoided because of his lowered resistance.

Medications.   Various drugs are used in treating the patient with colitis. Nearly all patients receive small, regular doses of a sedative to promote rest and relaxation and to alleviate some of the emotional stress so common to this disorder. Examples of sedatives that may be prescribed are amylobarbitone (Amytal), diazepam (Valium) and flurazepam (Dalmane).

Secondary infection of the raw ulcerated areas of the bowel is treated by the oral administration of an anti-bacterial drug, such as sulphasalazine, or an alternative antibiotic may be administered orally. The patient receiving a sulphonamide preparation is observed for side-effects such as skin rash, leucopenia, anaemia, nausea, vomiting and headache and requires a minimum of 2500 ml of fluid daily. If the infection extends deeply into the colonic wall, a parenteral antibiotic may be prescribed.

Anticholinergic drugs to reduce peristalsis may be used in some instances. Examples are propantheline (Pro-Banthine) and methanthelinium.

A corticosteroid such as prednisone is considered an effective anti-inflammatory drug in inducing a remission of severe colitis. Initially, the dosage is high (e.g. 40–60 mg daily) and is given in divided doses. As the diarrhoea and melaena decrease, the dose is gradually reduced. The doctor may keep the patient on a maintenance dose for 2–3 months or may discontinue it much earlier. If the patient is too ill to take the corticosteroid by mouth, an intravenous preparation (e.g. corticotrophin) may be used during the initial acute stage.

The patient who is receiving any corticoid preparation, particularly over a long period, must be observed for possible undesirable effects. He may develop sodium and fluid retention and ensuing oedema, hypokalaemia, hypertension, a false sense of well-being, lowered resistance to infection, a moon face and hirsutism.

Azathioprine (Imuran) may be prescribed for patients who do not respond favourably to sulphasalazine (Salazopyrin) and corticosteroids. The patient who is receiving it must be observed closely for signs of infection because of the drug's immunosuppressive effect.

Haematinics such as iron may be prescribed to aid in correcting the anaemia, and vitamin supplements may be necessary, as cited earlier.

Surgical treatment. A colectomy with a permanent ileostomy may be considered advisable in persisting colitis that fails to respond to medical treatment, or when there are frequent severe exacerbations which cause physical and psychological disability to the extent that the patient cannot lead a useful and independent life. Long-standing ulcerative colitis predisposes to malignant changes in the bowel. For pre- and postoperative care in intestinal surgery see Table 17.11.

Complications, such as haemorrhage and perforation of the bowel, are usually indications for emergency surgery.

For nursing care of the patient who has a colostomy and ileostomy see page 575.

Anorectal complications are common in patients with ulcerative colitis. Infection passes through the wall of the rectum and causes perirectal or perianal abscesses and fistulas that open onto the perineal area, discharging blood and pus. These complications require surgical treatment; the abscesses are drained, the fistula is excised and the area is left open to heal by granulation from within out to the surface.

Instructions. The possibility of a recurrence of the ulcerative colitis is reduced if the patient understands and respects certain care and precautions. The patient is encouraged to return to his occupation and to live as normal and useful a life as possible. A balance between rest, work and recreation is advisable. Assistance is given the patient in solving home or socioeconomic problems, since a relapse can frequently be attributed to a psychosocial disturbance. A social worker may be asked to see the patient or family to help solve existing problems, or a referral may be made to a welfare department or service organization from which help may be obtained. The family should be advised as to their role in supporting the patient.

Emphasis is placed on the importance of a nourishing diet with the elimination of certain foods that are found to be irritating to the colon. Chilling, exhaustion and contact with persons having a cold or infection are to be avoided since a relapse may follow.

Other disorders of the intestine

IRRITABLE BOWEL SYNDROME

This is a functional disorder of the colon which may be alluded to as *irritable colon, nervous diarrhoea* or *spastic colon.* The syndrome has a higher incidence in females, with the onset occurring usually between the ages of 20–40 years. The individual is generally tense, anxious and ill at ease.

Manifestations
The disorder is characterized by episodes of crampy abdominal pain and may take the form of diarrhoea or constipation, or alternating small hard stools and liquid stools. Exacerbations are frequently related to emotional stress caused by the individual's life situation. The abdominal pain tends to be colicky and may be fairly general or often may be referred to the left lower quadrant. The ingestion of food may initiate the urge to defecate which may lead to anorexia and loss of weight. Defecation may provide temporary relief of pain. Frequently abdominal distension and audible intestinal rumblings (borborygmus) are noted, and the patient complains of fatigue and weakness.

Investigation includes a barium enema and a sigmoidoscopy or colonoscopy. Stool specimens may be examined for organisms and parasites.

Management
Since this is a functional disorder usually associated with tension and psychological stress, the patient is encouraged to talk about her concerns. It may take several approaches to establish sufficient confidence to have the patient talk about that which worries her or why she is unhappy with her life situation. She has to realize that the listener appreciates her concerns and is willing to listen and help find a solution. Following the investigation, the doctor's reassurance that there is no inflammation, lesion or malignant growth reduces the patient's concerns.

A mild sedative or tranquillizer such as diazepam may be prescribed for a period of time but is not continued indefinitely. When constipation is troublesome, a bulk-producing laxative such as ispaghula husk (Fybogel) is recommended. The habit of taking laxatives is discouraged. The patient is encouraged to take a well-balanced diet with an increased amount of fibre-containing foods (e.g. bran).

An anticholinergic preparation may be given to reduce the colonic spasms that may occur.

INTESTINAL OBSTRUCTION

Obstruction to the passage of intestinal content may occur in the small or large bowel and is a serious, life-threatening condition that demands prompt attention.

Causes
The cause of the obstruction may be within the wall

or lumen of the intestine itself, or it may be extrinsic. It may be classified as mechanical, neurogenic or vascular and may be acquired or congenital (see Table 17.10).

Table 17.10 Causes of intestinal obstruction.

Mechanical	Non-mechanical
Inflammation and oedema of the intestinal wall	Neurogenic disturbances: Paralytic or adynamic ileus
Scarring of the intestinal wall	Dynamic ileus
Adhesions	Interrupted blood supply: Mesenteric thrombosis
Neoplasms (intramural and extramural)	Strangulation of blood vessels secondary to:
Foreign body	Incarcerated hernia
Incarcerated hernia	Volvulus
Volvulus	Intussusception
Intussusception	
Congenital stenosis and atresia	

Mechanical causes include inflammation, oedema and scarring of the intestinal wall; neoplasm of the bowel or of a neighbouring structure; adhesions, which are bands of fibrous scar tissue formed by the peritoneal tissue following inflammation and which may cause kinking and constriction of the intestine; occlusion by a mass, such as a hard, dry faecal accumulation, a large bolus of unchewed and undigested food, a gallstone or a foreign body; and intra-abdominal abscess.

Strangulated hernia, in which a loop of the intestine escapes from the peritoneal cavity through a defect in the abdominal wall, results in constriction of the lumen of the bowel and a blockage as well as compression of the blood vessels. The constriction may lead to gangrene of the protruding segment of the intestine.

Obstruction may result from *intussusception*, a condition in which a segment of the intestine is invaginated into the segment immediately below. This telescoping results in compression of the attached mesentery between the layers of intestine in the intussusception and interference with the blood supply to the bowel. Intussusception occurs mainly in infants and young children.

Volvulus, which is a twisting of a loop of bowel on itself, interrupts the passage of intestinal contents and the blood supply to the involved segment. Older persons are more often affected, and the twisted section of bowel is usually the sigmoid colon.

Congenital malformations may be responsible for intestinal obstruction in the newborn. The anomaly may be a stenosis or atresia in an area of the small or large intestine, or it may be an imperforate anus. The infant fails to pass meconium.

In *neurogenic obstruction*, peristalsis is inhibited by a disturbance in the normal nerve supply to the intestine. Often this is an imbalance in the autonomic innervation which results in a cessation of peristalsis. It may develop with peritonitis, pancreatitis, severe toxaemia as in pneumonia and uraemia, shock, or spinal cord lesions, or occasionally after extensive abdominal surgery. An electrolyte imbalance in which the blood potassium is below normal also predisposes to intestinal immobility. The inhibition of peristalsis due to impaired innervation causes the condition known as *paralytic* or *adynamic ileus*. Dynamic or spastic ileus occurs rarely in some toxic conditions and is associated with intestinal hyperactivity. The spasm of a segment is severe enough to obliterate the lumen.

Obstruction of vascular origin is due to interference with the blood supply to a segment of the intestine and may be secondary to mechanical obstruction, or it may be primary and itself cause failure of bowel activity. Thrombosis and occlusion of a mesenteric artery may occur, blocking the blood source to a large portion of the bowel and arresting peristalsis. The interruption in the blood supply may be secondary to an initial mechanical cause, as occurs in strangulated hernia, volvulus and intussusception.

Symptoms and effects
The symptoms and effects of obstruction depend on whether it is in the small or large bowel and whether or not the blood supply to the intestine is maintained.

The first symptom of mechanical obstruction is colicky abdominal *pain* due to the bowel spasms. The crampy pains are accompanied by high-pitched bowel sounds. In paralytic ileus, the pain is steady and is due mainly to the distension. There is an absence of bowel sounds in this type of obstruction. No faecal matter or gas is passed after that which was below the obstruction is evacuated.

In small bowel obstruction, *vomiting* begins earlier and is frequent; the vomitus at first consists of stomach content and then of fluid containing bile. Eventually it becomes dark brown and faecal in character as the intestine becomes distended with excessive fluids and gas which overflow into the stomach.

The *abdomen becomes distended* because of the accumulation of gas and fluids in the bowel. Intestinal secretions are increased and the loss of fluid and electrolytes in vomiting leads to *severe dehydration* and *electrolyte imbalance*. Extravasation of plasma from the capillaries adds to the accumulation of fluid in the intestine as the veins are compressed by distension. This depletes the circulating blood volume and causes *shock*.

The patient's general condition may deteriorate rapidly. Unless the bowel is decompressed and fluid and electrolytes are replaced, a serious state of *shock* develops, manifested by restlessness, anxiety, a rapid weak pulse, low blood pressure, subnormal temperature, greyish pallor and cold clammy skin.

If decompression of the intestine is not established, the pressure created within the intestinal lumen may increase until it exceeds venous and capillary pressure. This causes congestion, oedema and necrosis of the mural tissue and may lead to perforation of the intestine.

The colicky pain becomes continuous as peristalsis diminishes, and the intestine loses its tone because of the marked distension and strangulation. Bowel sounds diminish and the vomiting changes character; it is no longer preceded by nausea and retching; the vomitus comes up without effort (regurgitated).

Peritonitis may develop as the weakened intestinal wall becomes permeable to organisms. *Generalized abdominal tenderness* and rigidity become evident.

Obstruction of the large intestine is less acute, and the symptoms develop over a longer period of time. Complete constipation (obstipation) and crampy abdominal pain are the patient's first complaints. Distension of the large bowel develops more slowly since fluid is absorbed, but eventually the distension may be very marked as the segment of the bowel is closed off by the obstruction at one end and the ileocaecal valve at the other. The ileocaecal valve will permit the entrance of content from the ileum but not until the later stage does the content of the colon and caecum back up into the ileum. Vomiting and the attendant dehydration and electrolyte imbalance occur in this later stage.

Diagnosis

Diagnostic investigation in intestinal obstruction may include an x-ray examination of the abdomen in which the presence and levels of gas and fluid may be apparent without a contrast medium. Blood studies are made to determine the leucocyte and differential counts, since a leucocytosis may develop with certain causes of obstruction. Haemoglobin and haematocrit estimations are made since they rise as dehydration and haemoconcentration develop. Serum electrolyte determinations are made so that deficiencies may be corrected. Those usually requiring attention are sodium, chloride and potassium.

Bowel content eliminated from below the obstruction may be examined for blood which may be present if the obstruction is due to intussusception or to cancer of the large intestine.

Treatment

Intestinal obstruction other than that due to paralytic ileus is treated surgically. In simple mechanical obstruction without strangulation, the operation may be delayed for a brief period in which medical treatment is used to improve the patient's general condition. This treatment includes nasogastric and intestinal intubation and suctioning to remove the accumulation of gas and fluid and to relieve the vomiting, pain and distension.

Fluid and electrolytes are given intravenously to replace the losses; as much as 5–6 litres may be ordered daily as long as there is intestinal suctioning. An accurate record of all fluid output and intake is necessary. The doctor bases the electrolyte replacement as well as the amount of intravenous fluid on the volume of intestinal fluid lost in vomiting and aspiration. Glucose is included in the intravenous solution to provide calories. A blood transfusion may be used to increase the circulating blood volume and relieve shock, if present.

If there is evidence of interference with the blood supply to the obstructed intestine, emergency surgery is undertaken.

The surgical procedure used in intestinal obstruction depends upon the cause of obstruction and the patient's general condition. If the obstruction is due to adhesions, they are severed. It may involve resection of the affected area of intestine and anastomosis to restore continuity of the tract or a bypass of the lesion by anastomosing a part above the obstruction to a lower part (usually the colon). In the case of an incarcerated hernia, volvulus or intussusception, the obstruction is relieved and the intestine examined for viability. If the blood supply has been interrupted for some time or is not re-established, a segment of the bowel may be gangrenous, necessitating resection and anastomosis. The surgery may entail an ileostomy, caecostomy, or colostomy, which may be a temporary measure while an anastomosis heals or it may be done to establish drainage above the obstruction, making it possible to delay more extensive surgery until the patient's condition improves.[35] In some instances, the enterocutaneous fistula (colostomy or ileostomy) is permanent.

For nursing care of the surgically treated patient, see Chapter 11 and Table 17.11.

Intestinal obstruction due to paralytic ileus, as mentioned previously, is not treated by surgery. Intestinal intubation with a long weighted tube and suctioning are used to remove gas and fluid and reduce the distension. Fluid and electrolyte deficiencies are corrected; the serum potassium level receives special attention because hypokalaemia favours the peristaltic dysfunction. Paralytic ileus is most frequently a secondary condition; as the primary disorder improves and decompression occurs, peristalsis is usually re-established gradually.

---

[35] *Ileostomy* is an opening from the ileum onto the external surface of the abdomen. Intestinal content is eliminated through this opening.

Caecostomy is an opening through the abdominal wall into the caecum to provide elimination of the intestinal contents.

Colostomy is an opening through the abdominal wall into the colon. Faeces are diverted through this opening onto the external surface of the abdomen.

CANCER OF THE INTESTINE

The colon and rectum are leading sites of cancer and the incidence is very much higher than cancer of the small intestine. The discussion that follows relates principally to the large intestine. The most common site is the rectum; the sigmoid, caecum and ascending colon are next in order of frequency. Cancer of the colon or rectum may occur at any age but has its highest incidence in the fifth and sixth decades.

Conditions that frequently precede cancer of the bowel are ulcerative colitis that has been active for several years and multiple polyps (polyposis) in the bowel).

Types. The malignant growth may be papillary, soft and friable, or a firm nodular mass projecting into the lumen; it may be a ring-shaped (annular) mass of firm fibrous tissue, causing a constriction of the bowel, or it may be ulcerative and necrotic, leading to bleeding and perforation.

Metastases. The malignant cells from bowel cancer may be spread by blood and lymph and by direct extension to neighbouring tissue and structures. Frequent sites of secondary growths are the liver, stomach, bones, and peritoneal cavity. Direct extension may involve the bladder and reproductive organs.

Signs and symptoms

Manifestations vary with the location of the lesion in the intestine. If the neoplasm is in the *small intestine*, the symptoms develop insidiously and are vague and less noticeable. They include anorexia, nausea and vomiting, anaemia, loss of weight and strength, and occult blood in the stool. Obstructive symptoms appear gradually and the patient develops abdominal pain. If the tumour is in the duodenum, the manifestations may be similar to those of a peptic ulcer.

If the site of the neoplasm is in the *colon or rectum*, the commonest early signs are a change in bowel habit and blood in the stool. Any person manifesting either of these signs is urged to seek *prompt medical attention.*

There may be increasing constipation or perhaps alternating bouts of constipation and diarrhoea. The stool may gradually become smaller and ribbon-like in form and may be streaked with blood, mucus and pus. A continuous defecation urge and the feeling that evacuation is incomplete after passing a stool may be experienced. The patient presents a general picture of ill health with a loss of weight and progressive anaemia. Laboratory examination of the stool will probably reveal occult blood. In cancer of the large bowel, abdominal pain is usually a late symptom; at first the patient may have a vague discomfort, and later he may experience a colicky pain which gradually becomes more severe. Unfortunately, if the cancer is in the caecum or ascending (right) colon, the early symptoms are more insidious and difficult to detect until the mass is large enough to be observed by palpation. Occasionally, the first symptoms recognized are those associated with complications, such as obstruction or perforation of the bowel.

Diagnosis

A neoplasm in the *small intestine* may be recognized when barium sulphate is taken by mouth and the passage of the barium through the small intestine followed. Any delay at a given section may indicate narrowing of the lumen by a mass. The intraluminal contour of the small intestine is also recorded by x-rays.

Investigation of the large intestine involves a colonoscopy, sigmoidoscopy or proctoscopy. A biopsy of the lesion, if it is located, is done at the time of the endoscopic examination. X-ray is done with a barium enema providing a contrast medium. The patient's haematocrit and haemoglobin are checked for possible anaemia, and stool specimens are examined for blood, parasites and pus. Liver function tests may be done, especially if the neoplasm is in the small intestine, to determine if the malignancy has metastasized to the liver.

A carcinoembryonic antigen (CEA) test may be done. This antigen is produced within *some* malignant newgrowths and released into the blood. The test is not a reliable diagnostic measure since not all tumours produce the antigen. A normal level does not rule out carcinoma but a high level points to a problem. The test is of greater value in assessing the patient's progress following treatment; increasing levels indicate a progressive growth and spread of the disease. (Normal level, 2.5–3.0 ng/ml).

Treatment

If the neoplasm has precipitated an obstruction, intestinal intubation and suction are used to decompress the stomach and intestine. Fluid, electrolyte and blood deficiencies are corrected. Surgical treatment of the tumour in the small intestine is undertaken and involves wide resection, removal of regional lymph nodes and anastomosis or, if the cancer is considered inoperable, a bypass may be done. If a large portion of the small intestine is removed, absorption of nutrients may be so restricted that the patient will require intravenous nutrition (see p. 511).

Cancer of the colon is treated by resection of the bowel and an anastomosis. This operation may have to be preceded by an emergency colostomy or caecostomy for the relief of bowel obstruction. The resection is performed and the colostomy closed when the patient has recovered from the acute bowel obstruction. If the cancer involves the sigmoid colon and rectum, an abdominoperineal resection is done in which the entire anus, rectum and sigmoid are removed, leaving the patient with a permanent colostomy. Radiotherapy may be used postoperatively when the tissues have healed.

When the malignant disease is advanced and has metastasized to other structures, it may be considered inoperable. Treatment is then directed toward relieving the obstruction by a caecostomy or colostomy, correcting the anaemia, providing relief of pain and keeping the patient as comfortable as possible (see Nursing Care of Patients with Oncological Disorders, Chapter 9).

For nursing care of the patient who has bowel resection, see Table 17.11. For colostomy care, see p. 568.

Hernia

A hernia is a defect in the normal continuity of the wall of a cavity through which a structure contained in the cavity may protrude. It applies most frequently to a defect in the abdominal wall, the respiratory diaphragm or the pelvic floor. A pelvic hernia, or weakness of the muscle and fascia that support the pelvic structure may result in prolapse of the pelvic organs—the bladder, rectum and uterus. Pelvic herniation frequently occurs in the female following delivery of a child. Prolapse of the bladder is referred to as a cystocele, prolapse of the rectum as rectocele and that of the uterus is known simply as uterine prolapse.

Herniation of the diaphragm is discussed in the section on hiatus hernia.

Abdominal hernia

Unless qualified by diaphragmatic or pelvic, the term hernia refers to abdominal hernia. Various classifications and descriptive terms are used in relation to abdominal hernias (Fig. 17.10).

Congenital or acquired hernias
A hernia may be congenital, which implies that the defect in the abdominal wall was present at birth. The acquired hernia develops later in life and is most often due to heavy lifting and excessive strain on the abdominal wall or to a weakening due to surgery.

Inguinal, femoral and umbilical hernias
These terms denote the location of the hernia. The *inguinal hernia* may occur at the site at which either the left or right spermatic cord or the round ligament emerges from the abdominal cavity and enters the respective inguinal canal. Each canal proceeds obliquely through the abdominal muscles and terminates in the aponeurosis of the external oblique muscle. The spermatic cord passes from the canal and descends into the scrotum; the round ligament of the female emerges and inserts in the labium

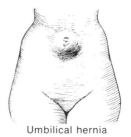
Umbilical hernia

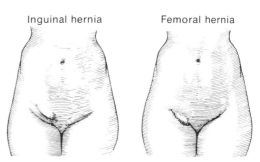
Inguinal hernia   Femoral hernia

Fig 17.10 Types of abdominal hernia.

majus. The opening through which the cord or ligament enters the canal is referred to as the *internal* or *deep inguinal ring*; the point of exit is called the *external* or *superficial inguinal ring*. These inguinal rings are weak areas and may become the site of a hernia when intra-abdominal pressure is increased. During fetal development, when the cord or ligament enters the canal, it pushes ahead of it a portion of the peritoneum (processus vaginalis) that normally becomes obliterated. In some instances it may persist and predisposes to the protrusion of a segment of intestine or omentum into the canal.

An inguinal hernia may be classified as indirect or direct. The term indirect is applied when there is a herniation of a portion of the peritoneum and a segment of bowel through the internal ring and inguinal canal. The hernia contents may continue into the scrotum or labium. The indirect hernia is considered to be basically congenital.

A direct inguinal hernia is usually acquired and is a herniation of peritoneum and bowel through a weakened area in the abdominal wall in the inguinal region. It develops as a result of continuous or frequent increased intra-abdominal pressure.

A *femoral hernia* occurs in the area of the abdominal wall through which the femoral artery passes from the abdominal cavity into the thigh. The femoral ring of each side is located in the groin. A portion of bowel or omentum may escape through the femoral ring, producing a swelling and mass in the groin.

An *umbilical hernia* is due to a failure of the fascia in the area of the umbilicus to close completely or heal firmly. It is usually recognized with the increased intra-abdominal pressure associated with crying, straining and coughing.

Reducible or irreducible (incarcerated) hernia

A reducible hernia is one in which the contents of the hernia can be manually replaced in the abdominal cavity. If the bowel or omentum cannot be returned to the cavity, it is referred to as an irreducible or incarcerated hernia. The irreducibility is determined by the size of the inguinal ring through which the viscera escaped and by the amount of intra-abdominal pressure.

Strangulated hernia

When a hernia is irreducible there may be compression at the internal ring of the blood vessels supplying the viscus within the hernia. Unless relieved promptly, the strangulated viscus becomes gangrenous.

Incisional or ventral hernia

Protrusion of a segment of intestine or omentum through an old incision may occur if there is incomplete or poor healing of the abdominal muscle and fascia.

Double hernia

If herniation occurs in both inguinal canals or both femoral rings it is said to be double, or bilateral.

Causes and incidence of hernia

Most abdominal hernias other than incisional are thought to occur primarily as the result of a congenital weakness at the site. The hernia may be evident early in life, or it may not develop until later when the weakened area is subjected to increased intra-abdominal pressure or to an increased relaxation or weakening of the abdominal muscles and fascial tissues. The increased intra-abdominal pressure may be due to severe coughing, straining at stool, vomiting, heavy lifting, obesity, pregnancy or a tumour. Loss of muscular tone and weakening of the fascial tissues may develop as the result of sedentary habits, prolonged illness or malnutrition.

Incisional hernia occurs most freqently following wound infection and drainage and is more likely to develop in patients who were very debilitated or obese at the time of operation.

Inguinal hernia has a much higher incidence in males, and femoral hernia is more common in females. Umbilical hernia that becomes manifest after infancy is seen more often in females.

An abdominal hernia is usually recognized first as a swelling at the site involved when the patient is upright or when he coughs. The swelling disappears when the person lies down and the hernia contents return to the abdominal cavity. Pain may be present due to traction on the viscus or local irritation of the peritoneum, and is relieved when the hernia is reduced. If the hernia cannot be reduced, impairment of the blood supply to the herniated bowel is likely to develop, causing strangulation, increasingly severe pain and symptoms of bowel obstruction. A strangulated hernia presents an acute surgical emergency.

Treatment and nursing intervention

The desirable and most effective treatment of hernia is surgical repair (herniorrhaphy). The hernia contents are replaced into the peritoneal cavity, the hernial sac is removed, and the weakened defective area in the abdominal wall is repaired by firm suturing of the muscular and fascial tissues over or around the openings. Precautions are taken in the repair of an inguinal hernia to avoid trauma of the spermatic cord or round ligament.

More conservative treatment may be necessary in some instances in which surgery would be too great a risk or the patient simply refuses operation. The hernia is reduced, and the patient is fitted with a truss, which is a firm pad that is placed directly to the skin against the hernia opening and held in place by a belt. It is fitted and applied while the patient is in the dorsal recumbent position. The truss is worn only during the day unless there is frequent coughing or vomiting that increases intra-abdominal pressure. The skin under the truss and belt should be bathed daily and lightly powdered to prevent irritation.

The truss is applied only if the hernia is reduced; otherwise, serious damage could be done to the hernia contents. The doctor advises the patient that he can probably reduce the hernia by lying flat with feet elevated and gently pushing the contents through the hernia orifice. If at any time he cannot readily reduce the hernia, prompt medical assistance should be sought. Overmanipulation in attempting reduction traumatizes the herniated viscera, causing swelling and oedema that further predispose to strangulation.

The nurse has an important role in encouraging persons with a hernia to accept the doctor's advice of surgical repair. The patient may find it difficult to submit to surgery when not experiencing any discomfort or disability. Left unrepaired, the hernia may become larger and restrict certain activities which could affect his employment. The repair becomes more difficult as the defect in the abdominal wall becomes larger, and there is an increasing risk of the hernia becoming irreducible and strangulated, which would necessitate emergency surgery.

Preparation for herniorrhaphy includes the usual considerations cited in the discussion of preoperative nursing care in Chapter 11. Close observation should be made to detect any signs of respiratory infection, since the increased intra-abdominal pressure associated with coughing could weaken or break down the repair postoperatively. Local skin preparation includes the abdomen, the pubis and the upper part of the thigh on the affected side.

If the hernia is irreducible and strangulated, demanding surgical intervention as quickly as possible, the preparation is the same as that for any emergency surgery (see p. 193) and will most likely include gastric or intestinal intubation and suctioning to relieve the vomiting and distension. Intravenous fluids may be given during the brief preparation and continued during the operation, as the patient may have lost much fluid. If signs of shock are present, a blood transfusion may be given to increase the circulating volume.

Postoperatively, the patient usually makes a rapid, uneventful recovery if the hernia was uncomplicated by strangulation at the time of repair. The male patient who has an inguinal herniorrhaphy may require a scrotal support in the form of a suspensory or elastic athletic support to reduce tension on the spermatic cord and possible oedema and swelling. The scrotum should be examined frequently during the first 2 or 3 postoperative days. Rarely, bleeding into the scrotum and the formation of a haematoma may occur, and swelling or discoloration should be reported. Application of ice bags to the scrotum may be suggested to relieve swelling and pain.

Urinary retention is a common postoperative problem and may necessitate catheterization. Excessive distension of the bladder is to be avoided because of pressure on the repair. In the case of a male, and if the patient's condition permits and the surgeon approves, he may be able to void more easily if he stands.

The patient who has had an inguinal or femoral herniorrhaphy is usually allowed out of bed the day after operation unless there is swelling of the scrotum, and is encouraged to move about. Before leaving the hospital, the patient is advised of the needed restriction in strenuous activities, such as lifting or pushing, and the importance of avoiding constipation and straining at stool. The doctor discusses the patient's return to his occupation; the length of time needed before he returns to work is influenced by the type of work he does, his age and the size of the hernia that was repaired. If his job involves heavy lifting and straining that might predispose a recurrence of the hernia, the surgeon may recommend a change of job. This may be a problem for the patient, and the assistance of a social or rehabilitation worker may be necessary to place the patient in less strenuous work. There could be a period of unemployment that creates hardships for his family; it may be necessary to arrange for the patient to see a social worker.

The *surgical* treatment of the *irreducible hernia* involves the release of the hernial contents and re-establishment of the blood supply to the bowel segment; the latter is encouraged by the application of warm moist towels. If the released bowel remains devoid of circulation and is gangrenous, it is resected and an end-to-end anastomosis is done. The hernia is repaired as quickly as possible. The nursing care involves the same considerations as for a regular herniorrhaphy as well as those necessary because of the bowel resection. For a discussion of care involved with a bowel resection, see later.

The repair of an *incisional hernia* involves the excision of the old scar, opening of the peritoneal sac, replacement of the protruding viscus into the abdominal cavity and firm closure of the peritoneum and fascia. Preparation of the patient for surgery may include the insertion of a nasogastric tube which is left in place for 1–2 days postoperatively to prevent vomiting and distension which would put a strain on the repaired area.

Treatment of an *umbilical hernia* in an infant will depend on the size of the fascial defect. The hernia may be treated by the continuous application of gentle pressure by means of elastic tape or a girdle-type of band made of crepe or elastic bandage. The mother should be instructed as to its purpose, and she is told to examine the area frequently to note any change. If the protruded area appears to be enlarging, the infant should be seen by the doctor. The child's increasing activity, sitting up, standing and walking strengthen the abdominal wall and a small hernia may close without surgical intervention. If the defect is relatively large and protrusion of the intestine is readily apparent under the skin, the surgeon may consider early surgical repair necessary to prevent the possibility of rupture of the hernial sac (peritoneum) and ensuing peritonitis.

Rectal and Anal Disorders

Haemorrhoids

Haemorrhoids are basically varicose dilatations of the veins lying under the mucous membranous lining of the anal canal. Accompanying the dilatation of the venous plexuses is an enlargement of the supporting tissues. This tissue and the dilated vein form the mass that is referred to as a haemorrhoid (Fig. 17.11). They are a very common distressing condition and may be classified as internal or external. *Internal haemorrhoids* underlie the upper portion of the anal canal which is lined by mucous membrane similar to that of the intestine. *External haemorrhoids* occur in veins in the lower portion of the canal, which is lined by smooth skin. The external haemorrhoids cause more pain and pruritus because the skin in that area contains pain receptors.

Aetiology

The cause of haemorrhoids is basically an increased back pressure of the blood in the rectal and anal veins, leading to dilatation. In many instances no cause of the increased pressure and dilatation is identified. They have a high incidence in persons with varicosities in the legs and seem to be influenced by heredity, for several members of the same family may be affected. Predisposing factors are

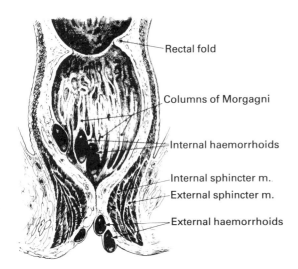

Rectal fold

Columns of Morgagni

Internal haemorrhoids

Internal sphincter m.
External sphincter m.

External haemorrhoids

Fig 17.11 Internal and external haemorrhoids.

chronic constipation, pregnancy, intra-abdominal tumours, portal hypertension and long periods of standing.

Symptoms
Manifestations of haemorrhoids are bleeding with defecation, protrusion of a small mass through the anus, pain (especially with and following defecation), itching, and a feeling of a mass or pressure in the anal canal. Protrusion of haemorrhoids usually occurs with defecation and, for a period of time, the individual may be able to replace them manually within the canal. The haemorrhoid may become so large that it may be strangulated on prolapse through the anus and become thrombosed by constriction of the anal sphincter. Oedema, inflammation and swelling ensue, and severe pain is experienced.

Management
Anyone who has pain or bleeding in the anorectal area is urged to see their general practitioner promptly, for these may be indications of a more ominous condition. Temporary relief in haemorrhoids may be obtained by the application of hot, moist compresses. An analgesic ointment such as Anusol cream or suppositories containing an analgesic and astringent may be prescribed. Bowel regulation is promoted by diet and increasing fluid intake. Constipation should be avoided; mineral oil or dioctyl sodium sulphosuccinate (Dioctyl) may be prescribed to keep the stool soft.

Haemorrhoids may be treated by surgical excision (haemorrhoidectomy), injection with a sclerosing agent, cryotherapy or ligation. Injection treatment is not used if there is an infection, severe prolapse or thrombosis of the haemorrhoids. The sclerosing agent may be phenol 5% in oil or a combined solution of quinine and urea. It is injected into the

submucosal tissue, not into the vein, causing a fibrosing and shrinking of the supporting tissues. Ligation of a haemorrhoid is achieved by the application of a special surgical rubber band. The tissue distal to the band becomes necrotic and separates. Cryotherapy involves freezing the upper part of the haemorrhoid causing necrosis; a similar result to ligation is achieved but with less pain.

Nursing Care of the Patient Requiring Intestinal Surgery

The preoperative, operative and postoperative care of the patient undergoing intestinal surgery includes that cited in Chapter 11. The special measures outlined in the nursing care plan (Table 17.11) are necessary considerations because of the actual entry into the intestine in the surgery.

The postoperative nursing intervention will vary somewhat with the different surgical procedures that may be done on the intestine and with the level of the intestine involved. The patient may have had a resection of a segment of the bowel and an end-to-end anastomosis to restore the continuity of the tract; alternatively the bowel may be retained, but an opening is made into the bowel through which the content is discharged onto the surface of the abdomen (colostomy or ileostomy). In cancer of the rectum or sigmoid colon, or in ulcerative colitis, the patient may have had an abdominoperineal resection in which the lower segment of the colon, the rectum and the anus are removed, and the remaining terminal part of the intestine is brought to the abdominal surface to establish a permanent colostomy.

ILEOSTOMY AND COLOSTOMY

The treatment of some intestinal disorders may necessitate surgery that establishes an opening into the bowel through which the intestinal content is discharged onto the surface of the abdomen. The opening may be temporary or permanent. A temporary diversion of the bowel content may be necessary while some abnormal condition below the level of the stoma is corrected or for quick decompression and drainage in obstruction. Later, the normal continuity of the tract is restored and the stoma is eliminated. If the opening is permanent, the portion of the bowel below is generally removed.

The operations performed are ileostomy, caecostomy and colostomy.

ILEOSTOMY

An ileostomy involves transection of the ileum and

Table 17.11 Care of the patient requiring intestinal surgery.

Potential problem	Goals	Nursing intervention	Expected outcomes
Preoperative preparation 1 Anxiety, related to lack of knowledge of the disease process, the surgery, impending alterations in body function; pain and discomfort; and possible malignancy	a Decreased anxiety b Understanding of the disease process, surgical procedure, expectations for the pre- and postoperative periods and consequences of the surgery for future functioning	a Encourage the patient to talk about his fears and ask questions. The nurse helps by being a willing listener and by indicating understanding and acceptance of his concerns. His questions are discreetly answered if possible without adding to his anxiety. Frequent visits to the patient and appropriate forms of diversion reduce his concentration on his condition b In talking with the patient and his family, socioeconomic or home problems may come to light for which the nurse may be able to suggest a solution or arrange for assistance from appropriate sources c The equipment and procedures that will be used postoperatively are briefly described, and their purpose and the patient's role are explained. The procedures most likely to be carried out include intestinal suction, intravenous therapy, frequent checking of vital signs, the withholding of oral fluids and food, frequent coughing, deep breathing and early ambulation. Knowing something of what to expect prevents fear and unnecessary concern for his condition	The patient: 1 Manifests decreased anxiety 2 Is more relaxed 3 Indicates understanding of the purpose and expectations of the surgical procedure 4 Practises deep breathing and coughing 5 Talks about expectations for postoperative care
2 Alteration in nutrition: less than body requirements related to inadequate intake and interference with digestion and absorption of food and fluids due to disease process	To improve fluid and nutritional status prior to surgery	a Assess the patient for signs of possible dehydration b Extra fluids are given for optimal hydration; parenteral solutions may be ordered to correct electrolyte disturbances or if the patient is unable to take sufficient quantities by mouth. A high-calorie, low-residue diet which includes extra protein and vitamins is desirable if it can be taken. If sufficient solid foods cannot be taken, a protein concentrate may be given in solution, and the necessary vitamins may be ordered in medicinal form c Blood transfusions may be given to correct existing anaemia and to improve the patient's general condition d Usually, only clear fluids are allowed during the 24–36 hours preceding the operation so that the intestine is empty. The sudden change in diet is	1 The patient's fluid balance is normal as determined by fluid intake and urinary output, serum haematocrit levels and skin turgor 2 Serum electrolytes and pH are within normal range

Table 17.11—*continued*

Potential problem	Goals	Nursing intervention	Expected outcomes
2 Alteration in nutrition (continued)		explained to the patient if he has been receiving a more liberal one	
3 Potential for injury (infection) related to surgical entry into the intestine and reduced resistance because of malnutrition and/or disease process	For the patient to be free from infection	**a** During the preoperative period, the patient may receive an oral antimicrobial drug to destroy intestinal organisms ('sterilization' of the bowel). Examples of drugs used for this purpose are succinylsulphathiazole (Sulphasuxidine), phthalylsulphathiazole (Sulphathalidine), and neomycin sulphate. If the drug used causes diarrhoea, it should be reported promptly, as the patient cannot afford loss of fluid and nutrients **b** A solution such as 'Golytely' is drunk until the rectal output is clear. Regular laxatives are given and the patient is allowed clear fluids only for 12 hours prior to surgery. For three days preceding surgery, a daily rectal washout is given. **c** Nasogastric intubation is usually required, and the tube is passed a few hours before the operation	**1** Preparation for intestinal surgery is carried out as ordered
Postoperative care **1** Potential for injury related to surgical intervention and incomplete healing process	**a** To promote healing **b** To prevent infection	**a** When a resection of the bowel has been done, decompression is continued until the anastomosis is partially healed and peristalsis is re-established The characteristics, as well as the exact amount, of the drainage are noted. It may be slightly coloured by blood at first but should clear in a few hours. Persistence of blood-coloured drainage or the appearance of large amounts of blood should be reported The intestinal suction tube may become obstructed by a small clot or by mucus and may require irrigation; a specific order as to the solution and the amount to be used is necessary. The suctioning may be discontinued for stated intervals the second or third postoperative day, and the patient's reaction is noted. The volume aspirated following each period of non-suctioning is carefully noted and recorded **b** Check dressing and wound area for early signs of haemorrhage. Inspect the incision at each dressing change for redness, oedema and drainage	**1** Body temperature and white blood cell count are within normal range one week postoperatively **2** The abdominal wounds are clean, dry and intact one week postsurgery **3** Any perineal wound is kept clean with minimal serous drainage

Table 17.11—*continued*

Potential problem	Goals	Nursing intervention	Expected outcomes
1 Potential for injury (continued)		**c** Monitor the patient's temperature regularly for several days. A sudden elevation of temperature may indicate infection **d** Following intestinal surgery, the patient will have 1–3 abdominal wounds: a drain will be inserted if there is any possibility of contamination of the peritoneum with intestinal secretions If the patient has an abdominoperineal resection there will be three wounds: a large abdominal incision, a colostomy stoma and a perineal incision. Once the colostomy is open, the abdominal incision is protected from possible contamination by covering the dressing with plastic or by using a waterproof dressing such as Op Site The perineal wound will have been sutured and usually has a drain in situ, attached to a continuous drainage bag. This is removed when the drainage is minimal and the patient is permitted to sit in a shallow bath	
2 Alteration in nutrition: less than body requirements related to intestinal surgery, decreased intestinal motility, and loss of fluids and electrolytes through intestinal drainage	To maintain adequate fluid and nutritional intake	**a** Nothing is given orally for the first few days; intravenous fluids are used to sustain the patient **b** Oral intake is started with specific small amounts of water. If there is no untoward response, the amount is gradually increased and other fluids are introduced During the initial introduction of oral fluids, the patient's response is determined. If the fluids are tolerated, the nasogastric tube is removed, and the diet progresses through fluids to soft foods and then to a light, bland diet. Carbonated fluids and gas-forming foods must be avoided **c** If a large portion of the small intestine has been resected, the patient may require parenteral nutrition. This may be a temporary means of providing adequate nourishment until the remaining small intestine adapts to the demand on it for increased absorption. In some instances, total parenteral nutrition becomes a permanent measure **d** An accurate record is made of the fluid intake and output which includes the intestinal drainage. Serum electrolyte	**1** Weight loss is less than 2 kg over the postoperative period **2** Urinary output is maintained within the normal range **3** Serum electrolytes and pH are within normal ranges **4** Bowel sounds are present within 5 days **5** Abdominal distension is absent **6** The ingestion of food and fluid is tolerated within one week postsurgery

Table 17.11—*continued*

Potential problem	Goals	Nursing intervention	Expected outcomes
2 Alteration in nutrition (continued)		determinations are made frequently; deficiencies commonly occur with prolonged gastrointestinal suctioning. Particular attention is given to the sodium, chloride, potassium and hydrogen carbonate levels. Central venous pressure may be monitored to provide a guide for the rate and volume of intravenous infusion which may be used safely (see p. 321). Too rapid infusion or an excessive volume may overload the individual's circulatory system, predisposing to pulmonary oedema and heart failure. The amount and types of solutions to be given intravenously may be estimated by the doctor on the basis of the records of the fluid balance, central venous pressure and laboratory reports. The abdomen is examined for distension and rigidity and, using a stethoscope, the abdomen may be examined for bowel sounds to determine if peristalsis is established	
3 Ineffective airway clearance related to incisional pain, abdominal distension and decreased mobility	To maintain normal respiratory function	**a** The patient is required to take five to ten deep breaths hourly to ventilate his alveoli fully and to cough several times to dislodge any mucus that may collect. The nurse supports the patient and may ease some distress by placing one hand lightly over the abdominal incision. A pillow held against the abdomen may help **b** The head of the bed is slightly elevated to decrease abdominal pressure on the diaphragm. The patient's position is changed hourly **c** Ambulation commences on the evening of surgery or the next morning. The patient should be referred to the physiotherapist	**1** The patient's respirations are regular, rhythmic and deep **2** Chest expansion is symmetrical **3** Crackles and wheezes are absent on auscultation of the lungs **4** Arterial blood gas concentrations (if measured) are within the normal ranges
4 Altered urinary elimination due to perineal surgery following abdominoperineal resection	To maintain adequate urinary elimination	The patient who has an abdominoperineal resection will have a retention catheter inserted into the bladder either preoperatively or immediately on completion of the operation. This is to prevent urinary retention, since most of these patients have difficulty in voiding. In the female patient, it protects the perineal wound from urine contamination	**1** Adequate urinary output is maintained
5 Alteration in bowel elimination related to decreased peristalsis, decreased mobility and ileostomy or colostomy	To re-establish bowel elimination	**a** In bowel resection and anastomosis, the passage of any gas by the rectum should be recorded; this probably indicates the re-establishment of	**1** Abdominal distension is absent **2** Bowel sounds are present on auscultation **3** Flatus is passed

Table **17.11**—*continued*

Potential problem	Goals	Nursing intervention	Expected outcomes
5 Alteration in bowel elimination (continued)		peristalsis. A small cleansing enema may be ordered on the fourth or fifth day **b** Elimination via an ileostomy or colostomy and the necessary care involved are discussed elsewhere in the text **c** Early ambulation is encouraged to promote the return of peristalsis	**4** Bowel elimination is re-established
6 Inadequate knowledge about diet, activity regimens and self-management of bowel elimination	**a** To acquire knowledge of necessary dietary modifications and appropriate activity **b** To develop skill in performing self-care activities (e.g. management of colostomy or ileostomy)	**a** The patient and family are taught the necessary dietary measures; gas-forming and high-roughage foods are avoided; the importance of an adequate fluid intake is stressed **b** Physical activity is gradually increased but the patient is taught to avoid lifting or other strenuous activity for the next few months. Walking is encouraged **c** Self-care skills required by the patient to care for a colostomy, ileostomy or to change a dressing are taught and opportunity for supervised practice is provided (see pp. 576 & 579) **d** A referral is made to appropriate community resources	**1** The patient describes a satisfactory home-care and follow-up plan **2** The patient demonstrates the ability to carry out dressing changes and the care of the colostomy or ileostomy **3** Appropriate use of available community resources is indicated **4** The patient describes plans to implement dietary modifications and to progressively increase activity without placing strain on abdomen

bringing the proximal end out to the abdominal surface to form a stoma. An ileal stoma usually protrudes 2–3 cm which makes the management easier than with a stoma that is level with the abdominal surface. The latter predisposes to seepage around the ileostomy appliance and excoriation of the skin. The removal of the distal severed portion of the bowel may be done at the same operation or may be postponed until the patient's condition is improved. If the lower part of the intestine is to be retained for a period of time, it is closed or, in some instances, the severed end may also be brought out to the abdominal surface.

An ileostomy is most frequently performed for Crohn's disease, or for colitis that does not respond to medical treatment and is incapacitating. It may also be necessary for patients with multiple polyposis of the colon or an intestinal obstruction in the upper portion of the colon.

A reservoir referred to as a pouch ileostomy or continent ileostomy, may be created by the surgeon to improve the quality of life for the patient (Fig. 17.12). Continent ileostomies are not usually performed on patients with regional enteritis (Crohn's disease) since the pouch may become affected.

The surgical procedure involves the formation of an internal pouch in the distal segment of the ileum. The pouch serves as a reservoir for the intestinal content. The pouch is drained at regular intervals by the insertion of a catheter through the stoma. The

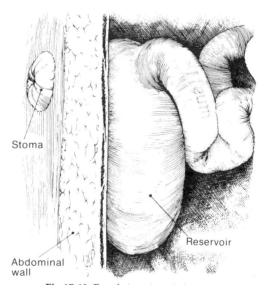

Stoma

Reservoir

Abdominal wall

Fig 17.12 Pouch (continent) ileostomy.

capacity of the reservoir gradually increases, and may reach 500–1000 ml over several months to a year. As the capacity increases, there is a corresponding decrease in the frequency of drainage required. Continuous discharge and leakage of the fluid or semifluid between evacuations of the pouch is prevented by the formation of a valve-like structure at the internal end of the ileum that leads from the stoma to the ileal pouch. Pressure of the contents of the pouch closes the valve, but it is structured so that it opens when the gentle pressure of a catheter is exerted against it on the stomal side.

The postoperative period for the pouch ileostomy is longer than that for the patient who has had the conventional ileostomy. It involves gastrointestinal drainage via a nasogastric tube, intravenous fluids and continuous catheter drainage of the pouch for several days while the pouch heals. In addition, the patient will probably have had a colectomy or an abdominoperineal resection of colon, rectum and anal canal. However, the advantages associated with an ileal pouch, such as the elimination of continuous drainage and the wearing of a bag, make the more involved procedure acceptable to the patient.

COLOSTOMY

A colostomy is an opening of the colon onto the surface of the abdomen. It may be in the ascending, transverse, descending, or sigmoid colon. If the colostomy is a temporary measure, the transverse colon is usually the segment used. A loop of the colon is brought to the abdominal surface, secured and left unopened until the peritoneum heals sufficiently to prevent faecal matter escaping into the peritoneal cavity. The bowel becomes adherent to the wound edges and an incision is then made into it in 2–4 days.

When the sigmoid colon, rectum and anal canal are removed, as in cancer of the sigmoid and rectum, the terminal end of the descending colon is brought to the abdominal surface to form a permanent colostomy.

CAECOSTOMY

Rarely, in large bowel obstruction, decompression of the distended bowel is achieved by a caecostomy. A small opening is made in the caecum through a small lower right abdominal incision and a fairly large tube is inserted through which the bowel content escapes to the exterior. The tube is attached to a drainage receptacle and remains in place until the patient's condition is such that he can withstand the more extensive surgery necessary to relieve the obstruction.

NURSING CONSIDERATIONS IN ILEOSTOMY AND COLOSTOMY

Differences between ileostomy and colostomy
Certain differences exist between an ileostomy and colostomy that result in different problems and necessitate different types of care. For example, control of the discharge is determined by the location of the stoma; drainage from the ileum is of liquid consistency and is rich in enzymes that cause excoriation

and erosion of the skin. It flows almost continuously, requiring the constant wearing of a receptive appliance unless an ileal pouch is constructed. There may be quiescent periods but they are not predictable and cannot be controlled. Complications are a more common occurrence with an ileostomy than with a colostomy, and odour presents a greater problem if there is continuous drainage. Irrigations are not used with the conventional ileostomy; the introduction of anything into the ileal stoma is discouraged for fear of injury to the intestine.

Colostomy drainage is usually more manageable and less irritating to the skin unless the opening is into the ascending colon; the drainage then is similar to that from an ileostomy. The colostomy is more often in the transverse or descending colon and much of the fluid and electrolytes have been absorbed from the faecal content, leaving it semisolid or solid by the time it reaches the stoma. Irrigations may be necessary but, in some instances, the sigmoid colostomy may be so well controlled that it resembles normal bowel movement, and the patient does not have to wear a receptive bag continuously.

Intestinal activity in the individual with a colostomy or ileostomy may be influenced by diet, fluid intake and emotions, just as in the normal person.

Psychological preoperative preparation
When the doctor advises the patient preoperatively that a colostomy or ileostomy may or will be necessary, the patient is emotionally disturbed. Obviously, if the colostomy is a temporary measure it will be accepted more readily but, if it is likely to be permanent, the patient may be more concerned about this than about the operation or his primary condition. His immediate response may be 'it would be better to die than have that'. He may become resentful or show marked depression, withdrawal and despair. He perceives this change in his body as making him unclean and unacceptable to society. There are fears because of odour and soiling. It is best to let the patient and his family express their feelings before attempting explanations. The nurse can help by being a willing listener, answering their questions and using every opportunity available to assure the patient that the 'ostomy' can be cared for without interfering with his work and social life. When the patient recovers from the initial blow, discussions may then be held as to how he will care for his ileostomy or colostomy.

General preoperative and postoperative care are similar to that for the patient who has intestinal surgery, see Table 17.11.

Nursing process

ASSESSMENT

Initial and continuous assessment is necessary of the following:

- The patient's perception of the ileostomy or colostomy
- The volume, colour, composition and consistency of the effluent (drainage)
- The patient's nutritional and hydrational status. The fluid intake and the quantity and composition of meals are noted. The patient's weight is recorded
- The condition of the stoma and surrounding skin surface
- The reaction to self-care
- The family's perception and reaction to the ileostomy or colostomy
- The patient's ability to manage the colostomy care

IDENTIFICATION OF PATIENT PROBLEMS

1 Alteration in bowel elimination: related to modifications in body function imposed by surgery and disease.
2 Potential impairment of skin integrity in the area surrounding the stoma due to irritating actions of the ileostomy or colostomy drainage.
3 Alteration in nutrition: related to changes in body functioning imposed by surgery.
4 Alteration in self-image: body image, self-esteem and role performance related to structural and functional changes in elimination and lack of control of bowel elimination and odour.
5 Lack of knowledge and misinformation related to ileostomy or colostomy management.

The *goals* are to:

1 Control intestinal discharge
2 Maintain the integrity of the peristomal skin
3 Control offensive odour
4 Adapt diet to meet altered needs
5 Cope with the change in body function
6 Acquire knowledge and skills for self-management of the altered body function

NURSING INTERVENTION

Containment and control of ileostomy and colostomy drainage

During the first few days following surgery, the stoma is swollen and oedematous and the volume of drainage is usually small. When the patient is permitted to take fluids and foods by mouth, peristalsis and secretion are stimulated and drainage increases.

Following surgery the skin is washed with warm water and dried. A washer of karaya gum, slightly moistened, is fitted snugly around the stoma to protect the skin and an open-ended, transparent, disposable plastic bag is applied. The transparency of the bag makes it possible to observe the stoma and the colour of the drainage at frequent intervals during the postoperative period. The bag is attached to an adhesive-backed square which secures the bag over the stoma. The size of the stoma is determined by a stoma-measuring card and bags of corresponding size are used. Too large an opening in the adhesive that attaches the bag exposes the skin to irritating drainage; too small an opening may traumatize or constrict the stoma. Non-allergenic adhesive or micropore tape is applied over the edges of the adhesive square that attaches the bag to maintain a seal. Several folds and a clamp or elastic bands are used to close the lower end of the bag securely.

During this initial period the bag is applied so that the lower end is at the patient's side, making emptying and rinsing possible while the patient is in bed. When the patient is allowed up, the bag is positioned so that it is suspended down over the lower abdomen toward his feet.

If there is a large volume of drainage, which may occur if the ileostomy or colostomy was an emergency measure, it may be necessary to attach a drainage tube to the bag. Elastic bands and adhesive are used to secure the bag around the tube. The latter drains into a closed drainage receptacle similar to that used for urinary drainage.

The disposable bag is emptied when it is one-third to one-half full; if allowed to fill it becomes too heavy and the pull on the bag may break the seal of the stoma and cause leakage. The lower end of the bag is opened and the contents allowed to drain into a receptacle. Using a syringe, the bag is then rinsed with lukewarm water. The volume and characteristics (colour, consistency and composition) of the drainage are noted and recorded. The appliance is changed daily until replaced by reusable equipment. A special solvent is available that enables the adhesive to be removed without damage to the skin. It may be applied with an eye dropper or an absorbent wipe. When the bag is removed, the skin is *gently* cleansed with warm water and thoroughly dried before reapplication of the karaya washer and a clean disposable pouch.

Continuing care. The patient is fitted for a reusable appliance as soon as the stoma shrinks to its permanent size (approximately 2–3 weeks) so that he can become familiar with its use and care before leaving the hospital. A well-fitting comfortable appliance means a great deal; the patient is likely to have more confidence and develop a more positive outlook. Several types of appliances are available from surgical supply companies; the surgeon or stoma nurse recommends the appliance most suited to the individual patient. The location and size of the stoma and the contour and firmness of the patient's abdomen are factors that must be considered in the selection and fitting of a reusable appliance. It should be simple and fit closely to prevent leakage without causing injury to the stoma or skin. The prevention of leaking is especially important for the patient with an ileostomy since the faecal drainage is liquid and cannot be controlled. With the colostomy patient, the drainage may be semiliquid and may have to be controlled by irrigations. The appliance should be inconspicuous, allow freedom of activity and be odour-proof. The essential parts include (Fig. 17.13):

1 A stoma-measuring card. The opening in the karaya washer (if used) and the double-faced adhesive disc must fit snugly to protect the skin; a margin of no more than approximately 2–4 mm is desirable.

2 A product to protect the skin. Examples of common preparations are karaya washers, karaya powder or ointment, Stomahesive or Coloplast wafers, Hollister skin gel or Orabase paste or powder.

3 A double-faced adhesive disc to secure the pouch to the skin. One side of the disc adheres to the skin and the other side attaches to the mounting ring (face plate).

4 A lightweight mounting ring (which may also be called face plate) made of plastic or rubber. One side of the ring has a rim around a centre hole. The side without the rim is secured to one adhesive surface of the double-faced adhesive disc. The pouch or rim side of the ring may have 'hooks' to which a belt may be attached.

5 A lightweight open-ended pouch that may be washed when removed and reused several times. The upper opening of the pouch is stretched over the rim of the mounting ring and secured by special rubber rings that are provided with the appliance. The lower end is tapered to form a narrower outlet. A clamp is also provided for closing the distal end of the bag. Until the colostomy patient develops control of the drainage by irrigation, an open-ended pouch is used. When control is developed a closed pouch is recommended.

6 A narrow, lightweight elasticated belt which attaches to the mounting ring or pouch may be worn.

7 Micropore or non-allergenic tape. This is applied over the edges of the ring for security and to prevent leakage.

8 A deodorizing agent such as Ostobon (a powder), Atmocol (an aerosol spray) or Nilodor (a solution) may be used. A tissue may be soaked with the agent and placed in the ileostomy pouch. Bags with charcoal filters are used to allow flatus to be released and also deodorized.

The reusable bag usually requires emptying several times daily, especially with an ileostomy. The lower end of the bag is opened and the contents drained directly into the toilet. Using a syringe the bag is then rinsed and closed. As noted with the use of the disposable bag, the bag should be emptied when one-third to one-half full to avoid loosening the disc by the weight.

The pouch may be removed daily from the rim of the mounting ring by some patients and replaced with a clean one. This must be done very carefully to maintain the seal by the disc. If the seal is broken or if the patient complains of any burning or itching, the complete appliance is changed immediately; other-

wise, the appliance is changed once or twice weekly by the ileostomy patient. A regular schedule should be arranged for emptying and changing the equipment; it should be at a time of day when drainage is at a minimum. This is determined by observation.

The colostomy appliance is changed every 4–5 days and whenever leakage occurs. When control develops, the pouch is changed daily and, if adhesive rings or squares are used, they are changed once or twice weekly. They are changed more often if they become soiled or if the patient experiences burning, itching or discomfort of the underlying skin.

In preparation for *application* of the reuseable appliance, the hole in the karaya washer (if used) is sized to fit the stoma and the washer is then lightly moistened with water. The pouch is placed over the rim of the mounting ring and secured. The pouch outlet is closed and clamped. The paper is peeled from one side of the double-faced adhesive disc and is then placed smoothly on the face of the mounting ring. The hole of the disc must be the same size as the hole in the ring and be directly over it.

When *removing* the appliance, a solvent is used sparingly on an absorbent wipe or with an eyedropper to remove the adhesive. The skin is washed *gently* and dried thoroughly. The skin and stoma are carefully inspected. If the skin is irritated or excoriated a product such as karaya powder or Stomahesive may be applied. When the skin is dry, the karaya washer is applied and the paper is peeled from the other surface of the double-faced adhesive disc. The latter is then centered over the stoma and applied with the outlet end of the pouch directed toward the patient's feet. Non-allergenic or micropore tape is then applied to the edges of the mounting ring to ensure a seal and for security. If the patient finds a belt necessary it is applied then, and is secured to the mounting ring or pouch.

The reusable ileostomy or colostomy appliance that was removed is cleansed immediately after application of the clean unit has been completed. The adhesive disc is removed from the mounting ring (face plate) and discarded. The ring is cleansed first with an adhesive remover and then with a brush under cool running water.

If the pouch is to be used again it is left attached to the mounting ring and flushed out with cool running water. The appliance is then left to soak for 30 minutes in a detergent solution, after which it is rinsed well and hung up to dry. A paper towel placed within the bag will keep the surfaces separated and facilitate airing of the pouch. When the appliance is dry, powder the pouch inside and out with talcum powder or cornstarch. Most bags are designed to be used only once. When the bag is full, both bag and contents are disposed of, and a new bag applied.

Colostomy irrigation.   A colostomy may be controlled entirely by diet, especially if the colostomy is in the descending colon or sigmoid; others may require an

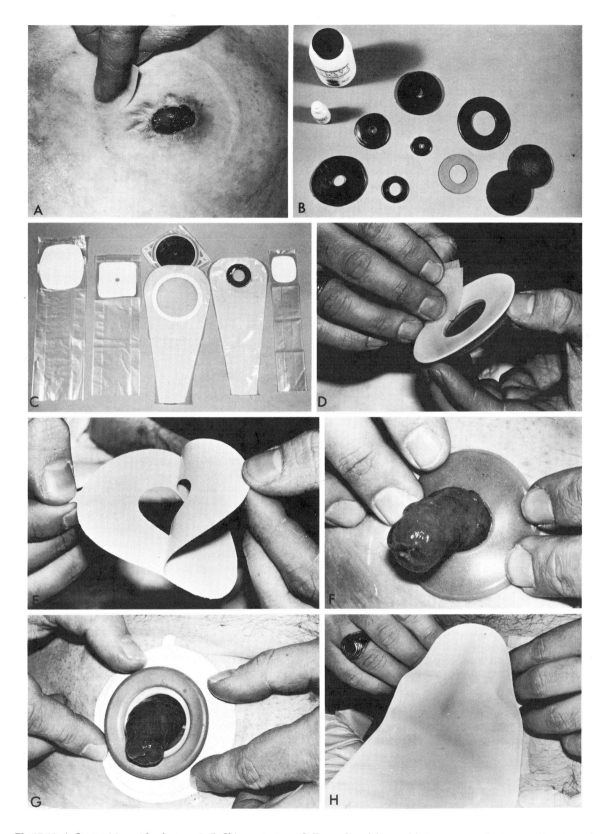

Fig 17.13 *A*, Stoma (sigmoid colostomy). *B*, Skin protectors. *C*, Examples of disposable temporary colostomy or ileostomy pouches. *D*, Mounting ring. *E*, Double-faced adhesive ring. *F*, Karaya washer in position around stoma. *G*, Mounting ring in position. *H*, Pouch being attached to mounting ring.

irrigation daily or every second day. Some controversy exists as to the benefits of, and the need for, irrigation. The procedure is popular in North America but is little used in Britain. The purposes of irrigating the colostomy are to remove faeces, gas and mucus from the intestine and establish a regular time of emptying the lower tract so that spontaneous, irregular drainage is less likely to occur and interfere with the person's activities and usual life-style.

If the patient is constipated it may be necessary to irrigate the colostomy. A funnel is attached to one end of a catheter; the other end is lubricated and placed about 10 cm into the colon. Warm water is placed in the funnel which is held above the level of the colostomy, and the water is allowed to run into the patient. The catheter is then removed and the outflow is collected in a suitable vessel. All the water must be returned before the process is complete. When evacuation is complete, the patient is left clean and dry, and a clean colostomy bag is applied. Drainage between irrigations may indicate that insufficient irrigating fluid was given or the fluid was given too quickly, or may be the result of constipation. If there is evidence of the latter, diet adjustment and increased fluid intake may be necessary.

A regular schedule should be set up for colostomy irrigation and for changing the colostomy appliance. The irrigation is most effective early in the morning, since this approximates the normal time of defecation. If bowel regularity is developed, irrigation every other day may be sufficient.

Care of a pouch ileostomy. General preoperative preparation is similar to that cited for intestinal surgery. The procedure of tube drainage of the ileal pouch, the nasogastric drainage and the withholding of food and fluids by mouth that follow the operation are discussed with the patient and family, and opportunities are provided for them to ask questions.

The patient is returned from the operation with a catheter inserted through the stoma and valve into the pouch. The catheter is connected to a closed drainage system. It is important to maintain continuous drainage and prevent an accumulation of secretions, gas and faecal matter in the pouch in order to promote healing and prevent complications. If the pouch becomes distended, ileal contents may seep through the suture lines and cause peritonitis. Regular, frequent irrigation of the tube may be required to promote drainage. Sterile normal saline or water may be used, and a directive is received regarding the exact volume that is to be introduced very gently with a syringe. Suction is not applied to withdraw the fluid; the return flow should drain by gravity through the catheter. If it is retained, the doctor is notified.

The colour of the drainage is checked frequently; it may be coloured by blood at first but the blood content progressively decreases over the first 2 days. If it does not, it is reported. The volume of the ileal discharge is also recorded. The faecal drainage eventually may become semiliquid as the diet is increased and the capacity and retention of the pouch increase. Thicker pouch content may cause a drainage problem since 'solid' particles may obstruct the drainage tube, necessitating irrigation, increased fluid intake and adjustment in the diet.

A lightweight dressing with a slit for the catheter covers the stoma and surgical wound. This is changed daily and the stoma inspected for colour, swelling and oedema.

The nasogastric tube is attached to low negative pressure to prevent the possibility of gastric secretions and gas accumulating and distending the gastrointestinal tract. The patient is not allowed anything by mouth until the tube is removed. He is sustained by the administration of intravenous fluids. The fluid balance and serum electrolyte levels are followed closely; the volume and composition of the intravenous fluids are based on these reports.

The catheter into the pouch is disconnected from the closed drainage system in approximately 10–12 days and is clamped. The clamp is removed hourly for drainage of the pouch. During the night the catheter is reconnected to the drainage system. The period between the drainages is gradually increased by 15-minute intervals and eventually, when the interval has been lengthened to approximately 3 hours, the catheter is removed. The pouch is then drained every 3 hours by reinsertion of the catheter.

The capacity of the pouch gradually increases and, in 6 months to a year, a capacity of 500–1000 ml is achieved. As the pouch progressively accommodates more and more, the frequency of the catheter insertion for drainage decreases, the objective being three or four times daily. Twenty-four-hour drainage is measured and recorded for many weeks. If the pouch does not drain freely when the tube is introduced, gentle irrigation with a prescribed volume is used.

When the nasogastric tube is removed, the patient receives small amounts of clear fluid exclusive of carbonated drinks. If these are tolerated without distension or vomiting the amounts are increased, followed by a progressive increase from more nourishing fluids through soft to a light normal diet. Food tolerance tends to be an individual matter; the introduction of 'new' foods one at a time makes it possible to identify those that are troublesome. Gas-forming foods, raw fruits and vegetables, foods with a high cellulose or fibre content, corn, celery, lettuce, beans, peas and cabbage are frequently among those not tolerated.

Maintenance of skin integrity
Each time the appliance is changed, the condition of the skin and stoma are noted. The latter should be bright red and moist; if it is bluish or grey or dry the

doctor is notified, as the change may indicate impaired circulation. The skin is examined carefully for possible excoriation or any break. Skin irritation is treated promptly and a more effective protective barrier is provided. Fewer skin problems are encountered by the colostomy patient than the ileostomy patient.

The peristomal skin is washed with mild soap and warm water, rinsed thoroughly and patted dry. Skin preparations that provide an effective barrier include karaya which comes in the form of washers, powder and ointment. The actual preparation used will vary with the hospital. Examples include Hollister skin gel, Orabase paste, Orahesive powder, Stomahesive wafers. Treatment of skin irritation and excoriation includes: cleansing of the skin daily with soap and water; the application of antacid solutions; and the use of protective skin barriers. Ulcerated areas are treated several times a day.

Control of odour
Odour is a constant source of concern to the ileostomy or colostomy patient and his family. It may be controlled by a clean, odour-free, well-fitting appliance, efficient emptying and flushing of the bag, and the use of a commercial deodorant. The deodorant (such as Ostobon) is placed on a tissue and put in the pouch. Household air freshener sprays can be used before changing or emptying a bag. Deodorant tablets of bismuth subgallate or chlorophyll are also available for oral administration but *should only be taken if prescribed by the doctor.* Bags should not be kept in use too long; eventually they absorb odours that are impossible to remove entirely. The bags that are now available make it possible to change them more often and prevent odour. The diet is adjusted to eliminate gas-forming foods. The environment should be kept well ventilated.

Alterations in nutrition
The ileostomy or colostomy patient usually starts out on a light, low-residue diet to which foods of a regular, normal diet are added gradually. Tolerance varies with patients but, by careful personal experimentation with foods, each person will recognize what he can and cannot take. The foods that most often have to be eliminated are those with a high-fibre or high-cellulose content. Nuts, prunes, celery, corn, pineapple, turnips, beans, cabbage and onions tend to be troublesome.

A well-balanced diet is encouraged and the person's weight followed. Patients are advised to eat slowly and to chew their foods well, which reduces the risk of a faecal bolus blocking the stoma. Emptying the pouch or changing the appliance just before mealtimes should be avoided.

Considerable water and salts are lost in ileostomy drainage, especially during the first 2 or 3 months. Gradually, the small intestine adapts to the lack of colonic function and absorbs more water and salts.

Until then extra water and foods rich in sodium and potassium should be taken. The patient may erroneously think that limiting his fluid intake will cause the intestinal drainage to be less fluid.

Coping with the change in body function
As soon as the patient has recovered sufficiently from the operation, the nurse concentrates on helping him to accept his 'ostomy' and on teaching him the necessary care and management. Although there may have been considerable discussion of the modified method of elimination preoperatively, when the patient is actually faced with it he may be filled with revulsion and become discouraged and depressed. The patient is again concerned about his future social acceptance. Acceptance comes first from the nurse, who willingly makes every effort to keep the patient clean and comfortable without any hesitation or aversion. Personal contact by touch, when bathing the patient and positioning and cleansing around the stoma for example, in a perfectly natural and matter-of-fact manner helps the patient to feel that he is acceptable. The nurse should encourage the patient and gradually introduce self-care with an understanding of the patient's reactions to the adjustments he must make. The patient may find it helpful to be visited by someone who has a stoma and is coping well. A visit by a stoma therapist may also be arranged.

Opportunities are created for the patient to interact and socialize with other patients on the ward. Return to normal activities and work are encouraged and may be achieved within 3 months.

The patient and partner are encouraged to ask questions about resuming normal sexual functioning. Literature and pamphlets are available that may be given to the patient and partner regarding sex. Further opportunity for discussion should be arranged after they have read the information and formulated their personal questions and concerns.

Self-care
A plan of instruction is developed to prepare the patient for assuming care of his ileostomy or colostomy and for living a healthy, active life. During the first few days after the operation, the patient's experience with pain and discomfort generally precludes concern about the stoma and his future care and activity. Gradually an awareness of the situation develops and the patient's reaction must be assessed. There may be a brief period of depression and withdrawal. Obviously, while reacting in this way, the patient is not receptive to any formal instruction. The nurse encourages expression of his concern by being a good listener and accepting his reactions and anxiety. The nurse's attitude is extremely important; any sign of distaste when caring for the patient or indication of haste to cut short the contact is likely to be interpreted by the patient that he is unacceptable. To him, this reflects what

will happen in his future, and fosters feelings of depression and resentment, making rehabilitation difficult.

The preparation for the patient's discharge from the hospital should include a member of the family. Participation of a person with an ileostomy or colostomy who may have already visited the patient may be very helpful in reinforcing the information. Teaching includes explanations, discussions and demonstrations related to the following factors:

Management of the ileostomy and colostomy. Active patient participation in stomal and appliance care is introduced gradually but as early as possible. By the time he leaves the hospital, the patient should be engaged in self-care and be confident in the fact that support and assistance are available to him in the hospital and at home.

At first, as the nurse cares for the ileostomy or colostomy, each step of the procedure is clearly described without minute details. Then, gradually, the patient is given the opportunity to perform part of the care. His participation is increased from day to day until eventually he is prepared to undertake complete care. This progressive, step-by-step approach takes time and patience but is less frustrating and discouraging for the patient. As he learns to assume self-care in the hospital, the nurse offers suggestions as to how he may manage the same procedure at home.

More formalized and detailed instruction includes directions for and demonstrations of:

1 The necessary equipment and supplies. In addition to discussing and demonstrating the various parts of the appliance, a written list is provided and information given as to how and where the products may be obtained.

2 Emptying of the pouch, care of the stoma and changing of the appliance. Planned discussions reinforce the learning that took place as the patient undertook, step-by-step, the daily care. It also gives him and the members of the family an opportunity to ask questions.

Additional directions for care and use usually accompany the appliance and should be read by the patient. Several useful booklets about ileostomy and colostomy care are usually available from the Colostomy Welfare Group[36] or the Ileostomy Association of Great Britain and Ireland.[37] The hospital may also issue printed directions which serve as a guide for the patient. The importance of establishing a regular schedule for care is emphasized.

3 Irrigation of the colostomy (if required by the patient). In addition to demonstrating and explaining the procedure and having the patient do it himself, written directions are given to him. Assistance may be necessary in deciding how the irrigation can be fitted in with his daily routine.

4 Care of the skin. The need for thorough but gentle cleansing of the skin is stressed, as is the use of a protective skin barrier because of the irritating effect of the enzyme-containing discharge. Inspection for redness and excoriation is described and advice given as to what should be done if either is present.

5 Care of the appliance. Cleansing of the mounting ring and reusable pouches (if used) are demonstrated and a written directive given.

6 Control of odour. The role of regular emptying, changing and thorough cleansing of the appliance in controlling odour is discussed. The use of a charcoal filter and deodorant in the bag is encouraged.

7 Problems or complications. Problems such as excessive drainage, blockage of the stoma, excoriation, burning sensation or itching of the skin are discussed as to possible causes, how they are recognized and the appropriate action.

Nutrition and fluids. The patient is advised that foods high in cellulose and fibre and some raw vegetables and fruits may be troublesome. A list of foods known to lead to a problem, and therefore to be avoided, is provided. The importance of a well-balanced diet and the taking of additional amounts of sodium, potassium and water is explained. It is suggested that one new food be added at a time so those that cannot be tolerated may be identified.

Bathing. The patient may take a shower or bath with the appliance in place or, if the discharge is at a minimum, the appliance may be removed and the stoma covered with a soft dressing and waterproof adhesive. Showering without the appliance is good for the skin. The patient must be sure that no soap residue remains, since this interferes with the seal provided by the adhesive disc. Bathing is usually done before applying a fresh appliance because the moisture is likely to loosen the adhesive disc.

Some people with stomas may have sufficient confidence to go swimming, since the appliance is concealed by a bathing suit.

Activity. Activity for the ileostomy and colostomy patient is normal except for heavy lifting, which predisposes to prolapse of the stoma and hernia, and body contact sports, which could result in injury to the stoma. The patient is encouraged to return to his occupation and recreational activities. Many people find that their general health is so much better than previously that they enjoy being able to participate in so much.

The patient may be concerned about sexual relationships; he is advised that the change in body

---

[36] 38/39 Eccleston Square, London SW1V 1PB
[37] Amblehurst House, Chobham, Woking, Surrey GV24 9PZ

image need not be a deterrent to satisfactory sex relations. If an abdominoperineal resection has been done, injury to parasympathetic nerves may very occasionally result in impotency. The female may experience some discomfort during intercourse for a period of time because of the perineal wound. This matter of sexual relationships is something the individual may wish to discuss freely with the stomatherapist. Further help may be available from the organization Sexual and Personal Relationships of the Disabled.[38]

Medications. Laxatives or other drugs should not be taken unless prescribed. If a medicine is ordered by a doctor other than the gastroenterologist, the patient should remind him of his ileostomy. Some preparations should be only in powder or liquid form to ensure absorption.

Sources of assistance. The patient is likely to be very apprehensive about leaving the protective hospital environment. A list of persons or associations from whom advice or assistance may be sought is provided with their telephone numbers. This list may include the stoma therapist, general practitioner or community nurse, and the relevant associations.

Care of the ileal pouch. As soon as the tube is removed, plans are made to teach the patient how to insert the catheter to empty the pouch. As cited earlier, the catheter is passed every 2 hours at first, and then the interval is gradually lengthened over the next 4–6 months. The patient is advised that if he experiences discomfort or a full sensation in the pouch, the pouch should be intubated to avoid distension and excessive pressure on the valve. The patient observes the passing of the catheter by the nurse, who explains the procedure as she does it and gives the patient the opportunity to ask questions. The patient then undertakes the passing of the catheter through the stoma and valve. The nurse remains during the procedure until assured that the patient is competent and sufficiently confident. He learns the details of carrying out the procedure, and may use a basin to receive the projectile drainage or may prefer to let it flow directly into the toilet. If the ileal outflow is slow, the patient is advised that he may bear down. Instructions are given as to the frequency and volume of drainage that would be considered inadequate, and what to do if this occurs. The doctor may want the patient to be taught to irrigate the pouch in the event of insufficient drainage.

Cleansing of the stoma and the skin and covering it with a small dressing (e.g. 5 cm² Band-Aid or a piece of gauze) are reviewed in preparation for discharge.

The necessary supplies are obtained for the patient and include a small case with two catheters, water-soluble lubricant for the catheter, a syringe, dressings and micropore tape. The sources for supplies are given and instructions supplied as to their care. The patient is instructed to wash the catheter in detergent solution thoroughly and rinse well.

It is important for the person with an ileal pouch to carry a card or wear a Medic Alert bracelet or pendant indicating his 'condition' and the need for drainage of the pouch. If he loses consciousness or is injured, this would be necessary to avoid excessive and dangerous distension of the pouch.

COMPLICATIONS

Potential complications of an ileostomy or colostomy include prolapse or retraction of the stoma, obstruction of the stoma, fluid and electrolyte imbalance, renal calculus and fistula.

In *prolapse of the stoma*, the mesentery of the remaining intestine is not secured sufficiently to the abdominal wall and/or the opening in the abdominal wall is too large. Increased intra-abdominal pressure results in a segment of the ileum or colon being forced out onto the abdomen. If several inches of the bowel is extruded, the patient assumes the dorsal recumbent position with the head and shoulders slightly raised and the knees flexed. A sterile towel or dressing moistened in sterile water or normal saline is placed over the area. The doctor may attempt manual replacement of the extruded segment or recommend surgical repair.

Retraction of the stoma occurs as the result of shrinking scar tissue in the supporting tissues of the abdominal wall. The opening becomes flush with the abdominal surface, making it difficult to protect the skin from the irritating effluent. Correction is by surgery.

Obstruction of the stoma may be caused by a faecal bolus formed as a result of insufficient mastication of food or the ingestion of fibrous or cellulose foods that are too bulky to pass through the stoma. Examples of such foods are corn, celery, bran, coconut and nuts. The blockage may be relieved by an irrigation given by the doctor. An obstruction may also be caused by a volvulus of the ileum near the stoma. If there is no ileal or colostomy discharge, the doctor is notified. Unless the obstruction is relieved, the patient will develop nausea, vomiting, crampy pain and abdominal distension.

Ileostomy dysfunction sometimes occurs, and is characterized by sporadic free liquid drainage with a very offensive odour. It is associated with peristomal scarring and stenosis which causes trapping of the intestinal contents until pressure and irritation result in the discharge. Dilation of the stoma may be necessary.

Normally, much of the water and electrolytes contained in the small intestinal content is reabsorbed in the colon. The person with an ileostomy loses considerable water, sodium and potassium in the ileal drainage and may develop *fluid and electrolyte imbal-*

---

[38] 25 Mortimer Street, London W1N 8AB.

ance. The patient is encouraged to drink a minimum of 1500–2000 ml of fluid daily, add salt to his foods and include potassium-containing foods (e.g. orange juice, banana, meat) in his diet. If the ileal drainage becomes excessive, fluids containing potassium and sodium are increased to compensate for the loss. Tomato juice, orange juice, tea with sugar and broth are fluids that may be used. If the excessive drainage cannot be controlled, the doctor should be notified. An antidiarrhoeal drug may be prescribed, serum electrolyte levels determined and intravenous fluids administered to correct dehydration and electrolyte imbalance.

The ileostomy patient is predisposed to the formation of a *renal calculus* (kidney stone) because of the water and sodium loss in drainage. This further emphasizes the importance of a greater fluid and electrolyte intake for the person with an ileostomy or colostomy, especially if the latter is on the right-hand side.

Rarely, an ileostomy or colostomy is complicated by a *fistula*. An opening develops in the ileum and the drainage forms a tract to the surface. This may be the result of a poorly fitting appliance or the recurrence of the primary disease. The drainage causes tissue irritation and erosion. Surgical intervention may be used to resect the tract and may include reconstruction of the stoma. Healing may necessitate complete rest of the intestine; the patient may receive total intravenous nutrition (parenteral nutrition) until the area is healed.

Herniation of the intestine due to a weakness of the muscular tissue at the site of the stoma may occur. It is recognized as a bulging area. Support may be provided by the ileostomy or colostomy appliance.

EXPECTED OUTCOMES

The patient:
1 Demonstrates an ability to cleanse the stoma and skin, inspect the peristomal skin, apply a suitable product to protect the skin, apply the appliance and drainage bag, clean the equipment, and remove the appliance.
2 Demonstrates, if relevant, the ability to irrigate the colostomy or to drain the ileal pouch.
3 Describes techniques to control odour from the ostomy.
4 Discusses a plan to adjust his diet (which should be well-balanced). This should include eliminating gas-forming foods, and, if he has an ileostomy, increasing his intake of fluids and salts.
5 Discusses plans for follow-up care.
6 States the community and other health resources that are available.
7 Feels able to resume daily activities, social interactions and return to work.

References and Further Reading

BOOKS

Bates B (1983) *A Guide to Physical Examination*, 3rd ed. Philadelphia: JB Lippincott. Chapters 9 & 12.

Braunwald E et al (1987) *Harrison's Principles of Internal Medicine*. New York: McGraw-Hill. Chapters 31–34, 36, 37 & 237.

British National Formulary (1986) British Medical Association and the Pharmaceutical Society of Great Britain, London.

Brocklehurst JC & Hanley T (1981) *Geriatric Medicine for Students*, 2nd ed. Edinburgh: Churchill Livingstone. pp. 85–89.

Davenport HW (1982) *Physiology of the Digestive Tract*, 5th ed. Chicago: Year Book Medical.

Fox JET & Monna K (1980) How to relieve your dysphagic patient's pain with a double swallow. In: RC Mackay & G. Silm (eds) *Research for Practice*. Halifax, Nova Scotia: Dalhousie University.

Guyton AC (1986) *Textbook of Medical Physiology*, 7th ed. Philadelphia: WB Saunders. Chapters 63, 64, 65 & 66.

Gwen BA & Simmons SJ (1979) *Gastroenterology in Clinical Nursing*, 3rd ed. St Louis: CV Mosby.

Howe PS (1981) *Basic Nutrition in Health and Disease*. 7th ed. Philadelphia: WB Saunders. Chapter 21, pp. 518–524 & 542–544.

Huskisson J (1985) *Applied Nutrition and Dietetics*, 2nd ed. London: Baillière Tindall. Chapter 4.

Jelliffe DB (1966) *The Assessment of the Nutritional Status of the Community*. Monograph No. 53. Geneva: WHO.

Jerzy GGB (ed) (1980) *Gastrointestinal Hormones*. New York: Raven Press. Chapter 2.

Johnston IDA & Lee HA (1978) *Developments in Clinical Nutrition*. Kent, UK: Medical Congresses and Symposia Consultants.

Kim MJ & Moritz DA (eds) (1982) *Classification of Nursing Diagnoses*. New York: McGraw-Hill.

Krause MV & Mahan LK (1984) *Food, Nutrition and Diet Therapy*, 7th ed. Philadelphia: WB Saunders. Chapter 6.

Krupp MA & Chatton MJ (eds) (1983) *Current Medical Diagnosis and Treatment*. Los Altos, CA: Lange Medical. Chapter 10.

MacKay RC & Silm G (eds) (1980) *Research for Practice*. Halifax, Nova Scotia: Dalhousie University. pp. 208–217.

Malasanos L, Barkauskas V, Moss M & Stoltenberg-Allen K (1981) *Health Assessment*, 2nd ed. St Louis: CV Mosby. Chapters 5, 17 & 18.

Miller S, Sampson LK, Soukup M & Weinberg SL (eds) (1980) *Methods in Critical Care: The AACN Manual*. Philadelphia: WB Saunders. pp. 307–352 & 415–440.

Pagana KD & Pagana TJ (1982) *Diagnostic Testing and Nursing Implications*. St Louis: CV Mosby. Chapter 2.

Polak JM & Bloom SR (1980) Neural and cellular origin of gastrointestinal hormonal peptides in health and disease. In: GGB Jerzy (ed) *Gastrointestinal Hormones*. New York: Raven Press.

Sabiston DC (ed) (1986) *Davis–Christopher Textbook of Surgery*, 13th ed. Philadelphia: WB Saunders. Chapters 27–33.

Smith LH & Thier SA (1985) *Pathophysiology*, 2nd ed. Philadelphia: WB Saunders. Section 14.

Vander AJ, Sherman JH & Luciano DS (1985) *Human Physiology: The Mechanisms of Body Function*, 4th ed. New York: McGraw-Hill. Chapter 14.

Wineck M (ed) (1980) *Nutrition and Gastroenterology*. New York: John Wiley.

PERIODICALS

Amato EL (1982) A nursing reference: gastrointestinal tubes and drains. Part I: intra-abdominal tubes and drains. *Crit. Care Nurs.*, Vol. 2 No. 6, pp. 50–57.

Anderson H, Bosaeus I, Falkheden T & Melkersson H (1979) Transit time in constipated geriatric patients during treatment with a bulk laxative and bran: a comparison. *Scand. J. Gastroenterology*, Vol. 14 No. 7, pp. 821–826.

Bachrach W, Boyce HW & Jackson D (1981) Problems in swallowing and esophageal carcinoma. *Heart Lung*, Vol. 10, No. 3, pp. 525–531.

Battle EH & Hanna CE (1980) Evaluation of a dietary regimen for chronic constipation. *J. Gerontol. Nurs.*, Vol. 6 No. 9, pp. 527–532.

Beck ML (1981) Preparing your patient physically for an esophogastroduodenoscopy. *Nurs. '81*, Vol. 11 No. 2, pp. 88–96.

Beck ML (1981) Three common gastrointestinal tests and how to help your patient through each. *Nurs. '81*, Vol. 11 No. 4, pp. 44–47.

Beck ML (1981) Three more gastrointestinal tests and how to help your patient through each. *Nurs. '81*, Vol. 11 No. 5, pp. 22–23 & 27.

Bragg V (1981) Extracolonic complications associated with inflammatory bowel disease. *J. Enterostomal Therapy*, Vol. 8 No. 1, pp. 14–16.

Breslin EH (1981) Prevention and treatment of pulmonary complications in patients after surgery of the upper abdomen. *Heart Lung*, Vol. 10 No. 3, pp. 511–519.

Carpenter CCJ (1982) The pathophysiology of secretory diarrhea. *Med. Clin. N. Am.*, Vol. 66 No. 3, pp. 597–610.

Cundy DW (1981) An artificial external esophagus. *J. Enterostomal Therapy*, Vol. 8 No. 1, pp. 17–20.

Fuller E (ed) (1981) When malabsorption follows gastrectomy. *Patient Care*, Vol. 15 No. 14, pp. 135–159.

Fuller E (ed) (1981) When the esophagus acts up. *Patient Care*, Vol. 15 No. 14, pp. 167–189.

Gallacher DV & Peterson OH (1980) Substance P increases membrane conductance in parotid acinar cells. *Nature*, Vol. 283 No. 5745, pp. 393–395.

Grant JP, Coster PB & Thurlow JT (1981) Current techniques of nutritional assessment. *Surg. Clin. N. Am.*, Vol. 61 No. 3.

Gross L & Bailey Z (1981) Enterostomal therapy: developing institutional community programs. *J. Enterostomal Therapy*, Vol. 8 No. 1, pp. 23–25 & 28–29.

Gruner OPN, Naas R, Gjone E. Flatmark A & Fetheim B (1981) Mental disorders in ulcerative colitis. *J. Enterostomal Therapy*, Vol. 8 No. 3, pp. 22–25.

Harford WV, Krejs GJ, Santa Ana CA & Fordtran JS (1980) Acute effect of diphenoxylate with atropine (Lomotil) in Patients with chronic diarrhea and fecal incontinence. *Gastroenterology*, Vol. 78 No. 3, pp. 440–443.

Hinson LR (1985) Nutritional assessment and management of the hospitalized patient. *Crit. Care Nurs.*, Vol. 5 No. 2, pp. 53–60.

Hughes RL, Freilich RA, Bytell DE, Craig RM & Moran JM (1981) Aspiration and occult esophageal disorders. *Chest*, Vol. 80 No. 4, pp. 489–495.

Hull C, Greco RS & Brooks DL (1980) Alleviation of consti-
pation in the elderly by dietary fiber supplementation. *J. Am. Geriatr. Soc.* Vol. 28 No. 9, pp. 410–414.

Ivey MF (1979) The status of parenteral nutrition. *Nurs. Clin. N. Am.*, Vol. 14 No. 2, pp. 285–304.

Johnson AC, Sessions JT, Snape WJ & Teichner VJ (1984) Constipation: is it functional, or . . .? *Patient Care*, Vol. 18 No. 4, pp. 128–133, 137, 140–143 & 146–147.

Johnson CK (1980) Health laxation and food habit influences on fiber intake of older women. *J. Am. Diet. Assoc.*, Vol. 77 No. 5, pp. 551–557.

Johnson LF (1981) New concepts and methods in the study and treatment of gastroesophageal reflux disease. *Med. Clin. N. Am.*, Vol. 65 No. 6, pp. 1195–1222.

Kasanof DM (ed) (1981) Current care for infectious diarrhea. *Patient Care*, Vol. 15, No. 3, pp. 149–175.

Kasanof DM (ed) (1981) Crohn's disease and ulcerative colitis? *Patient Care*, Vol. 15 No. 13, pp. 105–114.

Kennedy G (1981) Total parenteral nutrition, *Can. Nurse*, Vol. 77 No. 3, pp. 32–35.

Konstantinides NN (1985) Home parenteral nutrition: a viable alternative for patients with cancer. *Onc. Nurs. Forum*, Vol. 12 No. 1, pp. 23–29.

Lamy PP & Krug BH (1978) Review of laxative utilization in skilled nursing facility. *J. Am. Geriatr. Soc.*, Vol. 26 No. 12, pp. 544–549.

Lane B & Forgay M (1981) Upgrading your oral hygiene protocol for the patient with cancer. *Can. Nurse*, Vol. 77 No. 11, pp. 27–29.

Lewis B (1985) 'Streamlining the process of elimination. *Am. J. Nurs.*, Vol. 85 No. 7, pp. 774.

Liang T & Cascieri MA (1981) Substance P receptors on parotid cell membranes. *J. Neurosci.*, Vol. 1 No. 10, pp. 1133–1141.

Lindsey AM (1985) Building the knowledge base for practice. Part I: nausea and vomiting. *Oncol. Nurs. Forum*, Vol. 12 No. 1, pp. 49–56.

Lundberg JM, Anggard A & Fahrenkrug J (1981) Complimentary role of vasoactive intestinal polypeptide (VIP) and acetylocholine for cat submandibular gland flow and secretion. *Acta Physiol. Scand.*, Vol. 113 No. 3, pp. 317–329.

McConnell EA (1981) Curtailing a life-threatening crisis: GI bleeding. *Nurs. '81*, Vol. 11 No. 4, p. 70–73.

McNamara J (1982) Esophageal cancer. *Nurs. '82*, Vol. 12 No. 3, p. 64.

Maltz C (1981) A differential for diarrhea. *Emerg. Med.*, Vol. 13 No. 21, pp. 91–109.

Martyn PA, Hansen BC & Jen KLC (1984) The effects of parenteral nutrition on food intake and gastric motility. *Nurs. Res.*, Vol. 33 No. 6, pp. 336–342.

Mathews DM (1977) Protein absorption—then and now. *Gastroenterology*, Vol. 73 No. 6, p. 277.

May HJ (1982) Information for ileostomy patients. *J. Enterostomal Therapy*, Vol. 9 No. 1, pp. 10–13 & 21.

Millard MW & Millard ST (1981) When you suspect lower GI bleeding. *Patient Care*, Vol. 15 No. 5, pp. 62–106.

Miller JK & Miller RL (1980) Identifying and assessing oral ulcers. *Nurs. '81*, Vol. 11 No. 7, pp. 10–11.

Miller JK (1985) Helping the aged manage bowel function. *J. Gerontol. Nurs.*, Vol. 11 No. 2, pp. 37–41.

Moog F (1981) The lining of the small intestine. *Sci. Am.*, Vol. 245 No. 5, pp. 154–176.

Myers S, Walfish JS, Sachar DB et al (1980) Quality of life after surgery for Crohn's disease: a psychosocial surgery. *J. Enterostomal Therapy*, Vol. 7 No. 5, pp. 25–27 & 30–31.

Paulsen F (1981) Continuous escape and deodorizing of flatus. *J. Enterostomal Therapy*, Vol. 8 No. 3, pp. 26–29.

Rodman MJ (1980) Diarrhea: think twice before giving Medicine. *R.N.*, Vol. 43 No. 10, pp. 73–84.

Rodman MJ (1980) The drug interaction we all overlook. *R.N.*, Vol. 43 No. 12, pp. 58–62.

Ropka ME (1982) Hiatal hernia. *Nurs. '82*, Vol. 12 No. 4, pp. 126–131.

Saunders JF (1978) Lactulose syrup assessed in a double-bind study of elderly constipated patients. *J. Am. Geriatr. Soc.*, Vol. 26 No. 5, pp. 236–239.

Semmens S (1982) Nursing care plan for patient receiving total parenteral nutrition. *Crit. Care Nurs.*, Vol. 2 No. 5, pp. 86–89.

Shaw LM (1981) A teaching plan for Nissen fundoplication. *A.O.R.N. J.*, Vol. 34 No. 1, pp. 47–55.

Smith CE (1981) Abdominal assessment—a blending of science and art. *Nurs. '81*, Vol. 11 No. 2, pp. 42–49.

Smith RG et al (1980) A study of bulking agents in elderly patients. *Age Ageing*, Vol. 9 No. 4, pp. 267–271.

Volden C, Brinde J & Carl D (1980) Nasogastric intubation. *Nurs. '80*, Vol. 10 No. 9, pp. 64–67.

Warneke P (1981) Stress and psychological problems of patients undergoing APR. *J. Enterostomal Therapy*, Vol. 8 No. 6, pp. 14–15.

Wilpizeski MD (1981) Helping the ostomate return to normal life. *Nurs. '81*, Vol. 11 No. 3, pp. 62–66.

Wilson J & Colley R (1979) Meeting patients' nutritional needs with hyperalimentation. *Nurs. '79*, Vol. 9 No. 6, pp. 57–61.

Wilson J & Colley R (1979) Meeting patients' nutritional needs with hyperalimentation. *Nurs. '79*, Vol. 9 No. 8, pp. 56–63.

Wilson J & Colley R (1979) Meeting patients' nutritional needs with hyperalimentation. *Nurs. '79*, Vol. 9 No. 9, pp. 62–69.

Wilson J & Riedel G (1984) Lactose intolerance. *Can. Nurse*, Vol. 80 No. 1, pp. 27–29.

Wiseman IL (1981) A study of benign intestinal polyps. *J. Enterostomal Therapy*, Vol. 8 No. 5, pp. 15–18.

Yasko JM (1985) Holistic management of nausea and vomiting caused by chemotherapy. *Top. Clin. Nurs.*, Vol. 7 No. 1, pp. 26–38.

18

Nursing in Disorders of the Liver, Biliary Tract and Exocrine Pancreas

Physiology of the Biliary System

The biliary system consists of the liver, gallbladder and bile ducts.

LIVER

The liver is the largest organ of the body and is situated in the upper abdominal cavity immediately below the diaphragm. It is divided into four lobes and is highly vascular, receiving its blood supply from two sources. The portal vein carries blood from the stomach, intestines, spleen and pancreas into the liver. The hepatic[1] artery delivers blood from the aorta. The blood from both sources leaves the liver by a common pathway, the hepatic vein, which joins the inferior vena cava.

The liver tissue is organized in functional units called lobules. Each lobule consists of rows of cells radiating out from a central vein. Subdivisions of the hepatic artery and portal vein deliver blood into small spaces called sinusoids between the rows of cells, bringing the blood in direct contact with the hepatic cells. From the sinusoids it enters the central vein (Fig. 18.1). Large phagocytic, reticuloendo-thelial cells called Kupffer cells lie scattered within the sinusoids to ingest and destroy organisms and other foreign material within the blood. The central veins from the lobules empty into sublobular collecting veins, which unite to form the hepatic vein. Minute ducts into which bile is discharged are also formed between the rows of hepatic cells. The small lobular bile ducts are directed toward the surface of the lobules where they unite to form larger ducts. Eventually, the bile from the lobules is transmitted in one main channel, the hepatic duct, which joins the bile duct from the gallbladder (cystic duct) to form the common bile duct (Fig. 18.2).

FUNCTIONS OF THE LIVER

The liver performs a variety of very important complex functions. It is a vital organ, performing a

[1] From *hepar* the Latin word meaning liver.

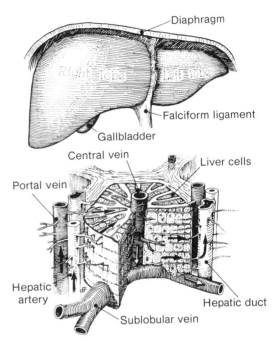

Fig. 18.1 The liver and an enlarged section of a lobule.

major role in total body metabolism. The liver synthesizes, processes and/or stores many of the substances that are essential to normal body functioning. It also processes and excretes some substances that would be harmful if left in their original form or retained.

Bile production and excretion
The liver cells secrete 500–1000 ml of bile daily into the hepatic ducts. It is a yellow-green or brownish fluid that is strongly alkaline and bitter to the taste. The constituents of bile are:

Water (90–97%). The water content is reduced when the bile is stored in the gallbladder where it is concentrated six to ten times.

Bile pigments. The pigments resulting from the breakdown of red blood cells and from foods are excreted as the bile pigments *bilirubin* and *biliverdin*.

Bilirubin is orange-red and is in greater concentration in man; biliverdin is green and predominates in those persons or species whose diet is mainly vegetable.

In the intestine, bile pigments are acted upon by bacteria and reduced to urobilinogen. Part of the urobilinogen is excreted in the faeces, giving them the normal brown colour. The remainder is reabsorbed through the intestinal mucosa into the blood. A small amount is excreted in the urine and the rest is returned to the liver where it is reconverted to bilirubin and again is secreted in the bile.

Bile salts. These are sodium and potassium salts of certain amino acids that function in digestion and absorption. The bile salts emulsify fats, increase the digestive action of the fat-splitting enzyme, and promote absorption of fats, fat-soluble vitamins and calcium salts. The bile salts are reclaimed from the intestine and returned to the liver by the portal circulation where they stimulate the hepatic cells to secrete bile. They are reused in the secretion.

Other constituents. Sodium and calcium salts, cholesterol, fatty acids and lecithin are other substances in bile.

Bile is discharged by the common bile duct into the duodenum through the sphincter of Oddi. The functions of bile may be summarized as follows:

Bile promotes the digestion and absorption of fats in the small intestine. Because it is alkaline, it neutralizes the acidic chyme when it moves into the small intestine. It stimulates peristalsis of the large intestine, which was the basis of the use of bile salts in preparations of laxatives. The reabsorbed bile salts stimulate hepatic cells to secrete bile. Bile is an excretory medium for some drugs, toxins, excess minerals (e.g. copper and zinc), pigments and cholesterol.

Metabolic functions
The liver has a role in the metabolism of *carbohydrates, proteins and fats.* Briefly, it converts glucose to glycogen and stores it (glycogenesis), reconverting it to glucose and releasing it into the blood when required in order to maintain an adequate blood sugar concentration. Glucose in excess of what can be converted to glycogen is converted to fat (lipogenesis) in the liver. The simple sugars, or monosaccharides, fructose and galactose cannot be utilized by the cells, so the liver changes the molecules to glucose.

Fats may be both synthesized and catabolized by the liver. Cholesterol, lecithin, phospholipids and lipoproteins are examples of substances that may be formed by the liver. Fats are desaturated or may be broken down into ketone acids or acetate.

Protein may be deaminized, a process in which the amine radical is removed and the remaining elements are used to form glycogen or other compounds to meet tissue needs. The amine radical is converted to urea and released into the blood for elimination by the kidneys. Amino acids are also used in the liver to form blood proteins, enzymes and structural compounds. Amino acids may be converted to carbohydrates to provide a source of energy.

Storage
The liver stores glycogen, vitamins A, D, E, K and B_{12}, iron, phospholipids, cholesterol, and a small amount of protein and fat.

Formation of certain blood components
In the fetus, the liver produces the erythrocytes. This activity gradually diminishes after midterm when erythropoiesis in the bone marrow increases. After birth, the liver stores vitamin B_{12} and releases it as necessary to promote the production of erythrocytes.

Heparin, and the blood proteins serum albumin, fibrinogen and alpha and beta globulins are formed by the hepatic cells. The liver also synthesizes most of the blood-clotting factors; it is the primary source of prothrombin, fibrinogen and Factors V, VII, VIII, IX, XI and XII.

Destruction of erythrocytes
The Kupffer cells break down the worn-out erythrocytes. The haemoglobin is released, the iron and globin are split off, and bilirubin is formed from the waste products and is excreted in bile. The iron is reclaimed, combined with a protein to form ferritin and stored until it is needed for the formation of haemoglobin.

Detoxification of harmful substances
Certain drugs and chemicals that could be harmful to tissue cells are changed by the liver and rendered harmless before being circulated and excreted by the kidneys. The liver detoxifies by conjugation, oxidation or hydrolysis. In conjugation, it combines the toxic substance with some other material to produce an inoffensive compound (e.g. benzoic acid is changed to hippuric acid). Barbiturates, nicotine and strychnine are drugs that are oxidized and completely destroyed by the liver. Laxative drugs and some nutrients such as vitamin D are neutralized in the liver.

The body itself produces certain chemicals (hormones) that, unless destroyed, would reach too high a concentration. Examples of physiological products that are destroyed in the liver are the antidiuretic hormone (ADH), progesterone and adrenocorticoid secretions. Some hormones such as insulin and glucagon undergo deamination (removal of amino acids) in the liver, which renders them inactive.

The Kupffer cells also protect the body by destroying organisms that may have been absorbed from the intestine.

Heat production
The liver is second only to muscle tissue in the pro-

duction of heat by its continuous cell activity. Under basal (resting) conditions, the liver is responsible for most of the body heat.

GALLBLADDER AND BILE DUCTS

The gallbladder is a sac on the undersurface of the liver with an average capacity of 40–50 ml. The cystic duct leading from the gallbladder merges with the hepatic duct to form the common bile duct. The latter unites with the pancreatic duct to form the ampulla of Vater, which opens into the duodenum. This opening is controlled by the sphincter of Oddi (Fig. 18.2).

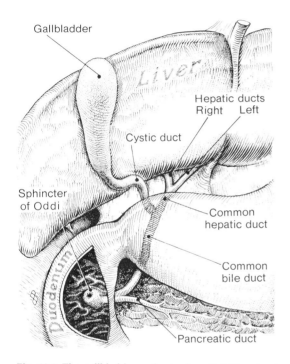

Fig. 18.2 The gallbladder and extra hepatic biliary tract.

Smooth muscle, connective tissue and a mucous membranous lining compose the walls of the gall-bladder and ducts.

The functions of the gallbladder are to concentrate and store the bile. When the stomach and duodenum are empty of food, the sphincter of Oddi remains contracted. During this period, the bile that is continuously secreted accumulates in the gallbladder. Contraction of the sac to eject the bile is dependent upon hormonal stimulation. When food containing fat and partially digested protein enters the duodenum, a hormone called cholecystokinin-pancreozymin (CCK-PZ or CCK) is secreted by cells of the duodenal mucosa. It is carried in the blood and, on reaching the gallbladder, stimulates the smooth muscle tissue to contract and eject bile. CCK

also produces relaxation of the sphincter of Oddi which allows the flow of bile into the duodenum.

Physiology of the Pancreas

The pancreas is a fish-shaped gland; the thicker portion, referred to as the head, lies in the curve of the duodenum, and the remainder extends to the left directly behind the stomach (Fig. 18.3). It has two distinct types of essential functional cells. Groups of one type secrete into small ducts which drain into a main channel running the length of the gland. This collecting channel is called the *pancreatic duct*, or the duct of Wirsung, and passes out of the head of the pancreas to unite with the common bile duct to form the ampulla of Vater. In a few people, the duct may have a direct entrance to the duodenum via the duct of Santorini. Because the secretion of this type of cell flows through ducts, it is classified as an *external* or *exocrine secretion*.

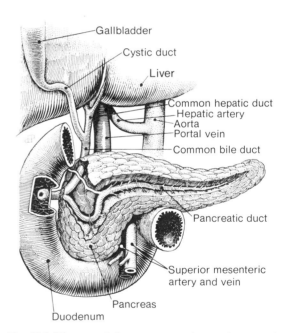

Fig. 18.3 Diagram of the pancreas and central pancreatic duct in relationship to the duodenum and common bile duct.

The other type of parenchymal cell is scattered in insular groups, forming what are known as the islets of Langerhans. These cells produce secretions which are classified as *internal* or *endocrine secretions* because they are absorbed into the blood and are not secreted into ducts.

EXOCRINE FUNCTIONS

The external secretion passes through the ampulla of Vater and sphincter of Oddi into the duodenum. It is strongly alkaline, owing to a high bicarbonate content. Several important digestive enzymes (trypsinogen, chymotrypsin, procarboxypeptidase, amylopsin and lipase) involved in the breakdown of proteins, carbohydrates and fats are contained in the exocrine secretion. Regulation of the secretion of these enzymes and their role in digestion is discussed under Digestion in the Small Intestine on page 489.

ENDOCRINE FUNCTIONS

The endocrine functions of the pancreas are the production of insulin, glucagon, somatostatin and pancreatic polypeptide hormones.

Insulin is secreted by the beta cells of the islets of Langerhans in response to a rise in blood glucose concentration. It has a major role in the metabolism of glucose and regulation of the blood sugar level. The transfer of glucose from the blood into most body cells is facilitated by insulin, but neurons and erythrocytes are not dependent upon it for the uptake of glucose. Insulin promotes utilization of glucose by the cells and the storage of glucose as glycogen in the liver. It also influences fatty acid synthesis (esterification) in fatty tissue and the uptake and conversion of amino acids into body proteins. It is rapidly removed from the blood and degraded by the liver.

Glucagon is formed by the alpha cells of the islets of Langerhans and by similar cells in the walls of the stomach and duodenum.[2] Glucagon functions to increase the blood glucose concentration by breaking down liver glycogen (glycogenolysis) and increasing the synthesis of glucose (gluconeogenesis) by the liver. It also promotes the breakdown of fats to fatty acids and glycerol and the release of potassium from the liver. Physical exercise, stress and the sympathetic nervous system also stimulate glucagon secretion thus mobilizing the body's energy stores.

The two main hormones, insulin and glucagon, secreted by the islets of Langerhans are opposite in effect. Insulin secretion increases during absorption of a meal high in carbohydrate in response to the increase in plasma glucose concentration. Absorption of a meal low in carbohydrate and high in protein increases plasma amino acid concentration which stimulates the release of glucagon as well as insulin, thus maintaining the plasma glucose level. Following absorption of a usual meal, the increase in plasma glucose and amino acid concentrations counteract each other and the result is an increase in insulin secretion with only a minimal change in glucagon.[3] During the post-absorptive period following a meal and during fasting, glucagon secretion increases and insulin secretion decreases as the plasma glucose concentration falls.[4]

Somatostatin, secreted by the delta cells of the islets of Langerhans, functions to maintain a relatively constant blood glucose level by inhibiting the secretion of insulin and glucagon.

Pancreatic polypeptide hormone is secreted by cells of the islets of Langerhans. Its function is not clear. Secretion increases following ingestion of protein, fats or glucose.

Nursing Process

ASSESSMENT

Disorders of the liver, biliary tract and pancreas affect overall body functioning. The body's energy balance is affected when the supply and storage of nutrients is altered, fluid and electrolyte balance is disrupted, bowel and bladder elimination is altered, blood clotting mechanisms are affected, and heat production diminishes. Patient assessment includes the collection of data on life-style, behaviour patterns, dietary habits and changes in physiological functioning of most body systems. Also, the nurse should have some understanding of the various examinations and tests carried out, and the implications of the results of these for the patient. Knowledge of the manifestations of disorders of the liver, biliary tract and pancreas will also help her to assess the patient and to plan nursing care.

History

1 *Activity and life-style*. Data are collected on: the type and extent of daily activities; how the patient feels following activity; how leisure time is used; the usual pattern and amount of sleep received; and the patient's perceptions of activities he is able to perform and not perform.
2 *Nutritional history* includes identification of daily food intake, eating habits, and factors affecting eating. Daily food intake is analysed for adequacy of essential nutrients, vitamins, fluid volume and kilocalories. How the individual responds to food is elicited as well as symptoms that occur following ingestion of food. The presence of nausea, vomiting, anorexia, excessive thirst and changes in body weight are determined. Use of alcohol and drugs is carefully recorded.
3 *Elimination*. The patient's usual bowel habits are determined and questions related to the nature, formation, colour and odour of stools are asked.

[2] Harper, Rodwell & Mayes (1979), p. 529.
[3] Vander, Sherman & Luciano (1985), p. 519.
[4] Vander, Sherman & Luciano (1985), p. 520.

The presence of steatorrhoea, melaena and clay-coloured stools is noted.

The volume and colour of urine and frequency of voiding are determined as well as the presence of nocturia.

4 *Changes in blood clotting* may be identified by questioning the patient about the presence of blood in urine or stools, petechiae in the skin, bruises, or cuts that bleed for an unusual length of time.

5 *Environmental and occupational history* includes the identification of factors in the patient's work and home environment that might be toxic to the individual.

6 *Pain and discomfort* are identified by questioning the patient about the location and duration of abdominal or epigastric pain or discomfort, pain referred to the right shoulder and factors which precipitate discomfort.

Physical examination

1 *General appearance.* Changes in posture or weight distribution as seen with abdominal ascites are observed, as well as the general colour of the skin and the sclera of the eyes.

2 *Height and weight* are measured and recorded. Changes in body weight are noted.

3 *Skin-fold thickness and body circumferences* may be measured to determine the amount of subcutaneous body fat (see p. 413 & 619).

4 *Temperature, pulse, respirations and blood pressure* are recorded. Body temperature reflects both liver function and cellular metabolism.

5 *The skin* is inspected for signs of petechiae or bruises, open lesions that have not healed, and jaundice as evidenced by a yellowish colour to the skin and sclera and itching of the skin. Skin turgor is assessed by lifting a fold of skin and observing for mobility of the tissue and the rate at which it returns to its previous position. Peripheral oedema is determined by pressing firmly for about 5 seconds with the thumb over a bony prominence such as the dorsum of the foot; on release of the pressure, the skin is observed and palpated for pitting or indentations and the rate at which it returns to normal. Observations are made for a decrease in axillary and body hair in both males and females.

6 *Examination of the liver.* The liver is situated in the upper right abdomen below the diaphragm. The size and position of the liver can be determined by percussion. Percussion begins in the right midclavicular line below the umbilicus and moves upward. The lower border of the liver is identified when the resonant abdominal sound changes to dullness over the solid liver tissue. The upper border of the liver is identified in a similar manner by starting at the midclavicular line over a resonant area of lung tissue and moving downward until dull sounds are heard at the edge of the liver. The liver borders are marked and measured. The liver size varies with the individual's body size. In an adult male the average size is about 11 cm at the midclavicular line and about 7 cm at the midsternal line.

Palpation of the liver requires a deep, bimanual technique. The examiner stands on the patient's right and places the left hand behind the lower left ribs and pushes upward with the hand to move the liver forward. The right hand is placed flat against the patient's abdomen parallel to the right costal margin and below the liver border. The patient is instructed to take a deep breath while the examiner presses the right hand gently in and up as the liver descends. The liver border normally feels smooth and regular in contour. Tenderness is not normally present.

7 *Abdominal ascites* is assessed by palpation with the patient in a supine position. The examiner places the palmar surface of one hand against one side of the abdominal wall and taps the opposite wall with the other hand. Fluid waves can be felt and may be observed moving across the abdomen if ascites is present. An assistant places the edge of one hand along the midline of the abdomen to decrease transmission of the waves to abdominal tissue. Fluid in the abdomen will also produce dullness on percussion. The area of dullness will shift downward when the patient is positioned on his side.

Inspection of the abdomen containing ascites will show distension, protrusion of the umbilicus and asymmetry when the patient shifts position.

8 *The pancreas and gallbladder* are not normally felt on palpation of the abdomen. The gallbladder may be detected if it is enlarged and tender.

Diagnostic tests

LABORATORY TESTS FOR LIVER, BILIARY AND PANCREATIC FUNCTION (SEE TABLE 18.1)

Blood tests

Plasma protein electrophoresis (serum albumin and globulin concentrations). Serum albumin is produced by the liver and, normally, is of greater concentration than globulin, most of which is produced by the lymphoid tissues. In disease of the liver cells, the amount of albumin decreases, and the ratio of albumin to globulin is reversed.

Normal: Total serum proteins, 60–80 g/l; albumin, 40–50 g/l; and globulin, 20–30 g/l.

Serum bilirubin. This test gives an estimation of the concentration of bilirubin in the blood and indicates whether it is conjugated or unconjugated. Normally, the liver cells extract the pigment from the blood and convert it to a water-soluble compound (bilirubin diglucuronide) before excreting it in bile. Unconju-

Table 18.1 Tests used to assess liver, biliary and exocrine pancreatic function.

Diagnostic test	Normal values	Description/discussion
Blood tests		
Plasma protein electrophoresis (serum albumin, and globulin concentrations)	Total serum proteins: 60–80 g/l Albumin: 40–50 g/l Globulin: 20–30 g/l A/G Ratio 3:1	Serum albumin produced in the liver is normally found in greater concentration than globulin which is produced by the lymphoid tissues With liver disease, serum albumin levels decrease and globulin levels increase.
Serum bilirubin: conjugated (direct), unconjugated (indirect), and total	Direct bilirubin: 2.0–8.0 μmol/l Indirect bilirubin: 0–12 μmol/l Total bilirubin: 3.5–20.5 μmol/l	Bilirubin is normally extracted from the blood and converted to a water-soluble compound in the liver before being excreted in bile In obstructive jaundice, the conjugated (direct) bilirubin level is increased In haemolytic jaundice, unconjugated or indirect bilirubin is increased
Serum alkaline phosphatase	35–105 iu/l at 37 °C or 5.0–13.0 King-Armstrong units	Alkaline phosphatase is an enzyme excreted in the bile by hepatic cells. Serum concentrations increase with liver disease or obstruction of the bile ducts
Prothrombin time (PT)	11–15 s	Prothrombin time is prolonged in liver disease as the liver cells cannot synthesize prothrombin
Liver enzyme tests Serum alanine aminotransferase (ALT)	ALT (SGPT): 1–12 iu/l (or 4–24 iu/l at 30 °C)	These enzymes are released when cells are damaged. Elevated levels provide an estimate of liver damage
Serum aspartate aminotransferase (AST)	AST (SGOT): 0–40 iu/l	
Gamma glutamyl transferase (GGT)	GGT: female, 8–55 iu/l male, 10–65 iu/l	
Pancreatic enzyme tests Serum amylase	0–130 u/l (or 50–150 Somogyi units/dl)	Elevated serum amylase and lipase levels occur when there is an obstruction of the pancreatic ducts and necrosis of cells
Serum lipase	0–160 u/l	
Serum calcium	2.2–2.6 mmol/l	Serum calcium increases with pancreatitis
Bromsulphalein (BSP) test	5% or less of the injected dye remains in the blood 45 minutes later	Used to detect liver cell damage and impaired function. Bromsulphalein is a dye normally excreted by the liver cells in the bile. Retention of the dye increases with liver cell damage or decreased hepatic blood flow
Blood lipids Serum cholesterol	3.9–7.2 mmol/l (or 150–250 mg/dl)	The cholesterol level in the blood falls in liver disease when cell function is impaired and rises in obstructive jaundice
Cholesterol esters	50–70% of total cholesterol	
Blood ammonia	47–65 μmol/l	Blood ammonia concentrations increase in severe liver impairment and may lead to hepatic coma
Hepatitis tests Hepatitis A antigen Anti-hepatitis A virus (anti-HAV) antibodies Hepatitis B surface antigen (HB$_s$ Ag) Hepatitis B core antigen (HB$_c$ Ag) Hepatitis 'e' antigen (HB$_e$ Ag) Anti-HB$_s$ Ag, anti-HB$_c$ Ag, and anti-HB$_e$ Ag antibodies	negative negative negative negative negative negative	These tests are used to identify the known antigens and antibodies associated with hepatitis virus A, hepatitis virus B, and non-A, non-B hepatitis viruses
Blood glucose	Fasting 3.9–6.1 mmol/l (or 70–110 mg/dl)	An elevated blood glucose may result from a decrease in insulin secretion if the cells of the islets of Langerhans are damaged

Table 18.1—*continued*

Diagnostic test	Normal values	Description/discussion
Leucocyte count	$4.0–11.0 \times 10^9$ per litre or 5000–10000 per mm^3	Elevated white blood counts occur with pancreatitis
Urine tests		
Urinary bilirubin	0	This bile pigment, normally absent in the urine, may be present in obstructive jaundice and hepatocellular jaundice
Urinary urobilinogen	0–6.8 µmol/dl (0–4.0 mg) in 24 hours or less than 1.0 Ehrlich unit per dl	In obstructive jaundice, when bile does not reach the intestine, conjugated bilirubin is not changed into urobilinogen and so urinary levels are decreased, as it is when oral antibiotics are administered When liver cells are damaged urinary urobilinogen concentrations increase
Urinary amylase excretion	260–950 King-Armstrong units/24 hours or up to 5000 Somogyi units in 24 hours	Elevations occur in pancreatitis with increases in the excretion of the enzyme amylase
Glycosuria	0	Glucose may be present in the urine with pancreatic dysfunction and decreased insulin production producing hyperglycaemia and glycosuria
Stool tests		
Faecal fat test	3–5 g in 24 hours	Elevated levels occur with obstruction of bile ducts

gated bilirubin is usually reported as 'indirect bilirubin' and the conjugated form as 'direct bilirubin'. In obstructive jaundice, the conjugate (direct) bilirubin level is increased. In haemolytic jaundice, unconjugated (indirect) bilirubin is the predominant pigment in the blood.

Normal: Conjugated (direct) bilirubin, 2–8 µmol/l; unconjugated (indirect) bilirubin, 0–12 µmol/l; and total serum bilirubin, 3.5–20.5 µmol/l.

Serum alkaline phosphatase. Normally this enzyme is excreted in the bile by the hepatic cells. The blood concentration may be increased when there is liver disease or obstruction in the bile ducts.

Normal: 5.0–13.0 King–Armstrong units or 35–105 iu/l at 37°C.

Serum enzymes (liver and pancreatic).
1 Liver enzyme tests. The liver cells contain the enzymes serum alanine aminotransferase (ALT), formerly referred to as serum glutamic-pyruvic transaminase (SGPT), and serum aspartate amino-transferase (AST), previously called serum glutamic oxaloacetic transaminase (SGOT). Since they are released into the blood when the cells are damaged, their concentration may be used to estimate liver damage.

Gamma-glutamyl transferase (GGT) is an enzyme found in greatest concentration in the liver and kidneys; it is released in response to alcohol.[5]

Normal: ALT (SGPT), 1–12 iu/l or 4–24 u/l at 30°C; AST (SGOT) 0–40 iu/l; and GGT, female 8–55 iu/l and male 10–65 iu/l.
2 Concentration of pancreatic enzymes.

Some of the enzymes secreted by the pancreas are normally absorbed into the blood and eventually are excreted in the urine. An elevation of the serum amylase and lipase levels occurs when there is an obstruction of pancreatic ducts and necrosis of cells.

Normal: serum amylase 0–130 µ/l (or 50–150 Somogyi units per dl); and serum lipase, 0–160 µ/l.

Serum calcium level. Pancreatitis causes a decrease in the blood calcium level. (Normal: 2.2–2.6 mmol/l.)

Prothrombin time. The liver is responsible for the synthesis of several clotting factors. The prothrombin time or activity reflects the effects of liver dysfunction on blood coagulation.

Normal: 11–15 seconds activity.

Bromsulphalein (BSP) test. Bromsulphalein is a dye normally excreted by the liver cells in the bile. The test is used to detect liver cell damage and impaired function. It is not used if obstruction in the bile ducts is suspected, because the dye would be retained in the body. Five milligrams of bromsulphalein for each kilogram of the patient's body weight is given intravenously, and a venous blood specimen is collected from another vein in 45 minutes. Normally, only 5% or less of the dye given remains in the blood.

[5] Tressler (1982), pp. 402 and 403.

Blood lipids. The concentration of cholesterol and cholesterol esters in the blood falls in liver disease, when cell function is impaired, and rises in obstructive jaundice.

Normal: serum cholesterol 3.9–7.2 mmol/l; cholesterol esters, 50–70% of total cholesterol.

Blood ammonia. In severe impairment of liver function, the ammonia concentration in the blood is elevated and may lead to hepatic coma.

Normal: 47–65 µmol/l (or 30–70 µg%).

Hepatitis tests. Viral hepatitis is caused by hepatitis virus A, hepatitis virus B, and non-A, non-B hepatitis viruses. Tests are available to identify the known antigens and antibodies associated with these viruses, which include: hepatitis A antigen; anti-hepatitis A virus (anti-HAV), a group of antibodies produced in response to the hepatitis A virus; hepatitis B surface antigen (HB_sAg); hepatitis B core antigen (HB_cAg); and hepatitis 'e' antigen (HB_eAg). Antibodies to these three latter antigens may also be detected at various stages of the illness (anti-HB_sAg, anti-HB_cAg, and anti-HB_eAg).

Normal: negative.

Blood glucose concentration. Damage to the islets of Langerhans may cause a reduction in insulin secretion and hyperglycaemia.

Normal: fasting, 3.9–6.1 mmol/l.

Leucocyte count. The white blood count is elevated in pancreatitis with a marked increase in the polymorphonuclear leucocytes in necrotizing and haemorrhagic pancreatitis.

Normal: $4.0–11.0 \times 10^9$ per litre.

Urine tests

Urinary bilirubin. A urinalysis may be requested for bilirubin. Normally, this bile pigment is not present in urine. Conjugated, or direct bilirubin, is water soluble and is present in the urine in obstructive jaundice and hepatocellular jaundice but is absent in haemolytic jaundice.

Urinary urobilinogen. Conjugated bilirubin is changed to urobilinogen by bacterial action when the bile reaches the small intestine. Most of the urobilinogen is then excreted in the faeces, and the remainder is absorbed. A small amount of the absorbed urobilinogen is excreted in the urine, but the larger portion is claimed by the liver to be excreted in the bile. If the liver cells are damaged they may not perform this latter function, and the amount of urobilinogen excreted by the kidneys is increased. The amount of the pigment in the urine may be decreased below the normal amount of obstructive jaundice when bile is not reaching the intestine or if the bacterial content of

the intestine is reduced, as it is in oral administration of antibiotics.

Normal: 0–6.8 µmol/dl (0–4.0 mg) in the urine per 24 hours (or less than 1.0 Ehrlich units/dl).

Urinary amylase excretion. Urinalysis may indicate an increase in the excretion of the enzyme amylase in pancreatitis.

Normal: 260–950 units in a 24-hour specimen (or up to 5000 Somogyi units in 24 hours).

Glycosuria. Dysfunction of the pancreas may incur a deficiency of insulin, resulting in hyperglycaemia and the excretion of excess glucose in the urine.

Stool test

Faecal fat test. Analysis of stool specimens made over a specified number of hours may be done to determine the quantitative fat content. Failure of the pancreatic lipase to reach the intestine results in undigested and unabsorbed fat.

Normal: 3–5 g in 24 hours.

X-RAY

A radiological examination is made of the abdomen. It may reveal gallstones, accumulation of gas in the duodenum or calcification in the pancreas.

PANCREAS SCAN

A scan may be done if tumours of the pancreas are suspected or to assess the extent of fibrosed, non-functional tissue. The patient receives selenium-75 (Se^{75}) tagged with methionine by intravenous injection. The radioactive substance is taken up by the pancreas; methionine is used in the formation of enzymes. The pancreas is then scanned with a scintillation counter; a graph is produced which indicates the *amount* of the radioactive tracer taken up by the different areas of the pancreas. Abnormal areas of tissue do not take up the radioactive selenium and so leave voids in the scan.

ULTRASOUND EXAMINATION OF THE PANCREAS

Ultrasonography of the pancreas provides a picture inside by the reflection of ultrasonic waves directed into the pancreas and is used in the diagnoses and localizing of tumours, abscesses and pancreatitis.

COMPUTERIZED AXIAL TOMOGRAPHY (CAT) SCAN

A CAT scan of the abdomen provides information about tumours or abscesses of the liver or pancreas, dilation of the gallbladder, bile ducts or portal vein.

ENDOSCOPIC RETROGRADE CHOLANGIOPANCREATOGRAPHY (ERCP)

A fibreoptic endoscope can be used to cannulate the

papilla of Vater in the duodenum. This gives access to both the bile and pancreatic ducts. Pancreatography is done to detect the presence of pancreatic disease, to delineate the pancreatic duct when a precise knowledge of its anatomy is needed for surgery, and to obtain histological or cytological evidence of disease. Retrograde cholangiography is performed to determine the cause of biliary problems, to diagnose cholestatic jaundice, and to remove gallstones which are obstructing the common bile duct. X-ray films are taken during the procedure.

When gallstones are removed by an ERCP and sphincterotomy, the patient will need his blood coagulation levels measured, and his blood typed and crossmatched. An antibiotic and intravenous fluid are administered prior to the procedure. The major problems that may occur are haemorrhage and infection, and the patient is assessed for any signs of these following investigation.

CHOLECYSTOGRAPHY

Radiography is also used in the diagnosis of gallbladder disease and the procedure may be referred to as cholecystography. A radiopaque organic iodine compound (e.g. Telepaque or Cholografin) that is eliminated in the bile is given orally or intravenously. The patient receives a fat-free evening meal which is followed by the administration of the 'dye' the night before the x-ray examination. Then, the patient must not take anything by mouth until after the first x-ray. The iodine compound is absorbed, excreted by the liver cells in the bile and, normally is concentrated in the gallbladder, since there was no fat in the meal to stimulate the emptying of the gallbladder. An x-ray film is taken in the morning (approximately 12 hours after the dye was given) to determine if the gallbladder has filled. Calculi are observed if present.

Following this first film, the patient is given a meal containing fat. A rich egg-nog or thickly buttered toast and an egg may be used. After one hour, a final x-ray is taken. Normally, after a fatty meal, the gallbladder contracts and empties bile into the small intestine via the common bile duct.

To summarize, cholecystography provides information as to whether the gallbladder fills and empties and whether it contains gallstones.

PERCUTANEOUS LIVER BIOPSY

A small specimen of liver tissue may be examined microscopically to assist in the diagnosis of liver disease. The specimen is obtained by aspiration with a special liver biopsy needle. Using a lateral approach, the needle is passed through the right eighth, ninth or tenth intercostal space, or may be introduced below the costal margin if the liver is enlarged.

Previous to the procedure, the patient's blood coagulation is evaluated by performing a partial thromboplastin time and platelet count. His blood is typed and crossmatched so that blood is available for transfusion if required. An explanation is made to the patient of the purpose of the biopsy and what will be expected of him during and after the procedure. He is required to sign a consent form. His pulse, respirations and blood pressure are noted by the nurse for comparison following the biopsy.

The patient is placed in the supine position close to the right side of the bed. The area is cleansed, and an antiseptic and sterile drape are applied. A local anaesthetic is then injected at the puncture site. The patient is instructed to take two or three deep breaths, and then to stop breathing following exhalation. The doctor quickly introduces the biopsy needle, aspirates and withdraws, taking only a few seconds.

Following the biopsy, absolute bed rest is necessary for 24 hours. The patient is required to lie on his right side with a small pillow under the costal margin. This position places pressure against the biopsy site, preventing the escape of blood and bile. Close observation is made of the patient for haemorrhage for 24 hours. The pulse, respirations, blood pressure, colour and general condition are noted and recorded every 15 minutes for 2 hours, then every 30 minutes for 2 hours. The interval is then gradually increased if there are no significant changes. Abdominal pain, tenderness and any rigidity are reported, since they may indicate irritation and inflammation of the peritoneum due to the leakage of bile from the liver. Severe pain and breathlessness are reported promptly as they may indicate that the lung or colon is perforated.

RADIOISOTOPE LIVER SCAN

A radioactive isotope known to be taken up normally by the liver may be given intravenously, and an estimation is then made of its uptake by means of a special external radioactivity detector. Rose bengal tagged with radioactive iodine (I^{131}), gold (Au^{198}) or technetium (^{99m}Tc) sulphur colloid may be used. The photoscan made by the detector indicates non-functioning and functioning areas of the liver tissue. Areas or lesions which do not take up the radioactive material appear as blanks or as much lighter areas in the recording of the scan.

OTHER STUDIES

A *barium swallow* under fluoroscopic examination (see p. 495) or an *oesophagoscopy* (see p. 496) may be done. The latter is used to detect venous dilation and varicosities in the oesophagus resulting from portal hypertension. A *splenoportogram* may be undertaken in which an opaque dye is injected into the spleen and an x-ray taken of the upper abdomen and lower chest. The dilated portal vein and its branches show up, and gastroesophageal varices may be recognized.

Manifestations of disorders of the liver and biliary tract

Liver function is essential to life and, fortunately, this large organ has exceptional functional ability and regenerative capacity. If liver disease is limited and tissue damage is localized to one area of the organ, the body is not likely to suffer serious impairment of function. If there is diffuse disease and parenchymal damage, dysfunction is more marked. Liver disease may be acute or chronic, and disturbed function may be reversible or irreversible, depending on the amount of tissue involved and the nature of the cause.

Disorders of the gallbladder and bile ducts interfere with the flow of bile into the duodenum. They may be acute or chronic and the intensity of the signs and symptoms parallels the severity of the condition. Like the liver, the pancreas has a large reserve capacity; a portion of the gland may be destroyed or become non-functional and the remainder will compensate sufficiently to maintain normal physiology.

Jaundice (icterus)
This is an indication of an excess of bilirubin in the blood, resulting in a yellowish staining of the tissues that may be seen in the sclerae, mucous membranes and skin. The cause may be intrahepatic or extrahepatic disease, and according to the cause, the jaundice may be classified as hepatocellular, obstructive or haemolytic.

The *hepatocellular type of jaundice* is associated with intrinsic liver disease and is due to failure of the hepatic cells to take up the bilirubin resulting from the breakdown of red blood cells and excrete it as bile. Jaundice may not be present in chronic liver disease (e.g. cirrhosis), especially in the early stages, since regeneration of the hepatic cells may parallel the damage.

Obstructive jaundice is caused by an interference with the flow of bile in the extrahepatic ducts. It is most often due to the impaction of gallstones in the common bile duct, but may occur as the result of a stricture in the duct or neoplastic disease in neighbouring structures (e.g. pancreas) compressing the duct. *Haemolytic jaundice* occurs when there is an inordinate destruction of red blood cells, resulting in excessive bilirubin formation.

The jaundiced patient's urine is likely to be dark because of the bilirubin or urobilinogen content. Urobilinogen is not present in obstructive jaundice, since it is formed in the intestine. The stools are pale grey in obstructive and severe hepatocellular jaundice.

Pruritus
The itching of the skin experienced by many patients

with jaundice is attributed to irritation of the cutaneous sensory nerves by the retained bile salts.

General constitutional symptoms
The patient complains of a poor appetite, vague digestive discomfort and flatulence, and loses weight. Lassitude, weakness and muscle wasting develop as a result of the impaired storage of carbohydrates and protein metabolism. A low-grade fever may be present.

Pain
Dull, aching pain in the right upper abdominal quadrant is a common complaint, especially in acute liver disease. Tenderness is manifested on palpation.

The pain associated with gallbladder or biliary duct disease may be felt in the right upper abdomen or midepigastric region, or is referred to the right scapular area. It may be a persistent, dull ache or very severe and disabling. The onset may follow a meal containing fatty foods. When it is very severe, causing the patient to writhe about, the pain is described as biliary colic.

Bleeding tendency
Inadequate production of prothrombin and other blood-clotting factors results in failure of the normal clotting process. Spontaneous bleeding may occur, manifested by purpura, epistaxis, bleeding of the oral mucous membrane, and/or melaena.

Ascites and oedema
An accumulation of fluid in the peritoneal cavity develops with progressive liver disease, such as cirrhosis. The hepatic tissue damage, obliteration of blood vessels, and compression by the fibrous tissue (scar) replacement produce a resistance to the inflow and outflow of blood from the portal vein. The resulting increase in the blood pressure within the portal vein and its contributaries promotes the escape of fluid into the peritoneal cavity.

Some patients also develop a generalized oedema because of the failure of the liver to produce sufficient serum albumin to maintain the normal colloidal osmotic pressure of the blood (see Chapter 6). Some blood protein is also lost in the transudate in ascites. Reduced liver activity results in increased concentrations of antidiuretic hormone and aldosterone (an adrenocorticoid secretion), further contributing to oedema. These secretions, normally destroyed by the liver, promote reabsorption of water and sodium by the kidneys.

Dilated veins and varicosities
The portal hypertension associated with liver disease is reflected in changes within the veins that drain into the portal vein. They become dilated and varicosities develop. The oesophageal and gastric veins are commonly affected and, because they are close to the

surface, one may rupture, resulting in massive haemorrhage manifested by haematemesis or melaena or both. Haemorrhoids develop because of the pressure and resistance to blood flow within the rectal veins.

Splenomegaly

The spleen enlarges because of the hyperplasia of the reticuloendothelial tissue and congestion, causing considerable discomfort for the patient.

Skin changes

In progressive chronic liver failure, several changes are likely to appear in the skin. Arterial spiders (spider angiomas or naevi) may develop in which a superficial arteriole gives rise to a series of fine, radiating branches readily visible on the surface. These lesions are seen predominantly on the face, neck, arms and chest, and are attributed to high oestrogen levels in the blood. Gynaecomastia and atrophy of the testicles may occur in males for the same reason. Normally, oestrogen is destroyed in the liver.

The palms of the hands are frequently mottled, bright red and warm because of capillary dilatation (palmar erythema). There is a loss of axillary and pubic hair in both sexes, and facial hair grows more slowly than usual in the male.

Neurological disturbances

Severe hepatic insufficiency leads to various mental changes. The patient may manifest irritability and behaviour not previously characteristic. He may become inactive, apathetic and forgetful. These symptoms may progress to confusion, lack of cooperation, stupor and eventually coma.

Twitching and a peculiar coarse tremor, referred to as flapping tremor, develop. Flapping tremor consists of a series of rapid, irregular alternating flexion and extension movements at the wrist and finger joints. The tremor may be referred to as *asterixis*. It occurs when the arms and hands are extended.

Ammonia toxicity is considered to be an important factor in producing the mental changes, coma and other abnormal central nervous system responses. The liver is unable to convert the ammonia that results from the breakdown of amino acids to urea.

Fetor hepaticus

In advanced liver disease, the breath has a faecal odour and the patient complains of a bad taste in the mouth. It is attributed to disturbed amino acid metabolism and abnormal bacterial action in the intestine.

Digestive disturbances

The patient with impaired bile transport may experience flatulence and an uncomfortable full feeling or nausea, especially after the ingestion of fatty or fried foods. Vomiting is usual if the patient has biliary colic or develops obstructive jaundice.

Fever

Chills and an elevation of temperature frequently accompany infection and inflammation within the gallbladder or bile ducts.

POTENTIAL PATIENT PROBLEMS

(See Table 18.2)
The potential problems that are related to the patient with manifestations of disorders of the liver and biliary tract include the following:
1 Alteration in nutrition: less than body requirements, related to impaired production and release of bile, impaired reabsorption of bile salts, altered metabolism of fats in the liver and altered body needs due to illness.
2 Potential for injury (bleeding) related to altered blood coagulation.
3 Potential for impairment of skin integrity related to pruritus, oedema, and altered metabolic state.
4 Alteration in comfort related to pruritus, ascites, generalized oedema, hepatomegaly, fever, chills and abdominal pain.
5 Alteration in thought processes related to neurological manifestations of hepatic insufficiency and ammonia toxicity.

1. INABILITY TO DIGEST AN ADEQUATE DIET

The *goals* are to:
1 Maintain adequate nutrition
2 Develop a plan to meet nutritional needs

Table 18.2 Identification of problems relevant to the patient with disorders of the liver and biliary tract.

Problem	Causative factors
1 Alteration in nutrition: less than body requirements	Impaired production and release of bile and reabsorption of bile salts Altered metabolism of carbohydrates, proteins and fats in the liver Altered body needs related to illness
2 Potential for injury (bleeding)	Altered blood coagulation
3 Potential for impairment of skin integrity	Pruritis and oedema of skin Altered metabolic state
4 Alteration in comfort	Pruritis Abdominal ascites Generalized oedema Hepatomegaly Fever, chills Abdominal pain
5 Alteration in thought processes	Hepatic insufficiency Ammonia toxicity

Nursing intervention

Patients with liver or biliary disorders require a diet high in kilocalories, protein and carbohydrate. The diet should contain 2500–3000 kcal per day; 110–150 g of protein; 300–500 g of carbohydrate; and low amounts of fat. Supplements of fat-soluble vitamins are required. Parenteral vitamin B_{12} is given once a month and vitamin K is required also. In certain liver diseases (for example cirrhosis) protein restriction may be required (see page 600).

The nurse and dietitian assist the patient and family to develop a plan to meet the patient's daily nutritional requirements. Small meals followed by periods of rest are recommended. Alternative routes of administering nutrients, such as tube feedings, may be necessary for short periods. Total parenteral nutrition may be considered for the acutely ill patient when oral intake is restricted. The diet is adjusted to the needs of the individual patient.

The patient and his family are taught which foods and fluids to avoid or restrict in the diet. Alcohol is contraindicated for all patients with liver impairment; sodium may be restricted and fats are limited to what the patient can tolerate or requires to make a meal palatable.

Expected outcomes

The patient and his family are aware of:
1 Daily nutritional and fluid requirements.
2 Foods to be avoided or limited.
3 Effective ways of meeting daily nutritional requirements.

2. INJURY (BLEEDING)

The *goals* are to prevent bleeding and/or to promptly identify episodes of bleeding.

Nursing intervention

Absorption of vitamin K, a fat-soluble vitamin, is impaired when bile salts in the intestine are decreased. Vitamin K, which is required by the liver to produce clotting factors, may be provided parenterally. When coagulation impairment is due to inability of the liver to synthesize clotting factors, bleeding may be controlled by the administration of fresh blood or platelets.

The patient should be assessed for signs of bleeding which include sudden bleeding episodes, petechiae, haematuria, melaena and haematemesis. Measures to control sudden oesophageal haemorrhage are discussed on page 602. Specific nursing interventions for the patient with an increased tendency to bleed are discussed in Chapter 13.

Expected outcome

Episodes of bleeding are absent and/or identified promptly.

3. SKIN DAMAGE

The *goal* is to maintain skin integrity.

Nursing intervention

The skin is cleansed frequently. The use of soap should be avoided if the patient is jaundiced and the bath water should be warm but not hot. The hot water and alkali in the soap tend to increase the pruritus frequently associated with jaundice. Emollient bath additive may provide relief from the itching. Calamine lotion may be applied following the bath. The fingernails are kept short and clean to prevent injury and infection of the skin in case of scratching. The nurse should provide emotional support to decrease the patient's level of anxiety; diversional activities are encouraged to divert the patient's attention from the itching.

Expected outcomes

The patient's skin is clean, intact and less irritating.

4. ALTERATION IN COMFORT

The *goals* are to:
1 Alleviate the discomfort
2 Control the pain

Nursing intervention

A mild analgesic such as paracetamol is usually sufficient to relieve pain and discomfort. The patient with severe intermittent or prolonged pain may require a narcotic analgesic for pain control (as in biliary colic for example). Nursing intervention related to assessment of the patient with pain and measures to control pain are discussed in Chapter 8.

Discomfort due to enlargement of the liver, abdominal ascites and generalized oedema is relieved by treatment of symptoms. Dietary restriction of sodium and diuretic therapy are generally recommended to alleviate fluid retention. If abdominal ascites reaches a volume that is causing respiratory distress, compression of the abdominal viscera and blood vessels, and considerable pain and discomfort, an abdominal paracentesis may be performed.

If an abdominal paracentesis is to be performed the nurse explains the aspiration procedure to the patient, and makes sure his bladder is empty. The head of the bed is elevated and the patient is supported with pillows. The doctor may wish to have the patient sitting on the side of the bed with a support for his back and feet. A sphygmomanometer is placed in readiness on one arm so that the blood pressure may be monitored during and after the paracentesis. The necessary sterile equipment and fluid receptacle are brought to the bedside. Following the application of an antiseptic and sterile towels, the doctor injects the site with a local anaesthetic before introducing the trocar and cannula. A tube is attached to the cannula to drain the fluid into the receptacle.

During the procedure, the nurse checks the patient's pulse, colour and blood pressure and provides necessary support. The doctor is alerted promptly if the pulse becomes rapid and weak, pallor is noted, or there is a fall in blood pressure. No more than 1 or 2 litres is withdrawn at one time. Removal of the fluid results in the loss of considerable plasma protein, especially serum albumin. Also, the sudden reduction of intraabdominal pressure results in a dilatation of the abdominal blood vessels and a pooling of a large volume of blood that may lead to circulatory collapse and shock.

A sterile dressing is applied to the site of the paracentesis when the cannula is withdrawn, and an abdominal binder is applied snugly. The patient is returned to the dorsal recumbent position, and the head of the bed is lowered. The amount and character of the fluid are recorded and a specimen of the fluid is labelled and sent to the laboratory for examination. The abdominal site is kept clean and dry to prevent infection and discomfort. The pulse, colour and blood pressure are checked at frequent intervals for several hours. A plasma or whole blood infusion may follow the paracentesis to replace the lost protein. Increased diuresis may be observed with the decreased pressure on the renal blood vessels.

Expected outcomes
1 The patient feels less discomfort.
2 Episodes of severe pain are absent.
3 Abdominal girth is decreased.

5. ALTERATION IN THOUGHT PROCESSES

The *goal* is to maintain cognitive function and level of awareness.

Nursing intervention
If the patient demonstrates signs of disorientation to time, place and person, irritability, altered behaviour patterns, apathy, twitching, tremors or other signs of neurological involvement, he is assessed regularly using the Glasgow coma scale (see p. 178). Nursing measures to maintain body functioning and prevent injury in the patient with altered consciousness are discussed in Chapter 10.

Expected outcome
The patient's level of consciousness, as measured by the Glasgow coma scale, increases.

Liver Disorders

Viral hepatitis

The most common inflammatory disease of the liver is due to viruses. Three types of hepatitis are currently recognized and they are referred to as hepatitis A (HA), hepatitis B (HB), and non-A, non-B hepatitis. Hepatitis due to the A virus (HAV) may be referred to as infectious (or epidemic) hepatitis; that caused by hepatitis B virus (HBV) was formerly referred to as homologous serum hepatitis. One or more additional hepatotropic viruses are known to exist and are referred to as non-A, non-B viruses (NANBV). The principle differences in the three types of hepatitis are in their mode of infection, incubation period, severity and chronicity.

Hepatitis A
This type of hepatitis accounts for the greater number of cases. The disease may be epidemic and has a higher incidence in children and young adults. It has an incubation period of 10–50 days and is included in the list of *reportable* diseases. It is an acute, self-limited disease which does not usually lead to chronic hepatitis or a carrier state.

Large amounts of the virus are eliminated in the faeces in the week preceding the onset of jaundice and for up to a week afterwards. Transmission is by the faecal–oral route and is therefore facilitated by poor hygiene. This disease may spread rapidly, especially in overcrowded and poor sanitary conditions.

Hepatitis B
Hepatitis B is caused by the virus B, which consists of an inner DNA core enclosed in a protein coat. Both the inner core and the large surface mass contain distinctive antigens. The principal mode of transmission is by the injection of infected blood and blood products. Syringes, needles and tubing used in parenteral administrations or for the withdrawal of blood or body fluids may provide the means of transmission if they are reused and not disinfected adequately. Because of this, hepatitis B is a common problem among drug addicts. The disease may also be spread by the faecal–oral route, although this is rare. The incubation period ranges from 6 weeks–6 months. It is more common in adults than children, while hepatitis A tends to have a higher frequency in children and young adults. Hepatitis B has an insidious onset; it may persist or become chronic, or produce a carrier state in which the individual may be asymptomatic but harbour the virus.

Non-A, non-B hepatitis
This term is applied to viruses causing syndromes similar to hepatitis A and B, but which have not yet been characterized in the laboratory; they can at present be diagnosed only by excluding the presence of HAV and HBV. One form of non-A, non-B hepatitis is spread in water supplies contaminated by sewage; this type resembles hepatitis A; another, more like hepatitis B, is transmitted by blood products such as Factors VIII and IX, thus putting haemophiliacs at special risk.

MANIFESTATIONS

The virus attacks the hepatic cells, and inflammation and necrosis follow. The swelling and congestion interfere with normal bile formation and flow, resulting in intrahepatic obstructive jaundice and elevated blood bilirubin levels. Serum enzyme levels [alanine aminotransferase (ALT) and aspartate amino transferase (AST)] rise sharply because of the necrosis, and the protein electrophoresis and serum albumin–globulin ratio may indicate a reduced formation of albumin and an increase in the gamma globulin. The latter points to the acute infectious nature of the disorder. Urinalysis reveals an excess of urobilinogen, especially in the initial stage. The blood is examined for the presence of hepatitis antigens and antibodies that have been identified [hepatitis A antigen and hepatitis A virus antibodies (anti-HAV) and hepatitis virus, B core antigen (HB$_c$Ag), hepatitis B surface antigen (HB$_s$Ag), and an 'e' antigen (HB$_e$Ag)], Antibodies to the core antigen can be detected when symptoms develop. Antibodies to the 'e' and surface antigens may develop within a month of onset of symptoms. Fortunately, in most cases complete regeneration of the liver cells occurs on recovery with a minimum of fibrous tissue formation and scarring. Very few patients experience residual impairment of liver function.

The signs and symptoms may vary in intensity from one individual to another. The onset is usually manifested by vague symptoms such as fatigue, loss of appetite, nausea, vomiting, headache, fleeting abdominal and joint pains, and fever. After several days, abdominal tenderness and pain in the right upper quadrant are more predominant, the urine becomes dark, either constipation or diarrhoea may be troublesome, the stools may be abnormally light in colour and jaundice becomes evident. Hepatitis B is usually more prolonged and debilitating. Table 18.3 lists the clinical manifestations of viral hepatitis.

DIAGNOSTIC PROCEDURES

Urine specimens are submitted for assessment of urobilinogen content. In viral hepatitis there is an excess of this substance in the initial stage of the disease. If the inflammatory process is widespread, intrahepatic biliary obstruction may result in the appearance of bilirubin in the urine and the disappearance of the urobilinogen.

The serum bilirubin level is elevated, serum flocculation tests are positive and the serum enzymes ALT (SGPT) and AST (SGOT) are elevated. Blood specimens are examined for the hepatitis A and B antigens and their associated antibodies. Specimens of faeces are examined for the hepatitis A virus.

TREATMENT AND NURSING INTERVENTION IN VIRAL HEPATITIS

Since there is no specific treatment for viral hepatitis,

Table 18.3 Assessment of the patient with viral hepatitis.*

Pathophysiological alterations	Clinical manifestations
1 Liver structure and function Hepatomegaly	The liver is tender and enlarged on palpation Abdominal discomfort
Altered bile production, excretion and reabsorption	Pruritus Jaundice of skin and sclerae Urine, dark orange in colour Stools, clay-coloured Diarrhoea or constipation
Altered metabolism of carbohydrates, proteins and fats	Nausea and vomiting Anorexia Flatulence Malaise, weakness and fatigue Irritability Weight loss Muscle wasting Fever
Altered production and destruction of blood components	Spontaneous bleeding Purpura Melaena Haematuria
2 Extrahepatic	Skin rashes Arthralgia Headache Sore throat, cough, coryza Depression

*Patton (1981), p. 24.

supportive therapy and attention to the patient's discomforts constitute the principal care.

Rest. The patient is kept on bed rest during the active stage of the disease until the extreme fatigue has abated. Prolonged bed rest has no scientific basis and has not been shown to prevent relapse or promote recovery and may be physically debilitating. The patient is encouraged to use the bathroom if his strength permits. Activity is resumed slowly, and the patient is observed for reactions. Liver function is monitored by repeated tests to detect any adverse effects of increased activity. The patient is helped to plan for regular rest periods.

Medications. Many drugs (such as barbiturates, oral contraceptives and morphine) which are normally inactivated by the liver are not prescribed. The patient is advised that he should not take any drug that has not been prescribed by the doctor during this illness.

Nutrition and fluids. In the acute stage, it is difficult for the patient to take sufficient fluids and food because of the nausea, vomiting and aversion to food. An increased fluid intake of at least 3000 ml is necessary because of the fever and to promote urinary elimination of the serum bilirubin. If the patient cannot tolerate fluids orally, glucose 5–10% may be given intravenously to sustain the patient. The patient is observed closely for signs of overhydration manifested by sudden weight gain, oedema and respiratory distress. Fluid intake and output are recorded. Parenteral administration of vitamin K may be recommended if blood coagulation is impaired as a result of impaired absorption of vitamin K when bile salts are decreased.

A high-calorie diet of 3000 kcal is recommended; nutritional deficiency retards the liver's ability to overcome the infection and regenerate functional tissue. As soon as the nausea and vomiting are controlled, the patient is offered small amounts of high-calorie foods frequently. These are gradually increased until the ultimate goal of 3000 kcal is achieved. The diet consists principally of protein and carbohydrate. The fat content may be restricted while there is jaundice but is increased, as tolerated, by the addition of whole milk, eggs and butter, which make the diet more palatable. Fried foods, fat meat and rich foods, such as pastries, usually are avoided for several weeks or months after recovery. The patient is advised not to take alcohol for at least 6 months.

The patient's weight is checked at regular intervals, since there may have been a considerable loss in the early phase of the disease.

Skin care. Frequent bathing and changes of linen during the period of fever are necessary. The use of soap is avoided; emollients may be added to the bathwater to relieve the itching. Calamine lotion may be used and fingernails are cut short and kept clean.

Prevention of the spread of infection. All patients with viral hepatitis are treated as potentially infectious and isolation precautions are observed. The type and extent of isolation precautions are variable but always include enteric and/or parenteral precautions. Patients with hepatitis A rarely need parenteral precautions unless they have a bleeding gastric ulcer or a similar problem. Personnel caring for the patient are informed of the possible sources of the infective organisms (faeces, vomitus, urine and blood) and of the fact that they are usually resistant to heat, antiseptics, and prolonged exposure to cold and freezing. A single room is necessary only if the patient is incontinent of faeces. A gown and gloves should be worn when direct contact with blood or faeces is possible.

The hands are scrubbed under running water with liquid soap after each contact. Bed linen contaminated with faeces or blood is placed in a clean bag at the bedside which is identified as an isolation bag. No special precautions are necessary regarding dishes or glasses. The use of disposable equipment for procedures involving penetration of the skin (e.g. needles and syringes) is recommended, and gloves should be worn by those handling them. Used needles and syringes are placed in a puncture-resistant container and labelled. If non-disposable syringes and needles must be used, they are disinfected after use by high dry heat or by autoclave. Blood, urine, faeces and sputum specimens should be clearly labelled 'Biohazard' to protect laboratory personnel.

If it is necessary to take the temperature by rectum, the nurse wears gloves while handing the thermometer, which is thoroughly disinfected after use.

The patient is advised of the importance of thorough hand-washing after going to the toilet. Gloves are worn when handling the patient's bedpan; excreta should be flushed promptly down the toilet. If the patient is being cared for at home, the patient and family are taught simple isolation techniques and the importance of good hand-washing.

Contacts. Known contacts of infectious hepatitis A are advised to consult a doctor as soon as possible. An intramuscular injection of human immune serum globulin may be given to provide protection. It is effective against the virus A organism. Hepatitis B immune globulin is available for contacts of hepatitis B virus. Its use is usually reserved for individuals exposed to hepatitis B virus through needle pricks or other accidental injection. The gamma globulin may not always provide immunity, but is found to lessen the severity of the disease should the person develop it.

Vaccines for active immunization against hepatitis are being developed and are recommended for high-risk groups, especially health professionals at risk of contamination with patient's blood (e.g. nurses in intravenous therapy or haemodialysis centres).

Follow-up. The patient is encouraged to continue medical supervision; laboratory and physical examinations are done to detect possible progressive or residual impairment of liver function. Supervision is usually continued for 1 year. The intervals between visits to clinic or doctor are gradually increased if the findings are favourable. The patient who has had hepatitis B, or non-A, non-B hepatitis, is advised that he should not serve as a blood donor.

Toxic hepatitis

Rarely, inflammation and degenerative changes in the liver occur as a result of a chemical. Carbon tetrachloride, phosphorus, sulphonamides, arsenical preparations and chloroform are examples of suggested offenders. The patient is treated by prompt withdrawal of the causative chemical, rest and supportive care.

Cirrhosis of the liver

The term cirrhosis denotes chronic diffuse degenerative tissue changes occurring in the liver. There is destruction of parenchymal cells and formation of excessive dense fibrous scar tissue. Blood, lymph and bile channels within the liver become distorted, compressed and effaced, with subsequent intrahepatic congestion, portal hypertension and impaired liver function. (For functions, see p. 585.) The fibrous tissue changes result in the liver becoming firmer. The surface is usually rough because of small projecting nodules of regenerated hepatic cells, and is frequently described as a 'hobnail surface'.

CAUSATIVE FACTORS

The mechanisms responsible for cirrhosis of the liver are not clearly defined.

Alcoholism. Cirrhosis of the liver is a common sequel to chronic alcoholism. Ingestion of moderate to large quantities of ethanol (ethyl alcohol) over several years can produce fatty infiltration of the liver and liver dysfunction. The toxic effects of ethanol on the liver develop more readily in the presence of malnutrition. Persons who become dependent on alcohol are often indifferent to food and consume less. Many persons show a marked improvement in the earlier stages of cirrhosis when alcohol ingestion is discontinued.

It is also thought that liver damage in the alcoholic may be related to an increased choline requirement incurred by the alcohol.

Hepatitis. Severe type B viral hepatitis in which there has been extensive necrosis followed by considerable scarring may lead to cirrhosis.

Chronic cholestasis. Degenerative changes characteristic of cirrhosis may also occur with prolonged cholestasis (obstruction to the flow of bile). The cause is usually partial obstruction by a stone or stricture within the extrahepatic bile ducts, but may be intrahepatic as a result of infection or inflammation and subsequent stricture of the small ducts within the liver.

Hepatic infiltration. Fibrotic changes in the liver may be associated with the infiltration of certain substances. Examples include excessive glycogen which accumulates in the liver in the individual with von Gierke's disease[6]; enlargement and fibrosis

develop. Similarly, Gaucher's disease[7] results from an abnormal reticuloendothelial cell content that incurs liver fibrosis and dysfunction.

CLASSIFICATION

Certain terms may be used to classify cirrhosis according to the cause and changes that occur. Cirrhosis associated with alcohol abuse accounts for 60–70% of the cases. When cirrhotic changes are a result of massive hepatic necrosis and subsequent fibrous scarring, the condition is known as *postnecrotic cirrhosis*. The term *biliary cirrhosis* is used to denote cirrhosis associated with cholestasis. Other forms include pigment cirrhosis (haemochromatosis), cardiac or congestive and rare forms of uncertain aetiology.

Cirrhosis may also be classified as micronodular, macronodular or mixed, according to the size and thickness of the nodules. Since it is generally a progressive disease, the size of the nodules progressively changes.

SIGNS AND SYMPTOMS

The liver has considerable reserve; early cirrhotic changes generally go unrecognized without apparent manifestations. With the characteristic insidious progress, signs and symptoms of impaired liver function appear gradually over a period of years. In the early stages the symptoms are vague digestive disturbances: the patient experiences anorexia, flatulence, nausea and loss of weight. Later, jaundice, dependent oedema, spider angiomas, anaemia and increased abdominal girth develop. Splenomegaly, neurological involvement (hepatic coma) and haemorrhage from oesophageal varices are characteristic of advanced cirrhosis and serious liver dysfunction.

The severity of liver dysfunction is determined by various liver function tests (see earlier) as well as by history, symptoms and physical examination. Palpation of the liver and spleen provides significant information. The liver is enlarged and firm and may have a rough surface; the spleen is enlarged owing to the resistance by the liver to the flow of blood from the portal vein.

TREATMENT AND NURSING INTERVENTION

The care required by the patient with cirrhosis depends upon the extent of the liver damage.

Nutrition. Since the progress of the disease is

---

[6] *Von Gierke's disease* is a congenital disorder characterized by excessive storage of glycogen in the liver which results in hypoglycaemia. The disorder is due to an enzyme deficiency.

[7] *Gaucher's disease* is an inherited disorder characterized by a deficiency of an enzyme that results in abnormal metabolism of glucocerebroside. Normally, this compound is broken down by the enzyme to useable glucose. When it is not, it accumulates in reticuloendothelial cells.

influenced by nutrition, a diet of 2500–3000 kcal, high in carbohydrates and vitamins is recommended. Protein may be high (110–150 g), but can be restricted to 40 g, or eliminated according to the severity of the disease. Sufficient fat to make the diet palatable is added if the patient can tolerate it and is not jaundiced. Three small meals with in-between snacks will probably be more acceptable than three large meals. Sodium intake is restricted because of the tendency to develop oedema and ascites. Low-sodium protein concentrate and low-sodium milk are available and may be used to assist with the protein intake. Total abstinence from alcohol is very important.

If the liver insufficiency is serious, and the patient is exhibiting neurological disturbances (e.g. depressed awareness, dulled mentation, confusion, asterixis and hyperreflexia) and an elevation in blood ammonia, protein is eliminated from the diet. The patient is sustained with carbohydrates. The disturbance of the nervous system is attributed to failure of the liver to metabolize the nitrogenous wastes; the ammonia level rises because it is not deaminized to form urea. If coma develops, intravenous infusions are used to support the patient.

Medications. Multivitamin preparations are prescribed. Parenteral vitamin K may be given if the prothrombin level is below normal and if a tendency to bleeding is manifested by petechiae, ecchymosis, epistaxis, melaena or haematemesis. Vitamin B_{12} injections may be necessary to correct anaemia.

Although the patient with cirrhosis usually develops oedema and ascites due to portal hypertension and decreased plasma oncotic pressure because of reduced liver production of blood proteins, the doctor may be reluctant to prescribe a diuretic because of the possible electrolyte imbalance and excessive reduction of intravascular volume. Diuretics that are given initially are potassium-sparing diuretics (e.g. spironolactone), as hypokalaemia may precipitate hepatic encephalopathy. Cirrhotic ascites is often refractory and requires the use of a combination of diuretics. Rapid acting diuretics waste potassium and necessitate frequent determinations of electrolyte and fluid balance.

Potentially toxic drugs normally inactivated by the liver are avoided. Examples of these are barbiturates, amobarbital, diazepam, oral contraceptives and opiates.

Rest and activity. If there is no ascites or signs of impending hepatic coma, the patient remains ambulatory, and a limited amount of activity that does not produce excessive fatigue is encouraged to promote appetite as well as circulation.

In more advanced liver impairment, bed rest is recommended. The patient's lassitude necessitates thoughtful nursing measures such as frequent change of position, special skin care and passive exercises to combat the effects of prolonged inactivity.

Assessment. The patient is weighed at the same time each day with the same amount of clothing and is observed for signs of oedema. The exact amount of nutrition taken daily is noted; resourcefulness on the part of the nurse is needed frequently to have the patient take nourishment. Physical weakness and lethargy may necessitate feeding the patient.

The daily fluid intake and output are measured and recorded. The abdomen is examined daily for evidence of developing ascites, and the girth is measured and recorded.

The nurse notes the patient's responses, orientation and level of awareness. Any indication of nervous system dysfunction is brought to the doctor's attention. Cot-sides are sometimes placed on the bed to protect the very lethargic, confused or comatose patient.

Prevention of infection. Resistance to infection is lowered in the patient with cirrhosis of the liver. Precautions are taken to prevent possible exposure to any source of infection.

Abdominal paracentesis. An abdominal paracentesis may be necessary if the fluid in the peritoneal cavity reaches a volume that is causing respiratory distress, compression of abdominal viscera and blood vessels and considerable pain and discomfort. (See procedure for abdominal paracentesis p. 596).

Peritoneovenous shunt. When ascites is consistent or recurring, a shunt may be surgically performed to relieve portal hypertension and ascites (see Fig. 18.6). The mortality rate from these procedures is high because the patients are such poor surgical candidates. A peritoneovenous shunt may be performed, which avoids the necessity of major surgical intervention. A tube is inserted into the superior vena cava and is connected by a one-way valve to a perforated collecting tube in the peritoneal cavity. The valve opens in response to pressure in the peritoneal cavity; ascitic fluid flows into the venous circulation and is transported by the venous tube from the peritoneal cavity into the superior vena cava. Infection is a major complication associated with this procedure.

Patient education. The patient who improves sufficiently to go home is informed of the extent he must restrict his usual activity. Strict adherence to his diet, total abstinence from alcohol, and the avoidance of infection and physical strain are stressed when interpreting the regimen to the patient and family. (If cirrhosis has been caused by alcoholism the nurse should suggest that the patient may be helped by a support group such as Alcoholics Anonymous.) Measures to prevent injury and abrasion to the skin and mucous membranes, because of his increased tendency to bleed, are emphasized. He will be required to visit his doctor or a clinic at regular intervals. A referral to the community nursing service or the primary health-care team may be necessary so that consistent supervision is ensured. They are advised of the recommended regimen and of the changes that may indicate regression, necessitating prompt medical care.

The prognosis for patients with cirrhosis depends on the degree of liver insufficiency. If treatment is instituted in the early stages and the patient is sufficiently motivated to adhere to the suggested care, he is likely to live a normal life span. If portal hypertension has developed with resultant ascites and oesophageal varices, the prognosis is grave.

COMPLICATIONS OF CIRRHOSIS AND THEIR MANAGEMENT

Hepatic encephalopathy and coma, and oesophagogastric varices are common complications.

Hepatic coma
Before the patient with cirrhosis of the liver develops coma, neurological disturbances are manifested. These include mental dullness, slow responses, forgetfulness and disorientation. Muscle reflexes are exaggerated, and muscular rigidity and asterixis (flapping tremor) are also present. The cause of the neurological involvement is failure of the liver to metabolize and detoxify nitrogenous substances; the toxic materials such as ammonia remain in the blood and are carried into the cerebral circulation. The failure may be due to hepatocellular necrosis or because portal blood bypasses the liver and reaches the central nervous system by being shunted directly into the systemic circulation.

Nursing measures used in the care of any unconscious person are applicable to the patient in hepatic coma (see Chapter 10).

Portal hypertension
The flow of blood from the portal vein through the liver may meet with resistance due to disease and cirrhotic changes in the liver. Pressure rises within the portal venous system, causing portal hypertension. The latter is defined as a portal pressure in excess of 30 cm of saline.[8] The increased pressure in the portal vein produces a back-up in the veins that normally empty into the portal system. Collateral circulatory channels develop between the portal vein and the systemic circulatory system to bypass the liver.

The veins most seriously affected by portal hypertension are those in the gastric cardia region and the lower part of the oesophagus. The veins become engorged and tortuous; the walls are weakened, pre-

[8] Braunwald et al (1987), p. 1346.

disposing them to rupture. These varicosed veins appear as large bulbous protrusions under the mucosa. The congestion in the mesenteric veins causes haemorrhoids and is also reflected in the apparent congested cutaneous veins around the umbilicus (caput medusae). In addition to varices, problems associated with portal hypertension include congestive splenomegaly and ascites.

The severity of portal hypertension may be assessed indirectly by evidence of oesophageal varices, which may be visualized using fibreoptic endoscopy or by liver scan. Direct measurement of portal hypertension requires surgical intervention and is rarely performed.

Bleeding oesophagogastric varices
The oesophagogastric varices are frequently the site of rupture of the vascular wall and severe haemorrhage. The perforation and bleeding may be caused by mechanical trauma from 'rough' food passing over a varicosity, erosion and ulceration of the mucosa and venous wall by gastric acid secretion, or sudden increased intra-abdominal pressure associated with coughing, vomiting, straining at stool or physical exertion. Severe haematemesis occurs; some blood will enter the intestine and eventually the person passes tarry stools.

Prompt emergency treatment and care of bleeding oesophagogastric varices are necessary; the excessive loss of blood is life-threatening.

Control of bleeding. Various measures are used to control bleeding and include the following:
● Balloon tamponade. A Sengstaken–Blakemore tube, a nasogastric tube with three or four lumens, may be inserted. One lumen ends in an elongated balloon that is inflated to exert pressure against the oesophageal wall; another ends in a small balloon that is positioned just within the stomach and, when inflated, compresses varices in the cardia and anchors the tube in place (Fig. 18.4); and the third lumen opens into the stomach, extending well beyond the balloon in the cardia. The third lumen permits drainage or aspiration of the gastric content; its proximal end is usually attached to suction. Removal of gastric contents reduces the amount of blood entering the intestine. Digestion of blood in the intestine produces nitrogenous wastes that, when absorbed, predispose the patient to hepatic coma. Some Sengstaken–Blakemore tubes have a fourth lumen which permits suction above the oesophageal balloon. Continuous suction is applied so as to aspirate any blood or secretions above the oesophageal balloon. Before the tube is inserted, the tube and balloons are tested for leaks. The nurse makes sure that the proximal end of each lumen is identified and clearly labelled to prevent possible error in inflation or deflation of tubes after insertion. The pressures to be maintained within the

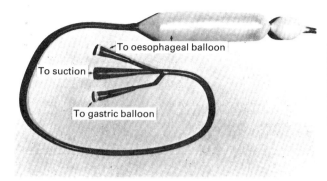

Fig. 18.4 A Sengstaken–Blakemore tube which is used in the treatment of bleeding oesophageal varices. The tube has three lumens. One leads to the longer inflatable balloon that is positioned in the oesophagus to provide pressure. A second lumen ends in the smaller balloon that lies just within the stomach. The third lumen opens into the stomach to permit gastric drainage.

balloons are indicated by the doctor and are usually 25–30 mmHg; excessive pressure can cause tissue ulceration (Fig. 18.5). Inadequate inflation is ineffective in checking bleeding and may also permit shifting of the tube. The gastric drainage is checked frequently for blood content which should progressively decrease following the insertion of the tube. In some instances, when the tube is in place and the balloons inflated, the doctor may lavage the stomach with ice water until the return flow is clear.

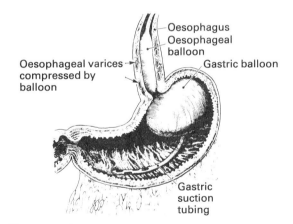

Fig. 18.5 A Sengstaken–Blakemore tube in position with the oesophageal and gastric balloons inflated.

A nurse remains in constant attendance; the patient is observed closely for any indication of respiratory distress. Saliva or blood escaping around the tube into the oropharynx may be aspirated. The patient is unable to swallow his saliva, so provision is made for suction or for expectoration into tissues or a basin.

The tube is positioned within the nostrils to exert a minimum of pull and pressure, and then secured. Frequent moistening and a very light application of a lubricant to the nasal mucosa may reduce the irritation. Some doctors position the tube via the mouth.

Compression by the inflated balloons is not usually continued longer than 48 hours. Pressure for a longer period could cause oedema, ulceration and perforation. The tube is left in position for continued gastric drainage and for the balloons to be reinflated readily if bleeding resumes. In some instances, the doctor may order deflation of the balloons for 5 minutes at regular intervals to reduce the risk of tissue damage.

- Gastric cooling. Rarely, a continuous application of cold to the oesophagus and cardia of the stomach may be used in an attempt to arrest variceal bleeding. A special double-lumen tube with balloons is inserted. By means of a mechanical pump, there is a steady circulation of a cold solution through the balloons and a refrigeration unit.
- Vasopressin infusion. Vasopressin (Pitressin) may be administered by a usual intravenous route or, with the assistance of angiography, may be given directly into the superior mesenteric artery. The vasopressin produces arterial vasoconstriction which reduces portal venous pressure by decreasing the volume of blood entering the portal system. The patient may experience crampy abdominal pain and be incontinent of stool.
- Sclerotherapy. This is the primary method of treatment. A coagulating substance is injected into the oesophageal varices. Visualization of the varices is achieved using fibreoptic endoscopy and a coagulating substance is injected. The patient is closely monitored following the injection. The patient will be required to have this procedure repeated at regular intervals for 1–2 years.
- Surgical treatment. If the measures cited above are not effective in checking the haemorrhage, emergency surgery may be performed to relieve portal hypertension. Different surgical procedures are used. A portacaval shunt in which an anastomosis is made between the portal vein and the inferior vena cava (Fig. 18.6B), a splenorenal venous shunt (Fig. 18.6C), an anastomosis between the superior mesenteric vein and the inferior vena cava (mesocaval shunt, Fig. 18.6D) or a transoesophageal ligation of the varices may

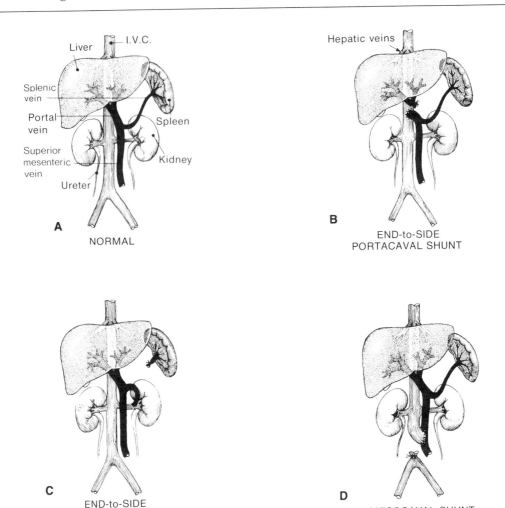

Fig. 18.6 Portal shunts used to relieve portal hypertension. *A*, normal portal system. *B*, Anastomosis of the portal vein and the inferior vena cava. *C*, Anastomosis of the splenic vein and the renal vein. *D*, Anastomosis of the superior mesenteric vein and the inferior vena cava.

be done. As an emergency measure, there is considerable risk. It is preferable if the patient's condition can be stabilized and surgery undertaken when bleeding is arrested.

Care following a surgical shunt is similar to that of patients undergoing any abdominal surgery. Close observation for haemorrhage and abdominal distension is important. If a nasogastric tube is passed to control vomiting and distension, a soft tube is selected and is introduced very gently to avoid precipitating haemorrhage by rupturing a varicosity. Specific orders are received from the surgeon as to how much the patient may move and whether deep breathing, coughing, and leg exercises are to be carried out. Similarly, the patient receives nothing by mouth until specifically ordered.

In the case of a splenorenal shunt, a retention catheter is inserted, and a close check is kept on the urinary output.

Vitamin K. Parenteral injections of vitamin K are prescribed to increase the patient's blood-clotting power.

Assessment. The patient requires continuous attention and on-going assessment.

The blood pressure and pulse are recorded every 15–30 minutes until the bleeding is controlled. The intervals are gradually increased as the patient's condition shows improvement and stabilization. The patient's respirations, colour and responses are noted; persisting grey pallor, rapid shallow respirations and dulling of awareness and responses are unfavourable signs.

The pressures in the balloons are checked at frequent intervals and corrected if necessary to the prescribed pressure. The gastric drainage is observed for amount and blood content. Persisting bright blood in the drainage is brought to the doctor's attention. The fluid intake and output are recorded, and the balance determined daily. Stools are examined for blood content.

Supportive measures. The patient with bleeding oesophagogastric varices is critically ill and needs physical and psychological support.

- Blood transfusion. Replacement of the blood lost is imperative. Fresh blood rather than stored is preferable in order to replace the thrombocytes lost.
- Nutrition and fluids. The patient is sustained for several days by intravenous infusion. Glucose in distilled water and plasma are solutions that may be used. An intravenous line is maintained until the patient is able to take fluids by mouth.

  Fluids may be introduced via the tube in the stomach before it is removed. When the tube is removed, small amounts of nutritious fluids are given. The diet is progressively increased to a light diet as tolerated. Roughage and raw fruits and vegetables are avoided. The patient is advised to chew his food well in small amounts so that the bolus is small and less likely to cause trauma to a vulnerable area in the oesophagus or cardia of the stomach.
- Rest and positioning. The patient is kept absolutely at rest. He may have to remain stationary to avoid displacing the balloons. Passive movements of the lower limbs and deep breathing are usually carried out to prevent circulatory stasis and to promote airway clearance. The head of the bed is elevated, unless contraindicated by shock. This position may reduce the flow of blood into the portal system.
- Psychological support. The haematemesis, emergency measures and rapid loss of strength are very frightening to the patient. His fears and concerns should be acknowledged, and reassurance provided that everything possible is being done and that someone will remain with him. Some explanation is calmly made as to what is happening and what is going to be done. Sedation may be necessary to allay the patient's tension and anxiety and provide rest. The patient may be less apprehensive and more relaxed if a family member is permitted to be with him when it does not interfere with treatments. The family is naturally concerned and should be kept informed about the patient's progress and what is being done.
- Mouth care. The inability to swallow saliva and to receive anything by mouth necessitates special mouth care. Suction may be necessary to remove secretions. Tissues or a basin should be provided into which the patient may expectorate. The mouth is cleansed with moist applicators and petroleum jelly, or cold cream is applied to the lips to prevent irritation that may develop with the repeated use of tissues.

Accidental injury to the liver

Rupture of the liver in accidents is not uncommon. Any interruption of the capsule enclosing the hepatic tissue carries the risk of severe internal haemorrhage that may prove fatal before surgical intervention is possible. A blood transfusion is given, and surgical repair undertaken. Control of the bleeding is of prime importance. The area may be sutured or packed, or oxidized cellulose (Oxycel) gauze may be applied. The latter supplies fibres on which the clot may form more easily. A drainage tube into the abdominal cavity or a sump drain attached to low suction may be used. In addition to the loss of blood incurred in injury, peritonitis may develop as a result of the chemical irritation caused by the bile that may escape from the liver. Destruction of liver cells may also follow the injury, resulting in impaired liver function.

Neoplastic disease

Benign and primary malignant neoplasms are rare in the liver, but it is a frequent site of metastasis, especially if the primary malignant neoplasm is in the abdominal cavity. The malignant cells may be transported to the liver via the portal venous or hepatic arterial blood or via the lymph. In many instances, secondaries in the liver are discovered before the primary source. The liver enlarges and signs of liver insufficiency develop. The patient experiences pain, food intolerance, anaemia, emaciation and ascites.

If a primary neoplasm is confined to one lobe of the liver, a hepatic lobectomy may be done. Following the operation, the patient is observed closely for possible haemorrhage and biliary peritonitis. More often, chemotherapy is used (see pp. 157–161). Drugs may be administered by direct hepatic arterial infusion.

Liver abscess

Infection with subsequent abscess formation occurs rarely and is most often associated with amoebic dysentery. The causative organisms (*Entamoeba histolytica*) are carried by the portal bloodstream from the bowel. The pyogenic infection may also be caused by staphylococcus, streptococcus or *Escherichia coli*. Along with manifestations of impaired liver function, the patient has chills and a high fever. There may be one or multiple small abscesses which frequently coalesce, forming one large cavity.

The patient is treated with antibiotics and also receives chloroquine or emetine hydrochloride (antiamoebic drugs) if the abscess is a complication of amoebiasis. The abscess is drained by aspiration followed by the injection of an antibiotic into the cavity. Open surgical drainage is avoided if possible because of the danger of dissemination of the infection within the peritoneal cavity and resultant peritonitis.

LIVER TRANSPLANTATION

Human liver transplants have been carried out since 1963. With improved surgical techniques, better means of preserving the donor liver and advances in immunosuppressive therapy, patients receiving liver transplants are surviving longer. The number of liver transplants being performed is increasing each year, although the procedure remains limited to a few centres. Patients considered for liver transplantation have chronic and fatal liver disease and are under the age of 55. The complex problems that are present preoperatively affect the patient's post-transplant recovery. Donor organs are generally matched to the recipient according to body size and blood type, as the liver is not as immunologically active as other organs. The recipient's immune system is suppressed usually with cyclosporine in combination with low dose corticosteroids.

Nursing intervention is directed at management of the side-effects of immunosuppressive therapy which include control of the resulting stomatitis and prevention of infection. The patient is instructed as to the actions, side-effects and prescribed regimen for maintenance immunotherapy as well as measures to prevent infection and actions to take if infection or signs of rejection occur. Patients and families require a great deal of emotional support and therapeutic intervention to help them deal with the transplant and the implications for the patient's life and the quality of life that can be anticipated. A team of nurses, doctors, social workers and possibly pastoral counsellors usually work collaboratively to help the patient and family through the decision-making period prior to transplantation, the wait for a donor liver, and the adjustment and often unexpected publicity that occurs following the procedure.

Disorders of the Gallbladder and Bile Ducts

Cholelithiasis

Cholelithiasis is the term used for stones in the gallbladder (Table 18.4). Their formation is not understood. They vary in shape and size and consist mainly of cholesterol and bile pigments. There may be one stone or many and, although they may develop in both sexes, they occur more often in middle-aged females. The incidence is high in individuals with regional enteritis.

Table 18.4 Nomenclature in disorders of the extrahepatic biliary system.

Cholelithiasis	Gallstones or calculi in the gallbladder
Cholecystitis	Inflammation of the gallbladder
Cholecystectomy	Surgical removal of the gallbladder
Cholestasis	Stoppage or suppression of the flow of bile
Cholecystostomy	Incision into the gallbladder and the insertion of a tube for drainage
Choledocholithiasis	Gallstone(s) in the common bile duct
Choledochitis	Inflammation of the common bile duct
Choledocholithotomy	Surgical removal of stone from the common bile duct
Choledochotomy	Incision and exploration of the common bile duct
Choledochoduodenostomy	Anastomosis of the common bile duct to the duodenum

SIGNS AND SYMPTOMS

Cholelithiasis may not give rise to any disturbance in many persons; in others, the stones cause signs and symptoms ranging from mild digestive disturbances following fat ingestion to all those previously cited under manifestations. Gallstones may cause acute or chronic inflammation of the gallbladder (cholecystitis), or cholestasis (stasis of the bile) within the liver leading to impaired function of that organ. Small stones tend to cause more acute problems, since they may escape into the ducts. They may pass into the duodenum, or may lodge in the cystic or common bile duct or the ampulla of Vater. Impaction of a stone in the common bile duct leads to obstructive jaundice and intense, incapacitating pain.

TREATMENT AND NURSING INTERVENTION

Cholelithiasis is treated surgically by removal of the gallbladder (*cholecystectomy*) and exploration of the common bile duct for a stone or stricture. The surgery is not usually done during an acute attack unless obstruction of the common bile duct persists. When impaction of a stone in the common bile duct occurs, leading to obstructive jaundice, the stone may be removed endoscopically (see p. 592).

During an episode of biliary colic, an antispasmodic drug such as atropine, propantheline (Pro-Banthine) or glyceryl trinitrate may be ordered to relieve the painful reflex spasm that occurs in response to the stone in a duct. Morphine or pethidine may also be prescribed in conjunction with one of the above drugs, but some doctors avoid their use because they oppose relaxation of the sphincter of Oddi.

Food and fluids by mouth are withheld, and the patient is given intravenous fluids. If vomiting and abdominal distension occur, a nasogastric tube is passed and regular aspiration is performed.

Following the acute episode and removal of the nasogastric tube, clear fluids are given and gradually increased to a light, low-fat diet as tolerated.

The patient is observed for signs of jaundice, and the colour of all stools is noted. The stools may be saved for examination for the presence of the stone that may have passed from the biliary tract into the intestine.

If the patient is jaundiced, and the stools are a pale grey, indicating an absence of bile in the intestine, a daily dose of vitamin K [menadiol sodium phosphate (Synkavit, phytomenadione)] is given parenterally to maintain prothrombin formation and prevent bleeding.

Cholecystitis

Inflammation of the gallbladder may be acute or chronic. Acute cholecystitis is most often associated with gallstones but may occur as a result of infection. The patient manifests pain and tenderness in the right upper abdominal quadrant or mid-epigastrium, fever, nausea and vomiting and leucocytosis. The severity of the symptoms varies with the degree of inflammation. Jaundice may develop if the inflammation involves the biliary ducts.

MANAGEMENT

The treatment includes bed rest, intravenous fluids, analgesics and antibiotics. If the condition persists or worsens, it may indicate suppuration (empyema of the gallbladder), necessitating prompt surgery. A *cholecystostomy* (drainage of the gallbladder) or a *cholecystectomy* (removal of the gallbladder) may be done.

Chronic cholecystitis is characterized by a long history of vague digestive complaints. The patient experiences abdominal discomfort and flatulence after a large rich meal or one high in fats. A dull, aching pain and nausea and vomiting may occur at times. The intensity and probably the frequency of the symptoms insidiously increase over months or years.

The chronic inflammation results in scarring and thickening of the wall of the gallbladder and cholestasis. If calculi are present, they progressively increase in size or number. The patient may have subacute or acute exacerbations in which he becomes incapacitated by nausea and vomiting, moderate fever and probably mild colic. The condition is usually treated surgically by removal of the gallbladder.

Bile duct disorders

Obstruction of the common bile duct may occur as a result of a gallstone that has escaped from the gallbladder (*choledocholithiasis*), inflammation (*choledochitis* or *cholangitis*), neoplasm or a stricture formed by scar tissue following trauma and inflammation. The duct above the obstruction dilates and obstructive jaundice develops.

In the case of an impacted stone, retrograde cholangiography may be done and the gallstone removed during the cannulation of the common bile duct (see p. 593). Surgery may be undertaken to open the duct and remove the calculus. When a stricture is present and the area is sufficiently small, it is resected and an end-to-end anastomosis performed. If the obstruction is due to primary carcinoma, excision may be undertaken and the duct stump anastomosed to the duodenum (*choledochoduodenostomy*) or the jejenum (*choledochojejunostomy*).

Extrinsic pressure on the bile ducts obstructing the flow of bile may occur with cancer of the pancreas or duodenum.

When surgery involves an extrahepatic bile duct, a T tube is inserted at the site of entry into the duct to maintain bile drainage during recovery of the tissues (choledochostomy). The stem portion of the tube is brought out on the abdominal surface through a stab wound or the incision and is attached to a drainage receptacle. Surgery on a bile duct is usually accompanied by a cholecystectomy, since the gallbladder is frequently the origin of the problem.

Nursing care of patients with extrahepatic disorders

Surgery is not usually done during an acute attack of cholecystitis or cholelithiasis unless the signs and symptoms are unremitting or progressive. The patient is kept at rest, and food is withheld. If there is vomiting, a nasogastric tube is passed and regular aspiration is performed (see Chapter 17). The temperature, pulse and respirations are recorded regularly; a sudden elevation is reported promptly. The patient is checked for signs of obstructive jaundice and abdominal distension.

When the vomiting is controlled and the nasogastric tube removed, oral fluids are given and graduated, as tolerated, to a light, bland, low-fat diet. If the patient is obese, the caloric intake is limited to approximately 1000 kcal daily.

PREOPERATIVE CARE

Preoperative preparation (see Chapter 11) for surgery on the extrahepatic biliary system includes close observation for jaundice and the administration of vitamin K to raise the prothrombin level. Special attention is given to having the patient understand the importance of the frequent coughing and deep breathing that he will be required to carry out after the operation. Because of the site of the surgery, the patient tends to take very shallow breaths to prevent pain and discomfort, predisposing to respiratory complications. A nasogastric tube may be passed before the patient is taken to the operating room.

POSTOPERATIVE CARE

General postoperative care as outlined in Chapter 11 is applicable. Close observation for bleeding is necessary, since low prothrombin levels may still exist.

The drainage tube (T tube) that is inserted in the common bile duct is generally clamped during the transfer from the operating room; after the patient is transferred, it is immediately attached to a drainage receptacle. The tubing leading to the receptacle is secured to the dressing and lower bed linen and should have sufficient slack to prevent traction and dislodgement. The patient is advised as to how to turn to avoid a pull on the tube and of the need to be sure that it is not kinked or compressed. The drainage is observed frequently during the first 24 hours in case of haemorrhage. There may be a small amount of blood mixed with bile in the first few hours, but persistent bleeding is reported to the surgeon. The character and daily amount of bile drainage are recorded. If there is a prolonged loss of bile, it may be given back to the patient through a nasogastric tube for the purpose of promoting more normal digestion and absorption in the intestine.

The dressing is checked frequently for possible bleeding or bile leakage. After a few days, the T tube is clamped for stated intervals and is removed when the surgeon considers the common bile duct is patent. Following removal of the tube, the dressing is observed for bile seepage. If the dressing is soiled with bile, it is changed frequently, the skin and wound are cleansed, and petroleum jelly gauze, an ointment or powder is applied to prevent excoriation and maceration of the skin by the strongly alkaline bile. The patient is also observed for signs of peritonitis; an elevation of temperature, abdominal pain, distension and rigidity are reported at once.

Until the procedures become less painful and the patient is less fearful, the nurse's assistance and support are required during the frequent, regular coughing, deep breathing and change of position.

Early ambulation is generally urged, and provision is made for a small drainage receptacle that may be attached to the patient's dressing gown if there is a T tube in the common bile duct.

The urine, stools, sclerae and skin are checked for any indication of obstructive jaundice.

The patient receives intravenous solutions of glucose and electrolytes until the nasogastric tube is removed and oral fluids and food are tolerated. The fat content of the diet is limited.

In preparation for discharge, the patient's diet is discussed. Generally, the surgeon will suggest that the patient gradually increases the fat intake and finds his level of tolerance.

Disorders of the Pancreas

Inflammation and neoplastic disease are the patho-logical conditions seen most frequently in the pancreas.

PANCREATITIS

Inflammation of the pancreas may be acute or chronic with recurrent acute episodes.

Acute pancreatitis

Acute pancreatitis is a potentially serious disorder; the severity of the inflammation varies. In the mild form the pancreas becomes swollen and oedematous and, with treatment, the patient is likely to recover within a few days. If the process is severe and persists, necrosis and haemorrhage ensue. Necrosis results from intrapancreatic activation of the proteinases and lipase, initiating autodigestion of the pancreatic tissue and blood vessels. Enzymes and blood may escape into the surrounding tissue and peritoneal cavity; peritonitis, paralytic ileus or ascites may develop.

CAUSE

Pancreatitis is considered to be the result of some factor or change within the pancreas that effects activation of the proteinases and lipase of the exocrine secretion, with subsequent breakdown of the ducts, parenchymal tissue and blood vessels. The causative factor may be an obstruction to the flow of the pancreatic secretion within the ducts. Continued secretion produces dilatation and back pressure, resulting in duct disruption and the escape of enzymes into the parenchyma. The obstruction may be due to a calculus in the pancreatic duct, a neoplasm, or fibrosis following some irritation within the pancreas.

A gallstone in the ampulla of Vater, compression of the ampulla by an extrinsic neoplasm, or spasm or oedema of the sphincter of Oddi may be the initiating factor. It is suggested that such an obstruction causes a reflux of bile into the pancreas, promoting activation of the enzymes and ensuing autodigestion.

Other possible aetiological factors are considered to be infection and injury of the pancreas. Pancreatitis is most frequently associated with biliary tract disease and alcoholism and has a higher incidence in middle-aged individuals.

MANIFESTATIONS

Acute pancreatitis has a sudden onset, being preceded usually by only mild, vague digestive disturbances. The principle signs and symptoms are pain, gastrointestinal disturbances, obstructive jaundice, shock and hyperglycaemia.

Pain. At first, constant severe incapacitating pain occurs in the upper abdomen, penetrating through to the back. It may be described as burning or boring. Later, with progression of the disease, the pain becomes more generalized in the abdomen.

Gastrointestinal disturbances.   Nausea and vomiting occur and persist. Constipation may be a problem. Abdominal distension and rigidity appear as a result of the development of peritonitis. The latter is caused by chemical irritation of the viscera and peritoneum by the enzymes that escape from the pancreas. Peristalsis diminishes, and eventually paralytic ileus and intestinal obstruction may complicate the patient's condition further.

Shock.   The patient has the appearance of being very ill: he becomes anxious and prostrated. Severe shock develops; the skin is pale, cold and clammy, the pulse is rapid and thready, and the temperature, which may have been elevated, falls to subnormal. Shock is attributed to the severity of the constant pain, the exudation of plasma into the peritoneal cavity that occurs with the peritonitis, and the loss of blood resulting from the erosion of vessels within the pancreas associated with necrotizing and haemorrhagic pancreatitis.

Vital signs.   The temperature may be elevated in the early stage but may become subnormal if peritonitis and shock develop. The pulse is rapid, and the blood pressure falls with the decrease in the intravascular volume due to dehydration and the concomitant shock. The patient is flushed at first, and then usually becomes pale. If peritonitis develops, he is likely to become a dusky or cyanotic colour.

Obstructive jaundice.   If the head of the pancreas is involved, it may compress the common bile duct and cause obstructive jaundice.

Blood changes.   With the escape of enzymes into the pancreatic parenchyma and peritoneal cavity, fatty tissue is broken down into glycerol and fatty acids. The latter combine with calcium to form insoluble calcium compounds. The serum calcium level falls and may be severe enough to produce tetany and affect heart action (prolonged diastole). The serum bilirubin level may be elevated after 2–3 days.

Haemoconcentration develops as a result of the loss of plasma. The prothrombin level falls because of the lack of absorption of vitamin K. Serum amylase and lipase levels are elevated.

Disturbance in glucose metabolism.   A deficiency of insulin may develop when the islets of Langerhans are involved in the pathological process, and hyperglycaemia and glycosuria (sugar in the urine) may be present.

TREATMENT AND NURSING INTERVENTION

The patient with acute pancreatitis is critically ill.

Care is directed toward the reduction of pancreatic secretion to a minimum, relief of pain, prevention of shock or correction if it has developed, correction of electrolyte and fluid imbalances and prevention of infection. Nursing responsibilities involve the following considerations.

Relief of pain.   Pethidine hydrochloride is used parenterally to relieve the patient's pain in preference to opiate preparations (morphine, codeine) since the latter tend to stimulate the contraction of the sphincter of Oddi. The patient is assisted in turning and moving and in finding the least painful position. Frequent attendance and verbal and non-verbal conveyance of an appreciation of the patient's suffering may contribute to making the pain less intolerable.

Assessment.   The patient's condition may change rapidly with progressive necrosis and resulting haemorrhage. The *vital signs* and the *general response and appearance of the patient* are observed frequently. A rapid weak pulse, a fall in blood pressure, pallor and increasing weakness may manifest haemorrhage or shock and are immediately brought to the doctor's attention. Frequent *haemoglobin* and *haematocrit estimations* may be requested by the doctor to detect haemoconcentration which would indicate the loss of plasma into the peritoneal cavity. An accurate record is kept of the *fluid intake* and *output*.

The *intensity and location of the pain* are noted, and the abdomen is examined for distension and rigidity. All *stools* are examined and, if they are bulky, greasy and foul-smelling or show other abnormalities, they are saved until seen by the doctor.

The *sclerae and skin* are observed for any yellow tinge that would indicate the development of jaundice.

Gastric drainage.   A nasogastric tube is passed and regular aspiration is performed. This relieves vomiting and distension and prevents the acid gastric secretion from entering the duodenum, which would stimulate the release of the hormones secretin and cholecystokinin-pancreozymin. The colour, consistency and 24-hour volume of the drainage are recorded.

Fluids and nutrition.   The patient receives nothing by mouth to avoid stimulating the secretion of the pancreatic enzymes. The restoration and maintenance of normal blood volume is very important to prevent or correct shock. Plasma or whole blood may be given intravenously, in addition to electrolyte and glucose solutions. A close check is kept on the blood chemistry, volume of gastrointestinal drainage, urinary output and amount of perspiration to determine the specific electrolyte and fluid needs. Total parenteral nutrition may be prescribed during the acute and convalescent phases of the illness.

When oral intake is permitted, fluids are introduced in small amounts. The principal nutrient given at first is carbohydrate; protein is added gradually, according to the patient's tolerance. Fats are avoided. The diet is progressively increased to a high-protein, high-carbohydrate, low-fat, light diet. Four or five small meals are recommended. A preparation of extract of pancreas (pancreatin) may be prescribed orally with meals to assist in digestion. Large meals are avoided, and total abstinence from alcohol is stressed.

Mouth and nasal care. Frequent cleansing and rinsing of the mouth are necessary during the period in which oral intake is restricted because the anticholinergic drug which the patient may be receiving suppresses salivary secretion. Oil, petroleum jelly or a cream is used on the lips to prevent cracking. The nostrils are cleansed with an applicator which has been slightly moistened with normal saline, and a light application of petroleum jelly or water-soluble lubricant is made to the nostril through which the tube passes to prevent irritation and excoriation.

Medications. As well as analgesics, the patient may receive an anticholinergic drug such as propantheline bromide (Pro-Banthine) and atropine sulphate by intramuscular or subcutaneous injection. These drugs inhibit vagal nerve stimulation of the pancreatic enzymes and promote relaxation of the sphincter of Oddi. If an anticholinergic drug is prescribed, the patient will experience a very dry mouth and close observations are made for the possible side-effects of urinary retention and paralytic ileus.

An antibiotic is usually ordered as a prophylactic measure since inflammation and necrosis make the pancreas very vulnerable to infection.

When the gastric drainage is discontinued, an antacid such as aluminium hydroxide gel or a combination of aluminium hydroxide and magnesium hydroxide (Maalox) may be given orally at frequent intervals to reduce the acidity of the chyme entering the duodenum.

Parenteral administration of vitamin K may be necessary to maintain normal prothrombin production and prevent bleeding.

Complications. If *paralytic ileus* and intestinal obstruction develop, a nasogastric tube may be passed into the stomach and decompression suction established (see Chapter 17). *Obstruction of the duodenum* may develop because of the swollen oedematous pancreas. Escaping pancreatic enzymes may digest an area of the gastric or duodenal wall, causing *severe haemorrhage* as well as perforation of the eroded organ.

Renal failure may develop within 24 hours of the onset of acute pancreatitis, necessitating dialysis.

Another complication that rarely develops in pancreatitis is the formation of one or more *pseudocysts.*

Accumulations of inflammatory exudate, liquefied necrotic tissue and secretions become walled off by a capsule of fibrous tissue. The cyst is atypical in that there is no epithelial lining characteristic of true cysts. This accounts for the term pseudocyst. A pseudocyst may form within or on the surface of the pancreas or in a neighbouring area into which pancreatic secretions have escaped. It may enlarge and impose on surrounding structures. The common bile duct may be blocked, the duodenum or stomach may be displaced, or the diaphragm may be elevated. The deviation and location are usually recognized in an x-ray.

The symptoms depend on the size and location of the cyst(s). In some instances resolution takes place spontaneously, or the cysts may produce persisting pain, digestive disturbances, anorexia, loss of weight and mechanical interference with other organs. Surgical drainage may be necessary and may be internal or external, depending on the location of the cyst. Internal drainage is achieved by anastomosing the cyst to the small intestine. If drainage is established through the skin, petroleum jelly gauze or a protective ointment or powder is essential to prevent excoriation of the skin by the enzyme content of the drainage.

Follow-up care. A long convalescence follows recovery from an acute episode of pancreatitis. The necessary care to avert an exacerbation is discussed with the patient and his family. The importance of strict adherence to the prescribed diet, total abstinence from alcohol and the avoidance of large meals are explained. Verbal and written instructions are given about the content and preparation of the recommended low-fat, high-protein, high-carbohydrate diet.

If anticholinergic drugs or antacids are to be continued, verbal and written directions are given which include advice as to early side-effects that should be reported to the doctor. To assist with digestion, the patient with chronic pancreatitis may need to continue to take extract of pancreas (pancreatin) orally with each meal.

Activities are gradually resumed and the individual may return to his former occupation in 1–2 months.

Surgical intervention. Surgery is not usually undertaken during an acute attack of pancreatitis unless there is increasing obstructive jaundice due to an impacted stone. The various operative procedures that may be used to treat the patient may be performed on the biliary tract or directly on the pancreas. They include exploration of the common bile duct and ampulla of Vater and the insertion of a T-tube for drainage, cholecystostomy, cholecystectomy, sphincterotomy to relieve obstruction caused by spasm of the sphincter of Oddi, anastomosis between the common bile duct and duodenum, or anastomosis between the gallbladder and the jejunum. Surgery on the pancreas may involve the removal of calculi in the pancreatic duct, drainage of a pseudocyst, or partial or complete pancreatectomy. Rarely, in severe chronic pancreatitis, sensory nerves (splanchnic nerves) which transmit pain impulses from the pancreas may be interrupted to relieve intractable pain.

The nursing care of patients having surgical treatment is similar to that required by patients having gastric surgery (see pp. 543–553).

Chronic pancreatitis

Chronic pancreatitis may develop following an initial acute episode or may develop insidiously. Recurrent acute exacerbations are likely to occur. It is frequently associated with alcoholism, chronic biliary tract disease, or hypercalcaemia due to hyperparathyroidism.

The chronic form of the disease is characterized by progressive fibrosing and calcification of areas in the pancreas following inflammation and necrosis. The degree of impaired function and the intensity of its signs and symptoms are proportionate to the amount of continuing inflammation or frequency of acute episodes and ensuing tissue damage.

MANIFESTATIONS

The patient with chronic pancreatitis experiences recurrent attacks of pain in the epigastric region and right upper quadrant which progressively becomes persistent. Anorexia, nausea, flatulence and constipation are common problems. Episodes are frequently precipitated by the ingestion of alcohol or a large meal with considerable fatty content.

As more and more of the pancreatic parenchyma becomes non-functional, a deficiency of enzyme secretion occurs in the intestine. Less fat and protein are digested; the patient's stools become bulky, greasy and offensive (steatorrhoea) and there is a progressive weight loss. A deficiency of insulin secretion may result in diabetes mellitus.

TREATMENT AND NURSING INTERVENTION

In some instances, slight impairment by chronic pancreatitis may be controlled by dietary adjustments and the avoidance of emotional stress, fatigue and infection.

A low-fat diet and four or five small meals rather than the usual three larger ones are recommended. The patient's fear of precipitating more severe pain may lead to a reluctance to eat and a resulting serious weight loss. He must be encouraged to take nourishing foods that he can tolerate. Impaired digestion due to insufficient quantities of enzymes in the intestine may be corrected by the administration of pancreatic enzyme supplements (preparation of pancreatic extract). Vitamin supplements, including vitamins A, D, K, folic acid and B_{12} may be required. Total alcohol abstinence must be respected to avoid precipitation of an acute episode.

Decreased insulin secretion may necessitate the giving of insulin to control glucose metabolism.

As the disease becomes more advanced, the pain experienced by the patient may indicate frequent doses of an analgesic. Not infrequently, this becomes complicated by the person's development of a tolerance for the drug, necessitating progressively larger doses; actual addiction may become a problem.

Rarely, surgical intervention may be used to drain pseudocysts or to relieve intractable pain. Partial pancreatectomy or anastomosis of the pancreatic duct with the jejunum may be undertaken.

NEOPLASMS OF THE PANCREAS

Carcinoma

Cancer of the pancreas usually arises from the ducts and, although it may occur in any part of the organ, it is most commonly seen in the head.

The patient experiences pain, progressive weakness and loss of weight. Jaundice develops if the neoplasm encroaches on the ampulla of Vater or common bile duct. The cancer may spread by direct invasion to adjacent structures and by metastasis to the liver.

TREATMENT

The condition is treated surgically if recognized sufficiently early and if it is the head of the pancreas that is involved. Neoplasms in the body and tail have usually metastasized by the time they are identified. Rarely, a pancreatoduodenal resection may be done; this procedure involves resection of the head of the pancreas, ampulla of Vater, duodenum and pylorus with anastomosis between the common bile duct and jejunum, anastomosis between the pancreas and jejunum, and a gastrojejunostomy. Palliative operations that may be used include a cholecystojejunostomy to relieve obstructive jaundice and a side-to-side anastomosis of the main pancreatic duct (duct of Wirsung) to the jejunum. Radiation therapy and/or chemotherapy may be used but have not been found to be very effective.

Preparation for surgery includes a high-calorie, low-fat diet if tolerated by the patient, intravenous infusion of glucose and electrolyte solutions, blood transfusions, and parenteral vitamin K if there is jaundice. Postoperative care includes gastrointestinal decompression to prevent distension of the jejunum and pressure on the sites of the anastomoses, The patient is supported by blood transfusions and intravenous electrolytes and glucose. Vitamin K administration may be continued.

Tumours of islet cells

A benign tumour may develop in non-beta islet cells and may become malignant. The tumour cells secrete gastrin freely, causing the Zollinger–Ellison syndrome, which is characterized by gastric hypersecretion and persisting peptic ulceration. The treatment is surgical removal of the tumours or total gastrectomy. Nursing care of the patient is similar to that cited under gastric surgery, pages 543–553.

Occasionally an adenoma develops from beta cells of the islets of Langerhans, causing an excessive secretion of insulin (hyperinsulinism) and hypoglycaemia. The adenoma is usually benign but, rarely, may be adenocarcinoma.

The symptoms presented by the patient are mainly due to the effect of the abnormally low blood sugar (50 mg or less per cent) on the brain cells. Brain cells are more sensitive to glucose deficiency than other body cells. The initial symptoms are hunger, restlessness and apprehension. These progress to weakness, loss of coordination, tremors, diaphoresis, disorientation, convulsions and coma. The manifestations appear during a fasting period (early morning) or following extreme exertion. Prompt administration of some form of glucose is necessary to raise the blood sugar. If the hypoglycaemia remains untreated, the glucose deficiency may result in permanent brain cell damage or death. When early signs are recognized, the patient is given sugar or orange juice with sugar. In the more advanced stage of hypoglycaemia, glucose 50% is given intravenously.

Surgical treatment may consist of excision of the adenoma or subtotal or total pancreatectomy. Preparation for the surgery includes a high-carbohydrate, high-protein diet and intravenous infusions of glucose solution to restore glycogen reserves. The glucose infusion is continued during the operation. Following surgery, close observation is made for a recurrence of hypoglycaemia. If a total pancreatectomy is done, the patient will receive supplemental insulin and pancreatic extract for the remainder of his life.

Diabetes mellitus is discussed in Chapter 20.

CYSTIC FIBROSIS

Cystic fibrosis is a congenital disease characterized by impaired functioning of the exocrine and mucus-secreting glands throughout the body. The secretions, especially those of the respiratory tract, are abnormally viscous. The sweat and saliva of affected persons have inordinate concentrations of sodium and chloride.

This disease is usually recognized in infancy because of the serious respiratory problems incurred by the thick, tenacious mucus. The secretions are retained, blocking bronchioles and alveoli, and the patient's vital capacity is reduced. As a result, he is very vulnerable to infection.

The viscous nature of the exocrine secretions of the pancreas causes a stasis and obstruction in ducts, which may result in cyst-like dilatations and degeneration of tissue and ensuing fibrosis. A deficiency of pancreatic enzymes in the intestine produces incomplete digestion and absorption as well as steatorrhoea. The islets of Langerhans are not usually affected. In severe disease, the newborn may fail to pass meconium because of intestinal obstruction, and an ileostomy may have to be done.

Cystic fibrosis is currently considered to be a hereditary disease (recessive trait) that is transmitted by a defective gene received from each parent. It is thought that the defect may result in the lack of a specific enzyme, causing interference with the cells' production of their secretions.

The child requires constant, intensive care and supervision. Special measures such as humidifiers and mist tents are used to keep the air in the patient's environment moist to help liquefy the respiratory secretions. Postural drainage, chest percussion and vibration, regular coughing and breathing exercises are also employed. Antimicrobial preparations may be prescribed to prevent infection. Obviously, any contact with persons who have an infection must be avoided.

The patient receives a high-calorie, high-carbohydrate, high-protein, low-fat diet. A preparation of pancreatic extract (pancreatin) is given to promote digestion and absorption. In warm weather, sodium and chloride depletion may occur as a result of increased sweating and may necessitate an increased intake of these electrolytes either orally or by intravenous infusion.

The family is referred to the community nursing service and to a branch of the Cystic Fibrosis Research Trust. The parents generally need considerable assistance in establishing a plan of care for the patient; the socioeconomic demands are great. The medications and therapeutic equipment are expensive, and there is a continuous demand on the parents' time in providing the necessary observation and care. Frequent visits to the clinic or surgery are necessary.

References and Further Reading

BOOKS

Anderson SVD & Bauwens EE (1981) *Chronic Health Problems*. St Louis: CV Mosby. Chapter 12.

Anderson LDMV, Turkki PR, Mitchell HS & Rynbergen HJ (1982) *Nutrition in Health and Disease*, 17th ed. Philadelphia: JB Lippincott. Chapter 33.

Avery Jones G & Jones L (1968) *Clinical Gastroenterology*, 2nd ed. London: Blackwell Scientific.

Boucher IAD, Allan RN, Hodgson HJF & Keighley MRB (1984) *Textbook of Gastroenterology*. Eastbourne; Baillière Tindall. Chapters 18 & 19.

Braunwald E et al (1987) *Harrison's Principles of Internal Medicine*, 11th ed. New York: McGraw-Hill. pp. 406–413.

Ganong WF (1985) *Review of Medical Physiology*, 12th ed. San Francisco, CA: Lange. pp. 406–413.

Harper HA, Rodwell VM & Mayes PA (1979) *Review of Physiological Chemistry*, 17th ed. Los Altos, CA: Lange. Chapter 34.

Krupp MA & Chatton MJ (eds) (1983) *Current Medical Diagnoses and Treatment*. Los Altos, CA: Lange. pp. 386–413.

Morson BC & Dawson IMP (1979) *Gastrointestinal Pathology*, 2nd ed. London: Blackwell Scientific.

Pagana KD & Pagana TJ (1982) *Diagnostic Testing and Nursing Implications*. St Louis: CV Mosby. Chapter 3.

Robbins SL, Angell M & Kumar V (1981) *Basic Pathology*, 3rd ed. Philadelphia: WB Saunders. Chapter 16.

Sabiston DC (ed) (1985) *Textbook of Surgery*, 13th ed. Philadelphia: WB Saunders. Chapters 34, 35, 36.

Sherlock S (1985) *Diseases of the Liver and Biliary System*, 7th ed. London: Blackwell Scientific.

Smith LH & Thier SO (1985) *Pathophysiology*, 2nd ed. Philadelphia: WB Saunders. Section 15.

Tresler KM (1982) *Clinical Laboratory Tests*. Englewood Cliffs, NJ: Prentice-Hall. pp. 401–414.

Truelove SC & Reynell PC (1972) *Diseases of the Digestive System*, 2nd ed. London: Blackwell Scientific.

Vander AJ, Sherman JH & Luciano DS (1985) *Human Physiology: The Mechanisms of Body Function*, 4th ed. New York: McGraw-Hill. Chapter 15.

PERIODICALS

Babb RR (1984) Ascites: differential diagnosis and treatment. *Hosp. Med.*, Vol. 11 No. 4, pp. 129–131, 135, 139–143.

Bradford KS (1983) Injection sclerotherapy in the management of bleeding esophageal varices. *Crit. Care Nurs.*, Vol. 3 No. 2, pp. 36–41.

Didich JM (1981) Gauging abdominal girth accurately. *Nurs. 81*, Vol. 11 No. 7, pp. 32–33.

Fredette SLF (1984) When the liver fails. *Am. J. Nurs.*, Vol. 84 No. 1, pp. 64–67.

Gannon RB & Pickett K (1983) Jaundice. *Am. J. Nurs.*, Vol. 83 No. 3, pp. 404–407.

Guenter P & Slocum B (1983) Hepatic disease: nutritional implications. *Nurs. Clin. N. Am.*, Vol. 18 No. 1, pp. 71–80.

Gurevich I (1983) Viral hepatitis. *Am. J. Nurs.*, Vol. 83 No. 4, pp. 571–586.

Jackson MM (1980) Viral hepatitis. *Nurs. Clin. N. Am.*, Vol. 15 No. 4, pp. 729–746.

Kieran T & Romgopal M (1979) Viral hepatitis: progress and problems. *Med. Clin. N. Am.*, Vol. 63 No. 3, pp. 611–619.

Kosel KG, Matas P, Seaborne L, & Westerberg J (1982) Total pancreatectomy and islet cell autotransplantation. *Am. J. Nurs.*, Vol. 82 No. 4, pp. 568–571.

Patton F (1981) Hepatitis: current concepts. *Crit. Care. Nurs.*, Vol. 1 No. 3, p. 24.

Robinson MK & Warden LS (1981) Hepatorenal syndrome. *Crit. Care Nurs.*, Vol. 1 No. 5, pp. 23–26.

Ropka ME (1981) Pancreatic insufficiency in the person with cancer. *Cancer Nurs.*, Vol. 4 No. 1, pp. 37–41.

Taylor DL (1983) Gallstones: physiology, signs and symptoms. *Nurs. 83*, Vol. 13 No. 6, pp. 44–45.

Thorpe CJ & Caprini JC (1980) Gallbladder disease: current trends and treatments. *Am. J. Nurs.*, Vol. 80 No. 12, pp. 2181–2185.

Traiger GL (1982) Drug-induced hepatotoxicity. *Am. J. Nurs.*, Vol. 32 No. 1, pp. 124–126.

Traiger GL (1982) New hepatitis B vaccine: a breakdown in hepatitis prevention. *Am. J. Nurs.*, Vol. 82 No. 2, pp. 306–307.

Traiger GL & Bohachick P (1983) Liver transplantation: care of the patient in the acute postoperative period. *Crit. Care. Nurs.*, Vol. 3 No. 5, pp. 96–103.

19
Nursing in Disorders of Nutrition and Metabolism

NUTRITION

Nutrition refers to the process of ingesting, assimilating and utilizing food. All living cells require a continuous supply of nutrients for survival. Body cells utilize the molecules from ingested food to provide the energy and materials necessary to maintain their structure and function. The cells, particularly those of the liver, are capable of converting the wide range of molecules from different foods to another type of molecule for use.

NUTRITIONAL REQUIREMENTS

Certain nutrients are considered to be *essential* and must be ingested in adequate amounts to meet body needs. These include: protein (eight of the twenty amino acids that cannot be produced in the body), some fatty acids, vitamins and minerals. To obtain essential nutrients, the individual must consume a daily diet composed of a variety of foods as no one food provides all essential elements. Tables of recommended daily allowances of essential nutrients have been developed to meet the nutritional needs of healthy individuals.[1,2]

A balanced diet consists of foods from each of the basic food groups of milk, meats, fruits, vegetables, and grains. An adequate daily diet for an adult includes: (1) two servings of milk or milk products such as cheese or yogurt; (2) two servings of meat, fish, poultry or lentils; (3) four servings of fruits and vegetables, including a citrus fruit, a dark green and a yellow vegetable; and (4) four servings of grain in the form of bread, or whole grain cereals.

Basic food group guides are useful in planning diets for healthy individuals and for adjusting diet to meet specific needs such as altered energy intake or increased or decreased intake of specific nutrients. Energy requirements are met primarily by carbohydrates (46%) and fats (42%), with about 12% provided by protein. For kilocalorie-reduced diets, it is recommended that fats (mainly) and carbohydrates be reduced and protein content remain the same (12% of the dietary kilocalories).

Energy requirement for an individual is determined by: (1) the amount of energy needed to maintain involuntary body functions at rest [basal metabolic rate (BMR)]; (2) the amount of energy required to metabolize food; and (3) physical activity. When kilocalorie intake equals kilocalorie use, body weight is maintained.

FACTORS WHICH INFLUENCE DIETARY PATTERNS

Dietary behaviour is influenced by physiological, psychological, sociocultural and environmental factors, as well as knowledge of food and food requirements. The consumption of food is usually a social activity; eating habits are very complex and are resistant to change as they become an integral part of the individual and family lifestyle.[3]

Physiological factors influencing nutritional needs and eating behaviour include the individual's metabolic rate, growth phase, body excretions, reproductive functions and level of daily physical activity. Increased energy and nutrients are required by the individual during periods of rapid physical growth, pregnancy and lactation, increased basal metabolic rate (e.g hyperthyroidism) and increased physical activity. Fewer kilocalories are needed by elderly individuals, because of their lower basal metabolic rate and decreased activity and by those with sedentary life-styles.

The hypothalamus and limbic system of the brain regulate food intake by influencing appetite, hunger and satiety. *Hunger* is a physiological phenomenon involving unpleasant sensations of abdominal discomfort and irritability which prompt the individual to search for food. *Appetite* involves the conscious desire to eat. *Satiation* is the pleasant feeling of being fully satisfied after a meal. *Anorexia* is the abnormal loss of the desire to eat which may be influenced by both physiological and psychological factors.

Emotions are important in determining eating behavior. Food has different meanings for each individual, and responses to stress or happiness are often expressed as changes in eating habits. Some individuals respond to stress and decreased self-esteem by overeating, while others have loss of appetite and decrease their food consumption. Eating habits are

---

[1] Howe (1981).
[2] DHSS (1979).

[3] Pender (1982) p. 278.

believed to be formed very early in life and become fixed and automatic responses.

Sociocultural factors influencing eating behaviour include religious and ethnic practices and the use of ethnic foods, which have special meaning for the individual and family. The 'mass-media' also play an important role in influencing food consumption; advertisements relating to specific foods have a great impact on individuals and families.

Environmental factors include the availability, cost and convenience of foods. The individual's income may be inadequate to meet the cost of the essential foodstuffs. The environment in which food is prepared and eaten also influences eating behaviour. Appetite is usually stimulated when eating takes place in a pleasant and relaxed social milieu.

Knowledge. Knowledge of dietary requirements and food values is an important factor in the individual's or family's eating patterns. In some instances, persons may not understand that in planning a balanced diet expensive food elements can usually be substituted by less expensive items that will meet the essential dietary requirements.

These non-biological influences on the use of food may contribute to the development of nutritional disorders and are important restraining factors when attempting to change eating habits.

METABOLISM

When food is absorbed it is taken from the blood by tissue cells. Some of it is used by the cells to meet material requirements for the construction of tissue, for growth and maintenance or for the production of substances such as hormones and enzymes. Much of the food is broken down to produce the energy required by the body to carry out its many functions. All cells require substances that furnish energy but, since those of different tissues vary in composition and function, the cells select materials to meet their special needs in respect to such differences. Glucose and fat are used mainly to supply energy, while requirements for cellular structure and chemical products are met principally by the amino acids and minerals.

When the foods are taken into the cells they undergo physical and chemical changes which comprise *metabolism*. When the cellular activity results in the synthesis of tissue substance, the process is referred to as *anabolism*, or anabolic metabolism. The processes that break down the materials into simpler forms and release energy are called *catabolism*, or catabolic metabolism.

Anabolism exceeds catabolism during the absorptive phase, following ingestion and digestion after a meal. Monosaccharides and amino acids are absorbed from the intestinal tract into the blood and are transported to the liver where the monosaccharides are immediately converted into glucose to supply the body's major source of energy during this absorptive period. Excess calories are stored in the liver and adipose tissue, mostly as fats.

During the post-absorptive period, which occurs about 4 hours following ingestion of a meal, during the night and during periods of fasting, energy is supplied by the stores of glycogen in the liver and muscles and by the breakdown of neutral fat stored in adipose tissue. When fasting is prolonged, body protein is catabolized to provide energy.

FATE OF CARBOHYDRATES IN THE BODY

Carbohydrates are absorbed as glucose, fructose and galactose and are the main energy source. Fructose and most of the galactose are converted to glucose by the liver. Some galactose remains as such and is one of the components of the myelin sheath found around many nerve fibres. The sheath is a fatty, insulating membrane that prevents the loss of the nerve impulse.

Glucose may be oxidized by the cells to provide energy; it is temporarily stored as glycogen in the liver or muscles or converted to fat and stored as such. It is also used in small amounts in the synthesis of tissue substances and secretions and is circulated in the blood for a period of time, providing what is known as the blood sugar. If it is in excess, some may be excreted in the urine.

Oxidation of glucose

The oxidation of glucose by the cells to acquire energy is a complex process involving a series of many chemical reactions. Each reaction is catalyzed by a specific enzyme with the final end products being energy, water and carbon dioxide.

It is not the intent to give the details here of the biochemical reactions that take place in the oxidation of glucose. If such information is desired, the reader should consult a textbook of biochemistry or medical physiology. The catabolism of glucose involves two main processes, glycolysis and the citric acid cycle (Kreb's cycle or tricarboxylic acid cycle).

Glycolysis splits the glucose molecule into two pyruvic acid molecules, at the same time releasing some energy. Ten successive chemical reactions are necessary to achieve glycolysis. The pyruvic acid molecules then embark on a series of chemical reactions which compose the citric acid cycle. Each of the ten chemical changes occurring in the citric acid cycle also requires a specific enzyme. The net result of the metabolism of one molecule of glucose is energy plus six molecules of carbon dioxide plus six molecules of water ($C_6H_{12}O_6 + 6O_2 \rightarrow E + 6CO_2 + 6H_2O$). Some of the energy that is released by the chemical reactions forms heat energy, and the remainder is stored in the cell as adenosine triphosphate (ATP). ATP is a compound with three phosphoric acid radicals; two of these radicals are connected to the compound by high-energy bonds which can be split off readily when energy is needed by the cell to promote other chemical changes. If one phosphate radical is released, the compound is changed to adenosine diphosphate (ADP). As energy is released by other chemical reactions, the energy is used to bond the free phosphate radical to ADP and then to regenerate ATP. These energy changes go on continually with the chemical processes that constitute metabolism.

The glucose that is not needed to maintain a normal concentration in the blood or for immediate oxidation is converted by several chemical reactions and enzymes to glycogen and stored as such. Most of the glycogen is found in the muscle and liver cells. The muscle cells store it for their own use for contraction. The liver stores it and, as the blood concentration falls, converts the glycogen back to glucose and releases it into the blood. The process by which the glucose is converted to glycogen is known as *glycogenesis*; the reconversion of the glycogen to glucose is called *glycogenolysis*.

Blood glucose
The blood sugar concentration is relatively constant, the normal being 3.9–6.1 mmol/l (80–110 mg/dl) of blood. It may rise to 7.2–8.0 mmol/l (130–140 mg/dl) after a meal, but falls to normal within 2 or 3 hours. Maintenance of the blood glucose level within normal limits is especially important for normal functioning and survival of the brain cells. A concentration of at least 3.9 mmol/l (80 mg/dl) of glucose in the blood is necessary in order to meet the needs of the cells.

A deficiency in the blood glucose concentration is quickly manifested by central nervous system disturbances. The person may become confused and lose muscle coordination and strength. If the deficiency is severe, loss of consciousness may occur and unless corrected, death may ensue. If the brain cells are deprived of glucose for even a very few hours they may suffer permanent damage.

Hypoglycaemia is the term given to a blood sugar concentration below the normal. If the concentration is above the normal, the condition is known as *hyperglycaemia*.

Regulation of the blood glucose concentration. Maintenance of the blood glucose within normal limits is done mainly by hormones. When the blood sugar concentration falls, the liver cells may be activated by two hormones, glucagon and adrenaline, to convert glycogen to glucose and release it into the blood. Glucagon is secreted by the pancreas when the blood sugar falls below the normal level. Adrenaline is secreted by the medulla of the adrenal glands. Sympathetic innervation to the adrenal glands is excited by a low blood sugar concentration, resulting in a release of adrenaline into the blood. Adrenaline also stimulates the breakdown of muscle glycogen to lactate which must return to the liver for gluconeogenesis to occur.

Insulin, a hormone secreted by cells in the islands of Langerhans of the pancreas, brings about a decrease in the blood sugar concentration by promoting the transport of glucose into the tissue cells. If the blood sugar level decreases toward or below the lower normal limits, there is a corresponding decrease in the secretion of insulin.

The adrenal cortex also secretes the hormones, glucocorticoids, that increase the blood sugar concentration. A decrease in the blood sugar stimulates the adenohypophysis (anterior pituitary gland) to release the adrenocorticotropic hormone (ACTH) which brings about the release of glucocorticoids. The increase in blood sugar is brought about by the glucocorticoids stimulating the liver cells to form glucose from non-carbohydrate substances. Protein and fats may be broken down and glycogen or glucose formed. This process may be referred to as glyconeogenesis or, if glucose is produced, as *gluconeogenesis*.

Similarly, the lowered blood sugar may cause the release of the thyroid-stimulating hormone (TSH) by the adenohypophysis and a resulting increase in the output of thyroxin, which promotes gluconeogenesis.

Lipogenesis
When the absorbed glucose exceeds what the cells use and what can be stored as glycogen, it may be converted to fat and stored in the fat depots of the body. Insulin plays an important role in stimulating the deposition of fat.

Excretion of glucose by the kidneys
As the blood flows through the kidney, about one tenth of the water in the blood and its associated solutes with a molecular weight of less than 67 000 are filtered by the glomeruli of the kidneys. Normally, all of the filtered glucose is reabsorbed by the tubules and the urine is sugar-free. If the blood sugar becomes abnormally high, not all the glucose is reabsorbed from the kidney tubule back into the blood; that which is not reabsorbed by the tubules passes out into the urine. The level of blood sugar at which glucose is excreted in the urine is referred to as the *renal glucose threshold* and is approximately 10 mmol/l (180 mg/dl) but this may vary with individuals. This excretion of the glucose, rather than its usual reabsorption, does reduce the blood sugar to some extent and is considered as a mechanism active in the regulation of the blood sugar.

FATE OF FATS IN THE BODY

Fatty acids and glycerol are absorbed into the microvilli of the intestinal cells. There they are combined to form triglycerides which are coated with phospholipids to become chylomicrons. The absorbed fat is carried into the major lymph channels and reaches the blood through the thoracic lymphatic duct. Fats may be used by the body cells to provide energy, synthesize fat compounds or be stored as fatty tissue.

In the use of fats to provide energy, the triglycerides are first broken down by the liver into glycerol and fatty acids. The glycerol is converted to glycogen which is then converted to glucose.

The fatty acids are split by a series of chemical changes, mainly occurring in the liver. In each reaction, two carbon atoms and energy are freed in an oxidation process, finally ending up with acetoacetic acid and smaller amounts of beta-hydroxybutyric acid and acetone. These acids, because of their chemical structure, may be referred to as ketone acids or ketone bodies and the process by which they are formed is called *ketogenesis*. The ketones move out of the liver into the blood and are transported to the cells in need of energy where they are metabolized via the citric acid cycle, releasing energy and ending up as carbon dioxide and water. Although 1 gram of fat has more than twice as much energy value (9.3 kcal or 38 kJ)[4] as does 1 gram of glucose (4.1 kcal or 17 kJ), as long as glucose is available to the cells, it is used in preference to fats.

The amount of ketones in the blood normally is very low and depends on a balance between the production by the liver and the assimilation by the tissue cells. Occasionally the rate of ketogenesis may exceed the rate at which the cells complete the

metabolism, resulting in an accumulation of ketone acids in the blood and ketonuria. The condition is called ketosis and may occur when there is an increased use of endogenous fat for energy, as in starvation, or if there is a deficiency of glucose or a disturbance in the metabolism of glucose, as in diabetes mellitus. Ketosis may also develop with a diet high in fats (ketogenic diet).

Fat is necessary in the body for the formation of some essential fatty compounds such as phospholipids, lecithin, steroids and cholesterol. These compounds are built into other tissues. For example, phospholipids and cholesterol are necessary components of cell membranes.

The fat that is not used for energy or for the synthesis of certain tissue substances is stored as fatty tissue in areas of the body called the fat depots. Most of the fat is deposited in the subcutaneous tissue, in the abdomen, especially on the mesentery and omentum, around the kidneys and between the muscle fibres.

A certain amount of stored fat is of value. The subcutaneous fatty tissue insulates the body against an excessive heat loss and against the cold of the external environment. Fatty tissue also provides a protective cushion for the body against trauma.

Following a meal not all the absorbed fat may enter the liver. Some of it moves directly into the fat depots so that the concentration of fat in the blood is quickly lowered. The fat in the tissues is mobilized when it is needed for energy. There is a constant movement of fat in and out of the fatty tissue (see Fig. 19.1).

As with carbohydrate metabolism, certain hormones produced in the body may influence fat metabolism. Most of them increase fat mobilization

---

[4] 1 kilocalorie (kcal) equals 4.184 kilojoules (kJ).

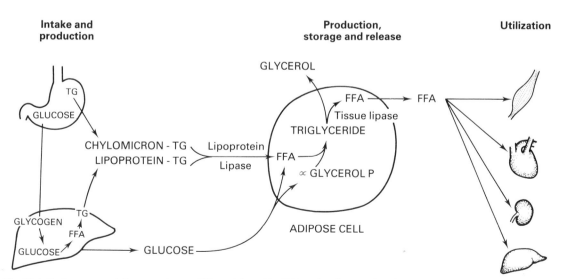

Intake and production **Production, storage and release** **Utilization**

Fig. 19.1 Fat homeostasis in normal man. TG = triglyceride. FFA = free fatty acids. The liver is a major site of the synthesis of fat, which is released as the triglyceride moiety of lipoproteins. The adipose cell is the major storage reserve of fat. Release of fatty acids from the adipose cell depends on the activity of a hormone-sensitive tissue lipase. The free fatty acids released to the circulation are largely oxidized by skeletal and cardiac muscle and to a smaller extent by kidney and liver.

and fat utilization by the cells. These hormones include the growth (somatotropic) hormone secreted by the anterior pituitary gland, thyroxine, cortisone secreted by the adrenal cortices, and adrenaline released by the medulla of the adrenals. Insulin increases lipid synthesis and utilization. Oestrogen secreted by the ovaries increases the deposition of fats in the tissues.

FATE OF PROTEIN IN THE BODY

The absorbed amino acids may be built into body tissue or used in the synthesis of cell products, such as enzymes and hormones, or the formation of protein compounds, such as plasma proteins. They may be converted to non-nitrogenous substances, such as carbohydrate or fat, which may be stored or oxidized to produce energy. From the large number of different amino acids, the cells select only those that they need to produce their particular type of protoplasm and cell products. Amino acids are very important to the child, whose protein requirement is more than twice that of the adult as he grows and amasses more tissue.

The amino acids that are not used by the cells for structure or cell products are taken into the liver where they may be stored or converted to a non-nitrogenous compound. By this means the liver prevents an excessive concentration of amino acids in the blood. Only a small amount can be stored but, when the blood concentration of amino acids falls, the liver releases the reserve.

Amino acids may be converted to glucose by the liver cells by a process called *deamination*. The amino radical is removed from the amino acid, forming ammonia. Since the ammonia would be toxic to tissue cells, it is combined with carbon dioxide to form urea. The urea is released from the liver into the general circulation and excreted by the kidneys.

The residual molecular elements of the amino acid are converted to glucose or fat and are oxidized to meet energy requirements. Normally, carbohydrate and fat provide the energy required by the cells. If these become deficient, protein is moved into the liver and is deaminized to meet the cells' energy needs. In starvation, this involves the use of blood proteins and tissue protein and deprives the cells of structural and functional amino acids. The cells' normal activities are disrupted and survival is threatened.

Some amino acids may be synthesized by the liver cells. The amino radical is removed from one amino acid and is attached to the molecule of a carbohydrate or a fatty acid. This process is called *transamination*.

Protein metabolism is influenced by certain hormones. The growth hormone, thyroxine, and testosterone (male sex hormone) stimulate the use of protein in the synthesis of tissue and cell products. The glucocorticoids promote mobilization of amino acids into the blood from the cells and their conversion to glucose.

Common Disorders of Nutrition and Metabolism

Assessment

The body's energy balance and body functions are affected when the supply or metabolism of nutrients is altered. Assessment of the patient with an actual or potential disorder of nutrition and metabolism includes the collection and analysis of data on lifestyle, behaviour patterns, dietary habits and changes in physiological functioning of most body systems (see Table 19.1).

HISTORY

1 *Age and sex.* The patient's age and sex are noted as these influence basal metabolic rate as well as life-style, activity and nutritional needs.

2 *Activity and life-style.* The amount of energy the patient expends daily is determined by finding out the type of occupation and extent of daily activities. How the patient feels following activity and his perception of activities he is or is not able to perform is also assessed.

3 *Rest and sleep* are assessed in relation to the patient's usual pattern.

4 *Nutritional history* includes identification of daily food intake, eating habits and factors affecting these. The patient may be asked to record his total food and fluid intake over a 24-hour period and include information about the time and circumstances under which the food was consumed, the method of preparing the food and the consumption of dietary supplements and snacks between meals. How the individual responds to food (has or has not an appetite for it, has strong likes or dislikes) is elicited as well as symptoms that occur following ingestion of foods. The patient's daily food intake is analysed for adequacy of the essential nutrients, vitamins and minerals, energy intake and fluid volume. The presence of nausea, vomiting, anorexia, excessive thirst and changes in body fat may be indicative of metabolic disorders. Food preferences, dislikes, food allergies and sociocultural factors which may influence his eating habits are documented.

5 *Elimination.* Bowel habits are determined, and information related to the nature, formation, colour, odour and frequency of stools is obtained.

The volume, frequency and colour of urine output is determined as well as the presence of nocturia.

Table 19.1 Assessment of the patient's nutritional status.

Data	Indications of good nutritional status	Indications of poor nutritional status
Health history		
Activity and life-style	Consistent daily activity	Sedentary life-style Sporadic excessive activity
Rest and sleep	Regular pattern	Inconsistent
Nutritional intake	Usual daily food intake contains basic food groups and all essential nutrients Fluid intake 1500–2000 ml/day Balanced calorie intake for size and activity	Some food groups and essential nutrients missing from diet Calorie intake less than or greater than required for body size and activity Fluid intake less than 1200 ml/day
Physical examination		
General body appearance	Stands erect Alert Abdomen flat	Drooped shoulders Inattentive Abdomen protruded
Weight	Constant In proportion to height and body size	Variable 10% or more under or over suggested weight for height and body type
Skinfold thickness	Within 90% of standard value for age and sex	10% or more above or below standard value for age and sex
Circumference measurement	Body muscle stores are within 90% of standard value for age and sex	Body muscle stores are 80% or less of standard value for age and sex
Skin	Clean, dry and intact	Dry, transparent, scaley with petechiae
Oral mucous membranes	Clean, moist and intact	Gums swollen and bleeding
Teeth	Clean, smooth, regular edges, straight and symmetrical and intact	Dental caries Discoloration Irregular edges Malpositioned and absent teeth
Lips	Smooth, intact	Red and swollen with fissures
Hair	Shiny and clean	Dull, listless and brittle
Nails	Smooth, shaped and intact	Brittle, ridged, irregular edges
Eyes	Clean, focused Conjunctiva pink and moist	Sunken Conjunctiva pale Discharge

6 *Socioeconomic factors* affecting the availability, storage and preparation of foods are identified.

PHYSICAL EXAMINATION

1 *General body appearance* is observed. The patient's general stature and posture, distribution of body fat and general state of alertness reflect his state of health.
2 *Height and weight* are measured and recorded, and changes in body weight over given periods are identified (e.g. weight-loss or gain over so many weeks or months).
3 *Skin-fold thickness*[5] is measured to determine the amount of subcutaneous body fat. Callipers are

used to measure the skin-fold thickness over the triceps, scapular region and upper abdomen.[6] Results are compared with a table of normal values for the individual's age and sex.
4 *Circumference measurements*[5] are taken bilaterally at mid-arm and mid-thigh level. The arm muscle circumference is determined by subtracting the triceps skin-fold measurement from the arm circumference measurement. Results are compared with a table of normal values for the individual's age and sex. These calculations provide information on the body's muscle stores.
5 *The skin* is inspected for rashes, lesions, petechiae, bruises and changes in colour. The presence of infections and lesions that fail to heal may indicate increased blood glucose levels, while indications of prolonged bleeding may reflect a vitamin K deficiency.

[5] Skin-fold thickness and circumference measurements are not routine observations but they are necessary with some patients (e.g. emaciated, debilitated).

[6] Buergal (1979), pp. 218–219.

DIAGNOSTIC TESTS (SEE SUMMARY, TABLE 19.2)

1 Blood and urine studies reflecting *carbohydrate metabolism* include:
   (a) *Blood glucose concentration.* Normal fasting levels are 3.9–6.1 mmol/l (or 70–110 mg/dl).
   (b) *Serum glucagon levels.* Normal: 50–100 ng/l.
   (c) *Serum osmolality test.* When the number of glucose particles in the serum increases, the serum osmolality increases. Normal: 280–300 mmol/kg.
   (d) *Urinalysis.* Urine is examined for the presence of glucose and acetone (ketone bodies); normally urine tests are negative for both. *Glucose* is present in the urine when the blood glucose level exceeds the renal threshold—10 mmol/l (180 mg/dl). *Acetone* is excreted in the urine during starvation and when hyperglycaemia is uncontrolled; on these occasions fatty acid catabolism occurs to provide needed energy because the cells cannot utilize glucose.

2 *Blood lipid studies* reflect *fat metabolism*. Tests carried out include determination of the levels of cholesterol, triglycerides and phospholipids.
   (a) *Total lipids.* Normal: 4.0–8.5 g/l.
   (b) *Cholesterol.* Normal: 3.9–7.2 mmol/l (150–250 mg/dl).
   (c) *Triglycerides.* Normal: <1.8 mmol/l (<160 mg/dl).
   (d) *Phospholipids.* Normal: 1.6–3.9 mmol/l (5–12 mg/dl).

3 Blood and urine tests for *protein metabolism. Serum protein* concentrations reflect changes in protein metabolism and liver function.
   (a) *Total serum proteins.* Normal: 60–80 g/l.
   (b) *Albumin.* Normal: 40–60 g/l.
   (c) *Globulin.* Normal: 20–30 g/l.
   (d) *Albumin/globulin* (A/G) ratio 3:1.
   (e) *Urine protein.* Normal: < 0.15 g/dl.
   (f) *Haemoglobin level* decreases with iron and protein deficiencies. Normal: males, 13–18 g/dl; females, 12–15 g/dl.
   (g) *Plasma amino acid fractionation* may also be determined to diagnose protein deficiencies.

4 *Vitamins.* Blood or urine studies may be done to determine levels of most vitamins. A decrease in blood levels of fat-soluble vitamins is indicative of impaired fat absorption.
   Prothrombin time studies reflect change in the absorption of vitamin K. Normal: 11–15 seconds.

Table 19.2 Diagnostic tests used to assess nutritional status.

Test	Normal values	Discussion
Carbohydrate metabolism		
Blood glucose	3.9–6.1 mmol/l (70–110 mg/dl)	Serum glucose and serum osmolality increase with obesity in relation to the decrease in insulin receptors
Serum glucagon	50–100 ng/l	The presence of glucose and ketone bodies in the
Serum osmolality	280–300 mmol/kg	urine indicates hyperglycaemia and fatty acid metabolism
Urine: glucose	negative	
ketone	negative	
Fat metabolism		
Total blood lipids	4.0–8.5 g/l	Low levels of lipids in debilitating stages of
Cholesterol	3.9–7.2 mmol/l	malnutrition
Triglycerides	<1.8 mmol/l	Elevated levels of lipids may indicate excessive
Phospholipids	1.6–3.9 mmol/l	intake of foods high in cholesterol, or diabetes mellitus
Protein metabolism		
Total serum proteins	60–80 g/l	Serum protein levels decrease with undernutrition
Albumin	40–60 g/l	and protein deficiency
Globulin	20 to 30 g/l	Haemoglobin levels decrease with iron and protein
A/G ratio	3:1	deficiencies
Urine protein	<0.15 g/dl	
Haemoglobin	Male: 13–18 g/dl	
	Female: 12–15 g/dl	
Vitamins		
Serum vitamin levels		Decreased levels of fat-soluble vitamins A,D,E and
Prothrombin time (PT)	11–15 seconds (75–100% activity)	K results from impaired fat absorption. Absorption of vitamin K is reflected by the prothrombin time. With a vitamin K deficiency, the prothrombin time is prolonged
Minerals		
Serum mineral levels	See Chapter 6	Decreased levels of minerals occur with specific dietary deficiencies

5 *Mineral levels* in the blood may also be determined to identify specific nutritional deficiencies (see Chapter 6 for normal concentrations).

Diet and health

Over the last 10 years, many reports have been produced linking our way of eating with health problems. These reports make recommendations on food and health in terms of prevention of diseases attributed to inappropriate food intake. Two recent reports should influence the advice given by nurses to patients and clients (see Table 19.3). These are the reports of the National Advisory Committee on Nutrition Education (NACNE)[7] and the report of the DHSS Committee on Medical Aspects of Food Policy (the COMA Report)[8]. A summary of their recommendations are as follows:

Guidelines for healthy eating

1 Maintain a desirable weight. Even mild overweight carries risk of ill-health.
2 Fat is implicated in heart disease. The reports

---

[7] National Advisory Committee on Nutrition Education (1983).
[8] DHSS Committee on Medical Aspects of Food Policy (1984).

recommend a reduction in the total amount of fat consumed to 30–35% of total energy intake, and to cut dairy fat and meat fat to between 5 and 10%. That is, to less than a third of total fat. (This is not, however, recommended for infants or children under 5 years.) This means less fried foods, eating more fish and poultry and less red meats and using skimmed or semi-skimmed milk.
3 Reduce sugar intake by half. At the moment, the average person in the United Kingdom eats 112 g (4 oz) of sugar per day and this should be reduced by cutting down on sweets, snacks and sugary drinks.
4 High blood pressure is a major risk factor in heart disease. Some individuals seem unable to cope with excess salt and it is recommended that salt is reduced from the present average of 2½ teaspoons a day to less than 2 teaspoons. This means less salt in cooking and adding less at table.
5 'Energy value should be maintained because more exercise is to be encouraged.' Reduction in energy as a result of cutting down fat and sugar should be balanced by more bread, potatoes, fruit and other vegetables.
6 Fibre intake should be increased on average from 20–30 g per head per day. This means increasing wholemeal bread, wholegrain cereals, fruit, vegetables and pulses.

Table 19.3 Nutritional guidelines for health education in Britain.*

Dietary component	Current estimated average intake	NACNE 1983 Recommended average intakes		COMA 1984 Individual recommendation
		Long term	Short term	
Energy intake	—	Recommended adjustments of types of food eaten and an increase in exercise output so that adult body weight is maintained within the optimal limits of weight for height		Obesity should be avoided
Total fat intake	38% of total energy (128 g)	30% of total energy (101 g)	34% of total energy (115 g) 10% reduction	35% of total energy
Saturated (S) fatty acid intake	18% of total energy (59 g)	10% of total energy (33 g)	15% of total energy (50 g)	15%
Polyunsaturated (P) fatty acid intake	—	No specific recommendations—if total fat intake is reduced to 30% then this will automatically tend to increase the P:S ratio		3.5–6.8%
Cholesterol	—	No recommendations		No recommendations
Sucrose intake	38 kg/head/year	20 kg/head/year (approx 50% reduction)	34 kg/head/year (approx 10% reduction)	No further increase
Fibre intake	20 g/head/day	30 g/head/day (50% increase)	25 g/head/day (25% increase)	No recommendation
Salt intake	8.1–12 g/head/day	Recommended reduction by 3 g/head/day	Recommended reduction by 1 g/head/day	No further increase Ways to decrease should be considered
Alcohol intake	4.9% of total energy	4% of total energy	5% of total energy	Excessive alcohol to be avoided
Protein intake	11% of total energy	No recommendations		No recommendations

*Janes (1986), p. 269.

Manifestations of alterations in nutrition and metabolism

Nutritional and metabolic changes affect all body systems and produce a variety of manifestations which vary according to the specific nutritional problems, extent of the deficit or excess and the duration of the change.

Table 19.4 lists the signs and symptoms manifested by a patient with alterations in nutrition that are less or more than body requirements. Nutritional status is reflected also in the individual's physical appearance as well as in his energy level and behaviour. Dietary deficits and excesses in nutritional requirements may be the result of specific disorders and are discussed in the relevant topics of other chapters.

Obesity

Obesity is a form of malnutrition that develops when the energy intake exceeds energy expenditure. It is characterized by an increase in fatty tissue throughout the body as a result of the excessive storage of triglyceride. Fig. 19.1 summarizes the process of the storage and release of fat in the body. Only a small amount of the excess kilocalories is stored as carbohydrate and there is only a very slight increase in the protein mass; the excess is stored as triglycerides in the form of adipose tissue. The individual is overweight when 10% over his normal weight and is classed as obese when his weight is 20% over his normal weight.

Obesity is a major health problem affecting a large percentage of the Western population. Even though these individuals are overweight, they are frequently undernourished in relation to one or more essential food factors. Metabolic changes associated with obesity include hyperinsulinaemia, impaired glucose tolerance, hyperlipidaemia (e.g. increased blood cholesterol level), hyperuricaemia and hypertension.[9] Chronic overeating may incur a chronic increase in insulin production which would eventually lead to a reduction in the number of insulin receptors in the target cells. The reduction in the number of receptors means that the insulin responsiveness of the target cells is decreased, which would result in an increased glucose concentration in the blood. Serum levels of free fatty acids are elevated with the constant movement of fats in and out of the fatty tissue. Obesity increases the risk of the individual developing cardiovascular disease, hypertension, diabetes mellitus, osteoarthritis, pul-

[9] Vander, Sherman & Luciano (1985).

Table 19.4 Patient's problems related to alterations in nutrition.*

Problem	Causative factors	Signs and symptoms

Nutritional intake of more than body requirements	Food intake in excess of energy output related to:
	    Failure to accommodate for changes in energy output
	    Psychosocial factors
	    Emotional stress
	    Availability of high-calorie foods
		Weight 10% or more above normal range
		Excessive body fat: above normal skin-fold and mid-upper arm circumference measurements
		Denial of overeating
		Nutritional history shows food intake greater than body needs and expenditure

Nutritional intake of less than body requirements	1 Food intake inadequate in relation to energy output related to:
	    Economic factors
	    Lack of knowledge of nutritional needs
	    Emotional disturbances
	2 Inability to ingest, digest or absorb nutrients due to physiological disorders
		Weight 10% or less of normal
		Lack of body fat
		Nutrition history shows food intake inadequate for body needs
		Anorexia, nausea and vomiting
		Aversion to eating
		Self-induced vomiting
		Feeling of satiety following ingestion of foods
		Oral mucosal inflammation
		Absence of teeth
		Difficulty swallowing
		Heartburn
		Abdominal pain, cramping or tenderness
		Abdominal distension and bloating
		Altered bowel sounds
		Abnormal loose, bulky, odourous stools
		Flatulence
		Weakness and fatigue
		Altered muscle tone
		Peripheral oedema

* Kim & Moritz (1982), pp. 300 & 330.

monary disturbances and psychosocial difficulties. The obese pregnant woman is predisposed to complications, especially during delivery.

Cause

The cause of obesity in most instances is considered to be overeating, but it may be underactivity or a combination of the two factors. Approximately 3500 kcal above the body's metabolic needs are consumed to gain 0.5 kg (1.1 lb) of fat.[10] The cause or causes of lack of food-intake control may not be known; eating habits, social customs, psychological stress in sedentary life-styles are contributing factors. Overeating in infancy and early life is believed by some to cause the production of an increased number of adipose tissue cells which persist throughout adult life and act as a stimulus for increased food intake.[11]

IDENTIFICATION OF PATIENT PROBLEMS

The problem is an intake of food which is in excess of energy output.

The *goals* are to:
1 Acquire knowledge of the food requirements of the body
2 Acquire knowledge of the relationship between food intake and energy expenditure
3 Acquire knowledge of the effects of excessive body fat and obesity on the body, and on health
4 Reduce body weight and body fat by decreasing kilocaloric intake and increasing energy expenditure
5 Maintain weight at a desirable level

NURSING INTERVENTION

Prevention of overweight and control of obesity are important nursing responsibilities. Public education should begin with parents and young children to promote the development of healthy eating habits. Changing life-long eating patterns in adults who are overweight is a difficult and long-term process.

Educational programmes for the obese require a holistic approach since the individual's food intake is influenced by social, cultural, religious, economic and genetic factors which influence his self-image and life-style. Fasting is rarely used and is likely to cause complications. Drug treatment, with appetite suppressants for example, is of limited value and usually provides only short-term results. Surgery in the form of a gastria stapling or reducing the intestinal absorptive surface is occasionally used on morbidly obese persons who do not respond to other forms of weight reduction and control.
1 The *knowledge* required by the individual relates to: (1) basic nutritional requirements of the body; (2) the relationship between food intake and energy

output; (3) the effects of obesity on health; and (4) the role of activity and exercise in control of weight.
2 *Approaches to reducing body fat.* Measures to prevent obesity begin with the education of parents during the prenatal period, and focus on developing healthy eating habits in infancy and childhood. Parents need help in assessing food requirements of developing infants. Obesity in children, with the increased number of fat cells in the body, tends to perpetuate the problem throughout life.

The nurse in the community can support parents in establishing healthy eating habits by carefully monitoring energy intake, eliminating excess fat and kilocalories from the children's diet, planning for the introduction of solid foods between 4 and 6 months of age, and using cuddling and other means of comfort when crying occurs, rather than relying on food to comfort an infant.

Family participation and support are essential for the success of any weight control programme for children or adults. Weight control programmes are available in most communities for individuals and groups. The person should be examined by a doctor who will recommend a programme based on the needs of the individual. Personal goals and objectives, factors which support behaviour change for that individual, and the degree of self-control or external control required to sustain change should be established.

Suggested approaches which may be included in an individualized plan include:
• *Self-monitoring*: the patient may prefer to keep records of food intake and daily activities and to monitor his own weight.
• *External control*: it may be more effective if a group or another person assumes responsibility for monitoring weight changes and provides positive or negative reinforcement for change, as indicated.
• *Use of reinforcement techniques* to provide motivation and support for success. Rewards may be selected by the patient to promote maximum motivation; for example, new clothes might provide strong motivation for one individual but make another feel that the goals are unrealistic.
• *Regular eating habits* can also facilitate weight management. Specific times and places should be established for eating; the individual sits down to eat and takes time to enjoy the food. This helps to increase awareness of the amount of food consumed and decreases the frequency of taking snacks. 'Junk' foods should be avoided and only low calorie snacks permitted. Meals served on a smaller plate may appear greater in quantity.

Diet is selected with guidance from health professionals to ensure that essential nutrients and fibre are included and that non-essential high energy foods are restricted. The rate of weight loss

---

[10] Howe (1981), p. 213.
[11] Mahan (1979), p. 229.

should be controlled and effects on the individual monitored.

• *Activity and exercise* are essential for weight control. Exercise serves to expend energy, to provide diversion from eating, to increase feelings of well-being and improve self-image. The amount of exercise needed to expend energy is greater than most people realize (e.g. walking at a rate of 2½ miles per hour for a 68 kg (10¾ stone) person expends 210 kcal per hour). Vigorous activities such as tennis, skiing and running expend 400, 600 and 900 kcal in one hour for the same individual.[12] Exercise and activity should be regular and selected to fit into the individual's daily routine and life-style. Simple measures like walking up the stairs at work rather than using the lift increases activity without being time-consuming for the individual. Walking is an activity which most individuals can accomplish. Social interaction during exercise may also provide the incentive needed to continue the activity.

Maintenance of weight control is a life-long process and depends largely on the establishment of healthy eating habits and an activity and exercise regimen. Family members and friends can do much to reinforce the habits initiated during a weight management programme. Individual and group counselling sessions are useful in initiating and supporting attitudinal and behavioural changes.

EXPECTED OUTCOMES

The patient:
1 States the components of a nutritionally balanced diet.
2 Describes the effects of excessive weight and excessive body fat on health.
3 Describes and implements a plan to increase daily physical activity.
4 Eats a diet containing essential food groups.
5 Consumes fewer calories than used in energy expenditure.
6 Shows a progressive decrease in body weight towards the normal range.
7 Shows a progressive decrease in body fat as measured by skin-fold thickness and body circumferences.
8 Describes a plan to continue weight reduction and to maintain a balanced diet containing essential nutrients.

Undernutrition

Humans normally ingest food intermittently throughout each day with the period of fasting varying from a few hours to 12–14 hours. A typical daily Western European or North American diet consists of 2000–3000 kcal in the form of 40–45% carbohydrate, 40% fat and 15–20% protein. (See Table 19.3

---

[12] Howe (1981), p. 215.

for the NACNE and COMA recommendations on healthy eating.) Daily requirements vary with body size, physical activity and growth. Fat storage in adipose tissue provides the largest fuel reserves, consisting of 15–25% of body weight in an adult male. Protein, consisting of 12–17% of body weight in men, is found primarily in muscle tissue. Carbohydrate reserves consist of glycogen stored in the liver, muscle glycogen and circulating blood glucose. These reserves are adequate to meet the needs of the brain and physiological processes during the usual intervals between meals and during short periods of exercise. If fasting extends beyond 18–24 hours, these reserves are rapidly depleted.[13]

Undernutrition occurs when the energy intake is less than the energy expenditure. Body fat is depleted for energy, and protein, mineral and vitamin deficiencies develop. The individual is underweight compared to ideal-weight charts.

Smith describes starvation as a continuum that can be divided into three phases: 'the post-absorptive state (9–15 hours after food intake); short-term starvation (lasting to 7 days); and prolonged starvation (2 weeks or longer).'[14] During the post-absorptive state, three quarters of the glucose used to supply the energy needs of the brain, muscles and vital organs is provided from the carbohydrate stored in the liver and muscle and from circulating blood glucose. The remainder is formed from the mobilization and breakdown of fat. The blood glucose level is maintained but the catabolic processes are initiated during the first 24 hours of fasting. Short-term starvation is characterized by the breakdown of fat deposits, since the glycogen stores are already depleted. Plasma insulin levels decrease and glucagon levels rise, stimulating glyconeogenesis and ketogenesis. Blood glucose levels drop and ketones function as fuel for the brain. The ability of the brain to utilize ketone bodies as well as glucose for its energy needs prolongs survival by decreasing the need for body protein to be utilized for glucose production.

Prolonged starvation is characterized by continued fat breakdown and mobilization, gluconeogenesis and proteolysis. The rate of protein breakdown decreases as fasting continues and ketones are utilized for energy; analysis of urine samples show that less urea is eliminated and more ammonia is excreted. The blood glucose level stabilizes at a low level. The liver produces less glucose but some additional glucose is produced by the kidney. Insulin levels remain low and glucagon levels remain normal.

Causes
Undernutrition may result from inadequate food intake or a pathophysiological condition. The cause

---

[13] Smith & Thier (1985), p. 364.
[14] Smith & Thier (1985), p. 364 & 365.

of inadequate food intake may be: (1) famine, un-availability of food; (2) poverty, which prevents the individual from obtaining sufficient food; (3) inability to shop for or prepare food, such as may occur in the elderly, disabled or housebound individual; (4) the lack of knowledge of essential nutritional needs; (5) the influence of the mass media promoting nutritionally unbalanced 'junk foods'; (6) emotional disturbance; or (7) pathophysiological conditions. These include those which: interfere with ingestion, digestion, absorption and/or metabolism of food; increase the body's requirements for energy; or result in loss of body fluids and their constituents.

IDENTIFICATION OF PATIENT PROBLEMS

The problem is a nutritional intake of less than body requirements.
   Goals related to inadequate food intake are to:
1 Acquire knowledge of basic nutritional needs of the body
2 Gain weight by increasing body tissue
3 Identify and alleviate underlying physical and/or emotional disturbances

NURSING INTERVENTION

Malnutrition from inadequate food intake due to socioeconomic factors is a world-wide problem, existing in industrialized countries as well as in developing nations. Alleviation of this problem requires increasing the world's food supply and its distribution as well as providing economic assistance to those in need. Individuals and families require knowledge of basic nutritional needs as well as assistance in the selection and preparation of foods to ensure an adequate diet within the limits imposed by their sociocultural and economic situations.

   For the individual who is underweight because of inadequate intake of food although it is available, nursing intervention includes: (1) providing information about basic nutritional needs of the body. This may be by discussion and the provision of pamphlets which outline a dietary plan containing the essential food principles (see Tables 19.1 and 19.2); (2) identifying the causes of inadequate nutrition; and (3) assisting the individual to develop a diet regimen that will promote the development of body tissue. Being thin may be currently fashionable and peer pressure tends to reinforce the idea. Simply increasing kilocalories may serve only to increase body fat; the diet should be balanced and contain extra protein as well as carbohydrates and fats. Meals should be regular and between-meal snacks of protein and vitamins encouraged. Moderate activity serves to build body tissue but adequate and regular rest is essential to conserve energy and promote weight gain.

   When emotional disturbances are the primary factor of malnutrition as, for example in the patient with anorexia nervosa or bulimia, intervention is focused on identifying and correcting the underlying emotional cause. This is a long-term process that requires counselling and psychotherapy for the patient and usually the family as well. The person needs help to acquire a realistic appraisal of self and body which may be distorted. Harmful and bizarre behaviours need to be identified and attitudes changed. The patient may have to be admitted to hospital initially. Environmental change may also be helpful to initiate changes in eating patterns and attitudes toward food. Maintenance of changes in eating patterns and self-image takes time and continuous therapy but long-term results are often effective.

   Undernutrition in the hospital patient is now being recognized as a major problem. Hinson states that there is convincing evidence that many patients in hospital are malnourished yet the condition frequently goes unrecognized and untreated.[15] Malnutrition is believed to contribute to the frequency of complications experienced by patients and to increase their stay in hospital. The illnesses leading to admission serve to reduce further the nutritional status of patients. A nutritional assessment should be made on admission and at regular intervals throughout the hospital stay. Measures are required to improve the nutritional status of many patients, especially in intensive care and during the post-surgery period. Discussion of feeding supplements and total parenteral nutrition is found in Chapter 17. The management plan for nutritional deficits is specific to each patient and plans are instituted to maintain nutritional well-being following discharge (see Table 19.5).

EXPECTED OUTCOMES

The patient:
1 Demonstrates understanding of basic nutritional needs of the body.
2 Gains weight progressively towards the normal range.
3 Expresses awareness of underlying emotional disturbances.
4 Complies with the prescribed dietary regimen and, if indicated, with a counselling or psychotherapy programme.

Anorexia nervosa

This is usually but not exclusively a disease of adolescents and young women that is characterized by excessive weight loss and vomiting which is often chronic and self-induced. The cause is attributed to an underlying psychiatric disturbance but also involves disturbances of the neuroendocrine system (hypothalamus), which also may be secondary to the profound weight loss.[16]

   The weight loss and absence of body fat, which

---

[15] Hinson (1985), p. 53.
[16] Smith & Thier (1985), p. 541.

Table 19.5 Suggested nursing intervention to promote nutritional health of patients in hospital.

1 Be aware of the patient population at risk for undernutrition
2 Include a nutritional assessment as part of the admission nursing assessment for all patients
3 Compare assessment findings with standards for age and sex to identify nutritional deficiencies
4 Document patient's daily calorie and protein intake and daily weight
5 In conjunction with the dietitian, assess the patient's daily energy expenditure taking into consideration body temperature, emotional stress and the disease process
6 Identify dietary restrictions that are temporary, such as those related to surgery, or permanent, such as sodium and protein restrictions related to end-stage renal failure, lactose intolerance or food allergies
7 Develop a nutrition plan in conjunction with the dietitian to meet the protein, vitamin, mineral and calorie needs of the individual patient during hospitalization
8 Reassess the patient's nutritional status regularly throughout hospitalization
9 Implement a teaching programme to assist the patient and family to meet long term nutritional needs
10 Refer the patient and family to relevant community resources

may progress to emaciation, are due to inadequate energy intake. Menstruation ceases, alkalosis may be present from the repeated vomiting, diarrhoea may occur when food is ingested and the person usually manifests apathy, weakness and irritability. Absorption of nutrients is not affected. The patient demonstrates an obsession with losing weight, refuses to eat and may conceal uneaten food or induce vomiting. The patient is usually admitted to hospital for initial restoration of nutritional status, which will involve attempts to re-establish normal eating habits under supervision. Long-term psychotherapy is usually necessary and should involve the family as well as the patient. The family can play an important role in supporting positive behaviour and in providing an environment conducive to change, especially in relation to meal-time and eating patterns. Taking of meals and improvement in appearance due to weight gain should be acknowledged.

Bulimia

Bulimia is an eating disorder characterized by episodes of increased hunger and overeating. It occurs most often in teenage girls and, as in anorexia nervosa, when eaten the food is rejected by induced secretive vomiting or purging with laxatives. The episodes may be sporadic or occur several times a week. The client is thin but does not become emaciated like the person with anorexia nervosa. Brockopp and Hall note that the disorder may cause complications which include gastric ulceration, erosion of the tooth enamel from gastric acid and renal problems associated with an electrolyte imbalance.[17] The teenagers with bulimia are usually 'loners', depressed and obsessed with eating and weight control.

Intervention is directed towards changing the individual's attitude to food and eating and to interruption of the overeating and vomiting or purging. To be helpful and provide the necessary support, a trusting nurse–patient relationship is necessary. Unobtrusive supervision during meals and the post-meal period may be required to curtail the overeating followed by the rejection of the food. Family members are given support and encouragement and are counselled on their role in assisting the client. Psychotherapy may be necessary to deal with the patient's low self-image and difficulties in socializing and in expressing her feelings.

Disorders of carbohydrate metabolism

Diabetes mellitus is a common disorder of carbohydrate metabolism that affects a large number of persons and is characterized by hyperglycaemia. The reader is referred to Chapter 20 for a detailed discussion of the disorder and the care of patients with diabetes mellitus.

Hypoglycaemia may result from inadequate food intake. It may also occur in response to endocrine disorders of the pancreas, disorders of ingestion or liver dysfunction.

Disorders of fat metabolism

Diabetes mellitus, obesity and underweight are examples of disorders involving fat metabolism. Atherosclerosis is a chronic degenerative disease of the blood vessels characterized by the development of fatty plaques in the intima of the vessel walls (see p. 327). Diabetes mellitus, obesity, diet, smoking and genetic factors may predispose the individual to the development of the disease.

Disorders of protein metabolism

Protein deficiency results primarily from inadequate intake of the essential amino acids which cannot be synthesized in the body. Anaemia, underweight, fatigue and retarded growth are signs of protein deficiency. Kwashiorkor results from a diet deficient in the quality and quantity of protein in infancy and childhood despite an adequate total energy intake. Protein-calorie malnutrition (PCM) occurs when the diet lacks both protein and calories. Protein deficiencies may occur with disorders of the digestive system and with serious illnesses when excessive protein is lost, for example, burns, draining wounds, pressure sores and some renal diseases in which there is a loss of protein in the urine. Immobility is a further cause of protein loss and occurs in debilitated patients on bed rest.

---

[17] Brockopp & Hall (1984), p. 32.

References and Further Reading

BOOKS

Anderson SVD & Bauwens EE (1981) *Chronic Health Problems*. St Louis: CV Mosby. Chapter 14.

Coates VE (1985) *Are They Being Served?* London: RCN.

Davidson S, Passmore R, Brock JF & Truswell AS (1986) *Human Nutrition and Dietetics*. Edinburgh: Churchill Livingston.

Department of Health and Social Security (DHSS) (1979). Recommended Daily Amounts of Food Energy and Nutrients for Groups of People in the United Kingdom. London: HMSO.

Department of Health and Society Security (DHSS) (1984) *Committee on Medical Aspects of Food Policy 'Diet and Cardiovascular Disease'*. Report of the panel on diet in relation to cardiovascular disease. Report on Health and Social Subjects No. 28. ('The Coma Report') London: HMSO.

Dickerson JWT & Booth EM (1985) *Clinical Nutrition for Nurses, Dietitians and Other Health Care Professionals*. London: Faber and Faber.

Fields WL (1983) *Introduction to Health Assessment*. Reston, VA: Reston Publishing. Chapter 4.

Guyton AC (1986) *Textbook of Medical Physiology*, 7th ed. Philadelphia: WB Saunders. Chapters 67, 68 & 69.

Howe PS (1981) *Basic Nutrition in Health and Disease*, 7th ed. Philadelphia: WB Saunders.

Huskisson J (1985) *Applied Nutrition and Dietetics*. Eastbourne: Baillière Tindall.

Jones DC (1975) *Food for Thought*. London: RCN.

Kim MJ & Moritz DA (eds) (1982) *Classification of Nursing Diagnoses*. New York: McGraw-Hill.

Krause MV & Mahan LK (1984) *Food, Nutrition and Diet Therapy*, 7th ed. Philadelphia: WB Saunders.

Krupp MA & Chatton MJ (eds) (1983) *Current Medical Diagnosis and Treatment*. Los Altos, CA: Lange. Chapter 20.

Malasanos L, Barkauskas V, Moss M & Stoltenberg AK (1981) *Health Assessment*. St Louis: CV Mosby. Chapter 5.

Moghissi K & Boore J (1983) *Parenteral and Enteral Nutrition for Nurses*. London: William Heinemann.

Muir BL (1980) *Pathophysiology*. New York: John Wiley. Chapters 17 and 18.

National Advisory Committee on Nutrition Education (NACNE) (1983) *Guidelines for Health Education in Britain*. London: Health Education Council.

Pender NJ (1982) *Health Promotion in Nursing*. Nowalk, CT: Appleton-Century-Croft. Chapter 11.

Robbins SL, Angell M and Kumar V (1981) *Basic Pathology*, 3rd ed. Philadelphia; WB Saunders.

Smith LH & Thier SO (1985) *Pathophysiology*, 2nd ed. Philadelphia: WB Saunders. Section 6 & 7.

Vander AJ, Sherman JH & Luciano DS (1985) *Human Physiology: The Mechanisms of Body Function*, 4th ed. New York: McGraw-Hill. Chapter 15.

PERIODICALS

Anonymous (1981) Overeating anonymous: a self-help group. *Am. J. Nurs.*, Vol. 81 No. 3, pp. 560–563.

Bayer LM, Bauers CM & Kapp SR (1983) Psychosocial aspects of nutritional support. *Nurs. Clin. N. Am.*, Vol. 18 No. 1, pp. 119–128.

Blackburn GL & Thornton PA (1979) Nutritional assessment of the hospitalized patient. *Med. Clin. N. Am.*, Vol. 63 No. 5, pp. 1103–1115.

Brockopp DY & Hall SY (1984) Eating disorders: a teenage epidemic. *Nurse Pract.*, Vol. 9 No. 4, pp. 32, 34 & 35.

Buergel N (1979) Monitoring nutritional status in the clinical setting. *Nurs. Clin. N. Am.*, Vol. 14, No. 2, pp. 215–227.

Ciseaux A (1980) Anorexia nervosa: a view from the mirror. *Am. J. Nurs.*, Vol. 80 No. 8, pp. 1468–1470.

Claggett MS (1980) Anorexia nervosa: a behavioural approach. *Am. J. Nurs.*, Vol. 80 No. 8, pp. 1471–1472.

Crocker K, Gerber F & Shearer J (1983) Metabolism of carbohydrate, protein and fat. *Nurs. Clin. N. Am.*, Vol. 18 No. 1, pp. 3–28.

Goodinson SM & Homes S (1986) Nutrition *Add-on J. Clin. Nurs.*, Vol. 3 Nos 7 & 8.

Groer M & Pierce M (1981) Anorexia–cachexia. *Nursing*, Vol. 11 No. 6, pp. 39–43.

Hinson LR (1985) Nutritional assessment and management of the hospitalized patient. *Crit. Care Nurs.*, Vol. 5 No. 2, pp. 53–60.

Janes EMH (1986) Changing our eating habits. *Add-on J. Clin. Nurs.*, Vol. 3 No. 7, p. 269.

Kawasaki G, Benz LA, Redder L & Provo SrL (1980) Solving the very big problems of the morbidly obese. *Nurs. '80*, Vol. 10 No. 11, pp. 40–43.

Langford RW (1981) Teenagers and obesity. *Am. J. Nurs.*, Vol. 81 No. 3, pp. 556–559.

Lehmann A (1982) Anorexia nervosa: emancipation by emaciation. *Can. Nurs*, Vol. 78 No. 10, pp. 31–33.

Lehmann A (1983) Nutrition Now. *Can. Nurs*, Vol. 79 No. 3, pp. 24–28.

Mahan LK (1979) A sensible approach to the obese patient. *Nurs. Clin. N. Am.*, Vol. 14 No. 2, pp. 229–245.

Malloy MJ & Kane JP (1982) Hypolipidemia. *Med. Clin. N. Am.*, Vol. 66 No. 2, pp. 469–487.

McNamara RJ (1982) The challenge of treating eating disorders. Part 1: the role of the nurse at the bedside. *Can. Nurse*, Vol. 78 No. 10, pp. 34–40.

Miller BK (1981) Jejunoileal bypass: a drastic weight control measure. *Am. J. Nurs.*, Vol. 81 No. 3, pp. 564–568.

Mogan J (1984) Obesity: prevention is the treatment. *Pat. Educ. Couns.*, Vol. 6 No. 2, pp. 73–76.

Mojzisik CM & Martin EW (1981) Gastric partitioning; the latest surgical means to control morbid obesity. *Am. J. Nurs.*, Vol. 81 No. 3, pp. 569–572.

Orr J (1985) Obesity. *J. Adv. Nurs.*, Vol. 10 No. 1, pp. 71–78.

Potts NL (1984) Eating disorders: the secret pattern of binge/purge. *Am. J. Nurs.*, Vol. 84 No. 1, pp. 32–35.

Richardson TF (1980) Anorexia nervosa: an overview. *Am. J. Nurs.*, Vol. 80 No. 8, pp. 1470–1471.

Sanger E & Cassino T (1984) Eating disorders: avoiding the power struggle. *Am. J. Nurs.*, Vol. 84 No. 1, pp. 31–33.

Stotts NA & Firesen L (1982) Understanding starvation in the critically ill patient. *Heart Lung*, Vol. 11 No. 5, pp. 469–477.

Stout K (1982) The surgical treatment of morbid obesity. *Nurs. Clin. N. Am.*, Vol. 17 No. 2, pp. 245–250.

White JH (1982) An overview of obesity: its significance to nursing. *Nurs. Clin. N. Am.*, Vol. 17 No. 2, pp. 191–198.

White JH & Schroeder MA (1981) When your client has a weight problem: nursing assessment. *Am. J. Nurs.*, Vol. 81 No. 3, pp. 550–553.

20

Nursing in Disorders of the Endocrine System

The Endocrine System

Introduction

A gland is an organ which extracts substances from the blood and produces one or more new chemical substances, referred to as secretions. Glands may be classified as exocrine or endocrine. The secretion of an *exocrine gland* is carried along a duct into a body cavity or to the external surface of the body. Examples of such glands are the salivary, gastric, mammary and sweat glands. *Endocrine glands* do not have ducts; their secretions, which are called *hormones*, pass directly into the blood and act on remote tissues.

The glands usually cited as composing the *endocrine system* are the anterior and posterior pituitary glands, thyroid gland, four parathyroid glands, two adrenal (suprarenal) glands, islets of Langerhans and two gonads (ovaries or testes) (see Fig. 20.1).

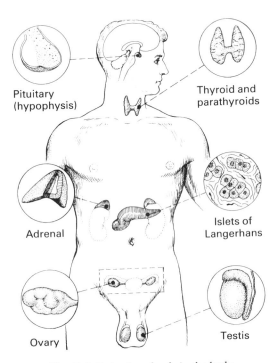

Pituitary (hypophysis)

Thyroid and parathyroids

Adrenal

Islets of Langerhans

Ovary

Testis

Fig. 20.1 Endocrine glands in the body.

Unlike other body systems in which the component organs are located close together and are connected, the glands are situated in various parts of the body. There are other organs which are known to demonstrate endocrine action through their liberation of chemical agents into the blood. They are not considered to be part of the endocrine system since they are a more integral part of other major systems. These include the gastrointestinal glands, which secrete gastrin, secretin and cholecystokinin-pancreozymin (see Chapter 17), and the kidneys, which secrete renin and the renal erythropoietic factor into the blood (see Chapter 21). The placenta, formed in pregnancy, also serves as an endocrine gland because of its production of progesterone, oestrogen and chorionic gonadotrophin.

Coordination and integration of the development and functions of the body that maintain homeostasis are dependent upon the nervous system and the endocrine system. The endocrine system is concerned mainly with growth, maturation, metabolic processes and reproduction. The action of each hormone is specific. One hormone may modify the activity of all body cells (e.g. thyroxine); others affect the activity of only one particular organ (e.g. adrenocorticotrophin). The site of action of any hormone is referred to as the *target organ or tissue*.

Target cells contain *receptors* for which specific hormones have an affinity. Some hormones are necessary for survival (e.g. adrenocorticoid); others are not essential to life (e.g. gonadal secretions).

MECHANISM OF HORMONE ACTION

Hormones are transported in the blood either freely in solution or in combination with a carrier protein. The water-soluble hormones, including the polypeptide and protein hormones, bind with the receptors on the surface of the target cells. The steroids and thyroid hormones require a carrier for transportation to the target cells and bind with intracellular receptors.

Hormones (the first messengers) which bind with surface receptors on the target cells act by altering a membrane-bound enzyme which stimulates the production of a 'second' messenger in the cell; the second messenger then activates enzymes within the cell to produce the specific cellular functions. The second messenger is believed in most instances to be cyclic adenosine monophosphate (CAMP).

Steroid hormones cross the membrane of cells containing their specific receptors and bind with the intracellular receptors. The receptor is altered by the hormone, allowing it to enter the cell nucleus and combine with the chromatin of certain genes. The messenger RNA is formed which migrates to the cell cytoplasm where it influences the synthesis of specific peptides and proteins. These peptides and proteins carry out the metabolic functions of the cells that were in the past attributed to the steroid hormones.

The precise mechanisms · for other hormone actions, such as the alteration of cell permeability to specific substances by insulin, the catecholamines and acetylcholine, are not known.[1]

REGULATION OF SECRETION

The production of endocrine secretions is generally controlled according to the need for their action; that is, production and release into the bloodstream are stimulated when their action is needed and are inhibited when the effect is achieved. Secretions by the pituitary gland are regulated by either hormonal or nervous signals originating in the hypothalamus. The control mechanism may be influenced by the blood concentration of the target organ, or by physicochemical processes. For example, regulation of secretion by the thyroid, adrenal cortices and the gonads is maintained by hormones which are produced by the anterior pituitary gland and are liberated in response to the blood concentration of the hormones of those glands. To illustrate, the anterior pituitary gland secretes a thyroid-stimulating hormone (TSH or thyrotropin), and the output of TSH is controlled by the level of thyroid hormones in the blood. This reciprocal arrangement is referred to as a *negative feedback mechanism*, in that the higher the level of thyroxine, the lower the level of TSH and vice versa. A hormone which stimulates the secretion of another hormone is referred to as a *trophic hormone*. An example of control by a *physicochemical process* is the influence of the osmotic pressure of the blood on the output of the antidiuretic hormone (see p. 631).

DYSFUNCTION

Disorders of an endocrine gland may incur an excess or deficiency of its hormone(s). Signs and symptoms of the disorder are predominantly manifestations of dysfunction in the target organ or tissues. Enlargement or outgrowths of a gland may also impose on neighbouring structures, interfering with their function(s).

PITUITARY GLAND (HYPOPHYSIS)

The pituitary gland is a very small gland located at the base of the brain in the sella turcica, a depression in the sphenoid bone. It lies just below the anterior part of the third ventricle and adjacent to the optic chiasm.[2] It is attached to the hypothalamus by a stalk, the *infundibulum*, which contains nerve fibres and blood vessels. The gland has two distinct parts: the anterior lobe, or anterior pituitary, and the posterior or neural lobe, (posterior pituitary). The anterior pituitary is an embryological outgrowth of the roof of the mouth and is completely separated from its origin. The posterior pituitary develops from the base of the brain, remaining connected to the hypothalamus by many nerve fibres (see Fig. 20.2).

The cells of the anterior pituitary are truly glandular in that they extract substances from the blood and secrete new chemicals (hormones). The posterior pituitary consists mainly of many terminal nerve fibres which originate with nerve cells (neurons) in the hypothalamus. The fibres are supported by non-secreting cells called *pituicytes*. The hormones released by the posterior pituitary are secreted by the neurons of the hypothalamus and are released at the nerve endings in the posterior pituitary.

Anterior pituitary lobe (adenohypophysis)

The anterior pituitary secretes the following hormones[3]:

- Thyroid-stimulating hormone (TSH)
- Growth hormone (GH)
- Prolactin (PRL), which affects lactation
- Adrenocorticotrophic hormone (ACTH), which stimulates the adrenal cortex
- ACTH-related peptides—beta lipotrophin (β-LPH) and alpha melanocyte stimulating hormone (MSH), and beta-endorphin (a substance with morphine-like actions). The MSH sequence of amino acids is found within LPH and ACTH. These molecules increase pigmentation of the skin and mucous membranes
- Follicle-stimulating hormone (FSH), which stimulates the development of mature Graafian follicles in women and stimulates spermatogenesis in men
- Luteinizing hormone (LH) which stimulates the development and maintenance of the corpus luteum in women; in men—where it is called interstitial cell-stimulating hormone (ICSH)—it affects secretion of testosterone

The cells of the anterior pituitary can be subjected to staining techniques which would histologically identify them as:

1 Eosinophil or acidophil cells. These cells produce GH
2 Basophil cells which are involved in the process of ACTH, lipotrophin (LPH) and beta-endorphin secretion. These cells are also involved in secretion of TSH, FSH, and LH

---

[1] Guyton (1986), pp. 880–881.

[2] For a description of the *optic chiasm* see Chapter 28.
[3] Dillon (1980), p. 215.

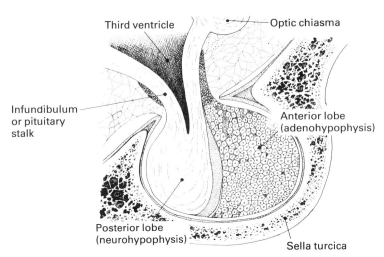

Fig. 20.2 The pituitary.

3 Chromophobe cells are probably non-secretory but are sometimes said to produce ACTH and LPH

Tumours are often classified according to this grouping, for example chromophobe adenomas.

More recently, cells have been reclassified by immunocytochemical and electron microscopic techniques as:

1 Somatotrophs—secrete GH
2 Corticotrophs—secrete ACTH, LPH and endorphins
3 Thyrotrophs—secrete TSH
4 Lactotrophs—secrete prolactin
5 Gonadotrophs—secrete LH and FSH

The hormones TSH, ACTH, FSH and LH stimulate other glands; GH, PRL and MSH act directly on tissues of the body.

A branch of the internal carotid artery supplies the anterior pituitary, but the blood is circulated through the lower hypothalamic tissue before entering the gland. It is carried from the hypothalamus in hypothalamic-hypophyseal portal vessels in the infundibulum (pituitary stalk) to the sinusoids of the anterior pituitary. Control of the various secretions is mediated by the hypothalamic releasing factors which are liberated by special hypothalamic neurons into the hypothalamic-hypophyseal portal system. On reaching the sinusoids, these substances influence the secretory activity of the respective glandular cells.

REGULATION OF ANTERIOR PITUITARY GLAND
SECRETIONS BY HYPOTHALMIC HORMONES

Hypothalamic hormones control, by stimulation or inhibition, the release of hormones from the pituitary gland.

The hypothalamic hormones comprise:
• Growth hormone releasing hormone (or factor) (GHRF)
• Growth hormone release inhibiting hormone (somatostatin; GHRIH)
• Thyrotrophin-releasing hormone (or factor) (TRH)
• Corticotrophin-releasing hormone (CRF)
• Gonadotrophin-releasing hormone (GnRH)
• Prolactin release inhibiting hormone (PIF)

FUNCTIONS OF THE ANTERIOR PITUITARY HORMONES

Fig. 20.3 depicts the metabolic functions of anterior pituitary hormones. The *growth hormone* is concerned with the growth of the body and plays an important role in determining a person's size. The most striking effect of the hormone is evidenced in the skeleton. Bones increase in length and thickness until late adolescence, the muscles enlarge and there is a corresponding growth of the viscera. Many metabolic processes are influenced by GH, and a positive nitrogen balance develops because of the increased use of proteins in tissue synthesis (i.e. fatty acids are mobilized from adipose tissue and used for energy). Growth is also dependent upon the secretion of normal amounts of other hormones. The thyroid hormones are necessary to maintain an adequate metabolic rate, and insulin must be available to promote glucose metabolism for the provision of energy. The growth hormone is diabetogenic; it increases the breakdown of glycogen in the liver, promotes the release of glucose into the blood and also produces an anti-insulin effect in muscles.[4] This promotes the synthesis and conservation of protein, conservation of glucose and utilization of fat.

The secretion of GH is controlled by the hypothalamus which produces two regulating hormones; one stimulates the release of GH and the other, somatostatin, inhibits the release of GH by the anterior pituitary. The secretion of GH is influenced by the

---

[4] Ganong (1985), p. 335.

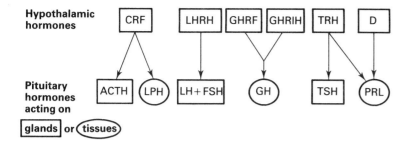

Hypothalamic hormones: CRF | LHRH | GHRF | GHRIH | TRH | D

Pituitary hormones acting on: ACTH | LPH | LH + FSH | GH | TSH | PRL

glands or tissues

Fig. 20.3 The principal direct relationships between the hypothalamus and the anterior pituitary. Hypothalamic releasing [R] and inhibiting [I] activities are described as hormones [H] when they have been chemically identified and synthesized, and as factors [F] while their recognition still depends upon biological activity only, as determined by *in vivo* or *in vitro* bioassay studies.
Key: CRF, Corticotrophin releasing factor; LHRH, Luteinizing hormone (follicle stimulating hormone) releasing hormone; GHRF, Growth hormone releasing factor; GHRIH, Growth hormone release inhibiting hormone (somatostatin); TRH, Thyrotrophin releasing hormone; D, Dopamine (Prolactin release inhibiting factor); ACTH, Adrenocorticotrophic hormone (corticotrophin); LPH, ß-lipotrophin; LH, Luteinizing hormone; FSH, Follicle stimulating hormone; GH, Growth hormone; TSH, Thyroid stimulating hormone (thyrotrophin); PRL, Prolactin.

state of nutrition; hypoglycaemia, fasting, exercise, stress and trauma increase its production. Hyperglycaemia and high concentrations of cortisol decrease the secretion.

Thyroid-stimulating hormone (TSH) promotes the growth and secretory activity of the thyroid gland, the function of which is the production of hormones which regulate the metabolic rate of all tissues. The production of TSH is regulated by a negative feedback mechanism. A decrease in the blood concentration of thyroid hormones increases the secretory output of thyrotropin; conversely, when the thyroid hormones reach a normal or above normal level, there is a reciprocal decrease in the release of thyrotropin.

Adrenocorticotrophic hormone (ACTH) has as its target organ the adrenal cortices, influencing their secretory output of several cortical secretions. ACTH secretion is regulated by an ACTH releasing factor produced in the hypothalamus in response to a decreased blood level of cortisone, or to nerve impulses initiated by biological stress (e.g. trauma, pain).

The *follicle-stimulating hormone (FSH)* causes the development of the ovarian follicle and the secretion of oestrogen. The secretion of FSH is reciprocally related to the blood level of oestrogen; FSH production is increased as the oestrogen level declines (see Chapter 23 for details of its role in the female menstrual cycle). In the male, FSH promotes the production of spermatozoa in conjunction with the male hormone testosterone.

Luteinizing hormone (LH) promotes ovulation and is necessary for the formation of the corpus luteum in the ruptured follicle. When the corpus luteum develops and secretes progesterone, the production of LH is suppressed. In the male, this hormone may be called the interstitial cell-stimulating hormone (ICSH) because it stimulates the production of the

male hormone testosterone by the interstitial cells of the testes.

Prolactin (PRL) stimulates the corpus luteum to secrete progesterone and initiates and stimulates the secretion of the mammary glands which have undergone preparatory changes in response to the oestrogen and progesterone blood levels. It is similar to luteinizing hormone. Its action in the male, if any, is undetermined.

An anterior pituitary hormone which is normally secreted in very small amounts in man is the *melanocyte-stimulating hormone (MSH)*, which increases skin pigmentation. Its chemical structure is similar to that of ACTH, and pigmentation of the skin may occur in the human with a high blood concentration of ACTH. Pigmented areas of the skin are frequently seen in persons with a deficiency of adrenocortical secretion which results in an increased, compensatory output of ACTH.

Posterior pituitary lobe

FUNCTIONS OF THE POSTERIOR PITUITARY HORMONES

Two hormones, the antidiuretic hormone (ADH) and oxytocin, are released by the posterior pituitary gland. ADH, also called vasopressin, increases the permeability of the distal and collecting tubules of the kidneys, resulting in increased reabsorption of water. Release of ADH by the posterior pituitary lobe is regulated by osmoreceptors in the hypothalamus. When the osmotic pressure of the blood is elevated (for example, because of dehydration or increased salt ingestion) the neurons sensitive to changes in the osmotic pressure of the blood transmit impulses to the posterior pituitary to release ADH into the circulating blood. Conversely, if the solute concentration of the blood is below normal, nerve impulses are not produced and release of ADH is inhibited.

The reduction in the blood concentration of ADH decreases the permeability of the renal tubules to water. A decrease in effective intravascular volume, regardless of osmolality, also results in a decrease in the secretion of vasopressin. This hormone plays an important role in maintaining normal fluid balance, and influences sodium ion concentration through its effect on the osmolality of the extracellular fluid. When it is present in large amounts, ADH stimulates a relatively transient, generalized vasoconstriction—hence the term vasopressin. Recent studies suggest that ADH plays a greater role in regulating blood pressure than was previously indicated.[5] ADH released into the general circulation is destroyed rapidly by enzymatic action, mainly in the liver and kidneys.

Oxytocin excites contractions of the pregnant uterus, especially during the latter part of gestation. The mechanism that prompts the release of oxytocin to initiate labour contractions is not known. Sensitivity of the uterine muscle to the hormone is thought to increase gradually throughout pregnancy, reaching a maximum at term. This hormone plays an important role in lactation; suckling initiates afferent nerve impulses which on reaching the hypothalamus bring about the liberation of oxytocin from the posterior pituitary gland. The hormone is carried by the blood to the mammary glands, stimulating the release and flow of milk. It is also suggested that oxytocin which is secreted during sexual stimulation of the female, promotes fertilization of the ovum by stimulating uterine contractions which propel the sperm towards the uterine tubes.[6]

THYROID GLAND

The thyroid is situated in the neck and consists of two lateral lobes, one on each side of the trachea immediately below the larynx. These lobes are connected by a band of tissue, the thyroid isthmus, lying across the anterior surface of the trachea (Fig. 20.4). The lobes contain numerous vesicles or follicles, and the walls of the follicles are composed of a layer of secreting cells. The follicles contain a clear, colloidal protein-iodine compound called thyroglobulin. The gland has an abundant blood supply; paired superior and inferior thyroid arteries arise from the external carotid and subclavian arteries.

Three hormones are produced and released into the blood. These are *triiodothyronine* (T_3) and *thyroxine* (T_4) which are produced by the follicular cells, and *calcitonin* (thyrocalcitonin, TCT) which is secreted by the parafollicular (C) cells. Thyroxine (T_4) occurs in greater amounts than (T_3). The thyroid hormones are formed by the combination of the amino acid tyrosine and iodine. The tyrosine mole-

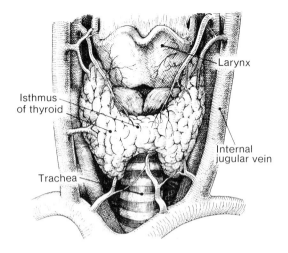

Fig. 20.4 The thyroid gland.

cule first combines with one or two iodine atoms to form monoiodotyrosine (MIT) or diiodotyrosine (DIT), respectively. Oxidative reactions, promoted by enzymes, combine these compounds to form T_3 and T_4 (MIT + DIT → T_3; DIT + DIT → T_4). T_3 and T_4 are stored in the thyroglobulin in the follicles. They are freed from the thyroglobulin and released into the blood as needed. In the blood most of the thyroid hormone combines loosely with a globulin fraction of the blood proteins from which it readily separates at cellular level.

The thyroid hormones (T_3 and T_4) increase the metabolic rate in most of the cells by stimulating oxidative processes. There is a notable increase in cellular activity, oxygen consumption and heat production. The hormones are essential for normal physical growth, maturation and mental development. The production and release of the thyroid hormones are controlled by TSH secreted by the anterior pituitary. It is also influenced indirectly by the nervous system through the hypothalamus, which is closely linked with the anterior pituitary via the hypothalamic-hypophyseal portal vessels. TSH promotes the uptake of available tyrosine and iodine as well as the release of the hormones from the thyroglobulin into the blood. A reciprocal or negative feedback relationship exists between TSH and the thyroid hormones. When the blood concentration of the thyroid hormones decreases, the hypothalamus produces a releasing factor (TRH) which alerts the anterior pituitary to release TSH. Production of TRH is influenced also by emotional factors and environmental temperatures. Conversely, with an increase in the thyroidal hormone concentration of the blood, a corresponding decrease of the TSH output occurs.

Calcitonin is secreted in response to an above-normal elevation in the blood calcium or an excess of glucagon in the blood. It lowers the serum calcium

---

[5] Guyton (1986), pp. 893–894.
[6] Guyton (1986), p. 895.

and phosphate levels by promoting their excretion in urine and movement into the bones.[7]

PARATHYROID GLANDS

The parathyroid glands are small oval bodies attached to the posterior surface of the lateral lobes of the thyroid (Fig. 20.5). The number may vary but is usually four. The principal secretion of the parathyroid glands is parathyroid hormone (PTH), which regulates the concentration of calcium and inorganic phosphorus in the blood through its action on the intestine, bone tissue and kidneys. It promotes absorption of calcium in the intestine and demineralization of bone and the movement of the calcium into the extracellular fluid. In the kidneys, the hormone increases the excretion of phosphorus by decreasing its reabsorption from the glomerular filtrate and conversely, the reabsorption of calcium is increased, decreasing its excretion in urine.

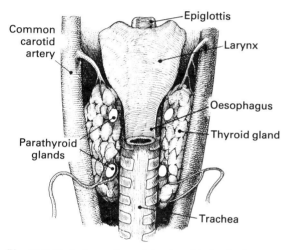

Fig. 20.5 Posterior surface of the thyroid gland, showing the parathyroid glands.

The parathyroid hormone, through its regulation of blood calcium and phosphorus levels, plays an important role in normal physiology. A normal concentration of calcium is essential for the normal structure of bones and teeth, coagulation of blood, maintenance of normal cardiac rhythmicity, normal neuromuscular excitability and cellular membrane permeability. The greater part of the absorbed calcium is deposited in bones. The optimal blood calcium level for meeting these functions is 2.2–2.6 mmol/l (8.5–10.5 mg/dl).[8] Phosphorus functions in cellular metabolism, bone structure and the maintenance of a normal pH of body fluids. The

normal blood concentration of serum phosphorus is 0.8–1.5 mmol/l (2.5–4.8 mg/dl).[9]

The rate of secretion of the parathyroid hormone is controlled by the concentration of calcium in the blood. When the calcium level rises above normal, the glands are inhibited and less hormone is produced. A fall in the blood calcium level stimulates the glands, resulting in an increased output of PTH.

Calcitonin is secreted by the C cells of the thyroid and has the opposite effect on blood calcium as that of PTH. Output is stimulated by an elevation in the calcium of the blood. It inhibits bone resorption and promotes the excretion of calcium and phosphorus in urine and the movement of calcium into the bones.

In summary, a feedback system exists between the parathyroid glands and the circulating blood calcium level. Following a decrease in calcium concentration there is an increased secretion of the parathyroid hormone. The hormone thus acts to: (1) raise the serum calcium level; (2) lower the serum phosphorus level; (3) decrease the urinary output of calcium; (4) increase the renal excretion of phosphate; and (5) promote the movement of calcium from the bones and the absorption of calcium from the intestine. A feedback mechanism also operates to regulate the secretion of calcitonin; hypercalcaemia stimulates its production.

ADRENAL GLANDS

The two adrenal or suprarenal glands are situated immediately above the kidneys. Each one is enclosed within a capsule and consists of two distinct parts, the cortex and medulla, which are functionally unrelated and are of different embryological origin. The cortex develops from germinal mesodermal cells. The medulla is derived from the ectoderm in close association with the sympathetic division of the autonomic nervous system with which it is functionally related. The adrenal glands have an abundant blood supply through branches of the aorta and the inferior phrenic and renal arteries.

The adrenal cortex

The cortex forms the outer part as well as the greater portion of the gland and produces hormones essential to life. These are steroids and collectively are called the *adrenocorticoids*, corticosteroids or corticoids. Cells of the cortex have a high cholesterol and vitamin C content which is used in the production of many steroid substances. Those secreted in physiologically significant amounts fall into three classes: mineralocorticoids, glucocorticoids and sex hormones. The steroids in each of these classes have some predominant characteristics or actions, but may overlap into another class. There are three zones

---

[7] Dillon (1980), p. 406.
[8] Macleod (1984), p. 906.

[9] Hassan (1985), p. 245.

or groups of cells: the outer one (zona glomerulosa) secretes the mineralocorticoids; the middle, thicker area of cells (zona fasciculata) secretes the glucocorticoids; and the inner layer of cells (zona reticularis) adjacent to the medulla secretes the adrenal sex hormones (androgens and oestrogen).

MINERALOCORTICOIDS

Mineralocorticoids are essential to life. The most significant one is *aldosterone*, which influences electrolyte concentrations and fluid volume. It stimulates the renal tubules to reabsorb sodium and excrete potassium, and it decreases the sodium concentration while increasing the potassium content of saliva, gastric secretion and sweat. An increase in the level of circulating aldosterone causes an increase in the serum sodium level, and that in interstitial fluid. The consequent elevation in their osmotic pressure causes an increased release of the ADH and a resultant retention of water. Conversely, a decreased output of aldosterone reverses these reactions.

The secretion of aldosterone is regulated in the interest of maintaining a normal sodium concentration and normal fluid volume. Factors which influence the amount of aldosterone released are the blood sodium and potassium levels and the blood volume. A decrease in the sodium concentration stimulates an increased output of aldosterone and, conversely, a rise in sodium to above the normal level decreases the output of the hormone. The effect of potassium is the reverse of that of sodium; that is, the adrenal cortices respond to an elevated potassium concentration by an increased secretion of aldosterone and vice versa. Decreases in renal arterial blood pressure such as occur in shock, physical trauma and haemorrhage increase renin secretion by the kidneys. The production of angiotensin II that results from the release of renin (see p. 690) stimulates the adrenal cortex to secrete aldosterone. The adrenocorticotrophic hormone (ACTH) also stimulates the secretion of aldosterone as well as glucocorticoids, but more is required than that necessary to initiate an output of glucocorticoids.

GLUCOCORTICOIDS

Several glucocorticoids have been recognized, but *cortisol* (hydrocortisone) is considered to be the most important, since it is more potent and is produced in much greater amounts than the other cortical hormones. Cortisol influences the metabolism of glucose, protein and fat, and is involved in the body's responses to physical and mental stress. Its actions are complex and not clearly understood; for example, it enables a person to deal more effectively with stress, but how this is achieved is not known. Cortisol elevates the blood sugar level and the liver glycogen stores are increased. Tissue protein is broken down and the amino acids are converted to

glycogen or glucose in the liver (gluconeogenesis). Fat is also mobilized, some of which is also converted to glucose.

Glucocorticoids are secreted in response to circulating ACTH. In turn, the production and release of ACTH by the anterior pituitary depends upon the release of corticotrophin-releasing hormone (CRH) which is secreted by the hypothalamus and delivered to the corticotrophs of the anterior pituitary. The production of CRH is influenced by a negative feedback mechanism; that is, a low concentration of adrenocorticoid secretions in the blood initiates the hypothalamic responses. With an elevation of blood glucocorticoids, the output of ACTH is depressed. Physical and psychological stress and hypoglycaemia also stimulate the release of CRH through impulses delivered from the cerebral cortex or midbrain to the hypothalamus. ACTH is secreted in diurnal rhythm; the secretory output is highest in the morning and lowest in the evening.

A concentration of cortisol in excess of the normal is of clinical significance because it suppresses local inflammatory responses to irritating substances (antiinflammatory effect), delays healing through depressed fibroplasia and reduces tissue sensitivity reactions to antigens (antiallergic reaction). Glucocorticoids have a tissue-wasting effect; they promote the breakdown of body proteins and tend to inhibit amino acid uptake and tissue synthesis. Other effects also associated with an excess of cortisol are atrophy of the lymphoid tissues, a decreased production of antibodies, an increased secretion of gastric hydrochloric acid and pepsinogen which predisposes to the development of ulcers, and increased cerebral excitability manifested by restlessness and euphoria. The glucocorticoids, as well as the mineralocorticoids, may also cause some sodium retention, resulting in a positive fluid balance.

ADRENAL SEX HORMONES

The adrenal cortices of both sexes secrete both male and female hormones—namely, *androgens, oestrogen* and *progesterone*. Oestrogen and progesterone are produced in lesser amounts than the androgens but, normally, the quantity of any of these hormones is considered to be physiologically insignificant compared with the amounts produced by the gonads. Occasionally, tumours of the adrenal cortex may result in an excessive production of the sex hormones, leading to precocious sexual development in childhood, masculinizing changes in the female adult or feminization in the case of an adult male.

Adrenal medulla

The medulla forms the central portion of each adrenal gland and is composed of specialized neurons (nerve cells) which secrete two hormones, *adrenaline* and *noradrenaline*. Because of their chemical composition, they are frequently referred to as catecholamines. During any stress or threat to the organism, the hormones are released and serve with the autonomic nervous system to produce defensive reactions throughout the body. Their production is controlled by nerve impulses transmitted to the medullae by sympathetic nerve fibres, and their effects are similar to those produced by sympathetic innervation. Approximately 80% of the secretion is adrenaline and the remainder is noradrenaline.

Adrenaline causes constriction of the peripheral and renal blood vessels and dilatation of the coronary and skeletal muscle vessels. The rate and force of contraction of the heart and skeletal muscle is increased. The smooth muscle of the bronchioles, gastrointestinal tract and urinary bladder relaxes. The dilator muscle fibres of the irises contract, resulting in dilatation of the pupils. The blood sugar is elevated by increased glycogenolysis (conversion of glycogen to glucose) in both the liver and skeletal muscles. The metabolic rate is accelerated, and there is an increased alertness and awareness due to stimulation of the brain. Adrenaline also promotes the release of ACTH, which in turn increases the secretion of glucocorticoids.

Noradrenaline causes a more generalized vasoconstriction and does not cause dilatation of any vessels. Because of this action, it is more effective in raising the blood pressure; both systolic and diastolic blood pressures rise.

PANCREAS (ISLETS OF LANGERHANS)

The pancreas is both an exocrine and endocrine gland. Its exocrine secretions are carried by a system of ducts to the duodenum and contain enzymes which play an important role in digestion (see p. 489). The islets of Langerhans form the endocrine component of the pancreas and consist of irregularly scattered groups of cells which are totally independent of the pancreatic system of ducts (see Fig. 20.6). The islets are highly vascularized and consist of four types of cells: alpha cells, which secrete the hormone glucagon; beta cells, which produce insulin; delta cells, which may secrete small amounts of gastrin and somatostatin (growth hormone-releasing inhibiting hormone) (GHRIH); and F cells which secrete pancreatic polypeptide. Insulin and glucagon are proteins and are rendered inactive in the gastrointestinal tract by the proteolytic enzymes: when prescribed, they must be administered parenterally.

SECRETIONS AND FUNCTIONS

Insulin
This hormone plays a dominant role in carbohydrate, fat and protein metabolism, especially in the liver and muscular and adipose tissues. Fig. 20.7

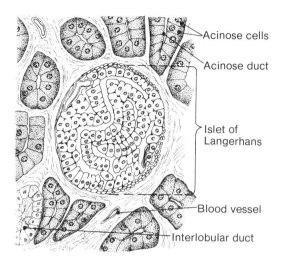

Fig. 20.6 Location of cells of islets of Langerhans between lobules of pancreas.

Acinose cells
Acinose duct
Islet of Langerhans
Blood vessel
Interlobular duct

depicts the production, release, transport and action of insulin on cells of peripheral tissues. Knowledge of the ways in which insulin promotes specific metabolic cellular activities is incomplete, but it has been established that it binds to receptors in cell membranes and stimulates the following actions: (1) the transfer of glucose into most cells and its metabolism by those cells[10]; (2) the formation of glycogen by the liver and muscle cells; (3) the synthesis of fatty acids and storage of fat in adipose tissue; (4) the uptake and incorporation of amino acids into cell proteins; and (5) an increased uptake of potassium by cells. These activities result in a lower concentration of glucose in the blood.

The chemical structure and composition of the insulin that is initially secreted by the beta cells is called preproinsulin.[11] This is rapidly broken down to form a large molecule called proinsulin. Proinsulin undergoes chemical changes which are activated by proteolytic enzymes within the cells to form insulin.

The secretion of insulin is regulated by a variety of stimulatory and inhibiting factors most of which are related to glucose metabolism or the cyclic AMP system. The concentration of blood glucose is the major controlling factor. An elevation increases the production of insulin and, conversely, a decrease below the normal blood level of glucose suppresses its secretion. Thus, a positive feedback mechanism is established which controls the output of insulin in order to maintain the blood sugar level within a normal range. Some amino acids have a similar effect on insulin secretion. Their action is enhanced when glucose levels are elevated. The synthesis of insulin

[10] Not all cells are *insulin-dependent* for the transfer of glucose. Notable in this respect are the brain cells, erythrocytes, kidney tubules and intestinal mucosa.
[11] Smith & Thier (1985), pp. 349–350.

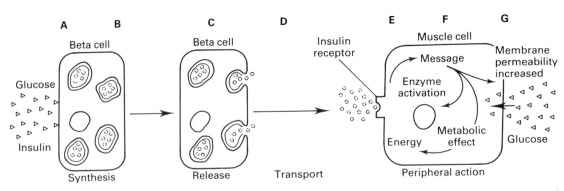

Fig. 20.7 Actions of insulin. The rise in blood glucose associated with a carbohydrate meal induces the beta cells in the islets of Langerhans to secrete insulin into the circulation. The insulin is then carried in the bloodstream to target cells throughout the body, where it binds to receptor molecules on the cell surface. This interaction triggers a series of events inside the cells that enhances the uptake of glucose from the blood and its subsequent breakdown for metabolic energy or storage as glycogen (animal starch) and fat. A defect anywhere along this pathway could result in diabetes. Possible causes include destruction of beta cells (a), abnormal synthesis of insulin (b), retarded release of insulin (c), inactivation of insulin in the bloodstream by antibodies or other blocking agents (d), altered insulin receptors or a decreased number of receptors on peripheral cells (e), defective processing of the insulin message within the target cells (f), and abnormal metabolism of glucose (g). Current evidence points to the beta cell as site of the primary defect in juvenile onset diabetes.

is also stimulated by an excess of growth hormone and glucocorticoids but somatostatin is an inhibitor of both insulin and glucagon secretion.[12] The glucocorticoid hormones act by decreasing intracellular AMP. The amount of insulin circulated in the blood increases when carbohydrate foods are ingested; this is attributed to the effect of the gastrointestinal hormones (e.g. gastrin, secretin, cholecystokinin-pancreozymin) on the beta cells. Glucose given intravenously does not produce the same effect as when it is taken orally.

Calcium ions are necessary for the release of insulin by the beta cells. Other factors that result in an increased insulin level include vagal nerve stimulation and oral hypoglycaemic agents.

Glucagon
This hormone may also be referred to as the hyperglycaemic factor, since its primary effect is stimulation of glycogenolysis (the conversion of glycogen to glucose) and its release into the blood by the liver to increase the blood glucose concentration. It also promotes gluconeogenesis, lipolysis, and secretion of the growth hormone and insulin. Its secretion by the alpha cells is stimulated by a low blood sugar level. An oral intake of proteins initiates an increased secretion of glucagon, greater than that seen in response to intravenous administration of amino acids. This suggests a gastrointestinal hormone that stimulates the secretion of glucagon. Sympathetic nervous stimulation of the pancreas also increases the glucagon output.[12a]

Somatostatin (growth hormone-release inhibiting hormone, GHRIH)
This hormone is found in cells of the hypothalamus, where it passes down the portal vessels to the anterior pituitary, gastrointestinal tract and islets of Langerhans. It inhibits the secretion of insulin, glucagon, pancreatic polypeptide, GH and various gastrointestinal hormones. It interferes with carbohydrate absorption and possibly with the absorption of protein and fat.[12b]

Pancreatic polypeptide
This hormone is known to decrease glycogen in the liver and may affect gastrointestinal secretion. Release of the hormone is stimulated by protein ingestion, fasting, exercise and hypoglycaemia.[12c]

BLOOD SUGAR LEVEL

The normal blood sugar (glucose) level 3–4 hours after a meal varies from approximately 6.5–7.5 mmol/l. Fluctuations occur as a result of energy expenditure and the ingestion of foods. The types of food taken also influence the degree of change; obviously, a meal high in carbohydrate produces a greater concentration of glucose for a period of time than a meal with a low carbohydrate content. An elevation of the blood sugar level above the normal is known as *hyperglycaemia*. A level below normal is referred to as *hypoglycaemia*.

As cited previously, the blood sugar level is regulated by the hormones of the islets of Langerhans (insulin, glucagon and somatostatin). It may,

[12] Keele, Neil & Joels (1982).
[12a] Smith & Thier (1985), pp. 357–358.
[12b] Smith & Thier (1985), p. 362.
[12c] Ganong (1985), p. 288.

however, be influenced by several other endocrine secretions. An excess of GH produces a tendency toward hyperglycaemia by decreasing the utilization of glucose and stimulating the production of glucagon. The release of glucocorticoids (cortisol) by the adrenal cortices promotes gluconeogenesis (formation of glucose from amino acids and the glycerol portion of fat), resulting in an elevation of the blood sugar. Adrenaline and noradrenaline stimulate liver glycogenolysis and the metabolism of muscle glycogen to lactic acid, which is then converted to glucose by the liver. The thyroid hormones also increase the blood sugar level by an acceleration of gluconeogenesis.

Endocrine Disorders

ASSESSMENT

Disorders of the endocrine system produce varied specific and non-specific manifestations. The effects are demonstrated by increased or decreased function of the target tissue. Assessment of endocrine disturbances requires a review of most body systems.

HISTORY

The history should include detailed information about the patient's past state of health, growth and development. Questions relate to changes in growth pattern, general rate of growth, development of secondary sex characteristics and abnormalities of secondary sex characteristics (for example facial hair in females, enlarged breasts in males). Changes in appetite, weight, memory retention, skin, hair and urinary elimination are determined. The patient is asked about past illnesses associated with the endocrine system including diabetes, thyroid disease, renal calculi, and hypertension. The menstrual pattern, age of onset and current changes are determined in the female. Family history related to endocrine disorders, growth and metabolic disorders are determined.

Information related to the patient's present state of health includes weight changes, appetite, the presence of obesity, tremors, palpitations, nervousness, sweating and weakness. How the patient usually responds to stressful physical and emotional events is elicited in detail and recent changes in these responses are also recorded. It would be helpful to know if there have been changes in sexual desire and activity.

Information about the patient's life-style includes occupation, degree of stress concerned with the job or at home, usual daily routine and effects of his or her present symptoms on daily activities and life-style.

PHYSICAL EXAMINATION

The presence of endocrine disorders generally requires an assessment of most body systems. The endocrine glands are not readily palpable, except the thyroid gland; physical assessment may provide information about the effects of the endocrine disorders on other systems of the body.

- *General appearance.* The patient's general appearance, body build and fat distribution provide valuable information about endocrine abnormalities and overall growth and development of the individual.
- *Body weight and vital signs.* The patient's weight and vital signs (temperature, pulse rate and rhythm, respirations and blood pressure) are recorded.
- *Skin, hair and nails.* The skin is observed and palpated for pigmentation, dryness, oiliness, elasticity, hydration, temperature and breaks in the integrity and any resulting discharge. The pattern of distribution and amount of body hair are observed and the texture and dryness noted. Nails are observed for thickness and changes in growth.
- *Genitalia and breasts.* The genitalia of the male and female are observed for size and shape and the breasts are examined to assess development and maturation.
- *Neurological examination* may be done in detail if degenerative changes are noted in the examination or history. Changes in sensation, pain, discomfort, reflexes and muscle tone are noted. The patient's speech is carefully listened to for huskiness, slurring, hoarseness, volume and pitch and rationality.
- *Achilles tendon reflex time.* This test may be carried out during the physical examination. The extent of the response of the foot to a tap on the Achilles tendon and the time involved in the rise and fall of the foot are measured by a special machine. The patient with an overactive thyroid records a more rapid and greater response; a lesser response over a longer period is characteristic of hypothyroidism.
- *Thyroid gland.* The thyroid gland is observed by facing the patient and having the patient extend his neck slightly and swallow a sip of water. The neck is observed for movement of cartilages and muscles and the shape and contour of any mass. Normally the thyroid gland is not observed and is not palpable. The gland is palpated using either a posterior or anterior approach by placing the fingers of both hands on the sides of the patient's neck with the finger tips meeting in the centre. The patient is asked to swallow to facilitate palpation during movement. If the gland is felt, the

degree of firmness of the tissue and the presence of any nodules are noted.

Tests used in assessing pituitary function (see Table 20.1)

Serum growth hormone (GH). Fasting levels of serum GH may be determined by radioimmunoassay.

Normal: adult male, 0–238 pmol/l (0–5 ng/ml); adult female, <380 pmol/l (<8 ng/ml); prepubertal child, <238 pmol/l (<5 ng/ml).

Growth hormone stimulation test. Base-line fasting blood levels of serum GH, glucose, cortisol and insulin are determined. The test consists of the intravenous administration of insulin followed by the determination of GH levels at 0, 15, 30 and 60 minutes. Other stimulation tests may be used, such as levadopa and glucagon.

Normally, GH levels increase in response to insulin stimulation.

Growth hormone suppression test. Glucose is administered orally or intravenously as in a glucose tolerance test. Normally, the level of GH will decrease.

Serum hormone levels for other pituitary hormones may also be determined.

Urine and serum osmolality tests. These tests are used to evaluate ADH regulation. Normally, urine osmolality is higher than serum osmolality. With an ADH deficiency, the urinary output increases and plasma concentrations of sodium increase.

Normal: serum osmolality, 275–295 mosmol/kg; Urine osmolality, maximum dilution 50 mosmol/kg, maximum concentration 800–1500 mosmol/kg.

Water deprivation tests (Mosenthal test). ADH secretion is normally stimulated when water is withheld and the urine output decreases. The test involves withholding fluids for up to 8 hours and measuring the urinary output and osmolality of each voiding. Plasma osmolality tests are made also, and the patient's weight loss is recorded. Failure to increase urine osmolality and the presence of increased plasma osmolality are characteristic of diabetes insipidus.

Serum and urine ADH concentrations. Levels of ADH in the serum and urine are measured by radioimmunoassay but these tests are not routinely available.

Radiological studies. These include x-rays of the sella turcica and computerized axial tomography (CAT) scan. Radiological examination of the sella turcica demonstrates changes in its size, shape and density. Tumours may be identified by a CAT scan.

Tests used in assessing thyroid function

Serum thyroxine (T_4). The total amount of the thyroid hormone in the blood is determined by radioimmunoassay.

Normal: 50–150 mmol/l (411 μg/dl).

Thyroid-stimulating hormone (TSH) radioimmunoassay. The serum level of the TSH is determined to detect if the problem is at the pituitary or thyroid level. This is a particularly valuable test if there is a deficiency of thyroid hormones.

Normal: 0–7 m μu/ml.

Serum triiodothyronine (T_3) concentration. Again, this is measured by radioimmunoassay.

Normal range: 1.2–3.1 nmol/l (80–200 ng/dl).

Radioactive iodine uptake. This test determines the rate at which the thyroid is removing iodine from the blood and using it. The patient receives a small (tracer) oral dose of radioiodine (I^{131}) in water. The amount concentrated in the thyroid over a given period of time is determined, for example, 8, 24 and 48 hours later by placing a Geiger counter over the neck. A hyperactive thyroid will have a high uptake, and an underactive gland will show a lower concentration than normal. The distribution of radioactivity may also indicate a difference in the degree of activity in different areas of the gland. Radioactivity of blood samples should be taken and compared with gland uptake. False results can occur if iodine has been taken prior to the test. This test is now used less often than it was.

Normal value: At 24 hours, 15–30% of that administered is absorbed by the thyroid.

T_3 suppression test. This test of thyroid function is based on the homeostatic balance between the production and release of thyroid hormones and their blood concentration which is regulated by the hypothalamus–pituitary–thyroid system. When a preparation of thyroid hormone is administered, raising the blood concentration of the hormone, the activity of a normal thyroid is suppressed; the output of hormones is decreased in order to establish the normal blood level. If the thyroid is hyperactive, the administration of thyroid hormone will not suppress its activity.

The suppression test involves a repeat radioiodine uptake test which is following the daily administration of T_3 for 7 days. The uptake of the normal thyroid will be considerably less in the second test. Failure of the increased blood concentration of the

Table 20.1 Diagnostic tests used in assessing endocrine function.

Diagnostic tests	Normal value	Description
Pituitary function		
Serum growth hormone (GH)	Adult: male, 0–238 pmol/l (0–5 ng/ml); female, < 380 pmol/l (8 ng/ml) Prepubertal child: < 238 pmol/l (< 5 ng/ml)	Fasting levels are determined by radioimmunoassay
Growth hormone stimulation test	GH levels increase in response to insulin stimulation	Insulin or another stimulant is administered intravenously. GH levels are made at 0, 15, 30 and 60 minutes and are compared to base-line levels
Growth hormone suppression test	The level of GH decreases in response to glucose suppression	Glucose is administered orally or intravenously
Serum and urine osmolality	Serum: 275–295 mosm/kg Urine: Maximum dilution, 50 mosmol/kg Maximum concentration, 800–1500 mosmol/kg	Used to evaluate ADH regulation With ADH deficiency, urine output increases and plasma concentrations of sodium increase
Water deprivation test	Increased urine osmolality and decreased urine output	Fluid is withheld for 8 hours and the volume and osmolality of each voiding is measured Serum osmolality is determined and weight loss is recorded
Serum and urine ADH concentration	Serum osmolality: 285 mosmol/kg (0–2 pg/ml) Urine osmolality: > 290 mosmol/kg (2–12+ pg/ml)	Levels of ADH in urine and serum are measured by radioimmunoassay
Radiological studies of the sella turcica		X-rays and computerized axial tomography (CAT) scans of the sella turcica show changes in its size, shape and density
Thyroid function		
Serum thyroxine (T_4)	50–150 mmol/l	The total amount of thyroid hormone in the blood
Thyroid stimulating hormone (TSH) radioimmunoassay	0–7 μu/ml	The serum level of TSH
Serum triiodothyronine test (T_3)	1.2–3.1 nmol/l	Radioimmunoassay to determine the serum level of T_3
Thyrotrophin-releasing hormone (TRH) test	Increased levels of TSH	The thyrotropic cells are normally stimulated by the intravenous administration of synthetic TRH to release TSH
Radioactive iodine thyroid uptake (RAIU)	At 24 hours: 15–30% absorbed	Determines the rate at which the thyroid removes iodine from the blood and uses it
T_3 suppression test	25% decrease in radioiodine uptake in the second test	A 24-hour radioiodine uptake is followed by daily administration of thyroid hormone for 7 days. The radioiodine uptake test is then repeated
T_3 resin uptake test	25–35%	T_3 tagged with radioiodine is added to a specimen of the patient's blood. The amount of binding by the erythrocytes is noted
Thyroid scan	Symmetrical with no areas of increased density	A scan is made of the thyroid following administration of a tracer dose of I^{131}
Achilles tendon reflex time	240–380 ms	The relaxation time is prolonged in hypothyroidism and more rapid and greater in hyperthyroidism

Table 20.1—*continued*

Diagnostic tests	Normal value	Description
Thyroid stimulation test	A normal radioiodine uptake and normal protein-bound iodine indicate the problem is related to secretion of TSH and not thyroid function	The response of the thyroid to an injection of TSH is measured by a radioactive uptake or a serum protein-bound iodine estimation
Thyroid antibody tests	Increased levels demonstrate involvement of immune system	Antibodies commonly measured are thyroglobin, thyroid microsomes, thyroid colloidal proteins and antinuclear antibodies
Parathyroid function		
Serum parathyroid hormone (PTH)	C-terminal PTH: 150–375 pgEq/ml Intact PTH: 163–347 pgEq/ml	Determine by two radioimunoassay tests
Serum calcium	Adult: 2.2–2.6 mmol/l (8.5–10.5 mg/dl)	Serum calcium increases with hyperparathyroidism and decreases with hypofunction of the parathyroid glands
Serum phosphorus	0.8–1.3 mmol/l (2.5–4.8 mg/dl)	Serum phosphorus levels increase with hypoparathyroidism and decrease with hyperparathyroidism
Urine calcium	25–75 mmol/24 h (100–300 mg/24 h)	The levels of calcium in the urine reflect changes in serum levels
Adrenocortical function		
Plasma cortisol concentration	a.m. specimen: 200–690 nmol/l (7.25 µg/dl) p.m. specimen: 8.0–220 mmol/l (3–8 µg/dl)	Plasma cortisol concentration is normally greatest 1–2 hours after awakening and is lowest 2–3 hours after going to sleep
Adrenocorticotrophic hormone (ACTH)	a.m. specimen: 2–18 pmol/l (10–80 ng/l) p.m. specimen: < 2 pmol/l (< 10 ng/l)	Fasting level of ACTH
ACTH stimulation	Increased level of plasma cortisol	ACTH is injected following the initial elevation of plasma cortisol and a second plasma level determined
Dexamethasone suppression test	50% reduction in plasma cortisol and 17-hydroxycorticosteriod in the urine	Dexamethasone, a synthetic glucocorticoid suppresses plasma cortisol and 17-hydroxycorticosteriod is decreased in the urine
Metyrapone test	The level of 17-hydroxycorticosteroid in the urine would be double the base-line level (base-line: male, 8–20 mg/24 h; female, 6–15 mg/24 h)	An accumulation of the precursor to cortisol (11-desoxycortisol) in the serum indicates that ACTH is being released and that the adrenal cortices are responding. Levels of 17-hydroxycorticosteroid in the urine are similarly elevated
Urinary excretion of 17-hydroxycorticosteroids	Adult: 28–90 µmol/l	Ketosteroids are metabolic products of androgens and glucosteroids. Their level is measured over 24 hours
Aldosterone concentration	Serum: 140–500 pmol/l (when patient is supine) Levels increase when the patient is upright Urine: 5–20 ng/24 h	Plasma levels of aldosterone alter in relation to ACTH, potassium and sodium levels. Urine measurement requires a 24 hour specimen
VMA (vanillylmandelic acid) concentration	9–34 µmol/24 h (1.8–6.8 mg/24 h)	This is the principle urinary metabolite of noradrenaline and adrenaline
Blood chemistry Sodium Potassium	Sodium: 135–145 mmol/l Potassium: 3.5–5.5 mmol/l Normal ratio Na:K, approximately 1:30	In adrenocortical insufficiency, the sodium level is below normal and the potassium level is elevated. The sodium/potassium ratio is decreased
Fasting blood sugar (glucose)	3.9–6.1 mmol/l (65–100 mg/dl)	Below normal with decreased adrenocorticoid secretion and above normal with hypersecretion

Table 20.1—*continued*

Diagnostic tests	Normal value	Description
Endocrine pancreas function		
Serum insulin	4–24 μU/ml	Determined by radioisotope immunoassay. It is useful in evaluating fasting hypoglycaemia
Urinalysis for glucose and ketone bodies	Glucose: negative Ketone: negative	The presence of glucose in the urine indicates the blood glucose level is above the renal threshold indicating either a low renal threshold or possibly diabetes mellitus. A negative reading indicates only that the blood glucose is below the patient's renal threshold
Blood glucose	Fasting range 3.9–6.1 mmol/l (65–100 mg/dl)	Provides the most accurate assessment of diabetic control
Glucose tolerance test	Blood glucose normally rises to 8.3 mmol/l returning to normal in 2 hours	Determines the patient's ability to clear the blood of excess glucose
Glycosylated haemoglobin (HbA$_1$)	4.82–5.09% of total haemoglobin	Increases occur in response to hyperglycaemia over the 120 day life span of the red cell

hormone to decrease thyroid activity and the iodine uptake indicates hyperthyroidism.

Normal: 25% decrease in radioiodine uptake by the gland in the second test. The test was more frequently used before development of radioimmunoassay and before the isolation of TRH.

T$_3$ resin uptake test. In this test T$_3$ tagged with radioiodine is added to a specimen of the patient's blood. The normal T$_3$-binding proteins are saturated and then the amount of binding of the remainder of T$_3$ by the erythrocytes is noted. In hyperthyroidism, the binding is high; conversely, it is low in hypothyroidism.

Normal value: 25–35%.

Thyroid scan. The uptake or lack of uptake of radioiodine by a limited area of the thyroid can be determined by a scan or scintigram. Following the administration of a tracer dose of radioactive iodine, a scanner is passed over the thyroid and automatically makes a graphic record of the radiation emitted, showing the distribution of the isotope in the gland. Areas of greater concentration show greater density on the record. This procedure is helpful in determining the presence of a localized hyperactive lesion such as an adenoma.

Thyroid stimulation test. This test is used to determine if the cause of hypothyroidism is within the thyroid or is secondary to a deficiency of TSH. The response of the thyroid to an injection of TSH is measured by a radioiodine uptake. Obviously, if the uptake of I^{131} remains abnormally low, the problem is primarily in the thyroid. If the radioiodine uptake is normal following TSH injection, the problem may

be attributed to a deficient secretion of TSH by the anterior pituitary.

Thyrotrophin-releasing hormone (TRH) test. Here the plasma TSH level is measured 30 and 60 minutes after an intravenous injection of TRH. In thyrotoxicosis the secretion of TSH by the anterior pituitary is suppressed.

Thyroid antibodies. Four types of thyroid antibodies commonly measured are antibodies to thyroglobin, thyroid microsomes, thyroid colloidal proteins and antinuclear antibodies. High antibody titres found with Grave's (hyperthyroidism) and Hashimoto's diseases demonstrate the role of the immune system in these disorders. It must be appreciated however, that antibodies can be identified in 10% of normal people.

Tests used in assessing parathyroid function

Serum parathyroid hormone (PTH). Two radioimmunoassay tests are available to determine serum levels of parathyroid hormone. Normal values depend on laboratory method and antisera used.

Serum calcium. This test measures both active, ionized calcium and the protein bound or inactive calcium in the serum. Serum calcium increases with hyperparathyroidism and decreases with hypofunction of the parathyroid glands.

Normal: 2.12–2.6 mmol/l (8.5–10.5 mg/dl).

Serum phosphorus. Serum phosphorus levels alter in reverse to those of ionized calcium; phosphorus levels are elevated with hypoparathyroidism and decreased with hyperparathyroidism.

Normal: 0.8–1.3 mmol/l (2.5–4.8 mg/dl)

Urine calcium. A 24-hour urine specimen is collected and the amount of calcium excreted in the urine is measured.

Normal: 25–75 mmol/24 h (100–300 mg/24 h).

Tests used in assessing adrenocortical function

Plasma cortisol concentration. A venous blood specimen is collected for estimation of the concentration of this principal glucocorticoid. Normally, plasma cortisol concentration is greatest approximately 1–2 hours after awakening and is lowest 2–3 hours after going to sleep. Determinations are made of the concentration at various times, usually 8 a.m. and 4 p.m.

Normal: a.m. specimen, 200–690 nmol/l (7.25 µg/dl); p.m. specimen, 8–220 nmol/l (3–8 µg/dl).

Adrenocorticotrophic hormone (ACTH). A fasting venous blood specimen is collected in a heparinized syringe and kept on ice during transport to the laboratory for estimation of serum ACTH.

Normal: a.m. specimen, 2–18 pmol/l (10–80 ng/l); p.m. specimen, < 2 pmol/l (10 ng/l).

ACTH stimulation. The initial evaluation may be followed by an injection of ACTH and a second plasma cortisol determination. Normally the level rises; if there is no increase, adrenocortical insufficiency is suspected.

Dexamethasone suppression test. The action of dexamethasone, a synthetic glucocorticoid, is similar to that of cortisol. ACTH secretion is suppressed when cortisol levels increase. Dexamethasone is administered at midnight and plasma cortisol levels are determined 8 hours later and a 24-hour urine specimen is collected and tested for 17-hydroxycorticosteroid content.

The expected result would be a 50% reduction in plasma cortisol and 17-hydroxycorticosteroids in the urine.

Metyrapone test. This drug blocks the formation of cortisol at the stage of 11-desoxycortisol; the latter is released and may be measured in the serum and urine. Normally, a low plasma level of cortisol stimulates the hypothalamus to deliver corticotrophin-releasing factor to the anterior pituitary to increase the output of ACTH. An accumulation of the precursor to cortisol (11-desoxycortisol) in the serum indicates that ACTH is being released and that the adrenal cortices are responding. The test procedure involves the oral administration of metyrapone.

Twenty-four-hour urine specimens are collected the day prior to the test, the day the metyrapone is given and the day following. The urine is examined for 17-hydroxycorticosteroid content. Blood specimens may be taken at intervals after the drug has been administered to determine the plasma ACTH or 11-desoxycortisol level.

The test evaluates both pituitary and adrenal functions. Normally the level of 17-hydroxycorticosteroid in the urine would be more than double the base line level. If 11-desoxycortisol is not produced and the plasma ACTH level is elevated, there is adrenal dysfunction. If the 11-desoxycortisol production is below normal and the ACTH level is low, the problem may lie in the hypothalamus–anterior pituitary system.

Urinary excretion of 17-hydroxycorticosteroids. An estimation of the concentration of 17-hydroxycorticosteroids in a 24-hour urine collection provides some indication of the secretory activity of the adrenal cortices. These hydroxycorticosteroids are metabolic products of androgens and glucocorticoids.

ACTH stimulation test. If the concentration is less than normal, an intravenous infusion of ACTH in normal saline is given slowly over 8 hours, and the urine is collected for a second 24-hour specimen. If the low level of 17-hyroxycorticosteroids still persists, it suggests dysfunction of the adrenal cortices. An elevation in the urinary steroids following the administration of the ACTH indicates a deficiency in the secretion of ACTH by the anterior pituitary.

Normal values: male, 11–30 µmol/l (4–11 mg/24 h); female, 8–28 µmol/l (3–10 mg/24h).

Aldosterone concentration. This mineral corticoid can be measured in the blood or urine. Plasma levels alter in relation to ACTH, potassium and sodium levels. Urine measurement requires a 24-hour specimen.

Normal: plasma, 140–500 pmol/l (50–200 ng/l); urine, 5–20 ng/24 h.

VMA (vanillylmandelic acid) concentration. This test is a measurement of the amount of VMA in a 24-hour urine specimen. VMA is the principal urinary metabolite of noradrenaline and adrenaline.

Normal: 9–34 µmol (1.8–6.8 mg)/24 h.

Blood chemistry. Blood electrolyte concentrations are determined, and the ratio of sodium to potassium is noted. In adrenocortical insufficiency, the sodium level is below normal and that of potassium is elevated, decreasing the ratio of sodium to potassium.

Normal values: sodium, 135–145 mmol/l; potassium, 3.5–5.5 mmol/l; potassium/sodium ratio; approximately 1:30.

The fasting blood glucose concentration is determined and is found to be below normal with decreased adrenocorticoid secretion and above normal with hypersecretion.

Normal blood glucose: 3.9–6.1 mmol/l (65–100 mg/dl).

Tests used in assessment of pancreatic endocrine function

Serum insulin. Radioisotope immunoassay of serum insulin levels is useful in evaluating fasting hypoglycaemia.

Normal: 4–24 µU/ml (but variable).

Urinalysis. A urine specimen is examined for the presence of glucose and ketone bodies (acetone, acetoacetic acid and hydroxybutyric acid). Normally, glucose is almost completely reabsorbed from the glomerular filtrate by the renal tubules, and what remains in the urine is insignificant and not detected by the usual tests. If sugar is present (glucosuria), the amount is noted on the basis of the intensity of the reaction and is indicated as a trace, one plus, two plus, and so on. Simple, quick methods of testing the urine for sugar have been devised in the form of a tablet, powder or strip of paper impregnated with the necessary reagent. Directions for their use and a colour comparison chart accompany each product. The colour chart indicates the characteristic colour change associated with certain glucose concentrations. The presence of glucose in the urine may only be suggestive of diabetes mellitus; for instance, the person may have a low glucose renal threshold. If glucose is found, blood sugar determinations are then made for more conclusive evidence.

A 24-hour urine specimen may be ordered to determine the amount of sugar the patient excretes in that period. The collection usually begins in the morning. The patient voids and that urine is discarded. The time is noted and all urine that is voided until that time the next morning is saved. The patient is asked to empty his bladder at the time the test is completed, and that urine is included in the specimen.

Ketone bodies may be present in the urine of a diabetic because of the mobilization and breakdown of fat. Ketonuria occurring with glucosuria generally indicates the presence of diabetes mellitus. Materials similar to those cited in testing for sugar are available for simple quick testing for ketonuria.

Blood glucose. A blood glucose determination is made from a specimen of venous blood following a period of *4–8 hours of fasting*. The normal range is 3.9–6.1 mmol/l.

Glucose tolerance test. This test determines the patient's ability to clear the blood of excess glucose following the ingestion of sugar and to return the blood sugar to a normal level. Preferably, the patient should receive approximately 150 g of carbohydrate in his diet for 3 days preceding the test. Food is then withheld overnight, and in the morning a urine specimen and venous blood sample are collected for glucose determinations. Instead of high-carbohydrate meals the patient is given 75 g of glucose dissolved in 250–350 ml of water (orally); it may be flavoured with lemon juice. Urine and blood specimens are collected ½, 1 and 2 hours after the ingestion of the glucose. These are examined for the glucose concentration. Normally, the blood sugar level rises to approximately 8.3 mmol/l but returns to normal within 2 hours. In the diabetic, the elevation in the blood sugar will be much higher and several hours (3–5) may be required for the original level to be attained. A blood glucose level above 10.0 mmol/l (180 mg/dl) at 2 hours is considered diagnostic of diabetes.

Normally, no sugar appears in the urine. In the diabetic the elevation in the blood sugar exceeds the glucose renal threshold and glucosuria occurs. With any glucose tolerance test, all medication that may affect the blood sugar level (e.g. thiazides, prednisone and oestrogen) should be withheld.

Glycosylated haemoglobin (HbA_1). This glucose linkage with haemoglobin is relatively stable throughout the body life span of the red cell so its concentration reflects the mean blood glucose level over the previous few months. It is thus a way of monitoring diabetic control.

Normal: 4.82–5.09% of total haemoglobin.

MANIFESTATIONS OF DISORDERS OF THE ENDOCRINE SYSTEM (see Table 20.2)

Signs and symptoms of endocrine dysfunction may be non-specific, resulting from changes in the widespread target tissues and are common to many disorders. They include the following:

1 *Alterations in growth.* Growth may be delayed or excessive. *Delayed growth* can occur from endocrine and metabolic disorders as well as genetic factors. Delayed growth from endocrine disorders usually occurs during a specific period of development. *Excessive growth* may result from endocrine disorders in which an excess of adrenal, ovarian or testicular or pituitary hormones is produced. Excessive pituitary secretion of growth hormone causes gigantism.

2 *Obesity.* Obesity can be associated with hormonal disorders and may be a causative factor (as in diabetes) as well as a result of a disorder.

3 *Appetite changes* include anorexia and polyphagia. Excessive eating (polyphagia) is most often seen with uncontrolled diabetes, hyperthyroidism and occasionally with a hypothalamic disorder.

Table 20.2 Endocrine glands, their hormones and associated disorders.

Gland	Hormones	Functions	Disorders
Anterior pituitary	Growth hormone (GH)	Growth; aids in determining size; accelerates metabolism; diabetogenic	Panhypopituitarism Gigantism—increase in GH in childhood Acromegaly—increase in GH in adulthood Short stature—decrease of GH in childhood
	Thyroid-stimulating hormone (TSH)	Promotes secretory activity of thyroid	Hyperthyroidism secondary to increase of TSH Hypothyroidism secondary to decrease of TSH
	Adrenocorticotrophic hormone (ACTH)	Stimulates secretion of adrenal cortices	Cushing's syndrome and excess TSH Addison's disease secondary to pituitary disorder Tumours
	Gonadotrophins Follicle-stimulating hormone (FSH)	In women: development of ovarian follicle and secretion of oestrogen In men: promotes production of spermatozoa	Amenorrhoea Infertility
	Luteinizing hormone (LH)	In women: induces ovulation, stimulates secretion of progesterone In men: stimulates production of androgens	
	Prolactin	Initiates and sustains lactation	Galactorrhoea Infertility
	Melanocyte stimulating hormone (MSH)	Pigmentation of skin cells	Increase in pigmented areas
Posterior pituitary	Antidiuretic hormone (ADH)	Increases permeability of distal and collecting tubules of kidneys (i.e. increases reabsorption of water)	Tumour
	Oxytocin	Contracts pregnant uterus; stimulates release and flow of milk	

Thyroid	Triiodothyronine (T_3)
	Tetraiodothyronine (T_4)
		Increases metabolic rate by stimulating oxidative processes; promotes normal physical growth, maturation, mental development	Hypothyroidism
			  Cretinism in child
			  Myxoedema in adult
			Goitre
			Hyperthyroidism
			Thyrotoxic crisis
			Thyroiditis
			Carcinoma

	Calcitonin	Promotes excretion of serum calcium and phosphate and movement into bones	
Parathyroid	Parathyroid hormone (PTH)	Controls concentration of calcium and inorganic phosphorus in blood	Hypoparathyroidism (tetany) Hyperparathyroidism
Adrenal glands Adrenal cortex	Adrenocorticoids (corticosteroids, corticoids)		Addison's disease (hypofunction of cortices) Cushing's syndrome (hyperfunction of cortices)
	Mineralocorticoids, aldosterone Glucocorticoids, cortisol (hydrocortisone) Sex hormones (androgens, oestrogen and progesterone)	Influences electrolyte concentration, fluid volume, blood pressure Influences metabolism of glucose, protein and fat; concerned with body's responses to physical and mental stress	Primary aldosteronism (increase of aldosterone)
Adrenal medulla	Adrenaline	Constricts peripheral and renal blood vessels; dilates coronary and skeletal muscle vessels; relaxes smooth muscle of bronchioles, gastrointestinal tract, urinary bladder; dilates pupils; elevates blood sugar; promotes release of ACTH; accelerates metabolic rate	Phaeochromocytoma (increase of production of both hormones)
	Noradrenaline	Generalized vasoconstriction	
Islet of Langerhans	Insulin	Active in carbohydrate metabolism	Diabetes mellitus Hyperinsulinism

4 *Polyuria and polydypsia.* Excessive urinary output and abnormal thirst are frequently the result of uncontrolled diabetes mellitus or diabetes insipidus.

5 *Weakness and exhaustion.* Excessive weight loss, muscle wasting, weakness and exhaustion may be seen in patients with uncontrolled disorders of the pancreas, thyroid or adrenal glands.

6 *Skin pigmentation.* Changes in skin pigmentation may develop in patients with disorders of the pituitary, parathyroid and adrenal glands.

7 *Hirsutism.* Changes in the distribution and texture of body hair occur with several endocrine disorders. Facial hair in the female may occur with adrenal or ovarian disorders.

8 *Sexual disturbances.* Impotence, menstrual disorders and infertility may be associated with endocrine disturbances. Impotence may occur in men who have had diabetes mellitus for several years. The onset of puberty and delay in the development of secondary sex characteristics may occur with deficiency of the growth hormone and gonadal dysfunction.

9 *Bone and joint disorders* accompany changes in the secretion of the growth and thyroid hormones and adrenocorticoids.

10 *Renal colic and stones* may be associated with bone disorders in patients with disorders of secretion of the thyroid and adrenal gland.

11 *Tetany and muscle cramps* occur in children with hypoparathyroidism.

12 *Personality changes* including lethargy, confusion, nervousness, restlessness, convulsions and coma may result from acute metabolic disorders associated with uncontrolled diabetes mellitus as well as with disorders of secretions of the pituitary gland, adrenal gland and thyroid.

Disorders of the pituitary gland (hypophysis)

Manifestations of disorders of the pituitary vary greatly, depending on which lobe is involved, the nature of the disease (hyperplasia, neoplasm or destruction of tissue) and the particular type of cell of the anterior pituitary that is involved. Dysfunction may be manifested in one or more of the gland's target organs, reflecting either an excessive or deficient output of one or more pituitary hormones. Secondary neurological disturbances may also occur as a result of pressure on neighbouring brain tissue by a pituitary neoplasm. For example, early symptoms may be persistent headache or visual disturbances. The visual disturbances frequently occur because of the proximity of the visual tract. Conversely, primary pathological lesions in the brain, especially in the hypothalamic region, may cause secondary involvement of the pituitary.

The more commonly recognized disease entities associated with the anterior pituitary include: gigantism, the result of an excessive secretion of GH in childhood; acromegaly, due to an excessive secretion of GH commencing in adulthood; dwarfism, resulting from a deficiency of GH in childhood; Cushing's disease, the result of a hypersecretion of adrenocorticotrophic hormone and Simmonds' disease (panhypopituitarism), which occurs with a deficiency of all the anterior pituitary hormones. Hyperthyroidism (Graves' disease) may also be secondary to an excessive production of TSH or an abnormal form of the hormone and is discussed in the section on disorders of the thyroid.

The most common disorder associated with the posterior pituitary is diabetes insipidus, which is a result of a deficiency of ADH.

GIGANTISM AND ACROMEGALY

An overproduction of GH before closure of the epiphyses causes a rapid overgrowth of the bones, producing the condition known as *gigantism.* It may commence in early childhood or not until adolescence. A person with this disturbance may attain a height of 7–8 feet. Most cases are attributed to an adenoma of the somatotrophs or acidophilic cells (alpha cells). When the person passes adolescence, acromegaly is superimposed on the gigantism.

If the adenoma develops after the epiphyses have closed, longitudinal growth cannot occur, but marked thickening of the bones occurs and *acromegaly* develops. Enlargement of the head, jaws, hands and feet becomes apparent. Increased growth of cartilage produces an increase in the size of the nose, ears, costal cartilages and larynx. Hypertrophy of the larynx may be accompanied by a deepening of the voice, and the change in the costal cartilages results in an increase in the thoracic circumference. The skin, subcutaneous tissues and lips thicken, the chin lengthens and the lower teeth separate because of the overgrowth of the mandible. Viscera enlarge and may become overactive, leading to disturbances.

As well as the evident skeletal changes and alteration in appearance, the patient experiences lethargy, weakness, increased metabolic rate and excessive sweating due to hypertrophy of the thyroid. Common complaints are joint pains, stiffness in the limbs, and tingling or numbness in the hands. Impaired carbohydrate metabolism and hyperglycaemia develop owing to the diabetogenic effect of GH. Pressure from the causative expanding neoplasm may cause headache, insomnia and loss of visual acuity and fields. Increased gonadal function may be associated with the early stage of acromegaly but, later, loss of libido and amenorrhoea are common. Osteoporosis, rarefaction of bones due to loss of calcium, may develop, especially in the vertebrae, and kyphosis (forward curvature of the spine) may be seen in the advanced stage. Hypertension is a common complication. The course of the disease varies considerably from one patient to another; it may develop slowly over many years in some, but in others it may prove fatal in 3 or 4 years. Destruction of pituitary tissue by progressive growth and spread of the tumour may cause a general hypopituitarism.

Diagnostic investigation involves x-rays of the skull in which the sella turcica is checked for widening. Laboratory studies include: serum inorganic phosphorus, which may be elevated; blood glucose level, which may be increased; and measurement of plasma GH concentration by radioimmunoassay which is elevated and remains elevated when glucose is administered.

Treatment
Gigantism and acromegaly may be treated by external or internal irradiation of the pituitary or by a hypophysectomy or transphenoidal microsurgery to remove the hyperfunctioning tissue. Internal radiation may be achieved by the implantation of radioactive gold (Au[198]) or yttrium (Y[90]) seeds in the pituitary. The gland is approached through the nasal cavity and sphenoid bone. Synthesized somatostatin (growth hormone release-inhibiting factor) has recently become available for treatment of acromegaly. Bromocriptine has also been administered orally when other forms of treatment have been ineffective. The disease is likely to cause emotional reactions and depression in the patient and his family. Support and counselling from the nurse may help them to accept and adjust to the situation. A high-calorie, well-balanced diet is necessary to meet the increased metabolic rate. With some, it may have to be modified because of the decreased carbohydrate metabolism. Substitution hormonal preparations are prescribed if a hypophysectomy is done or if the patient manifests insulin, thyroid, adrenal or gonadal insufficiency in the advanced stage of the disease. Treatment arrests further changes but the changes in bony structures are irreversible.

CUSHING'S DISEASE

A basophilic tumour of corticotrophs or disturbance in the hypothalamus may give rise to an excessive production of ACTH and, in turn, hyperactivity of the adrenal cortices. The adrenal cortices respond by hyperplasia and an excessive secretion of glucocorticoids, producing the characteristic features of Cushing's disease. The syndrome is more often a consequence of a primary disorder of the adrenal gland (see 661).

PITUITARY DWARFISM

A deficiency of GH in childhood produces short stature. Short stature due to a GH deficiency is differentiated from that due to a deficiency of the thyroid hormone (cretinism) in that the mental development is normal in the former. The deficiency in some patients may be limited to GH or it may involve other hormones. Sexual development and maturity may or may not be normal.

Another reason for shortness of stature may be malabsorption. Achondroplasia is a hereditary disorder of endochondral ossification characterized by normal sized head and trunk but failure of the long bones of arms and legs to grow properly.

PANHYPOPITUITARISM (SIMMONDS' DISEASE)

This disease denotes a deficiency of all the anterior pituitary hormones. The condition may be the result of a primary lesion, such as a tumour or cyst, within the anterior lobe itself, or it may be secondary to a space-occupying lesion in neighbouring structures or to interference with the blood supply to the gland. The latter may occur with thrombosis of the hypophyseal vessels rarely associated with postpartum shock (Sheehan's syndrome). Frequently the causative lesion is a craniopharyngioma which is derived from vestigial cells of Rathke's pouch.[13] This tumour occurs most often in children but may not give rise to symptoms until adulthood because it grows slowly. A second neoplasm that may be responsible for panhypopituitarism is an adenoma of the chromophobe cells. The cells of both these tumours are non-secreting and, as they enlarge, they compress and destroy the secreting cells. Surgical excision or irradiation of the gland for the purpose of suppressing the secretion of certain hormones in the treatment of carcinoma of the breast (see Chapter 24) or acromegaly may incur hyposecretion of all the adenohypophyseal hormones.

Manifestations
The multiple hormone deficiency results in a lack of stimulation to the thyroid, adrenal cortices and gonads. Secondary atrophy and a hyposecretion of their hormones ensue. If the condition occurs in childhood, failure of the secretion of GH along with the others produces dwarfism. Growth and development are arrested, the skin becomes wrinkled and the child develops an appearance characteristic of a 'wizened old person'.

In the adult, there is also a general wasting of all body tissues and the person exhibits emaciation and severe weight loss. The skin is dry and wrinkled and may assume a yellowish cast. The body hair becomes sparse. Decreased thyroid activity causes a reduction in the metabolic rate, leading to a subnormal temperature and extreme weakness. Arrested function of the gonads results in failure of ovulation and amenorrhoea in the female and an absence of spermatogenesis and impotence in the male. Concomitant hypoglycaemia and hypotension are seen and may lead to shock and coma. The low blood sugar is attributed to the decreased GH and adrenocorticoid secretions. If the panhypopituitarism is due to an expanding neoplasm, the posterior pituitary and the

---

[13] *Rathke's pouch* is the embryologic structure which arises from the roof of the mouth to form the adenohypophysis.

infundibulum (neural stalk) may become involved, manifested by polyuria and extreme thirst, which is characteristic of a deficiency of ADH. An expanding lesion may impose itself on the optic tract, impairing vision. The hypothalamus may also be affected and varied neurological disturbances become evident; for example, the patient may experience severe anorexia.

Treatment and nursing intervention

Treatment includes the administration of substitution hormones of the target glands. The patient receives corticosteroids and thyroid hormone in dosages adjusted to his individual needs. Thyroid hormone is prescribed only when the patient is receiving corticosteroids. Gonadal hormones may be prescribed, depending on the patient's age. Testosterone (male hormone) may be administered to both sexes for its anabolic effect. Oestrogen may be used with the female to preserve female secondary sex characteristics. Human GH, if available, may be given to children to increase height.

If the cause is a tumour, it is removed by transphenoidal microsurgery and/or treated by irradiation.

The nurse plays an important role in encouraging these patients to take a high-calorie, high-vitamin diet. Since anorexia is a frequent problem, resourcefulness is necessary to gain the patient's cooperation and to tempt him to take adequate nourishment. Various methods and approaches must be tried. It is usually helpful to provide small servings of high-calorie foods at frequent intervals rather than the usual three or four regular meals. Varying the foods, adding concentrates to fluids, determining the patient's preferences, having favourite 'dishes' prepared at home and brought to him, eating with others and a change of environment are just a few suggestions that may prove beneficial. If the patient is emaciated and inactive or confined to bed, bony prominences and pressure areas require frequent and special care to prevent pressure sores. The lethargy and apathy generally associated with Simmonds' disease predisposes to the patient's immobility. Prompting the patient to change his position and exercise within his tolerance is necessary to stimulate circulation and prevent complications.

DIABETES INSIPIDUS

The causative factor in this disorder may be a deficiency of ADH (vasopressin) or failure of the renal tubules to respond to ADH. In the latter, the disorder may be referred to as nephrogenic diabetes insipidus and is a rare sex-linked, recessive hereditary condition present at birth but may be acquired in adults secondary to renal disorders. A deficiency of ADH is most commonly due to hypoactivity or destruction of a part of the hypothalamic-posterior pituitary system resulting from primary or metastatic neoplasms or infection, such as encephalitis or meningitis. In some instances, no apparent cause can be identified.

Manifestations

Diabetes insipidus is characterized by a very large urinary output (polyuria) and extreme thirst (polydipsia). The daily output may range from 5–20 l and the patient may experience anorexia, headache, muscular pains, loss of weight and strength and electrolyte imbalance. The urine has an abnormally low specific gravity and does not contain any abnormal constituents. If fluid is withheld or does not keep pace with the output, an excessive loss of urine continues, leading to severe dehydration and shock. The persisting symptoms of polyuria and polydipsia day and night interfere with rest and normal activities.

Diagnosis

Investigation of the disorder usually involves water deprivation tests (see p. 638). Failure to increase the specific gravity of the urine and an elevation of plasma osmolality are characteristic of diabetes insipidus. Stimulation of ADH may also be achieved by parenteral administration of a hypertonic solution. If these studies are positive for diabetes insipidus, a trial dose of vasopressin (Pitressin) is given; if the polyuria and thirst are not relieved, nephrogenic diabetes insipidus is suspected and kidney function studies may be done.

Investigative procedures may also include neurological examination, x-rays of the skull, visual field tests and an encephalogram for detection of a possible brain tumour.

Treatment

The patient is treated by replacement therapy with hypotonic parenteral fluids and unlimited oral fluids; a preparation of posterior pituitary extract or vasopressin is prescribed. The preparations used include an aqueous solution of vasopressin (Pitressin), given daily by subcutaneous or intramuscular injection, and vasopressin tannate (Pitressin Tannate) in oil, given intramuscularly every 2 or 3 days. The latter preparation is absorbed more slowly and is usually administered in the evening. If the patient is allergic to the above animal vasopressin preparations, a synthetic substitute is available in the form of a nasal spray, lypressin (Syntopressin). One spray (or two may be necessary) is generally used in each nostril four times daily. The use of the nasal spray is more convenient but irritation of the nasopharyngeal mucosa may develop. Desmopressin (DDAVP) is a longer acting synthetic ADH substitute that may be inhaled intranasally. Chlorothiazide, an oral diuretic, has been found to be effective in some cases, possibly by causing sodium loss. Chlorpropamide and clofibrate have also been found to be effective in some cases.

The patient is usually hospitalized during diagnostic investigation and regulation of medication. It is difficult for the patient to accept the fact that he will most likely be dependent upon the drug for the remainder of his life. The nurse can help the patient to plan for necessary readjustments and should reassure him that he can resume a normal pattern of life.

The patient and a family member are taught the details of how to administer the drug, including care of the equipment. The instructions are also given in writing. They may require further explanation of the disorder to appreciate the importance of regular administration of the drug, and should be advised that in the case of vasopressin, it is ineffective if taken orally because it is inactivated by the digestive enzymes. The patient is advised to record his weight every 2 or 3 days and note the urinary volume. Water retention indicated by weight increase and scanty urine may necessitate a decrease in vasopressin dosage.

PITUITARY ABLATION

The anterior and posterior pituitary gland may be removed or destroyed because of hyperfunction or a neoplasm of the gland. Hypophysectomy is also employed in the treatment of diabetic retinopathy and cancer of the breast and prostate. Malignant disease of the latter organs in many instances is supported by the sex hormones oestrogens and androgens, respectively. Removal of the source of gonadotrophic hormones reduces support for the primary neoplasm and its metastasis. Withdrawal of the hormones does not cure the disease, but usually produces a remission for a period of several months.

Pituitary ablation may be carried out by radiation therapy, surgical excision or destruction by stereotactic radiofrequency or cryosurgery (freezing). Irradiation may be from an external source or radioactive yttrium-90 may be implanted. Access to the gland is usually by a nasal-transsphenoidal approach but a transfrontal approach may be used if the tumour is large and has spread. Transsphenoidal surgery involves the use of televised radiofluoroscopy and a binocular microscope. Hypophysectomy results in the withdrawal of ACTH, TSH, and probably ADH as well as the gonadotrophins. In some instances, the neural stalk, which transmits the nerve fibres from the hypothalamus to the posterior pituitary gland, may be preserved at operation, thus preventing diabetes insipidus. The patient requires cortisone, thyroxine and possibly ADH replacement for the remainder of his life. Gonadal function ceases, and the patient becomes infertile. If the surgery was done because of disease of the pituitary gland, the male patient may be given testosterone to prevent impotence.

Preoperative preparation
Because of the location and the infrequency of this particular operation, the patient and family are very apprehensive. The nurse should encourage them to talk about their fears and ask questions and provides necessary emotional support. The permanent results of the surgery will have been explained by the doctor but the nurse, knowing what the patient has been told, is prepared to answer their questions and explain the hormonal replacement.

Specific directions are received from the surgeon for the skin preparation. For transfrontal surgery, usually an area of approximately 5 cm from the hairline across the front of the head is shaved and cleansed. The patient is advised that there will be frequent recording of his blood pressure, temperature, pulse and respirations following the operation. Nasal packing will be inserted if a transsphenoidal approach is used. A corticosteroid preparation is usually given the day before operation and again before going to the operating room. A venous cannula is inserted, and continuous intravenous infusion is started to establish a route for the quick administration of drugs and fluids as needed.

Postoperative care
The care following a hypophysectomy is similar to that of any patient who has had intracranial surgery. Close observation is made for early signs of acute adrenal insufficiency (see p. 660) or fluid imbalance. An adrenocorticoid steroid is given intravenously until the patient can tolerate it orally. The dose is gradually decreased until the maintenance dose is established. Vasopressin (Pitressin) may be necessary to control the fluid loss; the dosage is adjusted to the urinary volume. Thyroid extract may be started orally on the second or third postoperative day.

The intravenous infusion is usually discontinued the morning following surgery. Oral fluids may be started the evening of surgery or the next morning. If a transsphenoidal approach was used, the incision will be above the front teeth. The patient is instructed not to brush his teeth until the incision is healed and the sutures are removed. Dental floss and mouthwashes are used to maintain dental and oral hygiene. The period of hospitalization is relatively short; instruction about the taking of the necessary hormones (cortisone, vasopressin and thyroxin) is carried out throughout the postoperative period and, if necessary, a referral is made for follow-up instruction and supervision by a community nurse.

Disorders of the thyroid

Disease of the thyroid may cause a hyposecretion or hypersecretion of the thyroid hormones and a change in the size of the gland. A deficiency in the secretion is called *hypothyroidism*; an excessive secretion is referred to as *hyperthyroidism*. The normally functioning gland is referred to as *euthyroid*.

HYPOTHYROIDISM

The effects and manifestations of a deficiency of thyroid hormone differ with the age at which it develops as well as with the degree and duration (see Table 20.3). The deficiency of thyroid hormones may be primary, due to a disorder in the thyroid itself, or may be secondary as a result of a pituitary or hypothalamic disturbance. If the dysfunction is congenital or develops in infancy or early childhood, it gives rise to cretinism. In the adult it produces myxoedema.

Cretinism
A deficiency of thyroid hormone in infancy or early childhood is characterized by the failure to achieve normal physical growth and mental development. The child may become a mentally handicapped dwarf. The symptoms of cretinism are rarely present in the newborn but more often appear gradually in infancy or early childhood. Suggestive signs include limpness and inactivity, feeding problems, pale, dry, cool skin, thick tongue, coarse features, coarse hair, and a puffy appearance. The circulation is sluggish, the temperature is usually subnormal and the pulse slow. Constipation is a common problem. The child's growth is stunted, and there is a distinct lag in the development of normal behavioural responses. If the deficiency is recognized in the early stages and a thyroid preparation administered, normal growth and development may occur. If the deficiency is allowed to persist, irreversible damage results, and both physical growth and mental development are retarded.

The fact that cretinism may be corrected if recognized and treated early emphasizes the nurse's role in promoting adequate infant and child supervision. Mothers should be taught the characteristics of normal growth and development. The mother is encouraged to take the child to well-baby clinics for regular examinations, or to consult with the health visitor.

Myxoedema
Adult hypothyroidism is known as myxoedema. The *symptoms* and the rate at which they develop correspond to the degree of thyroid inactivity (see Table 20.3). An abnormal decrease in thyroid hormone causes a general reduction in cellular metabolism, producing mental and physical sluggishness. The person gradually exhibits apathy and slowness in responses. An abnormal deposition of a mucopolysaccharide, which tends to hold water, occurs in the subcutaneous tissues, giving the person an oedematous appearance. The skin becomes dry and thick,

Table 20.3 Assessment of the patient with disorders of the thyroid.

Body system	Manifestations of hypothyroidism	Manifestations of hyperthyroidism
Cardiovascular	Pulse rate decreased Blood pressure low Cardiac enlargement and insufficiency	Pulse rapid and bounding Palpitations Widened pulse pressure (↑ systolic BP and ↓ diastolic BP) Cardiac arrhythmias widen
Respiratory	Dyspnoea Pericardial and pleural effusion	Shortness of breath on exertion Respiratory rate increased
Integumentary	Skin dry, thick and pale yellow Eyelids oedematous Lips and tongue enlarged Hair coarse and sparse Interstitial oedema	Increased sweating Skin warm and moist Eyelids retracted Hair loss
Gastrointestinal	Appetite poor Increased weight Constipation	Appetite increased Weight loss Diarrhoea
Musculoskeletal	Weakness and fatigue Slow movements	Weakness and fatigue Weakness of eyelid muscles
Nervous	Sensitivity to cold Slow mental processes Increased sleep and lethargy Speech hoarse, slow and monotonous Depression Mental disturbance	Sensitivity to heat Nervousness, apprehension, restlessness, irritability and emotional instability Tremor of hands Visual changes, difficulty focusing eyes Insomnia
Reproductive	Metrorrhagia Amenorrhoea Low sex drive Infertility	Oligomenorrhoea or amenorrhoea Low sex drive Impotence

the face (particularly the eyelids) appears puffy and the lips and tongue enlarge. The person experiences weakness, fatigue and an increased sensitivity to cold. His appetite is poor although he may show a gain in weight. The temperature, pulse and blood pressure may be abnormally low. Mental processes are retarded, and the patient sleeps a great deal. Impaired function of the reproductive system is manifested by menstrual disorders, such as metrorrhagia and amenorrhoea, and loss of sexual drive. Hoarseness and slow, monotonous speech may be noted. Because of his complacency and dull mental processes, the condition is of much less concern to the patient than to his family or friends witnessing the changes. Allowed to progress, the disorder may lead to arteriosclerotic changes, cardiac insufficiency, depression and psychosis with hallucinations and delusions ('myxoedema madness'), or pass into a comatose state.

Causes of myxoedema include destruction of the gland by a disease such as thyroiditis and Hashimoto's disease (autoimmune thyroiditis), irradiation, prolonged iodine deficiency, a disorder of the hypothalamic-anterior pituitary system which results in a deficiency of TSH, and complete thyroidectomy.

Treatment and nursing intervention
Hypothyroidism is treated favourably in uncomplicated cases with L-thyroxine. In cases where there are complications, such as ischaemic heart disease, triiodothyronine (T_3) may be given. T_3 acts very rapidly, but the effect is sustained for a shorter period than L-thyroxine which is not fully effective before 7–10 days. The dosage is usually small to start with and is gradually increased to guard against a too sudden and excessive demand on the heart by rapid acceleration of metabolism. The pulse is checked and recorded frequently until the maintenance dose is established. Reactions to overdosage include rapid pulse rate, palpitation, restlessness or hyperactivity, nervousness and insomnia. The maintenance dose is individualized on the basis of the responses observed and recorded.

It may be necessary for the nurse to explain the condition to the patient and his family and emphasize that replacement therapy must be continued indefinitely. The patient may neglect taking the medication when he feels better. During the myxoedematous state, it is important that the family appreciate that the patient's lethargy and dullness are a part of his disease. They may be prone to criticize and drive the patient. The nurse and his family must be patient and tolerant of his slowness. He should be encouraged and given time to complete responses and activities. Early indications of improvement and response to the drug therapy may be pointed out to them for reassurance that the physical condition is reversible although depression does not always resolve.

Much of the nursing care is symptomatic. For example, extra warmth is provided because of the patient's lower heat production and consequent decreased tolerance to cold. Without extra clothing and bedding, he may be uncomfortable in an environmental temperature that is comfortable to others. A minimum of soap is used on the patient's skin, and oily lotions or creams are applied to relieve the dryness. A low-calorie, high-protein diet is served with added roughage to combat the problem of constipation. Laxatives or enemas may be necessary to avoid impaction. The hypothyroid patient is seen at the outpatient clinic or by his general practitioner at regular intervals; adjustment of the drug dosage may be necessary from time to time.

Severe hypothyroidism may be complicated by coma which may be precipitated by exposure to cold, infection, trauma or the taking of medications which depress the central nervous system. Older persons with hypothyroidism are more predisposed to develop coma. Their temperature falls to hypothermic levels and respiratory insufficiency may develop. An endotracheal tube may be inserted or a tracheostomy may have to be done and mechanical respiratory assistance provided. Triiodothyronine and hydrocortisone are given intravenously along with glucose. Gradual rewarming by additional covers is used rather than the application of heat.

GOITRE

The term goitre simply indicates enlargement of the thyroid gland. It may be a compensatory hypertrophy as occurs in iodine deficiency or in cases in which there is an increased demand for the thyroid hormone, as in pregnancy and puberty. Enlargement may be the result of a neoplasm, thyroiditis or hyperplasia associated with pathological hyperactivity, as in Graves' disease (exophthalmic goitre). Rarely, it is due to a congenital defect in which a specific enzyme which is necessary in the process of forming the hormones is missing or defective. A goitre may be classified as: diffuse or nodular; endemic or sporadic, depending on the frequency with which it occurs in a given geographical area; and toxic, non-toxic or simple, depending on whether the enlargement is accompanied by hyperthyroidism.

Goitre most commonly refers to an enlargement that is endemic and due to a deficiency in the natural supply of iodine in the water and soil. It is seen most often in mountainous areas and inland areas distant from the sea (e.g. Rocky Mountains, the Alps and the Himalayas, and in Great Britain, Derbyshire). Terms used to describe it include simple endemic goitre, iodine-deficient goitre and simple colloid or non-toxic goitre. In most areas where the natural source is inadequate, the simple, inexpensive prophylactic measure of adding iodine to salt used in food has been adopted. Residents of such districts should be informed of the significance of using iodized salt.

The enlargement of the thyroid in iodine deficiency occurs because of stimulation by an increased release of TSH by the anterior pituitary in response to the low thyroxine concentration of the blood. The follicles increase in number and size and the thyroid becomes more vascular. If the iodine deficiency and excessive TSH stimulation are prolonged, the gland tends to develop nodules which contain greatly distended follicles that may eventually undergo degeneration.

The enlarged gland may cause disfigurement which creates embarrassment for the person. More serious symptoms are pressure on the larynx and trachea, manifested by a chronic cough and respiratory difficulty, interference with swallowing, and compression of nerves in the area.

The simple non-toxic goitre is treated with an iodide preparation (e.g. potassium iodide) or, if there is evidence of hypothyroidism, the patient receives a thyroid preparation. In the early stages, with an adequate supply of iodine, the goitre gradually becomes smaller. If the gland has been enlarged over a period of years and has become nodular, drug therapy is likely to be less effective. The gland remains large and surgical removal of a large portion may be indicated to relieve pressure on the trachea, larynx, oesophagus or nerves and to improve the patient's appearance.

HYPERTHYROIDISM

Hyperthyroidism implies an excessive secretion of the thyroid hormones and may be called *thyrotoxicosis*, *toxic goitre*, *exophthalmic goitre* or *Graves' disease*. The terms exophthalmic goitre, or Graves' disease are reserved for hyperthyroidism that is accompanied by exophthalmos and extreme nervousness.

The exact cause of hyperactivity of the thyroid in most patients is not clear. In many cases it is thought to be due to autoimmunity. Thyroid-stimulating immunoglobulins (TSI) are found in almost all patients with Graves' disease. These immunoglobulin G antibodies act on TSH receptors producing stimulation of the acinar cells of the thyroid.[14] Hyperthyroidism affects females more often than males, and is rare in childhood. Frequently, the onset is closely related to an emotional crisis in the person's life.

Manifestations
Some enlargement of the gland may be evident owing to a diffuse hyperplasia of the gland or the development of one or more adenomas. It may be readily seen to move upward with the larynx in swallowing.

The increased blood level of thyroid hormones accelerates the metabolic rate. The patient's appetite increases and, unless the food intake keeps pace with the rapid metabolic rate, there is a marked loss of weight. Lowered heat tolerance and excessive sweating are manifested. The hyperthyroid patient is uncomfortably warm in an environmental temperature quite acceptable to others.

Nervousness, apprehension, emotional instability and restlessness are evident, and the hands are warm and moist in contrast to the cold, moist extremities associated with anxiety. Although the patient is eating more, he complains of weakness and quick fatigue. The pulse is rapid and exhibits a sharp rise on exertion. The increased pulse rate is due to the increased metabolic demands and the effect of thyroxine on the sympathetic nervous system. Shortness of breath on exertion and palpitation are experienced as a result of the increased metabolic rate. The diastolic blood pressure is usually lower than normal because of widespread vasodilation. A fine, rapid tremor develops in the hands and is accentuated when they are outstretched. Diarrhoea, resulting from increased gastrointestinal activity, may be troublesome. Menstrual disorders, such as oligomenorrhoea (scant flow) or amenorrhoea, are common (see Table 20.3).

Eye changes may appear in hyperthyroidism (Graves' disease or exophthalmic goitre) which are unexplained. It has been suggested that increased sympathetic stimulation and autoimmune mechanisms contribute to its development.[15] Exophthalmos, a protrusion of the eyeballs, occurs as a result of an increase in the retro-orbital fat which pushes the eye forward. The upper eyelids are retracted, showing the upper sclerae. The lids fail to follow the movement of the eyes when the person looks down (lid lag).

Treatment
Hyperthyroidism may be treated by antithyroid drugs, radioactive iodine (I^{131}) or surgery.

Drug therapy. The drugs most commonly used suppress the formation of the thyroid hormones. They include carbimazole and methylthiouracil. The drug is generally taken over a prolonged period of 1–2 years if the patient remains free of side-effects. These antithyroid drugs are potentially toxic. Side-effects which may develop are dermatitis, agranulocytosis and fever. Rarely, hepatitis, joint and muscle pain and neuritis have been reported. The patient is advised to report promptly a sore throat, swollen tender 'neck glands,' fever, rash or jaundice. It is important that he understand the necessity for taking the drugs regularly and at the hours suggested in order to obtain the desired effect and prevent a remission. Some compensatory enlargement

[14] Robbins, Angell & Kumar (1981), p. 606.

[15] Dillon (1980), p. 354.

of the gland may occur and the patient is reassured that this is not serious.

The patient is followed closely; weekly visits to the general practitioner or clinic are usually required for 4–6 weeks and the interval is gradually lengthened. A blood specimen is taken for determination of serum levels of T_4, T_3 and TSH, and a leucocyte count is made on each visit. The reports may indicate a need for an adjustment in the dosage of the antithyroid drug.

Drug therapy may be given to reduce the hyperthyroid patient's nervousness and agitation; for example, propranolol a beta-adrenergic blocking agent may be prescribed to treat some of the toxic manifestations of hyperthyroidism. It decreases the heart rate and rapidly abates the fever of thyrotoxicosis.

Radiation treatment. If the patient is over 40 years old or if unable to tolerate the antithyroid drugs, radioactive iodine (I^{131}) may be administered. Treatment by radioiodine (I^{131}) is very simple. It is given orally and the radioiodine is trapped in the thyroid, where its radiations destroy tissue, reducing the functioning mass. Improvement is usually evident in 3 weeks and the metabolic rate is expected to reach a normal level in 2–3 months. Radioiodine is not generally given for therapeutic purposes to persons who are likely to want to have children, and is never given during pregnancy. The therapeutic dose is not considered large enough to constitute a radiation hazard to those in the person's environment.

The patient is observed closely for signs of aggravation of his disease and thyroiditis, manifested by tenderness and soreness in the area of the gland. Rarely, a thyroid crisis may develop (see p. 657). After receiving the I^{131}, regular visits to the clinic or the doctor are necessary. The patient is examined for remission of his disease and for possible hypothyroidism. The serum T_3, T_4 and TSH levels are determined. If hypothyroidism is indicated, a replacement preparation (e.g. a thyroxine preparation) is prescribed.

Surgical therapy. A partial thyroidectomy may be done if radioactive iodine is contraindicated: for example if the patient is young, if antithyroid drug therapy has failed, if sensitivity precludes its prolonged administration, or if the gland is very large, causing disfigurement or pressure on the respiratory tract or on the oesophagus. In hyperthyroidism, approximately three-quarters of the gland is removed; in the case of cancer of the thyroid, a complete thyroidectomy is done which necessitates continuous replacement drug therapy during the remainder of the patient's life.

Assessment
An accurate record of the patient's temperature, pulse and respirations is made at least every 4 hours,

and the patient's responses and degree of restlessness and agitation are noted frequently. This is necessary so that an early indication of increasing thyrotoxicosis and cardiac insufficiency may be recognized and receive prompt attention. The patient is told that his vital signs will be checked at regular intervals so he will not be unduly apprehensive about his condition because of the frequent checking. The doctor may request the recording of a sleeping pulse; in hyperthyroidism, the elevated rate persists during sleep. The patient is weighed daily or every second day to determine if his calorie intake is keeping pace with his metabolic rate. Reactions to visitors are noted; an elevation in pulse rate and increased agitation and excitement may indicate the need for additional limitations on visitors.

Identification of patient problems
The patient with hyperthyroidism is expending energy in excess of the body's ability to produce energy. Metabolic processes are increased, requiring more calories to prevent excessive weight loss. Environmental stimuli increase energy demands further.

Problems which may be experienced by the patient with hyperthyroidism include:
1 Increased anxiety and emotional lability because of the increased arousal associated with high blood levels of thyroxine
2 Alteration in nutrition due to the increased metabolic rate and excessive energy expenditure
3 Hyperactivity and fatigue because of increased energy expenditure
4 Intolerance of warm environments
5 Increased likelihood of injury to skin and eyes, due to increased sweating, weight loss, restlessness and possible exophthalmos
6 Altered body image related to changes in appearance (exophthalmos, tremors, weight loss)
7 Lack of knowledge related to the disorder, and/or medications

Nursing intervention

1. *Increase in anxiety.* The *goal* is to reduce anxiety.
• *Environment.* Because of the patient's nervousness and hyperexcitability, quietness and serenity of environment are very important. An established routine, so that he knows what to expect and what is expected of him at given times, may prevent unnecessary disturbance which only aggravates his condition. If the patient is being cared for at home, the family is made fully aware of these needs. They are advised that his irritability, restlessness and emotional lability are characteristic of his illness and that to argue with him or criticize him will worsen it.

In the hospital, the patient is placed in a single room; if this is not possible, careful consideration is given to his placement on the ward. Exposure to very ill, talkative or otherwise disturbing patients should be avoided.

- *Information*. The nurse explains all procedures and medical treatment to the patient and family and answers questions regarding care. They receive an explanation of the disease, the cause of symptoms, what to expect from treatment and are taught measures to relieve symptoms. The nurse works in a calm, quiet, competent manner and, whenever possible, the same nurse cares for the patient, since adjusting to strange personnel may be stressful.
- *Identification of additional stresses*. The nurse works with the patient and family to identify additional stresses that may have resulted from the patient's illness or existed previously. Referrals to community resources are made if relevant.
- *Visitors*. Visitors are restricted to those persons who do not excite the patient and who use judgement in their conversation with him. Obviously, those who focus on the patient's condition, transmit disturbing information, or are themselves excitable could aggravate the patient's symptoms. Visitors and family members require information on the need for limiting visitors and suggestions as to how they can best contribute to the patient's well-being.

2. Alteration in nutrition. The *goal* is to maintain or increase body weight.
- *Diet*. The patient requires a high-protein, high-carbohydrate, high-calorie diet (4000–5000 kcal) to prevent tissue breakdown by the high metabolic demand and to satisfy the patient's increased appetite. A snack between meals and at bedtime is provided. Tea and coffee are usually restricted to eliminate caffeine stimulation. Decaffeinated coffee may be used as a substitute.

- *Fluids*. The patient's excessive heat production and resulting perspiration increases his fluid loss, necessitating extra fluids. Also, there is an increased production of metabolic wastes, requiring dilution for elimination by the kidneys. A minimum intake of 3000–4000 ml daily is recommended, unless contraindicated by cardiac or renal dysfunction. An explanation of the importance of this amount of fluid is made to the patient to gain his cooperation, and a variety of fluids are provided.

3. Hyperactivity and fatigue. The *goal* is to decrease activity.
- *Rest and activity*. Activity is restricted because it increases the metabolic rate, but the patient's nervous excitability makes it difficult for him to rest. Efforts are made to provide some interest or occupational therapy that expends little energy. Depending on the severity of the patient's condition and his pulse rate, he may be allowed up,

since enforced confinement to bed may cause greater irritation and restlessness. He is discouraged from wandering about the ward aimlessly. Sedation may be ordered. A stronger preparation may be necessary at bedtime to insure adequate sleep.

The patient should be kept as comfortable as possible by frequent turning of the pillows and changing the bed linen and patient's gown when they become moist because of excessive perspiration. Situations which tend to annoy or frustrate the patient are avoided. Needs should be anticipated, and things that prove awkward for him because of tremor are unobtrusively done for him.

4. Intolerance of warm environments. The *goal* is to keep the patient comfortably cool.

Since the patient is producing more than the normal amount of body heat, he is only comfortable in an environment of lower temperature than normal persons tolerate. Scant, lightweight bedding is used and the room is kept well-ventilated and cool.

5. Damage to the skin and eyes. The *goals* are to maintain skin integrity and to prevent injury to the eyes.
- *Skin care*. A daily bath is necessary because of the profuse perspiration. If the patient is extremely restless, has lost weight and is confined to bed, special attention is given to the pressure areas. Talcum powder applied to the skin prevents friction.
- *Eye care*. If the patient has exophthalmos, the eyes should be protected from irritation by sunglasses. Methylcellulose (a conjunctival lubricant) drops (0.5–1%) may be recommended to prevent drying of the conjunctiva and cornea. The patient's vision is tested frequently, especially if the exophthalmos is progressive; compression of the optic nerve and artery may occur, with ensuing visual impairment.

6. Altered body image. The *goal* is for the patient to express concerns regarding alterations in body image.

Repeated explanations of the causes of the physical changes and assurance should be given. There is a prolonged phase of gradual improvement of the eyes once the hormone imbalance is corrected. It should be said, however, that the eyes may not return to the normal state. Good grooming and attractive dress promote self-confidence and the feeling of wellness.

7. Lack of knowledge about the disorder. The *goal* is to achieve self-management of the therapeutic regimen and self-care.

The patient and family are given information about hyperthyroidism, causes, manifestations and treatment. Learning needs are assessed and they are assisted in developing a plan for home care of the patient. The dietitian may be consulted regarding diet and meal planning.

Expected outcomes
The patient and/or family:
1 Are able to state the cause, manifestations and treatment of hyperthyroidism.
2 Are aware of the medication schedule, the expected responses and the indications of adverse reactions.
3 Understand the importance of a quiet, calm environment.
4 Feel less anxious.
5 Describe a plan for obtaining adequate nutrients and fluids.
6 Maintain or increase body weight.
7 Describe a plan to decrease physical activity and promote rest.
8 Keep his skin clean, dry and intact.
9 Demonstrate intact corneas and a usual degree of visual acuity.

NURSING THE PATIENT WHO HAS THYROID SURGERY

In caring for the patient who has had a thyroidectomy, pertinent factors to be kept in mind are: the *location of the gland in relation to the trachea and larynx; its proximity to the recurrent laryngeal nerve*, which controls the vocal cords; its *abundant blood supply*; and that the *parathyroid glands*, which influence neuromuscular irritability through their control of the blood calcium level, lie on the posterior surface of the thyroid. The nurse must be constantly alert for manifestations of disturbances due to these factors.

Preoperative preparation
The hyperthyroid patient who is to have surgery is given an antithyroid drug for several weeks prior to operation to reduce the metabolic rate, and return the gland to as near the euthyroid state as possible; alternatively propranolol in increasing dosage is given, until effective beta blockade has been achieved. During this period, whether at home or in the hospital, the care cited in the preceding section is applicable. The antithyroid drugs produce some compensatory enlargement of the gland and an increased blood supply. When the metabolic rate has been reduced to a satisfactory level, the drug is discontinued. Then, in a few days, a course of potassium iodide (Lugol's iodine) is commenced and continued for approximately 10 days. This reduces the size and vascularity of the gland, facilitating surgery and lessening the problem of bleeding. Since potassium iodide has a disagreeable taste and may also irritate the mucous membrane, it is well diluted in fruit juice (e.g. grape juice) or milk.

Preparation includes an electrocardiogram to obtain further information about the patient's cardiac status and blood typing and cross matching for transfusion. The female patient may have some concern for the cosmetic effect of the operation. She is assured that consideration is given to this and that the scar becomes barely perceptible in a few months. During the interval, it may be concealed by a scarf or necklace. Remembering that the hyperthyroid patient is hyperexcitable and apprehensive, judicious explanations are made of what may be expected after the operation. The patient is instructed to perform deep-breathing and coughing exercises. Demonstration and practice in supporting the head with the hands while turning in bed is carried out to decrease stress on the neck. Specific orders are received about the local skin preparation. For the female patient, the surgeon may require only thorough cleansing of the entire neck, upper shoulder aspect and upper chest. In the case of the male patient, shaving as well as cleansing may be indicated.

Preparation to receive the patient after operation
Special equipment to be assembled and ready for use when preparing to receive a patient following a thyroidectomy includes: (1) sandbags or small firm pillows to immobilize the head; (2) suction machine and catheters for clearing mucus from the throat; (3) sterile clip removers or stitch cutters in case of a haematoma at the site of surgery obstructing the trachea; (4) a humidifier to relieve tracheal and laryngeal irritation and facilitate the removal of mucus; (5) intravenous infusion equipment; (6) a sterile emergency intubation and tracheostomy tray in the event of respiratory obstruction; (7) equipment for obtaining a blood specimen quickly for blood calcium determination; and (8) ampules of calcium chloride or calcium gluconate, with the necessary equipment for intravenous administration in the event of the complication tetany (hypocalcaemia).

Postoperative care
A nurse remains in close attendance on the thyroidectomy patient, especially during the first postoperative 48 hours. He is usually very apprehensive, and serious complications may *develop rapidly*. Table 20.4 lists potential problems and their causative factors relevant to the patient following thyroid surgery.

Assessment. The blood pressure, pulse and respirations are recorded every 15 minutes; the frequency is gradually reduced if they remain stable. The axillary or oral temperature is recorded every 4 hours. The degree of restlessness and apprehension is noted and, if not relieved by the prescribed sedation, is brought to the surgeon's attention. Particular attention is paid to the patient's respirations; any complaint or sign of respiratory distress and cyanosis is reported promptly, since it may indicate laryngeal paralysis or compression of the trachea by accumulating blood. Some hoarseness is common and is due to irritation of the larynx by the surgery and the

Table 20.4 Identification of patients' problems following thyroid surgery.

Problem	Causative factors
1 Ineffective airway clearance	Haematoma pressing on trachea Tracheobronchial irritation from anaesthesia Difficulty in coughing up bronchial secretions because of oedema, pressure and pain at operation site, decreased head and neck mobility
2 Alteration in comfort: pain	Surgical intervention
3 Impaired mobility in head, neck and shoulders	Surgical intervention Pain and discomfort
4 Alteration in nutrition: intake of less than body requirements	Difficulty in swallowing
5 Potential for injury (haemorrhage, respiratory distress, loss of voice or tetany)	Surgical intervention to neck
6 Lack of knowledge about follow-up care	Lack of information, experience and resources

endotracheal tube used in administering the anaesthetic. The doctor is advised if the hoarseness and weakness of the voice persist beyond 3 or 4 days.

Potential patient problems (see Table 20.4)
1 Obstructed airway, because of:
  (a) Oedema, pressure and pain of the trachea, decreased head and neck mobility and tracheal-bronchial secretions from the anaesthetic, which all contribute to a difficulty in expectorating secretions.
  (b) Haematoma formation behind the wound site pressing on the trachea
2 Pain related to surgical intervention
3 Impaired mobility of head, neck and shoulders related to surgical intervention, pain and discomfort.
4 Inadequate nutrition because of difficulty in swallowing
5 Potential for injury (complications) as a result of the surgical intervention
6 Inadequate knowledge about follow-up care

Nursing intervention

1. Obstructed airway. The *goal* is to maintain respiratory function.
• The patient is assisted to a sitting position with support given to the head and neck in order to help the patient to cough and expectorate. Suction of the oropharynx is carried out if the accumulation of secretions is severe. Deep breathing and coughing should be encouraged several times each hour.
• The nurse should observe the wound and ensure free drainage from the wound drains is maintained (see below under Complications) to prevent the formation of a haematoma.

2. Pain. The *goal* is to control the pain.
Pethidine or morphine may be ordered to keep the patient comfortable and less apprehensive during the first 48 hours. Judicious use must be made of the narcotic; the drug is not repeated without consulting the

the drug is not repeated without consulting the doctor if there is evident depression of the respirations to 12 or less per minute or if there is increased difficulty in raising mucous secretions. On the other hand, unnecessary withholding of sedation increases the patient's metabolism and restlessness may precipitate tachycardia.

3. Impaired mobility of head, neck and shoulders. The *goal* is to promote wound healing and maintain range of movement of neck.
After recovery from the anaesthetic, the patient is placed on his back and the head of the bed is moderately elevated. The head and neck are supported by a pillow and are positioned in good alignment, preventing flexion and hyperextension. A sandbag or firm pillow may be necessary at each side of the head for immobilization. The patient is advised not to move his head but to relax, since it is adequately supported; he tends to develop tension in an effort to keep it still. Gentle massage of the back of the neck may promote relaxation and reduce his discomfort. When the patient's position is changed, the nurse lifts and supports the head, preserving good alignment. The patient is taught to lift and support his head by placing his hands at the back of his head when he wishes to move.

The patient often returns from the operating theatre with surgical drains inserted. These should be checked at intervals to ensure free drainage and, if a closed system, that the mechanism is functioning. While large accumulation of blood behind the wound site can cause respiratory obstruction, smaller haematomas can increase vulnerability to infection and delayed wound healing.

While the patient is confined to bed, foot and leg exercises are encouraged, as with other surgical patients. If the vital signs are stabilized and normal, the patient is assisted out of bed on the first post-operative day.

Following removal of the drains, the sutures or skin clips and firm healing of the incision, head exercises which include flexion (forward and lateral), hyperextension and turning are gradually introduced with the surgeon's approval. To prevent contraction of the scar, the patient may be taught to massage the neck gently twice daily, using lanolin, cold cream or an oily lotion.

4. Inadequate nutrition. The *goal* is to maintain adequate food intake.

Some difficulty in swallowing is usually experienced for a day or two, but fluids by mouth are encouraged as soon as tolerated. Intravenous fluids are given until an adequate amount can be taken orally. The patient progresses through a soft diet to a full diet in 2–3 days.

5. Potential for injury (complications). The *goal* is prompt identification and correction of complications.
- *Complications.* The nurse must be aware that haemorrhage, respiratory difficulty, loss of voice and tetany are serious complications which may occur following thyroid surgery. The first three may develop with startling rapidity and are usually seen within 48 hours of operation.
- *Haemorrhage* may be manifested by a rapid thin pulse, fall in blood pressure and evident bleeding. The bleeding may only be discovered by frequent checking of the dressing and by sliding the hands under the shoulders and behind the neck. Blood may collect quickly within the tissues and cause pressure on the trachea. The patient may complain of a choking sensation and shortness of breath; cyanosis and dyspnoea develop and, unless the pressure is relieved quickly, asphyxia may occur. The surgeon is notified immediately at the earliest sign of change. The dressing is loosened to promote freer, outward drainage. Instruments for removing the sutures or skin clips should already be at the bedside and the emergency tracheostomy tray is made ready, since the surgeon may consider an immediate tracheostomy necessary. On reporting the situation, the nurse may be instructed to remove the skin clips to allow the escape of blood. A thick sterile dressing is then applied until the surgeon arrives. The patient will probably be returned to the operating room to bring the bleeding under control. Blood replacement may be necessary.

Occasionally, *injury to one or both recurrent laryngeal nerves* may occur during thyroid surgery. These nerves control laryngeal muscles, the opening of the glottis and voice production. Injury to one nerve produces hoarseness and weakness of the voice but no serious respiratory disturbance. Bilateral nerve injury causes paralysis of muscles on both sides of the larynx, resulting in closure of the glottis and respiratory obstruction. The patient is unable to speak and stridor occurs (i.e. respirations become shrill and crowing), cyanosis develops and loss of consciousness ensues unless

respirations are quickly re-established. Prompt endotracheal intubation or emergency tracheostomy is done, and oxygen is administered via either tube. The injury and paralysis are rarely permanent; function is usually gradually restored, and the tracheostomy tube is removed.

During surgery, interference with the blood supply to the parathyroid glands or injury or removal of parathyroid tissue may occur which depresses secretion by the glands. Decreased parathyroid hormone concentration leads to *hypocalcaemia*, resulting in increased neuromuscular irritability and the condition known as *tetany*. Early signs of this complication include complaints of numbness and tingling in the hands and feet, muscle twitching and spasms, and gastrointestinal cramps. A change may be evident in the voice; it may become high-pitched and shrill because of spasm of the vocal cords. To confirm increased neuromuscular irritability due to hypocalcaemia, the patient is examined for a positive Chvostek's or Trousseau's sign. Chvostek's sign is demonstrated by twitching of the upper lip and contraction of the facial muscles in response to tapping of the facial nerve in front of the ear. Trousseau's sign is elicited by the inflation of a blood pressure cuff around an arm; if the blood calcium level is low, spasmodic contraction of the forearm muscles occurs, producing a claw-like flexure of the hand and fingers. A blood specimen is obtained for serum calcium determination with the appearance of early symptoms. Calcium gluconate 10% may be slowly administered intravenously by the doctor; then, an oral preparation is given until normal parathyroid function resumes. The patient is encouraged to take milk and calcium-containing foods.

Thyrotoxicosis or thyroid crisis rarely complicates the postoperative period following a thyroidectomy (see further on).

6. Inadequate knowledge about follow-up care. The *goal* is to develop a plan for post-hospital care and follow-up.

The patient's hospitalization is usually brief if no complications develop. Information as to the amount of activity he may resume is discussed with the patient. Extra rest will still be necessary, and the patient is advised to continue neck exercises until there is freedom of movement without any feeling of pulling. He is usually followed at the outpatient clinic or by the doctor for about a year, being examined for an residual laryngeal damage, hypoparathyroidism, recurring hyperthyroidism, or developing hypothyroidism. If no problems develop during that year, an annual checkup is then recommended.

Expected outcomes
The patient following thyroid surgery:
1 Is able to assume self-care.

2 Maintains body weight.
3 Demonstrates neck exercises satisfactorily.
4 Describes a plan to carry out neck exercises.
5 Describes a satisfactory plan for follow-up care.

THYROTOXIC CRISIS

This is a serious complication of hyperthyroidism that can prove fatal but, fortunately, it is rarely seen since the advent of antithyroid drugs and radioiodine. The crisis may be precipitated in a hyperthyroid person by a severe infection, such as pneumonia, or by an emotional crisis. It must also be kept in mind as a possible, but rare, complication of a subtotal thyroidectomy or radioiodine treatment. It is attributed to the sudden release of large amounts of the thyroid hormones into the circulation.

Manifestations
The metabolic rate rises rapidly and the patient manifests hyperpyrexia, an extremely rapid pulse, inordinate restlessness, disorientation, diarrhoea and vomiting, and eventually shock and coma due to heart failure and circulatory collapse.

Treatment
The patient receives a continuous intravenous infusion of glucose and electrolyte solutions. Hydrocortisone is given intravenously. An antithyroid drug such as carbimazole via a nasogastric tube may be administered. A sedative or tranquillizer such as chlorpromazine or diazepam is also given to reduce restlessness. Propranolol is prescribed to decrease tachycardia, Digoxin, given intravenously, is used if cardiac failure is present. Oxygen is administered and tepid sponging is carried out to reduce the patient's body temperature. Any underlying precipitating cause (such as infection) is treated. The patient requires constant observation and attention; a nurse remains in constant attendance.

THYROIDITIS

Inflammation of the thyroid occurs rarely and may be acute or chronic. Acute thyroiditis may be the result of viral or bacterial infection or may follow irradiation therapy of the gland. The thyroid area of the neck is tender, warm and reddened; the patient's temperature is elevated and signs of hyper- or hypothyroidism may develop. The patient is treated by bed rest if appropriate, and an antimicrobial preparation if the condition is of infectious origin, and local cold applications.

Chronic thyroiditis occurs in a form which may be referred to as *Hashimoto's disease*. This disease is an autoimmune reaction; that is, the patient develops antibodies in response to antigens originating in his own thyroid. It is suggested that substances which normally remain within the thyroglobin escape into the general circulation. The production of lymphocytes and plasma cells with antibodies is stimulated, and these cells infiltrate and attack the thyroid, resulting in destruction of the functioning tissue. The gland becomes swollen and congested, and eventually hypothyroidism develops. The condition may be treated with thyroxine, either alone or in combination with cortisone. Thyroxine is given for life, irrespective of whether or not the patient was initially hypothyroid. Thyroidectomy may be done but hypothyroidism rapidly ensues.

A type of chronic thyroiditis, which is extremely rare, is known as *Riedel's thyroiditis*. The cause is unknown. The condition is characterized by the slowly progressive involvement of the thyroid and adjacent tissues by dense, fibrous connective tissue. The affected areas become very hard and may cause pressure on the trachea and oesophagus. Surgical resection may be undertaken to relieve pressure, and various drugs used may include thyroxine, and corticosteroid and immunosuppressive drugs.[16]

CARCINOMA OF THE THYROID

The most common malignancy of the thyroid is adenocarcinoma. Signs and symptoms vary with the type of tumour but generally include rapid and progressive enlargement of the gland without an appreciable increase or decrease in thyroid hormone secretion, hardness and fixation of the gland, lymph node enlargement in the neck and supraclavicular areas, hoarseness due to involvement of the recurrent laryngeal nerve, dysphagia due to pressure on the oesophagus and respiratory distress because of pressure on the trachea.

The condition may be treated by total thyroidectomy. Full doses of oral thyroxine will be needed throughout the remainder of the patient's life. Thyroidectomy may include neck dissection to remove involved lymph nodes. If metastases are present, radioactive iodine (I^{131}) may be prescribed.

Parathyroid disorders

Primary disease of the parathyroid glands is rare; the disturbances seen are most often secondary to thyroid disease.

HYPOPARATHYROIDISM

Parathyroid insufficiency may be the result of idiopathic atrophy of the glands or surgery on the thyroid. In the case of surgery, there may have been interference with the blood supply to the glands, injury which inhibits secretion or, rarely, inadvertent removal of them.

---

[16] Dillon (1980), p. 373.

Effects
The deficiency of PTH causes hypocalcaemia, and symptoms of increased neuromuscular excitability and tetany are usually the first manifestations (muscle cramps, carpopedal spasms, laryngeal spasm affecting the voice, dysphagia, convulsions). Wheezy respirations may be heard due to broncho-spasm. Less calcium than normal is excreted in the urine because of the low blood calcium level, and the bones tend to become more dense. Renal excretion of phosphorus is reduced and the serum phosphate level is elevated, which predisposes the patient to acidosis. If the hormone deficiency is prolonged, calcium deposition may develop in the lens and con-junctiva of the eyes, the brain, lungs or gastric mucosa. The hair becomes thin and grey; areas of alopecia and loss of eyebrows are common. The skin becomes coarse and scaly and the nails are brittle and have horizontal ridges. Mental changes include depression, fatigue, psychosis, mental retardation and deficiency.

Treatment
The hypocalcaemia is corrected initially by the intravenous administration of calcium gluconate 10%. The patient is then given regular oral doses of a calcium salt, such as gluconate or lactate, along with a preparation of vitamin D to promote the absorption of the calcium. The patient is followed closely; fre-quent determinations of blood phosphorus and calcium levels are made in order to adjust vitamin D dosage. Overdosage may cause renal damage. Phosphorus-containing foods may have to be limited to avoid complications; these are principally dairy products. An alternative may be the prescription of aluminium hydroxide gel which binds the phospho-rus in the intestine, preventing its absorption. The patient is encouraged to take extra fluids to promote renal excretion of phosphorus.

HYPERPARATHYROIDISM

The cause of an excessive secretion of PTH is usually an adenoma but may rarely be hyperplasia or carci-noma of the glands.

Manifestations
The high PTH concentration in the blood causes decalcification of the bones, and hypercalcaemia occurs. The blood level of inorganic phosphorus falls as its renal excretion increases, and the concentration of calcium in the glomerular filtrate is higher than normal, predisposing to the formation of renal calculi. Neuromuscular excitability is depressed and loss of muscle tone is evident. Demineralization of the bones may be so marked that fibrous cystic areas develop which frequently lead to deformities and pathological fractures. In some instances bone tumours consisting of an overgrowth of osteoclasts develop. When bone changes occur, the disorder

may be referred to as *von Recklinghausen's disease* or *osteitis fibrosa cystica*, and the patient may experience tenderness and pain in the bones, especially with weight-bearing.

The patient with hyperparathyroidism may develop acute pancreatitis. He may complain of muscular weakness, loss of appetite, nausea, vomiting and constipation. The urinary volume is usually increased because of the excessive amounts of calcium and phosphorus to be excreted. Renal function may become impaired; the tubular epith-elium may be damaged by the excessive excretion of calcium or the formation of renal calculi. Frequently, the disease is only recognized when some deformity develops or a pathological fracture occurs.

Treatment
The patient with hyperparathyroidism should receive 3–4 l of fluid daily followed by the admin-istration of a diuretic such as frusemide (Lasix) to increase urinary excretion. If anorexia, nausea and vomiting are problems, intravenous infusions may be necessary to ensure an adequate intake. Fluid intake and output are carefully monitored. Foods containing calcium are restricted in the diet.

Hyperparathyroidism is treated by surgical exci-sion of the gland with the adenoma or, in the case of hyperplasia, removal of all the glands but one. Fol-lowing surgery, the patient is observed closely for the early signs of possible hypocalcaemia (tetany). Frequent serum calcium and phosphorus determina-tions are made. A diet high in calcium and phospho-rus may be necessary to restore normal bone structure.

Disorders of the adrenal cortices

As with other endocrine glands, dysfunction of the adrenal cortices may involve hyposecretion or hypersecretion of their hormones. Adrenocortical hypofunction produces Addison's disease. Hyper-function may cause Cushing's syndrome or primary aldosteronism.

ADDISON'S DISEASE (PRIMARY ADRENAL INSUFFICIENCY)

Primary failure of the adrenal cortices to produce corticosteroids is most often the result of atrophy of the glands but may also be caused by congenital adrenal hyperplasia, tubercular infection, adrenal haemorrhage or a neoplasm. Atrophy of the glands is attributed to an autoimmune reaction; specific antibodies to the adrenal glands are present in up to 60% of patients with primary adrenal insuffi-ciency.[17] Secondary hypofunction of the adrenal cortices occurs with hypopituitarism and the conco-mitant deficiency of ACTH and with excessive administration of steroids. The patient undergoes

---

[17] Dillon (1980), p. 510

various diagnostic procedures to distinguish between primary and secondary adrenocortical insufficiency. This is important since, in secondary insufficiency, the secretion of aldosterone usually remains normal and mineralocorticoids should not be administered.

Manifestations (see Table 20.5)

In Addison's disease there is a deficiency of cortisol which interferes with the maintenance of a normal blood sugar level; the body cannot compensate by gluconeogenesis, liver glycogen is depleted and hypoglycaemia develops, especially between meals. There is a general depression of metabolic activity and energy production. The ability to cope with even mild stress is greatly diminished and minor infections, slight injuries, exposure to extremes of temperature, or emotional problems that are relatively insignificant to the normal person may prove very serious to these individuals.

The patient complains of weakness and constant fatigue which becomes progressively more severe and incapacitating unless treatment is instituted. Listlessness, irritability and impaired mental ability may be manifested. Anorexia, nausea, abdominal pain and constipation alternating with diarrhoea are common complaints. Increased sensitivity to cold develops. The patient loses weight. The skin takes on a dusky, bronze hue and brown pigmented areas appear, especially in sites normally exposed to light, pressure or friction such as the backs of the hands (particularly over the knuckles), face, neck, axillae and 'belt' areas. Patchy areas of pigmentation may also be observed in the oral mucosa and conjunctivae.

The adrenocortical insufficiency causes an outpouring of the hormone ACTH. As noted earlier in this chapter, ACTH is similar in chemical structure to the melanocyte-stimulating hormone (MSH) and, in high concentration, may produce similar effects. As a result, pigmented areas of the skin are common to the patient with Addison's disease.

The aldosterone deficiency incurs decreased reabsorption of sodium by the renal tubules with a consequent excessive loss of water as well as sodium in the urine. Severe dehydration may develop, leading to a depletion of the intravascular volume and ensuing reduced cardiac output, hypotension and shock. There is not the normal exchange of hydrogen ions for reabsorbed sodium ions in the kidneys, and acidosis may develop. Increased reabsorption of potassium by the tubules produces an elevated blood level, and hyperkalaemia may develop (see Chapter 6) and cause cardiac arrhythmias. Hypotension is invariable and it would be unlikely that someone with a systolic blood pressure above 110 mmHg would have the disease. An infection or trauma may precipitate a slowly progressive disorder.

Treatment and nursing intervention

Addison's disease is treated by maintenance doses of corticosteroid preparations. The glucocorticoids are replaced by the oral administration of a cortisol preparation two or three times daily. The deficiency of mineralocorticoid (aldosterone) associated with primary adrenocortical insufficiency is met by giving fludrocortisone (synthetic aldosterone) orally once

Table 20.5 Summary of signs and symptoms associated with adrenal insufficiency and adrenocortical hyperfunction.

Addison's disease (adrenal insufficiency)	Cushing's disease (adrenal cortical hyperfunction)
Hypoglycaemia Weakness Constant fatigue Listlessness, irritability Impaired mental ability	Hyperglycaemia Weakness Backache
Anorexia, nausea Abdominal pain Constipation alternating with diarrhoea	Muscle wasting, pendulous abdomen Abnormal fat distribution
Weight loss	Weight gain
Skin: dusky, bronze with brown pigmentation	Skin: purple striae on abdomen, buttocks and thighs; atrophy and ecchymoses
Fluid loss; dehydration	Fluid retention; oedema
Electrolyte imbalances $\uparrow$ serum K^+ $\downarrow$ serum Na^+	Electrolyte imbalances $\uparrow$ serum K^+ $\downarrow$ serum Na^+
Hypotension	Hypertension
Cardiac arrhythmia	Cardiac dysfunction
	Secondary male sexual characteristics in females

daily or deoxycortone acetate intramuscularly. If the latter is used, after the maintenance dose is determined, a depot preparation may be given intramuscularly at intervals of 3 or 4 weeks instead of the daily dose. The patient with secondary adrenocortical insufficiency does not require the aldosterone replacement.

The nurse caring for a patient receiving corticoid preparations must be familiar with the potential adverse effects of these drugs. If the patient receives corticoids in doses even slightly in excess of the amounts normally secreted, certain changes are likely to occur, especially with prolonged administration. Constant observation is necessary for early signs of side-effects. Restlessness, insomnia, euphoria and swings in mood may be manifested. The patient's susceptibility to infection may be markedly increased by the drug's suppression of lymphocyte and antibody production and local inflammatory responses. Muscle wasting and weakness may occur as a result of an excessive protein breakdown and increased loss of potassium in the urine. Sodium and water retention may be evidenced by oedema. Increased fat deposition on the trunk and face may develop, changing the patient's general appearance. Increased fullness and rounding of the face produces the characteristic change referred to as the 'moon facies'. Females may develop secondary male characteristics accompanied by growth of hair on the face, and growth of the breasts in males is occasionally seen. Prolonged administration of corticoids in excess of normal secretion may produce hyperglycaemia and glycosuria. The patient also becomes predisposed to the development of gastrointestinal lesions, such as peptic ulcers.

The patient with Addison's disease is encouraged to take a high-carbohydrate, high-protein diet. The danger of hypoglycaemia which may occur with glucocorticoid deficiency may be offset by the patient taking nourishment between meals and at bedtime. In primary adrenal insufficiency the patient may require additional sodium chloride. A directive as to the amount of salt to be included in the diet should be received from the doctor; the average amount served with meals may be sufficient. The patient with secondary adrenocortical insufficiency will not require additional salt.

Acute corticoid insufficiency, which is also referred to as *Addisonian crisis*, may develop when corticoid replacement is inadequate or omitted, or it may be what brings the patient for medical attention before the disease is diagnosed. Frequently a crisis is precipitated by some physical or psychological stress such as infection, exposure to extremes of temperature, gastrointestinal upset (e.g. vomiting and diarrhoea), fever, profuse perspiration, strenuous activity, anxiety or grief. Acute insufficiency is serious and, unless treated promptly, can rapidly lead to death. Early symptoms are nausea, vomiting, diarrhoea, abdominal pain, fever and extreme weakness.

Severe hypoglycaemia and dehydration develop rapidly; the blood pressure falls, and shock and coma may follow. Blood glucose, sodium and cortisol levels are low and the potassium and urea concentrations are markedly elevated.

Addisonian crisis is treated by continuous intravenous infusion of dextrose in normal saline to which hydrocortisone (cortisol) is added for at least the first 24 hours. Hydrocortisone is also given orally or intramuscularly. The large doses of hydrocortisone which the patient receives usually exert a sufficient sodium-retaining effect, eliminating the need for supplementary administration of a mineralocorticoid preparation.

Frequent recordings of the blood pressure, temperature, pulse, respirations and level of response are made. The patient is kept at absolute rest to avoid expenditure of energy and is turned, bathed and fed by the nurse. He is kept flat and any change of position is made slowly because of the hypotension. Frequent, high-carbohydrate feedings are given as soon as they can be tolerated. When the patient's blood pressure and other vital signs have returned to normal and are sustained, and the condition which precipitated the crisis has been controlled, the corticoid dosage is gradually reduced to maintenance level.

Potential patient problem: lack of knowledge about disease management. The *goals* are to acquire self-regulation of the disease and to maintain a satisfactory level of functioning.

Nursing intervention. Since primary adrenal insufficiency requires life-long replacement therapy, an important nursing function is teaching the patient and his family about his disease and the necessary care. A simple explanation is given of the nature of the condition, and he is told that, although hormone replacement will be necessary during the remainder of his life, if the prescribed therapeutic regimen is followed, he can live a relatively normal life.

The importance of regular and adequate hours of rest, stopping activities short of fatigue and avoiding exposure to cold are stressed, indicating the effect of exposure and overexertion on cellular activity and the blood sugar level. No medications, including laxatives, except those ordered by the doctor should be taken. Explicit instructions are given regarding the taking of the prescribed corticoid preparations; directions are written clearly, and the importance of taking the exact amounts at the prescribed times is emphasized. The patient is warned that he should guard against being without his medication. Increased doses of medication may be recommended during periods of stress. If the patient is to have deoxycortone acetate intramuscularly every 3 or 4 weeks instead of fludrocortisone by mouth, a referral is made to a clinic or to the district nurse for the administration. The high-carbohydrate, high-protein diet with the amount of sodium recommended by the doctor is discussed in detail, explaining the need for nourishment between meals and at bedtime to maintain a normal blood sugar level.

The patient and family are advised of the need for avoiding contact with those with an infection as much as possible, and suggestions are made as to how this may be achieved. They should understand that a stressful situation or illness demands more corticoids. To prevent a serious crisis or acute corticoid insufficiency, prompt medical attention is necessary with any disorder such as a respiratory infection, vomiting, diarrhoea, fainting or sudden weakness. The role of worry and emotional situations in precipitating a crisis is emphasized. The patient with Addison's disease should always carry a steroid card or wear a Medic Alert bracelet or pendant which clearly indicates that he has a corticoid insufficiency and what should be done in the event of injury or sudden collapse.

In teaching, the nurse does not attempt to provide all the necessary information at one time. The instruction is planned to cover several sessions; salient points are clarified and reinforced by repetition, and opportunities are provided for the patient and family members to ask questions.

Expected outcomes
The patient and/or family are able to:
1 State the purpose of life-long steroid replacement therapy.
2 Describe a schedule for taking medications daily.
3 State the names, dosage, frequency, actions and side-effects of each prescribed medication.
4 State the effects of stress on his disease.
5 Describe a plan to minimize stress in daily living.
6 Describe actions to take to minimize the effects of stress when it occurs.
7 Discuss plans to minimize exposure to infection.
8 Describe symptoms that indicate Addisonian crisis and actions to take if symptoms develop.
9 Wear a Medic Alert tag and/or carry a steroid card identifying the disorder and medication plan.
10 Describe a plan for continuing health care.

CUSHING'S SYNDROME (ADRENOCORTICAL HYPERFUNCTION)

This is a rare disorder which is more common in females and results from an excessive secretion of adrenal corticoids. It may be due to primary hyperfunction of one or both of the adrenal cortices or may be secondary to a pathological hypersecretion of ACTH by the anterior pituitary gland. Primary hyperactivity of the adrenal cortex is usually caused by a neoplasm, most frequently an adenoma, but may also occur as a result of unexplained hyperplasia. A common cause is excessive administration of ACTH

Manifestations
These will vary in individual patients according to age and the amount of corticoid being produced in excess of the normal. The increased output of cortisol causes excessive protein catabolism, gluconeogenesis, an abnormal distribution of fat and atrophy of lymphoid tissue. The patient manifests a decreased glucose tolerance, hyperglycaemia, and muscle wasting and weakness. The appearance changes because of the increased deposition of fat on the trunk, thin wasted limbs, and a round, bloated-looking face ('moon' face). Purple striae may appear, notably on the abdomen, buttocks and thighs, and are due to increased fragility of the blood vessels and atrophy of the skin. Ecchymoses are common. The production of lymphocytes is suppressed, increasing the patient's susceptibility to infection. Osteoporosis may occur, usually in the vertebrae, because of calcium mobilization; the patient frequently complains of backache.

The excessive secretion of mineralocorticoids results in electrolyte, fluid and acid–base imbalances. Hypernatraemia, water retention and hypokalaemia develop. The increased reabsorption by the renal tubules of sodium ions in exchange for hydrogen ions (see Chapter 6) depletes the acid ions, producing alkalosis. The low blood level of potassium may cause extreme weakness and cardiac dysfunction. Hypertension due to the sodium and water retention is common.

As a consequence of the increased production of androgens, the female patient develops secondary male characteristics. There is a marked growth of hair on the face, the voice deepens, breasts atrophy, amenorrhoea occurs and the clitoris may enlarge. If the disease occurs in childhood, precocious sexual development is evident in the male. The female child manifests masculinization with marked enlargement of the clitoris.

If the disease is secondary to a hypersecretion of ACTH, the disturbances are associated principally with an excessive production of the glucocorticoids only.

Treatment and nursing intervention
The treatment of Cushing's syndrome depends upon whether the hypersecretion of corticoids is due to primary dysfunction of the adrenal cortices or is the result of a hypersecretion of ACTH. In the case of an adrenocortical neoplasm, the affected gland is removed. If the cause is hyperplasia, a bilateral adrenalectomy is usually done. The patient then receives hormonal replacement therapy as outlined under Addison's disease. If the condition is secondary to a pituitary tumour the tumour is usually treated by irradiation or surgical removal.

Nursing care of the patient with Cushing's syndrome is mainly symptomatic. If he is ambulatory, precautions are necessary to prevent accidental falls which may occur because of his weakness. The fluid intake and output are recorded to determine the amount of water retention, and the sodium intake is restricted. The blood pressure and pulse are taken at regular intervals so that early changes may be detected. Changes in mood and behaviour are common and should be recorded. Exposure to persons with infection is avoided because of the patient's lowered resistance.

PRIMARY ALDOSTERONISM

An excessive production of aldosterone occurs rarely and is usually caused by an adenoma or hyperplasia of the particular adrenocortical cells which secrete the hormone. The most striking features of the disease are the excessive renal loss of potassium, retention of sodium and hypertension. The patient experiences severe generalized muscular weakness due to the hypokalaemia. Depletion of the body potassium reduces the kidneys' ability to concentrate the urine, and polyuria occurs. Despite an increased retention of salt, there is no corresponding retention of water or oedema. This is attributed to an increased glomerular filtration rate and the polyuria. As a result of the hypernatraemia and polyuria, the patient usually experiences severe thirst. An elevation of arterial blood pressure is characteristic. In addition to hypernatraemia and hypokalaemia, laboratory investigation reveals elevated urinary and plasma aldosterone levels and normal renin concentration. Treatment consists of surgical removal of the adenoma or affected gland preceded by administration of potassium salts.

Secondary hyperaldosteronism due to an excessive secretion of renin by the kidneys may occur. It may be treated with spironolactone, an aldosterone antagonist, or renal surgery.

Dysfunction of the adrenal medullae

PHAEOCHROMOCYTOMA

Disease of the adrenal medullae is rare and most commonly occurs in the form of a neoplasm known as a phaeochromocytoma, which produces an excessive amount of adrenaline and noradrenaline. The tumour is usually unilateral and benign and causes hypertension, hyperglycaemia and hypermetabolism. The increased liberation of large amounts of the hormones is usually paroxysmal at first, lasting from a few minutes to hours, but is likely to eventually become persistent. The patient frequently complains of a pounding headache, nausea, vomiting, palpitation, air hunger, nervousness, tremor and weakness. Sweating, pallor, dilatation of the pupils, tachycardia and a sharp rise in the blood pressure are also manifested. The increased glucogenolysis and subsequent elevated blood sugar may result in glucosuria.

Tests used to establish the diagnosis of phaeochro-mocytoma include the estimation of the blood and urinary content of the hormones or their major metabolite, vanillylmandelic acid (VMA). Computerized axial tomographic (CAT) scanning and ultrasonography are more favoured because they are non-invasive.

The patient with phaeochromocytoma is treated by surgical removal of the tumour of the affected gland. Sympathetic blocking agents are administered preoperatively to decrease blood pressure and reduce other symptoms.

NURSING IN ADRENAL SURGERY

Surgery of the adrenal glands may be done on patients with hypersecretions of hormones due to hyperplasia or tumours of one or both glands. The procedure may involve the removal of both adrenal glands (bilateral or total adrenalectomy), the removal of one gland (unilateral adrenalectomy) or resection of a part of a gland (subtotal adrenalectomy). Bilateral adrenalectomy is occasionally undertaken in patients with cancer of the breast and occasionally in those with cancer of the prostate. Malignant disease of these organs is dependent to some extent on sex hormones, and, since the adrenal cortices produce both oestrogens and androgens, their removal eliminates a source of the supporting hormones. In the case of cancer of the breast, adrenalectomy is preceded by oophorectomy (removal of the ovaries). The patient with cancer of the prostate undergoes orchidectomy (removal of the testicles) before adrenalectomy is considered.

Preoperative preparation
Preparation of the patient for adrenal surgery includes the general preparation cited in Chapter 11. Blood studies are done to determine electrolyte concentrations, and corrections are made as indicated. Because of an excessive potassium excretion, a solution of potassium chloride may be ordered to restore the normal level of potassium in the blood. The blood sugar level and glucose tolerance are investigated. The patient is given a high-protein diet because of the protein depletion due to excessive glucocorticoid secretion. The fluid intake and output are measured, and the balance is noted. The blood pressure is recorded at least once daily to serve as a postoperative comparative base-line. The patient with hyperfunction of the adrenal cortices frequently has experienced hypertension for some time. Phentolamine (Rogitine) and/or phenoxybenzamine hydrochloride may be prescribed preoperatively to reduce vasomotor tone and hypertension because the anaesthetic and actual surgery may precipitate severe hypertension.[18]

If both adrenal glands are to be removed, the patient and his family must understand that constant

---

[18] Sabiston (1985), p. 685.

hormone replacement will be necessary for the remainder of the patient's life.

After operation, the patient's respirations tend to be shallow because the incision is close to the diaphragm. In discussions with the patient as to what he may expect postoperatively, emphasis is placed on the need for frequent deep breathing, coughing and early ambulation to prevent complications. He is taught how to cough.

The surgeon's approach to the adrenal gland is usually through a high flank incision or occasionally through the abdomen. When a bilateral adrenalectomy is done, two incisions are made unless the transabdominal approach is used. The entire trunk from the nipple line down to and including the pubis is cleansed. (This area *may* be shaved—see p. 191.) A nasogastric tube is passed before the sedative is given on the morning of operation. This prevents postoperative vomiting and abdominal distension.

Cortisol may be administered before and during as well as following the operation to prevent adrenal insufficiency in the immediate postoperative period. An intravenous solution is run slowly and continuously. This is in preparation for prompt administration of corticosteroids or a vasopressor as indicated.

Postoperative care

Assessment and management of medication and fluid therapy. During the first few postoperative days, and until the maintenance dosages of cortisol and deoxycortone or fludrocortisone are established in the case of adrenalectomy, special attention is paid to the patient's blood pressure, fluid balance and blood chemistry. Constant nursing care is necessary until the vital signs and the corticoid, sodium and potassium concentrations are stabilized. The blood pressure, respirations and pulse are recorded every 15 minutes for several hours and the interval gradually lengthened if they remain satisfactory. Any rapid or significant fall in the blood pressure, dyspnoea, or tachycardia is reported promptly. The fluid intake and output are accurately measured, and any imbalance is brought to the doctor's attention. Frequent checks are made of the blood sodium, potassium and glucose levels which influence the amount of corticoids given. Vomiting after the nasogastric tube is removed, increased weakness, dehydration, hypotension and an elevated temperature may indicate acute corticoid insufficiency.

As indicated previously, deep breathing and coughing are very important while the patient is confined to bed and are encouraged at least every 2 hours. The patient's position is also changed every 1–2 hours. Any complaint of chest pain is reported at once.

Intravenous corticoids are given continuously for a day or two with the dosage and rate of flow adjusted to the patient's clinical manifestations and the electrolyte and fluid balances. Oral doses of cortisol are started as soon as tolerated by the patient; a daily intramuscular injection of deoxycortone is also given and is usually replaced by oral fludrocortisone in a few days. The dosage of both corticoid preparations is gradually tapered off until maintenance amounts are established. When the intravenous corticoids are withdrawn, an intravenous infusion of glucose in water or normal saline is continued slowly even though the patient may be tolerating fluids by mouth. The purpose of this is to keep the route available for quick administration of corticoids or a vasopressor [e.g. metaraminol (Aramine) or noradrenaline acid tartrate (Levophed)] if needed. The patient's condition tends to be labile and may change quickly. The nurse must be constantly alert for signs of corticoid insufficiency or indications of excessive corticoid administration. When the nasogastric tube is removed, the patient is started on fluids containing glucose and progresses to a regular diet as tolerated.

When surgery is performed to remove a phaeochromocytoma, monitoring of the blood pressure is necessary every ½–1 hour for at least 36–48 hours; severe fluctuations may occur. A marked rise may occur during or immediately following surgery because of an excessive liberation of catecholamines from the tumour during removal. An adrenergic blocking agent such as phentolamine (Rogitine) is kept available for quick intravenous administration to neutralize the medullary hormones.

More often the problem following surgery is severe hypotension and concomitant shock. The blood pressure is maintained by giving a vasopressor such as noradrenaline acid tartrate or metaraminol in an intravenous solution. The rate of flow must be carefully controlled and adjusted according to frequent blood pressure recordings and the doctor's directives. The patient is kept flat, and any change in position achieved slowly.

When unilateral adrenalectomy or a subtotal resection of one or both glands is done, the patient may receive some cortisol following operation. Less will be required than in total adrenalectomy and it is gradually withdrawn.

Following adrenal surgery, the patient usually remains in bed until the blood pressure remains at a satisfactory level. Before commencing ambulation, the head of the bed is elevated and the blood pressure checked. When the patient is permitted to get out of bed a nurse remains with him, and the blood pressure is checked every 15 minutes the first time he is up. If a significant decrease in blood pressure occurs, the patient is returned to bed and kept flat. The application of elastic or crêpe bandages to the lower extremities may be necessary before getting the patient up in order to maintain a greater blood volume in vital areas.

Patient teaching. In preparation for discharge, the patient who has had a bilateral adrenalectomy receives the same instruction as the patient with Addison's disease (see p. 660). If he has had one gland removed or a subtotal resection done, he is cautioned to avoid overfatigue, exposure to extremes of temperature (especially cold), infections, and emotional disturbances as much as possible. It is possible that stress may precipitate an acute adrenal insufficiency or crisis because the remaining adrenal tissue cannot meet the increased hormonal demand. He is advised to contact his doctor immediately if he experiences weakness, fainting, fever, or nausea and vomiting, as he may require a corticoid supplement.

Following any adrenal surgery, the patient should resume activity very gradually and is followed closely at the clinic or by his doctor. Usually several months are required to adjust the hormonal replacement satisfactorily. The patient who has had hypertension due to phaeochromocytoma may not regain a stable blood pressure level for 3–4 months.

Expected outcomes for the patient following adrenal surgery are similar to those for the patient with Addison's disease.

Disorders of the islets of Langerhans

DIABETES MELLITUS

Diabetes mellitus is a heterogeneous group of disorders of carbohydrate, fat and protein metabolism characterized by chronic hyperglycaemia, degenerative vascular changes and neuropathy. It tends to accelerate degenerative changes throughout the body by widespread vascular changes in the large blood vessels and the microvessels.

Manifestations
As a result of a deficiency of insulin or inadequate insulin function there is an inadequate transfer of glucose into the cells; the utilization of glucose for energy and cellular products and its conversion to glycogen or fat and storage as such are depressed. Glucose accumulates in the blood, causing hyperglycaemia.

Fat may be mobilized from adipose tissue and broken down to provide a source of energy. The mobilized fat is withdrawn from the blood by the liver and broken down to glycerol and fatty acids. The fatty acids are oxidized by the hepatic cells to ketone bodies (acetoacetic acid, β-hydroxybutyric acid and acetone), which are then circulated and may be metabolized by cells to produce energy, carbon dioxide and water. Only a limited amount of ketone acids can be utilized by the cells. If ketogenesis proceeds rapidly, exceeding the rate at which they can be metabolized, the ketone acids accumulate in the blood, causing ketosis or ketone acidosis.

Tissue protein may also be broken down to amino acids which are used in gluconeogenesis, contributing to the hyperglycaemia. Both the uptake of amino acids by the cells and body protein synthesis are decreased.

Insulin-dependent diabetes mellitus (IDDM) usually has a sudden onset in a severe, acute form. In non-insulin-dependent diabetes mellitus (NIDDM) the onset is most often insidious, going undetected and untreated for a considerable period of time. Their diabetes may be recognized in a routine examination in which glucosuria is discovered, or eventually a distressing symptom presents which prompts them to consult a doctor.

The most striking symptoms are the result of abnormal carbohydrate metabolism and the resultant hyperglycaemia, but the syndrome is also marked by disturbances in protein and fat metabolism and degenerative changes, especially in the vascular system. The patient excretes an excessive volume of urine (polyuria) as a result of the increased concentration of glucose in the glomerular filtrate. The glucose increases the osmotic pressure of the filtrate, preventing the reabsorption of water. As a result of the excessive water loss, the patient experiences a persisting thirst (polydipsia), and dehydration and electrolyte imbalance may develop. The blood sugar concentration exceeds the capacity of the renal tubules to reabsorb it from the glomerular filtrate, and sugar is excreted in the urine (glucosuria). The maximum capacity of the renal tubules to reabsorb glucose represents what is referred to as the glucose renal threshold. The normal is 10–12 mmol/l (165 to 180 mg/dl).

Weakness and fatigue are common complaints because the glucose cannot be utilized to produce energy. There is a loss of weight which is attributed to the mobilization of fat from adipose tissue and the breakdown of protein. Some patients also experience an increased appetite (polyphagia).

Female patients may develop pruritus of the vulva, usually due to infection by fungi which thrive on the glucose deposit from the urine. The vulva becomes swollen and inflamed. In some instances it is this distressing condition that brings the patient to the doctor and leads to the diagnosis of her diabetes. Rarely, male patients develop pruritus and inflammation of the prepuce and glans penis.

Other manifestations generally associated with long-term disease are impaired vision due to retinal changes and opacity of the lens (cataract) and pain, numbness and tingling in the extremities due to peripheral neuritis.

Incidence
The two major types of diabetes are viewed as separate diseases and are discussed separately.

Insulin-dependent diabetes mellitus (IDDM) has its peak onset between 11 and 12 years of age. Studies of the incidence of IDDM lack standardization showing variability between countries and individual studies. Ranges vary from 0.07–3.5 per 1000 population.[19]

---

[19] Zemmet (1983), p. 454.

Seasonal variations occur in the onset of the disorder; the highest onset occurs in the autumn and winter and the lowest frequency in the summer, which supports the association of IDDM with viral infections.[20]

Non-insulin dependent diabetes mellitus (NIDDM) is one of the most common chronic disorders and is seen most often in middle-aged and older persons. While prevalence rates show variations in different studies, there is evidence of an increase of diabetes.[21] The incidence is higher in persons who are obese, among relatives of diabetics, and in persons of middle to upper socioeconomic groups.

Cause

The exact causes of the major types of diabetes mellitus are not known. A common factor in all types is hyperglycaemia.

Glucose metabolism. Diabetes mellitus can be caused by a variety of pathological processes that interfere with the metabolism of glucose. Such changes may occur anywhere along the insulin pathway depicted in Fig. 20.7. The dysfunction may occur in the pancreas and interfere with the production or secretion of insulin, in the bloodstream, or at the level of target tissue cells disrupting glucose uptake or utilization by the cells. Possible causes of diabetes include: (1) destruction of the beta cells; (2) abnormal synthesis of insulin; (3) retarded release of insulin; (4) inactivation of insulin in the bloodstream by antibodies or other agents; (5) altered insulin receptors or a decreased number of receptors on peripheral cells; (6) defective processing of the insulin message within the target cells; and (7) abnormal metabolism of glucose.[22] Defects in the beta cells appear to be the primary cause of insulin-dependent diabetes.

Heredity. It is now generally accepted that certain histocompatability antigens (e.g. HLA-B8, HLA-BW15 and HLA-BW18) occur more often in insulin-dependent diabetics than in healthy people. In NIDDM there is often a family history but this does not seem to be linked to HLA markers.[23] As a result the risk of development of diabetes cannot be accurately predicted. The sharing of a common diet and life-style by family members may also influence the incidence within a given family.

As many as 85% of newly diagnosed patients with IDDM have been found to possess an antibody which reacts with the alpha, beta and delta cells of the islets of Langerhans, suggesting an autoimmune factor is present. Islet cell antibodies have not been shown to be of any significance in patients with NIDDM. It is also suggested that a relationship exists between the HLA types and the development of microvascular disease and neuropathy in patients with IDDM.[24]

Obesity. The majority of diabetics who develop their disease after the age of 40 years are obese or have a history of obesity. It is believed that the number of insulin receptors on tissue cells is decreased with obesity and that the level of serum insulin increases. With weight loss and exercise, the number of cellular insulin receptors increase, insulin binding is more effective and the serum insulin level drops to a normal range. The association of diabetes with obesity is a very significant factor in considering prevention.

Infectious agents. There is increasing evidence that viral infections, especially in genetically predisposed individuals, may cause insulin-dependent diabetes. Indirect evidence of this association includes the seasonal variations found in the onset of the disease with the highest incidence in the winter and autumn and the lowest incidence in the summer. Onset of IDDM also increases following childhood viral infections. A Coxsackie virus has been isolated from human pancreatic tissue and other viruses have been demonstrated in the pancreatic tissue of laboratory animals.

Diagnostic procedures

Diagnostic tests for diabetes mellitus are used when the patient demonstrates the obvious signs and symptoms to rule out gestational hyperglycaemia and to identify individuals at risk of developing diabetes but not manifesting the typical symptoms. A *fasting blood glucose level* of more than 7.8 mmol/l is considered diagnostic of diabetes mellitus. *Urine tests* are of less value diagnostically as the blood glucose level must be above the renal threshold of 10–12 mmol/l (165–180 mg/dl) for glucose to appear in the urine. Other diagnostic tests include the *oral glucose tolerance test* and *measurement of glycosylated haemoglobin*. These tests are discussed on p. 643.

Classification of diabetes

Diabetes mellitus has been classified in a variety of ways. Classifications include: primary or secondary diabetes, juvenile or adult, and Types I, II or III.

The current international classification incorporates current knowledge of pathogenesis of the disease and patient characteristics. Table 20.6 outlines the clinical characteristics presented by patients with *insulin-dependent diabetes mellitus* (Type I) and *non-insulin-dependent diabetes* (Type II). Diabetes mellitus is categorized into three classes:

Insulin-dependent diabetes mellitus (IDDM), Type I. This

[20] Zemmet (1983), p. 455.
[21] Zemmet (1983), p. 458.
[22] Norkins (1979), p. 66.
[23] Hassan (1985) p. 93.

[24] Albin & Rifkin (1982), p. 1212.

Table 20.6 Classification of diabetes mellitus.†

	IDDM	NIDDM*
Synonyms	Juvenile onset	Maturity onset
Age of onset	Usually before 30 years	Usually after 40 years
Type of onset	Frequently sudden	Usually gradual
Presentation	Polydipsia, polyuria	Often asymptomatic
Body weight	Thin	Usually (80%) obese
Ketoacidosis	Ketosis-prone	Ketosis-resistant
Control of diabetes	Difficult; brittle	Generally easy
Control by diet alone	Not possible	Frequent
Control by oral agents	Not possible	Frequent
Long-term complications	Frequent	Frequent

*When present in youngsters (before age 20 years), non-insulin dependent diabetes is often referred to as maturity onset diabetes of youth (MODY).
†Smith & Thier (1985), p. 379.

group includes individuals who are usually but not necessarily, non-obese, develop diabetes suddenly, usually in youth, are likely to be linked to certain HLA types, and have a family history of the disease in only about 10% of cases. They are ketosis prone if insulin is withdrawn and therefore are insulin dependent. Antibodies to islet cells are frequently present and the cells are small.

Non-insulin dependent diabetes mellitus (NIDDM) Type II. Patients with Type II are generally obese, have a family history of NIDDM, develop the disease insidiously as adults, are non-ketosis prone and may demonstrate hyperinsulinism as well as hyperglycaemia. The insulin resistance may be due to a deficiency in the number of insulin receptors on the target cells or to postreceptor disturbances in the intracellular metabolism of glucose.

Other types (Type III). This class includes patients with diabetes mellitus associated with other identifiable causes. Causes include: pancreatic disease, hormonal disorders (e.g. Cushing's disease), drug or chemical causes, insulin receptor abnormalities and certain genetic syndromes.

Two additional subgroups included in the international classification are:

Impaired glucose tolerance (IGT). This group may be further divided into obese and non-obese. The prognosis can be improved if the individual stops smoking and loses weight.

Gestational diabetes (GDM). Glucose intolerance may have its onset during pregnancy.

Statistical risk groups. Included in this category are individuals at greater risk than the general population of developing diabetes. Risk factors may include: immediate family members with the disease, the presence of islet cell antibodies, and obesity.

Chronic complications of diabetes
The blood vessels of practically all diabetics undergo degenerative changes to some extent. These changes may be both microvascular and macrovascular. *Microvascular degenerative changes* are specific to diabetes; the basement membrane in the capillaries and arterioles thickens. The retinae, kidneys and skin are the areas most affected by *microvascular changes*.

Diabetic retinopathy occurs in the form of minute aneurysms in the retinal vessels. These dilatations are prone to rupture and cause a haemorrhage into the eye. The condition is only revealed by ophthalmoscopic examination. Diabetic retinopathy is a leading cause of blindness; visual loss varies with the location and proliferation of the lesions. Risk factors in the development of proliferative diabetic retinopathy include; poor diabetic control, increased diastolic blood pressure, impaired renal function, deterioration in motor nerve conduction and increased triglyceride levels.

Renal function may be slowly impaired by changes in the glomerular capillaries (intercapillary glomerulosclerosis or Kimmelstiel–Wilson syndrome) and by sclerotic changes in the larger renal vessels. The patient may manifest albuminuria and some degree of hypertension.

Macrovascular degeneration involves the development of atherosclerosis (deposits of the fatty substance cholesterol) in the arteries, narrowing their lumen. Atherosclerosis of the coronary arteries of the diabetic frequently leads to angina pectoris and myocardial infarction, especially in older persons.

Defective circulation due to vascular changes in the lower limbs may lead to gangrene. A small superficial injury may be a precipitating factor and the ensuing gangrene may necessitate the amputation of a toe, foot or leg. Restricted circulation may be manifested by abnormal coldness of the extremities, numbness, discoloration, muscular cramps, weakness, burning pain or a small ulcer that does not heal.

Management and nursing care of patients with vascular degenerative disorders are discussed in Chapter 14.

Diabetic neuropathy.[25] This complication affects all parts of the nervous system except the brain. Peripheral neuropathy is usually bilateral and worsens at night. The patient may experience muscular cramps, tingling and burning sensation as well as pain. Deep tendon reflexes are absent and the patient's vibratory and position senses may be impaired. Changes occur in the shape of the hands and feet; muscle atrophy and demineralization of bone occur. Joints deteriorate (Charcot's joints) and foot drop may develop. Autonomic neuropathy usually causes changes in gastrointestinal and oesophageal functioning. Impotence and retrograde ejaculation may occur in the male.

The causes of neuropathy in the diabetic are not understood. Treatment is symptomatic and good diabetic control is considered essential in limiting the progress of diabetic neuropathy.

Metabolic complications of diabetes are discussed on p. 678.

Prevention and screening

With the knowledge now available, preventive measures in diabetes mellitus are limited but measures can be taken to decrease side-effects of the disease by prevention and/or correction of obesity and stopping smoking. This is especially important for those with a family history of diabetes or a suggestive obstetric history. As indicated previously, the majority of non-insulin dependent diabetics are either obese at the time their disease is manifested or have a history of obesity. The incidence of diabetes among women who have previously given birth to an infant of 4.5 kg (10 lb) or more is sufficiently significant to recommend that they maintain their ideal weight and be checked annually for diabetes mellitus. The hospital and visiting nurse have a responsibility to advise persons who are overweight of the many adverse effects of obesity and that they are possible candidates for diabetes mellitus. Progress in defining genetic markers may soon lead to the ability to identify individuals at risk of developing insulin-dependent diabetes and the possibility of immunization or other measures to prevent the disease.

Programmes for screening and education of the general public about diabetes mellitus are organized by national diabetic associations in some countries. Routine urine testing at the time of health checks for job applicants, and when people are attending a hospital clinic for any reason, may unexpectedly uncover glycosuria. Women with a history of having had a large baby should be alert to the possibility of being a latent diabetic.

Informing the public as to the characteristics of diabetes mellitus, susceptibility factors (obesity and family history) possible consequences of undetected and uncontrolled diabetes by, for example, occupational health departments associated with the workplace is important.

Management

Management of diabetes mellitus is directed toward establishing and maintaining metabolic control by correcting the hyperglycaemia and glucosuria, maintaining the patient's normal weight and strength (and in the case of a child, normal growth and development), encouraging appropriate activity and the prevention of complications commonly associated with diabetes. The treatment of all patients includes a carefully regulated diet, moderate exercise and education about the disease and necessary self-care; for insulin-dependent diabetics it will include the administration of insulin. Patients with NIDDM may require oral hypoglycaemic agents. The plan of treatment for each patient is *determined on an individual basis*; the therapeutic requirements for control in the case of one insulin-dependent diabetic may be quite different from that of another. This also applies to non-insulin-dependent diabetics.

Transplantation of the whole pancreas or of the insulin-producing islet tissue is feasible. The mortality rate from whole organ transplant remains significant and complications from immunosuppression are serious. Transplantation of islets of Langerhans seems to provide greater hope as a future treatment modality. Rejection is decreased by culturing the transplant tissue in vitro prior to injection into the recipient. The supply of human islet tissue for transplantation is very limited, especially in relation to the potential demand.

Identification of patient problems

Patients with insulin-dependent diabetes mellitus and with non-insulin-dependent diabetes mellitus have similar problems. Differences in disease management for each group of patients are discussed with nursing intervention.

1 Alteration in nutrition and metabolism related to impaired glucose, fat and protein metabolism.
2 Alterations in activity/exercise tolerance, related to insufficient energy for usual and unusual activity.
3 Alteration in skin integrity related to vascular and neurological complications and altered metabolic responses.
4 Insufficient information about diabetes mellitus, including:
   (a) Knowledge of the disease process
   (b) Dietary, medication and activity regimens to control disease
   (c) Blood glucose monitoring and/or urine testing
   (d) Personal hygiene

---

[25] *Neuropathy* may be defined as non-inflammatory, non-specific pathological or functional disorder of the peripheral nervous system.

(e) Prevention of acute metabolic complications

Nursing intervention

1. *Alteration in nutrition and metabolism.*
   The goals are to:
   1 Achieve physiological metabolic control by appropriate dietary and medication regimens
   2 Adjust to alterations in demand for glucose and insulin during periods of increased stress or life-style changes.

- *Diet.* Diabetes does not preclude the need for all the essential food principles. Diet is a major factor in the control of diabetes, but the diet must be individualized and based on the type of diabetes, consideration of complications of the disease and cultural, social and ethnic preferences, as well as principles of good nutrition. The prescribed 'diabetic diet' has been replaced by an individualized diet regimen with the patient assuming responsibility for planning, implementing and adjusting the diet to his needs and life-style. The diet should be quite similar to that advocated for the non-diabetic and must provide sufficient variety to make it appetizing and palatable.

The *dietary plan* indicates the number of calories required each day and the proportions of these calories to be allocated to carbohydrate, protein and fat. The number of calories is determined by the patient's ideal and present weight, age, sex, activity and previous dietary intake. Initially, if the non-insulin-dependent patient is overweight, the number of calories must be lower than the figure indicated as needed for his ideal weight. The objective is to bring about a gradual and steady loss of weight until the normal weight is achieved. Appropriate increases in the food plan are usually made as the weight approaches normal. The insulin-dependent diabetic who is losing energy through glycosuria, has impaired protein and fat synthesis as well as inefficient use of glucose and so he requires an overall increase in calorie intake until better control achieves weight gain. Children require sufficient calories to meet their developmental and activity needs. Caloric requirements of asymptomatic diabetics are similar to those of non-diabetics but excessive calories are detrimental to all diabetics.

Generally, the proportion of prescribed calories allocated to each food type is approximately 50% carbohydrate, 15% protein and 35% fat. In providing the necessary carbohydrates, concentrated forms of simple sugars, such as sugar, sweets, jam, jelly, preserves, honey, ice cream, pastries, cake and sweetened beverages are strictly limited and then only permitted as part of a meal to prevent rapid increases in blood sugar levels. It is believed that fibre-enriched meals improve glucose tolerance, lower insulin-secretion and reduce glycaemia and glucosuria.[26] The mechanism of action of fibre in achieving these results is not entirely understood, but improvement in glycaemia and lipid regulation is widely reported. The carbohydrates most commonly used are whole grain bread, high fibre cereals, milk, fruit and vegetables. In the selection of fat, the substitution of unsaturated for saturated fats is recommended because of the diabetic's predisposition to the development of atherosclerosis and vascular lesions.

Food exchange information[26] provides help for patients and their families to select a varied diet. Diet alone can successfully achieve diabetic control in about one third of cases. Food intake is usually best divided into at least three main meals. If an oral hypoglycaemic drug or insulin is used, the carbohydrate intake is usually divided across meals and snacks distributed throughout the day and evening.

Careful education and the availability of good eating guides or exchange lists permit the diet to be varied and takes into account the availability of foods as well as the patients' preferences. Cookery books, extensive information about food values, and general dietary guidelines are available from the British Diabetic Association.[27] This material can be useful in supplementing the basic but individualized food plan that will be given to each patient on diagnosis by the local dietetic team.

It must be impressed upon the patient that all of his daily food allowance should be eaten, especially if he receives insulin or a hypoglycaemic drug. If the insulin-taking patient is unable to take his usual diet, the carbohydrate requirement is made up in some way (e.g. orange juice, milk). Meals should be taken regularly; the delay or missing of a meal may upset the blood sugar level and promote the breakdown of fat. The carbohydrate is distributed over the day to avoid abnormal fluctuation in the blood sugar concentration. Foods of no significant nutrient value or 'extra' foods which the patient may have as desired include clear broths and consommé, clear tea and coffee, and artificially sweetened carbonated beverage. Saccharin has long been used as a sweetening agent. It is 400 times as sweet as sucrose and has no energy value whatever. It is destroyed by heat. Newer sweeteners, Aspartame and acesulfane potassium, are increasingly used as artificial, non-nutritive sweeteners.

Sorbitol (a sugar alcohol) has been used as a sweetening agent, as has fructose (crystalline fruit sugar). Both are virtually all absorbed and metabolized but the rate of absorption from the

---

[26] British Diabetic Association (1982).
[27] British Diabetic Association, 10 Queen Anne Street, London W1M 0BD.

gut is slow and it has less effect on blood sugar than glucose. Both are often used in the manufacture of 'diabetic' jams, boiled sweets, biscuits and chocolate. Because they do not offer any energy savings they should not be used for slimming purposes, or by diabetics whose main therapeutic aim is to reduce weight.

The use of artificial non-nutritive sweeteners and the bulk nutritive sugar substitutes are not necessary in the management of diabetes, but many patients find their use improves the quality of their life and helps make dietary restrictions more acceptable.

The diabetic diet is very much an individual factor. Following the initial dietary plan, the patient is followed closely to determine if it is satisfactory; the blood glucose levels are checked several times a day, or urine may be checked for sugar, his weight is recorded daily, and general reactions (physical and psychological) are noted. Adjustments in the total calorie intake and distribution of food throughout the day are often necessary.

To summarize, the following are important points for individuals with diabetes mellitus to note:

1 The diet provides a balance of carbohydrate, protein and fat.
2 Total caloric intake will be adjusted as necessary, for the individual to achieve and maintain a desirable weight.
3 Caloric intake is adequate to provide for optimal growth and development (childhood, pregnancy).
4 Food is eaten at regular intervals throughout the day.
5 The carbohydrate foods eaten at various intervals should be consistent from day to day, unless medication or activity warrants changes.
6 The diet should consist of normal foods with a preference for foods which have a high fibre content.
7 Food intake is adjusted to accommodate changes in life-style (e.g. illness, physical activity, emotional stress, eating-out and travel).
8 Meal plans are individualized and consider social, cultural and ethnic values of the patient and family.

For the non-insulin-dependent diabetic, control of energy intake is of major importance. Ideally, the individual should eat three meals a day and follow a consistent eating schedule. Snacks are not usually necessary but can be accommodated provided the total energy is controlled. The importance of activity should be reinforced.

For the insulin-dependent diabetic, total caloric intake and carbohydrate intake should be relatively consistent and adequate to meet nutritional and developmental needs. The meal schedule should be adhered to and appropriate snacks taken consistently throughout the day and evening if required to prevent hypoglycaemia.

• *Insulin.* Insulin is prescribed for all insulin-dependent diabetics. Non-insulin-dependent diabetics are usually controlled by diet or by diet and oral hypoglycaemics together with exercise, but may require insulin during periods of stress (e.g. infection, surgery, pregnancy or emotional crisis). Insulin is prescribed for the individual whose plasma glucose cannot be controlled at acceptable levels despite weight control and adherence to dietary regulation, and for the treatment of keto-acidosis and non-ketotic hyperglycaemia.

Insulin (a protein) can be prepared from natural sources (i.e. pancreas of cattle and pigs) or synthetically by genetic engineering. Because it is a protein, insulin is destroyed in the gastrointestinal tract by proteinases; therefore, it must be given parenterally. Several types are available and may be classified as rapid-acting with shorter period of action, intermediate-acting with longer period of action, and long-acting with prolonged period of action. The *rapid-acting* preparations include unmodified, clear solutions such as soluble insulin and Actrapid. The *intermediate-acting* insulins include semilente insulins (e.g. Semitard) insulins and isophane insulins. Those which are *absorbed more slowly* and have a prolonged effect on lowering blood sugar are protamine zinc insulin and ultralente (e.g. Ultratard) insulin. See Table 20.7 for the onset and duration of action of each type of insulin. These figures are approximate, since individual differences in responses do occur.

Conventional insulins contain small amounts of pro-insulin units along with other impurities. Because these contaminants have been shown to be antigenic, attempts have been made to refine the insulin products. Most insulin presently produced by the major manufacturers is referred to as single-peak insulin and is over 90% pure insulin. Newer products are 99% pure insulin and are referred to as monocomponent insulins. These products are expensive and their use is reserved for individuals demonstrating antigenicity and resistance to the conventional insulin products. Pure pork insulin may also be used to decrease antibody production to insulin and for individuals resistant to other insulins; it more closely resembles human insulin and is less antigenic. Lipoatrophy may occur at the site of insulin injections; if this occurs a more purified insulin is used.

It is important that the nurse caring for or counselling diabetics be familiar with the action characteristics of the various types of insulin so that appropriate instruction can be given and the patients assisted in monitoring their medication.

(a) *Administration of insulin.* Insulin is measured in

Table 20.7 Examples of commonly used insulins.*

Category	Preparations	Molecular species	Onset (hours)	Peak (hours)	Duration (hours)
Short acting	Actrapid	Pork	0.5	2–5	8–10
	Human Actrapid	Human	0.5	2–5	8–10
	Humulin S	Human	0.5	2–5	8–10
	Velosulin	Pork	0.5	2–5	8–10
	Human Velosulin	Human	0.5	2–5	8–10
	Semitard MC	Pork	1	3–8	12–14
Intermediate	Humulin I	Human	1	4–10	16–24
	Insulatard	Pork	1	4–10	16–24
	Human Insulatard	Human	1	4–10	16–24
	Monotard MC	Pork	1	4–10	16–24
	Human Monotard	Human	2	6–16	24
	Humulin Zinc	Human	2	6–16	24
Long acting	Ultratard MC	Beef	4	8–30	36
Mixture of short and inter-	Initard 50/50	Pork	0.5	3–8	16–24
mediate acting insulins	Human Initard 50/50	Human	0.5	3–8	16–24
	Mixtard 30/70	Pork	0.5	3–8	16–24
	Human Mixtard 30/70	Human	0.5	3–8	18–24
	Rapitard MC	Pork and beef	1	3–15	20
	Lentard MC	Pork and beef	3	8–18	24

*Time course of action of insulin may vary in different patients at various times of the day and according to molecular species of the insulin. Human insulins can have a more rapid onset than pork or beef.

units. Each patient's regimen is determined individually in relation to a particular schedule and diet plan in an attempt to achieve a normal physiological level of glucose throughout a 24-hour period. The regimen is organized so that insulin action coincides with major meals and also provides action overnight. Diet and activity may have to be readjusted with the insulin routine to facilitate physiological control. Blood glucose levels are normally lowest during the night and begin to rise in the early morning hours. Newer insulin pumps can be adjusted to reduce insulin delivery in the early morning hours or patients may require a night-time snack. Most insulin regimens consist of combinations of regular and intermediate-action insulin with two to four daily injections: one being given in the morning and evening or one prior to each meal and at bedtime. A continuous subcutaneous insulin infusion by a portable pump facilitates achievement of physiological glucose levels. A continuous basal infusion of insulin is delivered with increased levels provided by a bolus delivered prior to meals, during unusual activity or illness. Most patients can be taught to adjust or supplement their insulin regimen in response to changes in their blood glucose levels, changes in activity, eating patterns, stress or illness.

Insulin is given by subcutaneous injection below the subcutaneous fat to prevent lipodystrophy. The arms, thighs and abdomen are the areas used, and the site is rotated (Fig. 20.8). Injections should be at least 2.5 cm (1 in) from a previous site and each site given at least 1 month to recover. Too frequent use of one site causes fibrosing and scarring which delay absorption as well as make the injection more difficult. Newer, non-detachable needles of finer gauge are less traumatizing to tissue and decrease the air

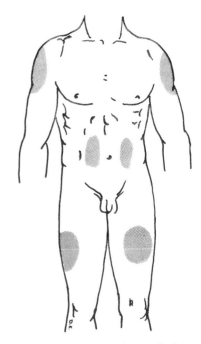

Fig. 20.8 Suitable locations for insulin injections.

bubbles in the syringe. With these shorter needles, the needle is inserted at a 90° angle rather than at the 45° angle usually used for subcutaneous injections. Cleaning the skin with alcohol prior to injection is now contraindicated. If the skin is not clean, then soap and water will suffice. Alcohol may be a contributory factor to hardening of the injection areas.

All insulin other than the soluble clear insulin must be thoroughly mixed before use to ensure uniform suspension and concentration throughout. This is done by rotating the bottle and inverting it slowly from end to end; vigorous shaking is avoided to prevent the formation of froth.

Some patients require a combination of fast-acting and slower-acting insulins. If soluble insulin and lente or isophane are to be combined for giving, the cloudy preparation (lente) is drawn into the syringe first and the clear preparation (soluble insulin) secondly. Accidental mixing can be readily identified; if any cloudy solution appears in the second vial, the vial should then be discarded. When both types are loaded, the syringe is then slowly tipped up and down until the two preparations are well mixed.

Each bottle of insulin bears an expiry date beyond which the content should not be used. Insulin should be kept in a cool place, preferably a refrigerator; freezing is avoided. Extremes of temperature and exposure to sunlight are likely to cause deterioration.

(b) *Insulin pumps.* A portable insulin infusion pump provides continuous, subcutaneous delivery of regular insulin to maintain a basal insulin level. Predetermined or self-regulated amounts of insulin to correspond with meals, unusual activity or illness are released (see Fig. 20.9). Some machines can be adjusted to decrease the rate of insulin delivery in the early morning hours. The goal of continuous insulin infusion therapy is to maintain blood glucose levels as close to normal physiological levels as possible;

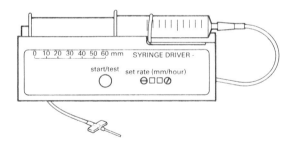

Fig. 20.9 Example of an insulin pump.

they fluctuate over a 24-hour period. Patients using these devices must be willing to be active participants in their disease management, follow dietary and activity regimens and monitor their blood glucose levels several times a day. Insulin pumps provide the patient with greater flexibility in travelling, the timing of meals and in participation in unusual activities. The pump may also be disconnected for 1–2 hours for swimming and bathing. Patient satisfaction is generally high although some individuals find the wearing of a pump is a constant reminder of having diabetes. Difficulties related to insulin pumps include battery failure, blocked needles and occasionally infection at injection sites.

(c) *Reactions.* Various local and general reactions to insulin may occur. The *local reactions* are minor in nature and include local sensitivity, lipodystrophy and fibrosis. Frequently, when insulin therapy is first started, sensitivity may be manifested at the site of injection because the insulin is a foreign protein and antigenic. The area becomes red, swollen and itchy but the response is generally temporary and disappears as the patient becomes desensitized by the repeated doses of insulin.

The local action of insulin on the adipose tissue cells may incur a swelling of the fatty tissue followed by atrophy which leaves a hollow space in the area. These atrophic areas are not serious but present an undesirable cosmetic effect. Management may consist of switching the patient to a more purified pork insulin. Frequent and repeated injections into one area of tissue may result in hypertrophy of tissue and eventual fibrosing. Fibrous tissue has poor vascularization which decreases the rate of absorption of insulin. This complication may be prevented by systemic rotation of the injection sites and avoiding the use of any one spot more often than once every 4 weeks. The nurse should also recommend that the injection site is not wiped with alcohol.

General insulin reactions include insulin resistance and hypoglycaemia. *Insulin resistance* is said to be present when diabetes cannot be controlled with less than 200 units of insulin per day.[28] It may occur secondarily to some other diseases, such as severe adrenocortical hyperfunction, acromegaly and thyrotoxicosis. As a primary condition, it is attributed to an antigen–antibody reaction. Antibodies are developed in response to the foreign protein (insulin). It is more likely to occur with insulin extracted from cattle than with that prepared from the pancreas of the pig. Insulin resistance usually develops insidiously several months after insulin treatment has begun. Treatment includes the use of purified porcine insulin, one of the newer monocomponent insulins or human insulins.

Hypoglycaemia is discussed on p. 681.

- *Oral hypoglycaemic drugs.* There are two groups of drugs which lower blood sugar—sulphonylurea compounds and biguanides (Table 20.8). The fact that they may be taken orally provides a distinct advantage. Their use is limited mainly to non-insulin dependent diabetics.

  The *sulphonylurea compounds* lower the blood sugar by stimulating the secretion of insulin and are usually used for non-obese patients. These preparations include tolbutamide, chlorpropamide and glibenclamide. The principal difference between these preparations is in the duration of their action; tolbutamide has a half-life

28 Braunwald et al (1987), p. 1795.

Table 20.8 Oral hypoglycaemic drugs.

Group	Half-life (hours)	Action
Sulphonylea compounds		Stimulates the beta islet cells of the pancreas to produce insulin
Tolbutamide	5–10	
Chlorpropamide	25—40	
Glibenclamide	10–15	
Biguanide preparations		Reduces absorption of carbohydrates from the gut
Metformin	2	May increase uptake of glucose in peripheral tissues

in lowering the blood sugar for 5–10 hours, chlorpropamide 24–40 hours, and glibenclamide for 10–15 hours. The biguanide preparation available is metformin which has a half-life of 2 hours. The action of the biguanide preparation is not clearly understood, but it is thought to improve glucose assimilation and insulin efficiency. They are less popular nowadays because of the higher incidence of side-effects, particularly gastrointestinal symptoms and the development of lactic acidaemia. They have been banned in some countries and Phenformin is no longer available in the United Kingdom.

It must be remembered that it is still important for the patient receiving oral hypoglycaemic agents to respect his prescribed diet, exercise and supervision. Although the risk of hypoglycaemia is less than with insulin therapy, it may occur, and the patient must be made aware of the early manifestations. Hypoglycaemia is more likely to occur in elderly persons and patients with renal or liver dysfunction, and with the concurrent taking of certain drugs. Examples of the latter are alcohol, aspirin, phenylbutazone, sulphonamides and methyldopa (Aldomet). Occasionally, oral hypoglycaemic agents produce some side-effects, such as gastrointestinal disturbances (heartburn, nausea, vomiting, diarrhoea), headache, skin rash and itching. Controversy has existed regarding cardiovascular effects of sulphonylurea preparations. Recent information indicates that this concern is probably unwarranted with current treatment changes, emphasis on diet and control of risk factors.[29] Long-term responses to these drugs (over 5 years) is unclear.

2. Alterations in activity/exercise tolerance. The *goals* are to:
1 Establish a daily activity and exercise pattern to promote physiological metabolic control
2 Adjust diet and medication to accommodate changes in activity level

[29] Lebovitz & Feinglos (1983), p. 606.

Diabetes should not interfere with the performance of daily activities. Physical activity promotes health and should be encouraged in moderation and at a consistent level for everyone. It promotes the use of glucose and may diminish the amount of insulin or oral hypoglycaemic needed to control the blood sugar level. It also stimulates and improves the circulation, helps to maintain muscle tone, prevents obesity and promotes a sense of well-being. Some diabetics have sufficient exercise in their occupation, but those in sedentary jobs or who are retired should have a planned programme which is introduced gradually. Since the prescription for diet and a hypoglycaemic agent is based on the patient's physical activity, the regimen should be approximately the same each day to minimize fluctuations in the blood sugar concentration. When variations in daily energy expenditure are necessary, adjustments in the diet may be needed. Extra carbohydrate in the form of fruit, milk or bread may be added if activity is increased, or even more concentrated carbohydrate forms may be required if activity is strenuous or prolonged. When the usual amount of activity is decreased for some reason (other than illness or infection), some decrease in the caloric and carbohydrate intake is usually indicated.

Active exercise at regular intervals is encouraged during hospitalization unless contraindicated for other physical reasons. With an anticipated increase of activity on discharge from the hospital, the insulin dosage may be decreased and the food plan amended accordingly. For the older diabetic a daily routine of walking and light home chores (house and garden) is recommended.

The aim is to maintain a balance between energy expenditure and the prescribed treatment (diet with or without insulin or oral hypoglycaemic). More than the usual amount of exercise lowers the blood sugar; less than the usual amount will raise it.

The diabetic participating in strenuous activity, particularly if he is on insulin therapy, should advise a colleague or, in the case of sports, a friend or sports supervisor that he is a diabetic in case of a hypoglycaemic reaction. He is instructed to increase his carbohydrate intake and/or decrease his insulin dose before he undertakes the increased energy expenditure. He should also carry sugar cubes or sweets which he can take at the first sign of weakness and hypoglycaemic reaction. When making a change in occupation that involves either a decrease or increase in activity, the diabetic should have his plan of therapy reviewed by his doctor.

3. Alteration in skin integrity. The *goal* is to maintain skin integrity.

Particular attention is paid to the patient's skin and feet, especially if he spends the greater part of the day in bed. The long standing or poorly controlled diabetic's skin is less resistant to pressure and irritation and, when broken, it readily becomes infected and is difficult to heal. This is attributed to the vascular changes. The skin is kept clean and dry; a mild soap is used for bathing, and a light application of lanolin or oil may be made to prevent cracking if the skin is dry. Foot soaks in *warm* water followed by oiling may be necessary to remove thick dry skin, calluses and corns. The toenails are cut to the shape of the toe to avoid ingrown toenails and possible infection. When the patient is in bed a footboard is used to relieve the weight of bedding on the feet, and a routine of frequent regular foot and leg exercises is established, especially with older persons. The areas vulnerable to pressure are protected by frequent turning and the placing of a square of synthetic sheepskin under the patient. Ambulation is encouraged and the patient is discouraged from sitting and standing for prolonged periods; brief periods of walking about, changing position and flexing and extending the limbs assist in improving circulation.

Exposure to infection is avoided since any infection tends to increase the demand for insulin and may interfere with the diabetic's normal food intake, predisposing him to ketosis. Any indication of a respiratory infection, gastrointestinal disturbance or skin lesion is promptly brought to the doctor's attention, since such conditions require more prompt and careful attention than in the non-diabetic.

4. Insufficient information about diabetes mellitus. The *goals* are to:
1 Acquire self-regulation of diabetes mellitus
2 Make knowledgeable decisions about health management
3 Prevent or identify promptly metabolic complications

The patient with diabetes mellitus has a chronic disease with which he must live the rest of his life. To achieve a state of health and an acceptable level of functioning, the patient must learn to coordinate his treatment regimen of diet, activity and medication into his daily routine of work or school and recreation to achieve and maintain normal physiological blood glucose levels. Knowledge about the disease and treatment plan are useless to a patient who has not been helped to apply the information. The diabetic is ultimately responsible for managing his health care. To do this, he must have adequate knowledge and skill to be able to make informed decisions about his current health problems and understand the implications of present actions on his future health status. The nurse with the doctor, dietitian and pharmacist is responsible for helping the patient set realistic goals, providing knowledge, teaching necessary skills and identifying learning resources. Teaching plans must be individualized to meet the unique needs of each patient and family.
- *Assessment of learning needs.* Assessment of what the patient already knows, what his goals are, how he learns, and life-style factors which will influence learning and compliance with the therapeutic plan is important before a learning plan can be developed. For a previously diagnosed diabetic, information is required about his usual diabetic routine at home, work or school, how his activities have changed, community resources used and what further information and skills he needs. Guidelines for assessing patients' learning needs are discussed in Chapter 2.

  The patient's responses to his diagnosis and treatment influence his readiness to learn. Initial responses to the diagnosis may include fear, withdrawal, or anger that this has happened to him. The nurse creates opportunities to listen to the patient and family members, facilitating expression of feelings while at the same time assessing learning needs. Most patients work through their immediate reactions reaching a phase in which they talk about their feelings and are prepared to listen and accept the reassurance that their disease can be controlled and that the necessary treatment and care can soon become a routine part of their life without seriously altering it.
- *Development of a teaching plan.* Once learning needs are identified, the nurse, with the patient and family, sets priorities. These may be dictated by the fact that the patient will be discharged in a few days and will be responsible for preparing his meals and/or administering insulin. The knowledge and skill necessary for safe functioning assumes priority and must be adjusted according to the readiness of the patient to learn. Information available from the British Diabetic Association may provide him with further support after discharge home.

  In planning the instruction, it is necessary to know the patient's background so that care can be adapted as much as possible to his accustomed way of life. The doctor and dietitian may participate in the programme, but the nurse should be familiar with their advice so that she can answer the patient's and his family's questions and reinforce certain areas when necessary. The amount of information given at one time depends on the patient's ability and willingness to receive it. Generally, brief periods of discussion are more effective than the presentation of a large amount of information at one time. Group instruction may be used in the hospital or clinic for some topics, but it must be remembered that each diabetic's treatment and life-style are unique. A large part of the discussion must be on an individual basis.

  Teaching is begun as soon as possible to avoid giving too much at one time, leading to confusion and discouragement, and to allow time for the patient to practise self-care, read and ask questions.

  Explanations are made in simple lay terms; and demonstrations are broken into steps, made slowly, repeated as often as necessary, and sufficient oppor-

tunity is provided for the patient to practise. Illustrations, films and written explanations and directions are used for clarification. Reading material (books, pamphlets) written for diabetics are made available; several publications are available from The British Diabetic Association.

• Content of learning plan. The instructions programme covers the following: (1) an explanation of diabetes; (2) diet; (3) insulin therapy or oral hypoglycaemic agents, if appropriate; (4) blood glucose monitoring; (5) urine testing; (6) metabolic emergencies; (7) diabetic identification card; (8) special personal care; (9) regular health supervision; and (10) sources of information and assistance.

(a) *What is diabetes mellitus?*   A simple basic explanation is made of the nature of diabetes, relating it to the symptoms experienced by the patient. To illustrate, the patient may be told that sugar and starches (such as bread and cereal) are converted by digestion to a simple form of sugar called glucose, which is the body's chief source of energy. In order for the cells to extract it from the blood and use it, the chemical insulin is necessary. There are two types of diabetes. In Type I or insulin-dependent diabetes, there is not sufficient insulin being produced to use the amount of sugar and starches being taken, so glucose accumulates in the blood in excess of the normal. The kidneys remove some of the excess, which is why the diabetic voids a lot of urine which contains sugar. The loss of large amounts of urine results in thirst. Weakness, fatigue and hunger occur because the sugar is not being 'burned' to produce energy. The body, in an effort to provide energy, may break down body tissue, causing a loss of weight. Daily insulin injections and dietary measures are necessary to control this disorder.

With Type II or non-insulin-dependent diabetes enough insulin to handle the amount of sugar may be produced but the cells cannot effectively utilize the glucose. Overweight often accompanies this type of diabetes which develops gradually in adults. This type of diabetes can usually be controlled by diet and activity to achieve a desirable body weight. Some patients may require an oral hypoglycaemic agent.

(b) *Diet.*   The prescribed diet must be clearly and carefully interpreted to the patient. The initial instruction is usually given by a dietitian, but considerable clarification and reinforcement by the nurse, who is with the patient more often and for longer periods, is usually necessary. The prescription, sample meal plan and food exchange lists are explained. The foods allowed each day, their division into meals and snacks, and the selection from the lists are reviewed several times. It is helpful to have the patient plan meals for several days. The purchase and preparation of food and how it may be worked in with the family meals are discussed. The following general principles which apply to the dia-

betic diet are cited and standard measuring cups and spoons are used; amounts used should be accurate and correspond with that indicated on the exchange lists; concentrated sweets such as sugar, confectionary, jams, jelly, preserves, honey, cake and pastries should be avoided; labels are carefully read when purchasing canned and prepared foods. To satisfy hunger, foods of no caloric value may be taken which include clear tea and coffee, consommé, clear broth, bouillon and artificially sweetened beverages; the daily food allowance should all be eaten, and meals should be taken at regular hours. The patient is advised that he should check his weight weekly and should be informed that obesity is a distinct hazard. The patient is encouraged to read and obtain for his personal use books and pamphlets which contain considerable detail on diabetic dietary plans. The dietitian will give more detailed advice and the British Diabetic Association literature can reinforce and extend the basic dietary education.

(c) *Drug therapy.*   If the patient is on *insulin* therapy, he is advised of the necessary equipment and where it may be obtained. An explanation is made of what insulin is, types available and the name and nature of the insulin prescribed for him, and how it is identified. Unit dosage is explained and measurement by units is demonstrated. The patient is encouraged to practice handling the syringe and needle and the measurement of his prescribed dose. Instruction and demonstrations are then given to familiarize him with the sterilization of the equipment (where non-disposable needles and syringes are used), aseptic handling, rotating of the vial to equalize the suspension of insulin, withdrawal of the required amount of insulin, the necessary rotation and preparation of sites for injection, the actual injection and the aftercare of the equipment. Storage and maintenance of an adequate supply of insulin are discussed. Insulin is only available on prescription. Automatic injectors are available which may be of assistance to those patients who find the injection of the needle difficult. The injector has a mechanically controlled spring which, when released, pushes the needle quickly through the skin. The need to plan and break down all this information into small logical teaching units or blocks is again emphasized. If discouragement and frustration are evident, further instruction is delayed and another approach considered.

If an *oral hypoglycaemic* agent is prescribed, the importance of taking the drug in the exact dosage at the times ordered is stressed. Written directions are given, and the patient is advised that if headache, nausea, vomiting or other disturbances are experienced, he should contact the doctor. The patient is reminded that he must not experiment with the dosage of the drug on his own and that adherence to the diet prescribed for him is most important even though he is receiving medication.

Adjustment of diet and medications in relation to increased stress and changes in life-style is important. Diabetic patients can be taught to adjust their diet and medication in relation to change in demand for glucose and insulin. Blood glucose monitoring by patients has made it possible for them to achieve good glycaemic control during illness and to be more flexible in their eating patterns, activity and travel.

Eating out and delayed meals may also necessitate changes in insulin administration. Whenever possible, diabetics should maintain their usual eating pattern, including the time of meals and the content of each meal. They quickly learn to select appropriate meals from menus or from the selection offered by friends and relatives. When eating out, the diabetic should be prepared for delays and the possibility of hypoglycaemia by carrying sugar lumps or other sources of quickly absorbable carbohydrate. When aware that meals will be delayed the patient is instructed to have a small snack before leaving home. Insulin-dependent diabetics with good understanding of their disease and its management, may be provided with guidelines from their doctor on the use of compensatory insulin supplements prior to large meals. Patients using insulin pumps and blood glucose monitoring quickly learn to take an extra bolus of insulin with an unusually large meal.

Illness will affect drug medication. Diabetics are instructed on how to manage their disease during illness. If nausea and vomiting are present, the diet plan may be converted to liquids. A balanced diet may still be obtained. Vegetables and fruit are ingested in the form of juices or soups. If oral intake is not possible, the doctor is consulted and parenteral fluids are administered. The insulin-dependent diabetic and patients on oral hypoglycaemics should continue to take their medication during an illness. Larger doses of insulin with more frequent supplementary doses may be required. Insulin dosage should be adjusted according to prescribed guidelines in relation to blood glucose determinations. If the patient is not using blood glucose monitoring, the doctor is consulted. Insulin may be switched to soluble, short-acting insulin for the duration of illness.

Non-insulin dependent diabetics may require insulin during periods of acute illness or surgery. The insulin is prescribed by the doctor and regulated according to blood glucose levels. In some instances, the hospitalized diabetic may receive insulin by continuous intravenous infusion.

Travel may also necessitate changes in drug therapy. The insulin-dependent diabetic needs to take precautions to avoid hypoglycaemia while travelling. If travelling by car, snacks or juices are kept available. On planes and train while meals may be obtained if delays occur, it is still important to carry some food in the handbaggage in case there are problems. Travelling through several time zones should not pose any difficulties, providing that a plan is developed ahead of time. The insulin-dependent diabetic must remember to carry insulin and syringes with him and be prepared to inject insulin wherever he is. It is important for the patient to take a sufficient quantity of insulin and supplies for insulin administration and blood glucose monitoring or urine testing for the duration of his stay, as products may vary or be difficult to obtain in different countries. Insulin should be refrigerated whenever possible but will be quite safe if kept in a small insulated container to prevent exposure to high temperatures and bright light.

(d) *Monitoring of blood glucose. Assessment of metabolic control of glucose* can be achieved by the patient on a continuous or intermittent basis by monitoring of blood glucose and/or the testing of urine for glucose and ketones.

The importance of *self-monitoring of blood glucose* is also explained. The relationship between poor metabolic control of diabetes and the development of microvascular and neurological complications is well documented. Urine glucose monitoring is not adequate to enable good control of glycaemia. It does not always identify hypoglycaemia and hyperglycaemia; the latter is detected only when the blood glucose levels exceed the renal threshold which is variable and may change in older diabetics and those with renal complications.

Blood glucose monitoring is a simple procedure, quickly mastered by most patients. It provides significantly accurate blood glucose determination, enabling the patient to achieve improved glycaemic control. Self-monitoring of blood glucose levels facilitates patient understanding of the diabetes and gives him an active role in the management of his disorder. Satisfaction is generally high; infections and other complications are negligible. The major disadvantage is the cost of the equipment and supplies. The yearly cost of blood glucose monitoring is about four times that of urine glucose monitoring. Self-monitoring of blood glucose is especially recommended for pregnant diabetics, patients with altered renal threshold, labile diabetics, patients in whom excellent control is desirable, individuals with frequent episodes of hypoglycaemia, all diabetics during illness, and any patients for whom urine testing is not possible.

Monitoring of blood glucose levels may be done: (1) continually, with diet, activity and insulin adjusted as indicated; (2) intermittently, with the patient using a blood glucose profile of a 'typical day' to assess glycaemic control; or (3) only during episodes of illness or when problems occur. The monitoring schedule will vary for each patient. A stable, non-insulin-dependent diabetic may take three to seven fasting tests per week while insulin-dependent diabetics continue to monitor glucose levels about four times daily.

The correct *technique of blood glucose monitoring* should be taught. Self-monitoring of blood glucose may be done with a reagent strip, with or without a machine. Both methods are sufficiently accurate for patient-monitoring but the machines are best used when meticulous control of glycaemia is desired. It is important to follow the manufacturer's instructions precisely, particularly as regards accuracy and timing. It is a common mistake to use the test strips after the recommended expiry date or to fail to store the strips in the airtight container.

The finger is cleansed and pricked with a single-prong lancet, either manually or using an automated device. A drop of blood is placed on a reagent strip left for the period of time recommended by the manufacturer; it is then washed or wiped off and the results interpreted either by comparing the strip with a chart or placing the strip into a machine which provides a digital read-out of the results. Most meters available today are small, portable and simple to use. Differences between machines include the method of calibration prior to use. If blood glucose monitoring is to be used, the patient is told about the sources where he may acquire information on the various types of equipment and receive instruction on their use. Practice with the equipment in hospital will help him to understand the differences and similarities of various products. Pamphlets, audiovisual presentations and individualized instruction are usually available from the supplier. The patient should begin to keep a record of the results of blood sugar tests while in hospital. The nurse and doctor discuss these with the patient each day, comparing results to the previous day and exploring factors which influenced any changes. The newly diagnosed diabetic patient will not grasp the significance of the results initially but including him in the decision making process about disease management will help him to gradually assume responsibility for his control.

He can discuss his daily records, actions taken and results obtained with the community health nurse, doctor and/or outpatient clinic staff.

Specific written instructions are provided to help the patient adjust insulin dosage according to the results of blood glucose tests when this is relevant.

(e) *Urine testing*. This provides a simple and convenient measurement of the concentration of blood glucose over the renal threshold level. Non-insulin-dependent diabetics are less likely to have glycosuria except occasionally following a large meal. Insulin-dependent diabetics may be required to test their urine for glucose four times a day (i.e. before meals and at bedtime or perhaps only once daily). The frequency of urine testing will be greater in the newly diagnosed diabetic and is decreased once control is achieved. Testing the urine for ketones is done if the glucose determinations are 2%, if symptoms of hyperglycaemia are present and when the patient is ill.

Urine should be tested on a 'double-voided' specimen. The first specimen, consisting of urine contained in the bladder for a period of time is discarded.

A second specimen for testing is obtained 30 minutes later. This fresh specimen more accurately reflects the urine glucose level at that time.

A variety of agents in the form of dip sticks and tablets are available for urine testing by the patient. Specific instructions are packaged with each product. Choice of product will depend on the patient's manual dexterity, the ease with which the product can be used while travelling, the colour scales of the product (many elderly patients with impaired vision have difficulty differentiating the blue–green colours resulting from urine reactions with Clinitest tablets) and the cost of the product.

(f) *Knowledge of metabolic emergencies* (hypoglycaemia and hyperglycaemia). The diabetic who is receiving insulin or an oral hypoglycaemic agent should know that under certain circumstances the blood sugar level may fall below normal, resulting in what is called an insulin or *hypoglycaemic* reaction. The patient and family should be familiar with the symptoms (see p. 681) and know what to do. The possible causes of hypoglycaemia are cited (see p. 681), and the patient is advised that on experiencing early symptoms he should immediately take carbohydrate. With more pronounced symptoms, a quick acting form of carbohydrate will be required, for example two or three cubes of sugar, tea or coffee with 2 or 3 teaspoonfuls of sugar, two or three small sweets, orange juice or grape juice (112 g or 4 oz) or 2 teaspoonfuls of honey or syrup may be used. If the symptoms do not disappear in 10 minutes, the administration is repeated. The patient on insulin is advised to always carry lump sugar or boiled sweets or glucose tablets with him.

The family should know that if the diabetic cannot swallow or retain sugar, glucagon should be administered or a doctor summoned at once, or he is taken as quickly as possible to a hospital emergency department. Friends and associates as well as the family should know that the diabetic receives insulin and may experience a reaction. The patient is advised that insulin reactions should be reported to the doctor; his insulin dosage or diet may require adjustment.

The patient should also be able to recognize early symptoms of uncontrolled diabetes, which causes *hyperglycaemia*. If it is not corrected in the early stage it may lead to the serious complications of diabetic ketoacidosis or hyperosmolar non-ketotic coma. Hyperglycaemia and dehydration with or without ketosis, develop more slowly than hypoglycaemia, usually over several days. The disturbance is usually manifested by loss of appetite, nausea, vomiting, thirst, weakness, drowsiness and general malaise. Sugar will be present in the urine and blood levels are greatly increased. They are frequently associated with infection or stress or may be due to prolonged dietary indiscretion or omission of insulin or oral hypoglycaemic agent. The patient is advised that his general practitioner should be contacted as soon as symptoms are experienced. Until medical attention is obtained he should remain in bed, keep warm, drink hot clear fluids *without sugar* freely and repeat them even if he vomits; if possible, someone should remain with him.

(g) *Diabetic identification card*. Every diabetic should carry a diabetic identification card at all times so that his condition will be made known quickly in the event of a reaction, illness or accident. Cards which carry appropriate information are available from the hospital, doctors, the diabetic clinic and the British Diabetic Association or its local branches; a written one may be carried temporarily.

(h) *Special personal care* (e.g. skin and foot care and eye care). The patient is advised that, because of his diabetes, he may be more susceptible to infections and will tend to heal more slowly when breaks occur in the skin. Any infection predisposes to uncontrolled diabetes, and persons whose disease is uncontrolled appear to develop infection more readily. The diabetic avoids contact with persons who have an infection as much as possible. The skin should be kept clean, warm and free of irritation and pressure as much as possible. Precautions are taken to prevent cracks and breaks in the skin. Scratches, cuts, abrasions and hangnails are cleaned and protected by a dressing. The use of strong antiseptics (such as iodine) and adhesive is avoided. Prolonged exposure to sunlight and the use of local heat applications (electric heating pad, hot water bottle) are discouraged. If heat applications are necessary, extra precautions are necessary because of some loss of sensation; a lower degree of heat and extra covers are used.

The adult diabetic's feet require regular special attention because of the increased susceptibility to circulatory disorders and loss of sensation. The patient is directed to bathe his feet daily with warm (not hot) water, using a mild antibacterial soap and a small amount of bath oil, and to dry them thoroughly, especially the areas between the toes, using gentle pressure rather than vigorous rubbing. Talcum powder may be used sparingly if the feet tend to be moist and perspire; if they are dry and scaly, a light application of lanolin or prescribed lotion is rubbed into the skin. The toenails are cut straight across with scissors. If calluses and corns cannot be controlled by rubbing them lightly with a pumice stone, they should be treated by a state registered chiropodist who is advised of the person's diabetes. The patient is cautioned against attempting to remove them by cutting or applying commercial preparations. Stockings or socks should fit well to avoid any constriction or wrinkles that might cause irritation or pressure and are changed daily. To prevent possible interference with the circulation, round garters are not worn. Shoes should be well-fitting so there is no irritation or pressure on any part of the foot, and new shoes are worn only for brief periods until 'broken in'. Walking barefoot and the application of heating appliances are discouraged. The feet should be examined daily for breaks in the skin, discoloration, dryness and drainage. Numbness, persisting coldness, discoloration, a burning feeling, pain or any unusual condition of the lower limbs is reported to the doctor.

It is advisable for the diabetic to have an annual *eye examination* because of the predisposition to visual change which can only be detected by an ophthalmologist. There is an increased tendency for retinal haemorrhage in diabetics which must be identified promptly and treated with laser beam.

(i) *Health supervision*. The newly diagnosed diabetic will be required to make more frequent visits to the general practitioner or the diabetic clinic. These will become fewer as his disease and treatment are stabilized. The nurse in either situation checks with him as to how he is managing and gives him the opportunity to ask questions. Some phase of his care may require repetition and reinforcement. Before leaving the hospital, the importance of keeping the scheduled appointments is stressed. In the case of older persons, assistance may be necessary in making some arrangements for transportation to the clinic.

(j) *Sources of assistance*. The patient and family are made aware of the available sources of help and information. These include the national and local diabetic associations. The services provided by the various organizations and recommended publications are cited. Patients are encouraged to join. This entitles them to the regular periodical and additional literature published by the association.

Expected outcomes

Knowledge of diabetes mellitus. The patient is able to:
1 Define diabetes mellitus.
2 Describe his particular type of diabetes mellitus in relation to other types.
3 Describe how diabetes affects his usual daily activities.

Diet. The patient is able to:
4 Describe a meal plan appropriate for his disease and usual life style.
5 Describe how the meal plan can be adjusted to accommodate illness and changes in activity.
6 List foods which should be limited or avoided.
7 Describe a plan to achieve or maintain desired body weight.

Medication (if applicable). The patient is able to:

8 State the name of the prescribed oral hypoglycaemic agent and its purpose.

9 Describe a plan to remind himself to take medication daily.

10 Describe side-effects of the prescribed oral agent.

11 Describe the action of insulin and its interrelationship with blood sugar and exercise.

12 State the name, dosage and time of administration of prescribed insulin(s).

13 Demonstrate the correct technique of preparing insulin for injection, rotation of injection sites, injection of the insulin and care and disposal of equipment.

14 State the prescribed medication routine for periods of illness and/or when the doctor should be notified during illness.

Blood glucose and/or urine monitoring. The patient is able to:

15 Demonstrate the technique of blood glucose monitoring (if applicable).

16 Demonstrate a technique of testing urine for glucose and ketones (if applicable).

17 Describe a plan for regular testing of blood glucose and/or urine.

18 Discuss the significance of blood glucose results in relation to time of day, associated food intake, recent activity and medication.

19 Suggest appropriate action for adjustment of diet, activity and/or medication plans in response to the test results.

Activity. The patient is able to:

20 State the reasons for maintaining regular exercise.

21 Describe how diet and insulin may be adjusted as activity levels change.

Skin integrity. The patient is able to:

22 State the need for regular skin care.

23 Demonstrate how feet are cared for.

24 Describe situations (infection, skin breakdown) requiring health supervision.

Acute metabolic emergencies. The patient is able to:

25 Define hypoglycaemia and hyperglycaemia.

26 Discuss causes of hypoglycaemia and hyperglycaemia that might apply to his personal situation.

27 Describe the symptoms experienced with (a) hypoglycaemia and (b) hyperglycaemia.

28 Describe a plan of action should symptoms of (a) hypoglycaemia and (b) hyperglycaemia occur.

Health management. The patient is able to:

29 List community resources available for diabetic patients and families.

30 Describe plans for attaining regular medical, dental and eye care.

31 Describe information to be provided to various health professionals.

32 State the importance of wearing an identification tag and/or carrying a card to identify the type of diabetes and medication plan.

The child diabetic

The care of the child or adolescent diabetic requires the understanding and cooperation of the entire family. Because of their growth and the vigorous activity characteristic of these young persons, closer medical supervision is necessary. They tend to be less stable, and more frequent adjustments in their insulin dosage and diet are necessary. The child is taught self-care and self-administration of his insulin as soon as possible. He must be able to recognize early symptoms of hypoglycaemia and know when to take the sugar cubes or a concentrated form of glucose that he always carries with him. It must be emphasized in discussion with the parents that the child be encouraged to assume responsibility for his own care and that he be permitted to live as much like a normal child as possible so that he and his associates will not think of him as being 'different'.

Throughout all patient and family education, emphasis is placed on the positive—that is, control can be maintained, permitting the diabetic to carry on an active satisfying life. Certainly they must be made familiar with signs of certain complications and know what action to take to avoid serious consequences, but one must guard against creating unnecessary anxiety and discouragement.

Acute metabolic complications

Metabolic dysfunction in the diabetic patient can lead to advanced hyperglycaemic states or to severe hypoglycaemia. Hyperglycaemia can progress to either ketoacidosis or hyperglycaemic, hyperosmolar non-ketotic coma.

Hyperglycaemia.

1 *Diabetic ketoacidosis*. Diabetic ketoacidosis is a serious metabolic complication which develops when there is too little insulin and an excess of glucose.

The cause of insulin deficiency may be due to inadequate production of insulin in the undiagnosed diabetic, inadequate administration of insulin or an increased need for insulin resulting from emotional or physical stresses such as infection. Excess glucose may result from increased hepatic production of glucose, decreased utilization of glucose by peripheral tissue and increased ingestion of glucose in the diet.

The production of *ketone bodies* involves processes occurring in adipose tissue, liver and muscle. The glucose in the blood cannot be utilized by the cells, and fat is broken down to provide energy. Fat is mobilized and broken down rapidly, producing ketone bodies (acetoacetic acid, ß-hydroxybutyric acid and acetone) in excess of the tissue cells' ability to metabolize them. Alterations in liver metabolism lead to further ketone production. This process is accelerated when glucagon levels rise. An associated decrease in the ability of muscle tissue to utilize these organic acids further contribute to ketoacidosis. The acids and acetone accumulate in the blood. At first the normal pH is maintained by the buffer systems, but eventually the alkali reserve becomes depleted and the pH of the body fluids falls, resulting in acidosis. At the same time, the increased concentration of glucose causes an increased output of urine (osmotic diuresis), and dehydration develops. The increased osmotic pressures of the extracellular fluid result in the movement of fluid out of the cells accompanied by electrolytes. Serious sodium, potassium and phosphate deficiencies develop.

Ketoacidosis has an insidious onset over several days, being preceded by *symptoms* characteristic of uncontrolled diabetes (polyuria, thirst, glucosuria, weakness). The symptoms related to the accumulation of ketones and reduced alkalinity of body fluids include anorexia, nausea, vomiting, deep and rapid respirations, drowsiness, weakness which progresses to prostration, and abdominal pain or muscular cramps. The skin and mouth are dry, and the eyeballs are soft because of dehydration. The patient may appear flushed in the early stages but later becomes pale owing to hypotension. The pulse is rapid and may be weak because of severe dehydration and the reduced intravascular volume. Unless the condition is recognized and treated promptly, the blood pressure falls, the patient becomes comatose, and his condition is critical. (Coma is uncommon in patients with known diabetes because of greater awareness through patient and family education leading to early adjustment of insulin therapy and prompt medical referrals.)

The patient's urine shows a high concentration of sugar and ketones. The blood sugar is elevated and the sodium and chloride blood levels are lower. The potassium level may be low at first owing to polyuria and vomiting; then it may become normal or elevated as the electrolyte moves out of the cells. The blood urea level is usually higher, and the leucocyte count is generally elevated. The carbon dioxide concentration and combining power are lowered as well as the pH. Plasma concentrations of blood ketones: β-hydroxybutyrate, acetoacetate and acetone are elevated.

The *treatment and nursing intervention* of the patient with diabetic ketoacidosis requires emergency care which is directed toward stimulating the utilization of glucose by the cells and decreasing the production of ketone bodies by the administration of insulin, and correction of dehydration and the electrolyte imbalance. Any causative disorder is also treated.

Immediate blood determinations are made of the glucose, carbon dioxide, potassium, sodium, chloride, phosphate, and urea concentrations. The haematocrit is also checked to determine haemoconcentration. An indwelling catheter may be inserted if the patient is comatose, to enable monitoring of urinary output. If the patient is stuporous or comatose, a nasogastric tube is passed to avoid risk of aspiration of vomitus. The patient receives repeated doses of regular (rapid-acting) insulin intravenously and/or a continuous intravenous infusion. The solution for the infusion and the dosage of insulin are based on the laboratory blood findings. Continuous cardiac monitoring is done to detect changes in heart action characteristic of an abnormal potassium blood level. Intravenous fluids are given to correct electrolyte deficits as well as dehydration. The initial solution used is usually normal saline; potassium chloride or potassium phosphate may be added to the solution. As cited previously, potassium moves out of the cells and at first the serum concentration may be normal or even elevated. With the administration of the intravenous insulin and solutions, plasma potassium moves into the cells and hypokalaemia may develop which may then necessitate the administration of a potassium solution. Repeated blood electrolyte, glucose and ketone determinations are necessary. When the blood glucose level approaches normal, the frequency of administration and the dosage of insulin are decreased, and an intravenous glucose solution (5% in water or saline) may be ordered. If the patient's blood pressure is low and shock is present, plasma or plasma expanders may be given. Unless the cause of the ketoacidosis was evident at the onset, efforts are made to determine why it occurred. The care plan in Table 20.9 describes nursing diagnoses, goals, nursing intervention and outcome criteria for the patient with diabetic ketoacidosis.

2 *Hyperglycaemic, hyperosmolar non-ketotic diabetic coma.* This serious metabolic complication is characterized by severe hyperglycaemia with no significant ketosis. Serum osmolarity is elevated; insulin is deficient but not absent; and severe dehydration and hypovolaemia exist.

Hyperglycaemic, hyperosmolar non-ketotic coma is most likely to occur in non-insulin-dependent diabetics who are controlled by diet and hypoglycaemic agents and who are elderly, institutionalized, physically or mentally incapacitated, or experience a precipitating stress such as infection. Renal insufficiency is frequently an underlying cause, with the kidneys failing to regulate glucose levels. When renal compensatory mechanisms are inadequate and dehydration also is present as may occur in the elderly who are infirm or ill, non-ketotic coma may develop.

The lack of ketosis in patients with this disorder has been attributed to the extreme dehydration which is believed to suppress the release of free fatty

Table 20.9 Nursing care plan for the patient with diabetic ketoacidosis.

Problem	Goal	Nursing intervention	Expected outcomes
1 Alteration in nutrition and metabolism related to hyperglycaemia and lack of insulin	To achieve metabolic control	**a** Administer insulin as ordered. Monitor rate of infusion **b** Determine blood glucose levels every 1–2 hours **c** Assess patient for signs of hypoglycaemia: sweating, pallor, apprehension, tremor, weakness, tachycardia, palpitation, dizziness, blurred vision and motor incoordination, convulsions	Serum glucose level is 5.6–7.8 (100–140 mg/dl)
2 Fluid volume deficit related to hyperglycaemia and osmotic diuresis	To replenish fluids	**a** Administer isotonic parenteral fluids as ordered **b** Accurately record fluid intake and output hourly **c** Assess patient for signs of fluid overload: dyspnoea, pulmonary crackles and wheezes, increased central venous pressure **d** Assess patient's blood pressure, pulse, respirations hourly **e** Record patient's temperature every 2–3 hours **f** Provide mouth care regularly **g** Turn and position patient every 1–2 hours	**1** Fluid intake and urine output are in physiological balance **2** Mucous membranes are moist **3** Skin turgor is present
3 Altered electrolyte balance related to osmotic diuresis producing decreased sodium, potassium, hydrogen carbonate and pH	To replenish electrolyte balance	**a** Administer potassium and other electrolytes as ordered in parenteral solutions **b** Assess serum electrolyte concentrations	**1** Serum potassium level is 3.5–5.0 mmol/l **2** Serum sodium level is 136–145 mmol/l **3** pH, 7.35–7.45; $[H^+]$, 44.7–45.5 mmol/l **4** Hydrogen carbonate level is 24–29 mmol/l
4 Altered level of consciousness related to metabolic alterations and dehydration	**a** To identify promptly changes in level of consciousness **b** To maintain personal safety **c** To maintain or restore sensory perceptual functioning	(See Chapter 10) **a** Assess level of consciousness and neurological status every 2 hours and record **b** Explain activities and procedures to patient **c** Position patient to maintain a patent airway **d** Keep cot-sides in place on patient's bed **e** Insert nasogastric tube as indicated	**1** The patient responds appropriately to the environment and to verbal commands **2** The patient's airway is patent
5 Lack of knowledge about the management of diabetes mellitus and disease management	To understand the disease process, measures to control diabetes and actions to take when metabolic complications develop	**a** Assess patient and family's level of understanding of diabetes, prescribed dietary, medication and activity regimen. Assess actions patient and family usually take to prevent, identify and act on metabolic complications **b** With the patient, family, dietitian, pharmacist, doctor and nurse, develop and implement a teaching plan for the patient and family **c** Evaluate patient and family's comprehension. **d** Inform patient and family of community resources and make referrals as indicated	Patient and family describe: **1** Causes of ketoacidosis **2** Prescribed dietary, medication and activity regimens **3** Signs of hyperglycaemia **4** Procedure to monitor blood glucose levels daily **5** Actions to take if hyperglycaemia occurs

acids from the adipose tissue and inhibit the pancreatic insulin response to glucose.[30]

The onset of hyperglycaemic, hyperosmolar non-ketotic coma is insidious, occurring over several days. The patient demonstrates weakness, polyuria and polydipsia. As intracellular dehydration progresses and fluid shifts to the extracellular spaces, symptoms of neurological involvement, lethargy, confusion, convulsions and eventually coma develop.

Treatment is directed toward reversing the hyperosmolar state with fluid replacement and correcting underlying causes. The prognosis for patients with this condition is generally poor but is improved with prompt treatment. Treatment differs in three ways from that of ketoacidosis: (1) Large volumes of hypotonic solutions are given intravenously instead of the isotonic solutions used to treat ketoacidosis; as many as 4–6 litres of hypotonic saline may be given during the first 10 hours. When the blood sugar is lower than 14.4 mmol (259 mg/dl), 5% dextrose in saline or water may be given. (2) Insulin is administered intravenously, but lower doses are required than for ketoacidosis. (3) Less potassium replacement is required. Other electrolytes are replaced as indicated by determination of blood levels. A nasogastric tube may be inserted to control gastric distension and prevent aspiration.

Nursing intervention is similar to that outlined in Table 20.9 for the patient with diabetic ketoacidosis. Careful monitoring and recording of the large volumes of hypotonic parenteral solutions that are administered is important. The patient is assessed for signs of fluid overload which include dyspnoea, pulmonary crackles and wheezes, and increased central venous pressure. The low doses of insulin prescribed are administered using an infusion controller to carefully regulate the dosage. Observations are made for signs of hypoglycaemia which are sweating, pallor, apprehension, tremor, weakness, tachycardia, palpitation, dizziness, blurred vision, motor incoordination, convulsions and coma.

Care of the patient with altered levels of consciousness is discussed in Chapter 10. Nursing intervention includes measures to maintain a patent airway and personal safety.

The patient and family's level of understanding of diabetes, the causes of metabolic complications, general disease management and actions to take when complications occur are assessed. An individualized teaching plan is developed, implemented and evaluated; referrals are made to the community nurse where appropriate. Attempts are made to determine the factors precipitating the episode and to institute measures to prevent future episodes of hyperosmolar, non-ketotic coma.

[30] Matz (1983), pp. 656 & 657.

Hypoglycaemia. Hypoglycaemia implies an abnormally low blood sugar concentration. Signs and symptoms usually begin to appear when the blood sugar level falls below 3.3 mmol (60 mg/dl). The onset of symptoms varies with individuals; some may develop symptoms at a higher level of blood sugar, while others may not manifest the disturbance until a lower level is reached. Adults tend to have symptoms earlier than child diabetics.

The *causes* of hypoglycaemia in the diabetic may be the delay or omission of a meal after having taken insulin or an oral hypoglycaemic agent, an undue amount of energy expenditure, an overdosage of insulin, a gastrointestinal disorder which produces anorexia, vomiting or diarrhoea, improvement in the diabetic's ability to utilize glucose, failure to adjust insulin dosage when significant loss of weight occurs, or it may occur following a gastrectomy.

The *manifestations* of hypoglycaemia are as follows: A hypoglycaemic reaction in a patient receiving regular insulin usually occurs approximately 2–6 hours after the injection. In the patient receiving an intermediate-acting insulin given in the morning, it happens more commonly in the afternoon or evening. Hypoglycaemic reaction to a slow-acting insulin generally occurs during the night or early in the morning of the following day.

It should be kept in mind that it is possible also for the patient receiving an oral hypoglycaemic agent to develop hypoglycaemia. It develops insidiously and may occasionally go unrecognized.

The signs and symptoms manifested by an abnormally low blood glucose are a reflection of its effect on the central nervous system. The brain is very dependent on a constant, adequate supply of glucose. Any deprivation, even for a relatively brief period, may seriously impair cerebral activity and result in permanent damage. Similarly, repeated occurrences of hypoglycaemia, even of short duration, especially in children, may incur some permanent cerebral impairment. The manifestations of hypoglycaemia vary from one patient to another but tend to be the same with each reaction for the same person, which makes it more easily recognizable by him. The earlier signs and symptoms include sweating, tremor, apprehension, hunger, weakness, tachycardia and palpitation. Symptoms usually do not appear until the blood glucose level is 2.8–3.3 mmol/l (50–60 mg/dl). More advanced symptoms are faintness or dizziness, blurring of vision or diplopia, headache, slow reactions, uncoordinated movement which occasionally leads to mistaking the patient's condition for alcohol intoxication, muscular twitching that may progress to convulsions especially in children, disorientation and confusion, stupor and eventual loss of consciousness. The urine is usually negative for sugar although occasionally, a trace may be found if the bladder has not been emptied for a few hours. The blood glucose is below 3 mmol/l. All diabetics, their immediate family and close associates should be familiar with the early signs and symptoms of hypoglycaemia and should know what to do.

If the patient can still swallow, he is treated by immediately being given some form of rapidly absorbable concentrated sugar. Ten to 15 g of carbohydrate are usually sufficient to restore the blood sugar level. Orange juice (120 ml) or other sweetened fruit juice or 2 teaspoonfuls of syrup, honey or sugar with a glass of water may be used. If there is no improvement in 5–10 minutes, the administration is repeated. If the patient is unconscious or uncooperative, a doctor is summoned and 30–50 ml of 50% glucose are given intravenously. Glucagon (1–2 mg) or adrenaline 1:1000 (0.5 ml) subcutaneously may be ordered to promote glycogenolysis and subsequent increase in blood glucose. A venous or capillary blood specimen is collected as soon as possible and is repeated at frequent intervals for blood sugar determinations until the patient is stabilized.

Following a reaction, the patient is encouraged to rest for several hours in order to decrease the utilization of his blood glucose. Carbohydrate administration may be repeated and some form of protein (cheese or milk) should be given the patient to provide additional glucose which is produced gradually as a result of protein metabolism. The nurse always checks with the doctor before giving the next scheduled dose of insulin. If the patient is at home, he is instructed not to take more insulin or hypoglycaemic agents at that time. Adjustments are usually made in the carbohydrate content of the diet and in the insulin dosage. The patient may learn from the experience if encouraged to examine the reaction in retrospect. A discussion of the possible cause and the early symptoms may be helpful in preventing further reactions and in having the patient recognize hypoglycaemia at the onset.

The *Somogyi effect* occurs in insulin-dependent diabetics who are treated too aggressively in an attempt to normalize blood glucose levels. The hypoglycaemia resulting from administration releases counterregulatory hormones, producing a rebound hyperglycaemia. The insulin produces a decrease in blood glucose which triggers the sympathetic nervous system to release ACTH. The liver releases glycogen and the blood sugar rises. Further administration of insulin causes a repeat of the cycle. Sudden falls in blood glucose levels followed by rebound hyperglycaemia are characteristic of the Somogyi effect. Treatment consists of gradually decreasing the insulin dosage. The phenomenon is less frequent in patients whose diabetes is controlled by insulin infusion pumps.

Surgery and diabetes mellitus

The emotional stress, physical trauma and physiological responses associated with surgery present a greater problem for the diabetic than for the normal person. A decrease in the utilization of glucose and an increased demand for insulin are likely to occur, predisposing the diabetic to acidosis. The diabetic who is to have elective surgery is usually hospitalized several days before the operation. During this period, his diabetes is thoroughly checked and brought under optimum control. The blood sugar level is brought within normal range, and the urine must be free of sugar and ketones. The patient undergoes a thorough investigation for complications of his disease (degenerative changes), and his fluid and electrolyte balances and nutritional status are assessed. For the insulin-dependent diabetic, on the morning of operation an intravenous infusion of regular insulin in normal saline is begun, with a second infusion of 5% dextrose in water. These two infusions are continued throughout surgery and postoperatively until the patient is able to take fluid orally. The rate of flow of each infusion is determined by serial blood glucose monitoring or one of the new glucose-controlled infusion systems may be used. This instrument adjusts the flow of each solution according to a preset blood glucose level. The patient's blood glucose concentrations are registered continuously with this system.

A diabetic who is not on insulin can often be managed with no special treatment other than careful postoperative observation of appearance, glycosuria, ketonuria and blood glucose concentration. In some instances, however, oral hypoglycaemic preparations are discontinued and an intravenous infusion with purified soluble porcine insulin is started the evening prior to surgery. This infusion may be stopped postoperatively or continued if the patient's blood glucose is elevated.

Postoperatively, constant nursing attention is necessary; responses and reactions vary greatly with individuals. The insulin requirement may increase sharply with some patients and not with others. The pulse, respirations and blood pressure are recorded frequently and for a longer period than usual, and a frequent check is made of the patient's level of consciousness. Blood specimens are obtained immediately after operation and are repeated every 2–4 hours; glucose and electrolyte levels are determined. The nurse must be constantly alert for signs of hypoglycaemia, ketoacidosis and non-ketotic hyperglycaemia.

Oral feeding is started just as soon as it can be tolerated. The sooner the patient is returned to his usual diet, the better. Frequent foot and leg exercises are especially important because of the diabetic's predisposition to vascular changes and circulatory problems. Precautions are taken to provide the maximum protection against infection; any slight indication of possible infection such as an elevation of temperature, cough or sore throat is reported immediately. Early ambulation is encouraged to promote greater utilization of glucose as well as to stimulate the patient's circulation.

Hypoglycaemic state

An abnormally low blood glucose may be due to a variety of factors. It may be fasting or postprandial.

An excessive secretion of insulin by the islets of Langerhans occurs rarely. It may be due to a functioning cell neoplasm in the pancreas involving the islet cells, or to an unexplained hyperactivity of the islets. The overproduction of insulin produces periodic hypoglycaemic episodes which are usually precipitated by fasting or exercise. The patient manifests the signs and symptoms cited on page 681. Because of the repeated attacks, changes in personality and reduced intellectual ability may be evident as a result of permanent brain damage. The patient is treated by surgical excision of the neoplasm or a subtotal pancreatectomy.

It may occur after a meal following a gastrectomy, or it may be functional and postprandial which is attributed to increased parasympathetic innervation to the beta cells of the islets of Langerhans by the vagus nerve resulting in an excessive secretion of insulin. It may be associated with a marked deficiency of cortisol or the growth hormone. In some instances, especially in children, it is idiopathic.

In postprandial hypoglycaemia, the protein and fat content of the patient's diet is increased to insure a more 'continuous' production of glucose (gluconeogenesis), since carbohydrate is used quickly from the blood. Glucagon may be prescribed for the patient; regular doses may be given subcutaneously. The patient is advised to take four or five regular meals and to carry sweets or sugar or a ready source of simple sugar.

References and Further Reading

BOOKS

American Diabetic Association (1982) *Diabetes in the Family* Bowie, Maryland: Robert J Brady.

Anderson SVD & Bauwens EE (1981) *Chronic Health Problems*. St Louis: CV Mosby. Chapter 13.

Braunwald E et al (1987) *Harrison's Principles of Internal Medicine*, 11th ed. New York: McGraw-Hill. Part 10. Section 2.

Canadian Diabetic Association (1981) *Standards and Guidelines for Diabetes Education in Canada*. Toronto: Canadian Diabetic Association.

Connaught Laboratories (1981) *Insulin in the Control of Diabetes*. Toronto: Connaught Laboratories.

Day JL (1986) *The Diabetes Handbooks. Non-Insulin Dependent Diabetes and Insulin Dependent Diabetes*. Wellingborough, New York: Thorsons.

Dillon RS (1980) *Handbook of Endocrinology*, 2nd ed. Philadelphia: Lea & Febiger.

Ellenberg M & Rifkin H (eds) (1983) *Diabetes Mellitus*, 3rd ed. New York: Medical Examinations.

Ganong WF (1985) *Review of Medical Physiology*, 11th ed. Los Altos, CA: Lange. Chapters 18–24.

Guyton AC (1986) *Textbook of Medical Physiology*, 7th ed. Philadelphia: WB Saunders. Chapters 74–79.

Harper HA, Rodwell VW & Mayers PA (1979) *Review of Physiological Chemistry* , 17th ed. Los Altos, CA: Lange. Chapters 21, 34 & 35.

Hassan T (1985) *A Guide to Medical Endocrinology*. London: Macmillan.

Keele CA, Neil E & Joels N (eds) (1982) *Samson Wright's Applied Physiology*, 13th ed Oxford: Oxford Medical.

Krupp MA & Chatton MJ (1983) *Current Medical Diagnoses and Treatment*. Los Altos, CA: Lange. Chapters 18 & 19.

Kwelowitz T & Berenson L (1981) *Diabetes: A Guide to Self-Management for Patients and Their Families*. Englewood Cliffs, NJ: Prentice-Hall.

Lebovitz HE & Feinglos MN (1983) Oral hypoglycemic agents. In: M Ellenberg & H Rifkin, *Diabetes Mellitus*, 3rd ed. New York: Medical Examinations.

Macleod J (ed) (1984) *Davidson's Principles and Practice of Medicine*, 14th ed. Edinburgh: Churchill Livingstone. Chapter 12.

Matz R (1983) Coma in non-ketotic diabetes. In: M Ellenberg & H. Rifkin, *Diabetes Mellitus*, 3rd ed. New York: Medical Examinations.

Pagana KD & Pagana TJ (1982) *Diagnostic Testing and Nursing Implications*. St Louis: CV Mosby. Chapter 7.

Robbins SL, Angell M & Kumar V (1981) *Basic Pathology*, 3rd ed. Philadelphia: WB Saunders. Chapter 19.

Sabiston DC Jr (ed) (1986) *Davis–Christopher: Textbook of Surgery*. Philadelphia: WB Saunders. Chapters 24–26.

Smith LH & Thier SO (1985) *Pathophysiology*. Philadelphia: WB Saunders. Section 8.

Steiner G & Lawrence PA (eds) (1981) *Educating Diabetic Patients*. New York: Springer.

Tresler KM (1982) *Clinical Laboratory Tests*. Englewood Cliffs, NJ: Prentice-Hall. Chapter 8.

Tridec (1981) *Diabetes Manual*. Toronto: Tri-Hospital Diabetic Education Centre.

Tridec (1981) *Diabetes Manual: Supplement for Insulin-Dependent Patients*. Toronto: Tri-Hospital Diabetic Education Centre.

Zemmet P (1983) Epidemiology of diabetes mellitus. In: M Ellenberg & Rifkin H (eds) *Diabetes Mellitus*, 3rd ed. New York: Medical Examinations.

PERIODICALS

Albin J & Rifkin H (1982) Etiologies of diabetes mellitus. *Med. Clin. N. Am.*, Vol. 66 No. 6, pp. 1209–1226.

Archangelo VP (1983) Simple goiter. *Nurs. '83*, Vol. 13 No. 3, p. 47.

Barkman PS (1983) Confusing concepts: is it diabetic shock or diabetic coma. *Nurs. '83*, Vol. 13 No. 6, pp. 33–34.

Borgatti RS (1980) Patient education: helping diabetics learn control habits. *Patient Care*, Vol. 14 No. 5, pp. 120–144.

British Diabetic Association (1982) Dietary recommendations for diabetics for the 1980s—a statement by the British Diabetic Association. *Hum. Nutr. Appl. Nutr.*, Vol. 36A No. 5, p. 378.

Burnett J (1980) Congenital adrenocortical hyperplasia: a boy with CAH. *Am. J. Nurs.*, Vol. 80 No.7, pp. 1304–1305.

Camunas C (1980) Transphenoidal hypophysectomy. *Am. J. Nurs.*, Vol. 80 No. 10, pp. 1820–1823.

Camunas C (1983) Pheochromocytoma. *Am. J. Nurs.*, Vol. 83 No. 6, pp. 887–891.

Chambers JK (1983) Save your diabetic patient from early kidney damage. *Nurs. '83*, Vol. 13 No. 5, pp. 58–63.

Cohen S (1980) Controlling diabetes mellitus. *Am. J. Nurs.*, Vol. 80 No. 10, pp. 1827–1850.

Cooper DS & Ridgeway EC (1985) Clinical management of patients with hyperthyroidism. *Med. Clin. N. Am.*, Vol. 69 No. 5, pp. 953–971.

Davidson MB, Mecklenburg RS, Pont A, Schneider AB, Bulger JJ & Bulger JT (1984) When you suspect severe hypoglycemia. *Patient Care*, Vol. 18 No. 3, pp. 177–179, 182, 183, 186, 187, 190, 191, 194, 195 & 197.

Dillman WH (1985) Mechanism of action of thyroid hormones. *Med. Clin. N. Am.*, Vol. 69 No. 5, pp. 849–861.

Donohue-Porter P (1985) Symposium on infections in the compromised host: insulin-dependent diabetes mellitus. *Nurs. Clin. N. Am.* Vol. 20 No. 1, pp. 191–198.

Forbes K & Stokes SA (1984) Saving the diabetic foot. *Am. J. Nurs.*, Vol. 84 No. 7, pp. 884–888.

Fredholm N, Vignati L & Brown S (1984) Insulin pumps: the patient verdict. *Am. J. Nurs.*, Vol. 84 No. 1, pp. 36–38.

Fuller E (ed) Making diabetes control a family affair. *Patient Care*, Vol. 14 No. 5, pp. 168–204.

Genuth S (1982) Classification of diabetes mellitus. *Med. Clin. N. Am.*, Vol. 66 No. 6, pp. 1191–1207.

Ginsburg J & Fink RS (1983) Diabetes mellitus. *Nursing* (Second Series), Vol. 2 No. 13, pp. 369–370, 374–378.

Guthrie DW & Guthrie RA (1983) The disease process of diabetes mellitus: definitions, characteristics, trends and developments. *Nurs. Clin. N. Am.*, Vol. 18 No. 4, pp. 617–630.

Heins JM (1983) Dietary management in diabetes mellitus: a goal-setting process. *Nurs. Clin. N. Am.*, Vol. 18 No. 4, pp. 631–643.

Herlihy B (1983) Glucagon and diabetes mellitus. *Crit. Care Nurs.*, Vol. 3 No. 1, pp. 38–43.

Hilton BA (1982) Diabetic monitoring measures: does practice make perfect? *Can. Nurs.*, Vol. 78 No. 5, pp. 26–32.

Hoffman JTT & Newby TB (1980) Hypercalcemia in pituitary hyperparathyroidism. *Nurs. Clin. N. Am.*, Vol. 15 No. 3. pp. 469–480.

Jackson C (1981) Diabetes: how your patient looks at it. *Nurs. '81*, Vol. 11 No. 5, pp. 82–83.

Jones SG (1982) Adrenal patients. Proceed with caution. *R.N.*, Vol. 45 No. 1, pp. 66–72.

Jones SG (1982) Adrenal patients, part II: kid-glove care in pheochromocytoma. *R.N.*, Vol. 45 No. 2, pp. 66–74.

Jones SG (1982) Adrenal patients, part III: bilateral adrenalectomy. Post-operative dangers to watch for. *R.N.*, Vol. 45 No. 3, pp. 66–68.

Kaplan MM (1985) Clinical and laboratory assessment of thyroid abnormalities. *Med. Clin. N. Am.*, Vol. 69 No. 5, pp. 863–880.

Khachadurian AK (1982) Diabetes: new systems for classification and diagnosis. *Geriatrics*, Vol. 37 No. 1, p. 111.

McCarthy JA (1981) Diabetic nephropathy. *Am. J. Nurs.*, Vol. 81 No. 11, pp. 2030–2031, 2033–2034.

McConnell EA (1985) Assessing the thyroid, *Nurs. '85*, Vol. 15 No. 5, pp. 60–62.

Manfredi C, Cassidy V & Moffitt BD (1977) Developing a teaching program for diabetic patients. *J. Contin. Educ. Nurs.*, Vol. 8 No. 6, pp. 46–52.

Metzger MJ (1983) A new test for blood sugar. *Am. J. Nurs.*, Vol. 83 No. 5, pp. 763–764.

Miller BK & White NC (1980) Diabetes assessment guide. *Am. J. Nurs.*, Vol. 80 No. 7, pp. 1314–1316.

Nangi AA & Campbell DJ (1982) Pheochromocytoma. Which Tests are Best? *Diagn. Med.*, Vol. 5 No. 6, pp. 52–56.

National Diabetes Data Group (1979) Classification and diagnosis of diabetes mellitus and other categories of glucose intolerance. *Diabetes*, Vol. 28 No. 12, pp. 1039–1057.

Norkins AL (1979) The causes of diabetes. *Sci. Am.*, Vol. 241 No. 5, pp. 62–73.

Pelczynski L & Reilly A (1981) Helping your diabetic patients help themselves. *Nurs. '81*, Vol. 11 No. 5, pp. 76–81.

Peter JB (1981) Thyroid autoimmunity. *Diagn. Med.*, Vol. 4 No. 5, pp. 19–25.

Plasse NJ (1981) Monitoring blood glucose at home: a comparison of three products. *Am. J. Nurs.*, Vol. 81 No. 11, pp. 2028–2029.

Podolsky S (1982) Management of diabetes in the surgical patient. *Med. Clin. N. Am.*, Vol. 66 No. 6, pp. 1361–1372.

Podolsky S (1982) Diagnosis and treatment of sexual dysfunction in the male diabetic. *Med. Clin. N. Am.*, Vol. 66 No. 6, pp. 1389–1396.

Raskin P (1982) Treatment of insulin-dependent diabetes mellitus with portable insulin infusion devices. *Med. Clin. N. Am.*, Vol. 66 No. 6, pp. 1269–1283.

Resler MM (1983) Teaching strategies that promote adherence. *Nurs. Clin. N. Am.*, Vol. 18 No. 4, pp. 799–811.

Rice V (1983) Problems of water regulation: diabetes insipidus and syndrome of inappropriate anti-diuretic hormone. *Crit. Care Nurs.*, Vol. 3 No. 1, pp. 64–82.

Rice V (1983) Magnesium, calcium and phosphate imbalances: their clinical significance. *Crit. Care Nurs.*, Vol. 3 No. 3, pp. 88–112.

Robertson E & Stevenson E (1983) Loss, stress and the diabetic surgical patient. *Can. Nurs.*, Vol. 79 No. 5, pp. 30–33.

Rubenfield S, Easley JD, Grossman RG & Jackson D (1982) Pituitary tumors and the Nobel prize. *Heart Lung*, Vol. 11 No. 6, pp. 581–587.

Sachs SR (ed) (1980) Caring for patients with Type II diabetes. *Patient Care*, Vol. 14 No. 5, pp. 146–162.

Sanford SJ (1980) Dysfunction of the adrenal gland: physiologic considerations and nursing problems. *Nurs. Clin. N. Am.*, Vol. 15 No. 3, pp. 481–498.

Schiffrin A (1982) Treatment of insulin-dependent diabetes mellitus with multiple subcutaneous insulin injections. *Med. Clin. N. Am.*, Vol. 66 No. 6, pp. 1251–1267.

Shenkman L (1982) The glandular emergencies. *Emerg. Med.*, Vol. 14 No. 3, pp. 26–51.

Skyler JS (1982) Self-monitoring of blood glucose. *Med. Clin. N. Am.*, Vol. 66 No. 6, pp. 1227–1250.

Soloman BL (1980) The hypothalamus and the pituitary gland: an overview. *Nurs. Clin. N. Am.*, Vol. 15 No. 3, pp. 435–451.

Sommers MS (1983) Nonketotic hyperosmolar coma. *Crit. Care Nurs.*, Vol. 3 No. 1, pp. 58–63.

Spoulding SW & Lippes H (1985) Hyperthyroidism: causes, clinical features and diagnosis. *Med. Clin. N. Am.*, Vol. 69 No. 5, pp. 937–951.

Stein C (1982) Psychological reactions to insulin infusion pumps. *Med. Clin. N. Am.*, Vol. 66 No. 6, pp. 1285–1292.

Stevens AD (1981) Monitoring blood glucose at home: who should do it and how. *Am. J. Nurs.*, Vol. 81 No. 11, pp. 2026–2027.

Strowig S (1982) Patient education: a model for autonomous decision-making and deliberate action in diabetes self-management. *Med. Clin. N. Am.*, Vol. 66 No. 6, pp. 1293–1307.

Surr CW (1983) Teaching patients to use the new blood-glucose monitoring products, part I. *Nurs. '83*, Vol. 13 No. 1, pp. 42–45.

Taylor DL (1983) Hypoglycemia: physiology, signs and symptoms. *Nurs. '83*, Vol. 13 No. 3, pp. 44–46.

Unger RH (1982) Benefits and risks of meticulous control of diabetes. *Med. Clin. N. Am.*, Vol. 66 No. 6, pp. 1317–1327.

Unger RH (1980) Diabetes in the 1980s: how different will management be? *Diagn. Med.*, Vol. 3 No. 2, pp. 30–52.

Valenta CL (1983) Urine testing and home blood-glucose monitoring. *Nurs. Clin. N. Am.*, Vol. 18 No. 4, pp. 645–659.

Wake MM & Brensinger JF (1980) The nurse's role in hypothyroidism. *Nurs. Clin. N. Am.*, Vol. 15 No. 3, pp. 453–467.

Weber CA & Clark AH (1985) Surgery for thyroid disease. *Med. Clin. N. Am.*, Vol. 69 No. 5, pp. 1097–1115.

Woolf PD (1985) Thyroiditis. *Med. Clin. N. Am.*, Vol. 69 No. 5, pp. 1035–1048.

Zinman B & Vranic M (1985) Diabetes and exercise. *Med. Clin. N. Am.*, Vol. 69 No. 1, pp. 145–157.

21

Nursing in Disorders of the Urinary System

The Urinary System

The urinary system consists of two kidneys, two ureters, the bladder and urethra. The kidneys are the primary functional structures in which urine is formed. The ureters are drainage tubes which transmit the urine from the kidneys to the bladder where it is temporarily stored. The urethra is a duct that carries the urine to the exterior surface of the body.

Structure of the kidneys

The kidneys are paired, bean-shaped organs that lie retroperitoneally against the dorsal abdominal wall. Each kidney is enclosed in a fibrous capsule and is embedded in fatty tissue. It consists of approximately 1 000 000 nephrons, many blood vessels and collecting tubules, and a pelvis. The kidney is anatomically divided into an outer, dark red portion called the *cortex* and an inner, lighter-coloured section lying between the cortex and the pelvis called the *medulla* (Fig. 21.1). The medullary tissue is arranged in *conical* or *pyramidal masses* separated by *renal columns* formed by projections of cortical tissue. The blood vessels, nerves and ureter enter or leave the kidney at the hilum, the indentation on the medial surface.

NEPHRON

The nephron is the functional unit of the kidney. It consists of a narrow, convoluted tubule and a tuft of capillaries referred to as a *glomerulus*. The upper end of the tubule is dilated and invaginated to envelop the glomerulus and is called *Bowman's capsule*. According to their position, the nephrons may be classified as superficial cortical or juxtamedullary nephrons. The latter lie deep in the cortex with their glomeruli and capsules close to the medulla and their tubules extending deep into the medulla.

The tubule is divided into three segments—the *proximal convoluted tubule*, the hairpin-like *loop of Henle* and the *distal convoluted tubule* (Fig. 21.2). A major function of the tubules is to convey water and solutes in either direction across the tubular cells between the interstitial fluid and the tubular content. The thickness and structure of the walls differ from one segment to another: this arrangement accounts for different substances being reabsorbed and secreted in different sections of the tubule.[1] Movement across the tubular membrane may be active (using cellular energy) or passive.

The proximal convoluted tubule is the longest portion of the nephron and has thin walls consisting of a single layer of cells. The intraluminal surface of the cells has minute finger-like extensions known as *microvilli*, forming what is called a brush border layer. The villi play an important role in reabsorption of glucose and amino acids. These absorptive cells rest on a basement membrane. At the brush border, the cells are joined by *tight junctions* which block communication between the intercellular channels and the tubular lumen (see Fig. 21.3).

The loops of Henle vary in length and lie mainly in the medulla. The walls in the descending limb become thinner as they approach the loop. Modifications in the cells result in the walls of the ascending

---

[1] In relation to kidney function, *reabsorbed* means the movement of substances from the tubular content to the interstitial fluid. *Secreted* implies the transport of substances from the interstitial fluid to the tubular lumen. *Endocrine secretion* indicates the cellular production of a substance and its release directly into the bloodstream.

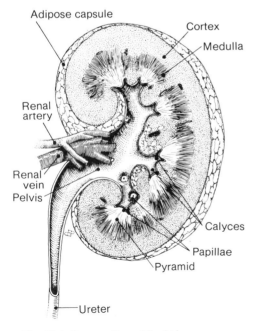

Adipose capsule
Cortex
Medulla
Renal artery
Renal vein
Pelvis
Calyces
Papillae
Pyramid
Ureter

Fig. 21.1 Cross section of the kidney.

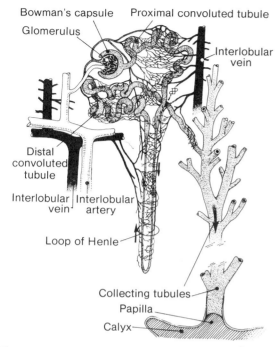

Fig. 21.2 A renal unit or nephron of the cortex of the kidney is shown with its blood supply and a collecting tubule.

limb of the loop being thicker. Its terminal portion approximates the glomerulus of the nephron, of which it is a part, and its afferent arteriole.

The distal convoluted tubule is shorter than the other portions of the tubule. In the area of the tubule where the distal tubule commences, the epithelial cells differ and form an area referred to as the *macula densa*. The cells in the remainder of the tubule are sensitive to the concentration of antidiuretic hormone (ADH) and adrenocortical steroids which influence reabsorption of substances by the distal tubule.

COLLECTING TUBULES

The distal tubules coalesce to form straight collecting tubules which unite to form progressively larger collecting tubules. Groups of the larger tubes come together to form a pyramid-like structure in the medulla. The apex of each pyramid is known as the *papilla* and contains the terminations of collecting tubules through which the urine passes into a cup-like pouch (calyx) of the renal pelvis.

RENAL PELVIS

When the ureter joins the kidney, it expands to form a funnel-shaped receiving basin for the urine delivered by the collecting tubules. It has numerous projecting pouches (calyces), each of which encases a renal papilla and is called a *calyx*.

BLOOD SUPPLY

The renal artery to each kidney arises from the abdominal aorta. When the artery enters the kidney, it progressively subdivides to become afferent arterioles. Each *afferent arteriole* enters a nephron to form a glomerulus. The glomerular capillaries unite to form the *efferent arteriole*, which terminates in a second capillary network in which the tubule is invested. The blood pressure in this second set of capillaries is much lower than that in the glomerulus. The blood is then collected into venules and eventually into a renal vein that carries it to the inferior vena cava.

A large volume of blood is continuously circulated through the kidneys. It is estimated that the renal blood flow averages about 1000–1200 ml per minute in an adult, approximately 23–24% of the cardiac output.

Just before the afferent arteriole becomes the glomerulus, the cells change and increase in the middle tissue layer of the vascular wall. These special cells are known as *juxtaglomerular cells*. They are responsible for the production of the chemical *renin*.

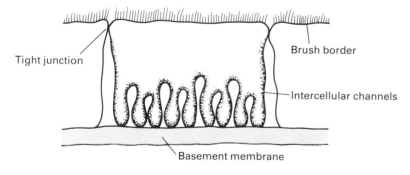

Fig. 21.3 Structure of the proximal tubular cells concerned with the reabsorptive process.

Sympathetic nerve fibres from the thoracolumbar autonomic nervous system transmit impulses to the afferent and efferent arterioles, causing vasoconstriction.

Renal functions

Normal functioning of the body cells is greatly dependent upon a relative constancy of the internal environment. The kidneys play a major role in maintaining this constancy by regulating the water and electrolyte content and the acid–base balance of the body; they *conserve* appropriate amounts of essential substances vital to normal cellular function (e.g. glucose) and *excrete* excesses, the waste products of metabolism, toxic substances and drugs in the urine. The kidneys also have an important *endocrine role*—the production of renin and erythropoietin, and their release into the blood when needed. The processes involved in these functions performed by the kidneys are filtration, selective reabsorption, the transport of substances from the interstitial fluid to the tubule and endocrine secretion (Table 21.1).

Table 21.1 Renal functions.

Overall function: Homeostasis—the maintenance of a suitable environment for optimum cellular function.
1 Regulation of fluid volume
2 Conservation of appropriate amounts of essential substances
3 Excretion of end products of metabolism, excesses, toxic substances and drugs
4 Regulation of the pH of body fluids by the elimination of non-volatile acids
5 Endocrine secretion of renin, erythropoietin and active vitamin D

FILTRATION

The permeability of the glomerular capillaries is greater than that of capillaries elsewhere in the body as a result of the unique three layer structure which permits most dissolved substances in the plasma to pass through into the Bowman's capsules. The same principles that govern the movement of fluid out of the arteriolar ends of the capillaries throughout the body are applicable to the filtration process in the glomeruli. The hydrostatic pressure of the blood in the glomerular capillaries is approximately 60 mmHg, which is considerably higher than that in the other capillaries of the body. This hydrostatic pressure is opposed by the osmotic pressure of the blood proteins (approximately 28 mm Hg) plus the hydrostatic pressure in Bowman's capsule (about 18 mmHg). The net filtration force is 14 mmHg (hydrostatic blood pressure [60] − colloidal osmotic pressure [28] – capsular hydrostatic pressure [18] = 14 mmHg).

The average volume of filtrate in both kidneys is estimated to be about 180 litres each day. The glomerular filtration rate (GFR) is directly proportional to the filtration force; the normal rate is approximately 125 ml per minute. Factors which may alter the glomerular filtration rate are:
1 Change in glomerular capillary hydrostatic pressure, which may be incurred by an increase or decrease in systemic blood pressure or by constriction or dilation of the afferent and efferent arterioles.
2 Increase or decrease in renal artery blood volume.
3 Increase or decrease in the hydrostatic pressure within Bowman's capsule due to compression by ureteral obstruction or disease within the kidney, causing swelling confined within the renal capsule.
4 Decrease or increase in the oncotic pressure (concentration of plasma proteins).
5 Increased glomerular permeability due to disease, such as nephrotic syndrome.
6 Decrease in glomeruli incurred by pathological destruction.

The glomerular filtration rate can be measured by determining the excretion volume and plasma concentration of a substance which is readily filtered through the glomeruli but not secreted or reabsorbed by the renal tubules.

Many solutes escape from the blood in the glomerular filtrate, but small amounts of only a few of them appear in urine. The formed elements and plasma proteins of the blood do not normally pass out of the glomeruli; the composition of the filtrate is the same as plasma minus the plasma proteins.

TUBULAR REABSORPTION

Reabsorption and secretion are complex renal activities. The composition and volume of the filtrate which enters Bowman's capsule differ markedly from those of urine. Of the 180 litres of filtrate produced in 24 hours, only about 1.5 litres are excreted as urine. Most of the water and many of the solid constituents of the filtrate are needed by the body to maintain homeostasis and normal cell metabolism. Other substances, such as urea, creatinine, uric acid, sulphates and phosphates are waste products of metabolism and are excreted in the urine. The tubule cells selectively reabsorb according to the body's needs. Certain substances, such as glucose and amino acids, are completely reabsorbed when their plasma concentrations are within normal range but appear in the urine when the normal is exceeded. About 99% of the water in the filtrate is reclaimed. Reabsorption of the inorganic salts (e.g. sodium, choloride, calcium, potassium, bicarbonate) is variable, depending mainly on their plasma levels. Reabsorption and secretion are carried out selectively, based on the preceding factors.

Some constituents of the filtrate are passively reabsorbed by diffusion or carrier-mediated transport through the tubular membrane. Others are reabsorbed by active cellular transport, which entails energy expenditure on the part of the tubular cells and the presence of certain enzymes. Active reabsorption of substances in the proximal tubule is believed to be in cotransport with sodium.[2] The location of reabsorption and secretion in the tubules varies with different filtrate constituents. The *proximal convoluted tubule* is responsible for the greatest amount of reabsorption. All of the glucose and amino acids and a large proportion of the water and other essential substances are reabsorbed here. Only about 35% of the total volume of filtrate enters the loop of Henle.

In the medulla there are branches of the efferent arterioles of juxtamedullary nephrons that form hairpin loops which approximate the loops of Henle. Each vascular loop of capillaries is called a *vasa recta*. The flow in the ascending limb of the vascular loop is sluggish, so ions diffuse out of the blood readily.

The vasa recta and the loop of Henle play an important role in concentrating the urine and conserving water by means of the countercurrent mechanism and determination of the peritubular osmolality. The countercurrent mechanism implies a U arrangement in which the fluid flows in opposite directions in the two limbs (ascending and descending) and there are interactions between them that alter the osmolality of the fluid along its course in the tube, with the modification being greatest at the base of the loop (Fig. 21.4).

The *loop of Henle* seems to be concerned principally with the transport of sodium chloride ions and water. The ascending limb (the thicker segment) is impermeable to water. It actively transports sodium and chloride ions out into the interstitial fluid, and the tubular fluid becomes hypotonic. The descending limb of the loop of Henle is permeable to water; water moves out to the interstitial fluid which has become hypertonic. At the same time sodium and chloride ions diffuse into the descending limb. The osmolality of the fluid within the descending limb progressively becomes more hypertonic as it approaches the base of the loop. The osmolality of the medullary interstitial fluid is increased, and sodium chloride diffuses into the blood in the descending limb of the vasa recta. But, as the blood flows in the opposite direction in the ascending limb, sodium chloride readily diffuses out again into the medullary interstitium; the osmolality of the blood as it leaves the medulla is only slightly higher than when it entered the vasa recta.

The maintenance of the volume and concentration of body fluids within a narrow normal range is largely controlled by the ability of the kidney tubules to concentrate or dilute the urine. When body fluids are diluted by an excess of water or diminished solute intake (especially sodium), the urine becomes dilute and the volume is increased. Conversely, if the concentration of body fluids is raised to above the

---

[2] Smith & Thier (1985), pp. 663–664.

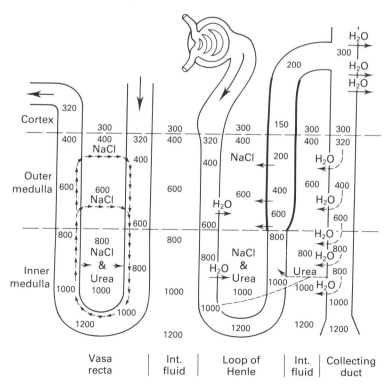

Fig. 21.4 The countercurrent mechanism for concentrating the urine.

normal level by an excessive intake of solutes or an extrarenal loss of water, water reabsorption from the filtrate is increased, concentrating the urine and decreasing the output volume.

The dilution and concentration of urine depend principally on two factors: first, the osmotic pressure of the peritubular fluid, which in turn is mainly dependent on the normal functioning of the loop of Henle and the distal convoluted tubules; and secondly, on the concentration of ADH in the blood.

The fluid entering the distal tubule is hypotonic, but the volume and osmolality are modified selectively as it proceeds through the distal and collecting tubules.

Reabsorption of water from the hypotonic filtrate in the distal convoluted and collecting tubules is regulated by ADH, which increases the permeability of their membranous walls. It is produced by the hypothalamus in the brain, and is stored and released into the blood by the posterior pituitary gland (neurohypophysis). Receptors in the hypothalamus are sensitive to changes in the osmotic pressure of the blood. When the pressure is increased to above normal (for example, by additional sodium), impulses are delivered to the posterior pituitary, resulting in the release of ADH which increases water reabsorption in the tubules. Conversely, if the osmotic pressure falls below the homeostatic level, the release of ADH is inhibited. The tubular membrane becomes relatively impermeable, restricting the reabsorption of water, and the urine is dilute.

The reabsorption of sodium by active cellular transport in the distal and collecting tubules is influenced by the adrenocortical hormone *aldosterone*. A high concentration of aldosterone stimulates the distal tubular cells to reabsorb increasing amounts of sodium. A deficiency of the hormone, such as occurs in Addison's disease, reduces the amount of sodium reclaimed, resulting in an excessive loss in urine. Aldosterone also affects the amount of potassium reclaimed and excreted. Increased concentrations of

the hormone promote excretion of potassium, and a deficient amount of aldosterone produces excessive retention of potassium.

TUBULAR SECRETION AND EXCRETION

Tubular cells are capable of actively transporting some substances from the blood into the filtrate—a reverse process to that of reabsorption. The potassium concentration of plasma is regulated by this process. Practically all of the potassium that escapes from the plasma into the filtrate is reabsorbed in the proximal tubule. Any excess in the blood is then actively secreted by the distal tubules and is excreted in exchange for sodium ions.

Cells of the distal tubules play an important role in maintaining a normal acid–base balance. They do this by secreting hydrogen ions into the lumen of the tubules in exchange for sodium ions and by forming ammonium ions that combine with chlorine ions to form ammonium chloride, which is excreted in the urine (see Chapter 6 for a discussion of the role of the kidney in the regulation of hydrogen ion concentration [H^+] and pH).

Some drugs are also excreted by active tubular removal from the blood into the tubules. These include diodone, amminohippuric acid and phenolsulphonphthalein, which may be used to investigate renal function.

ENDOCRINE RENAL SECRETIONS

The kidney produces two endocrine secretions, renin and erythropoietin.

Renin is a proteolytic enzyme that reacts with an inactive precursor fraction of the plasma globulin (angiotensinogen), producing a substance called angiotensin I which is converted to angiotension II by another enzyme in the lungs. As angiotensin II circulates it causes vasoconstriction of the systemic arterioles and stimulates the secretion of aldosterone and, to a lesser degree, glucocorticoids (Fig. 21.5).

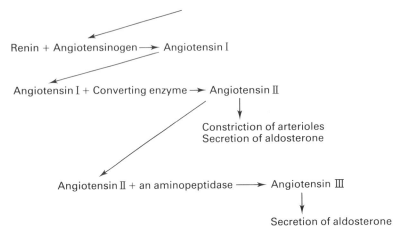

Fig. 21.5 Decrease in intravascular volume and/or fall in blood pressure, or stimulation of the macula densa by decreased sodium chloride content in tubular fluid entering the distal tubule.

Angiotensin II is changed to angiotensin III by an aminopeptidase in the red blood cells and many other tissues, including the adrenal gland. It is believed to stimulate aldosterone secretion.

Five mechanisms are suggested as influencing the production and release of renin: (1) the juxtaglomerular cells release renin in response to decreased arteriolar blood volume and pressure. (2) The macula densa is sensitive to sodium and chloride concentrations; a decrease in the sodium and chloride content of the tubular fluid entering the distal tubule brings about the release of renin. The release of renin and the ensuing formation of angiotensin II and III stimulates the release of aldosterone which promotes the retention of sodium ions. (3) Sympathetic stimulation of the juxtaglomerular cells may be associated with the production of renin. The stimulation may be mediated by the release of catecholamines (e.g. adrenaline) by the adrenal medulla or by renal sympathetic innervation. (4) Prostaglandins act on the juxtaglomerular cells to stimulate renin secretion. (5) Potassium concentrations also influence renin release by influencing sodium and chloride levels in the macula densa.[3]

A second hormone produced by the kidneys is the *renal erythropoietic factor* (REF, erythrogenin). It is produced and secreted into the blood in response to hypoxia, cobalt salts and androgens, and functions in the maintenance of normal erythrocyte production by the bone marrow. REF reacts with a plasma globulin to produce erythropoietin which stimulates the bone marrow to produce and release red blood cells.

A third hormone synthesized by the renal tubule cells is 1,25-dihydroxycholecalciferol (1,25-dihydroxyvitamin D_3). This is the active form of the hormone and is essential for the absorption of calcium from the small intestine.

Characteristics and composition of urine

When the filtrate flows into the main collecting tubules and renal pelvis, it becomes urine. The average volume excreted in 24 hours is approximately 1.5 litres but varies with fluid losses through other channels (e.g. sweat) and fluid intake. The reaction of urine is usually acid, with a pH of about 6.0, but may range from 4.5–8.5 with a varied dietary intake. The acidity increases with high protein ingestion and tissue catabolism, while a vegetable diet produces an alkaline urine.

The specific gravity, which gives a rough estimate of the concentration of solids, ranges from 1.003–1.040. The composition of urine varies with dietary intake and metabolic wastes produced. Normally, about 90–95% of urine is water. An average of 50 g of organic and inorganic solid wastes are eliminated daily. The chief solutes are urea, creatinine, uric acid and the chlorides, phosphates and sulphates of sodium, potassium, calcium, magnesium and ammonia.

Ureters, bladder and urethra

URETERS

Each of the two ureters is a tube 25–30 cm (10–12 in) in length, extending from a kidney to the bladder. They are situated behind the parietal peritoneum and enter the posterior wall of the lower half of the bladder obliquely. The slanted entrance forms a flap in the bladder wall that serves as a valve to prevent a reflux of urine as the bladder fills or contracts. Each ureter consists of an outer fibrous covering, a middle layer of muscle tissue, and a mucous membrane lining which is continuous with that of the bladder and the renal pelvis.

The function of these tubes is simply to convey urine from the kidneys to the bladder. Contraction of the ureteral muscular tissue produces peristaltic waves which move the urine along the tube and into the bladder in spurts.

BLADDER

The urinary bladder serves as a temporary reservoir for the urine, which it expels at intervals from the body. It is a collapsible muscular sac that lies behind the symphysis pubis. Three layers of plain muscle tissue form the bladder walls. The fibres are arranged in longitudinal, circular and spiral layers. Collectively, these layers are referred to as the *detrusor muscle*. The ureteral orifices in the posterior wall and the urethral opening outline a triangular area called the *trigone*. When the bladder is empty, the mucous membrane lining falls into folds (rugae) except in the area of the trigone (Fig. 21.6).

URETHRA

The *urethra* is a slender tube that conveys urine from the bladder to the exterior. It has a thin layer of smooth muscle tissue and is lined with a mucous membrane which is continuous with that of the bladder. The opening from the bladder is controlled by two sphincters: an internal one which is under autonomic (involuntary) nervous system control, and an external one which is voluntarily controlled by the cerebral cortex. The external urethral orifice is known as the urinary meatus.

In the female, the urethra is about 4 cm (1.5 in) long and lies anterior to the vagina. The male urethra is approximately 20 cm (8 in) in length and, on leaving the bladder, passes through the prostate gland. As well as conveying the urine, the male urethra receives the semen from the ejaculatory ducts of the reproductive system, transmitting it through the meatus (see Fig. 21.6).

---

[3] Ganong (1985), p. 379.

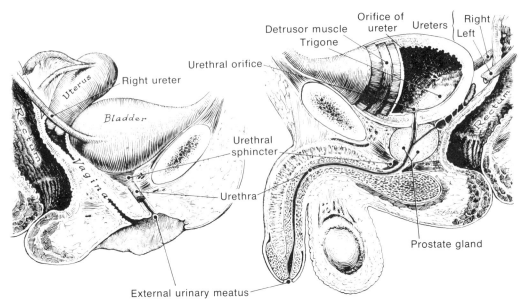

Fig. 21.6 The bladder, ureters, urethra and prostate.

Micturition

This is a term used for the elimination of urine from the bladder. The process involves both autonomic (involuntary) and voluntary nervous impulses. When 300–400 ml of urine collect in the bladder, receptors that are sensitive to stretching initiate impulses which are transmitted by afferent nerve fibres into the lower part of the spinal cord (Fig. 21.7). A reflex response via parasympathetic nerves to the bladder results in contractions of the detrusor muscle and relaxation of the internal sphincter.

The initial impulses from the stretch receptors are also relayed via a spinocortical tract to the cerebral cortex, producing an awareness of the need to void. When a person is prepared to empty the bladder, voluntary impulses are initiated which descend the cord and are carried out to the external sphincter, causing it to relax. With both sphincters relaxed, the detrusor muscle contracts and urine flows from the bladder through the urethra. Voluntary micturition

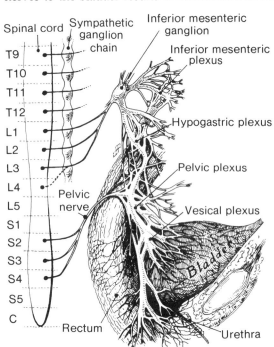

Fig. 21.7 A diagram showing innervation of the bladder.

may also be accompanied by relaxation of the perineal muscles and contraction of abdominal muscles. Infants and very young children empty their bladder whenever the micturition reflex is initiated, as they have not yet developed voluntary control over the external sphincter. Obviously, any interruption of the spinocortical impulse pathway interferes with control of the external sphincter, resulting in involuntary voiding or retention.

NURSING PROCESS

Assessment

Urinary elimination is a personal and private activity; social norms and personal habits influence how individuals respond when problems develop with urinary elimination. Patients may be uncomfortable and embarrassed discussing their problems and delay seeking medical assistance. When obtaining a health history and examining a patient with a urinary system disorder the nurse assesses each individual's level of anxiety, allows the patient to express feelings of discomfort and humiliation, acknowledges awareness of these feelings and reassures the patient that everything possible will be done to ease any embarrassment and provide privacy. It is also important to establish the terms and expressions used by the patient to describe the act of voiding and to ensure that the terminology used by the nurse is understood.

HISTORY

The patient is questioned about any *past history* of: (1) urinary system disorders, urinary tract infections, renal calculi or related surgical interventions; (2) diseases affecting the urinary system such as diabetes mellitus, hypertension, systemic lupus erythematosus, gout, streptococcal infections and venereal diseases; and (3) past use of drugs (either prescribed or bought over the counter).

Family history related to renal disease, congenital anomalies of the urinary system, and diseases such as diabetes mellitus, hypertension and connective tissue disorders is determined. Female patients should be asked about their obstetric history.

Specific information about the patient's usual and present *pattern of urinary elimination* is obtained. Information includes frequency of voiding, volume of urine excreted at each voiding and in a 24-hour period and usual times of voiding. Any changes in the usual pattern of elimination such as nocturia or frequency are identified. The patient is questioned about the colour, odour and clarity of urine and if there is any discomfort or pain associated with voiding.

Presenting symptoms. Clinical manifestations of urinary system disorders the patient may experience include:
1 Changes in the pattern of urinary elimination including frequency, nocturia, difficulty initiating the stream of urine, inability to control urinary output (incontinency) which may be associated with urgency or stress, bed-wetting
2 Changes in the volume of urinary output
3 Changes in the colour, odour or consistency of urine
4 Pain and discomfort associated with voiding
5 Sensory changes related to the urge to void
6 Chills and fever
7 General symptoms associated with renal impairment including hypertension, pruritus, oedema, headache, lethargy, fatigue, visual disturbances, loss of appetite and nausea

Factors influencing urinary system function.
1 *Past experiences and attitudes.* Urinary habits vary with each individual. The nurse discusses the patient's usual habits, attitudes to urinary elimination and experiences with toilet training which may have influenced present attitudes.
2 *Diet and fluid intake.* The volume of fluid intake has a direct effect on the urinary output. For patients with renal disorders it is important to identify usual eating habits and the relative amounts of protein and sodium in the daily diet.
3 *Life-style factors* that influence elimination include accessibility of toilet facilities, privacy and any unusual stresses associated with voiding.
4 *Activity, mobility and dexterity.* Physical activity is necessary to maintain muscle tone and normal amounts of calcium in the bones. Bed rest and immobility predispose to the formation of calculi. Impaired mobility and dexterity may interfere with the individual's ability to get to the toilet quickly enough to use it effectively.
5 *Level of awareness and orientation.* Confusion, disorientation and difficulty following directions may interfere with the individual's ability to respond appropriately to the urge to void as well as to meet fluid and nutritional needs.
6 *Medications.* The name, dosage, frequency and duration of use of any medications being taken is recorded. Some drugs are toxic to the kidneys while others alter the characteristics of urine; for example anticoagulants can produce haematuria and diuretics have a direct effect on urine production.

PHYSICAL EXAMINATION

General appearance. The patient is observed for general state of health, lethargy, fatigue and degree of alertness. Body weight, and any oedema of the face, abdomen or extremities are noted.

Skin and hair. The skin is observed for colour, general texture, broken areas, bruising or excoriation and any unusual odour is also noted. The hair is observed noting texture and dryness.

Urinary meatus and perineum.   The urethral orifice is observed for signs of drainage, oedema, redness or ulceration and underclothing is examined for urine or other stains. A vaginal examination may be done by the doctor on a female patient to identify possible uterine prolapse or cystocele; the prostate gland is palpated by rectal examination on male patients.

Bladder.   The bladder is not normally palpated but may be felt if it is overdistended. With the patient supine, the doctor gently palpates and percusses the area just above the symphysis pubis; the distended bladder feels smooth and firm. The degree of elevation above the symphysis pubis is measured. Palpation of a distended bladder causes increased discomfort for the patient.

Kidneys.   The kidneys are not usually palpable in adults. The lower pole of the right kidney may be felt in thin individuals or those with loss of muscle tone. With the patient supine and the examiner standing on the patient's right, the left hand is placed under the patient's right flank to elevate it. The right hand is used to palpate deeply through the abdominal wall at the costal margin. The lower pole of the right kidney will feel smooth and firm as it descends when the patient takes a deep inspiration. The left kidney is palpated in a similar manner with the examiner elevating the patient's left flank with the right hand and palpating with the left hand.

Neurological examination.   A complete neurological examination is done (see Chapter 22) in patients with neurological impairment and sensory losses such as absence of the sensation or urge to void.

DIAGNOSTIC PROCEDURES

The investigation of renal dysfunction may include examination of urine specimens (which may be voided or obtained by bladder or urethral catheterization), blood chemistry determinations, renal function tests, x-ray studies and ultrasound procedures.

Urine examinations
The specimen of urine submitted for analysis is *voided* unless the doctor requests that it be a *midstream* sample or collected by *catheter*. The voided specimen should be of the first voiding in the morning, if possible, since it provides some information about the kidneys' ability to concentrate wastes. Midstream and catheter samples are collected in sterile containers. All specimens are labelled clearly with the patient's name, time collected, method of collection and the examination required.
    Specimens collected for chemistry determination

should be examined in the laboratory within 2 hours of voiding. The colour and clarity of the urine are noted and the pH and specific gravity are determined.
    Routine ward testing of urine will identify the presence of protein, sugar, collective (but not specific) ketones, bilirubin, urobilinogen and blood. Other tests identify specific ketone bodies (acetone, acetoacetic acid, and hydroxybutyric acid), urea, potassium, chloride, bicarbonate, sulphates and phosphates. Microscopic examination of the urinary sediment, which is obtained by centrifuging the urine, may reveal abnormal constituents such as blood cells, casts, pus and bacteria. When equipment is available, the doctor may examine urinary sediment under a microscope for a preliminary diagnosis.
    If the urine is to be cultured, a midstream or catheter specimen is collected. Catheterization is avoided, if possible, because of the danger of introducing infection into the urethra or bladder. To obtain a midstream sample from a female, the perineum and meatus are cleansed the same as for catheterization to prevent possible contamination from the perineum and vaginal secretion. In the case of the male, the external meatus is cleansed before voiding. Following the cleansing, the patient is instructed to void, and the first 50 ml of urine are discarded to eliminate possible contamination by organisms that may be in the urethra. The subsequent urine is collected.
    A *24-hour collection* of urine may be requested for quantitative determination of the total solid content or of specific substances such as protein, glucose, certain electrolytes and hormones. When the collection is started, the patient voids and that urine is discarded. At the end of the 24 hours he voids and the urine is included in the specimen. The urine is refrigerated or kept in a cool place. If the patient is ambulatory, it is made clear to him that all his urine is to be saved during the designated period.

Blood chemistry determinations
Impaired glomerular filtration and loss of tubular ability to reabsorb and excrete discriminately lead to alterations in plasma composition. Blood specimens may be requested to determine the concentration of the following substances:
    Protein metabolic nitrogenous wastes
        Urea nitrogen (BUN)—Normal: 2.9–8.9 mmol/l
          (8–25 mg/dl)
        Creatinine—Normal: 60–120 µmol/l
          (0.5–1.5 mg/dl)
        Uric acid—normal: 0.22–0.48 mmol/l
          (3.7–8.2 mg/dl)
Electrolytes
        Serum sodium—Normal; 135–145 mmol/l
        Serum potassium—Normal: 3.5–5.5 mmol/l
        Serum calcium—Normal: 2.2–2.6 mmol/l
        Serum chloride—Normal: 100–106 mmol/l

Total serum base—Normal: 145–160 mmol/l
Serum phosphate (inorganic)—Normal:
    0.8–1.5 mmol/l (2.4–4.5 mg/dl)
Plasma Proteins—Normal: 60–80 g/l
Albumin—Normal: 40–50 g/l
Globulin—Normal: 20–30 g/l

Haematological tests

The haemoglobin concentration and haematocrit are determined, since anaemia is a common problem. If infection is suspected a leucocyte count is done, and a platelet count and prothrombin time may be needed in advanced chronic renal failure.

Renal function tests

Renal function tests may be classified according to the kidney function being evaluated. In renal function, the removal or clearance of substances from the blood is achieved by glomerular filtration and tubular cell activity. If a substance passes freely through the glomeruli, and is neither reabsorbed or secreted by the tubules, the quantity appearing in the urine is the same as that filtered by the glomeruli. By measuring the amount excreted in the urine in a specified period of time, information is obtained about the efficiency of glomerular filtration. The substances used for this evaluation may be creatinine or urea, which are naturally occurring metabolites, or inulin.

Glomerular filtration rate. For determining the glomerular filtration rate, the creatinine, inulin or Cr^{51}-EDTA clearance test may be used. Creatinine or Cr^{51}-EDTA clearance tests are used most frequently.

In the *creatinine clearance test*, the patient maintains normal but not excessive activity, since endogenous creatinine is produced in muscular activity. No special diet is necessary but excessive intake of tea, coffee and meat is avoided for a 24-hour period before the test. A 24-hour specimen of urine and a venous blood specimen are collected for creatinine concentration determinations. The rate of urinary excretion per minute is calculated. The normal amount of creatinine excreted in 24 hours varies with age; in an adult the normal is about 1.2–1.7 g, and in a child it is approximately 0.36 g. Calculations are made to determine the volume of plasma cleared of creatinine per minute, which is the glomerular filtration rate.

Cr^{51}-EDTA, a radioactive isotope, is given intravenously into one arm. Blood tests from the other arm are taken hourly for 3 hours and from the rate of clearance from the plasma, the GFR is calculated.

Inulin, a polysaccharide, is given intravenously and, normally, is readily filtered through the glomeruli but is neither secreted nor reabsorbed by tubular cells. The patient is encouraged to drink 500–1000 ml of water 1–2 hours preceding the administration of the inulin. The inulin clearance test is considered to be the most accurate method for measuring the GFR.

Tubular function. Assessment of tubular function involves testing the kidneys' ability to concentrate solid wastes, excrete phenolsulphonphthalein (PSP) and excrete acids in the urine.

In order to maintain homeostasis, normal kidneys are able to vary the concentration of solid wastes and the volume of urine according to the volume of body fluids. When there is an excessive loss of body fluid by other channels or a restricted intake, more water is reabsorbed by the renal tubules; the solid wastes are excreted in a smaller volume of urine and the specific gravity is high. Conversely, with a large fluid intake; less water is reabsorbed by the tubules, the volume of urine is greater and the specific gravity and osmolality are lower than usual. This ability to vary the volume and concentration of the urine appropriately is impaired in tubular damage and may be tested by a concentration or dilution test.

The *concentration test* is designed to determine the kidney's ability to concentrate urine when the fluid intake is restricted. Fluids are restricted over a specified period. Then, two or three urine specimens are collected, and the osmolality and specific gravity of each are determined. If the kidneys are normal, the specific gravity is not less than 1.024 and the osmolality is greater than 800 mosmol/kg of water and greater than the serum osmolality which should be unchanged. The procedure regarding the period of fluid restriction and the number of specimens collected varies in different institutions. The commonly used Fishberg concentration test involves restricted fluids with the evening meal (approximately 200 ml) and then no food or fluid until the test is completed the next morning. Three hourly urine specimens are collected in the morning (e.g. at 6, 7 and 8 a.m.). The time of voiding each specimen is indicated on the labels. *All the urine voided each time must be submitted to the laboratory.* Before the test is begun, the patient receives an explanation so he will understand the reasons for the fluid restriction and collection of specimens. This test must not be performed on patients with known renal impairment as dehydration may precipitate an acute deterioration in renal function.

Renal scan

Scans most frequently used are DTPA (diethylenetriamine penta-acetic acid) and DMSA (dimercaptosuccinic acid) scans. These compounds are both radioactively labelled and are injected intravenously. The renal areas are then scanned by a device sensitive to the gamma rays emitted from the compound to the kidney. DTPA is filtered and secreted but not absorbed. It is an especially useful test to monitor the perfusion of transplanted kidneys or of patients in acute renal failure.

DMSA is bound to renal tubules and may last in the kidney for several days. It is especially used to show scarring in the kidneys and may be used to calculate the percentage of function contributed by each kidney. The condition of the kidneys may also be studied by administering radioactive iodohippurate (I^{131}) intravenously and observing its distribution in the kidney and its elimination. A tracing (renogram) is obtained for each kidney. From the renograms the doctor is able to assess both renal artery and regional blood flows.

Voided urine specimens may also be collected following the injection, and are tested for the content of radioactive iodohippurate. Normally, about 75% is excreted within 30–40 minutes.

Intravenous urogram (Excretory urogram)
A radiopaque, iodine-based substance that is eliminated by the kidneys is given intravenously, and a series of x-ray films are made at intervals to note the concentration of the contrast medium in the renal pelves, ureters and bladder.

Preparation for an intravenous urogram includes an explanation of the procedure to the patient and questioning as to whether he has any allergies or has ever had asthma, eczema or a reaction to iodine. The doctor is advised if any sensitivity or allergy is indicated by the patient. No fluids are given for 8–10 hours preceding the examination to provide a better concentration of the radiopaque substance. Two bisacodyl (Dulcolax) tablets or another laxative may be ordered the day before, and an enema may be given 2–3 hours before the test to cleanse the intestines of gas and faeces which produce shadows on the film but is not usually necessary. The laxative is contraindicated if the patient has a gastrointestinal condition, such as peptic ulcer or colitis. Patients with renal impairment must not be severely fluid restricted nor dehydrated by vigorous bowel preparation. If hypovolaemia is induced the patient may suffer an acute deterioration in renal function which may not completely return. Care must be taken with transplanted patients who may have excellent function. The radiologist can give a larger dose of contrast medium to those inadequately prepared and take nephrotomograms.

The contrast medium which is given intravenously is an iodide preparation to which the patient may be sensitive. A set of emergency equipment should be readily available in the event of a reaction. The trolley should have adrenaline, intravenous antihistamine and adrenocorticosteroid preparations. Oxygen and a self-inflating resuscitation bag and mask should also be available. The patient is advised that he is likely to experience a salty taste and a sudden flush of warmth during the slow injection of the dye. He is observed closely for signs of respiratory distress, shivering, sweating and urticaria. These and any complaints of unusual sensations are promptly reported to the doctor.

Following the x-ray series, the patient is encouraged to take additional fluids to correct the dehydration incurred by the restriction of fluids and cleansing of the bowel.

Ultrasound
Ultrasonography is non-invasive and involves direction of an ultrasound beam to the tissues from a transducer held over the patient's body surface. The reflection or echo of the sound waves is converted to electrical impulses and displayed on an oscilloscope; the image may be recorded.

There is no preparation for an ultrasound scan of the kidneys, although a full bladder may be requested as it provides a good 'landmark' for the technician. The test is used to look at the size and structure of the kidneys and other organs.

Cystoscopy and retrograde pyelogram
Cystoscopy involves the passage of a cystoscope through the urethra into the bladder. The instrument is equipped with a light which permits direct visualization of the internal surface of the bladder. A long, fine catheter may also be introduced into each renal pelvis through the cystoscope (ureteric catheterization), and a urine specimen collected from each kidney. Ureteric catheterization may be used to obtain specimens from one or both kidneys for microscopic examination and culture, or in renal function tests when the function of each kidney is to be determined. For example, during cystoscopy and ureteric catheterization, phenosulphonphthalein may be given intravenously, and its appearance in the urine from each kidney noted and timed. Normally, it appears in 4–6 minutes following the administration. The specimens must be labelled as to right or left ureter.

A radiopaque iodide preparation may then be introduced into the catheters, and x-rays are taken which outline the renal pelves and ureters. This procedure is referred to as a *retrograde pyelogram*, and may be used in place of intravenous urography when the patient is sensitive to the intravenous contrast medium.

Preparation of the patient for a cystoscopy includes an explanation of the procedure. The patient's signature indicating his consent for the examination is required. He is given extra fluids for several hours preceding the examination to ensure a satisfactory flow of urine for specimens. He will receive a general anaesthetic, so food and fluid are restricted for 6–8 hours preceding and intravenous fluid is administered to ensure urinary flow.

If a general anaesthetic is contraindicated, the procedure may be performed under sedation. Increasingly, it is possible to perform cystoscopy with a flexible cystoscope under sedation without discomfort.

Upon completion of the examination, the patient rests in bed for a few hours. Discomfort in the back or bladder region may be relieved by local heat application (hot water bottle or electric heating pad) or a warm bath if the patient's condition permits. Additional fluids are encouraged. Any severe pain or persisting bright blood in the urine is reported to the doctor.

Computerized axial tomography

Computerized axial tomography is an x-ray technique which uses a computer to reconstruct an image of a layer of tissue in the body. A narrow x-ray beam which examines body sections from many angles produces images which are built up into a three dimensional picture of the organ. It is used for detection of tumours and cysts of the kidney. The patient must fast for 4 hours prior to the scan.

Renal angiography

Renal blood vessels may be outlined on an x-ray film following the administration of a radiopaque substance into the vascular system. The contrast medium may be injected directly into the aorta through a small catheter introduced into a femoral artery, and passed retrogradely into the aorta to just above the origin of the renal arteries. Since the patient may be sensitive to the radiopaque iodide preparation, the same precautions as cited for intravenous urography should be followed. Preparation of the patient is similar to that noted for the patient having intravenous urography. The site of catheter introduction into the femoral artery is observed frequently for bleeding for several hours. The site is also inspected for local swelling, redness and tenderness. The temperature of the lower limbs is noted and the popliteal and pedal pulses are checked. Any indication of impaired circulation is reported promptly.

Nuclear magnetic resonance imaging.

Nuclear magnetic resonance (NMR) employs radio frequencing, in the presence of a magnetic field, to produce anatomical sections of the body. It is non-invasive and can provide images in any anatomical plane. It is a very new technique and not widely used but has been shown to have an important role in the detection of abnormalities of renal tissue.

Percutaneous renal biopsy

A biopsy is a valuable test in diagnosis and assessment of the effects of treatment but carries with it the risk of haemorrhage. It is contraindicated if the patient has hypertension, a bleeding tendency, only one kidney, or suspected perirenal abscess. Before a patient is booked for renal biopsy, coagulation, bleeding and prothrombin times are determined. If these are satisfactory, the patient's blood is grouped and cross-matched, and compatible blood is kept available in the event of haemorrhage. An explanation is given to the patient of what he may expect. He is advised that he will be put in the prone position over a firm pillow (kidney elevator) for a brief period. The patient's written consent is required for the procedure.

The exact location of the kidney is identified by x-ray which may include an intravenous urogram or an ultrasound scan and the position indicated on the skin surface. The skin is cleansed and local anaesthesia is used. The patient is instructed to hold his breath during the insertion of the needle and the actual taking of the specimen. Following the removal of the biopsy needle, pressure is applied to the site for a few minutes.

The blood pressure and pulse are recorded every 15 minutes for 1 hour, then every 30 minutes for a period of 1–2 hours, and then every 4 hours for 24 hours. The patient is kept on bed rest in the dorsal recumbent position for 18–24 hours, or until the urine is cleared of blood.

Retrograde renal brush biopsy

This procedure involves brushing the tissue surface to obtain cells for cytological examination.

The patient receives a general anaesthetic and an intravenous infusion is started so that a contrast medium can be given to facilitate the movement of the brush. A cystoscopic examination is done and a whistle-tip urethral catheter is introduced through which the biopsy brush is passed into the renal pelvis. The urologist manipulates the brush into appropriate areas and moves the brush back and forth several times to pick up cells which become entrapped in the bristles.

A 24-hour collection of urine may be requested; it also undergoes cytological examination.

When the patient recovers from the anaesthetic, he is encouraged to take fluids freely or intravenous fluids are adminstered. The patient may experience colicky renal pain and require analgesia.

Urodynamic investigations

These studies provide information on bladder sensation and detrusor muscle and urethral sphincter function. The tests consists of: (1) urine flow studies, (2) filling and voiding cystometrography, (3) urethral pressure profile, and (4) synchronous pressure-flow cystourethrography and video recording.[4]

Urine flow studies measure the time and amount voided and usually include determination of the amount of residual urine in the bladder following voiding.

The cystometrogram is a method of recording the bladder's responses to increasing distension. A two-way catheter is inserted; the bladder is filled with fluid through one lumen while pressures are recorded via the second lumen. By this simple procedure, measurements are made of the volume of residual urine, resting intravesicular pressure, bladder capacity, intravesicular pressures during filling and at the point of emptying, the point at which sensation to void is felt, and the pressure and timing of any uninhibited contractions.

The synchronous video pressure flow cystourethrography is a newer, more sophisticated and expensive method of evaluating bladder and urethral func-

---

[4] Mandelstram (1986) p. 47.

tion; it provides information on the appearance of the bladder during the micturition cycle.

Manifestations of disorders of the urinary system

MANIFESTATIONS OF RENAL DYSFUNCTION

In impaired kidney function, the constancy of the internal environment (homeostasis), which is essential for the normal functioning of all body cells, is disrupted. The normal volume, composition and reaction of the body fluids may be altered by the inability of the kidneys to conserve essential substances and excrete excesses, metabolic wastes and toxic substances; disturbances in the functioning of other organs readily develop. Consequently, the signs and symptoms of renal insufficiency are varied, and many are not directly referable to the urinary system. Whether the disease is acute or chronic and whether it affects the glomeruli or the tubules will also vary the manifestations.

Abnormal urinary volume

Oliguria or anuria may develop, especially in acute and advanced renal failure. *Oliguria* means that less than 500 ml of urine is formed in 24 hours. *Anuria* implies a urinary output of less than 250 ml in 24 hours and is sometimes referred to as a renal shutdown. The diminished urine formation may be associated with decreased glomerular filtration due to renal disease (e.g. glomerulonephritis), hypotension as in shock and dehydration, decreased renal blood flow or an obstruction within the tubules.

Polyuria, a volume of urine in excess of the normal (over 2000 ml in 24 hours), may also indicate renal disturbance in which the ability of the tubules to reabsorb water and concentrate the solid wastes is limited. It is most often seen in chronic kidney disease or it may be secondary to diabetes insipidus as a result of a deficiency in the secretion of vasopressin (antidiuretic hormone). Polyuria may not be a manifestation of renal disease but may indicate a disorder elsewhere. Frequently, polyuria is the symptom that may cause an individual to go to a doctor where, on investigation, he is found to have diabetes mellitus.

Nocturia (voiding during the night) usually accompanies polyuria and the person becomes desperate for undisturbed sleep. Inability of the kidneys to reabsorb the normal amount of water and to concentrate the wastes may be referred to as *hyposthenuria*. As well as the excessive volume, a low specific gravity of approximately 1.010 of the urine persists because the impaired tubules cannot concentrate or vary the amount of solids.

Abnormal constituents in the urine

Abnormal constituents revealed in urinalysis vary with the underlying renal disease. They include protein (usually albumin), blood, casts, pus and organisms.

The large molecular structure of serum albumin inhibits its filtration through normal glomeruli. *Albuminuria* usually indicates inflammation and almost always indicates damage to the glomeruli. *Haematuria* denotes blood in the urine and may be macroscopic or recognized only by microscopic examination. It indicates some pathological process within the kidneys or postrenal structures.

Urinary casts are microscopic cylindrical structures formed in the distal and collecting tubules by the agglutination of cells and cellular debris in a protein matrix. They are moulded or cast in the shape of the tubule. Depending on their composition, casts are usually classified as red blood cell, epithelial, hyaline, granular or fatty. They point to the presence of some inflammatory or degenerative process within the tubules. Obviously, *pus and bacteria* in the urine indicate infection in the kidneys or urinary tract.

Abnormal urine colour

Abnormal discoloration of urine may be associated with infection within the urinary tract, but more often occurs with a disorder extrinsic to the kidneys and urinary tract. Examples of disorders in which the urine is discolored are: myoglobinuria, in which there has been a release of myoglobin from muscle cells, as happens in a crushing injury; haemoglobinuria which may develop following a blood transfusion reaction in which there is a breakdown of erythrocytes and the release of haemoglobin; porphyria, a genetic disorder in which normal use of porphyrin in the formation of haemoglobin does not occur, resulting in porphyrins being eliminated in the urine; and melanoma, a skin neoplasm characterized by excessive pigmentation.

It should be remembered that urine can sometimes be discoloured by the dyes used in intravenous x-ray examination, or by the eating of beetroot.

Uraemia

Metabolic wastes accumulate in the blood. Urea, creatinine and uric acid levels are elevated. In acute failure and anuria, the levels rise rapidly. In chronic kidney disease, even though there may be polyuria, the blood urea progressively rises.

Fluid, electrolyte and pH imbalances

Generalized *oedema* may be one of the early symptoms of renal insufficiency and usually becomes apparent first around the eyes. It may be due to decreased glomerular filtration and the retention of water and sodium, or to an abnormal permeability of the glomeruli to plasma proteins, especially serum albumin. The latter defect is associated with a condition known as nephrosis that occurs more often in children. The loss of plasma protein causes a decrease in the colloidal osmotic pressure of the blood, and an excess of water remains in the interstitial spaces. The urine is high in albumin, and the plasma protein is abnormally low.

In some instances of chronic renal failure due to impaired tubular function, the excessive volume of urine excreted (polyuria) may lead to *dehydration* unless there is a corresponding increase in the water intake.

Deficiencies or excesses of electrolytes may occur, depending on the nature of the renal disturbance and the degree of tissue damage. Failure of impaired tubules to secrete potassium ions is a serious development in renal insufficiency. Abnormal concentrations of sodium and calcium as well as hyperkalaemia may also develop, and may seriously affect cardiac function and threaten the patient's life.

Failure of the kidneys' capacity to excrete hydrogen ions by the formation and excretion of acid sodium phosphate and ammonia results in their accumulation in the blood causing *acidosis* (see p. 109 Chapter 6).

Vital signs

An elevation of blood pressure occurs in most patients with renal insufficiency associated with parenchymal disease of the kidneys. It is attributed to an increase in the blood volume as a result of the retention of sodium and water or a decrease in the renal blood flow and consequent secretion of renin by the juxtaglomerular cells. The renin results in the formation of angiotensin II and III which cause vasoconstriction of the arterioles and increased aldosterone release.

The pulse may become weak because of heart failure which may result from hypertension, excessive fluid load or electrolyte imbalance. Of the electrolyte disturbances, hyperkalaemia (elevated serum potassium) is the most serious (see Chapter 6).

The patient may experience dyspnoea due to pulmonary oedema. Kussmaul's breathing (deep rapid respirations), characteristic of acidosis, may be manifested. In advanced renal failure, the breath has an ammoniacal or 'uraemic' odour.

Fever is associated with infection in the kidneys or secondary infection, such as pneumonia, that may develop readily if pulmonary oedema is present.

Gastrointestinal disturbances

The patient experiences anorexia and, in the later stages of renal dysfunction, nausea and vomiting. Diarrhoea may also be troublesome in the acute stage. Hiccups may develop in advanced failure, and the oral mucosa may become sore and ulcerated.

Headache and pain

Headache is an early complaint as a result of the hypertension and cerebral oedema. Pain and tenderness in the back between the lower ribs and iliac crest occur in acute kidney disease because of the stretching of the renal capsule.

Visual disturbances

The patient may complain of 'spots before his eyes' or blurred vision which are attributed to oedema of the optic papillae (papilloedema). Loss of vision may actually occur as a result of a retinal haemorrhage.

Neurological manifestations

Signs of both irritation and depression of the nervous system appear in renal failure. The patient becomes irritable, lethargic and drowsy. He may become disoriented and progress to a comatose state. Muscular twitching may be noticeable and, in advanced kidney disease, may be an indication of ensuing convulsions.

Skin changes

In progressive renal insufficiency, the skin may take on a yellowish-brown discoloration. Dryness and scaliness are common with chronic disease and polyuria. The patient may complain of pruritus, and excoriated lesions may appear from scratching. In advanced failure, urea frost may be manifested, formed by deposits of small white crystals of urea excreted by the sweat glands. The frost is usually first seen around the mouth.

Haematological changes

Most patients with prolonged renal disease show a reduction in the production of red blood cells, a shortened red cell survival time with a resultant anaemia. Normal kidneys, as well as the liver, contribute erythropoietin which stimulates erythropoiesis. In renal dysfunction, this activity may be decreased.

With uraemia, the patient develops a bleeding tendency; the platelets are defective and the bleeding time increases. Petechiae, purpura or bleeding from mucous membranes may be present.

MANIFESTATIONS OF POSTRENAL DISORDERS

Manifestations of impaired bladder function and urinary elimination include abnormal constituents in the urine and alterations in the patterns of urination, (retention, frequency and urinary incontinence). Alterations in voiding may be related to infection in the urinary tract, emotional stress, a neurological disorder, bladder calculi, obstructive disease of the bladder or urethra and rarely, chemicals excreted in the urine.

Abnormal constituents in urine

Blood, pus, microorganisms and mucus may be present in the urine as a result of inflammation, tissue necrosis or a malignancy in the lower urinary tract. The urine may be cloudy or blood-coloured and have an ammoniacal odour.

Alteration in patterns of urinary elimination

Symptomatic changes in voiding include *frequency, urgency, dysuria, residual urine, alterations in the urinary stream, retention* and *incontinence*.

Frequency, urgency and dysuria. Irritation of the bladder or urethral mucosa may give rise to an abnormally frequent desire to void, urgency and painful micturition. The irritation is most frequently associated with infection in the lower urinary tract and less often with bladder calculi or chemicals excreted in the urine. The frequency of voiding may also be increased by nervous apprehension, the taking of a diuretic or increased fluids but is not considered abnormal. Frequency due to a urological disturbance is generally accompanied by an urgency which implies that there is an intense desire to void immediately. The normal voluntary control to retain the urine cannot be maintained, and some urine may escape before the patient can reach the toilet or use a bedpan.

When voiding is accompanied by pain or a burning, smarting sensation, the exact location and the time at which the discomfort occurs in relation to the flow of urine should be determined; that is, the patient must determine whether it is before, during or after the passage of urine that the pain occurs. This information may be helpful to the doctor in locating the problem. *Strangury* is a term used occasionally when the dysuria is unusually severe and there is increasing frequency of decreasing amounts of urine.

Residual urine. Micturition may not completely empty the bladder, leaving a residue of urine. This problem is diagnosed, and the amount determined, by catheterizing the patient immediately after he has voided. Residual urine is usually the result of an obstruction to the bladder outlet and causes a stagnation that predisposes to bladder and kidney infection and calculus formation.

Alterations in the urinary stream. The patient may have difficulty in initiating the urinary flow. This symptom of hesitancy is usually due to some obstruction in the bladder-urethral orifice or the urethra. Pressure within the bladder must be increased beyond the normal to force the urine past the obstructing lesion. This is most often seen in males as a result of prostatic hyperplasia but may also occur with malignancy or constrictions resulting from scarring and fibrosis. The inability to maintain a continuous stream and dribbling may develop as the lesion encroaches further upon the outflow passage.

Intermittent abrupt cessation of the urinary stream during voiding may occur if the bladder-urethral orifice is suddenly occluded by a calculus or a portion of a papillary tumour near the orifice. This may also occur as a result of fatigue of the detrusor muscle. Because of resistance to the urinary outflow, the muscle tires before the bladder is empty; after a few moments, it contracts again and voiding is resumed.

Retention of urine. The inability of a patient to void is a relatively common problem. It may be due to obstructive disease of the bladder or urethra, but occurs frequently after surgery, in acute illness and neurogenic disease, and as a complication after childbirth. The resulting distension of the bladder and stasis of urine predispose to the development of ureteric back pressure, reflux of urine into the ureters, and infection of the bladder and kidneys. The reaction of the bladder to progressive obstruction of the outflow is hypertrophy of the detrusor muscle. Diverticulae may develop; these are saccular protrusions of the mucosa between the muscle fibres. The sacs fill with urine which becomes stagnant and readily infected. Calculi may also form within the diverticula.

Retention of urine is suspected if the patient has had a normal fluid intake and has not voided within a period of 8–10 hours or if there is distension of the lower part of the abdomen. A distended bladder may also be present with frequent voiding of small amounts (30–50 ml), which is termed *retention with overflow.* The patient may experience a constant desire to void but efforts to do so are ineffective.

Urinary incontinence. The involuntary passage of urine is fairly common and is generally viewed as a social and hygienic problem; responses to it vary considerably from one person to another.

It may be related to: degenerative tissue changes, as seen in the elderly; neurological disease or injury which results in loss of bladder sensation or interruption of innervation to the detrusor muscle and sphincters; loss of cerebral awareness that may occur in any acute illness and in shock; relaxation of the pelvic floor muscles; infection or irritation of the bladder; or a congenital anomaly (e.g. hypospadias).

Types of incontinence include the following.[5]

1 *Reflex* incontinence, in which the filling of the bladder initiates reflex emptying, as occurs in infancy.
2 *Stress* incontinence, which may occur with coughing, sneezing, laughing or anxiety. The external urethral sphincter is less competent and any increased intra-abdominal pressure incurs the escape of urine.
3 *Urge* incontinence, associated with a strong desire to void, instability of the detrusor muscle or hypersensitivity of the bladder which interferes with normal capacity of the bladder.
4 *Overflow* incontinence, which occurs with urinary retention. Urinary retention causes the pressure within the bladder to exceed the pressure exerted by the urethral sphincters. A small amount (25–50 ml) of urine is eliminated at frequent intervals. It may be associated with urethral obstruction (e.g. prostatic hypertrophy), faecal impaction or impaired bladder innervation (e.g. neurological lesion).

---

[5] Mandelstram (1986), pp. 30–32.

5 *Enuresis* usually implies nocturnal urinary incontinence or bed-wetting. It most often occurs in children but may continue into adulthood in a few instances. The cause may be slow development of the child, or it may be associated with behavioural or emotional problems.

6 *Dribbling* or continuous urinary incontinence in conscious, alert persons usually results from damage to or degeneration of the urethral sphincter. Unawareness of dribbling is usually associated with a neurological condition.

7 *Post-micturition* dribbling causes soiling of clothing which is embarrassing for the person and those around him. It is more common in men of all age groups and may develop following urinary infection, an invasive procedure of the urinary tract or prostatectomy.

Identification of patient problems

Altered patterns of urinary elimination may include changes in volume, frequency and sensation (Table 21.2). The most common changes in patterns of urinary elimination are incontinence and retention. These two types of urinary disturbances are discussed separately below (see Tables 21.3 and 21.6). Disorders of the renal system produce disturbances in the formation of urine. Nursing diagnoses and intervention related to alterations in fluid volume, electrolyte and acid–base imbalances are discussed in Chapter 6. Further discussion is found later with nursing intervention related to patients with impaired renal function.

Table 21.2 Alterations in pattern of urinary elimination.

Problem	Causative factors	Signs and symptoms
Change in pattern of urinary elimination	Urinary tract infection Bladder calculi Emotional stress Neurological disorders Disorders of urine formation	Alteration in urine volume: Anuria—less than 250 ml in 24 hours Oliguria—less than 500 ml in 24 hours Polyuria—over 2500 ml in 24 hours Alteration in time, frequency and sensation Nocturia Frequency Urgency Dysuria Altered urinary stream Retention Incontinence

1. ALTERATION IN THE PATTERN OF URINARY ELIMINATION

Alteration of urinary elimination related to infection, bladder calculi, emotional stress, neurological disorders or disorders of urine formation is discussed below.

The *goal* is to establish and maintain a personally and socially acceptable pattern of urinary elimination.

Nursing intervention

Assessment. Assessment of the individual with alteration in the pattern of urinary elimination consists of taking a detailed history (as described earlier in this chapter). Alterations in urine volume may be caused by disorders of urine formation and cannot be altered by independent nursing intervention: medical diagnosis and treatment are essential. Nursing assessment of the patient's life-style and how the impairment is affecting the patient and his daily living is necessary to assist the patient to adjust to the problem and manage the prescribed treatment. A frequency–volume chart of the patient's urinary elimination and recording of fluid intake over several days are valuable in assessment.

Nursing intervention will be influenced by the cause of the disturbance. Factors to consider include the following:

Fluid intake. Adjustment of the patient's fluid intake may be necessary. Fluids are increased if the patient has oliguria or anuria with signs of dehydration (in the absence of heart failure or other contradictory factors) and for the patient with a urinary tract infection and dysuria. Fluids may be restricted in patients with decreased urine volume due to renal disease or when generalized oedema is present. Excessive intake is avoided prior to bedtime for patients with nocturia, as are fluids with a diuretic effect such as tea, coffee and chocolate. It is important to record accurately the amount and time of fluid ingested and excreted.

General measures to promote a satisfactory pattern of elimination are discussed with the patient. These measures include:

1 Establishing and maintaining a schedule for micturation

2 Maintaining adequate fluid intake unless contraindicated

3 Increasing physical activity

4 Assuming usual sitting or standing position for voiding

5 Providing privacy and a relaxed, quiet environment

Personal hygiene. The patient is instructed to cleanse carefully the perineal region, wiping from the pubic area towards the rectum to decrease the risk of urinary tract infection.

Medications. Antibiotics or sulphonamide preparations may be prescribed for patients with urinary tract infections. Fluid intake should be at least 2500 ml per day to prevent crystal formation when sulphonamide preparations are being given.

Antispasmodic agents such as propantheline may be prescribed to decrease bladder tone when it is the cause of dysuria.

Expected outcomes
1 The patient's urine is approximately 1200 ml per day and is in proportion to the fluid intake.
2 The patient's frequency of micturition is approximately six times daily.
3 The patient is able to voluntarily initiate voiding.
4 Micturition occurs without discomfort.
5 The patient's perineal skin is clean and intact.

INCONTINENCE OF URINE

Incontinence may be related to urethral sphincter incompetence, detrusor muscle instability, urine retention with overflow, fistulae, congenital anomalies or functional factors (see Table 21.3).

The *goal* is to control urination so that it occurs in an appropriate place and at an appropriate time.

Table 21.3 Alteration in pattern of urinary elimination—incontinence.

Problem	Causative factors	Signs and symptoms
Incontinence	Urethral sphincter incompetence Detrusor muscle instability Impaired neurological control of micturition Pelvic floor disorders Congenital anomalies of urinary system Loss of cerebral awareness Urinary tract infection	Involuntary passage of urine

Nursing intervention

Assessment. A detailed history is taken, as outlined earlier in this chapter, and urine examinations and documentation of voiding patterns are carried out. Medical urodynamic investigations may also be performed. It is necessary to identify the type of incontinence experienced by the patient, the duration and severity of the disorder and any relevant precipitating factors so that management of the incontinence can be planned. The person's 24-hour fluid intake is determined. The skin in the perineal area is examined for excoriation. The patient's

responses and feelings about the incontinence are explored as well as its effects on the patient's lifestyle.

Table 21.4 lists the basic skills required by an individual to achieve control of micturition. The nurse and patient collectively identify which of these basic skills the patient possesses, where difficulties are encountered in the course of daily activities, and what measures and techniques the patient uses to compensate for these deficits and their effectiveness.

Table 21.4 Basic skills required for socially oriented control of micturition.*

The ability to initiate micturition voluntarily at an appropriate time
The ability to delay, temporarily, the onset of micturition
Perception of the urge to urinate well in advance of reflex voiding
Awareness of socially acceptable places and/or circumstances to urinate
The ability to communicate needs and interpret oral directions and written signs to get necessary assistance or locate the toilet
The physical mobility and manual dexterity to reach the toilet, to assume and maintain body posture during micturition, adjust clothing, deal with doors, locks, flushing systems, seats and washing facilities

* Mandelstram (1986), p. 148

Analysis of medical and nursing assessments may demonstrate the need for further evaluation by other health professionals such as the occupational therapist and speech therapist. The occupational therapist will evaluate the home environment and toilet facilities in relation to the patient's mobility, dexterity and awareness. Difficulties manipulating clothing are also identified. The speech therapist will assess communication skills and recommend means by which the patient can communicate needs. The role of nursing staff and relatives in contributing to the patient's incontinence is also assessed, especially in the institutionalized, elderly and the disabled. Assistance to allow a schedule of regular voiding may be lacking, resulting in incontinence. Staff and family attitudes and relationships with the patient can be changed by helping them define expectations, set goals and develop strategies for dealing with the individual problem.

Management of incontinence. In some instances, the doctor can treat the cause directly and alleviate the disorder. In other cases, a multidisciplinary approach is required, using a variety of techniques to control the symptoms and help the individual to adjust and acquire socially and personally acceptable means to control the problem (see Table 21.5).

General measures directed to the alleviation of contributing factors include:
1 Weight reduction if the person is overweight
2 Maintaining a fluid intake of at least 2000 ml per day

3 Decreasing fluid intake if it has been excessive

4 Review of medication for possible contributing factors and adjustment of these medications if necessary

5 Adjustment of any diuretic therapy so that the action of the drugs occurs during the day

6 Decrease in alcohol intake

7 Institution of measures to suppress a chronic cough

8 Treatment of any underlying urinary tract infections

9 Increase in daily physical activity

10 Prevention or treatment of constipation

Table 21.5 Management of urinary incontinence.

To achieve control of micturition, the following skills are necessary:

Identify and alleviate contributing factors

Establish and maintain adequate fluid intake (2000+ ml per day)

Establish and follow a voiding schedule

Assume usual sitting or standing posture for voiding

Maintain desired physical activity

Practise pelvic floor exercises

Apply manual pressure over bladder to initiate voiding (Crede's manoeuvre)

Alter physical environment to provide ready access to toileting facilities

Adapt clothing

Maintain good hygiene; keep skin clean, dry and free of odours

Use protective measures and external devices when necessary

Intermittent catheterization

Medication is also used in the control of incontinence. Many drugs are available which influence the activity of the detrusor muscle and urethral sphincter but their use is limited because of the other generalized effects of these drugs and the unpleasant side-effects produced. Drugs which may be prescribed include:

- Cholinergic agents such as bethanechol chloride which stimulates detrusor contractions. These agents are used when the bladder is atonic or hypotonic.
- Anticholinergic agents which include propantheline (Pro-Banthine), belladona, and oxybutynin, decrease smooth muscle activity of a hypertonic bladder and may be used to treat urge incontinence related to neurogenic impairment.
- Alpha adrenergic agents such as adrenaline, phenylpropanolamine and imipramine (Tofranil) may be used to treat stress incontinence as they increase urethral sphincter resistance.
- Alpha adrenergic blocking agents e.g. phenoxybenzamine decrease urethral sphincter resistance in patients with overflow incontinence.
- Beta adrenergic blocking agents [e.g. propranolol (Inderal)] increase sphincter resistance and may be used to treat stress incontinence.

Physical exercises (pelvic floor exercises, Kegel exercises) to increase the tone of muscles involved in micturition may be taught to control stress incontinence in women. The patient sits with the feet on the floor and knees apart and is instructed to tighten the perineal muscles, as if stopping the flow of urine, and to hold the muscle contraction and then relax. This exercise is repeated several times every 2–4 hours throughout the day. During voiding, the patient is instructed to stop and start the urinary stream by contracting perineal muscles. A feedback device may be used for patients who lack sensory input as it provides them with pressure readings, demonstrating the effectiveness of the muscle contractions.

A *bladder training programme* is developed whenever possible with the active participation of the patient and family. A detailed chart of urine frequency and volume, fluid intake, the times of fluid intake and voiding and the circumstances surrounding incidents of incontinence is kept for several days. From this information, the nurse and patient can develop a voiding schedule and a plan that considers the patient's needs and daily activities. Voiding normally occurs on arising in the morning, before or after meals and before retiring in the evening. The voiding schedule may begin by having the patient void every 1 or 2 hours, with the intervals increased gradually as control is acquired. The patient's level of awareness and perception of the urge to void influence the degree of personal control that can be expected. When a patient is confused and disoriented, it is necessary for others to prompt them to follow the schedule and to provide assistance in tasks such as getting to the toilet and manipulating clothing.

Fluid intake of at least 2000 ml daily is maintained throughout the programme and physical activity is increased.

Toilet facilities, a commode chair, bedpan or urinal should be within reach of the patient and privacy provided. An assessment of the home environment is done and recommendations made if necessary for modifications to the home or the purchase or loan of a commode chair or bedpan. A night light should be provided. Voiding should always take place in the usual sitting posture for females and standing posture for males, with the nurse or a relative providing the necessary assistance.

For patients with flaccid, hypotonic bladders, Crede's manoeuvre is taught. The hands are placed flat over the abdomen below the umbilicus. Manual pressure is exerted over the bladder to initiate flow of urine. Suprapubic tapping or stroking of the thighs may also be used to stimulate reflex voiding when incontinence is the result of neurogenic dysfunction.

Suggestions are provided for adapting clothing for the patient with impaired manual dexterity or the individual who has minimal time between the sensation or urge to void and the act of voiding. The patient may need instruction and practice with the manipulation of zippers, buttons or other aspects of clothing.

Various aids are used in the management of incontinence. Self-control of continence cannot be achieved for every patient. Some may continuously require protective measures. Others may require protective measures during assessment and treatment or during periods of illness. Many protective devices and aids are available and include the following:

- *Protective pants and pads.* Underpads may be used on bed linen or furniture or pads are available to be worn by the patient. Various types of waterproof pants and diapers are also available. Each type is designed to meet a specific need and the absorbancy of the various pads vary. The marsupial pants (Kanga pants) are designed with a waterproof pouch to hold the pad in place. Most products are available in a variety of sizes and styles and some are disposable while others are washable. Use and selection of pants and pads must be individualized and requires the patient's interest and cooperation. Protection of clothing allows the patient to dress in his usual style and participate in social functions. The use of pads or plastic or rubber pants for adults may be demeaning and serve to promote feelings of dependence and withdrawal if their use is not discussed and agreed with the patient.

- *External urinary drainage devices.* A condom with an attached drainage bag is useful for male patients. It may be worn only at night or during the day under clothing; care must be taken to select an appropriately sized condom. The penis is checked frequently for oedema, redness or excoriation.

- *Catheter.* Catheterization as a means of controlling incontinence is not considered until other alternatives have been tried. An indwelling catheter may be used in some instances to permit increased independence for the patient. Intermittent catheterization is preferred to an indwelling catheter; the patient or a relative is taught to perform the procedure; the risk of infection is reduced with intermittent catheterization as opposed to an indwelling catheter. It is performed on a regular schedule which is determined in a similar manner to the bladder training schedule.

- *Electrical devices.* Electrical stimulators are receiving moderate attention as a means of increasing the tone of pelvic muscles. They create continuous contraction of the pelvic muscles which is relieved by releasing the electrical stimulation to facilitate voiding when desired.

- *Occlusive devices* are not satisfactory for long-term use. Penile clamps and an inflatable pad which applies pressure against the perineum to close the penile urethra are available for men.

Occlusive devices for females are vaginal tampons and an inflatable vaginal balloon which elevate the bladder neck and apply pressure on the urethra through the vagina and may be useful for minor stress incontinence or during periods of physical activity.

- *Surgery.* Surgical intervention for incontinence is directed to the correction of anatomical defects that contribute to the incontinence (for example: correction of obstructions in the urinary tract, repair of a cystocele, or uterine prolapse, or prostatic hypertrophy).

    Artificial urethral sphincters can be implanted in men and women. Various types of devices are available but they generally consist of a cuff filled with fluid and a mechanism for diversion of the fluid when voiding is desired.

Expected outcomes
1 The patient is continent or incidents of incontinence are less frequent
2 The patient and/or family discuss a plan for continuous management of incontinence
3 The patient and/or family are aware of what aids and resources are needed and how they can be obtained
4 The patient is able to mix socially with confidence
5 The skin in the perineal area is clean and intact
6 The odour of urine is absent

RETENTION OF URINE

Retention may be related to obstructive disease of the bladder or urethra, surgical intervention, or neurogenic diseases (see Table 21.6).

The *goal* is to establish and maintain a flow of urine from the bladder.

Nursing intervention

Assessment. The time of last voiding, the volume of fluid intake and the volume of urinary output are determined. Fluid loss by channels other than

Table 21.6 Alteration in pattern of urinary elimination—retention.

Problem	Causative factors	Signs and symptoms
Retention	Obstructive disease of the bladder or urethra Surgical intervention Neurological disease Embarrassment or fear	Frequent voiding of small amounts Absence of voiding in 8–10 hours with adequate fluid intake Bladder distension Urgency and persistent desire to void Restlessness Pain and discomfort in the region of the bladder and/or kidney

urinary is also considered. The patient's lower abdomen is examined for distension of the bladder. The patient may complain of low abdominal pain or the distress of feeling the need to void but being unable to initiate voiding.

Promotion of spontaneous voiding. Nursing measures used to induce voiding include increasing the fluid intake (unless contraindicated), providing privacy, pouring of warm water over the perineum, letting the patient hear running water, stroking of the inner portions of the thighs, and, unless contraindicated, assisting the patient to assume the normal position for voiding. Female patients may be supported in the sitting position in bed or may be allowed to use a commode at the bedside; male patients may be allowed to stand beside the bed. A warm bath may prove effective with some patients.

Urinary retention in a postoperative patient may result from incisional pain and discomfort. Analgesics are administered prior to offering the patient a bedpan or urinal or assisting them to a sitting position, commode chair or to the bathroom. Bethanechol chloride or neostigmine (Prostigmin), which are parasympathomimetic agents, may be prescribed to stimulate voiding. These drugs increase the tone of the detrusor muscle stimulating bladder contractions.

Urethral catheterization.   Emptying of the bladder by the insertion of a catheter into the urethra and bladder may be done on an intermittent basis using a straight French catheter, or a retention catheter (Foley) may be inserted to provide continuous drainage of urine. Urinary catheterization may be performed for reasons other than urinary retention; it may be necessary to assess urinary output accurately in a critically ill patient, to promote healing following surgery in the perineal region, to administer medications directly into the bladder or to measure the volume of residual urine remaining in the bladder following micturition.

The procedure and the purpose for it are explained to the patient and privacy is provided throughout the procedure. Precautions are taken to avoid the introduction of organisms and trauma of the mucosa; sterile gloves are worn, and strict aseptic technique is observed throughout the procedure. The catheter is handled with great care in order to minimize trauma. If the retention has been acute and severe, not more than 1000–1200 ml of urine are removed initially. The sudden, complete emptying of an overdistended bladder may result in an atonic bladder wall. The sudden release of pressure on the blood vessels in the bladder region causes a sudden inflow of blood and sometimes capillary bleeding may occur. Rarely, the patient may experience faintness. The catheter is clamped after 1000–1500 ml are removed and is then opened hourly to drain off 200–300 ml until the bladder is empty. It may be necessary to drain larger quantities if the patient is severely polyuric.

Management of an indwelling urethral catheter. A closed drainage system is used to maintain a continuous urinary flow and decrease the potential for the entry of organisms into the system. The catheter is attached to tubing and a collecting bag with a drainage valve or to a leg bag which contains a flutter valve to prevent backflow of urine into the bladder. The leg bag or regular drainage bag is kept below the level of the bladder and attached to a hanger or hook on the side of the patient's bed or chair. A leg bag is used for the patient who is mobile since it is less cumbersome and can be worn under clothing. The drainage system should not be disconnected unnecessarily.

The drainage system is assessed frequently for patency; kinks in the tubing and tension on the catheter and tubing are avoided. In the female patient, the catheter is taped to the inner thigh; in the male patient the catheter is taped laterally to the upper thigh or abdomen to prevent pressure on the penile-scrotal angle. The latter is an important preventive measure since erosion of tissue at the penile-scrotal angle may develop if tension is applied to the catheter and the resulting fistula can only be corrected by plastic surgery.

Indwelling urethral catheters are changed at varying intervals and may be left in place for 4–6 weeks depending on the type of material used in the catheter; information is usually available on the catheter package. Collecting tubing and drainage bags are changed every 2–7 days. Routine care includes washing the urinary meatus and perineum with soap, water and a clean cloth twice daily. Urethral catheters are inconvenient for the patient, but should not interfere with the performance of usual daily activities. Showers or baths are generally permitted.

Patient teaching.   Patients requiring retention catheters during periods of hospitalization require information about the purpose of the catheter and general principles of care and the importance of preventing infections. Patients are taught to keep the drainage bag below the level of the bladder, to prevent tension on the catheter and to maintain a closed system.

The patient requiring intermittent or continuous catheterization at home requires detailed instruction about the supply and care of equipment, and the performance of the procedure if necessary. Horsley, in reviewing the current literature on catheterization procedures, concludes that the use of clean intermittent catheterizations promotes improvement in urinary incontinence, urinary infections, renal function and bladder emptying and this is therefore the procedure of choice.[6] Frequency of catheterization is determined by the volume of urine.[7] Referrals are made to the district nurse to assist the patient and family in managing the catheter. At home, the drainage tubing and bag are cleaned with soap and water and soaked in sodium hydrochloride solution until it is next used (i.e. the night bag soaks during the day). The catheter is cleaned, stored dry in a clean polythene bag and used for 24 hours. Two catheters are in use for one week, one soaking for 24 hours while the other is in use. Bags and catheters are discarded and replaced after 7 days. Good medical asepsis is emphasized.

Management of the patient following removal of the catheter. An indwelling catheter is removed as soon as possible to lessen the trauma to urethral sphincters and the loss of muscle tone that ensues. After the catheter is removed, the patient is encouraged to pass urine hourly for a few hours and the time and amount of each voiding are recorded as well as the fluid intake. The patient is assessed for any discomfort, dribbling of urine due to dilatation of the sphincter by the catheter, sensation of urgency or stress incontinence. If the patient is unable to void in 6–8 hours and has had an adequate fluid intake, intermittent catheterization may be necessary. If only small amounts of urine are voided, catheterization may be done to measure the amount of residual urine.

Suprapubic catheterization. The insertion of a catheter into the bladder through the suprapubic area is a surgical procedure and requires local or general anaesthetic. Nursing care of the patient with a suprapubic catheter and closed drainage system is similar to that for the patient with an indwelling urethral catheter. The suprapubic catheter is sutured in place and is then taped to the abdomen to prevent tension on the catheter. The exit site is cared for as a surgical incision. Stomahesive is used to protect the skin around the insertion site or a transparent, sealed dressing (e.g. Op-Site) is used.

Expected outcomes
The patient:
1 Voids spontaneously.
2 Maintains a urine flow through a catheter.
3 Is free of urinary infection.
4 Understands the purpose and general management of retention catheters.
5 Is confident about home-care and self-management.

---

[6] Horsley, Crane & Reynolds (1982), p. 6
[7] Horsley, Crane & Reynolds (1982), p. 6.

Impaired Renal Function

Renal dysfunction may be due to a primary disease within the kidneys or may be secondary to a disorder elsewhere in the body. The body is dependent on the kidneys for the elimination of metabolic wastes and the maintenance of homeostasis. When kidney function is impaired, dysfunction of extrarenal systems ultimately develops. Similarly, primary dysfunction in other systems may readily affect renal function.

RENAL FAILURE

When the kidneys are unable to excrete metabolic wastes and perform their role in fluid, electrolyte and acid–base balance, renal failure exists. Homeostasis of the internal environment is no longer maintained. The retention of the waste and excess products normally excreted in the urine may be referred to as *uraemia*. The latter is not a disease but rather a syndrome or complex of symptoms reflecting failure of the kidneys to carry out their role in regulation of the fluid volume, acid–base and electrolyte balances and excretion of metabolic wastes. Renal production of renin, erythropoieten and vitamin D_3 is also disturbed. With failure of fluid volume regulation the patient becomes either oedematous or dehydrated and the acid–base imbalance leads to metabolic acidosis. Electrolyte imbalances occur and an accumulation of nitrogenous wastes produces elevated blood levels of non-protein nitrogenous substances such as urea, creatinine and uric acid. The disturbance in the secretion of hormones leads to alterations in blood pressure, erythrocyte production and calcium absorption by bone tissue. As renal efficiency diminishes, symptoms develop reflecting impairment of function in other body systems. Fig. 21.8 illustrates the systemic effects of renal failure. Renal failure may be acute or chronic.

Acute renal failure

Acute renal failure is a sudden, severe interruption of kidney function that in most instances is a complication of another disorder and is reversible.

CAUSES

The primary or initiating causes of acute renal failure are many, but the basic mechanisms causing the failure in most instances are tubular necrosis due to inadequate tissue perfusion and hypoxia, or acute inflammation of glomeruli. Causes may be classified as prerenal, intrarenal or postrenal.
    Prerenal refers to extrarenal disorders *which cause inadequate renal perfusion* as a result of a decrease in vascular volume or cardiac output or obstruction of a renal artery. The renal insufficiency is secondary to a

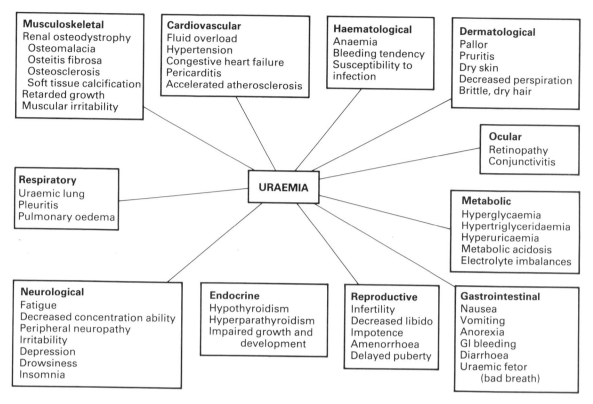

Fig. 21.8 Systemic effects of uraemia. (Lewis, 1981.)

condition which reduces the blood supply to the kidneys. The condition may be haemorrhage, dehydration, shock, cardiac failure, burns or renal artery occlusion by thrombosis or an abdominal mass.

Intrarenal refers to disorders in which there is actual renal tissue irritation and destruction which impairs renal functions; for example, acute inflammation of the glomeruli (glomerulonephritis), acute tubular necrosis and acute inflammation of the kidney tissue and renal pelvis (pyelonephritis). The primary renal tissue damage may be induced by a chemical or biological product or an infectious agent.

Renal failure may be the result of glomerulonephritis which is secondary to an *extrarenal Streptococcus haemolyticus* infection. The antigen complexes formed in response to the infection are trapped in the glomeruli and initiate the inflammatory process.

Nephrotoxic agents that are possible causes of a renal shutdown may be endogenous or exogenous in origin. Epithelial cells are destroyed; the tubular lumens are obliterated by swelling and oedema of the tissues as well as by casts formed from the sloughed cells. Examples of endogenous nephrotoxins are haemoglobin, released in haemolysis of erythrocytes following incompatible blood transfusion, and myoglobin, released from muscle cells in crushing injuries. The molecules of haemoglobin pass through the glomeruli and become concen-

trated in the tubules, obstructing the flow of filtrate. Similarly, the tubular necrosis that follows a crushing injury is attributed to the myoglobin accumulating in the tubules and causing an obstruction, as well as to shock. The individual who has been 'pinned down under a weight' for a period of time or who has been subjected to limb ischaemia may appear in satisfactory condition when released, but should be put to bed under close observation. He is likely to develop severe shock, acute renal failure and gross oedema of the injured part hours later.

Exogenous nephrotoxins may be poisonous chemicals or drugs. Poisons, which may be taken accidentally or with suicidal intent, include carbon tetrachloride, ethylene glycol (a constituent of antifreeze), bichloride of mercury, chloroform and lead. Common pharmaceuticals which may prove toxic and damaging to the tubules include sulphonamide preparations (e.g. sulphadiazine), salicylates, phenacetin, paracetamol, vancomycin, amphotericin B, cyclosporin, non-steroidal antiinflammatory agents, a cephalosporin and frusemide combination, and aminoglycoside antibiotics (kanamycin, gentamicin, tobramycin, etc.). Interstitial nephritis may be produced by methicillin and some analgesics. Obstructive disorders may result from cytotoxic drugs.

Postrenal causes of acute renal failure are conditions

which result in an obstruction to the outflow of urine. Calculi, a neoplasm or prostatic hypertrophy may obstruct collecting tubules, the pelvis, a ureter or the bladder; the accumulation of fluid within the kidney compresses blood vessels and nephrons, seriously reducing kidney function.

SIGNS AND SYMPTOMS

Patients in acute renal failure fall into two distinct categories: those who are oliguric, passing less than 400 ml of urine per day and those who are never oliguric but who continue to pass 1000–1500 ml of dilute urine per day. The effects of a decreased urinary output are retention of an excess of certain biochemical substances in the blood and a decrease in the pH of body fluids. Blood urea and serum creatinine, potassium and sodium chloride concentrations are elevated; the pH is decreased and hydrogen carbonate, haematocrit and haemoglobin levels are below normal.

The first sign of acute renal failure may be oliguria which may progress rapidly to anuria. The oliguric phase may last for 7–10 days and the urine contains blood and protein. An output of less than 30 ml per hour is an indication for concern and is reported immediately. If oliguria and anuria persists for a few days, manifestations of water retention and disturbances of blood chemistry are likely to develop. Sodium and water retention cause oedema and, unless the fluid intake is controlled, overhydration may lead to cardiac failure and pulmonary oedema. The serum sodium and chloride levels may not appear abnormal because of the dilution by the retained fluid.

The elevation in serum potassium becomes a serious threat to cardiac muscle. In addition to the fact that potassium is not being eliminated by the kidneys, haemolysis and the breakdown of tissue cells by the primary condition (trauma, burns, sepsis, etc.) increase the concentration of potassium ions in the blood. Metabolic acidosis which also develops in acute renal failure promotes the movement of potassium out of the cells. Hyperkalaemia may be manifested by depression of tendon reflexes, numbness, muscular weakness, flaccid paralysis and decreased respiratory rate and volume. Cardiac arthythmias are common, and cardiac arrest may occur.[8]

The rate of the accumulation of nitrogenous wastes (urea and creatinine) in the blood varies with the cause of the renal insufficiency. If there is rapid catabolism, as in infection, fever, and pathological destruction of tissue, the blood concentration of nitrogenous wastes may rise more quickly. The onset of the uraemic state is usually marked by mental changes, nausea and vomiting, and probably hiccups. The patient may complain of pruritus.

Metabolic acidosis develops because the hydrogen ions produced in metabolism are not being eliminated by the renal tubules. Respirations are increased in rate and depth, and an acidotic odour of the breath becomes noticeable.

Leucocytosis may be present; anaemia is likely to develop fairly quickly, and is manifested by a decrease in the haematocrit and haemoglobin. If the renal failure persists, the patient may develop a bleeding tendency. Ulcerated areas in the mouth are common and may bleed. Vomit and stools may contain blood, and petechiae and ecchymoses may appear. As the condition worsens, disseminated intravascular coagulation (DIC) may develop (see p. 286).

The patient becomes drowsy and may progress to a comatose state. Muscle twitching and convulsions may also develop.

The outcome in acute renal failure is unpredictable. Many patients do recover; tubular healing and repair occur within 2–6 weeks and there is no serious functional impairment. Those who do not recover do not necessarily die from renal failure alone; frequently, the cause of death is the seriousness of the underlying cause or the combination of several associated disorders and complications. The patient with renal insufficiency is very susceptible to infection, especially pulmonary. Fluid in the alveoli (pulmonary oedema) and the retention of secretions due to inability to cough because of weakness predispose to pneumonia. Early recognition of renal insufficiency and prompt treatment are important. The nurse may play an important role in early recognition by being familiar with the possible causes of renal failure and by being alert to any significant decrease in a patient's urinary output.

Diuretic phase

If the renal failure is reversible, the patient experiences a period of diuresis following the oliguric period; large volumes of urine are excreted. The tubules are unable to concentrate urine and serum creatinine and blood urea remain elevated. A diuretic phase may not be observed if the patient has been treated by dialysis.

Recovery phase

Improvement in renal function continues over 3–12 months. As it returns, the urine becomes more concentrated but some residual impairment often remains.

COMPLICATIONS

Complications which commonly develop in renal failure include hyperkalaemia, cardiac insufficiency, convulsions and coma.

---

[8] In hyperkalaemia, the electrocardiogram shows a prolonged QRS complex and increased amplitude and peaking of T waves.

Hyperkalaemia. Since potassium is liberated from the cells in tissue breakdown and cannot be eliminated in renal failure, the extracellular concentration may reach toxic levels. Cardiac function becomes impaired, and failure or sudden cardiac arrest may occur. The nurse is alert for possible clinical symptoms of potassium intoxication which include generalized muscular weakness, shallow respirations, complaints of tingling sensation or numbness in the limbs and around the mouth, a slow irregular pulse and a fall in blood pressure.

As well as ensuring that no potassium is ingested in fluid or food, preventive measures may include the oral or rectal administration of a cation exchange resin, such as calcium resonium. The resin preparation combines with the potassium in the gastrointestinal secretions, preventing its absorption. Care must be taken to give a stool softener with it, as constipation and occasionally bowel obstruction are complications. Potassium loss via the gastrointestinal tract is only effective if a regular and effective bowel habit is established. As cited earlier, if hyperkalaemia develops, an intravenous infusion of glucose with a dose of human soluble insulin may be given. This is to promote the deposition of the glucose as glycogen, a process which utilizes potassium. A solution of sodium bicarbonate or sodium lactate and probably calcium may be administered to counteract the effect of the excess potassium on the heart. An antiarrhythmic drug may also be prescribed. The only permanent and effective way for potassium to be removed from the body is by dialysis.

Cardiac insufficiency. Heart failure may occur as a result of the retention of sodium and water. The pulse may become weak and pulmonary oedema may develop, causing dyspnoea and moist respirations. If hypertension is associated with the renal failure, it may also be a factor in heart failure. Urgent fluid removal by ultrafiltration is required to ensure the safety of the patient. Only when this facility is not available should prescription of a vasodilating agent such as isosorbide dinitrate or reduction of intravascular volume by venesection be considered as a temporary measure until the patient can be transferred urgently to a dialysis unit.

Convulsions. Convulsions may occur and are usually preceded by muscular twitching, persisting severe headache, severe hypertension, increasing oedema and rising blood urea level. Padded sides are placed on the bed to prevent self-injury of the patient. During a seizure only sufficient restraint is used to protect the patient from injury. Benzodiazepines and diazepam (Valium) may be prescribed to control the seizures.

Coma. Increasing drowsiness may indicate increasing uraemia and may progress to disorientation and coma. The delirious patient requires constant attendance, and a sedative such as diazepam (Valium) may be prescribed. If the patient becomes comatose, the care appropriate for any unconscious patient is applicable (see Chapter 10). At this stage an urgent decision needs to be made either to refer the patient for dialysis or to institute palliative care.

MANAGEMENT

Medical management of acute renal failure is aimed at regulating fluid and electrolyte balance, controlling nitrogen imbalance, maintenance of nutrition and treatment of the underlying cause. Dialysis is initiated before the uraemic state develops to re-establish a normal homeostatic environment for tissue repair and restoration of renal function. Haemodialysis is considered preferable for the patient with acute renal failure. (See discussion of haemodialysis pp. 717–722 and peritoneal dialysis pp. 714–717). Daily dialysis is usually required but the frequency will vary according to the rate of catabolism and the fluid balance. Excess fluid may be removed by haemofiltration using continuous, slow ultrafiltration. The use of ultrafiltration filters (e.g. the Amicon or Gambro filter) permits continuous fluid removal from the patient's intravascular content without the side-effects of sudden fluid loss, and without altering serum osmolality as occurs with diffusion dialysis. Ultrafiltration can be monitored by the nursing staff in an intensive care unit and has the advantage of allowing intravenous fluids and medications to be given to treat the cause of the patient's acute renal failure while controlling the fluid balance.

Conservative treatment includes the administration of diuretics to increase urine output. Frusemide (Lasix) may be given intravenously. If the urinary output is not satisfactory after 1 or 2 doses, the drug is not usually repeated. Fluid intake is restricted to 500 ml plus the previous day's output. The dietary protein should not be limited to decrease the production of nitrogenous wastes but maintained to provide adequate resources for tissue repair and the patient should be dialysed as often as necessary to keep nitrogenous wastes at an acceptable level. This will often mean daily dialysis. The calorie intake is maintained by the administration of glucose. The electrolyte balance is closely monitored, sodium and potassium are restricted and dialysis is used to lower the potassium level.

NURSING PROCESS

Identification of patient problems
Table 21.7 lists actual and potential problems and patient goals for care relevant to most patients with acute renal failure.

Nursing intervention

Assessment. The patient with acute renal failure is

Table 21.7 Actual and potential problems of the patient with acute renal failure.

Problem	Contributing factors	Goals
1 Alteration in fluid volume: excess	Inability of the kidneys to excrete water	To achieve fluid balance
2 Alteration in nutritional status and needs: changes related to body requirements and retention of metabolic wastes	Inability of the kidneys to excrete catabolic nitrogenous wastes and excess electrolytes	To achieve and maintain adequate nutrition and electrolyte balance
3 Potential impairment of oral mucosa and skin integrity	Oedema and increased excretion of waste through the skin	To maintain the integrity of the skin and oral mucosa
4 Potential for infection	Effect of uraemia on the constituents of the blood	To prevent infection and bleeding
5 Anxiety	Sudden onset of illness, lack of knowledge and loss of control of events	To decrease anxiety
6 Potential for injury	Altered level of awareness	To prevent injury
7 Alteration in fluid volume: deficit	Fluid loss due to diuresis or diuretic therapy	To maintain fluid and electrolyte balance
8 Lack of knowledge about plans for discharge and follow-up care	Inadequate knowledge and/or misinformation	To develop plans for home management and follow-up care

seriously ill and requires constant nursing care and *close observation* for changes which may occur suddenly. An accurate record of the *fluid intake and output* is essential. As cited previously, an output of less than 30 ml hourly or 500 ml daily is ominous. Any evident sweating as well as vomiting is recorded and taken into consideration when estimating the volume of fluid the patient should be given.

The *pulse*, *respirations* and *blood pressure* are checked frequently. Cardiac function may be impaired by the retention of potassium and fluid or by hypertension which may accompany renal parenchymal disease. Blood tests are carried out at least daily to detect changes in the serum potassium level (hyperkalaemia). Continuous electrocardiographic monitoring may be established if the plasma potassium remains elevated.

Any oedema is noted, and the patient's weight is recorded daily. A weight loss each day of approximately 0.2–0.3 kg as a result of catabolism and the restricted intake is considered excessive. No loss or a gain usually indicates fluid retention. Breathing is observed for signs of developing pulmonary oedema, which may result from overhydration and cardiac failure. A noticeable increase in the volume and depth of respirations may point to acidosis.

The blood pressure is recorded at frequent regular intervals to provide information on the patient's progress. A progressive rise in excess of normal levels is reported to the doctor; it may point to increasing uraemia. The temperature is taken every 4 hours, even if normal, since a sudden elevation may occur and indicate complicating infection.

Muscular twitching, increasing drowsiness and disorientation are recorded, since they may be manifestations of uraemia, cerebral oedema and approaching convulsions and coma.

Frequent laboratory determinations of blood urea and serum creatinine and electrolytes are followed closely. The sodium and potassium levels are especially important in decisions relating to the types of solutions to be administered, and the patient's fluid balance and weight are used in determining the daily volume of fluid to be given.

The haematocrit and haemoglobin are noted. Patient responses to medications are carefully assessed. Administering a drug to a patient in renal failure requires knowledge of the metabolic and excretory course of the drug, that is, what happens to it within the body. Those drugs with which renal cells normally react or which are excreted by the kidneys are not given or, if used, are administered in smaller dosage than usually prescribed and levels monitored. Drugs containing potassium or sodium are not given.

Fluid volume excess. The daily fluid intake is limited to 500 ml plus an amount equal to the urinary output of the preceding 24 hours. The 500 ml replaces the obligatory loss through the skin and lungs. The fluid that may be given will depend on the laboratory findings. An explanation of the fluid restriction is made to the patient so he will understand why he may have only a limited amount distributed over 24 hours.

Nutrition. A minimum of 100–200 gm of potassium-free carbohydrate is given daily to reduce the amount of tissue protein and fat broken down for energy. Protein is not restricted to avoid a further rise in blood urea. Often patients initially do not tolerate large amounts of food and so are fed nasogastrically or intravenously until they have a desire to eat. If hyperkalaemia is present, 50 ml glucose 50% may be given intravenously with a dose of soluble insulin. This promotes the movement of potassium into the cells as well as providing calories.

Essential amino acids as well as hypertonic glucose may be provided by the administration of total parenteral nutrition (TPN) (see pp. 511–513). Adequate protein is necessary for synthesis of body tissues, enzymes and antibody production. The delivery of these nutrients requires the administration of a considerable volume of fluid, so parenteral administration of nutrients is used if the patient is treated by ultrafiltration or haemodialysis to remove the excess fluid and prevent overloading the heart.

Activity. Activity is not restricted but most patients are extremely ill and need help with every activity.

Skin and oral mucosa. In renal failure, the mouth requires special care. The tongue becomes coated, salivary excretion is reduced, and the mucosa and lips are dry and frequently encrusted. Ulcerative lesions may develop, and the patient may be distressed by the disagreeable taste frequently associated with uraemia. Sordes predisposes him to respiratory infection, local mouth infections and parotitis. Frequent cleansing of the mouth with hydrogen peroxide and rinsing with a mild antiseptic mouthwash are necessary, followed by a light application of mineral oil to which a few drops of lemon juice may be added. Petroleum jelly or cold cream is applied to the lips. The limited fluid intake and dry mouth are frequently a great source of distress to the patient. Resourcefulness on the part of the nurse may reduce the discomfort. Rinsing the mouth with ice-cold mouthwash or water is more acceptable than using lukewarm solutions. Occasional rinsing of the mouth with ice-cold fruit juice or ginger ale provides a change. Tart fruit or boiled sweets such as fresh pineapple or 'lemon drops' are helpful to stimulate secretions, reduce thirst and, at the same time, supply a little sugar.

The patient is bathed daily to remove the increased wastes that may be excreted in sweat and to provide comfort. Super-fatted soap is used in bathing and removed from the skin by thorough rinsing. His position is changed frequently, and pressure areas are protected by squares of sheepskin to prevent pressure sores.

Anxiety. Acute renal failure that is secondary to some serious disorder certainly heightens the patient's fear and anxiety. He requires an explanation of what is wrong and what is being done for him, as well as reassurance that someone will remain with him. Relatives are kept informed of the patient's progress and encouraged to visit the patient. They require support in understanding changes observed in the patient's behaviour and level of awareness.

Potential for injury. Cot-sides may be kept in position since the uraemic patient may become drowsy and disorientated. Uraemia frequently leads to convulsions and coma, but regular dialysis will prevent this.

Fluid volume deficit (diuretic phase). Improvement in renal function is manifested by a steady increase in the volume of urine. The latter may rise rapidly to as much as 6000–8000 ml in 24 hours. The diuresis is accompanied by marked losses of potassium, sodium and water because the tubules have not yet regained their ability to regulate the volume and composition of urine. Frequent serum electrolyte determinations continue, and necessary replacements are made either orally or intravenously. The fluid intake is increased to cover the volume lost. The nitrogenous waste concentration (BUN) decreases more slowly.

The patient is offered a soft diet and then a light diet. The nurse continues to record the intake and output, and renal concentration tests may be done to determine if there is some residual insufficiency due to tubular necrosis.

Patient education. Before being discharged from the hospital, the patient and family are advised that activity should be resumed gradually and that extra rest will be necessary for several weeks. Dietary instructions are given; the importance of avoiding infection is stressed, and suggestions are made as to protective measures to be used. The patient is given an outpatient appointment and is told that he will be expected to take with him a specimen of the urine voided on rising that morning. The prolonged convalescence frequently causes socioeconomic problems for the patient and family. The nurse may be able to assist by a referral to a socal worker.

Expected outcomes

1 The patient's weight is stable and within 2 kg of usual weight.
2 Fluid intake and output are balanced and within normal volumes.
3 Serum electrolyte concentrations, pH and osmolality are within the normal range.
4 Serum creatinine and blood urea nitrogen are within an acceptable range for the patient.
5 Urine electrolytes and osmolality are within the normal range.
6 Vital signs (blood pressure, pulse and respirations) are within the normal range for the patient.
7 Peripheral oedema is absent.
8 The patient understands his condition and is less anxious.
9 The patient is alert and oriented to time, place and person.
10 The patient's skin and oral mucosa are clean and intact.
11 The patient and family understand how to manage his convalescence.

Chronic renal failure

Chronic renal insufficiency is due to progressive disease of both kidneys. Irreversible damage to nephrons occurs which eventually leads to the retention of many waste and toxic products of metabolism, fluid and electrolyte imbalances, metabolic acidosis, anaemia, hypertension and decalcification of bone tissue (renal osteodystrophy).

CAUSES

The most frequent causes of progressive renal failure are the following:

Glomerulonephritis. This involves a variety of immunologically induced diseases which cause inflammation, fibrosis and destruction of glomeruli with tubular degeneration.

Polycystic kidney disease. Progressive enlargement of the cysts compresses functional renal parenchyma increasing renal insufficiency.

Nephrosclerosis. This is secondary to hypertension atherosclerosis and diabetes mellitus.

Other diseases which may cause chronic renal failure include chronic pyelonephritis, systemic lupus erythematosus, obstructive postrenal disease (e.g. calculi and neoplasms) and hyperparathyroidism.

Drug and analgesic abuse may lead to chronic interstitial nephritis and gold therapy can cause nephrotic syndrome.

MANIFESTATIONS

Regardless of the cause of the chronic renal failure, the disease progresses through three stages: (1) *diminished renal reserve* which is characterized by an asymptomatic decrease in renal function, (2) *renal insufficiency* demonstrating slightly elevated serum creatinine and blood urea nitrogen levels, and a glomerular filtration rate of about 25% of normal, and (3) *end-stage renal failure or uraemia* which occurs when the glomerular filtration rate is less than 10% of normal, and functional disturbances are apparent.

The patient may pass through the early stage of chronic kidney impairment without the renal disease being recognized. It may first be discovered in a routine physical examination, revealed by an elevation in blood pressure and by albuminuria. The rate of destruction of functional tissue varies among individuals and with the primary causative factor. Some persons live a normal active life for many years because the functioning nephrons compensate to some extent for those destroyed. Others, whose disease progresses rapidly, may enter the advanced uraemic phase in a matter of a few months. In compensation the glomerular filtration rate per nephron is increased as are the reabsorption and secretory functions of the tubules. However, a deficit still exists which progressively increases.

Gradually, with increasing nephron destruction, the patient enters the phase in which renal compensation can no longer maintain homeostasis, and symptoms become apparent. Filtration is impaired, and there is a loss of tubular ability to vary the composition and volume of urine according to the need to conserve or eliminate urinary solutes and water.

The signs and symptoms vary considerably in patients in the early stage of uncompensated insufficiency but tend to become similar in the more advanced stage (see Table 21.8). An elevation in blood pressure, lassitude, headache and loss of weight may be the earliest manifestations. Urinalysis reveals albumin due to increased permeability of glomeruli. The loss of plasma protein as the disease progresses may be severe enough to produce the nephrotic syndrome (see p. 739). As more and more nephrons are destroyed, decreased filtration results in the retention of metabolic wastes. The blood urea and serum creatinine levels rise. Creatinine and urea clearance tests show a decrease in ml per minute, and the severity of failure may be categorized as mild, moderate, severe, end-stage, or anuria on the basis of the clearance test findings. For example, if the creatinine clearance test is used, 50–84 ml per minute may be interpreted as mild failure, 10–40 ml per minute as moderate failure, less than 10 ml per minute as severe failure, and 0 ml per minute as anuria or end-stage failure.

Table 21.8 Physiological disturbances caused by chronic renal failure.

Fluid and electrolyte disturbances
   Volume overload or depletion
   Hyperkalaemia or hypokalaemia
   Metabolic acidosis
   Hypercalcaemia and hypocalcaemia

Cardiovascular and pulmonary disturbances
   Arterial hypertension
   Heart failure
   Pericarditis
   Pulmonary oedema

Neurological disturbances
   Fatigue, lassitude
   Headache, irritability
   Impaired cognition
   Fits
   Peripheral neuropathy

Gastrointestinal disturbances
   Anorexia, nausea and vomiting
   Weight loss
   Peptic ulcer
   Gastrointestinal bleeding

Haematological disturbances
   Anaemia
   Bleeding tendency
   Increased potential for infection

Musculoskeletal disturbances
   Muscular twitching and weakness
   Renal osteodystrophy

With a progressive decrease in glomerular filtration and the development of hypertension, the patient experiences increasing fatigue and lassitude, more severe headaches and loss of weight. Nausea, especially in the mornings, and anorexia become troublesome. Fat and glucose metabolism are impaired, as well as protein metabolism. Serum triglycerides increase and a moderate hyperglycaemia occurs as a result of increased sensitivity to insulin.

Initially, in chronic renal failure the 24-hour urinary volume is increased and the patient experiences nocturia as a result of tubular inability to concentrate the glomerular filtrate. The concentration of solutes in the urine is invariable, producing a fixed specific gravity. If the fluid intake does not cover the increased fluid loss, the patient develops a negative fluid balance and the retention of solid wastes is increased.

Tubular destruction causes electrolyte imbalances. There is usually an excessive loss of sodium which may produce hyponatraemia unless there is adequate replacement. Potassium retention is not usually a problem until the terminal oliguric phase. In moderately severe failure, metabolic acidosis develops and hypocalcaemia may also be a problem, contributing to muscular twitching and general weakness.

Eventually, the urinary output is reduced, hypertension becomes severe, and the nitrogenous waste and potassium blood concentrations rise sharply. The patient is pale, and the haematocrit and haemoglobin determinations indicate anaemia which accounts in part for the fatigue and reduced efficiency. In chronic renal failure a bleeding tendency is also manifested; the thrombocyte count is low and the prothrombin time is abnormal. Petechiae, ecchymoses and bleeding of mucous membranes may be observed.

The central nervous system is affected by the retained wastes; the person is irritable; memory, reasoning and judgement are impaired and the attention span is shortened. In the advanced uraemic stage, the patient manifests confusion, disorientation, drowsiness and stupor. Restlessness and twitching may be observed and frequently precede convulsive seizures. Retention of phosphate and decreased synthesis of the active metabolite of vitamin D by the kidney alter bone metabolism, producing renal osteodystrophy (osteomalacia, osteitis fibrosa, soft tissue calcification and osteosclerosis). Pruritis can be a severe problem for the renal failure patient, attributed to the precipitation of retained phosphates into the skin.

Cessation of ovulation and menstruation in the female with chronic renal failure is common, and the male patient may experience loss of libido and impotence.

Late symptoms are anuria, generalized oedema, persistent headache of increasing severity, nausea and vomiting, hiccups, diarrhoea, muscular twitch-ing, convulsions, ulceration of the mouth, fetid breath, rapid deep respirations indicating acidosis, drowsiness, disorientation and coma. As a result of the severe hypertension and water retention, a cerebrovascular accident or cardiac failure and pulmonary oedema may supervene.

MANAGEMENT

Care is directed toward having the patient live as useful, comfortable and satisfying life as possible within the limitations imposed by his disease. The primary cause of the renal failure is treated to retard the progression of his disease (e.g. hypertension, pyelonephritis). The therapeutic plan includes measures to correct the body biochemistry and modify symptoms.

Conservative treatment is reserved for those patients who can be maintained without dialysis or kidney transplantation. The dietary and fluid intake are adjusted to maintain water and electrolyte balance and to reduce the retention of nitrogenous waste. Dietary protein may be decreased and limited to proteins high in essential amino acids (i.e. eggs, meat, fish and poultry) and to proteins from vegetables and grains. Ideally, protein intake should be maintained and the patient dialysed for as long as is necessary to maintain nitrogenous waste at an acceptable level. Carbohydrate intake is increased to provide adequate calories and to prevent the catabolism of body protein. Polyunsaturated fats are recommended and cooking with fats is avoided. A normal sodium intake is maintained if the patient has no signs of oedema or hypertension, but is restricted if these symptoms develop. Dietary potassium is usually restricted and potassium exchange resins are prescribed if hyperkalaemia persists. Serum phosphate levels are controlled by the use of phosphate binders such as aluminium hydroxide gel. Multivitamin tablets are prescribed daily to prevent deficiencies of water-soluble vitamins which may develop when the diet is low in protein and potassium. Serum calcium is monitored closely and if generalized bone pain, muscle weakness or radiological evidence of bone changes are present, vitamin D in the form of 1α-hydroxycholecaliferol is given and calcium supplements may be prescribed if the phosphate level has been lowered.

The patient is closely monitored for symptoms of complications, and treatment is initiated promptly to control hypertension, fluid and electrolyte imbalances, metabolic acidosis, anaemia and altered bone metabolism.

When conservative treatment will no longer adequately control the blood concentration of wastes and the fluid and electrolyte balance within limits compatible with life, regular *dialysis* may be employed to maintain the patient and a kidney transplant is considered. A discussion of these forms of treatment follows.

Nursing intervention for a patient with chronic renal failure is discussed on pp. 729–737. Table 21.11 illustrates a care plan for patients with chronic renal failure.

DIALYSIS AND KIDNEY TRANSPLANTATION

Dialysis

When the patient with renal failure who is being cared for on a conservative therapeutic regimen manifests a steadily increasing blood urea level, a serum creatinine level of 800–1200 µmol/l or over, progressive hypertension, metabolic acidosis, hyperkalaemia or a threat to cardiac and respiratory sufficiency by the retention of sodium and water, dialysis may be instituted.

Dialysis is a physicochemical process which refers to the separation of two solutions by a semi-permeable membrane through which water and some solutes may pass. Molecules and ions of solutes which are small enough to permeate the membrane pass through along a concentration gradient from higher to lower until an equilibrium is established on either side. The size of the pores of the dialysis membrane permits only the transfer of small molecular solutes. Larger molecular substances such as proteins and blood cells do not pass through the membrane. The movement of water through the dialysing membrane is governed by the osmolality of the solutions; it passes from the solution of lower osmotic pressure to that of greater osmotic pressure. These physicochemical processes, diffusion and osmosis, always proceed toward a zero concentration gradient.

Dialysis is a therapeutic procedure used in acute and chronic renal failure to lower the blood level of metabolic waste products (urea, creatinine, uric acid) and toxic substances and to correct abnormal electrolyte and fluid imbalances. Two methods currently in use are *peritoneal dialysis* and *extracorporeal haemodialysis*. The latter dialysis occurs outside of the body using a dialysis machine that may be referred to as an 'artificial kidney'.

Although the procedures in the two types of dialysis differ, the purposes and principles are the same. In haemodialysis a semipermeable membrane separates the patient's circulating blood from a specially prepared solution known as the *dialysate*. In peritoneal dialysis, the peritoneum is the membrane which separates the dialysate from the patient's interstitial fluid; the dialysate is introduced into the peritoneal cavity.

The dialysate is generally a specially prepared aqueous solution of sodium, calcium, magnesium, potassium chloride, lactate or acetate and glucose. The composition of the solution varies according to the patient's serum electrolyte concentrations; for example, potassium may be omitted if the patient has hyperkalaemia. The glucose is added to provide a hypertonicity and osmotic pressure that moves water from the patient into the dialysate to relieve overhydration and hypertension. Lactate or acetate is included to raise the pH; it is converted to hydrogen carbonate ions within the body.

Urea, creatinine and uric acid are removed from the patient by dialysis because they are not present in the dialysing solution. Water is removed if there is overhydration, since the osmolality of the dialysate is greater than that of body fluids which are dilute because there is an excess. If the serum potassium is elevated, diffusion occurs in the direction of the dialysate until there is an equilibrium on both sides of the dialysing membrane.

A regular dialysis regimen has prolonged the life of many patients with chronic renal failure. It has permitted many of them to continue in their jobs and be independent, useful members of society. Although hospital dialysis units have increased in number in recent years, particularly in larger centres, the number of patients that can be treated is still limited. The hospital-based unit usually necessitates the patient being away from his work at least 2 days a week. Because of this, the units' limitations, and the distance of many patients from a centre, home dialysis has become a common form of treatment. Selection of the type of dialysis to be initiated is made with the patient's and family's participation and consideration of the needs of the individual patient and the available resources.

Peritoneal dialysis may be used for most patients with symptomatic renal failure and who have a healthy peritoneal surface area. It is most suitable as a treatment for patients who are independent, live alone or have limited living space. It imposes minimal strain on relatives.

In this method of dialysis, the dialysate is introduced into the peritoneal cavity. The peritoneum consists of two membranes; the parietal and the visceral which form a closed space and comprise the largest serous membrane in the body. The potential space between the two layers forms the peritoneal cavity and normally contains only a small amount of serous fluid. For substances to pass from the blood vessels into the peritoneal cavity they must pass through the mesothelium, or outer layer, and five thin layers of fibrous and elastic tissue that comprise the visceral peritoneum.[9]

The transfer of solutes and fluid across these layers takes place by diffusion and osmosis; osmotic pressure provides the force for the movement of fluid. Substances are also pulled across the membranes with the fluid; a process which is referred to as solvent drag.

----

[9] Sorrels (1981), p. 516.

Peritoneal catheters. A permanent peritoneal catheter is used with a patient who has chronic renal failure. A catheter with several openings in the tip, such as the Tenckhoff catheter or a modification of it is inserted into the peritoneal cavity (Fig. 21.10).

Tissue cells (fibroblasts) grow into the two Dacron cuffs on the subcutaneous section of the catheter in 2–3 weeks, stabilizing the catheter position and decreasing the incidence of infection and escape of fluid. The procedure is usually carried out in the operating theatre under either a local or a general anaesthetic.

Dialysates. Dialysates are commercially available in 1, 2 or 3 litre plastic bags and provide various options of dextrose concentration and osmolarity. Dextrose concentrations above 1.5% increase the osmolarity of the dialysate above that of the plasma and promote water removal. Additional electrolytes and medications are added to the dialysate according to the needs and serum electrolyte concentrations of the individual patient.

Dialysis cycles. Each exchange of dialysate is divided into three stages; the instillation time, dwell time and drainage time. The solution is warmed to body temperature and infuses fairly rapidly into the peritoneal cavity by the force of gravity. The *instillation time* for the 2 litres of solution usually used for an adult requires approximately 10 minutes. *Dwell time* is the period of time the dialysate remains in the peritoneal cavity. For intermittent dialysis this is approximately 15–30 minutes, with cycles repeated for a period of 12–13 hours about three times a week. The dwell time for continuous abdominal peritoneal dialysis (CAPD) varies from 4–8 hours and exchanges are carried out continuously, 7 days a week. Smaller molecules such as blood urea nitrogen equalize in 2–3 hours; larger molecules take longer to equalize. The osmolarity of the solution influences the dwell time required to remove water. Higher concentrations of dextrose (4.5%) remove larger volumes of water in less time than solutions of 1.5% dextrose. *Drainage time* is the third phase of the cycle which is the period in which the solution drains from the cavity and takes up to 20 minutes.

Methods of peritoneal dialysis

The two major methods of peritoneal dialysis are intermittent and continuous.

Intermittent peritoneal dialysis may be carried out in hospital or at home and may be performed manually or by using an automated system. Automatic cycling devices use commercially prepared dialysates and provide for 8–12 exchanges of warmed solution. The gravity-operated machines allow for presetting of filling time, dwell time and measurement of drainage volume. These machines are simple, noiseless, mobile and easily mastered by patients.

The second type of automated appliance is the reverse osmosis machine which produces sterile, deionized water from tap water, warms and stores the sterile water and mixes it with preset measured doses of electrolyte and dextrose solutions. The machine is fully automated, and has a high capital cost but low operating cost. It requires sterilization once a week and a formaldehyde solution is usually used for this.

Intermittent peritoneal dialysis is usually performed about two or three times per week for 12–18 hours for a total of about 36 hours per week. A typical cycle of 2 litres of dialysate would include 10 minutes for instillation, 3 minutes dwell time and 20 minutes for drainage.

With *continous cycling peritoneal dialysis* (CCPD) the patient may use an automatic cycle machine at home each night while sleeping.

Continuous ambulatory peritoneal dialysis is currently the treatment of choice for most patients because it permits independence from machines, a more varied diet and a more flexible life-style. It has proven to be effective in removing small and middle-sized molecules, sodium, potassium and water and in controlling hypertension and anaemia.[10] The procedure involves: (1) connection of the catheter to tubing from a plastic bag containing the dialysate solution; (2) instillation of the dialysate; (3) folding of the plastic bag into a waist, leg or pocket pouch worn under the clothing; (4) drainage of the peritoneal cavity by gravity into the plastic bag about 6 hours later; (5) disposal of the filled bag; (6) connection and instillation of a fresh bag of dialysate (see Fig. 21.9 and Fig. 21.10). Bags containing 2 litres of dialysate are exchanged approximately four times a day, 7 days a week. The exchange schedule may be adjusted allowing 6 hours between two exchanges, 4 hours between the next exchange and an 8 hour interval at night to permit uninterrupted sleep.

Complications of peritoneal dialysis

Peritonitis. This is the major complication of peritoneal dialysis. The causative organisms have been shown to colonize all catheters and peritonitis may be due to a sudden increase of organisms by contamination of equipment, or dialysate fluid, or a decrease in the patient's ability to clear the organisms. Reasons for this are not yet known. Symptoms include abdominal pain and tenderness, cloudy effluent, fever, and occasionally vomiting and paralytic ileus. The peritoneal effluent is cultured for identification of organisms and white blood cell count. Treatment may consist of peritoneal lavage; this may be performed by continuously flushing with dialysis solution, without dwell time, for a brief period or for up to 48 hours. This may be

---

[10] Areopoulos (1982), p. 191.

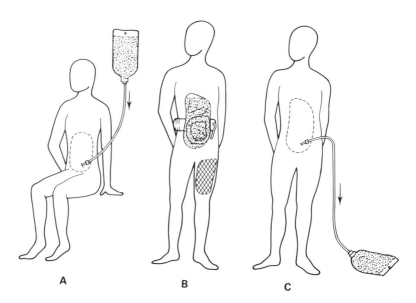

Fig. 21.9 Continuous abdominal peritoneal dialysis. *A*, Fluid flows from bag into peritoneal cavity through permanent access tube. *B*, Patient wears bag around waist or leg and resumes normal activity. *C*, Bag is lowered and fluid drains out. Bag is then discarded and procedure is repeated with fresh fluid.

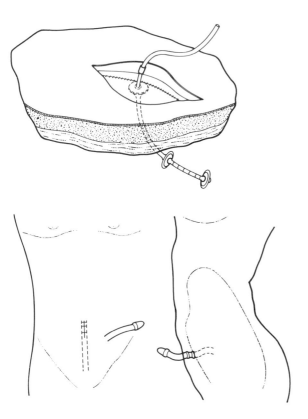

Fig. 21.10 Positioning of permanent peritoneal catheter.

followed by repeated exchanges with dwell times from 1–6 hours. Antibiotics are infused into the peritoneal cavity in the dialysate.

Catheter complications. Leakage around the catheter, obstruction of the catheter, retention of fluid and infection of the exit site are the most common complications associated with the catheter. Leakage occurs most often in the first 2 weeks following insertion of the catheter. Occlusion of the catheter may require the use of heparin in the dialysate to prevent or dislodge fibrin clots. Maintenance of regular bowel elimination helps to prevent problems with the flow of solution into the peritoneal cavity. Infection of the catheter site should be identified and treated promptly. Systemic antibiotics are given if positive cultures are obtained. Tunnel infections along the path of the catheter may necessitate replacement of the cathether.

Dehydration may result from use of large volumes of 4.25% dextrose dialysate. The patient will be hypotensive manifesting pallor, weakness, fainting and a rapid, weak pulse and will experience muscle cramps and may also be hyperglycaemic.

Pain. This may be due to the tip of the catheter pressing on viscera or overheating of the dialysate.

Disequilibrium syndrome. Rapid removal of nitrogenous wastes from the blood can produce a complication in which cerebral oedema develops causing severe headache, restlessness and disorientation. This is however very rare with peritoneal dialysis.

Protein catabolism and anorexia. The breakdown of tissue protein may occur because of loss of protein in the dialysate. Maintenance of adequate protein intake is necessary to prevent this complication.

Anorexia may occur initially, accompanied by a feeling of fullness when the dialysate is held in the peritoneal cavity. This problem usually disappears in a few months. When anorexia is present, the patient is assessed for signs of dehydration from excessive fluid loss.

Nursing intervention in peritoneal dialysis

Predialysis. Preparation of the patient involves evaluating the patient's understanding of dialysis; an explanation of the procedure and its purpose is given to the patient and family. Teaching should be carried out prior to the dialysis and reinforced and elaborated as the patient becomes more understanding and comfortable. Assessment includes determination and recording of the patient's blood pressure while lying and standing, pulse, respirations, temperature and weight. The serum creatinine, blood urea nitrogen and serum electrolyte concentrations are noted and the patient is assessed for signs of fluid overload, respiratory distress and dehydration. The abdomen is examined for distension and tenderness that might indicate peritonitis and the area around the exit of the catheter is observed for redness, drainage and infection.

During dialysis. Strict aseptic technique is observed in handling the catheter, tubing and dialysate. The solution is warmed and the type of dialysate and the time at which instillation commences are recorded. During the instillation and dwell periods, the patient is observed for both psychological and physiological reactions and the vital signs are monitored at frequent intervals. Blood chemistry studies are done periodically and changes evaluated. Any untoward symptoms such as abdominal pain, nausea, vomiting, sudden change in blood pressure, rapid weak pulse, pallor, headache, disorientation and change in level of consciousness require prompt intervention. The time at which the inflow of the dialysate is completed is recorded; this indicates the beginning of the dwell time. The abdomen is inspected for possible leakage around the tube. Mild abdominal discomfort may be alleviated by slowing the rate of the inflow, changing the patient's position or providing a snack. The patient may be more comfortable in an easy chair rather than in bed; being occupied by watching television, listening to the radio or reading usually helps the patient through the cycle. Lifting of food and fluid restrictions during dialysis prove pleasing to the patient as well as serving to replace protein that may be lost. Activity is encouraged as much as possible; equipment may be attached to movable poles, permitting a greater degree of mobility.

Drainage and post-dialysis period. A record is made of the times that the outflow is commenced and completed, the colour and volume of the fluid, the negative or positive balance (i.e. the difference between inflow and outflow volumes) and the patient's weight on completion of the dialysis cycle. The catheter is capped and an antiseptic or sterile occlusive dressing may be applied to the area around the entry site, or it may be left exposed.

If intermittent peritoneal dialysis is to be carried out at home or a schedule of continuous ambulatory peritoneal dialysis is to be established, the patient and family require detailed instruction before assuming responsibility for the procedure. Frequent supervisory visits by a nurse from the unit, or visits to the renal unit are necessary, especially during the initial period.

HAEMODIALYSIS

In haemodialysis, an extracorporeal flow of the patient's blood is separated from a specially prepared dialysate by a semipermeable membrane. Water and some solutes may move to or from the blood. The direction of movement is always toward reducing concentration gradients; water will move toward the solution of greater osmolality. Solid particles will shift by diffusion from the area of greater to lesser concentration in an effort to equilibrate the concentration on both sides of the membrane.

Haemodialysis is the more efficient method of dialysis but is a more complex procedure than peritoneal dialysis and requires more sophisticated equipment. As cited earlier, the principles in both methods of dialyses are the same but the procedure and equipment vary greatly. In haemodialysis, the blood from an artery is directed extracorporeally through an exchange unit and is returned to a vein. The components of the exchange unit include porous tubes through which the blood flows and a compartment containing the dialysate. A second essential unit is the dialysate supply system which mixes and delivers the solution to the exchange unit (Fig. 21.11). The membrane-like tube which transports the blood requires priming with blood or a prescribed intravenous solution to exclude all air before being connected to the patient's artery and vein. Heparin is added to the blood as it enters the dialysis machine to prevent coagulation.

Dialysers. Various models of haemodialysers are available; each type has individual features. They may vary in composition, structure and size of the dialysing unit, priming volume, ease of assembly, dialysate delivery system and whether or not the blood has to be pumped through the system. The types commonly used have a coil dialyser, flat parallel plate dialyser or a hollow fibre dialyser. Each functions on the same basic principles. The parallel plate (Gambro type see Fig. 21.11) and hollow fibre dialysers (Fig. 21.12) require lower blood volumes

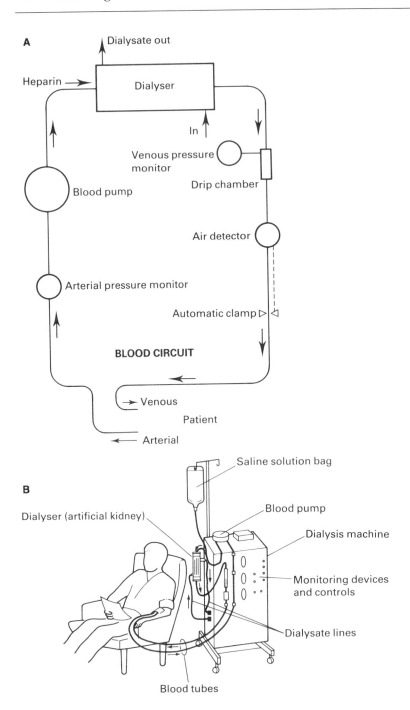

Fig. 21.11 Diagrammatic representations of haemodialysis.

and provide better control of ultrafiltration and for these reasons, they are most often used. Newer models are currently being developed which permit greater ultrafiltration of fluids and the filtration of middle sized molecules.

Ultrafiltration is the process of removing solutes and fluid through a membrane or filter. The pressure gradient across the membrane of a dialyser is influenced by the surface area and permeability of the membrane, the positive pressure of the blood, and the negative pressure of the dialysate. Excess fluid is removed in haemodialysis by the creation of a pressure gradient between the blood and the dialysate. Solute removal is facilitated by the use of a countercurrent flow which increases the concentration gradient. The blood and the dialysate move in

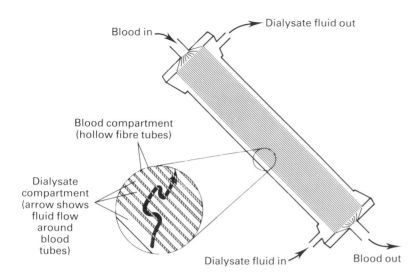

Blood in

Dialysate fluid out

Blood compartment
(hollow fibre tubes)

Dialysate
compartment
(arrow shows
fluid flow
around
blood
tubes)

Dialysate fluid in

Blood out

Fig. 21.12 Hollow fibre dialyser.

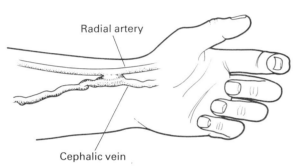

Radial artery

Cephalic vein

Fig. 21.13 An arteriovenous fistula.

opposite directions. The rate of flow of blood and dialysate can be regulated and is usually set with the blood flow through the dialyser at 200–250 ml per minute and the dialysate flow at twice this rate.

Blood is delivered to the dialyser via an established subcutaneous arteriovenous fistula or arteriovenous shunt. The *arteriovenous (AV) fistula* is surgically constructed by the side-to-side or end-to-side anastomosis of an artery and a vein (Fig. 21.14). The anastomosis may be between the cephalic vein and radial artery, or between the cephalic vein and brachial artery. A lower limb artery and vein may be the site of choice. A bruit can be detected over the fistula site, which indicates its patency. The fistula is usually established 6–12 weeks before use is anticipated to allow it time to 'mature'. The vein and its branches enlarge with the rerouting of the arterial blood.

Haemodialysis with an AV fistula involves the insertion of two needles into the *vein*. One needle is inserted at least 2 cm above the fistula and is connected to the outflow or arterial line of the dialyser. The second needle is inserted 3–4 cms above the outflow needle and is connected to the tube that returns the blood from the dialyser. Blood flows out from the

distal needle through the dialyser and back into the patient via the proximal needle (Fig. 21.13). A single-needle technique using a Y-connector to permit alternate arterial and venous flow may be used. *The limb in which an arteriovenous fistula is developed should not normally be used in taking blood pressure or blood specimens, as either may jeopardize their patency.*

The arteriovenous fistula access route in haemodialysis has several distinct advantages. It is completely subcutaneous, thus lessening the possi-

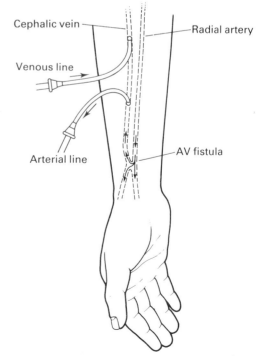

Cephalic vein

Radial artery

Venous line

Arterial line

AV fistula

Fig. 21.14 The position of needles when an arteriovenous fistula is established for haemodialysis.

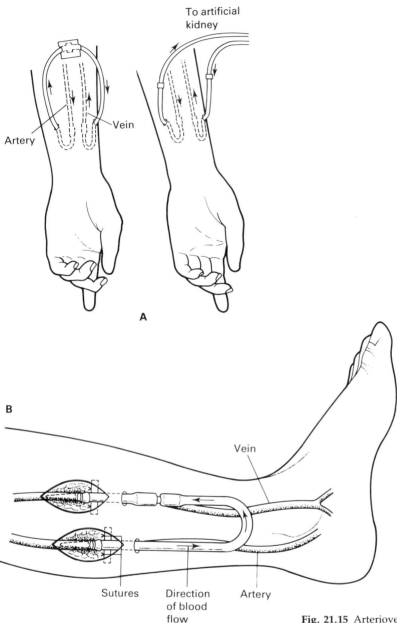

Fig. 21.15 Arteriovenous shunts, *A*, wrist. *B*, ankle.

bility of infection. Since it does not require a cannula and a bulky dressing, the patient's activity is less restricted and it also reduces the risk of haemorrhage and thrombosis.

An *arteriovenous shunt* is established by exposing an artery and an adjacent vein and implanting a cannula in each (Fig. 21.15). The ends of the cannula tubes are brought through the skin and are joined by a short connecting tube. The cannula and tubing are of inert synthetic materials (Teflon and Silastic) so reaction is avoided. The incisions are sutured around the tubes and a sterile dressing and bandage are

applied. Two small clamps are attached to the bandage at all times so that they are readily available should the tubes become disconnected and bleeding occur. The distal portion of the loop of the external U-shaped tube is kept covered with a light dressing at all times, but may be uncovered so that the patency of the shunt can be checked frequently.

To start dialysis the shunt-tubing is clamped and then the connecting tube on the AV shunt is removed; the arterial cannula is connected to the inflow (arterial) line of the dialyser and the venous cannula is attached to the outflow dialyser tube (i.e.

to the tube which returns the blood to the patient). The advantage of the AV shunt is its ready and painless accessibility for commencing dialysis. During the interval between dialyses, however, it requires frequent checking, dressing and protection. Since available sites for establishing an AV shunt are limited, precautions and care are necessary to prevent complications and maintain the patency of the shunt. The period of time that an AV shunt remains patent varies from 6–12 months, but may be several years.

The loop of the tube is checked frequently for blood flow. Clotting in the shunt system and obstruction of the flow may occur with kinking or malalignment of the tubes or pressure being exerted on them. The blood becomes dark red, and the bruit that is normally heard with a stethoscope over the venous side is absent. If clotting is suspected, no attempt is made to clear the tube by 'milking'. The problem is reported immediately to the doctor or dialysis unit. Efforts will be made to remove the clots by aspiration and the use of heparinized saline and declotting catheters.

The site is also checked for bleeding. If the tubing becomes disconnected, free bleeding is quickly recognized and the clamps previously mentioned are applied promptly to the tubing. Subcutaneous bleeding may result from the displacement of a cannula or erosion of the artery or vein. This is reported promptly; pressure is applied over the site and a tourniquet used.

The limb in which there is an AV shunt must not be used to determine blood pressure or administer intravenous infusions.

Other types of vascular access that may be used include *cannulation of large peripheral veins*, used when other routes are not available or for short-term dialysis, and *subclavian and right atrial catheters* which can be inserted and used for longer periods of time.

Vein grafts of synthetic material, autogenous veins or bovine grafts are generally used only when the patient's blood vessels are not suitable for the creation of a fistula.

Nursing intervention in haemodialysis
Nurses responsible for the care of patients receiving dialysis require specialized preparation. Dialysis is a complex therapeutic procedure used to correct a life-threatening body dysfunction. Staff nurses on general medical and surgical units should also have an appreciation of the implications for and the concerns of the renal patient and family. Personnel working in dialysis units usually assume responsibility for the specialized needs of dialysis patients being cared for in other areas of the hospital.

Factors to be considered in the nursing care plan for the haemodialysis patient include the following.

Emotional and socioeconomic concerns. When the patient's chronic renal failure necessitates hae-

modialysis, it is natural that the patient and family will be concerned and react. It is likely to have many implications; knowing that the disease has progressed to this stage and that his life becomes dependent upon the procedure is extremely threatening. Severe anxiety may be manifested due to concern for the future and life expectancy. Acceptance may be very difficult for some patients and they may manifest resentment and anger at first, followed by a period of depression. A regular schedule of dialysis two or three times weekly imposes modifications on the patient's and family's life pattern. Treatment may curtail his role in business; it may mean changing his occupation or giving up employment or, at best, working only part-time unless home dialysis can be provided. The adjustments that have to be made may cause both social and economic changes for family members, especially if the patient has been the main source of income or is the mother. Special diet requirements and transport to and from the dialysis unit or the need to accommodate dialysis equipment in the home may incur worrisome additional expense. A referral to a social worker may be helpful.

It is important for the nurse to be a willing listener and encourage the patient and family to reveal their concerns and problems; these vary from patient to patient and family to family. An understanding of their situation and recognition of their reactions are essential to providing the appropriate support and planning care, and in assisting them to accept the necessary modifications. A positive attitude on the part of the health care team promotes realistic patient and family acceptance and adaptation. Many patients obtain support and pleasure through socialization and the establishment of close relationships with other dialysis patients.

Gradually, as the uraemic toxicity is reduced, the patient experiences physical and emotional improvement and, by degrees, becomes more active and interested in living and may lead a relatively normal productive life.

Predialysis responsibilities. The patient and family receive a simply explanation of the purpose of dialysis and what to expect during the procedure. Many units have prepared brochures and audiovisual programmes to provide information and reinforce verbal explanations and instruction. If the patient is to be dialysed at home, an extensive home training programme is planned. Prior to the initial treatment, if the patient's condition permits, he visits the dialysis unit, meets the dialysis staff and may have the opportunity to chat with a patient on a regular dialysis programme. Such preparation is helpful in reducing the patient's fears. A consent form is signed by the patient or next of kin and an AV fistula or shunt is established.

For dialysis, the patient is positioned comfortably in a bed or a reclining chair with the limb with the AV fistula or shunt exposed and supported. His temperature, pulse, respirations, lying and standing blood pressure and weight are recorded before the dialysis is commenced. Blood specimens are obtained when the needles are introduced (or cannulae are opened) for laboratory determination of the haematocrit, electrolyte (K^+, Na^+), blood urea, and creatinine levels and clotting time. Anxiety is often greatly reduced if the patient and a relative are actively included even for the first dialysis. This might mean helping to set up the machine or preparation of the patient's dialysis access. A working knowledge of the equipment often greatly reduces fear.

The vascular access site is examined for signs of a haematoma or infection. Observations are made of the patient's colour and the condition of the skin (dryness, turgor, abrasions) and for oedema. His weight is compared with that recorded following the last dialysis; the difference in weight, as well as blood chemistry and physical findings determine the desired fluid loss and the appropriate dialyser, dialysate and flow-rate.

Responsibilities during dialysis. During dialysis the patient is monitored continuously for indications of the effectiveness of treatment and signs of complications. Each unit or home programme will have a schedule for observing and recording vital signs, equipment used, rate of flow, composition and temperature of dialysate, heparinization and blood clotting times, as well as on-going monitoring of the functioning of the equipment. The patient is closely observed for signs of dehydration or overhydration. Changes in blood pressure and respirations are recorded and the flow rate through the dialyser is regulated accordingly. If there is a rapid, excessive loss of water into the dialysate, the ensuing reduction in the intravascular volume causes a sharp fall in the blood pressure. Overhydration may be indicated by respiratory distress, moist sounds and an increase in the blood pressure.

Blood analysis for potassium and sodium levels may be repeated at intervals during dialysis. Adjustments may be necessary in the dialysate in accordance with the electrolyte values.

The clotting time is usually checked hourly by a simple ward-based test.

Headache, vomiting and twitching may develop if the patient becomes dehydrated and should be brought to the doctor's attention. The first dialysis should be short (i.e. 2–3 hours) to allow a gentle clearance of nitrogenous waste. This prevents the complication of cerebral oedema associated with disequilibrium syndrome which may present as disorientation or a convulsion.

Fluids are given, often in excess of daily allowance to give the patient a little more freedom, and the extra fluid may simply be removed throughout the dialysis. The patient's diet may be relaxed to some extent where possible, allowing free diet at least for the first 2 hours of dialysis. This still allows adequate time for metabolites to be dialysed out safely before the end of dialysis.

If the patient is on regular medication, the administration of these during dialysis is considered. Those which are dialysed out are often given post-dialysis, especially if taken in once-daily doses. Antihypertensive preparations are not given, since they may cause hypotension.

The temperature of the dialysate is monitored and automatically controlled on the newer machines. If the dialysate is too cool, the patient will complain of feeling cold. If the dialysate temperature is too high, haemolysis may occur.

The dialyser has an alarm to alert attending staff of malfunction; the fistula or shunt area is checked first to determine if a blood-line has become detached. Fast action is necessary to prevent a serious blood loss. A clamp may be placed on the line until it is reconnected.

The length of time the patient is kept on the dialyser varies with the patient's condition and type of machine used. The average range is 4–6 hours. The frequency also varies with patients. In acute renal failure, daily dialysis may be necessary until renal function is re-established. Patients with chronic renal insufficiency are dialysed two or three times weekly and may lead a relatively normal productive life the remainder of the week. The chronic dialysis programme may be long-term, extending over years, or may be a temporary measure for the patient who is awaiting a kidney transplant.

Postdialysis care. Upon completion of the dialysis the arterial line is clamped and as much blood as possible in the dialysing circuit lines is returned to the patient. The needles are removed or, in the case of a shunt, the dialysing lines disconnected and the cannulae reconnected. Dressings are applied and the area observed until there is no evidence of bleeding; it may be necessary to apply some pressure for a brief period. The patient's weight, blood pressure, lying and standing pulse and temperature are recorded.

Instruction. When a regular dialysis programme is recommended, the patient and a relative receive detailed instruction concerning diet and fluid intake, care of the fistula site or cannulae, activity, and recognition of disturbances that should prompt immediate notification of the doctor or dialysis unit. The brochure given out by the dialysis unit that explains dialysis also discusses these factors.

The diet prescribed varies from patient to patient and with doctors. The food intake must be balanced with the renal capacity to eliminate protein waste and prevent excesses of electrolytes (K^+, Na^+) and water. The protein content may be 60–80 g per day, allowing 0.75–1 g per kg of body if dialysis facilities are limited, otherwise a normal diet or a high protein diet is encouraged and dialysis hours adjusted to control nitrogenous waste.

Kidney transplantation

The development of donor selection by tissue typing and the steady progress that has been made in managing the rejection process, have resulted in an increase in the number of kidney transplants.

An advantage of a kidney transplant for the person who has severe renal failure is the discontinuance of the demanding dialysis schedule; considerable time is saved, and the individual's employment is uninterrupted and more productive. Dietary restrictions are lifted and constraint of activity is slight. The patient must be aware of the possible adverse effects as well as the benefits of transplantation prior to deciding on this mode of treatment. Some experience few complications and their quality of life is greatly improved. Others experience side-effects from the drugs used to control the rejection process and graft rejection. Transplantation requires major surgery and a life-long dependency on immunosuppressive drugs. Rejection of the transplant necessitates return to dialysis and consideration for retransplantation.

TRANSPLANT RECIPIENTS

The patient and family are informed of the available types of treatment of chronic renal failure and the risks and benefits of each, as well as the implications for their well-being and quality of life. Given such understanding, the patient makes the final decision whether to have the transplant or not.

The criteria for the selection of transplant candidates have become more liberal in the past few years. Uncontrolled infection and malignancy are the only firm contraindications at present. Treatment of the malignancy followed by a year without recurrence and an absence of infection for several months would make the person eligible for reconsideration as a candidate. The selection of candidates for kidney transplant is based on factors which will influence the outcome of the organ transplantation. These factors include: biological and physiological age, psychological status and the patient's primary disease process. If the renal failure is associated with diabetes mellitus, systemic lupus erythematosus, amyloidosis or scleroderma, the chances for success are decreased.

IMMUNOLOGICAL FACTORS

The greatest hazard associated with any organ or tissue transplant from another person is the incompatibility of the recipient's tissue with that of the donor, and the ensuing rejection process. Secondary to this are the effects of the immunosuppressive drugs used to depress the rejection process;

the most formidable is the recipient's increased susceptibility to infection.

The rejection process is an antigen–antibody reaction or immune response; the recipient's immune system recognizes the graft as a foreign substance, and specific antibodies and sensitized lymphocytes attack the foreign tissue.

The antigenicity and compatibility of the donor and recipient in tissue and organ transplants are determined by heredity. The antigens of concern, being determined by genes, are specific for each individual and are located on the surfaces of nucleated cells and red blood cells. Erythrocyte antigens compose the ABO antigen system used in blood typing and matching in blood transfusions, and may be present in vascular endothelium of the graft. Blood groups must be compatible in organ transplant.

The donor–recipient relationship is an important factor in influencing acceptance or rejection of a graft. The closer the relationship, the greater is the possibility of compatibility. Because cellular proteins and antigens are specific for each individual, donor tissue is rejected by the recipient's body unless it is taken from an identical twin. In this case, the transplant is compatible because the antigens of both the host and donor are identical, having been determined by the same genetic blue-print of a single fertilized ovum. Such a graft (with identical cellular proteins and antigens) is referred to as an *isograft*. A graft between two genetically dissimilar persons is known as an *allograft* or *homograft*.

The antigens located on the nucleated cells belong to the system designated HL-A (human leucocyte antigen). These antigens, present on cell membranes of most tissues, are easily detected on leucocytes which are readily accessible for tissue typing and clinical tissue tests for histocompatibility of potential donor tissue. Histocompatibility is defined as 'the quality of a cellular or tissue graft enabling it to be accepted and functional when transplanted to another organism.'[11]

The HLA complex is located on the sixth chromosome in man. Four major HLA loci (A, B, C, D) have been identified in this region with each locus having multiple alleles. Although over 77 antigens have been identified, each person possesses two antigens for each locus, one inherited from each parent. Locus D antigens which are subdivided into D and DR (D-related) are believed to be of particular significance in graft survival.

The principal methods used to determine the recipient's immunological response to potential donor tissue are: (1) tissue or HLA typing to identify the antigens at each HLA locus, (2) ABO blood-typing to identify compatability of red blood cells, (3) white blood cells cross-matching to detect the presence of preformed antibodies from previous

---

[11] Miller and Keane (1983).

exposure to an antigen, and (4) mixed lymphocyte culture to assess the degree of incompatibility between donor and recipient cells.

Tissue typing is the typing of antigens of the recipient and each potential donor. Antigens are identified by mixing lymphocytes with a series of standard sera which contain HLA antibodies. The reaction of the donor's and patient's cells to each serum is observed; lysis of the cells indicates that the antigen is specific to the known antibody. The patient's HLA typing is then compared to that of the donor.

ABO blood typing identifies the red blood cell antigens present in the recipient and donor. Antigens are identified when agglutination occurs on exposure of red blood cells to serum containing identified antibodies.

White blood cell cross-matching is performed by mixing blood from the recipient and donor and observing the reactions of the cells. Cell agglutination or lysis indicates a positive response; compatibility is indicated by a negative response.

The *mixed lymphocytes culture* involves making a culture of a mixture of the recipient's and potential donor's lymphocytes. The response of the recipient's lymphocytes to donor antigens is observed; reaction is demonstrated by the degree of change in the recipient lymphocytes in response to the other lymphocytes' antigens. The donor cells are treated before culturing to inhibit their response to the recipient's antigens. This test takes 5–7 days and can only be used with living donors.

DONOR

In early transplants, the kidney was always obtained from a live blood relative. Now, cadavers serve as the principal donor source. The cadaver is frequently an accident victim or someone who has had a sudden death and who is known to have been in good health.

If a living donor is used, he is usually related to the patient. As cited earlier, the donation is more likely to be successful if the relative is close (e.g. sibling, parent) than if the donor is a genetically non-related person (e.g. cousin, uncle by marriage).

Obviously, the living donor must be in good health. He undergoes a thorough investigation which includes an intravenous urogram and a renal angiogram to ensure normal kidneys with a normal vascular supply. He must have volunteered willingly and made the decision without pressure from others. The decision is a major one; it requires a mature, stable person. The immunological and other investigations preceding the operation to remove the kidney, the nature of the surgery, the inherent risk in being left with one kidney and the possibility of rejection of the graft by the recipient are explained and discussed freely with the prospective donor. He is informed of the time it will take, since it will

necessitate a period of absence from his job. A consent form is signed for the removal of the kidney following the investigation period.

Immediate preoperative preparation and postoperative care of the donor is similar to that cited in the section on nursing in renal surgery (see p. 743). The function of the remaining kidney is monitored closely. Blood urea and serum creatinine levels are followed for 2–3 weeks to assess compensatory efficiency. The patient's reactions are observed, since he may suddenly be alarmed by the risk he has taken and need support.

The demand for kidneys is much greater than the supply, and locally available kidneys may not be immunologically compatible. An established central service or register is maintained; persons with end-stage renal failure are registered with their tissue and blood types. When a locally available kidney is not compatible, one that matches may become available in another part of the country and is obtained through the United Kingdom transplant centre based in Bristol. Because of the demand for kidney transplants, various educational programmes have been organized to alert the public to the need for donors.

Legal and ethical considerations include the need for donation consent and the determination of death. In most areas, individuals can sign a form making a gift of any organ for the purpose of transplantation in the event of their death. The next of kin may also provide written authorization for the donation of organs if death is imminent. Laws in most countries, states and provinces define brain death and policies are established to ensure independence of the doctors treating the donor patient from the transplant team. Most regions now have a transplant coordinator who will be responsible for coordination of the organ transfer. She will often meet the potential donor, next of kin and ward staff and be responsible for feedback of information to them after the transplant. The coordinator also has a very important role in the education, not only of the medical and nursing staff, but also the general public to encourage greater referral of potential donors.

When death occurs, the kidneys are removed with their arteries, veins and ureters. The blood vessels are flushed out with an 'extracellular' electrolyte solution such as Ringer's lactate.

The organs are kept cool during transport and storage, until implantation. Transplantation should be done within 72 hours of obtaining the kidney from the donor. Storage up to 2–3 days requires pump oxygenator perfusion. When a cadaver kidney is used in transplant, the source remains anonymous to the recipient and his family.

TRANSPLANT PROCEDURE

The donor kidney is placed in the recipient's iliac fossa, usually on the side opposite to that from which it was taken—that is a left donor kidney is placed in the recipient's right iliac fossa. Its renal artery may be anastomosed to the host's hypogastric artery, and the renal vein of the graft is anastomosed to the common or external iliac vein (see Fig. 21.16). The ureter is implanted in the recipient's bladder via a submucosal tunnel; the latter prevents urinary reflux. A J-stent may be inserted into the transplanted kidney's ureter to prevent obstruction. It will normally be removed by cystoscopy after 3 months.

The patient's own kidneys are removed if there is recurrent infection or uncontrolled hypertension. Polycystic kidneys may need to be removed to provide room for the graft. Usually this will have been performed while the patient awaits transplantation.

In the case of a living donor, the removal of the kidney and the surgical implantation in the recipient are synchronized in adjacent operating theatres; this greatly reduces the period of ischaemia and the risk of tissue damage.

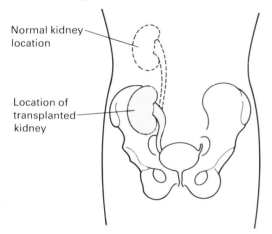

Fig. 21.16 Location of transplanted kidney.

PREOPERATIVE PREPARATION OF THE RECIPIENT

When a person is selected as a candidate for a renal transplant, the doctor discusses in detail all that is involved with him and his family. They are informed of what is entailed in the surgery—that the kidney graft may be rejected, necessitating the resumption of a maintenance haemodialysis programme; that continuous drug therapy and close supervision will be needed; and that precautions against infections will be necessary. He is encouraged to be as fit as possible whilst awaiting a transplant. This may involve taking calorie supplements to improve his nutritional status.

During the period before the operation, the patient's blood pressure, which is likely to be elevated, is monitored closely. If an antihypertensive drug is being administered, the nurse is alert for side effects and sharp pressure swings up or down. An accurate record is made of the fluid intake and output; the intake is regulated daily according to the

output of the previous day to avoid overloading the cardiovascular system and promoting electrolyte imbalances.

Efforts are made to improve the patient's nutritional status and to meet his caloric requirements. His diet is tailored to fit the protein and sodium restrictions prescribed.

Histocompatibility tests will have been completed prior to the scheduling of surgery. A detailed medical history and examination are done as well as a chest x-ray, electrocardiogram and other tests recommended as a result of the medical examination. Blood tests are extensive and include a full blood picture, serum electrolytes, creatinine, blood urea and blood coagulation determinations. Blood is cross-matched for the operation. If the serum potassium and creatinine and blood urea are elevated, the patient is dialysed prior to surgery.

If the patient's anaemia is severe, blood transfusions may be given. Controversy exists as to whether blood should be given; transfusions are believed to increase graft survival but may also cause presensitization.

The patient's and family's level of anxiety is assessed. The patient receiving a cadaver graft will have little notice prior to the actual surgery. Preparations must be done quickly but opportunity is provided for the patient to review his decision and to ask questions and share feelings.

Deep breathing and coughing are taught and practised and the patient is informed about what to expect postoperatively. If the patient is known to have respiratory problems, base-line blood gases will be measured preoperatively. A bath with a prescribed antibacterial agent added may help to minimize bacteria flora on the skin. A consent form is signed and a dose of an immunosuppressive agent of cyclosporin and antibiotics are given preoperatively. A central venous pressure line will be established under anaesthetic so the intravascular fluid volume can be monitored intra- and postoperatively. A retention (Foley) catheter is introduced into the bladder in the theatre under strict aseptic conditions for accurate monitoring of urine output.

NURSING INTERVENTION

The nursing care of the patient who has received a kidney transplant is similar to that cited on page 743, and includes measures to maintain fluid balance, kidney function, prevention of infection and assessment for possible graft rejection and other complications. The immediate care is the same as that for any patient recovering from anaesthetic.

Assessment. Vital signs, urinary output, fluid intake and electrolyte concentrations are monitored, and frequent observations are made for bleeding from the wound and early signs of infection and rejection. A renal scan is performed the day following surgery to provide a base-line for graft function.

Maintenance of fluid balance and kidney function
The retention catheter is connected to a sterile closed-drainage system; the urinary output is recorded hourly. Frequent urinalyses and cultures are made and 24-hour urine specimens may be obtained for measurement of creatinine clearance. Blood-stained urine may be expected at first but should progressively clear over a few days. Bleeding is due to the bladder incision made to implant the ureter in the bladder wall and the high vascularity of the bladder.

The transplanted kidney usually begins to excrete urine soon after the surgery. The volume may increase rapidly, resulting in profuse diuresis. Unless there is adequate replacement during this diuretic phase, dehydration, shock and electrolyte imbalance may develop. The patient may experience bladder spasm and pain with the large urine volume, because the bladder has not been used to receiving urine for some time preoperatively. If the transplant fails to excrete sufficient urine for several days, haemodialysis or peritoneal dialysis may be used until kidney function improves. If peritoneal dialysis is considered the surgeon must be consulted to ensure that the peritoneum was not damaged during the operation. Fluid and electrolyte restrictions are required until adequate urine volume is achieved. Once kidney function appears to be stabilized the hourly measurement can be discontinued. The catheter is removed, normally at about 4–5 days. The patient is encouraged to void frequently to avoid overdistension of the bladder and pressure on the ureteral implantation area. If the patient's own kidneys have been retained, consideration must be given to their usual output when assessing the function of the graft kidney. The patient's weight is recorded daily and changes noted.

The central venous pressure is recorded at least hourly initially. A regime of fluid replacement is normally prescribed to maintain the central venous pressure as 0–5 cmH$_2$0 measured at the sternal notch. This allows accurate assessment of fluid status and prevents dehydration or fluid overload. An increased intravascular volume places an increased demand on the pulmonary circulation, while dehydration may cause poor perfusion to the transplanted kidney and jeopardize its survival.

The fluid balance is determined every hour by comparing the total intake with total fluid loss and is assessed with other observations. The electrolyte composition of the intravenous fluids is based upon the laboratory reports.

Prevention of infection
The patient is receiving immunosuppressive medications and is at greater risk of infection. The application of good medical asepsis is stressed; thorough hand-washing is important before each contact with the patient. The patient is usually cared for in a transplant unit or area with consistent and specially pre-pared nursing staff. Protective isolation techniques used in the past are no longer believed necessary.

Because the patient's immune system is suppressed, normal inflammatory responses to infection may not occur. The patient's skin and oral mucosa are examined frequently for redness, swelling, drainage, warmth and tenderness. The temperature is taken every 4 hours and the patient is asked to report any pain or discomfort. The white blood cell count is monitored frequently and if severely depressed, protective measures may be instituted and immunosuppressive therapy decreased for a brief period.

The patient is required to carry out regular, frequent periods of deep breathing and coughing and ambulation is encouraged. The lungs are auscultated by the doctors for air entry and the presence of wheezes or râles. Patients are treated prophylactically with cotrimoxazole to prevent opportunistic lung infections and pneumocystis. Early removal of central venous lines and the urethral catheter eliminates potential sources of infection and facilitates ambulation. Mouth care is carried out regularly and includes antibacterial mouthwashes (e.g. nystatin); a soft toothbrush is recommended to prevent trauma to the gums.

Any invasive investigation must be covered with antibiotic treatment and any sign of infection investigated and broad-spectrum antibiotics given immediately. The appropriate antibiotic is identified quickly and given as the patient may develop septicaemia rapidly.

Rejection
The nurse must be constantly alert for early manifestations of the rejection process, which may occur as early as the second or third day. There may be swelling and increasing tenderness over the kidney, fever, general malaise, headache, an elevation in the leucocyte count, anorexia, decreased urinary output, hypertension, oedema and elevated levels of serum creatinine, sodium and potassium and blood urea.

The patient may become anxious at first and then appears gradually apathetic and lethargic. The kidney becomes swollen, oedematous and congested; thrombosis occurs in the renal blood vessels and tissue necrosis follows due to ischaemia.

The intensity of the rejection process and the rapidity with which it develops correspond to the degree of difference between the recipient's and donor's cellular antigens; the greater the difference, the more severe and rapid is the rejection. *Hyperacute rejection* occurs within minutes or hours of the transplant, due to preformed antibodies attacking the homograft. This severe type of reaction may be attributed to presensitization to donor antigens as a result of previous transfusions or several pregnancies. Widespread intravascular coagulation occurs in the transplanted kidney, and failure develops.

Acute or early rejection may develop in the postoperative or convalescent period or it may occur 1–4 months following the transplantation. Oliguria and increasing blood urea and creatinine levels are manifested. Rejection can usually be reversed by increased dosage of immunosuppressive drugs.

Chronic or late rejection develops insidiously after 3 or 4 months, or it may occur several years after the homograft was received. This type of rejection is characterized by arterial impairment due to intimal hyperplasia. It is attributed to chronic reaction between circulating antibodies and the antigens of the vascular endothelial cells. This process cannot be reversed with medication.

PREVENTION OF REJECTION

The administration of immunosuppressive drugs is resumed in the immediate postoperative period and continued. These drugs depress the body's responses to the donor kidney's antigens. The drugs which may be used are azathioprine (Imuran) and a corticosteroid preparation (prednisolone) (see Table 21.9) but cyclosporin A is currently the preferred immunosuppressive drug and is used with lower doses of steroids. Antilymphocytic globulin (ALG) may be given intravenously as an infusion in a progressively decreasing daily dose for 10 days if rejection is suspected.

The dosage of azathioprine and prednisolone are adjusted according to the leucocyte count and the patient's reactions to these drugs. It is necessary for the nurse to be familiar with their side-effects. Azathioprine may depress the bone marrow production of leucocytes and produce leucopenia. Reactions to prolonged administration of prednisolone may include the retention of sodium and water, an elevation of blood pressure, hirsutism, development of a round puffy face ('moon face'), euphoria, gastrointestinal ulceration, impaired liver and pancreatic function, and arrested growth in a child.

Cyclosporin A is severely nephrotoxic and so blood levels are closely monitored. It may also produce hepatic impairment and lymphomas. Patients often become hirsute and have tremors, especially in the early stages. This tends to disappear as the dosage is reduced. Since ALG is a serum, one must be alert for an anaphylactic reaction; an intracutaneous sensitivity test is done before the initial dose.

The signs and symptoms of rejection are cited above. When rejection is suspected the patient is given higher doses of prednisone; it may be given intravenously as well as orally. Plasma exchange may be carried out to remove antibodies and immune complexes and thus reduce the rejection response. This will depend on the patient's original disease. If the reaction is severe and there is marked fluid retention and elevation of serum potassium and creatinine and blood urea, dialysis may have to be resumed. Fluid intake and dietary restrictions may also be necessary.

If the rejection process is irreversible, the immunosuppressive drugs are discontinued and the graft may be removed. The patient may well become discouraged and the nurse should be prepared to offer support and reassure the patient that he may be considered for a second graft.

Other medications. Since most medications are eliminated through the kidneys, as few drugs as possible are given following a renal transplantation. Small doses of an analgesic may be prescribed, if necessary, for the relief of pain and discomfort when nursing measures do not provide adequate palliation.

PATIENT EDUCATION FOR HEALTH MANAGEMENT

The patient may become apprehensive about leaving the hospital and becoming independent. He is likely to become fearful as he learns he must follow a prescribed pattern of living indefinitely and be constantly alert for early signs of rejection and complications. He and a member of his family receive a planned series of instruction which provides them with the opportunity to become conversant with all aspects of his care. The hospital usually provides an outline of the information the patient requires in booklet or brochure form.

A social worker can be of considerable assistance to the patient and family in planning for the future. The social worker may provide assistance in finding suitable employment or, if work is not possible, may help in obtaining financial assistance for the patient and family. Suitable forms of recreation and sports in which he is interested are discussed.

The drugs which he must continue to take are discussed fully. It is helpful if a sample of each is attached to a card on which the name of the drug, its strength, and directions for taking are clearly printed. The nurse stresses the importance of these drugs, and that if they cannot be taken or retained because of illness, the patient must contact his general practitioner or the renal unit promptly. The cards are taken to the outpatient clinic or the general practitioner when visits are made so that if the dosage is changed the directions on the cards may be changed.

The patient is instructed to keep a daily record of his weight, fluid output and medications taken. Verbal and written explanations are made of the content and preparation of his diet. Since the prednisolone may increase his appetitte and promote sodium retention, the patient is advised to guard against exceeding his normal weight. Dietary restrictions are few and are individualized. Sodium intake may be restricted, and as cyclosporin may cause acidosis and hyperkalaemia in some patients, especially in the early days, potassium intake may need to be restricted.

Suggestions are made as to how he may protect himself as much as possible from infection. Close

Table 21.9 Immunosuppressive drugs.

Drug	Dosage	Action	Side-effects
Azathioprine (Imuran)	2–3 mg per kg body weight per day orally Regulated by leucocyte count	Inhibits the synthesis of nucleic acids in cell production Depresses the production of leucocytes (especially lymphocytes) and antibodies	Bone marrow depression; mouth ulcers; alopecia; and, rarely, hepatitis
Adrenocorticosteroid (e.g. prednisone, oral; methyl prednisolone, intravenous)	0.2–0.4 mg per kg body weight per day, orally Rejection normally treated with 1 g intravenously for 3 days	Suppresses the inflammatory response Suppresses lymphocyte and antibody formation	Lowered resistance to infection; gastrointestinal ulceration; bleeding; oedema and hypertension due to sodium retention; mood swings; weight gain; moon face and cataracts
Antilymphocyte globulin (ALG) and Antilymphocyte serum (ALS)	20–60 mg per kg body weight per day, 10 daily doses intravenously as an infusion. Dose decreases over the 10 day period. May be given prophylactically to patients with known antibodies to prevent rejection	Suppresses lymphocyte action	Anaphylaxis (patient requires very close observation); Alopecia; bone marrow suppression and haemorrhagic cystitis
Antithymocyte globulin (ATG)	Given intravenously as an infusion 2 mg per kg per day. Daily for 10 days. May be given prophylactically to patients with antibodies	Suppresses thymocyte action	Anaphylaxis; alopecia; bone marrow suppression and haemorrhagic cystitis
Cyclophosphamide (Endoxana)	1–5 mg per kg body weight, oral or intravenously (rarely used)	Suppresses cell reproduction	Bone marrow depression; alopecia and cystitis
Cyclosporin	5–16 µg per kg body weight orally or intravenously regulated by blood levels	Depresses humoral and cellular immunity	Nephrotoxicity, hepatic impairment, lymphomas, hirsutism and tremors

contact with persons with a cold or other types of infections should be avoided. Good hygienic practices in food handling and the frequent washing of the hands are stressed. Good personal hygiene is essential.

The early signs of rejection are reviewed with the patient and family. By this time the patient is usually quite familiar with them and realizes that prompt action is necessary. The patient and family are cautioned to report immediately a cold, sore throat, fever, dysuria, frequency or other disturbances which may indicate infection. The patient is also urged to contact the unit promptly if there is a sudden gain in weight (for example, 1 kg in a day), swelling of the ankles or puffiness of the face, pain, tenderness and/or swelling in the area of the graft, decrease in urinary output, headache, unaccounted for fatigue, or elevation in temperature.

Following discharge, the patient is followed closely by visits to the outpatient department at least once a week, since constant surveillance plays an important role in his progress and the development of acceptance of the situation with less fear. If his progress is satisfactory, and he indicates understanding and efficient management of his care, the intervals between visits are gradually lengthened.

COMPLICATIONS

In addition to infection and the rejection process, complications which may develop in the recipient after a kidney transplantation include the following:

Tubular necrosis. This is attributed to the ischaemia of the kidney during the period between its removal and grafting. It is manifested by oliguria and the effects of the retained metabolic wastes and excess fluid.

Gastrointestinal ulceration and bleeding.   These may be caused by the corticosteroid preparation which the patient receives to suppress the immune response to the graft. Any vomitus or faeces containing blood is reported to the doctor. An H_2 antagonist (cimetidine or ranitidine) is prescribed to all patients as prophylaxis. Dyspepsia is investigated promptly by endoscopy to detect erosions.

Cataracts.   These are also a side-effect of the prednisolone. Patients are advised to have their eyes examined annually.

Urinary fistula.   This may be due to failure of healing of the ureter at the site of anastomosis with the bladder.

Lack of wound healing.   This may be caused by the steroid medication or urine leakage.

Bone marrow depression.   This is due to the immunosuppressive drugs. Leucopenia develops, which predisposes the individual to serious infections; erythrocyte production is depressed, and the signs and symptoms of anaemia develop; normal coagulation may be impaired when the platelets are decreased, and bleeding from mucous membranes, petechiae and ecchymoses may become evident.

Nursing process in chronic renal failure

IDENTIFICATION OF PATIENT PROBLEMS

Table 21.10 lists actual and potential problems, contributing factors and goals common to most patients with chronic renal failure. Nursing care is individualized to meet the needs of each patient, his particular circumstances and treatment. Renal failure is a chronic progressive disorder; the needs of patients and their families will vary as the disease progresses.

Table 21.11 illustrates a sample care plan for patients with chronic renal failure.

1. Alteration in fluid balance: deficit or excess
Assessment of fluid balance is continuous. The patient and family are taught to identify signs of fluid excess or dehydration and to adjust fluid intake and prescribed therapy accordingly. In the early stage of chronic renal failure, tubular reabsorption of water is decreased so the intake must be increased accordingly. Generally a minimum of 2000 ml is required to prevent dehydration. When oliguria is present the fluid intake is limited to 400–500 ml plus the measurable loss (e.g. urine and vomit). Fluid restriction is minimal for the patient on continuous ambulatory peritoneal dialysis because fluid is continuously removed.

The nurse helps the patient to institute measures to control thirst and to adjust his daily fluid intake schedule to accommodate preferences and social activities.

2. Nutrition
The prescribed diet varies with the severity of the disease and the type of maintenance treatment used. In the early stages, protein restrictions may be based on the glomerular filtrational rate (GFR); for example, with a GFR of 20–25 ml/min, daily protein intake may be limited to 90 g and with a GFR of 10–15 ml/min, daily protein may be restricted to 50 g.[12] When the GFR decreases to 4–5 ml/min, protein restrictions are no longer effective in reducing the retention of nitrogenous wastes and dialysis is required. Protein is lost during peritoneal dialysis and the loss is greater if peritonitis develops. Less protein is lost during haemodialysis, but some free amino acids escape with this treatment. The protein intake must be adjusted to compensate for this loss and prevent catabolism of body protein; it is also increased with corticosteroid therapy because of the associated increase in catabolism. Calorie intake must be sufficient to permit activity without breakdown of tissue protein. The patient on continual abdominal peritoneal dialysis absorbs some glucose from the dialysate and so carbohydrate intake is limited.

Vitamin supplements are prescribed; vitamin D is given to prevent bone loss and also when the calcium level is low, and vitamin K is prescribed if the prothrombin is elevated. Zinc sulphate may also be prescribed to stimulate taste and appetite, as zinc is removed by dialysis.

Electrolyte balance is maintained by adjusting the dietary intake according to serum electrolyte levels. Since impaired tubular reabsorption results in an excessive loss of sodium, salt is not restricted in the diet unless there is oedema or hypertension. Dietary sodium is restricted following a transplant as corticosteroid therapy leads to sodium and water retention. Foods high in potassium are restricted for most renal patients because potassium is not effectively removed by impaired kidneys or by dialysis. Transplant recipients receiving diuretic therapy may require potassium supplements. The serum phosphate level is usually controlled by the use of phosphate binders such as an aluminium hydroxide antacid and avoidance of foods high in phosphorus.

Nutritional management in chronic renal failure is complex. Because of the multiplicity of factors to be considered in determining dietary modifications for each individual, patients experience some difficulty in understanding restrictions and in following the prescribed diet. Since diet is such an important part of disease management, the patient and family require considerable teaching and support over a period of time from the nurse as well as the dietitian.

Dietary management becomes more complex for

---

[12] Murphy & Cole (1983), p. 63.

Table 21.10 Actual and potential problems of the patient with chronic renal failure.

Problem	Causative factors	Goals
1 Alteration in fluid balance (deficit or excess)	Decreased formation of urine due to renal failure Effectiveness of dialysis therapy Fluid intake Corticosteroid therapy	To maintain fluid balance
2 Alteration in nutrition: nutritional intake lower than body requirements	Altered metabolism of protein, carbohydrates and fats Impaired elimination of nitrogenous wastes Altered absorption of calcium Protein loss through peritoneal dialysis Altered energy expenditure Altered bone metabolism Altered electrolyte and acid–base balance Nausea, vomiting and anorexia Loss of water soluble vitamins through dialysis	**1** To maintain adequate nutrition **2** To reduce retention of nitrogenous wastes **3** To maintain electrolyte and acid–base balance
3 Potential for infection	Effect of uraemia on bone marrow Effect of uraemia on circulating white cells Immunosuppressive drugs (when transplanted)	**1** To prevent infection **2** To observe for infection and treat promptly and effectively
4 Activity intolerance	Anaemia Constant fatigue and lethargy Muscular irritability Renal osteodystrophy Possible dyspnoea and cardiovascular complications associated with uraemia Peripheral neuropathy	To maintain an acceptable or the best possible level of daily activity
5 Impairment of skin integrity and alterations in oral mucosa	Increased coagulation time; fragility of blood cells Elimination of wastes through the skin Itching and scratching	To maintain the integrity of the skin and oral mucosa
6 Alteration in thought processes	Effects of uraemia on the nervous system	**1** To be aware of alterations in cognition and behaviour **2** To prevent injury
7 Inability to cope	Disruption of usual coping mechanisms Dependence Changes in roles and relationships Financial insecurity Altered body image Altered cognitive ability Loss of support systems Life-long nature of chronic illness	To achieve an acceptable quality of life within the constraints of a life-long state of chronic illness
8 Insufficient knowledge about: (1) kidney function, (2) methods of treatment (dialysis or transplant) (3) self-care measures (4) necessary alterations to life style	Lack of knowledge and experience Changes in treatment plan Lack of support systems Altered cognition	To acquire knowledge, skill and resources to safely manage health-care regimen

the patient with chronic renal failure who experiences sudden stress such as infection, surgery or trauma. Food and fluid intake must be closely monitored and adjusted to the manifested needs. Alpha-keto analogues of essential amino acids are useful during periods of stress and severe renal failure. Total parenteral nutrition may also be used to maintain adequate nutrition for the critically ill patient.

3. Preventing infection
Immunosuppressive drugs or uraemia affect white cell activity, making the patient prone to infection. Preventive measures and prompt treatment of infection are essential.

4. Activity intolerance
The patient with chronic renal failure experiences

considerable fatigue and lethargy; anaemia may contribute to the decreased energy. The anaemia may be due to decreased erythropoeitin production, depression of the bone marrow associated with uraemia, or to blood loss due to increased tendency to bleed and through dialysis. It develops gradually and may not be symptomatic at first.

In the early stage of the disease, kidney function may be adequate as long as the prescribed diet and fluid intake are followed and metabolic extremes are avoided. The patient is encouraged to remain active within the limits of his strength but is advised to avoid undue fatigue and excessive activity which increases serum creatinine and catabolism. The ability to continue to be a useful, independent member of society bolsters self-esteem and emotional well-being; the patient is encouraged to live as normal a life as his disease permits.

If the patient develops severe anaemia, periodic transfusions of whole blood or packed cells are given. The nurse working with haemodialysis patients takes precautions to minimize blood loss during dialysis. The taking of blood for laboratory tests is reviewed to limit the amount of blood taken. When the type of dialyser is selected, consideration is given to the patient's haematocrit level, and following haemodialysis residual blood can be reinfused.

The patient is questioned about joint and muscle pain and any changes in range of motion or mobility. The patient is also assessed for signs of hypocalcaemia; tetany, carpopedal spasm, seizures, numbness and tingling of extremities or confusion. When signs and symptoms of altered serum calcium and phosphorus develop, the patient's compliance with medication therapy and dialysis is assessed and changes made as necessary. An activity and exercise plan is developed to maintain muscle tone and mobility.

5. Skin and oral mucosa

Assessment of the skin of the patient with chronic renal failure may show pallor, a yellow-grey colour, dryness, bruising and decreased sweating. The patient complains of itching. The hair is dry, becomes brittle and the nails are rigid and dry. Uraemic frost on the skin from crystallization of urea deposits is rare except in terminally ill patients. The mouth is inspected regularly for signs of inflammation and bleeding.

The patient is taught to care for skin, hair and nails and to perform oral toilet frequently.

The patient is instructed to avoid factors which exacerbate itching and to follow the dietary regimen to control serum calcium and phosphorous levels.

The patient is taught to avoid falls or other injury that would cause bruising and bleeding and to obtain regular, preventive dental care.

6. Altered thought processes

Changes in the patient's level of awareness usually develop gradually as uraemia increases. Rapid progression of the disease produces severe disturbances in behaviour and cognition. Dialysis should be started before the progression of these neurological complications.

Early symptoms may include headache, lethargy, dizziness, euphoria, depression, apathy, sleeplessness, anxiety or drowsiness. Recent and remote memory and attention span are decreased and decision-making is impaired. In the late stages of renal failure, confusion, slurred speech, toxic psychosis, stupor, coma and convulsions may develop.

The patient is assessed for his orientation to time, place and person. Changes in behaviour as perceived by the patient and family are noted and relatives are helped to understand that the patient cannot always control his behaviour.

The patient's decision-making ability is determined before he is asked to perform complex tasks and cognitive abilities are evaluated before patient teaching is started. Explanations of procedures should be simple, broken down into steps and repeated frequently. It is possible that the patient's home environment may be able to be modified to promote safety.

Many of the behavioural and cognitive changes are reversible with dialysis. The importance of following the dialysis schedule is stressed and additional dialysis time may be planned when neurological symptoms indicate more severe renal insufficiency.

7. Inability to cope

Adaptation to chronic renal failure is a complex process and varies with each patient, the degree of loss of renal function, the type of treatment selected and support available.

Assessment of the patient's coping includes learning about pre-illness personality and the degree of dependence and independence assumed in daily life. The number and type of losses and changes required in the patient's life-style such as: loss of job and financial security; loss of position in the family; loss of freedom because of actual or perceived dependence on a machine; loss of stamina and sense of well-being; loss of self-esteem and self-worth; and reduced life expectancy.[13] Further changes in family roles and relationships are increased by decreased sexual function. Burns states that the previously independent person has the most difficulty adjusting initially, but measures to prevent feelings of helplessness and dependence can be effective. Selection of home dialysis or continuous abdominal peritoneal dialysis forces the patient to become an active participant in care while hospital dialysis may reinforce dependence and emphasize losses.[14]

Information about how the patient coped with stress in the past helps the nurse in assessing the

[13] Burns (1983), p. 14.
[14] Burns (1983), p. 15.

Table 21.11 Care plan for the patient with chronic renal failure.

Problem	Nursing intervention	Expected outcomes
1 Alteration in fluid balance: deficit or excess	**a** Record fluid intake and output **b** Assess: skin turgor; mucous membranes for moisture; oedema; weight gain or loss (daily and pre- and post-dialysis); BP (lying and standing); for dizziness, lightheadedness and nausea; respirations (rate, depth and character) **c** Teach patient and family to: record intake, output and daily weight; estimate fluid balance; adjust fluid intake to not more than 500 ml in excess of urinary output; develop a plan to limit fluid intake by identifying preferences, adjusting schedule to social activities, keeping mouth moist by sucking ice cubes, drinking chilled fluids in small amounts and rinsing mouth frequently with cool water or alcohol free mouthwash, and providing distraction (e.g. reading, radio); report significant increases or decreases in fluid balance; make adjustment in therapy as instructed to control identified fluid imbalance and/or inform health-care personnel	**1** The patient's weight is maintained within 2 kg of his optimal weight **2** Blood pressure, (lying and standing) is stable within the patient's usual range. Postural drop is absent **3** Generalized oedema, pulmonary râles and shortness of breath are absent **4** The patient and/or family states signs and symptoms of dehydration and fluid overload **5** The patient understands daily monitoring of fluid intake and output and body weight **6** The patient and family describe the relationship between weight changes and other signs of fluid imbalance with fluid intake **7** The patient and family describe actions to be taken when dehydration or fluid overload occur
2 Alteration in nutrition: nutritional intake lower than body requirements	**a** Monitor indicators of dietary compliance: daily weight; blood urea, creatinine and serum electrolytes **b** Administer antiemetics and antacids as prescribed and indicated **c** Inspect oral mucosa for dryness, ulceration and opportunistic infection **d** Provide regular mouth care; rinse mouth with a mild mouthwash or warm water; give small amounts of cool liquids to moisten mouth **e** Provide stool softeners as prescribed and indicated to treat or prevent constipation **f** Observe stools and vomit for blood **g** Instruct patient and family in dietary regimen in collaboration with the dietitian: —adjust protein intake as prescribed. Include protein foods of high biological value (e.g. eggs, meat, fish and poultry) in prescribed amount —adjust carbohydrate intake to provide adequate calories —limit fat intake. Use polyunsaturated fats **h** Provide supplements of water-soluble vitamins and ascorbic acid as prescribed **i** Control intake of foods high in potassium such as citrus fruits and juices, bananas and whole grain cereals **j** Administer phosphate binders as prescribed (aluminium hydroxide preparations) **k** Limit foods high in phosphorus such as dairy products, chocolate, dried fruits and vegetables, nuts and whole grain cereals **l** Reinforce instructions provided by dietitian **m** Explain the relationship between daily serum electrolyte, creatinine and blood urea results with food intake **n** When the test results change from the usual pattern, help the patient review his diet and make adjustments necessary to prevent recurrence	**1** The patient's weight is maintained at an optimal level defined for him **2** Weight loss due to catabolism of body protein does not occur **3** Anorexia, nausea and vomiting decrease or are absent **4** Serum levels of sodium, potassium, bicarbonate, pH, calcium, phosphorus and creatinine and blood urea nitrogen are maintained within acceptable ranges for the patient **5** The patient and family show understanding of dietary regimen. **6** The patient and family are aware of resources available to assist with understanding and compliance with diet **7** The patient understands signs and symptoms of inadequate dietary control, and how to correct it
3 Potential for infection	**a** It is important to be vigilant at all times for infection. Patients are taught the importance of reporting any minor elevation in temperature or inflammation **b** Immunosuppressed patients are taught that they must have prophylactic antibiotic cover for all invasive procedures	**1** The patient is free from infection **2** Potential infection is recognized and prevented **3** Infection is treated quickly and effectively **4** Invasive investigations are performed without sepsis

Table 21.11—*continued*

Problem	Nursing intervention	Expected outcomes
4 Activity intolerance	**a** The patient is encouraged to remain active **b** The patient is taught to: participate in moderate activity; avoid undue fatigue; develop an appropriate sleep pattern; plan daily routine to identify priorities (including rest periods and allowing for increased time to complete tasks); adjust his work schedule; prevent tissue trauma and bleeding; establish a daily activity schedule **c** Refer the patient to a social worker or an occupational health nurse to assist in planning adjustments to work routine, if the patient desires **d** Encourage patient to participate in recreational and social activities, as desired **e** Monitor patient's haemoglobin levels; administer blood transfusions as prescribed and indicated; take precautions during haemodialysis procedure to minimize blood loss and rationalize phlebotomy; administer prescribed iron and folate supplements if the dietary intake cannot be increased; assess the patient for muscular and joint pain and altered range of motion or mobility **f** Observe the patient's gait and for signs of tetany or confusion **g** Note presence of numbness or tingling in the extremities **h** Monitor serum calcium and phosphorus levels **i** Administer mild analgesics as prescribed and indicated for muscular or bone pain	1 The patient is able to perform essential activities of daily living 2 The patient plans daily activities to include important functions and obtain adequate rest 3 The serum haematocrit is maintained within a stable range for the patient 4 The patient states precautions to take in daily routine to prevent tissue trauma and bleeding 5 Muscular irritability and bone pain are absent or controlled
5 Impairment of skin integrity and alterations in oral mucosa	**a** Inspect mouth regularly for inflammation, bleeding and sores **b** Inspect skin for bruising, petechiae, scratches, dryness and scaling and colour **c** Inspect hair and nails for dryness and brittleness **d** Teach the patient to: keep skin clean; use oils or creams as appropriate; observe for signs of infection such as red areas on the skin, especially near fistulae, coughs and urinary tract infections; keep nails short and clean; avoid factors that exacerbate itching such as increased body heat, rubbing and scratching, rough textured or tight clothing; rub lanolin cream into skin as a substitute for scratching and rubbing; follow prescribed dietary measures to control serum calcium and phosphate levels and thus itching; prevent trauma to skin and prolonged pressure to bony prominences; perform mouth care using a soft toothbrush and using dental floss to remove plaque; inspect gums for bleeding; obtain regular, preventive dental care	1 The patient's skin and oral mucosa are clean and intact 2 Pruritus is controlled 3 The patient understands the need for good skin and mouth care 4 The patient understands how to recognize infection and the need to seek advice and treatment promptly
6 Alteration in thought processes	**a** Assess the patient's orientation to time, place and person and decision-making ability **b** Teach the family and patient: about the effects of uraemia on the nervous system; about the importance of complying with dialysis schedule to reverse or control confusion and alterations in cognition; to recognize any deterioration in cognition or behaviour which may indicate that dialysis is inadequate, and that the number of hours or frequency may need to be increased; a well dialysed patient should not suffer from central nervous system defects	1 The patient and family are aware of the effects of uraemia on cognition and behaviour 2 Personal injury as a result of decreased levels of awareness does not occur 3 The patient observes his dialysis schedule
7 Inability to cope (actual or potential)	**a** Assess the patient's: pre-illness personality and life-style; past responses to loss and change in function; response to present illness situation; family's response to present situation; support systems and their availability; cognitive functioning; level of fatigue and lethargy; understanding of chronic renal failure and its management	1 The patient performs his own activities of daily living 2 The patient and family express their feelings 3 Social activity increases 4 The patient complies with the agreed-to treatment regimen

Table 21.11—*continued*

Problem	Nursing intervention	Expected outcomes
7 Inability to cope (continued)	**b** Teach the patient and family: about chronic renal failure and its physical and emotional effects on the patient; about the treatment plan; about the role of patient and family as active participants in the decision-making process and disease management **c** Provide instruction before decisions are made about changes in treatment **d** Allow time for the patient and family to assimilate new information, and repeat as necessary **e** Provide opportunity for the patient to discuss his feelings, ask questions and explore alternatives **f** Provide support for decisions made, including the patient's right to refuse treatment **g** Inform the patient and family of support services (social worker, renal clinic) and make referrals as relevant	
8 Insufficient knowledge about: (a) kidney function, (b) types of treatment, (c) self-care measures, (d) necessary alterations in life style.	A patient and family teaching programme is implemented (see text)	**1** The patient and family state the functions of the kidneys and signs and symptoms of kidney failure **2** The patient and family agree to a plan for complying with the selected treatment modality **3** The patient receiving home intermittent or continuous peritoneal dialysis: (a) Demonstrates aseptic technique, changing of dialysate bags, measurement and recording of weight, blood pressure and fluid volume outflow (b) Describes the principles of dialysis and factors which can be altered to enhance or slow the exchanges (c) Assesses self for signs of fluid excess or dehydration, peritonitis or other complications (d) Describes the relationships between BP, weight, fluid intake and fluid loss with signs of fluid overload or dehydration (e) States actions to be taken when complications develop (f) States where to obtain equipment, supplies and assistance when needed **4** The patient receiving home haemodialysis: (a) Demonstrates aseptic technique, care of the vascular access, dialysis procedure, care of equipment and the recording of blood pressure and weight (b) Describes the basic principles of haemodialysis (c) Assesses self for signs of fluid and electrolyte imbalance, infection, clotting of vascular access or other complications (d) Observes precautions to prevent haemorrhage (e) States actions to be taken in the event of haemorrhage (f) States where to obtain equipment, supplies and assistance when needed

Table 21.11—*continued*

Problem	Nursing intervention	Expected outcomes
8 Insufficient knowledge (continued)		5 Following kidney transplantation, the patient states the name, dosage, method of administration, actions and side-effects of prescribed immunosuppressive agents 6 The patient and family understand the prescribed nutrition and fluid plan 7 The patient demonstrates ability to assess and record: signs and symptoms of fluid overload; uraemia; rejection and infection and to record weight, blood pressure and temperature 8 The patient and family actively participate in decision-making regarding care 9 The patient and family are helped to achieve continued employment 10 The patient and spouse (partner) share mutual concerns regarding their relationship 11 The patient develops and implements a regular activity schedule 12 Social interactions increase as desired 13 The patient and family are well informed about holiday planning

patient's present coping responses and in assisting him in developing new coping strategies. Many coping mechanisms used every day by individuals are dangerous when employed by the patient with chronic renal failure; denial and depression are detrimental when they interfere with compliance with treatment.

Changes in cognitive ability and behaviour affect the patient's perceptions of the illness, ability to comprehend what is happening, to understand and comply with treatment and make informed, rational judgements about care; dependency on others is increased. Chronic fatigue and lethargy further impair the patient's ability to cope.

The presence of family and other support groups enhances positive coping. The responses of family members and friends and their influence on the patient are evaluated. They require knowledge of the disease, understanding of the patient's responses and behavioural changes and understanding of the treatment plan so they can be informed participants. They will need help in developing new patterns of interacting with each other and new coping strategies.

Decisions about care are made with the patient and family as active participants and should be directed to achieving the goals of the patient. Doctors and nurses should avoid giving ambiguous messages to the patient and family by firstly expressing the desire for patient participation in decision-making and then imposing their own expectations of patient behaviour. Patient responses change as each new phase of treatment is encountered. The patient start-

ing dialysis must acknowledge dependence on machines to sustain life. Transplantation usually results in an initial state of euphoria which is followed by reactions to living with a foreign body, before eventual acceptance of the graft occurs. These patients live with a life-long need for medication and constant fear of graft rejection. Even with successful transplantation the patient needs help adjusting to the changes imposed by this life-long process.

8. Lack of knowledge
Since the patient and family must assume the responsibility for following the prescribed regimen, formal and informal instruction is planned. Patient education is started at the time of diagnosis and the teaching is adjusted as the patient's needs change with progression of the disease and revision of the treatment plan. The decision about home or institutional dialysis influences the degree of responsibility the patient and family assume for self-care and the resources needed to help them. Some patients and families learn to follow the treatment programme, make necessary observations, recognize significant changes, adjust care according to predetermined guidelines and seek help when needed. Other patients require a referral to community services because a regular support person is unavailable. Medical supervision is provided by the dialysis unit or treatment centre. If the patient is returning to work, the occupational health nurse at his place of employment should be advised of the situation so she may provide the necessary assistance and follow the patient's progress if he desires.

When a patient with chronic renal failure is admitted to hospital it is important that the nursing staff assess the patient's understanding of his care and support the patient's achievements in self-care by encouraging him in active participation. Taking away the patient's control each time he is admitted to hospital retards progress already made and contributes to feelings of dependency.

Goals for education are established for each patient and teaching methods vary with available resources. Many pamphlets are available for patient use. Renal centres will have instruction sheets, guidelines and audiovisual programmes which are useful to teach skills and reinforce demonstrations and practice sessions. Written instructions are given to each patient regarding his specific dietary modifications, medications, care of the fistula, shunt or catheter, and treatment schedule. Group teaching may be useful to impart general content and to allow patients and families to share experiences and to learn alternative coping strategies from each other.

A patient and family teaching programme includes: the function of the kidneys, types of treatment (dialysis or transplant), self-care measures, and life-style adaptations.

The function of the kidney. The healthy kidney regulates body fluid volume, excretion of waste and secretion of hormones to control blood pressure, red blood cell production and calcium absorption. When kidney insufficiency occurs, waste products and fluid are retained, blood pressure rises, anaemia develops and weakness of the bone structure occurs.

Types of treatment. When end-stage renal failure develops the patient becomes dependent on dialysis or receives a kidney transplant. Information is provided about: intermittent and continuous peritoneal dialysis; haemodialysis; types of vascular accesses available and the options of treatment at home or in a dialysis centre. The suitability, availability and implications of transplant are discussed.

A home peritoneal dialysis teaching plan includes knowledge and practice of the principles of asepsis, the techniques of changing dialysate bags, the catheter dressing procedure, the taking and recording of blood pressure and weight. It is necessary for the patient to have an understanding of the role of dialysis, the significance of weight changes and recognition of the signs of fluid overload, dehydration and peritonitis. Active patient participation and supervised practice sessions are essential.

A teaching programme for home haemodialysis includes knowledge of and practice in the principles of asepsis and care and assessment of the shunt or fistula. The patient learns to palpate the AV shunt, feeling for a 'thrill' and to use a stethoscope to listen for a bruit proximal to the venous insertion site resulting from the turbulence created by the high arterial pressure flowing into the vein. Safety measures to prevent haemorrhage are employed. The patient practises the dialysis procedure under supervision and learns to care for the equipment. Assessment of complications of fluid and electrolyte imbalance, infection, clotting of the vascular access are taught and actions to take when problems occur are discussed.

Following transplantation the patient has a life-long need for immunosuppressive drugs. Instruction includes the name, dosage, method of administration, action and side-effects of the medications. Sodium and fluid restrictions may be necessary with corticosteroid therapy.

Self-care measures
● *Nutrition and fluid.* Basic nutrition and the role of proteins, carbohydrates, fats and fluids in the body are discussed. The patient's diet plan is reviewed with him. Foods that contain protein of high caloric value which should be included are discussed and lists of foods that provide necessary calories without excessive protein, electrolytes and fluid are provided. The measurement and distribution of the required fluid intake over 24 hours are planned. The patient is instructed to record his weight daily and to do this at the same time each day with the same amount of clothing.

The dietitian helps the patient and family plan a meal schedule that includes foods the patient prefers, supplies recipes to allow for variety in meals and instructions on the preparation of foods. Reinforcement of compliance with dietary restrictions is provided by discussing and relating weight changes, the results of blood tests and blood pressure readings with the patient.
● *Medications.* The pharmacist or nurse provides instruction regarding medications. Participation in a self-administration of medications programme in hospital, provides opportunity for the patient to assume responsibility for his medication regimen, to adjust the schedule to his daily routine, and to begin to identify side-effects of the medications.
● *Monitoring of signs and symptoms of uraemia.* The patient is taught to identify signs of fluid overload and retention of nitrogenous wastes and to accurately measure and record weight, temperature and blood pressure as well as to understand the significance of changes and what to do when they occur.
● *Use of resources.* The patient is introduced to personnel involved in the nephrology programme and is provided with information on who to call when he has specific needs. As he works with the staff and learns more about his disease and its management, his rights as an active participant in the decision-making process about his care are emphasized. Referrals are made to visiting nurses in the community as necessary.

Patients are taught the importance of interpreting their treatment plan to other health professionals, especially when travelling or on admission to hospital for reasons other than for the renal programme.

Medic Alert tags and bracelets may be worn by patients and include identification of a vascular access or peritoneal catheter.

Necessary alterations to life-style. Helping the patient adjust his life-style is an individual process. The teaching programme includes consideration of the following:
- *Work.* The patient's treatment plan, chronic fatigue and lethargy may limit his ability to retain gainful employment. Cooperative efforts with employee health services and job counselling by a social service department help the patient plan changes in his work schedule to continue employment for as long as possible.
- *Sexuality.* Counselling of the patient and spouse or partner helps them to understand the reasons for the decreased libido in female patients and the intermittent impotence experienced by males. Participation in decision-making and care, and assistance in establishing and maintaining open communication within the family unit foster interpersonal and sexual relationships.
- *Holidays.* The patient and family are helped to plan holidays and are informed of resources available. These include portable machines which may be borrowed, a directory of renal units in other cities nationally and internationally, and trips and camping facilities available through the local or national Kidney Foundation.
- *Exercise.* The patient is helped to plan an activity schedule that includes moderate exercise within his physical ability and is taught that regular exercise improves circulation and appetite and promotes rest and a sense of well-being.
- *Social activities.* The patient is helped to adjust his daily routine when social activities are planned and to change social behaviours of eating and drinking to accommodate his treatment regimen. Support and encouragement from staff and families are needed for the patient to initiate and increase social interactions.

OTHER DISORDERS INVOLVING RENAL DYSFUNCTION

Glomerulonephritis

This disease is usually characterized by a diffuse, non-infectious inflammation of the glomeruli of both kidneys. Since the blood supply that supports the tubules normally passes through glomerular capillaries before reaching them, fibrous scarring and obliteration of some glomeruli lead to secondary degenerative changes in the associated tubules, blood vessels and interstitial tissues. Glomerulonephritis is more common in children and young adults and has a higher incidence in males. It may be acute or chronic.

CAUSE

The glomerular injury is usually caused by immuno-

logical processes. Three major immunological mechanisms are recognized. In one, antigen–antibody complexes formed extrarenally are trapped in glomeruli and initiate the inflammatory process; this is a common reaction responsible for glomerulonephritis. The second immune reaction involves antibodies that are formed against an antigen in or produced by the glomerular basement membrane, initiating glomerular inflammation. The third mechanism involves activation of the alternate compliment pathway.

A common cause of glomerulonephritis is the beta-haemolytic streptococcus (group A, Types 12, 4 and 1). The patient's history usually reveals that the renal disturbance follows an infection, such as a sore throat or respiratory infection of some form, by a latent period of 2–4 weeks. In some instances, the infection may have been so mild that little or no attention was given to it at the time. Post streptococcal glomerulonephritis is produced by immunological processes probably involving one or more of the above causative mechanisms.

Glomerulonephritis may also be associated with other diseases such as systemic lupus erythematosus, polyarteritis nodosa, scleroderma, diabetes mellitus, amyloidosis and bacterial endocarditis.

SIGNS AND SYMPTOMS

The onset is generally abrupt but in some instances may be insidious. The affected glomeruli are partially or completely obstructed, resulting in reduced filtration. Some glomeruli rupture, permitting the escape of blood into the tubules. The permeability of the glomeruli that remain patent is increased. The scant output of urine is cloudy and contains albumin, blood cells and casts.

Oedema develops and is usually seen first in the periorbital areas and ankles. The patient complains of pain and tenderness in the back, headache, and weakness. Visual disturbances may also be manifested. The blood pressure is elevated, and decreased filtration results in a gradual accumulation of nitrogenous wastes in the blood; the blood urea and serum creatinine levels may be elevated.

Nasal and throat swabs may be taken to determine if streptococci are still present. Examination of the blood may reveal an elevation in antistreptolysin O titre (ASO titre).

Neurological signs and symptoms corresponding to the degree of hypertension may be present (see Chapter 22). Unless the renal insufficiency is reversed, uraemia, pulmonary oedema and cardiac failure may ensue.

MANAGEMENT

The treatment of patients with acute glomerulonephritis consists mainly of rest, fluid and diet regulation, and chemotherapy to eliminate possible residual streptococcal infection. The daily fluid intake is restricted to 400–500 ml in excess of the urinary output of the previous 24 hours. The blood chemistry is followed closely and the sodium, potassium, and chloride intake regulated according to the findings. The patient receives a high carbohydrate diet to reduce the breakdown of tissue protein. Protein may be provided in the form of essential amino acid or keto analogues to achieve nitrogen balance. Similarly, salt restriction in the diet is regulated according to the degree of oedema and hypertension.

If the low output of urine is prolonged and the blood potassium and nitrogenous waste levels are progressively increasing, diuretic therapy is initiated or peritoneal dialysis or haemodialysis may be instituted (see pp. 714–722).

Plasma exchange may be carried out to remove antibodies and immune complexes since the disorder is usually caused by immunological processes. Precautions are necessary to protect the patient from exposure to infection. A superimposed infection could aggravate the disease or cause pneumonia that could prove fatal.

The frequent association of glomerulonephritis with respiratory infections emphasizes their potential danger and the importance of prevention and prompt, adequate treatment of such infections. Too often they are ignored, considered as unavoidably seasonal and treated very lightly. Women who have a history of acute glomerulonephritis are advised to consult a doctor before planning a pregnancy, since they are more likely to develop toxaemia and eclampsia.

According to the literature, the majority of patients with acute glomerulonephritis associated with infection (e.g. streptococcal) recover with no residual kidney damage. These patients generally show an increase in the volume of urine and a decrease in the blood pressure and BUN within 1 week. The albuminuria and microscopic haematuria may persist for much longer. A few patients progress through a subacute phase to chronic glomerulonephritis. Others may be asymptomatic for a period of months or years and then experience an insidious development of the chronic disease which may progress to chronic renal failure.

Pyelonephritis

This is an inflammation of the pelvis and parenchymal tissue of the kidney due to infection. The predominant causative organisms are the gram-negative enteric bacilli which have invaded the lower urinary tract and ascended to the kidney via the ureters. In rare instances, the pathogen, such as the staphylococcus or streptococcus, may be blood-borne.

Significant predisposing factors are defective urinary drainage and reflux of urine from the bladder into the ureters. Obstructions to the flow of urine from the kidney may be the result of a renal calculus, neoplasm, stricture of a ureter due to pressure, scarring or congenital anomaly. Stasis of urine in the lower urinary tract due to bladder or urethral dysfunction may increase the intravesical pressure sufficiently to produce a reflux into the ureters.

Pyelonephritis is more common in females than males. The incidence is relatively high in female infants and children, due perhaps to faecal soiling and *Escherichia coli* contamination of the urethral meatus. Its frequent occurrence in pregnant women is attributed to stasis of urine incurred by pressure from the enlarging uterus and atonia of the ureters due to the effect of progesterone. It may also occur following urethral catheterization; infection introduced into the bladder may ascend through the ureters to the kidney. Pyelonephritis in males in the later years of life is generally associated with defective urinary drainage as a result of an enlarged prostate.

MANIFESTATIONS

The onset is usually sudden. In children it may be accompanied by a convulsion. Manifestations include chills, fever, headache, nausea and vomiting, pain and tenderness in the loins, leucocytosis, and frequent and painful micturition (dysuria). The urine is cloudy and contains bacteria, pus, blood, and epithelial cells.

Treatment. The patient is encouraged to take liberal amounts of fluid unless there is complete obstruction of urinary drainage. An accurate record of the fluid intake and output is necessary. A culture may be made of the urine and the causative organism antibiotic sensitivity determined. Antibiotic therapy is prescribed. If nitrofurantoin (Furadantin) or a sulphonamide preparation is used, the patient is observed for possible reactions which usually appear in the form of nausea and vomiting and a skin rash.

Unless there is complete eradication of the infection, pyelonephritis may become chronic with insidious destruction of nephrons, leading to chronic renal failure and uraemia. Following the initial episode of acute pyelonephritis, the patient generally undergoes a thorough investigation for a predisposing obstructive lesion. Antimicrobial therapy and a high fluid intake are prolonged beyond the disappearance of acute signs and symptoms. Specimens of urine are examined and cultured at regular intervals after the antimicrobial drug is discontinued.

Tuberculosis of the kidney

Tubercular infection in the kidney is usually secondary to tuberculosis elsewhere in the body; most often the primary site is a lung or lymph node. The tubercle bacilli are carried by the blood to the kidneys.

Scattered characteristic granulomatous lesions (tubercles) develop, eroding renal tissue and leaving cavitations. The infection may involve pyramids and calyces, interfering with tubular drainage and leading to hydronephrosis. The infection may spread to involve the bladder.

The systemic symptoms characteristic of any tubercular infection are usually present – namely, low-grade fever, night sweats, loss of weight, fatigue and a positive tuberculin skin test. The urine contains pus and blood; smears and a culture reveal the presence of tubercle bacilli. The patient complains of back pain, which may become quite severe in advanced disease. An intravenous urogram is done to determine whether the disease is unilateral or bilateral.

The patient receives a prolonged, intensive course of antituberculous drugs. He is observed for possible reactions to the drugs which may take the form of dermatitis, fever, dizziness and impaired hearing. A nutritious full diet is encouraged without restrictions if there is adequate renal function to prevent oedema, hypertension and the accumulation of wastes in the blood. Frequent urine smears and cultures are made to determine the progress of the patient's disease. Treatment is continued for a period of 12–18 months even if the cultures become negative for tubercle bacilli.

The nephrotic syndrome (nephrosis)

The characteristic symptoms of the nephrotic syndrome are proteinuria (greater than 3.5 g of protein in 24 hours), hypoproteinaemia, generalized oedema and usually hyperlipidaemia. It may develop in a patient with primary renal disease, or it may be associated with other conditions in which kidney involvement is secondary. Systemic disorders (e.g. diabetes mellitus, systemic lupus erythematosus and amyloidosis), circulatory disturbances and infections are some of the causes.

The proteinuria, which is chiefly albumin, is the result of some change in the glomeruli that causes an increase in their permeability to the plasma proteins. Obviously, the loss of the proteins reduces the colloidal osmotic pressure of the blood, contributing to increased movement of fluid into the interstitial spaces as well as to its decreased reabsorption into the capillaries. The resulting decrease in intravascular volume leads to retention of sodium and water by the kidneys. The excessive concentration of serum lipids, which is determined by estimation of the cholesterol level, is not understood.

The urine is reduced in volume and usually contains casts as well as large amounts of albumin. In contrast with other forms of impaired renal function, the blood pressure and nitrogenous waste levels of patients usually remain within a normal range in the absence of advanced damage to glomeruli.

The severity of the nephrotic syndrome is variable.

In some, the oedema may cause only slight puffiness in the periorbital areas and ankles, yet in others it may be so extreme that ascites (accumulation of fluid in the peritoneal cavity) and pleural effusion develop. The oedematous areas are generally soft and readily pit on pressure. The patient is usually pale, may be breathless, complains of fatigue and may experience anorexia, which further complicates the problem of hypoproteinaemia. Susceptibility to infection increases and the incidence of venous thrombosis is greater as anticoagulant substances are lost in the urine. The onset may be insidious or abrupt.

TREATMENT

When the nephrotic syndrome is secondary, the treatment is directed toward inducing diuresis, reducing oedema, producing and maintaining a normal serum albumin level and reducing the lipid level in the blood.

The patient receives a low-sodium, high-protein full diet. The recommended daily protein is usually 1 g per kg of body weight plus an amount equivalent to the daily loss in urine. This implies that 24-hour collections of urine are made for estimation of the amount of protein excreted. Intravenous infusions of plasma or albumin may be given and infection is treated promptly with an antibiotic when it occurs. The patient may require anticoagulation with subcutaneous or intravenous heparin to cover the acute period.

The patient is particularly susceptible to infection because of the lowered resistance of oedematous tissues and reduced plasma gammaglobulin which is essential in the formation of antibodies. Precautions are necessary to avoid exposure to infection.

An adrenocorticosteroid preparation such as prednisone may be prescribed. It is usually given for a period of 3–4 weeks, with the dosage gradually being reduced until the minimum maintenance level is reached. It is then continued in that dosage. Immunosuppressive drugs such as azathioprine or cyclophosphamide may be given in combination with corticosteroid preparations to induce a remission.

A diuretic such as frusemide may be used in some instances if there is not a satisfactory response to the corticoid preparation and a reduction of the oedema.

The patient is not usually hospitalized after a satisfactory therapeutic regimen is established, nor is he confined to bed. Activity within his tolerance is encouraged. Treatment is generally required over a long period, and frequent medical check-ups are necessary.

Nephrolithiasis (renal calculi)

Stones or small concretions may develop in the collecting tubules, calyces or the pelvis of a kidney. They are formed by the precipitation of various substances in the urine; if retained, the initial precipitation forms a nucleus or matrix which promotes further precipitation and calculus enlargement. The substances commonly involved in calculus formation are calcium, oxalate, phosphate, uric acid, cystine, xanthine and ammonia, but most often the stones are of mixed composition (e.g. mixed phosphates and oxalates). They vary in size from tiny particles to large smooth or irregular masses. The irregular stone that forms in the pelvis and has projections into the calyces is referred to as a *staghorn calculus*. The usual composition of the latter type of calculus is phosphate.

CAUSE

The constituents of renal calculi are present in normal urine; any condition which increases their concentration, reduces their solubility or promotes retention of the urinary salts favours their precipitation and calculus formation and possible obstruction to urinary flow. Conditions favourable to their formation include hypercalcaemia, as occurs with hyperparathyroidism, excessive vitamin D, an excessive ingestion of milk or an alkali and prolonged immobilization. Other causes are hyperuricaemia associated with gout (an error in uric acid metabolism), cystinuria, resulting from a genetic metabolic disorder in which cystine and other amino acids are excreted in excess by the kidneys, dehydration, a highly acid urine and infection by Proteus (gram-negative bacteria usually associated with faeces). Proteus infection changes the urine to alkaline; this results in the precipitation of phosphates, forming what may be referred to as a struvite calculus.

SYMPTOMS

The manifestations of renal calculus depend upon the size of the stone and whether it remains stationary. It may remain latent over a long period, producing no symptoms. Small, gravel-like stones may be passed without any disturbance.

The majority cause some pain, haematuria, infection and, if large, kidney damage and renal insufficiency. Renal calculi may obstruct renal drainage by impaction of the tubules, by completely filling calyces and the pelvis, or by lodging in a ureter. The urine accumulates in the pelvis and tubules, dilating them and creating a back pressure; this condition is known as *hydronephrosis*. Compression of the blood vessels and nephrons by the mass of fluid leads to their destruction and obliteration and to renal insufficiency.

The patient may complain of pain in the back which may be caused by irritation of tissues by movement of the stone or the back pressure and accumulation of fluid if the stone is obstructing renal or ureteral outflow. A small stone may enter the

ureter and initiate *ureteric colic*. The patient complains of excruciating pain radiating from the back to the front along the groin into the genitalia. He becomes pale, sweats, is extremely restless and may vomit. Frequently he thrashes about, assuming unusual positions in an attempt to obtain some relief.

Haematuria results from injury to the membranous lining of the pelvis or ureter. Infection is frequently associated with a calculus and, if present, chills, fever, leucocytosis and pyuria are likely to be manifested.

Complete obstruction of the kidney outflow is eventually reflected in renal insufficiency and a palpable mass in the renal area as a result of the hydronephrosis. The total volume of urine is less than normal, and blood investigations indicate reduced elimination of waste products.

Investigation of the patient for nephrolithiasis includes a simple radiological study of the kidneys, ureters and bladder. Preparation for this x-ray usually involves an aperient the night before the x-ray followed by an enema in the morning. This is to prevent shadows on the film caused by faeces and gas in the intestine. Calcium, phosphate and cystine calculi will show up as dense areas. More detailed information is then obtained from intravenous urography (see p. 696). Uric acid stones are seen only following contrast injection. Serum calcium and uric acid levels are determined and renal function tests may be done (for the latter, see p. 695). Investigation includes examination of the urine for crystals, 24- or 48-hour serial pH analysis in which the pH of each voiding is recorded, and 24-hour quantitative calcium and magnesium determination.

TREATMENT AND NURSING INTERVENTION

If the urogram indicates that the calculus is small and may be passed by the patient, he is allowed up and encouraged to be active. Liberal amounts of fluids are given. All urine is strained through several layers of gauze or a filter paper and is observed. All sediment or solid particles passed are saved and submitted for identification of their composition.

During an attack of ureteric colic, the patient usually receives an analgesic, such as pethidine, to relieve the pain, and an antiemetic. When the pain subsides, he is allowed to rest in bed and encouraged to drink.

If the calculus is in the lower third of the ureter, a special ureteric catheter with a looped or corkscrew tip may be passed and an attempt made to withdraw the stone. This procedure is referred to as 'removal by instrumentation'.

When a stone in the kidney or ureter is too large to be passed, open surgery may be undertaken. Removal of a stone through the renal parenchyma is called a *nephrolithotomy*. Removal of a stone directly from the renal pelvis is known as a *pyelolithotomy*. The operation for extracting a stone from the ureter is a *ureterolithotomy*. If the calculus is in the lower part of the ureter, it is approached through an abdominal incision. When it is lodged in the upper part of the ureter, the approach is through an incision in the flank. For the nursing care of a patient undergoing renal surgery, see pp. 742–749.

More recently, renal calculi have been treated by lithotripsy. Electroshock waves are directed by a special machine (a lithotriptor) into the area of the stone. The calculus is broken up into small particles. The patient is then required to ingest a large quantity of fluid for several days to wash out the stone particles. Renal colic may be experienced intermittently for several days while the stone fragments are passed.

Calculi are prone to recur in patients with a history of previous episodes. In an effort to prevent the formation of new stones or the enlargement of existing stones, the pH of the urine is controlled according to the type of stone involved by a special diet and medication, and measures are used to eliminate any known or suspected infection. For the latter, an antibiotic or sulphonamide preparation is prescribed.

The patient is advised that a high fluid intake of at least 3000 ml daily is essential to maintain a dilute urine. A portion of this should be taken at bedtime and during the night to prevent the concentration of urine that normally occurs at night. If the climate or patient's occupation are such that there is an excessive loss of fluid in sweat, the intake should be increased by 1000 ml.

If the principal calculus component is calcium the prescribed diet is low in calcium and vitamin D. If the stone is of calcium phosphate, acidification of the urine with three to four glasses of cranberry juice daily is recommended. If uric acid is involved, alkalinization of the urine is important. Solubility is promoted by the administration of sodium bicarbonate or a citrate mixture. The pH of the urine is monitored and an effort made to maintain it at a level above 6.5. Allopurinol is prescribed to lower the serum uric acid level.

The formation of cystine stones is usually seen in children. Alkalinization of the urine and a diet low in methionine are recommended. For details as to the foods which are high and low in the different substances involved in calculus formation, the reader is referred to a diet therapy or urology text. A problem in relation to dietary restriction is that most stones are of mixed composition.

If the patient should become ill, prolonged immobility should be avoided. The patient is seen at frequent intervals by his doctor and closely monitored.

Neoplasms in the kidneys

Neoplasms in the adult kidney are of lower incidence than those in many other areas of the body. When they occur, they are usually malignant and are seen more often in males than in females. The most common form in adults is adenocarcinoma, which usually originates in the tubules. It readily invades the blood vessels, causing early metastases to bones, lungs or liver, which may be the lesion that brings the person to the doctor. Wilms' tumour is a highly malignant adenosarcoma which occurs in young children and may grow very large before being discovered.

MANIFESTATIONS

In the adult, the first symptom is usually haematuria. As the neoplasm enlarges, the kidney becomes a palpable mass and the patient experiences pain, abdominal discomfort from pressure, anorexia and loss of weight. Ureteric colic may occur as a result of a blood clot entering the ureter. Polycythaemia develops in some patients due to an overproduction of erythropoietin by the affected kidney. Others may have marked anaemia. In children, the neoplasm is frequently noted first as an abdominal mass or swelling by the mother.

A cystoscopy with ureteric catheterization is done to determine if the source of the bleeding is unilateral or bilateral. Radiological studies are made, using an intravenous or retrograde pyelogram to determine filling defects and the location of the neoplasm. A renal angiogram may also be done to assess the extent of blood vessel involvement.

TREATMENT

If the disease is localized to one kidney, a nephrectomy is performed, followed by radiation or chemotherapy or both. If the renal pelvis is involved, the ureter is removed along with the kidney (*nephroureterectomy*). For nursing care required following renal surgery, see pp. 742–744. When both kidneys are affected or the patient's condition is considered inoperable, radiation may be used. Chemotherapy is rarely effective. For the care of the patient receiving radiation and anticancer drug therapy, see Chapter 9.

Polycystic disease of the kidneys

This disorder is characterized by the widespread distribution of cysts of varying sizes throughout both kidneys. The disease is congenital and familial and affects both sexes. It is predominant in infants and adults over 40 years of age. In infants and young children, other abnormalities may be present. The disease is often found in more than one member of the family and in successive generations. Because of the distinct difference in the age of the groups in which the disease is manifested, it is suggested that there are two different genetic types. When it occurs in infants and young children, it is considered to be autosomal recessive, but the polycystic disease which becomes manifest in adults is autosomal dominant.

The adult form is more common and progresses slowly; the patient remains asymptomatic during the first three to four decades of life. As the cysts enlarge, functional tissue and blood vessels are compressed and, eventually, serious renal insufficiency develops. Pressure on abdominal viscera may interfere with normal functioning and cause discomfort. The symptoms are intermittent gross haematuria from the rupture of blood vessels, pain in the back and abdomen and a palpable mass. The patient may experience episodes of ureteric colic due to blood clots entering the ureters. The degree of compression and damage of parenchymal tissue by the cysts determines the length of survival of the kidneys. With progression of the disease, he gradually manifests signs of increasing renal failure. The blood pressure and blood nitrogenous waste levels rise, electrolyte and fluid imbalances and anaemia develop, and the patient eventually develops end-stage renal failure.

Conservative treatment of the patient is similar to that for chronic renal failure. The patient may be maintained and kept active by regular haemodialysis and is considered a candidate for renal transplantation.

Since polycystic disease of the kidneys is an inherited disorder, when a patient is discovered to be affected, other members of his family should seriously consider whether they wish to be screened. There is no treatment for polycystic disease as nothing can arrest the progression but confirmation of the condition may adversely affect an individual's career prospects. Regular monitoring and control of blood pressure is essential for all those possibly affected. Screening is advisable when pregnancy is being considered so that a couple may decide whether to risk having an affected child.

Trauma of the kidneys

Accidental blows and injury to a kidney are not uncommon and may cause contusion or laceration or rupture of the capsule. In laceration and rupture, haemorrhage and the escape of urine into the surrounding tissues are serious problems. Gross or microscopic haematuria occurs and there is pain and tenderness in the kidney region. If the injury is severe and massive haemorrhage occurs, shock develops rapidly. Blood transfusions are given, and surgical intervention is used promptly to bring the bleeding under control. The kidney may be repaired, or a partial or complete nephrectomy may be necessary, depending on the damage revealed.

Contusion of the kidney will usually heal spontaneously. The patient is kept at rest, the fluid intake and output are recorded, and a frequent check is made of the urine for blood. If the damage is extensive, nephrons may be replaced by fibrous scar tissue, resulting in residual impaired function and renal hypertension.

NURSING IN RENAL SURGERY

The more common surgical procedures used in the treatment of kidney disease include the following: *nephrectomy* (the removal of a kidney – may be partial or complete), *nephrolithotomy* (the removal of a calculus from the parenchymal portion of the kidney), *pyelolithotomy* (the removal of a calculus through an incision into the renal pelvis), *nephrostomy* (an incision into the kidney and the insertion of a tube for drainage), and *nephroureterectomy* (the removal of a kidney and its ureter).

Preoperative preparation

Surgery on a kidney is preceded by a period of investigation of kidney function and the patient's general condition. If a nephrectomy is anticipated, the ability of the opposite kidney to compensate and assume the full responsibility for renal function must be determined. The patient and his family are generally very apprehensive of this major surgery. Aware of this, the nurse observes their behaviour to determine their level of anxiety, concerns, and the reassurance needed. By showing an interest in them, providing opportunities for them to express their feelings, answering their questions and explaining what may be expected, the nurse helps to reduce the patient's and family's anxiety and promotes their confidence in those responsible for his care. They are advised by the surgeon that the removal of the kidney is necessary but need reassurance that normal function can be maintained by one kidney.

The physical preparation is similar to that cited in Chapter 11. Unless contraindicated by a condition such as uraemia, the fluid intake is increased to promote the maximum excretion of metabolic wastes before surgery as well as optimal hydration. Since the incision is usually made in the flank of the affected side, the surgery will be performed with the patient in a hyperextended side-lying position which may produce muscular aches postoperatively. A nasogastric tube may be passed at operation because renal surgical patients are prone to develop a reduction or cessation of peristalsis and severe abdominal distension. Table 21.12 outlines a care plan for a patient following renal surgery.

Disorders of the Postrenal Urinary System (Bladder, Ureters and Urethra)

Normally, the adult voids approximately 5 or 6 times daily; the volume of urine is in proportion to the fluid intake and losses by other channels (e.g. skin, intestine). The average daily output is 1200–1800 ml. The person is able to initiate voiding voluntarily and micturition occurs without discomfort.

Table 21.12 Care plan for the patient following renal surgery.

Problem	Goals	Nursing intervention	Expected outcomes
1 Alterations in pattern of urinary elimination related to renal surgery and possibly urethral catheter	To maintain adequate urinary output	**a** The volume of urinary drainage from the indwelling catheter is noted every hour in the immediate postoperative period **b** The urine is checked for signs of blood and sediment **c** Urine drainage from a nephrostomy tube is measured and recorded as part of the urinary output **d** An accurate record of the daily fluid intake and output and the patient's weight is made and fluid balance determined	1 Urinary output is greater than 30–50 ml/h 2 Haematuria is absent after the first few days
2 Ineffective airway clearance related to pain from incision and possible removal of 12th rib	To maintain respiratory function	**a** The patient is assisted to perform deep breathing and coughing **b** Medication for pain is offered prior to deep breathing and the affected side is 'splinted' with hands and a pillow while the patient breathes deeply and coughs 8–10 times **c** The patient is assisted to turn every few hours. The patient may be on either side unless a nephrostomy tube is in place **d** With each change of position, avoid displacing the drainage tube or leaving it compressed, kinked or with traction on it **e** Encourage ambulation by the first postoperative day	1 Crackles and wheezes are absent on auscultation of the chest 2 Respirations are symmetrical, rhythmic and regular
3 Alteration in comfort: pain related to surgical incision and abdominal distension	To minimize the pain	**a** Analgesics are administered every 3–4 hours for the first few days. Medications should be given before pain becomes severe **b** The patient is assisted to turn every 2 hours and to walk to a chair to relieve muscle tension and discomfort from the hyperextended lateral position used during surgery **c** The patient is assessed for return of bowel sounds, passage of flatus and abdominal distension **d** Early ambulation is encouraged	1 Episodes of severe pain do not occur 2 Bowel sounds are present, flatus is passed and abdominal distension is absent
4 Alteration in nutrition and fluids: less than body requirements related to surgical intervention and abdominal distension	To maintain fluid balance and nutritional status	**a** The patient is sustained by intravenous infusions for 36–48 hours. Serum electrolyte determinations and the fluid balance serve as a guide to the volume and composition of the fluids used **b** Oral intake is resumed when intestinal peristalsis is established **c** Clear fluids may then be given orally in small amounts and increased gradually as tolerated **d** Solid food is introduced when tolerated	1 The patient's weight is stable at usual weight
5 Impairment of skin integrity related to surgical intervention	To promote wound healing	**a** The operative site is checked at frequent intervals for bleeding. If the kidney was removed, the wound may be sealed with only a tissue drain inserted. If the kidney remains, a tube may have	1 The incision is clean, dry and intact 2 Drainage is absent after a few days

Table 21.12—*continued*

Problem	Goals	Nursing intervention	Expected outcomes
5 Impairment of skin integrity (continued)		been inserted, necessitating frequent observation for patency and characteristics of the drainage **b** The tube may become obstructed by a clot, causing back pressure unless promptly cleared. Irrigation with a small amount (approximately 10 ml) of sterile normal saline may be ordered to remove clots **c** If the tube is connected to a drainage receptacle, the amount is measured and recorded every 4 hours **d** The dressing is observed for drainage which may be extensive following renal surgery except after nephrectomy **e** Moist dressings are changed frequently **f** The incision is assessed for redness and drainage	
6 Inadequate knowledge about post-hospital care	To develop a plan for follow-up care	**a** Necessary limitations of activity, any dietary restriction, and the optimal fluid intake are discussed in detail with the patient and a family member before hospital discharge **b** If the wound still requires a dressing, the patient and a family member are taught how to care for it, or a referral is made to a district nurse	**1** The patient and family understand how to perform self care at home and where to seek advice

DISORDERS OF THE BLADDER

Cystitis

This is an acute or chronic inflammation of the urinary bladder characterized by frequency, urgency, dysuria and abnormal urinary constituents. It is most often due to infection caused by the ascent of organisms by way of the urethra, but it may also be associated with the administration of certain drugs (e.g. cyclophosphamide) and radiation therapy of the lower abdomen. Predisposing factors in infective cystitis are trauma of the tissues, stagnation of the urine, and distortion or compression of the bladder by an enlarged neighbouring organ. The latter condition is a factor in the cystitis that not infrequently develops in the pregnant woman, especially in the last trimester; the enlarging uterus compresses the bladder. Cystitis has a higher incidence in females; this is attributed to the shorter urethra of a relatively wide calibre. Organisms from rectal and vaginal discharge can enter readily. In the male, it is usually secondary to prostatic hyperplasia or infection or to congenital malformation (e.g. hypospadias).

The inflammation is generally confined to the mucosa and submucosa which are hyperaemic and oedematous. Scattered haemorrhagic areas are present, and small ulcerative lesions may develop as a result of sloughing of the lining tissue. The urine contains blood cells, pus, bacteria and mucus. If cystitis becomes chronic, the inflammation may extend into the detrusor muscle. Fibrosis of the tissues occurs with persisting inflammation, which reduces the bladder capacity and increases the problem of frequency.

TREATMENT

In some instances, cystitis is of brief duration, being resolved spontaneously. There is always the danger that the infection may ascend via the ureters and cause pyelonephritis. The infection is treated by the administration of an antibiotic or urinary antiseptic such as co-trimoxazole or amoxycillin. A urine specimen obtained before any antimicrobial drug is given may be cultured to determine the infective organism and its drug sensitivity. A specific antibiotic may then be ordered. Sodium bicarbonate or sodium citrate may also be prescribed for the purpose of making the urine alkaline to decrease the bladder irritation and dysuria. Warm baths may reduce bladder spasm and provide considerable relief. The patient is encouraged to drink liberal amounts of fluids which should include citrus fruit juices.

If the condition persists, the cystitis is suspected of being secondary. The patient is then investigated for a primary condition which might be pyelonephritis, a bladder calculus, urethral stricture or, in the case of the male, an enlarged prostate.

Since cystitis is frequently the result of an ascending infection and occurs readily in females, good personal hygiene and efficient cleansing of the perineum, especially after defecation, are extremely important and require emphasis in health teaching. Adequate cleansing is often very difficult for the ill person who is weak or handicapped and confined to bed. It becomes the nurse's responsibility to see that the patient is thoroughly cleansed.

Bladder calculi

Stones in the urinary bladder are rare. They nearly always form as a result of urinary stasis as occurs in prostatic hypertrophy, neurological disease or injury that has resulted in the loss of voluntary bladder control or interruption of the sacral reflex arc, bladder diverticula, urethral stricture or prolonged immobility. They can also be caused by the presence of an indwelling catheter for a prolonged period of time.

The patient may complain of sudden cessation of the urinary flow before the bladder is emptied which is due to occlusion of the bladder-urethral orifice by the calculus. He may find that he is able to void only in certain positions, which are those that keep the stone away from the outlet. Irritation of the mucosa by the stone may result in haematuria, and infection is usually present. Small fragments of bone may pass into the urethra and become lodged there, causing urinary obstruction and severe pain. A bladder calculus may be recognized on an x-ray film of the bladder or visualized by cystoscopy (see p. 696). The stone(s) may be removed by mechanical crushing of the stone or ultrasonic lithotripsy may be used to crush the calculus. For nursing care following a cystotomy, (see pp. 748–751). The patient is given large amounts of fluids to help wash out the bladder.

The condition causing the stasis of urine which promotes calculi formation should be treated to avoid recurrence. If the patient has an obstructing prostate, it may be removed at the same time that the stone is removed. Patients who are immobilized must be turned and moved about frequently; a bed that can be tilted at different angles may be used. The patient who spends most of his day immobile in a wheelchair is equally as susceptible as the bed patient and should receive attention.

Bladder injury

Accidental injury of the urinary bladder, causing perforation and ensuing extravasation of the urine (escape of urine from the bladder), is not uncommon. It may occur when the pelvis is fractured or as a result of direct blows to the lower abdomen. If the bladder is full and distended at the time of accident, it is more vulnerable.

If the laceration occurs in the upper portion, the rupture is intraperitoneal. Urine escapes into the peritoneal cavity and produces peritonitis. The patient becomes shocked (see Chapter 15) and experiences abdominal pain and tenderness, with a rigid distended abdomen and usually a paralytic ileus (see Chapter 17).

Rupture of the lower part of the bladder is usually extraperitoneal; urine escapes into the surrounding tissues, and infection, cellulitis and necrosis of tissue may ensue. Occasionally an abdominal or perineal fistula develops.

When there is a history of an injury or blow to the lower abdomen followed by pain and tenderness, injury to the bladder is suspected. A urine specimen is obtained promptly, either by having the patient void or passing a catheter, to determine if there is haematuria. If blood is present in the urine, a cystogram may be done to confirm the diagnosis and locate the laceration.

TREATMENT

The injury is a serious threat to life and requires prompt treatment. The shock and haemorrhage are treated with a blood transfusion and intravenous infusions. An indwelling catheter is inserted into the bladder, and the patient is prepared for abdominal surgery. The site of injury is repaired and a temporary cystostomy (incision of the bladder and introduction of a suprapubic catheter) done to establish urinary drainage and prevent the possibility of pressure on the repair suture line. If the rupture was intraperitoneal, the extravasated fluid is aspirated before closure.

Following surgery, the patient is observed closely for signs of infection. Antibiotics may be administered immediately. An accurate record of the fluid intake and all drainage is very important. (See section on nursing care of the patient having had a cystostomy, pp. 748–751). For the care of the patient with peritonitis and paralytic ileus, (see Chapter 17).

Exstrophy of the bladder

This is a developmental defect in which the anterior wall of the bladder has failed to fuse. The degree of failure of fusion varies. The opening may be small, forming a fistula that opens and drains urine onto the external surface of the abdomen, or the entire anterior bladder wall may be absent, accompanied by a wide defect in the abdominal wall, resulting in full exposure of the bladder interior. Urine spurts onto the abdominal wall from the ureters. The more extensive defects are nearly always associated with other anomalies in the genitourinary system. The pelvic bones may fail to meet to form the symphysis pubis. Epispadias (absence of the anterior wall of the male urethra) is a frequent counterpart. In the female, the urethra may be lacking. Exstrophy of the bladder is more common in males than females.

Infection of the bladder usually supervenes and may extend to the kidneys, seriously impairing their function. The corrective procedure used depends on the extent of the malformation and concomitant defects. If the exstrophy is not extensive, the bladder opening and the abdominal fistula are closed. If the defect is extensive, permanent urinary diversion may be undertaken (see pp. 747–754). The defective bladder is removed and the abdominal wall repaired. The surgery is usually undertaken early in the child's life in order to prevent kidney infection and chronic renal failure.

Bladder neoplasms

Neoplasms in the bladder may develop at any age but occur more frequently after the age of 50 and have a high incidence in males. The majority arise from the epithelial lining as papillomas and may be benign or malignant. Those that are benign and recur tend to become malignant eventually. Others appear as ulcers which are usually malignant and are more invasive of deeper tissue layers. Prolonged occupational exposure to aniline dyes is recognized as a predisposing factor. It is recommended that the period of working with these chemicals should be limited to 3 years and that during this period such persons should have routine Papanicolaou smears (Pap tests) made of the urine. Workers are also advised of the importance of prompt reporting of any blood in the urine or slight bladder irritation. Smoking has also been cited as a predisposing cause of bladder cancer.

The first symptom is usually intermittent painless haematuria, or cystitis may be the initial factor that brings the patient to his general practitioner. The lesion may encroach on the urethral orifice, giving rise to hesitancy and a decreased force and calibre of the urinary stream. Suprapubic pain and a palpable mass generally indicate that the condition is in an advanced stage. The patient may experience pain in the flank region if the growth obstructs a ureteral orifice which causes hydronephrosis. The lesion ulcerates, which accounts for the haematuria, and readily becomes infected. If the infection is severe and anaemia has developed, the patient manifests weakness and loss of weight.

Diagnostic procedures include a cystoscopy and biopsy. A cystogram will identify filling defects of the bladder and CAT scans and ultrasound examination of the pelvis may be done. Cytological studies may also be made of a urine specimen.

TREATMENT

The treatment used depends upon whether the neoplasm is benign or malignant and, in the case of malignancy, upon the stage and the depth of the tissue involved. Surgery, radiation, chemotherapy, or a combination of these may be used. Small papillomatous growths may be treated by transurethral resection followed by electrocoagulation of the base tissue. An indwelling catheter is inserted in the bladder on completion of the operation, and the urinary drainage is observed frequently for possible bleeding. Bladder spasm and irritability may cause considerable discomfort which may be reduced by a warm bath. The patient is encouraged to take a minimum of 2000 ml of fluids daily.

Since papillomas, benign as well as malignant, tend to recur, these patients are followed closely for 5–6 years. They are advised to report any bleeding or bladder irritability promptly. A cystoscopic examination is usually done every 3 months during the first year following the resection, every 6 months during the second year, and then annually for 3 or 4 years.

If the neoplasm is malignant, a segmental resection of the bladder or total cystectomy (removal of the bladder) may be done.

Segmental resection
A partial cystectomy is only used if the cancer is in the upper part of the bladder well above the urethral orifices. At operation, a tube or catheter is placed in the bladder and brought out through the incision, and an indwelling catheter is also introduced through the urethra. Removal of a part of the bladder obviously reduces its capacity. Adequate drainage in the postoperative period is necessary to prevent distension and possible disruption of the suture line. The tube in the incision may be connected to gentle intermittent suction. The length of time it remains in the bladder will depend on the rate of healing.

The urethral catheter usually remains in place for approximately 2–4 weeks. On its removal, frequency becomes a problem for the patient because of the reduced bladder capacity. He is likely to become discouraged and depressed at this time, and understanding support from the nurse is essential. He may attempt to reduce the frequency by cutting down his fluid intake, which must be guarded against. The importance of a minimum fluid intake of 2000 ml and the spacing of the fluids so the intervals between voiding may be increased during certain periods (e.g. at night) are discussed with him. The traumatized bladder gradually becomes less irritable and increases its capacity.

Cystectomy
A total cystectomy with ureteric transplantation for permanent urinary diversion is used when the cancer is situated in the lower part of the bladder or is quite extensive. Permanent urinary diversion may be achieved by cutaneous ureterostomy, ureterointestinal anastomosis, or the formation of an ileal conduit (Fig. 21.3).

In *cutaneous ureterostomy*, the detached ends of the ureters are brought through the abdominal wall and secured at skin level. This is rarely the procedure of choice. Maintaining the patency of the ureters is difficult because strictures tend to develop. If catheters are placed in the ureters to maintain drainage, they readily block and are difficult to keep in place.

Cutaneous ureterostomy

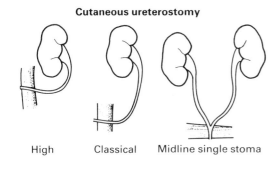

High   Classical   Midline single stoma

Ileal conduit

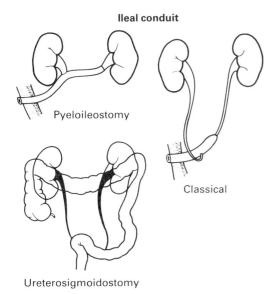

Pyeloileostomy

Classical

Ureterosigmoidostomy

Fig. 21.17 Methods of permanent supravesical diversion.

Chronic kidney infection is a frequent complication with subsequent renal failure.

Ureteroenterostomy
Ureteroenterostomy (*ureterosigmoidostomy*) provides a completely internal diversion. The ureters are implanted into the sigmoid colon and the urine and faeces leave the body via a common channel – the rectum and anus. The urine drainage from the ureters is retained in the lower bowel until approximately 200 ml accumulate. The 'defecation' impulse is initiated and the urine is expelled by voluntary relaxation of the anal sphincters. This is a more acceptable procedure to the patient; it provides continence and eliminates an abdominal orifice, skin problems and the constant use of special drainage appliances. Unfortunately, the direct connection with the bowel predisposes the patient to ascending infection of the kidneys and subsequent renal insufficiency and to disturbances in blood chemistry.

The latter are attributed to the absorption of substances from the accumulating urine in the intestine. Acidosis is a frequent problem, resulting from the reabsorption of chlorides.

The *ileal conduit* (*ureteroileostomy*) currently appears to be the procedure most favoured. A segment of the ileum with its mesentery and blood supply is removed. The open ends of the ileum left by the resection are anastomosed to re-establish intestinal continuity. One end of the resected ileal section is closed. The open end is brought through the abdominal wall to the skin surface and secured. The detached ends of the ureters are implanted in the ileal segment near its closed end.

For the nursing care of a patient with urinary diversion, see pages 748–754.

Radiation
Internal or external radiation may be used in treating cancer of the bladder. It may be used alone, as an adjunct to surgery, or with chemotherapy. Intracavitary radiation may be achieved by the enclosure of a radioisotope (e.g. Co^{60}, Au^{198}) in a catheter balloon which is placed within the bladder. The catheter is connected to a drainage receptacle, and all urine is saved and sent to the radioisotope department. In some instances, radon seeds or radiotantalum (Ta^{182}) needles may be implanted around the lesion. Safety precautions are necessary in the handling of these radioactive materials and are cited in Chapter 9. Internal radiation causes cystitis, and the patient usually experiences considerable bladder spasm and discomfort. Fluids are given freely and analgesics may be necessary. The application of heat over the bladder region may provide some relief.

External radiation therapy is usually reserved for those patients whose cancer is deeply invasive and highly malignant. When it is used, the patient is likely to experience some gastrointestinal disturbances (nausea, vomiting and diarrhoea) as well as cystitis, since the intestine proximal to the bladder will be exposed to the rays. For care of the patient receiving external radiation therapy, the reader is referred to Chapter 9.

In advanced carcinoma of the bladder and when metastases are suspected, chemotherapy may be used as well as surgery and irradiation (see Chapter 9).

BLADDER SURGERY

Operative procedures used in the treatment of bladder disease may be transurethral or by open surgery. Open surgery involves an incision through the abdominal wall. Transurethral operative procedures may be performed to obtain a biopsy, remove a neoplasm or calculus, or resect the prostate gland. The resectoscope, which is used to resect tissue, is similar to a cystoscope but has insulated walls and is equipped with a wire loop which is activated by a high frequency current to cut tissue and control haemorrhage by electrocoagulation (diathermy). The procedure is referred to as a transurethral resection (TUR). For resection of the prostate, see Chapter 23. A lithotrite, which is a special crushing instrument, is used to remove a stone, and the procedure is called litholapaxy.

Open surgery on the bladder may be undertaken for repair of a perforation or laceration, the removal of a neoplasm, calculus, or the prostate gland, or a segmental resection or removal of the bladder. The open operative procedures include *cystotomy* (an incision into the bladder and closure without a drainage tube), *cystostomy* (an incision into the bladder and the insertion of a drainage tube which is brought out on to the abdominal surface), *segmental resection* (the removal of a section of the bladder) and *total cystectomy* (the removal of the bladder, involving ureteral transplantation and urinary diversion). A suprapubic approach is most commonly used in open bladder surgery, with the bladder being opened below the peritoneum.

Nursing care of the patient having a cystotomy, cystostomy or segmental bladder resection

PREOPERATIVE PREPARATION

Unless the bladder is injured or there is acute retention that cannot be relieved by urethral catheterization, the patient who is to have bladder surgery usually undergoes several days of investigation and preparation. Kidney function is assessed and certain blood chemistry levels are determined (e.g. urea, creatinine, potassium, sodium, chloride, calcium). The urine is examined microscopically and, if infection is present, a urinary antiseptic or an antibiotic is prescribed. The patient is encouraged to take 2500–3000 ml of fluid daily unless a large amount of fluid is contraindicated by cardiac or renal insufficiency. The fluid intake and output are recorded and the balance noted. The patient's nutritional status frequently requires attention. Many of these patients are elderly and the existing condition may have contributed to their lack of interest in food, resulting in deficiencies. In encouraging the patient to take nourishment, its importance in his recovery is explained. Dietary adjustments and supplements may be necessary to meet his nutritional needs.

During the preparatory period, an indwelling catheter may be used to provide adequate drainage and reduce the residual urine. The patient is usually allowed to remain ambulatory. If there is an indwelling catheter, he is given a plastic drainage receptacle that may be attached to his thigh or gown while he is up. He should understand that it must be kept low enough to accommodate gravity drainage of the urine.

When the patient has been advised of the necessity for surgery, the nurse is alert to his need for psycho-

logical support. Opportunities are provided for him to express his feelings and concerns and to ask questions. He and his family are advised as to what may be expected following the operation. If the patient is to have a partial cystectomy, this explanation will include a discussion of the frequency of voiding that will be experienced when the tubes are removed because of the reduced capacity of the bladder. Reassurance is given that this gradually becomes less troublesome. If the period of waiting for the surgery is prolonged, some form of occupational therapy in which the patient is interested may be provided, and his family is encouraged to visit regularly. If the patient's anxiety is interfering with his rest and he is unable to sleep, the doctor is consulted and a sedative may be ordered.

The immediate preparation for open bladder surgery is similar to that for any patient having abdominal surgery (see Chapter 11). Skin preparations and shaving should extend from the lower costal margin to midthighs and include the perineal area. If the operation is scheduled for late in the morning or for the afternoon, an intravenous infusion may be given earlier in the day to prevent preoperative dehydration.

POSTOPERATIVE NURSING INTERVENTION

Preparation to receive the patient after operation includes the assembling of sterile tubing and drainage receptacles ready for prompt connection to an indwelling urethral catheter and a cystostomy tube. A tray of sterile equipment and solution (sterile water or normal saline) for irrigating the catheters in the event of obstruction by clots should be readily available. Nursing diagnoses and goals for the patient following a cystotomy, cystostomy or segmental bladder resection are listed in Table 21.13.

1. Maintenance of urinary elimination. The patient returns from the operating theatre with an indwelling urethral catheter which is secured to the upper thigh to prevent traction. It is connected to sterile tubing leading to a closed sterile drainage receptacle. The length of the tube should allow for turning and moving the patient without tension being exerted on the catheter. The excess tubing lies free on the bed and is secured so there is no loop between the bed and drainage receptacle; that is, the tube must hang straight from the edge of the bed for gravity drainage.

If there is a cystostomy as well, a tube is anchored in the bladder by a suture at the time of operation. This tube may be a special right-angled tube with a mushroom, winged or straight tip, or it may be a straight tube which requires a right-angled glass connecting tube. The cystostomy tube is attached to a sterile tube and receptacle, and the same precautions are necessary as those cited in the previous paragraph.

Table 21.13 Identification of problems relevant to the patient who has just had a cystotomy, cystostomy or segmental bladder resection.

Problem	Goals
1 Alteration in pattern of urinary elimination related to bladder incision, urethral catheter and cystostomy tube	To maintain urinary elimination
2 Ineffective airway clearance related to anaesthesia and decreased mobility	To maintain respiratory function
3 Impairment of skin integrity related to surgery and possible leakage of urine	To promote healing
4 Alteration in comfort: pain related to surgical intervention and bladder spasms	To control pain
5 Alteration in nutritional and fluid balance related to surgery and discomfort	To maintain nutritional status and fluid balance
6 Alteration in bowel elimination related to surgery and discomfort	To avoid straining at stool
7 Inadequate knowledge about fluid intake, catheter care and health supervision	To acquire knowledge, skill and resources to manage health care

Both drainage systems are checked frequently (at least hourly for the first 36–48 hours) for patency. The characteristics (colour, consistency, and content or sediment) of the drainage are noted at the same time. The urine will be blood-stained for the first 2–3 hours, gradually becoming lighter. The drainage is best examined at the glass or plastic connecting tubes before it becomes mixed with what is already in the receptacles.

The cystostomy tube, urethral catheter or tubing may become obstructed by a blood clot. The drainage system is checked for patency. If blockage of the tubing is indicated, it may be 'milked' or changed. If the obstruction is within the catheter tube in the bladder, an order may be given to irrigate with sterile normal saline. Fifty to 75 ml of the fluid are introduced; if the initial fluid does not return, no more fluid is instilled and the surgeon is consulted. Adequate postoperative drainage is very important to prevent bladder distension and pressure on the suture line.

The drainage from each system is measured and recorded every 4 hours. Care of the tubing and drainage bag varies with local policy. It may be replaced daily with a fresh sterile set or changed every second day or twice weekly.

The cystostomy tube usually remains in place from 4–7 days, depending on the patient's healing. The urethral catheter is generally left for a few days longer or until the incisional opening in the bladder heals. When the cystostomy tube is removed, some urine will escape onto the dressing for a few days until the fistula heals over.

Following the removal of the urethral catheter, a close check is made of the patient's frequency of voiding and the volume of the daily output for several days. If the patient is up and about, he is asked to record the necessary information. When a urethral catheter that has been in place for several days is removed, dribbling is a frequent problem because the bladder–urethral sphincters have been continuously dilated for a period of time. Frequent perineal exercises, which consist of contracting the abdominal, gluteal and perineal muscles while continuing to breathe normally, may help the sphincters recover their tone and control. Occasionally, a patient may not be able to void and catheterization may be performed if he has not voided within 8 hours.

A permanent cystostomy is sometimes done as a palliative measure for a patient who has an inoperable obstruction of the urethra (e.g. advanced carcinoma of the urethra, bladder neck or prostate). A urethral catheter is not inserted in this patient; bladder drainage is entirely dependent upon the cystostomy tube.

- *Assessment.* As well as frequent checking of the drainage system(s), the patient's blood pressure, pulse, colour and level of consciousness are noted and recorded at frequent intervals, which are gradually lengthened if the vital signs are satisfactory. Haemorrhage and shock are common complications following either transurethral resection or open bladder surgery. Bleeding may be evident in the drainage, but the dressing, surrounding skin areas and groins are also examined.

  The daily fluid intake and output are recorded for a longer period than with most surgical patients. The ratio of the intake to the output is examined by the nurse so that she is alert to possible renal insufficiency or retention of urine. The characteristics of the urine are noted for a period of 10–14 days. The appearance of sediment, blood, shreds of mucus-like material, cloudiness or the presence of an unusual odour is reported. Sloughing and ensuing bleeding may occur 8–10 days following the removal of a lesion.

2. Maintenance of airway clearance. The patient is urged to take five to ten deep breaths and cough every 1–2 hours to prevent pulmonary complications until he becomes ambulatory and active. Active flexion and extension of the feet and lower limbs are encouraged three or four times daily to prevent venous stasis. If these cannot be carried out actively, passive movement of the limbs through the normal range of motion is done by the nurse.

The patient is allowed out of bed as soon as his condition permits, and ambulation is encouraged to prevent complications. When the patient is up, the drainage tubes may be connected to smaller plastic receptacles which may be attached to the patient's thigh or dressing gown. When the patient becomes more independent in his activity, he must be advised that when he returns to bed, the drainage receptacle is transferred to the side of the bed in order to maintain gravity drainage.

3. *Impairment of skin-integrity.* Compared with other abdominal surgery, the dressing is changed earlier and more frequently for patients who have had open bladder surgery. There is almost certain to be some leakage of urine through the incision and around the tube. The skin is cleansed of urine frequently and is kept as dry as possible to prevent excoriation and infection. Following each cleansing, an application of a protective preparation such as petroleum jelly, zinc oxide ointment or karaya gum powder is made to the skin. The lower back, buttocks, groin, inner thighs and perineum are examined each time the dressing is changed. If any areas are moist with urine drainage, they are washed and thoroughly dried to prevent excoriation. The bedding is changed as often as is necessary to ensure dryness and comfort.

4. *Control of pain.* Bladder trauma and irritation cause bladder spasms which are very painful, and the patient may also experience the desire to void frequently, even though the bladder is emptied by tube drainage. In the case of the sensation of frequency, it may be necessary to explain to the patient that the bladder is empty and that trying to void only increases bladder spasms and pain. An analgesic such as morphine or pethidine is usually necessary at intervals during the first 48 hours. If the pain and discomfort persist, the surgeon is consulted. Either the catheter or cystostomy tube may require adjusting to relieve the contact and pressure of its tip on the bladder wall.

5. *Maintenance of fluid balance and nutrition.* A daily fluid intake of at least 2500–3000 ml (unless contraindicated by other coexisting disease) is necessary to ensure adequate irrigation of the bladder as well as to maintain satisfactory hydration. Most of it usually has to be administered by intravenous infusion the first day or two. A soft diet is given and is progressively increased to a regular diet as tolerated.

6. *Maintenance of bowel elimination.* The patient may be given a mild laxative after 2 days, or an enema may be given. Constipation and straining at stool are prevented, since they tend to increase the patient's pain.

7. *Patient education.* Most patients who have had a cystotomy or cystostomy remain in the hospital until the wound is healed and normal micturition is re-established. The nurse discusses the resumption of their previous activities with them and explains any restrictions indicated by the doctor. They are advised to continue taking a minimum of 2000–2500 ml of fluid daily. Some may require reassurance that no special care of the wound is necessary and that they may resume baths.

If the cystostomy is permanent or a urethral catheter is to remain in place, the patient and a family member are given detailed instruction about the necessary care. This instruction is given over several days and should be completed soon enough for the patient to carry out the care himself before going home. This gives him confidence and provides the opportunity to clarify certain points. Verbal and written instructions will include an explanation of the necessary equipment, its use and maintenance, how it may be acquired, and any precautions to be observed in its use. An inconspicuous, oval-shaped, plastic or rubber urinal (drainage receptacle) that may be strapped to the thigh is available. The inlet tube which is attached to the upper end of the bag is connected to the catheter or cystostomy tube by means of a plastic connecting tube. The other end of the urinal has a screw stopper or clamp which permits emptying of the bag into the toilet at necessary intervals. The importance of thorough washing of the hands with soap and running water before connecting or disconnecting the equipment is stressed to reduce the possibility of ascending infection. The patient and a relative are also taught how to anchor the tube that is in the patient to the abdomen or thigh to prevent traction on it.

The bag and tubing are cleansed daily with a detergent and warm water, flushed with vinegar thoroughly rinsed with water, and aired. They are advised to have two sets, if possible, so that one set may be well aired after the cleansing. This helps to prevent odour which could cause considerable embarrassment and discouragement for the patient. The patient is reminded of the need to continue taking at least 2000–2500 ml of fluid daily to provide adequate bladder irrigation. Odour is likely to be less of a problem with more dilute urine, and there is less danger of infection with constant washing out of the bladder.

A referral may be made to the district nurse for assistance and supervision when the patient goes home. This is likely to be needed when the patient is elderly and finds it difficult to cope with the necessary care. The patient and family are advised how often the bladder tube or catheter is to be changed at the clinic or by the general practitioner and of the need to contact the general practitioner promptly if the tube slips out of the bladder.

Expected outcomes
1 The volume of urinary output is in balance with fluid intake.
2 Respirations are regular, rhythmic and symmetrical.

3 Crackles and wheezes are absent on chest auscultation.

4 The surgical incision is clean, dry and intact.

5 Episodes of severe pain are absent.

6 Bladder spasms and irritation decrease in severity and frequency.

7 The patient's weight is maintained at his usual weight.

8 Bowel function is maintained.

9 Straining at stool does not occur.

10 The patient and family understand how to manage convalescence.

The cystectomy and ureteral transplantation patient

Complete removal of the bladder necessitates establishing a new urinary outlet; this may be achieved by cutaneous ureterostomy, ureteroenterostomy (ureterosigmoidostomy) or ileal conduit (ureteroileostomy). For a description of these procedures, see page 747.

Following operation, the patient who undergoes a cystectomy and ureteral transplant is seriously ill. The amount of surgery usually involved predisposes the patient to severe shock. Frequently, considerable surrounding tissue is resected with the bladder (e.g. lymphatics, prostate gland), and if the ileal conduit procedure is used, an intestinal resection and anastomosis are done. The patient will have a large vertical or transverse incision through which the bladder is removed, the ureters are freed for transplant, and the intestine is resected. The stoma through which the urine will drain is made separately in the right abdominal wall. Care of the patient requires consideration of the needs incurred by the cystectomy, the intestinal surgery, the ureteric transplantation and urinary diversion as well as the individual patient's psychological and physiological responses to such radical surgery.

PREOPERATIVE PREPARATION

The operative procedure and the permanent change in urinary drainage that will ensue are explained to the patient and his family by the surgeon and the stoma therapist. This is likely to produce considerable anxiety and despair and will prompt many questions. The nurse observes the patient closely for his reactions and conveys her acceptance and appreciation of his concerns. Opportunities are provided for him and his family to express their feelings and ask questions and, when they are ready, the necessary adjustments and care associated with urinary diversion are outlined in simple terms. They are told that a relatively normal, active life is possible. This may be reinforced by having a person who has had a permanent urinary diversion and has made a successful adjustment talk with them. If such a person is not available, someone with an ileostomy may prove helpful. The nurse who is willing to take time

to talk freely with the patient, help him to make plans for his future, and is patient in repeating answers and reinforcing what has probably already been said can provide immeasurable support. A rapport is developed that contributes to acceptance of the situation and the development of positive attitudes on the part of the patient and family.

There will be several days of investigation and preparation. Kidney function is assessed and the blood levels of nitrogenous wastes, potassium, sodium and chloride are determined. The patient usually receives a blood transfusion during and probably following the surgery, so typing and cross matching are necessary. At least 2500 ml of fluid daily are given unless contraindicated by cardiac insufficiency or urinary obstruction.

If the intestine is to be entered, the patient receives a low-residue diet for 3 or 4 days, then clear fluids only for 2 days before operation to reduce the faecal content. The reasons for these restrictions are explained in order to gain the patient's cooperation and acceptance. Laxatives and enemas are also used for cleansing purposes, and a course of an antimicrobial drug that is poorly absorbed from the gastrointestinal tract is given orally to destroy intestinal organisms (e.g. silver sulphadiazine, neomycin). The skin preparation includes the abdomen, upper thighs and perineum. A nasogastric tube is passed at the operation to provide drainage of secretions and prevent intestinal distension after the surgery. The remainder of the preparation is similar to that for any major abdominal surgery (see Chapter 11).

The operation is a lengthy procedure; if the members of the family decide to go home, they are assured that they will be called as soon as the operation is over and advised of the patient's condition. If they choose to remain in the hospital, they are directed to a room where they may wait. A brief visit with them at intervals by the nurse and suggestions made as to where they may have a cup of coffee or lunch are appreciated and indicate a sympathetic understanding of their anxiety and concern.

MANAGEMENT OF THE PATIENT WITH A URETEROILEAL CONDUIT

Preparation to receive the patient after operation includes the assembling of a sterile urinary drainage receptacle with tubing, gastrointestinal suction machine, intravenous infusion standard, sterile irrigation equipment and sterile normal saline.

A large part of the required care is essentially the same as that for any patient having an intestinal resection, cited in Chapter 17). Table 21.14 lists nursing diagnoses and goals relevant to the patient with a ureteroileal conduit.

1. *Maintenance of urinary elimination.* On completion of the operation a disposable plastic ileostomy bag is secured to the skin around the stoma by means of an

Table 21.14 Identification of problems relevant to the patient with a ureteroileal conduit.

Problem	Goals
1 Alteration in pattern of urinary elimination related to formation of a ureteroileal conduit	To maintain urinary elimination
2 Potential impairment of skin integrity (stoma and peristomal skin) due to surgical intervention and irritation	1 To maintain integrity of stoma and peristomal skin 2 To prevent infection
3 Alteration in mobility related to surgical intervention and pain	To maintain physical function
4 Alteration in nutrition and fluid balance related to surgery on intestine, bladder and ureters	To maintain nutritional status and fluid balance
5 Inadequate knowledge about care of stoma and peristomal skin, changes and care of appliance, identification of potential problems, daily fluid intake, sources of equipment and supplies	To acquire knowledge, skills and resources to manage health-care regimen

adhesive disk. The lower end of the bag is then connected to the tubing and drainage receptacle. With this arrangement, the ileostomy bag is examined when checking the drainage. The bag may require moving to empty any accumulation of urine into the lower bag. A cessation of drainage may indicate occlusion of the stoma by mucus or by swelling and oedema of the tissues, and the surgeon is notified immediately. A sterile catheter may be inserted periodically to determine if there is residual urine. The temporary ileostomy bag is changed during the first 24 hours to examine the stoma and surrounding skin. Once the oedema subsides and the stoma shrinks, the patient is fitted with a permanent ileostomy which may be left in place for 5–7 days.

2. Maintenance of integrity of stoma and peristomal skin. When the bag is removed, the stoma is covered with sterile wipes while the skin is gently washed and thoroughly dried. The skin is likely to show some irritation, particularly during the first few weeks. A protective coating of Stomahesive or karaya gum powder may be applied after each cleansing and before a new bag is applied. If excoriation of the skin persists or is severe, the fit of the face-plate is checked and the appliance is changed more frequently. The stoma is inspected regularly for signs of oedema, bleeding, other drainage or discoloration.

Abdominal pain, distension or rigidity, nausea, vomiting or fever is reported promptly. Any of these symptoms may indicate peritonitis, resulting from the escape of intestinal content from the site of the intestinal anastomosis or from a leakage of urine from the ileal conduit or ureters into the peritoneal

cavity. The nurse is also constantly alert for a positive fluid balance, fever and any complaint of back pain, which might indicate renal infection or insufficiency. Ureteric infection is prevented by maintaining a high fluid intake, regular emptying of the drainage appliance and use of a bedside drainage bag at night.

3. Maintenance of mobility and physical function. The patient is turned every 1–2 hours. Since the ileal conduit opens onto the right side of the abdomen, more complete drainage occurs when he is on his right side or back with the trunk elevated. With each change of position, the bag and tubing are checked for any kinks or compression.

Early ambulation is encouraged to foster adequate drainage and prevent complications. The plastic drainage receptacle may be carried by the nurse or may be attached to the patient's gown. If an ileostomy bag is applied to the stoma, the drainage tube may be detached while the patient is out of bed.

4. Maintenance of nutritional status and fluid balance. The nasogastric tube remains in place for 3–4 days and the patient is given intravenous fluids. The patient is observed for any signs of distension. Small amounts of water are given and the tube is clamped. If the water is tolerated and bowel sounds indicate the re-establishment of peristalsis, and there is no distension, the nasogastric tube is removed. The intake of clear fluids is gradually increased and the diet progresses through soft foods to a light solid diet. Gas-forming foods are avoided for 4 to 6 weeks and then added gradually as tolerated.

5. Patient education. The patient and a family member are taught the care of the stoma, skin and appliance following the same plan as that outlined under instruction of the ileostomy patient in Chapter 17. Emphasis is placed on the precautionary measures necessary to prevent infection. The patient should have his permanent appliance and the opportunity to develop complete familiarity with the necessary care, before being discharged from the hospital. During this period, he is advised of the importance of continuing a daily intake of 2500 to 3000 ml to keep the ureters and ileal conduit patent. The patient and family are cautioned that the doctor is to be consulted immediately if there is a decrease in urinary drainage, abnormal constituents such as blood in urine, fever, pain in the back or abdomen, severe skin excoriation or general malaise. The patient is followed closely after hospital discharge. A referral may be made to the district nurse, and the patient is seen at regular intervals at the clinic or by his general practitioner. These visits may be frequent at first, and the intervals are gradually increased to 3 to 6 months if the patient's progress is satisfactory.

Expected outcomes
1 The urinary output balances fluid intake.

2 The peristomal skin is clean, dry and intact.

3 The stoma is pink, moist and intact.

4 The ureters are patent and draining urine.

5 Signs of infection, pain, discomfort, elevated temperature, malaise and drainage are absent.

6 The patient is up and about.

7 The patient's weight is maintained at his usual level.

8 Fluid intake is 2500–3000 ml per day.

9 The patient and family demonstrate the ability to change and care for the appliance and peristomal skin.

10 The patient and family understand how to implement self-care following discharge.

THE PATIENT WITH CUTANEOUS URETEROSTOMY

This method of urinary diversion is used less often than the others because it is difficult to maintain adequate drainage. Stenosis of the ureters is prone to develop. The detached end of each ureter is brought out to the skin surface and everted to form a slightly protruding ureteric bud. The patient comes from the operating theatre with a catheter secured in each ureter. They are labelled right and left corresponding to the ureters, and are connected to separate drainage receptacles which are also labelled, respectively, right and left. The drainage is checked frequently and, if either catheter stops draining, the surgeon is notified and sterile equipment is prepared for irrigation. The catheters are left in place 7–12 days to minimize the urinary flow over the stomata while healing of the ureters to the abdominal wall takes place. The surgeon may order the application of normal saline compresses to the stomata around the catheters to prevent drying of the mucous membrane of the ureteric buds.

When the catheters are removed, an ileostomy bag may be applied over the stomata. The free end of the bag has an opening by which the urine drains into a connecting tubing and larger drainage receptacle. When the patient is up and about the tubing may be connected to a plastic urinal strapped to the patient's thigh. There is also a special ureterostomy cup available, which is placed over the ureteric buds and may be held in place by a strap around the patient or by adhesive disks similar to those used with ileostomy bags. The cup is connected to a plastic urinary bag that can be attached to the patient's thigh. The urinal bag is replaced at night by a drainage receptacle at the side of the bed. The bag or cup is changed every 2 or 3 days, and the connecting tubing and bags are changed daily. If an adhesive disk is used to hold the appliance in place, it is removed with a special commercial solvent available from the companies supplying the equipment. The skin around the ureteric buds requires frequent examination and attention. It is washed and thoroughly dried with each change of the appliance, and requires the application of a protective preparation such as Stomahe-

sive, karaya gum powder or zinc oxide ointment. If the skin becomes excoriated, the stoma therapist is consulted.

The patient and a relative are given detailed instruction in the care of the stomata, skin and appliance. Two sets of equipment are desirable to allow efficient cleansing and airing. Opportunities are provided for the patient to become competent in the necessary care before he is discharged from the hospital. As with other methods of urinary diversion, the importance of a daily fluid intake of 2500–3000 ml is stressed. There is always the danger that a patient may restrict his fluids so he will have less drainage to cope with, not realizing the need for continuous internal irrigation of the ureters. The patient and his family are cautioned to get in touch with the doctor at once if drainage from either stoma stops, fever develops, or pain in the back or abdomen is experienced. Continuous drainage of urine from both ureters is necessary to prevent back pressure and ensuing hydronephrosis as well as ascending infection of the kidneys. The patient is followed closely; the stomata may require periodic dilatation. A referral to the district nurse for frequent supervision is recommended and the patient is seen regularly by the clinic, or by the general practitioner.

SUMMARY CONCERNING URINARY DIVERSION

Factors to be considered in caring for a patient who undergoes permanent urinary diversion, regardless of the method used, include the following:

The patient's psychological reaction to a change in body image and normal pattern of function requires thoughtful understanding on the part of the nurse, with sincere efforts to reduce the patient's despair and promote acceptance and motivation.

Preoperative cleansing and 'sterilization' of the bowel are necessary if the operative procedure involves resection of or entry into the intestine.

Maintenance of continuous, adequate urinary drainage from the ureters postoperatively is essential to prevent renal complications.

Drainage of urine through an opening onto the skin necessitates special skin care to prevent excoriation and maceration.

A daily fluid intake of 2500 to 3000 ml of fluid is important to provide good internal irrigation of the renal pelvis and ureters.

A planned programme of instruction in the care of the stomata, skin and appliance is given to the patient and a relative. It should take place over a period of time that will allow them to acquire a satisfactory understanding and competence by the time the patient leaves the hospital. The instruction includes an explanation of the need for ample fluids and prompt reporting of decreased urinary drainage and significant symptoms.

Information about the patient's previous employment is obtained, and consideration is given as to whether it is suitable for him to resume his work or whether a referral to a social worker would be of assistance in finding other employment.

The patient requires a close follow-up. Frequent home visits by a district nurse, especially during the first few weeks after leaving the hospital, can provide assistance and considerable support to the patient and his family. Regular visits to a clinic or the general practitioner are necessary.

URETERIC DISORDERS

Primary disorders of the ureters occur less frequently than disease of other parts of the urinary system. A congenital anomaly or rarely a neoplasm may occur in a ureter. The commonest anomaly is a defect at the opening of the ureter into the bladder; normally, urine can only flow from the ureters into the bladder. The ureterovesical defect permits a urinary reflux—a backward flow of urine into the ureter from the bladder. This predisposes to pyelonephritis. Surgery is carried out to correct the defect. Primary neoplasm of the ureter is quite rare and entails extensive surgery.

Ureteritis occurs with pyelonephritis; for treatment, see p. 738. Severe or prolonged inflammation of the ureter may incur considerable scarring and narrowing of the passage or a calculus may become lodged within a ureter causing an obstruction to the flow of urine as well as severe pain. Surgical intervention may be necessary to remove the obstruction.

DISORDERS OF THE URETHRA

Urethritis

Inflammation of the urethra is most often due to infection but may also follow trauma. The patient complains of dysuria and frequency. The causative organism may be identified by cultures and smears of the urine or discharge from the urinary meatus. A urinary antiseptic or an antibiotic (depending on the causative organism) is prescribed, and the patient is encouraged to drink copious amounts of fluids.

Urethral stricture

Stricture of the urethra may be congenital or acquired. A congenital stricture may go unrecognized for a period of time and only be discovered when it causes retention and stasis of urine that lead to urethritis or cystitis. An acquired stricture is usually the result of infection or trauma which has caused inflammation and ensuing fibrous scarring. The patient with a stricture may experience hesitancy in initiating voiding and a small, slow urinary stream.

Treatment consists of gradual dilatation by the introduction of bougies or catheters weekly or every 2 weeks over several months. In some instances, a catheter may be left in place to maintain dilatation or to provide adequate urinary drainage. Rarely, a temporary cystostomy is necessary because of severe retention.

Urethral caruncle

A caruncle is a small, vascular, benign tumour that develops on the urethral wall near the urinary meatus. It occurs in females, usually appearing after the menopause. It bleeds easily and may be very sensitive. The patient may complain of pain on voiding and while sitting.

The caruncle is removed by cautery or excision. An indwelling catheter may be inserted and left in place for 24–48 hours because oedema of the urethral tissues may interfere with voiding. The patient may find the pressure of the catheter on the site very uncomfortable. For this reason, some doctors avoid the use of a catheter unless acute retention develops. A dressing of petroleum jelly is applied to the site to avoid irritation and friction until the area heals.

References and Further Reading

BOOKS

Anderson SVD & Bauwens EE (1981) *Chronic Health Problems*. St Louis: CV Mosby. Chapter 15.

Areopoulos DG (1982) Peritoneal dialysis. In: JE Castro (ed), *The Treatment of Renal Failure*. Lancaster: MTP Press.

Braunwald E et al (eds) (1987) *Harrison's Principles of Internal Medicine*, 11th ed. New York: McGraw-Hill. pp. 1139–1221.

Brockelhurst JC & Hanley T (1982) *Geriatric Medicine for Students*, 2nd ed. Edinburgh: Churchill Livingstone. Chapter 8.

Cameron S (1981) *Kidney Disease—The Facts*. Oxford: Oxford University Press.

Castro JE (ed) (1982) *The Treatment of Renal Failure*. Lancaster: MTP Press.

Ganong WF (1984) *Review of Medical Physiology*, 11th ed. San Francisco: Lange. Chapters 24, 38 & 39.

Gutch CF & Soner MH (1983) *Review of Hemodialysis for Nursing and Dialysis Personnel*, 4th ed. St Louis: CV Mosby.

Guyton AC (1986) *Textbook of Internal Medicine*, 7th ed. Philadelphia: WB Saunders. Chapters 34 & 35.

Horsley J, Crane J & Reynolds MA (1982) *Clean Intermittent Catheterization* (CURN Project). New York: Grune & Stratton.

Jamison RL & Kriz W (1982) *Urinary Concentrating Mechanism: Structure and Function*. New York: Oxford University Press.

Kidney Foundation of Canada (1983) *Living with Your Kidney Disease: A Patient Manual*. Montreal: Kidney Foundation of Canada.

Krupp MA & Chatton MJ (1983) *Current Medical Diagnosis and Treatment*. Los Altos: CA: Lange. Chapter 15.

Lancaster LE (ed) (1984) *The Patient With End-Stage Renal Disease*, 2nd ed. New York: John Wiley & Sons.

Leaf A & Cotran R (1980) *Renal Pathophysiology*, 2nd ed. New York: Oxford University Press.

Levine DZ (1983) *Care of the Renal Patient*. Philadelphia: WB Saunders.

Mandelstram D (ed) (1986) *Incontinence and Its Management*, 2nd ed. London: Croom-Helm.

Miller BF & Keane CB (1983) *Encyclopedia and Dictionary of Medicine, Nursing and Allied Health*, 3rd ed. Philadelphia: WB Saunders.

Roberts SL (1985) *Physiological Concepts and the Critically Ill Patient*. Englewood Cliffs, NJ: Prentice-Hall. Chapter 10.

Robbins SL, Angell M & Kumar V (1981) *Basic Pathophysiology*, 3rd ed. Philadelphia: WB Saunders. Chapter 14.

Sabiston DC (ed) (1986) *Textbook of Surgery*, 12th ed. Philadelphia: WB Saunders. Chapter 47.

Smith K (1980) *Fluids and Electrolytes: A Conceptual Approach*. New York: Churchill Livingstone.

Smith LH & Thier SO (1985) *Pathophysiology*, 2nd ed. Philadelphia: WB Saunders. Section 10.

PERIODICALS

Barrett N (1981) Cancer of the bladder. *Am. J. Nurs.*, Vol. 81 No. 12, pp. 2192–2195.

Barrett N (1981) Ileal loop and body image. *AORN J.* Vol. 36 No. 4, pp. 712–722.

Benz CC (1982) Chronic renal failure and the common denominator theory: a practical application. *Neph. Nurs.*, Vol. 4 No. 4, pp. 4–12.

Bradshaw TW (1983) Making male catheterization easier for both of you. *R.N.*, Vol. 46 No. 12, pp. 43–45.

Braren V, Workman CH, Johns OT, Brooks AL & Rhamy RK (1980) Use of the umbilical area for placement of a urinary stoma. *J. Enterost. Ther.*, Vol. 7 No. 2, pp. 8–10.

Bruce GL, Hinds P, Hudak J, Mucha A, Taylor Sr MC & Thompson CR (1980) Implementation of ANA's quality assurance program for clients with end stage renal disease. *Adv. Nurs. Sci.*, Vol. 2 No. 2, pp. 79–95.

Burns P (1983) Learned helplessness in the renal patient. *Neph. Nurs.*, Vol. 5 No. 1, pp. 14–16.

Buszta C (1981) Patient evaluation pre- and post-transplant. *Neph. Nurs.*, Vol. 3 No. 3, pp. 38–42.

Buszta C (1981) The nurse, the transplant patient and the family. *Neph. Nurs.*, Vol. 3 No. 6, pp. 4–8.

Carpenter CB & Strom TB (1982) Renal transplantation: immunologic and clinical aspects. Part I. *Hosp. Pract.*, Vol. 17 No. 10, pp. 125–134.

Carpenter GI (1981) The aging kidney. *Geriatr. Med.*, Vol. 11 No. 8, pp. 19–23.

Castleden CM & Dufferin HM (1981) Guidelines for controlling urinary incontinence without drugs or catheters. *Age Aging*, Vol. 10 No. 3, pp. 186–190.

Catanzaro M, O'Shaughnessy EJ, Clowers DC & Brooks G (1982) Urinary bladder dysfunction as a remedial disability in multiple sclerosis: a sociologic perspective. *Arch. Phys. Med. Rehab.*, Vol. 63 No. 10, pp. 472–474.

Ceccarelli CM (1981) Hemodialytic therapy for the patient with chronic renal failure. *Nurs. Clin. N. Am.*, Vol. 16 No. 3, pp. 531–550.

Chambers JK (1981) Assessing the dialysis patient at home. *Am. J. Nurs.*, Vol. 81 No. 4, pp. 750–754.

Cunio JE (1981) Plasma exchange therapy. *Neph. Nurs.*, Vol. 3 No. 5, pp. 35–38.

Davis V & Lavandero R (1980) Nursing update. Part 2: caring for the catheter carefully before during and after peritoneal dialysis. *Nurs. '80*, Vol. 10 No. 12, pp. 67–71.

Ford M & Wasilewicz (1981) Bridging the gap between hospital and home. *Can. Nurs.*, Vol. 77 No. 1, pp. 44–47.

Freed SZ (1981) Urinary incontinence in the elderly. *Hosp. Pract.*, Vol. 17 No. 3, pp. 81–94.

Grant SA (1981) Urine alkalinity and the long-term complications of ileal conduits. *J. Enterost. Ther.*, Vol. 7 No. 4, pp. 20, 21 & 24.

Harris RB, Hyman RB & Woog P (1982) Survival rates and coping-styles of maintenance hemodialysis patients. *Neph. Nurs.*, Vol. 4 No. 6, pp. 30–39.

Hodgson S (1980) Anemia associated with chronic renal failure and chronic dialysis. *Neph. Nurs.*, Vol. 2 No. 3, pp. 43–46.

Houlihan PJ (1982) When your patient is a transplant recipient. *Can. Nurs.*, Vol. 78 No. 7, pp. 40–44.

Kennedy AP & Brocklehurst JC (1982) The nursing management of patients with long-term indwelling catheters. *J. Adv. Nurs.*, Vol. 7 No. 5, pp. 411–417.

Killion A (1982) Reducing the risk of infection from indwelling urethral catheters. *Nurs. '82*, Vol. 12 No. 5, pp. 26–30.

Kurtzman NA (1982) Chronic renal failure: metabolic and clinical consequences. *Hosp. Pract.*, Vol. 17 No. 8, pp. 107–122.

Lancaster LE (1982) Kidney transplant rejection: pathophysiology, recognition and treatment, *Crit. Care Nurs.*, Vol. 2 No. 5, pp. 50–53.

Lancaster LE (1983) Renal failure: pathophysiology assessment and intervention. *Neph. Nurs.*, Vol. 5 No. 2, pp. 38–41 & 51.

Lane T, Stroshal V & Woldorf P (1982) Standards of care for the CAPD patient. *Neph. Nurs.*, Vol. 4 No. 5, pp. 34–45.

Lavandero R & Davis V (1980) Caring for the catheter carefully before, during and after peritoneal dialysis. *Nurs. '80*, Vol. 10 No. 11, pp. 73–79.

Lazarus JM (1982) Dialytic therapy: principles and clinical guidelines. *Hosp. Practice*, Vol. 17 No. 10, pp. 111–133.

Lewis SM (1981) Pathophysiology of chronic renal failure. *Nurs. Clin. N. Am.*, Vol. 16 No. 3, pp. 501–513.

Long ML (1985) Incontinence: defining the nursing role. *J. Geront. Nurs.*, Vol. 11 No. 1, pp. 30–35 & 41.

Mars DR & Treloar D (1984) Acute tubular necrosis—pathophysiology and treatment. *Heart Lung*, Vol. 13 No. 2, pp. 194–201.

McConnell EA (1982) Urinalysis: a common test but never routine. *Nurs. '82*, Vol. 12 No. 2, pp. 108–111.

McFarland SC (1981) Nursing management in continuous ambulatory peritoneal dialysis. *Neph. Nurs.*, Vol. 3 No. 2, pp. 48–51.

McGreal MJ, Vigneaux AM & Young JM (1982) Continuous ambulatory peritoneal dialysis: treatment of choice for some children. *Can. Nurs.*, Vol. 78 No. 1, pp. 21–25.

Merritt JL, Lie MR & Opitz JL (1982) Bladder retraining of paraplegic women. *Arch. Phys. Med Rehab.*, Vol. 63 No. 9, pp. 416–418.

Murphy LM & Cole MJ (1983) Renal disease: nutritional implications. *Nurs. Clin. N. Am.*, Vol. 18 No. 1, pp. 57–70.

Orr ML (1985) Pre-dialysis patient education. *J. Neph. Nurs.*, Vol. 2 No. 1, pp. 22–24.

Paganini EP & Nakamoto S (1980) Continuous slow ultrafiltration in oliguric acute renal failure. *Trans. Am. Soc. Artif. Intern. Organs*, Vol. 26, pp. 201–204.

Pawlowski J (1984) Percutaneous nephrolithotripsy: a nursing care plan. *AORN J.*, Vol. 39 No. 5, pp. 779–781.

Pickering L & Robbins D (1980) Fluid electrolyte and acid-base balance in the renal patient. *Nurs. Clin. N. Am.*, Vol. 15 No. 3, pp. 577–592.

Powers AM (1981) Renal transplantation: the patient's choice. *Nurs. Clin. N. Am.*, Vol. 16 No. 3, pp. 551–564.

Prowant BF & Fruto LV (1980) Continuous ambulatory peritoneal dialysis. *Neph. Nurs.*, Vol. 2 No. 1, pp. 8–14.

Rainone AM & Littman E (1981) The use of the amicon filter in dialysis-related complications. *AANNT.*, Vol. 8 No. 3, pp. 32–33 & 37.

Reckling JB (1982) Safeguarding the renal transplant patient. *Nurs. '82*, Vol. 12 No. 2, pp. 47–49.

Reid SB (1982) Giving more than dialysis. *Nurs. '82*, Vol. 12 No. 4, pp. 58–63.

Restor FC & Cogan MG (1980) The renal acidoses. *Hosp. Practice*, Vol. 15 No. 4, pp. 99–111.

Rice V (1982) The role of potassium in health and disease. *Crit. Care Nurs.*, Vol. 2 No. 3, pp. 54–74.

Richard CJ (1980) Peritoneal dialysis—a nursing update. Part I: physiological aspects and nursing responsibilities. *Neph. Nurs.*, Vol. 2 No. 5, pp. 38–43.

Richard CJ (1980) Peritoneal dialysis—a nursing update. *Neph. Nurs.*, Vol. 2 No. 6, pp. 4, 5, 8, 46, 49 & 52.

Rodriguez DJ & Hunta VM (1981) Nutritional intervention in the treatment of chronic renal failure. *Nurs. Clin. N. Am.*, Vol. 16 No. 3, pp. 573–585.

Sorrels AJ (1981) Peritoneal dialysis: a rediscovery *Nurs. Clin. N. Am.*, Vol. 16 No. 3, pp. 515–529.

Stark JL (1982) How to succeed against acute renal failure. *Nurs. '82*, Vol. 12 No. 7, pp. 26–33.

Stone L (1984) Percutaneous nephrolithotripsy: an advancement in kidney stone extraction. *AORN*, Vol. 39 No. 5, pp. 773–778.

Taber SM, Lee HA & Slapak M (1982) A rehabilitation assessment of renal transplantees (based on United Kingdom experience). *Neph. Nurs.*, Vol. 4 No. 5, pp. 9–14.

Thomas B (1980) Problem solving: urinary incontinence in the elderly. *J. Gerontol. Nurs.*, Vol. 6 No. 9, pp. 533–536.

Thompson P (1981) Acute renal failure—a challenge for all nurses. *Neph. Nurs.*, Vol. 3 No. 5, pp. 4–8.

Toner M (1982) Urinary obstruction: the hidden threats in treatment. *RN*, Vol. 45 No. 5, pp. 58–63.

Ulrich B (1980) The psychological adaption of end stage renal disease: a review and a proposed new model. *Neph. Nurs.*, Vol. 2 No. 3, pp. 48–52 & 58.

Wells JM (1981) Hypotension during hemodialysis: physiological mechanisms involved. *Neph. Nurs.*, Vol. 3 No. 3, pp. 20–27.

Williams ME & Pannill FC (1982) Urinary incontinence in the elderly. *Ann. Int. Med.*, Vol. 97 No. 6, pp. 895–907.

22

Nursing in Disorders of the Nervous System

Introduction

The nervous system is an integrated multipurpose system made up of many parts. It contains the higher human functions such as memory and reasoning, controls and coordinates all parts of the body and provides a complex communication system between the body's internal and external environments.

Structurally, the nervous system is composed of two parts: the *central nervous system* (CNS) and the *peripheral nervous system*. The CNS consists of the brain and the spinal cord, while the peripheral system consists of the spinal and cranial nerves.

The two functional divisions of the nervous system are the *somatic* or *voluntary nervous system* and the *autonomic* or *involuntary nervous system*. The somatic system is primarily concerned with the transmission of impulses (coded messages) to and from the non-visceral parts of the body such as the skeletal muscles, bones, joints, ligaments, skin, eyes and ears. Its activities are usually conscious and willed responses. The autonomic system is concerned with regulation of the activities of visceral muscles and glands.

Division of the nervous system into discrete parts is useful for discussion purposes in the abstract. However, in the body, the activities of each division are *interrelated*, and the nervous system and the endocrine system work in concert to harmonize the many complex functions of the total system.

This section focuses on some of the major structural and functional components of the nervous system which have implications for nursing. Muscle tissue is also considered, because disturbances in movement such as paralysis and spasticity due to nervous system dysfunction are relatively common. Few primary disorders of muscle activity are encountered in nursing practice. With the exception of cardiac and intestinal muscle, the nervous system initiates and coordinates contraction of muscle tissue to produce body movements, including visceral activity.

Neuron

The neuron, or nerve cell, is the structural and functional unit of the nervous system (Fig. 22.1). Each neuron consists of a cell body and cytoplasmic processes. The cell body contains a nucleus and other structures and masses concerned with cell maintenance and activity. The cytoplasmic processes include a single axon and one or more dendrites.

The *axon* is a tubular process which conducts nerve impulses away from the cell body, out to the dendrites of other neurons or to muscles and glands. Near its end, the axon divides into numerous fine branches, each of which has a specialized ending called the presynaptic terminal. *Dendrites* are short, thin projections which branch profusely as they extend from the cell body. They receive stimuli and carry impulses generated by the stimuli toward the nerve cell body. Most stimuli affecting nerve cells are chemical messengers (neurotransmitters) that are secreted from one neuron to an adjacent neuron. The profuse branches of dendrites increase the surface area over which impulses may be picked up.

The processes (axons and dendrites) may be referred to as *tracts* if they are inside the CNS or a nerve if outside the CNS. The latter is formed by a bundle of neuronal processes. The term *ganglion* refers to a collection of cell bodies outside the brain and spinal cord. Within the brain and spinal cord, such a collection may be referred to as a nucleus.

Neurons may be classified according to their function: *motor* (efferent or effector) neurons, *sensory* (afferent or receptor) neurons, and *connecting* (internuncial) neurons. The axons of motor neurons transmit impulses from the CNS to stimulate muscle or glandular tissue. Axons of sensory neurons transmit impulses to areas of the brain or spinal cord from the periphery. One or more of the sensory neuron's dendrites ends in a peripheral receptor, such as the eye or the ear, to receive incoming stimuli. Connecting neurons, which occur only in the grey matter of the brain and spinal cord, convey incoming stimuli to neurons of various integrating centres of the CNS. The connecting neurons form the association areas in the cerebral cortex. They have an important role in the CNS because they 'decide' the responses to the incoming (sensory) impulses and promote the initiation of the appropriate motor neuron response.

Neurons are designed to initiate, receive and react to stimuli, transmit impulses, process and store information. Neuronal activity results in a wide variety of responses ranging from a simple reflex to complex behaviour requiring central coordination.

Unlike most body cells, neurons lose their ability to undergo mitosis early in life and they lose their viability if denied a supply of oxygen or glucose for more than a few minutes. When neurons are destroyed in the peripheral system, neuronal pro-

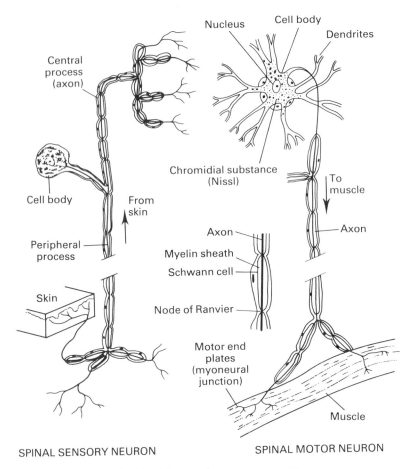

Fig. 22.1 Motor and sensory neurones.

cesses may be replaced under favourable conditions. However in the CNS neurons are not replaced. These unique properties of nerve tissue have important implications for the nursing care of patients with neurological dysfunction.

Nerve impulse

The functions of the nerve cells are to receive, initiate and conduct 'messages' known as nerve impulses. An impulse is a combination of physical and chemical processes which are initiated at the point of stimulation. It occurs as the result of a mechanical, chemical or electrical change at some point in the immediate environment of the neuron. This change temporarily alters the permeability of the cell membrane at that point and is referred to as the stimulus. The series of events that result from the change in membrane permeability produces an electrical current (Fig. 22.2).

When a normal neuron is in a resting state, the outer surface of its membrane is electropositive, but the inner surface is electronegative. As a result, it is said to be polarized. This electrical polarity is attributed to the selective action of the cell membrane by which a higher concentration of sodium ions is maintained outside the cell. The positive sodium ions, which are normally attracted to the negative ions within the cell, are not allowed to cross the membrane; if they do so, they are ejected by the cell membrane. The electronegativity within the cell is mainly due to the non-diffusible protein anions and retained chlorine anions. When the stimulus occurs, the membrane becomes permeable to sodium. The influx of cations depolarizes the membrane; a reversal of the electrical potential develops as the outer surface of the membrane becomes electronegative and the inner surface becomes electropositive. This change alters the electrical relationship of the excited area to the adjacent portions; the shift of ions acts as a stimulus, and a wave of depolarization passes along the length of the neuronal process. In a fraction of a second, following depolarization, the membrane recovers its normal permeability and the resting electrical polarity is restored. The electrical currents that are generated as impulses sweep over the fibres and may be recorded and used in assessing function (e.g. electroencephalogram).

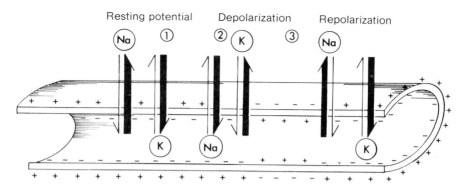

Fig. 22.2 Resting state, depolarization and repolarization.

During the conduction of impulses, the neurons consume oxygen and glucose and produce heat and carbon dioxide. The velocity of impulse transmission is determined by the diameter of the neuronal process (nerve fibre) and the presence or absence of a *myelin sheath*, a white lipid and protein insulating cover. Nerve fibres enclosed in a myelin sheath are referred to as myelinated. Larger, myelinated fibres conduct more quickly than smaller, unmyelinated ones. Neural impulses move at a maximum of 100 metres per second in large fibres.

SYNAPSE

A synapse is the junction, or discontinuity, between the axon of one neuron and the dendrite of another. A release of chemicals at the synapse provides for the transmission of impulses from neuron to neuron. The termination of a nerve fibre in a muscle cell is called a *neuromuscular junction*. This is basically similar to the synapse between two neurons. The synapse of each axon terminal of a motor neuron on a voluntary muscle cell is referred to as a *motor endplate*.

Chemicals released from the terminal portion of the axon can have an excitatory or inhibitory effect on the transmission of impulses across a synapse. There is evidence that about 30 different neurotransmitter substances exist. The chief excitatory transmitter is acetylcholine. Glutamic acid, secreted in some of the sensory pathways is also an important excitatory transmitter. Noradrenaline and adrenaline cause excitation in some areas but inhibition in others. The chief inhibitory substances are gamma-aminobutyric acid (GABA), glycine, dopamine and serotonin (5-hydroxytryptamine). The transmitter acetylcholine is destroyed by the enzyme cholinesterase within about one millisecond of its release, and others transmitters are similarly destroyed or reabsorbed into the axon. In this way, rapid, repetitive, discrete stimulation (or inhibition) of neurons is possible; this is an essential factor in the function of the nervous system.

REFLEX ARC, RECEPTOR, EFFECTOR

A large amount of body activity occurs at an unconscious, involuntary level in response to particular types of stimuli. Reflex arcs are the involuntary, fixed motor responses to sensory stimuli. The reflex arc includes a sensory or receptor neuron (afferent limb), an integrating centre within the CNS at any level below the cerebral cortex and a motor neuron (efferent limb). A reflex is often a defence mechanism that permits quick, automatic responses to painful potentially harmful situations. Its basic purpose is to maintain total body integrity.

A receptor consists of bare nerve endings or specialized structures sensitive to specific stimuli. An effector is muscular or glandular tissue. When a receptor is stimulated by a change in its environment (e.g. pressure, temperature, chemical, stretching), it evokes an impulse in the nerve fibres. The impulse is carried through the cell body of the sensory neuron and along its axon into the CNS. Here, it may pass through one, several or many connecting neurons before it excites a motor neuron whose axon (efferent or motor fibre) carries the impulse out of the CNS to the effector tissue or organ. The terminal portion of the efferent fibre releases a chemical at its junction with the effector, initiating its response. For example, this response is contraction in the case of muscle, and is secretion if it is a gland that is innervated. (See reflexes p. 776.)

Neuroglia

The nervous system is composed of two types of cells, namely, neurons and neuroglia (glia). The *neurons* are the essential units of the conduction system of the nervous system while *neuroglial* cells provide structural support for the neurons.

Neuroglial cells lack axons (Fig. 22.3). They are generally divided into five major classes:
1 *Astrocytes* (astroglia) are star-shaped and are implicated in providing essential nutrients for neurons, in the blood-brain barrier concept, in information

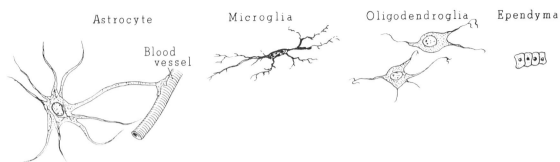

Fig. 22.3 Neuroglial cells of the central nervous system.

storage processes, and in the maintenance of bioelectrical potentials of neurons.

2 *Oligodendrocytes* form and maintain the myelin sheaths of axons in the CNS.

3 *Microglia* are phagocytic cells which are related to the macrophages of the connective tissues. They remove disintegration products of the neurons.

4 *Ependymal cells* line the ventricular system and the choroid plexuses (see p. 766). They are involved in the production of cerebrospinal fluid.

5 *Schwann cells* form the myelin sheath around the axons of the peripheral neurons.

Neuroglial cells comprise about 40% of the total volume of the brain and spinal cord. Since strong intracellular substances such as collagen and elastin are lacking in neuroglial cells, fresh brain and spinal cord tissue appears soft and jelly-like. In contrast to neurons, neuroglial cells retain their mitotic abilities throughout the life span of the individual. From a clinical viewpoint, neuroglial cells are important because they are the most common source of primary tumours in the nervous system.

THE CENTRAL NERVOUS SYSTEM

Brain

The human brain is the organ concerned with thought, memory and consciousness. It is also concerned with a range of sensory experiences, with motor activity, the regulation of visceral, endocrine and somatic functions and with the use of symbols and signs that underlie communication. For descriptive purposes the brain may be subdivided into the cerebrum, basal ganglia, thalami, hypothalamus, midbrain, pons, medulla oblongata and cerebellum.

CEREBRUM

The cerebrum is the most important part of the nervous system. It accounts for 80% of the total weight of the brain. It is divided into two hemispheres by the *longitudinal fissure*. The two hemispheres are joined at their bases by bands of neuronal fibres collectively

forming the *corpus callosum*. It is believed that the corpus callosum transfers information from one hemisphere to the other. A fold of dura (see p. 767) called *falx cerebri* lies between the two hemispheres.

In selected higher functions, one cerebral hemisphere appears to be the 'leading' one and is referred to as the *dominant hemisphere*. Cerebral dominance tends to be most complete in relation to the complex aspects of language. Handedness also is related to cerebral dominance although its relationship is less clear-cut than previously believed. In true right-handed persons it is nearly always the left hemisphere which is dominant and governs language; but the converse of this is not necessarily true. The degree of cerebral dominance appears to vary among individuals and with respect to different functions. Recent research indicates that each hemisphere, independently, contains the ability to learn but that the right hemisphere has a superior role in intuitive and creative responses and in spatial perception. The concept of cerebral dominance has implications for nursing care of patients with stroke or head injury in which there is damage in one hemisphere.

Each cerebral hemisphere is subdivided into four anatomically distinct regions called lobes: the frontal, parietal, temporal and occipital (Fig. 22.4). The

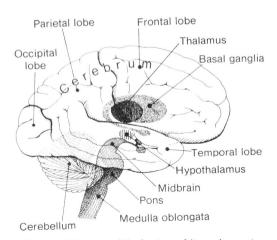

Fig. 22.4 Diagram of the brain and its major parts.

frontal lobe is separated from the parietal lobe by the central fissure. The temporal lobe is separated from the parietal and frontal lobes by the lateral fissure of Sylvius and the occipital lobe is separated from the parietal and temporal lobes by the parieto-occipital fissure. These four regions underlie the skull bones which have the corresponding names. Some texts refer also to insular and limbic lobes but neither are true lobes. The insular cortex lies in the depth of the lateral cerebral fissure. The limbic lobe is based largely upon a physiological concept.

The brain contains areas of grey and white matter. The *grey matter* is a collection of neuronal bodies and unmyelinated processes. *White matter* consists primarily of myelinated fibres coming off cell bodies. Grey matter, which forms the surface of the cerebrum, is called the *cerebral cortex*. The cortex is believed to contain about 100 billion neurons. It is 2–5 mm thick and is arranged in a series of convolutions or coil-like elevations called gyri. Shallow crevices between the gyri are called sulci (see Fig. 22.5). The folding into gyri and sulci appears to be a means of increasing the surface area of the brain. Sulci that are particularly deep are called fissures.

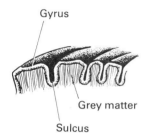

Fig. 22.5 The surface of the cerebrum.

The cerebral cortex is a highly specialized area whose functions are not precisely understood at present. It is known to have an essential role in consciousness, mental ability, and memory. Some texts refer to the cerebral cortex as the neocortex in the belief that it appeared fairly late in vertebrate evolution.

The cerebral cortex of each hemisphere is made up of primary sensory areas or centres, primary motor areas or centres and association areas. Primary *sensory areas* are receptive areas for incoming impulses. Primary *motor areas* are concerned with dispatching outgoing impulses to prompt action responses in peripheral structures (Fig. 22.6). *Association areas*, which are areas that do not perform primary functions, lie around the sensory and motor areas. They occupy the greater portion of the cortex and have multiple connections with the sensory and motor centres. The functions of the association areas are somewhat general but nevertheless are very important. Functional loss of sensory association areas greatly diminishes the ability of the brain to

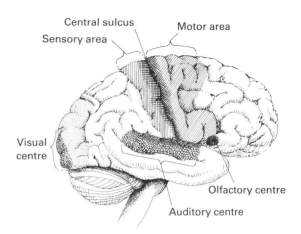

Fig. 22.6 Major centres of the cerebrum.

analyse characteristics of sensory experience, to give them meaning and make decisions as to appropriate responses. Responses involving storage of perception in memory or stimulation of motor centres to bring about body movement or speech could be adversely affected.

The primary sensory and motor centres occupy certain areas of the cerebral cortex and perform highly specialized functions. The motor area that initiates all voluntary movements of the body occupies the strip of the frontal lobe immediately anterior to the central fissure. In general, the motor area in one hemisphere controls the movements on the opposite side of the body. The various muscles are spatially represented on the motor strip so that the feet are located in the area of the longitudinal fissure and the muscles of chewing are located at the opposite end of the motor strip (see Fig. 22.7). The size of the cortical area representing the body parts is proportional to the complexity and functional importance of the part. The area anterior to the primary motor area is known as the *premotor* or *secondary motor* area. It is believed to be concerned with control and coordination of skilled movements of a complex nature. It has direct connections with the primary motor area and lower levels of the brain.

The sensory impulses that enter the cerebral cortex are transmitted to specific areas of the cortex, depending on their origin. Impulses concerned with the *somataesthetic senses* such as touch, pressure, temperature, pain and the sense of body position and its parts are transmitted to the parietal lobe immediately posterior to the central fissure. As with the motor areas, sensations from the lower part of the body are received at the medial portion lying within the longitudinal fissure. Impulses from the head are received at the lower part of the strip (see Fig. 22.7). Sensations originating in the right side of the body are transmitted to the left hemisphere and those originating in the left side are received in the right hemisphere.

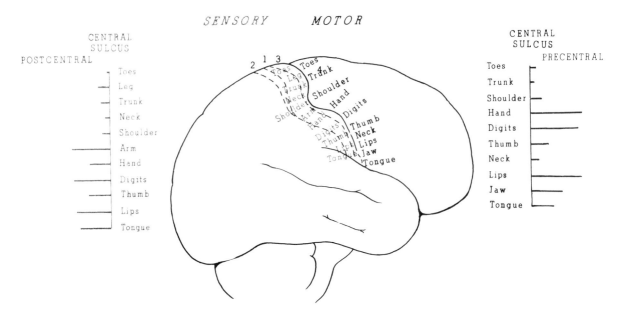

Fig. 22.7 Lateral view of the brain showing somataesthetic and primary motor areas. The amount of brain surface related to a specific part of the body is not proportional to the size of the part but to the extent of the activity.

The primary receptive area for vision is located in the posterior part of the occipital lobe. The *visual centre* in the right occipital lobe receives impulses from the right half of the retina of each eye and, conversely, the left cerebral visual centre receives impulses from the left half of each eye. Visual association areas are immediately anterior to the primary receptive area for vision. With destruction of the visual association area, the person can clearly see objects but he will be unable to recognize or identify them. This disability is known as *visual agnosia*.

The *primary auditory receptive areas* or *centres for hearing* are located in the superior parts of the temporal lobes. Impulses from both ears are received in both the right and left auditory centres. The auditory association area occupies a part of the temporal lobe immediately below the primary areas. It is known as Wernicke's area. Damage to Wernicke's area results in receptive *aphasia*. This means that the person hears words but they are not meaningful to him. The person would be able to speak but because of comprehension failure would make errors in speech content. The *olfactory sense* or *sense of smell* is also represented in the temporal lobes.

At the junction of the lateral fissure where temporal, parietal, and occipital lobes meet is a very important area called the *interpretive area*. This area provides an integration of the somatic, auditory, and visual association areas, and plays the greatest role of any area of the cerebral cortex. Any destruction of tissue in this area will result in impaired intellectual ability.

The frontal lobes contain the motor area described above. Other areas in the frontal lobes are the premo-tor cortex, the prefrontal areas, and Broca's area. The premotor cortex is also known as the motor association or secondary motor area. It plays a role in the activities of several cranial nerves. The prefrontal areas of the frontal lobe provide additional cortical area for cerebral function. They are concerned with memory and ability to concentrate, and ability to think in abstract terms. They are also concerned with personality, emotional reactions, initiative and sense of responsibility for socially acceptable standards. *Broca's* area is categorized as an association area because it aids in the formulation of words. Injury to this area results in the inability of the person to speak in sentences; his vocabulary is limited to 'yes' and 'no'.

Beneath the grey cerebral cortex, the cerebrum is mainly composed of white matter. Myelinated neuronal processes are arranged in functionally related bundles called tracts. These are classified as commissural, association, and projection tracts. The *commissural tracts* transmit impulses between the two hemispheres. The *association tracts* carry impulses from one area of the cortex to another in the same hemisphere. *Projection tracts* are ascending and descending pathways from one level of the central nervous system to another. One of the most important of these is the internal capsule. The *internal capsule* is a massive bundle of efferent and afferent nerve fibres that connect the various subdivisions of the brain and spinal cord.

BASAL GANGLIA (NUCLEI)

Basal ganglia are groups of nerve cell bodies deeply

embedded within the white matter of each cerebral hemisphere. Anatomically, they are very complex. Physiologically, the parts include four main nuclei. These are the *lenticular nucleus* (composed of the globus pallidus and putamen), the *caudate nucleus*, the *amygdaloid body*, and the *claustrum*. The lenticular nucleus and the caudate nuclei are collectively called the *corpus striatum* (striate body). Major portions of the thalamus, reticular formation, and red nuclei (pigmented grey matter) operate in close association with these and are part of the basal ganglia system for motor control.

The functions of the basal ganglia are complex and not clearly understood. The system actually operates, along with the motor cortex and cerebellum, as a total unit, and individual functions cannot be ascribed solely to the various parts of the system (Fig. 22.8). One of the general functions of the basal ganglia is inhibition of muscle tone throughout the body. With widespread destruction of this system, muscle rigidity occurs throughout the body. The resultant phenomenon is known as *decerebrate rigidity*. The corpus striatum helps to control gross intentional movements which are normally performed unconciously. It is believed that the principal function of the globus pallidus (see above) is to provide background muscle tone for intended movements.

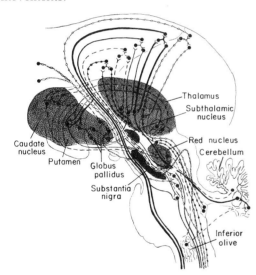

Fig. 22.8 Pathways through the basal ganglia and related structures of the brain stem, thalamus, and cerebral cortex.

A number of clinical syndromes with implications for nursing result from damage to the basal ganglia. Chorea or St Vitus' dance, a condition in which random, uncontrolled, continuous movement patterns occur, result when the caudate and putamen neurons that secrete the inhibitory transmitter GABA are greatly reduced in number or activity. *Athetosis*, a disorder characterized by slow, writhing

body movements, occurs with injury to the globus pallidus. *Parkinson's disease*, also known as paralysis agitans, results from widespread destruction of the substantia nigra (pigmented grey matter within the midbrain) (Fig. 22.8). Abnormal motor activities in Parkinson's disease are related to a lack of dopamine secretion in the caudate nucleus and putamen due to destruction of the substantia nigra. Dopamine is a neurotransmitter which is believed to inhibit the activity of acetylcholine-producing neurons in normal persons. The same basal ganglia that are inhibited by dopamine are excited by acetylcholine-secreting neurons. Therefore, anticholinergic drugs such as scopolamine can benefit the patient with Parkinson's disease by decreasing the level of activity in the basal ganglia.

THALAMI

The thalami are a pair of egg-shaped masses of grey matter at the base of each hemisphere. Each mass is referred to as a thalamus and forms part of the lateral walls of the third ventricle. The thalami form the main relay centre for sensory impulses and cerebellar and basal ganglia projections to the cerebral cortex (Fig. 22.8). Impulses are 'sorted' in the thalami and forwarded to appropriate cerebral cortical areas. *Encephalins and endorphins* (compounds with morphine-like action) have been found in some nuclei of the thalami. It is believed that these substances may have a role in pain relief such as occurs with extreme fear, placebos and transcutaneous electric nerve stimulation.

HYPOTHALAMUS

This is an important grey mass which lies beneath the thalamus. It forms the floor and part of the wall of the third ventricle. It contains nuclei of the autonomic nervous system for the control of most of the body's involuntary functions as well as many aspects of emotional behaviour. There are neuronal links between the hypothalamus and the posterior pituitary gland. The hypothalamus exerts a control on vasomotor tone and heart rate. It is concerned with regulation of body temperature, and it regulates body water. Body water regulation is achieved by creating the sensation of thirst and by controlling the excretion of water in the urine. Neurons in the hypothalamus serve as osmoreceptors (cells sensitive to changes in osmotic pressure of body fluid) and regulate the production and release of the antidiuretic hormone (ADH), which plays an important role in maintaining or restoring body fluid balance. ADH causes reabsorption of water in the kidneys. thereby decreasing water loss in the urine. The hypothalamus is also concerned with gastrointestinal and feeding regulation. Hunger centres and a satiety centre have been identified in this grey mass. In addition, it activates feeding reflexes such as lick-ing the lips and swallowing. The cells of certain hypothalamic nuclei secrete the hormone oxytocin which is concerned with uterine contraction and with the expulsion of breast milk for infant feeding. The hypothalamus also plays an important role in the secretion of hormones by the anterior pituitary gland. It is also known to affect responses such as pleasure and fear. Endorphins, which are believed to function as excitatory transmitters that activate portions of the brain's analgesic system, have been found in abundance in the hypothalamus.

MIDBRAIN

This is a short segment of the brain that is below the thalami and the pons where the third and fourth cranial nerves originate. It is sometimes considered the upper part of the brain stem. A narrow canal (aqueduct of Sylvius) passes through the centre connecting the third and fourth ventricles. The midbrain contains many ascending and descending nerve fibre tracts and it is a relay station for sight and hearing. Centres (groups of neurons) for postural and righting reflexes also occur in the midbrain.

BRAIN STEM

The brain stem is composed of the pons varolii and the medulla oblongata, although the midbrain may be considered as the upper part. The *pons varolii* is located between the midbrain and medulla. It consists of numerous tracts which link various parts of the brain and serve as conduction pathways. The pons also contains portions of the reticular formation and groups of neurons (nuclei) which give rise to cranial nerves V–VIII (inclusive).

The *medulla oblongata* lies between the pons and the spinal cord. It is composed of ascending and descending conduction pathways. Autonomic centres that regulate such vital functions as breathing, cardiac rate and vasomotor tone as well as centres for vomiting, gagging, coughing and sneezing reflex behaviours are located in the medulla. Cranial nerves IX–XII have their cell bodies in this area.

CEREBELLUM

This part of the brain lies beneath the posterior portion of the cerebrum, posterior to the pons and medulla. It is separated from the cerebrum by a fold of meningeal membrane (dura mater) called the tentorium cerebelli. Three pairs of cerebellar peduncles attach the cerebellum to the midbrain, pons, and medulla. These peduncles receive direct input from the spinal cord and brain stem and convey it to the deep cerebellar nuclei and cerebral cortex. The result is both an excitatory and inhibitory influence on the cerebellar nuclei, with a pre-

dominance of excitatory influences. An excitatory effect on the brain stem and on the thalamic nuclei maintains a tonic discharge to the motor system.

The cerebellum is integrated into many connective pathways throughout the brain for the provision of muscle coordination in the body. All sensations are relayed through the cerebellum, thus providing information about muscle activity. For example, afferent impulses are delivered to the cerebellum from the labyrinth of each internal ear. These impulses prompt reflex muscle responses to maintain balance of position or postural equilibrium. The functions of the cerebellum are essentially to control fine movements and balance, to control coordination of movement, and maintain feedback loops to correct movement, and to coordinate the action of muscle groups. Dysfunction of the cerebellum can result in gait disturbance, equilibrium ataxia (overstability or understability), and tremors.

RETICULAR FORMATION (RETICULAR ACTIVATING SYSTEM, RAS)

This is a diffuse system of motor and sensory fibres and nerve cells which forms the central core of the brain stem (Fig. 22.9). It has widespread afferent

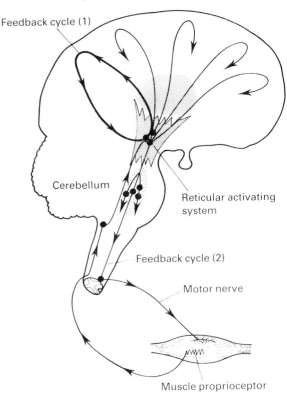

Fig. 22.9 Feedback mechanisms of the reticular activating system (RAS). (1) Impulses carried to the cerebral cortex and back to the RAS. (2) Impulses to peripheral muscles and back to RAS.

connections, receiving sensory impulses from all over the body. The cerebral cortex can stimulate this system. The actual function of the RAS continues to be the subject of research and speculation. However, it is known to be associated with initiation and maintenance of wakefulness and alertness which make perception possible. The neurons of this area learn to be selective, making judgements as to whether the cortex should be alerted or not. For example, a mother may sleep through hearing traffic noise but she is aroused by the slightest whimper from her infant. When specific areas of the reticular formation are damaged severely, as occurs in diseases such as encephalitis lethargica (sleeping sickness), or when a brain tumour develops in this region or serious haemorrhage occurs, the person becomes comatose and is resistant to normal awakening stimuli.

BLOOD SUPPLY TO THE BRAIN

The ever-active brain receives about one fifth of the blood pumped by the heart and it consumes about 20% of the oxygen utilized by the body. Approximately 800 ml of blood flows through the brain each minute, with 75 ml present in the brain at any given time. The brain requires a continuous flow of blood since it can store only minute quantities of glucose and oxygen and derives its energy almost exclusively from the metabolism of glucose delivered by the blood. Its blood requirement is the same whether one is mentally active or sleeping.

Brain cells are extremely sensitive to hypoxia, particularly those of the cerebral cortex. Interruption of blood supply to the brain produces loss of consciousness in seconds. Irreversible brain damage occurs if the blood supply is interrupted for 2–6

minutes. Brain stem neurons are less sensitive to hypoxia than cortical cells; individuals experiencing prolonged hypoxia may survive because the vital centres in the medulla are more resistant and recover, but irreversible cortical damage persists, resulting in mental deficiency.

Various built-in protective mechanisms of the brain act to increase blood flow and nutrient supply when the need arises. These mechanisms include arterial anastomoses and autoregulatory mechanisms which: (1) increase cerebral blood flow even in profound hypotension; and (2) help to extract greater amounts of glucose and oxygen from perfusing blood. Even after other organs are deprived of blood and can no longer function, blood flow within the brain may remain near normal levels. Factors which affect cerebral blood flow include arterial and venous blood pressure at brain level, conditions of the vessels (e.g. atherosclerosis), intracranial pressure, viscosity of the blood, and, to a lesser extent, constriction and dilatation of cerebral vessels.

The arterial blood supply to the brain is derived from *two internal carotid arteries* and *two vertebral arteries* (Fig. 22.10). The vertebral arteries originate from the subclavian arteries and unite at the junction of the pons and medulla to form the *basilar artery*. The basilar artery continues to the midbrain level where it divides to form the paired posterior cerebral arteries. In general, the vertebral arteries and their branches (posterior cerebral arteries) supply blood to the lower third of the diencephalon (thalamus and hypothalamus), the cerebellum, and the occipital region of the cerebral hemispheres. The internal carotid arteries arise from two different vessels. The left common carotid artery originates in the aorta directly while the right common carotid artery arises

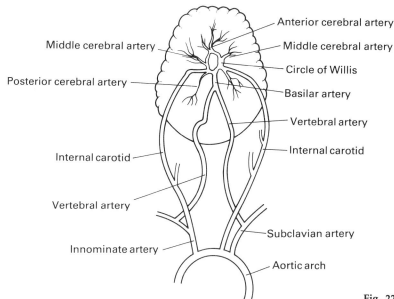

Fig. 22.10 Blood supply to the brain.

from the innominate artery which originates in the aorta. The common carotid arteries branch to form the external and internal carotid arteries. The internal carotid arteries supply blood, via the anterior and middle cerebral arteries, to most of the hemispheres excluding the occipital lobes, the basal ganglia, and the upper two thirds of the diencephalon.

Although the vertebral basilar arterial tree and the internal carotid arterial tree are essentially independent, some anastomotic connections between the two systems exist. Small posterior communicating arteries connect the two systems to form an arterial crown known as the cerebral arterial *circle of Willis*. The anterior communicating artery which connects the two anterior cerebral arteries completes the circle. It allows an adequate blood supply to reach all parts of the brain even after one or more of the four supplying vessels is obstructed.

The veins draining the brain stem and cerebellum follow the arteries to these structures. Veins draining the cerebrum have short, stocky branches which come off at angles and drain into superficial venous plexuses and the *dural sinuses*. Dural (venous) sinuses are valveless channels located between two layers of dura mater. Most venous blood drains into the internal jugular veins at the base of the skull.

Blood–brain barrier
This is a unique relationship between the capillary walls in the brain and the glial cells. It is believed that the blood–brain barrier limits entry of substances, which may be harmful, into the extracellular space of the brain around the neurons. This barrier phenomenon effectively keeps microorganisms out of the brain. However, it is equally effective in keeping most antibiotics out, thus complicating therapy for intracranial infections. The brain cells of infants, particularly if premature, are readily permeable to some substances (e.g. bilirubin, radioactive phosphorus) that are prevented from reaching the neurons when the glial cells are mature or fully developed. Techniques for reversibly opening the blood–brain barrier and the synthesis of therapeutic agents that can cross the barrier are areas that are currently under study.

VENTRICLES AND CEREBROSPINAL FLUID

The ventricular system is a series of cavities within the brain (Fig. 22.11). Each cerebral hemisphere contains a *lateral ventricle*, each of which communicates with the *third ventricle* by means of an intraventricular foramen (foramen of Munro). The third ventricle is a slit-like space between the thalami and it is continuous with the fourth ventricle through a narrow channel called the cerebral aqueduct (aqueduct of Sylvius). The *fourth ventricle* is located between the pons and the cerebellum and is continuous with the subarachnoid space (see Meninges) and with the central canal of the medulla and the

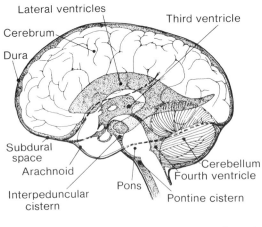

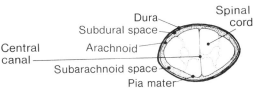

Fig. 22.11 A diagram showing the ventricles, meninges and spaces.

spinal cord. The foramen of Magendie, the medial opening of the fourth ventricle, allows cerebrospinal fluid (CSF) to circulate around the cord. Two lateral openings (foramina of Luschka) channel fluid around the brain. This distribution of CSF provides a protective cushion for the brain and cord.

The ventricular system is lined by ependyma (see p. 760) and is filled with CSF. Each ventricle contains a *choroid plexus* which is a rich network of blood vessels covered by a layer of ependymal cells which constantly secrete CSF. The CSF is a clear, colourless, water-like fluid with a specific gravity of 1.007. It contains occasional lymphocytes and traces of the minerals and organic materials found in blood. The glucose concentration is normally 2.8–4.5 mmol/l (50–80 mg/dl) and protein concentration is 0.1–0.4 g/l (10–40 mg/dl) at the lumbar level. Protein varies in different parts of the system since it is affected by gravity. The total volume of CSF in the adult ranges from 125–150 ml. Normal pressure is 40–180 mmH$_2$O.

The CSF circulates through the ventricular system and around the brain and cord in the subarachnoid space. It is steadily reabsorbed into the *arachnoid villi*, which are projections from the subarachnoid space into the venous sinuses of the brain. Any interruption within the CSF circuit, such as occurs with a congenital absence of openings between the fourth ventricle and subarachnoid space, results in an excessive accumulation of fluid within the ventricles. The condition is referred to as hydrocephalus. The brain tissue becomes compressed between the skull and the expanding volume of fluid.

MENINGES

The soft brain and spinal cord are surrounded by three layers of connective tissue membranes known as the meninges. The three meninges, from the outermost layer inward, are the dura mater, the arachnoid mater, and the pia mater. The *dura mater* ('hard mother') is a thick, tough, inelastic, collagenous double membrane. One layer of the dura is attached to the skull while another is adjacent to the arachnoid. Two potential spaces associated with the dura are the epidural (or extradural space) and the subdural space. *Epidural space* refers to the potential space between the cranium and the periosteal layer of the dura. *Subdural space* describes the potential space between the dura and the arachnoid, and is said to contain a thin film of fluid. However, recent electron-microscopic findings indicate that when the dura and arachnoid appear to separate, the separation actually occurs within the innermost cellular layer of the dura. In several places the inner dural layer is reflected as sheet-like protrusions into the cranial cavity. These are called dural septa. The principal dural septa are the *falx cerebri*, between the two hemispheres, and the *tentorium cerebelli*, between the cerebral hemispheres and the cerebellum. The tentorium cerebelli separates the superior surface of the cerebellum from the occipital lobes, defining the *supratentorial* and *intratentorial cranial compartments*. The opening in the tentorium through which the brain stem passes is known as the *tentorial notch* or *tentorial incisura*. This notch is of clinical significance when intracranial pressure increases.

The *arachnoid* ('spider-web-like') is a thin, avascular, delicate membrane. It conforms to the general shape of the brain. A subarachnoid space, filled with CSF, is present between the arachnoid and pia mater. Several large spaces referred to as cisterns occur in the subarachnoid space and can be useful radiological landmarks. The *pia mater* ('gentle mother') is a thin, vascular, elastic membrane which adheres closely to the brain and spinal cord, following every sulcus and gyrus. The choroid plexuses arise from the vascular structure of the pia mater. The arachnoid and pia mater are sometimes collectively referred to as the *leptomeninges*.

Spinal cord

The spinal cord is a long, cylindrical structure of grey and white matter within the vertebral column. It is continous with the medulla oblongata, originating at the foramen magnum of the skull and extending to the first or second lumbar vertebrae. It tapers off into a fine, non-neural cord called the *filum terminale* which continues inferiorly (caudally) to its attachments in the coccyx. A small canal (central canal) extends the full length of the cord. It contains CSF, and the upper (rostral) end opens into the fourth

ventricle. The cord is surrounded by the three meninges which are continuous with those encapsulating the brain. The meninges extend to the level of the fifth lumbar vertebra.

The grey matter (cell bodies) in the spinal cord is concentrated in its interior, roughly in the form of an H. White matter, composed of nerve tracts and fibres, surrounds the H-shaped grey matter (see Fig. 22.12). Afferent impulses are received by neurons in the posterior columns or horns of grey matter. Efferent impulses are discharged by neurons in the anterior columns or horns of the grey matter. The grey matter also contains neurons which may transmit impulses from one lateral half of the cord to the other, from posterior to anterior and to other levels of the CNS.

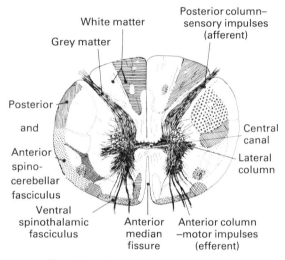

Fig. 22.12 Cross-section of the spinal cord.

Nerve fibres emerge from the spinal cord in uninterrupted series of posterior (sensory or afferent) and anterior (motor or efferent) rootlets which unite to form 31 pairs of posterior and anterior roots. In the area of an intervertebral foramen, a posterior and an anterior root meet to form a *spinal nerve* (Fig. 22.13) which supplies innervation to a segment

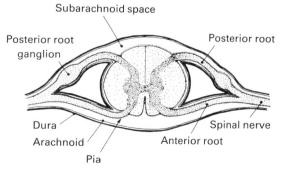

Fig. 22.13 The spinal nerve: its posterior root ganglion, posterior root and anterior root.

of the body. The cord has two enlargements: cervical and lumbar. The cervical enlargement (plexus) is associated with nerve roots which innervate the upper limbs, and the lumbar enlargement (plexus) innervates the lower limbs.

The spinal cord has three major functions: (1) It carries impulses via sensory nerves through ascending tracts up to the brain. (2) It carries impulses from the brain via motor nerves through descending tracts to nerves supplying effector organs (muscle and glands). (3) It functions as a centre for reflex actions (see p. 776).

Nerves and tracts

Nerves are bundles of neuronal processes which extend beyond the CNS, while tracts are bundles of processes within the CNS. Nerves consisting only of afferent fibres, which transmit impulses from the periphery to the CNS, are called *sensory nerves. Motor nerves* are composed entirely of efferent fibres, which transmit impulses from the CNS out into the periphery. Many nerves, for example, all spinal nerves, contain both efferent and afferent fibres and are known as *mixed nerves.*

Structurally, three types of nerve fibres or processes occur. One type known as a medullated or myelinated fibre is enclosed in a lipoprotein sheath (myelin) and an outer membranous sheath called the *neurilemma* (sheath of Schwann). Another type has no myelin sheath but does have a neurilemma and is referred to as a non-myelinated or non-medullated fibre. Most non-myelinated fibres belong to the autonomic nervous system, which is concerned with visceral activity. A third type of neuronal process has a myelin sheath but lacks the neurilemma. All fibres within the CNS, as well as the optic and auditory nerves, are of this type. Neuronal processes lacking the neurilemma cannot regenerate following injury.

Nerve tracts transmit impulses that are usually similar in origin, termination and function. The origin and destination may be determined from the name of the tract. For example, the corticospinal tract carries impulses originating in the cerebral cortex to the spinal cord; the spinothalamic tract transmits sensory impulses from the spinal cord to the thalamus.

NERVE RÉGÉNÉRATION

Unlike most cells in the body, the adult nerve cells cannot reproduce by mitosis to replace any that are destroyed. Some, however, can respond to injury by reconstitution. If a nerve fibre's connection with its cell body is interrupted, the fragment distal to the cell body ceases to function and degenerates. If a neurilemma sheath is present however, the fibre may regenerate and restore function. Nerve fibres within the CNS have no neurilemma and cannot regenerate to re-establish function. If research could solve this problem many tragic effects of stroke or

trauma of the CNS could be relieved. Spinal cord reconstruction has been attempted in recent years (see Reference section).

When a fibre with a neurilemma is damaged, the fragment distal to the nerve cell body disintegrates and the debris is removed by phagocytic glial cells. The neurilemma (Schwann) cells in the proximal end near the interruption and in the distal stump divide mitotically to form continuous cords of neurilemma cells. The distal ends of the proximal axons branch into numerous sprouts which grow into the interruption and distal stump along neurilemma cords which guide them to the sites of the nerve endings. This is a slow process. Non-myelinated fibre regenerate more rapidly than those that must form a myelin sheath.

Interruption of a peripheral nerve is followed by loss of sensation and movement in the part served by the affected nerve. If the two cut ends of the nerve are approximated and sutured, less scar tissue forms, favouring the regeneration process. Occasionally, because of fibrous scar tissue, a branch or bud of viable fibre stump may not find its way into the 'tube' of Schwann cells which is essential to the growing fibres. In such an instance, multiple growing tips may be produced by the fibre stump and may form a small mass referred to as a neuroma.

THE PERIPHERAL NERVOUS SYSTEM

The peripheral nervous system is composed of nerves and ganglia. The nerves may be divided into two main groups—*cranial* and *spinal* nerves—according to whether they emerge from the central nervous system at the cranial or spinal level.

Cranial nerves
There are 12 pairs of cranial nerves that are considered to be part of the peripheral nervous system. They emerge from the undersurface of the brain and are numbered according to the sequence in which they arise from the front to back. For example, the first cranial nerve is located most anteriorly in the frontal lobe, and the twelfth is located most posteriorly in the medulla. Cranial nerves are also named according to their function or distribution. Some of the cranial nerves consist mainly of afferent (motor fibres), three are comprised of afferent (sensory) fibres, and others are made up of both motor and sensory fibres and are referred to as mixed nerves. Cell bodies of the motor fibres form nuclei within the brain stem. With the exception of the olfactory nerves and the optic nerve, sensory fibres originate in ganglia (groups of cell bodies outside the CNS). Olfactory fibres originate in the nasal mucosa and optic fibres arise from the retina of the eyeball. The origin and functions of cranial nerves are described in Table 22.1.

Spinal nerves
Thirty-one pairs of nerves arise from the spinal cord.

Table 22.1 Origin and functions of cranial nerves (12 pairs).

Number	Name	Origin of main nerve fibres	Function
I	Olfactory	Sensory fibres: neurons in nasal mucosa	Olfactory sense (sense of smell)
II	Optic	Sensory fibres: neurons of retina	Vision
III	Oculomotor	Motor fibres:* nucleus in midbrain	Movements of the eyeball and upper eyelid; size of the pupil of iris (i.e. constriction and dilation of pupil to regulate amount of light admitted); control of ciliary muscle to regulate degree of refraction by the lens
IV	Trochlear	Motor fibres: nucleus in midbrain	Movement of eyeball by superior oblique muscles

V	Trigeminal
	
	Largest cranial nerve; has three sensory divisions—ophthalmic, maxillary, mandibular
		Motor fibres:
		    nucleus in pons
		Sensory fibres:
		    gasserian or semilunar ganglion in temporal bone
			Motor function: mastication
			
			Sensory function: sensations (pain, touch, temperature) of the face, nose, teeth and mouth

VI	Abducens	Motor fibres: nucleus in pons	Movement of the eyeball by lateral rectus muscle

VII	Facial	Motor fibres:
		    nucleus in pons
		
		Sensory fibres:
		    geniculate ganglion in temporal bone
			Motor function: contraction of facial and scalp muscles (facial expression); secretion of saliva by submaxillary and sublingual glands
			Sensory function: taste (from anterior two-thirds of tongue)

VIII	Auditory (acoustic)
	Has two divisions:
	    vestibular
	    cochlear
		Sensory fibres:
		    vestibular branch: vestibular ganglion in internal ear
		    cochlear branch: spiral ganglion in internal ear
			Sensory function:
			    vestibular branch: equilibrium (position balance)
			    cochlear division: sense of hearing

IX	Glossopharyngeal	Motor fibres:
		    nucleus in medulla
		
		Sensory fibres:
		    jugular and petrous ganglia
			Motor function: swallowing reflex control of blood pressure through connection with carotid baroreceptors; salivary secretion by parotid glands
			Sensory functions: taste and oral and pharyngeal sensations

X	Vagus
	Has very wide distribution
		Motor fibres:
		    nuclei in medulla
		
		Sensory fibres:
		    jugular and nodosa ganglia
			Motor function: muscles of pharynx, larynx, thoracic and abdominal viscera (e.g. regulates gastrointestinal motility of peristalsis; influences cardiac rate); secretion by gastric, intestinal and pancreatic glands
			Sensory function: sensations in pharynx, larynx, and thoracic and abdominal viscera

XI	Accessory	Motor fibres: nucleus in medulla and the spinal cord	Movement of shoulder and head by trapezius and sternocleidomastoid muscles
XII	Hypoglossal	Motor fibres: nucleus in medulla	Movements of the tongue

*Most motor nerves are considered to also contain some sensory fibres by which information as to the existing conditions in the muscles concerned (proprioceptive data) is transmitted into the central nervous system. The proprioceptive impulses result in appropriate motor responses to facilitate the required pattern of movement.

They are numbered and named according to the order in which they arise and the vertebral level at which they emerge. There are *eight cervical, twelve thoracic, five lumbar, five sacral pairs*, and *one coccygeal pair*.

All spinal nerves are mixed (sensory and motor) and each one has two origins which are referred to as anterior and posterior roots (Fig. 22.13). The anterior roots carry two types of motor fibres: (1) the *general somatic efferent fibres* which have axons originating from lower motor neurons (anterior horn cells in the spinal cord) and which innervate voluntary striated muscles; and (2) the *general visceral efferent fibres* (autonomic nerves) which innervate visceral and cardiac muscle, and regulate glandular secretions. The posterior roots convey sensory input via two types of sensory fibres: (1) the *general somatic afferent* fibres which carry impulses for pain, temperature, touch, and proprioception from the body wall, tendons, and joints into the central nervous system; and (2) *general visceral afferent fibres* which carry sensory impulses from the viscera into the central nervous system.

After emerging from the vertebral canal, each spinal nerve divides into two major branches: the anterior and posterior rami. The *posterior rami* divide into smaller branches which go directly to the muscles and skin of the posterior portions of the head, neck and trunk. The *anterior rami* supply all the structures of the extremities and lateral and anterior portions of the trunk.

The branches of the anterior rami tend to form intricate networks of interlacing nerve branches before proceding to the structures they innervate. These networks are referred to as *plexuses*. Spinal nerves lose their individuality after passing through a plexus and they emerge as peripheral nerves. Four major plexuses are formed by the anterior rami of spinal nerves—the cervical, brachial, lumbar and sacral plexuses. The *cervical plexus* gives rise to peripheral nerve branches that innervate muscles of the neck and shoulders. It also gives rise to the phrenic nerve which supplies the diaphragm. Important peripheral nerves which arise from the *brachial plexus* are the musculocutaneous, median, radial and ulnar nerves, all of which supply the upper limbs. The *lumbar plexus* generates the femoral, saphenous and obturator nerves which innervate the lower abdominal wall, external genitalia, and parts of the thigh and leg. The nerves leaving the *sacral plexus* supply the buttocks, perineum and lower extremities. The most important nerve derived from this plexus is the sciatic, the longest and largest nerve in the body.

Ganglia

A ganglion is a group of nerve cell bodies located outside the CNS. Many important drugs known as ganglion blocking agents exert their effects by inhibiting impulse transmission in this area.

Ganglia associated with the sensory fibres of the cranial nerves are named specifically [e.g. the gasserian ganglion is formed by the three sensory divisions of the trigeminal (V) nerve]. The ganglia which form the posterior or sensory roots of the spinal nerves lie just outside the spinal cord within the vertebral column. These are the spinal or posterior root ganglia.

The ganglia associated with the autonomic (visceral) nervous system may be divided into three groups according to their location. The vertebral, sympathetic, or lateral ganglia occur in two chains. One chain of 22 ganglia lies on each side of the vertebral column. A second group of autonomic ganglia is called the collateral or paravertebral ganglia. These lie in front of the vertebral column and close to large arteries from which they are named (e.g. iliac, mesenteric). A third group is referred to as the terminal ganglia. They lie close to or within the viscera which the nerve fibres supply.

The autonomic nervous system

The autonomic nervous system controls the visceral functions of the body. This system helps to control such phenomena as arterial blood pressure, gastrointestinal motility and secretion, urinary bladder emptying, sweating and body temperature. It carries only efferent impulses and the responses are involuntary.

The autonomic system is largely activated by centres located in the spinal cord, brain stem and hypothalamus. In addition, parts of the cerebral cortex can transmit impulses to the lower centres and in this way influence the autonomic system. For example, chronic emotional stress can result in excessive stimulation of the autonomic system, which in turn may contribute to the development of gastric or duodenal ulcers or other stress-related problems. Often, the autonomic system operates by means of visceral reflexes. That is, sensory signals enter the centres in the CNS and these in turn transmit appropriate reflex responses back to the organs via the autonomic system to control their activities.

The autonomic nervous system is divided into the *parasympathetic* and *sympathetic* systems. Most viscera have a nerve supply from each division; impulses delivered from one system excite visceral activity, and those originating with the other division inhibit activity (see Table 22.2).

THE PARASYMPATHETIC NERVOUS SYSTEM

The parasympathetic fibres leave the CNS through several cranial nerves (75% are in the vagus nerve) and through the pelvic nerves. For this reason, the system may also be referred to as the craniosacral division. This system has both preganglionic and postganglionic fibres. With only a few exceptions, the preganglionic fibres pass uninterrupted to the ganglia which are located within or close to the

Table 22.2 Autonomic effects on various organs of the body.*

Organ	Effect of sympathetic stimulation	Effect of parasympathetic stimulation
Eye: Pupil	Dilated	Constricted
Ciliary muscle	Slight relaxation	Contracted
Glands: Nasal	Vasoconstriction and slight	Stimulation of thin, copious secretion
Lacrimal	secretion	(containing many enzymes for
Parotid		enzyme-secreting glands)
Submaxillary		
Gastric		
Pancreatic		
Sweat glands	Copious sweating (cholinergic)	None
Apocrine glands	Thick, odoriferous secretion	None
Heart: Muscle	Increased rate	Slowed rate
	Increased force of contraction	Decreased force of atrial contraction
Coronary arteries	Dilated ($ß_2$): constricted (α)	Dilated
Lungs: Bronchi	Dilated	Constricted
Blood vessels	Mildly constricted	? Dilated
Gut: Lumen	Decreased peristalsis and tone	Increased peristalsis and tone
Sphincter	Increased tone	Relaxed
Liver	Glucose released	Slight glycogen synthesis
Gallbladder and bile ducts	Relaxed	Constricted
Kidney	Decreased output	None
Bladder: Detrusor muscle	Relaxed	Excited
Trigone	Excited	Relaxed
Penis	Ejaculation	Erection
Systemic blood vessels:		
Abdominal	Constricted	None
Muscle	Constricted (adrenergic α)	None
	Dilated (adrenergic $ß$)	
	Dilated (cholinergic)	
Skin	Constricted	None
Blood: Coagulation	Increased	None
Glucose	Increased	None
Basal metabolism	Increased up to 100%	None
Adrenal cortical secretion	Increased	None
Mental activity	Increased	None
Piloerector muscles	Excited	None
Skeletal muscle	Increased glycogenolysis	None
	Increased strength	

*Guyton (1981), p. 223.

viscera they innervate. Postganglionic fibres of this division are short and are located within the respective organs (Fig. 22.14).

The responses to parasympathetic stimulation are localized and specific for parts of the body.

Generally, parasympathetic innervation promotes a normal state; it is concerned with the restoration and conservation of body energy and elimination of body wastes (see Table 22.2).

THE SYMPATHETIC NERVOUS SYSTEM

The sympathetic nerves originate in the thoracic and lumbar regions of the spinal cord. Because of these origins, the system is also referred to as the thoracolumbar nervous system. The sympathetic nerves leave the spinal cord via the anterior roots and form the white communicating rami (called the thoracolumbar outflow of the spinal nerves) of the thoracic and lumbar nerves. Through these, nerves

reach the trunk ganglia of the sympathetic chain. Upon entering the chain, these preganglionic fibres may synapse with a host of ganglion cells, pass up or down the sympathetic chain to synapse with ganglion cells at a higher or lower level, or pass through the trunk ganglia and out to the tissues and organs that are innervated by these nerves (Fig. 22.15).

The sympathetic system produces generalized physiological responses rather than specific, localized ones. It responds to stress, strong emotions, severe pain, cold, or any threat. The purpose of the responses induced is to mobilize the body's resources for defensive action ('fight or flight') (see Table 22.2).

Stimulation of the sympathetic nervous system results in stimulation of the adrenal medullae. Increase in secretion of adrenaline and noradrenaline results, and this augments the body defence responses mediated by the sympathetic nervous system.

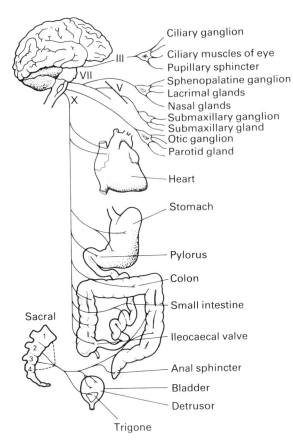

Fig. 22.14 The parasympathetic nervous system.

Chemical mediators

In both the sympathetic and parasympathetic nervous systems the transmission of impulses from the preganglionic fibres to the ganglia is dependent upon the release of *acetylcholine* by the preganglionic axon terminals. Acetylcholine is rapidly deactivated by *cholinesterase*. The postganglionic fibres of the parasympathetic system also release acetylcholine at their junction with the effector organs to facilitate the transmission of their impulses. The neurotransmitter that is released by the postganglionic nerve terminals in the sympathetic system is *noradrenaline* which is deactivated by enzymes (e.g. monoamine oxidase, catechol-O-methyltransferase) or taken up again by the nerve terminals.

MUSCLE TISSUE AND ACTIVITY

Muscle tissue comprises up to 50% of the total body weight. This tissue performs activities which are critical to survival such as respiration, circulation of the blood, and peristaltic movement of food through the gastrointestinal tract. It is also responsible for movements of body parts as well as the mobility of the body as a whole. The capacity of the body to carry out its vital activities is dependent upon the specialized physiological properties that are unique to muscle tissue (see Table 22.3).

During muscle contraction, the chemical reactions which occur liberate both mechanical and heat energy. The heat energy contributes to the maintenance of body temperature. At rest, most of the body heat is produced by metabolic activities such as occur in the liver.

Muscle cells, because of their elongated shape, may be referred to as muscle fibres. In most muscles, the fibres extend the entire length of the muscle. The cell membrane of the muscle fibre is called *sarcolemma*. Three types of muscle tissue with different types of control are present in the body to meet its need for varying degrees of muscular activity. These are *cardiac, smooth (visceral or involuntary)*, and *striated (skeletal or voluntary)* muscle tissue. Cardiac muscle tissue is discussed in Chapter 14.

Smooth muscle tissue is present in walls of blood vessels and most hollow viscera. The cells are smaller and are arranged in sheets or layers and their

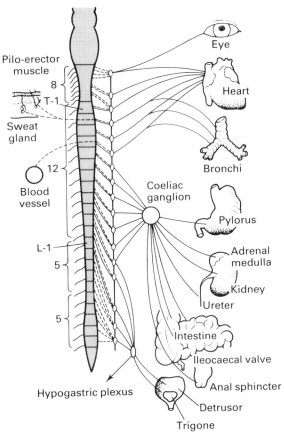

Fig. 22.15 The sympathetic nervous system (dashed lines represent postganglionic fibres in the grey rami leading into the spinal nerves for distribution to blood vessels, sweat glands, pilo-erector muscles).

Table 22.3 Physiological properties of muscle tissue.

Property	Description
Contractility	The shortening and thickening of muscle cells as a result of their ability to convert chemical energy to mechanical energy
Disability	The capacity to stretch
Spasticity	The ability to resume original length after a stretching force is removed
Excitability Sensitivity	The capability to respond by contraction to a change in the environment which may be initiated by a nerve impulse, pressure, stretching, chemical changes (e.g. calcium concentration) or temperature changes (e.g. cold stimulates contraction)
Clonus	The sustained partial contraction maintained by groups of muscle cells contracting in relays in response to nerve impulses from the spinal cord. This is a state of readiness for action

sarcolemmae are not as well defined as in skeletal muscle. Smooth muscle has inherent, rhythmic contractile activity and is under autonomic control.

Skeletal muscle tissue forms the muscles which are attached to bones and is responsible for external body movements and the maintenance of position against gravity. It is called striated because of variations in protein concentration which are evident with light microscopy. Its cytoplasm, which may be called *sarcoplasm*, contains hundreds or thousands of myofibrils and its sarcolemma is well defined. Unlike most body cells, each skeletal muscle fibre has several nuclei. A skeletal muscle is composed of both muscle and connective tissue. Groups of muscle fibres are arranged in bundles (fasciculi) and are held together by connective tissue. Groups of these bundles are bound together and the entire muscle is encased in a tough sheath of connective tissue (epimysium) and may also have a tough fibrous coating, called *fascia*. (Fig. 22.16). The muscle sheath contains

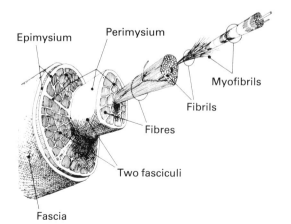

Fig. 22.16 Cross-section of a skeletal muscle.

blood and lymph vessels and nerve fibres. Prolongations of the connective tissues extending beyond the actual muscle fibres form the tendonous attachments to bones. Each skeletal muscle has an *origin*, which is the stationary attachment of muscle to skeleton, and an *insertion*, which is the attachment to the moveable part. When the muscle contracts, the insertion is pulled toward the origin. The thick part of the muscle consisting of the bundles of fibres may be referred to as the *body* of the muscle. Individual skeletal muscles are usually named according to action (e.g. flexor or extensor), location or origin.

MOTOR AND SENSORY INNERVATION OF SKELETAL MUSCLES

Contraction of skeletal muscles normally only results from impulses discharged by motor neurons within the CNS and transmitted along peripheral nerve fibres to the muscle. Since the motor centres lie within the cerebral cortex, contractions are usually voluntarily produced. Involuntary (unwilled) contractions do occur in the form of reflex responses (see p. 776).

The process whereby a nerve impulse is converted into a muscle action current is referred to as *neuromuscular transmission*. Each nerve fibre terminates at a specialized region of the muscle fibre, called *myoneural* or *neuromuscular junction* or *motor-end-plate*. The end-plate is a localized specialization of the sarcolemma. Essentially, the release of acetylcholine at the end-plate and its rapid destruction by the enzyme cholinesterase is at the basis of electrical and chemical reactions and the release of mechanical and heat energy in the contraction of muscle fibres.

It has been estimated that at least 40% of nerve fibres innervating a given muscle are sensory rather than motor end-organs. Three major types of end-organs (receptors) that are sensitive to changes in muscle fibres and that initiate impulses which are transmitted by afferent nerve fibres from skeletal muscles to the CNS are known to exist. These are muscle spindles, golgi bodies and free nerve endings. *Muscle spindles* lie between muscle fibres. They are excited by stretching and are associated with the stretch reflex. *Golgi bodies* are proprioceptors located in tendons and are sensitive to tension; when the tension becomes excessive, impulses are initiated which result in inhibition of muscle contraction. *Free nerve endings*, which are mainly associated with blood vessels in muscle tissue, give rise to pain impulses.

CHEMICAL COMPOSITION AND CONTRACTION

Skeletal muscle is composed of 75% water, 20% protein, and 5% inorganic material, organic 'extractives' and carbohydrates (glycogen and its derivatives). The proteins myosin, actin, tropomyosin, troponin and myoglobin give muscle fibres their elasticity and contractile power. The major inorganic constituents of muscle include potassium, sodium, magnesium, and calcium. Phosphate chloride and small amounts of sulphate are also present. Compounds which can be extracted from muscle include creatine and phosphocreatine, adenine, quanine, uric acid and adenylic acid (from adenosine triphosphate or ATP).

Almost everything discussed regarding initiation and conduction of action potential in nerve fibres applies equally well to skeletal muscle fibres (see p. 758). Energy for muscle contraction is generated by a series of chemical reactions within the fibres. Briefly, these include the following: the motor nerve impulse causes depolarization of the sarcolemma, leading to the sudden breakdown of adenosine triphosphate (ATP) to adenosine diphosphate (ADP) and the release of phosphate and energy; the energy promotes the interaction of actin and myosin filaments which produces the actual shortening and thickening of the muscle (contraction); phosphocreatine is hydrolyzed and gives up phosphate, which combines with ADP to quickly restore the ATP so that a constant source of energy for contraction is maintained; glycogen is then broken down, releasing phosphate and lactic acid; the phosphate molecules combine with creatine to replenish the phosphocreatine; about one-fifth of the lactic acid is oxidized to energy, carbon dioxide and water; and the remainder of the lactic acid is reconverted to glycogen. The initial reactions which provide instantaneous energy for contraction do not utilize oxygen (anaerobic). The oxidation of lactic acid requires oxygen and the energy released is utilized in the resynthesis of the basic compounds used during contraction. In hypoxaemia or in strenuous exercise, the oxygen supply is generally inadequate to oxidize lactic acid and provide the required energy for resynthesis. Lactic acid accumulates and the condition is said to have incurred an oxygen debt; that is, the oxygen provided was not sufficient to keep pace with the production of lactic acid.

The initial source of energy for muscle contraction is oxygen and the basic food substances, particularly the metabolism of carbohydrates and fats. Therefore, interruption of blood flow through a contracting muscle quickly leads to muscle fatigue.

The *strength of the contraction* of a muscle depends on the number of fibres excited, the length of the fibre, and the size of the muscle. When stimulated, each fibre contracts to its fullest capacity (all-or-none law) and when the stimulus is maximal or intense, all fibres are involved. The force of contraction of a fibre increases proportionately with its length up to a certain point, after which it decreases. The larger the muscle mass, the greater amount of energy produced. A muscle responds to repeated, increased demands by hypertrophy of individual fibres, and to decreased demands by atrophy.

Muscle contractions are referred to as twitch,

tetanic, isotonic, and isometric. A single stimulus to a muscle produces a quick, brief contraction referred to as a *twitch*. *Tetanic contraction* occurs when a muscle is stimulated at progressively greater frequency and a sustained contraction results due to a fusion of successive contractions. Muscle contraction is said to be *isometric* when the muscle length does not change during contraction but its tension is increased. It is said to be *isotonic* when muscle shortens and produces movement but the tension in the muscle remains constant.

Muscles are arranged to function in pairs; the contraction of one of the pair is accompanied by relaxation of the other (reciprocal inhibition). For example, if the biceps is to contract to flex the forearm, the triceps must relax. The muscle which contracts is called the agonist, and the one which relaxes at the same time is known as the *antagonist*. Other muscles may be necessary in certain patterns of movement and may be classified as *synergists* or *stabilizers*. They facilitate the work of the agonist.

Voluntary movement

Normal voluntary movements are the result of controlled contraction and relaxation of groups of muscles. All willed movements depend upon excitation of neurons within the cerebral cortex (upper motor neurons) as well as at a lower level (lower motor neurons). Those at a lower level may be the motor components of cranial nerve nuclei in the brain stem or they may be in the spinal cord. Two major neuronal pathways in the CNS are involved in voluntary muscle activity. These are referred to as the pyramidal tract and the extrapyramidal system.

PYRAMIDAL TRACT (CORTICOSPINAL TRACT)

The pyramidal tract arises in the sensorimotor cortex of the cerebrum and is one of the major pathways whereby motor signals are transmitted from all the motor areas of the cortex to the anterior motor neurons of the spinal cord.

Voluntary movement begins with the stimulation of a discrete area of neurons in the motor area of the cerebral cortex. If the movement applies to only muscles on one side of the body, only the motor area of the cerebral hemisphere on the opposite side will be involved. As the axons of the motor neurons of each hemisphere descend, they converge to form a compact mass referred to as the *internal capsule*. The fibres continue downward through the brain stem and in the lower medulla approximately 90% decussate (cross over) to form the pyramids of the medulla (Fig. 22.17). These fibres descend in the lateral corticospinal tract of the cord and terminate in posterior horns of cord grey matter. Fibres which did not decussate earlier, continue ipsilaterally in the anterior corticospinal tracts and cross over further down the cord.

At various levels in the cord, the fibres synapse with neurons in the anterior horns of grey matter. The axons of these neurons form the motor fibres of the peripheral nerves whereby the impulses are delivered to muscle fibres. Some fibres in the tract

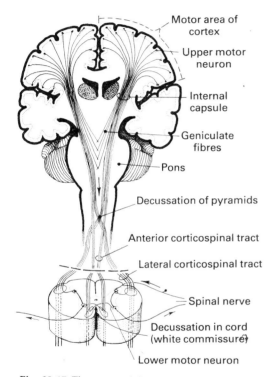

Fig. 22.17 The pyramidal tract (corticospinal tract).

may synapse in the brain stem with nuclei of cranial nerves. The impulses are then carried out to a muscle by motor fibres of a peripheral cranial nerve.

The neurons of the cerebral cortical motor area are referred to as the upper motor neurons. Those with which the axons of upper motor neurons synapse are called *lower motor neurons*. The cell bodies of lower motor neurons reside within the CNS and their axons carry the impulses to skeletal muscles in the periphery.

Interruption of the pyramidal tract at any level produces muscle paralysis. Spastic paralysis occurs with damage of an area above the lower motor neurons. The muscles controlled by the affected

upper motor neurons resist passive movement and exhibit increased tone and exaggerated reflexes, because the inhibiting influence of higher centres is interrupted. Injury to lower motor neurons or their axons results in flaccid paralysis in the respective muscles, loss of tone and reflexes and wasting (atrophy) of the muscles.

EXTRAPYRAMIDAL SYSTEM (EXTRAPYRAMIDAL TRACTS)

This system includes all the tracts exclusive of the pyramidal tract, that transmit motor signals from the brain to the spinal cord (Fig. 22.18). Unlike the pyramidal tract, which is a direct link from the cerebral cortex to the spinal cord, the extrapyramidal system conveys its influences to the cord via multi-neuronal and multisynaptic linkages involving the cortex, basal ganglia, thalami, cerebellum, brain stem and related structures. Extrapyramidal impulses are initiated in several areas of the brain below conscious level and all are transmitted by reticulospinal tracts to lower motor neurons. The lower motor neurons provide the final common pathway for all the afferent impulses (both pyramidal and extrapyramidal) to skeletal muscles. Inhibition, facilitation, and coordination, essential for smooth, precise muscle activity is normally provided by the extrapyramidal system.

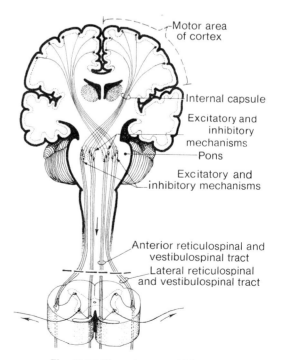

Fig. 22.18 The extrapyramidal tract.

An imbalance in the interactions within the complex circuitry of the extrapyramidal system occurs with malfunction of various nuclear complexes. The motor disorders resulting from the improper functioning of the extrapyramidal system and associated nuclei include various abnormal movements such as paralysis agitans, athetosis and choreas.

Voluntary muscle activity involves the pyramidal and extrapyramidal tracts in concert. The pyramidal tract transmits the impulses which are consciously initiated to produce a given movement. The other essential components of the movement such as reciprocal relaxation of certain muscles, correlation, stabilization and adjustment in posture are automatically contributed by the extrapyramidal system.

The following activity illustrates the role of the pyramidal and extrapyramidal tracts in voluntary movement. If a person who is standing reaches out to pick up a pen from a table, he consciously concentrates on the action of his fingers and thumb necessary to grasp the object. Several muscle responses are involved as well as the flexion of fingers and thumb. The forearm is extended to reach the pen (the biceps relaxes and the triceps contracts); muscles contract to stabilize the shoulder and wrist; leaning forward to reach the pen may be necessary, so the trunk flexes and shifts the centre of gravity, necessitating muscle action in the trunk and lower extremities to ensure maintenance of the upright position.

Reflexes

A reflex is an involuntary, stereotypic response mediated by the nervous system. It serves as a defence mechanism and it may involve the contraction of muscle tissue or the secretion of a gland. Although reflexes occur without voluntary or willed initiation, the person usually becomes conscious of the reflex activity because the impulses reach the cerebral cortex and are interpreted as sensation. The pathway over which nerve impulses pass is called a reflex arc (Fig. 22.19). The arc is comprised of receptors (e.g. proprioceptors in a muscle, special sense organs), an afferent pathway (sensory nerve fibres), CNS connections (e.g. connecting or internuncial neurons of the spinal cord), motor neurons (e.g. lower motor neurons in anterior columns of spinal cord), efferent pathway (motor nerve fibres), and effector organ (muscle fibres or glandular cells). The simplest reflex arc consists of two neurons—a sensory and a motor neuron. The patellar reflex ('knee-jerk') which is elicited by tapping the tendon of the quadriceps femoris muscle is an example of this type of reflex.

Reflex responses are either protective or postural. *Protective reflexes* are produced in response to irritating or painful stimuli. Examples include: the closing

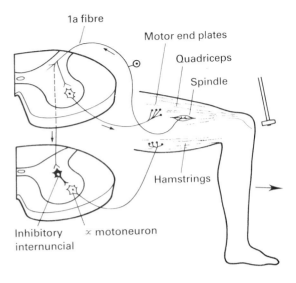

Fig. 22.19 The spinal reflex arc—response to knee tap (knee jerk).

of the eyelid when the cornea is lightly touched (blink reflex); rapid withdrawal of a hand from a hot stove (withdrawal reflex); and contraction of superficial abdominal muscles and movement of the umbilicus in the direction of the skin area stimulated in response to light, rapid stroking of the cutaneous surface of the abdomen (abdominal reflex).

Postural reflexes maintain an appropriate degree of muscle tone which is essential in supporting the body against gravity and maintaining an upright position. The body can stay upright because muscles exert a continual pull on bones in the opposite direction to ever-present gravitational forces. Reflex mechanisms which regulate the muscle contraction necessary to provide the antigravity force are the stretch (myotatic) reflex and impulses originating in the internal ear. With a change in position, movement of the fluid in the semicircular canals in the ears elicits sensory impulses which are conveyed by the vestibular fibres of the eighth cranial (auditory) nerve to nuclei in the brain stem. From here, impulses are transmitted via vestibulospinal tracts to motor neurons which discharge impulses to appropriate muscles, producing an increase in their tone in support of the body's upright position.

Reflexes which are clinically important may be organized into four groups: (1) superficial (or skin and mucous membrane) reflexes, (2) deep (or myotatic) reflexes, (3) visceral (or organic), and (4) pathological (or abnormal). The nasal (or sneeze) reflex and the pharyngeal (or gag) reflex are examples of *mucous membrane reflexes*. The abdominal reflex and the plantar reflex are *skin reflexes*. *Deep reflexes* include those in which receptors are located in deeper tissue such as tendons. The biceps reflex, which is flexion at the elbow when the biceps tendon is struck, is a deep reflex. *Visceral reflexes* include pupillary reflexes such as constriction in response to light stimulus, the oculocardiac reflex (slowing of the heart rate in response to pressure over the eyeballs), and the carotid sinus reflex (decrease in heart rate and blood pressure in response to pressure over the carotid sinus in the neck).

Pathological reflexes are usually elicited only when neurological disease is present. Primitive defence responses, normally suppressed by cerebral inhibitory influences are frequently present in these reflexes.

Neurological Assessment

Neurological assessment (evaluation) may include: a neurological history or interview, the neurological examination, assessment of the effect of neurological dysfunction on daily living, emergency assessment—craniocerebral and spinal testing, continuous intracranial monitoring, observations, and diagnostic studies.

NEUROLOGICAL HISTORY (INTERVIEW)

The neurological history is part of the general health history. It usually includes demographic data, a description of the patient, the history of the present disorder, past history, a review of systems and family and social history. Since neurological illness frequently affects mental status, the patient's mental condition and his perception of his problem are evaluated. If the patient is unable to provide reliable information, the history may be obtained from a relative or friend who is familiar with the patient. The source of the data is included in the history.

NEUROLOGICAL EXAMINATION

The neurological examination is that part of the physical examination which evaluates the function of the cerebrum and the cranial nerves as well as the motor and sensory status, reflex status and the status of the autonomic nervous system.

Cerebrum

Evaluation of cerebral function includes information obtained from observing the patient, evoking responses and from family and friends. It relates to the appropriateness of the individual's appearance, behaviour, level of consciousness, mood, attitude and flow of speech. Cognitive functions such as orientation, speech comprehension, general intelligence, attention and concentration, memory

retention and immediate recall, vocabulary, judgement and abstract reasoning are also evaluated. Deterioration in one or more of these functions commonly occurs with cerebral dysfunction.

The patient's family may report a change in his appearance, particularly facial expression, posture and personal grooming. Disordered emotional reactions may be evident in the patient's fluctuating attitudes. There may be inappropriate laughing, crying, irritability or unprovoked expressions of anger. Sharp mood swings may occur; the patient who is withdrawn and depressed or anxious may suddenly become excited or euphoric. Impaired reasoning, unjustified fears, distortion in perception and loss of memory may occur. The attention span may be abnormally short and there may be inability to do very simple calculations or to identify normally familiar objects or sounds. Confusion or disorientation as to time, place or person may occur with a cerebral lesion. The patient's response to stimuli may vary from a coherent verbal response to no response of any sort, even to painful stimuli.

Speech dysfunctions which occur with cerebral lesions vary with the location, size, and nature of the lesion. Aphasia, dysphasia, agnosia, apraxia, and dyslexia are examples of speech disorders which may occur.

Aphasia refers to the loss of ability to understand words or to use them to communicate. Difficulty in using words to communicate due to lack of coordination and ability to put words in order occurs more commonly and is referred to as *dysphasia*. Aphasia may be classified as *motor (expressive, Broca's)* or *sensory (receptive)*. Motor aphasia implies the person understands spoken and written words and knows what he wants to say but cannot speak the words. Motor aphasias include any loss of communication by writing, speaking or making signs. Sensory aphasia implies that the comprehension of written and spoken words is affected. A patient may suffer auditory aphasia (word deafness) which is the inability to make sense of sound because of an inability to comprehend symbolic communication associated with sound. Some may experience visual aphasia ('word blindness') which means loss of ability to understand the symbolic content of written words or figures and even though they can see them they cannot read them. In many instances of aphasia, elements of both expressive and receptive communication are lost.

Certain areas of the cerebral cortex are essential to the recognition of objects by sight, sound, feeling, smell and taste. Cerebral dysfunction may result in the inability to recognize objects through any of the senses and is referred to as *agnosia*. Agnosia may be visual, auditory or tactile. A cerebral lesion may also result in *apraxia* which is the inability to carry out purposeful, useful, or skilled acts in the absence of paralysis, or use objects correctly. *Dyslexia* means inability to comprehend written words.

Cranial nerves
Cranial nerves are referred to by specific name or number (see Table 22.1). Most arise from the brain stem, and much information can be obtained by testing cranial nerve function. Evaluation of cranial nerve function involves the following:

Olfactory (cranial nerve I). The patient is asked to close his eyes and to identify a series of odorous substances such as coffee, peppermint, oil of cloves. Each nostril is tested separately. Inability to identify the substances (in the absence of a cold or allergy) may suggest a lesion in the frontal lobe such as a basal skull fracture or a tumour of the olfactory groove.

Optic (II). This test includes ophthalmoscopic examination and evaluation of visual acuity and visual fields. Visual acuity may be grossly evaluated by asking the person to read from a printed page or distant sign both with and without corrective lenses if such are used. See assessment in Chapter 28, Nursing in Disorders of the Eyes.

Ophthalmoscopic examination may reveal papilloedema (sometimes referred to as choked disc), which is oedema of the area where the optic nerve and blood vessels enter and leave the eyeball, and is a classical sign of increased intracranial pressure. Optic atrophy, the opposite of papilloedema, indicates a decreased blood supply.

Oculomotor (III), trochlear (IV) and abducent (VI). These nerves are usually tested together since they are all involved in the muscles that rotate the eyeball, constrict the pupils and elevate the eyelids. On examination, pupils should be round and equal in size and shape. Each pupil is tested, in a darkened room, for the direct light reflex. A light is directed into each pupil and the response is observed. The normal pupil constricts briskly in response to light stimulus. The consensual light reflex is also tested. This is a slightly weaker constriction of one pupil when the other is stimulated by light. Accommodation is tested by asking the person to look at a distant spot and then to follow the examiner's finger to within 15 cm (6 in) of the person's nose. Visualization of a distant object causes pupillary dilatation while viewing a near object produces constriction and convergence. The acronym PERRLA may be used to denote 'pupils equal, round, reactive to light and accommodation'. Abnormal pupillary responses suggest neurological dysfunction. The range of ocular movements is evaluated by asking the person to follow the examiner's finger as it moves up, down, medially and laterally. Inability to move the eyeball in a particular direction may result in *diplopia* (double vision). Normal eyes move conjugately (track together). Disconjugate movement implies failure of function of one or more of the eye muscles. Abnormal eye movements can result from injury to the nerves

themselves or their nuclei in the midbrain and pons. During examination of ocular movements, observations for *nystagmus* are made. This is an involuntary rhythmic movement of one or both eyes in a lateral or vertical direction. It may occur in normal persons with severe myopia or fatigue or it may occur with neurological disease. *Ptosis* (drooping) of the eyelid may occur with paralysis of the levator palpebrae muscle due to damage of cranial nerve III.

Trigeminal (V). The trigeminal nerve has *sensory* and *motor* components. The sensory function is assessed by testing both sides of the face and mouth for touch, temperature and pain sensations while the person's eyes are closed. The motor function is evaluated by having the person make chewing and biting movements. The jaw reflex is tested by tapping the midchin when the jaw is slightly ajar and the mouth closed. The ophthalmic branch of the trigeminal nerve controls the corneal reflex. If this reflex is intact, the person blinks briskly when the cornea of each eye is lightly touched with a wisp of cotton wool. The corneal reflex is one of the last to disappear when the patient's condition is deteriorating.

Facial (VII). The facial nerve has a sensory and motor component. The sensory component is tested by seeing if the person can recognize the taste of bitter, sour, sweet and salty substances respectively when applied to the tongue. The motor divisions are tested by asking the person to use the facial muscles in such expressions as smiling, frowning, closing the eyes tightly and puckering the lips.

Acoustic (auditory) VIII. This nerve has two divisions, the cochlear nerve and the vestibular nerve. The cochlear nerve is tested for hearing acuity by whispering in one ear, using a ticking watch and a tuning fork (see Chapter 29). Loss of hearing or reports by the patient of constant or abnormal recurring sounds described as roaring, ringing, buzzing or swishing should be recorded and reported to the doctor. The vestibular nerve, concerned with equilibrium reflexes, is tested by rotating the patient and performing the caloric test (see p. 786). Dizziness and loss of position balance (equilibrium) may occur with disturbance in the semicircular canals of the internal ear, of the vestibular part of the auditory nerve, or pathway within the brain.

Glossopharyngeal (IX) and vagus (X). These nerves are usually examined simultaneously because of their overlapping innervation of the pharynx. In response to touching of the pharynx with a tongue depressor, a brisk gag reaction should be elicited. Ability to swallow water is assessed and the posterior third of the tongue may be tested for taste. Absence of the gag or swallowing reflex occurs in neurological damage and it renders the person vulnerable to aspiration. To assess the vagus nerve, the ability to speak and to cough is evaluated. Ineffectual cough and a weak, hoarse voice suggest possible vagal involvement.

Spinal accessory (XI). This nerve is tested by inspecting the sternocleidomastoid muscle and the upper portion of the trapezius muscle for symmetry, atrophy and strength. The person is asked to elevate the shoulders with and without resistance from the examiner's hand, and to rotate the head to each side against the pull of the chin to the midline by the examiner's hand.

Hypoglossal (XII). This nerve is assessed by observing various movements of the tongue and examining it for symmetry, atrophy and tremor when protruded.

Motor function
This is evaluated by examining muscle symmetry, size, shape, tone and movement. Muscle function, balance accuracy, and muscle strength are assessed. Inspection and comparison of muscles on both sides of the body, palpation and measuring the circumferences of areas with a tape measure provides information about size and shape and can reveal abnormalities such as atrophy or hypertrophy. Muscle tone is assessed by palpating muscles at rest and noting the resistance to passive movement. Excessive resistance (*spasticity*), a constant state of resistance (*rigidity*) and decreased muscle tone (*flaccidity or hypotonia*) are examples of abnormal muscle tone.

Movements are examined for 'fine' and 'gross' abnormalities. Fine muscle abnormalities are *fasiculations* which are involuntary ripples, or twitches, which occur when the person is relaxed. They suggest lower motor neuron disease. Gross abnormal movements may indicate extrapyramidal disease and include athetoid, choreiform and distonic movements, spasms, myoclonus, tics, and tremors.

Athetoid movements are involuntary, repetitive, slow and writhing. They may be unilateral or bilateral and follow a definite pattern in the individual patient, ceasing only during sleep. Athetosis is commonly seen in persons with cerebral palsy.

Choreiform movements are involuntary, rapid, rhythmic and jerky. They begin abruptly, are variable in pattern and distribution and may occur during sleep. The limbs, face and tongue are most often involved, and difficulty in speaking, chewing and swallowing may be present. The forcefulness of the movements may lead to injury unless protection is provided. *Spasms or cramps* are sudden, violent, involuntary contractions of a muscle or muscle groups which result in pain, interference with function and voluntary movement. Muscles of the limbs and neck are most frequently affected. The cause may be a lesion within the CNS (e.g. degenerative changes in the extrapyramidal system, a deficient blood supply to the muscle(s), overstretching and injury of the muscle fibres or, a blood calcium or sodium defi-

ciency). *Dystonic movements* involve spasms in portions of the limbs as well as the trunk. The result is usually slow, grotesque, twisting movements and abnormal posture. *Myoclonus* is shock-like contractions of a portion of a muscle, an entire muscle or group of muscles restricted to one area of the body or appearing synchronously or asynchronously in several areas (seen most commonly in epilepsy). Tics are frequently of psychogenic origin. They are stereotyped, repetitive, purposeless movements which vary from individual to individual. Twitching of a cheek is an example of a tic. *Tremors* are involuntary shaky movements, particularly of the limbs, which may have a physical or psychological aetiology. A fine, rapid tremor, particularly of the hands, may be associated with anxiety, fatigue or toxic conditions such as thyrotoxicosis, uraemia and alcoholism. *Intention tremor (cerebellar tremor)* occurs when a voluntary movement is initiated and progressively intensifies especially with precision movements. A *resting (static) tremor* is one that diminishes with voluntary movement and disappears during sleep.

Muscles are further evaluated by putting all the joints through a full range of passive movement. Pain, contractures and muscle resistance are abnormal findings.

Muscle strength may be assessed by flexion and extension and other movements, first without resistance and then with the examiner offering resistance. In addition, the person may be asked to hold the arms straight in front of him with the palms up and his eyes closed, for 20–30 seconds. If one arm moves downward or one hand begins to pronate, a *drift* is said to be present, suggesting muscle weakness in that arm. Drift can be tested in the lower limbs by asking the person to raise both legs off the bed while in a supine position.

Coordination, balance and *accuracy* of muscle function is largely mediated by the cerebellum. These attributes may be assessed by point-to-point tests (e.g. with the eyes open, then repeated with the eyes closed, the person repeatedly touches the examiner's finger and then his own nose). Coordination and balance may also be assessed by observing the person's gait while his eyes are open and again when closed. Locomotion depends upon a normal degree of tone, close integration and coordination of the involved muscles of the lower limbs and trunk. These factors are primarily dependent upon normal innervation.

Various abnormal gaits may be observed in the presence of neurological dysfunction. The *ataxic gait* is an unsteady, uncoordinated walk. With the feet placed far apart to provide a wide base for support, each foot is lifted abnormally high and slapped down with each step. The steps are unsure, unevenly spaced and may deviate to one side. Ataxic gait is associated with a loss of proprioceptive sense and a lack of coordination of muscle action. It tends to be more pronounced in the dark, as visual influences diminish. The *stepping gait* (foot drop gait) is characterized by foot drop due to paralysis of the anterior tibial muscles usually secondary to lower motor neuron disease. The person looks as though he is walking upstairs, because he lifts his advancing leg abnormally high to avoid dragging the foot and stumbling. *Cerebellar ataxia* is staggering, unsteady and wide-based. Turns are made with difficulty. The person is unable to stand steadily with the feet together, whether the eyes are open or closed. It is associated with damage in the cerebellum or related tracts. *Parkinson's gait* is characteristic of patients with the basal ganglia defects of Parkinson's disease (see pp. 844–845). With this gait, the trunk is stooped forward, the knees are slightly flexed, steps are short and often shuffling and the speed of walking progressively accelerates. Turning occurs stiffly and as if 'all in one piece'.

Paralysis or loss of motor function is a common occurrence in neurological disease or injury. Paralysis may be partial and exhibited by weakness (*paresis*) or complete and may be classified according to the extent of the involvement. *Monoplegia* refers to paralysis of one limb. *Hemiplegia* means paralysis of one side of the body . There is loss of muscle power in the limbs and the muscles of the face on the same side. If the side of the face opposite to that of the paralyzed limbs is affected, the term *alternate hemiplegia* may be used (Fig. 20.20A). *Paraplegia* denotes paralysis of the legs or the lower half of the body (Fig. 22.20B). *Quadriplegia* or *tetraplegia* refers to paralysis of the trunk and all four extremities (Fig. 22.20C). Isolated paralysis indicates the loss of the contractile ability of one muscle of a group. It is frequently associated with peripheral nerve damage and is usually accompanied by loss of sensation in the area supplied by the injured nerve.

Paralysis may also be classified as that due to an upper or lower motor neuron lesion. Damage to the motor areas of the cerebral cortex or their projection pathways (corticospinal or pyramidal tracts) produces paralysis due to an upper motor neuron lesion or what may also be termed *spastic paralysis*. Since the lower motor neurons and reflex arc are intact, the affected muscles are still capable of reflex movements and exhibit hypertonicity (spasticity) as well as exaggerated reflexes. There is increased activity of postural (stretch) and protective reflexes. Paralysis resulting from injury of the motor neurons in the nuclei of cranial nerves or in the anterior horns or columns of grey matter in the spinal cord or damage to their axons in the periphery may be referred to as that due to a *lower motor neuron lesion* or as *flaccid paralysis*. Flaccidity occurs because the reflex arc is interrupted; there is a lack of reflex innervation and responses.

Serious abnormal postures which may develop with some cerebral and brain stem disorders are *decerebrate rigidity* and *decorticate rigidity* (see p. 807). Normally, primitive reflex spinal mechanisms which initiate involuntary muscular responses are kept inactive by cerebral control. These primitive involuntary responses may be referred to as spinal automatisms. When control from the higher centres is abolished, sustained rigid posturing develops, which may be decorticate or decerebrate.

Sensory function
This includes assessment of the visual, auditory, olfactory, gustatory, touch, proprioceptive, pain and temperature senses. Most of these have been discussed in conjunction with assessment of the cranial nerves. The body areas usually tested for touch, pain and temperature are the face, hands, arms, trunk, thighs, feet, perineal and perianal regions. The patient is asked to close his eyes, and each side of the body is compared to the other. Sensitivity to touch (a wisp of cotton wool), superficial pain (a pin prick), deep pressure pain, heat and cold, vibration and position is tested. In addition, the patient is asked to differentiate among various textures.

Sensory tests are often difficult to evaluate and a great deal depends upon the cooperation of the patient. Neurological lesions more often result in a diminution of sensation than in total anaesthesia. A sensory disturbance may be localized in one particular area of the body because of the different sensory pathways being associated with different parts. Hypo-or hypersensitivity in the area may provide information about the location of a lesion.

Reflex status
Evaluation of reflexes provides valuable information about the nature, location and progression of neuro-

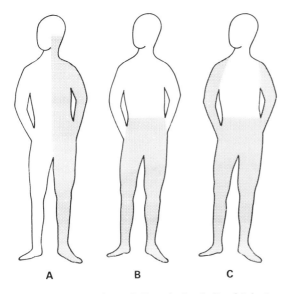

Fig. 22.20 *A*, Hemiplegia. *B*, Paraplegia. *C*, Quadriplegia.

logical disorders in both the conscious and unconscious patient. Exaggeration or diminished responses of normal reflexes and the presence of pathological reflexes are frequently among the earliest indications of neurological disturbance. Reflexes most commonly tested are the deep tendon or muscle-stretch reflexes, superficial reflexes and pathological reflexes. The part of the body tested should be relaxed and the stimulus applied with the same intensity to each side of the body. Rapidity and strength of the muscle contractions are noted.

The *deep reflexes* are tested by tapping briskly on a tendon over a bony prominence, evoking an instantaneous stretching of certain muscles and their resulting contraction. The maxillary, biceps, brachioradialis, triceps, patellar and Achilles reflexes are the most common tested. *Superficial reflexes* are elicited by light, rapid stroking of a particular area of the skin or mucous membrane with an object. The corneal and pupillary reflexes, the pharyngeal or gag reflex, abdominal, cremasteric, plantar, perianal and gluteal are the common superficial reflexes tested. The cremasteric reflex is elicited in males by light stroking of the upper, inner surface of the thigh. The normal response is elevation of the testicles and scrotum. The perianal or gluteal reflex response is contraction of the external anal sphincter. These reflexes depend upon an intact upper motor neuron pathway. Diminished superficial reflex responses occur on the opposite side of the body when lesions are present above the decussation of the corticospinal tract. Loss of these reflexes occurs on the same side as the lesion when the lesion is below the corticospinal tract decussation.

The *Babinski reflex* is the most valuable *pathological reflex* suggestive of neurological disease, particularly of the pyramidal tract. In response to light stroking of the lateral aspect of the sole of the foot, an extension or dorsiflexion of the big toe and fanning of the other toes occurs. Other pathological reflexes are Chaddock and Oppenheim. Each of these will produce the same type of response as the Babinski reflex, with stimulation of different areas of the lower leg.

Autonomic nervous system status
Evaluation of this system concerns the involuntary (vegetative) functions. Local or general flushing, alterations in patterns of perspiration, faulty body temperature regulation (e.g. hypothermia or hyperthermia) and urinary or faecal incontinence suggest autonomic system dysfunction.

ASSESSMENT OF THE EFFECT OF NEUROLOGICAL DYSFUNCTION ON DAILY LIVING

Six general categories constitute a practical guide for assessment of the effect of neurological dysfunction on daily living. These are consciousness, mentality, movement, sensation, integrated regulatory function and coping with disability. Examples of specific functions which may be tested in each functional category related to four of the general categories are outlined in Table 22.4. The general category integrated regulatory function refers to those functions commonly thought of as autonomic or with a large autonomic component. It can be evaluated by identifying dysfunctions in the area of eating (ingesting, digesting), eliminating, breathing, circulation, temperature control, sexual responses and emotion. The general category coping with disability refers to the functions of adapting, coping, supporting, and growing. It can be evaluated by identifying how the person perceives his problem, how he usually deals with problems and what he is doing with this one.

Mitchell and Irvin[1] suggest that the entire neurological examination can be incorporated into the process of helping a patient with a bed bath if the nurse systematically plans to test functions during the activity. They also suggest that an entire neurological examination can be performed in 5–7 minutes if the patient is independent in most activities of daily living. They state that observation of gait and symmetry will yield information about motor and cerebellar function and position sense. Responses to questions such as 'Why are you here?' and 'Has your ability to take care of yourself changed?' will yield information about perception, expectations, orientation, language clarity and changes in self-care. Asking the patient to read a headline, to explain its meaning and to recall it later on can test visual acuity, language ability and recall. Asking the patient to take a glass of water in his right hand, swallow, and return the glass to the examiner can evaluate ability to follow a command which has three parts: (1) identifying the right from left; (2) crossing the midline; and (3) swallowing.

Observing the patient dress and undress, and simultaneously observing language and eye movements can provide information about motor, sensory and cerebellar functions. Difficulty in any area of activity would suggest that more detailed examination is necessary in order to identify the nature and extent of dysfunction.

EMERGENCY ASSESSMENT

In emergency situations or when the patient is seriously ill, neurological assessment includes measures to save life. First, breathing is assessed. Next, bleeding is controlled and circulation is maintained. Thirdly, brain and spinal cord function are assessed. Assessment of the brain in these circumstances may be referred to as craniocerebral assessment. The term neurological signs refers to the clinical evidence of neurological dysfunction.

Craniocerebral testing includes assessment of

---

[1] Mitchell & Irvin (1977), pp. 23–28.

level of consciousness, eye signs, motor and sensory status, and vital signs. Although each of these parameters may be observed independently of each other, neurological evaluation requires that the results be interpreted in relation to each other. Recording and interpretation of neurological data are facilitated by a structured chart (see Fig. 10.3). Change in neurological status can be rapid and dramatic or slow and subtle. The patient's condition will determine frequency of craniocerebral testing.

Level of consciousness
Decrease in responsiveness to stimuli indicates progressive deterioration in brain function. The chance of complete recovery decreases with increase in the duration of impaired consciousness; decrease in responsiveness to stimuli must be reported immediately in order that measures can be implemented to reduce the risk of irreversible neurological dysfunction or death. The patient whose level of consciousness is decreasing may become progressively lethargic, irritable or restless, disinterested in the environment and eventually disoriented. Orientation to time is usually lost first; loss of orientation to place occurs next and lastly, orientation to person.

The Glasgow coma scale (see p. 178) offers a standardized method for assessing the level of consciousness and for communicating practical information about the patient's progress and needs. A patient with a Glasgow coma score below the normal of 15 will need close observation for deterioration of consciousness. A score that is over 10 requires no invasive monitoring or support measures. A score of 7 or less is commonly accepted as definite coma. If the score is in the 8–4 range, active and invasive measures such as intubation, ventilation and intracranial pressure monitoring are instituted. If the score is 4 or less and 12 hours or more have elapsed since head injury occurred, only palliative care may be given. A score of 3 is the lowest score, compatible with brain death but not necessarily indicative of brain death.

Eye signs
The pupils are observed for size, shape, equality and reaction to light stimulus. An abnormality exists when one or both pupils are dilated or constricted relative to lighting conditions or when pupillary reaction to light stimulus is sluggish or absent (nonreactive or fixed pupil). This suggests increased intracranial pressure or localized cerebral dysfunction and should be reported immediately. Pupillary changes are considered in conjunction with other neurological assessment data. Drugs, metabolic and other factors which may alter pupillary reactions are taken into account.

If the eyes are swollen and the patient is unable to open them, it may be necessary to have one nurse gently open the eyelids while another examines the pupils. If the eyelids cannot be opened, this is noted on the chart.

The position and alignment of the eyes and evidence of involuntary eye movements are noted when the pupils are examined. Eye movements may be checked (see p. 778). In addition, the *oculocephalic response* (doll's head eye phenomenon), a reflex ocular movement, is usually checked by the doctor. This reflex can only be elicited in patients with decreased responsiveness. It helps to pinpoint the area of dysfunction. With the patient's eyes open, the head is moved rapidly from side to side or up and down. Pathology is present if the eyes deviate to the left when the head is turned to the right and vice versa.

Motor status
In the conscious patient, motor function is evaluated by asking him to move his limbs. Observations are made for evidence of abnormalities such as paresis and asymmetry in movement. Muscle strength in the upper extremities is assessed by asking the patient to squeeze the nurse's middle and index finger with each hand. The patient's hand grips should be strong and equal and the nurse should have difficulty pulling her fingers out of the grip. The patient should be able to release the grips spontaneously or immediately upon request. The lower limbs are tested for strength by asking the patient to push with his feet against resistance offered by the nurse's hands. Motor status can also be evaluated by testing for drift (see p. 779). In the unconscious patient, the motor response to various stimuli (e.g. sound, touch, pressure, pain) is observed. To distinguish a reflex grip from a command grip the nurse asks the patient to grip and release her fingers repeatedly.

Sensory status
This is evaluated by touching or stroking the patient's limbs, while his eyes are closed, and asking him what he feels. Anaesthesia or paraesthesia suggest neurological dysfunction. The ability of the patient to distinguish between the sharp and dull ends of a pin applied separately to each side of the body while the patient's eyes are closed also provides information about sensory status. In the patient with decreased level of consciousness, the appropriate response to pain stimulus is withdrawal from the stimulus or attempts at pushing it away.

Vital signs
Serial monitoring of arterial blood pressure, peripheral pulse and respirations is recorded because changes in these parameters may indicate specific problems. An elevated systolic pressure, widening pulse pressure and slowing of the pulse occurs with increased intracranial pressure. Respiratory rate, depth patterns, and changes (e.g. Cheyne–Strokes, hyperventilation, ataxic breathing) are noted and

recorded. Change in respiratory pattern may represent further increase in intracranial pressure and must be reported.

The body temperature is an important consideration, since an elevation increases cellular metabolism and oxygen demand; measures to restore normal temperature must be implemented. The temperature is taken orally in most instances. If the patient breathes through his mouth and the axillary temperature is not satisfactory, the temperature is taken rectally. If a mercury thermometer is used, the temperature will need to be taken in the axilla in the seizure-prone patient, the confused patient and the patient with reduced consciousness. These patients should not be left unobserved while the thermometer is in place.

Spinal status
In emergency assessment, this is done to detect evidence of cord compression, spinal nerve or nerve root compression. It includes observation of the chest for evidence of asymmetry of respiratory movements which occurs if there is paralysis or weakness of any of the chest muscles. Motor and sensory function and bladder and bowel control are assessed. Motor assessment includes movement of extremities and muscle strength as cited under motor status. Sensory assessment involves determining the level of feeling in the limbs and trunk and any sensory loss (e.g. temperature, pain, light touch, pressure) that is present. Assessment of reflexes may also provide valuable information.

CONTINUOUS INTRACRANIAL MONITORING

Continous or direct intracranial monitoring is an invasive procedure which is used in selected situations. It can provide reliable information indicating changes in intracranial pressure before such changes are clinically evident. It does not replace non-invasive clinical monitoring of neurological signs. It is valuable in patients whose 'neurosigns' cannot be readily assessed because they have been given drugs such as tubocurarine chloride (which blocks the myoneural junctions) so that they can be mechanically ventilated, or in those with induced hypothermia.

Several different intracranial monitoring devices are available. They may be intraventricular, subarachnoid, subdural or epidural. Each device is complex, works differently, has a different set of advantages and disadvantages and requires different nursing considerations. Since the pressure in one compartment of the brain is normally not necessarily the same as that in another one, the values obtained with each device will vary.

Intracranial pressure monitoring involves a pressure sensor and transducer implanted inside the skull. The transducer converts mechanical impulses to electrical impulses and a recording device converts these into visible tracings on an oscilloscope or on graph paper. *Nursing care* includes maintenance of sterility, observing the dry sterile dressing around the insertion site for drainage, positioning the patient and the equipment properly, keeping the system intact and operational, and interpreting intracranial pressure waves.

Intracranial *pressure waves* are defined as abnormal spontaneous alterations in intracranial pressure. Three wave patterns have been identified but only the plateau, or A waves, are considered to have clinical significance because of the cerebral ischaemia and brain damage which they incur. Plateau waves are sudden, transient waves lasting 5–20 minutes. They usually begin from a base-line of already elevated intracranial pressure. They increase ventricular fluid pressure and intracranial pressure by 50–100 mmHg (normal intracranial pressure is 4–15 mmHg or 60–160 mmH$_2$O).

Transient, observable, clinical symptoms of plateau waves are called pressure wave symptoms. These symptoms may be associated with deterioration in consciousness, abnormal respiratory patterns and pupillary reactions, altered motor function such as paresis, characteristic changes in vital signs, headache, nausea and vomiting, dysphasia, and other symptoms of cerebral dysfunction. Early recognition of any of these changes and early intervention to control the pressure can prevent permanent brain damage or even death.

Identification and control of factors which initiate these plateau waves are important considerations. These factors include: hypercapnia, hypoxaema, cerebral vasodilating agents, Valsalva's manoeuvre, prone position, neck and hip flexion, isometric muscle contractions, coughing, sneezing, rapid eye movement, arousal from sleep, and emotional upset.

OBSERVATIONS

The patient responses which may suggest neurological changes and which need to be observed, recorded and reported are discussed below.

Focal signs. These are signs of neurological dysfunction which are related and limited to a specific cortical area of origin. They may be motor, sensory or psychological. For example, a lesion or pressure on the motor strip or the visual pathway will produce signs of motor or visual deficits which reflect interference in these areas. Focal signs may include such phenomena as paralysis of one limb, facial paralysis and loss of sensation, loss of hearing or vision, aphasia, ataxia, seizures, changes in personality and disorientation.

Lateralizing signs. These are signs of neurological dysfunction which are confined to one side of the body. For example, paralysis of one side of the body as occurs in stroke.

Restlessness. This may range from slight increase in activity with decreased level of consciousness to severe agitation in the alert individual. The cause needs to be identified and the patient protected from injury. Restlessness in the neurological patient may be the first sign of increasing intracranial pressure. It may be due to irritation or injury of brain tissue, airway obstruction and respiratory insufficiency, returning consciousness, pain, malposition, full bladder or rectum, tight dressings or other restraints. Restlessness may precede a seizure.

Fits or convulsions. These are common in patients with discrete lesions involving the frontal or parietal lobes and in patients with increased intracranial pressure. Seizures are sudden episodes of disturbances in consciousness which may be accompanied by uncoordinated, purposeless muscle contractions and changes in sensations or behaviour. Those which place the patient at risk of injury and require immediate intervention are those which involve the entire body in tonic and clonic movements and when there is loss of consciousness. *Tonic* refers to sustained muscle spasm while *clonic* means alternate contraction and relaxation of muscle. Seizures are due to excessive, neuronal discharges within the brain. They should be prevented if possible since they may worsen the patient's condition and/or cause injury.

Specific information about the patient's fits may help to identify the cause and to localize a brain lesion. The patient's level of consciousness and his activity before, during and after the seizure are recorded. In addition, answers to the following questions are sought and documented: Where did the fit begin and what was the initial activity? Did the patient cry out? What was the progression of the seizure activity? What body parts were involved? Was the activity tonic, clonic, localized or generalized and did the movements change in character during the fit? Was there deviation of the head or eyes and to which side? Were the eyes open or closed? Did the pupils change in size? Were the pupils equal and did they react to light? Was there incontinence of urine or faeces? Was there thick salivation of mucus (frothing at the mouth)? What was the patient's colour? What was the respiratory status throughout the seizure? What was the duration of the seizure activity? Did the patient experience a warning prior to the seizure? Was it auditory, visual, olfactory, tactile or other? Was there any weakness or paralysis of the extremities after the episode?

Headache. This may be due to inflammation or traction on pain-sensitive structures such as blood vessels, cranial nerves and dural attachments and it is an important symptom of increasing intracranial pressure. The location of the headache, its duration and severity are recorded as well as the position the patient assumes for maximum comfort. The headache of neurological origin is usually intermittent, deep, aching and pressure-like and it is intensified by coughing, straining and change in posture. Other characteristics will depend upon the location of the lesion.

Nuchal rigidity. This is an involuntary stiffness of the neck muscles and is assessed by asking the patient to flex his head. Pain in the neck and rigidity may indicate cervical spine injury, meningeal irritation, or subarachnoid bleeding.

Posturing. Decerebrate or decorticate posturing (see p. 807) may suggest worsening of the patient's neurological status.

Vomiting. This occurs particularly during the night or early morning. It may be due to direct pressure on the vomiting centre in the medulla. Nausea is usually absent and the vomitus is precipitous and forcefully ejected (projectile vomiting).

Cerebrospinal fluid leakage. This may occur from a head wound, from the posterior pharynx, the nose, or the ear. CSF leakage is potentially serious since microorganisms may enter the subarachnoid space and give rise to meningitis or brain abscess. To determine whether drainage from the nose is CSF or mucus, a glucose indicator may be used. CSF is a dialysate of blood and is positive for glucose. Another method to test for CSF is the 'halo ring' method. A gauze pad is held under the dripping fluid and if blood and CSF are both present the two will separate on the pad, a red drop will form in the centre with a serous ring around it indicating the presence of CSF.

Incontinence of urine and faeces. This is common in disease of the brain and spinal cord.

NEUROLOGICAL DIAGNOSTIC PROCEDURES

Neurodiagnostic procedures supplement and add precision to clinical data. As with any procedure, the patient needs both *physical and psychological preparation* to promote confidence in unfamiliar personnel and procedures. During procedures the patient needs privacy, support and encouragement. Following completion of the procedure he requires comfort, observation for complications and protection from injury or complications. Neurodiagnostic procedures may be classed as invasive or non-invasive.

Non-invasive neurodiagnostic procedures
Non-invasive procedures pose minimal risks to the patient. A signed consent is not usually required prior to the test, but if a contrast medium is injected intravenously during the procedure, a signed consent is required.

Neuroradiography. X-rays of the skull and spine are among the first and most common neurological investigations ordered. They are used to detect changes in bone structure such as destruction, healing and calcification. Fractures, abnormal bone development, vascular diseases, bone diseases and tumours may be demonstrated. *Tomography* involves layered radiological exposures at measured depths which permits examination of single layers of tissues and provides some idea of the two-dimensional shape of the defects.

Non-invasive cerebral blood flow. This procedure is used in selected situations to substantiate other test results. A radionucleide isotope is administered rapidly by intravenous injection. With the patient positioned in front of a gamma camera, pictures of the radioactivity are taken every 1.5 seconds. The blood flow is calculated by computer. Following analysis of the pictures, films become available for permanent record. The patient requires a full explanation of the test since anxiety may alter cerebral blood flow through stimulation of the sympathetic nervous system. The patient should know that he will be required to lie quietly during the procedure, that the isotope used has a very short half-life and that a very low dosage is used.

Non-invasive regional blood flow. This is a recent development which is not yet widely used. Its purpose is to estimate both brain perfusion and brain function. It has been used to evaluate the vasodilating property of drugs on the cerebrovascular system. Its advantage is that it does not initiate vasospasm by changing the patient's physiological and/or psychological status. The patient lies on a padded table, clips are placed on his nose, probes are placed on the scalp and he is instructed to breathe through a mouthpiece. A radioactive gas (xenon) is inhaled. The non-invasive regional blood flow is calculated by computer following analysis of radioactivity counts picked up by the probes. The gas is exhaled after a single pass through the peripheral circulation. The patient will be required to lie quietly during the procedure and to cooperate with the technician.

Brain scan (radioisotope uptake). This procedure is used to determine the presence of a space-occupying lesion. The procedure is the same as for non-invasive cerebral blood flow (above) except that pictures are taken 60 minutes following an istotope injection. In certain pathological conditions, the blood–brain barrier is disrupted, and all tissues, both normal and abnormal, will take up the isotope. The isotope accumulates in abnormal tissue and is retained in greater concentration. The patient should be assured that the amount of radiation received is less than with ordinary skull x-rays and that the radioisotope will be excreted from the body within 24 hours.

Computerized axial tomography (CAT scan). This procedure has dramatically reduced the use of dangerous invasive procedures. It may be performed with or without an intravenous injection of contrast medium. In preparation wigs and clips are removed from the head, and food and fluid may be withheld for 6 hours preceding the test because the contrast medium may cause nausea. The patient is asked if he has any allergies. An explanation of the test is essential since the machine may be frightening for the patient. The patient will be asked to lie perfectly still in the supine position. The head is placed comfortably in an opening in the scanner. The patient is alone during the procedure but has both visual and auditory contact with a technician through a large window and an intercom system. A portion of the scanner rotates slowly around the patient's head while radiographic readings are taken. The machine is periodically adjusted. Computer images can be seen on a screen immediately and they are available for permanent record. Differences in radiation absorption and differences in tissue densities that are too subtle to be picked up by conventional x-rays may be detected by tomography. The entire procedure takes less than an hour and it can be done on an outpatient basis. The amount of radiation the patient receives is approximately equivalent to that received with a skull x-ray.

Carotid doppler study. This non-invasive diagnostic study is used to assess the blood flow through the carotid arteries and the extent of sclerotic vascular change that may be partially or completely obstructing the normal flow of blood to the brain. The study may be done on persons who are considered at risk of stroke because of attendant signs and symptoms (e.g. transient ischaemic attacks).

The study involves the placing of a probe over the carotid area. The probe gives off ultrasound waves and receives them back as they rebound from erythrocytes flowing through the carotid arteries. The probe is connected to an oscilloscope which indicates the difference between the frequency of the waves given off by the probe and those that rebound. The difference is known as the Doppler shift.

Positron emission (transaxial) tomography (PET scan or PETT). This new technique is similar to the CAT scan but has other advantages. Minute doses of radioactive tracers prepared in a cyclatron are inhaled or injected into a vein. The radioactive emissions (positrons) of the tracer are picked up by sensitive detectors around the head as it distributes in the brain. The PET scan provides safe, rapid scanning of blood flow in the brain as well as biochemical mapping. It can be used to study diseases related to chemical changes in the brain and to localize the area of action in the brain.

Nuclear magnetic resonance (NMR). This is a newer technique which is not widely available. Giant magnets are used for diagnostic purposes. Radiofrequency pulses, directed at the patient, enable a changing pattern of hydrogen nuclei in the body to be recorded.

Electroencephalography (EEG). The EEG is a recording of the brain's electrical activity. Several small electrodes are superficially placed on the scalp in standard positions. The electrodes are attached to an amplifier and recorder. It is believed that the electrical activity of neuronal dendrites of the superficial layers of the brain are responsible for the low-voltage electrical waves. If the patient has been prescribed an anticonvulsant drug it is usually withheld for 24 hours or more prior to the test. The patient needs assurance that an electric shock will not occur during the test and that the machine cannot 'read the mind'. The technician cleans the scalp and applies the electrodes with collodion. In some instances needle electrodes are inserted into the scalp, which necessitates cleansing the scalp before the needles are inserted. The patient lies or sits in a quiet dimly lit room. In order to evoke or accentuate certain abnormal wave patterns the patient may be asked to hyperventilate or the technician may flash bright lights before the eyes. Some abnormalities only become evident during sleep; therefore, a sedative may be prescribed and recordings made before, during, and after sleep.

The EEG may take up to an hour to complete. Following the test the patient may need assistance in using acetone to remove the collodion from the hair and scalp. The EEG is particularly useful in evaluating seizure disorders and it may help to localize tumours.

An ambulatory EEG may be performed over a 24-hour period, using a portable recorder attached to the patient's waist. This is used to diagnose petit mal, temporal lobe epilepsy, seizures of unknown origin or suspected hysterical fits.

Echoencephalography (echogram). This has been largely supplanted by the CAT scan but is still used where the scan is unavailable. It is a simple procedure which uses ultrasonic waves to indicate deviation of midline structures. Probes are placed on the temporal bones to transmit an ultrasonic beam which travels through the patient's skull. Midline structures, particularly the walls of the third ventricle and the pineal gland, send back echo waves which are recorded and projected on a screen or recorded on a chart. Displacement of midline structures by intracranial lesions can be visualized.

Electromyography (EMG). This is a record of the electrical currents produced by skeletal muscles. Small needle electrodes are inserted into a muscle and the electrical currents are recorded with the muscle at rest and during activity. The test is useful to monitor changes in peripheral nerve dysfunction, to determine types of primary muscle disease and to identify defective transmission at the myoneural junction. The patient usually experiences some discomfort when the needle electrodes are inserted and if many muscles are tested some discomfort may persist.

Nerve conduction study. This is frequently done with the EMG (above). It studies the excitability and conduction velocities of motor and sensory nerves to help diagnose disease of peripheral nerves. During the procedure the patient may experience a mild electrical shock.

Caloric test. This test evaluates the function of the vestibular portion of the eighth cranial nerve. It helps to differentiate lesions of the brain stem and the cerebellum. Normally, stimulation of the auditory canal with hot water produces a rotary nystagmus toward the side of the irrigated ear. The nystagmus is away from the irrigated ear when ice-cold water is used. Nystagmus does not occur if pathology is present. The patient needs to know that he may experience vertigo, nausea, and vomiting but that a nurse will be available to assist him.

Neuropsychological tests. These tests are done when deficits in adaptive abilities are suspected. Motor, perceptual, language, visual–spatial, cognitive and other abilities can be assessed to determine the extent of impairment in brain functions. The tests measure deficits in coping skills by evaluating these skills directly rather than indirectly. They require several hours to complete and they may result in recommendations concerning educational and vocational placement.

Invasive neurodiagnostic procedures
Invasive procedures may be very complex and the patient may experience pain and discomfort. Invasive procedures carry a risk of morbidity and mortality. Prior to each of these procedures, craniocerebral testing is done in order to provide base-line information for comparison during and after the test. A signed consent form must be obtained prior to many of these procedures.

Lumbar puncture (LP, spinal tap, spinal puncture). This involves the insertion of a spinal needle into the lumbar subarachnoid space of the spinal canal by the doctor. The needle is passed through the intervertebral space between the third and fourth or fourth and fifth lumbar vertebrae, stopping at a safe distance from the cord.

The puncture may be performed to determine the pressure of CSF, to obtain specimens of the fluid for examination (for normal CSF see p. 766), or to remove blood and pus from the subarachnoid space and thereby reduce pressure if it is dangerously high. It is also used to inject drugs for anaesthesia or other purposes.

The patient assumes the lateral recumbent position, with his back on the edge of the bed, and flexes his knees on his chest so that they touch his chin, in order to widen the interspinous spaces. The nurse may need to support the patient behind the neck and knees. Asepsis is emphasized to prevent infection in the spinal canal which could be serious and even fatal. The skin is prepared, local anaesthetic injected and a spinal needle inserted. If the needle contacts one of the dorsal nerve roots, pain down one leg occurs. Needle removal rectifies this and the patient is assured that no damage has occurred. The fluid pressure is measured with a manometer and several samples of CSF are collected in sterile tubes for examination. Following needle removal a small sterile dressing or dab of collodion is applied to the site.

Normal CSF pressure in the recumbent position is 40–180 mm H_2O. Abnormally low pressure may indicate an obstruction in the spinal subarachnoid space above the puncture site. Elevated pressure may signify infection, or a space-occupying lesion such as a brain tumour or blood clot. Generally, LP is contraindicated in the presence of a space-occupying lesion because the rapid reduction in pressure caused by the removal of CSF can cause the brain to shift downward and herniate in the foramen magnum ('coning'). This, in turn, compresses the vital centres in the medulla and could cause sudden death. Should sudden collapse occur, airway establishment and resuscitation are necessary. Removal of CSF from the lateral ventricles may also be required.

Nursing care following LP includes keeping the patient flat in bed for 6–24 hours (depending on policy and presence of headache), monitoring neurological signs, checking the puncture site for abnormalities and leakage and encouraging fluids (unless contraindicated). When increased intracranial pressure is present, herniation of the brain does not necessarily occur during or immediately after LP but rarely may occur several hours later. The patient should have frequent neurological checks for several hours post-LP and adverse changes should be reported to the doctor.

It has been estimated that various post-LP problems occur in one out of four patients. These problems may be transient difficulty in voiding, temperature elevation due to meningeal irritation, pain, oedema, or haematoma at the puncture site and pain radiating to the thigh due to nerve root irritation. Post-LP headache may also occur. This is normally attributed to the removal of CSF during the test or to later leakage of the fluid into the tissues. The headache is typically frontal and suboccipital and is relieved when a horizontal position is assumed. The patient lies flat, a cold compress or ice-bag may be applied to the head, and a mild analgesic may be prescribed.

Cisternal puncture. This is done if an LP is contraindicated or if there is a block in the spinal subarachnoid space. A short needle is inserted into the cisterna magna (a small sac of CSF between the cerebellum and medulla) just beneath the occipital bone. Because this puncture is close to the brain and the patient's cooperation is necessary, anxiety-reducing and supportive measures are essential. The nape of the neck is shaved, the patient is positioned on his side and his head is flexed forward and held firmly by the nurse, or he may be sat upright, resting his arms on pillows on a bed-table. Observation is necessary for signs of respiratory difficulty which may suggest that the needle has made contact with the medulla. Usually the patient resumes normal activity soon after the procedure.

Cerebral angiography (arteriography). This is a radiographic visualization of the brain's vascular system by injection of a radiopaque material into the arterial system. It evaluates structure but not function. The approach may be direct injection into the carotid or vertebral arteries. Ninety per cent of the time the indirect route by way of the femoral artery is used because it is easier on the patient. A local or general anaesthetic is used, a needle is inserted and a catheter is threaded through the needle under fluroscopic control into the descending aorta and from there into the desired vessels in the head. During injection of the contrast material, rapid, sequential x-rays are taken. Following removal of the needle, a sterile gauze pad is applied over the injection site and firm pressure is applied for 5–10 minutes to prevent haemorrhage and haematoma formation.

In preparation for the procedure, information about allergies the patient may have should be recorded in a conspicious place and brought to the doctor's attention. A skin shave is required, food and fluid are withheld for up to 6 hours , and dentures, contact lenses, spectacles, make-up and jewellery are removed. Sedation is usually prescribed 1 hour before the procedure. The nurse should explain to the patient that he should lie very still during the test and that a burning sensation may be felt through the neck and face for a few seconds.

Following the angiogram the patient remains on bed rest for at least 8 hours. The head of the bed is elevated if a carotid artery puncture was done. Neurological observations are carried out frequently and the pressure dressing is checked for bleeding. A cold compress or ice-bag may be applied to the injection site to control oedema and discomfort and to reduce the possibility of bleeding. If a limb was used for the puncture site (e.g. femoral artery), the distal part is checked for colour, temperature, and presence of a pulse. It is important to assess the adjacent extremity because vasospasms, thrombosis or formation of a haematoma can occur, obstructing the blood supply to the distal part.

Rarely, cerebral angiography may precipitate a stroke, seizure, allergic reaction to the contrast substance, or other serious complications. Any signs of deterioration in the patient's condition must be reported to the doctor immediately.

Myelography. This is an x-ray examination of the spinal cord and vertebral canal following injection of a radiopaque contrast substance into the spinal sub-arachnoid space. It is used to detect and localize lesions which may be compressing the spinal cord or nerves. The medium is injected through a lumbar puncture and its flow is observed using an image intensifier and x-rays are taken.

As with all procedures, an explanation is given to the patient so that he will know what to expect and can cooperate more fully. A history of any allergy is recorded and brought to the doctor's attention. Food and fluid are withheld up to 6 hours prior to the test and sedation may be prescribed 1 hour prior to the procedure. The lumbosacral area of the back is shaved if necessary.

Following the myelogram, if an oil-based contrast medium is used, such as iophendylate (Myodil), the patient is kept flat in bed for 24 hours. If a water-soluble contrast medium is used, e.g. metrizamide (Amipaque, Dimer X), the patient must be sat upright for at least 6 hours. The injection site is inspected, neurological signs are assessed, fluids are encouraged, and fluid intake and output recorded. Persistent headache, pain and stiffness of the neck upon flexion are reported.

Tissue biopsy. Brain, muscle and nerve tissue may be biopsied for accurate diagnosis. *Brain biopsy* is commonly done during intracranial surgery. Sometimes it is obtained to provide information essential to genetic counselling and to determine a prognosis for the patient. A number of inherited disorders, dementias, and other progressive conditions may be diagnosed through brain biopsy. Since most patients subjected to this procedure already have advanced disease, with problems such as seizures and motor dysfunction, it may be difficult to anticipate complications. But in all instances, since a surgical wound is involved, observation for haematoma formation, wound drainage and maintenance of a sterile dressing are essential. The patient receives the necessary explanation and support and his neuro-logical status and vital signs are evaluated and com-pared to preoperative values.

Tissue for *muscle biopsy* is taken from an area not previously traumatized by injections or EMG needles, since these would produce changes char-acteristic of inflammation. The patient receives thorough explanation, since his cooperation is needed throughout the procedure, and the area is cleansed and may require shaving. He will experi-ence pain when the anaesthetic is injected locally and again when the muscle itself is cut because the tissue that is sampled cannot be anaesthetized since this would produce artifacts. Following the procedure,

nursing care includes comfort and observation for bleeding or infection.

Nerve biopsy, usually carried out in conjunction with muscle biopsy, is done to establish an accurate diagnosis of peripheral neuropathy. Preparation of the patient is similar to that described for muscle biopsy. Following the procedure, the patient usually experiences mild sensory loss in the surgical area for a short period.

NEUROLOGICAL DISORDERS

The highly complex nature of the nervous system is revealed through its numerous and diverse dis-orders. The dysfunctions which result depend pri-marily on the area(s) of the nervous system affected, the extent of the lesion, and, to a lesser degree, the nature of the pathological process. This section presents a discussion of only those disorders which are most commonly encountered in nursing practice.

Cerebrovascular Disorders

Cerebrovascular disorders are among the most common of all neurological disorders. The greater number may be classified as ischaemic or hae-morrhagic. *Either may cause a cerebrovascular infarction which is commonly known as a stroke* or may also be referred to as cerebrovascular accident (CVA).

CEREBRAL-ISCHAEMIC DISORDERS

Cerebral atherosclerosis

This is a chronic degenerative process of the cerebral arteries in which the intimal layer gradually develops atheromas (fibrous fatty plaques). These narrow the vascular lumen, damage the underlying layer of tissue media and tend to undergo calcification, ulcer-ation with overlying thrombosis and intraplaque haemorrhage which worsen the luminal narrowing or cause total occlusion. These degenerative changes result in interference with cerebral perfusion. Although the brain represents only about 2% of the body's weight, it consumes 20% of its oxygen. Since the brain cannot store energy nor temporarily exist by anaerobic metabolism, deprivation of oxygenated blood for even a very few minutes leads to neuronal death.

Atherosclerosis affects the larger vessels at the base of the brain first, particularly at the points of vessel branching and tends to develop silently. The incidence increases with increasing age. Its presence is manifested when it is well advanced by: (1) the development of ischaemia of vital organs (e.g. deterioration of mental faculties); (2) episodes of local neurological dysfunction, which are referred to as transient ischaemic attacks; (3) predisposition to thrombosis which may give rise to emboli; (4) weakening of an arterial wall resulting in an aneurysm. Occasionally, on routine physical examination, a noise or bruit may be heard through a stethoscope placed over the eye or carotid artery when there is turbulent blood flow due to irregularities in the vessel wall.

Since the cause of atherosclerosis continues to elude scientists, therapy is directed to reducing the risk factors. Risk factors amenable to modification include: (1) diets high in cholesterol and saturated fat, (2) hypercholesterolaemia, (3) hypertension, (4) cigarette smoking, and (5) diabetes. Controversy continues with regard to the control of atherosclerosis by modification of diet and blood lipid values. In addition, some defend and others deny a role for control of blood sugar in the progression of atherosclerosis, but the desirability of controlling hypertension and cigarette smoking is unquestioned. An anticoagulant (e.g. aspirin, warfarin) may be prescribed.

Surgical therapy for atherosclerosis causing cerebral ischaemia involves a carotid endarterectomy or cerebral artery bypass (see p. 790).

Cerebral thrombosis

This is the most common cause of stroke and is usually due to atherosclerosis of the carotid, vertebral or larger cerebral arteries. The narrowing of the lumen of the vessel by atherosclerotic plaques leads to thrombus formation, occlusion of the artery and ischaemia of the respective brain area. Inadequate delivery of blood to the brain and subsequent thrombosis may be secondary to cardiac insufficiency, shock or to reduced intravascular volume as occurs in haemorrhage and severe dehydration. Anticoagulant therapy may be prescribed.

Cerebral embolism

Embolic material which may be a thrombus or atherosclerotic plaque which becomes free in the bloodstream, lodges in a cerebral artery, occluding the vessel and resulting in a cerebral infarction (stroke). The middle cerebral artery is the most frequent location. The occlusion occurs suddenly; there is no warning or time for the development of collateral circulation. Anticoagulant therapy may be prescribed to prevent a recurrence and a second stroke.

Transient ischaemic attacks

A large percentage of patients with an atherothrombic stroke have a history of transient ischaemic attacks which may be referred to as *little strokes*. These episodes of local neurological dysfunction may last a few seconds to several hours; most last 5–10 minutes. There may be only a few attacks or as many as several hundred before an actual stroke. These transient attacks are due to focal ischaemia incurred by temporary occlusion of an artery by vasospasm microemboli or insufficient blood supply. They are usually associated with atherosclerosis.

Transient attacks are warning signs of impending complete stroke. Manifestations include transient paresis or hemiplegia, visual deficits (decreased vision in one eye), difficulty in or loss of speech, difficulty in comprehension, dizziness, unsteadiness and sudden falls.

Lack of knowledge in the patient experiencing transient ischaemic attacks is a major concern. It is a nursing responsibility to assess the patient's understanding of the episodes and urge prompt, medical attention. Timely and appropriate therapy can reduce the number of these attacks and may reduce the risk of a disastrous stroke in the near future.

The therapeutic regimen may involve a low fat diet, control of hypertension, no smoking and an anticoagulant such as warfarin or aspirin. Selected patients are treated surgically by a carotid endarterectomy or cerebral artery bypass.

ENDARTERECTOMY

Endarterectomy of the internal carotid involves the removal of the atheroma from the intima. A venous graft or dacron prosthesis may be necessary to reinforce the vascular area from which the plaques are removed.

Not all patients with atherosclerosis or experiencing transient ischaemic attacks are candidates for surgery; those who are very elderly and have extensive vascular disease or who have serious heart or renal problems are a high risk.

Nursing intervention
Preoperative preparation of the patient for an endarterectomy includes an explanation of the procedure and what may be expected immediately after the operation. The patient receives an anticoagulant such as Nicoumalone (sinthrome) or heparin. Baseline neurological information is recorded for postoperative comparison. The care is the same as for a general preoperative preparation (see Chapter 11) except that a specific directive may be received concerning skin preparation.

Postoperative nursing care as with any patient who might develop neurological complications, involves frequent craniocerebral testing which is necessary to detect early evidence of neurological deficit (see Table 22.4). Frequent monitoring of the blood pressure is essential: an elevation may place stress on

Table 22.4 Organization of a functionally oriented nursing neurological evaluation.*

General category	Functional category	Examples of specific function which may be tested
Consciousness	Arousing (reticular activating system)	Arousability, response to verbal and tactile stimuli
Mentation	Thinking (general cortical function plus specific regional functions)	Educational level Content of conversation Orientation Fund of information Insight, judgement, planning
	Feeling (affective)	Mood and affect Perception and reaction to ability, disability
	Language	Content and quantity of speech Ability to name objects Ability to repeat phrases Ability to read, write, copy
	Remembering	Attention span Recent and remote memory
Motor function	Seeing (cranial nerves, II, III, IV, VI)	Acuity Visual fields Extraocular movement Pupil size, shape, reactivity Presence or absence of diplopia, nystagmus
	Eating (cranial nerves V, IX, X, XII)	Chewing Swallowing Gag (if swallowing impaired)
	Expressing (facially) (cranial nerve VII) Speaking (cranial nerves VII, IX, X, XII) Moving (Motor and cerebellar systems)	Symmetry of smile, frown Clarity, presence or absence of nasality Muscle tone, mass, strength Presence or absence of involuntary movements Coordination: heel-to-toe walk, observing during dressing Posture, gait, position
Sensory function	Smelling (cranial nerve I) Blinking (cranial nerve V) Hearing (cranial nerve VII) Feeling (sensory pathways)	Ability to detect odours Corneal reflex Acuity, presence or absence of unusual sounds Pain-pinprick Touch, stereognosis Temperature–warm, cold

Note: *Examples of specific functions that may be tested in each functional category are shown. The structures involved in each of the functions categorized are indicated in parentheses.*
*Mitchell & Irvin (1977).

the operative site and cause severe haemorrhage. Hypotension predisposes to thrombus formation within the artery at the surgical site. Frequent observation of the operative site for evidence of bleeding or oedema in the area is necessary. The neck circumference is observed frequently for swelling due to internal bleeding. Respiratory distress is reported promptly; swelling due to oedema or clot formation may compress the trachea and interfere with respirations. Observations are also made for signs of any intracranial functional changes.

The patient is kept at rest and quiet with a minimum of stimuli during the first 24 hours; all exertion on his part is avoided. After this period, the patient is gradually mobilized if his vital signs are satisfactory and stable.

An anticoagulant is prescribed and is usually continued for about 6 months following the surgery. Regular checking of prothrombin time is necessary.

On discharge from the hospital, the patient is advised to report any blood in the urine or stool, bleeding of gums or discoloured bruised areas (ecchymoses). Former activities are resumed very gradually.

CEREBRAL ARTERY BYPASS

Cerebral artery bypass surgery may be performed on patients who have lesions in the smaller arteries inside the skull which cannot be corrected by endarterectomy. Using microsurgical techniques and a craniotomy just above the ear, a large scalp artery (e.g. superficial temporal) is anastamosed to a blocked artery in order to supply blood beyond the stenosis.

Nursing intervention
Nursing care postoperatively is similar to

postendarterectomy. Frequent craniocerebral testing allows for early detection of neurological changes suggestive of compromised cerebral blood flow or increased intracranial pressure.

The major complications following bypass surgery include interruption of blood flow through the graft, stroke and subdural haematoma due to bleeding at the surgical site. The patient is positioned off the operative side with the head of the bed elevated 30°. Anticoagulant therapy may be continued for several months following surgery. Long-term benefits and indications for cerebral bypass have not been firmly established but there is some evidence of decreased stroke rate and improvement in the quality of life of those patients who have had a bypass.

CEREBRAL HAEMORRHAGIC DISORDERS

Cerebral aneurysm

An aneurysm is a saccular dilation of an arterial wall (see Fig. 22.1) thought to be caused most often by the congenital absence of muscular and elastic tissue in the wall of that area of the vessel. It may also develop as a result of degenerative vascular changes. The most common cerebral aneurysm is referred to as a *berry aneurysm* because it is a rounded, outpouching on a stem (Fig. 22.21). The majority occur at the base of the brain in the circle of Willis at points of bifurcation. The lesion does not always produce symptoms and may be single or there may be several.

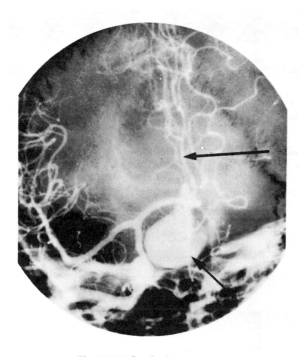

Fig. 22.21 Cerebral aneurysm.

Aneurysms are the cause of death in over 50% of all fatal cerebrovascular lesions in persons under the age of 45 years. Although the weakness in the arterial wall is congenital, actual distension of the vessel occurs much later in life. The distension may produce localizing symptoms by pressure on adjacent structures (e.g. paralysis due to pressure on cranial nerves). Rupture of the artery is the most serious consequence. It may be preceded by a series of small leaks over several weeks manifested by headache and stiffness of the neck but more often the rupture occurs without any warning. The most vulnerable persons are those who are 35–60 years of age and those with hypertension or polycystic disease of the kidneys. Rupture may be precipitated by physical or emotional exertion and the bleeding may occur into the subarachnoid space, cerebral substance or both these areas.

Assessment

Signs and symptoms. Rupture of a cerebral aneurysm forces blood under arterial pressure into the brain tissue and subarachnoid space giving rise to an explosive headache, nausea, vomiting and in some, rapid loss of consciousness. Symptoms of meningeal irritation will also be present, which include pain and nuchal rigidity, positive Kernig's sign (inability to extend the knees without pain while in supine position with hips flexed), positive Brudzinski's sign (person in supine position bends the knees to avoid pain when the neck is flexed), photophobia, blurred vision, irritability, restlessness and possible temperature elevation. The presence and severity of symptoms are determined by the location and extent of the bleeding.

Investigation. When an aneurysm is suspected on the basis of the presenting symptoms, cerebral angiography is done and will demonstrate an aneurysm in most of the patients. A CAT scan may be done to detect intracranial collections of blood. A lumbar puncture usually reveals the presence of blood in the CSF as well as an increased pressure. When the diagnosis is confirmed, the clinical data are used to grade the aneurysm which is used as a guide to therapy and to establish the prognosis (see Table 22.5).

Prognosis. The prognosis following the initial bleed of a cerebral aneurysm is grave; many patients succumb at this time. Of those who survive the initial onset, a large number (approximately 42%) die of a recurrence of bleeding within a few days or weeks. Others may die as a result of cerebral infarction due to severe vasospasm. Survivors of a cerebral aneurysm haemorrhage may recover with few neurological deficits but many are partially or totally disabled due to paralysis, mental deterioration and/or seizures.

Table 22.5 Classification of cerebral aneurysms.

Classification	Patient response
I, Minimal bleed	Alert, minimal headache, neurological deficits absent
II, Mild bleed	Alert, mild to severe headache, neck rigidity, minimal neurological deficits (e.g. oculomotor palsy)
III, Moderate bleed	Drowsy or confused, neck rigidity, may have mild focal deficit such as limb weakness
IV, Moderate to severe bleed	Responds only to painful stimuli; neck rigidity, major neurological deficits (e.g. hemiparesis), possible early decerebation
V, Severe bleed	Unresponsive, decerebrate rigidity, moribund appearance

Medical management
The patient with a cerebral aneurysm requires prompt treatment. Those categorized as grade III, IV or V are managed conservatively until they progress to grade I or II. Only those classified as grade I or II are considered to be candidates for surgery.

Conservative treatment includes a hypotensive agent to lower the blood pressure, a mild sedative to reduce agitation and anxiety, a mild analgesic (usually codeine) to relieve pain, and a steroid preparation, for example dexamethasone (Decadron), to control cerebral oedema and intracranial pressure. Analgesics and sedatives are used cautiously since they tend to mask neurological changes and symptoms. To reduce the risk of a rebleed, an antifibrinolytic agent such as tranexamic acid (Cyclokapron) may be administered orally or parenterally; its action prevents the dissolution (lysis) of the clot that was formed.

Surgical treatment. This involves microsurgical technique because of the critical location, size and fragility of some aneurysms. If the aneurysm can be clipped, a metal, self-closing, spring clip or ligature is applied to the neck of it to occlude the aneurysm. Those which cannot be occluded may be wrapped in a special gauze-like material and coated with an acrylic substance to reinforce the vascular walls to prevent another leak or rupture. Another procedure may involve proximal and distal ligation of the aneurysm which embolizes it. If the lesion is surgically inaccessible, gradual occlusion of the common carotid artery on the affected side by the application of a Selverstone clamp may be done; the blood supply to the affected side of the brain is gradually reduced. This latter procedure places the patient at risk of hemiplegia.

NURSING PROCESS

Assessment
Vital signs and neurological status are assessed at frequent intervals (15 or 30 minutes) during the acute stage; see assessment p. 782). A decrease in the level of consciousness, disorientation or other neurological changes are recorded and reported promptly to the doctor. The blood pressure is followed very closely since an elevation may increase the bleeding or precipitate rebleeding. If receiving a hypotensive drug, there is the risk of the pressure falling to a level that incurs ischaemia of the brain tissue; in addition there is the risk of rebleeding, vasospasm and secondary hydrocephalus. The latter may develop as a result of interference with the normal absorption process of the CSF by the accumulation of blood in the subarachnoid space into the venous sinuses (see p. 806). Hydrocephalus compresses the brain, giving rise to signs of increased intracranial pressure.

Identification of patient problems
The problems of the patient treated *conservatively* include:
1 Potential for continued intracranial bleeding or for recurrence of bleeding
2 Alteration in self-care activities: restricted
3 Alteration in comfort: headache
4 Anxiety and ineffective coping. Fear of the circumstances and concern for the outcome
5 Potential for injury secondary to altered level of awareness, disorientation and immobility
6 Alteration in food and fluid intake due to nausea, vomiting and restricted fluid intake
7 Alteration in urinary and bowel elimination secondary to reduced level of awareness, decreased intake and enforced immobility
8 Potential for complications: rebleeding, hydrocephalus and vasospasm
9 Potential for residual mental and/or physical impairment resulting in need for rehabilitation

The *goals* are to:
1 Prevent further bleeding
2 Relieve the headache
3 Reduce anxiety
4 Prevent injury and complications
5 Rehabilitate the patient to maximum potential (if disabled)

Nursing intervention
Those treated conservatively are usually patients

categorized as grade III, IV or V (see Table 22.5). If the patient is unconscious, nursing measures will include those which apply to any unconscious patient (see Chapter 10).

1. Control of bleeding and the prevention of a rebleed. The patient is kept on complete bed rest with one pillow under the head or the head of the bed elevated about 15–20° to promote venous drainage and prevent increased intracranial pressure. As cited above, the blood pressure is monitored frequently; it is important that it remain within the extreme low range of normal. The patient is kept very quiet and exposed to a minimum of stimuli (lighting is subdued, no radio or television and door closed). The reason for this is explained in a manner that will not alarm him if he is sufficiently alert. Visitors are limited; family members are informed that they may sit quietly with the patient and that conversation is discouraged.

Because self-care requires exertion which increases the blood pressure predisposing to rebleeding, bathing, feeding and change of position are done by the nurse. In change of position and when getting on and off the bedpan, the patient is cautioned against physical effort and also against straining at stool.

If the patient is unable to rest, a mild sedative may be prescribed; as cited previously the use of sedation is used judiciously because it may mask neurological changes and symptoms. The essential immobility predisposes to venous stasis and thrombophlebitis; the application of anti-embolic stockings to the lower limbs may be recommended. They are removed and reapplied according to manufacturers instructions.

Vomiting and coughing are controlled because they increase the intracranial pressure. If the patient is nauseated and vomiting, oral fluids and food are withheld and an antiemetic prescribed. Deep breathing is encouraged at regular intervals and the administration of oxygen may be prescribed to prevent cerebral hypoxia.

2. Alteration in comfort. The severe headache which the patient experiences causes restlessness, nausea and vomiting. Nursing measures include keeping the patient at rest and as quiet as possible. Cold applications to the head may help and a mild analgesic (e.g. codeine) is usually prescribed.

3. Anxiety and ineffective coping. The patient is very fearful and concerned for his future; much of this is aroused by the enforced immobility, the frequent assessments being made and the restrictions on visitors. The serial assessments, procedures, enforced immobility and restrictions are explained if the patient is alert. Reassurance of adequate and efficient care is given. A calm, reassuring approach can be therapeutic.

The family's perception of the illness, their expectations and coping patterns are assessed. Their role in keeping the patient quiet and at rest is explained to them. They are kept informed as to the patient's progress, and opportunities are provided for expression of feelings and for questions. Tests and procedures are explained to them.

4. Potential for injury. Impairment of awareness may occur resulting in disorientation. Cot-sides are kept up and frequent close observation made for confusion and restlessness; a mild sedative may be necessary. Physical restraints are not used. It may be necessary to have someone remain constantly with the patient to avoid personal injury.

When the comatose patient regains consciousness, frequent orientation to place and circumstances is necessary as well as reassurance as to care and progress.

5. Potential pressure sores. The enforced immobility incurs the potential for skin breakdown. The patient's position is changed at least every 2 hours. The bed is kept dry and free of wrinkles, and vulnerable pressure areas may be protected by aids such as a sheepskin and the use of an alternating pressure (ripple) mattress. (See Chapter 27) for details of potential decubitus ulcer.)

6. Fluid and food intake. When tolerated, the patient receives a soft diet and is not usually permitted to feed himself. The fluid intake may be limited to a specific volume per 24 hours to promote a reduction in cerebral oedema and in the intracranial pressure. An accurate record of the fluid intake and output is maintained.

7. Urinary and bowel elimination. Rarely, the patient has difficulty voiding in the supine position and requires catheterization. In some instances an indwelling catheter may be used in the acute phase to prevent the expending of exertion in using a bedpan, to protect the skin if the patient is incontinent or to closely monitor the urinary output.

A mild laxative or stool softener may be prescribed after 3 or 4 days to prevent constipation and straining at stool. Enemas are contraindicated.

8. Potential complications. As well as the danger of a recurrence of bleeding by the aneurysm, the patient is at risk of developing vasospasm of cerebral vessels. Initially the spasm occurs in vessels in the region of the aneurysm, then spasms may become more extensive through the brain. The patient manifests symptoms of cerebral ischaemia. The nurse should be alert for the symptoms of paresis, paralysis, speech impairment and disorientation. If the spasm persists, infarction of the brain tissue occurs, causing serious neurological deficits.

Secondary hydrocephalus may develop as a result of interruption of the normal drainage of CSF into the general circulation system, by the residue of blood in the fluid blocking absorption by the arachnoid villi. The accumulation of CSF causes increased ICP and compresses the brain. See p. 807 for signs of increased ICP.

Treatment may involve a cranial burr hole and the placing of a tube in a ventricle (ventriculostomy) for external drainage of the CSF. If the hydrocephalus persists, a permanent ventriculoatrial or ventriculo-peritoneal shunt may be done to drain the CSF.

9. *Residual impairment.* The patient may recover and may be left with brain damage that results in reduced physical and/or mental capacity. Assistance is necessary in planning a change in the life-style of both patient and family. See Chapter 3 on Rehabilitation.

The patient treated by surgery
Generally, only patients classified as grade I or II are considered as surgical candidates.

Most surgeons wait several days before operating to allow time for the postrupture oedema of the brain to reduce. The greatest challenge to the nurse may be the patient in grade I or II category during this waiting period. He may be a young person who is worried about being away from his work and family. He may not feel particularly ill and finds it very difficult to understand why he must be kept immobile and treated as though he is helpless. The nurse spends time talking quietly with him, explaining and reassuring, and making every effort to prevent incidents that are likely to increase his blood pressure and initiate rebleeding.

A specific directive is usually received from the surgeon as to the preoperative preparation; other-wise it is similar to that cited for intracranial surgery (see p. 811).

Postoperative care is that outlined for the patient having intracranial surgery. If no complications arise, ambulation is started within 2 or 3 days after operation. Progression from lying to the sitting posi-tion and then to standing is made very slowly as the patient will have been on complete bed rest for a period before the surgery.

The integrity of the surgical procedure may be checked by a postoperative cerebral angiogram.

Expected outcomes
1 There is an absence of rebleeding, vasospasm and hydrocephalus.
2 Intracranial pressure and vital signs return to normal.
3 The patient is comfortable, free of headache, nausea and vomiting.
4 The patient's level of anxiety is reduced.
5 Food and fluid intake meets normal requirements.
6 Bowel and bladder elimination patterns return to normal.
7 Skin integrity is maintained.
8 If the patient has residual impairment, the patient

and family indicate a satisfactory plan for rehabilitation and home management.

Stroke (cerebrovascular accident)

A stroke or CVA involves an interruption of the blood supply to a part of the brain and the develop-ment of neurological deficits. If the ischaemia per-sists, necrosis of the deprived area follows, the infarcted area eventually liquefies and is absorbed and the neurological deficits remain. The cause of the stroke may be atherosclerosis, cerebral thrombosis or embolism, or intracranial haemorrhage. Cerebral haemorrhage as a cause of stroke may be petechial or massive. The artery that ruptures is usually vulner-able due to degenerative vascular changes (athero-sclerosis) or the presence of an aneurysm. A haemor-rhagic stroke may be precipitated by an elevation of blood pressure and is usually associated with some physical or emotional stress.

According to the rate of development and per-manence of the neurological effects, a stroke may be categorized as transient ischaemic attacks (little strokes), stroke in evolution or completed stroke. Transient ischaemic attacks are discussed earlier, on p. 789. Gradual development of stroke symptoms over a period of several hours or days is usually associated with a cerebral thrombosis or slow leak in a cerebral artery. This type of stroke is referred to as a stroke in evolution. A stroke is classified as a com-pleted stroke when the neurological deficits remain longer than 3 or 4 days.

Incidence
Strokes are a leading cause of death and disability. They have their highest incidence in those over 60 years of age. The chief risk factors are hypertension, atherosclerosis, obesity, congenital aneurysm, ischaemic heart disease and diabetes mellitus. Birth control pills have also been implicated.

NURSING PROCESS

Assessment

Manifestations and effects. These vary greatly, being determined by the location and size of the infarction, the type of lesion (thrombosis, embolism or haemor-rhage), and the rate at which cerebral oedema and infarction develop. The damage may be so severe that death ensues within a few hours or days, or the injury may be so slight that the symptoms are transient and may even go unrecognized. Between these extremes are many variants. Many survivors have little or no disability; the remainder have some potential for recovery of function as the pressure and oedema subside in the area of the lesion.

● *Premonitory manifestations.* Premonitory symptoms may be experienced which might include persistent headache, dizziness, fleeting loss of consciousness or 'blackout', brief confusion, blurring of vision in one or both eyes, slurring of speech, and transient local motor and sensory deficits. Any of these symptoms should serve as a warning especially if the client is known to be at risk.

- *Alteration in level of consciousness.* The patient may experience only a decrease in responsiveness to stimuli, confusion or clouding of consciousness while others may suddenly or gradually become unconscious. The coma may last a few hours to days; the gravity of prognosis tends to increase if the coma extends beyond 36 hours.
- *Headache and vomiting.* If the patient remains conscious, he may complain of severe headache as a result of increased intracranial pressure. Vomiting frequently occurs with the initial onset and may be recurring in the conscious patient.
- *Neuromuscular deficits.* The immediate onset may be accompanied by convulsive movements which may be local or general. The effects of the impairment of neuromuscular control by stroke vary from only a muscular weakness to complete paralysis. Hemiplegia (paralysis of one side of the body) is one of the most common effects of a stroke and indicates interruption of motor pathways. The interference with impulses usually involves the internal capsule in the affected hemisphere. The axons of motor neurons which initiate willed movements in each hemisphere converge into the internal capsule (see p. 775). The motor fibres from each hemisphere decussate in the medulla; as a result, paralysis of one side of the body indicates that the cerebral lesion is contralateral; that is, a stroke in the right side of the brain causes paralysis of the left upper and lower extremities. For a few days, there is a marked loss of tone in the affected muscles and an absence of normal reflexes. Even though the patient is in coma, a greater loss of tone in the affected limbs is recognizable (when flexed the limb falls more quickly in a limp, lifeless manner). Later this flaccidity is replaced by spasticity; deep tendon reflexes and the Babinski's sign are present.

One side of the face may be paralysed which causes the alternate abnormal distension and retraction with each respiration. The mouth is also drawn to one side.

When conscious, the patient may experience difficulty in swallowing (dysphagia) indicating some paralysis of the swallowing muscles.

- *Incontinence.* Urinary and bowel incontinence are common in the early stage. The bladder is atonic and the patient does not experience the desire to void. Later, tone returns and the bladder may become spastic and the patient experiences frequency and urgency. Unless the cerebral damage is extensive, involving both hemispheres, bladder control is re-established with training. The patient may be insensitive to the defecation reflex, resulting in incontinence.
- *Eye changes.* The pupils may be unequal in size; the larger of the two is on the side of the lesion. The eyes as well as the head tend to turn to the side of the lesion in the early stage; later the deviations may be reversed. Hemianopia (loss of vision in half of the visual field) occurs and may be temporary. In the unconscious patient, the corneal and pupillary reflexes may be absent and the fundus may reveal papilloedema due to increased intracranial pressure or hypertension.
- *Impairment of speech.* There may be complete or partial loss of the ability to communicate. The speech centre is in the dominant cerebral hemisphere; if the stroke occurs on that side, aphasia is likely to occur. The left hemisphere is dominant in the majority of persons. The patient may not only be unable to communicate verbally but may manifest some impairment of comprehension of either or both written or verbal communication.

The aphasia may take various forms (see Table 22.6). In motor or expressive aphasia, the person understands and knows what he wants to say but cannot utter the words. In receptive aphasia the person does not comprehend either written or spoken words. If there is total loss of speech and communication it is referred to as global aphasia and indicates a serious, massive lesion.
- *Mental impairment.* A stroke may impair the patient's memory, comprehension and the ability to reason and make judgements. There may be inability to recognize previously familiar objects or

Table 22.6 Common types of aphasia

Auditory aphasia	Inability to comprehend spoken word. May be referred to as *word deafness*
Expressive aphasia	Individual understands spoken and written words and knows what he wants to say but cannot speak the words. Also referred to as *motor or Broca's aphasia*
Global aphasia	Complete aphasia involves both the sensory and motor functions that provide all forms of communication
Receptive aphasia	Inability to comprehend spoken, written or tactile speech symbols. Also referred to as *sensory aphasia*

sensory impressions (agnosia) and to use objects correctly (apraxia).

Emotional lability is common; the patient may cry or laugh inappropriately.

- *Vital signs.* The respirations are usually slow and stertorous or may be Cheyne–Stokes. The pulse is usually slow, full and bounding in the initial phase. The temperature may be normal during the first few hours and then becomes elevated. Hyperpyrexia is an unfavourable sign.

Diagnostic procedures. When a stroke occurs, procedures may be carried out to identify the underlying cause because the therapy for an ischaemic stroke differs from that of a haemorrhagic stroke. Diagnostic procedures also may reveal the extent and location of involvement. They may include the following:

1 A CAT scan may be done; a collection of blood, cerebral oedema or an infarcted area will show up because of its increased density. It will also demonstrate the displacement of tissue.
2 An EEG may be used to determine the amount of brain wave activity and differentiate a thrombotic or haemorrhagic stroke. High-voltage slow waves are characteristic of a haemorrhagic stroke; if the cause is thrombosis, the tracing usually shows low-voltage slow waves.
3 Rarely, a lumbar puncture is done, and in the case of a stroke and infarction there is an elevation in the leucocyte count in the CSF; the presence of blood in the CSF indicates haemorrhage.

On-going assessment. An initial assessment of the vital signs and neurological status establishes a base for on-going evaluations and prompt recognition of changes. During the acute phase, vital signs, level of consciousness and motor and sensory functions are monitored at frequent intervals. The chest is observed for range of movement and symmetry in inspiration and may be auscultated for air entry and the presence of secretions. Blood gas analysis is done to determine the need for oxygen. Frequent observations are made for: signs of increased intracranial pressure, fits or convulsions, shock and progressive loss of neuromuscular functioning.

Following the acute stage, the patient's motor functions and level of awareness are assessed daily. Some improvement may occur day to day as the cerebral oedema and pressure are reduced and collateral circulation is established. The regaining of function tends to follow a pattern in which the facial and swallowing muscles recover first, then those of the lower limbs. Usually, speech and arm function return more slowly and less completely. Observations are made frequently for early signs of complications such as contractures and pressure sores.

Identification of patient problems
1 Altered level of consciousness: coma

2 Alteration in respiratory process:
  (a) Weakness and irregularity in respiratory muscle function
  (b) Ineffective airway clearance
  (c) Deficient gas exchange
3 Potential increased intracranial pressure secondary to cerebral oedema and haemorrhage
4 Headache and vomiting due to increased intracranial pressure
5 Alteration in elimination processes:
  (a) Possible urinary retention with overflow
  (b) Incontinence
  (c) Potential constipation, faecal impaction and bowel incontinence
7 Alteration in fluid and food intake: deficit due to coma, vomiting and/or dysphagia. The taking of food may also be influenced by difficulty with mastication as well as swallowing
8 Potential for injury secondary to neurological deficits, confusion or fits
9 Potential pressure sores due to immobility and incontinence
10 Self-care deficits due to coma, paralysis, impaired cognition and awareness
11 Impaired verbal communication: aphasia
12 Impairment of mobility: occurs in varying degrees ranging from weakness to complete paralysis
13 Cognitive dysfunction: impaired awareness, confusion, loss of memory, reasoning and judgement
14 Emotional lability: inappropriate responses, for example inappropriate outbursts of anger, crying and laughing. If awareness is not impaired, the patient usually manifests the characteristics of the grieving process (denial, anger, depression, gradual acceptance and resolution)
15 Lack of knowledge about rehabilitation and home management

In the acute phase the *goals* are to:
1 Maintain vital functions and help the patient to survive the cerebral assault
2 Prevent complications and increasing disability
3 Lessen anxiety and discomfort

In the convalescent and rehabilitative phase the *goals* are to:
1 Prevent complications
2 Help the patient regain his independence to his maximum potential
3 Provide support for the patient and family during their adjustment to the changes in their life situation

Nursing intervention
The most important therapeutic measures relevant to stroke involve sustained and adequate treatment and respect for risk factors.

The degree of recovery following a stroke is

determined by the size of the haemorrhage and infarction and is influenced by the patient's age, available rehabilitation programmes and the individual's personality and behavioural responses. Improvement can occur but deficits which are present after 6 months are usually permanent. Early, sustained and intensive therapy for the highly motivated patient with strong professional and family support frequently results in independence and a very satisfying recovery and quality of life.

Treatment and nursing care of a patient with a thrombotic stroke will differ somewhat with that of a haemorrhagic stroke and of course it varies with the degree of cerebral damage and ensuing neurological deficits. In the case of a thrombotic stroke, in evolution, an anticoagulant such as heparin may be administered and efforts are directed to maintaining a normal level of blood pressure. The patient is kept on bed rest with a minimal of disturbance and environmental stimuli to reduce the potential for haemorrhage. Surgical removal of the thrombus may be undertaken. When the stroke is due to a cerebral haemorrhage, therapy and nursing involve efforts directed towards relief of the increased intracranial pressure, life-support measures, relief of hypertension to prevent further bleeding and the prevention of complications.

The care required by the stroke patient during the acute phase following the initial onset differs from that required during the convalescent and rehabilitative phase. The care will also vary with the severity of the cerebrovascular accident and extent of brain damage. During the acute phase, intervention is principally directed towards maintaining life and preventing increased neurological deficits and complications.

1. Altered level of consciousness. When the patient is comatose, the principles which apply to the care of any unconscious patient will apply; see Chapter 10.

2. Altered respiratory process. The stroke patient may have slow, stertorous respirations or Cheyne–Stokes respirations. If the stroke is massive, the respirations may be slow, irregular and shallow. Secretions accumulate because of depressed cough reflex and ineffective airway clearance. Intermittent suctioning may be necessary to clear the upper airway. Prolonged periods of suctioning, more than 15 seconds, increases intracranial pressure. Intubation and mechanically assisted ventilation may be necessary. Oxygen administration by mask or nasal cannulae may be prescribed. Regular, frequent (2 hourly) turning of the patient and chest physiotherapy promote mobilization of secretions and lessen the risk of respiratory complications. If the patient is sufficiently alert, deep breathing is encouraged.

3. Increased intracranial pressure. In some instances, the patient is required to lie on the side of the lesion and minimal activity is prescribed for several hours to reduce the possibility of intracranial bleeding and increased pressure. The head of the bed may be elevated and good alignment of the head is maintained to avoid compression of the neck vessels; flexion may interfere with cerebral venous drainage and promote cerebral congestion, bleeding from the lesion and increased intracranial pressure. If hyperthermia develops, tepid sponging may be prescribed. Light bedclothes and clothing are used and an electric fan may be placed near the patient's bed.

4. Alteration in comfort. The conscious patient may complain of severe headache. Reduced lighting and minimal environmental stimuli may help and a cold compress or ice-bag may be applied to the head. A mild analgesic (e.g. paracetamol) may be prescribed, but strong analgesics are withheld because they mask neurological symptoms. If the patient vomits, he should be on his side and assistance provided to prevent aspiration, bearing in mind that the normal reflexes are usually depressed in the initial stage.

5. Alteration in elimination processes. If the patient is unresponsive a catheter may be inserted to prevent retention with overflow and incontinence or to measure the urinary output accurately. The retention catheter is left in for as brief a period as possible to avoid infection and allow retraining to commence as soon as possible.

The enforced inactivity associated with a stroke frequently gives rise to constipation and impaction. When the patient's condition has stabilized, a stool-softener may be administered or glycerine suppositories may be used to stimulate defecation; straining at stool should be avoided.

6. Alteration in fluid and food intake. If the patient is unconscious, a specified volume of fluid may be administered intravenously over 24 hours. The rate of flow and volume are carefully controlled to avoid a rapid increase in intravascular volume and blood pressure with subsequent increased intracranial bleeding and pressure. If coma is prolonged or the patient has dysphagia, nasogastric tube feeding may be introduced to provide sufficient nutrients (see Chapter 17). An accurate record of the patient's fluid intake during the acute phase is necessary.

When consciousness is regained, the gag reflex is tested before giving any fluids orally. If the patient can swallow, a soft diet is given and progressively increased to a full balanced diet as tolerated. The hemiplegic patient may have to be fed at first if his dominant arm is affected, but with the necessary assistance, he is encouraged to feed himself as soon as possible to establish independence.

If one side of the face is paralysed, food is placed in the opposite side of the mouth. Mouth care is then given following each meal to remove retained food particles from the affected side to prevent aspiration and the development of ulcers.

7. *Potential for injury*. Protection from injury is necessary due to the motor deficits and possible seizures. Contractures and deformities may develop because flexor muscles take over and loss of range of joint movement occurs. Limbs are supported in a natural position. Passive movements of all joints are carried out at regular intervals, for example when changing the patient's position.

Sensory function may also be impaired; as well as a reduced sensitivity to pressure, pain and temperature, there may be loss of the ability to know the location of parts of his body in space (impaired spatial perception). Cot-sides are kept up; the patient may be disoriented and also if turning in bed, may not have the normal reflexive muscular responses that would maintain his balance and prevent falling from the bed. When allowed up, precautions are taken to prevent falls and accidents (sufficient assistance, hand-rails, walking frames or sticks). Convulsion precautions should be observed (see p. 854).

8. *Potential pressure sores*. To maintain the integrity of the skin while confined to bed, the patient is turned every 2 hours and vulnerable pressure areas (sacral and lateral hips, heels, malleoli, knees, elbows, shoulders, scapular areas and head) are kept clean and dry. A protective lotion or emollient may be applied if the skin is dry. Aids such as an air (ripple) mattress and synthetic sheepskins may be used to protect pressure areas.

When the patient is allowed out of bed, precautions are necessary to prevent prolonged periods of sitting; he must be taught to stand or shift his weight from one hip to another at frequent intervals to relieve compression of vessels in the area.

9. *Self-care deficits*. During the acute phase, the nurse bathes, feeds and provides the necessary personal care for the patient. During this phase and as long as the patient complains of headache or manifests neck rigidity, the patient is kept on bed rest. As soon as his condition has stabilized, opportunity is provided for the patient to carry out the activities of daily living; active assistance is gradually withdrawn while giving support and encouragement. The call light or buzzer, water, toilet articles and other needed items are placed within the patient's reach. The nurse should encourage the patient to be aware of and to use his affected side if possible.

10. *Medications*. If the blood pressure is elevated, an antihypertensive drug or diuretic may be prescribed. The blood pressure is monitored at frequent, regular intervals; a low normal blood pressure is desirable.

If there is a confirmed diagnosis of cerebral thrombosis or embolism, an anticoagulant such as heparin may be prescribed. Prothrombin time is done frequently (normal: 11–15 seconds) and observations made for possible bleeding.

11. *Anxiety*. The patient as well as the family may experience considerable anxiety and concern due to the loss of body functions (motor, communication), dependence and change in roles and appearance. Plans for rehabilitation and available home services are outlined with both the patient and his family.

Rehabilitative phase following stroke
Rehabilitation really commences with the initial onset and acute phase: certain aspects of the care received in the early stage of the illness play an important role in the patient's rehabilitation. As soon as the patient is well enough, an assessment is made of residual disabilities and remaining capacities. A multidisciplinary team then becomes involved in plans to assist the patient to develop his maximum potential, independence and to assist the family with the necessary adjustments. Both patient and family should participate in setting achievable goals. Attainment of the goals usually requires months of perseverance and patience. The patient and family naturally experience periods of frustration, depression and pessimism. Activities are taken in steps so that achievement is experienced. Complete restoration to previous functional ability may not be possible but much can be done to restore the patient to a degree of independence that makes life more tolerable for him and his family.

Aphasia. The aphasia associated with a stroke most often is expressive in type although variants do occur (see Table 22.6). The sudden loss of the ability to communicate creates fear and frustration in the patient; feelings of isolation, insecurity and loneliness develop. The nurse endeavours to allay some of the anxiety by anticipating the patient's needs as much as possible, acknowledging his difficulty and concern and indicating time and willingness to work through his problem. He is likely to benefit psychologically from knowing that someone understands and will help. Many aphasic patients can recover the ability to communicate to some degree. It is not possible to predict this at the onset; speech is usually recovered very gradually and slowly and requires the assistance of those around the patient. The nurse avoids conveying what may be false optimism at first but reassures the patient and family that special assistance will be given to minimize speech and other neurological deficits. In the early stage, gestures to indicate needs and wishes may be encouraged but should not be accepted indefinitely since established use of them inhibit efforts to speak.

If the services of a speech therapist are available, a retraining programme is planned. In many situations, the nurse will be mainly responsible for helping the patient recover the ability to communicate. It is necessary, as soon as possible, to determine whether the patient can express his ideas verbally or by written work and whether he understands the spoken and written word. His comprehension may be limited to short simple phrases or single words. Rarely, intellectual impairment occurs (e.g. receptive aphasia) which precludes speech rehabilitation. It is important to talk normally and with ease to the patient; auditory stimulation and socialization can play important roles and are considered as valuable as structured remedial drills. It must be remembered that the fact that he cannot speak is no indication that his intelligence, comprehension and hearing are impaired. The patient should be included in the conversation taking place in his presence. Short simple sentences, kept at functional level relating to his present and immediate needs and environment are used if there is evidence of difficulty in comprehension. When encouraging the patient to try, emphasis is placed on nouns and simple responses such as 'yes' and 'no' at first; then progression through verbs and adjectives to short sentences is made. The necessary retraining in many instances is much the same as the process used with the young child learning to communicate. The use of several sensory avenues is usually more effective than the use of just one at a time. Hearing words in direct association with the objects and the printed words that represent them contributes to recovery.

During speech therapy, the patient should be rested and relaxed and in a quiet undistracting setting. The periods of instruction are kept brief as the patient tires easily and his attention span is likely to be short. He should never be pressured to the point of frustration which leads to discouragement and withdrawal. Emphasis on exact pronunciation is avoided.

Early in the illness, the family members and others are helped in understanding the patient's communication problems and their role in his recovery of speech. The importance of conversing normally with him, expecting a response, making every effort to understand and giving him plenty of time to respond are emphasized. The methods and details related to periods of instruction and their participation are discussed with the family. At least one member should be given the opportunity to observe a teaching session carried out in the hospital or rehabilitation unit. The need for patience and the need for providing opportunities for the patient to practise and use what speech he has are stressed. The family is advised that progress may be slow and are cautioned against making excessive demands on the patient. Progress should be acknowledged because it encourages and prompts motivation for continued effort.

Pamphlets and booklets on aphasia are available from the Chest, Heart and Stroke Association; these may be reviewed with the family and clarification of details made if necessary.

Motor deficits. As cited earlier (p. 795), the muscles of the affected limbs are flaccid for a few days then became spastic. The paralysed arm becomes adducted and flexion occurs at the elbow, wrist, fingers and thumb joints. The lower limb assumes a position of external rotation at the hip, flexion of the thigh and leg and plantar flexion of the foot (Fig. 22.22). With immobility, muscles atrophy and the collagen fibres of the connective tissue of the tendons, ligaments and joint capsules tend to shorten and become dense and firm. The process may be hastened by circulatory stasis, oedema and trauma. As a result, if the affected limbs are permitted to remain immobile in the positions they automatically assume, contractures and reduced range of joint motion may become permanent. Deformities are created which actually increase the person's disability and make rehabilitation difficult. Liaison with the physiotherapist is essential when caring for the stroke patient. In many units, the Bobath techniques are implemented during the patient's rehabilitation period, and the nurse should familiarise herself with these.

Maintenance of joint motion, support to prevent the pull of gravity on joints and subsequent subluxation, and positioning to prevent contractures and maintain good alignment are essential from the onset of the stroke.

When lying on the unaffected side, the patient's unaffected shoulder is brought slightly forward and the arm should lie straight, in line with the trunk. The unaffected leg should be straight. A pillow is placed under the affected arm, which is straightened at the elbow; the hand is straightened, with the

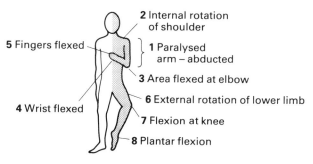

2 Internal rotation of shoulder

5 Fingers flexed

1 Paralysed arm – abducted

3 Area flexed at elbow

4 Wrist flexed

6 External rotation of lower limb

7 Flexion at knee

8 Plantar flexion

Fig. 22.22 Contractures which develop with hemiplegia. 1, Paralysed arm. 2, Internal rotation of shoulder. 3, Area flexed at elbow. 4, Wrist flexed. 5, Fingers flexed. 6, External rotation of lower limb. 7, Flexion at knee. 8, Plantar flexion.

fingers spread over the upper part of the pillow. The affected leg is flexed at the knee and hip, with a pillow underneath for support. A pillow is placed along the back of the patient, onto which he is lightly rolled and supported.

When the patient is lying on the affected side, a reverse similar position is adopted, except that the unaffected arm is flexed at the elbow, with the hand towards the edge of the bed. The affected leg is flexed slightly at the knee. Pillows are this time placed under the unaffected, not the affected, limbs for support and to prevent friction and pressure. A pillow at the back should support the patient, but he is not rolled back towards the pillow.

Marked spasticity of the affected hand may necessitate the application of a padded splint, especially at night, to prevent flexure contractures of the wrist and fingers. A support may be provided to prevent foot drop.

The limbs are passively moved through a full range of movements 2 or 3 times daily. While the patient is dependent and confined to bed, his position is changed and passive movements carried out every 2 hours.

The stroke patient is usually assisted out of bed for progressively increasing periods as soon as his condition has stabilized. His balance should be assessed and improved (if possible) before walking is commenced. Being up reduces the possibility of complications and promotes a more positive attitude on the part of the patient toward his future. When the patient is up, support of the affected arm in a sling may sometimes be necessary to prevent subluxation of the shoulder joint. A pillow may be used to support the arm when sitting in a chair. Most hemiplegic patients fortunately experience extensor spasm of the affected knee and hip muscles with weight-bearing which stabilizes the leg as the unaffected leg carries through a forward step. Some patients do experience spasm of flexor rather than extensor muscle spasm in the affected leg and as a result when the patient attempts to walk, the knee and hip flex and do not support him. This necessitates the application of a leg brace for stabilization. When assisting the patient who is walking, the nurse or family member supports him from the affected side. He may require an aid, such as a walking frame, to assist him to regain independence. If plantar flexion and toe-dragging interfere with walking, a drop-foot splint may be used. A few hemiplegic patients suffer ataxia and loss of balance which may preclude ambulation and the patient remains in a wheelchair.

As soon as possible the retraining for self-care is begun; the initial focus is on personal care and activities of living. Retraining carried out by the occupational therapist and the nurse includes the simple useful functions on which every person is dependent in normal living. Examples are dressing and undressing, opening doors, using the tele-phone, writing and the handling of various articles (e.g. cutlery, wallet). The hemiplegic patient is taught how to change his position in bed (turn, sit up, transfer to a chair, stand up). The bed is lowered and made stationary when transfer techniques are carried out. A schedule of exercises is established to strengthen the trunk and unaffected limb muscles. The programme includes the affected limbs; if the muscles are weak, active assistive and active exercises are used. If the muscles are unresponsive, passive movements are carried out to prevent contractures and ankylosis. Ice-baths or heat treatment may be used if limbs are stiff and painful.

Sensory deficits. The patient is assessed for possible impairment of sensory functions such as pain, pressure and temperature. There may also be loss of the ability to know the location of parts of his body in space (proprioception deficit) making the judging of distances and movements more difficult. The patient's vision may also be impaired by the loss of function in the corresponding halves of the visual fields (homonymous hemianopia) in both eyes. The inability to recognize objects by touch, sight or hearing may be manifested. The necessary precautions are established to prevent accidents such as falls and burns and become an important part of the rehabilitation programme.

Prevention of recurrence. The patient may be required to continue taking an anticoagulant and he and the family are advised of its purpose and the importance of prompt reporting of signs of bleeding. A balanced diet with less fat content may be recommended and a dietary plan reviewed with the patient and family that will meet his caloric needs according to his weight and energy expenditure. If necessary the patient is strongly advised against smoking. It is recommended that female patients should not take contraceptive pills.

Family and home management. The total care and rehabilitation programme is fully discussed with a member of the family. The importance of encouraging and permitting the patient to do things for himself is emphasized. Family and friends find it difficult to stand back while the patient struggles and perseveres with activities. Prior to discharge, the patient may be encouraged to spend 1 or 2 days at home, e.g. at the weekend, and a home assessment may be carried out by appropriate personnel. Following his discharge from hospital, both patient and family still require considerable support and assistance; referrals should be made to appropriate support and community services. Modifications of the environment may be necessary to facilitate the development of independence and prevent accidents. Handrails in the bathroom, placement of articles for ready accessibility, making the bed stationary and the removal of scatter rugs and wax from floors are a few examples of adjustments that may be made in the environment.

The assistance of social services may be necessary to help solve the problems imposed by the illness and residual disabilities. Early signs of resentment of the dependency of the patient on the part of some family members may be recognized. By listening to their points of view, by explaining the patient's condition and unusual patterns of behaviour and by helping the family organize themselves so that all share in the increased responsibility, complete rejection of the patient may be prevented.

The Chest, Heart and Stroke Association has several helpful publications that should be made available to the stroke patient and his family.

Socialization. The patient is encouraged to develop interests and worthwhile hobbies and to gradually assume responsibility for home chores within his capacity. The performance of some useful tasks promotes the patient's morale and greater harmony within the family.

Friends are encouraged to visit and the patient is included in the social activities of the family.

Expected outcomes

The acute phase.
1 The patient regains consciousness.
2 Vital functions return to normal.
3 The patient is free of respiratory, urinary and skin complications and has not had any fits.
4 The patient tolerates a soft diet, and swallows without difficulty.

The convalescent and rehabilitative phase.
1 The patient manifests a positive, cooperative attitude toward the rehabilitation programme.
2 Self-care activities and mobility are progressively being achieved.
3 The patient is taking a balanced diet with sufficient calories to meet his energy expenditure in the exercise programme and his mobility.
4 The patient regains normal elimination patterns.
5 The family and patient make an acceptable, informed plan for home management.
6 The family supports the patient, shares responsibility and cooperates in changing roles and in making the necessary adjustments

Trauma of the Nervous System

HEAD INJURIES

Accidents on the highways, in industry and sports, and violence on the streets and in the home are the major causes of head injury which ranks high on the list of causes of morbidity, mortality and permanent disabilities. Frequently, head injury is only one of the major problems seen in the traumatized patient and priorities of care are established on the basis of the assessment of the patient as a whole person.

Head injuries may be classified as open or closed, coup or contrecoup, and primary or secondary. *Closed head injury* refers to injury in which there is no break in the tissues (scalp and skull) which separate the intracranial cavity from the external environment (e.g. subdural haematoma). *Open head injury* means that a break exists in the tissues which separate the intracranial contents from the external environment (e.g. compound or perforating skull fracture).

Coup and contrecoup injuries result from direct trauma to the head in which the sequence of intracranial events resembles an acceleration–deceleration phenomenon. *Coup* refers to bruising of the brain tissue which directly underlies the site of impact and which rebounds against that portion of the cranium. *Contrecoup* is brain injury on the side opposite to the site of impact. It is due to the wave of pressure created by the impact, compressing the brain substance against the bony ridges and opposite wall of the cranium. For example, a fall on the back of the head may cause injury to the frontal and temporal cerebral lobes. Injury to the nerve fibres, blood vessels and tendons in the brain stem results from the stress of shearing forces.

Primary head injuries

SCALP LACERATIONS

These alone are considered minor injuries although the bleeding may be profuse due to scalp vascularity. These wounds require the same attention as any other open area; they are cleansed thoroughly, underlying bone is examined for fractures, sutures applied if necessary and a sterile dressing applied. Reassurance should be given, relating to the blood loss.

FRACTURE OF THE SKULL

When it is suspected or is known that an accident victim received a blow to the head, x-rays are made of the skull and examined for possible fracture. A skull fracture is not considered serious unless brain tissue is bruised, compressed or lacerated, cranial blood vessels or meninges are torn or there is a leakage of CSF.

A skull fracture may be classified as linear (hairline), depressed, basilar, comminuted or compound (see Table 22.7). 'Pond' fractures may occur in babies and young children (see Table 22.7).

No specific treatment is used for a simple linear or comminuted skull fracture but the patient is kept at rest and under close observation because of potential

Table 22.7 Types of skull fractures.

Type	Description
Linear or simple	A fracture in which the two fragments remain in apposition (i.e. are not displaced). Patient may experience headache or be unconscious because of concomitant intracranial injury (e.g. subdural haemorrhage, concussion)
Depressed	Fragments of the skull are driven inward, compressing or piercing the meninges and brain. As well as direct injury to cranial content at fracture site, there is likely to be a rapid increase in intracranial pressure affecting total brain functioning
Basilar or basal	Fracture of the base of the skull which is thinner and less resistant. Cause is usually indirect force incurred by a fall from a height with the person landing on his feet or buttocks; impact of spine against the base of the skull may produce a serious fracture. More hazardous because it may open into paranasal sinuses or middle ear, predisposing to infection. Drainage of CSF from the nose and ear may occur. Emerging cranial nerves may be injured. If fracture is adjacent to the medulla, vital centres may be damaged
Comminuted	Multiple linear fractures occur but the fragments are not displaced
Compound	There is a laceration of the scalp as well as a fracture of the skull. Potential for infection of bone and cranial contents is greater
'Pond'	A depression in the skull, which occurs in babies and young children, before ossification is completed. The skull may not fragment

bleeding and haematoma. Meningeal blood vessels may have been torn and incur extradural, subdural or subarachnoid haemorrhage. Concussion or contusion of the brain is a frequent result.

Early surgical exploration is indicated when the depressed fracture occurs. Skull fragments are elevated and splinters and debris removed. Severe fragmentation and depression may necessitate removal of that area of the skull. Later, a cranioplasty may be done; a plate of inert material (e.g. titanium) is inserted to protect the brain and improve the patient's appearance.

BRAIN INJURY

Injury to the brain may result from a blow to the head and may or may not be associated with a fracture of the skull. A head injury may cause concussion, cerebral contusion or laceration, haemorrhage and/or compression.

A brain injury may be mild and reversible or may be severe and irreversible, leaving residual neurological deficits if the patient survives. Oedema of the brain and intracranial haemorrhage increase intracranial pressure which, if severe, may compress the brain stem and its vital centres (supratentorial herniation). Initially, *every head injury is considered serious*; it must be emphasized that regardless of outward appearance, the person requires close observation for evidence of developing secondary brain damage which could result in permanent disability or death.

Concussion may be described as a temporary cerebral paralysis as a result of a blow to the head. It is characterized by a brief period of unconsciousness due to jarring of the brain and its sudden forceful contact with the rigid skull. The period of unconsciousness varies from a few minutes to hours or days depending on the severity of the injury. When the patient regains consciousness, he may be confused, dazed and restless and is unable to recall events which preceded the accident. Headache is a common complaint. If there is no haemorrhage or brain tissue damage, no abnormal neurological findings are present; normal reflexes and muscle tone return.

Nursing care for concussion includes observation for evidence of neurological deterioration, and ensuring that a reliable person is available. The responsible person is instructed to remain with the patient, rouse and observe him hourly. If the patient becomes increasingly drowsy or difficult to rouse or, if he experiences headache, vomiting, visual disturbances, fits or a reduction in limb strength, the doctor must be notified immediately. It is advisable to provide instructions in writing for the responsible person since anxiety may affect the ability to recall what has been said. The patient is advised to rest quietly and apply a cold compress or ice-bag to the head for relief of the headache. Recovery following an uncomplicated concussion occurs within a short period of time and usually no further problems arise.

Cerebral contusion and laceration refers to bruising and tearing of superficial brain tissue. The multiple areas of tissue damage may give rise to a wide variety of patient responses. It must be emphasized that a head injured patient can have significant trauma and still be alert. Loss of consciousness is not a requirement for a diagnosis of severe head injury. Aphasia may result with a frontal–temporal contusion. A temporal lobe contusion may give rise to agitation, confusion and 'foul-mouthed' responses. Lesions of the brain stem are usually of the more serious type. Level of consciousness may be altered for several hours or weeks. A variety of other neurological abnormalities are usually present on both sides of the body. If neurological signs are present on one side of the body, it is probable that a secondary event such as the development of a haematoma has occurred. The tissue injury is usually accompanied by brain swelling and oedema. Recovery may be a lengthy process; permanent tissue damage and scarring may result in permanent disability if the patient survives.

Secondary events following head injury

INTRACRANIAL HAEMORRHAGE

Haemorrhage within the cranium and the formation of a haematoma following a head injury frequently leads to rapid deterioration in the patient's condition. The bleeding may be extradural, subdural, subarachnoid or intracerebral. The signs and symptoms presented are due to increased intracranial pressure and compression of areas of the brain (see p. 806).

An *extradural haematoma* is an accumulation of blood between the dura and skull (see Fig. 22.23A) and is a serious complication. Since the meningeal artery is frequently torn, extradural bleeding is at arterial pressure. The brain is compressed and displaced and the intracranial pressure rises rapidly. The patient may be comatose for a brief period, regain consciousness, then gradually develop serious neurological symptoms (disturbed vision, dilated pupil and loss of reflex to light in the eye on the affected side, severe headache, confusion, decreased motor and sensory function, seizure, vomiting) and loss of consciousness. Prompt treatment is essential. If an extradural haemorrhage is not recognized and promptly treated, the rapidly increasing intracranial pressure may cause tentorial herniation, pressure on vital centres and death within a few hours.

Subdural haemorrhage is a relatively common complication of head injury. Blood accumulates in the subdural space (see Fig. 22.23B), gradually forming a haematoma which compresses the brain and increases intracranial pressure. The bleeding may occur following a seemingly minor head injury. Since the bleeding is usually at venous pressure, the development of symptoms may be delayed and vague but progressively worsen and eventually,

increasing intracranial pressure and brain compression lead to coma.

As cited previously, all head injuries should be treated initially as serious and a potential threat to life.

Subdural haemorrhage may be subacute or chronic in patients of advanced age or with cortical atrophy. In these patients, evidence of increased intracranial pressure usually appears very gradually and intermittently.

Subarachnoid haemorrhage is bleeding of cerebral vessels into the space between the arachnoid and pia mater. The signs and symptoms are similar to those presented by the patient with a subdural haemorrhage and depend on the area of the brain involved. The patient complains of severe headache and examination usually reveals neck rigidity, dilation of the pupil and loss of reflex in the eye on the affected side, loss of motor and sensory function on one side and blood in the CSF (see Fig. 22.23C).

Intracerebral haemorrhage is bleeding resulting from a torn or diseased vessel within the cerebrum. It may occur as a result of a contrecoup injury, a penetrating wound such as a gun-shot or stabbing or, cerebral atherosclerosis (stroke). The symptoms depend on the particular vessel and cerebral area (see Fig. 22.23C).

BRAIN SWELLING AND OEDEMA

Infection, brain injury and cerebral haemorrhage and infarction cause brain swelling and oedema and consequent increased intracranial pressure which may lead to tentorial herniation. Oedema develops as a result of an inflammatory response; the swelling occurs when there is oedema or an accumulation of blood in the brain tissue. Infection such as meningitis or brain abscess develops most commonly with an open head injury or basilar skull fracture.

TENTORIAL HERNIATION

This is a very critical condition which may occur with brain injury and is not compatible with life. The tentorium is a fold of the tough dura mater that lies below the cerebrum separating it from the cerebellum and brain stem. As the brain stem ascends to join the cerebrum, it passes through a space referred to as the tentorial hiatus. The rigid skull prevents outward expansion of the contents of the intracranial cerebral area; as a result a space-occupying lesion such as a haematoma or cerebral swelling and oedema may precipitate the herniation of a portion of the cerebrum through the tentorial hiatus. This leads to compression of the brain stem and its vital centres.

SUMMARY

To summarize, the signs and symptoms associated with a head injury depend on the area of the brain

A

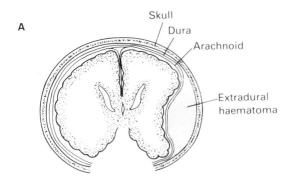

B

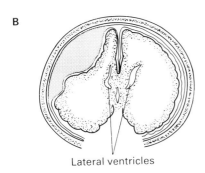

Lateral ventricles

C

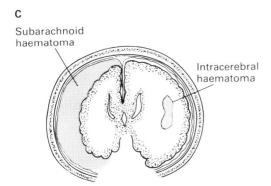

Fig. 22.23 *A*, Extradural haematoma. *B*, Subdural haematoma. *C*, Subarachnoid haematoma; intracerebral haematoma.

involved and the nature and severity of the tissue damage. They may appear immediately following the injury or several hours afterward as a result of intracranial haemorrhage, cerebral oedema and swelling of the brain and the ensuing compression and elevation of intracranial pressure.

The symptoms may include: loss of consciousness which may develop at the time of injury and last for a varying length of time; recurrence of unconsciousness following a lucid interval; drowsiness and stupor progressing to coma; severe headache or dizziness; disturbed vision; dilation and failure to react to light of one or both pupils; motor and

sensory deficits, seizures, nuchal rigidity, speech impairment, disorientation, changes in vital signs indicative of increasing intracranial pressure (see p. 807); and the escape of CSF from the ear or nose.

Complications and events which may develop in head injured patients include those associated with immobilization (e.g. contractures, pressure sores, thrombi and emboli). In addition, these patients are at risk of the development of such problems as post-traumatic epilepsy, stress ulcers, intracranial CSF fistula (drainage of CSF from the nose or ear) diabetes insipidus (inappropriate ADH release), carotid artery occlusion, and psychiatric disorders. Loss of social restraint, intellectual deficits and marked memory deficits are among the problems which may follow serious brain trauma.

Emergency care

As in all emergencies, the first consideration is the establishment of a clear airway. The brain cells are very dependent upon a continuous oxygen supply and, if injured, adequate provision becomes even more imperative. A clear airway is also important because obstruction tends to increase cerebral venous congestion and intracranial pressure. It should be kept in mind that serious intracranial damage can occur without external signs of a head trauma. An assessment is made of:
- Vital signs
- Level of consciousness
- Pupil size, equality and reaction
- Motor function in limbs
- Response to commands
- Sensory response to painful stimuli
- Orientation

If signs of shock (pallor, cold moist skin, slow capillary and venous filling, hypotension, weak pulse, shallow respirations, restlessness, dulling of consciousness) are observed in the patient with a head injury, an examination is made for the presence of other injuries; for example, shock in the adult trauma patient is not usually a result of the head injury. If unconscious, the victim is turned to a lateral or semiprone position to minimize the danger of obstruction of the airway and aspiration. The spine is kept straight and the head aligned; flexion and hyperextension of the head must be avoided.

An open scalp wound is covered with available clean material. The victim is covered and kept quiet and undisturbed while arrangements are made to transport him to the emergency department of the hospital.

Assessment

On admission to hospital, further consideration is given to supporting respiratory function and the patient's physical status and neurological status are assessed. A record of the initial findings serve as a base for on-going comparative assessment so that even slight changes may be readily recognized.

The neurological observations are repeated at half-hour to hourly intervals for at least 24 hours. The doctor is promptly notified of changes such as clouding or loss of consciousness, cannot be roused, increased blood pressure, inequality of pupils, change in respiratory pattern and loss of strength in one or more limbs; a change may indicate an increasing intracranial pressure. The interval between assessments is gradually lengthened depending on the basis of the patient's progress. Hourly recordings are made of the temperature if hyperthermia develops.

When consciousness is regained following a head injury, the patient is aroused every hour when he goes to sleep to determine his level of consciousness and to assess him for changes.

DIAGNOSTIC PROCEDURES

Investigative procedures to determine the nature, location and severity of the damage may include skull and cervical x-rays, CAT scan, lumbar puncture and cerebral angiography. An EEG may also be done to demonstrate increased or decreased brain wave activity.

MEDICAL MANAGEMENT

This will depend on the nature and severity of the head injury; the patient may or may not require surgical intervention. For the care of the patient having intracranial surgery (see p. 811).

If there is a cerebral haemorrhage, cerebral oedema or a depressed fracture there is concern for the potential of increased intracranial pressure, brain compression and infarction. In minor injuries, the most significant factor in care is observation for 24–36 hours for signs of intracranial haemorrhage and increased intracranial pressure (see p. 806). For more serious head injuries, the management of the patient is essentially the same as that outlined for the patient with increased intracranial pressure.

The escape of blood and CSF from an ear or nasal passage may occur with a fracture of the base of the skull and tearing of the dura mater between the brain and the ear or nasal passage. The drainage may be confirmed as CSF by a simple test (see p. 784). Such injury creates a potential for intracranial infection such as meningitis or brain abscess. The drainage is allowed to flow freely; the patient is positioned on the affected side. A dry sterile towel is placed under the head or a dry sterile dressing placed loosely over the orifice and changed frequently since moisture provides a most favourable environment for growth of organisms. Those caring for the patient should wash their hands well before working in the area of the drainage. The patient is cautioned not to blow his nose and not to suppress a sneeze. Under no circumstances should the drainage passages be packed and suction to the nasal passages is never performed if CSF leakage is suspected. The patient is observed closely for signs of infection; and a prophylactic antibiotic may be prescribed.

Identification of patient problems

1 Respiratory dysfunction secondary to:
   (a) Loss of patency of airway
   (b) Injury to or compression of the respiratory centre in the brain stem
2 Alteration in level of consciousness
3 Alteration in comfort when conscious: mild to severe headache
4 Motor and sensory deficits due to brain compression and damage
5 Alteration in level of awareness of self and environment
6 Potential for injury related to reduced level of consciousness, confusion, motor and sensory deficits or seizures
7 Impairment of skin integrity secondary to scalp wound, immobility or seizures
8 Alteration in fluid and food intake secondary to comatose state, fluid intake restrictions per 24 hours, or anxiety
9 Alteration in elimination patterns:
   (a) Urinary (incontinence, retention)
   (b) Bowel—constipation and potential impaction
10 Self-care deficits secondary to unconsciousness, enforced immobility or motor deficits
11 Anxiety related to confusion and loss of memory of previous events
12 Lack of knowledge about diagnostic and therapeutic procedures, condition, hospitalization and post-hospital care

The *goals* are to:
1 Regain consciousness and normal awareness
2 Ensure that vital signs return to normal limits
3 Complete motor and sensory functioning: no residual disabilities
4 Relieve the patient's headache
5 Maintain the integrity of the skin and make sure the scalp wound heals without infection
6 Normalize the patient's nutritional and hydrational status

Nursing intervention

If the patient is comatose, the care is the same as that described for the unconscious patient in Chapter 10. The patient is also at risk of increased intracranial pressure.

The head-injured patient is at risk of infection if an open scalp wound is present; the wound is cleansed, débrided if necessary and dressed. A reinforcing dose of tetanus toxoid may be prescribed as a prophylactic measure or human tetanus immunoglobulin may be given.

Loss of the corneal reflexes, periorbital oedema and ecchymoses are common problems with a head injury. If the corneal reflex is absent, the eyelid may be taped shut with non-allergic tape to protect the cornea from dryf the corneal reflex is absent, the eyelid may be taped shut with non-allergic tape to protect the cornea from drying and abrasions. The tape is removed every two hours and the eye irrigated with normal saline and artificial tears (e.g. hypromellose) instilled before retaping. If the eyelids are swollen, it may be necessary for a second nurse to hold the lids open while pupillary reflexes are assessed. If the lids cannot be opened, the doctor is notified; it is important that pupillary changes be detected in sufficient time to institute treatment.

The patient with a head injury may develop seizures. During a seizure, the pillow is removed and the patient is placed in a lateral or semiprone position. He is restrained only sufficiently to prevent injury. It is important to note: the parts of the body involved and which area was involved first; if the head and eyes are turned to one side; the duration of the convulsion; and the condition of the patient following the seizure. An anticonvulsant drug such as phenytoin (Epanutin) may be prescribed—even if the patient has not exhibited any seizures—as a prophylactic measure.

Hyperthermia may develop following head injury due to a disturbance of the temperature-control centre in the hypothalamus or to infection. A progressive elevation of temperature is an unfavourable sign. The patient is covered only with a light cotton sheet and the temperature of the room is reduced. Other measures to reduce temperature may be employed.

The recovery process following head injury may require intensive rehabilitation to restore independence even to minimal levels. Regardless of the cause of injury, if there are residual disabilities the rehabilitative needs are similar to those of other neurologically impaired patients (see Chapter 3).

Expected outcomes

The expected outcomes are similar to those outlined for the patient with a stroke, see p. 801.

Increased intracranial pressure

The cranium, which, in the adult is a rigid vault allowing practically no expansion of the content, contains the brain, CSF and blood. An increase in the volume of any one (brain, blood or CSF) causes an increase in the intracranial pressure and a comparable decrease in the volume of one or both of the other contents. The response may be:
1 Displacement of CSF.
2 A compromise in cerebral blood supply which causes cerebral ischaemia. The latter leads to

hypoxia, hypercapnoea and acidosis at cellular level, resulting in interruption of cell metabolism.
3 Displacement of brain tissue (*herniation* of brain tissue). This occurs when the other compensatory mechanisms fail. Brain displacement may occur in the supratentorial compartment or infratentorial compartment. The tentorium is a fold of the dura mater which lies below the cerebrum, separating it from the cerebellum and brain stem. As the brain stem ascends to join the cerebrum, it passes through a small space referred to as the tentorial hiatus or notch. Increasing intracranial pressure may cause a downward displacement of the cerebrum through the hiatus, causing a supratentorial herniation or what is referred to as coning. It causes compression of the brain stem; the patient becomes comatose and respiratory and circulatory failure may develop rapidly. A lesion in the temporal lobe compresses the mid-brain and third cranial nerve, first causing dilation of the pupil. This is referred to as a lateral or lineal herniation.

Infratentorial herniation involves displacement of brain stem or cerebellar tissue through the foramen magnum. Coma, motor dysfunction and respiratory depression develop.

Causes of increased intracranial pressure. The causes of increased intracranial pressure are swelling of the brain, increased CSF volume and increased blood volume.

Swelling of the brain may be due to a tumour (increased mass of tissue cells), abscess, inflammatory exudate, or cerebral oedema. An increase in the cranial volume of CSF is usually associated with a disturbance in the absorption or the outflow of the fluid; it accumulates in the ventricles, compressing brain tissue and blood vessels. An increase in the intracranial blood volume may be due to compression of the venous sinuses or jugular veins or to vasodilation of the cerebral vessels.

NURSING THE PATIENT WITH POTENTIAL OR ACTUAL INCREASED INTRACRANIAL PRESSURE

Treatment may be medical, surgical or a combination of both. Surgical intervention usually deals with the specific cause and may involve ventricular drainage. Medical treatment includes the intravenous administration of osmotic diuretics (e.g. mannitol) and the corticosteroid, dexamethasone.

ASSESSMENT

The defining characteristics of increased intracranial pressure are related to the location of the lesion, the nature of the lesion (e.g. tumour, haemorrhage) and the speed of development. The pressure may increase very rapidly, as with an extradural haemorrhage, or it may increase very gradually, as with a slow-growing tumour. If the pressure increase is rapid and diffuse, the compensatory mechanisms fail, brain function is compromised and clinical signs of increased intracranial pressure appear.

Early symptoms include headache which progressively becomes more severe, drowsiness, slowing of responses and vomiting, which may not be preceded by nausea. With further development there is decreasing consciousness, an increase in the systolic blood pressure with a widening pulse pressure, change in respiratory pattern, eye changes (pupillary dilation, loss of reflex to light stimulus), papilloedema and bradycardia (Table 22.8).

Table 22.8 Symptoms of increased intracranial pressure.

Headache
Restlessness, disorientation
Changes in responsiveness (decreased level of
  consciousness)
Changes in vital signs:
    ↑ systolic blood pressure
    widening pulse pressure
    ↓ pulse rate
    altered respiration rate and rhythm
    may develop periods of apnoea
    ↑ temperature (later sign)
Vomiting—usually projectile
Changes in pupillary size, equality and reflex responses
Change in posture—rigidity may develop
Loss of motor function
Loss of sensory function

The patient's vital signs and neurological status are assessed frequently to detect changes and early signs of deterioration. Craniocerebral testing is done and the vital signs are recorded. Evaluation of the patient's neurological status also includes observations for involuntary movements (twitching, tremors or convulsion), restlessness, rigidity and posturing (decerebrate or decorticate rigidity) (see Fig. 22.24).

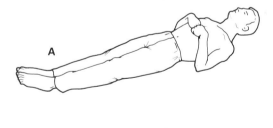

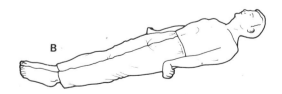

Fig. 22.24 *A*, Posture in decorticate rigidity. *B*, Posture in decerebrate rigidity.

The chest is auscultated for air entry and the pooling of secretions. The colour and condition of the skin (moist or dry, temperature, integrity) and fluid balance also are noted. If the patient is conscious his alertness, orientation, speech and ability to move his limbs are checked; he is roused to his maximum level of alertness with each assessment. The required frequency of these observations may be indicated by the doctor but usually begins with 15–30 minute intervals which are gradually lengthened to 1 hour then 4 hours if the evaluations indicate stability. A blood specimen may be taken for blood-gas analysis; the frequency is determined by the reports.

Evidence of confusion, disorientation, stupor, unequal pupils and absence of pupillary response to light, decreasing motor and sensory functions, rigidity increasing systolic pressure, elevated temperature, change in respiratory pattern and restlessness should be reported promptly to the doctor.

As an on-going assessment a system for continuous monitoring of intracranial pressure may be established. A special sensor (catheter or screw form) is passed through a burr hole in the skull and placed in the epidural, subdural or subarachnoid space or in a ventricle. A tubing with a stopcock is attached to the sensor and externally to a transducer which converts the pressure waves to electrical impulses which appear on an oscilloscope or a graph paper. Strict asepsis must be observed. There are various types of monitoring equipment and the procedure is complex. It must be managed and supervised by experienced persons who fully understand the type of monitor being used and the pressure values for the area in which the sensor is placed. The pressure in one compartment (e.g. ventricle) is different to that in another compartment such as the subdural space.

IDENTIFICATION OF PATIENT PROBLEMS

1 Alteration in respiratory function related to:
  (a) Ineffective clearance of airway
  (b) Injury or compression of the respiratory centre
  (c) Obstruction of the airway by the tongue and lower jaw, if unconscious
  (d) Aspiration of mucus or fluids secondary to absence of the pharyngeal reflex or impairment of the swallowing muscles
2 Potential for injury:
  (a) Increased intracranial pressure
  (b) Disorientation and impaired awareness
  (c) Restlessness
  (d) Seizures
3 Alteration in comfort; severe headache
4 Alteration in body temperature; potential hyperthermia
5 Alteration in cardiac function secondary to compression and ischaemia of vital centres in the medulla
6 Potential for skin breakdown related to immobi-

lity and possible restlessness and hyperthermia
7 Potential fluid imbalance related to osmotic diuretic, inadequate intake and vomiting
8 Nutritional deficit related to inadequate intake and increased metabolic rate with hyperthermia and injury
9 Alteration in elimination; bowel and urinary
10 Self-care deficit secondary to reduced level of awareness or loss of consciousness and motor and sensory changes
11 Lack of knowledge deficit related to care and progress

The *goals* are:
1 To reduce intracranial pressure to the normal level
2 Absence of dysfunctions incurred by increased intracranial pressure (elevated blood pressure, respiratory dysfunction, decreased awareness, hyperthermia, loss of consciousness, vomiting)
3 To relieve the patient's headache
4 Absence of restlessness and seizures
5 To maintain skin integrity
6 To be able to have and tolerate a normal nutritional and fluid intake

NURSING INTERVENTION

1. Respiratory dysfunction
The patient is positioned to maintain a clear airway; if unconscious the lateral or semiprone position, unless contraindicated by the location of the intracranial lesion or surgery, is used to prevent obstruction of the pharynx by the relaxed lower jaw and tongue, and also to facilitate drainage of secretions. If secretions are a problem, it may be necessary to use gentle suction to avoid initiating the gag or cough reflex; the latter causes an elevation in intracranial pressure. Suction to the nose is not performed. Suction is limited to 15 seconds (see Chapter 16 for suction procedure). Hyperventilation of the lungs with 100% oxygen for 2–5 minutes before suction may be prescribed.

If the patient is sufficiently alert, he is cautioned not to cough and sneeze and is prompted to take several deep breaths at regular intervals (every 2 hours). Physiotherapy may be used to help mobilize secretions.

The administration of oxygen by mask or nasal cannulae may be indicated by the blood-gas analysis. If respiratory insufficiency develops due to weak ventilatory function, endotracheal intubation or a tracheostomy may be done and the patient supported by a mechanical ventilator (see Chapter 16). Hyperventilation and a lowered PCO_2 level is desirable to reduce cerebral vasodilation and promote cerebral venous return, reducing cerebral blood volume and intracranial pressure.

When oral fluids are permitted, only a very small amount is given at first to test the swallowing reflex to prevent choking, coughing and aspiration.

2. Potential for injury

Increased intracranial pressure. Planning and implementation of care must take into consideration the prevention of *further increase* in the intracranial pressure as well as the reduction of the existing increased intracranial pressure.

Positions and activities which raise the intracranial pressure are avoided. The head of the bed is usually elevated about 30°; the patient with potential or actual increased intracranial pressure is never placed in a head-low position but is positioned to prevent any impediment of cerebral venous return. The head is aligned with the spine; flexion and twisting of the head, anything tight around the neck that might compress the jugular veins and extreme hip flexion are avoided. When moving or changing position, the conscious patient is instructed not to push with his feet or push or pull with his arms and to breathe out through his mouth. The latter prevents the Valsalva manoeuvre which quickly raises the intracranial pressure.

The fluid intake is usually restricted to a stated volume distributed over 24 hours to maintain slight dehydration which reduces the extracellular volume and intracranial pressure. Intravenous fluids are infused slowly and must be closely monitored; rapid infusion could cause a serious, rapid rise in the intracranial pressure. A sign placed in a conspicuous place on the patient's bed alerts personnel and family to the fluid restriction.

An osmotic diuretic may be prescribed to dehydrate the brain; the drugs administered for this purpose are principally hyperosmolar solutions which are given intravenously. They promote the transfer of fluid from the brain tissue into the vascular compartment by osmosis and increase the urinary output. Solutions used include mannitol and, less commonly, urea and glucose (e.g. Ureaphil). The corticosteroid dexamethasone (Decadron) is commonly used to help reduce the intracranial pressure; the exact mechanism of the action is unclear. The patient receiving dexamethasone is observed for possible side-effects and complications since corticosteroids suppress the immune response, making the patient more susceptible to infection and also may cause gastrointestinal bleeding. An antacid (e.g. Maalox) or an antisecretory agent such as the H_2 receptor antagonist cimetidine (Tagamet) may be prescribed to protect the stomach and intestine.

Disorientation and impaired cognitive function. The patient's orientation, judgement, level of consciousness and mobility may change quickly. Protection from injury is necessary. Cot-sides are kept in position unless someone stays at the bedside with the patient. This applies for a considerable period of time even though the patient is conscious and oriented. Following an intracranial disorder and increased intracranial pressure, patients frequently are subject to spells of dizziness, lapses of orientation, or may be slow in regaining their postural reflexes.

Restlessness. This may be due to cerebral hypoxia or increasing elevation of the intracranial pressure but it should be kept in mind that restlessness may also be associated with retention of urine, pain, an uncomfortable position, the regaining of consciousness, or fear and concern about the situation. Restraints are not used. The cot-sides are padded for protection. Efforts are made to determine the cause if the patient is restless and to eliminate it if possible. If there are neurological symptoms and changes in vital signs that indicate a further increase in the intracranial pressure, they are reported promptly so that further treatment may be undertaken. If the restlessness occurs with the regaining of consciousness, the patient is reoriented to the situation; if the cause of the restlessness is thought to be the patient's anxiety, he is encouraged to express his concerns and receives explanations and reassurance.

Narcotics and strong sedation are not given to a patient with increased intracranial pressure; they mask neurological signs and depress respirations. Nursing measures such as position change, warm drink, and staying with the patient and encouraging expression of concerns may promote comfort and reduce restlessness. The environment should be quiet and the lighting subdued. In extreme restlessness a mild sedative may be prescribed to prevent exhaustion.

If the patient is extremely restless, the skin will require additional care. Friction areas are lightly oiled at frequent intervals and the elbows and heels may have to be padded for protection.

It should be remembered that the patient with reduced consciousness may be able to hear and comprehend although not able to respond; hearing is the last sensation to be lost. It is important that those caring for the patient continue to communicate with the patient and guard against inappropriate conversation. Verbal communication provides cerebral stimulation and information; it can be comforting and reassuring to the patient. Non-verbal communication by touch and presence is also reassuring to both patient and family. Family members are advised of the possibility of the patient hearing and are encouraged to communicate with the patient even though he is unresponsive.

Seizures. Compression of the brain associated with increased intracranial pressure may cause seizures which may be preceded by restlessness and twitching or may occur suddenly without warning. An anticonvulsant such as phenytoin sodium (Epanutin) may be prescribed and may be administered parenterally to prevent fits.

If a seizure occurs, pillows are removed and the patient turned on his side as soon as possible to prevent obstruction of the airway and to facilitate the drainage of oropharyngeal secretions. Only sufficient restraint to prevent injury is used. The patient is not left alone but someone is dispatched to notify the doctor. (For the observations to be made and patient care during a seizure see p. 806).

3. *Alteration in comfort*
The patient usually experiences headache with the onset of increased intracranial pressure which progressively becomes more severe as the intracranial pressure rises. A mild *non-narcotic* analgesic such as paracetamol may be prescribed. The patient may find that cold applications provide some relief. As the intracranial pressure increases and the patient loses consciousness pain perception diminishes. A quiet room, subdued lighting and a minimum of environmental stimuli are important. Jarring of the bed and sudden movements are avoided. The patient is turned and moved slowly and gently.

4. *Alteration in body temperature*
Compression of the temperature regulating centre by increased intracranial pressure may result in a marked elevation of the temperature and, at the same time, the normal physiological heat dissipating mechanisms are suppressed (dilation of superficial blood vessels and perspiration). The metabolic rate is increased in proportion to the fever; with a temperature of 40.5°C (105°F), there is an increase in metabolism of approximately 50%. Oxygen demands are increased and carbon dioxide production increases.

The room is kept at 18–20°C (65–68°F) and a light cotton sheet used to cover the patient. If the temperature is elevated, the sheet is arranged to cover only the lower half of the body. Tepid sponging may be ordered and an electric fan directed on the patient to help cool the body surface. Ice-packs may be placed over the axillae and groins. An antipyretic such as aspirin, administered by rectal suppository, may be prescribed. If these measures are not successful in controlling the temperature, a hypothermia blanket or mattress may be used. The patient should not be cooled too quickly; shivering must be prevented since it increases metabolism, oxygen consumption and the production of carbon dioxide and other metabolites which increase intracranial pressure.

5. *Alteration in cardiac function*
The compression and ischaemia caused by increased intracranial pressure may seriously affect the cardiac and vasomotor centres. Close monitoring of the pulse for irregularity and changes in the rate and volume is necessary. A decrease in cardiac output reduces cerebral perfusion to a greater degree, resulting in ischaemia, increased Pco_2 and vasodilation and an ensuing increase in the intracranial pressure. Changes in the pulse are brought promptly to the doctor's attention; continuous cardiac monitoring may be established and an antiarrhythmic drug prescribed if necessary. The excessive loss of

body fluid as a result of osmotic diuretic therapy may cause a reduction in intravascular volume and a corresponding reduction in cardiac output. Cardiac failure is more likely to occur if the patient has a pre-existing cardiac problem.

6. Potential for skin breakdown

Maintenance of skin integrity requires special attention because of the patient's immobility and possible restlessness and hyperthermia. The patient's position is changed from side to back (only if conscious) to side every 2 hours unless contraindicated by the location of the patient's intracranial lesion or surgery. For example, if a relatively large space-occupying lesion has been removed, the patient is not permitted to lie on the operative side to prevent a shifting of the brain into the remaining space.

When the patient is repositioned, he is turned slowly and gently. Bony prominences and pressure areas receive special attention to maintain skin integrity. The bedding must be kept dry and free of wrinkles. An alternating air pressure (ripple) mattress may be used and pieces of soft resilient material (synthetic sheepskin) are placed under vulnerable areas.

7. Potential fluid imbalance

As cited previously, the fluid intake and output are monitored very closely. A slight negative balance is considered desirable to reduce intracranial pressure; but, with a greater negative balance (i.e. greater output than intake), the intravascular volume is decreased resulting in a reduced cardiac output. Fluid intake is usually calculated each 8–12 hours according to the output; 400–500 ml are added to the output volume to cover insensible loss. Intravenous infusion is usually necessary owing to an inability to take sufficient fluid orally because of nausea, vomiting or coma.

8. Nutritional deficit

The headache, nausea, vomiting or loss of consciousness results in the patient's inability to take adequate food, which is reflected in changes in his strength and muscle mass. Nasogastric feeding may be given every 4 hours to provide necessary fluid and calories. If the patient is febrile, the increased metabolic rate requires more calories; if the caloric requirement is not met, the patient becomes seriously debilitated. The dietitian may be consulted in order to plan a suitable feeding regime.

9. Alteration in elimination

Bowel elimination. For the patient with a potential for, or with actual, increased intracranial pressure, bowel elimination is usually disregarded for 3 or 4 days. The absence of a bowel movement is related to immobility, reduced fluid and food intake and decreased awareness; also, the patient is discouraged from trying to have a movement since the effort involved raises intracranial pressure. A mild bulk laxative or stool softener may be given or a bisacodyl (Dulcolax) suppository may be used. The unconscious patient may be incontinent; prompt cleansing of the patient and changing of the bed are essential. The conscious patient is cautioned against straining at stool. It may be necessary to examine the patient for faecal impaction if he has had no bowel movement for several days.

Urinary elimination. If the patient is unresponsive, incontinence is a problem, making a retention catheter and a closed drainage system (i.e. not open to the air) necessary so that an accurate assessment can be made of the output, as well as to maintain skin integrity. The output is noted every 1–2 hours to evaluate the effectiveness of the osmotic diuretic.

The fluid intake and output are monitored for oliguria and water retention or an excessive volume of urine with a low specific gravity. The retention or excessive output may develop as a result of a disturbance in the secretion of ADH by the posterior pituitary lobe. An increase in ADH incurs a decreased urinary output while a deficiency of ADH causes large volumes of urine to be excreted necessitating the administration of vasopressin (Pitressin).

The urinary output is also a good indicator of the patient's cardiac and circulatory status and his ability to maintain renal perfusion. There is concern if the output per hour is less than 20 ml.

When a urinary catheter is retained, the patient is at risk of infection and cystitis. Catheter care seems to vary from one unit to another. The area around the meatus is cleansed every 4 hours with an antiseptic solution or soap and water. The doctor may order irrigation of the bladder twice daily. Strict asepsis is observed when irrigating or changing the tubing and receptacle. The urine is observed for cloudiness, sediment and offensive odour. A specimen of urine is obtained at least every other day for culture so that infection may be detected and prompt treatment instituted. The catheter is removed as soon as possible.

10. Self-care deficit

The reduced level of awareness or loss of consciousness and the motor and sensory changes that occur with increased intracranial pressure result in self-care deficits. The nurse provides the personal care that the patient would normally carry out himself such as bathing, cleaning of teeth and mouth, combing of the hair and feeding. Nursing care (e.g. bathing, suction, mouth care, eye care and position change) should be carried out with undisturbed intervals between them. Clustering of activities in a short period of time results in a cumulative increase in intracranial pressure. If the eye reflexes are absent, the eyes may be irrigated with sterile normal saline and hypromellose drops (artificial tears) instilled 3 or

4 times daily to keep the surface of the eye clean and moist. If one or both eyes remain open a protective shield is applied.

If permitted, the limbs are moved slowly and gently through their range of motion to preserve joint movements.

11. Lack of knowledge

If the patient is sufficiently alert, he will be concerned about his condition; the frequent neurological assessment and recording of vital signs and fear of loss of body functions and independence arouse considerable anxiety which increases intracranial pressure. Procedures are explained and the patient is advised that everything possible is being done. Anxious relatives also require reassurance; they are informed from time to time of the patient's progress and what is being done. They should receive accurate information without unfounded reassurance.

EXPECTED OUTCOMES

1 The intracranial pressure has decreased to a safe level; this is indicated by:
    (a) Improved neurological status; more responsive, eye reflexes normal, continence.
    (b) Vital functions within normal limits.
    (c) Absence of headache.
    (d) Orientation to time, place and person.
    (e) Increasing interest in condition, environment and self-care.
2 The patient takes and retains adequate fluid and sufficient calories.
3 The patient's skin is intact.
4 Seizures are absent.
5 The patient is more relaxed and less anxious. He indicates understanding and acceptance of explanation of procedures and progress.

BARBITURATE THERAPY

This is a relatively new form of treatment for increased intracranial pressure. Its use is controversial and is not widely used at present in the United Kingdom. It involves the administration of large doses of a barbiturate such as pentobarbitone sodium (Nembutal) which rapidly induces coma.

Prior to the administration of the drug, the patient is intubated and placed on a mechanical ventilator. An intracranial monitoring device (see p. 807) and a central venous line (see Chapter 14) are in place and other emergency support devices readily available.

The mechanism by which this form of treatment reduces intracranial pressure is unclear; it is thought that the barbiturate has a constrictive effect on cerebral vessels, reducing the pressure and at the same time diverting blood from well-perfused areas to ischaemic areas. It is also suggested that barbiturate coma reduces brain metabolism and the oxygen demand, allowing the cells to rest in a dormant state.

VENTRICULAR DRAINAGE IN INCREASED INTRACRANIAL PRESSURE

A ventricular puncture may be done and a tube inserted into a ventricle to establish drainage of CSF to lower the intracranial pressure. Externally, the tube is attached to a sterile closed system. The level at which the tubing and bag are placed is prescribed by the doctor. The bed is usually kept flat unless otherwise indicated by the doctor. The rate of drainage is monitored very closely; too rapid drainage is to be avoided and blockage of the tube is to be reported promptly. Strict asepsis must be observed in handling the tubes and the dressing at the burr hole. The patient may be given an antibiotic as a prophylactic measure. If the patient complains of severe headache or a neurological disturbance (e.g. disturbed vision) develops that was not experienced before the ventricular puncture, the doctor is notified.

INDUCED HYPOTHERMIA IN INCREASED INTRACRANIAL PRESSURE

The use of a deliberate lowering of the patient's temperature to below the normal body temperature to reduce intracranial pressure is controversial. The rationale for this treatment is that with the decreased body temperature, brain activity decreases and the cells can survive longer periods with reduced amounts of oxygen and nutrients than would otherwise be possible. In addition, there is a reduction in the metabolic by-products carbon dioxide and lactic acid, both of which are potent cerebral vasodilators.

Hypothermia may be achieved by using a hypothermia blanket or mattress or by packing the patient in ice (see Chapter 7 for the procedure).

Nursing the patient treated by intracranial surgery

PREOPERATIVE PHASE

Assessment

If the preoperative period extends over several days, the patient is observed for possible neurological changes from day to day which may indicate a worsening of his condition. The vital signs are followed closely; pupils are checked regularly for size, equality and reaction to light, and the patient's alertness, orientation, sensory perception, motor ability and strength of limbs are noted.

Vital signs and neurological observations are recorded to provide a base-line for measuring progress in the postoperative period.

Identification of patient problems

1 Anxiety related to the surgery and the outcome
2 Lack of knowledge related to the operation, and pre- and postoperative events
3 Potential for infection secondary to interruption of the integrity of the scalp and cranium

4 Potential nutritional deficit related to decreased food intake as a result of condition (tumour, aneurysm, abscess, injury)

5 Fluid deficit secondary to inadequate intake, restricted intake or the administration of an osmotic diuretic because of increased intracranial pressure

6 Potential increased intracranial pressure

7 Potential for respiratory depression and thrombophlebitis

8 Embarrassment and concern related to the shaving of the head

The *goals* are to:

1 Have the patient and family informed as to the reason for the operation

2 Provide an insight into preoperative and anticipated operative and postoperative events and to promote acceptance of the situation with less anxiety

3 Have the patient physically and psychologically prepared for the surgery

Nursing intervention

1. Anxiety. Any impending surgery is perceived as a threat to the person and generates anxiety, but that involving the brain is even more threatening. The alert patient and the family are usually very fearful of a fatal outcome or permanent changes, disability and a loss of intellect and competence. Expression of doubts and concerns is encouraged; time and opportunities for questions and answers are provided. The patient is not left alone for long periods; contact with others interrupts concentration on the operation and provides the opportunity to express his fears. Visits are limited to family members and friends who can control their anxiety and show a quiet, reassuring presence with the patient. If necessary, the services of a chaplain or other appropriate personnel (e.g. clinical nurse specialist) may be called on for additional reassurance.

2. Inadequate knowledge. It is the doctor's responsibility to inform the patient and the family initially of the need for the surgery, the nature of the procedure, risks and possible outcome. The nurse should be familiar with what they have been told so she can amend knowledge deficits, answer questions, clarify misconceptions and refer special problems that are revealed to the doctor.

Preoperative preparation and anticipated intraoperative and postoperative events are explained.

The family is advised that the patient may have temporary oedema and discoloration of the face and eyes and possible neurological deficits such as facial paralysis and aphasia after the operation.

3. Potential for infection. Because of surgical interruption of the integrity of the scalp and cranium, the head must be cleansed and prepared to minimize the possibility of infection. Unless it is an emergency, the hair is washed the day before the operation and the required area of the head shaved with an electric razor a few hours before the surgery, leaving, if possible, some hair to cover the scar. In some instances, the entire head is shaved to provide adequate and safe exposure. Any rash, infection or abrasion of the scalp is brought to the surgeon's attention.

4. Nutritional deficit. If the patient has not been able to take adequate nourishment because of his condition (e.g. semicomatose, pain, vomiting, anxiety), supplements may be administered to restore electrolyte balance and improve his nutritional status. No solid food is given orally within the 6 hours preceding the surgery.

5. Fluid deficit. Usually, there is concern if a preoperative patient manifests dehydration and efforts are made to re-establish normal tissue hydration. A fluid deficit in the patient who is to have intracranial surgery may be an important therapeutic measure. A restricted fluid intake may be necessary to control intracranial pressure or he may have received an osmotic diuretic such as mannitol to reduce increased intracranial pressure.

No attempt is made to increase the fluid intake without a specific directive. The patient may have water up to 4 or 5 hours before the operation unless otherwise indicated.

6. Potential for increased intracranial pressure. Frequent assessment of neurological and vital signs is made during the preoperative period to detect early signs of increasing intracranial pressure (see p. 807). The patient does not receive the usual preoperative cleansing enema. A mild laxative may be prescribed 2 days before the surgery if necessary. The patient is cautioned not to strain when defecating. An enema is usually contraindicated because of the risk of increasing intracranial pressure with straining at stool.

7. Potential for respiratory and circulatory complications. The patient is encouraged to remain ambulatory during the preoperative phase if his condition permits. If his intracranial lesion is such that his balance and mobility are impaired, safety precautions are taken to prevent falls and injury.

The patient with swelling or oedema of the brain and increased intracranial pressure is predisposed to circulatory and ventilatory depression. For this reason the patient does not receive the usual preoperative sedative. Atropine sulphate may be prescribed to reduce tracheobronchial secretions during the inhalation anaesthesia. It also reduces the vagal influence on the heart (i.e. slowing of the heart) incurred by the operative procedure.

If lengthy surgery is anticipated (more than 2 hours), anti-emboli support stockings may be applied to the lower limbs to promote venous return and the prevention of thrombus formation.

A urinary catheter may be inserted so that the output may be monitored during surgery as a reflection of the person's circulatory status. Normally, the renal output is approximately 60 ml per hour. Less than 20 ml per hour indicates a serious reduction in perfusion of the kidneys.

8. Embarrassment and concern relating to loss of hair. Cutting of the hair and shaving of the head can be quite disturbing to the patient and his family since it alters his appearance. Before starting the procedure, an explanation is made as to why it is necessary. Suggestions are made about the wearing of a scarf, turban or hairpiece until the hair grows again.

Common intracranial surgical procedures
Intracranial surgery necessitates an opening in the skull. The size and location of the opening depend upon the nature and site of the lesion and the amount of exposure needed for the operation. If the lesion is in the cerebrum, it is referred to as being *supratentorial* and the incision is well above the hairline. If it is in the cerebellar or brain stem regions, it is designated as *infratentorial* and the incision is usually in the occipital region.

The surgical procedures include:
- *Burr hole.* This is a small circular opening into the cranium made with a bone drill. The purpose may be to obtain tissue for a biopsy, aspirate CSF from a ventricle, or relieve pressure caused by swelling and oedema of the brain or a tumour.
- *Craniotomy.* In this procedure a scalp incision and two or more burr holes are made over the area to be explored. The bone between the burr holes is incised allowing elevation of a *bone flap* to provide access to the brain. The opening is curved so the scalp and bone flap can be folded back to expose the affected brain area.
- *Craniectomy.* This involves excision of a portion of the skull and may vary from a small burr hole to a sizeable area of several centimetres. The craniectomy may be done to remove shattered bone or to relieve pressure by expanding cranial contents.
- *Cranioplasty.* This is a replacement of a section of the cranium with a synthetic material such as titanium to re-establish the contour and integrity of the skull. In some instances, the bone flap that was initially separated from the skull is replaced; this is referred to as an *osteoplastic craniotomy*.

POSTOPERATIVE PHASE

Immediately following intracranial surgery the patient may be transferred to a recovery room, a surgical intensive care unit or a neurosurgical observation area according to his needs and the facilities which are available. In preparation for receiving the patient, the full range of support equipment for neurosurgical emergencies must be available. This includes: emergency drugs and intravenous solutions, oxygen and suction, tracheostomy tray and lumbar puncture tray. In some instances, a ventilator may need to be available. The frame at the head of the bed should be low or removed, if possible, so that the patient's head is readily accessible.

Since all patients suffer some elevation of pressure inside the cranium following brain surgery, the nursing care described for increased intracranial pressure on p. 807 as well as the care of the unconscious patient (see Chapter 10) are applicable in the postoperative phase.

Assessment
Vital signs and neurological status are determined when the patient is returned from the operating room against which progress can be assessed. The blood pressure, pulse, respirations and temperature are recorded and pupillary size, equality and reaction and level of consciousness noted. The chest is auscultated at regular intervals for air entry and the accumulation of secretions. A blood specimen may be taken for determination of blood-gas concentrations; the frequency of this analysis is determined by the reports. If the patient is conscious, his alertness, orientation, speech and ability to move his limbs are checked. The required frequency of these observations may be indicated by the neurosurgeon but usually begins with 15–30 minute intervals which are gradually lengthened to 1 hour then 4 hours if the evaluations indicate stability.

Evaluation of the patient's status includes observations for involuntary movements (twitching, tremor, seizure), restlessness, rigidity and posturing (decerebrate rigidity or decorticate rigidity—see p. 807). The colour and condition of the skin (moist or dry, temperature and integrity) and fluid balance are also noted.

The head dressing is examined for security, for moistness suggesting leakage of CSF and for evidence of bleeding. There may be a drain attached to a gentle negative-pressure system.

Identification of patient problems
Following intracranial surgery, much of the care cited for the patient with increased intracranial pressure (p. 807) and for the unconscious patient (Chapter 10) is applicable. Consideration is also given to the following problems:
1 The potential for further increased intracranial pressure due to the reaction to the trauma imposed by the surgery
2 Alteration in tissue perfusion (shock) secondary to loss of blood or body fluid or to cardiac failure
3 Potential for injury (risk of injury due to malpositioning or disorientation)

4 Potential for infection due to open wound and lowered resistance
5 Self-care deficits
6 Hyperthermia secondary to the disturbance of the temperature-regulating centre.
7 Lack of knowledge. The patient and family require assistance in making necessary adjustments and planning home management

Nursing intervention

1. Potential for Increased Intracranial Pressure. All patients experience some elevation of intracranial pressure following brain surgery due to the oedema and swelling resulting from the trauma and inflammation incurred by surgery. (See p. 806 for a discussion of increased intracranial pressure.) Frequent vital signs and neurological evaluations are necessary to recognize significant changes indicating increased intracranial pressure (see Table 22.8).

The head of the bed may be elevated about 30° to promote cerebral venous return unless contraindicated by shock or a specific directive from the surgeon. A small pillow may be necessary under the head to maintain good neck alignment which promotes cerebral venous return. Following infratentorial surgery (cerebellum or brain stem) the bed is generally kept flat for 2–3 days to prevent pressure on the brain stem and its vital centres.

The fluid intake is usually restricted to a stated volume distributed over 24 hours to maintain slight dehydration which reduces extracellular fluid and intracranial pressure. Intravenous fluids are infused slowly and closely monitored; rapid infusion could cause a rapid rise in intracranial pressure. A sign placed conspicuously on the patient's bed will alert personnel and family to the fluid restriction.

An osmotic diuretic may be prescribed to dehydrate the brain. The drugs administered are principally hypertonic solutions.

2. Alteration in tissue perfusion (shock). Deficient tissue perfusion may develop as a result of haemorrhage, excessive loss of body fluid or cardiac failure; the latter is more likely to occur if there was a pre-existing heart problem. The excessive loss of body fluid, resulting in reduced intravascular volume may be associated with osmotic diuretic therapy.

The manifestations include rapid thready pulse, fall in blood pressure, restlessness, change in level of consciousness, and pale, cold clammy skin. The respirations may be increased or remain normal in the early stage but if the shock is not reversed, respiratory depression develops.

3. Potential for injury. Following intracranial surgery, the patient is at risk of injury from malpositioning. The required position depends on the patient's level of consciousness and the location and nature of the surgery.

While unconscious he is positioned to promote cerebral venous return as well as to prevent obstruction of the airway and aspiration of secretions. The limbs are positioned and supported as described for the unconscious patient in Chapter 10. The head of the bed may be elevated 25–30° and the head aligned with the spine. The patient with potential or actual increase in intracranial pressure is never placed in a head-low or prone position. Flexion or twisting of the head and extreme hip flexion are voided.

If a relatively large space-occupying lesion has been removed, the patient is not permitted to lie on the operative side in order to prevent a shifting of the brain into the remaining space. Following infratentorial surgery, the patient lies on either side using a small pillow under the head to maintain alignment. Keeping the patient off his back for 2–3 days prevents pressure on the incision as well as possible forward flexion on the incision. A specific directive as to positioning may be given by the surgeon.

The position is changed at regular intervals (e.g. every 2 hours) from side to side to back to side unless contraindicated. When the patient is repositioned, he is turned slowly with adequate support for the head, so that it and the trunk are turned as if they were one unit. Sudden movement and jarring are avoided at all times. Bony prominences and pressure areas are inspected and receive care each time the patient is turned.

Trauma to the brain stem may depress the gag and swallowing reflexes predisposing to aspiration. When oral fluids are permitted, only a very small amount is given at first to test the swallowing reflex.

4. Potential for infection. Following intracranial surgery the risk of infection arises from the open wound, from the patient's lowered resistance as a result of the illness and its related stresses and from the possible administration of a steroid preparation (e.g. dexamethasone). Since infectious processes increase metabolism, waste products such as carbon dioxide and lactic acid are produced in greater amounts. Waste products in increased amounts cause cerebral vasodilation which increases intracranial blood volume and pressure. Strict asepsis is essential when the head dressing is changed. The wound is inspected for redness, swelling, offensive odour and drainage; signs of infection are reported promptly and a swab of the wound drainage is taken for culture purposes. Immediate treatment to prevent meningitis, encephalitis or brain abscess is essential; an antibiotic is prescribed.

5. Self-care deficits. Following intracranial surgery, the patient is dependent upon the nurse for complete care (bathing, repositioning, toileting, feeding) for a few days. As soon as he is well enough, the patient is encouraged to perform self-care activities. The patient may be lethargic and require prompting to resume activity. He may show no interest in appearance and need urging to improve his grooming and to dress when he is well enough to be up most of the day. The female patient, particularly, may be very self-conscious about the loss of her hair. She is encouraged to use a turban, headscarf or wig.

6. *Hyperthermia*. The patient may develop an elevation of temperature. To counteract this tendency, the room temperature is kept at 18–20°C (65–68°F) and only a cotton sheet and bedspread are used as covers. If hyperthermia develops, a sheet is arranged to cover only the lower half of the body. An antipyretic (e.g. acetylsalicylic acid) is prescribed and administered by rectum. If the temperature continues to rise, tepid sponging is given and an electric fan is directed on the patient.

7. *Lack of knowledge*. In some instances, there may be some residual neurological deficit following some intracranial surgical procedures. A rehabilitation programme is planned and instituted as soon as possible with the goal of restoring the patient to independent useful living within his potential. This may involve the physiotherapist, speech therapist, occupational therapist and social worker as well as the doctor and nurse. The patient may have to relearn the performance of ordinary daily activities and progress from the simple to the more complex much as a child learns. It is frequently a slow process and both the patient and family are likely to have periods of depression and discouragement. The nurse assists them in making their plans for home management and the necessary activities and exercises. A referral is made to appropriate support services so that support and guidance are continued.

Expected outcomes
1 The patient is alert and has resumed self-care activities.
2 The surgical wound has healed and is free of infection.
3 Vital signs are normal.
4 The patient participates willingly in the prescribed exercise programme.
5 The patient and family make informed decisions about home management.

SPINE AND SPINAL CORD INJURY

Spinal cord injury is a major cause of serious disability, particularly in males between the ages of 15–30 years. The incidence of spinal injury associated with a fractured spine is 500–600 per annum in Great Britain.[2] Motor vehicle accidents continue to be a major cause of spinal injuries and frequently alcohol and drugs are involved. The nurse has a unique

opportunity to identify people, especially children, at risk of maladaptive or violent behaviours and to initiate the process of channelling aggressiveness into satisfying but safe activities.

TYPES OF INJURIES

A spinal injury may or may not involve injury to the cord. Fracture of one or more vertebrae may occur and with no displacement of fragments, the cord may not be affected. Spinal cord injury is most commonly associated with the fracture of one or more vertebrae in which one or more fragments compress or penetrate the cord. The fracture may be the result of: (1) sudden forceful angulation of the spine (hyperextension, hyperflexion, or hyperextension–hyperflexion); (2) excessive force applied along the axis of the spine causing shattering fractures and vertical compression (e.g. landing on the feet or buttocks from a height); (3) a direct blow to an area of the spine; or (4) the tearing of supporting ligaments resulting in rotation or displacement of the vertebrae with the cord being trapped between two displaced spinal segments or fracture fragments.

EFFECTS OF SPINAL INJURIES

Injuries to the vertebrae may result in spinal cord contusion, laceration and compression. Bleeding into the tissues and oedema occur, causing swelling and compression of nerve tracts. The damage may be slight and completely reversible or it may leave a minor degree of residual impairment. Oedema and bleeding in the cervical cord area is very serious; compression may interrupt innervation of the diaphragm incurring respiratory failure. A laceration which transects the cord or causes severe compression may result in complete, irreversible interruption of ascending or descending tracts. Destruction of the cord resulting in interruption of its tracts is not always due to transection. Injury may incur haemorrhage, circulatory stasis, extravasation of fluid and blood cells, ischaemia and necrosis of the tissue. Interruption of ascending tracts causes loss of sensation below the site of injury. This means that pain, pressure and temperature sensation may be dulled or lost and the patient may be unable to appreciate the position of affected limbs due to interference with proprioception impulse pathways. Interruption of descending tracts results in paralysis of the parts deriving their innervation from the cord below the level of the lesion. Flaccid paralysis and an absence of reflexes occur first and are usually followed by spastic paralysis and exaggerated tendon reflexes. Bladder, bowel and autonomic nervous functions are disturbed.

When the spinal cord is suddenly transected, a phenomenon known as *spinal shock* develops in which all cord functions including involuntary reflex

[2] Bromley (1981).

responses are depressed; there is the sudden loss of all motor, sensory, reflex and autonomic responses below the site of cord injury. This occurs due to the sudden interruption of the initiative and regulatory impulses between the higher centres and the cord below the site of injury; that is, impulses are no longer being passed to or from neurons below the lesion. The result is loss of muscular tone (flaccid paralysis), an absence of reflexes and loss of sensation below the lesion. Cord reflexes for voiding and defecation are suppressed and retention and overflow incontinence occur. Vasomotor tone is lost and the blood pressure falls. Body temperature control is affected since there is no perspiration below the lesion; hyperthermia may develop. Spinal shock may subside in a few days or may persist for a much longer period. The loss of autonomic impulses and tone in the intestine may cause distension and paralytic ileus (see Chapter 17). Occasionally, recovery of reflex activity following spinal shock is characterized by hypersensitivity of the spinal neurons; for example, spasticity of the muscles develops and the bladder becomes hypertonic resulting in diminished capacity and frequent reflex voiding.

The victim with injury to the spine without cord involvement retains motor and sensory functions and complains of pain at the site of the trauma and in parts innervated by that area. Later this may change; bleeding into the tissue and oedema may occur causing swelling and compression of the cord. *Initial management of spine-injured patients is on the basis of potential cord damage.*

The spinal cord and its tracts are not capable of regeneration but regeneration of the nerve roots (outside of the cord) can occur if the neurilemma is not severely damaged (see p. 768). Some recovery of function may occur in the first few weeks as oedema subsides and neurons, which were compressed but not destroyed, resume activity. However, recent work on spinal cord reconstruction, by a number of neurosurgeons, has been encouraging (see reference section).

The paralysis which occurs with spinal cord injury may be complete or partial (paresis) and may be paraplegia or quadriplegia. *Paraplegia* refers to paralysis of the lower limbs, which may include the lower part of the trunk and loss of the bladder and rectal control. *Quadriplegia or tetraplegia* means paralysis of the lower extremities and trunk and varying degrees of paralysis of the upper extremities depending upon the level of injury. If quadriplegia is complete there may be no voluntary control of function below the neck and very little potential for independence in self-care. With incomplete quadriplegia, voluntary control of selected muscles in the upper limbs may be restored and independence in many areas of self-care may be possible. Respiratory insufficiency or failure is a major concern in quadriplegia since there is usually some involvement of the nerve supply to the diaphragm and intercostal muscles.

MANIFESTATIONS OF SPINAL CORD INJURY

As cited previously these depend on the level and degree of damage.

1 *Respiratory insufficiency.* Those with injury at cervical level are particularly at risk of respiratory failure, since the phrenic nerves which innervate the diaphragm pass through the third, fourth and fifth cervical segments of the spinal cord. Intercostal muscle innervation is derived from the thoracic region of the cord. Injury above this level of the cord leaves the patient totally dependent upon diaphragmatic respirations.

2 *Loss of motor function.* The paralysis may be complete or partial (paresis).
   (a) Paraplegia, which implies paralysis of the lower limbs, may include the lower part of the trunk with loss of bladder and bowel control.
   (b) Quadriplegia (tetraplegia), which implies paralysis of the lower extremities and trunk and varying degrees of paralysis of the upper extremities (complete or partial) depending on the level of cervical injury.

3 *Hypotension.* There is a loss of vasomotor function in the affected parts resulting in vasodilation and a fall in blood pressure—owing to dysfunction of the sympathetic chain.

4 *Loss of sensory function.* Pain, temperature, pressure and proprioception sensations are absent below the level of cord injury (in areas corresponding to those paralysed). The patient may experience some pain at the site of injury in the acute phase.

5 *Flaccidity of muscles.* There is a complete loss of muscle tone during the early stage. Later, this is replaced by spasticity.

6 *Absence of reflexes.* The areflexia is usually followed by hyperexcitability of the spinal neurons initiating the reflex responses.

7 *Distended urinary bladder.* The detrusor muscle becomes atonic and the sensation of 'the need to void' is absent. Retention of urine with overflow develops.

8 *Loss of gastrointestinal tone.* Vomiting and abdominal distension may develop due to cessation of peristalsis. If prolonged, paralytic ileus develop.

CARE OF PATIENT WITH SPINAL INJURY

Care of the spine-injured patient involves three phases—namely, the emergency, acute and rehabilitative phases.

Emergency intervention

Spinal cord injury and permanent disability may be minimized with accurate assessment and appropriate care immediately following the accident. Injury to the spinal cord is suspected if the victim is unable to move his limbs, if numbness or peculiar sensations are present, or if there is unexplained shock. The victim may also be having difficulty breathing if the injury is cervical. Wounds about the head or shoulders, pain, tenderness or deformity adjacent to the vertebral column or unconsciousness following injury also suggest spinal cord injury. If there is doubt regarding the presence of cord injury, the patient should be managed as if one were present.

Usually the spinal cord injured victim is conscious. He should be kept flat to permit free diaphragmatic breathing and he should be advised to keep his head still; neck flexion or side to side rotation could seriously aggravate an injured cervical spine. A quick assessment is made for other injuries and the more immediate emergencies of respiratory insufficiency and bleeding. Airway obstruction and inadequate ventilation have first priority but in establishing an airway or in providing assistance, extension of the neck must be avoided. If the patient is unconscious, the modified jaw thrust may be used to open the airway; two fingers are placed at the angle of the lower jaw to lift it forward. With cervical cord injury, the chest wall muscles may be paralysed and entire respiratory function is dependent on the diaphragm; respiratory assistance and suctioning may be necessary.

A firm flat stretcher is used on which to transport the victim; he must be moved as a rigid single unit; even slight flexion, extension or twisting of the spine may cause irreversible cord damage. All movements should be smooth and well coordinated. Immobilization of the head and neck are essential before the victim is moved. A firm cervical collar or sand bags taped to each side of the head may be used if available. Gentle manual traction may be applied to the head to stabilize it if satisfactory equipment is not available. In some instances it may be advisable to await the arrival of qualified emergency personnel before attempting to move the victim.

Care during acute phase

ASSESSMENT

1 A brief history of the accident is obtained from the victim or person who was at the site.
2 An immediate assessment is made of the vital signs and continuous monitoring established if necessary.
3 If the client's condition permits, or a family member is available, a brief review is made of his health history so that significant factors such as allergies, pre-existing disorders and medications being taken are identified.
4 The patient is examined for injuries and a neurological evaluation is made to identify spinal cord damage. An assessment is made of:
(a) Level of consciousness

(b) Orientation
(c) Motor and sensory functions (e.g. movement of the limbs; levels of sensation)
(d) Reflexes (e.g. patellar, abdominal)
(e) Condition of the skin: cold or warm, moist or dry all over or above or below a certain level.
5 The spine is x-rayed to identify vertebral fractures and dislocation and their level.
6 Blood-gas analyses are made to determine the need for respiratory assistance and the administration of oxygen.
7 A data base is established from the initial assessment for comparison with the *on-going assessments*. Frequent evaluation (15–60 minutes depending on condition) is necessary; the patient's systemic and neurological status may change rapidly in the first 24–48 hours due to bleeding and/or increasing oedema at the site of the injury. Repeated assessments are essential to detect the development of further cord compression and involve:
(a) The recording of vital signs
(b) Evaluation of respiratory function by chest auscultation for air entry and the presence of secretions, tidal volume and vital capacity determinations and serial arterial blood-gases analyses. Diaphragmatic activity may be assessed by asking the patient to sniff
(c) Inspection and percussion of the abdomen for gastrointestinal distension and listening with a stethoscope for bowel sounds
(d) Observation for the level of awareness
(e) Observation for changes in motor and sensory functions: the level of loss of sensation is noted. Changes in such as motor function and strength, level of sensation, evidence of respiratory insufficiency or distress, fall in blood pressure and weakening of the pulse, reduced awareness and vomiting and abdominal distension must be reported promptly to the doctor.

MEDICAL MANAGEMENT

The treatment of the spine-injured patient depends on:
• Whether there is cord injury and neurological deficits or not
• The level of the injury
• The nature of the injury (e.g. fracture fragments compressing the cord, laceration of the cord)

Immediate efforts are directed towards sustaining life and preventing cord damage or, where it has occurred, preventing further injury. The spinal lesion is treated by immobilization of the spine. Realignment of vertebrae and relief of pressure on the cord or spinal roots may be achieved by traction. In some instances surgery (decompresion laminectomy) is undertaken to relieve pressure on the cord, remove vertebral fragments which are hazardous to the cord or to realign dislocated vertebrae which do not respond to traction or hyperextension. The surgery may include spinal fusion (see Table 22.9) or wiring of the spinous processes to stabilize the spine.

Cervical spine injury
If there is no neurological deficit or fracture-dislocation, a cervical collar may be applied. When there is a fracture-dislocation with or without neuro-logical deficit, skeletal traction is applied by means of Crutchfield tongs, a halo traction device or a halter.

Tongs are inserted into the skull at approximately the midlateral line, a short distance above the ears. The areas are prepared for the insertion by shaving, cleansing and the injection of a local anaesthetic. A very small incision is made in the scalp and small holes made in the skull with a drill to accommodate the tongs. The scalp may require sutures before a dressing is applied. The sites of insertion of the tongs are inspected daily for signs of infection, the areas are cleansed with an antiseptic and fresh sterile dressings are applied. Traction of 4.5–13.2 kg (10–40 lb) may be applied and is achieved by a rope that overlies a pulley; one end is affixed to the tongs and the other hangs free with the prescribed weight attached. The prescribed weight depends on the size of the patient and the amount of displacement. It is usually moderate at first and increased as indicated by x-ray or manifestations; that is, realignment of the vertebrae or fragments is not occurring the weight is increased.

The patient may be placed on a turning bed (e.g. Egerton–Stoke Mandeville electrical turning and tilt-ing bed) which is fitted with a pivoting device; this permits turning without interference to the traction. An ordinary bed with a fracture board, if necessary, beneath the mattress and the head board removed to allow clearance for traction may be used. The head of the bed is elevated to enable the body to act as counteraction for the weights and prevent the patient sliding toward the head of the bed. When realignment of the vertebrae or fragments and suffi-cient healing are achieved, the patient is fitted with a plastic collar or neck brace to provide cervical immo-bilization and support and is gradually ambulated.

The *halo traction device* involves the application of a metal ring to the head which is secured to the skull by the insertion of four pins (similar to the application of tongs). The sites of insertion into the skull are anter-ior, posterior and lateral. The ring is firmly anchored to a body cast or special vest by metal rods. This form of cervical immobilization and traction allows the patient to be ambulatory (Fig. 22.25).

If only slight traction is required, a halter-like arrangement may be used in place of the tongs. The halter is arranged to place traction under the chin and occipital area. Prolonged continuous application usually causes considerable discomfort and skin irritation for the patient by the pressure and pull, especially under the chin.

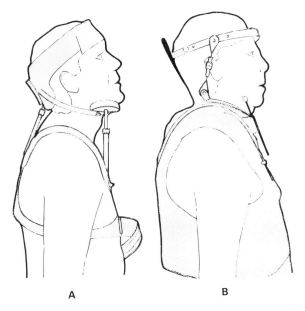

A   **B**

Fig. 22.25 Halo traction (used in cervical vertebral fracture). *A*, Four poster brace. *B*, Halo jacket.

Thoracic or lumbar spinal fracture
Where there is a fracture of the spine in the thoracic or lumbar region without dislocation and compres-sion of the spinal cord the patient may be placed flat on a firm mattress on a bed with a firm base, or on a fracture board on an ordinary bed, or on a turning bed for several weeks. If the ordinary bed is used, specific directions are received as to whether the patient must remain on his back at all times. If turning is permitted, precautions are taken to ensure good alignment and avoidance of movement and displacement of the framents ('log-rolling'). When there is sufficient healing, the patient is gradually ambulated. A brace, plaster jacket or firm corset may be necessary for several months to provide support and immobility of the spine.

A *fracture dislocation* of thoracic or lumbar vertebrae may be treated by hyperextension of the spine which may be achieved by various methods. One method is the placing of a firm roll or sandbag across the bed under the mattress to provide the required angu-lation. Fracture boards are placed on the bed if it has a sprung base, and a very firm mattress is used on which a sponge rubber mattress is placed, since the patient must remain in the supine position.

In some instances a plaster cast is used to immobi-lize the spine following a fracture in the thoracic or lumbar region. It usually extends from the shoulders to below the hips. An opening may be cut in the cast over the abdomen to prevent pressure and discom-fort in that area. The cast edges are bound by the stockinette, which is under the cast, being turned back and secured with adhesive. The skin areas at the borders of the cast are examined daily for possible irritation. The cast is cut back over the buttocks sufficiently to accommodate the use of the bedpan without soiling of the cast. Extra precautions are taken to protect it by the use of pieces of waterproof material such as plastic.

THE PATIENT WITH SPINAL INJURY *WITHOUT* CORD INVOLVEMENT

Identification of patient problems
1 Potential for spinal cord injury secondary to vertebral fracture fragments and spinal instability
2 Potential for complications secondary to immobility:
   (a) Ineffective airway clearance
   (b) Pressure sores
   (c) Ankylosis and muscle atrophy and contractures
   (d) Hypercalcaemia: urinary tract calculi
   (e) Infection
3 Alteration in comfort due to some pressure on spinal nerves
4 Alteration in nutritional requirements
5 Alteration in bowel elimination due to immobility
6 Altered self-image and anxiety
7 Self-care deficits due to immobility and traction
8 Lack of knowledge about management following hospitalization.

The *goals* are to:
1 Prevent spinal cord and nerve damage
2 Promote alignment and healing of vertebral fracture
3 Prevent complications
4 Regain mobility and independence

Nursing intervention

1. Potential for spinal cord injury. The potential for cord injury is present as long as the spine is unstable. Frequent systematic assessment for possible cord compression becomes an important nursing aspect (see pp. 817 and 821). The vertebrae must be *aligned* and *immobilized* until sufficient healing takes place to stabilize the spine.

If it is a cervical lesion and tongs with traction are used to reduce dislocation and immobilize the spine, the equipment is inspected several times daily to make sure the tongs are in position, that the equipment is secure and that the rope and prescribed weight hang free. *Traction must be maintained continuously.*

The patient with a spinal fracture is usually cared for on a turning bed (e.g. Egerton–Stoke Mandeville, Stryker or circoelectric bed) which facilitates turning the patient from the supine to prone position and vice versa with minimal risk of movement of the vertebrae. It also reduces the discomfort and strain for the patient in the process. A turning frame allows for more frequent turning to protect the skin and also facilitates the use of a bedpan without raising the patient. The turning bed cannot be used if hyperextention is required to treat a fracture of the spine. Patients have reported intense fear of falling off the frame during the turning. The importance of maintaining spinal alignment and immobility, the purpose of the particular frame and the turning process is fully explained to the patient and family. A small pillow may be used to fill in space between the patient and the frame for support. Unnecessary exposure is avoided; the pubic area is covered with a towel or draw sheet that can be easily removed after turning. Straps are secured tightly around the frames so that the patient feels supported and secure. When the locks are released, the frames are turned quickly and smoothly. The spring locks, which automatically lock when the frame bearing the patient is in the correct position, must be tested for security before the turners' holds are released.

Sufficient light-weight top bedding is used to keep the patient comfortable. A thin layer of sponge rubber on each frame may be permitted by the doctor if the patient finds the canvas too hard and uncomfortable.

Following each turning, the extra support pieces must be put in place. In the supine position, a footboard attaches to the frame to support the feet; a *small* rubber or towel roll may be necessary to fill in the space under the knees *without flexion* and padded arm rests are provided. A mirror at the head allows a wider view of the environment. In the prone position, the head is supported by a strip canvas on which the forehead rests leaving the face free. A rack is placed below the head on which personal articles (e.g. book) or the meal tray can be placed. A pillow is used under the ankles, and the feet are suspended over the end of the canvas. The arm rests are replaced.

Immobilization of the spine to promote tissue healing may be achieved by maintaining the patient in a supine position on an ordinary bed with a fracture board, if necessary, under a firm mattress. *If permitted*, the patient may be turned from side to side safely if a sufficient number of personnel are available to maintain alignment and stability of the spine; the patient is turned as one rigid unit (in log-rolling fashion). The patient is cautioned against making any effort to participate; his arms are folded on his chest or abdomen before turning and firm pillows and sand bags are used to maintain alignment in the lateral position. If the patient must remain on his back continuously, a thin sponge rubber mattress may be placed on top of the mattress. This facilitates the giving of frequent back care and the changing of the lower bed linen. A nurse on each side of the bed working from the head down uses one hand to depress the mattress while caring for the skin or changing the linen with the other one.

2. Potential for complications. Nursing care is concerned with the prevention of the following complications to which the immobilized spine-injured patient is predisposed.

(a) *Reduction in pulmonary tidal volume and effective airway clearance*. The immobilized patient's respirations tend to be shallow, resulting in reduced volumes in respiratory gas exchange as well as ineffective clearance of secretions. The patient is encouraged to practise frequent, brief periods of deep breathing. If auscultation indicates the presence of secretions and limited air entry, a regimen of coughing at regular intervals is introduced. A high fluid intake (e.g. 3000 ml daily) assists in mobilizing the secretions and in more effective clearance. Frequent turning of the patient if permitted also promotes drainage of pulmonary secretions. The nurse should liaise with the physiotherapist who may carry out chest care.

(b) *Pressure sores*. Frequent skin care must be a part of the nursing care as long as the patient is immobilized. The most vulnerable areas are those over body prominences such as the sacrum, scapulae, heels and ankles. If the patient is not on a turning bed the occipital area is also susceptible. The skin is kept clean and dry. The patient is turned every 2 hours day and night. The bedding is kept free of wrinkles, crumbs, tissues, etc. Resilient materials such as synthetic sheepskin or sponge rubber may be used under pressure areas. If the patient is on an ordinary bed, an alternating pressure (ripple) mattress is helpful. If the skin is dry, an oily lotion may be useful.

If a decubitus ulcer develops, nursing goals include the prevention of infection and promotion of healing see Chapter 27.

(c) *Ankylosis, muscle atrophy and contractures*. Immobility leads to stiffening of the joints, muscle wasting and contracture which limit the range of motion. An active and/or passive exercise programme may be established. The limbs are *gently* moved through their full range of motion and isotonic and isometric active exercises may be gradually introduced. These activities are important in maintaining joint mobility and muscle tone and in stimulating circulation which reduces venous stasis, lessening the possibility of phlebothrombosis. The physiotherapist is usually involved in this aspect of care.

(d) *Hypercalcaemia*. Prolonged immobilization prevents normal weight-bearing and muscle pull on the bones. This causes the movement of calcium out of the bones, resulting in increased urinary excretion of calcium that predisposes to the formation of renal or bladder calculi. An exercise routine and a daily fluid intake of 3000 ml are important. The amount of calcium-containing foods (e.g. milk and milk products) in the diet may be restricted.

(e) *Infection*. If tongs are used in providing traction, the sites of insertion are inspected daily for signs of inflammation and infection. Following cleansing with an antiseptic, fresh sterile dressings are applied. The application of an antibiotic ointment may be prescribed as a prophylactic measure.

3. *Pain*. Fracture and dislocation in spinal injury may cause pressure on spinal nerves causing pain at the site and in parts innervated by those nerves. Mild analgesics are prescribed; strong analgesics are avoided because they mask neurological changes that would indicate cord involvement. Change of position, gentle massage and passive exercises of the limbs may provide relief for the patient.

4. *Alteration in nutritional requirements*. A well balanced diet high in protein is recommended to promote healing, prevent tissue breakdown (decubitus ulcer, muscle atrophy) and maintain resistance to infection. If the patient is overweight the caloric intake may be reduced to lessen the weight-bearing for the spine when he is ambulatory. If a serology test shows hypercalcaemia, calcium-containing foods may be restricted as cited above. Dietary modification may be necessary to prevent or treat constipation; roughage content is increased with emphasis on whole grain cereals and bread and fresh fruits and vegetables.

5. *Alteration in bowel elimination*. Constipation and faecal impaction occur frequently with immobilization. Increased dietary roughage, a high fluid intake of at least 3000 ml and exercises if permitted assist in promoting bowel function. A mild laxative or a suppository may also be necessary. Unless the patient is on a turning bed, a slipper bedpan is used for defecation; the patient is turned as a rigid unit (log-rolled) on and off the pan.

For a discussion of faecal impaction see Chapter 17.

6. *Anxiety and alteration in self-image*. The sudden immobilization and dependence are a severe shock to the patient with a spinal injury. The loss of the ability to function as a normal independent, productive being is a threat even though it is for a limited time while the spine heals. The individual's self-image is altered with enforced immobility. He is encouraged to express his concerns as he searches for meaning in what he is experiencing. His thinking is directed to positive aspects and an explanation of the therapeutic and anticipated rehabilitative programmes is likely to be helpful. Specific expressed concerns should be addressed and assistance provided to find a solution.

7. *Self-care deficit*. Assistance with feeding, bathing and toileting is necessary during immobilization. Self-help measures such as simple activities like feeding self, washing the face, hands and arms, and

cleaning the teeth are initiated as soon as the patient's condition permits. The fact that the patient's reach is limited must be remembered; any attempt to obtain something beyond that reach may result in vertebral dislocation and cord injury.

8. Rehabilitation. When realignment and healing of the vertebrae have occurred, the spine is allowed to gradually resume weight-bearing by having the patient assume the sitting or upright position and start walking. Prolonged inactivity, especially in the recumbent position may cause postural hypotension. Someone should remain with the patient when he first begins to assume the upright position.

Management at home is discussed with the patient and family. They are advised of the prescribed exercise programme that is to be continued and the recommended amount and type of activities and those to be avoided until approved by the doctor are outlined. For example, he may be cautioned against lifting and flexion of the head or trunk depending on the location of the injury. The patient with a spinal injury without cord damage is usually able to return gradually to his pre-injury life-style.

Expected outcomes
1 The patient does not experience any pain or hypotension when upright.
2 The patient regains self-care ability and mobilization.
3 The patient and family indicate an understanding of the necessary care following hospitalization.
4 Informed decisions are made for home management by the patient and family.

THE PATIENT WITH SPINAL INJURY *WITH* CORD INVOLVEMENT (PARAPLEGIA AND QUADRIPLEGIA)

Identification of patient problems
1 Alteration in breathing pattern: respiratory insufficiency due to interruption of normal innervation of the diaphragm and/or intercostal muscles
2 Hypotension and impaired tissue perfusion secondary to spinal shock and dysfunction of the autonomic nervous system
3 Potential for further cord injury
4 Potential for pressure sores as a result of immobility and impaired tissue perfusion
5 Alteration in urinary elimination: retention with overflow or incontinence, due to disturbed innervation
6 Alteration in bowel elimination: distension, constipation, incontinence secondary to spinal shock and immobility
7 Alteration in food and fluid intake secondary to gastrointestinal distension, anxiety and difficulty in eating caused by immobility and position

8 Self-care deficits due to paralysis and enforced immobility
9 Alteration in comfort: pain and spasticity
10 Potential for infection
11 Potential for complications: muscle contractures, deformities, osteoporosis and thrombophlebitis
12 Inability to control body temperature secondary to dysfunction of the autonomic nervous system
13 Disturbance in sleep pattern due to impact of accident, dependency and permanent disability
14 Patient and family reactions to change in patient's role, his loss of mobility and independence
15 Potential for injury secondary to paralysis, immobility, muscle spasm, loss of sensation
16 Sexual dysfunction
17 Lack of knowledge: requires new coping patterns because of altered body image and limitations. Alteration in role and home management

The *goals* are to:
1 Prevent further spinal cord damage
2 Support and strengthen existing resources (e.g. respiration)
3 Prevent the complications of immobility
4 Rehabilitate the patient to his maximum potential

Nursing intervention

1. Respiratory dysfunction. In the *acute phase,* the patient with cervical or high thoracic cord injury is at risk of respiratory failure, reduced gas exchange and ineffective airway clearance. Initially, diaphragmatic function may appear to be adequate, but during the first 48 hours, oedema develops in the area of the injury. Its progress in the patient with a cervical injury may compromise vital centres in the medulla; respiratory failure develops as well as hypotension and weakening of the pulse. Chest trauma or preexisting respiratory disease seriously complicates respiratory function.

Endotracheal intubation or a tracheostomy and oxygen administration may be necessary. Suction is applied to the airway at regular intervals to remove secretions (see Chapter 16). If ventilatory muscle function is not adequate to maintain sufficient pulmonary gas volumes and blood-gas levels, mechanical respiratory assistance is provided, (see Chapter 16 for care of the patient with respiratory insufficiency). Chest physiotherapy and increased humidity of inspired air and oxygen are provided to mobilize the secretions.

When the patient recovers sufficiently and the blood-gas analyses indicate satisfactory levels, mechanical respiratory assistance is discontinued and a regime of deep breathing and coughing is established.

The patient continues to be at risk of respiratory insufficiency and complications in the post-acute phase. Abdominal muscle function may be weak or lacking, and, as a result, the cough is weak in the paraplegic and absent in the quadriplegic. Suction equipment should be readily available and intensive physiotherapy provided to help the patient develop an effective cough if possible, as well as to mobilize secretions. During the period that they must remain flat while the spine heals and stabilizes, spinal cord-injured patients are predisposed to bronchopneumonia and atelectasis.

2. Impaired tissue perfusion and hypotension. The widespread vasodilation and spinal shock associated with a spinal cord injury in the acute stage requires immediate attention. The vasodilation and fall in arterial blood pressure impairs tissue perfusion. The patient is kept flat and the lower limbs raised on pillows to increase the blood volume to the heart and brain. The foot of the bed *is not raised* to avoid elevation of the trunk which would incur upward pressure on the diaphragm causing further respiratory difficulty. Vasomotor tone generally returns to normal in 1 or 2 weeks.

Following the period of immobilization, the patient may experience the problem of postural hypotension when the upright position is assumed, the patient faints as a result of a precipitous fall in blood pressure and cerebral ischaemia. This occurs as a result of failure of vascular reflexive responses which normally increase vasomotor tone and prevents the sudden rush of blood and pooling in the vessels in the abdomen and lower extremities when the patient becomes upright. Postural hypotention decreases the volume of blood returned to the heart. If the condition is not corrected promptly, the inadequate cerebral perfusion and hypoxia may cause permanent brain damage. In the quadriplegic, even slight elevation of the head of the bed may result in a drastic reduction in blood pressure.

Postural hypotension may be corrected gradually. Progressive elevation may be used to gradually increase tolerance of the upright position safely. The patient's blood pressure is monitored in the elevated position and he is observed for pallor, perspiration and complaints of nausea. If hypotension develops, the patient is promptly lowered until flat. A vasopressor agent may be prescribed.

3. Potential for further cord injury. Alignment and immobilization of the spine are necessary to prevent further injury to the cord and further disability. If there is cervical vertebral displacement, tongs and traction are usually applied. During the period of immobilization, the patient may be cared for on a turning bed. The degree of dependency depends on the level of cord injury. Obviously, paraplegic patients are less dependent than quadriplegics but the latter have varying degrees of paresis in the shoulders and arms.

If traction with tongs and/or a turning bed is used, the same principles as cited previously apply.

4. Potential for pressure sores. The changes in vasomotor tone and the resulting impairment of tissue perfusion, the enforced immobility and the loss of cutaneous sensation contribute to tissue breakdown. If a decubitis ulcer occurs, healing is difficult in patients with spinal cord injury and rehabilitation is delayed.

Frequent skin care should begin within a few hours of the injury; decubiti can develop with startling rapidity in these patients. The skin must be kept clean and dry. The patient is turned or lifted every 1 or 2 hours, day and night. The bedding is kept dry and free of wrinkles and crumbs. Resilient material such as synthetic sheepskin is used under pressure areas. An alternating pressure (ripple) mattress may be used in some instances.

With each turning, the skin is inspected for signs of impending decubiti: early signs are redness which persists beyond 15 minutes after the pressure is relieved and increased localized warmth. The change is brought to the doctor's attention and efforts increased to protect the areas. For a more detailed discussion of preventive measures see Chapter 27. If a decubitus ulcer develops, nursing goals are to prevent infection and promote healing (see Chapter 27).

The patient needs to understand the importance of keeping the skin intact and his role in maintaining its integrity. Following the period of immobilization to stabilize the spine, as the patient begins to assume the self-care within his potential, the importance of shifting of pressure is explained and he is taught how to change his position at frequent regular intervals in bed and in a wheelchair. The patient is taught to inspect the vulnerable areas at least once daily using a mirror.

Most patients with paraplegia or quadriplegia are eventually mobilized by light-weight wheelchairs. The patient is taught transfer from bed to chair and from chair to toilet and that at regular intervals he must shift his body weight. He learns to lift his trunk by pushing with his arms and hands on the chair arms or seat in order to relieve constant pressure on the buttocks and sacral region. Aids such as sheepskins and cushions filled with polyester granules may be provided.

5. Alteration in urinary elimination. During the spinal shock, the bladder is atonic and there is retention of urine with overflow. The stasis of urine predisposes to infection and the distension may cause fissures or areas of pressure necrosis in the bladder wall. Ureteral openings are dilated allowing reflux of urine into the kidneys. An indwelling catheter or intermittent catheterization is introduced soon after admission to prevent overdistension of the atonic bladder. The prevention of incontinence also assists in protecting the skin from irritation and breakdown. If continuous catheter drainage is required, a sterile closed drainage system is used; precautions must be strictly observed to prevent infection. Frequent antiseptic cleansing of the meatus and surrounding tissue is necessary. Renal complications (e.g. pyelonephritis, calculi) are the major cause of mortality in cord-injured persons. The atony of the bladder remains for a varying length of time before hyperreflexia takes over and the bladder becomes hypertonic, resulting in frequent automatic emptying of small volumes. To counteract the hypertonicity and diminished bladder capacity, if an indwelling catheter is used, the catheter is clamped for stated intervals, or if intermittent catheterization is used, the intervals are gradually increased. Catheter use is discontinued as soon as possible because of the risk of infection and a bladder training programme is initiated. The reflex emptying of the bladder and incontinence are very distressing to the patient; he may resist an adequate fluid intake with the thought that it may at least lessen the frequency of involuntary voiding. This is dangerous since it predisposes to infection and the formation of calculi. Some patients become dependent on catheter use on a permanent basis, and may have to be taught intermittent self-catheterization. Ideally a bladder training programme should be introduced as soon as possible to avoid dependency on a catheter. The patient is taught to initiate the reflexive emptying of the bladder by the Credé manoeuvre or the Valsalva manoeuvre. With some patients, stretching of the anal sphincter by the insertion of a gloved finger into the anal canal in combination with the Valsalva manoeuvre is more effective. The bladder may not completely empty and stasis of urine predisposes to infection. Periodic catheterization may be done to determine residual volume; less than 75–100 ml is usually acceptable. A specimen of urine is submitted for analysis at regular intervals and also if the urine has an offensive odour, is cloudy or there is blood or sediment.

6. Alteration in bowel elimination.   With spinal shock the gastrointestinal tract becomes atonic; severe distension and vomiting without effort may develop (paralytic ileus). Gastrointestinal aspiration via a nasogastric tube may become necessary until peristalsis is re-established; abdominal distension causes respiratory embarrassment by pressure on the diaphragm.

The spinal cord injury interrupts impulses from the higher centres of awareness and control. The sensation of the need to defecate is lost and the rectal and anal sphincters function reflexly (automatic spinal cord response). Because of the immobility and dietary changes the patient experiences constipation, and impaction develops readily. When bowel sounds are present, a mild laxative or suppository (glycerin or bisacodyl) may be used to evacuate the bowel at first then, as the patient's condition improves and he is taking a more normal diet, invo-

luntary defecation occurs. A diet high in fibre is usually necessary to prevent constipation. The diet is adjusted to the stool consistency and frequency. As soon as the patient is able to sit in a chair, training for bowel elimination by conditioned reflex begins. A regular hour for bowel elimination may be established; morning is the normal time for most patients. The procedure involves a warm beverage, followed in one-half hour by the insertion of a glycerin or bisacodyl (Dulcolax) suppository and stimulation by inserting a lubricated gloved finger every 10–15 minutes until defecation occurs. Digital stimulation may be necessary following the bowel movement to ensure complete rectal evacuation. Once a pattern of regular reflex evacuation has been established the patient may find that digital stimulation alone or the use of a device to massage the anal canal may be effective.

The patient is assisted to a commode or toilet at the same time each day or every other day. Privacy should be provided. A member of the patient's family should be involved in the bowel training programme as part of the preparation for home management.

7. Alteration in food and fluid intake.   During the initial phase oral food and fluid are withheld. Some degree of paralytic ileus develops in most spinal cord-injured patients due to spinal shock. Fluids are administered by intravenous infusion to maintain hydration. A nasogastric tube may be inserted and aspiration established to relieve gastric and intestinal dilation. Unless treated, the distended gastrointestinal tract interferes with the diaphragmatic excursion, compromising respirations. When peristalsis is re-established, fluids are administered orally and, if tolerated, solid foods are added. A high calorie, high protein diet is important to combat the tendency toward a negative nitrogen balance which is commonly associated with immobility. An adequate nutritional intake also plays a role in promoting tissue healing and resistance to breakdown (e.g. decubitus ulcer) and provides energy for exercises and the rehabilitative programme. A diet which meets the patient's nutritional needs may be a problem because of his emotions, inactivity and what may be the awkward position he is in for immobilization (e.g. prone on Stryker frame). Dietary supplements between meals may be necessary. Later, calorie intake may have to be reduced to prevent overweight which complicates rehabilitation and increases the risk of complications. Bulk and roughage are necessary in the diet to promote bowel elimination.

Calcium intake (milk and milk products) may be restricted to prevent urinary calculi which may develop as calcium moves out of immobilized bones. A fluid intake of at least 3000 ml a day is encouraged to prevent concentration and stasis of urine. Grape and apple juices are preferable to citrus fruit juices;

they produce an acid urine which reduces the precipitation of calcium and the formation of calculi as well as reducing the risk of infection. Organisms are less likely to grow in an acid environment.

Some cord-injured patients develop stress ulcers (gastric or duodenal). The aetiology has yet to be fully determined; hyperacidity due to histamine release following the trauma, or mucosal ischaemia, are among the leading theories at present. Cimetidine (Tagamet) parenteral or oral medication may be prescribed as a prophylactic measure. Dietary adjustments may be necessary to meet these patients' tolerance.

Food must be placed readily within reach and the patient encouraged to feed himself as soon as his condition permits. Initially those with quadriplegia will require assistance with feeding until appropriate assistive devices are available. Swallowing may be difficult in the recumbent position and inhalation may occur. The patient is instructed to take only small amounts at a time and swallow frequently. Suction equipment should be readily available in the event of inhalation. The patient is permitted to exercise some choice over the food that is served and the feeding experience made as pleasant as possible.

If the partial quadriplegic has motor function in the triceps and biceps muscles, self-feeding may be accomplished. With flexion at the elbow and the fitting over the hand of a wide elastic band with a pocket, self-feeding may be achieved. Special utensils such as a spoon fit into the pocket.

8. *Self-care deficits*.   During the acute phase, the paraplegic patient is bathed and fed but as soon as his condition permits he is encouraged gradually to assume self-care. The patient with complete quadriplegia is deficient in self-care and activities of daily living. The patient with partial quadriplegia has varying degrees of deficiency in self-care. The patient becomes increasingly aware of his limitations and dependency; personal care must be provided with sensitivity to the patient's feelings. It is difficult to convince the patient in the early stages that eventually it is possible that he will regain considerable independence.

In order to regain even minimal independence in self-care, the individual must be able to move about and be able to have some grasp in at least one hand. Paraplegic persons do have the distinct advantage of having the use of both hands and are capable of achieving self-care. The quadriplegic is dependent on head movements, assistive devices and care provided by others.

9. *Alteration in comfort*.   The patient with a spinal cord injury may experience pain which radiates along the spinal nerves that originate at the level of injury. Spasticity of the muscles below the level of the cord injury is also a source of severe discomfort in paraplegia and quadriplegia and may lead to con-

tractures and deformities. The pain is severe and fatiguing and may be embarrassing at times for the patient. It may retard rehabilitation. The muscle spasms are hypersensitive reflexes which develop after spinal shock subsides. The stimulus may not even be obvious. Examples of stimuli which may initiate the spastic response include light touching of the skin, jarring of the bed, turning, cold, fatigue, a distended bladder and emotional reactions. Regular passive moving of the limbs through their range of motion is beneficial especially when done under water. Drugs such as muscle relaxants, for example dantrolene (Dantrium), are only partially effective and their use is discouraged because of the toxic side-effects, dependency and drowsiness. Rarely, severe painful spasticity is treated by surgery; various procedures have been done and include severing of tendons, transection of a nerve root (rhizotomy) and neurotomy (cutting of nerves).

Narcotics and strong analgesics are not used with the patient with high cervical injury because of the depressing effect on respiration.

10. *Potential for infection*. If tongs are used in providing traction, the sites of insertion are inspected daily for signs of inflammation and infection. Following cleansing with an antiseptic, fresh sterile dressings are applied. The application of an antibiotic ointment may be prescribed as a prophylactic measure.

Patients with cord involvement and paralysis, develop urinary tract infection readily which may become chronic and life-threatening through extension to the kidneys. Preventive measures include strict asepsis when intermittent catheterization or a closed drainage system is used and a minimal daily fluid intake of 3000 ml. Fluids which produce acidity of the urine are recommended (e.g. apple and grape; see above). Regular periodic culture of urine is done so that early detection of infection can be made and treatment instituted promptly.

11. *Potential for complications*: muscle contractures, deformities, osteoporosis and thrombophlebitis. Patients with spinal cord injury and the resulting paralysis develop muscle and tendon contractures and ankylosis of the joints unless preventive measures are observed. The shortening of the muscles and tendons may cause serious deformities which restrict his rehabilitation. For example a flexure contracture of the thigh at the hip joint may inhibit the patient's use of a wheelchair. Wrist drop and foot drop develop readily in paralysed limbs unless preventive measures are instituted. Immobility, muscle spasticity and poor alignment in positioning the patient are contributing factors. Preventive measures include frequent change of position and maintenance of good body alignment using sand bags, trochanter rolls and pillows if necessary, regular passive range-of-movement exercises and a

physiotherapy programme as soon as the patient's condition permits.

The health of bones normally depends on stress due to muscle pull and weight bearing. When these are lacking, as with paralysis and prolonged immobilization, bone demineralization and osteoporosis occurs. Therefore, weight bearing is started as soon as possible to stimulate osteoblastic activity and prevent demineralization. The head of the bed is gradually elevated as tolerated, and, when safe, the patient is positioned upright on a tilt table. Weight bearing for at least a few minutes each day may also help to prevent contractures, particularly in the hips.

Regardless of intervention, eventually atrophy of paralysed muscles does occur to some degree. This is primarily due to absence of nerve impulses to the muscle.

Thrombophlebitis is a common problem in a paralysed patient, particularly in the first 3 months following injury. Absence of the pumping action of contracting muscle and poor skeletal muscle tone which results with paralysis and immobility leads to pooling of blood in the lower viscera and extremities and a reduced venous return. This predisposes to thrombophlebitis. Localized oedema, redness, warmth, tenderness and red streaks of an extremity suggest thrombophlebitis. Deep venous thrombosis is particularly serious since it may lead to pulmonary emboli. Deep vein thrombosis is evident when calf tenderness, Homan's sign (discomfort behind the knee on forced dorsiflexion of the foot) and oedema of the entire limb are present. Because of loss of sensation, pain and tenderness are not perceived. Assessment for venous thrombosis, done daily, includes calf observation, gentle palpation for calf firmness and measurement of the circumference of the thigh and calf. The tape measure is placed at the same level above and below the knee each time. Management to prevent thrombosis includes a regular schedule of range of movement and exercises (these activities act as a mechanical pump to increase circulation), frequent change of position, elevation of the legs 15° for stated periods and the wearing of anti-emboli stockings while in bed. Anticoagulant therapy (e.g. acetylsalicylic acid) may be prescribed as a prophylactic measure.

12. Inability to control body temperature. This is a common problem for patients with a spinal cord injury. Dysfunction of the autonomic nervous system occurs and there is decreased ability to lose or conserve heat in the paralysed parts of the body. Room temperature is controlled to meet the patient's need since he is mainly dependent on environmental temperature for control. When experiencing a rise in body temperature, tepid sponging, light clothing and bedding and the use of fans are helpful. If the patient is cold, additional covers and warm drinks are recommended. Perspiration is a common occur-

rence if the patient is experiencing some stress such as a full bladder or rectum, discomfort or pain.

13. Disturbance in sleep pattern. This is a common problem as a result of the psychological impact of the traumatic event and enforced immobility and dependency. The cord-injured patient may experience frightening dreams in which the accident is relived. Discomfort and the necessary frequent repositioning as well as a high level of anxiety may disrupt the patient's sleep.

Lack of adequate rest and sleep depletes the person's energy and endurance which are essential for healing and rehabilitation.

Nursing care involves the provision of a quiet environment, comfort measures such as position change, warm drinks and remaining with the patient, encouraging him to discuss his anxieties and feelings and to provide reassurance that he is not alone. Regular rest periods are scheduled to prevent exhaustion. Some sedation may be necessary, but caution is observed to avoid drug dependency and respiratory depression.

14. Patient and family reactions. It is understandable that a spinal injury which results in paralysis is a very traumatic psychological experience. Suddenly, the victim is changed from an independent person with control of his activities to dependence on others for even very personal care. He feels alone and desperate and his self-image is completely changed. Responses and adjustment to the loss of body functions usually parallel the grief reaction.

Initially, shock and denial of reality help the victim to maintain self-control and survive. Consistent, high-quality nursing care is supportive in this phase. Gradually, a beginning awareness develops and the patient responds with anger and resentment that this has happened to him. The nurse, understanding why the patient is behaving as he is, listens and accepts his responses; support at this time may help to strengthen the patient's tenuous grasp of reality. Anger may be followed by a period of despair and depression in which the patient may eat or drink very little and does not manifest any interest in his rehabilitation, his family or those around him. Close observation of his reactions and comments indicate to the nurse when to encourage conversation or when presence alone is preferable to the patient. At the appropriate time, the nurse verbally acknowledges recognition of how the situation looks to the patient. The patient may raise questions that relate to concerns such as independence, financial support and sexuality in his future. Anxiety may escalate in proportion to the unknown; anxiety depletes energy and tends to distort reality. The patient is assured that everything possible will be done to help him regain the ability to do some things for himself. Reassurance should be realistic; offering false hope must be avoided. The quadriplegic patient poses the greater challenge to the nurse. About the third or fourth day, the patient may become confused and experience sensory hallucinations. This appears to occur with greater frequency when the patient is on a turning bed. Perhaps this is due to the fact that not only is he unable to feel any portion of the bed but, because of its narrowness, he cannot see what he is lying on. The room appears abnormal because only the ceiling and floor are seen unless a mirror is provided. Constant support and reassurance are necessary throughout this phase to help the patient hold on to reality.

Gradually, the patient begins to see things realistically and explore the possibilities for his future. In this reorganization phase, learning to cope with body changes predominates. Assimilation of the changes in body image and pattern of life takes considerable time; periods of withdrawal and depression are to be expected from time to time. Such reactions are accepted but with expectation that efforts will be resumed. Thinking is directed to the positive, to things he can do and realistically can learn to do. As soon as his condition permits, the patient is encouraged and expected to do the things that his functional motor capacity allows. The acknowledgment of improvement and achievement helps to sustain motivation. The development of a sense of worthiness and self-esteem essential for resocialization greatly depend on the positive attitude, appreciation and reliance conveyed by professionals and significant others.

The victim's injury and the possible implications of disability are difficult for family members to accept. As well as concern for the patient, the situation may involve a complete change of life-style for them. They may be faced with financial hardships and a disruption of home management. Role functions change, responsibilities are shifted and plans and goals may be shattered.

Family bonds may become greater as they face the situation together; new strengths, capabilities and determination to cope with their problems may be revealed. In other instances, the reaction of some family members after the patient's acute phase may be resentment for the individual whose accident has altered their life. The patient is rejected and his feelings of loneliness, fear and depression are increased.

The nurse takes time to talk with the family; they are kept informed of the patient's progress and of the therapeutic and rehabilitative programmes. Their role in supporting the patient is discussed. Time is given to learning of their problems and suggestions made that assist them in planning and resolution. For example, a referral to a social service worker, a chaplain or a rehabilitation officer may be helpful.

Family and friends are encouraged to spend time with the patient to provide support and reinforce the impression that they are not rejecting him as useless. Encouraging the patient to do things for himself and letting him do them are emphasized.

15. *Potential for injury*. Limited sensation in the paralysed parts, limited mobility, muscle spasm and dependency place the paralysed patient at risk of injury and complications. It is necessary for the patient to develop the necessary strength in the unaffected parts to mobilize and control the affected parts in order to prevent complications incurred by immobilization and falls. The bones in paralysed limbs are easily fractured due to osteoporosis. A waist strap is used while the patient is in a chair until he is strong enough to control his trunk. Consistent use of wheelchair brakes during transfers is essential for safety.

Any local heat application is used judiciously; loss of cutaneous sensation predisposes to burns. The skin is inspected daily for abrasions, bruises, pressure ischaemia and irritated areas.

16. *Sexual dysfunction*. The potential for sexual fulfilment is a major concern of the patient with permanent disability. Some patients may express this concern directly but more often concern is present long before it is expressed. One paraplegic reported: 'It is such a personal thing. If someone else had brought up the subject I might have felt more comfortable about asking the questions I had.' If the patient brings up the topic of sexuality, his concerns are acknowledged and he is encouraged to express them freely. Factual information is provided without embarrassment.

The cord-injured patient needs to know that meaningful and satisfying relationships are still attainable and that even though he may no longer be able to function sexually in the same ways as before the injury, he can be helped to learn new ways of giving and receiving sexual satisfaction. The patient needs to understand that sexuality of an individual involves the total person and that one's self-image is an important dimension in the resocialization process in disability.

The question of fertility and ability to procreate may also be raised by patients with a spinal cord injury. Male infertility is not uncommon following a cord injury because of testicular atrophy, decreased production of sperm and infrequency of ejaculation. The female with cord injury is usually able to conceive and deliver a child with few adaptations being necessary. Since there exists a vast body of knowledge specific to sexuality in disability, it is appropriate to discuss other resources of information with the patient. Referral to a qualified counsellor or agency may be advisable. Issues such as parenting, adoption, contraception and artificial insemination as they relate to the physically disabled are currently receiving attention and are being studied.

17. *Rehabilitation*. As soon as the patient is well enough, an active rehabilitation programme is planned and instituted. The patient and family participate in the planning and scheduling of the pro-

gramme to meet their knowledge deficits and adjustments. Family members should be involved in order to support the patient and maintain consistent care. Rehabilitation begins with simple self-care activities, progressing to more complex as skill is achieved. With increasing independence, the paraplegic learns to turn, transfer from bed to chair and chair to toilet. Progress is slow and requires persistent effort and repeated encouragement; recognition of even the slightest gain prompts motivation. Planned periods of rest and diversion are necessary to offset intensive exercises and prevent exhaustion. The family are cautioned against fostering dependence by doing things for the patient for which he has the capacity to do or learn to do for himself.

A guide which offers suggestions for planning an individualized teaching programme was developed by Welnetz[3]. The format also provides a means of recording what the patient and family have been taught, and also may serve to summarize the learning achieved. The reader is referred also to Chapter 3 on Rehabilitation.

Expected outcomes

1 The vital capacity and respiratory pattern are normal.
2 There is a satisfactory pattern of urinary and bowel elimination.
3 The patient takes a balanced diet of sufficient calories to maintain his normal weight.
4 The patient assumes self-care, requires minimal assistance and manages wheelchair activities.
5 The patient shows an excellent response to the rehabilitation programme.
6 The skin is intact and is in good condition.
7 The patient and family have accepted the change in their pattern of living and are making informed decisions about the future.

RUPTURED OR HERNIATED INTERVERTEBRAL DISC

Intervertebral discs consist of a tough, fibrocartilaginous outer capsule (annulus fibrosus) and a central core of resilient, semi-solid material (annulus pulposus). The discs lie between the bodies of the vertebrae and serve as cushions and shock absorbers. The capsule of each disc is attached to the bodies of the adjoining vertebrae and the anterior and posterior longitudinal ligaments. If injury or degenerative change causes tearing or a weakened area in the capsule, the nucleus pulposus extrudes resulting in a protrusion that may irritate or press on a spinal nerve root or the cord giving rise to signs of nerve or cord compression. If untreated, serious disability may result.

Ruptured or herniated intervertebral disc may occur at any level of the spine but the lumbar and lumbosacral discs are most frequently affected (98%)

because this area of the spine is subjected to considerable weight and pressure and is frequently the site of degenerative changes. When the condition develops suddenly, it may be referred to as acute low-back syndrome or pain; if the symptoms gradually and progressively develop, the condition may be referred to as chronic low-back syndrome or pain.

Aetiology. Causes include: trauma due to lifting of heavy objects with the trunk flexed; back injury (e.g. fall); slipping that incurs excessive strain on the supporting ligaments; congenital anomaly; and degenerative process associated with arthritis or ageing.

Assessment

Manifestations. The patient experiences pain in the back and in the area of distribution of the involved nerve. Affected lumbar or lumbosacral discs cause pressure on the sciatic nerve giving rise to sciatica. The patient complains of low back pain which radiates into the respective buttock and down the posterior aspect of the thigh and leg. The pain is aggravated by bending, lifting, straight-leg raising, coughing, sneezing and straining at stool. Muscle spasm develops increasing the discomfort and postural deformity may be evident due to the spasm. Continued pressure may produce degenerative changes in the involved nerve; decreased or absence of deep tendon reflexes, diminished sensation in the area of distribution of the affected nerve roots, weakness of the urethral sphincter and muscular weakness may develop.

Disc herniation in the cervical area causes shoulder pain which radiates down the arm. Muscle spasm causes neck stiffness, limiting range of movement. Sensory changes may also develop.

Diagnostic procedures. Confirmation of the diagnosis and location of the lesion may involve an x-ray of the spine, a discogram, a myelogram (see p. 788) and rarely, a lumbar puncture to determine if the disc protrusion is blocking the flow of CSF.

On-going assessment. Periodic assessment of sensory and motor functions below the level of the disc lesion is necessary. Any decrease in sensation or motor strength, change in pattern of respiration or elimination is brought promptly to the doctor's attention. Emergency surgical intervention may be indicated to prevent permanent disability.

If pelvic or head traction is used a frequent check is made of the equipment to ensure function. The patient is observed also for correct body alignment. The skin under the halter or pelvic appliance is examined at frequent intervals for excoriation; the iliac crests are particularly susceptible to pressure and irritation from the pelvic girdle.

---

[3] Welnetz (1981).

Medical management
The patient with a ruptured or herniated disc may be treated conservatively or by surgery. Surgery is usually reserved for those patients who do not respond to conservative therapy and are experiencing persistent or recurring episodes of pain and increasing signs of nerve or cord compression and disability.

Conservative treatment includes rest, heat applications (diathermy, ultrasound, or hot packs), the administration of a muscle relaxant and an analgesic, exercises, traction and then some form of back support (brace or therapeutic corset) on ambulation.

Surgical therapy involves a laminectomy followed by decompression of nerve roots or the cord by excision of the herniating disc tissue. This may be followed by the fusion of the spinous processes of the regional vertebrae for stabilization and immobilization of the area. The grafts may be taken from an iliac crest or a lower limb.

If a fusion is done, the patient's movement following the operation is more restricted so that the bone grafts will heal and immobilize the area. The patient learns to adjust to this area of immobility but the adjustment is greater for the patient who has had a fusion of the cervical spine; a collar is usually worn for a period of time following the surgery.

Prevention of disc problem
There is a high incidence of low-back syndrome in persons between 30 and 50 years of age in the work force. The disorder is frequently the result of poor body mechanics. The nurse has the responsibility to practise and teach good basic body mechanics which contribute to the prevention of excessive strain on back muscles and ligaments.

Significant factors in the prevention of undue strain on back muscles and ligaments include the following:
- Good posture should be maintained and a general exercise regimen followed to prevent muscle weakness. When sitting, the hips should be well back in the chair so that the weight is on the thighs and lower part of the buttocks and the back is kept straight. Exercising the trunk muscles (especially the abdominal and gluteal) to promote strength and tone contributes to the patient's ability to function with a minimal risk of strain and injury to the discs.
- Heavy objects should be carried close to the body
- When lifting a heavy object from a lower level, the knees and thighs should be flexed with the back straight as this places the greater strain on the thigh and buttock muscles rather than on the back
- Bending at the waist with the knees straight and twisting of the spine should be avoided
- Objects with which one is working should be at a comfortable level and close enough to avoid the strain of reaching
- Pulling taxes the muscles less than pushing

- If standing for long periods, broaden the base (feet apart) and periodically shift weight from one foot to the other for a brief period.

Identification of patient problems

The patient with rupture or herniated disc—treated conservatively.
1 Impaired mobility secondary to pain, muscle spasm and therapeutic immobilization
2 Potential nerve or cord injury due to nerve or cord compression by the disc protrusion
3 Alteration in comfort secondary to pressure on the nerve roots or cord and muscle spasm
4 Potential for complications:
   (a) Impairment of skin integrity due to immobility, the abrasive effect of traction equipment or collar and diminished sensation in parts below the level of the affected disc
   (b) Respiratory dysfunction: shallow respirations and retention of pulmonary secretions
   (c) Muscle atrophy and joint stiffness due to immobility
   (d) Thrombophlebitis secondary to venous stasis
5 Alteration in elimination: constipation secondary to inactivity and prescribed medications (analgesic, muscle relaxant)
6 Self-care deficit
7 Alteration in food intake: reduced calorie intake to correct overweight
8 Lack of knowledge: the patient requires an understanding of the condition and how to prevent recurrence by good biomechanics and exercises. Assistance may be necessary to make a change to employment that will be less demanding on his back.

Nursing intervention

1. Impaired physical mobility. In the acute phase, the patient is placed at rest on a firm mattress on a firm-based bed; a fracture board is used if the bed has a sprung base. The purpose of bed rest is to reduce weight and strain on the lesion and lessen irritation of the nerve roots. The patient is usually more comfortable with the head of the bed slightly elevated (about 20°) and some support under the knees. A *small* roll or pillow may be placed under the knees but must be small enough to avoid flexion and pressure on the popliteal nerve. An alternative may be a pillow under the length of the lower limbs. Repositioning at frequent intervals is necessary; the patient is taught to roll like a log, keeping the spine straight and the uppermost leg flexed when turning. He is warned to avoid sudden movements and twisting of the spine and is advised of the importance of maintaining good body alignment. Articles that the patient may need should be kept within easy reach to avoid undue reaching and stretching.

2. Potential nerve or cord injury. Traction may be

used to relieve pressure on the nerve roots or cord and to immobilize the regional spine. In the case of a cervical disc herniation, a collar may be worn to immobilize the neck, or a halter may be applied which is attached to a rope over a pulley and weight and the head of the bed is elevated so that the body weight counteracts the traction. If a lumbar disc is affected, pelvic traction (Pugh's traction) may be applied and the foot of the bed is elevated.

3. Alteration in comfort. These patients experience considerable pain and muscle spasm which may necessitate the administration of an analgesic and muscle relaxant. A mild analgesic, such as paracetamol, may provide the necessary relief, but some patients may need a stronger preparation such as codeine. A muscle relaxant such as diazepam (Valium), dantrolene sodium (Dantrium) or methocarbamol (Robaxin) may be prescribed. Change of position frequently will provide some relief; care to avoid any extension of the back or stretching of back muscles is important.

4. Potential for complications
(a) *Pressure sores.* If traction is used or the patient experiences pain on moving, the prolonged periods of immobility and limited movement may cause decreased tissue perfusion in pressure areas. Vulnerable pressure areas such as shoulders, sacral area and heels require frequent care to prevent pressure sores. A sheepskin under these areas or an alternating pressure (ripple) mattress may be necessary. A directive is received from the doctor as to how frequently a cervical collar or traction appliance may be removed and the skin under it cared for and the patient's position changed.

The application of heat in the form of diathermy, ultrasound or infrared lamp is commonly used to treat these patients. Precautions must be used against burning; sensory nerve root involvement may incur diminished sensation resulting in the patient being unaware of excessive heat. Also, the use of heat tends to make the skin more susceptible to pressure and breakdown.
(b) *Respiratory dysfunction.* During the period of bed rest, the patient is prompted to take several deep breaths every 3–4 hours to promote normal pulmonary gas exchange and to prevent retention of secretions. The latter predisposes to infection and pneumonia.
(c) *Muscle atrophy and joint stiffness.* A range-of-movement exercise regimen is established to prevent limited joint movement and muscle weakness. At first the exercises may be limited to the upper limbs with lumbar disc involvement; lower limb exercises are gradually introduced as pain and muscle spasm become less severe. With a cervical lesion, arm exercises may be restricted for a period of time.

As soon as possible, a specific flexion exercise programme to strengthen the back muscles is planned by a physiotherapist. The exercises are carried out frequently and may be in the pool in the physiotherapy department.
(d) *Thrombophlebitis.* If the period of bed rest is prolonged and the patient is not able to carry out range-of-movement exercises of the lower limbs, antiemboli stockings may be worn to reduce venous stasis. This is especially important if the patient has varicosities.

5. Alteration in elimination. The patient with low back pain may experience constipation due to the inactivity and the prescribed analgesic and muscle relaxant. Constipation increases intraabdominal pressure and necessitates straining at stool which further increases the back pain. Dietary roughage and fluid intake are increased and a stool softener or bulk-producing laxative is given to promote regular defecation without straining. If use of a commode is not possible, a slipper bedpan is used; a folded towel or small pillow is placed behind the bedpan to provide support to the back and reduce the strain on the back muscles. The patient is assisted to log-roll on and off the pan.

6. Self-care deficits. Assistance with feeding, hygiene, grooming and toileting is necessary because of the pain and immobility. As the pain and muscle spasms subside, increased activity is encouraged.

7. Alteration in food intake. If the patient is overweight, the caloric intake is usually restricted to 1000–1200 kcal. An explanation of the effect of extra weight on the spine is made to the patient and support and encouragement given for adherence to the prescribed diet.

8. Knowledge deficit. An explanation of the disc problem is made to the patient, including the relationship of the pain he experiences to nerve pressure. A diagram is useful for clarification and opportunities are provided for questions and further information. The principles of good biomechanics to be observed in posture and activities are taught and demonstrated. He is advised to always use a straight-back chair, to avoid quick jerky or twisting movements and to sleep on a firm mattress; a fracture board under his mattress at home may be recommended. When mobile, the patient may be required to wear a brace or therapeutic corset to provide support and restrict movement. The importance of carrying out the prescribed exercises in the prevention of recurrence of the pain is emphasized when preparing the patient for managing at home.

In some instances, the doctor may advise the patient against resuming his former occupation. This may cause considerable anxiety for the patient. A referral to the social service department may be necessary to provide assistance in obtaining suitable employment or in making adjustments in his current place of employment.

The patient with a cervical disc problem may resume activities gradually while wearing a cervical collar for support and to limit neck movements.

(For nursing care following spinal surgery to treat a herniated or ruptured disc see the section that follows.)

Expected outcomes

The patient:

1 Indicates an understanding of the spinal disorder and the cause of the pain he experienced
2 Is free of pain and muscle spasm
3 Indicates an appreciation of what comprises good body mechanics and has demonstrated satisfactory application of these
4 Makes constructive plans for readjustment in occupation activities and home management which respect the recommended limitation of certain movements.

Nursing the patient treated by spinal surgery

Spinal surgery may be performed to: remove a neoplasm, a herniated or ruptured disc or bony fragments following an injury; reduce a fractured vertebra; decompress the spinal cord following an injury; relieve intractable pain or spasticity; or suppress involuntary movements. For common spinal surgical procedures see Table 22.9.

PREOPERATIVE PHASE

Assessment

1 An assessment is made of the patient's perception of the surgery he is to have, his expectations and knowledge deficit.
2 A preoperative assessment is made of the patient's physical status (see Chapter 11).
3 The patient's motor and sensory functions are evaluated.

A summary is made of the vital signs and sensory and motor status to serve as a base-line in assessing the patient's postoperative progress.

Identification of patient problems

1 Insufficient knowledge about the condition, the surgical procedure and the anticipated postoperative period
2 Physical preparation required: instruction in deep breathing; isometric exercises; log-rolling for change of position and maintenance of spinal alignment. Blood grouping and cross-matching because of potential for shock
3 Potential for infection due to interruption of continuity of the skin.

Nursing intervention

1. Lack of knowledge. Fear is a common patient response when advised of the need for spinal surgery. The patient is frequently fearful of pain, paralysis and dependency. The nurse determines what the patient and his family have been told by the doctor so that misconceptions may be clarified and certain problems brought to the doctor's attention. A staff member is made available to the patient and family to answer their questions and provide factual information as necessary. If there is a risk of permanent change in functional ability or appearance associated with planned surgery, it is explained by the doctor. The nurse listens to the concerns expressed in response to this, indicates appreciation of their anxiety and recounts the possible assistance and solutions that will be available, emphasizing the positive aspects. If there are socioeconomic concerns, a referral may be made to social service personnel for assistance in solving the problems. Less apprehension and fewer worries contribute to relaxation and more favourable progress postoperatively.

The patient is helped to accept the fact that he will probably experience pain because of nerve root

Table 22.9 Spinal surgical procedures.

	Procedure	Conditions in which used
Laminectomy	Partial or complete removal of the vertebral arch by the two laminae. It precedes other spinal operations to provide access to the canal	Chronic low back pain (disc problems) Spinal fracture (to remove fragments) Cord decompression Removal of a neoplasm
Discectomy	Excision of an intervertebral disc	Ruptured or herniated disc
Spinal fusion	Application of bone grafts to two or more adjoining vertebrae to ankylose them	Ruptured or herniated disc Relieve nerve or cord compression
Rhizotomy	Division or transection of a nerve root either outside or within the spinal canal	Chronic pain
Cordotomy	Division of the pain-conducting pathways (spinothalamic anterolateral tracts) in the spinal cord. Percutaneous cordotomy involves the insertion of a needle (under x-ray) into the spinal cord (See text)	Intractable pain (usually associated with malignant disease)

irritation and oedema, that these will gradually diminish and that support will be available. The possibility of some temporary muscle spasm is discussed; it is less alarming when it occurs if it has been explained previously. The patient is advised how his various needs (food, fluids, elimination etc.) will be met.

2. *Physical preparation* (see Chapter 11). Deep breathing and muscle conditioning exercises (isometric and active) that the patient will be required to do postoperatively are taught and the patient is required to practise these activities. The importance of maintaining spinal alignment following the surgery and how it is achieved are explained and demonstrated; turning as though the body were one unsegmented unit (log-rolling) is practised. If a turning bed is to be used, its purpose and operation are explained and demonstrated to the patient and family.

Spinal operations are usually lengthy procedures, causing the patient to be at greater risk of shock. The patient's blood is grouped and cross-matched and blood is made available. A rigid support such as a back brace, therapeutic corset or bivalve plaster of Paris cast (anterior and posterior shells) may be prepared so that it will be available for early ambulation of the patient.

Local skin preparation entails shaving and cleansing of the back from the shoulders to the lower border of the buttocks and from side to side. Surgery in the cervical region necessitates higher preparation and may require removal of the lower hair and shaving of the lower posterior scalp. If a fusion is planned, similar preparation of the donor area will be necessary (either an iliac crest or a leg is usually the donor site).

INTRAOPERATIVE PHASE

Spinal surgery is usually performed under general anaesthetic. The patient is placed in the prone position, except in an anterior cervical fusion, the skin is prepared and a vertical incision is made. Shock is a potential hazard; the patient usually receives intravenous fluid and blood transfusion. An indwelling urinary catheter may be inserted before the surgery so that an assessment can be made of the general circulation by the rate of urine output by the kidneys.

POSTOPERATIVE PHASE

The care following spinal surgery varies with the particular surgery done, the patient's response to it and the surgeon's preferences. For example some patients are immobilized for weeks while others are ambulated a day or two following the procedure. An understanding of what was done and specific directives are necessary in planning care, especially in relation to positioning and movement. The major principles to be observed with all patients in moving and positioning are the maintenance of proper spinal alignment, the avoidance of any twisting, angulation and jerky movements of the spine and the prevention of strain on the back muscles.

Assessment

The patient's vital signs and responses are monitored at frequent intervals (1–2 hours) for the first 24–48 hours; the interval is gradually lengthened if the patient's condition is stabilized. The chest is auscultated for air entry and retention of pulmonary secretions.

When the surgery is below the thoracic region, assessment includes an evaluation of sensation and motor ability in the lower limbs. The colour and temperature of the limbs and leg and foot pulses may be checked since vascular problems may develop. If the surgery was cervical or high thoracic, close observation of the person's respiratory pattern is necessary as well as sensorimotor responses of the arms. Hoarseness of the voice and ineffective cough may develop due to injury of the recurrent laryngeal nerve.

Wound area(s) are checked for possible haemorrhage, leakage of CSF and contamination. The urinary output is recorded and the abdomen examined for distension.

Any deterioration in vital signs or neurological deficits are brought promptly to the doctor's attention.

Identification of patient problems

1 Potential for spinal injury. Even slight angulation or tension or jerky movements may injure the spine and cause nerve or cord damage
2 Potential for respiratory insufficiency secondary to cord and nerve compression in cervical spinal surgery, immobility and shallow respirations because of the pain
3 Alteration in comfort due to oedema in the operative area, irritation and trauma of nerves at the time of surgery and muscle spasm
4 Alteration in elimination pattern—retention of urine, paralytic ileus, constipation.
5 Potential for wound haemorrhage or infection
6 Alteration in food and fluid intake
7 Potential impairment of skin integrity due to immobility and later due to the wearing of a brace or corset
8 Impairment of mobility: enforced immobility and maintenance of spinal alignment
9 Lack of knowledge. Information is required to prevent recurrence of the back problem and assistance is needed in planning the necessary adjustments in the resumption of activity and management at home.

Nursing intervention

1. *Potential for spinal injury.* A turning bed (e.g. Stryker frame) is prepared to receive the patient. If the regular bed is to be used, it is prepared with fracture boards (if required), a firm mattress and a turning sheet. The latter extends the full length of the spine and buttocks. At least four people are necessary to transfer the patient to the bed to ensure adequate support and good alignment of the spine. Movements must be gentle, smooth and in unison. The patient is positioned flat in the supine position unless a directive is received indicating a specific position (prone, lateral) other than supine. The surgeon usually states the period of time the patient remains in that position before being turned. In the supine position, a small pillow is used to support the head, and pillows are placed under the *full length* of the lower limbs to reduce the strain on the back muscles.

When repositioning is permitted, it is usually done every 2 hours and the patient is reminded of the instructions received preoperatively and is cautioned not to attempt to take an active part in the turning. The patient's arms are folded across his chest and the turning sheet is rolled tightly toward the patient from each side and, with the lifters keeping the sheet taut to provide the necessary support, the patient is eased to one side of the bed. The sheet on that side of the bed is grasped by the persons on the other side of the bed and steadily and gently pulled to roll the patient toward them. An adequate number of personnel is necessary so that one may turn the lower limbs and support the uppermost leg in a slightly flexed position until it can be supported on a pillow. One pillow is placed firmly against the patient's back for support and one placed in front of the patient provides support for the arm that is uppermost.

An alternative method to using a turning sheet is to have three people standing on the same side of the bed who place their hands under the shoulders, back, buttocks and legs and lift the patient over to the side of the bed. Then one nurse moves to the other side of the bed and together they log-roll the patient on to his side. After the first day, some patients are able to turn themselves.

In the case of high thoracic or cervical spinal surgery, a pillow under the head is not permitted in order to avoid even slight flexion of the neck. A small folded towel or piece of sponge rubber may be allowed under the neck for support. The head and neck may be immobilized with sand bags until the patient is fully aware of the importance of not moving his head.

The patient is cautioned against reaching and against pulling on the bed rails. The call-bell and articles needed by the patient are kept within easy reach of him.

2. *Potential for respiratory insufficiency.* If the patient has had surgery in the cervical region of the spine, respiratory difficulty may develop due to postsurgical oedema and compression of nerve pathways carrying impulses to the diaphragm and intercostal muscles. Suction and mechanical respiratory assistance may be required; the necessary emergency respiratory equipment should be readily available (suction apparatus, Ambu bag, intubation tube and ventilator). Rarely, the recurrent laryngeal nerve is also affected and the patient's cough is ineffective in removing secretions. Compression of this nerve also results in temporary hoarseness or loss of voice.

The patient is required to breathe deeply several times at regular frequent intervals; he may find this painful because of the strain placed on the operative site. Its importance is stressed and support provided. When possible it may be timed with the administration of the prescribed analgesic to reduce the discomfort. Coughing is contraindicated. The chest is auscultated frequently for air entry and pulmonary secretions.

3. *Alteration in comfort.* Following spinal surgery, the patient usually experiences considerable pain in the back and in areas to which nerves arising from the affected area are distributed. The pain results from the surgical tissue trauma and ensuing oedema. Spasms of the back and leg muscles frequently occur contributing to the patient's discomfort. If a fusion was done, the donor site may also be painful for several days.

Nursing care includes the administration of the prescribed analgesic, repositioning of the patient, sufficient support of the lower limbs to prevent any strain on the back and good spinal alignment. If the patient required medication for relief of pain for a prolonged period prior to surgery, he may require it more frequently for the first few postoperative days because of his drug tolerance. The patient who has had cervical spinal surgery may also experience a sore throat, temporary loss of voice and dysphagia due to oedema and trauma of the recurrent laryngeal nerve. An oral spray may be prescribed to provide some relief but frequent use of lozenges or the spray which dull or numb oral sensation is avoided because choking and inhalation may occur which cause aggravation of the patient's pain.

4. *Alteration in elimination patterns.* The frequency of voiding and the volume of urinary output are recorded. Urinary retention may occur during the first day or two following spinal surgery. The immobility and positioning contribute to the patient's problem in voiding. Catheterization may be necessary but it should first be determined whether the surgeon would prefer to let the patient out of bed to void rather than use catheterization.

Constipation must be avoided since straining at stool increases pain and CSF pressure. A bulk-producing laxative or stool softener may be prescribed to facilitate defecation without effort. The patient is log-rolled on to a slipper bedpan and a small pillow is used behind the pan to support the back or, the patient may be permitted to use a commode beside the bed. A raised toilet seat is helpful in keeping the spine erect and in reducing discomfort when using a commode or toilet.

5. *Potential for wound haemorrhage or infection.* If the wound dressing remains dry, it usually is left undisturbed for several days or until the sutures are removed in 7–10 days. A pressure dressing (extra padding) may be applied to prevent leakage. In the case of a fusion, the first dressing may be done by the surgeon. If the dressing becomes moist or there is evidence of bleeding or leakage of CSF, the dressing is reinforced and the surgeon notified. If the patient develops an elevation of temperature or there is reason to suspect wound infection, the dressing may be removed earlier for wound inspection. One or more vacuum drains may be inserted into the surrounding tissues. These are emptied and recharged as necessary (e.g. 6–12 hourly), the contents observed and the amount of drainage recorded. The drains are removed after 2–3 days. Protection of the back incision by a dressing may be used for a longer period than with other wounds because of the pressure it is subjected to when the patient is in the supine position or is wearing a brace or therapeutic corset.

6. *Nutrition and fluids.* The patient is allowed sips of fluids the evening of the operation day. The diet is increased over the next 2–3 days as tolerated. Nausea and vomiting, abdominal distension and an absence of bowel sounds may develop following lumbar spinal surgery due to disturbance of autonomic innervation. These symptoms should be reported promptly; a nasogastric tube may be passed and intermittent aspiration or low continuous suction established for gastrointestinal decompression. The patient is sustained by intravenous fluids.

7. *Potential pressure sores.* Because of the immobilization, the skin requires special attention. Vulnerable areas are protected each time the patient is repositioned. Resilient material may be placed under pressure areas for protection as long as it does not interfere with spinal alignment. The under-bedding is kept dry and free of wrinkles and crumbs.

The patient is reminded to move his limbs gently at frequent intervals to reduce possible venous stasis. Elastic or anti-emboli stockings may be recommended especially if the patient has varicosities.

8. *Exercises and ambulation.* Even passive movements of the limbs may be restricted for the first few days. When they are medically approved, they must be done gently and smoothly to prevent any jerking and torsion of the spine. A specific directive is received as to active exercises; these may be started quite early with some patients, whereas with others, especially fusion patients, active exercises are avoided for several weeks. After the sutures are removed and the wound is firmly healed, the patient may be lowered into a warm pool for active and passive exercises under the supervision of a physiotherapist. This type of therapy is particularly helpful if the patient is experiencing considerable muscle spasm.

Except with fusion patients, early ambulation is usually encouraged. If the patient is experiencing pain or is very fearful of moving, it may be advisable to administer the prescribed analgesic 10–20 minutes before getting him up. Two or three persons are required to ensure sufficient support when getting the patient on to his feet, especially the first time. He is gradually reintroduced to a sitting position in bed, to avoid postural hypotension.

When getting out of bed, the patient is brought up into the upright position while his lower limbs are lowered over the side of the bed. The patient is supported while standing and when taking a few steps. His reactions are observed closely: weakness, dizziness and fainting are not uncommon. Only a few steps may be tolerated initially. Sitting may not be permitted for several days; when it is, a firm straight-back chair is used and the periods of sitting are restricted to 10 or 15 minutes. The frequency and length of the 'up' periods are gradually increased. Activities and self-care are introduced and increased according to the doctor's directive and the patient's capacity and responses. Some patients will be required to wear a brace or therapeutic corset while out of bed. The patient should wear a firm walking shoe rather than bedroom slippers.

9. *Inadequate knowledge.* Preparation for discharge to home, the required rehabilitation programme and the resumption of former activities must be individualized on the basis of the nature of the surgery that was done, the patient's response and capacity and whether there are residual disabilities. The activities the patient may do and those he should not do, the important body mechanics in these activities and the exercises to be followed are outlined. Detailed explanations of these are made to the patient and family and assistance is given with their planning of necessary adjustments in home management. If the patient is required to wear a brace or corset, he is advised of the protection of his skin under it as well as the care of the support.

Activity as defined by the surgeon is encouraged; in many instances the patient is fearful of resuming activities and tends to become overdependent. The nurse must be alert for this reaction and provide the necessary reassurance but should expect him to carry out the permitted activities. The patient should be advised that residual pain may be present for some months, especially when he is tired. The importance of keeping the back straight when lying and sitting to lessen stress on the back muscles is stressed. The patient is advised to use a firm mattress (with a board under it if necessary) and when side-lying to place a pillow between his flexed knees. The prone position should always be avoided because of spinal extension and increased strain. The patient is also reminded that his normal body weight should be maintained to prevent stress on his spine.

The patient is followed closely by regular visits to the doctor or outpatient department for a period of 6 months to a year. When the patient goes home, a referral to the community nurse, physiotherapist or rehabilitation unit may be made for on-going guidance and supervision.

Expected outcomes
1 The patient is comfortable and free of pain and muscle spasm
2 Self-care activities and mobility (within the prescribed limits) are resumed
3 The patient complies with the recommended body mechanics and prescribed exercise regimen
4 The wound(s) are dry and healed

5 The patient indicates awareness of the need to prevent overweight, continue the prescribed exercises and follow the instructions about positions and support.

Neoplasms of the Nervous System

INTRACRANIAL NEOPLASMS

Intracranial tumours may be primary or secondary (metastatic), may occur at any age and in any part of the brain. *Primary* neoplasms may be benign or malignant and commonly arise from the neuroglial tissue, meninges, cerebral blood vessels, hypophysis and nerve fibres are named according to their tissue origin (see Table 22.10). Most primary intracranial tumours are gliomas. Unlike neoplasms elsewhere in the body, primary neoplasms of the brain rarely metastasize. *Secondary* intracranial tumours commonly originate in the lungs or breast.

Table 22.10 Intracranial tumours.

Name of neoplasm	Origin	Most frequent sites	Comments
Gliomas	Neuroglial tissue		Commonest type of intracranial neoplasm; rate of growth varies with type of glioma
Astrocytoma	Astrocytes	Adults–cerebrum Children–cerebellum	Most common glioma; grows very slowly; infiltrates surrounding tissue
Glioblastoma	Undifferentiated glial cells	Frontal, parietal and temporal lobes	Highly malignant
Medulloblastoma	Undifferentiated glial cells	Cerebellum	Rapid extension; highly malignant
Ependymoma	Ependymal cells of the lining of the ventricle and aqueducts	Fourth ventricle	Rare; frequently papillomatous; may obstruct flow of CSF
Oligodendroglioma	Oligodendrocytes	Cerebral hemispheres	Rare; grows very slowly; tends to calcify
Meningioma	Meninges	Along the course of the intracranial venous sinuses	Are extracerebral, causing compression of brain tissue; usually encapsulated; grow slowly
Haemangiomas Angioma	Blood vessel wall	Middle cerebral artery	(Not a true neoplasm) Congenital mass of tortuous, enlarged vessels; benign, but may interfere with adjacent tissues
Angioblastoma	Blood vessel wall	Cerebellum	Tendency to form cysts
Pituitary Adenomas Chromophobe adenoma	Adenohypophyseal glandular tissue	Anterior pituitary lobe (adenohypophysis)	Encapsulated; compresses pituitary gland tissue and optic nerves, leading to hypopituitarism and impaired vision
Chromophil adenoma (acidophilic adenoma)	Adenohypophyseal glandular tissue	Anterior pituitary lobe (adenohypophysis)	Seen less often than chromophobe adenoma; causes hyperpituitarism (gigantism or acromegaly)
Craniopharyngioma	Embryological defect in craniopharyngeal duct	Anterior to the pituitary stalk	Produces pressure on surrounding structures, interfering with function
Acoustic neuroma	Eighth cranial (acoustic) nerve		Encapsulated

Brain tumours vary in size, location and pattern of growth. The glioblastomas are highly malignant and invasive while others like the meningiomas are benign and compressive. This accounts for the great variability in the development of symptoms and in the prognosis following surgery. Most brain tumours in the adult tend to occur in the supratentorial compartment (above the brain stem and cerebellum).

ASSESSMENT

Manifestations

Any intracranial neoplasm is a space-occupying lesion; as it grows, intracranial content and pressure increase within the rigid cranium. Signs and symptoms result from gradual or rapidly developing compression, invasion and infiltration of brain tissue; cerebral oedema, ischaemia and destruction of the tissue surrounding the neoplasm may develop due to compression. The manifestations reflect the location; neurological deficits (sensory and/or motor) and behavioural changes appear as the tumour imposes on specific cerebral areas, some deficiency in mental capacity may develop and seizures may occur due to alterations in the electrical potential of cells. Hydrocephalus may develop if there is interference of the normal flow and absorption of CSF, and endocrine imbalances may occur associated with the compression or invasion of the pituitary gland.

The signs and symptoms change and intensify as the tumour expands and intracranial pressure progressively increases. Symptoms include:

- Papilloedema and visual changes such as diplopia, reduced acuity and field of vision, absence of normal reflexes
- Impairment of motor function: loss of coordination, weakness, rigidity of one side, paralysis
- Sensory dysfunction: loss or distortion
- Impairment of speech
- Headache which may be localized or generalized and is worsened by any activity which increases intracranial pressure such as coughing, vomiting, bending over and straining at stool
- Fits/seizures
- Changes in mental functioning: loss of memory and ability to reason, lethargy, reduced attention span, drowsiness, disorientation, change in personality, emotional lability, hallucinations, psychotic episodes. There may be loss of consciousness in the later stage
- Sudden vomiting (without preceding nausea) which usually occurs early in the morning or with a position change
- Vital signs change as the intracranial pressure increases; the blood pressure increases, the pulse is slower and the respiratory pattern changes

All intracranial neoplasms are potentially lethal due to the destruction of brain tissue and the increased intracranial pressure; brain herniation may occur due to the increased intracranial pressure.

Diagnostic procedures

An extensive neurological examination is made and investigative procedures include ophthalmological tests (examination of the fundus and visual acuity and fields), brain scan, electroencephalogram, echoencephalogram, lumbar puncture and spinal fluid studies, and cerebral angiogram. Endocrine studies may be done to determine if there is involvement of the pituitary gland. Chest x-rays are made to rule out metastasis from the lungs. The skull may also be x-rayed; if an intracranial mass is present, a pineal shift may be evident. When surgery is done, a biopsy is obtained to determine the type of neoplasm and whether it is benign or malignant. Details of previous history may indicate a metastatic tumour (i.e. former diagnosis of primary lung or breast cancer).

MEDICAL MANAGEMENT

The treatment used for a brain tumour depends on the location and type of neoplasm and the condition of the patient. It may involve surgery, radiation and/or chemotherapy. Whenever possible, surgical excision of the neoplasm is the method of choice but in some instances it may be inaccessible or involve vital areas (e.g. brain stem) making removal impossible. Non-encapsulated neoplasms infiltrate surrounding tissue, making surgery less effective. In some instances, surgical decompression is indicated to relieve compression symptoms by a craniotomy (see p. 813). If the lesion is obstructing the CSF and is inoperable a palliative shunt may be done involving the placement of a tube between the lateral ventricle and the subarachnoid space in the posterior fossa below the brain (cistern magna) or between the ventricle and the superior vena cava or the peritoneal cavity. Radiotherapy is employed with tumours which are surgically inaccessible or which cannot be entirely excised. It is effective in slowing the progress of some primary neoplasms (e.g. gliomas) and metastases, improving the quality of the patient's life as well as lengthening it. Radiation may cause temporary cerebral oedema and an increased intracranial pressure; a corticosteroid preparation may be administered to lessen these side-effects. Hair loss may result from irradiation to the head.

Certain chemotherapeutic drugs, for example carmustine (BiCNU), lomustine (CCNU), may be used alone or in combination with surgery or radiation. However, many of the cytotoxic drugs are unable to penetrate the blood–brain barrier, if it remains intact.

Nursing the patient with a brain tumour

Assessment

An initial evaluation is made and recorded of the

patient's motor and sensory functions, speech ability, orientation, behavioural responses, pupillary reactions and any complaints of headache, dizziness and tingling or numbness of a part. Assessment is an on-going process through successive contacts so that changes and newly developed symptoms may be recognized promptly. The nurse's recognition and recording of physical and behavioural changes may play an important role in the diagnosis and localization of the intracranial tumour. Knowing that a space-occupying lesion is suspect, the nurse is especially alert for signs of increasing intracranial pressure (see p. 807). The patient's and family's understanding of the condition and reactions are evaluated in order to plan how they may be assisted and supported and to establish a helping relationship.

Identification of patient problems
Nursing care is planned according to the patient's needs which are determined by the disturbances, dysfunctions and dependence caused by the intracranial lesion. These generally include the following nursing diagnoses:
1 Potential for injury due to sensory and motor deficits, impaired cognitive functioning and seizures
2 Fear and depression due to what is perceived as a threat to independency, appearance, life-style and life itself
3 Alteration in comfort: headache due to cerebral oedema and increased intracranial pressure
4 Alteration in food and fluid intake secondary to the patient's fear, lethargy, drowsiness and inactivity
5 Self-care deficits due to sensory and motor deficits and lethargy.

Nursing intervention

1. Potential for injury. The patient is at risk of injury because of changes in motor and sensory functions, disorientation, impaired vision and possible convulsions. Nursing care includes safety precautions such as padded cot-sides on the bed, convulsion precautions (see p. 854), assistance if necessary in ambulation and close observation for behavioural disturbances. An anticonvulsant drug such as phenytoin (Epanutin) may be prescribed to control fits. Frequent repetition of information may be necessary to maintain the patient's orientation as much as possible.
The patient is kept mobile and active in self-care, if his condition permits, to prevent the complications of immobility.

2. Fear and depression. The patient with a brain tumour who is able to comprehend his condition may experience fear of mutilation, loss of mental functioning and independence, disability and death. No single intervention can entirely relieve his con-

cern but an understanding and supportive approach helps. Acknowledging the patient's fear as understandable, encouraging him to talk about his concerns, express his feelings and ask questions may ease the situation somewhat for him. Information is provided to prepare the patient for investigative procedures and treatment and, when appropriate, the patient is involved in making decisions which concern him.
The family's anxiety is understandable. Their strengths and weaknesses that may have implications for the patient's progress are identified. They are kept informed about the patient, what is being done for him and how they may support him. Opportunities are provided for them to ask questions and express their concerns. In some instances, it may be necessary to suggest to the family that they avoid conveying their emotions to the patient. Information about the hospital chaplaincy service may be useful to the patient and family.

3. Alteration in comfort. The patient with an intracranial neoplasm is likely to experience severe headache. The head of the bed is elevated about 30° to promote cerebral venous drainage and an ice-bag or cold compresses applied. A mild analgesic such as acetylsalicylic acid (aspirin) or paracetamol may be prescribed. Stronger analgesics are avoided unless the pain becomes very severe and uncontrollable, because they tend to mask neurological changes that might occur. To reduce intracranial pressure, osmotic diuresis may be induced by the intravenous administration of mannitol (Osmitrol) or a hypertonic solution of glucose and urea (Ureaphil). These preparations are not reabsorbed by the renal tubules, and, by their osmotic action, they reduce the amount of water reabsorbed from the glomerular filtrate and increase the urinary output. A corticosteroid preparation such as dexamethasone may be given to reduce cerebral oedema and relieve the headache. A reversal of some symptoms may also occur with the decrease in intracranial pressure. Corticosteroids suppress the immune response and lower the patient's resistance to stress and infection. Precautions are used to protect the patient and close observations made for early indications of infection. If the administration of a corticosteroid preparation is prolonged, gastric irritation may develop; an antacid may be prescribed and the drug is given with food.
The nurse changes the patient's position at frequent intervals or prompts the patient to make the change, if he is lethargic, listless or drowsy. Repositioning contributes to his comfort as well as protects the skin from prolonged pressure and breakdown.

4. Alteration in food and fluid intake. Nutritional and fluid deficits may occur. The patient's fear, lethargy, drowsiness and inactivity decrease desire for and interest in food and fluids. Dietary preferences are identified and the preferred foods offered in small servings four or five times a day. Foods that are high in calories and provide the essential food elements are selected. It may be necessary to increase the roughage content if constipation is a problem because of inactivity and analgesics. The fluid intake and output are recorded and the fluid balance determined every 8 hours.

The patient may require assistance with his meals to ensure an adequate intake. This may also apply in relation to the fluid intake.

5. Self-care activities. The patient may have to be assisted with personal care, meals and toileting. In order to keep the patient mobile, it may be necessary to have the patient change position, stand and walk at intervals; assistance may be necessary to prevent falls.

For preoperative and postoperative nursing care of the patient being treated by surgery see p. 811. If radiation and/or chemotherapy is used see Chapter 9.

Expected outcomes
1 Intracranial pressure is reduced
2 Headache is relieved
3 The patient is more alert, oriented and assuming self-care activities
4 The patient is free of seizures
5 Nutritional and hydrational status is improved.

SPINAL NEOPLASMS

Spinal tumours may be benign or malignant, primary or secondary (metastatic) and may be classified according to their location as extradural or intradural. Primary spinal tumours are less common than those of the brain. *Extradural neoplasms* occur in the vertebrae, the extradural space or paraspinal tissue. They are usually metastases from the lungs, breast, kidney, prostate or gastrointestinal tract. As they enlarge they encroach on the cord because of the limited space, causing pressure on the cord and nerve roots. *Intradural* neoplasms are extramedullary (outside the cord within or under the dura), intramedullary which arise within the cord or, intradural–extramedullary. The latter type constitute a large majority of spinal neoplasms and may arise from the meninges (meningioma), nerve roots (neuromas or neurofibromas) or blood vessels (haemangiomas). Gliomas comprise the majority of intramedullary neoplasms. Fifty per cent of all spinal tumours occur in the thoracic area.

ASSESSMENT

Manifestations
The effects of spinal neoplasms develop as a result of mechanical irritation and compression of spinal nerve roots, compression and displacement of the spinal cord and compression of blood vessels, reducing the blood supply to the structures. The symptoms are similar to those which occur in spinal injury but the sensory and motor dysfunctions develop more slowly. The parts of the body affected depend on the level of the lesion. In the case of nerve root involvement, the affected areas correspond to those innervated by the nerve fibres derived from that particular nerve root. Involvement of cord tracts and neurons may interfere with functions in all parts on one or both sides of the body which derive their innervation below the level of the neoplasm.

The pathological progress may occur in three stages. In the first stage unilateral nerve root irritation causes abnormal sensations and pain. The pain is intensified by coughing, sneezing or with certain movements. This stage may be referred to as the radicular syndrome because of its association with spinal nerve roots.

In the second stage, cord compression begins causing muscle weakness and atrophy possibly progressing to paralysis on the same side of the body as the neoplasm. Muscle spasms may occur. There is also a progressive sensory impairment in corresponding areas (loss of sense of touch, pressure and proprioception). For example, the patient may be unable to identify the position of his affected limbs. Deterioration in the pain and temperature sensations occurs on the contralateral side of the body.

In the third stage, signs of complete cord transection occurs manifested by complete paralysis and loss of sphincter control below the level of the lesion. Sensory loss is more marked.

In summary signs and symptoms of a spinal neoplasm include:
- Abnormal sensations (e.g. tingling, 'pins and needles') and pain
- Progressive muscle weakness and atrophy
- Flaccid paralysis
- Exaggerated deep tendon reflexes
- Muscle spasms
- Loss of sensations (for example, pressure, pain, temperature, proprioception)
- Bladder and bowel dysfunction

Diagnostic procedures
An extensive examination is made to evaluate neurological functioning. Investigative procedures include spinal x-rays, a myelogram (see p. 788) and electromyogram (see p. 786). A lumbar puncture and a Queckenstedt's test are done to determine if there is an obstruction to the flow of CSF. A CSF specimen may be analysed for cellular and protein content.

MEDICAL MANAGEMENT

Spinal neoplasms may be treated by surgery, radiation and/or chemotherapy.

Primary extramedullary neoplasms are removed by surgery as soon as diagnosed; unnecessary delay may result in permanent cord damage and paralysis. Intramedullary newgrowths are more difficult to remove without seriously damaging the cord and interrupting motor and sensory tracts. When the neoplasm is inoperable or metastatic, relief of compression of the cord by laminectomy and possibly partial resection of the tumour may be undertaken. Radiation therapy of the involved area or chemotherapy may be used as an adjunct to surgery or alone.

Patient's problems and nursing care are parallel to those cited for the patient who has had spinal surgery on p. 830.

Degenerative Disorders

Commonly occurring degenerative disorders of the nervous system include Alzheimer's disease, multiple sclerosis, Parkinson's disease, myasthenia gravis and motor neurone disease.

ALZHEIMER'S DISEASE

Alzheimer's disease is a *presenile dementia* of unknown aetiology and is the most common degenerative brain disorder.[4] A history of familial incidence is considered to play a role in the development of the disease. Approximately 20% of all institutionalized psychiatric patients have the disease and it is estimated that 5–10% of the remainder of the population over 65 years of age is also affected.[5] The disease is eventually fatal.

Alzheimer's disease is indistinguishable from senile dementia (loss of intellectual capacity) except that the age of onset is earlier, beginning between 45 and 65 years of age. Both males and females are equally affected. The frontal and temporal lobes are most affected but gradual progressive atrophy of the entire brain occurs. Microscopically, there is widespread loss of nerve cells.

Clinical course and effects
In the progress of the disease three stages may be identified. The first stage lasts 2–4 years and is characterized by subtle changes which may be dismissed as inattention or carelessness. Eventually, there are recognizable changes in personality, loss of memory for recent and remote events, apathy, loss of spontaneity and initiative, neglect of personal hygiene and appearance, and a suspiciousness of other's motives with a tendency to blame them for one's incapacities. Loss of spatial orientation is seen in the inability to put on a garment without confusion as to top and bottom and sleeve and neck. Weakness, muscular twitching or seizures may occur, and motor aphasia (the person cannot recall words he wishes to say) and speech slurring may become evident. Indifference to social customs and graces develops.

In the second stage of the disease, the changes of the first stage intensify. Disorientation is complete; emotional lability increases and there may be restlessness at night. Memory loss becomes so severe that even close friends and relatives are not recognized and the patient may not recognize himself in the mirror. Movements are slow and simple writing, reading, mathematical skills and reasoning deteriorate seriously. Other deficiencies such as inability to recognize objects by way of the senses become obvious. Motor dysfunction may progress from unsteady gait to inability to stand or walk. The person loses weight due to poor nutrition; he shows no interest in meals.

In the final stage of the disease movements become stereotyped, there is inability to use language, urinary and bowel incontinence, abnormal reflexes and muscular rigidity develop and eventually, there is flexion of the lower extremities and the individual becomes bedridden and totally helpless. There is a marked tendency to grasp objects and put them to the mouth. The disease may last for several years. Death usually results from bronchopneumonia or infected pressure sores.

ASSESSMENT

The diagnosis of Alzheimer's disease is made on the basis of the neurological history and examination. Extensive investigative procedures are usually done to rule out treatable conditions. There is no known treatment for the disease but tranquillizers may be prescribed to minimize the more abnormal behaviours.

IDENTIFICATION OF PATIENT PROBLEMS

1 Ineffective coping because of altered cognitive functioning
2 Potential for injury due to loss of memory, impaired motor and cognitive functioning
3 Self-care deficits in relation to adequate rest, nutrition and personal hygiene
4 Alteration in elimination patterns: urinary and bowel incontinence
5 Potential for social isolation secondary to loss of interest, initiative and memory (friends and relatives not recognized)
6 Potential for complications:
   (a) Respiratory dysfunction secondary to inactivity and lowered resistance to infection
   (b) Impairment of skin integrity secondary to immobility, incontinence, malnutrition and injury.
7 Inadequate knowledge.

[4] Adams & Victor (1981), p. 796.
[5] Dewlis & Bauman (1982), p. 33.

NURSING INTERVENTION

1. Ineffective coping. In the early stage, the patient and particularly the family require considerable counselling. Expectations of the patient's abilities should be lowered. The patient needs to be understood and accepted as he is because his memory cannot be restored nor his behaviour changed. A written outline of the activities of daily living to be carried out may prove helpful. For example, if the person is to carry out an errand away from home, it may be useful to him to refer to a written directive.

Each day, the patient identifies a few essential tasks on which to focus since coping with more than these is too difficult.

2. Potential for injury. The environment is kept free of hazards and stress as much as possible. As disorientation develops and as body movements become increasingly more awkward the risk of falls increases. The patient may forget that a cigarette is burning or that a stove burner has been turned on. With progressive loss of memory, the person requires close supervision. It is important that he carries identification in case of wandering off and becoming lost and exposed to the elements. It should be remembered that restlessness and disorientation are likely to be worse at night when sensory stimuli are minimal and there is some decrease in cerebral perfusion.

The patient can usually manage for a longer period and be capable of doing more if in the familiar surroundings of his home where a 'mechanical like' routine is established.

3. Self-care deficits. Regular periods of rest are planned for the person: fatigue tends to aggravate the manifestations of deterioration. Some patients respond to relaxation therapy tapes. The daily food and fluid intake are noted and the patient is weighed at regular intervals. In the early stage of Alzheimer's disease, the patient gradually loses the appreciation of nutritional needs. The home-maker becomes unable to shop and prepare food and eventually skips meals. Prompting and assistance with meals and in-between snacks are necessary to ensure that the patient gets sufficient. High calorie foods and supplements are used when necessary. Plans are made to provide hygienic care as neglect becomes obvious. Provision is made for bathing, grooming, dressing, the wearing of incontinence pads if necessary and frequent change of washable clothing.

4. Alteration in elimination pattern. With progression of Alzheimer's disease, the patient develops urinary and bowel incontinence. A schedule for prompting the patient to go to the toilet at intervals determined by customary elimination frequency may help in avoiding incontinence. When the patient is incontinent, the perineum and surrounding area are cleansed and dried promptly to prevent excoriation. Constipation may be a problem due to the immobility and reduced food intake. The roughage content of the diet may be increased and a mild laxative (bulk-producing or stool softener) administered. If the constipation is not recognized and corrected, faecal impaction develops readily.

5. Potential for social isolation. The patient tends to avoid social situations as his cognitive and communicative skills diminish. Efforts should be made for his exposure to human interaction and for socialization just as long as they have even the slightest meaning. Including the person in short social events and in small-group affairs could be helpful.

6. Potential for complications. Because of the inactivity and malnutrition, the patient is predisposed to respiratory infection. An exercise programme, walking, deep breathing and coughing, adequate nutrition as well as protection from exposure to those with an infection contribute to the prevention of respiratory infection.

As the immobility, helplessness and malnutrition worsen, the patient becomes more and more predisposed to pressure sores. Regular bathing, careful observation and protection of vulnerable areas, repositioning at regular intervals and prompt changing of clothing or bedding following incontinence are necessary. Injury to the skin may occur as a result of a fall; any abrasion or laceration is cleansed with an antiseptic and protected.

7. Inadequate knowledge. Some major adjustments in the life-style and relationships of the family, as well as the patient, are necessary as the disease advances. Planning for these at an early stage of the disorder facilitates the change process as it becomes necessary. Although the life span of the person with Alzheimer's disease cannot be protracted, the quality of the life of all those concerned can be enhanced through early professional intervention, counselling and effective planning. It is helpful to introduce the family to the local branch of the Alzheimer's Society.[6] The association provides family support through meetings, pamphlets and community referrals. The Society also provides education for the general public.

In the early stages, the family is advised of ways to help the patient maintain independence and carry on at home. The family is informed of signs of progression of the disorder and how members can best cope with increasing dependency of the patient. They are alerted to the hazards that may develop with the increasing dementia. When the affected person is no longer productive, roles and relationships must change. It is particularly difficult when a formerly

[6] Alzheimer's Disease Society, 3rd Floor, Bank Building, Fulham Broadway, London, SW6 1EP.

responsible and productive person becomes dependent upon others for decision-making and personal care. The process of adjustments is slow and requires understanding and acceptance of the patient's condition. The family's reactions may indicate the need for a referral for professional counselling.

In the later stages of the disorder, management focuses on helping the family cope with extremely problematic situations. Institutionalization of the patient usually becomes necessary and the family may need considerable persuasion and support in making this decision.

EXPECTED OUTCOMES

1 The patient:
   (a) Is able to carry out self-care activities, is mobile and continent and responds to family and friends and participates in selected social functions.
   (b) Maintains adequate nutritional intake as evidenced by body weight.
   (c) Is free of complications.
2 The family members:
   (a) Are understanding and accepting of the situation.
   (b) Plan and make informed decisions and adjustments to assist the patient to be independent for as long as possible.
   (c) Make the necessary adjustments and arrangements for care as changes occur in the patient's condition.

MULTIPLE SCLEROSIS (MS, DISSEMINATED SCLEROSIS)

Multiple sclerosis is a chronic, progressive, degenerative disease that is characterized by patches of demyelination throughout the brain and spinal cord. Myelin is the lipoprotein sheath surrounding the axons of the neurons and enables impulses to travel much faster along the fibre than is possible in unmyelinated fibres. The destruction of areas of myelin is followed by a proliferation of neuroglial cells. Scar tissue forms as hardened (sclerotic) white elevations known as plaque. Nerve fibres (axons) eventually degenerate; there is loss of impulse transmission and focal deficits occur which in some instances may be permanent. The optic nerves and the cervical spinal cord tend to be most vulnerable to this degenerative demyelinating process in the initial episodes.

Incidence and population at risk
Multiple sclerosis has a worldwide distribution and affects 40–60 people per 100 000 of the population. People are twice as likely to be stricken if they live in cold damp climates. The United Kingdom has been recognized as a high risk zone; in north-east Scotland and Ulster, the incidence is 100 per 100 000 popu-

lation, and in the Shetlands and Orkney, 300 per 100 000.[7] The onset of the disease is highest amongst persons aged 17–30 years with a slightly higher incidence among women. A familial tendency has been recognized but a definite genetic pattern has not been identified.

Aetiology
The specific cause of multiple sclerosis continues to elude scientists; current evidence suggests that genetic factors, environmental factors, viruses and the individual's immune system may be collectively implicated. The view that viral infection and an immunological abnormality interact to induce the central nervous system damage is particularly favoured.

ASSESSMENT

Clinical course and manifestations
Multiple sclerosis is characterized by remissions and relapses. The course and the effects vary widely from one person to another and are unpredictable. Spontaneous remissions of varying lengths are common particularly in the early years of the disease, and in some instances appear to be permanent. Rarely multiple sclerosis takes a fulminating, malignant course in which a combination of cerebral brain stem and cord manifestations develop suddenly; the patient becomes comatose; there is no remission and death may occur within a few weeks.

Most patients survive more than 20 years after the initial onset and lead active productive lives for many of those years. A lesser number experience a steady progression of their disease with frequently recurring relapses leading to a chronic incapacitated state, dependency and complications.

The initial onset of symptoms of multiple sclerosis usually develops suddenly (within a day or two) but with some, may develop slowly over several weeks. The initial onset of exacerbation usually coincides with a stressful experience such as anxiety, trauma, infection, excessive fatigue, exposure to an extreme of temperature and pregnancy.

Since the location and extent of the demyelinization are so variable, the signs and symptoms also are highly variable from one patient to another. They may include the following:
● Extreme fatigue
● Visual dysfunction (e.g. diplopia, blurring of vision, nystagmus)
● Transient tingling sensations or numbness (paraesthesia) or loss of sensation
● Intention tremor
● Ataxia
● Muscular weakness in one or both arms and legs
● Paraparesis

---

[7] Matthews (1978).

- Bladder and bowel dysfunction
- Impairment of speech (scanning)
- Emotional lability: alternating periods of euphoria, depression and irritability
- Personality changes
- Cognitive dysfunction; loss of memory and confusion

Deficits which persist beyond 3 months are usually permanent. Weakness of the respiratory muscles and cough reflex may develop, predisposing the patient to pulmonary complications.

Diagnosis
At present there are no specific diagnostic tests for multiple sclerosis. Several procedures such as CAT scan, spinal and skull x-rays and myelogram may be done to rule out other causes. A lumbar puncture may be done and the CSF analysed for increased gamma globulin and protein levels which are characteristic of most patients with multiple sclerosis. The ability of the eyes to react to flashing lights is evaluated (visual evoked response) or other evoked responses may be tested (e.g. auditory). Delayed or less than the expected response is considered suggestive of demyelinization.

MEDICAL MANAGEMENT

There is no cure for multiple sclerosis; the treatment is symptomatic and supportive which increases in amount and complexity as the patient's disease progresses. Corticosteroids have been used to reduce the intensity and duration of relapses but this therapy is controversial. There is no consensus on the role of any specific dietary measures. Physiotherapy is prescribed for most patients to promote activity and independence as long as possible.

IDENTIFICATION OF PATIENT PROBLEMS

1 Inadequate or inaccurate knowledge about the disorder, health maintenance and management of a remission
2 Alteration in self-image and fear due to the potential change in life-style, disability and dependence
3 Potential remissions; adjustments in activities to maintain health
4 Impaired mobility secondary to muscular weakness, fatigue, ataxia and/or paralysis
5 Potential for injury because of difficulty in walking
6 Potential sensory deficits: abnormal vision and diminished cutaneous sensation may occur
7 Alteration in pattern of elimination:
    (a) Urinary frequency, urgency or incontinence
    (b) Constipation
8 Alteration in nutritional status due to loss of appetite secondary to anxiety and depression,

weakened mastication and swallowing muscles and/or inability to prepare meals
9 Self-care deficits due to muscular weakness or paralysis, immobility and depression
10 Impairment of verbal communication secondary to weakness or paralysis of the muscles involved in producing speech
11 Potential for complications:
    (a) Impairment of skin integrity
    (b) Respiratory insufficiency and infection

NURSING INTERVENTION

Nursing *goals* are to:
1 Promote understanding and acceptance of the disorder
2 Promote patient understanding of the importance of avoiding precipitating factors
3 Maintain patient independency as long as possible
4 Assist with the necessary adjustments in the home
5 Prevent injuries and complications

Good counselling and care may contribute to the prevention of relapses as well as help to keep the patient active and independent for as long as possible. Institutional care usually becomes necessary when complete dependence has been reached or when secondary conditions such as bladder or pulmonary infection or pressure sores intervene.

1. Inadequate knowledge.   The patient and his family are informed about multiple sclerosis, the nature of the disease, effects, the fact that relapses of varying length occur and the potential precipitating factors in relapses. They are advised that it is not possible to predict the course of the disorder. Management is discussed in detail with emphasis on continuing former activities and gainful employment and the necessary modifications in life-style to avoid those factors known to contribute to a recurrence of symptoms. Important factors in the prevention of potential injuries and complications are outlined.

Community resources of assistance are made known to the patient and family. These include the Multiple Sclerosis Society,[8] social services and community nurses. During relapses, or as the disorder progresses leaving residual disability, assistive devices (e.g. wheelchair), asssistance with physical care and/or home management, financial assistance and support and encouragement may become necessary. The local branch of the Multiple Sclerosis Society is an excellent source of information and assistance. For example, it helps in securing assistive devices, transporting patients to the physiotherapy department or clinic and contacting other resources for assistance (e.g. Social Service Department) if

---

[8] Multiple Sclerosis Society of Great Britain and Northern Ireland, 286 Munster Road, London, SW6 6AP.

necessary. The society also has voluntary workers who make home visits and arrange occupational and recreational programmes for multiple sclerosis patients. If the patient's former occupation is too strenuous or stressful, vocational retraining may be appropriate so that the person can return to gainful employment during remissions. The Action for Research into Multiple Sclerosis[9] is also a useful society.

2. Alteration in self-image and fears. The changes in body function and capacity and increasing loss of independence alter the patient's image of self. Roles and relationships change and responsibilities shift. Sensory and motor deficits which occur with multiple sclerosis frequently lead to impaired sexual functioning which may affect relationships. Fear of the long-term consequences of the disease, increasing dependency and the reactions of others are threatening. Both patient and family are likely to experience the stages of grief reaction as they come to grips with the realities of the situation. Nursing care involves acceptance of their reactions, supportive understanding and open discussion of concerns. Anxiety and depression on the part of the patient and family may delay the process of acceptance of the diagnosis and imposed adjustments and limitations. Efforts to assist them with their planning for management may not be effective. Psychiatric counselling may be appropriate.

3. Maintenance of health. In early remissions when the residual effects are likely to be minimal, the patient is encouraged to resume his usual pattern of life, modifying it as necessary to avoid overfatigue, emotional stress and infections since these may precipitate a relapse. Regular and adequate rest, a well-balanced diet and learning to accept what cannot be readily changed to avoid emotional stress reduce the risk of an exacerbation.

In the case of the female patient, menstruation and fertility are unaffected but she is advised of the increased risk of a relapse incurred by pregnancy. In addition, delivery may be complicated by spasms of the hip adductor muscles. Contraceptive pills may aggravate symptoms of multiple sclerosis. Intrauterine devices are not usually recommended because pelvic inflammatory disease or other problems could remain undetected as a result of impaired sensation.

4. Impaired mobility. Muscle spasticity and weakness, especially in the lower limbs, is a common disabling factor in multiple sclerosis. A carefully controlled physiotherapy programme is instituted within the patient's tolerance to keep him active and prevent muscle contractures and atrophy. Exercises

in a warm pool reduce the spasticity. Close observation is made for signs of excessive fatigue and a rest period should follow the exercise period.

A walking stick or crutches may be necessary to assist the patient in maintaining mobility. Walking between parallel bars may be helpful. When walking becomes impossible, a wheelchair is provided and the patient is taught to transfer himself from the bed to chair and from chair to toilet if he has sufficient strength in his arms. Instruction is given in manoeuvring the chair from room to room and outside if possible to widen the patient's horizon and prevent isolation. In the case of the home-maker, adjustments in the kitchen and around the home may be made to permit the patient to continue usual activities. An occupational therapist will assess the situation and make work simplification suggestions.

Family members require instructions on how to transfer the patient from the wheelchair to the bed and vice versa if the patient is experiencing weakness or motor deficit in the upper limbs.

A period of rest between activities is imperative; overexertion and fatigue reduce functional reserve and increase the patient's frustration and depression. Tolerance for all activities increases with regular activity alternated with regular periods of rest and sleep.

Muscle spasticity may become a painful problem in the disabled limbs. Passive movements of the affected limbs may reduce the spasticity and prevent contractures. A muscle relaxant, for example dantrolene sodium (Dantrium), may be prescribed. The patient's response to the drug is observed; the dosage is decreased if the patient becomes drowsy.

5. Potential for injury. The patient is at risk of injury especially as walking becomes increasingly more difficult. In order to prevent falls, floors are kept clear of scatter rugs, stools, electric flexes and other articles over which the patient might trip. Hand-rails in appropriate places facilitate safer mobility. Shoes that provide firm support and have non-slip soles are worn. Articles that are needed for self-care and the performance of chores are kept within easy reach. As disability increases judicious use of safety devices such as cot-sides is necessary.

6. Potential sensory deficits. Sensory deficits such as impaired vision and diminished temperature and pressure sensations increase the patient's potential for injury. If a portion of the visual field is affected, the patient learns to turn his head in order to bring objects into the range of his vision. Diplopia may be relieved by the wearing of an eye patch on one eye and then periodically placing it on the other eye. The patient and family are taught safety measures to prevent burns; for example control of the temperature of food and beverages as well as bath water. Areas of diminished sensation are inspected daily for irritation and injury.

---

[9] Action for Research into Multiple Sclerosis (ARMS), 71 Grays Inn Road, London, WC1X 8TR.

7. *Alteration in pattern of elimination.* Urinary frequency and urgency are common problems for the patient with multiple sclerosis. Later, as the disease progresses, loss of sphincter control and incontinence develops. The patient is advised to set up a regular schedule for going to the toilet to avoid the distress caused by urgency and dribbling or incontinence. If the patient's mobility is impaired, a prompt response to the patient's request for assistance is necessary.

Some patients experience urinary retention or may not completely empty their bladder when voiding. Methods to facilitate voiding are employed (see Chapter 21). The use of catheterization is avoided if possible because of the risk of ascending urinary tract infection. If catheterization becomes necessary, strict asepsis is observed, a high fluid intake is encouraged (3000 ml daily) and regular assessment is made for infection (temperature, culture of urine).

Constipation is a frequent problem as a result of the reduced mobility. The roughage and bulk content in the diet is increased as well as the fruit juice and water intake. A bulk-producing laxative or stool softener may be necessary to prevent faecal impaction. If the patient does not have adequate defecation for 3 days, measures to promote evacuation are instituted.

8. *Alteration in nutritional status.* The patient's weight is recorded at regular intervals since the food intake is frequently reduced due to a poor appetite which develops due to the patient's anxiety, immobility, weakness in mastication and swallowing, or the patient's inability to shop and prepare meals.

Well-balanced meals that are easily digested are necessary; the food intake is monitored. High-calorie fluids and blender foods may be necessary in order to meet the patient's requirements for energy, tissue maintenance and resistance. If the patient is overweight, a decreased caloric intake is prescribed to reduce the burden on weakened muscles.

9. *Self-care deficits.* Nursing care includes repeated assessments of the patient's ability to complete self-care which may become increasingly difficult as the disease progresses and the provision of the care needed. For example, muscular weakness or paralysis of the arms may prevent the patient from cleaning his teeth and combing his hair. Food particles and mucus may accumulate in the mouth if swallowing is difficult, necessitating mouth care after each meal.

10. *Impairment of verbal communication.* The speech may progressively become slower and more difficult as muscular weakness increases, creating frustration for both the patient and those caring for him. Time should be allowed for him to communicate and every effort made to understand him. Referral to a speech therapist may be helpful. Nursing care includes support and reinforcement of the therapy, talking with the patient and encouraging his verbal response and acknowledging even slight achievement.

11. *Potential for complications.*
(a) *Pressure sores.* As mobility and sensory perception deteriorate, the potential for skin breakdown increases. Frequent change of position, keeping the skin clean and dry and careful observation and protection of vulnerable areas are necessary. The prescribed exercise regimen helps to promote tissue perfusion which contributes to the prevention of pressure sores. Vulnerable areas may be protected by pieces of sheepskin or an alternating air pressure (ripple) mattress.
(b) *Respiratory insufficiency and infection.* Immobility and weakness of respiratory muscles resulting in shallow respirations and difficulty in expectorating secretions predispose the patient to pulmonary infection. Respiratory volumes are assessed and the chest is auscultated at regular intervals to determine respiratory status. The patient is instructed to take several deep breaths and to cough at regular intervals. Frequent repositioning is also encouraged to prevent stasis of pulmonary secretions. Progressive weakness of the respiratory muscles and increasing immobility necessitate oropharyngeal suction and chest physiotherapy. Contact with those who are potential sources of infection is avoided (e.g. family members or friends with upper respiratory infection).

EXPECTED OUTCOMES

1 The patient and family indicate understanding of:
  (a) The nature of the disease and the potential course and outcome.
  (b) Factors which may precipitate a relapse.
  (c) Potential complications and their prevention.
2 Informed decisions are made to utilize appropriate resources (e.g. local branch of Multiple Sclerosis Society) and make the necessary adjustments for home management and to maintain potential patient independence.
3 The patient shows signs of a remission of the disease process; maintains self-care, mobility and socialization according to functional level; maintains normal weight; communicates effectively; participates actively in the prescribed exercise programme; and has control of voiding and defecation. The patient also shows an interest in vocational retraining.
4 The patient is free of complications.

IDIOPATHIC PARKINSON'S DISEASE (PARALYSIS AGITANS)

Parkinson's disease is a complex clinical syndrome associated with a decreased concentration of the chemical dopamine and its major metabolite. Dopamine is produced by the substantia nigra (black substance), a nucleus of highly pigmented cells in the midbrain which function as a part of the extrapyramidal system. The chemical is delivered via the neuronal axons to the basal ganglia where it appears to be essential for normal neurotransmission and functioning of the basal ganglia. Dopamine exerts an inhibitory effect on movements by opposing or lessening the stimulating effect of acetylcholine. When a deficiency of dopamine occurs, tremors, rigidity, slowness and limited voluntary movement become evident.

Types, aetiology and incidence
Several forms of Parkinson's disease occur. They are classified according to the cause and include: post-encephalitic, drug-induced, atherosclerotic, toxic, post-traumatic and idiopathic Parkinson's disease. Other than the idiopathic form of the disease, those cited rarely occur.

As the term implies, the cause of idiopathic Parkinson's disease is unknown. A consistent finding is a decreased concentration of dopamine and its major metabolite in the substantia nigra and basal nuclei. The degree of deficiency relates closely to the extent of cell loss in the substantia nigra.

Parkinson's disease affects one person out of 1000 in the United Kingdom, with 1 person in every 100 affected in the 60–70 year age group. Men and women are affected equally.[10] There is no evidence of familial influence nor is the disorder more prevalent in any part of the world.

ASSESSMENT

Clinical course and manifestations
Parkinson's disease may be described as progressing through several stages according to the disability experienced.

First stage. Tremor and muscular rigidity develop insidiously, and at the onset are usually unilateral when the part is at rest, disappear with voluntary movement and sleep, and become more pronounced with fatigue and stress. The tremor initially usually develops in the fingers and thumb producing the characteristic pill-rolling movement. The arms are adducted and semiflexed and the normal arm swing associated with walking is absent. Movements are slowed (hypokinesia) and a monotone becomes evident in the speech. If the tremor involves the dominant side, the person's handwriting is small and cramped reflecting the tremor and rigidity.

Second-stage. In this stage, the effects are bilateral and

more pronounced but the person is able to function. There is increasing slowness (bradykinesia), the trunk and head are flexed forward, the patient may have difficulty in starting to walk and in turning and his gait is slow and shuffling. Rigidity of the facial muscles and unblinking eyes produces a mask-like inexpressive appearance referred to as Parkinson's mask.

Third stage. The patient's gait and mobility are notably disturbed. He becomes more stooped and when walking there is a progressive acceleration of his steps producing what is known as a festination gait, making stopping difficult and predisposing to falls. There is difficulty in changing position (e.g. turning in bed, sitting down). The patient has difficulty with tasks involving finger movements (e.g. tying shoe laces, opening or closing zippers).

Drooling occurs due to the decrease in automatic swallowing of saliva. Disturbances in autonomic innervation may develop; there may be excessive, or an absence of perspiration, and disordered temperature regulation. Excessive lacrimation, ptosis and/or pupillary constriction may develop. Gastrointestinal activity may be slowed, causing constipation.

Pain and fatigue are experienced due to the continuous increased traction of muscles on their attachments. Speech becomes weak, slurred and devoid of any inflections as the muscles concerned with articulation become more involved.

Fourth stage. The patient becomes disabled to a greater degree because of the inability to initiate voluntary movement. Dependency is greatly increased. Speech becomes incoherent and difficulty in mastication and swallowing develops. The respiratory volumes are reduced and the ability to cough is diminished, predisposing to respiratory complications.

Up to now, the patient's intellectual functioning is unaffected, but at this later stage dementia may become evident in some patients.

Diagnosis
The diagnosis of idiopathic Parkinson's disease is based on the history and neurological examination. Several investigative procedures may be done to rule out other disorders.

MEDICAL MANAGEMENT

Currently, medication and physical therapy comprise the most common form of treatment for Parkinson's disease. Medication may not be prescribed until the patient's manifestations are pronounced and disabling, since its effectiveness tends to diminish after 2–5 years of use. The drugs and dosages that are useful vary from patient to patient. Relief of symptoms is usually partial.

The most commonly prescribed drug is levodopa

---

[10] Stern & Lees (1982).

(L-dihydroxyphenylalanine or L-Dopa) which is effective in reducing symptoms in 80% of patients. Initially the dose is small and then is gradually increased until the desired therapeutic levels are reached. Levadopa is converted to dopamine in the basal ganglia which reduces the patient's tremor, muscular rigidity and bradykinesia. Some patients experience side-effects of varying intensity manifested in gastrointestinal and/or cardiovascular disturbances. The patient is observed for anorexia, nausea, vomiting, marked weakness, behavioural changes, hypotension and cardiac arrhythmia.

A decarboxylene inhibitor such as carbidopa (Sinemet) is given which promotes the entrance of levodopa into the brain (across the blood–brain barrier) and lessens side-effects. Long-term side-effects tend to develop and include decreased attention span, loss of memory for recent events, mood swings, athetosis and behavioural changes.

Anticholinergic drugs are believed to inhibit the transmission of abnormal impules responsible for the excessive muscle tone. An anticholinergic preparation such as benzhexol hydrochloride (Artane) and benztropine mesylate (Cogentin) may be used with levodopa or alone for selected patients. The incidence and severity of side-effects vary with the anticholinergic preparation and from one patient to another. They include dryness of mouth and skin, headache, visual blurring, tachycardia, dizziness, palpitation, urinary retention and constipation.

Antihistamine preparations such a diphenhydramine hydrochloride (Benadryl) and orphenadrine hydrochloride (Disipal) may be prescribed in the early phase of the disease for patients who do not tolerate other drugs. Side-effects of antihistamine include drowsiness and light-headedness; the patient is advised of necessary safety precautions (for example, he should not drive).

Amantadine hydrochloride (Symmetrel) is also used in treating the patient with Parkinson's disease. Its action is not known but it is helpful with the patient who does not tolerate levodopa. Restlessness and changes in cognitive function may develop.

Surgical treatment of Parkinson's disease is seldom used; it is usually reserved for younger patients with unilateral involvement who do not tolerate or respond to medication therapy. A stereotactic pallidotomy or thalamotomy is done in which a destructive lesion is produced in the globus pallidus or the ventrolateral area of the thalamus by cryosurgery (freezing), electrocoagulation or the introduction of absolute alcohol.

IDENTIFICATION OF PATIENT PROBLEMS

Continuous assessment is very important in order to recognize the patient's response to the prescribed medication and physiotherapy, symptoms of progression of the disease, reduced ability for self-care and increasing disability and dependency.

1 Inadequate or inaccurate knowledge about the Parkinsonian syndrome, its characteristics, prescribed treatment and management
2 Muscular dysfunction due to impairment of extrapyramidal control: tremor, rigidity, slowness and lack of coordination
3 Potential for injury due to muscular dysfunction
4 Altered body image and loss of self-esteem secondary to incapacity, change in role, appearance and dependency
5 Nutritional deficit due to difficulty in eating, mastication and swallowing, anorexia and nausea caused by the prescribed medication
6 Impairment in communication. Speech difficulty secondary to the rigidity of the muscles involved in speech and reduced pulmonary volumes
7 Potential for complications:
   (a) Respiratory complications due to respiratory muscle dysfunction, causing reduced pulmonary volumes and the inability to cough to remove secretions
   (b) Break in skin due to immobility and falls
   (c) Impairment of eye function due to diplopia or due to drying and injury of the cornea caused by a reduction in blinking and moistening of the surface of the eye
   (d) Medication reaction (see side-effects, above); medication withdrawal.

The *goals* are to have the patient and family accept and adjust to the situation and have the patient maintain independence, accustomed role and a relatively normal life-style for as long as his condition permits.

NURSING INTERVENTION

The patient with Parkinson's disease is managed at home on a drug programme until the advanced stage of the disorder causes marked disability and dependency. The clinic or community nurse assumes the major role in assessing the patient's needs and providing the necessary counselling and guidance for the patient and family at the onset and through successive months and years. It is important that the nurse recognizes the emotional, physical and socioeconomic problems incurred by the disease. The fact that the *patient's intellect is unimpaired* must be kept in mind as well as his tendency to become very self-conscious, depressed and withdrawn because of his appearance and limitations.

The patient is advised to contact the national Parkinson's Disease Society[10a] and avail himself of the services and group activities they provide. Socialization in structured groups of persons with similar problems is helpful.

[10a] Parkinson's Disease Society, 36 Portland Place, London, W1N 3DG.

1. *Inadequate knowledge.* An explanation of the disorder and the prescribed therapy is made to the patient and family. Opportunities are provided for discussions in which they can ask questions and express their feelings and concerns. They are assisted in planning how to maintain a satisfactory lifestyle, role functions and socialization. The patient is encouraged to be independent and carry out self-care activities. Those around him are advised that the patient's intellectual ability is unimpaired; it should be emphasized that he needs to be treated normally, to socialize and to do things for himself even though he may take much longer. The environment should be cheerful and free of haste and confusion.

2. *Impairment of physical mobility.* A physiotherapy programme is established involving range-of-movement exercises and posture and gait training. The nurse should be familiar with the prescribed programme and prompt the application of the recommended movements and posture.

The patient tends to sit for prolonged periods and, when in bed, may be unable to change his position because of the muscular rigidity. This immobility places the patient at risk of circulatory stasis and pressure sores. Prompting, and assistance if needed, to move and change position are necessary to prevent prolonged periods of immobility. Assistive devices such as a rope secured to the end of the bed or suspended from an overhead bar may help the patient to raise himself. When up, a chair with arms permits him to raise himself to a standing position.

As finer movements become increasingly difficult, clothing with zippers, velcro or ties rather than buttons, and pull-on shoes instead of those with laces are provided so that independence in dressing and undressing can be maintained. By being able to achieve these tasks he is more likely to be more interested in his personal appearance.

3. *Potential for injury.* The patient's flexion of the trunk, shuffling gait and slowness of the righting reflexes to maintain his balance predispose him to falls. Simple modifications within the environment may prevent such accidents. Areas of activity should be well lighted and hand rails on the walls in appropriate places are helpful. The floors should be non-slippery and hazards such as scatter rugs, electric flexes and small stools over which the patient might trip are removed. A raised toilet seat and hand-rails in the bathroom facilitate self-care and prevent falls.

Well-fitting walking shoes with non-slip soles are recommended; a wide-based stance is encouraged to help maintain balance when walking or standing.

Precautions are necessary if the patient is to handle hot liquid, particularly if his tremor involves the dominant side. Additional protective measures may be required according to specific deficits.

4. *Altered body image.* Loss of normal smooth, coordinated mobility, change in appearance, loss of the capacity for gainful employment and self-care and loss of accustomed social interaction result in the patient's altered self-image, loss of self-esteem and depression. The patient is encouraged to express his feelings, to take an active role in setting realistic goals and planning management. The patient is inclined to develop an acute sense of humiliation, and he may withdraw and become isolated.

The patient's strengths and potential capacity are emphasized and independence encouraged; socialization and group activities are arranged. The nurse indicates expectation of efforts on the part of the patient to maintain good grooming; assistance with the activities of daily living is provided as needed.

The expertise of other professionals may be required to provide counselling, motivation, guidance and support, particularly during the adjustment period. Involvement in the local branch of the Parkinson's Disease Society may promote acceptance and adjustment.

5. *Nutritional deficit.* The patient may not be taking adequate nourishment because of the difficulty in feeding himself due to his tremor, difficulty in mastication and swallowing due to rigidity and/or anorexia and nausea incurred by the prescribed medication. Not infrequently, these patients' dentures become a source of discomfort and are poorly fitting because of the muscular contraction and loss of weight. The quality and quantity of food taken by the patient and his body weight are followed closely. Only a small amount of his meals may be taken because of fatigue and depression. The patient is encouraged to feed himself and provision is made for the fact that he takes longer and spills food. Food that can be easily managed and which appeals to the patient should be provided. Oral care before meals will moisten the mouth and reduce the unpleasant taste that some patients experience when receiving levodopa. Following a meal, mouth care is repeated to remove food particles that frequently remain because of the difficulty with swallowing. Soft or blender food in frequent, small helpings may be more acceptable. The patient may be less self-conscious and take more if privacy is ensured and he is given plenty of time while he is eating. Protection for his clothing is provided so that traces of his incapacity do not remain to increase his concern. The patient is advised to flex his head forward to facilitate swallowing.

In advanced stages of the disease the patient will require more assistance, especially with fluids. Aspiration may occur as dysphagia worsens; suction equipment should be readily available.

6. *Alteration in elimination.* Constipation is a common occurrence because of the decreased activity, decreased food (bulk) intake and decreased fluid in the gastrointestinal tract due to an inade-

quate intake and the loss of saliva (drooling). The drug therapy may also contribute to the problem.

The fluid, roughage and bulk intake are increased. A stool softener or bulk-producing laxative (e.g. bisacodyl) may be necessary to prevent faecal impaction. The patient is encouraged to establish a regular time for defecation and a raised toilet seat will make it easier for him.

Urinary dribbling and incontinence may occur; the cause may be the inability of the patient to reach the toilet soon enough. A regular toileting schedule is arranged and the patient prompted and assisted if necessary. A commode or urinal is kept readily available for use at night.

7. Alteration in comfort. The patient experiences the discomfort of continually contracted muscles and readily becomes fatigued. Physiotherapy, avoidance of prolonged periods in one position and planned rest periods contribute to comfort.

As a result of disturbed autonomic nervous system control, excessive perspiration may occur. Daily bathing and frequent change of clothing may be needed to promote comfort and control body odour.

8. Impairment in communication. The rigidity of the muscles involved in speech and the reduced pulmonary volumes which may develop interfere with the patient's enunciation and volume of speech. He is prompted to deliberately speak loudly and exaggerate pronunciation. Deep breathing with slow exhalation, singing and speech classes in groups help to improve speech. Facial exercises such as smiling, blowing out, grimacing, eye movements and neck extension performed before a mirror may lessen facial rigidity.

9. Potential for complications
(a) *Respiratory insufficiency and infection.* As a result of diminished respiratory movements and volumes, decreased ability to cough and immobility, pulmonary secretions are retained and readily become infected. Frequent deep breathing and helping the patient to cough are necessary. Suction is used to assist in removing secretions. If the patient is confined to bed, the head of the bed is elevated and he is repositioned at regular frequent intervals. A humidifier in the room and a daily minimal fluid intake of 3000 ml unless contraindicated by the patient's cardiovascular status are helpful in liquefying the secretions.
(b) *Break in skin.* Frequent inspection and care of the patient's skin are essential because of the immobility and potential falls. If able, he is taught to change his position and shift his weight at frequent intervals.

Excessive salivation and difficulty in swallowing may cause drooling which is very uncomfortable as well as embarrassing for the patient. The skin around the mouth and on the chin may become irritated. An adequate, available supply of soft tissues, skin care using a protective lotion or ointment and frequent changes of clothing and pillow cover are necessary.
(c) *Impairment of eye function.* The patient may experience prolonged exposure and drying of the surface of the eye due to a reduction in the normal frequency of blinking. This may lead to corneal irritation. The instillation of artificial tears (e.g. methylcellulose) may be prescribed and the patient and/or a family member is taught how to instil the solution. Diplopia may become a problem. A patch on one eye may help.
(d) *Medication reaction.* The patient is observed for his reaction to the prescribed medication. An assessment is made for positive responses as well as for undesirable side-effects. For example: Is the tremor less? Has the patient's gait improved? The potential side-effects in relation to the drugs have been cited previously (see Medical Management, p. 845). If side-effects develop, the doctor is notified; an adjustment in dosage may be necessary or another drug prescribed.

Sudden withdrawal of an antiparkinsonian drug or severe emotional disturbance may precipitate a reaction referred to as a Parkinsonian crisis. It is characterized by a marked aggravation of tremors, rigidity and akinesia. Tachycardia, increased respirations, acute anxiety and diaphoresis also occur.

The reaction is a medical emergency requiring prompt treatment. Treatment includes respiratory and cardiac support, the administration of an antiparkinsonian preparation and the parenteral administration of a sedative such as phenobarbitone may be necessary.

EXPECTED OUTCOMES

1 The patient and family:
   (a) Indicate a satisfactory understanding of Parkinson's disease
   (b) Are able to express their concerns about necessary adjustments and the future
   (c) Have made precautionary environmental changes to ensure safety.
2 The patient:
   (a) Tolerates the prescribed medication without serious side-effects
   (b) Complies with the exercise regimen
   (c) Is free of complications
   (d) Has maintained his body weight
   (e) Has contacted the Parkinson's Disease Society.

MOTOR NEURONE DISEASE (AMYOTROPHIC LATERAL SCLEROSIS)

This is a progressive chronic disease in which there is a degeneration of motor neurons in the spine (anterior horn cells), brain stem and/or cortical motor areas.

The cause of motor neurone disease is unknown. The onset of the disorder occurs most often between the ages of 40 and 60 years. The muscles innervated by the affected neurons lose their ability to contract, and atrophy.

ASSESSMENT

Clinical course and effects
The first symptom is usually weakness of the hands and arms; finer movements are lost and articles are dropped. Twitching and hyperreflexia develop along with the spasticity and weakness of the lower limbs. As the disorder progresses, speech, swallowing and respiration are impaired as motor neurons at higher levels are involved. The diagnosis is made on the patient's symptoms and their progressive nature. Electromyographic studies are done to confirm the loss of innervation to the muscles. The course is usually progressively retrograde; rarely is there a remission.

TREATMENT AND NURSING INTERVENTION

There is no specific treatment for motor neurone disease. When the disease is diagnosed, the patient and family are advised by the doctor of the expected progression and fatal outcome of the disorder. They require support, opportunities to express their feelings and ask questions, explanations and assistance in planning home management. The nurse can advise them to contact the Motor Neurone Disease Society[11] or Muscular Dystrophy Group.[12] The patient is encouraged to remain active within his potential muscular ability. It should be kept in mind that in motor neurone disease, the cognitive ability remains unaffected. Simple assistive devices are provided that will help the patient to maintain his potential level of independence. For example, velcro fasteners on clothing, cutting the patient's food, and ankle and foot supports that prevent dragging the foot and tripping are helpful measures. Obviously the rehabilitation and home management must be individualized because of the variability of symptoms and stages of the disease in patients. Progression of the disease and increasing dependency eventually necessitates the use of a wheelchair.

Those caring for the patient must give frequent attention to the positioning of paralysed limbs to prevent contractures and injuries. Assistance in frequent repositioning is necessary to lessen the patient's discomfort and prevent pressure sores. The patient's sensory functions are not impaired. For further details of nursing intervention in paraplegia and quadriplegia see p. 821.

---

[11] Motor Neurone Disease Society, 25 Rickfords Hill, Aylesbury, Bucks, HP20 2RT.
[12] Muscular Dystrophy Group of Great Britain, Nattrass House, 35 Macaulay Road, London, SW4 0QP.

When respiratory muscle functioning becomes involved, a tracheostomy and mechanical respiratory assistance are necessary.

EXPECTED OUTCOMES

1 The patient carries out self-care and maintains independence within his physical, social and vocational potential.
2 The patient and family progress through grief reactions to acceptance of the diagnosis and make informed decisions about home management.
3 The patient is free of complications (respiratory, contractures and decubitus ulcer).
4 In the terminal stage, family members are supportive of the patient and each other.

MYASTHENIA GRAVIS

Myasthenia gravis is not a degenerative condition but is included here because of its chronic, progressive nature. It is a neuromuscular disorder characterized by weakness and easy fatigability of voluntary muscles due to interference with impulse conduction at the neuromuscular junction.

The *cause* is unknown. It has been suggested that there is a deficiency of either acetylcholine or the enzyme cholinesterase. In addition, a deficiency in the number of acetylcholine-sensitive receptors in the motor end-plate has been identified. There is some evidence that autoimmune and genetic factors are implicated in the disease. Abnormalities of the thymus gland and increased antibodies that react against muscle tissue elements have been identified in some patients with myasthenia gravis. The incidence of the disease is higher in families than would occur by chance alone.

Incidence. It is not a common disorder. The incidence is highest between 20 and 30 years of age, and women are affected more frequently than men at this age. In later years, men and women are equally affected.

ASSESSMENT

Clinical course and effects
The onset of myasthenia gravis may be insidious with the symptoms of fatigue and weakness being associated with muscular activity. Initially, only the extrinsic ocular and levator palpebrae muscles may be involved resulting in ptosis of the eyelids) and diplopia. This may be referred to as ocular myasthenia. More generalized muscle involvement (generalized myasthenia) with progression of the disease produces the following manifestations: an expressionless appearance due to weakness of facial muscles; difficulty with mastication and swallowing; nasal voice tone that loses volume as the patient talks; limb weakness, which becomes evident with

the patient experiencing difficulty with self-care management (e.g. bathing, brushing the teeth, combing the hair); respiratory difficulty; and loss of control of bladder and rectal sphincters.

Muscle weakness is most noticeable at the end of the day and following exercise. Some recovery of strength is evident upon rising in the morning or following a period of rest. Mild atrophy may occur in the affected muscles and some aching may be present. Usually, sensation is unchanged.

There is great variability in the course of the disease; spontaneous remissions may occur. Factors which may aggravate symptoms include infection, temperature extreme, exposure to sunlight, emotional stress and physical exertion. Weakness of the diaphragm and intercostal muscles is serious; respiratory insufficiency and complications may be fatal.

Diagnostic tests
The diagnosis of myasthenia gravis may be made on the basis of the history of weakness in specific muscle groups. A test may be used which involves the intravenous injection of a preparation of a cholinesterase antagonist such as edrophonium chloride (Tensilon). If myasthenia gravis is present, the patient's generalized muscular strength increases and symptoms such as ptosis and voice tone and volume improve. When edraphonium chloride is given the patient is observed closely for cardiac arrhythmia (bradycardia) and a syringe and solution of atropine sulphate for parenteral administration should be readily available to correct the adverse response. Neostigmine bromide (Prostigmin) may be used instead of endrophonium chloride; the response here is slower.

Electromyographic studies may also be done in the process of diagnosing the disease. With repetitive stimulation the amplitudes of the muscle response are reduced.

MEDICAL MANAGEMENT

There is no known cure for myasthenia gravis. Treatment includes the administration of drugs, plasmaphaeresis and surgery. The drug most commonly used is a cholinesterase antagonist preparation such as neostigmine (Prostigmin) or pyridostigmine (Mestinon). The patient is usually hospitalized and observed for his reaction to the drug. The dosage varies with each patient; starting with a very small dose, it is gradually increased to the level that seems most effective. Side-effects include excessive salivation and perspiration, abdominal cramps, nausea and diarrhoea.

If the patient does not respond to the anticholinesterase, the corticosteroid prednisone may be given for its antibody suppressant effect, on the basis that the disorder is an abnormal immune response. The patient is observed for side-effects of prednisone which include retention of sodium, hypertension, hypokalaemia and increased blood glucose level.

In plasmaphaeresis, blood is removed and processed to remove antibodies before being reinjected. This form of treatment is used in conjunction with an immunosuppressive drug. The plasmaphaeresis may need to be repeated over a period of time.

Surgical therapy involves thymectomy (the removal of the thymus gland). Hyperplasia occurs in many of the patients, or a thymic tumour may be present, and removal of the gland results in a marked improvement in some and complete remission in others. Surgery is used mainly in younger patients in the early stages of the disease.

IDENTIFICATION OF PATIENT PROBLEMS

1 Inadequate knowledge about myasthenia gravis, its characteristics, treatment and home management plan
2 Impaired ability to perform usual activities due to muscular weakness and fatigue
3 Impairment of vision due to weakness of ocular muscles
4 Nutritional deficits secondary to difficulty with mastication and swallowing and generalized weakness
5 Impairment of verbal communication secondary to weakness of muscles involved in speech and reduced vital capacity
6 Respiratory insufficiency: hypoventilation due to weakness of diaphragm and intercostal muscles
7 Potential for complications:
 (a) Physical injury due to muscular weakness and visual disturbance
 (b) Pressure sores due to immobility secondary to weakness
 (c) Myasthenic or cholinergic crisis due to either a deficiency or an excess of the prescribed anticholinesterase preparation

NURSING INTERVENTION

Most patients with myasthenia gravis are managed in the home. Hospitalization may be necessary for evaluation, establishing the required medication dosage, exacerbation of symptoms, respiratory failure or myasthenic crisis. Nursing management is primarily concerned with maintenance of muscle strength and the prevention of complications and muscle atrophy.

1. Knowledge deficit. The patient and family require information concerning the nature of the patient's disorder, factors which may aggravate symptoms, the importance of adequate and planned rest and the prescribed medication.

The patient and family, with the assistance of the nurse, make a plan for rest periods, a medication regimen, and the best times to carry out certain activities. The latter are less difficult if performed early in the day and after a dose of the prescribed cholinesterase antagonist rather than preceding its administration.

The patient and a responsible family member should know the function of the prescribed drug(s), the importance of taking them precisely on time and the possible side-effects. The patient may be told by the doctor to adjust the dosage to meet his particular needs; his needs and the adjustment to make must be clearly understood by the patient. Taking drugs for myasthenia gravis half an hour before or after the time scheduled is not effective in symptom control and a myasthenic crisis may occur. Many drugs can cause a worsening of myasthenia gravis; the patient is advised not to take any medication that has not been prescribed by his doctor.

The patient and family are made aware of the factors which may aggravate symptoms (see p. 849). They should also be informed about the potential myasthenic and cholinergic crises, what they are, causes, symptoms and the necessary action. If the patient has indicated a tendency to develop a crisis, suction equipment and a manual resuscitation bag (e.g. Ambu bag) may be recommended as being available in the home and the family taught when and how to use them.

Contact with the British Association of Myasthenics[13] is recommended and the patient is advised to wear a Medic Alert identification tag at all times.

2. Impaired ability to perform usual activities. The patient is assessed for potential strength in order to establish the assistance required. The patient, if he is able, is helped to plan a schedule for self-care, taking meals, and carrying out desirable activities such as socializing that will prevent overfatigue. The activities are spaced and separated by periods of rest.

Bed rest and the provision of personal hygiene care and feeding are necessary during the period when the medication regimen is being established or if the patient does not respond to therapy.

3. Impairment of vision. The ptosis and diplopia interfere with the patient's visual acuity. If ambulatory, the visual disturbance places them at risk of injury. The double vision may be relieved by the wearing of a patch over one eye. If both eyes are affected the patch is alternated from day to day on the two eyes. Covering the eyes during rest periods may be helpful.

4. Nutritional deficit. The potential for inadequate nutrition arises because of dysphagia and development of fatigue when eating. The scheduling of a rest period and the anticholinesterase drug half an hour before meals makes the taking of food less difficult. A

substantial breakfast is encouraged because weakness is less in the morning. High calorie foods in soft or liquid form also make it easier for the patient. When feeding the patient, brief rest periods are necessary throughout the meal. If dysphagia is severe, nasogastric feedings may be necessary. Suction equipment should be readily available in case of aspiration. The patient's body weight is recorded once or twice weekly.

5. Impairment of verbal communication. The difficulty in speaking may be minimized by encouraging the patient to speak slowly and use short sentences. Alternative methods of communication may be necessary at times (writing, signs).

6. Respiratory insufficiency. The patient is observed closely for hypoventilation, indicating weakening of the respiratory muscles. Vital capacity may be determined when the patient attends clinic or is hospitalized. Restlessness, tachycardia and dulling of mental responses may indicate hypoxia. Mechanical respiratory assistance may be necessary until drug regulation takes over.

7. Potential for complications
(a) *Physical injury.* The patient is at risk of falls. A supportive walking shoe is recommended and the environment freed of hazards such as scatter rugs, foot stools and electric flexes. Hand-rails in the bathroom and rooms inhabited by the patient provide greater security for the mobile patient.
(b) *Pressure sores.* The weakness discourages change of position. When in bed the patient's position is changed at regular intervals and vulnerable areas inspected and given care each time. If the patient is up in a chair, he is prompted, and assisted if necessary, to shift his weight frequently.
(c) *Crisis reaction to drugs.* The patient who requires high doses of an anticholinesterase drug is at risk of developing a *cholinergic crisis*. This is a life-threatening reaction resulting from over-medication necessitating prompt emergency treatment. A dramatic increase in myasthenic symptoms occurs in about one hour, the patient experiences extreme weakness, blurred vision, nausea, vomiting, intestinal cramping, diarrhoea, increased salivation and bronchial secretions, respiratory insufficiency, bradycardia, constricted pupils and increased perspiration.

Treatment involves withholding the anticholinesterase. Endotracheal intubation, mechanical respiratory assistance and frequent suction are necessary to prevent severe respiratory failure, hypoxia and death. Atropine sulphate may be prescribed to lessen the secretions. Following the cholinergic crisis, regular dosage of the anticholinesterase is decreased.

A crisis may also develop due to *undermedi-*

---

[13] British Association of Myasthenics, 91 Cartlow Hall, Oswaldtwistle, Lancashire.

cation which is referred to as *myasthenic crisis*. The symptoms are similar to those that occur in a cholinergic crisis but develop three or more hours after taking the anticholinesterase drug. An anticholinesterase preparation is given as well as supportive treatment as indicated (e.g. respiratory assistance). Regular dosage of the anticholinesterase is increased.

In order to determine whether the crisis is cholinergic or myasthenic, edrophonium chloride may be administered intravenously by the doctor. If the crisis is myasthenic the patient's muscle weakness is reversed and regular. If the muscle weakness is increased, cholinergic crisis is indicated and anticholinesterase drug preparations are withheld and atropine sulphate may be prescribed as an antidote for anticholinesterase.

SURGICAL THERAPY—THYMECTOMY

If the patient is treated by thymectomy, nursing intervention includes those considerations cited in Chapter 11. In addition, the patient requires respiratory support by suction, chest physiotherapy and oxygenation. Frequent assessment is made of the patient's vital capacity and for air entry and the retention of pulmonary secretions. Muscular strength, speech and ocular functions are also assessed at regular intervals.

EXPECTED OUTCOMES

1 The patient experiences improved muscle strength, improved vision and communication ability.
2 The patient and family indicate: an understanding of myasthenia gravis; acceptable plans for the prescribed treatment; an awareness of the importance of punctuality with medication, the signs of a crisis reaction and the action to be taken.
3 Plans are made by the patient to adjust his lifestyle to his symptoms (e.g. plans activities when his strength is greatest and to rest after an activity).
4 Contact is made with the Myasthenic Association and arrangements made to obtain and wear a Medic Alert identification.

Paroxysmal Disorders

EPILEPSY (SEIZURES/FITS)

A seizure is the manifestation of abnormal, rapid and uncontrolled neuronal electrical discharges within the brain. It is characterized by sensory, motor, and autonomic disturbances and change in level of consciousness. The term *epilepsy* refers to a chronic disorder characterized by recurring seizures of unknown causation. In the normal brain, a certain stability exists between excitation and inhibition. When a seizure occurs, the ability to suppress abnormal neural activity may be impaired or lost, or there may be increased excitation within the neurons. The abnormal activity may occur in a small group of neurons and remain relatively localized or may spread to involve extensive areas of neurons. In some seizures, no focal origin of abnormal electrical discharges can be identified; large areas of the brain appear to be involved simultaneously.

Incidence and cause
The disorder characterized by recurring seizures and commonly referred to as epilepsy represents one of the most common neurological problems affecting individuals irrespective of geographical location, sex and race.[14] About one person in 20 has a seizure of some type during his life and in the population at large, about one in 200 has epilepsy (recurrent seizures).[15] Most of those who develop idiopathic epilepsy do so before the age of 20 years.

Epilepsy may be *idiopathic* (without known cause) or *symptomatic*. The latter type of seizures are secondary and may be caused by almost any intracranial pathological condition and by many general systemic disorders. Symptomatic seizures may occur with increased intracranial pressure or brain damage associated with a head injury, cerebral oedema, or an intracranial space-occupying lesion, haemorrhage or infection. They may be a sequel to brain injury or infection that has resulted in brain damage and scar tissue formation. General systemic conditions in which seizures most commonly occur include hypoglycaemia, hypocalcaemia (tetany), renal insufficiency (uraemia), hypoxia, high fever (especially in children), toxaemia of pregnancy and chemical poisoning (e.g. alcohol, strychnine, amphetamine, lead, some insecticides).

There is no known specific cause of primary (idiopathic) epilepsy but an inherited predisposition to hypersensitivity and dysrhythmia of the neurons is considered to play a role.

ASSESSMENT

A detailed history of the patient and family and complete physical and neurological examination are necessary. A description of what happens with a seizure is obtained from an observer and the patient questioned as to preceding events and experiences. Particular attention is paid to the age of an individual at the onset of seizures since idiopathic epilepsy usually develops before the age of 20 years. Symptomatic or secondary epilepsy usually develops later in life.

---

[14] Van Meter (1982), p. 11.
[15] Sweezey (1982), p. 17.

CAT scan, skull x-ray, laboratory studies of blood and CSF and an electroencephalogram (EEG) are done. The EEG is useful in locating the focus of the abnormal electrical cerebral activity (Fig. 22.26). Investigative procedures such as the scan and laboratory studies are done to rule out organic lesions.

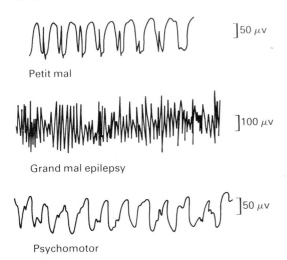

Petit mal   ]50 μv

Grand mal epilepsy   ]100 μv

Psychomotor   ]50 μv

Fig. 22.26 Electroencephalogram in different types of epilepsy.

Classification of seizures
A seizure is manifested by sensory, motor, cognitive and autonomic changes that interfere with normal functions of the individual. Seizures vary in form and length depending on the origin of the abnormal neuronal activity and the extent and course of its spread within the brain. The manifestations of a seizure may include loss of consciousness, changes in behaviour, involuntary uncoordinated movements, abnormal sensations and alterations in visceral function. The seizure may vary in length from a brief transitory phase of a few seconds to several minutes.

Certain factors tend to precipitate seizures in some persons. These may be external stimuli such as sudden loud noises; intermittent flashing lights and prolonged television, particularly if it is exciting. Excitatory factors also include emotional stress, fatigue, ingestion of alcohol, fever, and menstruation.

Clinically, seizures are commonly classified as partial or focal seizures or as generalized seizures.

Partial (focal) seizures. This type of seizure may be manifested by motor, sensory or a complex of disturbances depending on the cerebral area involved. Neuronal hyperactivity remains confined to the initial focal area or may spread to neurons in the adjacent areas but does not involve the whole brain. Partial seizures may be classified as Jacksonian or psychomotor.

A *Jacksonian* seizure is generally considered symptomatic of an organic brain lesion. There is usually a well-defined focal origin in the cerebral cortex. The manifestations are usually motor but may be only sensory or a combination of both. Clonic movements (alternate contraction and relaxation of voluntary muscles) begin in one part of the body, the most common sites being the thumb and fingers, the angle of one side of the mouth and the great toe. The movements spread to involve the entire extremity or face and other parts of the same side.

A *psychomotor seizure* may also be referred to as a temporal lobe seizure because of its focal origin. It is characterized by automatism, psychosensory disturbances and a clouding of the consciousness. The person, in a trance-like state, usually carries out a stereotyped, inappropriate action which may be quite bizarre. Rarely, violent or unlawful acts may be performed. Following the attack, the victim is totally unaware of what took place. The psychosensory symptoms may include hallucinations of hearing, smell, taste or vision, a disordered sense of reality and a sense of detachment from the surroundings, a feeling that what is happening at the present moment has been experienced before, or a sense of strangeness with familiar persons, objects or events, or an abnormal sense of well-being or fear. The attack may last from one to several minutes. During the psychomotor disturbances the patient is unresponsive to any effort on the part of the observer to check his actions.

Generalized seizures. The hyperactive neuronal discharges spread throughout the brain. Generalized seizures may be classified as grand mal (major) or absence (petit mal) seizures.

Absence (petit mal) seizures are characterized by sudden cessation of activity with a momentary absence of consciousness (5–30 seconds). The person stares blankly into space and the eyes usually roll upward. Objects being held may be dropped. Occasionally a few involuntary movements and falling may occur. More often, the episodes are unnoticed and the person resumes his activity, unaware that there has been an interruption.

Absence seizures may occur as often as a hundred times in a day. Attention and learning are affected with frequent occurrence. They usually have their onset in infancy or early childhood and either cease during adolescence or develop into grand mal seizures.

Grand mal seizures may also be referred to as major motor or tonic–clonic seizures. They represent about 10% of all seizures and may occur in children and adults. The seizure may develop with or without warning to the patient. Some patients experience irritability, tension or headache for a period before the episode. A brief sensory or perceptual aberration, referred to as an aura, may immediately precede the impending seizure. The aura may be auditory, visual, gustatory, olfactory or numbness or tingling in an area of the body. The aura is related to the focus of origin of the seizure and is specific for each patient.

The seizure begins with sudden loss of consciousness and the tonic phase of the seizure. The person falls to the floor; the tonic spasm of the muscles causes rigidity and distortion of the body. An involuntary cry is heard. The latter is caused by the sudden contraction of the thoracic and abdominal muscles forcing air through the spastic glottis. Respirations are arrested temporarily and cyanosis may develop. The jaws are fixed, hands clenched, the eyes opened widely and the pupils dilated. The initial tonic phase may last up to 60 seconds and is followed by a clonic phase of irregular jerky movements. Breathing is re-established and is stertorous, blowing out frothy saliva which cannot be swallowed due to spasms. There may be some bleeding caused by biting of the tongue, lips and oral mucosa. Urinary incontinence is common and rarely, faecal incontinence occurs.

The clonic movements gradually subside and consciousness is regained soon after. The patient may be confused, dazed or respond normally; he then falls into a deep sleep for several hours, awaking with no memory of the seizure and the brief conscious interlude. During the postseizure (postictal)[16] period, the patient may be disorientated or may complain of headache, fatigue and muscular soreness. In rare cases, the patient may become aggressive or violent.

Status epilepticus. This is a serious form of epilepsy in which seizures occur in such rapid succession that

recovery of consciousness between the episodes does not occur. Hyperpyrexia develops, coma deepens and permanent brain damage occurs due to anoxia. Complete exhaustion and death occur, if the patient is not treated.

The most common cause of status epilepticus is considered to be abrupt discontinuation of an anticonvulsant drug. Untreated or inadequately treated seizures may also lead to this emergency condition.

MEDICAL MANAGEMENT

When the seizures are a symptom of an identifiable organic disease (e.g. brain tumour, uraemia, poisoning), treatment is directed toward eliminating the cause and may include the prescription of an anticonvulsant drug. Regular administration of anticonvulsant drugs remains the most effective method of treating patients with epilepsy. This does not cure the disease but, with the majority of patients, seizures are sufficiently controlled to permit them to be self-supporting and live a relatively normal life. The patient's ability to accept his condition and his lifestyle play an important role in successful control.

Some of the more commonly prescribed drugs are listed in Table 22.11. The dosage is very much an individual factor; the drug regimen commences with a small dose and is increased if seizures occur. Tolerance for the antiepilepsy drugs and the side-effects vary with patients. With some the side-effects may reflect reaction of the nervous system by drowsiness, change in mood or behaviour, visual disturbance, ataxia and impaired cognitive function. Some drugs may cause bone marrow depression and/or bleeding tendency in some patients; many patients experience gastrointestinal disturbances. The patient is

---

[16] *Ictus* means seizure or sudden attack.

Table 22.11 Anticonvulsant drugs.

Drug	Side-effects and comments
Phenytoin (Epanutin)	Nausea, ataxia, diplopia or nystagmus, slurring of speech, gingival hyperplasia, rash and hirsutism Drug should be taken with meals. Good oral hygiene, gum massage and regular dental supervision are necessary
Carbamazepine (Tegretol)	Bone marrow depression, nausea, vomiting, headache, urinary retention, oedema, rash and drowsiness Blood cell counts and haematocrit should be done at least monthly
Phenobarbitone (Luminal)	Incapacitating drowsiness, rashes
Primidone (Mysoline)	Depression, irritability, dizziness, ataxia and, rarely, impotence If used with symptomatic seizures, dosage decreased gradually before withdrawal
Ethusuximide (Zarontin)	Gastrointestinal irritation, drowsiness and headache Should be taken at meal-time with a large amount of fluid. Primarily for use in petit mal epilepsy
Temazepam (Normison, Euhypnos)	Drowsiness, anorexia and changes in behaviour Taken with meals
Sodium Valproate (Epilim)	Gastrointestinal irritation, bleeding tendency and liver dysfunction Drug should be taken with meals. Frequent blood cell counts and bleeding times should be done

observed closely for side-effects and dosage adjusted as indicated or another anticonvulsant preparation prescribed to replace the one causing the side-effects.

Biofeedback, which is based on operant conditioning,[17] may be used for patients who do not respond to drugs. There is evidence that patients have been able to decrease seizures by learning to increase their sensorimotor rhythms which are displayed in EEG patterns.

Surgery may be used in the treatment of a small number of selected patients. Selection is based on the following criteria: (1) the seizures seriously affect the patient's life and they cannot be controlled by other means; (2) abnormal neuronal activity is localized and surgically accessible; (3) the region to be excised will not result in significant impairment or increase disability which already exists. Results of resection of a focus in the anterior temporal lobe (temporal lobectomy) have been most successful. In rare instances a hemispherectomy (removal of one hemisphere) has been done with varying results.

IDENTIFICATION OF PATIENT PROBLEMS

1 Potential for injury due to the loss of consciousness and uncontrolled strong muscular contractures
2 Lack of knowledge about the disorder, the treatment and necessary modifications in life-style which may be necessary
3 Alteration in self-image due to anxiety, and the stigma which a segment of society attaches to epilepsy

The *goals* are to:
1 Control the seizures
2 Accept the disorder that gives rise to the seizures
3 Comply with the medication regimen and recommended modifications in life-style
4 Cope with the situation

NURSING INTERVENTION

1. Potential for injury
When a patient has a seizure, the most important function is to protect the patient from injury. When a patient is known to be subject to seizures or is suspect because of his condition, precautions include: (1) having the patient near the nursing station, or where he can be readily observed; (2) providing a small firm pillow; (3) keeping the bed low; (4) having suction equipment readily available; (5) taking the temperature by axilla; (6) having padded sides in place on the bed; (7) staying with the patient during a bath or shower; (8) supervising the patient if he smokes; and (9) in some situations where it is

[17] *Operant conditioning* implies learning control by eliciting a particular desirable response to a stimulus.

approved, having a padded tongue depressor or disposable airway at the bedside.

During a seizure, the nurse stays with the patient; his safety and the observations and recording of events are paramount. Observations may be helpful in distinguishing between primary or secondary epilepsy and in localizing the seizure focus. A seizure cannot be stopped once it has begun; it is self-limiting and no immediate treatment will shorten it. If the patient is in bed, the pillow is removed and the top bedding turned down so that the patient's responses can be observed. If the patient is up, and has not already fallen, he is eased to a semi-prone position and a folded blanket or towel placed under the head to prevent injury during the clonic phase. Restrictive clothing at the neck is loosened and the immediate area cleared of anything that might contribute to injury (e.g. furniture, electric fan, lamp). No attempt is made to insert anything between the teeth as the teeth are clenched and there would be a risk of pushing the tongue into the oropharynx, obstructing the airway. In addition, injury to the teeth and soft tissue may occur; aspiration of blood or a broken tooth may become a possibility. As soon as the clonic phase begins to subside, the patient is turned on his side to promote drainage of secretions and prevent aspiration. Suction may be necessary. The patient is protected as much as possible from exposure to others.

During the seizure, the following *observations* are made:
• The mode of onset; did the patient indicate an aura? Was there a cry? Is there deviation of the head and eyes—if so, to what side? In what part of the body did the initial phase start?
• Are the seizure movements localized or generalized? If generalized, are they symmetrical or asymmetrical?
• Is the patient cyanosed?
• Are the teeth clenched and is there frothing at the mouth?
• Is there incontinence of urine or faeces?
• How long did the seizure last?

Following the seizure, the patient's condition is assessed.
• Is he oriented?
• Is he able to move his extremities and, if so, is the motor power normal?
• Is his speech normal?
• Is there any injury that was sustained during the seizure?
• Is he comfortable or does he complain of headache or weakness?
• When questioned, does he recall experiencing an aura, unusual sensation or anything unusual? What was he doing just before the seizure?
• Did the patient sleep following the seizure?

After a seizure, the patient is made comfortable

and usually sleeps for several hours; he is fatigued following the strenuous muscular activity. Close observations are made since seizures may recur. When the patient wakens, reorientation may be necessary as well as an explanation of the event.

In the interest of safety and the prevention of injury for self and others, the person with epilepsy may not be allowed to drive a motor vehicle, operate certain machines or work at heights or where there is loud noise or flashing lights. The doctor may also advise the patient against swimming, climbing, riding, cycling and participation in contact sports. Decisions regarding activities are based on the type, frequency and severity of seizures and the patient's response to the prescribed drug.

Family members are taught what to do when a seizure occurs so that they can respond effectively.

Information provided also includes the following. Moderation and normality in the individual's lifestyle is stressed; regular activity without fatigue is encouraged since it tends to inhibit seizures; regular patterns of rest and sleep should be observed; and a well-balanced diet is recommended with a limited intake of tea and coffee. Alcohol should not be taken. Total fluid intake should be reduced during the premenstrual period.

The doctor's advice is sought regarding occupations and recreational activities that are considered safe for the patient and others. Restrictions that are initially imposed may be lifted if the patient is seizure-free for a stated period of time. For example, laws pertaining to a driver's licence vary from one country to another. In some instances, a permit is issued if the person is seizure-free for 2 or more years.

2. Knowledge deficit

The person with epilepsy and his family require help in assuming management of the disorder. An explanation of the disorder, methods of controlling seizures, factors which may precipitate a seizure and the rationale for any restrictions imposed. They are advised that the individual's seizure threshold and compliance with the prescribed treatment determine the success of seizure control and that usually the anticonvulsant drug is necessary throughout life.

Information about the prescribed anticonvulsant drug is provided. The client and family should be alerted to the potential side-effects and are advised to get in touch with the doctor if they occur. They should know that if the drug is not tolerated that there are others that will be prescribed until optimal control of fits with minimal side-effects is achieved. It is emphasized that the drugs must be taken at the prescribed frequency even though there are no seizures; effective blood levels of the drug must be maintained by compliance with the prescribed dosage and frequency. Drug doses must not be altered except with the doctor's approval; the drug is prescribed on an individual basis according to the

type, severity and frequency of the seizures and the individual's response. The patient is cautioned against the taking of any non-prescription drug.

The importance of regular visits to the doctor is emphasized. Blood serum levels of the anticonvulsant drug are determined and dosage adjustment made if indicated. Since a blood dyscrasia is a potential side-effect of many of the drugs used, blood cell counts, haematocrit and bleeding time are evaluated regularly.

The patient and family are requested to keep a record of seizures which includes antecedent events or any known or suspected precipitating factor(s). Information is provided about The British Epilepsy Association[18] and its services and membership in the local branch is urged. A Medic-Alert identification bracelet or pendant should be worn so that appropriate care can be given during a fit or an emergency. The patient should always carry the names, addresses and telephone numbers of persons to be contacted.

3. Alteration in self-image

Patients express anxiety and embarrassment and see themselves as being 'different and inferior', having to adjust to potentially disruptive seizures and dependency on medication. Acceptance of the diagnosis is difficult for the patient who may respond with denial, anger, resentment and despair before acceptance and adaptation. The nurse listens, answers questions and indicates acceptance and understanding of the patient's reactions.

Assessment of the epileptic patient may reveal deep-seated fears concerning the condition and concerning potential rejection by uninformed others. Fears and anxieties which are unexpressed and unrelieved may result in ineffective coping. A thorough evaluation of the patient's attitude toward epilepsy and his expectations concerning health maintenance is essential. The attitudes and expectations of family members should also be evaluated since their understanding and support is crucial to the patient's ability to adjust to his condition. The book by Shelagh McGovern[19] can be a valuable resource for those faced with the need to adjust to epilepsy.

Epilepsy is not yet clearly understood and there is no known cure. Because of this, and the historical context, fear of the disorder is widespread. At one time the disorder was thought to be caused by the possession of a person by devils, and even today, myths, misunderstandings and social stigma still exist. As a result, the patient may fear rejection by peers and employers and refuse to disclose his health problem even though it would be wiser to do so. Concerns about the epileptic's intellectual abilities,

---

[18] British Epilepsy Association, Crowthorne House, Wokingham, Berkshire.
[19] McGovern (1982).

psychological stability and ability to perform efficiently on the job have been expressed by educators and employers. It is important for the nurse to be aware of potential prejudices which may be encountered by the patient and his family. The fact that mental capacity and abilities are as varied among epileptics as in any cross-section of society and that epilepsy is not synonymous with mental retardation or psychosis requires emphasis. There is no characteristic personality associated with epilepsy; the same range of personality differences exists among those with epilepsy as non-epileptics. Personality and behavioural aberrations are more likely to be associated with seizures caused by an organic lesion. Too often, the traits observed in the so-called epileptic personality are usually the result of injustice, rejection and/or frustrations experienced by the individual at the hands of the uninformed public.

The patient and family are informed that the condition is not incompatible with normal or even superior intellect, independence and a satisfying lifestyle. The family must guard against overprotection of the person since it impedes the adjustment process.

It is often useful to remind the patient, prejudiced persons and ourselves, that many famous and productive people throughout history were subject to seizures. The long list of such persons include Julius Caesar, William Pitt, Lord Byron, Charles Dickens, Martin Luther, Vincent Van Gogh, Ludwig van Beethoven, George Handel, Peter Tchaikovsky and Alfred Nobel.

Public education is necessary to promote a greater understanding and acceptance of persons with epilepsy. The Epilepsy Association should be supported in its efforts to counsel and support epileptics and their families, and to educate society about epilepsy and that epileptics are acceptable as normal. Special segments of society who should be informed include teachers, employers, police and transportation personnel.

The nurse encourages the patient and family to actively participate in 'Action for Epilepsy' Campaign of the Epilepsy Association (a network of self-help groups), and to socialize and replace restricted activities or sports with those considered safer for the individual. In the case of a young person still in school, the parents are encouraged to have him continue his education. The teacher should be advised of the student's condition and supplied with literature prepared by the Epilepsy Association. The school is notified of any restrictions made by the doctor on sports.

Marriage and procreation are possible for the epileptic. Some controversy exists concerning genetic predisposition to epilepsy. It is considered by some authorities to be greatest when epilepsy develops early in childhood and when both parents are epileptics. Genetic counselling may be advisable for the young married epileptic and spouse.

NURSING CARE IN STATUS EPILEPTICUS

The patient requires constant observation and attention. Respiratory support is necessary by suction between seizures and the administration of oxygen; endotracheal intubation may be necessary to maintain an adequate airway. The patient is positioned in the prone or semi-prone position to promote drainage of secretions and prevent aspiration. The cot-sides are padded to prevent the patient injuring himself. External stimuli are reduced to a minimum; sudden noises and movements may precipitate a fit.

The vital signs are recorded frequently; fever commonly develops and respiratory and cardiac failure may occur as a result of extreme exhaustion. Intravenous diazepam (valium) may be administered by the doctor.

An intravenous line is established by which anticonvulsant and sedative preparations are administered as well as fluids and nutrients (e.g. glucose).

The skin requires special attention because of the friction to which it is subjected. Soft undersheets are used and may be powdered to lessen friction.

EXPECTED OUTCOMES

Following a seizure:
1 There is an absence of symptoms of physical injury.
2 The patient responds normally and has no apparent motor impairment.
3 The patient is cooperative in describing preseizure activities and experiences.

In relation to on-going management:
4 The patient and family relate and discuss the seizure disorders, precipitating factors, precautionary measures for safety and the drug treatment.
5 The patient's and family's anxiety is at an acceptable low level and they appear prepared to accept and to admit to epilepsy.
6 Family members express confidence in themselves to respond effectively during a seizure.
7 Plans are made for the patient to resume satisfying activities, to become a member of the Epilepsy Association and to obtain and wear a Medic Alert identification.
8 The patient takes the prescribed drug regularly, has no side-effects and indicates plans for regular, on-going medical supervision.

Infections of the Nervous System

MENINGITIS

Meningitis is an acute inflammation of the pia and arachnoid meningeal membranes (leptomeninges) of the brain or spinal cord. The cause is usually bacterial or a virus. Almost any bacteria can cause meningitis but the most common are the meningococcus, pneumococcus and the haemophilus influenzae. Acute viral meningitis may also be due to mumps virus (myxovirus) or one of the picornviruses; the latter include the enteroviruses and those causing the common cold (rhinoviruses). Meningitis is frequently secondary to infection of the sinuses, ears, or respiratory tract. A less common form, mainly in the immigrant population, is tuberculosis meningitis.

ASSESSMENT

Signs and symptoms
The onset of meningitis tends to be insidious when caused by a virus. The bacterial type is more sudden and acute, manifested by headache, irritability, nausea, vomiting, back pain, chills and fever and symptoms of meningeal irritation. Photophobia is a common complaint. The classic signs of meningeal irritation include neck (nuchal) rigidity (stiffness of the neck and severe pain with forceful flexion), positive Kernig's sign (inability to straighten the knee when the hip is flexed), and positive Brudzinski's sign (hip and knee flexion in response to forward flexion of the neck). Signs of increased intracranial pressure such as blood pressure elevation, pupillary changes, changes in respiratory patterns, seizures, bradycardia, confusion, drowsiness and coma may develop. Focal neurological signs rarely occur.

Diagnosis
The diagnosis of meningitis is made on the basis of clinical signs and symptoms and is confirmed by isolating the organism from the CSF. The CSF is under increased pressure, is cloudy or purulent, and has an increased leucocyte count, a high protein content and a reduced concentration of glucose. Blood, nose and throat cultures are done to assist in identifying the organism and x-rays may be done of the chest, skull and sinuses to detect areas of inflammation.

Meningitis requires emergency treatment, since delay may result in cerebral damage and disability or death. It includes elimination of the source of infection, massive doses of an appropriate antibiotic and an anticonvulsant drug if seizures occur. The antibiotic may be administered intrathecally as well as parenterally. There is no specific treatment for viral meningitis.

IDENTIFICATION OF PATIENT PROBLEMS

1 Alteration in comfort due to the headache, back pain and fever
2 Potential for increased intracranial pressure secondary to the intracranial inflammatory process
3 Fluid and nutritional deficit secondary to nausea,

vomiting, headache, fever, confusion and decreased awareness
4 Potential for injury due to seizures, disorientation or coma
5 Potential spread of infection to others, particularly if the causative organism is meningococcus
6 Self-care deficits secondary to discomfort, reduced awareness, weakness or coma
7 Inadequate knowledge about management of the convalescent period and residual disabilities

NURSING ASSESSMENT

The nurse should establish a data base in relation to the level of consciousness, orientation and motor and sensory functions. Frequent regular assessment is made for any signs of neurological deterioration and the vital signs are monitored frequently and recorded; retrograde changes in the neurological status or in vital signs are reported promptly to the doctor.

NURSING INTERVENTION

The patient with meningitis is at risk of developing increased intracranial pressure and ensuing seizures and coma. For this reason, nursing care may include the nursing aspects related to: increased intracranial pressure, p. 808; the unconscious patient, Chapter 10 and seizure precautions and care, p. 854 as well as the following considerations.

1. Alteration in comfort. A major problem of the patient with meningitis is *discomfort* due to headache, back pain, fever, photophobia and anxiety. Nursing care includes provision of emotional support, reassurance that help is available and an explanation of all nursing activities. Irritability due to increased reaction to sensory stimuli is minimized by maintaining a cool, quiet, darkened environment, by approaching the patient gently with a soft, calm voice and by keeping communication simple and direct.

The head of the bed is elevated 30°; an ice-pack may help to relieve the headache and an analgesic is usually necessary to relieve the pain. Frequent mouth care is necessary because of the fever and vomiting. Excess bedding is removed, cooling washes may be given to reduce the fever and an antipyretic is usually prescribed.

2. Fluid and nutritional deficit. An adequate fluid and nutritional intake may be a problem because of nausea, vomiting and the headache. Fluids are usually administered intravenously; the 24-hour volume may be limited to a specific amount if there are manifestations of increased intracranial pressure. The fluid intake and output are monitored. As soon as tolerated, the patient is encouraged to take frequent, small, high-calorie feeds to combat the infection and fever. These are increased to regular meals as indicated by the patient's tolerance.

3. *Potential for the spread of infection to others.* The spread of the patient's infection to others must be considered. The hospital infection control department is consulted; it may be necessary to use isolation procedures.

The nurse has a role in preventing meningitis by teaching respiratory care to the public since meningitis can be spread by droplet infection. The proper use and disposal of tissues and the importance of handwashing should be emphasized as well as the prevention of upper respiratory tract infection.

4. *Self-care deficits.* The patient will require bathing, feeding, assistance with changing position and getting on and off the bedpan because of the headache, pain and weakness. Because of fever, reduced awareness and the tendency to remain immobile, vulnerable skin areas are inspected and given care at frequent intervals.

5. *Potential for respiratory complications.* The patient is encouraged to breathe deeply at regular intervals. Respiratory rate, and volume, air entry are assessed frequently. In the early phase of meningitis the patient is at risk of ineffective airway clearance and respiratory dysfunction due to brain stem and innervation involvement.

6. *Inadequate knowledge.* Following meningitis the patient is usually debilitated and readily fatigued and may have some residual neurological deficits. Several weeks or months may be needed for the patient's convalescence and rehabilitation. Following the initial acute phase, a highly nutritious diet is encouraged and a regimen of range-of-movement exercises is established to prevent weakness, contractures and joint ankylosis, and to promote circulation.

Minor disabilities may reverse with time while others may be residual and require detailed evaluation and an intensive rehabilitation programme. The nurse, familiar with the programme, plays a role in supporting the patient and interpreting it to the family and in assisting them in making plans for adjustments and home management.

EXPECTED OUTCOMES

1 Laboratory reports and the patient's vital signs return to normal.
2 The patient is comfortable, well hydrated and is increasing nutritional intake and has resumed self-care activities.
3 The patient and family indicate satisfactory plans for home management.

ENCEPHALITIS

Encephalitis is an inflammation of the brain. It may be caused by one of various organisms but is most commonly due to arboviruses or the herpes simplex virus (*Herpesvirus hominis* type I). The arbovirus multiplies in a blood-sucking vector such as the mosquito and tick. These viruses have a predilection for nerve tissue. The viruses which cause meningitis (e.g. *Haemophilus influenzae*) may invade the brain tissue and give rise to acute encephalitis. The disorder rarely develops as a complication of chicken pox, measles and mumps.

ASSESSMENT

Clinical course and effects
Viral encephalitis gives rise to symptoms of an acute febrile illness, signs of meningeal irritation and changes in cognitive functioning, consciousness and motor status. With the arbovirus type, the onset of symptoms is gradual, beginning with headache, nausea, vomiting and fever and progressing in a few days to convulsions, neck rigidity and coma. The herpes virus gives rise to the symptoms described above and, in addition, olfactory and gustatory hallucinations, aphasia, bizarre psychotic behaviour and occasionally hemiparesis may occur. This is because certain parts of the frontal and temporal lobes are affected. Transtentorial herniation due to severe oedema may result in coma and death.

With arbovirus encephalitis, if the patient survives, there may be neurological signs that subside within two weeks but there may be irreversible central nervous system changes. With herpes virus encephalitis, the mortality rate is high and severe neurological and mental deficits (e.g. fits, aphasia, dementia) are common sequelae.

Diagnosis
The diagnosis of viral encephalitis is difficult. CSF and blood studies are done and a detailed history of the antecedent events and contacts taken. A brain biopsy for culture may be done.

IDENTIFICATION OF PATIENT PROBLEMS AND NURSING INTERVENTION

The patient with encephalitis is acutely ill and requires intensive nursing care. Very frequent assessment of the patient's neurological status and vital functions is necessary.

The *actual and potential problems, nursing interventions* and *expected outcomes* are similar to that cited for the patient with meningitis. The patient with encephalitis is usually more restless than the meningitis patient; his confusion and bizarre behaviour may lead to injury unless safety precautions are taken (e.g. padded cot-sides in position at all times).

If the patient survives, a prolonged, intensive rehabilitation programme is usually necessary to assist the patient to cope with the residual disabilities and the alteration in his self-image. (See Chapter 3 for rehabilitation.)

HERPES ZOSTER (SHINGLES)

Herpes[20] zoster is an infection of the nervous system caused by the varicella virus (the same virus that causes chicken pox). It causes inflammation of the spinal and cranial sensory ganglia and along their nerve distribution. In some instances, areas of the posterior column of grey matter of the cord may be involved. It is believed that in many cases, the virus is reactivated after having remained dormant in the body for varying lengths of time. The disease rarely occurs in children and increases in incidence and severity in persons over 40 years of age. Those with a chronic debilitating disease such as cancer and those receiving immunosuppressant therapy are particularly susceptible.

ASSESSMENT

Clinical course and effects
The most common sites of involvement are thoracic sensory nerve roots (ganglia) and nerves (T5–T10) and the ophthalmic division of the trigeminal (V) cranial nerve. With the onset of the infection, the patient experiences fever, malaise and hypersensitivity, itching and pain along the area of the distribution of the sensory nerve fibres. After 3 or 4 days, vesicular eruptions appear along the course of the nerves; they become crusted, dry and scaly in a few days but the areas remain sensitive and painful for much longer. The lesions are generally unilateral. With ophthalmic involvement corneal ulceration and ensuing scarring may occur leading to some permanent visual impairment.

NURSING INTERVENTION

Nursing care is directed toward relief of pain and the prevention of infection of the skin lesions. The patient is not usually confined to bed unless the fever is high but extra rest is required. The application of wet dressings or lotions (e.g. calamine lotion, corticosteroid preparation) which have a drying, cooling and antipruritic effect may provide some relief. The application of tincture of benzoin or collodion to intact vesicles may be prescribed. Acyclovir (Zovirax) is an antiviral agent which is active against varicella zoster virus and herpes simplex virus. It is available as a cream and as an intravenous preparation.

The hypersensitive areas are protected from clothing by a light, soft, cloth or dressing. An analgesic such as aspirin, paracetamol or a combination of one of these with codeine is prescribed for the relief

of pain. If the eye is involved, antibiotic and corticosteroid preparations are instilled. Acyclovir cream must not be used in the eyes.

Care should be taken when bathing the patient or when washing and combing his hair to protect the eyes and affected areas.

The patient is encouraged to take a high-calorie nutritious diet to increase body resistance. The acute phase of herpes zoster lasts from 10–14 days but pain and hypersensitivity may persist for months. Postherpetic neuralgia is not responsive to treatment; there is a danger the patient may become very dependent on drugs. A referral to a pain clinic may be necessary.

EXPECTED OUTCOMES

1 Pain and irritation decrease.
2 Skin lesions heal.
3 The patient is not as readily fatigued.
4 Nutritional status improves, as evidenced by weight gain.

BRAIN ABSCESS

A brain abscess is a collection of pus that may be free or encapsulated within the brain tissue. It usually occurs by direct extension of a purulent infection of the ear, mastoid, or nasal sinuses, or it may follow an open head injury or intracranial surgery. The most common causative organisms are streptococci and staphylococci and the abscess may occur in any area of the intracranial cavity.

ASSESSMENT

Signs and symptoms
The general clinical manifestations are the same as those that occur with a space-occupying lesion of the brain (see p. 835). Symptoms of acute infection are not necessarily present. Headache is often an early symptom, as well as drowsiness, confusion and sometimes transient focal neurological signs. These general manifestations tend to fluctuate in intensity and may be followed by signs of increased intracranial pressure, including fits and decreased level of consciousness. Specific neurological signs depend upon the location and extent of the pus accumulation; for example, an abscess of the parietal lobe may cause a variety of focal sensory abnormalities.

The mortality rate with brain abscess is high; those who survive experience a lengthy and frustrating recovery period. Approximately 30% suffer permanent sequelae. Seizures are the most common residual problem.

Diagnosis
A detailed health history is made in an effort to identify a possible focal source of the infection (e.g. ear infection). A CAT brain scan is done to rule out

---

[20] *Herpes* implies an inflammatory skin disorder caused by a herpes virus and characterized by clusters of small vesicles.

other types of lesions and locate the abscess. A lumbar puncture is done to obtain a CSF specimen for culture and analysis. A cerebral arteriogram may also be done in an effort to locate the abscess.

MEDICAL MANAGEMENT

Large doses of an antimicrobial agent (antibiotic) are prescribed. If the abscess is well localized, surgical removal or drainage may be undertaken, or repeated aspiration of the exudate followed by injections of an antimicrobial agent may be done.

IDENTIFICATION OF PATIENT PROBLEMS

Nursing the patient with a brain abscess is similar to that cited for the patient with meningitis. If surgery is used, the reader is referred to nursing care for the patient having brain surgery (see p. 811).

Nurses have a role in reducing the incidence of brain abscess through formal and informal health education. Maintaining body resistance to infection and early treatment of dental, sinus and ear infections and other infectious disorders are emphasized.

POLIOMYELITIS (ANTERIOR POLIOMYELITIS)

Poliomyelitis is an acute infectious disease caused by a group of viruses which have a predilection for the motor neurones (anterior horn cells) of the spinal cord and brain stem. The causative virus is found in the nasopharyngeal secretions and faeces of infected persons. The infection may be spread by personal contact or by contaminated food, milk or water. The incubation period is 7–14 days and the most communicable period is during the latter part of this incubation and the first week of the acute illness. Antibody formation may confine the viruses sufficiently to prevent serious invasion of the nervous system.

ASSESSMENT

Clinical course and effects
The severity and course of poliomyelitis vary depending on the severity and level of involvement. Early symptoms are non-specific and include headache, fever, malaise, sore throat and gastrointestinal disturbances. The infection may go unrecognized at this time or may be suspected only by reason of known contact. The disease may not progress beyond this stage or the symptoms become more intense. The patient manifests restlessness, limited spinal flexion and tenderness in the muscles and complains of pain in the back and limbs: Positive Kernig's and Brudzinski's signs, characteristic of meningeal irritation, are demonstrated (see p. 857). Examination of the CSF reveals an increase in leucocytes and protein content. The symptoms may subside within a week or two without further devel-

opment of the disease and the patient is said to have had *non-paralytic poliomyelitis.*

If the disorder is not reversed it goes on to the *paralytic phase* in which paralysis of one or more parts occurs as a result of dysfunction or destruction of motor neurons. The muscles which lose their innervation vary with the level of the lesions. When motor neurons in the brain stem are involved, the disease is classified as *bulbar poliomyelitis.* The neurons of various cranial nerve nuclei and regulatory centres of vital functions (respiratory, cardiac, vascular) become involved in bulbar poliomyelitis. The patient may experience respiratory insufficiency, inability to cough, cardiac arrhythmia and dysphagia.

Involvement of the motor neurons in the *lumbar portion of the cord* may cause paralysis of one or both lower limbs and weakness of the lower abdominal and back muscles. Voluntary control of the urinary bladder may also be affected. Disease at the *thoracic level* of the cord may produce weakness of the chest and upper abdominal and back muscles. The affected thoracic muscles interfere with normal pulmonary function. Infection at the *cervical level* is critical since it interferes with innervation of the diaphragm and muscles of the neck, shoulders and arms. The patient may develop respiratory insufficiency.

The paralysis in poliomyelitis may be temporary or permanent. Neurons may recover as the disease process is arrested. The return of muscle power may take place slowly over several months or years. If the neurons are irreversibly damaged and replaced by scar tissue, the disability is permanent. The muscles atrophy and the affected limbs become flail-like.

INCIDENCE AND PREVENTION

Persons of all ages can develop poliomyelitis unless protected by natural or acquired immunity. Fortunately there has been a sharp decline in the incidence of the disease due to the widespread immunization programmes. There has been some concern recently that absence of the disease has caused some indifference to, and neglect of, immunization. Control measures include immunization (see Chapter 5) and isolation of infected persons.

TREATMENT

There is no specific therapy for poliomyelitis. The care is symptomatic and is directed toward relieving the patient's pain, preventing deformities, minimizing the paralysis and promoting maximum rehabilitation.

IDENTIFICATION OF PATIENT PROBLEMS

1 Anxiety due to concern about the outcome of the disease
2 Potential spread of infection to others because of the communicability of the virus

3 Alteration in comfort as a result of the muscle spasticity and immobility
4 Potential respiratory insufficiency due to involvement of motor neurons at cervical or brain stem level
5 Impaired mobility due to pain and paralysis
6 Inadequate knowledge: the patient and family require assistance in planning long-term care, home management and rehabilitation

NURSING INTERVENTION

1. Anxiety. Fear and anxiety about the outcome of the poliomyelitis on the part of the patient and family are understandable. They are encouraged to express their concerns and are reassured that everything possible is being done. Procedures are explained so that the patient knows what to expect and the family is kept informed about the patient's progress. They are advised that the paralysis may not be permanent but that it may take several months for the return of function.

2. Potential spread of the infection. Isolation procedures are usually required until the temperature returns to normal. Precautions with excreta are necessary since the nasopharyngeal secretions and faeces may be a source of the virus.

3. Alteration in comfort. Much of the pain experienced by the patient is due to muscle spasm. When the affected limbs are passively moved, they must be handled very gently to prevent precipitating a spasm. Avoid grasping the limbs in the area of the muscles. The application of heat may be prescribed to reduce the pain due to muscle spasm. Hyperextension which stretches muscles is avoided when positioning the patient.

4. Respiratory insufficiency. If bulbar poliomyelitis develops, the patient is at risk of respiratory failure, and aspiration of secretions; constant nursing attention is necessary. Positioning to promote drainage and suctioning may be necessary. If respiratory insufficiency develops, a tracheostomy is done and mechanical respiratory assistance provided (see Chapter 16).

5. Impaired mobility. The patient whose disease progresses to paralytic poliomyelitis is nursed on a firm mattress and good body alignment is maintained to prevent contractures and deformities. Appropriate supports (pillows or bolsters) are used to maintain a neutral position to promote relaxation of the paralysed muscles and prevent foot drop, outward rotation of the lower limb, hyperextension of the knee and wrist drop.

The patient is turned at regular intervals and skin areas vulnerable to pressure are inspected to prevent pressure sores.

An exercise programme is begun as soon as the acute pain and muscle tenderness subside, and the temperature remains normal. Passive movements, assisted and active exercises and exercise against resistance are used in and out of water to strengthen weakened muscles and minimize muscle atrophy. Residual disabilities such as a foot drop may require the assistance of a brace to facilitate walking.

6. Lack of knowledge. The rehabilitation of the patient and re-education of his muscles following paralytic poliomyelitis will take considerable time. He will need long-term care and will be faced with many of the physical, psychological and socioeconomic problems cited in the discussion of rehabilitation of the handicapped in Chapter 3.

EXPECTED OUTCOMES

1 The patient is free of muscle contractures and deformities.
2 Adequate ventilation is maintained.
3 The patient is compliant with the exercise and hydrotherapy programme.
4 Informed decisions can be made about home management. Family members are supportive of the patient.

RABIES

Human rabies[21,22] is common in some parts of the world, for example Asia, Africa and parts of North America, but is rare in the United Kingdom. It is a life-threatening viral infection of the nervous system (neurotropic rhabdovirus) which is communicated to man through the bite (or rarely, lick or scratch) of an infected animal. A wide range of animals are affected. The most common vectors in Europe are infected foxes (sylvatic rabies). Human infection is usually from domestic dogs or cats which have been bitten by foxes. A small number of human infections have been attributed to corneal transplant from an unsuspected infected donor. The rabies virus, present in the animal's saliva, travels along peripheral nerves to the central nervous system.

Following a bite by an animal, the wound is cleansed thoroughly with water and soap or detergent, for at least 5 minutes, and the person is seen by a doctor. The animal is confined, if possible and observed for signs of rabies. If the animal is found to be rabid it is destroyed. If the animal was not found but rabies is suspect in the district the person is given antirabies vaccine promptly before the rabies virus reaches the central nervous system. Human rabies immunoglobulin (HRI) is given intramuscularly and infiltrated around the wound. If the disease progresses to the central nervous system,

---

[21] Ball (1982).
[22] Edmond, Bradley & Galbraith (1982).

hydrophobia, seizures and paralysis occur and are usually followed by death.

If rabies is confirmed, the patient is kept in isolation. Heavy sedation and analgesia are given. A tracheostomy and intermittent positive pressure ventilation may be required. Rabies is a notifiable disease and must be reported to the health authority.

Potential incidence is reduced by the rabies vaccination of all imported family pets. Contact with strays should be avoided; particularly if they do not appear normal, do not act as one would expect, or if saliva is frothing and escaping from the mouth.

Rabies is uncommon in the United Kingdom (10 cases were reported between 1960 and 1980, all infected outside the country). This is attributed to the controlled importation and quarantining of animals. Those people at risk of coming into contact with infected animals, for example veterinary personnel, quarantine workers, laboratory technicians, health care staff in rabies units, should be vaccinated. Human diploid cell vaccine is given intramuscularly, 6 doses over 3 months.

Advice on rabies can be obtained from the Communicable Disease Surveillance Centre (England and Wales), the Communicable Diseases (Scotland) Unit, and the DHSS (Northern Ireland).

TETANUS

This acute, life-threatening disease is due to the exotoxin released by tetanus bacilli (*Clostridium tetani*). The effects of the toxin on the nervous system cause severe hypertonicity of the skeletal muscles and recurring attacks of intense tonic spasms.

The tetanus bacillus is spore-forming and anaerobic and and may be found in the faecal discharge of animals and man as well as in soil. The spores or bacilli enter the body via a wound where they germinate and multiply in anaerobic conditions. Deep penetrating wounds, wounds contaminated with soil and those in which there is necrotic tissue and a reduced oxygen concentration are more prone to develop tetanus. The organisms remain localized but produce the exotoxin which is absorbed into the bloodstream. The toxin acts on the neuromuscular junction and anterior horn cells (motor) of the spinal cord. The incubation period, which may vary from 2 days to several weeks, usually ranges from 6–14 days. The disease is not communicable except by transmission of discharge from the patient's wound to an open wound of another person.

Prevention
Tetanus may be prevented by immunization, prompt thorough cleaning of wounds and debridement of necrotic tissue. Active immunization is developed by a series of doses of tetanus toxoid. It is now usually given to children in combination with other vaccines (see Chapter 5). If a patient has a wound that is heavily contaminated with soil and

has not had a booster dose within the past 5–6 years, 250–500 units of human tetanus antitoxin (HTAT; human tetanus immunoglobulin) may be prescribed to confer passive immunization.

ASSESSMENT

Persons at risk are those not immunized, drug addicts, persons at risk of contact with animal faeces, and neonates in countries where it is not uncommon to find unqualified persons attending births.

Manifestations
The first symptom is usually hypertonicity of the jaw muscles; the patient has difficulty in opening his mouth and in chewing. This progresses to painful spasms and rigid clamping of the jaws (lockjaw). Spasticity of the facial muscles distorts the patient's expression and involvement of the throat and tongue makes swallowing and speech difficult. Eventually, tonic rigidity spreads to involve all skeletal muscles. Periodic spasms of increased intensity occur and are extremely painful and exhausting. During these attacks, the head is hyperextended and the back may be arched off the bed (opisthotonus), respirations are arrested because of spasm of the larynx and respiratory muscles, cyanosis develops and there is danger of asphyxiation. Fever and diaphoresis develop due to the excessive energy expenditure. The patient remains conscious and oriented unless severe exhaustion, hypoxia or a complication such as pneumonia intervenes.

The paroxysmal muscle spasms gradually decrease in frequency and severity after 7–10 days but it may take several months before normal muscle tone returns.

Diagnosis
The diagnosis is usually made on the clinical manifestations but if a debridement is done, an excised tissue specimen is used for culture. Inoculation of an animal with the patient's serum may be done; the animal will react to the presence of the exotoxin.

MEDICAL MANAGEMENT

The patient receives human tetanus immunoglobulin, 3000–6000 units, to counteract the tetanus toxin. An antibiotic (e.g. penicillin, tetracycline) is prescribed to destroy the tetanus bacilli. Sedatives, tranquillizers and muscle relaxants are prescribed to control the convulsive spasms.

A tracheostomy is usually done because of laryngeal spasm; it facilitates suctioning and respiratory assistance.

IDENTIFICATION OF PATIENT PROBLEMS

1 Potential for asphyxiation due to laryngeal and respiratory muscle spasm and aspiration of secretions

2 Potential for physical injury resulting from violent muscular spasms

3 Alteration in nutritional and hydrational status due to the patient's inability to open his mouth, chew and swallow

4 Potential damage to skin because of the patient's immobility, interference with tissue perfusion and profuse sweating

5 Alteration in elimination:
   (a) Urinary—retention of urine
   (b) Bowel—constipation

6 Lack of knowledge. The patient's and family's fear and apprehension develop because of the nature of the disease. The family are advised by the doctor that it may be fatal.

The *goals* are to:

1 Reduce the frequency and severity of the convulsive spasms.

2 Prevent injury from spasm activities.

3 Maintain adequate respiratory function.

4 Maintain intact skin.

5 Improve nutritional and hydrational status.

NURSING INTERVENTION

The patient with tetanus requires constant nursing attention in a quiet room with subdued lighting.

1. Potential for asphyxiation. If a tracheostomy is not done, frequent suction is necessary to remove oropharyngeal secretions. If a tracheostomy is established to maintain an airway, the care cited in Chapter 16 is applicable. Involvement of the respiratory muscles may necessitate mechanical respiratory assistance (see Chapter 16).

2. Potential for injury. The violent convulsive spasms may cause physical injury. Padded cot-sides are in place. External stimuli are kept to a minimum; disturbances such as a sudden noise, jarring of the bed and handling of the patient may precipitate a tonic spasm and the accompanying severe pain. Everything must be done as gently as possible. A calm low voice is used when speaking to the patient or within his hearing. He is advised when he is going to be touched or moved. Patient care (e.g. bathing mouth care, tube feeding) is carried out following the administration of a tranquilliser or muscle relaxant to reduce the possibility of precipitating a convulsive spasm.

3. Alteration in nutrition and hydration. In severe tetanus, the patient is unable to chew or swallow because of the muscular spasms. Profuse sweating results in dehydration, and electrolyte imbalance also occurs. Intravenous fluids are given to correct the electrolyte imbalance and replace the fluid loss. Nasogastric feeding is commenced when the muscular spasms are under control. The feeds should have a high calorie content because of the energy expended due to the muscle contractions. Oral fluids and food are introduced when the patient's condition improves.

4. Pressure sores. The patient's immobility and profuse sweating predispose to irritation of the skin particularly over pressure areas. These vulnerable areas are kept dry and inspected frequently. This is done following the administration of the prescribed tranquilliser or muscle relaxant to lessen the possibility of a spasm. An alternating air pressure (ripple) mattress is helpful as well as squares of sheepskin under the susceptible areas.

5. Alteration in elimination patterns. The fluid intake and urinary output are monitored. Catheterization may be necessary due to retention of urine. Constipation is a common problem because of the muscle spasticity; a stool softener or rectal suppository may be prescribed when the patient's spasms are fewer and less severe.

6. Lack of knowledge. The patient and family or significant others experience considerable fear and apprehension because of the nature of the disorder. Quiet, reassuring presence and gentle handling are helpful. Procedures are explained before they are commenced. The incapacity and immobility are of concern as to the outcome; they are advised that the disability is not permanent.

When the convulsive spasms have ceased, the patient is encouraged to move his limbs *very slowly and gently* through their range of movement. The increased muscle tone and immobility may have caused some decrease in range of movement.

EXPECTED OUTCOMES

1 Convulsive tonic spasms have ceased.

2 The tracheostomy tube is removed and the patient's airway remains patent.

3 The skin is intact.

4 Joint range of movement is normal.

5 Bowel and urinary bladder elimination are normal.

6 Nutritional status has improved.

Peripheral Nerve Disorders

Disorders of the cranial nerves may be secondary to other diseases but a few are primary to specific nerves. The more common of these are trigeminal neuralgia and Bell's palsy. Peripheral nerve dysfunction may be incurred by direct local trauma (pressure, severance, infection and inflammation) or may be secondary to a variety of general conditions such as malnutrition, alcoholism and chemical poisoning.

TRIGEMINAL NEURALGIA (TIC DOULOUREUX)

Trigeminal neuralgia is a very painful disorder of the

sensory fibres of the trigeminal (fifth cranial) nerve. The nerve has three main divisions, the ophthalmic, maxillary and mandibular and its motor fibres are concerned with mastication while the sensory fibres carry sensory impulses (pain, touch, temperature) from the face, nose, teeth and mouth. The sensory fibres of all three divisions pass to the gasserian ganglion which lies in a fold of the dura mater in the temporal region. From the ganglion, the sensory impulses are transmitted to a nucleus in the pons. The motor fibres originate in a small nucleus of neurons also situated in the pons and join the sensory fibres of the mandibular division just beyond the ganglion (see Fig. 22.27).

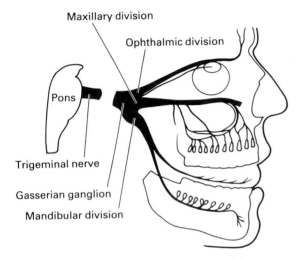

Fig. 22.27 Distribution of the sensory fibres of the trigeminal nerve.

Defining characteristics
Trigeminal neuralgia is characterized by recurring episodes of excruciating pain along the distribution of one or more divisions of the nerve. The mandibular branch is most often affected. Abnormally hypersensitive areas, referred to as trigger zones, occur along the pathway of the nerve. On very slight stimulation, the trigger zones initiate pain. During the intense pain, twitching, grimacing, frequent blinking and tears from the eye on the affected side may be observed.

The attack is brief, lasting from seconds to 2 or 3 minutes. The episodes recur frequently, day or night for several weeks at a time. The onset of an episode may occur spontaneously or may coincide with touching or movement of the face or exposure to cold or a draught. The patient may relate the precipitation of pain to eating, talking, cleaning the teeth, or washing or shaving the face. The recurring incapacitating pain has been known to cause severe depression and even suicide.

Cause and incidence
The cause of the neuralgia is unknown. In rare instances it is a manifestation of multiple sclerosis, herpes zoster or a tumour. The disorder occurs in middle-aged and elderly persons and has a greater incidence in women.

Diagnosis
The diagnosis is made on the basis of the patient's history and a neurological examination. The sinuses, teeth and mouth are examined for possible infection or tumour as an aggravating factor.

MEDICAL MANAGEMENT

The patient may be treated by medication or surgery. There is no specific drug for the disorder. Anticonvulsant agents such as phenytoin (Epanutin) or carbamazepine (Tegretol) may suppress or shorten the painful episodes. These drugs may produce side-effects (see Table 22.11). An analgesic may be prescribed; if a narcotic is used, there is the risk of addiction. Drug therapy may provide relief at first but, usually, gradually loses its effectiveness.

Injection of alcohol into the affected nerve branch may be done to interrupt the sensory impulses and usually provides relief for several months. During this period of effectiveness, the patient has loss of sensation in the areas of distribution of the injected nerve branch.

Surgical procedures may be peripheral or intracranial. Resection or avulsion of the involved branch may be done but the relief may not be permanent if the nerve fibres regenerate. A more popular surgical measure is percutaneous radiofrequency thermocoagulation. An electrode is advanced into the ganglion. Lesions are produced in the gasserian ganglion and preganglionic fibres destroyed. This procedure, with the patient conscious, permits destruction of the pain sensory fibres and leaves the neurons and fibres concerned with other areas and the corneal reflex intact.

The more common major procedures which involve a craniotomy include vascular decompression of the trigeminal nerve and retrogasserian rhizotomy. The latter is used less often now; it involves resection of the sensory trigeminal root between the ganglion and brain. Unfortunately, there is residual loss of sensation in the face or cornea depending on the branch affected. If the ophthalmic division is involved, the loss of the corneal reflex predisposes the patient to drying of the cornea, keratitis and ulceration. The vascular decompression for the relief of trigeminal neuralgia is a complex microsurgical procedure in which a loop of the blood vessel which is pressing on the nerve is lifted off the nerve. A small plastic device is implanted to prevent recurrence of pressure on the nerve. Sensation is not impaired with this type of surgery.

NURSING ASSESSMENT

Efforts are made to identify pain-precipitating factors, the nature and exact location of the pain, duration of episodes and how the patient copes with the pain. The patient's nutritional and hydrational status and oral condition are noted.

IDENTIFICATION OF PATIENT PROBLEMS

1 Alteration in comfort due to the recurring severe pain
2 Fear of precipitating an episode
3 Nutritional deficit. Normal nutrition is not maintained because of fear of precipitating pain
4 Self-care deficits secondary to fear of precipitating pain
5 Lack of knowledge. The patient needs to be informed of potential precipitating factors and the possible side-effects of prescribed anticonvulsant drugs. If there are residual effects following surgery, the patient is advised of the necessary care.

NURSING INTERVENTION

The *goals* are to:
1 Control painful episodes
2 Prevent recurring attacks
3 Provide support
4 Prevent complications following invasive treatment

1. Alteration in comfort. The patient receives the prescribed analgesic or anticonvulsant. Warm moist applications may reduce the severity of pain and exposure to cold and draughts avoided. The patient is supported during the episode and advised that it is usually self-limited.

2. Fear of recurring pain. The patient is constantly in fear of precipitating pain. Factors which are likely to initiate pain are avoided. Exposure to cold is avoided; lukewarm food and fluids are taken; foods requiring mastication may be replaced by puréed foods. During an exacerbation of the disorder, the patient remains quiet and undisturbed; jarring of the bed and unnecessary activity around him are avoided.

3. Nutritional deficit. Fear of pain prevents normal food intake; the patient develops nutritional deficiencies and loses weight. Soft or puréed foods are offered and liquid concentrates may have to be added to increase the patient's calorie intake. Extremes of temperature in food and fluids are avoided.

4. Self-care deficits. Again, because of fear of pain, the patient may neglect personal hygiene (e.g. washing the face, cleansing teeth, bathing, combing of hair, shaving). He may become inactive, withdrawn and fully occupied with preventing an episode. It may be helpful to provide warm water and a very soft cloth of absorbent cotton and suggest that he might like to wash his face. The importance of mouth hygiene in preventing complications is explained and a warm mouthwash provided. The opportune time for these activities may be following the administration of an analgesic. The patient is encouraged to move about and participate in some physical exercise and activities.

5. Inadequate knowledge. The avoidance of potential precipitating factors is discussed with the patient. Emphasis is placed on the importance of nutrition and ways of increasing calorie intake suggested. Normal activity is encouraged between episodes of pain. If the patient is receiving an anticonvulsant preparation, he is advised of the potential side-effects and the need for regular medical supervision.

If surgery incurred loss of corneal sensation and reflex, the patient is taught to irrigate the affected eye or instil a prescribed solution 3 or 4 times daily and to voluntarily close the eyelid frequently to keep the surface moistened. Protective glasses should be worn. If there is loss of maxillary or mandibular sensory function, the patient is instructed to take food into the unaffected side of the mouth. Food may be trapped on the affected side due to the diminished sensation. The teeth should be cleansed and a mouthwash used after meals and at bedtime. Hot foods and beverages which could burn the oral mucous membrane are avoided. Dental problems on that side will not produce the usual warning of pain; the importance of a visit to a dentist at least twice a year is stressed.

Pre-and postoperative care
If a surgical procedure is to be performed, *preoperative nursing care* includes emotional support, explanation of what is to be done and potential permanent effects if these are anticipated (e.g. loss of sensation on the affected side of the face, numbness, stiffness and heaviness) and the protective measures that will be necessary. A minimal amount of hair will be shaved to prepare the scalp for surgery.

In the *postoperative phase* of trigeminal nerve surgery, the general principles of postoperative care are applicable (see Chapter 11). Specific intervention will depend upon the type of procedure that is done. Following intracranial surgery, intervention will be similar to that following craniotomy (see p. 811). If a suboccipital approach is used for vascular decompression, intervention will include particulars related to infratentorial surgery (see p. 814). The patient is observed for: (1) signs of difficulty in mastication due to possible interference with the motor fibres of the mandibular branch of the trigeminal nerve; and (2) temporary facial paralysis on the operative side which may result from trauma of the facial (seventh cranial) nerve. It is not unusual for the patient to develop herpes simplex (cold sores) around the mouth because of trauma to the gasserian ganglion, hyperthermia or dehydration. These lesions usually heal spontaneously but may be treated topically.

If function of the ophthalmic branch of the trigeminal nerve is interrupted, the corneal reflex will be absent on that side. Irrigation of the eye or the instillation of a prescribed preparation is necessary to moisten the eye and wash out dust and foreign particles. The patient is requested to voluntarily close the eyelid frequently to moisten the surface of the eye. If the sensory functions of the maxillary or mandibular branch of the trigeminal nerve are interrupted, eating may be difficult (see the discussion under Inadequate Knowledge).

EXPECTED OUTCOMES

The patient:
1 Discusses fears and concerns and on being reassured that assistance is available, demonstrates a lower level of anxiety.
2 States factors which precipitate pain and indicates management of the episodes.
3 Understands the potential side-effects of the prescribed anticonvulsant drug.
4 Understands the precautions necessary to prevent complications following surgery.
5 Is free of pain.
6 Resumes normal activity and food intake.

BELL'S PALSY (PERIPHERAL FACIAL PARALYSIS)

Bell's palsy is a disorder of the motor component of one of the facial (seventh cranial) nerves and is characterized by loss of the ability to move the muscles on one side of the face.

ASSESSMENT

Manifestations and course
The condition is most common in persons between 20 and 40 years of age. The patient may experience pain behind the ear or in the face for a day or two prior to the onset of paralysis. When paralysis occurs, a drawing sensation on the affected side is experienced. There is flaccidity, drooping of the mouth, drooling, flattening of the nasolabial fold, widening of the palpebral fissure and inability to completely close the eye on the affected side. There may be watering of the eye. The individual is unable to smile, whistle or grimace. The taste sensation is lost over the anterior two-thirds of the tongue on the respective side. Herpes lesions may appear on or in the corresponding ear. In 80% of the victims, muscle tone begins to return in a few weeks and movement is usually restored over a period of months.

Diagnosis
Bell's Palsy is diagnosed on the basis of the patient's history and the neurological examination.

MEDICAL MANAGEMENT

Treatment is usually provided on an outpatient basis. It may include analgesics for discomfort due to herpes, or application of acyclovir (Zovirax) cream, a corticosteroid preparation to relieve oedema and inflammation, application of moist heat and gentle facial massage and electrical stimulation of the facial nerve to maintain muscle tone. The sagging facial muscles may be supported with a facial sling or adhesive strips. If the condition does not improve, rarely, surgery is performed to re-establish closure of the eye during sleep and restore tone to facial muscles. The surgical procedure involves the anastamosis of the peripheral part of the nerve with another nerve.

IDENTIFICATION OF PATIENT PROBLEMS

1 Fear as a result of the sudden appearance of the symptoms
2 Potential for injury to the cornea (keratitis, ulceration) secondary to exposure of the eye and drying
3 Nutritional deficit secondary to inability to chew food on the affected side, inability to control saliva and drooling, emotional involvement and the awkwardness and embarrassment associated with eating
4 Alteration in comfort due to the sensation of stiffness and heaviness
5 Alteration in self-image as a result of the change in appearance and drooling

NURSING INTERVENTION

Nursing care emphasizes patient comfort and the prevention of complications. The patient's concerns are assessed, and his condition explained. Reassurance is given that he has not had a stroke and that most patients recover within a few weeks. The nurse instructs the patient in the use of the prescribed artificial tear solution to protect the eye and advises the use of sunglasses during the day, an eye-patch at night and periodic *gentle* manual closure of the eye.

Frequent small feedings of soft food that can best be managed by the patient are recommended in order to promote nutrition. The patient is instructed to place food in the unaffected side of the mouth for mastication. Oral hygiene after each meal is emphasized to prevent accumulation of residual food in the affected side of the mouth. The face should be protected from extremes in temperature. A mild analgesic may be prescribed if the patient is experiencing discomfort.

The patient is self-conscious about his appearance; his desire for privacy should be respected, especially during meals. The family is cautioned against demonstrating surprise at the patient's appearance and against comments that embarrass the patient and remind him of the change.

EXPECTED OUTCOMES

Nursing care is effective when the patient with Bell's Palsy:
1 Expresses understanding of potential hazards and the necessary preventive measures.
2 States plans for coping with facial paralysis for its duration.
3 Is free of complications.

POLYNEURITIS (MULTIPLE PERIPHERAL NEURITIS)

Although the term neuritis implies inflammation, it is more often applied to any neuropathy where there is dysfunction and pain of peripheral nerves from any cause. Polyneuritis is a disorder in which there is pain and impaired function along the distribution of many peripheral nerves. It is usually symmetrical and both motor and sensory disturbances occur.

MANIFESTATIONS AND CAUSE

The symptoms generally start in the parts innervated by the distal portions of the nerves and spread proximally. The patient first experiences pain, pins and needles, tingling and weakness in hands and feet ('glove and stocking' effect) then, a progressive loss of sensation, diminished tendon reflexes and inability to perform finer movements. The areas are tender and sore when subjected to even light pressure.

The causes include toxicity, nutritional deficiencies (especially vitamin B complex), metabolic disorder and cell-mediated immunological response. In some instances the cause is not identified.

Some of the more common polyneuropathies are diabetic polyneuritis, vitamin deficiency polyneuritis associated with alcoholism, arsenic or lead polyneuritis, malnutrition polyneuritis and acute idiopathic polyneuritis (Guillain–Barré syndrome).

GUILLAIN–BARRÉ SYNDROME (ACUTE IDIOPATHIC POLYNEURITIS)

The Guillain–Barré syndrome is an inflammatory disease of the spinal nerve roots within the dural sheath, peripheral nerves and may also involve the cranial nerves. The loss of nerve impulse conduction that occurs is due to compression, demyelination and nerve degeneration as a result of the inflammation and oedema.

Incidence and aetiology
It may occur at any age but the incidence is greater in persons 30–40 years of age. Men and women are equally affected. The cause of the disorder is unknown but viral infection and immunological reaction are both suspect. Frequently, the patients give a history of having 'just had' an upper respiratory infection or a gastrointestinal disturbance.

Clinical course and effects
The onset of Guillain–Barré syndrome is usually abrupt. Bilateral muscle weakness, beginning in the legs, may ascend to involve the trunk, arms and cranial nerves. Paraesthesia may precede the weakness. Within a few days, the weakness is followed by flaccid motor paralysis with weakness of the respiratory muscles. If the cranial nerves become involved, inability to swallow, talk, or even close the eyes develop. Muscle tenderness or sensitivity of the nerves to pressure may be experienced. Autonomic changes include sinus tachycardia and hypertension in the acute phase followed by hypotension.

Guillain–Barré syndrome is life-threatening due to potential respiratory and vasomotor failure if mechanical ventilation and vasopressor drugs are not promptly available. The mortality rate is estimated at 10–20%; death may result from a superimposed infection. Complete spontaneous recovery within weeks or months is usually anticipated in the survivors.

Diagnosis
Guillain–Barré syndrome is diagnosed on the basis of the clinical picture, the abrupt onset of bilateral weakness, paralysis and absence of muscle atrophy. The protein content of cerebrospinal fluid is usually elevated due to the inflammation of the nerve roots.

Treatment
In some instances steroids may be used to counteract the inflammation. Treatment is mainly supportive.

IDENTIFICATION OF PATIENT PROBLEMS

1 Anxiety due to the sudden development of dependency and paralysis
2 Potential respiratory insufficiency due to weakness of the diaphragm and intercostal muscles
3 Self-care deficits due to muscular weakness and paralysis
4 Impairment of mobility secondary to weakness or paralysis
5 Potential dysphagia and aspiration secondary to weakness of the muscles concerned with swallowing and diminished gag reflex
6 Impairment of communication as a result of reduced ventilatory volume and motor deficits or endotracheal intubation
7 Lack of knowledge about the disorder, the procedures being used, and home management

NURSING INTERVENTION

Guillain–Barré syndrome is a life-threatening disorder. Frequent assessments are necessary; increasing nerve involvement and paralysis may develop over a short period. A data base is established so that progress can be evaluated.

motor functions are very threatening to the patient. An explanation of events and procedures is made to the patient. Continuous support and reassurance are necessary. Frequent visits to the bedside should be made; if left alone for long periods, the patient becomes very apprehensive because of his help-lessness.

2. *Potential respiratory insufficiency.* Frequent obser-vation is made of the patient's respirations, and blood-gas concentrations are determined at regular intervals. The chest is auscultated for air entry and the retention of pulmonary secretions. Endotracheal intubation and mechanical respiratory assistance may be necessary (see Chapter 16).

3. *Self-care deficits.* The patient may be dependent on the nurse for total hygienic care (bathing, cleaning of teeth, toileting) feeding and change of position. Demands on the patient's energy are kept to a mini-mum during the acute stage. The nurse must be particularly sensitive to non-verbal responses and unexpressed needs, since the patient's weakness or intubation may restrict his communication.

4. *Immobility.* The patient's position is changed at regular intervals and the limbs positioned to prevent deformities, strain on tendons and ankylosis. Cot-sides should be kept in place as a safety precaution. Range-of-movement and other exercises are not instituted until the postacute stage. Following the acute stage when the condition has stabilized, range-of-movement exercises are introduced and gradually increased according to the patient's progress in regaining motor function and strength. Immobility creates the potential for pressure sores. Vulnerable areas are inspected with each repositioning. Sheepskin or an alternating air-pressure (ripple) mattress may be used under the patient.

5. *Alteration in comfort.* The involved parts are handled very gently and are subjected to a minimum of pressure because of the sensitivity and soreness.

6. *Potential dysphagia and aspiration.* Before giving the patient food or beverage, the gag reflex and his ability to swallow are tested with a very small amount. Foods that do not require chewing may be more readily tolerated. The head should be raised during the meal to prevent choking and feed slowly. Suction equipment should be readily available in case of aspiration. If endotracheal intubation is necessary, the patient is sustained by intravenous infusion or nasogastric feedings.

7. *Inadequate knowledge.* The patient and family are informed about the disorder and treatment. They are advised that the patient will require considerable rest and a prolonged convalescent period when he returns home. They are assisted in planning a daily regimen for the patient and home management.

EXPECTED OUTCOMES

The patient:
1 Is free of complications.
2 Has resumed self-care activities.
3 Has no residual loss of motor function and is regaining strength.
4 Has a normal vital capacity.
5 Feels optimistic about his recovery.
6 Is compliant with the recommended rest, exercise and activity programme.
7 Is taking adequate nutrients and has regained some of the weight lost in the acute stage.

References and Further Reading

BOOKS

Adams RD & Victor M (1981) *Principles of Neurology.* Toronto: McGraw-Hill.
Albrecht G (ed) (1976) *The Sociology of Physical Disability and Rehabilitation.* Pittsburgh: University of Pittsburgh Press.
APBI (1985–86) *Data Sheet Compendium.* London: Data-pharm Publications.
Ball AP (1982) *Notes on Infectious Diseases.* Edinburgh: Churchill Livingstone.
Bannister R (ed) (1985) *Brain's Clinical Neurology,* 6th ed. New York: Oxford University Press.
Bobath B (1978) *Adult Hemiplegia—Evaluation and Treatment,* 2nd ed. London: William Heinemann Medical.
Braunwald E et al (eds) (1987) *Harrison's Principles of Internal Medicine,* 11th ed. New York: McGraw-Hill.
Bromley I (1981) *Tetraplegia and Paraplegia—A Guide for Physiotherapists,* 2nd ed. Edinburgh: Churchill Liv-ingstone.
Budassi SA & Barber JM (1981) *Emergency Nursing.* St Louis: CV Mosby.
Carpenter MB (1978) *Core Textbook of Neuroanatomy,* 2nd ed. Baltimore: Williams & Wilkins.
Chusid JG (1982) *Correlative Neuroanatomy and Functional Neurology,* 18th ed. Los Altos: Lange Medical.
Conway-Rutkowski BL (1982) *Carini and Owens' Neurological and Neurosurgical Nursing,* 8th ed. St Louis: CV Mosby.
Edmond RTD, Bradley JM & Galbraith NS (1982) *Infection—'Pocket Consultant'.* London: Grant McIntyre.
Fitzgerald MJT (1985) *Neuroanatomy: Basic and Applied.* Eastbourne: Baillière Tindall.
Guyton AC (1981) *Basic Human Neurophysiology,* 3rd ed. Phi-ladelphia: WB Saunders.
Hickey JV (1986) *The Clinical Practice of Neurological and Neu-rosurgical Nursing.* Philadelphia: JB Lippincott.
Hudak CM et al (1982) *Critical Care Nursing.* Philadelphia: JB Lippincott.
Jacob SW, Francone CA & Lossow WJ (1982) *Structure and Function in Man,* 5th ed. Philadelphia: WB Saunders.
Jennett B & Teasdale G (1981) *Management of Head Injuries.* Philadelphia: FA Davis.
Kinash RG (1978) *Nursing Needs and Experiences of Patients With Spinal Cord Injury.* Saskatoon, Canada: University of Saskatchewan Press.
McGovern S (1982) *The Epilepsy Handbook.* London: Sheldon Press.

Matthews WB (1978) *Multiple Sclerosis—The Facts*. Oxford: Oxford University Press.

Noback CF & Demarest RJ (1981) *The Nervous System: Basic Principles of Neurobiology*, 3rd ed. New York: McGraw-Hill.

Nolte J (1981) *The Human Brain*. St Louis: CV Mosby.

Pallett PJ & O'Brien MT (1985) *Textbook of Neurosurgical Nursing*. Boston: Little, Brown.

Purchese G & Allan D (1984) *Current Nursing Practice— Neuromedical and Neurosurgical Nursing*, 2nd ed. London: Baillière Tindall.

Robbins SL et al (1981) *Basic Pathology*, 3rd ed. Philadelphia: WB Saunders.

Stern G & Lees A (1982) *Parkinson's Disease—The Facts*. Oxford: Oxford University Press.

Swift N & Mabel RM (1978) *Manual of Neurological Nursing*. Boston: Little, Brown.

Taylor JW & Ballenger S (1980) *Neurological Dysfunctions and Nursing Intervention*. New York: McGraw-Hill.

Van Meter MJ (ed) (1982) *Neurologic Care: A Guide for Patient Education*. New York: Appleton-Century-Croft.

Walter JB (1982) *An Introduction to the Principles of Disease*. Philadelphia: WB Saunders.

Way LW (ed) (1985) *Current Surgical Diagnosis and Treatment*, 2nd ed. Los Altos: Lange Medical. Chapter 39.

Wilson SF (1979) *Neuronursing*. New York: Springer.

Weiner WJ & Goetz C (eds) (1981) *Neurology for the Non-Neurologist*. Philadelphia: Harper & Row.

PERIODICALS

Agee BL (1985) Helping your patient survive the perils of CNS infection. *Nurs. '85*, Vol. 15 No. 5, pp. 11–13.

Agee BL & Herman C (1984) Cervical logrolling on a standard hospital bed. *Am. J. Nurs.*, Vol. 84 No. 3, pp. 314–318.

Allmond BJ (1981) Management of cervical and thoracic spine/cord injured patients. *J. Neurosurg. Nurs.*, Vol. 13 No. 2, pp. 97–101.

Allwood AC & Lundy C (1980) Cerebral artery bypass surgery. *Am. J. Nurs.*, Vol. 80 No. 7, pp. 1284–1287.

Banning J (1982) Epilepsy: Kathy's story. *Can. Nurs.*, Vol. 78 No. 4, pp. 37–41.

Barbeau A (1982) Parkinson's disease—the Canadian story. *Future Health*, Vol. 4 No. 1, pp. 11–12.

Beniak J (1982) Patient education in epilepsy. *J. Neurosurg. Nurs.*, Vol. 14 No. 1, pp. 19–22.

Blanco KM (1982) The aphasic patient. *J. Neurosurg. Nurs.*, Vol. 14 No. 1, pp. 34–37.

Booth K (1982) The neglect syndrome. *J. Neurosurg. Nurs.*, Vol. 14 No. 1, pp. 38–43.

Bowers SA & Marshall LF (1982) Severe head injury: current treatment and research. *J. Neurosurg. Nurs.*, Vol. 14 No. 5, pp. 210–219.

Bregman C et al (1983) Agitated aggressive patient. *Am. J. Nurs.*, Vol. 83 No. 10, pp. 1409–1412.

Byers V & Gendell H (1982) Using metrizamide for lumbar myelography: adverse reactions and nursing implications. *J. Neurosurg. Nurs.*, Vol. 14 No. 6, pp. 315–317.

Carlson CE (1980) Psychosocial aspects of neurologic disability. *Nurs. Clin. N. Am.*, Vol. 15 No. 2, pp. 309–320.

Chung HO (1982) Infective polyneuritis (Guillain–Barre syndrome). *Nurs. Times*, Vol. 78 No. 8, pp. 315–319.

Craven R & Sharp B (1972) The effects of illness on family functions. *Nurs. Forum*, Vol. 9, pp. 182–183.

Crate M (1965) Nursing functions in adaptation to chronic illness. *Am. J. Nurs.*, Vol. 65 No. 10, pp. 72–76.

D'Alton JG & Norris JW (1983) Carotid doppler evaluation in cerebrovascular disease. *Can. Med. Assc. J.*, Vol. 129, pp. 1187.

Dewis ME & Bauman A (1982) Alzheimer's disease: the silent epidemic. *Can. Nurs.*, Vol. 78 No. 7, pp. 32–35.

Farrell J (1978) Caring for the laminectomy patient: how to strengthen your support. *Nurs. '78*, Vol. 8 No. 5, pp. 65–69.

Feustel D (1981) Alterations in neuron innervation associated with spinal cord lesions. *J. Neurosurg. Nurs.*, Vol. 13 No. 2, pp. 48–52.

Fischbach FT (1978) Easing adjustment to Parkinson's disease. *Am. J. Nurs.*, Vol. 78 No. 1, pp. 66–69.

Fournier L (1985) Carotid doppler. *Can. Nurse*, Vol. 81 No. 10, p. 27.

Gehrke M (1980) Identifying brain tumors. *J. Neurosurg. Nurs.*, Vol. 12 No. 4, pp. 203–205.

Goldsmith HS et al (1984) Vascularization of brain and spinal cord by intact omentum. *Appl. Neurophysiol.*, Vol. 47 No. 1–2, pp. 57–61.

Goldsmith HS et al (1985) Early application of pedicled omentum to the acutely traumatised spinal cord. *Paraplegia*, Vol. 23 No. 2, pp. 100–112.

Guin PR (1983) Radiofrequency lesions—a treatment for trigeminal neuralgia. *J. Neurosurg. Nurs.*, Vol. 14 No. 4, pp. 192–194.

Hachinski V (1982) Should all TIAs be seen by a neurologist? *Mod. Med. Can.* (Neurology-Psychiatry), Vol. 37 No. 6 (Supplement), pp. 99–101.

Hader WJ (1982) Prevalence of multiple sclerosis in Saskatoon. *Can. Med. Assn. J.*, Vol. 127, pp. 295–297.

Hahn K (1982) Management of Parkinson's disease. *Nurse Pract.*, Vol. 7 No. 1, pp. 13–25 & 50.

Hargrove R (1980) Feeding the severely dysphagic patient. *J. Neurosurg. Nurs.*, Vol. 12 No. 2, pp. 102–107.

Hart G (1980) Perceptual distortion . . . post CVA. *Can. Nurse*, Vol. 76 No. 5, pp. 44–47.

Holland NH, McDonnell M & Wiesel-Levison P (1981) Overview of multiple sclerosis and nursing care of the MS patient. *J. Neurosurg. Nurs.*, Vol. 13 No. 1, pp. 28–33.

Hrovanth M (1982) Myasthenia gravis: a nursing approach. *J. Neurosurg. Nurs.*, Vol. 14 No. 2, pp. 7–12.

Jones CC & Cayard CH (1982) Care of ICP monitoring devices: a nursing responsibility. *J. Neurosurg. Nurs.*, Vol. 14 No. 5, pp. 255–261.

Kao CC (1982) Basic considerations in spinal cord reconstruction. *J. Am. Paraplegia Soc.*, Vol. 5 No. 1, pp. 9–12.

Kelly-Hayes M (1980) Guidelines for rehabilitation of multiple sclerosis patients. *Nurs. Clin. N. Am.*, Vol. 15 No. 2, pp. 245–256.

Kimball CD & Belber CJ (1979) Protocol for intravenous barbiturate therapy in increased intracranial pressure in a community hospital. *J. Neurosurg. Nurs.*, Vol. 11 No. 3, pp. 144–147.

King RB & Dudas S (1980) Rehabilitation of the patient with a spinal cord injury. *Nurs. Clin. N. Am.*, Vol. 15 No. 2, pp. 225–243.

Louis MC & Povsee SM (1980) Aphasia and endurance: considerations in the assessment and care of the stroke patient. *Nurs. Clin. N. Am.*, Vol. 15 No. 2, pp. 265–282.

Lyons MC & Wilson DA (1981) Regional cerebral blood flow—a newer non-invasive neurodiagnostic test. *J. Neurosurg. Nurs.*, Vol. 13 No. 6, pp. 286–292.

Malasanos LJ (1982) Tremors: associations and assessment. *J. Neurosurg. Nurs.*, Vol. 14 No. 6, pp. 290–294.

McNairn N (1978) About multiple sclerosis. *Can. Nurse*, Vol. 74, pp. 35–40.

Miller J (1985) Inspiring hope. *Am. J. Nurs.*, Vol. 85 No. 1, pp. 22–25.

Miller L (1979) Neurological assessment: a practical approach for the critical care nurse. *J. Neurosurg. Nurs.*, Vol. 11 No. 1, pp. 2–5.

Mitchell PH (1981) A nursing perspective on neurological evaluation: nursing assessment for nursing purposes. *Axon*. The Canadian Ass'n of Neurological and Neurosurgical Nurses, Vol. 2 No. 8, pp. 1–5.

Mitchell PH & Irvin N (1977) Neurological examination: nursing assessment for nursing purposes. *J. Neurosurg. Nurs.*, Vol. 9 No. 1, pp. 23–28.

Mitchell PH, Oxuna J & Lipe ME (1981) Moving the patient in bed: effects on intracranial pressure. *Nurs. Res.*, Vol. 30 No. 4, pp. 212–218.

Mittal B & Thomas DGT (1986) Controlled thermocoagulation in trigeminal neuralgia. *J. Neurol. Neurosurg. Psychiat.*, Vol. 49 No. 8.

Norman S (1982) The pupil check. *Am. J. Nurs.*, Vol. 28 No. 4, pp. 588–591.

Polhopek M (1980) Stroke: an update on vascular disease. *J. Neurosurg. Nurs.*, Vol. 12 No. 2, pp. 81–87.

Reier PJ (1985) Neural tissue grafts and repair of the injured spinal cord. *Neuropathol. Appl. Neurobiol.*, Vol. 11 No. 2, pp. 81–104 (Ref 115).

Ricci MM (1979) Intracranial hypertension: barbiturate therapy and the role of the nurse. *J. Neurosurg. Nurs.*, Vol. 11 No. 4, pp. 247–252.

Rimel RW & Thyson GW (1979) The Neurologic examination in patients with central nervous system trauma. *J. Neurosurg. Nurs.*, Vol. 11 No. 3, pp. 12–19.

Ross AJ et al (1979) Neuromuscular diagnostic procedures. *Nurs. Clin. N. Am.*, Vol. 14 No. 1, pp. 107–121.

Scharf R (1980) When is a head injury concussion? *Can. Fam. Phys.*, Vol. 26, pp. 948–951.

Sheahan S (1982) Assessment of low back pain. *Nurs. Pract.* Vol. 7 No. 5, pp. 15–19, 23.

Smith J & Geist BL (1978) Evaluation and care of the acute craniotomy patient. *J. Neurosurg. Nurs.*, Vol. 10 No. 3, pp. 102–111.

Speers I (1981) Cerebral edema. *J. Neurosurg. Nurs.*, Vol. 13 No. 2 pp. 102–115.

Spinal Cord Reconstruction (1984) Proceedings of the Seminar on Spinal Cord Reconstruction, Naples (Oct 21–22 1983) *J. Neurosurg. Sci.*, Vol. 28 No. 3–4, pp. 115–240.

Stewart C (1981) Principles of patient education for the patient with an altered neurological status. *J. Neurosurg. Nurs.*, Vol. 12 No. 4, pp. 179–183.

Sweezey E (1982) Epilepsy. *Future Hlth.*, Vol. 4 No. 1, p. 17.

Tarling C (1985) Aids to patient mobility. *Clin. Nurs.* (Second Series), Vol. 2 No. 33, pp. 974–979.

Tilton CN & Maloof M (1982) Diagnosing the problems in stroke. *Am. J. Nurs.*, Vol. 82 No. 4, pp. 596–601.

Trekas J (1982) Managing epilepsy. Don't forget the patient. *Nurs. '82*, Vol. 12 No. 10, pp. 63–65.

Walleck C (1978) Neurological assessment for nurses—a part of the nursing process. *J. Neurosurg. Nurs.*, Vol. 10 No. 1, pp. 13–16.

Welnetz K (1981) Health teaching for spinal cord injured patients and families during acute hospitalization. *Axon* (Canadian Association of Neurological and Neurosurgical Nurses), December.

Whitney FW (1985) Alzheimer's disease: toward understanding and management. *Nurs. Practit. Am. J. Primary Health Care*, Vol. 10 No. 9, pp. 25–28.

Wing S (1981) Brain abscess. *J. Neurosurg. Nurs.*, Vol. 13 No. 3, pp. 123–126.

Woodward ES (1982) The total patient: implications for nursing care of the epileptic. *J. Neurosurg. Nurs.*, Vol. 14 No. 4, pp. 166–169.

Young MS (1981) A bedside guide to understanding the signs of intracranial pressure. *Nurs. '81*, Vol. 11 No. 2, pp. 59–62.

Zegeer LJ (1982) Nursing care of the patient with brain edema. *J. Neurosurg. Nurs.*, Vol. 14 No. 5, pp. 268–275.

Embryology

The reproductive system is unique in mammals in that it differs markedly between sexes. Sex is determined at the time of fertilization by the inclusion of the XX chromosomal pair of the female or the XY genotype of the male. In this early period of human development, sex differentiation can be determined microscopically by the presence or absence of Barr bodies in a cell nucleus which has been taken from the embryo. These Barr bodies, which are always one less than the number of X chromosomes, indicate the genotype of the embryo.

As the embryo grows, a genital ridge develops but remains undifferentiated in either sex until the seventh week of intrauterine life. At this time sex differentiation can be made morphologically because the genital ridges of the embryo, accompanied by the primordial germ cells, have grown and differentiated into a rudimentary testis or ovary, depending on the sex of the cell.

An elaborate bilateral duct system also develops. In the male much of this duct system degenerates, and the remaining portion forms the epididymis and ductus deferens, which then join the male urethra. In the female the duct systems develop bilaterally and, as growth continues, the two ducts meet and fuse in the midline. The portion which fuses becomes the uterus, cervix and vagina. This process of fusion take some weeks to complete and, indeed, may never occur, giving rise to paired uteri and vaginas. Fusion may be incomplete, causing some abnormalities of the uterus (Fig. 23.1).

While internal development proceeds the external genitalia are also becoming differentiated. In the 'neuter' phase of development three small protuberances appear caudally on the external surface of the embryo. These protuberances consist of the 'genital tubercle' and, on either side of this tubercle, the genital swellings. In the male the tubercle becomes elongated and develops into the male phallus while the genital swellings become the scrotal tissue. These two swellings must develop, descend and fuse, closing the urethra in the male penis and forming the pendulant scrotum. Should fusion not be complete on the dorsal surface, a condition known as hypospadias occurs (Fig. 23.2). Epispadias, a rarer malformation, may also occur. Here the failure of the urethra to fuse completely occurs on the ventral side of the penis. From these swellings, the prepuce, or

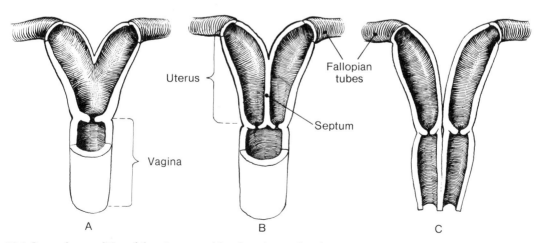

Fig. 23.1 Some abnormalities of the uterus resulting from incomplete fusion of the ducts. *A*, Bicornate uterus. *B*, Uterus septus and a double cervix. *C*, Double uterus, cervix and vagina.

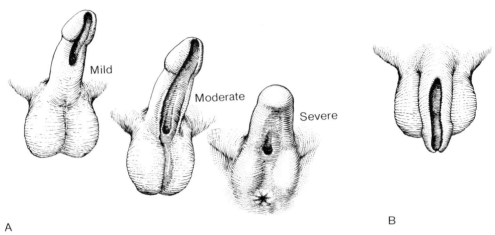

A

B

Fig. 23.2 *A*, Hypospadias—mild, moderate and severe. In severe hypospadias note the similarity to the female. *B*, Epispadias.

foreskin, of the penis also arises. The foreskin is attached to the penile shaft at the base of the glans. The foreskin then drops down like a hood over the glans and remains partially fixed until sometime between birth and 3 years of age. During this time the congenital adhesions break down and the prepuce is then easily retractable over the glans penis.

The female genitalia arise from the same three ridges. The tubercle becomes the clitoris, and the genital swellings develop into the labia majora and minora. As the labia meet anteriorly, they form a loose-fitting, hood-like fold over the clitoris. This fold is similar to the prepuce of the male penis. Posteriorly, the labial folds fuse just before the anus. Thus, male and female reproductive systems have homologous counterparts.

By the sixteenth week of embryologic life the sex of the infant can be determined externally. At this time the testes of the male, which normally reside in the scrotum, are not there. In early development the testis and ovary are abdominal organs. As further growth takes place, they descend over the pelvic brim in the case of the ovaries or into the scrotum in the case of the testes. The descent of the testes appears to be in response to hormonal and mechanical control. As the fetal testes begin to produce testosterone, in about the seventh month of fetal life, descent occurs, and they pass through the inguinal canal and the external inguinal ring to enter the scrotum by the ninth month. During descent the testis is surrounded by a tube of peritoneum known as the processus vaginalis. After descent has occurred, this tissue generally becomes obliterated, leaving the testis covered by the tunica vaginalis. Following descent, the testis shows a decline in its production of testosterone until puberty. As in all processes, descent may not occur or may occur imperfectly. This may result in undescended testes.

Physiology

THE MALE REPRODUCTIVE SYSTEM

The system consists of the paired testes, epididymis, vas deferens, common ejaculatory ducts, urethra, penis and the scrotum. The accessory organs are the seminal vesicles, prostate gland and the bulbourethral glands (Fig. 23.3). A cross section of the testis (Fig. 23.4) demonstrates the relationships between the seminiferous tubule, rete testis, efferent ductules, epididymis and vas deferens.

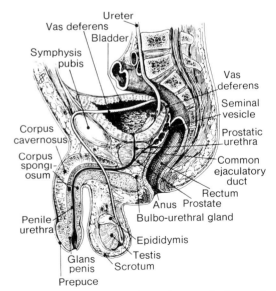

Fig. 23.3 Sagittal view of the male reproductive system and pelvis.

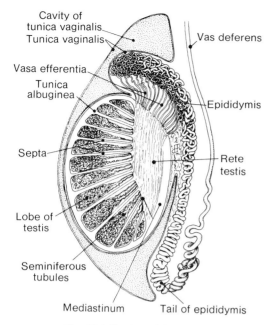

Fig. 23.4 Section of the testis.

The testes

Each lobe of the testis contains a seminiferous tubule surrounded by tissue. In this tissue are interstitial, or Leydig, cells, which are endocrine in action, producing the male hormones of which testosterone is the most prominent. These cells become activated to produce some androgens in the fetal period but remain nearly dormant until puberty. At puberty, under the complex control of the hypothalamus and pituitary glands, the testes are stimulated to produce male hormones. Under the influence of these androgens, the body begins the process of puberty. The external organs of reproduction grow and develop. The distribution of body hair changes to that of the adult male. The larynx and musculoskeletal systems develop and change. Concurrently, the testes begin to produce sperm. Puberty ends with the sexual and reproductive maturity of the individual.

Spermatogenesis
Spermatogenesis begins in the seminiferous tubule (Fig. 23.5). Here a basilar membrane around the lumen of the tubule is lined with two major cell types which project into the lumen of the tube. The first of these, the germ cells, are called spermatogonia. These cells undergo growth and multiplication to become primary and secondary spermatocytes and then spermatids. Until this phase is complete the cell appears to have sufficient nutrients in itself. Now, however, the second type of cell, the Sertoli or sustentacular cell, is apparently necessary to provide nutrition for the spermatid. The spermatid is engul-

fed by the Sertoli cell and begins a metamorphosis which produces viable spermatozoa.

When growth is complete, the sperm is released into the lumen of the seminiferous tubule and is rapidly transported to the epididymis and thence through the duct system. Although sperm may appear to be mature at the time of release into the tubule, they do undergo further maturation, increasing in fertility and vigour as they progress through the ducts. Sperm removed from the tail of the epididymis rather than the head are more fertile. If sperm are not ejaculated, they degenerate and are absorbed. Spermatogenesis is continuous and a sperm requires approximately 75 days to mature. This is in contrast to the female, who does not produce ova throughout her lifetime but merely matures ova present from her own primordial germ cells.

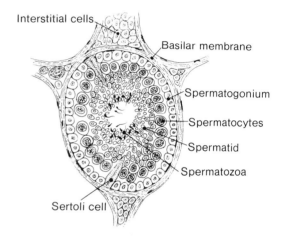

Fig. 23.5 Transverse section of a seminiferous tubule in the interstitial tissue of the testis.

Spermatogenesis is also sensitive to heat, and occurs at a temperature a few degrees lower than body temperature. It is for this reason that the testes are suspended in the scrotum, allowing the temperature of the testes to be regulated by the body. The dartos muscle within the scrotum contracts or relaxes in response to varying temperatures. Coldness causes it to contract, bringing the testes closer to the body for extra warmth. The reverse is true in heat. It is also known that men with uncorrected cryptorchism remain sterile, because body temperature intra-abdominally is incompatible with successful spermatogenesis.

A feedback mechanism controls the production of sperm and testosterone (see Fig. 23.6). The anterior pituitary gland, when stimulated by the gonadotrophin releasing hormone (GRH) of the hypothalamus, releases two hormones: the follicle-stimulating hormone (FSH) and luteinizing hormone (LH). FSH stimulates the semineferous tubule to begin spermatogenesis and the Sertoli cells to produce

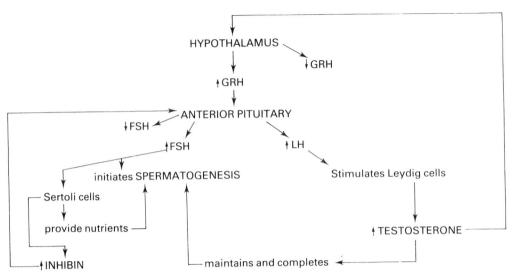

Fig. 23.6 Feedback mechanism for spermatogenesis and production of testosterone.

nutrients for the sperm. The Sertoli cells also release a hormone named inhibin which signals the anterior pituitary to reduce production of FSH.

The luteinizing hormone stimulates the interstitial cells of the testes to produce testosterone which maintains and completes spermatogenesis. Spermatogonia will proceed to the spermatocyte stage under the influence of FSH but testosterone is necessary to complete the step from spermatocyte to fertile spermatozoa.

High levels of testosterone exert an inhibitory effect on the hypothalamus. When testosterone reaches a low level it no longer exerts this inhibitory effect and more GRH is released, repeating the cycle.

Duct system and accessory glands

The viable sperm must be transported from the testis to the penis and thence to the female reproductive tract so that fertilization may take place. Here the duct system and the accessory glands play a major role. As the vas deferens ascends into the pelvic cavity, it widens into a broad ampulla. The duct of each seminal vesicle and the ampulla of the adjacent vas deferens meet to form the common ejaculatory duct. As a secretory organ, the seminal vesicle does not store sperm but rather produces a fluid which is rich in nutrients and prostaglandins. These nutrients provide for the sperm until fertilization. The prostaglandins are believed to aid fertilization by reacting with cervical mucus to make it more penetrable by sperm and to induce contractions in the uterus and tubes which help sperm to reach the ovum.

The prostate gland, which is fused to the neck of the bladder, is divided into three lobes which surround the urethra. The prostate develops in puberty and is easily palpable on rectal examination.

During the years of sexual maturity the prostate secretes a thin, milky-looking fluid which contains among other substances a clotting enzyme and a pro-fibrinolysin. The fluid is alkaline and is believed to reduce the acidity of seminal fluid and vaginal secretions. This is an important reproductive function, as the motility and viability of sperm are greatly reduced in an acid solution. Sperm are more motile in a neutral or slightly alkaline solution.

Further fluid is added to the semen by the bulbourethral glands. These paired glands lie posterior to the urethra and discharge their fluid into it when they contract at ejaculation. This fluid seems to function merely as a lubricant and fluid medium for the sperm.

Deposition of the semen in the vagina of the female is one function of the penis. The penis also serves as an excretory organ. In order to obtain intromission, the penis must move from its normally flaccid state to one of erection. Such a change is due to engorgement with blood of the corpora cavernosa and the corpus spongiosum.

Semen is a milky, viscous fluid varying at one ejaculation from 2–7 ml in quantity and containing about 60 000 000 to 100 000 000 sperm per millilitre. The alkaline fluid is rich in nutrients and minerals to support the sperm. It coagulates a few minutes after ejaculation and then reliquefies later. The clotting enzyme of the prostatic fluid acts on the fibrinogen of seminal vesicle fluid to form a coagulate. This coagulate spontaneously dissolves some 15–20 minutes later under the influence of the fibrinolysin formed from the prostatic profibrinolysin. During this time the sperm are immobile; following reliquefaction they are highly motile. The sperm, which are now actively motile by lashing their tails, move rapidly up through the uterus into the outer third of the uterine (fallopian) tube where fertilization usually takes place. It is believed that the acrosome or projection on the head of the sperm releases hyaluronidase, an enzyme which dissolves the outer wall of the ovum. This allows a sperm to enter the ovum and fertilization to take place.

THE FEMALE REPRODUCTIVE SYSTEM

The female reproductive tract consists of paired ovaries, uterine tubes, a uterus and vagina (Fig. 23.7). Externally, the labia, clitoris, and Skene's and Bartholin's glands are part of the reproductive system (Fig. 23.8). The external area may be collectively referred to as the vulva, perineum or pudenda. Generally, perineum refers to the area stretching from the symphysis pubis laterally to the thighs and posteriorly to the tip of the coccyx. This is arbitrarily divided into the anterior and posterior perineum by an imaginary line drawn between the ischial tuberosities. Anteriorly, this contains the urogenital triangle and posteriorly the rectal triangle, including the perineal body. The area between the labia majora is referred to as the pudendal cleft. That area which lies between the labia minora and extends from the clitoris to the fourchette is referred to as the vestibule. Bartholin's glands, whose ducts open into the vestibule, may be referred to as the greater vestibular glands, Skene's being the lesser.

The female reproductive system functions to produce the female hormones (oestrogen and progesterone), to ripen ova for fertilization, and for inter-course which permits fertilization of ova and the release of sexual tension. In addition, the organs of reproduction incubate the human conceptus, providing it with safety and nourishment until the fetus is expelled from the uterus to continue its growth and development externally.

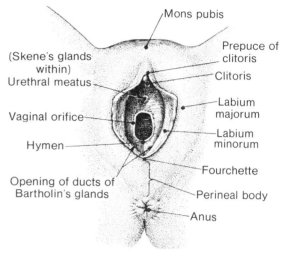

Fig. 23.8 Female external genitalia.

The ovary

The ovary is a small, almond-shaped organ lying posterior to the broad ligament of the uterus and attached to it by the mesovarium. Cross sections of

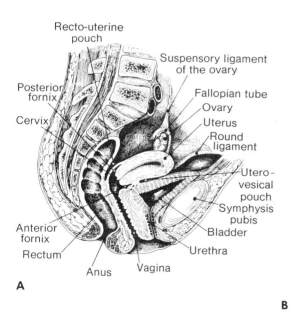

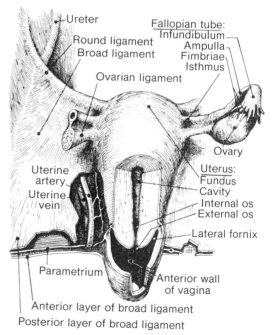

Fig. 23.7 *A*, Median sagittal section of the female pelvis. *B*, Uterus and adnexa, posterior view (uterus, cervix and vagina wedge sectioned).

the ovary show a cortex and a medulla. The cortex, or outer layer, is composed of connective tissue and cells, among which are scattered the ova and developing follicles. Over this outer layer of the cortex is a thin layer of germinal epithelium. The medulla is composed of connective tissue containing blood vessels and smooth muscle fibres.

The fetal ovary is recognizable very early. By the fourth month of intrauterine life some cells in the ovary have differentiated enough to be recognizable as primary oocytes. Initially these oocytes number in the millions but most degenerate. At birth less than two million are present; at puberty there are about 300000, and of these only 400–500 will develop to ovulation. By the menopause few primordial follicles remain and they soon degenerate. Throughout childhood certain of these oocytes develop but never reach maturity and ovulate. Then, under the influence of the maturing hypothalamus, which stimulates the anterior lobe of the pituitary to produce hormones, puberty begins.

The secondary sex characteristics begin to develop. First there is growth and development of the breast tissue. Pubic hair appears and the internal and external organs of reproduction become fully developed and functional. The vagina, under the influence of oestrogens, thickens and develops several layers of squamous epithelium. This makes it more resistant to infection. Previously, the vaginal pH had been neutral or alkaline; now it becomes acidic. This is largely due to Doederlein's bacillus which oxidizes the glycogen which has been deposited in the vagina to form lactic acid. Concurrently, the ovaries are developing and menarche, or the beginning of menstruation, occurs.

As in the male, GRH stimulates the anterior pituitary gland to release two hormones: FSH and LH. Under this hormonal influence, primordial follicles in the ovary begin to develop. Each primordial follicle is composed of an oocyte and surrounding granulosa cells. As growth occurs the oocyte or ovum enlarges and there is an increase in the number of granulosa cells. Growth is eccentric and the ovum comes to lie at one side of the group of granulosa cells. Fluid, rich in oestrogens, collects between these cells and the ovum. A clear membrane, the zona pellucida, develops and surrounds the ovum. As the follicle grows, cells begin to form around it and are called thecal cells. These thecal cells, stimulated by the FSH and LH, produce oestrogens.

Many follicles in both ovaries start to ripen but usually only one follicle continues on to ovulation. The others undergo degeneration. The mechanism of this atresia is still unknown. The thecal cells surrounding these degenerated (atretic) follicles continue to produce oestrogens. The mature follicle may now be termed a graafian follicle, after de Graaf who first described it in 1672 (Fig. 23.9).

As the graafian follicle approaches ovulation, it comes to lie close to the surface of the ovary. The

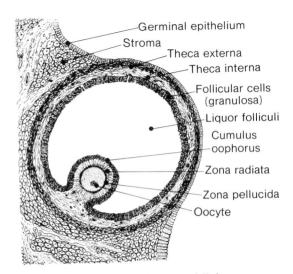

Fig. 23.9 Mature graafian follicle.

tissue over it becomes thin and taut. Soon the follicle wall ruptures and the ovum, surrounded by the zona pellucida and attached cells, is expelled into the abdominal cavity. The time of rupture is designated as ovulation and marks the end of the preovulatory (proliferative or follicular) phase.

The ovary now embarks on the luteal (secretory) phase of its cycle. Immediately following ovulation, the wall of the follicle collapses inward and some haemorrhage may occur into this cavity. In a few hours the remaining granulosa cells hypertrophy and begin to show the characteristic yellow of the corpus luteum. These yellowed granulosa cells are now called luteal cells. The luteal cells are stimulated by LH to become the corpus luteum and to begin producing progesterone. Oestrogen continues to be produced as well. The corpus luteum reaches full maturity by about the ninth day following ovulation. At this time it is easily recognizable on the surface of the ovary as a raised yellowed area and may constitute nearly half the volume of the ovary. Near this time the corpus luteum may receive a message that the ovum has been fertilized. If it does so, the corpus luteum is maintained and becomes known as the corpus luteum of pregnancy. If fertilization does not occur, the luteal site begins to degenerate, and progesterone production drops. As the site degenerates, so do the thecal cells. Oestrogen production from this source declines. The luteal site shrinks to form a small mass of whitish scar tissue on the surface of the ovary which is known as the corpus albicans.

Hormones and the ovarian cycle. In response to the falling oestrogen and progesterone levels, the hypothalamus signals the anterior pituitary gland to release FSH and LH. Under this stimulus the follicles begin to develop and the thecal cells produce oestrogen. The rising levels of oestrogen exert a negative feedback effect on the hypothalamus to reduce the amount of GRH released and hence the amount of FSH and LH, for the levels of FSH and LH fall slightly following the initial rise in oestrogen levels (Fig. 23.10). As oestrogen peaks, it is thought to exert a positive feedback effect on the hypothalamic–pituitary axis that results in a surge of LH and, to a lesser extent, FSH. This surge of LH occurs about 24 hours before ovulation (Fig. 23.11).

In cycles where the LH surge does not occur or is of insufficient magnitude, ovulation fails to occur. Exactly how the LH surge affects ovulation is unclear except that it is necessary for completion of the cycle. Follicles will grow and develop under FSH stimulation but will fail to ovulate without the surge of LH.

Ovulation occurs in a climate of falling oestrogen, LH and FSH levels and a rising progesterone level, as LH stimulates the follicular site to begin production of progesterone. As the preovulatory cycle is one of high oestrogen level, the postovulatory phase is one of high progesterone level. The other hormones continue to be produced but at lower levels. These levels of FSH and LH are too low to stimulate development of new follicles.

The cells of the corpus luteum are organized to enlarge, proliferate, secrete and then degenerate. The surge of LH seems to be the main organizing factor for this. This stabilizes the corpus luteum and the length of the postovulatory phase of the cycle. As the 12 day old corpus luteum degenerates and becomes a corpus albicans the levels of progesterone and oestrogen drop, signalling the hypothalamus to begin releasing GRH again, thereby repeating the cycle.

In response to this cycle, the endometrium of the uterus also undergoes cyclic phenomena. These phenomena are known as the uterine cycle. The two cycles, uterine and ovarian, are intimately related and occur simultaneously.

The uterus

The uterus is a thick-walled, muscular, pear-shaped organ about 7.5 cm (3 in) in length in the adult virgin. It is held in position by its ligaments and by the pelvic floor. The uterus is composed of three layers: (1) an inner mucous layer, or endometrium; (2) a middle muscular layer, or myometrium; and (3) an outer serous layer which covers the entire body of the uterus except where it is reflected up and over the bladder. The uterus is divided into two distinct parts, the body and the cervix.

The cervix projects into the vagina. It appears to be mainly connective tissue, and only 10% is muscle. The endometrial lining of the body of the uterus extends downward, undergoing certain modifications in the cervical canal and terminating just above the external os of the cervix where it meets the stratified squamous epithelium of the vaginal wall.

The uterine cycle

In the uterine cycle the endometrium plays a major role. The endometrium is a thin, pink membrane which is attached directly to the underlying muscle layer. It is composed of surface epithelium, uterine glands and connective tissue, and is richly supplied with blood vessels and tissue spaces. The thickness of the endometrium varies with the cycle. At the beginning of a new cycle it is probably about 0.5 mm thick. In response to the oestrogens of the preovulatory phase of the ovary it begins to proliferate and continues to do so throughout the cycle until it reaches a peak of proliferation and secretion several days following ovulation. In addition to the effect of oestrogen, the progesterone released in the luteal phase of the ovary further promotes the secretory activity of the endometrium. In this secretory stage the endometrium is oedematous, the glands are large and sacculated, the arteries have developed their typical coiled, tortuous pattern and some connective tissue has undergone hypertrophic stages. The rich, succulent endometrium now contains much glycogen. At this time the endometrium may be 5–6 mm in depth. In short, all is ready for the implantation of the fertilized ovum, should it appear. In perfect timing the endometrium reaches its peak development approximately 7–8 days following ovulation, or just when the fertilized ovum should appear in the uterine cavity ready for implantation.

If the ovum has been fertilized and the corpus luteum is continuing to secrete progesterone, the endometrium is maintained and implantation may occur successfully. However, should the corpus luteum not receive this message, it begins to degenerate. Oestrogen and progesterone production decline. This decline in hormone level causes the endometrium to retract and degenerate. Vasoconstriction of blood vessels occurs and the uterus becomes ischaemic. Shortly thereafter the endometrium begins to slough away and menstruation begins. The process of sloughing takes from 3–7 days, with each woman usually establishing her own pattern. Menstrual flow is composed of endometrial tissue, mucus and some blood. As the tiny arterioles constrict and relax, bleeding occurs. Usually not more than 50–60 ml of blood per menstrual period is lost. This blood does not clot because of the action of fibrinolytic enzymes released into the uterine cavity during menstruation. Occasionally, a heavy menstrual loss neutralizes the available fibrinolysins and clots occur. At the completion of menstruation the endometrium has returned to its unproliferative state. It is now ready to respond again to the rising oestrogen levels.

Ovulation

The menstrual cycle

The uterine and ovarian cycles are often referred to

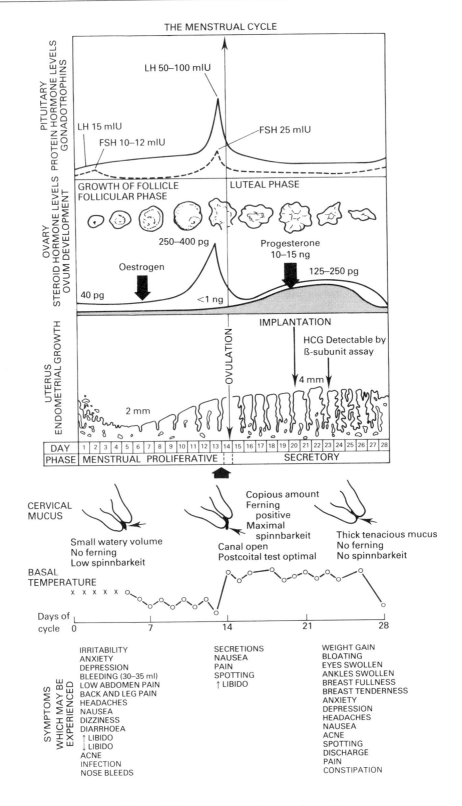

Fig. 23.10 Summary of menstrual cycle events.

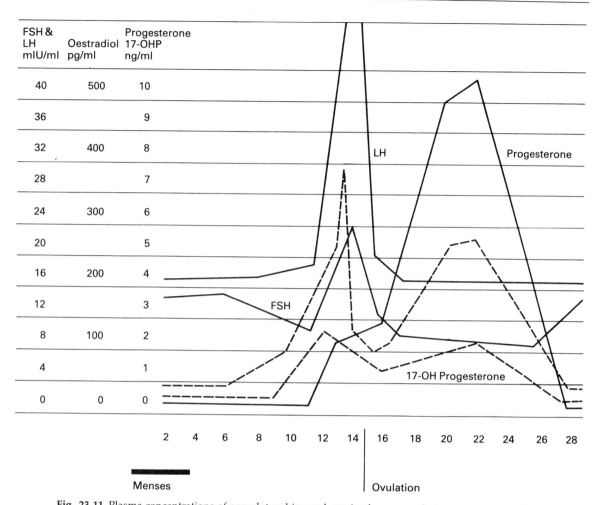

FSH & LH mIU/ml	Oestradiol pg/ml	Progesterone 17-OHP ng/ml
40	500	10
36		9
32	400	8
28		7
24	300	6
20		5
16	200	4
12		3
8	100	2
4		1
0	0	0

LH

Progesterone

FSH

17-OH Progesterone

2   4   6   8   10   12   14   16   18   20   22   24   26   28

Menses

Ovulation

Fig. 23.11 Plasma concentrations of gonadotrophins and ovarian hormones during one ovarian cycle.

as the menstrual cycle. This cycle begins on day one, which is the day menstruation begins, and continues until the day before menstruation begins again. Ovulation occurs on or around the fourteenth day of a 28-day cycle. However, this is subject to many factors, and the timing of ovulation in any one woman is a matter of considerable variation (see Fig. 23.12).

The menstrual cycle is divided into two independent sections: the pre- and postovulatory phases. The two phases are independent because the length of one does not control the length of the other. Ovulation is the dividing factor signalling the end of one phase and the beginning of the next.

Not all cycles are ovulatory and it is known that women can have an anovulatory cycle and still menstruate. The precise mechanism for this phenomenon is not clearly understood. The most common explanation is that a follicle develops, there is a failure of the LH surge and the follicle degenerates. Anovulatory cycles are most common in adolescent girls in whom the first menstrual periods may be anovulatory and in women at the menopause.

Follicles do not mature at the same rate each month. This produces a month to month variation in the timing of ovulation and the length of the preovulatory phase in any one woman. This variation in timing is evident by variation in the onset of menstruation.

The onset of menstrual flow is controlled by the corpus luteum of the ovary. Once ovulation occurs, menstruation follows 14 (±1) days after and this time relationship is constant. Fluctuations in the length of the cycle arise in the preovulatory phase.

These events produce a natural variation in cycle length from month to month. Each woman establishes her own rhythm and this may differ from other women. When expressed as an average, one woman will have an average cycle length of 22 days and another of 32 days. Each is normal for that individual and is the result of physical differences between women as well as the influence of environmental factors.

Age is an important physical influence on cycle length in women. The menstrual pattern throughout life is divided into three zones: two of transition and a central period of increasing stability. The two transition periods (postmenarche lasting about 5–7 years, and premenopause lasting about 6–8 years) are characterized by variation in cycle length.

As a girl ages, her average cycle length shortens and variation in cycle length reduces. The younger the girl experiences menarche the sooner she begins to develop a more 'regular' cycle.

The central period, from age 20–40 years, shows a continued reduction in variation and a shortening cycle interval. The average cycle length shortens between 0.1 and 0.18 of a day per year. Maximum stability is reached from age 35–39 years (Table 23.1).

Transitory variation in cycle length occurs in response to significant life events. Events associated with excitement, stress, a change of environment or anxiety can delay the ripening of a follicle and, consequently, ovulation. An area of the posterior hypothalamus seems to allow psychological impressions to enhance or decrease the secretion of GRH. Without GRH, FSH and, particularly, LH are not released by the pituitary. This delays the ripening of a follicle or prevents a sufficient surge of LH to take place. Fig. 23.12 demonstrates the effects observed in the cycle in response to these life events. If the event occurs in the follicular phase of the cycle it may either inhibit (anovulatory cycle) or delay ovulation. If ovulation is inhibited, the cycle in which the event occurred could be shorter in length, normal in length or prolonged in length. If ovulation is delayed, the cycle is prolonged in length. If the event occurs in the luteal phase of the cycle that cycle is unaffected but the succeeding cycle may show the expected effects.

Cervical, vaginal and tubal cycles

Changes also occur in the cervix, vagina, and uterine tubes in response to stimuli from the ovary. Oestrogen prompts the endocervical glands to respond by increasing their secretions and becoming longer and more tortuous. This is accompanied by increased vascularity and tumescence of the cervix. From about the seventh day of the menstrual cycle to about the twenty-first the cervical mucus gradually increases in amount. The mucus contains an increasing concentration of sodium chloride, which causes it to show a typical ferning pattern when allowed to dry on a slide. During the other periods of the cycle and during pregnancy the dried cervical mucus shows a beaded pattern. The mucus reaches its peak of production at ovulation. The consistency changes at ovulation and becomes thinner and can be drawn out into long, thin threads; this is called spinnbarkeit. These changes demonstrate the timing of the body as the mucus will permit easy entry of the sperm at ovulation, the most logical time. Indeed, it appears that the cervical mucus permits passage of sperm through the cervix only at this particular time.

Changes in the vagina and uterine tube are minimal compared to the changes in the ovary, uterus and cervix. The vaginal epithelium proliferates and reaches a peak at ovulation time. The uterine tube becomes swollen. Its secretory cells enlarge and project beyond the ciliated cells. Maximum development is timed to occur simultaneously with ovulation and the passage of the ovum through the tube. The ovum is also assisted in its passage by the wave-like contractions of the uterine tube and the beating

Table 23.1 Mean cycle interval in days of successive 5-year age groups from three studies. (N = numbers of women recording menstrual cycles; SD = standard deviation.)*

Age (years)	Gunn, 1937 Mean	SD	N	Chiazze, 1968 Mean	SD	N	Shields-Poë, 1981 Mean	SD	N
15–19	32.1	3.64	3	30.8	3.38	436	—	—	—
20–24	30.1	3.84	59	30.5	3.99	257	29.6	2.56	5
25–29	29.9	5.71	63	29.6	2.68	266	29.4	2.46	17
30–34	27.6	2.74	34	29.0	2.92	505	29.4	2.51	17
35–39	27.4	2.44	25	28.5	2.58	550	27.9	3.02	13
40–44	27.0	2.55	24	28.3	2.77	302	26.2	4.55	11

*Shields-Poë DA (1981).

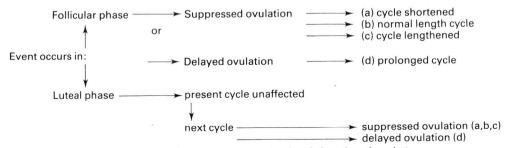

Fig. 23.12 Effects of life events on menstrual cycle length and ovulation.

of the tubal cilia toward the uterus. These contractions appear to be under the influence of oestrogens. The uterine tube secretes fluids, which provide nutrients first for the ovum and then for the conceptus until implantation occurs.

Sexuality

Sexuality is broadly defined as the becoming and being of a man or a woman. As such, adult sexuality has four major divisions (Fig. 23.13).

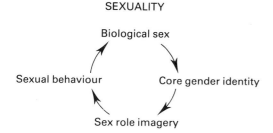

Fig. 23.13 Divisions of adult sexuality.

Biological sex refers to the individual's physical attributes. This is based in the genotype (XX, XY or other combinations) and includes internal and external genitalia with the corresponding underlying hormonal, neural, vascular and physical components.

Core gender identity refers to one's inner sense of being a man or a woman and is established early in life, usually by 3 years of age. At this age, the child knows he is a boy or a girl. In most cases the core gender identity corresponds to the physical attributes of the individual.

Sex role imagery refers to the learned behaviour that the particular society subscribes to their men and women. Sex or gender role imagery is complex because it includes the myriad beliefs about what is labelled feminine or masculine in a society. It also conveys the image of appropriate sexual conduct for particular social groups. Some examples of these beliefs are: trousers are worn by men, skirts by women; nursing is a woman's profession; women are passive, men are active. Sex role imagery is of great interest because it represents much of the learned behaviour which influences human choice and life-style. Much stereotyping of human behaviour has resulted from the need for society to set up expectations by which to guide and judge sex role behaviour. The learning of sex role imagery begins in infancy and continues throughout most of life. This learned behaviour, combined with personal experience, is internalized and becomes the individual's personal belief about sexuality.

Sexual behaviour refers to sexual expression and is the acting out of sexual feelings and beliefs. It includes a broad spectrum of human behaviour and varies from how one walks, to how and with whom one performs the sex act. For example, is the individual heterosexual in outlet and object? Does the person indulge in a variety of sexual practices, for example masturbation or fellatio?

These four aspects of sexuality are interrelated and reinforcing. Biological make-up and learning promote a core gender identity which influences acceptance of specific sex roles. Sexual expression reflects biology, gender identity, sex role and behaviour.

PHYSIOLOGICAL ASPECTS OF SEXUAL RESPONSE

Human sexual response occurs as a result of stimulation. The ability to respond physiologically to this stimulation exists in all healthy persons. The stimulation which elicits a response varies from purely mental images such as fantasy, dreams or remembered events to stimulation received through the senses. Touch is probably the most important source of stimulation and certain areas of the body appear to be more sensitive as stimulators of sexual arousal than are others. These sensitive areas vary for each individual but the sexual organs (penis in the man and clitoris, labia and vagina in the woman) are usually the most sensitive of the areas.

Learning modifies the emotional and physiological responses of people to sexual stimuli. As a result of prior learning or past experience similar sexual stimuli may elicit a wide range of response. However in all situations the appropriate psychological stimuli for that individual will increase pleasure in and ability to perform the sex act.

The response of the body to sexual stimulation is a total one, but the most noticeable changes are seen in the primary sexual organs. Tables 23.2 and 23.3 outline these responses. The sexual response cycle has been divided into four progressive phases. The phases do not differ between the sexes and depend in each sex on the same physiological mechanisms. The first is the excitement phase, in which the person becomes sexually aroused. It occurs in response to any source of stimulation, somatogenic or psychogenic or any combination of these. This phase is quite sensitive to outside influences and if the stimuli are interrupted or not intense enough the excitement phase may be prolonged or aborted.

As sexual arousal continues to mount, the individual enters the plateau phase. Sexual tension is intensified and reaches the preorgasmic level. Alteration in stimuli may also cause this phase to be prolonged or to revert to the pre-plateau level of sexual arousal.

Orgasm is the phase of release of sexual tension and is accompanied by ejaculation in the male. It is experienced as an involuntary subjective feeling of

Table 23.2 General body reactions during the sexual response cycle.*

Male		Female
	Excitement phase	
Nipple erection (30%)		Nipple erection (consistent)
		Sex-tension flush (25%)
	Plateau phase	
Sex-tension flush (25%)		Sex-tension flush (75%)
Carpopedal spasm		Carpopedal spasm
Generalized skeletal muscle tension		Generalized skeletal muscle tension
Hyperventilation		Hyperventilation
Tachycardia (100–160 beats per minute)		Tachycardia (100–160 beats per minute)
	Orgasmic phase	
Specific skeletal muscle contractions		Specific skeletal muscle contractions
Hyperventilation		Hyperventilation
Tachycardia (100–180 beats per minute)		Tachycardia (110–180 beats per minute)
	Resolution phase	
Sweating reaction (30–40%)		Sweating reaction (30–40%)
Hyperventilation		Hyperventilation
Tachycardia (150–180 beats per minute)		Tachycardia (150–180 beats per minute)

*Katchadourian & Lunde (1975).

pleasure or relief. This feeling is concentrated in the clitoris, vagina and uterus of the woman and in the penis, prostate and seminal vesicles of the male. There is much individual variation in the intensity and duration of orgasm; generally this relates directly to the degree of sexual arousal which preceded the orgasm.

Following orgasm the individual enters the resolution phase or period during which the body returns to its pre-excitement state. Within this resolution phase the male passes through the refractory period, a time during which the male cannot be restimulated to orgasm. The length of the refractory period varies with sexual episodes and may vary from a few minutes to several hours in the same individual.

Most of the observed responses during sexual excitement and resolution are due to two physiological mechanisms: vasocongestion and myotonia. Vasocongestion occurs as the muscular walls of the arterioles relax and expand allowing blood to rush in. This marked influx of blood into the area exceeds the ability of the veins to remove it and a period of vasocongestion occurs. Myotonia is increased muscle tension. During sexual activity, both smooth and skeletal muscles are affected.

Vasocongestion is a vascular phenomenon triggered by a nervous impulse. Effective stimulation activates the parasympathetic nervous system and inhibits the sympathetic fibres. The parasympathetic nerve fibres cause the arterioles to relax and expand allowing blood to rush in. Vasocongestion and penile erection result. At orgasm the sympathetic fibres are stimulated causing the arterioles to constrict, reducing blood flow to the area, and the muscles to contract rhythmically. These impulses are transmitted through the spinal cord to the brain where they are experienced as pleasure.

A simple reflex arc also exists in the spinal cord.

With genital stimulation, erection and ejaculation will occur after the spinal cord has been severed if the area of spinal nerve damage was above the sacral and lumbar areas governing erection and ejaculation. Because pleasure is experienced through the sensation passed to the brain, the sexual response is not felt by the individual.

The influence of sexual hormones on sexual response in humans cannot be clearly separated from learned responses. High circulating levels of hormones are important in stimulating the adolescent to overcome the latency period of childhood and become sexually oriented. Surgical removal of ovaries or testes later in life is not associated with a marked decrease in sexual interest in most adults. Adrenal hormones seem to be important to the continued sex drive or libido.

MALE SEXUAL RESPONSE

The most dramatic change in the male during sexual excitement is the erection of the penis. This is due to engorgement with blood of the corpora cavernosa and the corpus spongiosum. Erection of the penis may be partial but it is considered to be functionally erect if vaginal penetration can be achieved. Following full erection, further engorgement of the corona of the glans penis occurs just before orgasm. Concurrent with penile erection, the scrotum becomes contracted and thickened. This tightening of the scrotal sac assists in the elevation of the testes. The testes increase in size and are elevated until they are pressed against the body. Under parasympathetic nervous control, the bulbourethral glands secrete a few drops of fluid which is seen at the urethral orifice (Fig. 23.14).

Ejaculation occurs in two phases: the first phase or emission involves the upper part of the male repro-

Table 23.3 Reactions of sex organs during the sexual response cycle.*

Male	Female
Excitement phase	
Penile erection (within 3–8 seconds)	Vaginal lubrication (within 10–30 seconds)
As phase is prolonged:	*As phase is prolonged:*
Thickening, flattening, and elevation of scrotal sac	Thickening of vaginal walls and labia
As phase is prolonged:	*As phase is prolonged:*
Partial testicular elevation and size increase	Expansion of inner two-thirds of vagina and elevation of cervix and corpus
	As phase is prolonged:
	Tumescence of clitoris
Plateau phase	
Increase in penile coronal circumference and testicular tumescence (50–100% enlarged)	Orgasmic platform in outer third of vagina
Full testicular elevation and rotation (orgasm inevitable)	Full expansion of two-thirds of vagina, uterine and cervical elevation
Purple hue on corona of penis (inconsistent, even if orgasm is to ensue)	'Sex-skin': discoloration of minor labia (constant, if orgasm is to ensue)
Mucoid secretion from Cowper's gland	Mucoid secretion from Bartholin's gland
	Withdrawal of clitoris
Orgasmic phase	
Ejaculation	*Pelvic response (no ejaculation)*
Contractions of accesory organs of reproduction: vas deferens, seminal vesicles, ejaculatory duct, prostate	Contractions of uterus from fundus toward lower uterine segment
Relaxation of external bladder sphincter	Minimal relaxation of external cervical opening
Contractions of penile urethra at 0.8 second intervals for 3–4 contractions (slowing thereafter for 2–4 more contractions)	Contractions of orgasmic platform at 0.8 second intervals for 5–12 contractions (slowing thereafter for 3–6 more contractions)
Anal sphincter contractions (2–4 contractions at 0.8 second intervals)	External rectal sphincter contractions (3–4 contractions at 0.8 second intervals)
	External urethral sphincter contractions (2–3 contractions at irregular intervals, 10–15% of subjects)
Resolution phase	
Refractory period with rapid loss of pelvic vasocongestion	Ready return to orgasm with retarded loss of pelvic vasocongestion
Loss of penile erection in primary (rapid) and secondary (slow) stages	Loss of 'sex-skin' colour and orgasmic platform in primary (rapid) stage
	Remainder of pelvic vasocongestion as secondary (slow) stage
	Loss of clitoral tumescence and return to position

*Katchadourian & Lunde (1975).

ductive tract; the second expels sperm and semen from the body. At ejaculation the seminal vesicles contract and seminal fluid is forced into the common ejaculatory ducts and into the urethra. The muscular layers of the prostate gland contract rhythmically forcing prostatic fluid into that portion of the urethra near the prostate. Simultaneously with these contractions of prostatic muscle, the fibres at the neck of the bladder continuous with muscle fibres in the prostate gland also contract, closing the internal urethral orifice. The contracting ampulla of the vas deferens discharges its contents into the prostatic urethra. When all fluids are pooled in the prostatic portion of the urethra the first phase of ejaculation has been completed. The man is aware of ejaculation coming and he can no longer control or delay the process.

The second phase is accomplished by rhythmic contractions that force the semen along the length of the urethra and expel it from the urinary meatus under pressure. The man responds with pleasure to the contractions of the penis and accessory organs and the feeling of fluid volume escaping. Generally, the first few expulsive contractions and a greater volume of ejaculate are associated with greater pleasure.

FEMALE SEXUAL RESPONSE

The vagina, a fibromuscular tube from 7.5–10 cm (3–4 in) long, is the female organ of intercourse. Here sperm are deposited. It also serves as a passage for the fetus from intrauterine to extrauterine life. The

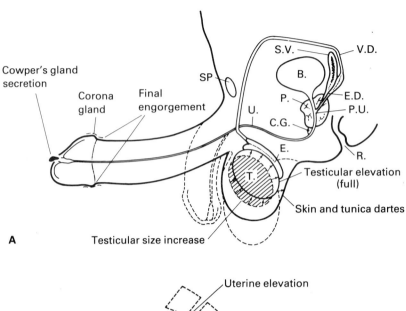

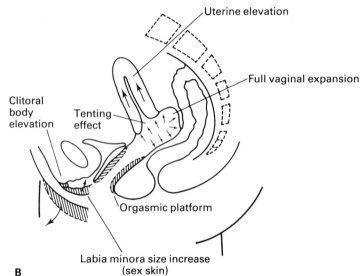

Fig. 23.14 *A*, Male pelvis—plateau phase. *B*, Female pelvis—plateau phase. [Key to *A*: SP, symphysis pubis; SV, seminal vesicle; VD, vas deferens; B, bladder; ED, ejaculatory duct; P, prostate; PU, prostatic urethra; CG, Cowper's gland (bulbourethral gland); U, urethra; E, epididymus; T, testis; R, rectum.]

vagina is protected by the labia, which usually remain in close approximation over the introitus. During sexual excitement the labia become engorged and swollen and gape, thus exposing the vestibule.

Under neural stimulus, Bartholin's glands secrete a fluid which serves to lubricate the vaginal introitus. However, the mucus these vulvovaginal glands secrete is minimal and not of sufficient quantity to lubricate the entire vagina. Hence, most vaginal lubrication arises from the vaginal walls themselves. Very quickly following sexual stimulation the vaginal walls exhibit a 'sweating'-like appearance as beads of mucoid material appear throughout the rugal folds. Soon the droplets run together to form a complete coat of lubrication over the inner surface of the vagina. Since there are no glandular elements in the vaginal wall, it is hypothesized that the exudation is a result of marked dilatation of the venous system which surrounds the vagina. The cervix, once thought to be the source of much of the lubrication of the vagina, also appears to play a relatively minor role. This seems to be confirmed by the fact that little or no secretory activity of the cervix has been observed during sexual activity. Also, women who have undergone total hysterectomy and bilateral salpingo-oophorectomy produce reasonable vaginal lubrication in response to sexual stimulation. Indeed, the same response will develop in artificially constructed vaginas, and the source of the lubricating material is presumed to be the same.

The vagina also responds to sexual stimuli by enlarging. The inner two-thirds of the vagina expand and lengthen, forming a basin for the seminal pool which will form in the posterior fornix of the vagina just below the cervical os. The outer third of the vagina becomes engorged and constricted, serving to assist the vagina to form a reservoir for the semen. Engorgement of pelvic organs also results in a slight elevation of the uterus and cervix.

An orgasm may occur as a generalized systemic feeling, with sensation localized in the clitoris, and rhythmic muscular contractions of the outer third of the vagina and the uterus. With orgasm, pelvic engorgement of blood vessels is rapidly resolved. This causes the uterus to return to its normal position, placing the cervix very near to or in the seminal pool, thus facilitating movement of sperm through the cervix.

The clitoris seems to be a unique organ in human anatomy. As the primary focus of sensual response, it appears to serve no other function. Made of fibrous tissue with two corpora cavernosa and richly innervated, it undergoes engorgement and enlargement when the female is sexually stimulated either physically or mentally. The tumescent clitoris then retracts against the symphysis pubis and becomes difficult to see or feel.

The subjective experience of orgasm is synchronous with orgasmic platform contractions and the pleasure associated with orgasm is related to their number and intensity.

Following orgasm the woman enters the resolution phase. Unlike the male, a woman, if provided during this phase with sufficient further stimulation, may return to the orgasmic level.

Menopause

The reproductive functions of the male and female continue throughout adult life. Given health and opportunity, the male's sexual and reproductive capabilities are life-long; the only major change is a slowing of sexual response and a gradual reduction in libido (sexual drive).

Women, however, present a different picture. Reproductive function, usually demonstrated by menses, continues until middle age. Then, at the average age of 50, women cease menstruating. The cessation of menstruation is perhaps the most obvious sign of menopause, or 'change of life'. Actually menopause, in onset and duration, resembles puberty, which was a gradual awakening of reproductive function over a period of 6 months to 2 years. This transitional period is known as the climacteric. The climacteric may take a few months to several years and is the result of altered ovarian function. Ovarian follicles cease to ripen. The endometrium does not respond as richly, and menstruation becomes scantier and shorter in duration. The women may have several anovulatory cycles, just as

she may have had in puberty. Eventually the menses may become irregular and finally cease. Menopause is said to be complete when the woman has had no menses for 1 year. As the perimenopausal woman may ovulate erratically, family planning advice is important to her. She cannot assume she will not become pregnant until menopause is complete, after which the risks of pregnancy occurring are very slight.

Decreasing oestrogen levels stimulate gonadotrophic hormones (FSH, LH) which show a proportionate rise, but the ovary does not respond fully. The vascular system, once functioning smoothly under hormonal control, begins to respond to these imbalances and the woman may experience 'hot flushes', feelings of tingling and faintness. She may have periods of sweating, especially at night. Hypertension may develop, for oestrogen appears to have inhibiting effects on the development of atherosclerosis. Osteoporosis has also been linked to declining oestrogen levels. She may feel depressed and experience swings in mood for no apparent reason. Much of this may be unsettling to the woman, especially when accompanied by cessation of reproductive function and fears of advancing age and of loss of usefulness, sexual function and love of her husband.

Most women accept the changes with some minor disturbances. It would seem that an understanding of menopause and some reassurance of her usefulness and worth will help most women. Only about 25% of women require hormone replacement treatment. This is in the form of short-term therapy with oral oestrogens. The dosage is individualized to relieve the symptoms and is continued for 2–3 months, at which time a reassessment is made to decide whether to continue or stop treatment. Because the prolonged use of oestrogens in the perimenopausal women is associated with an increased risk of cancer of the endometrium, women should be alerted to the risks of long-term oestrogen therapy.

It should be understood that all oestrogen production does not cease at menopause. The ovaries do not appear to be inert postmenopausally, and it is thought that they continue to excrete small amounts of hormones. This is in addition to oestrogens from the adrenal gland. Over the years oestrogen production declines further and the development of other organ changes occurs. The vulva becomes atrophic and thin from a resorption of fatty tissue. The uterus decreases in size; the endometrium becomes thin and atrophic. The vaginal epithelium thins out and is more susceptible to injury and infection. Lubrication of the vagina may require supplementation so that dyspareunia (painful sexual intercourse) need not occur.

Sexual function can continue with little change in the vast majority of postmenopausal women. The most important factors in the continuance of sexual function appear to be the opportunity for and the frequency of intercourse, so that the changes of menopause themselves do not mean this phase of a woman's life must cease. Indeed, relief from fear of pregnancy may make the experience a more enjoyable one.

Disorders of the Reproductive System

NURSING PROCESS

Assessment

Assessment of a patient with a disorder of the reproductive system includes taking a history and a physical examination.

HISTORY

Information is obtained about the following:
1 History of any disorders, illnesses, injuries, surgery and diagnostic investigations of the reproductive system.
2 History and character of menstruation (including: menarche, last menstrual period, length of cycle, duration of flow, amount of flow, menopause and last cervical smear test).
3 History of reproductive events [including: number of pregnancies and the outcome of these (abortion, premature, full-term), delivery (types), children

(any stillbirth or neonatal death and cause if known), present health status, complications of pregnancy, history of infertility and cause if known, and present and past use of contraception].
4 Review of function. In reviewing a system questioning should elicit:
  (a) Any changes or disturbances in function (for example, dysmenorrhoea, dissatisfaction with sexual functioning or birth control).
  (b) The presence of any symptoms of disease. If symptoms are present they are explored in order to determine their location, character, duration and severity. The common manifestations of disorders are: pain, lesions, discharges, itching, non-cyclic bleeding, swellings and masses.

PHYSICAL EXAMINATION

The physical examination includes:
1 General physical examination.
2 Inspection of secondary sexual characteristics (see Fig. 23.15 for an example in women).
3 Inspection and palpation of internal and external genitalia (see Figs. 23.16 and 23.17).

The vaginal examination is often a source of anxiety for women. The examination is personal and invades body boundaries and there is a sense of exposure. For these reasons the individual having

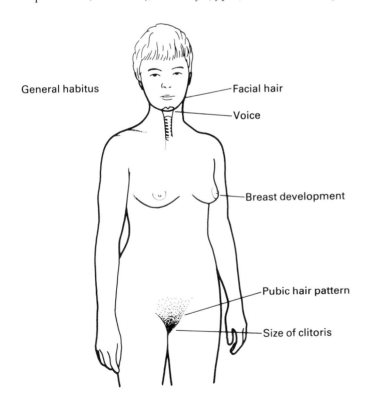

General habitus

Facial hair

Voice

Breast development

Pubic hair pattern

Size of clitoris

Fig. 23.15 Inspection of secondary sex characteristics forms part of this examination. (A deep voice, facial trichosis, hypoplastic breasts, a tendency to male escutcheon, and an enlarged clitoris suggest the need for studies to exclude a masculinizing lesion of the pituitary, adrenals, or ovaries.)

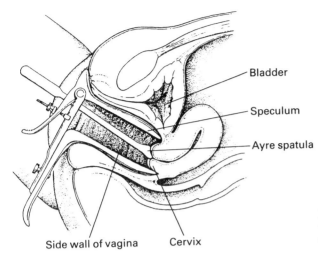

Bladder

Speculum

Ayre spatula

Side wall of vagina   Cervix

Fig. 23.16 Internal vaginal examination demonstrating the position of the speculum and ayre spatula used to obtain cervical cells for a smear test.

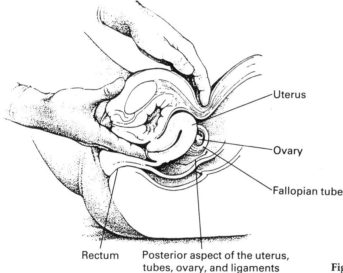

Uterus

Ovary

Fallopian tube

Rectum   Posterior aspect of the uterus, tubes, ovary, and ligaments

Fig. 23.17 Bimanual vaginal examination.

her first vaginal examination should be prepared in advance for what is involved. The examination procedure is described and she is shown the equipment. The patient undergoing a vaginal examination may have a sense of physical and emotional exposure; the nurse can help to reduce these feelings by her sensitive and supportive approach.

Identification of patient problems

The patient with a disorder of the reproductive system presents some special concerns for the nurse. In many ways a human being is defined by his sex. Knowing he or she is a man or a woman gives the person a set of behaviours, culturally and physiologically determined, which help to guide his or her actions. The normal functioning of the reproductive system gives constant reassurance of a person's essential maleness or femaleness. The distortion or interruption of these processes may prove very disturbing to the individual and family.

The person may experience problems in relation to his or her self-image and have fears about future sexual performance and attractiveness. Body parts that contribute to self-esteem and identity have a high psychological investment. The threat posed by loss of these body parts depends on:
1 Their meaning to the individual
2 His or her stage of development of body image and self
3 The reactions of the social group to which he belongs, including the spouse

The person may fear loss of reproductive function. The ability to reproduce is seen by many as a criterion of usefulness and sexuality. The loss of function may be followed by feelings of uselessness or of being only half a person. These feelings can be particularly distressing to the woman who has defined herself in terms of her reproductive and sexual function. To her the removal of her uterus or ovaries may be tantamount to removing her femaleness. Because she may feel less a woman, she fears her husband will see her as less a woman. Indeed, in some unfortunate situations, he may. Thus, to the fear of loss of reproductive function may be added the fear of loss of a loved one. For some the fear of loss of libido as well as sexual function may be very frightening and can cause the patient much anguish.

Also, most patients have been culturally conditioned to the idea that these areas of the body should not be discussed, much less exposed, in examination or discussion. Such experiences may disturb the individual and produce shame that may be enhanced by lack of privacy and exposure of the body in examinations or during care. Other patients may feel guilt over their illness. Venereal disease, abortion and cancer arouse guilt feelings in certain individuals which may be expressed as a feeling of 'being punished for past deeds'.

The nurse deals with patients who experience anxiety and fear, shame, guilt, diminished self-esteem or re-awakened anxieties over personal identity.

When caring for such patients the *goals* are to:
1 Promote feelings of self-worth at both the personal and sexual level
2 Assist the individual to a resolution of dysfunctional sexual problems
3 Avoid practices that contribute to shame
4 Relieve guilt
5 Help the individual overcome body image disturbances
6 Increase the patient's knowledge of relevant anatomy and physiology
7 Dispel misconceptions

Nursing intervention

These goals may be achieved by the following nursing interventions. The nurse should:
1 Assess the degree of threat posed by loss of function or body parts to the individual and plan, give and evaluate nursing care for that individual based on the assessment.
2 Give physical nursing care which
   (a) Promotes feelings of dignity, self-worth and attractiveness by attention to personal hygiene and grooming
   (b) Promotes the return of health, control over body functions and independence
3 Reduce fear and guilt by:
   (a) Acknowledging and discussing feelings
   (b) Anticipating the need for explanations and interpretations
   (c) Clarifying and correcting misinformation about causes of illness, physiology and the consequences, if any, of treatment on present function
   (d) Maintaining a confident, non-judgemental approach to the patient
   (e) Assisting in acknowledging the loss, if any
   (f) Obtaining appropriate additional sources of spiritual or emotional help for the patient

Expected outcomes

Interventions are successful if behavioural changes have occurred, although behavioural changes may be difficult to document in areas such as self-concept, anxiety and guilt. The patient:
1 States that he feels better, less frightened or happier.
2 Takes an interest in his appearance and renews interests in his social life, which may also indicate a return to a more positive outlook toward the future.
3 Demonstrates an understanding of his illness, treatments and any residual changes in function to the level of his ability or willingness.
4 Demonstrates a knowledge of the risk factors which may lead to a recurrence of the problem and the actions which may reduce or eliminate the risk factors, if appropriate.
5 Discusses his altered body with the nurse and so indicates a willingness to begin to deal with the problem or to accept it with appropriate adjustments.

Adjustment to many of these changes requires some time and complete resolution is rarely seen in hospital. Expectations of resolution and effectiveness of intervention must be realistic.

SEXUAL ISSUES ASSOCIATED WITH GIVING NURSING CARE

Several issues involving sexuality may arise in the course of nurse–patient interactions. They reflect the changing role of the patient and involve confusion over the meaning of nursing or patient actions. The most common arise from the intimate level of care involved in nursing and acting out sexual behaviour by the patient.

Touch
The nurse may feel uncomfortable at having to touch the genitals or breasts of patients. The patient may also experience discomfort at being cared for so intimately by the nurse. It reinforces for many adults the dependent child-like role associated with nursing care. On the other hand, touch may be a source of great comfort to patients. Touch should be used

discriminately and its purpose should be understood by both patient and nurse.

Prior to giving nursing care the nurse gives an explanation of what will be done so that the patient is not surprised and has time to adjust. The nurse's movements should be firm, purposeful and reflect a knowledge of the procedure; her manner should be 'matter-of-fact'.

Touch for the purpose of comfort is offered as seems appropriate to the situation and patient. Many patients are grateful for a hand to hold during frightening or stressful procedures or times. Other patients would be uncomfortable offered that form of comfort. A knowledge of and sensitivity to the patient assists the nurse in judging what forms of comfort are helpful to which patients.

Male erection

The erections which occur during the delivery of nursing care are most often the result of the stimulation of the spinal reflex arc. The stimulus from a full bladder or perineal care may produce this non-sexual or non-psychological erection. Should this occur during care it is important for the nurse to remain calm, acknowledge the situation and finish care. A flustered nurse who 'runs away' from the patient may increase his confusion, shame and guilt. The patient also needs to understand the nature of reflex, non-sexual erections.

Sexual acting out

A patient may act out sexually to test his or her sexual image, to gain control of the situation, or to attract attention. Examples of sexual acting out in this context include touching the nurse inappropriately, improper suggestions or gestures toward the nurse or exposing himself. The nurse addresses the situation directly and unambiguously. The nurse–patient relationship is defined and any misconceptions about role and function are clarified. Limits are set, clearly defined and enforced.

Meanwhile the patient is helped to explore his anxiety and fears. As these are identified and appropriately dealt with, the sexual acting out usually ceases.

DISORDERS OF SEXUALITY

Disorders of sexuality can occur in each of the four areas of sexuality (see Fig. 23.13) but most disorders are psychosexual in origin. Only a few arise from physical illness and trauma or congenital error. Most become obvious through difficulties in sexual expression.

Variations in sexual expression are classified by object choice and sexual aim. Object choice refers to problems such as homosexuality, paedophilia, incest, animal contacts or fetishism (inanimate objects). Variations in sexual aim refers to problems such as voyeurism, exhibitionism and sado-masochism.

Transsexuality is a problem in which the individual appears to have a gender identity at odds with his or her physical self. This results in cross dressing but is not the same as homosexuality. These individuals seek out sex change therapy because of a deep need to have a body similar to their gender identity. Most frequently they are men who deeply believe themselves to be women.

Occasionally a child reaches puberty and is then discovered to be genetically and internally different from his or her external genitalia. Because the child has been socialized in the sex role defined by the external genitalia, it is usually advised they continue in the sex assigned at birth. It is usually more successful to alter the physical state than to attempt to reverse gender identity and several years of gender role learning. Parents of a child born with ambiguous genitalia should understand the necessity to delay sex assignment until careful physical and genetic screening indicates the true sex of the infant.

Sexual concerns

Many persons experience doubts over their inner feelings of being a man or a woman. This may be more prominent in adolescence when the final development of gender identity takes place, but may recur throughout the individual's life. Since sexual identity is considered to be an important component of overall identity, this may stimulate concerns over self-identity.

Concerns over performance are also prevalent. The individual may doubt whether he or she has the necessary physical attributes, experience or appeal to attract, satisfy and keep a sexual partner.

Sexual dysfunction

Sexual dysfunction in the male is most frequently associated with the inability to achieve an erection (impotence) and to delay ejaculation until both partners achieve a sense of satisfaction (premature ejaculation).

In the female, sexual dysfunction is associated with inhibition of or lack of response (frigidity). Some women may not become sexually excited or, if aroused, do not experience orgasm with intercourse. Women may also complain of painful intercourse (dyspareunia) or a strong contraction of the outer one-third of the vagina (vaginismus) which makes insertion of the penis extremely difficult.

Sexual dysfunction can be the result of psychological, interpersonal or physical factors. Psychological causes may be: anger, depression, anxiety, ignorance, or deeper psychosexual conflicts. Interpersonal factors involve conflicts with the partner or an inability to establish interpersonal relationships. Physical causes include illness, injury or drugs.

Diagnosis and treatment involve a history, physical examination and laboratory tests to ascertain the most likely cause. Nurses may be involved in all stages of assessment but are most frequently involved in history taking and case finding.

During history taking the patient is asked if he or she has any sexual complaints. This makes sexuality an acceptable topic to discuss should the patient have a problem or develop one in the future. If the patient does present with a sexual problem, it is discussed in a frank, open manner, maintaining a broad, objective attitude toward the patient's sexual beliefs and practices. The patient is not urged to disclose more information during a session than he is comfortable in revealing. The patient's sexual concerns are assessed in the context of his other problems and in the context of his value systems.

Once the nature of the problem has been identified, treatment commences. Annon[1] has described four levels of sexual counselling. The four levels are: (1) permission, (2) limited information, (3) specific suggestions, and (4) intensive therapy. Permission involves reassurance that the patient is normal and may continue doing what he has been doing. Limited information involves providing information specific to the patient's concern or problem. This frequently allows the patient to make appropriate changes in behaviour. These changes in behaviour usually involve the patient following a suggested course of action. This may vary from the treatment of organic disorders to the relearning of sexual behaviours through more in-depth education and sexual exercises. The fourth level, intensive therapy, is highly individualized, in-depth therapy provided by professionals who have advanced experience and knowledge in the sex therapy field.

It is the responsibility of the nurse to create an atmosphere conducive to the identification of sexual problems; if unable to provide the appropriate intervention she should refer the patient to another professional. Nurses with the requisite knowledge and skills and who are comfortable with the subject function in levels one and two, providing reassurance and knowledge of human sexual response and practice in health and illness. Nurses with additional and advanced preparation and experience in sexual therapies may function at higher levels.

RAPE TRAUMA SYNDROME

Rape is a sexual assault which by means of force violates the individual's right to personal body integrity and to engage in sexual activity only with consent. Sexual intercourse need not be full penetration but involve only contact between the genitalia of the victim and rapist. The legal definitions of rape and sexual assault vary between legal jurisdictions. In the United Kingdom rape is legally defined in the 1976 Sexual Offences (Amendment) Act as when a man 'has unlawful sexual intercourse with a woman with-

out her consent and at the time he knows that she does not consent to the intercourse or is reckless as to whether or not she consented to it.' By defining rape as a form of assault the primary motivating factors of anger, aggression and need for power are acknowledged.

Sexual assault is considered a crisis in the life of the victim. It contains the elements of suddenness, arbitrariness and unpredictability: three factors associated with crisis and with rape. A crisis demands psychological and physical adaptation or response from the individual. Crisis is recognizable by the disruption of regular patterns of behaviour and thought which occur in the individuals involved. The degree and nature of the response will vary from one individual to another. Several key factors should be kept in mind in assessing both an individual's initial response to crisis and eventual resolution of crisis. They are:

1 How the individual perceives and understands the incident and her/his feelings about the incident.
2 The emotional stability of the individual prior to the crisis.
3 The coping skills possessed by the individual.
4 The presence or absence of support systems such as family, friends, and colleagues who will be available to assist the individual in the next few days and weeks.

The person in crisis is acutely sensitive to the responses of the individuals around them. The type of intervention a person experiences immediately after sexual assault may either aggravate the crisis or ameliorate it. As the effects of sexual assault may be long-lasting if the crisis is not resolved in a positive manner, it is important for the professionals in contact with the victim to attempt to alleviate the situation. The victims of such assaults have the right to expect to be treated with dignity and respect in a manner that does not take away personal control and to receive prompt physical and emotional support.

In order to provide such services many areas have established rape crisis centres. These centres ensure that the victims are treated in a knowledgeable, caring manner. Some rape crisis centres are independent clinics; others are designated as a part of the emergency department of a hospital. All personnel associated with them should understand and be experienced in dealing with the social, emotional, legal and medical issues surrounding rape and sexual assault.

REACTION TO SEXUAL ASSAULT

Three phases of response to this form of physical and psychological trauma have been identified. There is an acute or impact phase, a recoil or adjustment phase and finally a post-traumatic or re-integration phase.

---

[1] Annon (1978), pp. 1–15.

Acute phase

In the acute phase the victim presents a variety of reactions. Initially many will appear very upset; others will appear calm and controlled. The state of seeming control and calm may be an indication of the state of shock the person is in rather than the intensity of their eventual reaction. The individual may express disbelief, fear, anxiety, guilt, shame, helplessness, anger, or rage. Some may be highly irritable and moody; all seem to share a fear of death, fear the attacker will return and fear that it will happen again. They are concerned over why it happened. Some will see their behaviour as contributing to the event; they feel guilty and worry that somehow they encouraged the attack. Occasionally society, with its biases, may support this view. The victim expresses anger toward the assailant and some may convert their anger and helplessness into depression and further guilt.

Physically these women complain of disturbances in eating and sleep patterns, increased headaches, fatigue and gynaecological symptoms and general body pain. Socially, they are fearful and may shun going out. They have increased dependency needs and may find decision-making difficult. Much anxiety may centre around the decision to press charges against the individual or to tell family, friends, and colleagues because of fear of misunderstanding by family members and others of their role in the event. Sexually they may retreat from encounters and be unable to enjoy or even tolerate sexual contact for a period of time. This is further aggravated by any physical trauma they have suffered. This phase lasts from a few days to a few weeks.

Adjustment phase

As the victims progress from the initial shock of the acute phase, defence mechanisms emerge and most of the disturbances of that phase decrease. They return to their normal activities of work, school or home and appear outwardly composed. Most will now attribute the rape to chance or some other societal cause but not to self. They see little need to continue professional counselling or to continue talking about the situation. This is healthy and to be expected and should be encouraged. Most women will pass into this phase. Others will show a maladaptive response such as excessive self-blame, severely altered self-image or agitation and depression. The adjustment phase can last a few weeks to years.

Integration phase

Following the adjustment phase most individuals will feel a need to discuss their experiences. This need is usually triggered by some event, such as an anniversary of the rape. The person may feel emotionally upset, depressed, fearful, angry and may need to talk about the experience.

During this phase the person resolves feelings about the rapist and her role in the rape. She develops a new self-image which allows for the episode of rape. Following this period of sorting-out, the individual is free to take control of her life, accepting the feelings surrounding the assault in a more dispassionate manner. Some patients may never reach this stage.

ASSESSMENT

An accurate and precise history of the event and a physical examination are the first steps in care. Before proceeding, the doctor must obtain a signed consent form from the woman or guardian. The consent, which must be witnessed, obtains permission to do a complete physical and pelvic examination, and to collect the necessary specimens.

The history and physical examinations are used to assess the extent of trauma but are also used to collect evidence that may be used for forensic purposes. Because of the need to collect legal evidence there is usually a well-defined protocol to follow which outlines the information to be obtained and the specimens that are to be collected. Nurses involved in emergency departments must be familiar with the protocol for the assessment of rape victims applicable in their setting.

Most protocols include: a detailed history and description of the assault and the assailant; a recent sexual and menstrual history; a precise description of the physical findings; laboratory tests for infections, sperm, pregnancy and any identifying markers, for example hair which the attacker may have left. The woman's emotional state is also assessed and described.

TREATMENT

The patient receives immediate treatment appropriate to the injuries identified during examination. Follow-up care is equally important in order to prevent undesirable sequelae.

Extragenital and genital bruising and lacerations are the most common injuries suffered. Bruises are usually not evident at initial examination but will be identified at a follow-up visit. A few patients will be more severely injured and require immediate and extensive medical and nursing care. Occasionally a patient may require a pelvic examination under anaesthesia, with suturing and repair of injury. Most patients, however, will receive treatment for trauma in the emergency department.

The possibility of infection, both venereal and non-venereal, must not be overlooked. Cultures are made. If the patient is unable to return for follow-up or appears unlikely to return, prophylactic antibiotic therapy is given. Some centres administer it routinely. In any case, the patient is asked to return for repeat cultures for venereal disease in 48 hours and again at 6 weeks for a blood test for syphilis.

Pregnancy is a potential sequela of rape. Prophylactic treatment is instituted at the discretion of the doctor. A careful sexual, menstrual and birth control history is mandatory in assessing risk. If there is a possibility of pregnancy the patient may receive hormone therapy ('morning-after-pill') to prevent it. A combined oestrogen/progestogen preparation is used, for example two tablets of Eugynon or Ovran (equivalent to 100 mg ethinyloestradiol plus 500 mg levonorgestrel). It is given within 72 hours of unprotected intercourse and repeated once 12 hours later. The use of combined oestrogen and progestogen has fewer side-effects when compared with the use of oestrogen alone. The patient is also requested to return in 6 weeks for a pregnancy test so that she may be offered an abortion or pregnancy counselling if it is required.

PSYCHOLOGICAL SUPPORT

Intervention and assessment go hand in hand in the treatment of sexual assault patients. Although separated in this format, the integration of emotional support with assessment and treatment is imperative in the care of these patients. Immediate interventions should include the following:

1 Assume the patient is telling the truth.
2 Go out of your way to demonstrate concern.
3 Advise them not to bathe, douche, or clean up in any way and to seek medical attention immediately.
4 In the emergency room, give the patient as much privacy and priority as is possible.
5 Allow a supportive person to remain with the patient.
6 Do not take away personal control.
7 Be gentle in word and deed.
8 Explain clearly the reasons for all examinations and collection of specimens.
9 Assess the extent of the emotional crisis for the individual. For example: What is his/her manifest emotional state? Is he/she able to make decisions? What evidence of coping is there? What personal supports does the person have?
10 Allow the expression of feelings.
11 Listen supportively.
12 Explain follow-up and counselling services.
13 Give teaching about tests and follow-up care.

The spouse and family may have a variety of emotions about the assault. Some will be supportive to the victim; others may not. Most families require help in understanding the processes of the examination and emotional reaction of the patient. They should be included in the care by the nurse.

CONGENITAL ANOMALIES OF THE REPRODUCTIVE SYSTEM

Maldescent of testes
Approximately 4% of newborn males will exhibit

some form of maldescent of the testes. Unilateral maldescent of testis is about four times as prevalent as bilateral maldescent. The condition is usually the result of hormonal deficiency or mechanical malfunction. The majority of testes descend during the first 3 months of extrauterine life. Many more descend at puberty under the influence of rising testosterone levels. Probably less than 1% of men remain with undescended testes following puberty. The principal sign is an inability to palpate one or both testes in the scrotal sac.

It is important to distinguish between three possible types of maldescent. Retractile testes are those which, under the influence of a strong muscular reflex, are drawn up to the external inguinal ring. This gives a false impression on palpation that the testes are not in the scrotum. No treatment is required. Ectopic testes are those which have descended to an abnormal site. Commonly this is the superficial inguinal pouch but may be almost anywhere near the normal path of descent. Cryptorchidism is a condition in which the descent of the testis is interrupted anywhere along the normal path of descent.

Because histological changes are observed in the undescended testes as early as 4 years of age, treatment is initiated early to ensure maximum functioning of the testes. Orchiopexy (surgical placement and fixation of the testes in the scrotal sac) is the primary method of treatment and should be completed by the age of 1 year. Hernioplasty may also be done to repair the inguinal hernia which is often present in these cases. The patient will be on complete bed rest with restricted activity for several days. Thereafter, excessive physical activity should be avoided for about 6 weeks. Hormone therapy in the form of chorionic gonadotrophins may be given in cases of bilateral undescended testes to stimulate production of testosterone in the testes. Successful descent usually indicates that these testes would probably have descended spontaneously at puberty. Hormone therapy is less successful with unilateral conditions.

Should the condition not be diagnosed until after puberty, orchiopexy is indicated even though the man may be sterile. First, the Leydig cells of the testes continue to produce male hormones which will sustain the secondary sex characteristics. Secondly, such testes have a higher incidence of malignancy than do normally positioned testes and can be more easily examined yearly for malignancy in the scrotum than in the abdomen. In unilateral conditions, the extrascrotal testis will be removed to reduce the possibility of malignancy further. This leaves the man with one functioning testis as a source of sperm and male hormones.

Absence or duplication of organs (male)

Congenital absence of the penis, scrotum and vas

deferens is very rare. However, in certain genetically determined syndromes, the testicular tissue may be absent or non-functioning. One such example is Klinefelter's syndrome. The person with this syndrome has an XXY genotype; this produces atrophic testes and sterility. The person may also have eunuchoid development, and mental retardation may or may not be present. Androgens are administered to prevent feminization. Other examples are hermaphrodites, or persons who have some characteristics of both sexes. This could be genetically determined as true hermaphroditism or could be due to a feminizing lesion, producing pseudohermaphroditism.

Hypospadias

Hypospadias arises from a failure of the folds to fuse (Fig. 23.2). Chordee, a curvature of the penis, usually accompanies hypospadias and epispadias. Since the sex of the child may be doubtful, chromosome and endocrine studies will be carried out and treatment based on the results of these findings. In mild cases of hypospadias, no treatment is necessary, as function is usually not impaired. In more severe cases, surgical repair will be necessary. This repair will straighten the penile shaft so that normal intercourse is possible. In addition a urethra will be formed which extends as near as possible to the tip of the glans so that semen is deposited deep in the vagina. Surgery is usually not immediately indicated and may be done in a series of operations beginning at about the age of 2 in a child in whom the condition has been detected early. In a few unfortunate cases the child is assumed to be female from birth, and these extreme cases may not be discovered until puberty and the development of secondary sex characteristics. For this reason, it is important that the nurse carefully examine the external genitalia of the newborn and report to its doctor any baby which she feels does not appear normal.

Epispadias

Epispadias is much rarer than hypospadias and is often associated with exstrophy of the bladder (Fig. 23.2B). Because of the possible bladder involvement, the patient may be incontinent as a result of imperfect or absent urethral sphincters. Surgical repair provides the child with a functioning penis and urethra.

Preoperatively, a cystostomy may be done. The patient may also return from the operating room with a splinting catheter in the urethra until healing takes place. If the patient is discharged home with a cystostomy, the parents will need instruction in the care of the child.

Absence or duplication of organs (female)

The uterus, cervix and vagina can undergo duplication or incomplete fusion (Fig. 23.1). The exact incidence of such anomalies is unknown, since they are largely asymptomatic. Some may cause sterility in women or an increased risk of abortion. Rarely an organ is completely absent. Also, as in the male, some absence (agenesis) or maldevelopment of tissue (dysgenesis) is genetically determined. Ovarian agenesis may be the result of an XO genotype (Turner's syndrome). The patient with this genotype may present a characteristic appearance from birth with a webbed neck, multiple anomalies, small birth weight or irregularities of the hairline. However, in others, the patient may present in adolescence because of the failure of the menarche to appear. Treatment is usually oestrogen replacement therapy, with 20 μg being given every day for 3 weeks, followed by withdrawal combined with norethisterone, 5 mg daily on days 12–21. Withdrawal of oestrogen permits the endometrium to slough away, thus simulating a menstrual period. The addition of progesterone prevents endometrial hyperplasia due to oestrogen stimulation. Because the ovaries do not exist, the patient remains sterile.

Imperforate hymen

Normally the hymen is patent. Rarely, it may not be. Usually the condition is not discovered until adolescence when the girl may present herself because of absence of menstrual flow. Menstruation occurs but the menstrual blood is retained behind the closed hymen. The patient may complain of crampy, lower abdominal pain occurring monthly. She may also notice dysuria, frequency, and urinary retention as the growing mass of retained menstrual blood accumulates in the vagina, putting increasing pressure on the bladder and urethra. Treatment consists of a cross-shaped incision of the hymen which allows drainage of the debris. This debris is often a thick, chocolate-like material. Because of this old blood, the risk of postoperative infection is greatly increased. Antibiotics are usually ordered. The nurse must pay careful attention to good aseptic technique postoperatively to reduce the risk of infection further. She must see that adequate drainage is maintained, frequent cleansing of the perineum occurs, and perineal dressings are changed frequently.

The hymen may also be rigid. This is usually discovered when the patient presents with a complaint of dyspareunia. In mild cases the patient will be instructed to dilate the hymen digitally, usually while sitting in a bath of warm water. If this does not succeed, vaginal dilators may be inserted by the doctor or nurse and later by the patient. In difficult cases, hymenotomy is performed. This is one rationale for a premarital examination. The discovery of a rigid hymen and its treatment premaritally may be of great importance to a newly married couple.

FERTILITY AND INFERTILITY

Control of fertility

Perhaps one of the greatest problems facing the world today is the control of fertility. One is bombarded with news of overpopulation and its implications for the future of the world. These implications have usually been stated in terms of the developing nations, but have taken on a global context. In addition, contraception is considered a matter of personal decision—it can exercise an important liberalizing potential for the family or the single person. In the light of these discussions the health professional has a responsibility to extend the knowledge and availability of contraception to anyone who requests it. With more birth control clinics available the nurse has a major role in the control of fertility.

Nursing responsibilities

Generally, the nursing responsibilities include referral of the patient to the appropriate clinic or doctor and education and interpretation. Depending on the nurse's situation and knowledge, these may be taken care of in an initial interview (or group discussion) with a patient (or a group of patients) seeking birth control advice. The nurse can assist the patient or couple in making a decision by presenting concise, factual information about the methods available. The couple should choose a method which will be most compatible with their personal circumstances. Most certainly this should be the one they will use and feel comfortable in using. No method of birth control is effective unless it is used constantly. This final decision is usually made with medical counsel. As the doctor reviews the patient's history, he may make other recommendations which will affect the person's or couple's choice. The patient or couple will need counselling in the proper use of the method they have chosen and what to expect in the period of initial adjustment. The nurse should validate the patient's real understanding of the method chosen and provide explanations and interpretations if necessary. In a simple fashion the knowledge of an alternative emergency method should be provided as well, for it is this which may prevent a pregnancy. The patient should leave the clinic or hospital with knowledge of an alternative method. Usually, the use of spermicidal foam or the use of a condom by the husband will overcome these situations. The nurse is responsible for gaining sufficient knowledge of the complex subject of contraception to be able to present factual knowledge to couples and to discuss the pros and cons of each method. In addition, the nurse will need to understand much of the emotional, social and religious aspects of contraception. A detailed presentation of family planning is beyond the scope of this work, but a brief outline of methods follows.

Methods of contraception

Coitus interruptus

This method consists of the male withdrawing his penis from the vagina before ejaculation occurs and ejaculating outside the vagina. Coitus interruptus, or withdrawal, is better than no attempt at birth control but is still very unreliable. Care must be taken not to ejaculate on or near the vulva, as the sperm may make their way into the vagina and pregnancy can result. The method requires the man to have advance awareness of ejaculation. This control and knowledge may be difficult to establish and may require more sexual experience than the man or couple possesses. Also, some sperm may escape before ejaculation occurs. The method has also come under considerable criticism for its psychological effects. These have been associated principally with frustration as a result of unresolved sexual tensions on the part of one or both partners. However, if the method is accepted by the couple and orgasm and ejaculation do occur, the resulting psychological stresses are probably minimal.

Condom

The condom is a thin rubber sheath which is placed over the penis before intromission. It prevents pregnancy by acting as a mechanical barrier to the sperm. Proper use includes application before intromission to avoid the possibility of a pre-ejaculatory emission of semen into the vagina and careful withdrawal of the penis and condom following intercourse to be sure that some semen is not lost into the vagina or over the vulva. Some doctors advise the use of a spermicidal jelly as a lubricating agent over the condom. This is a method of additional safety, particularly if the condom should be defective. However, newer methods of manufacture have greatly reduced this hazard. The condom is reasonably priced and is available without prescription. This greatly increases its availability and makes it one of the most widely used methods in the world.

Some couples find it objectionable as a method of birth control because it may interrupt sexual foreplay, it can lessen sensation, and its effective use relies heavily on the motivation of the male. These objections can be overcome if it is used by a highly motivated man who is taking mature responsibility for his behaviour.

Diaphragm

The diaphragm is a thin rubber cap which is inserted into the vagina by the woman and placed over the cervical os. The cap provides a mechanical barrier to the sperm. In addition a spermicidal jelly is placed on both sides of the cap. When the diaphragm is in place the spermicidal jelly will be in touch with the cervix and vagina.

The diaphragm is not dispensed without a prescription and requires individual fittings by a doctor initially, after a few months of use and following pregnancy or miscarriage. The woman also requires careful teaching in the proper insertion and care of the diaphragm. The diaphragm is inserted manually or with an inserter which is provided. The position of a diaphragm should be checked following each insertion. The woman stands with one foot elevated or squats. The diaphragm is squeezed between two fingers, thus narrowing it, and the woman slips the diaphragm into her vagina. In its proper position, the diaphragm cups the cervix with its anterior side behind the pubic bone and its posterior side in the posterior fornix of the vagina. Following insertion, the woman must be taught to check the position of the diaphragm to see that it is properly situated. Properly positioned, it is not felt by either partner. It can be left in place for 24 hours but should then be removed and cleansed with soap and water. Removal should not take place until at least 6 hours postcoitus to ensure death of all sperm present in the vagina.

Used by well instructed, highly motivated women it is a highly effective method of birth control. Some women find it distasteful to insert the diaphragm and to check its position; for these women it is probably a poor method of birth control.

Spermicidal preparations

In more recent years chemicals with a spermicidal action have been placed in gels, creams, aerosol foams, suppositories and foam tablets. These are inserted into the vagina about ½ hour before intercourse. The foam or jelly coats the cervix and inner vaginal walls. It should remain in the vagina for at least 6 hours to be sure that all sperm are dead. Used consistently, the method can be effective, particularly for the older woman approaching the menopause. Objections to the method revolve around the messiness which can result after coitus. Some men may complain of a slight urethral irritation when some foaming types of preparations are used.

Douche

The vaginal douche or irrigation may be used for cleanliness following coitus or may be considered to be a method of birth control by those who are under the impression that it 'washes the sperm away'. In fact, it may force the sperm into the uterine cavity and merely speed them on their way. It is not a method of contraception.

Breast-feeding

Under the stimulus of breast-feeding many women remain anovulatory for several months. Others quickly regain their fertility. Hence, breast-feeding should not be considered a method of birth control.

The rhythm method

This method requires temporary abstinence from coitus during the possible ovulation time of the woman. It is the only method of birth control officially sanctioned by all religions. The rationale of the method is based on several assumptions. First, a woman is only fertile at the time of ovulation, which occurs once monthly at a predictable time, and the ovum lives for approximately 24 hours. Secondly, sperm will survive in the genital tract for only 3 days. Placing these facts together, and allowing 3 days before and after ovulation for the life span of the sperm, we arrive at 6 days. Since we know that the time of ovulation varies in any one woman we must allow 1 or 2 days for extra safety on either side. This now gives us a fertile period of approximately 8 days' duration, falling near the middle of the menstrual cycle.

The crux of the problem is the timing of ovulation. Since no anticipatory method of timing ovulation has been discovered, we must rely on a retrospective view of the time of ovulation in any one woman. Under the influence of the rising progesterone levels following ovulation, the basal body temperature in women shows a rise. This rise should be noticeable within the first 24 hours following ovulation. The temperature remains slightly elevated for the remainder of the cycle (Fig. 23.18). Also, at the time of ovulation, the cervical mucus changes. There is an increase in amount and a reduction in viscosity. Woman can be taught to recognize and record these changes. Most doctors will attempt to predict the time of ovulation for any one woman after she has carefully recorded the dates of her menstrual periods, the mucus changes, and her temperatures taken daily at a uniform time. Depending on the woman, doctor or clinic, this may be done for 3–6 months. An average is then calculated from these dates and her individual period of likely fertility is plotted. In the graph (Fig. 23.18) the fertile period can be seen for a regular 28-day cycle. The calculated fertile period should be reviewed at specified intervals. At periods of her life when ovulation is being established or re-established, during postpartum and lactation or menopause and during periods of emotional stress the method is highly unreliable. In women of very regular periods and with high motivation the method has had success. However, until a foolproof method of anticipating ovulation is achieved, this method is unreliable.

The intrauterine device

An intrauterine device (IUD) is an object placed inside the uterus which remains in the uterus and prevents pregnancy. The action is not completely understood. Some doctors believe that IUD creates a hostile intrauterine environment either for sperm or for the fertilized ovum. Others feel that it is implantation which is prevented.

The IUD ranks as a very effective method of birth control in about 80% of the women who try it. Most IUDs used today are made of a flexible plastic and are

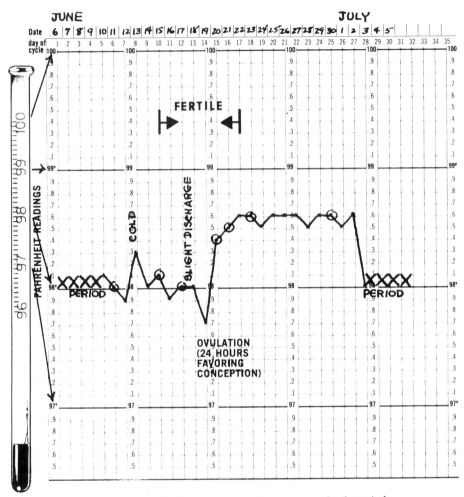

Fig. 23.18 Basal body temperature chart showing fertile period.

in several shapes. The addition of copper to the IUD produces a more effective device.

The device must be inserted by a doctor or other suitably trained person. It is a sterile procedure. First, the doctor will sound the uterus, confirming its depth and position. Then, having threaded the IUD into the inserter, he will insert this through the cervix, push down the plunger and retract the inserter. The use of the uterine sound and the skill of the person greatly reduce the risk of perforating the uterus. Uterine perforation during insertion remains a rare complication. Insertion of an IUD may be painful in the nullipara because of the tightness of the cervical os. Insertion is tolerated well by a majority of women.

Many devices are equipped with strings which hang into the vagina just below the cervix. The woman is taught to check for the presence of these strings monthly after her menstrual period. The IUD device can be expelled from the uterus, and this is most likely to occur during the menstrual period.

Women who have never been pregnant have an increased tendency to expel the device, as have women who have previously expelled it. If the woman notices that the IUD appears to have been expelled, she should report this to the doctor so that he can confirm this. The use of an alternative form of birth control would be advisable in the interim.

Removal of the device is carried out by a doctor. A woman should be discouraged from removing her own IUD. Some are difficult to remove because of their shape.

Complications and contraindications of the use of an IUD include increased menstrual loss and cramping. These are the most common side-effects and approximately 15% of women will require removal of the IUD for these reasons.

Pregnancy does occur in about 3% of women using an intrauterine device. If the patient wishes to continue with the pregnancy, the IUD is removed if possible. The risk of spontaneous abortion is about 50% with the IUD in place and there is an increased risk of infection. These risks vary with the type of IUD and its location in the uterine cavity.

The IUD may contribute to the development of pelvic inflammatory disease in about 2% of women. If neglected, the IUD contributes to sterility. The only sign of this infection may be irregular intramenstrual bleeding and complaints of pain. If an infection is suspected, the IUD is removed and the infection treated. The IUD is contraindicated in women with a pelvic infection or those at high risk of one.

Rarely an IUD can pass silently through the uterine wall into the abdominal cavity. This may be discovered when the woman cannot locate the strings, gets pregnant, or experiences abdominal or pelvic symptoms. It is removed during laparotomy.

Oral contraceptives
Birth control pills are synthetic chemical hormones whch resemble the female hormones of the ovary. In suppressing ovulation they mimic the action of pregnancy. The high hormone levels depress the hypothalamus, which in turn inhibits the release of pituitary gonadotrophins which stimulate ovulation. Thus, the woman is anovulatory. Protection is established as soon as the woman begins taking the pills, if she starts taking them on day 1 of the menstrual cycle.

The pills are divided into two types, the combined pill and progestogen pill. The combined pill contains synthetic oestrogen and progesterone hormones in each pill. This pill is more effective in preventing pregnancy because it induces changes in the cervix, making the mucus thicker and more impenetrable by sperm. Also, changes occur in the endometrium which would discourage implantation should fertilization occur.

The progestogen or 'mini-pill', contains a progestational agent and no oestrogen. It should not be confused with the low-dose (30 µg oestrogen) combined pill. Many of a woman's menstrual cycles while on the progestogen pill may be ovulatory. This pill depends on the effects of progestogen to produce changes in cervical mucus, the endometrium and hormonal levels to inhibit fertilization. Because of the reduced oestrogenicity of the pill it has fewer major side-effects than the combined pill but is slightly less effective in preventing pregnancy. This makes the low-dose combined pill the pill of choice

initially. The risk of pregnancy in both types of pills is minimal if taken as prescribed.

The combined pill is taken once a day for 21 days (sometimes 20) and no pill for the next 7 days, regardless of the woman's period. Initially, the first pill is taken on the first or fifth day of the woman's menstrual period. Now the pill will regulate her menstrual cycle and she takes them as prescribed. It is wise for her to cross them off on a calendar or devise a method of knowing when to start again because each succeeding 21-day series of pills is begun on the basis of when she took the last pill, not on her subsequent menstrual period. She begins again regardless of the state of her menstrual period. Progestogen pills are taken every day without omission. This does make it easier for women to follow, for no timing, counting or remembering other than to take the pill is required. Also, to maintain consistently high hormonal levels in the body, the pill should be taken at approximately the same time each day.

Withdrawal bleeding is regulated by the pill and occurs regularly at some time during the 7 pill-free days. This withdrawal bleeding simulates true menstruation. With the withdrawal of the high hormone levels, the endometrium sloughs away. However, menstruation is usually scantier and shorter, since the endometrium is thinner and scantier. A woman may miss one period but, should she miss two, this should be reported to the doctor immediately.

Much discussion has occurred over the possible side-effects or complications attendant on the use of oral contraceptives. For many women, adjustment to oral contraceptives may take some months (Table 23.4). During that time she may experience nausea, fullness and tingling in her breasts, headache, some spotting between menstrual periods, weight gain, chloasma or masking of pregnancy, acne, loss of libido or changes in vaginal discharge. On the other hand she may feel better, have relief from menstrual cramps and have an increased libido. Sometimes changes in dosages or in the timing of taking the pill helps. If she takes the pill with supper or lunch, she may feel less nauseated later.

The missed pill is cause for concern in many women. The woman should take the pill when she remembers it and take the next pill as she is accustomed to do. This may mean taking two pills in one

Table 23.4 Side-effects of birth control pills.

Oestrogen	Progestogen	Oestrogen and progestogen
Breakthrough bleeding	Acne	Weight gain
Nausea	Depression	Post pill amenorrhoea
Headaches	Dry vagina	Increased breast size
Chloasma	Loss of libido	Breast tenderness
Increased vaginal discharge		
Cervical erosion		
Cystic breast changes		

day. Should more than one pill be missed, then the couple should use an alternative form of birth control for the remainder of that cycle. If several pills are missed, the doctor should be consulted, as the cycles may be sufficiently interrupted as to require some further regulating under medical supervision.

The major complications of the pill are rare but not inconsiderable. For some women the hazards of the pill are still less than the hazards of a pregnancy or an abortion. Major concern revolves around the increased incidence of diseases of the circulatory system in women using the pill. The major circulatory diseases include thromboembolic disease, coronary artery disease, cerebrovascular accidents and hypertension. The risks rise with age, cigarette smoking, and duration (over 5 years) of pill use. Thus the smoking woman who has been using oral contraceptives for 5 years or more and is over 35 is placing herself at considerable risk if she continues use of the pill. Such women should be counselled to give up smoking and if unable to do so, to consider another method of birth control.

The long-term taking of pills (5–7 years) with high oestrogen content is associated with an increased risk of developing a rare, benign tumour of the liver. These tumours may cause rupture of the liver capsule with subsequent haemorrhage.

These complications have brought prolonged use of oral contraceptives into question. However, medical opinion still supports widespread use of the pill for carefully chosen women. The role of the family planning doctor and nurse is of great importance. The factors of past health, age, and smoking history are important, as is the duration of use.

Women on a contraceptive pill should see a doctor every 6 months to have their blood pressure and weight monitored and for an assessment of their general health. Pelvic examination is carried out annually and a cervical smear test is performed at least every 3 years. They are taught to seek prompt medical care if they experience severe or recurrent abdominal pain, chest pain and shortness of breath, severe headaches, eye problems such as blurred vision, flashing lights or tenderness and warmth over veins in the legs.

Safe birth control, compatible with the woman's life-style, will demand the use of several different methods of birth control throughout her life. The pill is best during periods of high risk for pregnancy and a strong desire to avoid pregnancy; the IUD, diaphragm, or condom for periods of higher risk but less desire to avoid pregnancy or to space children; finally, sterilization for those who wish no more worries in this direction.

Sterilization

Sterilization means the termination of reproductive capacity. As the social and emotional barriers to sterilization have altered, it has increased in popularity. When family size is complete, many couples choose sterilization as the method of birth control. In other cases, when the hazards of pregnancy are life-threatening, it may be strongly indicated.

Removal of any or all of the major organs of reproduction in either male or female results in sterility. Generally that is considered too extreme. A simple method of mechanically barring sperm and egg from meeting is required which will neither reduce natural hormone levels nor affect sexual capacity.

Vasectomy. In men vasectomy will accomplish this purpose. This simple operation can be done on an outpatient basis or at a clinic. On the surface of the scrotum the ascending spermatic cord is palpated and identified. Under local anaesthetic a small incision is made slightly to one side of each cord. The vas deferens is exposed, severed and electrocoagulated. Thus, new sperm are barred from reaching the vagina. Other sperm are still present in the tract above the ligation. For this reason a man is not considered sterile until he has had two negative sperm counts postoperatively.

The first sperm count is done after 10 ejaculations and is repeated following a further series of ejaculations until a negative sperm count is obtained.

In the immediate postoperative period the man may expect some minor bruising and discomfort for 24–72 hours. The discomfort is relieved by a simple analgesic, rest and wearing a scrotal support. Protected intercourse is resumed when he feels comfortable to do so. Few major side-effects, either physical or emotional, are reported following the procedure. Some cases are recorded of reconstructing the vas deferens. However, the rate of successful reconstruction is low. This is partly due to extravasation of sperm which causes the development of sperm antibodies following vasectomy. Even though physical reconstruction of the vas deferens might be possible, the antibodies continue to destroy the sperm. Vasovasostomy (repair of the separated vas deferens) produces fertility in only 22% of men. Thus, the patient should regard a vasectomy as irreversible.

Tubal ligation. Tubal ligation is the comparable operation in women. It can be done vaginally but is usually done abdominally. Under a general anaesthetic two small incisions are made in the abdomen. The uterine tube is dissected, a loop of tube is lifted up, ligated, and above the ligation is either crushed with a clamp or severed. In some operations the uterine end of the tube may be turned back and embedded in the posterior wall of the uterus. Various names for these techniques include Madlener, Pomeroy and Irving, respectively. Tubal coagulations, in conjunction with a laparoscopy, may also be done. The surgeon identifies the tubes through the laparoscope and then applies the heat source which coagulates the tube. In the hands of a skilled operator the procedure is safe and associated with few side-effects. Cups and rings can also be used to achieve sterilization. These methods are less damaging to the tubes than cauterization. As in the male, the tubes can be reconstructed, but the incidence is not high. Thus, the patient should see the operation as irreversible. The operation is not entirely harmless. Rare major complications postoperatively can be pulmonary embolism and later tubal pregnancy. These make the operation a more hazardous procedure than a vasectomy.

Nursing responsibilities in both operations include regular pre- and postoperative care. However, in addition to the consent for operation, there is a separate consent form for sterilization which must be signed before the operation.

Infertility

Infertility is defined as the failure to conceive after 12 months of adequate exposure without the use of contraceptives. Primary infertility refers to a couple who have never conceived. Secondary infertility refers to a couple who have had a previous pregnancy but now cannot conceive. Approximately 10% of couples prove infertile. Of this 10% about 40% of the problem rests with the man, 40% with the woman and from 5–10% with the couple as a unit.

CAUSES OF INFERTILITY

The possible causes of infertility are too numerous to list. However, the major causes can be grouped under several headings. Any impairment of ovarian function which interrupts ovulation creates infertility. This may be caused by hormonal imbalances or may be due to some intrinsic defect in the ovaries themselves. The same is true of the testes. The conducting system may not be patent. Infections leading to adhesions are a major cause in both men and women. Malformations or displacements of the organs of the reproductive tract may contribute to infertility. The problem may arise because of unique factors particular to the union. Vaginal secretions may not be compatible with the seminal fluid, causing the sperm to die.

ASSESSMENT AND DIAGNOSIS

The investigation usually begins when the woman presents herself to the gynaecologist with a complaint of failure to conceive. By this time the problem may have become a nagging fear for both her and her husband. Often reassurance and ventilation of the anxiety seem to help the patient, for many patients are reported as returning shortly thereafter as pregnant. A persistent infertility case will require thorough investigation. Many gynaecologists prefer to see the couple together so that both partners may receive an outline and discussion of the approach which will be used. The doctor's assessment of the possible cause of the infertility will

guide the direction of the investigation. Some techniques which are used in investigating infertility are described.

Medical history and physical examination
A detailed medical history and physical examination are done for both partners. Particular attention will be paid to the development of the secondary sex characteristics and any evidence of virilizing or feminizing effects. Any history of infections, and injuries involving the genitourinary tract will be carefully noted. In addition the doctor will take a marital history to gain an adequate picture of the couple's sexual pattern. The woman will be asked to give a detailed menstrual history. At this point some education in human reproduction may help the couple.

Before other tests are begun, infections, particularly cervicitis and prostatitis, are likely to be treated, as they may contribute to infertility. Anaemia, poor health, exhaustion, overwork, stress and other psychological situations all may be causative factors, and the doctor often tries to relieve these first if they seem of sufficent magnitude to be affecting the sexual adjustment of the couple.

Ovulation
Whether or not ovulation occurs monthly may have to be established. The patient is asked to keep a basal body temperature chart. This also helps the doctor to estimate hormonal levels. The woman is asked to come to the surgery or clinic near ovulation time. Cervical smears will be taken and tested for spinnbarkeit and ferning. Respectively, these tests help to time ovulation and indicate how receptive the cervical mucus is to sperm. If ferning appears to be unsatisfactory, the patient may be requested to return for serial vaginal smears, which give indications of ovulation.

Plasma assay will be done to assess the levels of FSH and LH. Plasma progesterone levels are sampled one week after the biphasic shift in the basal body temperature graph, or day 21 in the 28-day cycle. These results, together with the graphs and other tests, permit an outline of the events of the menstrual cycle that are occurring in the woman.

Urinalysis
Urine tests may be done to measure urinary oestriols and, if the doctor feels it is warranted, the presence and amount of 17-ketosteroids.

Endometrial biopsy
This is done to indicate whether or not a healthy endometrium is present. If it is not, then the problem may be one of failure of the fertilized ovum to achieve successful implantation. Occasionally tuberculosis, hitherto unsuspected, is discovered, and may be the cause of the infertility.

Laparoscopy. Laparoscopy allows the direct visualization of pelvic contents and an opportunity to perform ovarian biopsies if necessary. It may also be combined with a hysterosalpingogram.

Hysterosalpingogram. A hysterosalpingogram is the injection of a radiopaque dye into the genital tract. It serves to outline the uterine cavity and uterine tubes. The patient may not be anaesthetized. The test is done in the x-ray department under sterile technique. The patient is usually asked to move from side to side after the injection in order to promote spilling of the dye into the abdominal cavity. This test provides information about the exact location of any abnormality.

Possible complications of tubal patency tests. Pain, collapse and vomiting may be experienced shortly after the test is done, especially in women who were not anaesthetized. The patient should be observed for these signs for approximately 3 hours following a test. Helping the patient to assume a knee-chest position for a few minutes before standing up may prevent further discomfort. Cramps and vomiting may be more prevalent following cervical dilatation.

Other complications may include exacerbation of pelvic infections, air embolism or sensitivity reactions to the dye and inadvertent abortion.

On the other hand, either of the tests may be therapeutic because they may have opened the tract. This is supported by many patients who conceive with no further treatment.

Sims–Huhner postcoital test

Postcoitally, a specimen of seminal fluid from the posterior fornix of the vagina and the cervical canal is aspirated. The specimen is examined for motility of the sperm and their ability to survive in the cervix or vagina. The test is best performed at the time of ovulation. The patient will be instructed not to douche or use lubricants for 2 days before the test. Following intercourse she will remain supine, hips elevated on a pillow for 30 minutes. Within the next 2–4 hours she will come to the doctor's surgery or the fertility clinic, at which time the specimen will be taken. A reading will assess how many live, motile sperm are in the specimen. Should the sperm not be present, the investigation may be directed toward the male. Does he have sperm? If he does, why is he not capable of depositing them near the cervix? If they are dead or non-motile, the vaginal environment may be hostile to them. One such reaction is due to the stimulus a foreign protein (sperm) evokes in the woman's body. Consequently, antibodies develop. The antibodies in the female inactivate the sperm before fertilization can take place. Following a 3- to 6-month period of abstinence or the use of a condom by the male, circulating antibodies may be sufficiently reduced to permit sperm to live in order to fertilize.

Crossed hostility

This test is carried out when the postcoital test is negative. A drop of ejaculate is placed on a slide with a drop of cervical mucus. Sperms should be seen actively invading the mucus. If not, the mucus may be impenetrable for several reasons or the sperm may have low motility. If the problem is with the mucus, any infection which is present is treated and oestrogen may be given from day 1 to day 10 of the menstrual cycle to produce a more water penetrable mucus.

Semen analysis

A specimen of seminal fluid will be examined for volume and the number, morphology and motility of sperm. Ideally, 2–5 ml of fluid should be present. The fluid should gel and then reliquefy after 15–20 minutes. The sperm should number above 60 million per millilitre of ejaculate, and 60% should still show vigorous activity when examined at room temperature 2 hours after ejaculation. Not more than 20% of the sperm should show abnormal forms.

The specimen is collected after a 3-day period of abstinence from coitus. It is collected in a dry, sterile jar by masturbation or coitus interruptus and is brought to the clinic for examination within 2 hours of collection.

If no sperm are present in the ejaculate, the patency of the duct system may be assessed by a vasogram. Testicular biopsy may be indicated. If the biopsy shows living sperm, then the failure of the sperm to arrive in the seminal fluid may be due to a blockage in the tube. Hormone assays of FSH, LH and testosterone will also be done. (In most clinics this is the first investigation carried out.)

TREATMENT

Surgery

In both male and female, surgery is aimed at restoring function. Adhesions may be released; the ducts are reconstructed. In certain cases polyethylene tubes are inserted into the uterine tubes to help maintain patency. Cysts and tumours are removed as indicated. The nursing care is the same as that for any pelvic operative procedure.

Hormone therapy

Clomiphene. Hormones may be administered to induce ovulation. Clomiphene (Clomid) is an anti-oestrogenic substance which stimulates the hypothalamus to stimulate the pituitary to increase the output of FSH and LH. By displacing the circulating oestrogens, the hypothalamus is released from the inhibiting effects of high levels of oestrogen. In addition, clomiphene may increase ovarian sensitivity to FSH and LH.

Treatment consists of administering 50–200 mg pills daily for 5 days. These tablets may be started on the fifth day of the cycle or at any time if no cycles are occurring. Ovulation is expected 7–12 days following treatment. The patient must be instructed to monitor her basal body temperature carefully, as a rise in temperature is expected with ovulation. Coitus should occur close to ovulation. Treatment may be repeated several times until pregnancy occurs or the treatment is judged ineffective. Good rates of success are recorded. Clomiphene is more successful when used in situations of altered function, such as amenorrhoea following the oral contraceptives or anovulation in Stein–Leventhal syndrome.

The drug does stimulate the growth of benign ovarian cysts which usually disappear after its use. The incidence of multiple births is increased in couples using this medication. There do not appear to be any long-term effects.

Gonadotrophins. The gonadotrophins may be supplied artificially. Hypothalamic-releasing factors may be given to stimulate the pituitary. Human pituitary gonadotrophins made from freeze-dried human pituitaries may be administered. These are, in effect, the FSH and LH hormones. The patient receives injections of FSH to ripen a follicle and then LH to stimulate ovulation. The process is complex, necessitating close monitoring of the patient for ovulation and for overstimulation of the ovaries. Ovarian cysts follow its use, as do multiple pregnancies. Like clomiphene, good pregnancy rates have been achieved. Because of abortions and high fetal wastage associated with prematurity and multiple births, the overall success rate in terms of live children is lower.

Bromocriptine (Parlodel). Occasionally, a woman experiences amenorrhoea due to elevated prolactin levels secondary to pregnancy, steroid contraceptives, pituitary tumours or other drugs and treatments. High prolactin levels inhibit the effect of FSH and LH on the ovary. Bromocriptine is an ergot derivative which inhibits release of prolactin from the pituitary. As the prolactin levels fall FSH and LH stimulate the ovary to ovulate. About two-thirds of patients treated become ovulatory. The major side-effects are nausea and dizziness.

Hormone therapy may also be instituted in the man. Gonadotrophins may be prescribed and have achieved some success in raising the sperm counts of men with low counts. Sometimes vitamin B will be prescribed to ensure the normal inactivation of oestrogens by the liver. Varying doses of testosterone may be tried with varying rates of success.

NURSING RESPONSIBILITIES

Most infertility investigations and treatments are done on an outpatient basis or during short hospitalization. Some nurses may be involved in infertility clinics; others may see the patient only during a brief visit to hospital to have an investigative test. Depending on the nurse's involvement, she may be expected to:

1 Provide education in human reproduction and sex education.
2 Teach the patient how to accurately perform certain tests or treatments.
3 Prepare the patient physically and emotionally for the procedure.
4 Assist the patient and doctor during investigative procedures.
5 Monitor the patient's physical and emotional status post-treatment for the development of complications.
6 Respond appropriately to changes in patient condition, for example if the patient experiences vomiting, nursing measures for dealing with vomiting are used.
7 Realize that the patient may come to the investigation with a sense of failure and decreased self-esteem. She should respond in ways which do not increase the sense of failure or further decrease self-esteem.

DISORDERS OF THE MENSTRUAL CYCLE AND MENSTRUATION

Mittelschmerz

Mittelschmerz is a feeling of lower abdominal pain on one side on or near ovulation day. It is thought to be caused by fluid or blood escaping from the ruptured follicle site and causing peritoneal irritation. It occurs in about 25% of women. Occasionally when the right side is involved, fear of appendicitis may bring the woman to the doctor.

Premenstrual tension

This syndrome is probably experienced by most women in mild forms. However, extreme cases are seen. The symptomatology includes a feeling of fullness or heaviness in the lower abdomen, backache, painful breasts, irritability, headache, weight gain premenstrually, nervousness, depression and insomnia.

The absence of normative data on the physical and emotional changes in the menstrual cycle mean that the syndrome has not been clearly defined. No single aetiology has been identified and several theories of aetiology exist. Diuretics are now considered to have been over-used and the theory relating all symptoms to fluid retention has not been supported.

What seems clear is that somatic and psychological symptoms exist; they occur cyclically but in varying degrees with each cycle. There is usually an abrupt onset and departure of the symptoms and the woman tends to be 35 years of age or older.

Among the treatments that are usually tried are: birth control pills, pyridoxine (vitamin B_6), progesterone and bromocriptine. Any of these treatments may help some women. For patients suffering severe psychological symptoms, psychotherapy may be recommended both to provide support and to distinguish between other emotional disturbances which may be present and masking as premenstrual tension.

Treatment consists in taking a sympathetic and understanding approach, as the patient may be very upset by the changes of mood and behaviour which she experiences. Women are taught to chart their symptoms to reduce the unexpectedness of them, to talk about these changes with husband and family in order to increase family understanding, to eat nutritious, regular meals, and to reduce stress during the latter half of the menstrual cycle.

Further research into the complex neuroendocrinological relationships of the menstrual cycle is needed before all the symptoms associated with the menstrual cycle can be fully understood and effectively treated.

Dysmenorrhoea

Dysmenorrhoea is defined as pain with menstruation. Two types, primary and secondary dysmenorrhoea, are commonly distinguished.

PRIMARY DYSMENORRHOEA

Primary dysmenorrhoea is a spasmodic type of pain, occurring at the onset of the menstrual period and lasting from 1–24 hours. It is most common among young girls, rarely beginning with the menarche and fading away spontaneously around 24 years of age or following the delivery of a full-term infant. No pathology in pelvic structures is associated with this type of dysmenorrhoea. In addition to the cramps, there may be shivering, a feeling of tension, nausea, vomiting, pallor and fainting.

The aetiology remains unclear but current theory supports prostaglandins as the cause of the increased myometrial activity and subsequent pain experienced. Excessive quantities of prostaglandins are synthesized during the breakdown of the secretory endometrium. They cause increased muscular contractions, uterine ischaemia and are also responsible for the symptoms of nausea, vomiting and pallor by their influence on smooth muscle.

Dysmenorrhoea is also associated with ovulation, as anovulatory cycles are rarely accompanied by dysmenorrhoea. This probably explains why the first cycles are pain-free and dysmenorrhoea in some girls is synchronous with ovulation. Also, the daughters of women who have suffered dysmenorrhoea are more frequently dysmenorrhoeic. Whether this is learned or inherited is still disputed. In any case the psyche can play a role in aggravating the symptoms but is very rarely the sole explanation. A woman's personal tolerance for discomfort undoubtedly affects her response to any pain, dysmenorrhoea being no exception.

Treatment includes a kind and sympathetic approach by all members of the health team. Prostaglandin inhibitors such as acetylsalicylic acid (aspirin) and mefenamic acid (Ponstan) may be prescribed. The addition of analgesics is useful for some women and the doctor may prescribe a course of oral contraceptives. This induces anovulatory periods and may be followed by very good results. It may also be diagnostic. Should dysmenorrhoea continue, the doctor may look for other causes. In more extreme cases, surgery may be chosen. The cervix is dilated with varying success. A presacral sympathectomy or, in desperation, a hysterectomy may be done.

Nursing intervention

The school and occupational health nurses commonly deal with the girl or young woman suffering from dysmenorrhoea. She may present herself in their office, or the nurse may be asked to interview the girl or woman who frequently misses school or work because of dysmenorrhoea. Frequent, severe dysmenorrhoea should always be investigated by the gynaecologist, and it is the nurse's responsibility to suggest this to the patient and assist her in obtaining this care.

In regard to general care, the patient may need instruction in the normal anatomy and physiology of menstruation. This serves to eradicate misconceptions and lessen the fear and anxiety which may be associated with her periods. She may need some instruction in menstrual hygiene so that her period does not seem distasteful and restricting. This may simply mean a switch from sanitary pads to tampons and frequent bathing. The patient may need to be encouraged to get more exercise and be sure that she is not constipated before her period.

Immediate care involves providing a sympathetic, understanding approach, a place to lie down, a blanket for warmth, application of heat to the lower abdomen and a mild analgesic. When the symptoms are relieved, the girl often continues with her work. If the patient requires medication for relief, she should be instructed to take the tablet before dysmenorrhoea becomes acute. This will prevent the symptoms and the girl or woman feels that she has some control over the events which are happening to her rather than being totally subject to them.

SECONDARY DYSMENORRHOEA

Secondary dysmenorrhoea is a constant type of pain which often starts 2–3 days before the period and persists well past the first day. It may continue for a day or two following the period. Pain may radiate through the abdomen into the back and down the thighs. It occurs after several years of normal painless menses and is frequently associated with pelvic pathology. The most frequent causes are tumours, inflammatory diseases, endometriosis and fixed malpositions of the uterus. It is essentially a symptom of disease. Should the nurse be consulted by a woman describing these symptoms, the woman should be referred to a gynaecologist immediately.

Amenorrhoea

Amenorrhoea, or absence of menstruation, may be primary or secondary. Secondary amenorrhoea is that which occurs after several months or years of normal menses.

Menorrhagia

Menorrhagia is excessive bleeding at the time of normal menses.

Polymenorrhoea

Polymenorrhoea refers to cyclic bleeding which is normal in amount but occurs too frequently.

Epimenorrhagia

Epimenorrhagia is cyclic bleeding which is both excessive and too frequent.

Metrorrhagia

Metrorrhagia refers to any bleeding which occurs between menstrual periods. Any bleeding per vaginam at any time other than normal menses is included, even if it amounts only to slight staining.

Dysfunctional uterine bleeding

True dysfunctional uterine bleeding refers to that which occurs in the presence of endocrine dysfunction rather than organic disease. It may be seen as chronic epimenorrhagia or as an episode of acute bleeding. Some episodes of haemorrhage are caused by high levels of oestrogen in the proliferative phase of the cycle. These high levels depress the hypothalamus–pituitary complex and no ovulation occurs. Because there is no ovulation, no progesterone is produced and the endometrium remains proliferative and becomes cystic. As oestrogen levels fall, usually after a 6- to 8-week period of amenorrhoea, bleeding occurs. This disorder is associated with the older woman.

Other episodes of bleeding are related to fluctuating oestrogen levels produced by an imperfectly functioning hypothalamus–pituitary–ovary feedback mechanism. Follicles are stimulated to partial maturation; some oestrogen is produced but then the level falls, producing intermittent irregular and possibly prolonged bleeding. The causes are related to immaturity or ageing of the feedback mechanism and to imbalance induced in the system from physical or psychologial factors.

In most cases treatment consists of administering the combined oral contraceptives. They exert a regulating and inhibiting effect on the endometrium and feedback mechanism. Three to six cycles of hormonal therapy are usually required to re-establish the normal menstrual pattern. A dilatation and curettage may be done initially. The endometrium is scraped, a biopsy done and then hormone therapy is initiated. If required, adjunctive therapy such as iron replacement is also started. More severe cases are treated with higher and more complex doses of oestrogens and progestins, in combination or sequence. In some cases when hormone therapy does not succeed, a hysterectomy may be necessary.

Endometriosis

Endometriosis is the location of endometrial tissue outside the uterine cavity. Although the location may be varied, the most frequent locations are in or near the ovaries, the uterosacral ligaments and the uterovesical peritoneum. Extrapelvic sites may be as varied as the umbilicus, an old laparotomy scar, vulva or even lungs. The tissue responds to the hormones of the ovarian cycle and undergoes a small menstruation just like the uterine endometrium. Statistics vary, but perhaps 5% of all patients seen by the gynaecologist suffer from endometriosis.

AETIOLOGY

Causes may be varied. Two major theories are prevalent. One concludes that small bits of endometrial tissue are forced or regurgitated back up the uterine tube and escape into the abdomen during menstruation. The other theory points out that the peritoneum and reproductive tract derive from the same early embryological tissues. Some of the tissues may be misplanted from that early time. Under sufficient stimulation, these cells respond and differentiate into a functioning endometrial tag. Rare cases seem to be caused by small pieces of endometrium being transported to other parts of the body through the lymphatics or by the blood. This seems to be true of endometrial tissue in the limbs or in lung tissue. As the ectopic endometrium menstruates, the blood collects in little cyst-like nodules which have a characteristic bluish-black look. Usually they are pea-sized but may be much larger. Those in the ovary and uterosacral area often attain a size of 3–6 cm. These ovarian cysts are sometimes termed 'chocolate cysts' because of the thick, chocolate-coloured material which they contain. The cysts become surrounded by fibrous tissue which makes them easy to palpate, as they feel firm and well defined. Frequently the cyst perforates and spills its sticky contents into the abdomen. The resulting irritation promotes the formation of adhesions which readily fix the ovary or the affected area to the broad ligament or other pelvic structures.

The disease is seen most frequently in the nulliparous woman, aged 30–40. It occurs more commonly in the upper economic and social groups, presumably because of less frequent and later childbearing.

The patient may have no symptomatology, and the disease may only be discovered incidental to abdominal surgery. More commonly, the patient complains of pain. Secondary dysmenorrhoea may appear, with pain becoming severe 1–2 days before menstruation. The pain gradually becomes worse and may be described as 'boring'. This is due to the distension and pain of the swollen, shedding areas contained within the fibrous capsule of the cysts. The patient may also complain of backache, dyspareunia of a deep nature localized in the posterior fornix of the vagina or persistent lower abdominal pain occurring throughout the cycle. Pain may be of an acute nature, localized in the abdomen when a cyst ruptures. The gynaecologist may suspect endometriosis when a patient is infertile, since this is a common symptom of this group. Sometimes the adhesions become severe enough to cause a bowel obstruction or painful micturition.

Diagnosis is frequently confirmed on bimanual examination when firm nodular lumps are felt in the adnexa. Visualizing the typical bluish nodules may be done by culdoscopy, laparoscopy or during a laparotomy. Diagnosis is confirmed by biopsy when endometrial glands and stroma are seen microscopically.

Laparoscopy.   The gynaecologist may feel that direct viewing of the pelvic organs is necessary. Examination under anaesthesia involving colpotomy, culdoscopy and culdocentesis may be used but these procedures are now being replaced by laparoscopy. It provides better lighted, direct visualization of the anterior aspect of the tubes and ovaries. The procedure is done under a general anaesthetic and aseptic conditions.

To avoid damage and to obtain better visualization of the abdominal and pelvic contents, the cavity is distended by the introduction of carbon dioxide. The abdominal wall is lifted by the gas above the underlying organs. The patient is tilted head downwards to about a 45° angle, shifting the abdominal contents up and away from the site of insertion of the laparoscope and from the pelvis. Through a small incision in the lower rim of the umbilicus a trocar and cannula are inserted on an angle; the trocar is then withdrawn and the endoscope inserted. It enters the peritoneal cavity approximately half-way between the umbilicus and the symphysis pubis. The contents of the abdomen and pelvis are observed and the uterus may be manipulated from below by a clamp in the cervix—this changes angles and brings the organs into better view. At the end of the procedure the endoscope is withdrawn, the gas expressed from the abdomen through the cannula and the incision closed with a clip or stitch which is removed in 24–48 hours.

There are few complications, but cardiac arrhythmias, collapse and death have been recorded. The patient may complain of some mild abdominal or shoulder pain following the procedure. This is usually abdominal gas which collects beneath the diaphragm and is not intestinal colic. The gas is absorbed gradually over a few days, but a change of position may help. Severe pain or signs of abdominal tenderness or tightness should be reported.

The patient receives pre- and postoperative care, but does not require a shave preparation. She is ambulatory on return from the recovery room and generally returns to a full diet immediately.

This is based on the age of the patient, her desire for more children and the severity of the disease. Pregnancy relieves the symptoms and may be advised if the couple want more children. Pseudopregnancy may be achieved by the administration of progesterone for varying periods of time, or danazol 200–800 mg daily for 6 months.

Treatment may be surgical and is directed at preserving reproductive function. Affected areas are removed, and fixed organs released. Infertility often ceases following surgery. In severe cases a hysterectomy may be done. Depending on the extent of the cystic involvement, oophorectomy may also be performed. The symptoms usually disappear at menopause as ovarian atrophy begins and hormonal stimulation declines.

Adenomyosis uteri

This condition is similar to endometriosis in that it is characterized by endometrium within the muscular wall of the uterus or the uterine tube. The cause is unknown. In any case, the uterine endometrium appears to grow downward between the muscle bundles of the myometrium. This produces a uniform, moderate enlargement of the uterus. The patient may complain of menorrhagia and dysmenorrhoea. Often pelvic endometriosis is also present. Then the uterus may be fixed (frozen) in the pelvis, and pelvic nodules may be palpated. The patient may complain of pain in the sacral or coccygeal area as well.

INTERRUPTIONS OF PREGNANCY

Abortion

An abortion is the termination of a pregnancy before the 28th week of pregnancy. 'Miscarriage' also refers to abortion but is the lay term for designating lack of criminal involvement.

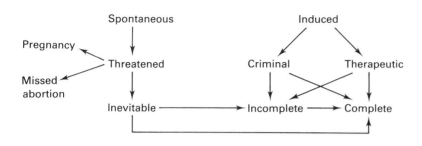

Table 23.5 Classification of abortion.

The incidence of abortion is difficult to state accurately but between 10 and 20% of all conceptions are thought to abort. See Table 23.5 for classification of abortions.

CAUSES

Most known causes can be separated into three major groups: fetal, maternal and faulty environment. Fetal causes are often associated with chromosomal or other abnormalities which are incompatible with life. This has been considered to be as high as 40% of all causes of abortion. Maternal and faulty environment causes are more varied. Endotoxins, as a result of severe infections in the mother, may invade the fetus, usually causing its death and later expulsion. Drugs ingested by the mother may damage the fetus directly or may damage the placenta and hence the nutrition of the fetus. Hormonal imbalances may be the cause of some abortions, especially in cases in which the thyroid gland is involved. Lack of progesterone may result in a poorly developed endometrium. As a result, nidation does not occur or does so ineffectively. Anatomical uterine defects or uterine pathology causes some abortions. Nutritional factors are linked to abortion and premature labour, for adequate nutrition of the woman bears an important part in her reproductive capacity. The emotional state of the woman is also considered a possible contributing factor. This often centres on fear, grief or emotional trauma in susceptible women. Physical trauma can also induce an abortion. This may be true of surgery performed during pregnancy.

A threatened abortion is one in which the threat to the pregnancy is slight. With care, the woman may carry the pregnancy to term. Since any bleeding, however minor, per vaginam is abnormal in the pregnant woman, any evidence of such bleeding is taken as a sign of threatened abortion until proven otherwise. In addition, some backache or mild intermittent lower abdominal pain may be present. If the abortion is not to be immediate, cramping and bleeding may stop. It becomes inevitable when bleeding continues, cramps become stronger and regular, the cevix dilates and the membranes rupture. The inevitable abortion becomes the complete abortion when all products of conception are expelled. This usually occurs before the twelfth week of gestation. The abortion is incomplete when some of the products of conception are retained. This is usually the placenta and membranes and is more frequent following the twelfth week, when the placenta is more firmly embedded. The umbilical cord breaks, leaving the placenta and membranes in utero. A missed abortion is one in which the fetus dies; symptoms of abortion cease and the products of conception are retained in the uterus for 2 or more months. Following this, the uterus is not observed to increase in size. Indeed, it begins to regress slightly as the amniotic fluid is absorbed. No fetal heart is heard. The patient remains amenorrhoeic, and the breasts regress. The abortus is usually expelled spontaneously but may be retained for many months or years. In such cases it becomes a shrivelled sac with areas of dense calcification.

A woman is considered to be an habitual aborter when she aborts three or more consecutive pregnancies. The causes can be any of the causes of a single abortion but persist through several pregnancies. In addition, an incompetent cervix is frequently sited as a cause of habitual abortion. Possibly because of inherent problems in the cervix or trauma to the cervix, the cervix dilates easily and will not retain the pregnancy. Loss of the pregnancy usually occurs later at about 16–20 weeks. Dilation of the cervix is rapid, with little pain and bleeding. Rupture of the membranes occurs, followed by the expulsion of the fetus.

TREATMENT AND NURSING CARE

Threatened abortion
The treatment of threatened abortion is aimed at preserving the pregnancy. Every pregnant woman should be told the danger signs of pregnancy. Often this instruction is the responsibility of the nurse in either the clinic or the surgery. Thus, the woman should recognize bleeding as abnormal and be aware that she should notify her doctor immediately. She should then go to bed and rest unless otherwise instructed by her doctor. If the bleeding is slight, the

patient is managed at home and advised to get extra rest for a few days. For some patients this may be impossible, and admission to hospital is necessary.

On admission to the hospital, the patient is placed on bed rest. Temperature, pulse and blood pressure are noted as frequently as the patient's condition warrants. All the pads, linens and clothing stained with blood are kept for inspection by the doctor. This helps in the estimation of blood loss. In addition, the patient is observed for any increased bleeding or cramping which would indicate a change in status. A diet low in roughage is usually ordered with supplementary iron and vitamin C. Purgatives and enemas are not given in order to avoid stimulation of the uterus. Rectal and vaginal examinations are contraindicated. Bleeding usually ceases within 24–48 hours if the pregnancy is going to continue. At this time the doctor will probably perform a careful speculum and bimanual examination, since other possible causes of bleeding must be ruled out. These causes could be carcinoma or other complications of pregnancy.

On discharge home the patient is instructed to get extra rest and to avoid strenuous exercise, heavy lifting, excitement or fatigue. Coitus may be restricted for a period of 2 weeks or longer. Should bleeding recur, the patient is advised to notify her doctor and remain in bed.

Missed abortion
The patient will be followed by her obstetrician to see that the pregnancy progresses normally. If it does not and a persistent brownish discharge recurs, missed abortion may be suspected. A positive pregnancy test may only indicate that placental tissue still remains living. An ultrasound examination of the fetus usually confirms the diagnosis. The obstetrician is faced with the choice of interfering to evacuate the uterus or waiting until it is done spontaneously. Physically, there is usually no pressing need. Emotionally it is very distressing to the woman and her family to know that she is carrying a dead fetus. The danger from disseminated intravascular coagulation (DIC) as a complicating factor to intervention by the obstetrician increases as the dead fetus is retained. Presumably this occurs as some of the degenerating products of the fetus enter the maternal bloodstream. This danger appears to be most serious about 4–6 weeks after fetal death. Coagulation studies may be done before intervention is attempted.

For these reasons the obstetrician usually intervenes approximately 2 weeks after death of the fetus. The dead fetus may be aborted by means of suction evacuation if death occurs before 12 weeks of gestation or by prostaglandin administration if it occurs during the second trimester. The procedure is emotionally and physically exhausting for the patient. She requires much supportive nursing care. Also, the contractions are painful, and some analgesic should be administered. Since no danger can result to the fetus, the mother need not suffer unduly. Close observation of the patient's condition for overhydration is necessary because of the danger of overhydrating her with large amounts of fluid containing synthetic oxytocin, which has an antidiuretic action. An intake and output record should be kept.

Inevitable abortion
The treatment of an inevitable abortion is similar to that of a threatened abortion. The patient is placed on bed rest. Blood will be taken for haemoglobin, typing and cross-matching. The amount and character of the bleeding is observed carefully. Blood pressure and pulse may need to be taken every 10 minutes if bleeding is profuse, and the patient must be observed for other signs of shock. Any tissue or suspicious clots are saved to be examined for traces of fetus and placenta. Good perineal care is maintained by frequent cleansing of the vulva to reduce the risk of infection and to promote the patient's comfort. Procedures for perineal care will vary. Generally, soap and water are sufficient. The perineum is swabbed from the pubes to the perineal body (front to back) and from the vulva out to the thigh. The rectal area is washed last. This is to prevent the spread of bacteria from the rectum upward into the vagina and thence to the endometrium. A perineal shave may be ordered. If the abortion seems to be approaching a conclusion, it is not assisted. However, with the membranes ruptured, the cervix dilated and contractions tapering off, the process may be hastened by the administration of intravenous oxytocin.

If the abortion has been complete and the obstetrician is satisfied of this, the woman is treated similarly to the postpartum patient. If the patient is Rh negative blood group, she receives Rh_0 (anti-D immunoglobulin) to prevent complications in further pregnancies. A slight lochial discharge is expected and the woman must be taught perineal care. She will be discharged home in 3–4 days, depending on the state of her health. To reduce the risk of infection, coitus is contraindicated until lochial discharge has ceased. This usually occurs within 2 weeks.

When the products of conception are retained, the uterus must be emptied. Two of the major causes of bleeding associated with pregnancy result from the partially separated placenta and retained fragments of conception. The uterus cannot contract effectively; the torn blood vessels remain open and bleed. Also, the risk of infection is much increased by the debris lying in the uterus. If the bleeding is acute, the patient is usually taken to the operating theatre and an emergency dilation and curettage (D and C) is done. Under a general anesthaesia, the cervix is gently dilated until the passage of a curette is possible. Dilation is accomplished by using the dilators or by the use of a special vibrating dilator. The curette is used to scrape the tissue from the walls of the uterus.

Following this operation the patient receives perineal care and is observed for signs of haemorrhage and infection. She may receive an intravenous oxytocic solution to help involution of the uterus. Because of the danger of accidental perforation of the uterus with the instruments, the patient is observed postoperatively for signs of peritoneal irritation or abdominal (concealed) haemorrhage. Packing may or may not have been inserted in the vagina to help control or prevent haemorrhage. This should be carefully noted on the chart. If packing was inserted, the nurse observes the patient even more carefully for signs of shock, since any bleeding may be concealed by the packing. If there is packing, it is removed within several hours to allow free drainage of lochia and thus help prevent infection. By altering urethrovesical relationships, vaginal packing increases a woman's inability to void postoperatively. Inability to void with subsequent bladder distension should be avoided, either by removing the packing or inserting a catheter.

Incompetent cervical os

The patient who has had several abortions will probably receive a thorough assessment between pregnancies in an attempt to ascertain her problem. Should the cause be considered an incompetent cervical os, the obstetrician may attempt to tighten the cervix with a suture. This is usually done during the twelfth to sixteenth week of pregnancy. The Shirodkar technique consists of running a non-dissolving suture around the cervix like a drawstring or purse string.

On return from the operating theatre, the pregnant patient is observed for signs of labour and imminent abortion. Should the abortion appear inevitable, the suture must be removed or serious tearing of the cervix might occur. At 38 weeks, the suture is removed and vaginal delivery follows, or the suture is retained and delivery is by caesarean section.

Emotional response to spontaneous abortion

Response to early abortion. Early pregnancy is characterized by feelings of unreality while the mother strives to confirm that the pregnancy is real. The first trimester is also a stage of ambivalence toward the pregnancy and its timing. Emotional energy appears to be invested in accepting and acknowledging the pregnancy and this is true both of planned and unplanned, wanted and unwanted pregnancies. The fetus is rarely described at this time as a baby. Consequently most women do not appear to be deeply attached to the fetus. About a third of women in the first trimester exhibit attachment and relate to the fetus as a baby. Most women respond to a spontaneous abortion with a sense of loss. To some, it will be the loss of a pregnancy but to others the loss of a baby.

The response to the loss may be surprise, disappointment, grief, guilt and anger in differing proportions depending on the meaning of the loss at that time. The woman who has had several abortions may be experiencing this loss and also the threat of the loss of ability to ever bear a live child.

Most women express surprise at the abortion. They are unprepared for the pain, loss of blood and if recognizable or noticed, the sight of the fetus. It seems that the concept of a baby is so vague in their minds at this time that such real evidence of a fetus is unexpected. Because of the ambivalence of the first trimester many feel guilt associated with the negative thoughts they may have had about the pregnancy or its timing.

Response to late abortion. By mid-gestation, the pregnancy usually has been accepted as real and the fetus becomes a baby to the majority of women. Most couples have begun to establish a relationship with the baby and loss at this stage is usually perceived as the loss of a baby. There may be more desire to see the fetus, to know the sex and weight and to identify the baby by name even though it may legally be an abortion. Emotional response may be more intense and appear more painful if there is no 'object' to attach the pain to. Seeing the infant or keeping a picture of the baby may assist with grieving and the resolution of the loss for some parents. Others will not choose or require such a method of relating to the fetus.

Parents will exhibit immediate responses similar to those with an early spontaneous abortion. Questions of 'Why me?' and 'What did I do?' will also surface as they search for an explanation for the event. The associated physical discomforts seem to make the stress worse for the mother. The father, who usually becomes the supporter and planner at this stage, may feel overlooked and his grief unacknowledged. The couple may mourn unequally and in different ways, making it difficult for them to support one another.

The reactions of parents who have chosen therapeutic abortion for genetic reasons are similar to these parents. Guilt may be increased in some. Others are fearful of the censure and disapproval of hospital staff. Immediate nursing interventions are aimed at acknowledging the loss, accepting the feelings and wishes of the parents and reinforcing reality. This assists in promoting the long-term goal of resolution of normal grieving, which takes a few months.

The patient experiencing the loss of a desired child derives little consolation from being told that she can have other children or that she has children at home. It is the loss of this child which she feels; she needs sympathy, understanding and someone to listen. She requires factual information about the events, the baby and future childbearing. If the couple wish to see the baby, they are prepared verbally for what they will see. For example, the baby is shown to them wrapped in a blanket. If deformed, it is wrapped to cover all but the face. After preparation, the baby may be unwrapped to reveal the body if they wish. This is an area where the nurse must use judgement and discretion. Some parents like a short time alone with the baby. If the parents do not wish to see the baby, their decision is respected. It is not a positive or necessary step for all parents.

A brief review of the grieving process with the parents is helpful so that they will understand the feelings of grief, irritability and fatigue which may come. The value of rest, sleep and exercise in coping with grieving is stressed. Unequal patterns of grieving and ways of obtaining support are discussed.

Baptism of fetus

If the patient who aborts is Roman Catholic, the fetus must be baptized. In addition, some Protestants may feel strongly that the fetus should be baptized. The nurse may ascertain this by tactfully inquiring what the patient's wishes are. Baptism may be performed by any person, regardless of his religious beliefs. If a clergyman is immediately available, he should be asked to perform this rite. In his absence, the nurse may have to baptize the fetus. Clear water must be poured over the head of the fetus while the nurse pronounces the words 'I baptize you in the name of the Father and of the Son and of the Holy Spirit'. The water must come into direct contact with the fetus. Therefore, if the fetus is still in the amniotic sac, the sac must be broken before the baptism is performed. The procedure is similar for all religions. If the fetus is very small, it may have to be immersed in water to ensure that water reaches the head. Sometimes a conditional baptism is given with the words, 'If thou art living, I baptize thee . . .' This is done in cases in which the fetus may have died before delivery, but the exact state is unknown.

Therapeutic abortion.

The past few years have seen an explosive increase in the number of therapeutic or induced abortions performed throughout the world, in response to the liberalization of abortion laws. It is estimated that legal abortion for social and medical reasons is now available to over half the world's population, making the therapeutic abortion one of the most common medical procedures performed.

Because an abortion concerns the life and death of at least two people, it is governed by religious and legal codes. Complex issues surround the topic of induced abortions and a discussion of all of them is beyond the scope of this work. Only a brief discussion of the law and medical and nursing management is presented here.

The laws governing abortions vary from country to country and from state to state. In all nations legal codes exist defining the conditions under which an abortion may be done. They outline who may do an abortion, where it may be done (in or outside the hospital), and when it may be done in relationship to the length of gestation. The law also defines the social and medical conditions which constitute cause for an abortion. In the United Kingdom, the Abortion Act (1967) gives indications and restrictions for therapeutic abortion (see Table 23.6). All abortions performed outside the limits of the legal condition are illegal. In many countries assisting a patient to procure an abortion outside the law is also punishable by law. For these reasons the nurse should be acquainted with the law pertaining to the area in which she practises.

Table 23.6 Indications for therapeutic abortion under the Abortion Act (1967).

1 The continuance of the pregnancy would involve risk to the pregnant woman greater than if the pregnancy were terminated

2 The continuance of the pregnancy would involve risk of injury to the physical or mental health of the pregnant woman greater than if the pregnancy were terminated

3 The continuance of the pregnancy would involve risk of injury to the physical or mental health of the existing child(ren) of the family of the pregnant woman greater than if the pregnancy were terminated

4 There is a substantial risk that if the child were born it would suffer from such physical or mental abnormalities as to be seriously handicapped

The restrictions

1 That one or more of the above conditions are believed to be present in the opinion of two doctors, who are acting together in good faith and in full knowledge of the facts

2 That this opinion be notified to the DHSS

3 That the operation be carried out in a NHS hospital or an approved establishment

4 That the doctor carrying out the operation notify the DHSS

5 That the consent of the woman be obtained. If the patient is under the age of 16 the consent of the parents is also necessary

Abortions can be divided into two groups on the basis of risk to the woman and her future childbearing potential. Low-risk or early abortions are those done before 12 weeks of gestation. Late or high-risk abortions are done from the thirteenth week of gestation onward. As the upper limits of abortion are defined by the law they will vary from 20–28 weeks of gestation, depending upon the jurisdiction. An abortion may carry greater risk if the patient has a serious accompanying medical condition.

Early abortions.

Most abortions performed before 12–14 weeks of gestation are done by suction dilation and curettage (D and C). If done before 8 weeks of gestation the cervix usually does not require dilation but it is more difficult to ensure complete evacuation of the products of conception. The procedure is most commonly done on an outpatient basis. A general anaesthetic may be given, but many abortions, particularly those not requiring cervical dilation, may be done without anaesthesia or with a local anaesthetic such as a paracervical block. Some surgeons administer intravenous oxytocin (Syntocinon) before suctioning to ensure a strong firm contraction of the uterus; others do not feel this is necessary.

Following these initial steps the doctor determines the size, shape and position of the uterus by bimanual examination. The cervix is then visualized and immobilized by forceps and the cervical canal sounded for direction and the uterus for depth. Should the cervix require further dilation, it will now be done to the size of the cannula required to perform the D and C. The size of the cannula is determined by the length of gestation. A flexible plastic suction tip is then slipped through the cervix. It is attached to a vacuum source which sucks out the uterine contents. The pressure of the pump is carefully regulated to achieve evacuation while avoiding damage to the walls of the uterine cavity. The doctor judges when the uterus is empty by the grating feel of the denuded uterine walls, the contractions of the uterus and the content and character of the aspirated fluid. The aspirated tissue is caught in a gauze trap to facilitate recovery for immediate inspection and for examination by the pathologist. Immediate identification of fetal tissue is important to confirm the diagnosis of an intrauterine pregnancy which has been completely evacuated. As the operator becomes more experienced, the need for postsuction curettage of the uterus declines but may still be performed in cases of doubtful complete emptying of the uterus. It is necessary to confirm the intrauterine pregnancy to avoid an ectopic pregnancy continuing unnoticed. Immediate inspection and, later, pathology reports may confirm a molar pregnancy which, if left undetected, would deprive the patient of important follow-up care.

Following the procedure the patient recovers as determined by the anaesthetic she received. Many patients experience some cramping postabortion, which is normal. The cramps are frequently gone by the time the effects of the anaesthetic, either general or paracervical, are over, but may persist for longer. A mild analgesic may be required. The patient is then observed for a few hours more or allowed to go home with instructions, depending upon her condition.

Late abortions. When the pregnancy is more than 12–14 weeks a D and C becomes more difficult. Other methods must be selected by the gynaecologist. He may decide to induce labour by the use of an intraamniotic injection. The technique and preparation are similar to a paracentesis, but an amniocentesis is done. With strict sterile technique the patient's abdo-

men is prepared and draped. A skin wheal is made with a local anaesthetic agent. Then a needle is inserted through the abdomen, and into the amniotic cavity. One of several agents is injected into the uterine cavity—urea, glucose, hypertonic saline, and prostaglandins have all been used. Hypertonic saline and prostaglandins seem to be the most commonly used. If the drug chosen is saline, some amniotic fluid is withdrawn and replaced by an equal amount of 20% saline solution. The fetus dies, and the uterus is apparently irritated and begins to contract. The contractions may need to be assisted with an oxytocic medication given intravenously.

Later pregnancies of 16–20 weeks' gestation may be terminated by the performance of a hysterotomy. This means that an incision is made into the uterus and the contents removed. It is a miniature caesarean section. The pre- and postoperative care is similar to abdominal surgery. Postoperatively, the fundus must be checked for firmness and position. Lochia is observed for colour, amount and odour, since haemorrhage or infection may occur postoperatively. Vulval care is carried out.

Prostaglandins. Prostaglandins are naturally occurring fatty acids which were first isolated in semen and thought to arise in the prostate gland. Since then they have been found in all tissues. One of their actions is the ability to make smooth muscle contract. This ability is pronounced in relation to uterine muscle. Two forms of prostaglandins, E_2 and $F_{2\alpha}$ are used therapeutically. E_2 is several times stronger than $F_{2\alpha}$. The most common side-effects described are nausea, diarrhoea, pyrexia and local tissue reactions at the site of injection. Synthetic analogues of both F and E groups are now made. They produce fewer side-effects and still stimulate uterine contractions. One of their major uses is to induce abortion and to stimulate labour in full-term pregnancies.

Prostaglandins may be given in an intravenous drip which is carefully regulated by an infusion pump. The dosage is started at very low levels; the responses of the patient, fetus and uterus are carefully monitored. The dose is gradually increased until the uterus is contracting satisfactorily. Labour and delivery or abortion will follow for most patients in 12–24 hours. If the stimulation is not sufficient, additional stimulation with oxytocin may be given. This is associated with an increased risk of rupture of the cervix and uterus, so the response of the contracting uterus must be carefully monitored. The patient's complaints of discomfort or pain should be carefully heeded.

Intraamniotic injections of prostaglandins may also be given. The procedure is similar to the injection of saline. The prostaglandins are absorbed and the uterus begins to contract. Delivery usually occurs about 20 hours after the injection. Occasionally additional stimulation with an oxytocin (Syntocinon) drip is required. The use of oxytocin reduces the time to abortion by 6–8 hours.

Side-effects include nausea, vomiting and diarrhoea. Because the action is directly on smooth muscle, antinausea pills which act on the central nervous system are only partially successful. Diphenoxylate (Lomotil) does reduce the diarrhoea and is usually given. Prostaglandins may produce bronchospasm in asthmatics.

Extra-amniotic injection with prostaglandins is another common method of inducing abortion. A polyethylene tubing or a Foley catheter is passed under aseptic conditions through the cervix, and is directed between the uterine wall and the membranes. The bag of the Foley catheter is inflated to help retain the catheter in the uterus. The tube is attached to further tubing attached to a syringe containing the solution. The rate of infusion is controlled by an infusion pump. Small amounts are injected and the uterine response observed. The dose is gradually increased. Abortion occurs in anywhere from 12–24 hours.

Nursing interventions. The therapeutic abortion is not a totally benign procedure. Physical and mental complications can arise. Thus, the decision to perform an abortion is a weighty one for the gynaecologist as well as for the woman. She and her family will need support and acceptance. Some patients will benefit from counselling beforehand, especially those for whom the abortion involves conflict. All patients require an explanation of the procedure. Unfortunately, many patients are so driven by the overriding need to have the pregnancy terminated that detailed explanation or teaching is not absorbed. Most patients appear less tense, more relaxed and less hostile once they know that the pregnancy is terminated. They are then more receptive to teaching and explanations about follow-up. Anxiety, loneliness and fear are the problems expressed by patients waiting for their contractions to start. Some have told no one, and have no friends or family to support them through the procedure. The nurse can be an important factor in their experience of the event.

Postoperatively the patient is nursed similarly to the patient who has had a spontaneous abortion and a D and C to complete the process. In late abortions the patient requires more intensive nursing care. While the intra-amniotic injections are being given the patient must be observed for reactions to the drug injected. Hypertonic saline may be absorbed into the circulatory system. To avoid this a small amount is injected, the patient's response assessed, and then the remainder injected. If saline is being absorbed intravascularly she may complain of confusion, heat sensations, headache, tinnitus, a dry mouth and tachycardia. In this event the saline is stopped and the injection site altered. When the injection is completed, the patient then awaits the beginning of contractions. To reduce the risk of infection, oxytocin is usually begun within 12 hours if uterine contractions are not adequate. The patient may express some thirst during this period of waiting. All patients who have been given saline absorb a portion of it, thus producing some electrolyte imbalance. Fluid is required and she should be allowed to drink. The patient experiences labour and requires the support and nursing care which is given to a labouring patient. The contractions are distressing, especially since they appear to be for a negative purpose. Analgesia is required by some patients and should not be withheld. Bed rest is usually maintained after active labour begins or after administration of a sedative. In extra-amniotic injection of prostaglandins the catheter may be expelled as the uterus contracts and the cervix dilates. Oxytocin stimulation may be required to maintain labour.

As progress is difficult to assess, the patient frequently aborts in bed alone or with the nurse in attendance. If previously warned she may call the nurse when she feels pressure. However, the patient herself frequently receives little warning.

All products of conception are retained for examination by the doctor and the pathologist. Often the placenta is retained and only the fetus expelled. The nurse should clamp and cut the cord and remove the fetus. Now the patient enters one of the hazardous periods during an abortion, and requires close observation by the nursing staff. Severe haemorrhage may result from the partially separated placenta or the retained products of conception. Haemorrhage may take several forms: the sudden gush, a steady trickle, or small gushes interspersed with periods of minor loss. In all cases the nurse must assess the cumulative loss as well as the immediate one. Individual episodes of bleeding might not alert the nurse to haemorrhage but she must assess the loss over the period of time from the beginning of bleeding to the present. In this way morbidity is reduced, since evacuation of the uterus is begun before the patient has suffered severe loss. If the placenta is not expelled spontaneously within 2 hours and bleeding does not indicate immediate removal, the patient will be scheduled for a D and C for a convenient time within a few hours. Meanwhile, frequent observations of the lochia must be maintained, as the patient's status may change at any time. Following the D and C she is nursed as other patients postabortion who have had a D and C.

Infection may develop, and the patient is monitored for signs of pelvic infection every 4 hours during the hours when she is aborting. Regular daily checks of temperature, general well-being and the character of the lochia follow.

Most abortion patients are discharged within hours of being aborted or within 1 or 2 days. They need clear discharge instructions so that they may take care of themselves in the days that follow. Each patient should be told:

1 To resume normal activities, except for hysterotomy patients who as postoperative patients may do so more gradually.

2 To expect intermittent menstrual-like discharge for the next week or two, but no heavy, bright-red bleeding.

3 To use sanitary pads as long as bleeding occurs. The use of tampons is inadvisable.

4 Some cramping may occur but should not persist or be severe.

5 To report any fever or unusual discomfort.

6 To expect her menstrual period within 4–5 weeks after the procedure. If it does not occur, it may indicate a continuing intra- or extrauterine pregnancy or a new pregnancy. Ovulation occurs as early as 18 days following an abortion and pregnancy is possible immediately. Birth control advice and teaching should be given to the patient as necessary.

7 It is wise to limit coitus while the menstrual-like flow continues to reduce the risk of infection.

8 To contact her doctor or clinic immediately if any of the unusual signs should occur.

9 When she is to return for a follow up visit.

While the therapeutic abortion is now associated with low maternal morbidity and mortality statistics (lower than pregnancy in many countries), it does carry some serious risks which need to be considered. Psychiatric sequelae are rare but do occur. The main concern appears to be an increased incidence of spontaneous abortion and premature labour in those women who have had a prior abortion. The risk is greatest with the older methods of dilation and curettage, and is greater still when damage to the cervix has been documented. It is important to educate women to seek abortion as early as possible so that the need for dilating the cervix will be reduced. Prevention is better than cure, and birth control should be seen as the first line of defence. Nursing has an important role to play by providing knowledge of and access to birth control to those who need it.

Criminal abortion

The criminal abortion is a dangerous procedure. Often women attempt to abort themselves by the use of strong douches or instruments which they insert into the uterus. Frequently, the instrument used punctures the posterior fornix of the vagina, the cervix or perforates the uterus. The bowel may be involved should the instrument be inserted far enough. Conditions are furtive, untrained people frequently officiate, and sterility is not maintained. These patients frequently contract an infection and present a grave situation. The situation is known as a septic abortion. Infection is essentially an endometritis, which may spread to peritonitis or to septicaemia.

Ectopic pregnancy

Implantation of the fertilized ovum anywhere outside the uterine cavity is considered an ectopic pregnancy. Most frequently this occurs in the ampullary portion of the uterine tube, but it may be ovarian, abdominal or cervical. Ectopic pregnancies are estimated as occurring once in every 250 pregnancies. Women with a history of one ectopic pregnancy have an increased risk of having a second one.

An ectopic pregnancy results when the passage of the zygote to the uterine cavity is impeded or slowed. Any blocking of the tube or reduction in tubal peristalsis will achieve this. Former salpingitis, tumours and hormonal imbalances may all play a part.

As implantation occurs, the chorionic villi burrow into the thin tubal wall. Eventually, they burrow into a blood vessel, and bleeding occurs. If the bleeding is sufficient, the fetus dies. This is the fate of most. The abortus may be retained in the tube as a tubal mole or may be extruded through the end of the uterine tube as a tubal abortion. Occasionally, the trophoblast burrows through the wall of the tube and out into the peritoneal cavity. This is known as a ruptured tubal pregnancy and often occurs as the result of a pregnancy in the narrow isthmus of the tube. A secondary abdominal pregnancy may follow if the chorionic villi settle elsewhere in the abdominal cavity and begin to grow. This is rare.

SIGNS AND SYMPTOMS

The accurate diagnosis of an existing ectopic pregnancy or a recently aborted ectopic pregnancy may be difficult. Fortunately, ultrasonography has simplified the task. These women may first be seen in the emergency department or in the clinic with a variety of symptoms.

The woman has a history of the early signs of pregnancy, including amenorrhoea usually of 6–10 weeks' duration. Soon after her first missed period she may have complaints of a localized pain on one side, due probably to the distension of the tube. Following that she may have sharper intermittent pain in the same area. This may be due to strong peristaltic waves of the tube attempting to pass the embryo or abortus along the tube. At some point the patient may experience a sharp, severe pain. This is probably synchronous with separation of the embryo and some haemorrhage. The sharp pain may be followed by generalized abdominal discomfort as blood spills into the abdomen. Referred shoulder pain may occur. Four or 5 days following this episode there is bleeding per vaginam due to falling hormone levels, which occur following the death of the fetus and cause the endometrium to regress and menstruation to occur.

ACUTE RUPTURED TUBAL PREGNANCY

Sometimes the patient reports no early symptoms

but experiences one episode of acute abdominal pain shortly after her missed period. This acute pain is often accompanied by vomiting and fainting. Some vaginal bleeding may be present but appears too minimal to warrant the reaction of the patient. The patient may rapidly go into shock with a drop in blood pressure, rapid weak pulse, pallor, sweating, low temperature and cold extremities. The abdomen is distended with blood and may be tight and tender to the touch. A pelvic examination of the patient may be difficult because of the exquisite tenderness. The patient presents as an emergency situation.

When the diagnosis of a tubal pregnancy is confirmed, a salpingectomy (removal of the uterine tube) with the removal of the fetus is performed. This is usually done within 24–48 hours of diagnosis unless the situation is acute, in which case it is done immediately.

Ectopic pregnancies in other locations will be investigated in a similar fashion. Treatment is usually surgical removal of the fetus. However, abdominal pregnancies have carried to term and been delivered by laparotomies.

Tumours of the trophoblast

Trophoblastic tumours are a group of neoplasms which arise in the chorionic villi of the fertilized ovum during the trophoblast stage. The condition is rare in Europe and North America, occurring about once in every 2500 pregnancies. It is more prevalent in the Far East. The reason for this is not known. The tumours range from benign to malignant (Table 23.7). Not all benign tumours become malignant, nor are all malignant tumours preceded by a benign stage.

Table 23.7 Trophoblastic tumours.

Benign ⇄	Intermediate ⟶	Malignant
Hydatidiform mole	Metastasizing mole Chorioadenoma destruens	Choriocarcinoma (chorionepithelioma malignum)

HYDATIDIFORM MOLE

Hydatidiform mole is an abnormal development of the chorionic villi of the conceptus. It begins to form about the fifth week of embryonic life. The mole appears to occur when the fetal cardiovascular structure fails to develop, but an intact trophoblast and a functioning maternal structure remain. As the fluid accumulates, the chorionic villi distend into small clear vesicles, clinging to thin threads of connective tissue in a grape-like pattern. Few blood vessels are present in the mass. Characteristically, there is no fetus. Rarely, some mole-like degeneration may be present on one part of an otherwise normal placenta.

The condition is the most common of all the tumours. Thus, the majority of women who have a molar pregnancy do not need to fear malignancy. Only 3–7% of benign moles will proceed to malignancy.

The intermediate stages are characterized by an increased ability to invade uterine musculature and to send bloodborne deposits of trophoblast cells throughout the body. However, in some cases, the host, or pregnant woman, seems able to contain the spread of the tumour and it disappears. The intermediate stage is frequently not identified clinically, but is obvious only on pathological examinations of specimens of tissue. This means that all moles must be treated as potentially malignant until demonstrated otherwise.

Signs and symptoms
The patient exhibits the signs and symptoms of early pregnancy. Vomiting may be more frequent. The uterus is often much larger than expected for the weeks of gestation. About the twelfth week, some vaginal bleeding may occur, and this is often the first sign of some abnormality. No fetal movements are reported by the mother, and no fetal parts can be palpated. On palpation the uterus may have an elastic consistency. There is an increased incidence of pre-eclampsia. Urine tests for the quantity of chorionic gonadotrophins excreted show very high titres which persist and do not fall as is usual in a normal pregnancy. These high levels also stimulate the formation of theca lutein cysts in the ovary. The cysts regress following the abortion of the mole.

Treatment and nursing responsibilities
The patient is usually admitted to the hospital and nursed as a threatened abortion until proven otherwise. All perineal pads are carefully inspected for pieces of the mole, as this would be diagnostic. Thyroid function tests may be ordered, for high levels of chorionic gonadotrophins may exert a thyroid-stimulating effect.

An ultrasonic scan of the abdomen is done. The scan plots a 'snowflake' pattern, which is typical of a mole and is considered diagnostic. In preparation for an ultrasound scan the patient is instructed to drink 6–8 large glasses of water in quick succession. The bladder fills within 15–20 minutes, after which the scan is done. The full bladder pushes the bowel away from the uterus and tubes, permitting better penetration of sound waves. At the same time the uterus is pushed up and away from the symphysis pubis, allowing better visualization. The full bladder provides a water path or window through which to look, a landmark in the abdomen, for it is clearly outlined, and an internal reference standard for density comparisons.

In scanning soft tissue, two types of measurements are done; one outlines tissue and the other estimates density of the tissue outlined. The snowflake pattern of a mole reflects an irregular shaped mass with areas of alternating density. Because sound waves can be dispersed or lost, a contact gel is used between the transducer and the skin of the patient. This keeps the sound waves on track as it were. The area is carefully mapped out as the transducer is moved in lines 1 cm apart up and down and across the area. The findings are displayed on a monitor screen. Print-outs can be obtained for permanent record.

Ultrasound is being used increasingly in gynaecology for the localization of foreign objects in the uterus, the diagnosis of tumours of the uterus, ovary and tubes, ectopic pregnancy, and as a device to outline precise areas for irradiation. The patient suffers no discomfort save that of a full bladder during the procedure.

Often the mole is partially aborted spontaneously. Haemorrhage may be acute. Oxytocics will be given to control the bleeding, and a careful and complete evacuation of the uterus will be done. Because of the danger of perforating the uterus in areas weakened by the erosion of the mole, a curette is not used. Instead, the cervix is dilated and suction equipment used to evacuate the uterine contents. Postoperatively the patient is observed for signs of haemorrhage.

Because of the possibility of a malignancy occurring, the patient receives close follow-up care during the next 12–18 months. The first signs of the recurrence of the mole or the development of a malignancy is a rising chorionic gonadotrophin level. Therefore, the urinary levels of gonadotrophin will be monitored at regular intervals. Amenorrhoea, metrorrhagia or persistent cystic ovaries may alert the gynaecologist to look for rising hormone levels. The patient is advised against pregnancy during this period, as early pregnancy also produces high chorionic gonadotrophin levels which could mask the signs. Cytotoxic drugs (such as methotrexate) are given in all intermediate cases, and may be given as prophylaxis to all women who have had a molar pregnancy.

CHORIONEPITHELIOMA MALIGNUM

Chorionepithelioma is a malignant tumour of the embryonic chorion and is marked by invasion of the uterine musculature by malignant trophoblastic cells which have lost their original villous pattern. Destruction of uterine tissues with accompanying necrosis and haemorrhage is the result. The growth quickly metastasizes, and the most frequent site is the lung. The condition is extremely rare but because of its rapid advancement is considered to be one of the most malignant of all pelvic neoplasms. Death usually occurs within 12 months unless the patient receives early treatment. Fifty per cent of all cases of chorionepithelioma are preceded by a mole. The others are preceded by a normal pregnancy or abortion. Because of careful follow-up of patients who

have had a molar pregnancy, the number of deaths from this disease have been reduced.

The chemotherapeutic agent methotrexate is the treatment of choice but may be combined with surgery. The drug is a folic acid antagonist and may be administered orally or parenterally for 5 consecutive days and then withdrawn for a week. The course may need to be repeated several times if chorionic gonadotrophin titres do not regress. Actinomycin D may also be used alone or in combination with methotrexate.

INFECTIONS OF THE REPRODUCTIVE TRACT

Infections in the male

BALANITIS

Balanitis[2] is an infection of the glans penis. Many different organisms may be causative. It is generally associated with poor personal hygiene in the uncircumcised male, but it may be due to venereal diseases. Symptoms include redness, swelling, pain and a purulent discharge. The disease may be chronic and may cause the formation of adhesions and scarring.

Treatment
The infection is treated with the appropriate antibiotic following culture and sensitivity tests. Once the inflammatory process is controlled, circumcision, the excision of the prepuce, is advised.

On return from the operating theatre, the patient has a small petroleum jelly gauze dressing which is changed following each voiding. The patient may be taught to do this and how to care for the dressing at home.

Should bleeding occur, a pressure dressing is applied. The dressing may make voiding impossible or difficult. Usually the dressing can be removed within a short period of time.

Phimosis
Phimosis is a condition in which the preputial orifice is too small to permit retraction over the glans. It may be congenital but is most frequently a sequel to infection or trauma. Circumcision is advised.

Paraphimosis
Paraphimosis occurs when a narrowed prepuce is either forced back over the glans or is gradually retracted over it. It then forms a tight, constricting band around the glans; venous return is impaired, and swelling and pain follow. Usually pain is too severe to permit manipulation, so a general anaesthetic is given, and the foreskin is pulled forward.

---

[2] *Balanos* is the Greek word meaning acorn; in reference to the glans, it is a combining form indicating relationship to the glans penis.

Occasionally the foreskin may have to be incised, and a slit is made up the dorsal surface. This is usually followed by circumcision after the treatment of any infection which may have been present.

PROSTATITIS

Prostatitis is usually an ascending infection of the genitourinary tract, but it may also be the result of the haematogenous spread of the organism. It is often secondary to urethritis or instrumentation of the urethra, as occurs in the use of an indwelling catheter.

In the acute stage, fever and chills are accompanied by haematuria, frequency and dysuria. A urethral discharge may be noted. Rectal examination usually reveals an enlarged, tender, 'hot' prostate. Since infection of the seminal vesicles almost invariably accompanies prostatitis, the seminal vesicles can be palpated as well. Prostatic massage and instrumentation of the urethra are avoided to prevent possible spread of the infection to the epididymis, bladder and kidney. Exceptions are made only to relieve acute urinary retention, which may be a sequel to the enlarged prostate. A small urethral catheter will be used. In severe cases, drainage may be by suprapubic cystostomy rather than by catheterization. Prostatic abscesses may develop and usually drain through the urethra. Occasionally, excision and drainage are required.

The patient is placed on bed rest. Appropriate drug therapy is prescribed; this is usually co-trimoxazole (Bactrim). The patient is in considerable pain. The nurse often sees a tense, anxious and frightened patient who needs reassurance and support. Explanations to clarify that the infection is not venereal may be necessary. Analgesics, warm baths and rectal irrigations help to relieve the pain and bladder spasms. The irritable bladder may require special attention, and antispasmodics and bladder sedatives are frequently ordered.

In cases in which treatment is early, excellent results usually follow. However, the acute picture may become chronic. The symptoms are mild and include a low-grade fever and some bacteria and pus in the urine. Fertility and potency are not affected unless complications ensue. The chronic infection may stubbornly resist treatment. Prostatic massage every 7–14 days is done by the doctor and helps by draining the bacteria away. Sexual intercourse or masturbation accomplishes the same purpose. Daily baths also help resolve the infection.

EPIDIDYMITIS

Epididymitis may be caused by any pyogenic organism. It frequently follows prostatitis and may be a complication of prostatectomy. Fever, malaise and chills accompany swelling and pain in the scrotum. The patient may be so uncomfortable that he may walk in a waddling fashion. Symptoms of cystitis may be present, and a hydrocele often develops. The swelling and irritation cause congestion of the testes which impedes the circulation of blood. Sterility follows from necrosis of the tubular epithelium and fibrosis which occludes the ducts.

The patient is placed on bed rest. The scrotum is elevated on towel rolls. Local applications of heat or cold may be ordered. Warm baths often relieve symptoms of congestion and pain. After the patient is ambulant, a roomy scrotal support is worn.

Antibiotics are given but are not usually curative. If the disease is diagnosed early, a local anaesthetic agent is injected into the spermatic cord above the testes. Symptoms are usually absent in a day or two following this treatment. Chronic epididymitis may follow an acute episode. If the involvement is bilateral, sterility follows.

ORCHITIS

Inflammation of the testes may follow any infectious disease or may be acquired as an ascending infection from the genital tract. Most commonly it follows mumps parotitis. The mumps virus is excreted in the urine; therefore, the spread to the testes in this case appears to be by descent. The onset is sudden, manifested by pain and swelling of the scrotum followed by fever and prostration. Urinary symptoms are usually not present. A hydrocele may develop, and the involvement may be unilateral or bilateral. Sterility probably follows death of the spermatogenic cells from ischaemia. Bed rest, scrotal support and local applications of heat or cold are ordered. A padded athletic support may be worn continuously.

Antibiotics are used in some situations but are not of value against the mumps virus. Local infiltration of the spermatic cord with a local anaesthetic may relieve the symptoms. The prevention of mumps in the postpubertal male has some value. If a man who has not been immunized as a child against mumps or who has not previously had mumps has been in contact with the virus, gamma globulin is usually administered.

Infections in the female

BARTHOLINITIS

Bartholinitis is an infection of the greater vestibular gland and may or may not be gonorrhoeal in origin. The infection is an ascending one, progressing up the ducts to the gland. Symptoms are usually those of an acute infection—pain, swelling, inflammation and a purulent discharge. Cellulitis of the surrounding tissues aggravates the situation, but the infection may localize and become an abscess. This is usually excised and drained. Sometimes the infection subsides, leaving the duct scarred and occluded.

This may be followed by a cyst filled with the secretions of the gland which now cannot escape. The cyst is usually a painless swelling in the lower third of the labium minus. Treatment is to excise the cyst and gland. Alternatively, a marsupialization (conversion of the duct into a pouch) of the cystic duct may be done. This leaves the functioning gland in place.

Hot baths, saline soaks and/or the use of a bidet may be ordered following surgery. The patient should be advised on frequency of bathing and how to perform adequate vulval toilet before she is discharged.

VAGINITIS

Physiological leucorrhoea
Physiological leucorrhoea is a normal whitish discharge which helps to keep the vagina moist. It is composed of endocervical secretions, leucocytes, desquamated epithelial cells and other normal flora of the vaginal tract. The pH is normally 4–5 but varies during the life-cycle of the woman. At birth, it may be as low as 5 under the hormonal stimulus of the mother. As a child it is 6–7. At menarche the pH becomes acidic again, and assumes the adult pH of 4–5. Postmenopausally, oestrogen is withdrawn, and the pH rises to 6–7 again. The quantity of the discharge also varies among women, during stages of the menstrual cycle and during pregnancy. An increase is usually noticed at ovulation, during sexual stimulation and during pregnancy. The most characteristic symptom of a vaginitis is a change in the normal vaginal discharge.

Trichomoniasis
The most common cause of vaginitis is a flagellated protozoon, known as a trichomonad. Trichomonads may be found in the large bowel and occasionally in the bladder and vestibular glands. They can be transmitted to a man at intercourse and from him can be communicated to other women or serve as a source of reinfection. In men, trichomonads may be harboured in the urethra, bladder or prostate.

The woman presents with symptoms of a heavy, greenish-yellow, frothy discharge which has a slight odour. This heavy discharge may be irritating to the vulva, causing pruritis and excoriation. The vaginal mucosa is reddened and is slightly oedematous. The patient may complain of dyspareunia and, if the bladder is involved, of dysuria and frequency. As the condition becomes chronic, the woman has fewer symptoms. Diagnosis is confirmed when trichomonads are seen microscopically in a vaginal smear.

Men frequently have few symptoms. There may be some urethral itching and a slight discharge. Invasion of the bladder may produce frequency and burning on micturition. Wet smears are made of the urethral discharge, and the protozoa seen microscopically confirm the diagnosis.

Treatment is usually the oral administration of metronidazole (Flagyl) 250 mg three times a day for 10 days. Repeat smears will then be done, and a repeat course of therapy may be necessary. During the treatment, a condom should be worn until both partners are considered cured. Woman may be given vaginal suppositories instead of oral therapy. A suppository is inserted morning and night daily for 4–8 weeks. This is continued through the menstrual period, for the menstrual flow is alkaline and provides an excellent medium for the protozoa. Insertion is like that of a vaginal tampon. The patient is instructed to remain flat for about 10 minutes following insertion.

Monilial vaginitis
Monilial vaginitis occurs when the vagina is invaded by the fungus *Candida albicans*. The vaginal pH is usually 5–7. Pregnant women and diabetics are predisposed because of glycosuria and the increased glycogen present in the vagina during pregnancy. Contamination may be from the rectum. A thick, white, curdy vaginal discharge is present which frequently causes pruritus and irritation of the vulva. The vaginal walls are reddened and covered with typical white patches. When the patches are swabbed off, bleeding may occur. Diagnosis is confirmed microscopically from a vaginal smear.

The patient is instructed in careful perineal care and hand washing to avoid reinfection and spread of the fungus to others, especially children. Nystatin vaginally or in the form of pessaries achieves good results. It may be given to pregnant women.

Atrophic vaginitis (senile)
Because of hormonal changes following the menopause, the pH rises and the glycogen stores are reduced in the vagina. The vagina loses its rugae and becomes smooth and shiny. It is now more susceptible to invasion by organisms. A sticky, mucoid discharge may appear. The patient complains of a burning in the vagina, dyspareunia and pruritus of the vagina. Occasionally, the discharge is blood flecked, as areas of the vagina ulcerate and adhesions develop and tear. Severe infection is controlled by the use of systemic antibiotics or sulpha drugs. Oestrogens are administered orally or vaginally. When the vaginitis is relieved, medication is stopped, and the patient may be advised to have cleansing vinegar douches periodically.

TOXIC SHOCK SYNDROME

Toxic shock syndrome is a rare systemic disease occurring as the result of circulating toxins produced by *Staphylococcus aureus* (*S. aureus*) bacteria. The organisms produce two toxins; enterotoxin F, which affects intestinal mucosa causing gastroenteritis, and exotoxin C, which is pyrogenic. Signs and symptoms occur following the introduction of toxins into the bloodstream. The disease varies from a subclinical form to a severe septicaemia.

Signs and symptoms commonly include a high fever, rash, vomiting, diarrhoea, headache, sore throat and muscle pain. Hypotension progressing to shock occurs within 48 hours in severe cases. Laboratory results indicate renal, hepatic and haematological involvement. Diagnosis is confirmed by swabs positive for *S. aureus* taken from the patient's nose, throat, vaginal discharge and tampon, where applicable.

The disease is associated with intravaginal tampon use but is not caused by them. A significant number of women in the severe state are menstruating and using tampons. It is related to the fact that women have *Staphylococcus aureus* present in the vagina. Tampons act as a dam to vaginal flow providing ideal conditions for bacterial growth. Some tampons were found to carry the organisms and have now been withdrawn from the market. The new synthetic material tampons aggravate the situation by their greater drying effect. They may create microulcerations in the vaginal mucosa, allowing microorganisms to escape into the bloodstream.

Treatment is supportive, aimed at relieving the symptoms and curative by eradicating the source of toxin production. If associated with tampon use, the tampons are removed and the vagina cleansed with a disinfecting solution and daily saline douches. The patient receives systemic medication to which the organisms are sensitive. These measures prevent further development of the bacteria but are ineffective against the already-circulating toxins.

Patient teaching is aimed at prevention of a recurrence. The patient with toxic shock syndrome associated with tampon use is advised to discontinue the use of tampons entirely or until she has three negative vaginal cultures for *S. aureus*, each culture a month apart. The patient then follows general instructions for the use of tampons.

1 Use only one tampon at a time.
2 Use the tampon of the absorbency that will control the flow; that is, never use one of super absorbency when a regular one would do. This reduces the chance of vaginal drying with subsequent trauma and ulceration.
3 Change the tampon frequently (every 4–6 hours).
4 Do not forget a tampon; always check by finger insertion in the vagina if you think you may have forgotten one.
5 If you suspect an infection, immediately remove the tampon and consult your doctor.

CERVICITIS

The cervix is the main barrier against ascending infections of the genital tract. As such it is exposed to many insults. The majority of these are small lacerations which occur during childbirth or injuries associated with surgery, instrumentation or venereal disease. Bacteria invade these slits in the cervix. When the cervical epithelium is damaged, the infection easily spreads to the endocervix. Congestion and oedema follow. An increase in cervical mucus results in an elevation in vaginal pH. The cells of the endocervix begin growing out around the external os. This outgrowth of cells produces a red, granular raised lesion. As the cervix is exposed to further trauma, the eroded areas become infected again and again. Chronic cervicitis results.

The symptoms vary. Usually a heavy vaginal discharge exists. The patient may notice deep dyspareunia or some bloodstained discharge following intercourse or douching.

The diagnosis depends on the characteristic appearance of the lesion. Cytological studies are usually done to distinguish cervicitis from early carcinoma. When carcinoma is ruled out, the condition is generally treated by cautery of the endocervix. After cautery the old tissue sloughs away, followed by the regeneration of the new from the outside edges of the lesion. The patient should expect a brownish discharge for 1–2 weeks as the old tissue sloughs away.

Often patients with cervicitis need to be taught proper perineal care. The use of strong, irritating douches should be discouraged, and perineal hygiene is stressed.

PELVIC INFLAMMATORY DISEASE (PID)

Pelvic inflammatory disease has come to mean all ascending pelvic infections once they are beyond the cervix. Many organisms may be responsible for the symptoms. However, among the most frequent are the gonococcus and *Staphylococcus aureus*. On occasion, tuberculosis and anaerobic bacteria can be causative. Symptoms may follow labour and delivery, a criminally induced abortion, surgical procedures, or a contact with gonorrhoea or cervicitis. The condition may be acute or chronic.

Signs and symptoms
The typical picture is one of a systemic infection with fever, chills, malaise, anorexia, nausea and vomiting. This is usually accompanied by lower abdominal pain which is either unilateral or bilateral. In more chronic cases, this pain is increased before and during menstruation. Pain is experienced on movement of the cervix. Leucorrhoea is present. With gonorrhoeal or staphylococcal infections the discharge is usually heavy and purulent; streptococcal infections cause a thinner, more mucoid discharge.

Spread of the infection occurs by two typical routes, which are demonstrated in Fig. 23.19. Symptoms depend on which route the infection follows. In Route I the bacteria spread along the surface of the

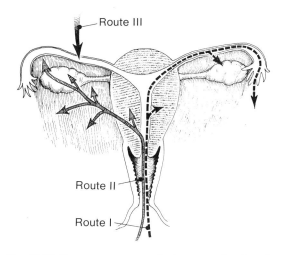

Fig. 23.19 Common routes of the spread of pelvic inflammatory disease. Route I: commonly gonococcus and staphylococcus. Route II: frequently streptococcus. Route III: tuberculosis, usually a descending infection from another source.

endometrium to the tubes and into the peritoneum. The consequences of this route may be adhesions or cysts of the tube, with consequent infertility. In more advanced cases abscesses develop about the ovary or in the cul-de-sac. Infection following Route II is spread mainly through the lymphatics and produces a pelvic cellulitis in contrast to the more localized endometritis or salpingitis (infection of the uterine tube) of Route I. Thrombophlebitis may follow this cellulitis. Advanced and virulent infections admitted by either route may become systemic and may show all the signs of septicaemia.

Treatment and nursing care
The patient with an acute episode is usually admitted to the hospital. She may or may not be isolated, depending on the cause of her infection. The patient is placed on bed rest in semi-Fowler's position to promote drainage of pus into the vagina and the cul-de-sac. Vulval toilet should be done as needed to keep the patient clean and comfortable. Douching is usually avoided, since it may only advance the infection further. Heat to the lower back and abdomen may be soothing. Analgesics and sedation may be ordered. The patient will receive antibiotics following culture and sensitivity studies. In some cases blood cultures may be obtained. Surgical treatment is deferred, if possible, until the infection is controlled. A culdocentesis or colpotomy may be done to drain a pelvic abscess. Tubo-ovarian abscesses may require an abdominal approach. In cases of prolonged, debilitating infections which are resistant to conservative treatment, salpingectomy or hysterectomy may be done.

VENEREAL DISEASE

The most common venereal diseases are non-specific urethritis, gonorrhoea and syphilis.

Gonorrhoea

The specific organism causing gonorrhoea is *Neisseria gonorrhoeae*, and it is transmitted almost exclusively by sexual intercourse. The organism dies quickly when not harboured in the human body.

SIGNS AND SYMPTOMS

Symptoms appear 2–10 days after the initial contact. In the male urethritis occurs, heralded by a purulent urethral discharge. Some itching and burning about the meatus are also present. The urethral meatus is red and oedematous. The infection may remain localized and in about 10% of men is asymptomatic. An ascending infection involving the prostate, seminal vesicles, bladder and epididymus may result. If adhesions develop, they may damage the urethra and duct system with consequent urethral stricture and infertility.

Diagnosis is confirmed when the gonococcus is seen microscopically in smears or cultures taken from the site of infection. If urethral discharge is slight, the first urethral washings may be used. These are obtained by collecting the first portion of a voided urine specimen. The penis is not swabbed off before collecting the specimen.

In the adult female the vagina with its layers of squamous epithelium is resistant to the gonococcus. Therefore, the vulnerable areas are the vestibular glands, the urethra and the endocervix. The glands become red, swollen and sore. A purulent discharge may drain from the urethra and the ducts of the glands. Leucorrhoea is present in cases in which cervicitis accompanies the picture. Dysuria and frequency often occur. In about 50% of women the symptoms may be mild and vague. The infection may ascend above the cervix and may form the characteristic picture described in pelvic inflammatory disease.

Diagnosis is made on the basis of organisms seen in smears or cultures. To obtain these specimens the patient is instructed not to void or douche for approximately 2 hours before the cultures are taken. The vulva are not cleansed first. With the patient in a lithotomy position, smears are taken from the urethra, cervix and the ducts of the vestibular glands.

TREATMENT

Treatment with antibiotics, notably penicillin, is highly successful and has succeeded in reducing the incidence of complications.

In 1976 a drug-resistant strain of *Neisseria gonorr-*

hoeae was identified; this strain of the organism produces an enzyme (penicillinase) that inactivates penicillin. Patients infected with this resistant strain are treated with spectinomycin or a cephalosporin. Treatment is successful in cases in which repeated cultures are judged to be negative.

Non-specific urethritis

Non-specific urethritis is an infection of the male urethra. The man complains of mild gonorrhoea-like symptoms which may become severe. It is important to rule out gonorrhoea as a cause. The onset of the symptoms is frequently related to coitus, often during menstruation when vaginal bacteria are increased, but in other cases no obvious link exists.

The infection may be due to one of several agents, but in 40% of cases is the result of a chlamydial infection. Chlamydia are a group of organisms which multiply like bacteria but do so only in the host cell, like viruses. Several strains exist: L_1–L_3 cause lymphogranuloma venereum; A, B and C cause trachoma; D–K may cause urethritis, cervicitis, salpingitis, and pneumonitis and conjunctivitis in the newborn.

The infection frequently coexists with gonorrhoea but may persist as a postgonococcal urethritis following successful treatment of the gonorrhoea. This can be anxiety producing for the patient. Reassurance and teaching about the complaints are helpful in relieving anxiety.

Cultures for *Chlamydia trachomatis* are made from swabs of the anterior urethra and from first urethral washings. Tetracycline is the treatment of choice. Those unable to take tetracycline, including pregnant women and children, are treated with erythromycin. Sexual intercourse is contraindicated during the acute stage as it prolongs the symptoms. Repeat cultures are made to confirm the effects of treatment.

The infection may progress to a chronic state or to epididymitis, prostatitis and rarely Reiter's disease. In women the organism contributes to non-specific cervicitis, vaginitis and pelvic inflammatory disease. The newborn may acquire the infection during delivery through the vagina. For these reasons many doctors treat the female partners of infected men. It is hoped this will prevent later development of chlamydial related pelvic disease in these women and reduce the incidence of newborn eye and chest infections. Unlike syphilis and gonorrhoea, reporting and identification of contacts is not mandatory.

Syphilis

Syphilis is a more serious disease and, fortunately, is less common than gonorrhoea. The causative organism is the spirochaete *Treponema pallidum*.

SIGNS AND SYMPTOMS

Incubation varies between 10 and 90 days. In most cases the disease is spread by sexual intercourse. As with the gonococcus, the spirochaete does not survive outside the host. In the untreated condition, three stages are distinguished. The stages may overlap or be widely separated. The primary lesion is a small, painless chancre or ulcer. It is deep and has indurated edges. Usually, this chancre heals spontaneously, giving the false impression that the disease is cured. This primary lesion appears most commonly on the penis of the male. In the female, it may appear on the labia, vagina or cervix. The secondary stage is usually characterized by a rash appearing over the body. This rash may be accompanied by condylomata lata on the female vulva. This is a cauliflower-appearing collection of flat, grey vulvar warts. As are all lesions of syphilis, these are teeming with spirochaetes and are highly infectious. The rash is usually accompanied by malaise and fever. In a short period the rash regresses and the patient enters the latent stages. Latency refers to the absence of symptoms in the infected individual. Pregnant women can still infect their fetus in utero, thus demonstrating the infectiousness of the blood. However, progress of the disease in the individual seems arrested and only rarely can others be infected in this stage. Three outcomes are now possible: (1) the patient proceeds immediately or after a delay of 10–30 years to the third stage; (2) the disease remains latent for the rest of the person's life; or (3) a spontaneous cure occurs. In the tertiary stage the bones, heart, and central nervous system, including the brain, can be affected. Personality disorders arise and the typical ataxic gait of the tertiary syphilitic appears. A large, ulcerating necrotic lesion known as a gumma now occurs. Rarely is it seen in the genital tract, but it may occur on the vulva or in the testes. At this stage the disease may be arrested but not reversed.

Diagnosis is made by a careful history, clinical findings, and cultures or biopsies from the lesions. Blood serology is also assessed. Since blood serology is not positive for about 4 weeks after the onset of the disease, the early diagnosis is made from scrapings of the lesions. They can be seen on dark-field examination. These scrapings are made before antibiotic therapy is initiated so that the diagnosis can be confirmed.

TREATMENT

Treatment is by antibiotic, and penicillin is the drug of choice. A series of injections is necessary; oral medication is not effective. The Jarisch–Herxheimer reaction is a local and systemic reaction which may occur after beginning antisyphilitic therapy. Fever, sweating and headache appear 2–12 hours after treatment. The reaction should be differentiated from a penicillin reaction.

Most cases of venereal disease are treated on an outpatient basis, and the patient must be taught how to protect himself and others. First, the nature and transmission of the disease should be understood. No immunity develops and reinfection can occur easily. Strict personal and perineal hygiene should be observed. Hand washing following any handling of the genitalia is imperative, as the gonococcus can be readily carried to the eye, which quickly becomes infected. Blindness may ensue if treatment is not received. Women who are handling small children need to be especially careful. The vagina of a pre-pubertal girl is sensitive to the gonococcus because it lacks the protective layers of squamous epithelium. A form of vulvovaginitis may occur as a result of con-tamination from a family member. Sexual inter-course is to be avoided until the doctor notifies the patient he or she is cured. The nurse must practise all she teaches by following strict medical asepsis while caring for patients who are in the infectious stages of the disease. All equipment must be sterilized follow-ing use, and dressings or swabs are disposed of in a safe way. The disease may be transmitted by direct contamination with living spirochaetes of a lacer-ation. For this reason, the nurse who has a break in her skin must be very careful when dealing with the lesions of syphilis. Gloves may be indicated. Once therapy has been initiated, the patient is usually non-infectious within 48 hours.

The disease may be very distressing to the patient. The patient may experience guilt feelings, and mari-tal difficulties may arise when one partner infects the other. The disease carries a social stigma. For these reasons, confidentiality must be maintained by the nurse at all times; the issue is protected by law and the disease is reportable. Contacts must be identified and discreetly followed by the health advisor. The nurse, by explaining the nature of the disease, usually obtains the patient's cooperation in identi-fying contacts. In addition, the nurse should include venereal disease in any lectures she prepares on gen-eral health education in the schools so that the popu-lation may become more aware of the signs and symptoms as well as the modes of transmission of these diseases.

DISPLACEMENTS AND RELAXATIONS OF THE FEMALE GENITAL ORGANS

Retroversion and retroflexion of the uterus

The normal position of the uterus is one of some anteversion and anteflexion (Fig. 23.20). It is not a fixed organ. The filling of the bladder or bowel may cause a change in uterine position. On occasion, the uterus assumes a retroverted or retroflexed position. When retroverted, the fundus points toward the sacrum and the cervix toward the anterior vaginal wall. Retroflexion refers to the position of the fundus of the uterus in relation to the cervix. In retroflexion the fundus bends back over the cervix (Fig. 23.21).

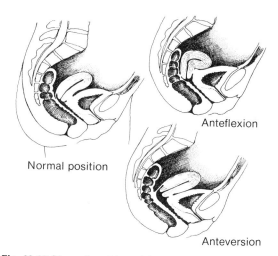

Fig. 23.20 Normal position of the uterus, anteflexion, and anteversion.

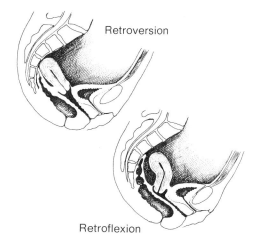

Fig. 23.21 Retroversion and retroflexion of the uterus.

Degrees of retroversion and retroflexion are possible so that the case may be mild or extreme.

The aetiology appears to lie in a weakness of the supporting structures which may be either congeni-tal or acquired. The acquired weakness is frequently due to injuries during the maternity cycle. Adhe-sions and tumours may pull or push the uterus into this position.

The patient may complain of backache, infertility, dyspareunia or dysmenorrhoea, but she is fre-quently symptomless unless the situation is extreme. Backache and dysmenorrhoea are probably associ-ated with pelvic congestion. Infertility may arise because the cervix does not reach the seminal pool. Frequently, the ovaries prolapse into the cul-de-sac and become congested and enlarged. Because of this, intercourse may be painful.

TREATMENT

Usually the uterus is manually replaced, and a vaginal pessary is inserted to hold the uterus in place. The pessary functions by holding the cervix in a posterior position. This in turn rotates the uterus forward. When the pessary is properly in position, the patient is unaware of its presence and no difficulty is experienced on voiding or during intercourse. The patient will return in about 4–6 weeks to have the pessary checked and removed for cleaning. The gynaecologist may then give the patient a 6-week trial period without the pessary to see if she remains free of symptoms. If not, a further trial with the pessary may be given.

All pessaries are irritating, especially those which are rubber and have some degree of movement. An offensive-smelling leukorrhoea usually develops, and chronic ulceration may occur.

In other cases the uterus will be surgically suspended by shortening the round ligaments. This is done when the pessary does not correct the situation.

Prolapse, cystocele and rectocele

Uterine prolapse refers to the downward displacement of the entire organ. Prolapse (Fig. 23.22) may occur in varying degrees. First-degree prolapse describes the condition existing when the uterus descends within the vagina. Second-degree prolapse occurs when the cervix protrudes through the introitus. Procidentia, or third-degree prolapse, refers to the entire uterus protruding through the introitus with total inversion of the vagina.

Cystocele, urethrocele, rectocele and enterocele refer to herniations or relaxations of the bladder, urethra, rectum and small bowel into the vagina (Fig. 23.23). They may occur singly or in combinations with some degree of uterine prolapse.

The single most important aetiological factor in the development of these conditions is thought to be injury at childbirth. The pelvic floor and supporting structures may be stretched and torn during the process of delivery and are thereby weakened. Further relaxation results after menopause as the tissues atrophy following oestrogen withdrawal. Large intra-abdominal tumours may also place an added strain on already weakened tissue. In some rare cases, the structures seem to be congenitally weak.

The patient with a prolapse often complains of a feeling of 'something coming down'. She may have a dragging or a heavy feeling in the pelvis, accompanied by backache and bladder symptoms of either retaining or losing urine. She may have recurrent cystitis. When the cervix protrudes through the introitus, it may become ulcerated from constant friction. This may produce pain and bleeding. The patient with a cystocele frequently has symptoms of stress incontinence.

Diagnosis is usually confirmed by bimanual and rectal examinations. The patient will be asked to bear down, cough or strain while the doctor estimates the degree of prolapse or herniation.

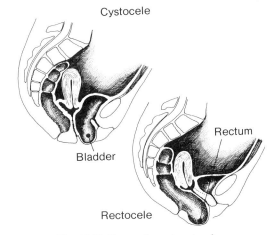

Fig. 23.23 Cystocele and rectocele.

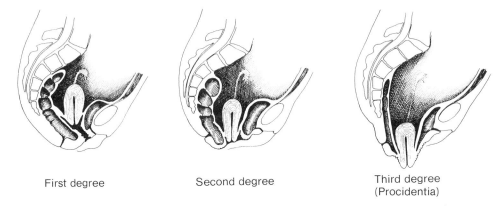

First degree   Second degree   Third degree (Procidentia)

Fig. 23.22 Uterine prolapse, showing first, second- and third-degree (procidentia) prolapse.

The best treatment is prevention. Better care during the maternity cycle has helped to reduce the incidence of these complications. Exercises should be taught by the physiotherapist and encouraged by the nurse to all patients in the postpartum period and the same exercises may be taught to help relieve mild prolapse. These consist of alternately tightening and relaxing the gluteal and perineal floor muscles. Practising starting and stopping the stream of urine also helps the patient regain good perineal muscle tone. She should continue to practise these exercises several times a day for several weeks.

In situations in which surgery is contraindicated, the use of pessaries may be employed. A variety are available for different degrees of prolapse.

Surgical intervention is frequently necessary to correct the situation. An anterior and posterior colporrhaphy and perineorrhaphy repair a cystocele and rectocele, respectively.

In some women where prolapse of the uterus is present and future childbearing is not an issue, a Manchester repair may be done. This combines the amputation of an elongated cervix and shortening of the cardinal ligaments with an anterior and posterior repair. Although childbearing is not precluded by an anterior and posterior repair, delivery by caesarean section is usually recommended in order to retain this repair. Vaginal hysterectomy with an anterior and posterior repair is usually performed for more severe uterine prolapse. The uterine tubes and the uterus with all or part of the cervix will be removed. The ligaments and blood vessels are ligated, and a cuff is made in the upper portion of the vagina.

The nursing care of these patients is similar to that given to any patient undergoing surgery. The patient receives a perineal shave preparation. Orders may be given outlining special perineal or vaginal preparations. The nurse assists the patient in understanding the limitations, if any, surgery will impose on sexual and reproductive capacity, since misunderstandings frequently occur.

During surgery the patient may receive an intravenous vasoconstrictor to reduce the danger of haemorrhage. Blood loss during vaginal surgery tends to be heavy and is heavier still in premenopausal women.

The patient's legs are carefully lifted together to be placed into and removed from the stirrups. No one should lean or apply pressure on the anaesthetized leg to avoid thrombus formation. These measures reduce postoperative discomfort, avoid strain on the repaired perineal muscles and help reduce the incidence of postoperative emboli. These same measures should be used whenever a patient's legs are placed in stirrups.

Following vaginal surgery, the nurse observes the patient for signs and symptoms of haemorrhage, urinary tract infection, thromboemboli and infec-tions at the surgical site. Haemorrhage may be frank, oozing or in the form of a large haematoma. The oozing of blood may not be readily noticed by the patient or the staff; therefore, the nurse must be careful to observe the estimated blood loss over a period of time, not just each time she checks the patient. A haematoma is a form of concealed haemorrhage; the blood vessels bleed into the tissue of the vagina or perineum. The patient complains of discomfort or pain over the site. The tissue bulges and may be so taut as to glisten. The nurse should notify the doctor immediately and be prepared to assist with treatment and the possible return of the patient to the operating theatre. Blood transfusions may be required. The clot may be evacuated, the bleeding vessels ligated or the site firmly packed. An antibiotic may be ordered to lessen the chance of infection.

Postoperatively the patient returns with a suprapubic drain. This is a small polyethylene tube which has been threaded through a needle into the bladder. The abdomen is surgically prepared, the bladder filled with sterile water, and the needle inserted. The tube is taped or caught with a stitch to the skin to avoid accidental removal and attached to a sterile drainage system. It drains freely for 3–4 days and the patient voids as she can. Seventy per cent of women void spontaneously before the tube is clamped, starting on the fourth day. If the tube leaks, tape may be placed around the base. The tube can be used to obtain residuals, but occasionally a catheter may have to be used. Suprapubic drainage has reduced the incidence of postoperative urinary tract infections by reducing the need for catheterizations. They also reduce the emotional tension surrounding first voiding.

In some cases the patient may have catheter drainage. She is catheterized preoperatively, and the catheter remains in place for 7–9 days until the oedema has been resolved. The catheter is clamped and released for periods of time, finally removed, and then the patient attempts voiding. She is usually catheterized twice daily for residual urine during the first 24–36 hours without the catheter. If the amount of urine remaining in the bladder is above 75–100 ml, a Foley catheter may be reinserted or the cystostomy tube opened.

Voiding in sufficient quantities should occur at least every 6 hours. To induce the patient who is unable to void to do so requires all the nurse's skill in an attempt to avoid catheterization. Patients are usually encouraged to move about early and getting up to void helps. If the use of a bidet or vulval toilet is allowed, it usually helps if these are encouraged immediately before the patient attempts to void. When catheterization is necessary, the strictest aseptic technique should be followed.

Perineal care is important to the prevention of infection. Depending on the extent of the surgery, sterile technique may be required. It should be as frequent as necessary to keep the perineal area clean and dry. General principles of working from front to back are followed. In addition, sterile pads are applied. Vulval toilet may be ordered with sterile or plain water or some solutions. The nurse or patient runs the solution from a bag and tubing over the perineum into a basin. If the patient is well enough, she is taught how to do these procedures.

Straining at stool is avoided by a low residue diet and the avoidance of constipation.

On discharge the patient may receive further instructions; some doctors definitely restrict heavy lifting and prolonged standing, walking and sitting. Intercourse is contraindicated for approximately 6 weeks.

Stress incontinence

Stress incontinence is the involuntary loss of small amounts of urine when a woman coughs, sneezes or otherwise suddenly increases the intra-abdominal pressure and, therefore, the intravesical pressure. It should be distinguished from urge incontinence and frequency.

Continence is thought to be maintained at the junction of the urethra and bladder by continuous spiral muscles from the base of the bladder to the upper urethra. Assistance is also received from the muscles surrounding the urethra, as well as a tight supporting perineal floor. In the continent woman these relationships can be demonstrated radiologically by observing that the angle between the urethra and posterior wall of the bladder is approximately 90° (Fig. 23.24). Normally, this angle is only obliterated at micturition (Fig. 23.25) when an increased intra-abdominal pressure combines with a relaxed urethrovesical muscle and perineal floor to lower the base of the bladder. However, in stress incontinence, the slight effort of straining, coughing or sneezing is sufficient to reduce this angle, and an involuntary loss of urine occurs. This explanation is thought to describe about 90% of cases of stress

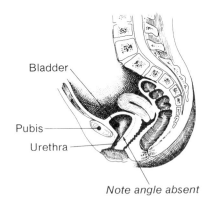

Note angle absent

Fig. 23.25 The bladder during micturition.

incontinence. A woman may have a cystocele (Fig. 23.24) and still be continent if the relationships demonstrated by the angle are maintained. However, many women with a cystocele also have accompanying stress incontinence.

Occasionally, stress incontinence follows a cystocele repair. This is probably due to elevation of the bladder to a position which obliterates the angle. For this reason many surgeons check the angle following repair to be sure it will be adequate.

The symptoms may become distressing to the woman. Frequent small dribbles of urine cause wetness, irritation and an offensive odour. The woman may have to wear a perineal pad or plastic pants continuously. Gradually she may become shy of social contacts and confine herself to home.

Diagnosis is made following a physical examination and a urodynamic evaluation. A pelvic and modified neurological examination is done to diagnose any underlying pelvic or neurological disease. The urodynamic evaluation, which includes a series of tests, helps to distinguish true stress incontinence from other conditions. The series of tests usually requires a day at the hospital and is done on an out-

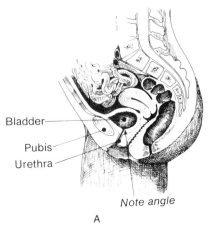

Note angle

A

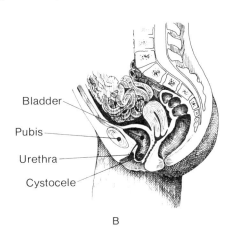

B

Fig. 23.24 *A*, The bladder at ease—no stress incontinence. *B*, Cystocele without stress incontinence.

patient basis. In preparation the patient is instructed not to void or take self-medication for 6–8 hours before going to the urodynamic laboratory. This provides a full bladder for testing and avoids drug effects on nerve conduction.

Initially uroflowmeter readings are done. The patient is instructed to void into a funnel connected to a flowmeter. This meter is an electronic device which calculates the rate at which urine flows, the time taken to void and the volume voided. The results are printed on a graph (Fig. 23.26). An abnormally high rate of flow is associated with stress incontinence. Immediately following this the patient is catheterized for residual urine. This test may be followed by a cystometrogram. During this latter procedure a catheter is passed, attached to a transducer and the bladder is filled with fluid, usually water. The patient is asked to tell the doctor when she feels a sense of fullness and when her bladder actually feels full. She is told to void and then asked to stop voiding. The transducer meanwhile records on a graph the changes in bladder pressure associ-

ated with these events. The doctor can assess how the patient perceives and responds to these sensations and requests. Normally bladder pressure increases when voiding as the bladder is contracting and drops when voiding ceases and the bladder relaxes. This may be combined with a urethral pressure profile. Urethral pressure is recorded as the catheter is slowly withdrawn at a constant rate through the urethra.

More elaborate tests may be done such as electromyograms to measure response and strength of bladder muscle, videorecordings and measurements of intra-abdominal pressure by rectal electrodes. They are used less often in stress incontinence. These tests may be followed by cystourethroscopy in which the urologist directly visualizes the interior of the bladder and urethra. In this procedure a dye outlines the urethra and bladder, demonstrating the state of the angle at rest, during straining and if possible, on micturition.

These procedures, with the exception of the uroflowmeter, require sterile equipment, appro-

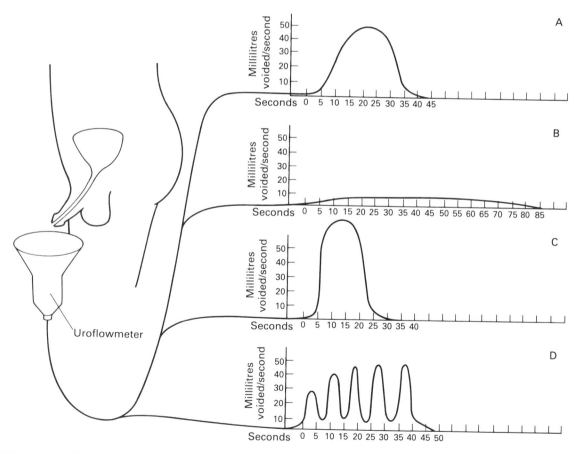

Fig. 23.26 Uroflowmeter flow curves. *A*, Normal flow pattern; normal rate and peak flow. *B*, Obstructed flow pattern; long voiding time and low peak. *C*, Superflow pattern; short voiding time and high peak. *D*, Abdominal flow pattern; voiding occurs only during periods of increased intraabdominal pressure (i.e. straining).

priate preparation of the patient and sterile gowning and gloving of the staff. A few patients may require an anaesthetic.

Treatment begins with prevention of injury and ensuing incontinence by good maternity care and the practise of postpartum exercises in the immediate postpartum period.

Stress incontinence is aggravated by chronic urinary tract infections, obesity and chronic coughing. Prevention includes the education of women about stress incontinence and the aggravating factors. Any urinary and vaginal tract infections are treated; the obese patient is advised to lose weight and an appropriate diet is discussed to assist her with this. The heavy smoker is advised to reduce or stop smoking as a means of reducing coughing, and is also instructed about stop-smoking programmes designed to help in this. The patient is assisted to re-establish a normal voiding pattern and bladder control. She is usually provided with a bladder drill and exercise regimen.

Bladder drill involves routines related to voiding. The patient is instructed to void each hour by the clock whether she feels the need to or not. When she has kept herself dry this way for three or four days she increases the time interval between voidings by one-half hour every three days until she can comfortably hold urine for three hours. She is instructed to drink plenty of non-stimulating fluids (e.g. caffeine-free) during the day, to drink nothing for 2 hours before going to bed and to empty her bladder completely before going to sleep. She is also instructed to empty her bladder before and after sexual intercourse.

The exercises consist of always giving an extra push at the end of voiding to make sure all urine is expelled. She also is instructed to practise tightening the buttocks and pelvic floor muscles and stopping and starting the stream of urine during micturition. The exercises are practised several times a day. If the patient is unsure whether or not she is practising them correctly, she can be taught to insert two fingers into the vagina and contract the vaginal muscles to grip the fingers as tightly as possible. This provides the patient with a direct measure of her progress. Once she has learned the technique, it can be practised without inserting her fingers.

Various smooth muscle relaxants which inhibit detrusor activity and increase bladder capacity may be prescribed while the patient is practising the bladder drill and re-establishing a voiding pattern.

If this regimen is unsuccessful, and in cases of prolapse with urethral incompetence, surgery may be necessary in order to support the urethra and restore the proper urethrovesical relationship.

Two types of operations are commonly used. In the Aldridge sling operation the surgeon makes a sling of fascia. This sling is then attached to the anterior abdominal wall. This serves to support the urethra, which can be demonstrated by observing the restoration of the angle. The approach may be abdominal, vaginal or both. Occasionally, the sling is too tight and the patient has difficulty micturating and emptying the bladder properly. Cystitis and other complications may occur. Teaching the patient to bend her body forward when attempting to void postoperatively helps. This relaxes the muscles of the abdomen, thereby loosening the sling and lowering the base of the bladder.

The Marshall–Marchetti–Krantz operation supports the urethra by suturing the anterior vaginal wall on each side to the periosteum of the pubic bone and the anterior wall of the bladder to the pubic bone.

The two most common operations performed in the United Kingom are the Burch colposuspension (which has an estimated 85% success rate) and the anterior vaginal repair operation (with an estimated 30% success rate).

In the Burch colposuspension operation the procedure is carried out abdominally. The vagina is lifted by means of two sutures inserted into each side of the bladder and then attached to the iliopectoral ligament.

Fistulae

Fistulae may occur between the vagina or uterus and the bladder, urethra or rectum (Fig. 23.27). They can occur as a sequel to injury during labour and delivery, surgery, and disease processes, such as carcinoma, and radiation therapy.

When urinary fistulae develop, some urine leaks into the vagina or uterus. Rectal fistulae causes the escape of flatus and faeces into the vagina. In both instances, irritation to the tissues occurs. An offen-

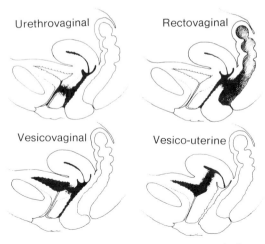

Fig. 23.27 Fistulae: urethrovaginal; rectovaginal; vesicovaginal; and vesicouterine.

sive odour develops and causes much embarrassment for the patient. Since many fistulae spontaneously heal within a matter of several weeks, treatment may be postponed. During that period nursing care is very important to the patient. Frequent perineal care is required to keep the patient clean. Cleansing and deodorizing douches may be ordered. High enemas may be given to reduce the constant flow of faeces. Care should be taken to go above the fistula with the rectal tube. If the fistula does not heal spontaneously, surgery may be indicated. Following surgery involving the bladder, the patient may return from the operating room with a urethral as well as a suprapubic catheter. Drainage must be maintained so that pressure on the repaired area is kept at a minimum. Repair may also include implantation of the ureters elsewhere. Rectal fistulae may be repaired and a temporary colostomy established in order to provide time to heal. Ambulation may be postponed for a few days. The woman may be discharged home on restricted activity until the doctor advises that the repair is complete.

BENIGN AND MALIGNANT DISORDERS OF THE REPRODUCTIVE TRACT

In the male

SPERMATOCELE

A spermatocele is a cyst of the spermatic cord which contains sperm in a thin white fluid. It lies above the testis and is separate from it. The mass will transilluminate. Usually a spermatocele requires no treatment. Sometimes it may become large enough to be confused with hydrocele and to be aggravating to the patient. Then it may be excised. The aetiology is unclear.

VARICOCELE

Varicocele is the dilatation of the venous plexus about the testis. It occurs most frequently on the left side. Its appearance on the right side may indicate that a tumour is occluding the vein above the level of the scrotum. Some testicular atrophy may occur if the circulation is impeded for long periods of time. This may result in subfertility. On palpation behind and above the testis the doctor feels a mass of tortuous veins which empties when the patient lies down.

Treatment may consist of a scrotal support which relieves the dragging sensation. If fertility is an issue or the condition is severe, the internal spermatic vein may be ligated. The results are usually excellent. A scrotal support may be worn for 4–5 days following surgery, since scrotal oedema may be present.

HYDROCELE

A hydrocele is a collection of fluid in the tunica vaginalis. It may occur following local injury, infection or a neoplasm and may be unilateral or bilateral. More often it is chronic, and the cause is unknown. In newborn babies, the cause is usually a late closure of the processus vaginalis. This frequently closes spontaneously. In some young men a chronic type exists because the processus vaginalis never closes completely, and a connection remains between the peritoneal cavity and the tunica vaginalis.

Treatment is not required unless the testis cannot be palpated to rule out abnormality, circulation to the testis is impaired or the hydrocele becomes large, unsightly and uncomfortable. Then the hydrocele is aspirated, and a sclerosing drug may be injected. In chronic cases the tunica vaginalis is excised (hydrocelectomy). Postoperatively the scrotum is elevated on a pillow or bridge dressing, and a pressure dressing is applied. Depending on the operation, there may or may not be a drain present in the incision. The patient must be observed for haemorrhage which may be concealed in the hydrocele sac. When ambulatory the patient usually requires a fresh scrotal support daily. Immediately after the operation he may need a larger support than usual.

TORSION OF THE TESTIS

Torsion of the testis occurs when the testis rotates within the tunica vaginalis. Often this is due to spasm of the cremaster muscle which rotates the testis in what is usually an abnormally large vaginalis. The young man experiences a sudden severe pain in the area of the testis which is unrelieved by rest or support. Because the torsion reduces the blood supply to the testis, testicular atrophy follows rapidly. Sometimes under local anaesthesia the surgeon will attempt to reduce torsion. If this is unsuccessful, surgical reduction follows.

BENIGN HYPERPLASIA OF THE PROSTATE

The reason benign enlargement of the prostate gland occurs is unknown. However, it is estimated that over 50% of men over 60 show some signs of prostatic enlargement. Of these, about 25% will require treatment.

In the young adult male the prostate gland is encased in a thin capsular membrane which is closely adherent to the underlying tissue. Gradually tissue begins to enlarge by new growth (hyperplasia) and the capsule of the prostate becomes thick and is loosely attached to the underlying tissue. This inner tissue can now be easily stripped away, leaving the thickened capsule intact.

There is debate about what actually happens in a prostate gland undergoing hyperplasia. One theory states that the hyperplasia occurs in the periurethral glands (Fig. 23.28), which then press the true prostatic tissue outwards to form the thick capsule. In this

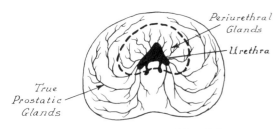

Fig. 23.28 Transverse section of the adult prostate.

case a procedure which leaves the capsule intact is not a prostatectomy. Others reason that the growth is primarily prostatic tissue, with periurethral glands included. Here prostatectomy is indeed performed, but only partially, as the posterior prostatic lobe which forms part of the capsule is not removed (Fig. 23.29). In any case the enlarging prostate encroaches on the urethra and the base of the bladder, producing certain symptoms.

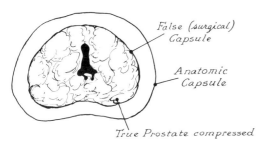

Fig. 23.29 Transverse section of a hyperplastic prostate.

Signs and symptoms
Gradually, the man may experience hesitancy in beginning the flow of urine. The stream of urine is reduced in force and size. Incomplete emptying of the bladder produces residual urine which reduces bladder capacity so that urgency and frequency result. Nocturia occurring three or more times in one night is a good indication of frequency. Often, cystitis occurs as well. In severe cases, the bladder becomes overdistended, and hypertrophy and small diverticula follow as weakened areas of bladder mucosa bulge out between the bands of muscle fibres. The back-up of urine causes hydroureter or even hydronephrosis. Over long periods of time renal function may be impaired.

Frequently, the patient does not seek medical attention until acute retention of urine occurs. Overdistension of the bladder is usually the precipitating factor. The patient is catheterized and decompressed. Decompression allows for the slow release of urine from the bladder. This prevents a sudden release of pressure in the abdomen which could cause shock and haemorrhage. Shock follows the rush of blood from vital centres to fill the newly released blood vessels. This sudden filling may cause

small blood vessels in the bladder mucosa to rupture. The catheter remains in place for 2–3 days, after which normal voiding patterns usually return. The patient is then encouraged to maintain regular ejaculation to relieve prostatic congestion. He is cautioned to avoid an excessive intake of fluid in a short period of time, as this rapidly distends the bladder, precipitating retention. He should void frequently when he has the urge to do so in order to avoid overdistension of the bladder. If followed, these instructions should help the individual to avoid acute retention. However, one should remain alert for the patient with retention with overflow who voids frequent small amounts of urine. This may be seen in the chronic case with progressive upper urinary tract involvement.

Backache and sciatica may also bring the patient to the doctor, since the enlarged prostate exerts pressure on nerves.

Surgical treatment
Surgery is indicated to relieve the symptoms and to prevent infections of the urinary tract and renal damage. If the amount of residual urine in the bladder is above 75–100 ml, the surgeon may feel surgery is necessary even though the symptoms are not severe. Residual urine is estimated in several ways. Immediately after voiding, a catheter may be passed and any remaining urine is drawn off and measured. A radiopaque dye can be injected into the bladder. The man is then asked to void and postvoiding films are made. Direct visualization of the bladder may be done by cystoscope, and any bladder changes will be noted. Intravenous pyelograms will indicate the extent of ureter and kidney involvement. Renal function tests may be ordered as well.

A period of preoperative preparation may be necessary. Residual urine and hydroureter are treated by catheterization for a period of 1–2 weeks. The patient is prepared for surgery by explaining what may follow the operation so that the postoperative period is not so traumatic.

Several operations are commonly used to treat this condition. The choice of operation seems to depend on the size of the prostate, the condition of the patient and the preference of the surgeon. A prostate in excess of 50 g is considered by most surgeons to be too difficult to remove transurethrally. Therefore, an open route is chosen.

Transurethral prostatectomy
This procedure is the most frequently performed operation and is the closed method. Postoperative recovery is usually rapid; sexual potency is maintained and urinary results are good. The operation is performed with a resectoscope, an instrument similar to a cystoscope but equipped with cutting and cauterizing attachments. This slender instrument is inserted up the urethra to the prostatic urethra, and the enlarged prostate is chipped away. The capsule

remains intact. During the operation, the bladder and urethra are continuously irrigated with a sterile, isotonic, non-conductive clear fluid. In this manner, debris and blood are washed away. Following removal of the intracapsular tissue, a Foley catheter with a 30 ml bag is passed. The catheter bag is pulled down into the prostatic fossa where it exerts pressure on blood vessels and helps to prevent haemorrhage. The catheter is usually attached to straight drainage, but it may be attached to medium or high decompression drainage. If haemorrhage has been a problem, the patient may have a cystostomy tube attached to continuous irrigation. This acts as a safety valve should clots plug the catheter.

The decompression drainage aids haemostasis by keeping constant pressure on the prostatic fossa. Also, the partially full bladder may help reduce bladder spasm. However, care should be taken to check that the catheter is draining and that the bladder is not full. A full bladder may cause haemorrhage by 'milking' the blood vessels in the fossa.

Immediately after the operation the catheter drainage is bloody. The nurse must be alert for signs of haemorrhage by paying close attention to the blood pressure and pulse of the patient and the amount of drainage. The drainage is watery and blood-tinged for 24–48 hours postoperatively. A thick, bright red drainage with clots forming indicates bleeding. Frequent irrigations of the catheter are usually ordered. If the catheter becomes plugged, the doctor is notified.

The fluid used to irrigate the bladder during the operation may be absorbed, causing haemodilution. The signs and symptoms of this may be those of sodium deficiency or excessive blood volume. Complaints of headache, nausea, vomiting or muscle weakness should not be ignored by the nurse but must be reported. Hypertension, restlessness, apprehension, shortness of breath or blurred vision likewise should be reported. If the surgeon expects that the operation may be more than 2 hours long, fluid intake may be restricted for 12 hours before the operation. Following the operation, 200–300 ml of normal saline may be given intravenously over 2 hours. The nurse must observe the patient for signs of pulmonary oedema.

Complaints of spasmodic, intermittent pain by the patient in the suprapubic region or a constant desire to void are related to bladder spasms. In severe cases the patient will need medication to obtain relief. The nurse should explain bladder spasms and catheters to the patient and instructs him not to try to void. These instructions and explanations are best given preoperatively so that the patient is prepared for the postoperative period; they are then reinforced postoperatively.

Complaints of persistent pain in the suprapubic area may be due to an overdistended bladder from a catheter which is not draining properly or from haemorrhage into the bladder. Rarely the bladder may have been perforated during the operation and blood and urine seep into the abdominal cavity. First the nurse irrigates the catheter and patency is established. The pain should diminish proportionately; if not, other causes must be ruled out. Pain medication may be given to the patient to give some relief during this period but pain medication does not provide relief from an overdistended bladder.

Because haemorrhage remains a threat, even in the later postoperative period, care is taken to prevent its occurrence. The patient is cautioned against straining to pass stool, and a light diet is usually ordered. Enemas, rectal tubes and rectal thermometers are contraindicated during the first postoperative week.

Because of the danger of a urinary tract infection, a prophylactic antibiotic may be prescribed. The catheter is removed 3–7 days postoperatively and, for a short period following this, the patient is usually instructed to record and measure each voiding. If difficulty in voiding is still present, the catheter may be reinserted. The nurse should watch for signs of incontinence which may follow or signs of urinary retention which may indicate a urethral stricture. Before being discharged the patient should be told that an episode of bleeding may occur about the second to fourth week postoperatively. In that event, he should contact his doctor and come to the emergency department of the hospital. Also he is warned to avoid any straining, heavy lifting or vigorous exercise for about 1 month postoperatively.

Suprapubic prostatectomy

This operation may be chosen when the prostate is large and when some bladder surgery is indicated as well. Sexual potency is maintained following the operation.

A small abdominal incision is made above the pubis and directly over the bladder. The bladder is opened and, through another incision into the urethral mucosa, the prostate is excised. The prostatic capsule remains intact. Various methods of draining the bladder and applying pressure to the operative site may be used postoperatively. A Foley catheter with a large bag and a cystostomy tube may be used. Sometimes a cystostomy tube with packing or a haemostatic bag in the prostatic fossa is used. Traction to maintain pressure on the haemostatic bag is achieved by attaching it to a birdcage apparatus which is placed between the patient's thighs. The packing and the haemostatic bag may have to be removed in the operating theatre at a later date. Sometimes only a Penrose drain in the suprapubic incision is all that is judged necessary. It is usually removed after 36 hours. If a cystostomy tube is present, it is removed 3–4 days postoperatively. The indwelling catheter usually stays until the incision is nearly healed. The suprapubic incision may take time to heal. Bladder spasm is a frequent difficulty to these patients. Usually the muscles become fatigued in 24–48 hours and the bladder spasms become fewer. These patients also have incisional pain necessitating the administration of analgesics. This type of pain is differentiated from bladder spasm and an overdistended bladder by increasing in severity with movement. Recovery may be prolonged, since ambulation is slower.

Retropubic prostatectomy
This method is preferred by some surgeons. Urinary results are excellent and potency is maintained. An abdominal incision is made above the bladder. The bladder is not incised, but the surgeon dissects down between the pubis and the bladder to reach the prostate. The capsule is opened and the tissue is removed. A large Foley catheter is inserted postoperatively. Since the bladder has not been opened, discharge on the abdominal dressing should not contain urine. If it does, the surgeon should be notified. The postoperative care is the same as for any prostatectomy patient. These patients seem to have fewer bladder spasms and less difficulty voiding.

Perineal prostatectomy
In a perineal prostatectomy the surgeon excises the prostate through a semicircular incision in the perineal body. The prostatic capsule is opened and the gland is removed. The pre- and postoperative care resembles that of other prostatectomies. A perineal shave preparation will be necessary. Because of the risk of rectourethral fistula, the large bowel may be surgically prepared preoperatively. Unfortunately, after this operation is performed the patient may be impotent, and some difficulty may be experienced in establishing urinary continence following surgery.

Cryosurgery
For patients unable to tolerate regular surgery, cryosurgery is being performed. The patient is prepared as though he were going for a cystoscopic examination. A local anaesthetic with sedation is used. To protect the bladder walls the bladder is distended with sterile water or air. Then the probe with the freezing agent, either liquid nitrogen or nitrous oxide, is inserted into the prostatic urethra and the tissue destroyed. The patient returns to the ward with a self-retaining catheter attached to straight drainage until he can void on his own. This usually occurs within 10–21 days. The advantages of the method include little haemorrhage and early ambulation. However, there is some danger of retaining the sloughed tissue and damage to the surrounding tissues.

CARCINOMA OF THE PROSTATE

Carcinoma of the prostate gland is one of the most common tumours seen in men. Perhaps 16% of all malignancies in the adult male are due to prostatic lesions. The tumour most often arises in the posterior prostatic lobe and in 85% of cases is hormone-related, depending upon androgens to retain its integrity. The tumour also causes an increase in the secretion of acid phosphatase which is normally high in prostatic secretions. This increased production is reflected in blood serum levels and may indicate a prostatic tumour. Cancer of the prostate is frequently seen in association with benign hyperplasia but does not result from it. In addition, surgery for benign hyperplasia is not prophylactic against cancer as the posterior prostatic lobe is retained.

Because of its frequency and the fact that early diagnosis can be made in most cases by a rectal examination, all men should be advised to have an annual check-up after the age of 40. Nurses are advised to include this advice whenever it is related in their health teaching to the community.

Signs and symptoms
The symptoms are essentially those of benign enlargement of the prostate. On rectal examination, the examiner palpates a hard nodule. Since the nodule may resemble other conditions, a biopsy is often done. Two types are commonly used. A *needle biopsy* is safely done on an outpatient basis. The perineum is cleansed and draped. The surgeon palpates the nodule with one finger in the rectum, and simultaneously guides a needle, passed through the perineum, to the site. Several samples are usually collected. On discharge, the patient is told that blood-stained urine is to be expected for a short time and is instructed to watch the injection site for signs of redness, pain and swelling and to report their occurrence to his doctor. This technique is not judged to be as complete as *direct biopsy*. Under anaesthesia, the perineum is cleansed, and a small incision is made. Direct biopsy of the prostate is made and sent to the laboratory. If immediate results are positive, a prostatectomy may be done before the patient leaves the operating room. If negative, the incision is closed, and the surgeon awaits the more extensive laboratory report. Because of the possibility of an immediate prostatectomy, the patient is prepared for the operating room as if he were undergoing major surgery.

Classification
Carcinoma of the prostate is classified into four stages. These stages are based on the results of rectal examinations, serum acid phosphatase levels, x-rays of the skeleton and metastases. Stage I, or carcinoma in situ, is often called latent, or focal. Usually there are no symptoms. In Stage II the nodule may be palpated on rectal examination, and serum acid phosphatase levels are normal. When Stage III is reached, the growth has spread to the seminal vesicles, the base of the bladder and outside the prostatic capsule, but no distant metastases are present. Seventy-five per cent of men will show elevated serum acid phosphatase levels. With Stage IV carcinoma excessive

levels of serum acid phosphatase circulate in the bloodstream. Previously, the thick prostatic capsule has kept the lesion localized and prevented spread into the abdominal cavity. Now the blood and lymphatics have carried the disease to distant sites. The bones of the pelvis are most frequently affected, and elevated serum alkaline phosphatase levels reflect this spread. Also, because of bone and liver involvement, severe anaemia may occur, accompanied by the other symptoms of a terminal disease.

Treatment and nursing intervention
Stages I and II are treatable. Stages III and IV usually receive palliative therapy. Treatment is by radical prostatectomy by the retropubic or perineal routes. The entire gland and seminal vesicles are removed. The bladder neck is sutured to the urethral stump. A large Foley catheter is inserted which serves as a splint for the urethra as well as a drain for the bladder. Drains may be placed in the incision lines as well. Pre- and postoperative care are similar to that of any prostatectomy.

Incontinence may follow temporarily or on a longer basis. The patient is usually greatly relieved to be assured that this is usually temporary and that control can be regained by practising perineal floor tightening and relaxing a few times periodically throughout the day when permitted.

If the perineal route was used, care must be taken to avoid infection. The incision is cleansed two to three times daily and following bowel movements. A heat lamp and warm baths may be ordered for several days postoperatively. The scrotum may be elevated on an adhesive bridge in order to acquire adequate exposure of the incision. In the presence of haemorrhoids, a heat lamp is usually contra-indicated.

In Stages III and IV, therapy includes radiation therapy and the administration of oestrogens. Radiation therapy is used in Stage III in higher doses to achieve a cure and in Stage IV in lower doses to achieve palliation. The course of treatment extends over 5–6 weeks. Oestrogen suppresses the production of androgens upon which the tumour is dependent. The patient experiences relief, and life is prolonged. However, the side-effects may be severe, so that oestrogen is usually reserved for patients with metastases. Some doctors may give lower doses of oestrogens in the earlier stages to shrink the tumour before surgery. The side-effects include oedema of the ankles, tender gynaecomastia, some nausea and vomiting, impotence with loss of libido, and a significant increase in the incidence of death from thromboembolic disease. The patient on oestrogens is observed for these side-effects. Sodium intake is reduced in order to prevent oedema. Eventually the effect of the oestrogens is reduced, and an orchiectomy (removal of testes) may be done to reduce the amount of androgens in the body.

This combination of oestrogens and orchiectomy

may produce good results for about 18 months. Then the adrenals seem to recover from the oestrogen-induced hormonal imbalance and begin producing androgens again. Cortisone may be given now in an attempt to depress this source of androgens. In extreme situations an adrenalectomy may be performed. Deep x-ray therapy reduces discomfort from bone metastases. Radioactive phosphate given orally or intravenously also lodges in the bone, bringing relief from pain. In the case of a bladder obstruction, a transurethral prostatectomy is done. Since the operation is merely palliative, no attempt is made to remove all of the growth.

The patient will require nursing care related to the special needs of the cancer patient and to the aforementioned prostatectomy therapies.

CARCINOMA OF THE TESTES AND PENIS

Most tumours of the testes are malignant. Only about 1% of all malignancies occur in this area. Men between the ages of 18–35 are at greatest risk. Because the organ is palpable and early detection is possible, all men should be taught how to examine the testes. This is especially important for men with a history of cryptorchism, whether surgically corrected or not, as they are at increased risk of the disease. Caucasians are at highest risk for the condition. Although the tumour is rare, and this should be stressed in teaching, each man should be alert to possible changes in his testes. Any painless lump felt in the testis should be examined by a doctor. The man should also be alert to a testis that feels enlarged, is firm, gives the impression of heaviness, and when squeezed, fails to elicit the deep visceral pain that is usually associated with testicular pressure. Textbooks on physical assessment provide the nurse with guidelines and pictures of testicular examination. If either the nurse or the patient is uncomfortable with the teaching, the nurse should arrange for the patient to see an acceptable instructor, either a male nurse or doctor.

Diagnosis and treatment
Five distinct types of neoplasms have been identified and the tumour may occur as one type or as a mixed one. Some tumours contain embryonal or chorio-carcinomatous elements and if so produce elevated serum levels of alpha-fetoprotein and the beta sub-unit of human chorionic gonadotrophin (β-HCG). As in all cancers the type of neoplasm and stage of the disease will govern treatment. Treatment is bilateral orchiectomy and, for some types of tumours, the surgery is followed by radiation therapy to the lumbar lymph nodes. Other types will receive chemotherapy postsurgery.

Malignancies of the penis are essentially malignancies of the skin. The glans and prepuce are nearly always affected. The disease is less frequent among circumcised men. Treatment is by excision of the affected areas or by partial or total amputation of the penis.

In the female

POLYPS

Polyps are common benign growths occurring mainly in the endometrium and cervix. The polyp has a characteristic smooth, shiny surface and is pink to deep red in colour. They are small in size, seldom exceeding more than 3 cm in length. The cause is unknown. No symptoms are usually present, but occasionally postcoital bleeding occurs. Treatment is by surgical excision of cervical polyps and may be followed by dilation and curettage to remove endometrial polyps.

MYOMAS OF THE UTERUS

A myoma (fibromyoma, leiomyoma) is a benign tumour of the uterus composed of myometrium and fibrous tissue. Colloquially, myomas are known as 'fibroids'. At least 25% of women over 35 years of age show some evidence of myomas. The cause is unknown, but oestrogen stimulation is thought to play a part.[3,4]

Myomas occur mainly in the uterine body. According to their position they are classified as subserous, submucous and intramural (Fig. 23.30), and may become pedunculated. A pedunculated fibroid in the uterine cavity may be referred to as a fibroid polyp. This may be extruded through the cervix and may come to lie in the vagina. Myomas in the broad ligament or cervix are recorded, but these locations are rare. Several fibroids of varying sizes may be present in any one uterus. As the fibroids

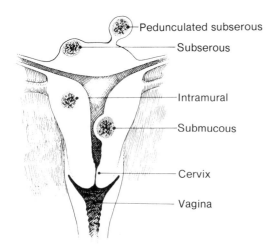

Fig. 23.30 Uterine myomas.

---

[3] Llwellyn-Jones (1986).
[4] Dewhurst (1986), Chapter 47.

become larger, their blood supply may be reduced, causing some degeneration. The most common is a hyaline degeneration in the middle of the myoma. This causes a loss of cellular structure and, in extreme cases, a collection of gelatinous fluid lies at the centre. Sometimes the tumour shows signs of fatty changes and may even become calcified (womb-stone). A so-called red degeneration may occur, usually in association with pregnancy. The tumour looks like raw beef on the inside. The patient shows signs of malaise with fever, rapid pulse and pain over the fibroid. Following menopause all myomas atrophy and show slight shrinkage.

Signs and symptoms
Symptoms vary with the size and location of the tumour. Frequently, with small tumours, there are no symptoms. Occasionally hypermenorrhoea occurs. Pain is rarely a symptom but most frequently is associated with torsion of a pedunculated myoma. Sometimes the myoma passing through the cervix causes cramps. Dysmenorrhoea may occur as a result of mechanical interference. Large myomas can cause frequency or retention of urine. Pressure on veins, lymphatics, and nerves of the pelvis may cause varicosities, unilateral or bilateral oedema of the lower extremities, or a radiating pain through the thighs. Occasionally, these tumours may be the cause of abortions or infertility. Some tumours become infected.

Treatment
Treatment depends on the age of the woman, her desire for more children and the size of the myoma. In the young woman who wishes children, a myomectomy is usually done. This is the enucleation of the myoma, but the uterus is retained. Blood loss during the operation may be extensive as the surgeon excises multiple myomas from a large uterus which may not contract efficiently. Persistent oozing of blood may occur postoperatively for the same reasons. The nurse should be alert to this possibility. In cases of very large myomas the treatment is hysterectomy.

In the young woman, myomas are not a contraindication to pregnancy and usually cause no difficulty. Rarely, they may obstruct labour or cause a postpartum haemorrhage.

TUMOURS OF THE OVARY

Tumours of the ovary are many and varied. The aetiology of most is unknown. For purposes of clarity they are roughly divided into non-neoplasms and neoplasms. Only a few are described in each group.

Non-neoplasms
Non-neoplasms are usually simple cysts or collections of fluid surrounded by a thin capsule. They do not grow but expand only as more fluid accumulates.

These physiological cysts are seen mainly during the reproductive years. The follicular cyst is the most common of this group. Corpus luteum cysts may occur as well. Theca lutein cysts develop under the stimulation of high levels of chorionic gonadotrophins.

Occasionally, the Stein–Leventhal syndrome or polycystic disease of the ovary occurs. The syndrome appears in the late teens and early twenties with variable symptoms. These may include a history of sterility, secondary amenorrhoea, hirsuitism and cysts bilaterally in the ovary. The ovary shows some enlargement and presents a glistening white appearance. Microscopically, many atretic follicular cysts are present. The syndrome is thought to follow an endocrine imbalance, probably arising in the ovary but affecting the hypothalamus. The ovaries produce an excessive amount of androgens which inhibit maturation of a follicle with subsequent disturbance of the ovarian-hypothalamic relationships. What triggers the imbalance is unknown. Medical treatment consists of a course of the drug clomiphene, with or without gonadotrophins, to produce an LH surge and ovulation. Surgical treatment is known as a wedge resection of the ovary. About half the ovarian tissue is removed in a wedge shape. This reduces the amount of tissue producing high androgen levels, which subsequently fall and ovulation takes place. Medical treatment appears to be replacing surgical treatment.

Neoplasms
Pseudomucinous cystadenomas are the single most common neoplasms, occurring in about 40% of patients with a neoplastic ovarian growth. They may attain the largest size of any ovarian tumour. The tumour is characterized by multiple pockets filled with a thick fluid called pseudomucin. They may be bilateral and may become malignant.

Serous cystadenoma is the second most common of this group and appears to arise from germinal epithelium. The cyst contains a serous fluid. These cysts are frequently bilateral and often become malignant.

The dermoid cyst or teratoma may be cystic or solid. When it is soft, the cyst is filled with sebaceous material, hair and ordinary skin. The solid cyst frequently contains cartilage, bone, teeth, thyroid, and similar material. Rarely is the cyst malignant. It occurs most frequently in young women and may be bilateral.

Neoplasms of the ovary may also be divided into those which have some hormonal effect and those which do not. One tumour with no hormonal effect is a *dysgerminoma*. It arises from the primitive germ cells and is usually malignant. A *fibroma* is a benign solid neoplasm occuring most frequently in the postmenopausal patient. The fibroma arises from connective tissue in the ovary and may be associated with Meigs' syndrome, which is characterized by ascites and pleural effusion.

Those tumours which have hormonal effects may be further subdivided into feminizing and virilizing lesions. The most common of the rare feminizing tumours is the *granulosa cell tumour*. The tumour produces oestrogen and may induce precocious puberty or cause hypermenorrhoea or postmenopausal bleeding. It may be malignant or may be associated with carcinoma of the endometrium. The most common of the even rarer masculinizing tumours is *arrhenoblastoma*. By the production of androgens, presumably from the primitive male cell elements in the ovary, the woman is masculinized. In about 15–25% of cases it proves to be malignant.

CARCINOMA OF THE OVARY

Primary carcinoma of the ovary is usually the common adenocarcinoma. However, a review of ovarian growths is indicated, as almost any one of them has the potential to become malignant. The most common malignancy arises from the serous cystadenoma. Only one ovary may be affected but the other quickly follows, apparently because of the close lymphatic connections. About 5% of all cancers in the female arise in the ovary.

Secondary tumours represent metastases from almost any other cancer. The Krukenberg tumour deserves mention. In this case bilateral, equal involvement is usually secondary to tumours in the stomach. Back-up of the lymphatic drainage appears responsible for this particular tumour, especially since other metastases usually occur later.

Signs and symptoms
The ovarian tumour in its early stages is often symptomless. At regular yearly check-ups, palpation of the adnexa will reveal a mass. Often this may be the first discovery of the tumour. The symptoms result from the size of the tumour or its position. An increase in girth may be noticed but ignored. Pressure on the bladder causes frequency or a feeling of fullness. Constipation, oedema of the legs, anorexia and a full feeling in the abdomen may be present. Pain may be associated with stretching of the tissues as the tumour enlarges. Ascites may be present, accompanied by difficulty in breathing.

Treatment
Because of the danger of malignant growth, any ovarian mass is observed suspiciously. A rule of thumb says that any soft mass below 5 cm may be watched closely for 2–3 months. If no further growth occurs, then conservative treatment may be considered. Other tumours demand biopsy, and a laparotomy is indicated. Following diagnosis, the surgeon strives to preserve as much ovarian function as is possible. In premenopausal women benign growths, if size permits, will be enucleated and ovarian function retained. Malignant growths are treated with total hysterectomy and bilateral salpingo-

oophorectomy (removal of the tubes and ovaries). Surgery is followed by chemotherapy. Unfortunately, many malignancies have metastasized before discovery of the tumour. Prognosis is poor and surgery may be only palliative. Further treatment is directed toward relieving the symptoms of the terminally ill patient. Recurrent ascites may be a problem, and frequent paracentesis may be indicated.

Complications of ovarian tumours
Torsion or twisting of the growth on its stalk frequently occurs. Circulation is impeded, and necrosis may follow. The patient usually feels a sudden severe pain in the lower abdomen. Treatment is by excision of the tumour at an immediate laparotomy.

The cyst may rupture. Often the 'chocolate cyst' of endometriosis ruptures and drains fluid into the abdomen. Again the patient may present with an 'acute abdomen.'

Haemorrhage and infection occur in tumours as well. Usually, they are more common in the malignant tumour.

Postsurgical menopause is the result of a bilateral oophorectomy. The symptoms are similar to those of the regular menopause, but may be more severe because of the sudden withdrawal of hormones. Replacement therapy with oestrogens may begin before the patient leaves the hospital if it is not contraindicated by malignancies which are aggravated by oestrogens.

CARCINOMA OF THE CERVIX

Carcinoma of the cervix is a common malignancy in women. The woman who has borne children or had an early sex life with several partners is more apt to develop the disease.

Cancer of the cervix is a complex disease which is preceded by several earlier cervical changes (Table 23.8).

These changes usually occur at the squamocolumnar junction of the cervix (Fig. 23.31), and initially are evident only on histological examination. They reflect a varied pattern of development. Some cases arise with no known precursor stage, while others appear to have gone through all the changes or any

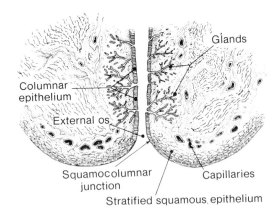

Fig. 23.31 Squamocolumnar junction of the cervix.

combination of them. The earlier changes may be reversible, and so do not always herald cancer. How many of these will reverse is unknown, but about 50% of women with carcinoma in situ are thought to develop invasive cancer; this development may take an average of 10 years. The cervical smear is the best method of early detection of these changes. Combined with treatment of these changes it is largely responsible for the declining mortality rates associated with cervical cancer.

Because 5-year survival rates are excellent in those cases which are discovered early, the Royal College of Nursing and the Royal College of Obstetricians and Gynaecologists both recommend that all women who are sexually active or over 25 should have cervical smear tests at least every three years. The nurse has a responsibility to disseminate this knowledge. The nurse emphasizes the hopeful aspects of cure following cases of early recognition. This may encourage more women to seek medical attention by reducing their anxiety. Fear of what she may discover often seems to prevent the patient from consulting her doctor. The nurse should do her utmost to persuade the woman confiding irregular bleeding to her to seek medical attention immediately.

Signs and symptoms
A small lesion develops which, in the early stages,

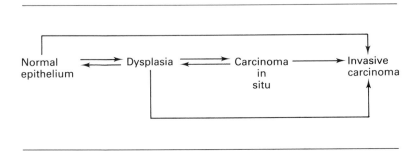

Table 23.8 Patterns of development of cancer of the cervix.

can be confused with other cervical conditions. The early stages may be asymptomatic, but eventually some bleeding from the vagina occurs. An unusual vaginal discharge may be present which may have an offensive odour. Pain is a late symptom and is followed by weight loss, anorexia and cachexia.

Carcinoma of the cervix is divided into stages. Stage 0 is carcinoma in situ, or focal carcinoma. There is an intact basement membrane containing the malignant cells. Stage I is invasive cancer, which means that the basement membrane has been breeched and the cells are invading the surrounding tissue. Stages IA and IB refer to degrees of this invasion which is still within the confines of the cervix. Unfortunately, about 20% of Stage I will already have spread to the lymphatics. A small lesion similar to an erosion may be present on the cervix. In Stage II the carcinoma has spread to close adjacent structures, and the upper third of the vagina may be involved. By Stage III invasion has reached the pelvic walls and lower vagina. Stage IV is marked by extensive pelvic involvement, including the bladder or bowel, and distant metastases may be present.

Treatment
Treatment is usually guided by the stage assigned to the situation by the gynaecologist. Since the main method of diagnosing Stage 0 carcinoma is the cervical smear test, the results of this test help to guide treatment. The smear results are organized into five classes. In Classes I and II the cells are nonmalignant, and no treatment is necessary. Class III is suspicious and arouses concern. The patient is asked to have repeat smears done in 3 months or a biopsy is done. Classes IV and V are positive, indicating that definite changes are present which require biopsy.

Biopsy. A *punch biopsy* may be done with special punch biopsy forceps. Because of the paucity of nerve endings in the cervix, the biopsy may be done with relative comfort for the patient. She may feel something like a pinch when the biopsy is taken. A Schiller test can be done. Normally the cervix contains glycogen. This is depleted in areas of abnormal

cell change. When Lugol's solution (iodine in potassium iodide) is swabbed on the cervix, the normal epithelium stains a dark brown. Glycogen-deficient areas are a pale colour by contrast, and these are the areas requiring biopsy.

Further treatment may be a *cone biopsy*. It is an operative procedure in which a cone-shaped segment of the central cervix is removed. The internal os remains intact (Fig. 23.32). On examination the section may contain all of the malignant area. In these cases the biopsy may be considered sufficient treatment. Pre- and postoperative care for the patient is similar to other vaginal surgery such as a D and C. The major difference is that these patients face the threat of a malignant disease and may be extremely anxious. Considerable skill in providing supportive nursing will be demanded of the nurse. Haemorrhage is a threat, and the patient should be warned of this. Bleeding from the biopsy site may occur up to a week after the biopsy when the patient is at home. The nurse should inform the patient of this possibility before discharge so that she will notify her doctor and not be unduly alarmed. Sometimes the haemorrhage is severe enough to necessitate readmission to hospital and a blood transfusion.

The biopsy results may indicate normal cells, dysplasia, carcinoma in situ or invasive carcinoma. Many situations contribute to dysplasia, and the patient is usually treated for these and followed closely with repeat cervical smears. Some of these will revert back to normal epithelium. If they do not, a cone biopsy may be performed or, in the older woman, a hysterectomy. Carcinoma in situ may be treated with a cone biopsy if the woman wishes more children or by total hysterectomy. All carcinoma in situ must be treated to ensure prevention of most invasive carcinoma. Invasive carcinoma of the cervix will be treated according to the stage in which it is classified.

Surgery and radiation therapy. Stages IA and IB and some early Stage II's are treated by radical surgery (modified Wertheim's hysterectomy), which attempts to eliminate the cancer, and radiation

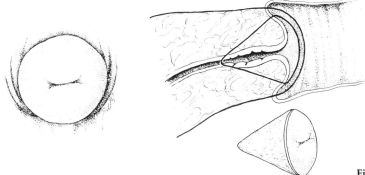

Fig. 23.32 Cone biopsy of the cervix.

therapy. There is much debate over the optimum approach. Some prefer radiation alone; others prefer surgery with or without radiation. In major medical centres, with highly qualified surgeons and sophisticated radiation equipment and radiologists, higher cure rates have been recorded with a combination of surgery and radiation. In smaller centres lacking highly experienced surgeons some quote higher cure rates for radiation alone. Most seem to agree that Stages III and IV are best treated by radiation and some palliative surgery. In cases where the surgeon feels that the tumour is surgically excisable a pelvic exenteration is done. Surgery is used in cases of a radioresistant tumour.

The patient who is having a total hysterectomy (Fig. 23.33) for carcinoma in situ will have the uterus, cervix and upper third of the vagina removed. The ovaries are conserved in most cases of the premenopausal woman but may be removed in the older woman. The patient is prepared as for abdominal surgery. A perineal shave preparation may be ordered as well, and the mons pubis, vulva, perineal body, and the upper third of the thighs are shaved. Postoperatively, any vaginal discharge must be observed. Some staining may occur from the vaginal cuff. A Foley catheter may be inserted and may remain in place for 1 or 2 days postoperatively. The nurse is alert to possible signs of hormonal imbalance following removal of the ovaries as well as signs of a urinary tract infection and thromboemboli.

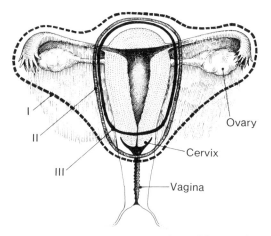

Fig. 23.33 Types of hysterectomy. I: total hysterectomy with bilateral salpingo-oophorectomy. II: total hysterectomy. III; subtotal hysterectomy.

In a Wertheim's hysterectomy, the uterus, ovaries, broad ligaments, surrounding tissue, upper half of the vagina and pelvic lymph nodes are removed. Sometimes the ovaries will be retained, especially in a younger woman. In a more extensive Wertheim's operation, the pelvic fascia and further lymph tissue will be removed. Preoperatively the patient has a cystostomy examination and her ureters are cath-

eterized. This allows them to be easily identified during the extensive pelvic dissection. The patient's vagina and cervix are painted with an iodine solution to identify any glycogen-deficient areas which would indicate further vaginal resection.

Nursing intervention
When the patient returns to the ward she will require general postoperative care. Two Redivac drains may have been inserted, one in either lower quadrant, and attached to a drainage system. These are removed when there is no drainage. Drainage is usually more extensive if no radiation has been given before surgery, and less if radiation has been given. Occasionally two rubber drains, one on either side, may be draining into the vagina. They are shortened about the third postoperative day and removed about the fifth day if drainage has ceased. If oozing of blood was a problem during surgery, the pelvis may have been packed with a gauze pack, the tail of which is brought out through the vaginal cuff into the vagina. This is usually advanced in 48 hours and removed in 72 hours. The ureters and bladder have been handled during surgery and may be atonic. Care must be taken to see that the catheter is draining properly and that bladder distension does not occur. The catheter should drain clear urine. Observations are made for signs of thromboemboli postoperatively; the femoral areas as well as the calves are examined. Early ambulation is encouraged, but does not merely mean sitting in a chair by the bedside for extended periods of time. Better venous return is achieved by having a patient lie in bed with her legs elevated to about 15° than by sitting for long periods of time in a chair at the bedside. Ambulation refers to movement—getting up to sit in a chair for 10–15 minutes, back to bed with feet slightly elevated, getting up to walk to the bathroom, getting up to eat lunch and back to bed to rest. Leg exercises, coughing and deep breathing are important in promoting good circulation.

Fistula formation is a hazard and the risk is greater if radiation therapy has been given prior to surgery. Because these fistulae are a result of poor blood supply and the sloughing of tissue they are a later development, usually appearing in the second postoperative week. The most common are vesicovaginal and ureterovaginal. Thus, any unusual drainage of urine must be noted. In addition, any unexplained fever or lower quadrant or flank pain should alert the nurse. The fistula is usually not repaired immediately, but postponed until a more favourable time.

A pelvic exenteration includes all of the Wertheim's hysterectomy plus a total vaginectomy and removal of portions of the bladder or bowel, depending upon the spread of the disease. The patient may return postoperatively with an ileostomy, a colostomy or an ileal conduit. Nursing care for such conditions is elaborated in Chapter 17. In these operations preoperative bowel preparation is done. Postoperatively, drains may be left in areas of node dissection to prevent the pooling of blood and serum which may easily lead to infection. The drains may be draining freely or may be attached to suction. Usually they are advanced daily and removed by the fifth postoperative day.

The postoperative adjustment to life may be difficult. Preoperative discussions with the doctor and nurse should help to prepare the patient. In pelvic exenteration sexual function of the vagina is lost; in a Wertheim's operation it may have to be modified. Menopause may occur as oestrogen therapy is frequently contraindicated. The care of the colostomy or ileostomy must be learned and accepted. The patient will require much understanding and support from the nursing staff while the nurses gently encourage her to retain as much independence as is compatible with her situation.

Frequently, external and internal radiation therapy is used in conjunction with, or instead of, surgery for these patients. Because a high oxygen concentration in the tissues and blood increases the radiosensitivity of the tumour, anaemia and low circulating blood volumes are corrected before radiation therapy by medication or blood transfusions. Radium in special containers is inserted into the cervical canal and into the lateral fornices of the vagina. The insertion of the radium is an operative procedure. The patient receives a cleansing enema the day before and a perineal shave preparation. During the procedure a urinary catheter with a small bag is passed. This prevents a distended bladder from coming into contact with the radium, which would greatly increase the chance of a vesicovaginal fistula. After the radium is inserted, packing is placed in the vagina and may be sutured in place to maintain the position of the radium. Because the tight packing prevents voiding, the catheter drains the bladder. The patient's temperature is monitored, as radiation may stimulate a latent infection. The patient remains on bed rest with head and shoulders nearly flat. A slipper bedpan is used, and straining at stool is discouraged. The catheter is checked to see that it is draining. These measures help to ensure that the radium remains where it has been placed. Complaints of pain and any bloody discharge should be reported to the doctor. The time for removal should be carefully observed. Removal may be uncomfortable for the patient because of the tight packing, and the patient may need an analgesic for this. For further information on the care of the patient consult the section on care of the patient receiving radium inserts, p. 156.

CARCINOMA OF THE ENDOMETRIUM

This is a frequently occurring malignancy which appears to be increasing in incidence. Since it is a disease largely of older women, this may be due to a lengthened life span. Oestrogens aggravate the tumour and prolonged oestrogen therapy, especially in the premenopausal or postmenopausal woman, has been implicated as a contributing cause of endometrial cancer.

The first symptom is a painless, bloody vaginal discharge. Thirty to 40% of women with postmenopausal bleeding have cancer of the endometrium. Bleeding postmenopausally should therefore never be ignored but investigated immediately. A careful endometrial biopsy is usually done. The growth is usually in the fundus of the uterus, but may arise in or spread to the isthmus. The thick body of the uterus contains the growth and it metastasizes late in its growth.

Treatment is by intracavitary radiation followed by a careful total hysterectomy and bilateral salpingo-oophorectomy. Care is taken to pack the vagina or suture the cervix, and tie the tubes to prevent spread by seeding from the uterus. Surgery is often followed by radiation of the vagina as well in order to reduce the risk from stray malignant cells spread during surgery. Some surgeons may do the hysterectomy first and follow with radiation. More advanced cases are treated with combinations of external and internal radiation with surgery to relieve symptoms. Where radium is inserted, several containers attached to strings may be placed in the body of the uterus to irradiate the endometrium. Cure rates are excellent when the tumour has been discovered early.

Progesterone therapy retards the growth of the tumour and metastases. Treatment in the form of medroxyprogesterone acetate (Provera) may be started before surgery and continued for two years afterwards.

CARCINOMA OF THE VAGINA

In recent years there has been an increase in clear cell adenocarcinoma of the vagina in girls and young women. This is a result of in utero exposure to diethylstilboestrol (DES), a synthetic non-steroid oestrogen compound. DES was first synthesized in 1938; by 1940–41 the drug was prescribed for women to help prevent or treat threatened spontaneous abortion, which was thought to be due to low progesterone levels. Unlike natural oestrogens, it stimulated the body to increase the production of progesterone. The drug was withdrawn from use for this purpose in 1971. Between 1940 and 1971 many thousands of women received treatment with DES. Prior to its withdrawal it had been shown to be a transplacental teratogen and carcinogen, producing a wide range of congenital anomalies of the genital tract in the offspring and a rare vaginal cancer in a few daughters of such pregnancies (Table 23.9). During organogenesis, exposure to DES affected Muellerian duct tissue. This tissue remained inappropriately or, in many women, is in the wrong place. Time of exposure was more important than amount of exposure. Disorders following DES exposure in utero include physical anomalies, adenosis and carcinoma of the vagina. Estimates vary

Table 23.9 Effects on children of exposure to diethylstilboestrol (DES) in utero.

Women
1 Congenital anomalies:
  (a) Cervix—hooded, ridged, ringed by fibrous tissue
    —hypoplastic
  (b) Uterus—abnormally shaped, small, internal adhesions, constrictions
  (c) Vagina—transverse ridges
    —stenosis
  (d) Adenosis or ectopic tissue by vagina and cervix
    —this may disappear by age 30
    —not cancer precursor but usually present when cancer occurs
2 Cancer of the genital tract:
  Usually clear cell adenocarcinoma
  Commonest between ages 14–20
  Rare, incidence 1–4 per 1000 at-risk women
3 Increased reproductive difficulties
  Secondary to abnormalities of cervix and uterus
  (a) Primary infertility
  (b) Spontaneous abortion
  (c) Ectopic pregnancy
  (d) Premature labour and delivery

Men
1 Congenital anomalies:
  (a) Testis—undescended
    —hypoplastic
  (b) Epididymis—benign cysts
  (c) Penis—microphallus
    —urethral stenosis
2 Fertility problems related to:
  Decreased sperm counts
  Alterations in density, motility and penetrating ability of sperm
3 Possible increased cancer risk:
  Testicular

but from 65–95% of at-risk women have cervical and uterine anomalies and about 90% have adenosis. By contrast the risk of developing cancer is small; perhaps 0.5% of women affected by DES exposure. There is less information concerning sons of women treated with DES but they appear to be at less risk of abnormalities. Perhaps 30% of 'DES sons' have testicular abnormalities. Although DES induces breast cancer in male mice, there is no evidence at present to indicate that it does so in either sex in humans.

Treatment and nursing intevention
The regular follow-up and screening visits of those who were exposed to DES begins with the first menstrual period or at age 14 years, whichever is first. Early monitoring of the girl to detect changes at the cellular level involves regular examinations every 6 months including cervical smears, Schiller's test to determine areas of change and hence areas for biopsy, and possibly a colposcopy examination. Cervical smears are only about 75% effective in detecting change in this condition and the cellular screening must be more rigorous and extensive. Women who have not been involved in this early

screening programme present with bleeding or a suspicious lesion in the vagina.

Treatment is radical vaginal surgery followed by irradiation and possibly chemotherapy.

Nursing interventions are directed to case-finding by public education and by questioning of appropriate age groups during history taking. Once a case of DES exposure is suspected, teaching about the condition, attendant risks and necessary follow-up is done and the patient is referred to a doctor. The patient and the mother usually require support from professionals and from others in a similar situation.

Adenosis. The signs and symptoms of *adenosis* include complaints of a heavy clear mucoid discharge, dyspareunia and postcoital bleeding. On inspection, small bright red papillary or granular lesions may be seen on the smooth pink vaginal mucosa. Alternatively, large diffuse red patches may be seen. Numerous small cystic nodules beneath the epithelium are felt on the anterior and posterior vaginal walls. During palpation care must be taken to inspect and palpate the entire vagina as the blades of the speculum may obscure the adenosis. Most adenosis requires no treatment. Extensive adenosis may need cryotherapy or partial vaginectomy with skin grafting.

CARCINOMA OF THE VULVA

Carcinoma of the vulva is a less frequent malignancy, occurring mainly among women in their fifth and sixth decades of life. It is frequently preceded by vulvar changes.

Dystrophy of the vulva
Dystrophy of the vulva refers to changes in vulvar epithelium which are most often associated with ageing but may occur in the younger woman. Most are benign but some are premalignant. Because premalignancy must be assessed at the cellular level a biopsy is done on all lesions.

The patient complains of a shrinking of vulvar structures which progressively narrows the introitus. Dyspareunia, pruritus and soreness are frequent complaints. Smooth red or white patches of thick or thin epithelium may be evident. They may be only in the vestibule or scattered over the vulva and perineum. These patches crack easily, and fissures and excoriated areas develop. Pruritus is common and secondary infection of the scratched lesions occurs. Ulceration may develop.

Mild symptoms usually respond to improved perineal hygiene, control of pruritus and infection and topical application of oestrogen. Patients with more severe symptoms are admitted to the hospital. Nursing care will then involve keeping the vulva dry, cool and clean by daily baths. No pants or pyjamas are worn. The patient is nursed as much as possible with her legs apart and a bed cradle over the perineum to keep it dry and cool. A hair dryer may be used at intervals to blow cool dry air over the perineum. This helps relieve pruritus and promotes healing. It is wise to avoid powders and creams. Medication to reduce the pruritus may be needed as well. If the condition resists treatment or recurs, a simple vulvectomy may be done. Those patients who show signs of cellular changes consistent with an increased risk of developing cancer will have periodical examinations and biopsies done or a simple vulvectomy.

In addition the nurse must observe the vulva and perineum of any patient for whom she cares in order to identify changes which would require further investigation. She should encourage patients who confide symptoms in her to seek medical attention.

Treatment
Carcinoma of the vulva is treated by radical vulvectomy. Here the dissection is extensive for the clitoris, labia and all the perineal subcutaneous tissue; all the perineal glands and the femoral and inguinal lymphatics are removed.

Nursing intervention
Preoperative preparation includes all the measures common for perineal and abdominal surgery. The patient and nursing staff may react with repugnance at the thought of this surgery. It is frequently seen as mutilating. However, the results of the operation are quite favourable. Sexual function is retained, as the vagina is not removed. Young women have conceived following simple vulvectomy and have been delivered by caesarean section.

Postoperatively, the patient returns to the ward with an indwelling catheter. Much oedema is present and great care must be taken not to dislodge the catheter. It may be very difficult to replace. The operation may be done in two stages or all at once. In the former, the patient returns with an open area, requiring future skin grafting. Barrier isolation may be required for this patient both before and after skin grafting. A bed cradle over the pubic area will keep bed linen away. When the procedure is completed in one operation the patient may return with a bulky pressure dressing held in place by a T binding. In other cases there are bilateral stab wounds near the iliac fossa containing drains which are attached to suction; this arrangement may replace the pressure bandage. Thus, the fluid is drained away and the skin flap is kept in close approximation to the underlying tissue so that it becomes firmly attached to the tissue. Some necrosis along the incision lines may be expected, and occasionally skin grafting may be necessary to replace a necrotic area. The stitches are usually not removed for 2–3 weeks. Close observation is maintained for thromboemboli. Once ambulation is begun, the patient may need elastic stockings to avoid swelling of her legs. Standing for long periods of time should be avoided.

References and Further Reading

BOOKS

Borg S & Lasker J (1981) *When Pregnancy Fails.* Boston: Beacon Press.

Broome A & Wallace L (1984) *Psychology and Gynaecology Problems.* London: Tavistock.

Clayton S, Lewis T & Puker G (1986) *Gynaecology by Ten Teachers*, 14th ed. London: Edward Arnold.

Dennerstein L, Wood C & Burrows G (1982) *Hysterectomy.* Oxford: Oxford University Press.

Dewhurst J (1984) *Female Puberty and its Abnormalities.* Edinburgh: Churchill Livingstone.

Dewhurst J (1986) *Dewhurst's Integrated Obstetrics and Gynaecology*, 4th ed. London: Blackwell Scientific. Chapter 47.

Garry M, Govan A, Hodge C & Callander R (1978) *Gynaecology* (Illustrated), 2nd ed. Edinburgh: Churchill Livingstone.

Glover J (1984) *Human Sexuality in Nursing Care.* London: Croom Helm.

Guillebaud J (1986) *Contraception: Your Questions Answered.* Edinburgh: Churchill Livingstone.

Guyton AC (1986) *Textbook of Medical Physiology*, 7th ed. Philadelphia: WB Saunders.

Hatcher RA et al (1980) *Contraceptive Technology*, 10th ed. New York; Irvington.

Hogan R (1980) *Human Sexuality, A Nursing Prospective.* New York: Appleton-Century-Croft.

Houghton D & Houghton P (1984) *Coping with Childlessness.* London: George Allen & Unwin.

Huffman JW, Dewhurst CJ & Capraro VJ (1981) *The Gynecology of Childhood and Adolescence*, 2nd ed. Philadelphia: WB Saunders.

Jeffcoate N (1975) *Principles of Gynecology*, 4th ed. London: Butterworths.

Katchadourian HA & Lunde DT (1987) *Fundamentals of Human Sexuality*, 3rd ed. New York: Holt Rinehart and Winston.

Lerner J & Khan Z (1982) *Manual of Urologic Nursing.* St Louis: CV Mosby.

Llewellyn-Jones D (1986) *Fundamentals of Obstetrics and Gynaecology*, 4th ed., Vol. 2. London: Faber and Faber.

Lumley J & Astbury J (1980) *Birth Rites and Birth Rights.* Melbourne: Thomas Nelson.

Masters WH & Johnson VE (1966) *Human Sexual Response.* Boston: Little, Brown.

Masters WH & Johnson VE (1970) *Human Sexual Inadequacy.* Boston: Little, Brown.

Meltzer AS (1981) *Sexually Transmitted Diseases.* Westmount, Quebec: Eden Press.

Pepperell RJ, Hudson B & Wood C (1980) *The Infertile Couple.* Edinburgh: Churchill Livingstone.

Reynolds M (1984) *Gynaecological Nursing.* London: Blackwell Scientific.

Rosenthal SN & Bennett JM (eds) (1979) *Helping the Victims of Sexual Assault.* Toronto: Provincial Secretariat for Justice.

Rosenthal SN & Bennett JM (eds) (1981) *Practical Cancer Chemotherapy.* Garden City, New York: Medical Examination Publishers.

Shields-Poë DA (1981) Spontaneous abortion as an index of exposure to carcinogens. Unpublished Master's Thesis, University of Toronto, Department of Medicine and Biostatistics, Toronto, Ontario, Canada.

Simons W (1985) *Learning to Care on the Gynaecological Ward.* London: Hodder & Stoughton.

Singer A (ed) (1985) Cancer of the cervix: diagnosis and treatment. *Clinics in Obstetrics and Gynaecology,* Vol. 12 No 1, London: WB Saunders.

Speck P (1984) *Loss and Grief in Medicine.* London: Baillière Tindall.

Speroff L, Glass RH & Kase N (1983) *Clinical Gynecologic Endocrinology and Infertility,* 3rd ed. Baltimore: Williams & Wilkins.

Sweet B (1987) *Mayes Midwifery,* 10th ed. London: Baillière Tindall.

Tschudin V (1987) *Counselling Skills for Nurses,* 2nd ed. London: Baillière Tindall.

Webb C (1985) *Sexuality, Nursing and Health.* Chichester: John Wiley.

PERIODICALS

Annon JS (1978) The PLISSIT model: a proposed conceptual scheme for the behavioural treatment of sexual problems. *J. Sex Educ. Ther.,* Vol. 2, pp. 1–15.

Cavanagh D (1969) The vaginal examination. *Hosp. Med.,* Vol. 5 (Jan.) pp. 35–51.

Chamberlain G (1981) Aetiology of gynaecological cancer *Royal Soc. Med. UK,* Vol. 5, pp. 246–261.

Chiazze L et al (1968) The Length and variability of the human menstrual cycle. *JAMA,* Vol. 203 No. 6, pp. 377–380.

Cubykjam BHL (1983) Toxic shock syndrome and other tampon related risks. *JOGNN,* Vol. 112 No. 2, pp. 94–99.

Davison R (1984) Health education—cervical cancer. *Nurs. Mirror,* Vol. 159 No. 16, pp. 32–33.

DeCherney A & Lake Polar M (1984) Evaluation and management of habitual abortion. *Br. J. Hosp. Med.,* (April) pp. 261–268.

Endacott J & Whitehead M (1983) Female and male climacteric nursing. *J. Clin. Nurs.,* Vol. 2 No. 4, pp. 399–403.

Fish S (1983) Hormone replacement therapy. *Nurs. Mirror,* (Supplement), Vol. 157 No. 6.

Gottesfeld KR (1978) The use of ultrasound in gynecologic diagnosis. *Applied Rad.,* Vol. 7, pp. 132–140.

Gunn D, Jenkin P & Gunn JE (1937) Menstrual periodicity: statistical observations on a large sample of normal cases. *J. Obs. Gyn. Br. Emp.,* Vol. 44, pp. 839–879.

Hassey K (1985) Demystifying care of patients with radioactive implants. *Am. J. Nurs.,* Vol. 85 No. 7, pp. 788–792.

Hill G (1984) The nurse's role. Cervical Cancer 4. *Nurs. Times,* Vol. 159 No. 15, pp. 26–28.

Hulme H (1983) Therapeutic abortion and nursing care. *Nurs. Times.* Vol. 79 No. 41, pp. 56–59.

Kemp J (1984) Attitudes to abortion. *Nurs. Mirror,* Vol. 158 No. 17, pp. 34–35.

Kinch RAH (1982) The premenstrual syndrome. *Ann. RCPSC,* Vol. 15, pp. 469–474.

Lehmann A (1983) DES: a living legacy: what nurses can do about it. *Can. Nurse,* Vol. 79 No. 11, pp. 34–39.

Martocchis B (1985) Grief and bereavement. *Nurs. Clin. N. Am.,* Vol. 20 No. 2, pp. 327–341.

Matsumoto S et al (1968) Environmental anovulatory cycles. *Int. J. Fert.,* Vol. 13, pp. 15–23.

McNeil S, Paradis A & Wig P (1984) Nursing grand rounds: toxic shock syndrome. *Can. Nurse,* Vol. 79 No. 4, pp. 38–41.

Miles PA (1984) Sexually transmitted diseases. *J.O.G.N.N.,* Vol. 13 No. 2, p. 102–124.

O'Brien PMS (1986) Premenstrual syndrome. *Br. J. Sex. Med.* (March) pp. 78–82.

Reid RL & Yen SSC (1981) Premenstrual syndrome. *Am. J. Obst. Gynecol.,* Vol. 139, (Jan.) pp. 85–104.

Rutter M (1984) Intermenstrual bleeding. *Nurs. Times,* Vol. 80 No. 9, pp. 29–32.

Schuster EA (ed.) (1982) Symposium 1: sexuality and nursing practice. *Nurs. Clin. N. Am.,* Vol. 17 No. 3, pp. 343–448.

Smith K (1985) Dysfunctional uterine bleeding. *Br. J. Hosp. Med.* (Dec.) pp. 352–354.

Treloar A et al (1967) Variation of the human menstrual cycle through reproductive life. *Int. J. Fert.,* Vol. 12 No. 1, pp. 77–126.

Webb C & Wilson-Barnett J (1983) Hysterectomy: dispelling the myths—1. *Nurs. Times.* Vol. 79 No. 30, pp. 52–53.

Webb C & Wilson-Barnett J (1983) Hysterectomy: dispelling the myths—2. *Nurs. Times.* Vol. 79 No. 31, pp. 44–46.

Webb C (1985) Barrier to sympathy. *Nurs. Mirror Res. Forum,* Vol. 160 No. 1, pp. 6–7.

Willis H (1982) Hormonal status of women. *Nurs. Mirror,* Vol. 155 No. 16, pp. 54–56.

Woods NF, Most A & Dery GK (1982) Toward a construct of premenstrual distress. *Res. Nurs. Health,* Vol. 5, No. 3, pp. 123–136.

The Normal Breast

The breasts, or mammary glands, lie on the anterior chest wall. The base of each rests on the fascia of the pectoralis major muscle, and supporting ligaments extend from the skin through the breast to the fascia. The breasts are undeveloped in both sexes until puberty. At this time, the female breasts enlarge and develop secreting cells and ducts in response to increased concentrations of ovarian and certain adeno-hypophyseal (anterior pituitary) hormones. Oes-trogen is responsible for the growth of the duct system, and the luteotropic hormone and progester-one are considered the chief stimulants for the devel-opment of the secreting cells. The cylindrical projec-tion on the skin surface forms the *nipple*, which is perforated by duct orifices. The pinkish area of skin around it is referred to as the *areola*; it becomes mark-edly pigmented during pregnancy and retains the darker colour following delivery. The male breasts remain rudimentary throughout life.

Following growth and maturation, the female breast is composed of 15–20 lobes, each with a duct that opens onto the surface of the nipple. Each lobe consists of clusters of secreting cells which form lobules (Fig. 24.1). The main ducts (lactiferous ducts) are formed by the union of smaller ducts which drain the lobules. They are dilated just before entering the base of the nipple to form reservoirs, or ampullae, for the milk during active secretion. The lobes and ducts are separated and supported by areolar, fibrous and fatty tissues. The size of the breasts is mainly determined by the amount of fatty tissue rather than by glandular tissue.

The blood supply to the breasts is abundant and is derived from the internal mammary arteries and branches of the thoracic and intercostal arteries. A large proportion of the lymph in the breasts is chan-nelled through the axillary lymph nodes; the remainder drains through mediastinal nodes (see Fig. 24.2).

The breasts are subject to menstrual cyclic changes associated with alterations in the concentrations of various hormones. Varying degrees of enlargement, tenderness and discomfort develop during the few days preceding menstruation and disappear in a day or two.

During pregnancy, the lobes and ducts enlarge in preparation for the secretion of milk. Lactation is the function of the breasts and occurs only after the birth of a child, continuing as long as the milk is with-drawn. After menopause, the lobes and ducts undergo some atrophy and replacement with fibrous tissue.

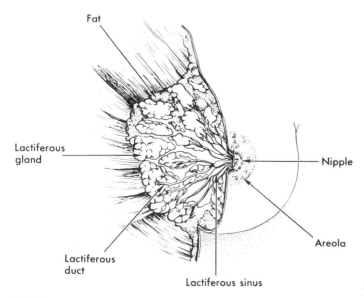

Fig. 24.1 The female breast.

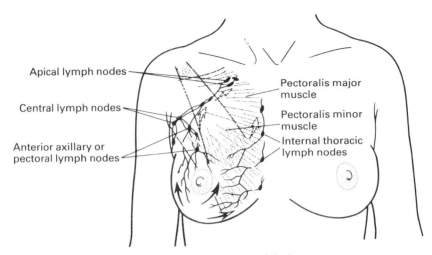

Fig. 24.2 Lymphatic drainage of the breast.

Apical lymph nodes

Central lymph nodes

Anterior axillary or
pectoral lymph nodes

Pectoralis major
muscle

Pectoralis minor
muscle

Internal thoracic
lymph nodes

Nursing Process

Assessment

HISTORY

A detailed history is taken of the individual's: (1) age; (2) health history; (3) family history of illness and disorders of the breasts; (4) parity and nursing of infant(s); (5) menstrual history (age of onset, regularity, menopause); (6) date of discovery of lesion; (7) symptoms (detailed description) that prompted patient's visit to the doctor; (8) knowledge of risk factors associated with breast cancer; (9) breast self-examination practices; and (10) feelings concerning the meaning of the breast to the individual's femininity.

PHYSICAL EXAMINATION OF THE BREASTS

Inspection. With the patient uncovered to the waist, the breasts are observed with the patient sitting upright, leaning forward and lying down. In each position the patient is asked to place the arms first at the sides and then to raise them above the head. The breasts are observed for: (1) nipple inversion, retraction and discharge; (2) retraction or dimpling of an area; (3) redness, excoriation, discolouration, oedema; and (4) changes in contour and symmetry.

Palpation. The breasts are palpated with the patient in the supine and then sitting position. Palpation begins with the patient's arms at the sides and is repeated with the arms raised over the head. The entire breast is examined in a systematic manner, beginning in one quadrant and moving around until the starting point is again reached. The palmar

surface of the fingers is used, with the examiner's hands moving from the outer circumference toward the nipple or in concentric circles from the nipple outward. With the patient in a sitting position, the breast is supported in one hand while being palpated with the other. The normal breast varies in consistency and may feel granular in older individuals. If any masses are discovered they are palpated for size, shape, consistency, mobility, discreteness of borders, location and tenderness. The infraclavicular, cervical and axillary areas are palpated for enlarged lymph nodes.

DIAGNOSTIC TESTS

Prompt, thorough medical investigation is indicated when any changes or symptoms are observed.

Mammogram. This is an x-ray procedure used in breast examination without the injection of a contrast medium. A series of x-rays of the breasts is made from two planes, from above and lateral. The films are examined for any areas of increased density and, if present, their characteristics (location, size, shape, regularity of borders). A lesion may be detected in a mammogram that is not palpable.

Xerograph. Xerography involves the use of an aluminium plate with an electrically charged coat of selenium. On x-ray exposure, an electrostatic image is transferred to paper by a special process. The xerogram provides more accurate, detailed information about the soft tissues of the breast than the mammogram.

Thermogram. The skin over some tumours of the breast is warmer than that over normal areas. A thermogram may be made of the breast with an infrared camera to detect these areas of higher temperature. The thermography is carried out in a room in which the temperature is controlled at 21°C or 70°F; the patient is brought to the room 30 minutes before the thermogram is made.

Biopsy. Biopsy provides a specimen of tissue for cytological examination; the specimen may be obtained by aspiration, resection or excision. In the case of breast tumours, most surgeons prefer an excision biopsy, since it permits an examination of the complete tumour.

Bone scans. In patients with malignant tumours of the breast, especially when axillary lymph node involvement is identified, bone scans are done to identify bone metastases.

MANIFESTATIONS OF BREAST DISORDERS

Symptoms of breast disorders may be insidious and may include: alterations in the size and/or shape of the breasts; palpable masses in the breast tissue and discharge from the nipples. The size and shape of breasts vary among individual females and with age. Very large breasts may cause physical discomfort by the weight they impose on shoulders and other parts. Attitudes towards breast size are individual and are greatly influenced by social values, clothing styles and the person's self-image and femininity. Changes in the symmetry of the breasts may be caused by pathological processes. Palpable masses in the breasts may not be tender but frequently are discovered by women during self-examination of their breasts. Disorders of the breast in males are less common than in females but alterations in size and shape do occur as a result of hormonal influences and abnormal tissue growth.

BREAST SELF-EXAMINATION

Regular self-examination of the breasts plays an important role in easy detection of a breast lesion.

Identification of patient problems
The problem is lack of knowledge about: (a) the importance of breast self-examination; and (b) the techniques of breast self-examination.
    Breast cancer is the most common malignancy in women, accounting for approximately 26% of newly diagnosed carcinomas in females each year.[1] Greenwald's study estimated that the mortality from breast cancer could be reduced by 18.8% if breast self-examination was carried out.[2]
    Many women do not examine their breasts routinely. Stromberg found the reasons for inconsistent monthly breast self-examination were: (1) fear

and anxiety about cancer of the breast; (2) lack of specific knowledge about the technique of breast examination and confidence in how to do it; (3) ignorance of the importance of monthly breast self-examination as a necessary supplement to physical examinations; and (4) modesty and embarrassment.'[3]

Goals for women who lack knowledge of the importance of breast self-examination and the techniques involved are to:
1 State breast cancer risk factors relevant to self
2 Perform breast self-examination each month

Nursing intervention
All women from their early teens onward should be taught to examine their breasts monthly and to see a doctor promptly if any changes are observed. Annual physical examinations are recommended for all women and twice yearly examinations for women over 30 with a family history of breast cancer.
    Every nurse has the responsibility, as well as frequent opportunity, to teach patients and friends the importance and procedure of regular self-examination of the breasts. It should not be assumed that women have been taught the procedure or that they perform self-examination of the breasts thoroughly and routinely.

Teaching resources. A variety of resources are available for teaching breast self-examination. Pamphlets outlining the process are published by the Health Education Council for England and Wales, the Health Education Group in Scotland and similar groups in Europe, also the Mastectomy Association and other Cancer Societies. These are available for distribution, usually free of charge, from local branches. Films demonstrating the procedure are often available from the same sources. Other films, video programmes, slide tapes, charts and pamphlets are available also from commercial suppliers. Screening centres are being seen as more and more important. Some private clinics provide examination services for women and free facilities for screening are available in the United Kingdom at Family Planning Clinics, Well Woman Clincs, and through the General Practitioner services.

Teaching strategies. Olenn's study of 174 women who were instructed in breast self-examination showed that those who perceived the importance of the practice were more likely to comply.[4] Awareness of breast cancer risk factors was found to increase motivation. Olenn also found that a lack of confidence in performing breast self-examination impeded compliance. Practice sessions in an area

---

[1] Silverberg (1982), p. 15.
[2] Greenwald et al (1978), pp. 271–273.

[3] Stromberg (1981), p. 1652.
[4] Olenn (1981), p. 1656.

that provides privacy is recommended. Breast models also provide an opportunity for the tactile experiencing of various breast changes; immediate feedback on what the woman is feeling is obtained. Pamphlets provide pictorial and written instructions that the individual can use when performing breast self-examination at home.

Suggested content for teaching programme. Instruction on breast self-examination should include: (1) information on the importance of the practice; (2) content on breast cancer risk factors; (3) opportunity for tactile practice on self and/or models, with immediate feedback; and (4) distribution of printed material depicting and describing the procedure for on-going reinforcement of the correct techniques at home.

1 *The importance of monthly breast self-examination.* Women should be aware that 90% of breast tumours are initially identified by women themselves. A high percentage of breast carcinomas are palpable and can be detected early at a size of about 1 cm. Routine breast examination increases the likelihood of early detection and thus improved prognosis, as the chance of metastasis is decreased in the early stages of the disease.

2 *Risk factors.*[5] Breast cancer is more likely to occur to women who: are older (the incidence increases sharply with age until menopause and again 5 years post-menopause); live in North America or northern Europe; have fibrocystic disease of the breast; have no children, or who have their first child after the age of 30 years; have a family history of breast cancer; are Jewish; and have an early menarche or a late menopause, or both.

Risk factors are assessed in relation to the individual and are re-evaluated with age and changes in health status.

3 *Self-examination of the breast.* The examination should be made regularly each month, a few days after menstruation, and should be continued after menopause. It involves inspection before a mirror and palpation while bathing and then in the supine position. See Fig. 24.3 for a description and diagram of the techniques of breast self-examination.

---

[5] Robbins, Angell & Kumar (1981), p. 589.

How to examine your breasts

In the shower:

Examine your breasts during bath or shower; hands glide easier over wet skin. Fingers flat, move gently over every part of each breast. Use right hand to examine left breast, left hand for right breast. Check for any lump, hard knot or thickening.

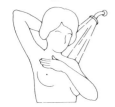

Before a mirror:

Inspect your breasts with arms at your sides. Next, raise your arms high overhead. Look for any changes in contour of each breast, a swelling, dimpling of skin or changes in the nipple.

Then, rest palms on hips and press down firmly to flex your chest muscles. Left and right breast will not exactly match—few women's breasts do.

Regular inspection shows what is normal for you and will give you confidence in your examination.

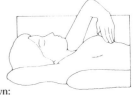

Lying down:

To examine your right breast, put a pillow or folded towel under your right shoulder. Place right hand behind your head—this distributes breast tissue more evenly on the chest. With left hand, fingers flat, press gently in small circular motions around an imaginary clock face. Begin at outermost top of your right breast for 12 o'clock, then move to 1 o'clock, and so on around the circle back to 12. A ridge of firm tissue in the lower curve of each breast is normal. Then move in an inch, toward the nipple, keep circling to examine *every part of your breast,* including nipple. This requires at least three more circles. Now slowly repeat procedure on your left breast with a pillow under your left shoulder and left hand behind head. Notice how your breast structure feels.

Finally, squeeze the nipple of each breast gently between thumb and index finger. Any discharge, clear or bloody, should be reported to your doctor immediately.

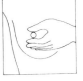

Fig. 24.3 Self-examination of the breast.

Expected outcomes
The individual:
1 Is able to list risk factors for breast cancer that apply to her.
2 Demonstrates the technique of breast self-examination on herself and/or a model.
3 Performs breast self-examination every month.

DISORDERS OF THE NIPPLE

Drainage from the nipple in a non-lactating breast is usually a result of an intraductal papilloma, carcinoma, mammary dysplasia or ductal ectasia (distension). The discharge is usually serous or bloody but may be milky, brownish or purulent and may be unilateral or bilateral. It may be spontaneous or occur with manipulation. The breasts are assessed for a mass, and a history is taken to determine whether there is any relationship between the drainage and menstruation and if the patient is taking oral contraceptives or oestrogen therapy for postmenopausal symptoms.

An *intraductal papilloma* is a benign, wart-like growth usually involving a single collecting duct. It is located near the areola, is non-tender, may be soft or firm and bleeds or produces a yellow, pink or bloody drainage on pressure or with trauma. Treatment involves surgical excision of the papilloma and the involved duct.

Ductal ectasia is a form of fibrocystic mastitis characterized by dilation of multiple and usually bilateral ducts in the subareolar area. Signs and symptoms include burning and itching, pain and swelling of the nipple and areolar area of the breast. Treatment may involve surgical excision of the involved ducts.

FIBROCYSTIC DISEASE AND BENIGN EPITHELIAL HYPERPLASIA

These are relatively common disorders of the female breast and are characterized predominantly by fibroplasia, epithelial hyperplasia and the formation of cysts. The lesions are influenced by a hormonal imbalance, are usually bilateral and occur most often in women 30–50 years of age, with a higher incidence in those approaching menopause. A painless mass is usually the first and only manifestation; occasionally there may be some tenderness. The patient may experience more severe soreness and pain of the breasts than is usual in the premenstrual period.

The cysts may be aspirated under local anaesthesia. If a solid mass is encountered or the aspirated fluid contains blood, an incisional biopsy may be done to rule out carcinoma. Following the initial aspiration, the patient is re-examined periodically and aspiration of recurrent or newly formed cysts may be necessary. Fibrocystic disease is believed to increase the risk of breast cancer.[6] The disease regresses with the onset of menopause.

---

[6] Robbins, Angell & Kumar (1981), p. 587.

FIBROADENOMA

Fibroadenoma is a benign tumour which develops most frequently in young women. It generally occurs singly, but rarely there may be more than one. Although it is not usually encapsulated, it remains localized and is freely movable and usually painless. Medical authors indicate no increased tendency to subsequent carcinoma in patients who have had a fibroadenoma.

The treatment consists of local excision of the tumour, which is submitted for cytological examination for confirmation of the diagnosis of non-malignancy.

Potential patient problems

It must be realized that patients admitted for biopsy and confirmatory diagnosis of a benign breast growth have very specific nursing needs related to their diagnosis.

The potential problems of these patients include:
1 Failure to adjust to the diagnosis and to accept that the lump is benign.
2 Inability to appreciate the need for regular breast self-examination.
3 Non-acceptance of the results of treatment (or non-treatment—for example scarring, disfigurement and discomfort.

Patients who are offered surgical removal of the growth are potentially at risk of developing many of the problems associated with surgery of malignant growths, especially those concerning self-image and the development of appropriate coping mechanisms.

Nursing intervention

Nursing intervention for patients with *benign breast* disorders includes assessment of the patient's emotional responses to the disorder and biopsy, instruction regarding breast self-examination and measures to reduce the physical symptoms.

The emotional response of individuals to the diagnosis of a benign breast tumour or scarring and possible disfigurement from a biopsy varies with the individual and the degree of the perceived threat to her self-image and femininity. The nurse assesses the patient's response and allows opportunity for the patient to express her feelings and concerns. A referral may be made to the general practitioner and a community nurse.

Breast self-examination is taught to all patients and the importance of regular, monthly examination is stressed.

Measures which may help alleviate the physical symptoms of the disorder are explained if relevant to the individual. Such measures include: (1) wearing a brassiere 24 hours a day to provide firm support for the breast and to ease discomfort associated with movement; (2) use of heat or cold applications or mild analgesics to relieve discomfort; and (3) altering diet to eliminate caffeine, theophylline and theobromine.

Expected outcomes

The patient with a *benign breast* disorder is able to:
1 Express her emotional responses to the experience.
2 Demonstrate breast self-examination.
3 State the importance of regular breast self-examination.
4 State measures to relieve physical symptoms of the breast disorder.

CARCINOMA

The breast is the most common site of cancer in the female. It rarely occurs under the age of 25, and the incidence progressively increases with age. The greatest number of patients develop their disease between the ages of 40 and 50.

Most breast cancers originate in the epithelial tissue of the ducts; the remainder arise from the secreting cells of the lobules. Fifty per cent of breast carcinomas develop in the upper outer quadrant, 10% in the lower outer quadrant, 10% in the upper inner quadrant, 5% in the lower inner quadrant and 25% in the central portion of the breast.[7]

The cause of breast cancer is unknown. Three factors presently being considered are: (1) hormonal, (2) viral, and (3) genetic.

Many malignant tumours of the breast appear to be influenced by ovarian hormones, especially oestrogen. It has been demonstrated that some patients with cancer of the breast have a remission of their disease when the oestrogen concentration is reduced by oophorectomy, adrenalectomy, hypophysectomy or by the administration of anti-oestrogenic agents.

The discovery that a virus, which is transmitted in breast milk, causes breast cancer in mice is a recent development that has stimulated a search for a possible viral cause of the cancer in humans.

Factors influencing the risk of development of breast cancer are listed above. Age, hereditary predisposition and a prior history of breast cancer are the most significant of these factors.

The rate of growth of the cells of the neoplasm may depend on the immune response or resistance of the individual. See Chapter 4 for a discussion of the immune response.

MANIFESTATIONS

The earliest symptom is generally a single, painless, non-tender mass which is poorly circumscribed and may have a nodular surface. It is usually discovered by the patient when bathing or during a routine self-examination of the breasts. Other symptoms which may develop include change in the size or contour of the affected breast, retraction of the nipple or an area of the skin over the breast, bleeding or discharge from the nipple, a scaly rash around the nipple, enlargement of axillary or infra- or supraclavicular lymph nodes or a bleeding, ulcerated area on the breast surface.

As the cancer grows, it spreads to adjacent tissues, such as the skin and underlying fascia and muscle. Retraction is due to involvement of the supporting fibrous tissue; there is a proliferation of fibroblasts and ensuing scar tissue within the breast and fascia of the chest muscles. The breast becomes firmer and cannot be moved as freely. Ulceration is associated with advanced disease which has spread to involve the skin.

METASTASES

Cancer of the breast may spread directly into adjacent structures or may metastasize to distant structures by emboli of tumour cells being transported through the lymphatics or the blood vessels. The axillary, supraclavicular or mediastinal lymph nodes are usually the first site of secondary involvement. Other structures which frequently become the site of metastases are the lungs, liver, spine, pelvic bones and femora.

Records show that progress relative to cure and survival of persons with cancer of the breast has been disappointing. It is suggested that a majority of the women have metastasis at the time of diagnosis and primary treatment.[8]

TYPES OF BREAST CANCER

Cancers of the breast may be classified according to the primary breast tissue involvement or according to certain tissue changes. The most common type is *scirrhous carcinoma* characterized by marked fibrosing and hardness. The *medullary breast cancer* grows rapidly, forming a larger mass which is softer in consistency than the scirrhous type. There is less fixation of the breast. A third type which occurs rarely is the *inflammatory carcinoma*, which involves the skin and more superficial tissues as well as the lymphatics. *Lobular cancer* involves primarily glandular tissue and is less invasive than other types. *Intraductal carcinoma*, which has a high incidence, originates in the epithelial tissue of one or more mammary ducts. *Papillary carcinoma* is characterized by small papillary growths within the duct system and usually causes bleeding from the nipple. *Paget's disease* is also an intraductal cancer that extends to involve the nipple and areola; a scaly rash and erosion of the nipple accompany this type.

---

[7] Robbins, Angell & Kumar (1981), p. 590.

[8] Fisher (1977), pp. 953–961.

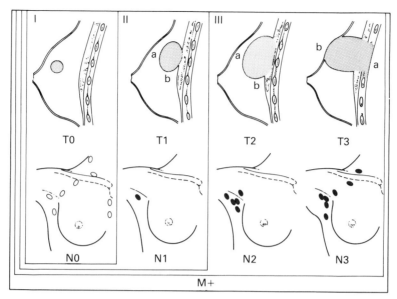

Fig. 24.4 Anatomical staging for breast cancer. *Tumour (T) categories*: Primary advancement in the T category is designated by size, i.e. T1 < 2 cm, T2 > 2–5 cm T3 > 5 cm. Each has a subcategory of a. vs. b. reflecting extension into pectoral muscle and fascia that acts as the organ capsule. The most advanced stages consist of extensive skin and chest wall invasion, resulting in complete fixation. Pathological categories have been created for smaller lesions often detected by mammography that are less than 2 cm in size. *Node (N) categories*: The *number*—not size—of nodes and then *location* determine advancement. One to 3 nodes (N1) carries a better prognosis than 4 or more (N2) in axillary dissections rather than palpation. Nodes in pectoral, supraclavicular or external mammary areas are indeed poor prognostications if associated with axillary nodes, but the latter group could be a location of primary tumour. *Stage grouping*: Stages, in part, reflect curability by local/regional modes of surgery and radiation therapy. The equivalence of T and N categories are, prognostically: T2 = N1, T3 = N2, T4 = N3.

The patient's disease may be classified by location, and whether it is infiltrating or non-infiltrating, or in stages (clinical staging) according to the characteristics of the primary breast *tumour*, regional lymph *node involvement* and *distant metastasis*. This classification is referred to as the TNM system[9] (see Fig. 24.4):

Tumours
TO — No demonstrable tumour
TIS — Pre-invasive carcinoma
T_1 — Tumour of 2 cm or less. No skin involvement
T_2 — Tumour over 2 cm
T_3 — Tumour greater than 5 cm in size
T_4 — Tumour of any size with skin infiltration, ulceration, peau d'orange (skin dimpled similar to that of an orange), skin oedema, or pectoral muscle or chest wall attachment

Nodes
NO — No palpable axillary lymph nodes
N_1 — Palpable axillary lymph nodes that are not fixed. Metastases suspected
N_2 — Palpable fixed axillary lymph nodes
N_3 — Homolateral supra- or intraclavicular nodes considered to contain metastases. Oedema of the arm

Metastases
MO— No distal metastasis
M_1 — Clinical and radiographical evidence of metastasis other than those to homolateral axillary or intraclavicular lymph nodes

A second classification that may be adopted to indicate the stage of the individual's disease uses the following categories:

Staging[10]
Stage I   A tumour less than 5 cm in diameter without nodal involvement and no metastases
Stage II   A tumour less than 5 cm in diameter with movable axillary nodes and no metastases
Stage III All tumours of any size with or without skin involvement or fixation, and with or without nodal involvement but without metastases
Stage IV   All tumours of any size with or without skin involvement or fixation and with or without nodal involvement but with metastases

TREATMENT

The forms of treatment used in carcinoma of the breast are surgery, radiation, alteration of hormonal concentrations (either by administering certain

---

[9] Sabiston (1986), p. 551.

[10] Robbins, Angell & Kumar (1981), p. 593.

hormones or by removing hormone-producing structures), chemotherapy and combinations of these. There is no unanimous opinion as to the best method of treatment; the search continues for treatment that will provide more encouraging statistics than those currently recorded.

Currently, the choice of treatment is influenced by the stage of the disease, the age and general condition of the patient and the existing knowledge of the mechanisms of spread of the neoplasm. Even when the tumour is confined to the breast, metastases may become apparent 10–20 years later. Consideration of the systemic nature of the disease influences treatment. Radical mastectomy may be advocated, or a modified radical or simple mastectomy may be the procedure selected, combined with radiation or chemotherapy. The initial treatment of surgery and/or radiation and chemotherapy is believed to increase the body's level of immunity.

Surgical treatment
Radical mastectomy is the operation adopted by many surgeons and involves removal of the complete breast, the underlying pectoralis (major and minor) muscles and the axillary lymphatics and lymph nodes. A large area of the overlying skin is removed and, if the remaining skin flaps cannot be approximated without a good deal of tension, a skin graft is done. The anterior surface of the thigh is the usual donor site.

A *modified radical mastectomy* is a more conservative procedure which removes the breast, axillary lymphatics and lymph nodes and leaves the pectoral muscles. This is frequently the operation performed when the patient's disease is found to be in Stage I or II. Removal of the breast leaving the axillary lymphatics, lymph nodes and pectoral muscles intact comprises a *simple mastectomy*.

A *lumpectomy* involves removal of the tumour, leaving the breast intact.

Radiation implantation. Devita[11] notes that as early as 1924 surgeons were attempting to treat breast cancer with local implantation, but that until recently results were vastly better using external beam treatment. However, he confidently reports on recent clinical trials where the patient had local tumour removal leaving the breast intact, removal of the draining lymph nodes, whole breast and lymph node irradiation and direct radiation using interstitial implants of iridium-192 to the tumour site, with marked improvement in results.

Radiation therapy
External radiation therapy may be used as an adjunct to surgery or alone in cases in which the disease is advanced and inoperable, or in which there is a local

recurrence after surgery. For the care of the patient receiving radiation therapy, see p. 155.

Chemotherapy
There is an increasing use of chemotherapeutic agents as an adjunct to mastectomy in the treatment of breast cancer. Combinations of anticancer drugs are usually used. An example of a combination used in therapy is CMF, which is cyclophosphamide (Endoxana) (C), methotrexate (M) and fluorouracil (F). The schedule for administration may vary with patients; if a single drug is used it is usually given intravenously daily for 5 consecutive days every month. In the case of CMF, cyclophosphamide may be taken orally for 2 weeks and the other two drugs (methotrexate and fluorouracil) are given intravenously on certain days.

Adjuvant chemotherapy is prescribed over a long term—one or more years. The drugs are circulated in the blood throughout the body, reaching areas of metastatic disease. They are toxic to many normal cells in addition to cancerous cells, and have severe side-effects. It is important that the nurses caring for patients receiving these drugs be familiar with the action and side-effects, and be prepared to provide the patients with the necessary support and guidance. Adequate instruction may mean the difference between the patient coping with the chemotherapy with minimal interference to her accustomed way of life and being a chronic invalid. See Chapter 9 for side-effects of these chemotherapeutic agents and the nursing responsibilities.

Hormone deprivation
As cited earlier, some patients with carcinoma of the breast experience a remission of their disease when the concentration of certain hormones (mainly oestrogen) is reduced. Their cancer is said to be hormone-dependent. Cells in some breast cancers have a high affinity for oestrogen; these cells are referred to as oestrogen-receptor cells. Moetzinger indicates that approximately 60% of breast cancers are oestrogen-receptor positive.[11] Those patients whose breast cancer tissue has a high oestrogen-receptor content are considered candidates for hormone deprivation by endocrine ablative surgery or anti-oestrogenic chemotherapy.

Oestrogen receptor assays are indicated on all breast cancer tissue at the time of initial diagnosis. It is suggested that the presence of progesterone receptors, in addition to the oestrogen receptors, in breast cancer cells increases the response to hormone depreciation therapy.[11]

The patient may have an oophorectomy (removal of the ovaries), especially if she is premenopausal. This reduces the production of both oestrogen and progesterone. An adrenalectomy or hypophysectomy may also be done to decrease the production of oestrogen if the patient has shown a favourable response to an oophorectomy. The patient who has

---

[11] Devita, Hellman & Rosenburg (1985).

an adrenalectomy will require cortisone replacement therapy (see p. 662 for care following adrenalectomy). If a complete hypophysectomy is done, the administration of cortisone and thyroid extract will be necessary because of the removal of the respective tropic hormones (ACTH and TSH), as well as a vasopressin (Pitressin) preparation to replace the antidiuretic hormone (ADH).

The administration of an androgen (male hormone) may be prescribed alone or in conjunction with one of the above surgical procedures. Androgen therapy is likely to cause masculinization; there is a deepening of the voice, growth of hair on the face and the development of other secondary male characteristics. Cortisone may be ordered even though no adrenalectomy is done; it suppresses adrenocortical activity, thus reducing the secretion of sex hormones by the adrenal glands. Nonsteroidal anti-oestrogen drugs such as tamoxifen citrate (Nolvadex), which bind with oestrogen receptors, may be administered along with the standard chemotherapeutic agents and may be the treatment of choice in post-menopausal women.

BREAST CANCER IN THE MALE

Carcinoma of the breast is relatively rare in the male, usually occurring in the fifth or sixth decade. The course of the disease is similar to that in the female; it readily metastasizes to regional lymph nodes and other structures. It is often unrecognized and neglected in the early stage because of the low incidence in men; as a result, metastases have frequently developed when the patient is first seen. Treatment involves radical mastectomy and radiation therapy or chemotherapy. A bilateral orchidectomy (removal of the testes) and hormonal therapy may also be used.

Preoperative care

POTENTIAL PATIENT PROBLEMS

Potential problems of the patient going to have breast surgery (see Table 24.1) are:
1 Lack of information about hospital routines, the surgical procedure, pre- and postoperative care.
2 Anticipatory grieving related to the loss of a breast, potential threat to life, potential disfigurement and the potential or actual diagnosis of cancer and alteration in body image and femininity.

NURSING INTERVENTION

1. Lack of information
The *goal* is to help the patient understand the hospital routines, the surgical procedure and pre- and postoperative care.
The nurse explains hospital routines and pro-

cedures to the patient and family and, if possible, introduces them to a member of the nursing staff of the operating theatre. The patient and family are told what the preoperative physical preparation will involve; what to expect on arrival in the operating room; and the routine assessment of blood pressure, pulse and level of consciousness that will take place in the post anaesthetic recovery period. Family members are informed of the services available to them during the surgery and how they will be informed about the patient's progress.

Deep breathing, coughing and arm exercises are demonstrated by the nurse and opportunity is provided for the patient to practise them.

The patient is informed that fluids will be administered intravenously postoperatively, what measures will be provided to relieve pain and how the nurse will assist her with deep breathing and coughing and in performing arm exercises. The type of drainage system to be used in the incision is also described.

The nurse assesses the patient's understanding of the diagnosis and operative procedure, reinforces information provided by the surgeon and allows the patient and family to ask questions, express concerns and explore the implications of the surgery for them.

If there has not been a previous biopsy to determine if the mass is benign or malignant, the patient may be uncertain of the extent of surgery to be performed. Before operation, the surgeon explains to the patient and the family the procedure that will be followed and the operative consent form indicates 'biopsy and possible radical mastectomy'.

The patient must be informed of the possibility and must sign the consent form for a mastectomy, or the mastectomy will be performed at a later date following the biopsy. The patient is then able to make an informed decision about the extent of the surgery to be performed.

2. Anticipatory grieving
The *goals* are to:
1 Reduce anxiety and fear
2 Express feelings and concerns

The general public has become more aware of cancer but, unfortunately, many persons do not realize that a large number of cancer patients who receive early treatment are cured. To many, the word cancer only implies suffering, mutilation and death. In many instances fear of learning the truth leads to delay in seeking medical advice.

The impact of being advised of the need for a biopsy and possible radical mastectomy if the mass is cancerous understandably evokes fears and emotional reactions in the patient. Her anxiety may be focused upon suffering, disfigurement, loss of femininity, or death. How she will react is unpredictable; responses and behaviour are individualized, depending on background and previous experi-

Table 24.1 Identification of problems and needs relevant to the patient having breast surgery.

Problem	Causative factors	Goals
Preoperative		
1 Knowledge deficit related to hospital routines, the surgical procedure, pre- and postoperative care.	Lack of knowledge Anxiety	To acquire understanding of hospital routines, the surgical procedure, pre- and postoperative care
2 Anticipatory grieving	Potential loss of breast Potential threat to life Potential disfigurement Potential or actual diagnosis of cancer Potential alteration in body image and femininity	
Postoperative		
1 Potential for injury	Surgical intervention Potential complications Incomplete healing process	To maintain body functioning To prevent complications To promote healing
2 Alteration in comfort: acute pain	Surgical intervention Anxiety	To control pain and discomfort
3 Ineffective breathing pattern	Surgical intervention Pain and discomfort	To maintain respiratory functioning
4 Alteration in nutrition: less than body requirements	Decreased oral intake following surgery and anaesthesia Increased body needs for repair and healing	To maintain nutritional and fluid status
5 Ineffective individual coping mechanisms	Loss of a breast The threat of death Altered self-image	To reduce emotional distress To develop constructive coping skills
6 Impaired mobility of the affected arm	Surgical procedure and removal of axillary lymph nodes Pain and discomfort Oedema of arm	To restore normal functioning of the affected arm
7 Disturbance in body image	Loss of a breast	To identify the impact of disease and surgery on body image and sexuality To restore feelings of attractiveness To discuss ways of maintaining sexual identity
8 Lack of knowledge about wound care, protection and use of the affected arm and follow up health care	Lack of knowledge Anxiety, denial or anger	To understand the treatment plan, wound care and exercises To be aware of community resources To develop a plan for continuing care and therapy

ences. One patient may appear quite unconcerned but actually is in turmoil underneath her composure. Some may be withdrawn and unresponsive, others are angry and resentful that this should happen to them, and a few may be actually disorganized. The patient may have feelings of helplessness, loneliness and abandonment. Each patient requires the support of a nurse who understands and appreciates what the implications of the situation may be for the woman and her family.

The nurse needs to know what the surgeon has told the patient and should observe her closely for her reactions. The patient is encouraged and is given opportunities to talk about the situation and ask questions. In this way, the nurse learns of the patient's particular concerns and can discuss them, appropriately clarifying misconceptions. Being able to express her fears openly and being aware of the nurse's understanding and available support generally help to reduce the patient's level of anxiety and promote acceptance of the situation. A highly anxious patient will have difficulty processing the volume of information she is faced with preoperatively. Information is introduced gradually, repeated and reinforced to assist the patient in making critical decisions that will affect her future.

Physical preparation
Usually, there is a minimal period of preparation; the surgery is considered urgent in order to prevent spread of the disease if possible. Investigation to detect metastases may include a chest x-ray, liver and bone scanning and determination of the alkaline phosphatase concentration in the blood. The patient's blood is typed and cross-matched, and blood is made available for transfusion. Her general condition is assessed, and erythrocyte and haemoglobin estimations are made. If anaemia is present, a transfusion may be ordered preoperatively. The fluid intake is increased to ensure optimum hydration.

The local skin preparation (shaving and cleansing) is ordered by the surgeon. It usually extends from above the clavicle to the umbilical level, and from the nipple line on the unaffected side to the back on the affected side, and includes the axilla and the arm to the elbow. If the surgeon anticipates the need for skin grafting, preparation of an indicated donor site will be necessary. A sedative is generally given the night before operation to ensure adequate rest. The remainder of the preparation conforms to general preoperative preparation (see Chapter 11).

EXPECTED OUTCOMES

1 The patient and family indicate an understanding of the surgery and implications for the patient.
2 The patient and family show a general understanding of hospital policies, preoperative care and immediate postoperative management of the patient.
3 The patient and family express feelings and concerns regarding the implications of the diagnosis and surgery.
4 The patient demonstrates deep breathing, coughing and arm exercises.

Postoperative care (see Table 24.1)

If the patient's surgery involves only resection of a tumour and not mastectomy, nursing intervention related to the patient's physiological needs is minimal. A nurse remains with the patient until she recovers from the anaesthetic; she is then made comfortable and is left to rest. The doctor visits to advise her of the pathological findings. She may be permitted to be up later that day or the next morning and, if no further surgery is required, she is usually discharged from the hospital on the second or third postoperative day. The sutures are removed in 5–7 days in the doctor's office or surgical clinic.

If a mastectomy was done, the following potential problems should be taken into consideration:

POTENTIAL PATIENT PROBLEMS

1 Potential for injury and complications due to

surgical intervention and incomplete healing process
2 Alteration in comfort: acute pain related to surgical intervention and anxiety
3 Ineffective breathing pattern related to surgical intervention, pain and discomfort
4 Alteration in nutrition: less than body requirements, related to decreased oral intake following surgery and anaesthesia, and increased body needs for repair and healing
5 Ineffective individual coping mechanisms, related to loss of a breast, the threat of death and altered self-image
6 Impaired mobility, pain, discomfort and oedema of the affected arm related to the surgical procedure
7 Disturbance in self-image related to loss of breast
8 Lack of knowledge about wound care, protection and use of the affected arm and follow-up health care

1. Potential for injury and complications
The *goals* are to:
1 Maintain body functioning
2 Prevent complications
3 Promote healing

Assessment. The breast has an abundant blood supply, which increases the blood loss during surgery and the risk of postoperative haemorrhage. Close observation of the patient is maintained during the first 36–48 hours to detect early signs of shock or haemorrhage. The dressings are inspected for blood, and the bedding under the affected side is also checked, since blood may not be visible on the dressing because of its flow over the patient's side or from the axillary area. The space between the chest wall and the skin may be drained by a tube brought out through a stab wound and attached to a wound suction receptacle (Redivac). The amount and colour of the drainage are noted at frequent intervals, and any indication of bleeding is reported at once. The removal of the serosanguineous fluid promotes healing as the underlying space is reduced and the skin flaps are brought into apposition with the chest wall.

The patient's blood pressure, pulse, colour and responses are recorded at frequent intervals. Her reaction to the mastectomy is also noted, since emotional disturbance may contribute to shock. Throughout the patient's hospitalization, the affected arm is checked frequently for oedema and, after 48 hours, the range of motion.

Positioning. When the patient is responding fully, the head of the bed is gradually elevated to promote wound drainage. The patient is turned on the unaffected side every 2 hours. The affected arm is immobilized for 24 hours to prevent haemorrhage and wound strain. The immobilization is usually achieved by enclosing the arm within the strapping or binder that is used to hold the dressings in place. The arm is supported and elevated on a pillow above the level of the right atrium to promote lymphatic and venous drainage. The hand is raised so that it is higher than the elbow. When moving or turning the patient, the arm is *gently* lifted, and any abduction and extension that might increase wound tension are avoided. Arm exercises are started early in the post-operative period, beginning with movements of the hand, wrist and elbow. The patient tends to hold the arm close to the trunk, predisposing to contracture and limited range of shoulder movement. To prevent this a firm pillow is placed between the trunk and the arm to maintain abduction.

Wound care. The dressing is quite bulky and, unless there is bleeding, is usually left undisturbed for several days. The drainage tube may be removed the second or third day, depending on the amount of drainage. Sutures are removed in 7–9 days; the surgeon may remove every other one, leaving the remainder for a few days longer, depending on the healing that has taken place and the degree of tension on the incision. If a skin graft has been done, the donor site dressing may be removed in 3–4 days, leaving the area exposed. It may be quite sensitive and require protection from the bedding. The patient is encouraged to view the wound while it is being dressed so that she gradually becomes accustomed to the permanent change in her appearance prior to discharge from hospital.

Before the patient is discharged from hospital, she is taught how to care for the wound area. It may be bathed as usual but should be gently patted dry; vigorous rubbing is discouraged to prevent wound separation. Gentle massage of the area with petroleum jelly or lanolin may be suggested to increase the elasticity of the skin, which is generally drawn very tightly over the chest wall. The patient is cautioned that if any irritation, redness, open sore or swelling of the wound or swelling of the arm (oedema) occurs she should see her general practitioner.

2. Alteration in comfort
The *goal* is to control pain and discomfort.

An analgesic such as morphine or pethidine is prescribed for the relief of pain during the first 48 hours. A milder analgesic such as codeine is then used if necessary. Turning the patient, slightly changing her position and alternate flexion and extension of the fingers and hand and forearm of the affected arm to promote relaxation or adjustment of supporting pillows may also contribute to the relief of discomfort.

3. Ineffective breathing pattern
The *goal* is to maintain respiratory functioning.

The respirations are likely to be shallow because of the chest wound. To prevent pulmonary complications, the patient is encouraged to take several deep breaths and cough at frequent intervals during the first few days postoperatively. Gentle support to the affected side while deep breathing and coughing may lessen the discomfort and be reassuring to the patient.

4. Alteration in nutrition
The *goal* is to maintain nutritional and fluid status.

There is a considerable loss of blood and fluid during a radical mastectomy. A blood transfusion is frequently given during the surgery or immediately after. Fluids are given intravenously the day of operation to replace the loss and may be continued until sufficient quantities are taken orally. The patient is given fluids by mouth as soon as she can tolerate them and is progressed to a regular diet accordingly.

5. Ineffective individual coping mechanism
The *goals* are to:
1 Reduce emotional distress
2 Develop constructive coping skills

The patient who has had a mastectomy requires a great deal of support and needs to know that someone understands her problems. The psychological impact of having cancer and experiencing the loss of a breast is great and, even though the patient was well prepared before operation, shock and depression follow, especially when the dressing is removed and the operative area is seen. The nurse indicates a willingness to listen to the patient, acknowledging and accepting her reactions. If she is withdrawn, efforts are made to have her talk and express her despair.

Graydon, in summarizing the results of studies of how women cope with breast cancer, found that the period of distress for most women is not immediately after the surgery but 2 or more months later.[12] Denial and other coping mechanisms break down over time and awareness of the loss increases. Most women cope effectively with the experience within 3 months to a year following surgery.

Nursing intervention to help women cope following breast surgery for cancer includes identification of the coping strategies used by the individual, and support of the most effective of these. The nurse can provide support initially following surgery by listening to the patient, acknowledging and accepting her reactions.

Long-term support for the patient is necessary; identification of people who the patient feels can provide support throughout hospitalization and recovery is important.

Friends provide additional support for the patient, as do women who have had a mastectomy. The patient is informed of community health services available to her, The Mastectomy Association and

[12] Graydon (1982), p. 49.

local self-help groups such as 'Coping with Cancer' and BACUP.[13] These groups enable patients to give and receive support as well as to share experiences.

It is helpful to talk with the family, especially the husband, to alert them to the patient's depression and fear of rejection and to seek their cooperation. The family should tactfully show that their relationships have not changed and that the patient is still acceptable to them. The husband is advised of the marked change in his wife's physical appearance and told that this can be corrected by prosthesis.

6. Impaired mobility of the affected arm
The *goal* is to restore normal functioning of the affected arm.

The patient is usually assisted out of bed the day after the operation if her vital signs are stable. The affected arm is supported to decrease tension, oedema and discomfort caused by movement and dependency. A nurse remains with her to determine her reaction and provides support when she is walking or going to the toilet because her balance and accustomed pattern of movement are interfered with by the immobilization of the arm.

Exercise of the affected arm is necessary soon after the operation to promote circulation and lymph drainage, prevent contracture and limited range of movement and restore normal function.

During the first few days, the patient is encouraged to alternately flex and extend the fingers, hand and forearm several times, three or four times a day. Squeezing a soft rubber ball is also a very useful exercise. Then gradual abduction of the arm and raising it over the head are introduced when indicated. The purpose of the exercises is explained, and the patient is advised that to regain the full use of her arm she must begin to use it now. The initial exercises are begun slowly; the frequency, vigour and range of movement are progressively increased from day to day according to the patient's tolerance. Using the affected arm in the performance of self-care activities such as washing the face, bathing, cleansing the teeth and brushing and combing the hair is encouraged by the nurse. See Fig. 24.5.

A more formalized programme of exercises is planned and started for the individual patient or for a group of patients in hospital at the same time. These generally include pulley motion, rope-turning, pendulum-swinging, climbing the wall with the hands, and rod raising. Additional exercises may be included later.

Pulley motion is achieved by throwing a rope over a shower curtain rod or overhead bed bar. The patient takes an end of the rope in each hand, stands straight with arms abducted and extended and pulls the rope up and down in seesaw fashion. When one arm is pulling the rope down, the other arm is raised.

The rope-turning exercise involves circumduction of the arm. A 7- or 8-foot rope is tied to a door knob or a firm, stationary object. The loose end of the rope is held in the hand of the affected arm, which is kept straight. The rope is then swung around in circles as one turns a skipping rope. The range may be limited at first, but the patient is encouraged to progressively make larger circles.

In pendulum-swinging, the patient bends forward from the waist, allowing her arms to fall forward in front of her. They are then swung from side to side in a pendulum motion.

Climbing the walls with the hands requires the patient to stand close to and face a wall and place the palms of her hands against it at shoulder level. Using the fingers in a crawling motion, the hands are moved up the wall as far as she can reach and then down again to shoulder level. The objective is to reach full extension of the arm.

In the rod-raising exercise, a rod (similar to a broom handle) approximately 4 feet long is grasped with the hands as far apart as possible. It is raised over the head, lowered behind the head, raised again and returned to the original position. An exercise which may be substituted for this one entails raising the arms out from the sides to shoulder level, placing the hands behind the neck, extending the arms again, and then lowering them to place the hands behind the lumbar region of the back.

All exercises are done only twice the first day; then, gradually, they are increased from day to day until each is repeated 10 times two or three times daily. When the patient is discharged a written outline of the exercises which she is expected to continue is prepared for her and reviewed by the nurse. The Mastectomy Association[14] have a booklet which illustrates and gives directions for postmastectomy exercises and activities as well as useful information on prostheses. A supply of these booklets should be kept available on the surgical ward for use by the nurse in teaching the patient exercises. A copy is also given to the patient.

Oedema of the arm. The removal of axillary lymphatics and lymph nodes in radical mastectomy predisposes to oedema and swelling of the arm after operation. If it develops, an elastic or crêpe bandage is applied, extending from the wrist to the shoulder. The patient may be fitted with a pressure gradient elastic sleeve. The arm is elevated on pillows during the night. During the day, it is recommended that the patient rest the arm several times on the back of a sofa or a table or something comparable for a brief period.

7. Disturbance in self-image
The *goals* are to:
1 Identify impact of disease and surgery on body image and sexuality.

---

[13] Clement-Jones (1985), pp. 1021–1023.

[14] Mastectomy Association, 24 Harison Street, King's Cross, London WC1.

General instructions

1 Stand erect with head high and arms at sides
2 Place feet hip width apart for balance
3 Flatten abdomen — avoid hollow back
4 Wear comfortable low-heeled shoes or do the
exercises in your stocking feet

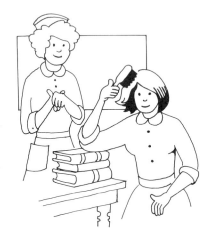

Hair brushing exercise

1 Sit beside a table. In the beginning rest your arm (on the operated side) on a few books. Comb and brush your hair keeping your head erect

2 One side will do to start. Little by little, release your arm from its resting position and work the brush around your head until you are covering the entire scalp

3 Rest whenever you feel the need to, but be persistent. (Your hair will benefit from this too!)

1

Hand and wall climbing

1 Start in a standard position, facing wall, with toes as close to the wall as possible

2 Bend elbows and place palms against the wall at shoulder level

3 Work both hands up the wall parallel to each other until arms are fully extended

4 Work hands down to shoulder level

5 Return to standard position. Rest and repeat

(It will relax you a bit if you rest your head against the wall)

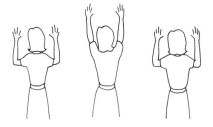

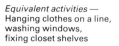

Equivalent activities —
Hanging clothes on a line, washing windows, fixing closet shelves

2

Fig. 24.5 Exercises for the post-mastectomy patient.

2 Restore feelings of attractiveness.
3 Discuss ways of maintaining sexual identity.

Reintegration of body image following mastectomy occurs gradually. Supporting the woman in looking at, feeling and touching the incision helps her to become aware of, and acknowledge, the change in her appearance.

The patient is encouraged to be fitted for a brassiere with a prosthesis. The improvement it makes to her general appearance will raise her morale. The various types of prostheses (e.g. sponge

**Try to work naturally, using your arms
as you always have, when you:**

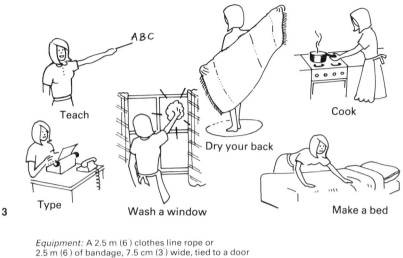

ABC

Teach

Cook

Type

Dry your back

Wash a window

Make a bed

3

Equipment: A 2.5 m (6) clothes line rope or
2.5 m (6) of bandage, 7.5 cm (3) wide, tied to a door
knob with a double knot. This exercise may
seem difficult to do at first but will be
easier in a few days

1 Stand 1.2 m (4) away from the door
in standard position. Face door

2 Take the loose end of the rope in the hand
on your operated side. Make a knot to put
between your third and fourth fingers

3 Place the other hand on your hip
to help your balance

4 Extend arm forward on your operated
side. (Do not bend elbow or wrist.) Turn
rope in small circle at first and gradually
work into as wide a swing as possible

5 Rest and repeat given number of times.
(Try the same exercise with your other
arm occasionally)

Rope turning

4

Fig. 24.5 Exercises for the post-mastectomy patient (continued).

rubber, silicone, or padding) may be described and a list of reliable supply firms with experienced fitters is given to the patient. Prosthesis manufacturers have brochures that should be kept available for exploration by the patient. The nurse shows the patient how to pad the brassieres she has with absorbent cotton covered with soft cotton so they can be used until a properly fitted prosthesis can be worn. The surgeon will indicate when the wound is sufficiently healed that she may wear a prosthesis. The nurse may utilize opportunities to discuss the appearance of the wound with the patient and her partner and explore their feelings about this alteration in her appearance and the effects on sexuality. Nipple stimulation will be absent and oophorectomy and hormone therapy may alter sexual responses. The nurse can provide information, foster open communication between the patient and spouse and encourage them to discuss ways of expressing sexuality and maintaining sexual identity. Breast reconstruction may be possible and should be discussed with the surgeon.

Pulley motion

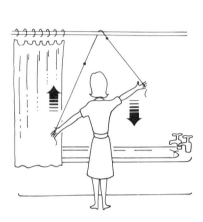

Equipment: A 2.5 m (6´) rope or 2.5 m of bandage, 7.5 cm (3″) wide; a shower rod or similar rod above your head. Place knots in rope at ends and at two intervals (see drawing)

1 Toss the rope over the rod

2 Stand directly behind the rope in a standard position

3 Hold the ends of the rope in each hand with knots between your third and fourth fingers and raise arms sideways

4 Using see-saw motion and with arms stretched sideways, slide the rope up and down over the rod, until the knots in the rope touch the rod

5 Return to standard position, rest and repeat

6 Do not bend at the waist. Keep your feet flat on the floor during this exercise

Equivalent activities: Drying back with bath towel, pulling venetian blinds, or adjusting window shades

5

Elbow pull-in

1 In standard position, extend arms sideways to shoulder level

In rhythm:

2 Bend elbows clasping fingers at back of your neck

3 Pull elbows in toward each other until they touch

4 Return to position (2) with elbows bent — fingers clasped at back of neck

5 Unclasp fingers and extend arms sideways at shoulder level

6 Return to standard position. Rest and repeat

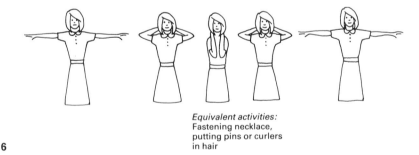

Equivalent activities: Fastening necklace, putting pins or curlers in hair

6

Fig. 24.5 Exercises for the post-mastectomy patient (continued).

If the wound is not completely healed and requires cleansing and dressing, the patient or a member of her family is taught the necessary procedure, or a referral may be made to the district nurse. A district nurse may also be helpful in supervising the patient's exercise programme and care during radiation therapy if it is given.

8. Lack of knowledge
The *goals* are to:
1 Understand the treatment plan, wound care, arm protection and exercises and availability of community resources
2 Develop a plan for continuing care and therapy

Back scratcher

1 Start in standard position

2 Place hand of unoperated side on your hip for balance

3 Bend elbow of arm on operated side until your fingertips reach your shoulder blade — opposite side

4 Return to standard position Rest and repeat

7

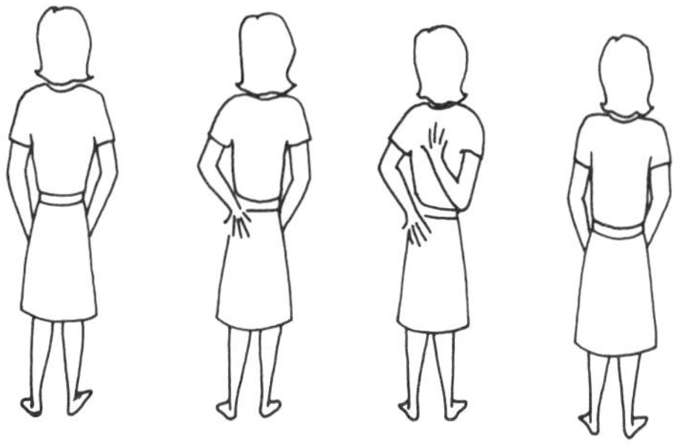

Equivalent activities: Buttoning a blouse which fastens in the back, fastening your bra, washing your back

Paddle swing

1 Start in standard position

2 Bend forward from the waist, allowing arms to hang toward the floor by gravity

3 In this position, place right arm forward over your head; place left arm back. Do not bend elbows

In rhythm:

4 Swing right arm back while left arm comes forward, then allow arms to hang forward as in position (2)

5 Return to standard position. Rest and repeat

It will help you when you do this exercise if you lean on a table or desk, built up with cushions. Rest one side of your body (the unoperated side) on the cushions. It will free the other side for easy swinging. This means that you will only swing the arm on the operated side

8

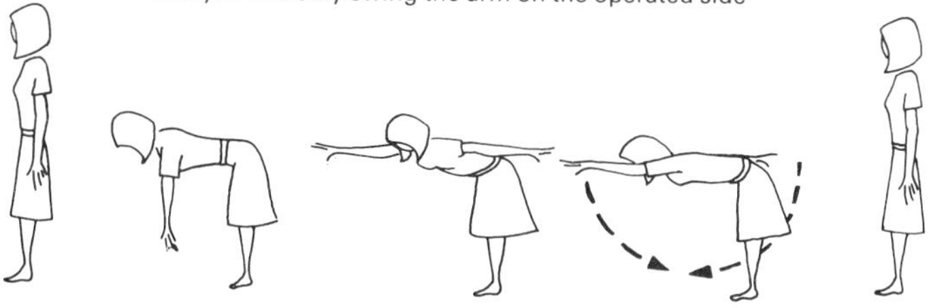

Fig. 24.5 Exercises for the post-mastectomy patient (continued).

The patient is advised that extra precautions should be taken to protect the arm on the operative side. This is necessary because of the loss of the defence mechanisms (lymph nodes, and the lowered resistance associated with the disease), irradiation and chemotherapy. Cuts, scratches, burns and constrictions (e.g. blood pressure cuff or watch with elastic strap) should be avoided. The arm is protected by carrying the purse and heavy articles on the other arm. The arm should not be used for the withdrawal of blood specimens or receiving injections. Jewellery (watch, bracelet, rings) should be worn loosely in case the arm or hand becomes oedematous, resulting in constriction and difficulty in removing rings or a bracelet. The identification card carried by the individual should indicate that needle injections and constriction should not be used on the affected arm, and why (mastectomy lymphoedema). A Medic

Pendulum swing

1 Start in standard position. Bend forward from the waist, allowing arms to hang toward the floor by gravity

2 Swing both arms together, describing an arc from one shoulder to the other. Do not bend elbows. Keep arms parallel

3 Return to standard position and allow arms to fall to sides. Rest and repeat

Equivalent activities:
Sweeping

9

Forehead touch

1 In standard position, face wall at arm's length distance. Place hands against the wall at shoulder level, parallel to each other

2 Slowly bend elbows, leaning forward until forehead touches wall

3 Straighten elbows slowly, pushing body away from wall

4 Return to standard position. Rest and repeat

NOTE: Keep head, trunk and legs in straight line throughout exercise

10

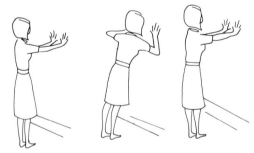

Fig. 24.5 Exercises for the post-mastectomy patient (continued).

Alert pendant or bracelet may be obtained that indicates the need for caution.

If a series of radiation treatments or chemotherapy is to be given, the surgeon discusses this with the patient and advises her when the treatment will commence. It is not usually instituted until the wound is healed, and it may be given on an outpatient basis. The doctor also informs the patient as to when she may resume her household activities or return to her former occupation. The resumption of former activities is encouraged just as soon as the patient is well enough. It relieves her depression and leaves her less time to concentrate on her disease. Use of the involved arm is encouraged and arm exercises should be carried out daily as scheduled.

A close follow-up is necessary; the patient is

Arm bending

1 In standard position extend arms sideways to shoulder level

In rhythm:

2 Bend elbows, touching fingers at back of neck

3 Extend arms sideways to shoulder level

4 Bends elbows, touching fingers at back of waist

5 Return to standard position, rest and repeat

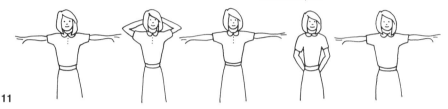

Equivalent activities — Drying back with bath towel

11

Fig. 24.5 Exercises for the post-mastectomy patient (continued).

required to make frequent visits to her doctor or the cancer clinic during the first year or two. Then, if there has been no evidence of recurrence of her disease, the interval between examinations is lengthened to 6 months or 1 year.

All patients are taught self-examination of the breast and are informed of the importance of examining the remaining breast each month.

A series of tests including liver and bone scans and blood tests are performed to rule out the presence of metastasis. The nurse prepares the patient for these tests and explains the purpose of the adjuvant therapy.

Once chemotherapy has begun, the patient requires information about the actions and side-effects of the drugs and measures that help prevent or alleviate adverse reactions. If the patient experiences nausea, an antiemetic is given with each treatment. Fluid intake is increased to prevent bladder irritation from cyclophosphamide. Relaxation techniques may be taught to decrease the nausea following treatment. The nurse helps the patient establish a schedule for medication that is least disruptive to her life-style. For example, medications may be given on Friday afternoons for women who are working, allowing her to remain at home over the weekend when adverse effects from the drugs are most likely to occur.

EXPECTED OUTCOMES

1 The incision is clean, dry and intact.
2 Pain and discomfort are controlled or absent.
3 Respirations are normal in rate, depth and rhythm.

4 Weight loss is less than 2 kg (5 lb).
5 The patient describes and demonstrates arm exercises.
6 Range of motion in the affected arm and shoulder are within normal range.
7 The patient selects a comfortable, correctly fitted breast prosthesis.
8 The patient expresses feelings of satisfaction with her appearance.
9 The patient begins to participate in usual social activities.
10 The patient resumes usual sexual relations.
11 The patient describes plans for a health maintenance programme:
  (a) Treatment schedule
  (b) On-going tests and medical follow-up
  (c) Measures to prevent infection
  (d) Arm and shoulder exercises
  (e) Protection of the affected arm
  (f) Self-examination of the remaining breast.

INFECTION OF THE BREAST

Infection of the breast causes acute mastitis and most commonly occurs during lactation. The causative organism enters through a fissure or abrasion of the nipple which might have been prevented by careful cleansing and protection. The patient's temperature is elevated, and the breast becomes firm, red, painful and very tender. The patient is given an antibiotic and kept at rest. The baby is taken off the breast temporarily, and hot or cold applications may be ordered. Unless the infection is checked in the early stage, suppuration may develop, necessitating surgical drainage.

Mammoplasty

Mammoplasty is surgical intervention to alter the size and shape of the breasts. *Augmentation mammoplasty* is done to enlarge the breasts and involves the placement of a silastic[15] prosthesis in a surgically constructed pocket between the capsule of the breast and the pectoral fascia.

Breast reduction involves removal of breast tissue to construct breasts that are more normal in size and shape.

The breast holds significance for all women and has a profound impact on one's self-image and sexuality. Breasts that are too small or too large by cultural or individual standards do affect how the individual views herself and how she relates to others. Rationale for the surgery is very individualistic.

Large breast reduction surgery is also done to relieve backache and shoulder pain. Large breasts may also interfere with activities such as driving a car, or operating machines. They can be equally as embarrassing to the individual as small breasts.

Breast reconstruction[16] may be done following mastectomy. Newer techniques enable the creation of a breast that resembles the natural breast in size, shape and feel. The patient's nipple may be implanted in the inguinal area at the time of the mastectomy and later used in the breast reconstruction.

---

[15] *Silastic*: a silicone substance with rubber-like properties. It is biologically inert.
[16] Dinner & Bateman (1985), pp. 490–496.

References and Further Reading

BOOKS

Bouchard-Kurtz R & Speese-Owens N (1981) *Nursing care of the Cancer Patient*, 4th ed. St Louis: CV Mosby, Chapter 16.

Brain MC & Carbone PP (1985) *Current Therapy in Hematology—Oncology*. St Louis: CV Mosby. pp. 162–178.

Cahoon MC (ed) (1982) *Cancer Nursing*. Edinburgh: Churchill Livingstone. Chapter 3.

Coombes RC et al (1981) *Breast Cancer Management*. London: Academic Press.

Devita VT, Hellman S & Rosenburg SA (1985) *Cancer: Principles and Practice of Oncology*, 2nd ed. Philadelphia: JB Lippinncott.

Fields, WL & McGinn-Campbell KM (1983) *Introduction to Health Assessment*. Reston, Virginia: Reston. Chapter 12.

Graydon JE (1982) Physiological and psychosocial aspects of breast cancer. In: MC Cahoon (ed), *Cancer Nursing*. Edinburgh: Churchill Livingstone.

Krupp M & Chatton MJ (eds) (1983) *Current Medical Diagnosis and Treatment*, Los Altos, CA: Lange Chapter 11.

McLean M (1980) *If You Find a Lump in Your Breast*. Palo Alto: Bull Publishing.

Robbins SL, Angell M & Kumar V (1981) *Basic Pathophysiology*, 3rd ed. Philadelphia: WB Saunders. pp. 585–594.

Rubin P (ed) (1983) *Clinical Oncology: A Multidisciplinary Approach*. The American Cancer Society. pp. 120–140.

Sabiston DC (ed) (1986) *Textbook of Surgery*, 13th ed. Philadelphia: WB Saunders. Chapter 22.

Sims R & Fitzgerald V (1985) *Community Nursing Management of Patients with Ulcerative/Furgating Malignant Breast Disease*. London: RCN.

Tait A & Maguire P (1987) *Caring for Patients with Breast Disease*. Beaconsfield, England.

The Royal Marsden Hospital (1984) *Manual of Clinical Nursing Policies and Procedures*. London: Harper & Row.

The Royal Marsden Hospital (1986) Patient education leaflet. *Breast Self-Examination*. Available from Haigh Hochland Booksellers, Oxford Road, Manchester.

PERIODICALS

Buchanan-Davidson DJ (1980) *Is breast cancer the same in men and women? Cancer Nurs.*, Vol. 3 No. 2, pp. 121–130.

Bullough B (1981) Nurses as teachers and support persons for breast cancer patients. *Cancer Nurs.*, Vol. 4 No. 3, pp. 221–225.

Calnan M (1985) An evaluation of the effectiveness of a class teaching breast self-examination. *Br. J. Med. Psychol.*, Vol. 58 No. 4, p. 317–329.

Cohen RJ (1984) Diagnosis: breast cancer. *Hosp. Med.*, Vol. 20 No. 7, pp. 81, 82, 86, 88–89, 92–93, 96–98, 102.

Clement-Jones V (1985) Cancer and beyond; the formation of BACUP (British Association of Cancer United Patients and their Families and Friends). *Br. Med. J.*, Vol. 291, pp. 1021–1023.

Dinner MI & Bateman C (1985) Breast reconstruction: use of autogenous tissue. *AORN J.*, Vol. 42 No. 4, pp. 490–496.

Eich SJ (1985) Promising early breast cancer treatment without mastectomy. *Cancer Nurs.*, Vol. 8 No. 1, pp. 51–58.

Ellerton ML & Smillie CL (1983) Do you believe in screening. *Cancer Nurs.*, Vol. 79 No. 2, pp. 34–36.

Fisher B (1977) Adjuvant chemotherapy in primary management of breast cancer. *Med. Clin. N. Am.*, Vol. 61 No. 5, pp. 953–965.

Flynn KT & Durivage HJ (1982) Anti-estrogen therapy for breast cancer: focus on Tamoxifen. *Onc. Nurs. Forum*, Vol. 9 No. 4, pp. 21–25.

Frank DI (1981) Sexual counseling to a mastectomy patient. *Nurs. '81*, Vol. 11 No. 1, pp. 64–67.

Ginsberg SJ (1982) Timely detection: key to optimal management of breast cancer. *Geriatrics*, Vol. 37 No. 1, pp. 97–106.

Greenwald et al (1978) Estimated effect of breast self-examination and routine physician examinations on breast cancer mortality. *N. Engl. J. Med.*, Vol. 299 No. 6, pp. 271–273.

Hassey KM, Bloom LS & Burgess SL (1983) Radiation: alternative to mastectomy. *Am. J. Nurs.*, Vol. 83 No. 11, pp. 1567–1569.

Hirshfield-Bartek J (1982) Health beliefs and their influence on breast self-examination practices in women with breast cancer. *Onc. Nurs. Forum*, Vol. 9 No. 3, pp. 77–81.

Kinnie DW (1982) Opinion: the case of the one-step biopsy procedure for breast cancer. *Ca-A Cancer. J. Clin.*, Vol. 32 No. 1, pp. 46–50.

Knobf MKT (1984) Breast cancer: the treatment evolution. *Am. J. Nurs.*, Vol. 84 No. 9, pp. 1110–1120.

Lamb MA & Woods NF (1981) Sexuality and the cancer patient. *Cancer Nurs.*, Vol. 4 No. 2, pp. 137–144.

Lindsey AM, Norbeck JS, Carrieri VL & Perry E (1981) Social support and outcomes in postmastectomy women: a review. *Cancer Nurs.*, Vol. 4 No. 5, pp. 377–383.

McMaster V (1985) Evaluation of breast self-examination teaching materials in primary care setting. *J. R. Coll. Gen. Pract.*, Vol. 35 No. 12, p. 578–580.

Margolese RG (1982) Response: the case for the two-step biopsy procedures for breast cancer. *Ca-A Cancer J. Clin.*, Vol. 32 No. 1, pp. 51–57.

Marszalek EJ & Solomon JS (1981) A breast counseling service. *Am. J. Nurs.*, Vol. 81 No. 9, pp. 1658–1659.

Michalek AM, Walsh D, Burns P & Mettlin M (1981) Report on a BSE educational program for lay audiences conducted by nurse health educators. *Cancer Nurs.*, Vol. 4 No. 5, pp. 385–388.

Moetzinger CA & Dauber LG (1982) The management of the patient with breast cancer. *Cancer Nurs.*, Vol. 5 No. 4, pp. 287–291.

Morthouse LL (1982) Coping with mastectomy crises. *Top. Clin. Nurs.*, Vol. 4 No. 2, pp. 57–65.

Nail L, Jones LS, Giuffre M & Johnson JE (1984) Sensations after mastectomy. *Am. J. Nurs.*, Vol. 84 No. 9, pp. 1121–1124.

Northouse LL (1981) Mastectomy patients and the fear of cancer recurrence. *Cancer Nurs.*, Vol. 4 No. 3, pp. 213–220.

Oberst MT (1981) Testing approaches to teaching breast self-examination. *Cancer Nurs.*, Vol. 4 No. 3, p. 246.

Olenn MB (1981) Motivating BSE. *Am. J. Nurs.*, Vol. 81 No. 9, pp. 1656–1657.

Reich SD (1981) Estrogen receptors and advanced breast cancer. *Cancer Nurs.*, Vol. 4 No. 3, pp. 247–248.

Reynolds SA, Sachs SH, Davis JM & Hall P (1981) Meeting the information needs of patients on clinical trials: a new approach. *Cancer Nurs.*, Vol. 4 No. 3, pp. 227–230.

Schwarz-Appelbaum J, Dedrick J, Jusenus K & Kirchner CW (1984) Nursing care plans: sexuality and treatment of breast cancer. *Onc. Nurs. Forum*, Vol. 11 No. 6, pp. 16–24.

Scott DW (1983) Quality of life following the diagnosis of breast cancer. *Top. Clin. Nurs.*, Vol. 4 No. 4, pp. 20–37.

Silverberg E (1982) Cancer statistics 1982. *Cancer*, Vol. 32 No. 1, p. 15.

Smith P (1985) Breast models: a useful tool for instruction. *Occup. Hlth. Nurs.*, Vol. 33 No. 10, pp. 513–514.

Stromberg M (1981) Screening for early detection. *Am. J. Nurs.*, Vol. 81 No. 9, pp. 1652–1657.

Townsend CM (1980) Breast lumps. *Clin. Symp.*, Vol. 32 No. 2, pp. 3–30.

Valanis BG & Rumpler CH (1985) Helping women to choose breast cancer treatment. *Cancer Nurs.*, Vol. 8 No. 3, pp. 167–175.

Warren B (1979) Adjuvant chemotherapy for breast disease: the nurse's role. *Cancer Nurs.*, Vol. 2 No. 1, pp. 32–37.

Wilcox PM (1981) Benign breast disorders. *Am. J. Nurs.*, Vol. 81 No. 9, pp. 1644–1651.

Wiley KR (1981) Postbiopsy care. *Am. J. Nurs.*, Vol. 81 No. 9, pp. 1660–1662.

Wilson CA & Strohl RA (1982) Radiation therapy as primary treatment for breast cancer. *Onc. Nurs. Forum*, Vol. 9 No. 1, pp. 12–15.

Wissing VS (1984) Breast cancer: the hormone factor. *Am. J. Nurs.*, Vol. 84 No. 9, pp. 1117–1119.

25

Nursing in
Bone Disorders

Structure and Function of Bones

BONE TISSUE

Bone is a rigid connective tissue consisting of bone cells, calcified collagenous intercellular substance and marrow. Each bone, except at joint surfaces, is covered by a tough, supportive membrane called the *periosteum*. It is firmly attached to the underlying bone by penetrating fibres, and its blood vessels give off many branches which enter the tissue to provide the essentials for growth, repair and maintenance. The inner layer of the periosteum gives rise to the osteoblasts, which function in the development and replacement of bone. The shaft of the long bones is hollow and is lined with a comparable membrane referred to as the *endosteum*. Although approximately two-thirds of bone tissue is inorganic mineral substance, which gives it the characteristic hardness and inert appearance, it is viable tissue undergoing constant metabolic processes, just as other tissues.

Bone tissue contains a network of minute anastomosing canals and spaces which contain blood vessels, lymphatics, lymph and bone cells. The rigid intercellular substance is formed in scale-like sheets or layers (lamellae) around the canals and spaces. It is composed of a tough collagenous network of fibres which becomes impregnated with mineral salts, principally tricalcium phosphate and calcium carbonate.

There are three types of bone cells—osteoblasts, osteocytes and osteoclasts. The *osteoblasts* are found beneath the periosteum on the surface of growing bones and in developmental or ossification areas within the bones. They are responsible for the formation of the collageneous fibres, the organic bone matrix and the deposition of the mineral salts. The *osteocytes* are matured osteoblasts which become imprisoned in small spaces by the calcification. It is believed these regulate bone metabolism. The *osteoclasts* are considered responsible for the breaking down and reabsorption of bone tissue. Normally, there is a constant turnover of the mineral deposits. This continuous breaking down, reabsorption and new bone formation is necessary, since old bone becomes weak and brittle. The bone cells respond by internal reconstruction according to the forces acting upon the tissue. The mineralization and strength of the bones are influenced by the amount of weight-bearing and muscle pull to which the bones are subjected. Those of the active person and of an athlete are stronger and more resistant to stress than the bones of non-active persons. One of the complications of prolonged bed rest is the decalcification and weakening of the bones; the calcium is excreted by the kidneys and there is therefore a risk of the formation of renal calculi. In older persons the bones tend to become brittle and less resistant to stress, increasing the possibility of fractures. This is due to the general decline in cell reproduction which results in a slower rate of production of the collagenous matrix and mineralization as well as of reabsorption.

Types of bone tissue

Each bone is composed of two types of tissue—compact and cancellous. Outer layers consist of dense, *compact tissue* (cortical bone), and the interior is of a spongy or porous nature (*cancellous*). The numerous larger spaces of cancellous tissue contain *red bone marrow*. The thickness of each type of tissue varies in different bones as well as in parts of the same bone.

In the long bone (e.g. humerus, tibia, femur), the extremities have a thin outer layer of compact tissue enclosing a larger mass of cancellous tissue (see Fig. 25.1). The shaft is formed mainly of two thick layers of compact bone separated by a small amount of porous tissue. The central hollow portion of the shaft forms the medullary canal, which is filled with fatty, *yellow marrow*. Flat bones (e.g. skull bones, scapula, ribs) have a thicker layer of cancellous tissue lying between two relatively thinner layers of compact tissue. Short and irregular bones such as those of the wrist and ankle have a thin shell of compact tissue enclosing a fair thickness of cancellous tissue.

Functions of bones and contained marrow

The bones are bound together by ligaments and collectively form the skeleton, which provides a supporting framework for the body and protection for vital structures. They assist in body movement by providing attachment for muscles and leverage for their action. The bones also serve as the body's store of calcium. A constant level in the blood and tissue fluid is necessary for several physiological processes (e.g. blood clotting, normal muscular activity, normal heart action). If the blood calcium falls below the normal level, the deficit may be met by the withdrawal of calcium from the bones. Conversely, much of the excess in the blood is desposited in bone tissue.

The red bone marrow is a highly vascular haemopoietic tissue contained within the spaces of cancellous tissue. It produces erythrocytes, granulocytes and thrombocytes (blood platelets). During childhood, all cancellous tissue contains red marrow. In the adult, much of this is replaced by yellow marrow, and the cancellous tissue of the ribs, sternum, skull bones, vertebrae, pelvic bones and the proximal ends of the long bones play the major role in haemopoiesis. Yellow bone marrow consists mainly of fat cells and blood vessels; the largest amount is found in the medullary canals of long bones.

The development and growth of bones

The development of the bones begins early in embryonic life and is not normally completed until the late teens or early twenties. They are composed of membranous connective tissue or cartilaginous tissue, which is gradually replaced by bone in the process of ossification.

The cranial bones and the mandible (lower jaw) develop by *intramembranous ossification*. There is a marked increase in the vascularity of the membranous tissue. This is followed by the appearance of localized centres of ossification from which bone formation proceeds to the periphery. Radiating bundles of fibres and osteoblasts appear between the blood vessels, followed by the development of the collagenous fibrous matrix which becomes impregnated with calcium salts. The original membrane becomes the periosteum. As the conversion to bone proceeds outward, the edges of the membranous tissue continue to grow. When ossification overtakes the growth of the membranous tissue, the full size of the bone has been reached. The continued growth of the membranous tissue of the cranial bones accounts for the 'soft' areas or fontanelles in the skull in the infant.

The bones which are preformed of cartilage undergo *intracartilaginous (endochondral) ossification*, which involves destruction of the cartilage and its replacement by bone tissue. Osteoblasts develop at the surface of the cartilage and initiate the formation of surface layers of bone tissue by producing a collagenous fibrous matrix in which mineral salts are deposited. Then osteoblasts, osteoclasts and blood vessels invade internal areas of the cartilage, setting up ossification centres around which cartilage is progressively removed and replaced by bone tissue.

In long bones (Fig. 25.1), an ossification centre appears within the shaft (*diaphysis*) and later in each end (*epiphysis*). As ossification proceeds, growth of the cartilage continues, resulting in a persisting thin

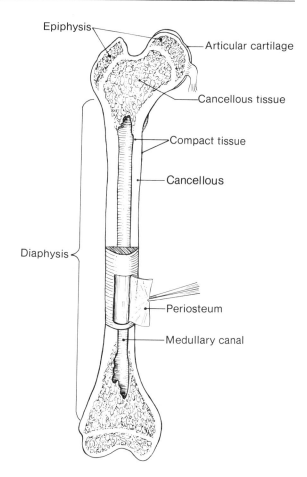

Fig. 25.1 Diagram of a long bone.

strip of cartilaginous tissue between each epiphysis and the diaphysis, which is referred to as the *growth or epiphyseal plate*. The bones continue to grow as long as new cartilage develops to maintain this plate. Cessation of growth occurs when it becomes ossified, and the epiphyses are fused with the diaphysis. Bones grow in circumference by the formation of layers of bone beneath the periosteum.

FACTORS IN BONE DEVELOPMENT, GROWTH AND REPAIR

Several factors influence the development, growth and maintenance of normal bone structure. A diet which is adequate in calcium and phosphorus is essential for ossification and the constant formation of new bone to replace that which is reabsorbed. Vitamin D is necessary for the absorption and utilization of the minerals. A deficiency of any one of these substances in children may lead to *rickets*, which is characterized by soft deformed bones, failure of closure of the fontanelles, soft and poorly developed teeth, bleeding tendency and muscle spasms. In adults, a deficiency of calcium and phosphorus or vitamin D may cause a weakening of bone structure referred to as *osteomalacia*. Milk and milk products provide an abundant source of the minerals. Vitamin D may be formed by exposure of the skin to sunlight, which acts on a sterol (7-dehydrocholesterol) that is a component of the skin. To ensure an adequate supply of vitamin D, a preparation of fish liver oil (e.g. cod liver oil) or of ergosterol which has been exposed to ultraviolet rays (calciferol) may be administered to infants and children. The nurse must be cognizant of the fact that excessive amounts of vitamin D can cause hypercalcaemia, which may be manifested by anorexia, nausea, vomiting, drowsiness, headache, heart irregularity, bladder irritation and renal calculi. Liver and kidney functions are necessary to convert the inactive vitamin D to the active metabolite dihydroxycholecalciferol.

Adequate dietary amounts of protein and vitamin C are necessary to bones for the formation of the collagenous, fibrous, intercellular matrix in which the minerals are deposited. Vitamin A, which is essential to all tissue growth, is also necessary.

Bone growth and ossification are also influenced by certain hormones—namely, the somatotrophic or growth hormone produced by the anterior pituitary, thyroid and parathyroid hormones (see Chapter 20). Bone metabolism is also affected by oestrogen, androgens and calcitonin.

In addition to the above factors, the demand placed on the bones by weight-bearing and muscle pull plays an important role. Inactivity and less than the normal demand weaken the structure; calcium and phosphorus are lost from the bone, and the condition known as oesteoporosis may develop. Osteoblastic activity is slowed, and bone deposition is depressed. Muscle pull and the degree of stress also influence the shaping of the bone. For example, processes such as the greater and lesser trochanters of the femur, the tibial tuberosity of the tibia, and the deltoid tuberosity of the radius develop as the result of muscle pull when the bones are developing and growing.

Assessment

Assessment of the patient with bone disorders focuses on the major functions of the bones, which are to provide a supporting framework for the body, protect the vital organs and assist in movement. The haemopoietic functions of bone tissue are discussed in Chapter 13.

HISTORY

The initial health history obtained from a patient with a bone disorder will vary with the circumstances. Accidental trauma to the skeletal system may limit the amount of information available prior to treatment. If possible, the nurse should determine the cause and circumstances of the injury, when it occurred and actions taken since the injury. The conscious patient is questioned regarding the characteristics and severity of pain and any resulting changes in sensation, movement or appearance.

Assessment of *pain* includes identifying the: (1) location, (2) duration, (3) severity of the pain, (4) radiation or localization of the pain, (5) factors or circumstances causing or aggravating the pain, and (6) measures which are effective in alleviating the pain.

The patient's perceptions of changes in the structure of the body area such as swelling, muscular atrophy or physical deformity are determined. The health history also identifies the patient's usual patterns of physical activity, recent changes in the usual pattern, and the effect of the present problem on daily physical functioning. Measures used by the patient to compensate for any physical losses, stiffness, or weakness also are identified.

The past medical history includes information on congenital defects, trauma or surgery to the musculoskeletal system and diseases, such as poliomyelitis, arthritis, gout, renal failure, joint and collagen diseases, malnutrition or neuromuscular disorders that may affect bone structure and function.

A detailed list of drugs taken by the patient, their dosage, frequency and duration of use is obtained.

The occupational history identifies physical activities related to the job, such as heavy lifting, pushing or prolonged standing or sitting.

PHYSICAL EXAMINATION

Inspection and palpation are the primary techniques used to examine the skeletal system. Physical examination of joints is discussed in Chapter 26. Since examination of bones is incomplete without assessment of joint movement, the reader is referred to pp. 1002–1008.

Inspection begins by observing the patient's general appearance, posture, gait and the manner in which the patient performs basic activities. General body build, musculature, body fat and ease of movement are observed. Examination of the skeletal system should progress from head to toe, with the examiner comparing the symmetry of structures and movement. The body part being examined must be appropriately exposed to permit good visualization without unduly compromising the patient's privacy. Normally, extremities appear smooth and symmetrical without deformity, swelling, bony protrusions or masses. The length of the extremities or individual bones is measured with a tape-measure and compared with the opposite side. With the patient lying on a firm surface, the arm is measured from the acromion process of the shoulder to the tip of the middle finger. Lower extremities are measured for real shortening from the lower edge of the anterior superior iliac spine to the medial malleolus of the leg on the same side and this is repeated for the other leg. Apparent shortening is assessed by measuring from a fixed point in the midline of the body (e.g. the umbilicus) to each medial malleolus in turn.

Symmetry, size and tone of muscle mass are observed; disuse causes atrophy of muscles and pain leads to contraction of the involved muscle.

Palpation of bones may require adjustment of the position of the part to relax adjoining muscles to permit the examiner to feel the bones. Bones normally feel firm and smooth. Any pain, tenderness on pressure or irregularity of contour are noted.

If abnormalities are detected, further neurological examination may be warranted. Neurological examination includes assessment of sensation, reflex response and motor function (see Chapter 22).

Gait. To assess the patient's gait, the examiner asks the patient to walk: the movements are observed from all angles. Examination of the patient's gait is performed for both diagnostic and therapeutic purposes. Human locomotion or movement of the body from one place to another is complex and requires a series of measurements throughout the entire cycle. The normal gait has two phases, the *stance* phase and the *swing* phase, with each step approximately 38 cm (15 in) in length. The stance, which is 60% of the cycle, consists of the following: (1) the heel strikes the ground with the knee extended; (2) the foot is placed flat as the knee begins to flex; (3) the knee flexes and weight is evenly distributed over the foot flat on the ground; and (4) the heel raises from the floor (see Fig. 25.2). The opposite leg is in the swing phase. During the swing phase, the leg moves forward from push-off with the knee and hip flexed (acceleration); this is followed by mid-swing where the knee remains flexed and the foot is dorsiflexed and the limb moves forward past the other extremity. Deceleration occurs as the muscles contract and prepare for the heel-strike of the stance phase.

During the gait cycle, the observer is alert for the length of the stride, displacement of the centre of gravity, rhythmicity and symmetry of movement, pelvic rotation, foot, ankle and knee movements and muscle activity during each component of the cycle. Arm and trunk movements associated with locomotion are also noted.

Observation of the gait provides information on the structure and functional ability of the patient. Gait assessment using computerized photography to analyse all of the body events occurring during each step of the gait cycle is possible in some hospitals.

DIAGNOSTIC TESTS

Radiological examinations include standard x-ray studies to assess density, continuity, texture and contour of a bone. The x-rays are usually taken from both the anteroposterior and lateral angles. Contrast medium x-rays are taken for examination of some of the soft tissue structures by administering a radiopaque dye (e.g. myelography).

Bone scan is performed to detect and interpret the degree of bony destruction or repair which is taking place in the skeleton. It is particularly helpful in the diagnosis and location of bone metastases. A radioisotope (e.g. technetium) is administered to the patient via intravenous injection. This substance is taken up by the bone, causing rays to be emitted which are detected by a scanner.

Bone marrow biopsy is performed to assess the haemopoietic function of the bone marrow (see Chapter 13).

Blood studies include those related to mineral metabolism and blood cell counts. They include: (1) alkaline phosphatase, which is an enzyme necessary for mineralization of the organic bone matrix. Serum levels are measured to assess bone formation activity (normal: 8–27 i.u/l). (2) The serum calcium level reflects the ability of the bone to store calcium and is useful in diagnosing diseases which cause changes in bone density [normal: 2.2–2.6 mmol/l (8.5–10.5 mg/dl)]. (3) The serum phosphorus changes are associated with altered bone density level in relation to calcium metabolism [normal: 0.8–1.5 mmol/l (2.5–4.5 mg/dl)].

MANIFESTATIONS OF BONE DISORDERS

Pain and discomfort
Pain is a common manifestation of a bone disorder. It is usually severe, boring and poorly localized and

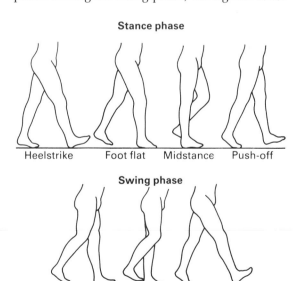

Stance phase

Heelstrike   Foot flat   Midstance   Push-off

Swing phase

Acceleration Midswing Deceleration

Fig. 25.2 Phases of normal gait.

may be referred to other areas of the body. For example, degeneration in the hip may cause pain on the inner side of the knee, and a spinal disorder may result in referred pain down the legs. The pain may be persistent in nature, aggravated by movement and the associated muscular spasm increases the patient's discomfort. Reactions to pain include restlessness, frequent change of position and splinting or immobilization of the affected part. If the joint is immobilized for a prolonged period, joint stiffness and contracture deformity of the joint can develop. Detailed information on pain control may be found in Chapter 8.

Physical deformity
Changes in physical appearance result from swelling, muscular wasting, joint contractures or structural deformity of bone tissue.

Decreased movement
Alterations in movement as a result of bone disorders or their treatment may be localized or generalized. Movement may be restricted, decreased or absent temporarily or permanently and cannot be controlled by the individual. The severity of the immobility is determined by the effect on daily functioning and body position. The extent and duration of impairment of physical movement and altered body posture in relation to gravity influence the potential for development of complications and permanent impairment. Musculoskeletal changes begin immediately with segmental or general immobilization. Demineralization of bones occurs as a result of decreased stress on the bones. Bone reabsorption increases and is greater than bone formation, producing decreased density of bone; the risk of fractures is therefore increased with prolonged immobility. Muscles decrease in mass and strength, reducing work capacity. Joints may become less stable and range of motion is limited, reducing the patient's activity.

Cardiovascular changes may develop quickly with limited mobility especially if body position is altered in relation to gravity. The changes include decreased venous flow, postural hypotension and decreased work capacity, venous stasis, the formation of thromboemboli and decreased activity tolerance. Retention of respiratory secretions and decreased ventilation may lead to atelectasis and pneumonia. Constipation, urinary retention and renal calculi are problems frequently associated with loss of mobility. Areas of the skin may be exposed to prolonged pressure producing ischaemia and skin breakdown.

Identification of patient problems

Problems common to many patients with a bone disorder include:
1 Alterations in comfort: pain
2 Impaired function and mobility (see Table 25.1)

LOSS OF FUNCTION AND IMPAIRED MOBILITY

Loss of function and impaired mobility is related to localized or generalized skeletal impairment, loss of a part or limb, pain and discomfort, physical deformity, decreased activity tolerance and muscle strength, and treatment modalities.

The *goals* are to:
1 Maintain existing functional mobility.
2 Prevent further impairment.

Nursing intervention

Assessment. Identification of the effects of impaired function and mobility requires information about past and present functioning of the patient's cardiovascular, respiratory, urinary and renal, gastrointestinal and neurological systems and condition of the skin, as well as assessment of the musculoskeletal system. Knowledge of the specific bone disorder causing impaired function and mobility and of the medical treatment are necessary before interventions specific to the individual patient can be planned. The plan of care utilizes the patient's existing resources and potential.

Intervention discussed in this chapter emphasizes

Table 25.1 Identification of problems relevant to the patient with a bone disorder.

Problem	Causative factors	Goals
1 Discomfort/pain	Disease process Muscle spasm and weakness Physical deformity Trauma	To control the pain during acute and chronic phases of illness
2 Impaired mobility	Skeletal damage Loss of a limb Pain and discomfort Decreased ability to tolerate activity Muscle weakness Methods of treatment	To promote activities of daily living and optimal functioning

the preservation and promotion of function and mobility and the prevention of potential complications. Nursing interventions related to the effects of impaired mobility on the cardiovascular, respiratory, urinary and renal and gastrointestinal systems and the skin are discussed in respective chapters but it must be remembered that intervention which promotes mobility has a favourable effect on body functions. Maintenance of joint movement is discussed in more detail in Chapter 26 but is also applicable to the intervention discussed below.

Physiotherapy and the orthopaedic patient. Decreased function or mobility, whether localized or generalized, requires a planned exercise programme regardless of the duration of the problem. Table 25.2 provides a list of exercises from which an individualized programme may be devised. Exercises selected to slow bone demineralization include activities which transmit forces along the shaft of long bones. Isotonic and resistive exercises (in which the length of the muscle shortens on contraction but the muscle tension remains the same), and ambulation are effective in creating forces along a bone. These exercises are performed by pushing or pulling against a stationary object such as a footboard, trapeze bar or the foot of the bed. Isotonic and isometric exercises increase muscle strength and promote venous blood flow. Isometric exercises produce changes in muscle tension without an increase in muscle length or movement of the body part. They involve alternate contraction and relaxation of the muscle.

Selection of exercises and the target muscle groups will depend on the needs of the patient. When one limb or area of the body is immobilized, exercises are planned to maintain physical functioning of the remainder of the body and minimize loss of muscle mass and strength throughout the body as well as in the affected part. The physiotherapist is an active participant in planning and carrying out the patient's exercise programme. If the patient's lower limbs are immobilized, a monkey pole or overhead trapeze is installed over the bed and exercises planned to strengthen the upper extremities in preparation for walking with crutches, sticks or walking frame or for manipulation of a wheelchair. Exercises are active whenever possible; passive exercises are performed for specific muscle groups and when active exercise is not possible. Exercises should be scheduled following rest periods and repeated at planned intervals throughout the day.

Positioning. The patient's position is changed frequently whether in a bed or chair to prevent skin breakdown, increase comfort and maintain good body alignment. The upright position is used whenever possible for the beneficial effect of gravity on blood pressure. When the position is changed from lying to standing, support stockings and instructing the patient to contract muscles in the lower extremities may help to decrease postural hypotension. A tilt table may be used to help the patient adjust to postural changes.

A patient confined to bed is taught to use a monkey pole or ropes to shift position and elevate the buttocks off the bed to relieve pressure. The patient in a chair is taught to raise each leg alternately and to rock back and forth and sideways to shift his weight and relieve pressure.

Mobilization. If possible, walking is encouraged to maintain muscle tone, strength and mass and to prevent demineralization of bone and joint stiffness as well as to maintain a sense of well-being. It also lessens the development of pressure sores. Exercises assist in preparing a patient for mobilization. When walking, the patient wears shoes that provide firm support and have low, non-skid heels. When a walking aid or wheelchair is required, it is necessary to strengthen the extensor muscles of the upper arm (triceps). Exercises can be performed by the patient on bed rest as preparation for walking with crutches, sticks or walking frame. The patient lies on his abdomen and lifts his chest off the bed using both arms; he lies flat on his back and alternately flexes and extends his forearms several times while holding a

Table 25.2 Exercise programme for the patient with impaired mobility.*

Exercise programme	Rationale
Dorsiflexion and plantar flexion—10 times, four times daily to 10 times per hour	Muscle pump; aids venous return
Quadriceps femoris muscle contraction Abdominal muscle contraction Gluteal muscle contraction—10 times, four times daily	Isometric exercises maintain muscle strength, mass and joint stability. They also help to maintain cardiac work capacity
Pushing feet against footboard—10 times, four times daily	As above, and promotes longitudinal stress on long bones to reduce demineralization
Active and passive exercises—four times daily	Maintains range of joint movement
Simulated crutch-walking—three times daily	Strengthens triceps muscles

*Lentz (1981), p. 735.

weight in each hand; or he may sit on the side of the bed with his feet dangling over the edge and press down on the mattress with both hands lifting his hips off the bed. Quadriceps muscles may be strengthened by isometric contractions or by lifting his leg off the mattress.

The patient in lower-limb traction strengthens arms and shoulders by using a trapeze bar and lifting sandbags.

Exercises may be planned to promote flexion and extension of the hips, knees, ankles and toes and to strengthen abdominal muscles in preparation for walking.

The physiotherapist usually assumes responsibility for assisting the patient in walking and works with the doctor and nurse to select appropriate walking aids for the patient or a wheelchair if indicated for short-term or permanent use. The nurse is responsible for reinforcing teaching done by the physiotherapist in relation to use of aids, encouraging the patient to walk, assessing the patient's gait and providing constructive advice to promote development of a satisfactory gait.

● *Mechanical aids for walking*. Crutches, sticks, walking frames, splints, braces and limb prosthesis may be used to facilitate walking; a wheelchair may be used for mobility when walking is not possible or requires excessive energy expenditure that interferes with the achievement of other activities.

1 *Crutches*. Crutches are used when the patient is unable to bear weight on one or both legs. The initial instruction in the use of crutches is usually carried out by a physiotherapist with support, assistance and reinforcement of instructions by the nurse; the nurse may occasionally assume full responsibility in instructing the patient. In either situation, it is necessary to understand the principles involved in crutch-walking and have a knowledge of the various gaits which may be used. There are three main types of crutches: axillary, elbow and gutter crutches. Selection of crutches to suit the individual is of utmost importance, as is initial supervision and assessment of how the individual is coping.

One method of measuring for axillary crutches is to measure the patient while he is lying flat with his arms at his sides, from the axilla to a point 15 cm (6 in) out from the side of his foot, allowing 2 cm (¾ in) that will be added by the crutch tip. Another is to subtract 40 cm (16 in) from the patient's height. With children who require prolonged use of crutches, they must be changed periodically to allow for normal growth. The hand bars on which the palms of the hands bear the weight must allow for flexion of the elbow at a 30° angle, or almost complete extension of the arm. A third factor in the selection of axillary crutches is to allow space between the cruch top and the axilla. Undue or prolonged pressure here can cause severe, and occasionally permanent, paralysis of the radial nerve. The axillary bar may be padded with material

such as sponge rubber wrapped in soft cloth.

Elbow crutches are less cumbersome but provide less stability than axillary crutches. Adjustment of the length of the crutch between the hand grip and the lower end is by means of a spring-loaded double-ball catch. Some crutches may also be adjusted in length between the hand grip and arm band. The length of the crutches is assessed with the patient standing and wearing shoes. The tips of the crutches should be on the ground 15 cm (6 in) in front of and lateral to the toes. The patient should be able to stand up straight with his shoulders depressed and elbows in 30° of flexion.

Gutter crutches are used when there is weakness of the muscles controlling the elbow joint or hand, fixed-flexion deformity of the elbow joint or a deformity in the hand causing difficulty in gripping. Adjustment of the length of the crutch is by the same means as for elbow crutches. The forearm is secured into the gutter by velcro fastenings; the patient is asked to stand up as straight as possible; the tips of the crutches should be on the ground 15 cm (6 in) in front of and lateral to the toes; and the height of the crutch is adjusted so that the elbow is in 90° of flexion.

Some minor adjustments may be necessary after the patient becomes more skilled in crutch walking. Good quality rubber tips on the ends of the crutches are imperative for safety. These must be checked frequently. A suction cup tip is available which is particularly helpful for those who are severely disabled and must place their crutches at a wide angle for good balance.

The efforts of all concerned are directed toward assisting the patient to use crutches to walk smoothly and evenly while maintaining good posture. The patient's disability and strength will determine which gait he is to use—the swinging, the four-point, three-point or two-point. Lessons should be given in an environment that avoids crowding, has a smooth floor surface, is free of hazards such as electric cords or rugs, and is equipped with a full-length mirror, if possible.

When only one leg can bear weight, or both legs can bear body weight but are not able to be moved individually by the patient due to lower limb paralysis, the patient may use the swing-to gait. Both crutches are placed at an equal distance in front while the patient is resting his weight on his good leg. Placing his weight on the hand bars of the crutches, he swings ahead so his legs are in line with the crutches, and then repeats the sequence. Smoothness and speed increase with practice, and emphasis is placed on the maintenance of good balance and a short stride. In using the swing-through gait, both crutches are moved forward, the person places his weight on the hand bars and, lifting the body, then swings through the crutches to a position ahead of them. This gait is used by paraplegics and those with a fused or immobile hip.

The four-point alternate gait is used when both lower limbs are affected and all or part of the body weight can be taken on each foot. One crutch is brought forward, then the opposite leg, then the second crutch and finally the other leg. Having the patient count to four may aid in achieving smoothness. This method provides stability since there are always three points of contact with the floor. As the patient's balance improves, he may progress to the two-point crutch gait. Body weight is taken through both lower limbs. Weight is borne on one crutch and the opposite leg while the other crutch and leg advance; then the weight is shifted to the latter pair, and the process is repeated.

If one leg is affected but partial weight-bearing is allowed, the three-point crutch gait may be taught. Both crutches and the weak leg are brought forward, and then the good leg is advanced. By using the three-point crutch gait the body weight taken by the affected leg can vary from none to partial to full. Emphasis is placed on taking steps of equal length to avoid a limp that may persist even after crutches are discarded. As his strength increases, the patient may progress to the two-point gait, which is more rapid and appears closer to the normal.

2 *Walking sticks.* A walking stick provides support and facilitates balance. Types of stick include: the straight-legged or single stick, the tripod stick which has three leg prongs, and the quadruped cane with four prongs. Three and four pronged sticks aid balance. The length of the stick should permit the patient to extend the elbow and bear weight on the hand holding the stick when it is one stride ahead of the patient. The stick is used on the side opposite the impaired lower limb and rubber tips are essential to prevent skidding. Walking with two sticks involves use of the two- or four-point gait described under crutch-walking.

3 *Walking frame.* The standard frame has hand grips on the horizontal tubes on each side. Gutter and pulpit frames are available; these provide forearm and underarm support respectively. The underarm supports are adjusted according to the patient's height, so as to prevent axillary pressure. Frames on wheels are available for those who are unable to lift the frame. A walking frame provides stability and a sense of security, but has the disadvantage of hindering achievement of a normal gait. The patient is generally encouraged to progress to the use of a stick.

4 *Splints and braces (orthoses).* These are appliances used to provide support and joint stability or prevent or correct a deformity. They are made by an orthotist for the individual patient. The patient is taught to apply the splint correctly, to care for and protect the skin under the appliance, and to care for the appliance.

5 *Lower limb prosthesis* is used following an amputation to facilitate balance and support body weight during ambulation (see pp. 992–995).

6 *Casts* are applied following a fracture or soft tissue injury; they can also be used in the prevention or correction of deformities. The function of a cast is to support and immobilize the affected part at rest and during mobilization (see pp. 971–972).

7 *Wheelchair mobility.* A wheelchair is an acceptable form of mobility when the patient is handicapped or when other aids are not appropriate or satisfactory. The preferable wheelchair has removable arm rests as well as removable leg rests that extend and elevate. Wheelchair management requires the same upper extremity strengthening as for the patient using crutches or a walking frame.

Expected outcomes
1 The patient follows the planned exercise programme.
2 Muscle tone, strength and mass are maintained or increased in the affected and unaffected limbs.
3 Range of movement is maintained or increased.
4 Good body alignment is maintained.
5 The patient mobilizes safely.
6 Muscle spasms decrease or abate.
7 Contracture deformities of joints do not occur.
8 The skin is intact.
9 Bone demineralization does not occur, as evidence by absence of changes in bone density on radiological examination, and serum levels of calcium and phosphorus are within the normal range.

Nursing in Bone Disorders

FRACTURES

A fracture is a break in the continuity of a bone, separating it into two or more parts, which are referred to as *fragments*. The soft tissues in the area are also injured.

Causes

The majority of fractures are due to violence incurred by falls, blows or rotational forces. The force, in excess of the bone's resistance, may be applied directly or indirectly. In direct violence, the fracture occurs at or near the site of the applied force. When indirect violence is the cause, the force is applied at a point remote from the site of the fracture. For example, in a fall on the outstretched hand, the stress may be transmitted to the radius, ulna, humerus or clavicle. A fracture rarely may be due to a sudden forceful contraction of attached muscles.

A fracture can occur as the result of disease of the bone which has weakened its structure to the point that it cannot withstand the normal degree of stress.

Metastases, primary tumours (e.g. sarcoma, osteitis fibrosa cystica due to hyperparathyroidism), osteogenesis imperfecta (a congenital condition affecting the formation of osteoblasts) and osteoporosis are examples of diseased conditions of bone that may lead to spontaneous fracture. Prolonged stress may also cause a fracture in certain bones. For example, a long march may cause a metatarsal fracture.

Types of fractures[1] (see Fig. 25.3A–K)

Traumatic or pathological.   The fracture may be designated as traumatic when it is the result of violence or as pathological or spontaneous if it is due to disease of the bone.

---

[1] *Note:* Injury and fracture of the spine and skull are discussed in Chapter 22 because of the serious neurological involvement.

Complete or incomplete.   A fracture is complete if the bone is separated into two distinct parts or incomplete if the break is not all the way through the bone. The greenstick fracture seen in children is an incomplete fracture in which the bone is broken on one side and bent or crumpled on the opposite side.

Open (compound) or closed (simple).   An open or compound fracture is associated with a wound in the overlying skin which establishes communication between the fracture site and the outside air. This type of fracture is potentially infected. The skin wound may be produced by the force that inflicted the fracture or by a fragment of the bone. Conversely, in a closed (simple) fracture the overlying skin remains intact and there is no communication with the outside.

Complicated.   Other vital structures are involved with the fracture, for example blood vessels, nerves or organs.

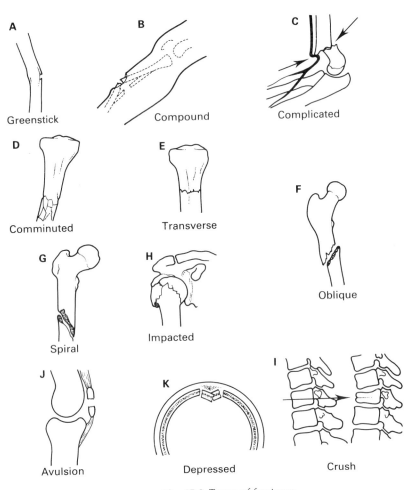

Fig. 25.3 Types of fractures.

Comminuted.   There is more than one line of fracture and more than two fragments in this type of fracture.

Transverse.   The line of fracture is at right angles to the long axis of bone.

Oblique.   The fracture runs at an angle of less than 90° to the long axis of bone.

Spiral.   The fracture line curves in a spiral fashion around the bone.

Impacted.   A fracture is impacted when one fragment is driven into another. Cancellous bone is usually involved.

Crush or compression.   The fracture occurs in cancellous bone which is compressed beyond limits of tolerance.

Avulsion.   This occurs when a ligament or tendon under excessive stress fractures or tears away its bony attachment.

Depressed.   A segment of cortical bone is depressed below the level of the surrounding bone.

Special.   Several fractures have been named after surgeons. The commonest of these are the Colles' and Pott's fractures. In a *Colles' fracture,* a break occurs in the distal portion of the radius and possibly in the styloid process of the ulna. A *Pott's fracture* involves a break through the distal ends of the tibia and/or fibula. An *epiphyseal separation* or fracture occurs when the break is through the epiphyseal or growth plate.

Effects and manifestations

LOCAL EFFECTS

A fracture is always accompanied by some degree of damage to the contiguous soft tissues. Blood vessels within the bone, the periosteum and surrounding tissues are torn, resulting in haemorrhage and then the formation of a haematoma. The periosteum at the site may be stripped from the underlying bone tissue, interrupting the blood supply into the area and thus contributing to the death of bone cells. There may also be haemorrhage into adjacent muscles and joints and damage to ligaments, tendons and nerves. Soon after a fracture occurs the muscles in the area go into spasm, causing severe pain and possible displacement of a fragment due to tendon pull.

Depending on the location of the fracture, visceral injuries may occur, which may threaten the patient's life. Examples of such injuries are rupture of the bladder by a fractured pelvis and rupture of the spleen or perforation of a lung by a fractured rib.

SYSTEMIC EFFECTS

The patient suffers some degree of shock which is influenced by the severity of the injury, the amount of soft tissue damage, associated disorders or multiple injuries, and the patient's age and general condition at the time of injury. (See Chapter 15 for predisposing factors and manifestations of shock.) Usually a slight elevation of temperature and leucocytosis occur in the first 2 or 3 days.

MANIFESTATIONS

The symptoms of a fracture vary with its location, type, the amount of displacement of the fragments and the degree of damage to soft tissue structures.

The patient or an observer usually relates a history of a fall, blow or sudden forcible movement, and the victim may actually say that he heard the bone break. Sudden severe pain at the site is experienced which may or may not persist. Frequently, because of injury and shock, nerve function is impaired, and pain may be absent for a brief period following the injury. As function returns, muscle spasm in the area, as well as tissue damage, accounts for much of the pain, which becomes worse with any movement. Obvious deformity may be present as a result of displacement of the fragments, and there may be shortening of the affected limb due to contraction of attached muscles. Impaired mobility and loss of mechanical support occur, and, in the case of long bones, there may be obvious movement in a part that is normally rigid. Complete loss of function may result from nerve compression by displaced fragments; this is usually restored when the fracture is reduced and the fragments are placed in normal apposition and alignment.

Crepitation (grating sound produced by movement of the ends of the fragments) may be noted if the patient moves the part. Under no circumstances should any attempt be made to elicit the symptom of crepitus because of the possibility of further serious damage to soft tissues (e.g. blood vessels and nerves), unnecessary displacement of fragments and the production of an open fracture. Swelling may develop rapidly over the site of the fracture because of bleeding and the escape of fluid into the tissue. After 2 or 3 days this area frequently becomes discoloured (ecchymosis).

In the case of the rupture of viscera by a fragment, symptoms of impaired function of the damaged organ appear. With rupture of the bladder by a fractured pelvis, extravasation of urine gradually becomes evident, and blood appears in the urine. Rarely, perforation of the intestine is associated with pelvic fracture and causes severe shock and peritonitis; the abdomen becomes distended and board-like. A serious complication of a rib fracture may be puncture of a lung. The patient manifests severe shock, respiratory distress, coughing and haemoptysis.

Some fractures, especially those which are incomplete, or impacted, or of short bones, may produce few signs and symptoms. The fracture may be suspected only on the basis of the history of violence, tenderness on pressure over the site or the patient's complaint of pain upon use of the part or weight-bearing on it. Again, no attempt should be made by the person administering first aid or a nurse to elicit symptoms by having the person move or stand. The patient is treated as having a fracture if there is any doubt.

The surgeon bases his diagnosis of a fracture on the history of the accident, physical examination of the patient and roentgenograms of the affected part.

Fracture healing

Bone is different from many of the specialized tissues because of its ability to regenerate and bridge a gap to unite broken bones. Many tissues heal by laying down non-specialized fibrous scar tissue.

Immediately following a fracture, the space between the fragments and around the fracture line is filled with blood and inflammatory exudate. The haematoma and the exudate are invaded by fibroblasts and capillaries from adjacent connective tissue and blood vessels, forming granulation tissue. Simultaneously, osteoblasts proliferate, mainly from the inner surface of the periosteum (and endosteum in a long bone), and invade the granulation tissue. Calcium salts are deposited, forming a loosely woven, bone-like tissue referred to as a callus. It forms a 'collar' around the bone at the fracture site, giving it greater thickness than the original bone. The callus unites and helps to stabilize the fragments but is not strong enough to bear weight or withstand stress. If the blood supply is poor, or if it is disturbed by excessive mobility at the fracture site, cartilage may be formed instead of bone. As the osteoblasts increase, the callus is gradually restructured by ossification (production of a collagenous fibrous network which becomes impregnated with mineral salts) to form bone tissue. Remodelling is the final stage of fracture healing. The external bulbous bony area is remodelled by the action of osteoclasts.

In some instances, a fracture is complicated by malunion, delayed healing or non-union. *Malunion* implies healing of the fracture in an abnormal position. There may be angulation of the bone or overriding of the fragments which alters the shape and length of the limb. Function may be impaired. The cause is usually ineffective reduction and/or fixation during healing. *Delayed healing* simply implies that the fracture is not healing as rapidly as is normally expected. In *non-union*, the granulation tissue that formed between the fragments following the fracture is converted to dense fibrous tissue instead of normal callus and bone tissue. Causes of delayed union or non-union include too wide a gap between the fragments, the interposition of soft tissues or a foreign body between the fragments, poor blood supply to the site, loss of the initial haematoma by the escape of blood through an open wound or surgical intervention, infection of the bone, malnutrition and disease of bone, e.g. bone metastases.

The serum alkaline phosphatase level is a good indication of bone formation; it is secreted by osteoblasts which promote the deposition of calcium. The serum level of phosphatase rises with the increased osteoblastic activity during bone repair.

General principles and methods of treatment of fractures

EMERGENCY CARE

The patient's general condition and the extent of his injuries are quickly assessed and priorities are set. Respiratory insufficiency, haemorrhage or shock may be evident and take precedence over injured bones.

The first aid treatment that the patient with a fracture receives is very important; movement of the patient or improper handling may cause serious tissue damage and increased pain, haemorrhage and shock. If a fracture is obvious or suspected, care at the site of the accident and during transportation to a hospital is directed toward reducing pain and preventing further tissue damage, visceral injury, and a closed fracture becoming open. The patient should receive a minimum of handling; unless there is danger of further injury, he is left where he is until lifted onto a stretcher or into a vehicle for transportation to the hospital. The patient is told what is going to be done and why, and that he should remain immobile. Before moving the patient, the fracture site and the joint above and below are immobilized. Inflatable air splints of clear plastic come in various sizes and provide good support. If these are not available, a splint can be made from whatever is available (e.g. a board, two or three thicknesses of cardboard, a folded quilt or blanket, pillows). In the case of a board, the surface applied to the patient must be padded (towels or clothing may be used) to prevent pressure. If the limb is in an abnormal position, it is splinted in that deformed position; no attempt is made to reduce the fracture or restore the limb to a normal position. If splint material is not available, a lower limb may be immobilized by placing a pillow or folded blanket between the legs and tying them together. The uninjured limb serves as a splint. In the case of an arm, it may be secured against the trunk by binders or bandages. If it is an open fracture, the wound is covered with the cleanest material available (e.g. a clean handkerchief). If the bone is protruding from the wound, no attempt is made to replace it or reduce the fracture. Nothing is given by mouth in case a general anaesthetic will be necessary.

When the patient arrives at the hospital a quick

assessment is made of his general condition, and if there is respiratory insufficiency, bleeding or shock, appropriate treatment is instituted before the fracture receives attention. When the general condition is satisfactory, roentgenograms are made of the fracture area. Clothing is removed from the uninjured side of the body first.

TREATMENT

The treatment of a fracture usually involves reduction, fixation (immobilization) of the part, protection while the bone heals, and rehabilitation during and following the healing process to restore normal function. When possible, bone stress is utilized to increase the process of repair. The bone fragments are mechanically fixated to enable immediate use, creating stress at the fracture site which accelerates osteoblastic activity. Some fractures, such as those of distal phalanges of the fingers and toes, may heal without reduction and immobilization equipment. Analgesics are given for relief of pain, as prescribed.

Reduction
This is the procedure by which fragments are brought into their preinjury position so that the normal shape and length of the bone are restored and union is promoted. Obviously, reduction is only necessary if there is some displacement of the fragments (Fig. 25.4). It is carried out as soon as possible. A delay makes it more difficult to obtain satisfactory alignment because of the rapid organization of the blood clot and the development of associated muscle

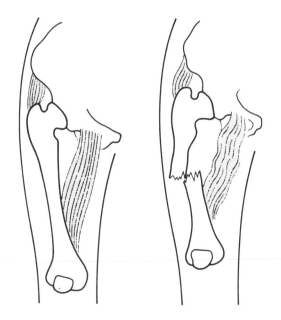

Fig. 25.4 Fracture of the femoral shaft. The pull by the adductor muscles causes a displacement of the fragments.

spasm. Also, there is likely to be less tissue trauma with early reduction.

A fracture may be reduced by a number of methods, with the use of general or regional anaesthesia or an analgesic such as pethidine or papaveretum. Methods for reducing fractures include closed manipulative reduction, traction applied distal to the fracture, or open (internal) reduction. In *closed reduction*, the surgeon manipulates the fragments into position by manual traction, pressure, and/or rotation. In fractures in which one fragment is overriding the other and there is considerable muscle pull, continuous *traction* may be applied to the distal fragment to bring it into apposition and to maintain the alignment. This method of reduction is used most often in fractures of the femur because the pull of the strong thigh muscles tends to displace the fragments and cause overriding. The traction may be applied to the skin (skin traction) or directly to bone (skeletal traction). In some fractures, reduction can only be achieved through an *open surgical incision*.

Reduction may necessitate a general anaesthetic. The nurse determines from the patient when he last had food and fluid and what was taken. This is reported to the surgeon. Reduction may have to be delayed a few hours to allow the stomach to empty and reduce the risk of vomiting and aspiration.

Immobilization or fixation
Various methods are used to maintain reduction and fixate the fragments. They may be categorized as external fixation, external skeletal fixation traction or internal fixation. The method used depends upon the particular bone (e.g. location—short, long or flat), the type of fracture and the muscles involved.

External fixation is most commonly achieved by enclosing the part in a cast. A *plaster cast* is most widely used and is made by the application and moulding of moist plaster of Paris bandages to the affected part. The bandages are strips of cotton material impregnated with gypsum (anhydrous calcium sulphate). They are immersed in warm water, 21–24°C (70–75°F), for a few seconds and then are lightly compressed by pushing both ends toward the middle to remove excess water before application and to prevent telescoping of the bandage. The addition of water to the bandage causes the gypsum to crystallize. While wet it is possible to mould the soft moist bandage to the affected body part. As it is applied, each layer is rubbed with the palms of the hands into that below to prevent separation of the cast into layers. As the water evaporates from the bandages, the plaster hardens and the application becomes rigid.

Before the cast is applied, the skin is cleansed and examined for any contusions or abrasions. The part is then enclosed in circular stockinette for skin protection. Extra padding is used over bony prominences or to fill in spaces which might weaken the cast. It is also applied when swelling is anticipated.

When the application of the plaster bandages is completed, the stockinette which extends beyond the cast is turned back over the cast edges and is secured by incorporation into the cast or with adhesive tape. Newer cast materials are available that are light-weight, strong, do not soften in water and set faster. Such materials include: low temperature thermoplastics, which become pliable when heated and harden when cooled; fibreglass with photosensitive resin, which becomes rigid when exposed to ultraviolet light; fibreglass with polyurethane prepolymer which is activated by contact with water. The cast applied to a limb may be referred to as a cylinder. A *walking cast* may be applied with stable fractures of the tibia and fibula. A stump or walking iron may be incorporated into the cast which encloses the leg and most of the foot. This device permits the patient to be up, walk and bear his weight on the limb. If a stirrup is not used, additional layers of plaster on the sole may be used. A *spica cast* is applied to the trunk and one or both lower or upper limbs (e.g. shoulder spica, hip spica). A cast which is applied to the trunk is called a *jacket* or *body cast*. A *bivalve cast* is one which has been moulded to the limb or trunk, allowed to dry, and then cut down each side so it may be removed for brief periods to allow skin or wound care or other treatment. The sections are held in position by bandages, velcro or straps. When swelling of the limb is expected a plaster back slab may be applied rather than a cylindrical cast. This is made by the application of slabs of plaster of Paris to the posterior aspect of the limb which are then secured in position by cotton bandages. See the discussion of nursing care of the patient with a cast on pp. 979–981.

A *splint* is occasionally used as a means of immobilization and may be of metal, plastic or moulded plaster of Paris. It should be long enough to immobilize the joints immediately above and below the fracture and is shaped or moulded according to the part to which it is applied. Padding is placed between the skin and the splint to prevent irritation and pressure. The splint is secured by straps or firm bandages. Precautions are necessary in order to have the splint held stationary without interfering with circulation. Any swelling, discoloration, coldness or numbness of the distal parts of the limb is reported immediately so the splint may be loosened.

External skeletal fixation. With this method of treatment the bone fragments are held in alignment by skeletal pins. Two or more pins are inserted into each fragment either side of the fracture and the fracture is reduced. The pins are then held in proper relation to one another by an external support; plaster may be used but more commonly a rigid mechanical system of clamps and connecting rods is employed (Fig. 25.5). External skeletal fixation may

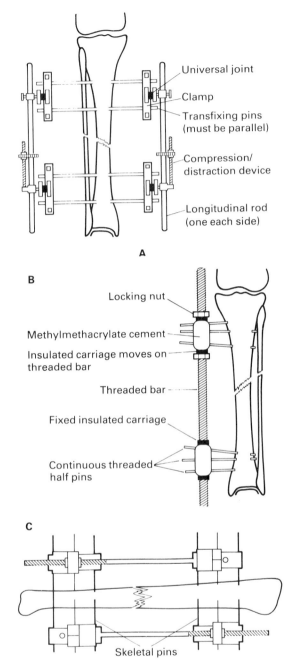

Fig. 25.5 External skeletal fixation systems. *A*, Universal day frame. *B*, Portsmouth external fixation bar (Denham external fixation compression). *C*, The Belfast fixator.

be used in the treatment of fractures associated with extensive damage to the soft tissues where traction is not suitable and internal fixation would carry a high risk of introduction of foreign material into the wound. It may also be used in the management of infected fractures, in multiple fractures (to allow the treatment of other fractures by traction) and in pelvic fractures with disruption of the symphysis pubis. External skeletal fixation is designed to hold the fracture without a plaster cast until union, and allow access to any wounds. The disadvantages are the risks of pin-track infections, the loosening of the pins, and delayed union, as external callus formation may be suppressed by tissue trauma and rigid immobilization of the fracture.

Traction[2] is most commonly used to reduce and maintain reduction in fractures of the limbs by overcoming the effects of gravity and muscle pull. It involves the application of a force along the long axis of the bone distal to the fracture. For this force to be effective, a force in the opposite direction is required (countertraction). Countertraction is necessary and is usually provided by elevating the foot of the bed in the case of a lower limb; the weight of the body on the incline supplies the required countertraction. It is important that the patient's mattress is supported on a firm base. An important use of traction is to overcome the deforming muscle pull that is associated with many fractures. For example, a fracture in the femur is accompanied by marked displacement of the fragments due to the contracture of the very strong muscles of the thigh and hip. The adductor muscles produce a lateral bowing (see Fig. 25.4). The appliance used may produce fixed traction or balanced (sliding) traction, with or without suspension of the affected limb.

Fixed traction is traction between two fixed points, for example a lower limb is supported in a Thomas' splint (a metal splint with a medial and lateral bar and a leather-covered ring which surrounds the thigh at the groin); traction is exerted by either skin extension tapes tied to the distal end of the splint or by passing a pin through the tibia and pulling directly on the bone. Countertraction is obtained by the thrust of the ring against the ischial tuberosity (see Fig. 25.6).

In *balanced* or *sliding traction* there must also be two opposing forces (traction and countertraction). The forces are balanced and mobile, allowing the patient to move about the bed without disturbing the desired line of pull. Traction is applied by the use of a weight and pulley system. A cord passes over the pulley to the weights and is attached at the proximal end to skin extensions in skin traction, or to a skeletal pin which passes through the patient's bone in skeletal traction. Countertraction is obtained by elevation of the foot of the bed by approximately one inch to one pound of weight. Gravity together with the patient's body weight provide the required countertraction (Fig. 25.7).

The limb in fixed or balanced traction may be suspended off the bed surface, allowing the patient greater mobility in bed. Suspension of the lower limb is achieved by supporting the limb in a splint (e.g. Thomas' splint); this is suspended to an overhead frame by means of cords, weights and pulleys (Fig. 25.8) or by springs.

As cited in reduction, fixed or balanced traction may be applied to the skin or directly to the bone.

Skin traction is established by application of adhesive or non-adhesive tapes to the medial and lateral surfaces of the limb. These are secured by a firm encircling crêpe or elasticated bandage. The skin extension tapes extend beyond the foot and attach to a spreader, which must be wide enough to prevent the tapes from contacting the malleoli and sufficient distance from the foot to allow for plantar flexion. A cord, connected to the spreader, passes over a pulley on a cross-bar at the foot of the bed and suspends a prescribed weight (usually 5–8 lb for an adult) to exert the traction force (Fig. 25.9). The disadvantage of skin traction is the limited number of pounds of traction weight that can be used without damaging the skin. The choice of the type of skin extension tapes to be applied is dependent on the condition of the patient's skin, hypersensitivity to adhesive strapping and the surgeon's preference. Non-adhesive skin traction kits with foam rubber or foam-backed skin extensions are available. If adhesive strapping is to be applied the surgeon may or may not want the leg shaved. Some consider that shaving removes epithelium, leaving the skin more vulnerable to irritation by the adhesive. An application of tincture of benzoin may be ordered to protect the skin and provide better adherence of the tapes. The adhesive is not applied over the malleoli or foot. The bandage must not be applied tightly around the limb as this may cause skin or vascular complications.

Skeletal traction is obtained by the insertion of a metal wire (Kirschner wire) or pin (e.g. Steinmann or Denham pin) through the bone distal to the fracture. By this means traction is applied directly to the skeleton. A special traction stirrup, U-loop or bow is fastened to the protruding wire or pin (Fig. 25.10); cord is attached to this which leads to a weight and pulley system. Countertraction is obtained by gravity and the patient's body weight on an inclined bed. The limb in traction is then usually suspended off the bed surface.

Various arrangements are used in applying traction to the lower limb. Those commonly employed are Buck's traction (or extension), Bryant's (Gallow's) traction, Hamilton Russell traction, Perkin's traction and balanced skeletal traction with a Thomas' splint and knee flexion piece.

Buck's traction involves simple skin traction (as previously described). The leg is supported on a soft pillow to keep the heel clear of the bed. Particular care is

---

[2] *Note: Traction* may also be employed to correct a deformity, relieve pressure on a spinal nerve or prevent a contracture deformity in cases in which there is muscle spasm.

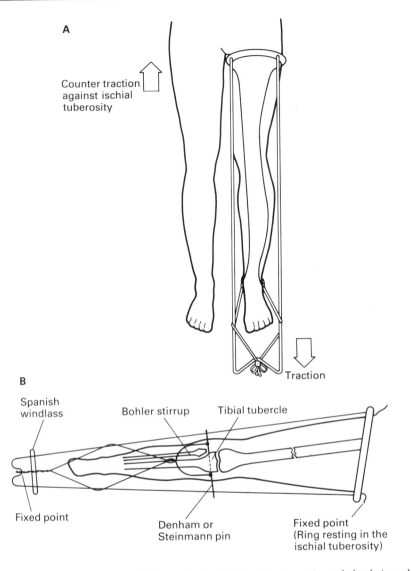

A

Counter traction
against ischial
tuberosity

Traction

B

Spanish
windlass

Bohler stirrup   Tibial tubercle

Fixed point

Denham or
Steinmann pin

Fixed point
(Ring resting in the
ischial tuberosity)

Fig. 25.6 *A,* Fixed traction using skin traction and a Thomas' splint. *B,* Fixed traction using a skeletal pin and Thomas' splint.

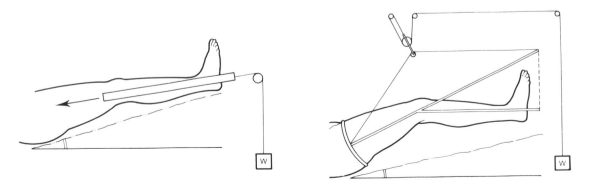

Fig. 25.7 Balanced (sliding) traction.

Fig. 25.8 Suspension of a Thomas' splint.

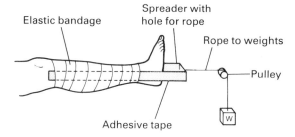

Fig. 25.9 Skin traction of a lower limb.

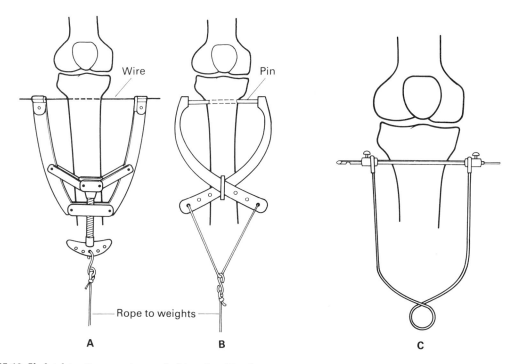

Fig. 25.10 Skeletal traction may be applied by: *A*, a Kirschner wire and traction stirrup; *B*, a Steinmann pin and traction stirrup; or *C*, a Steinmann pin and Böhler stirrup.

taken to avoid pressure from tight bandaging over the fibula head to prevent compression of the peroneal nerve which lies close to the surface. Damage to the nerve could result in interference with normal ankle movement. Countertraction is obtained by elevating the foot of the bed. Buck's traction is used for the temporary management of fracture of the femoral neck, for the management of fractures of the femoral shaft in older and larger children, for undisplaced fractures of the acetabulum and for the correction of minor fixed flexion deformities of the hip or knee (Fig. 25.11).

Bryant's or *Gallow's traction* is used in the treatment of a fracture of the femoral shaft of a young child (under 4 years). The traction may be fixed or balanced. Skin traction is applied to both legs which are then suspended at right angles to the body. For fixed traction the traction cords are tied to an overhead

beam and the cord tightened sufficiently to raise the child's buttocks just clear of the mattress; countertraction is supplied by the weight of the pelvis and lower trunk. The traction may be balanced by means of weight and pulley systems (Fig. 25.12).

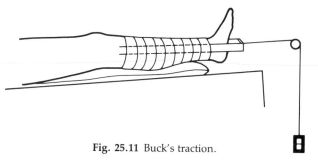

Fig. 25.11 Buck's traction.

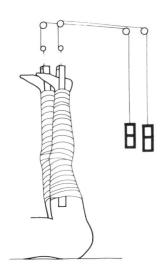

Fig. 25.12 Bryant's traction.

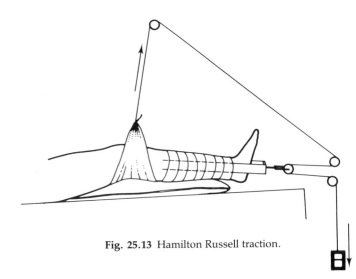

Fig. 25.13 Hamilton Russell traction.

Frequent observations on the state of the circulation in both limbs must be made, especially in the first 24–72 hours after the application of the traction, as vascular complications may occur in either limb. Any discoloration, fall in skin temperature, oedema, impaired or loss of motion or sensation of the feet must be reported immediately. All bandages and strapping are removed.

Hamilton Russell traction is also used in the treatment of a fracture of the shaft of a femur. Vertical traction is applied at the knee; at the same time a horizontal force is exerted on the tibia and fibula. The pull on the leg bones is exerted to counteract the contraction of thigh muscles (quadriceps femoris and hamstring) which insert on the leg bones. Considerable spasm of these strong muscles occurs with a fracture of the femur, causing displacement and overriding of the fragments. The horizontal force is exerted on adhesive tapes or non-adhesive tapes applied to the medial and làteral surfaces of the leg. The tapes are applied from just below the knee to about 2.5 cm (1 in) above the malleoli. They are carried beyond the foot and attached to a spreader. A circular bandage is used to secure the tapes as in Buck's extension. The lateral tapes are terminated just below the head of the fibula to avoid compression of the peroneal nerve. Fig. 25.13 illustrates Hamilton Russell traction.

An overhead bar (Balkan beam) is attached to the bed in line with the affected limb. A crossbar is provided at the foot of the bed to hold the necessary pulleys. One pulley is attached to the overhead bar in line with the tubercle of the tibia, two are secured to the bar at the foot of the bed, one several inches above the other, and a fourth is attached to the spreader plate to which the traction tapes on the leg are attached. A sling or hammock is placed under the knee and attached to a traction cord that leads vertically to the overhead pulley and then to the uppermost one on the crossbar. From there the traction cord passes over the pulley on the foot spreader and back to the lower pulley on the crossbar. It then attaches to weights which hang suspended well above the floor. The weight used with an adult patient is usually 8–10 lb. The level of the pulleys on the bar at the foot of the bed is such that the heel is kept clear of the bed to prevent a pressure sore.

The force exerted by the sling is that of the weight at the end of the rope. The horizontal pull on the leg is approximately twice that exerted on the knee by virtue of the pull of the two parallel traction cords at the foot. The vertical and horizontal tractions are exerted on the same point and together produce a resultant force in line with the femur. A thin pillow is usually placed lengthwise under the thigh; precautions are taken not to increase the slight flexion of the thigh. A second pillow is used under the leg, leaving the heel suspended. A foot support may be provided to prevent footdrop. The foot of the bed is elevated to provide countertraction. The popliteal area is padded to protect it from the pressure of the sling, and the colour and temperature of the foot are checked and recorded frequently to determine if there is any interference with circulation. The patient is encouraged to flex and extend the toes. A monkey pole is attached to the Balkan beam, enabling the patient to move when he wishes.

Perkin's traction involves balanced skeletal traction without any form of external splintage. Active movements of the limb are commenced as soon as possible. Perkin's traction can be used in the management of fractures of the femur from the trochanteric region distally (Fig. 25.14). A split bed in which the distal one third of the mattress and base of the bed can be removed is used when the patient has a fracture of the femur managed by Perkin's traction, as this will facilitate flexion of the knee.

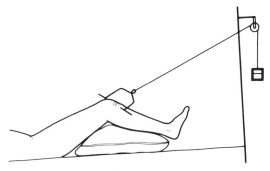

Fig. 25.14 Perkin's traction.

Balanced skeletal traction with a half- or full-ring Thomas' splint with a Pearson's knee flexion piece is commonly used to obtain reduction of a fracture of a shaft of a femur and to maintain reduction until union occurs. (Fig. 25.5).

Firm cotton slings are secured to the upper part of the Thomas' splint to support the thigh and to the Pearson's knee flexion piece to support the leg. The Thomas' splint extends from the groin to beyond the foot in line with the femur. The knee is in 10–20° of flexion to control rotation and prevent stretching of the posterior knee capsule and ligaments and subsequent joint instability. Some provision may be made to support the foot to prevent footdrop. The skeletal traction is usually applied to the proximal area of the tibia. The pull is exerted in line with the femur by means of a traction cord attached to the bow or stirrup that is fitted to the protruding ends of the pin that passes through the bone. The traction cord passes over a pulley and suspends a weight. The proximal and distal ends of the splint are suspended by separate cords, pulleys, and weights. Countertraction is obtained by elevating the foot of the bed. When the patient moves up or down in bed the splint moves with him, and traction is maintained. The patient has greater freedom of movement and is usually more comfortable in this system of traction. It also has the advantage of allowing a certain amount of movement in adjacent joints. (See nursing care of the patient in traction on pp. 982–984).

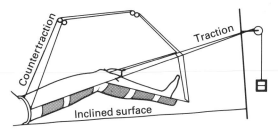

Fig. 25.15 Balanced (sliding) skeletal traction using a Thomas' splint and a Pearson's flexion piece (knee).

Internal fixation. Some fractures require *internal surgical reduction and fixation.* Various types of internal fixation devices are used. These include stainless steel or vitallium wire, screws, plates, rods, and pins and bone grafts. They may be secured to the sides of the bone, placed through the fragments or passed through the intramedullary cavity of the bone. Internal fixation may be reinforced after the wound is closed by the application of a cast or splint. However, new devices of such strength and design are being made that external splintage is not required, thus allowing immediate joint freedom, early weight bearing and short term hospitalization. This system of fracture fixation has been developed by the Association for the Study of Internal Fixation (ASIF or AO).

Special internal fixation devices are used to immobilize the fragments in a hip fracture or fracture of the femoral neck. Three-flanged nails (Smith-Petersen pins or nails), Neufeld nail or a McLaughlin nail and plate or a compression hip screw may be used (see Figs. 25.16 and 25.17). In a few patients, especially the elderly with an intracapsular fracture through the neck of the femur, reduction may not be possible and there may be a risk of avascular necrosis of the femoral head; in these cases a hemiarthroplasty is performed by replacing the head of the femur with a metallic prosthesis (A discussion of hip fracture occurs later in this chapter.)

(See nursing care of patients who have had bone surgery on p. 984.)

Following any method of reduction and fixation, roentgenograms are made periodically to determine whether reduction is satisfactory and healing is occurring. In the case of traction, some adjustment in the amount of weight being used may be necessary. For instance, the x-ray may demonstrate too wide a separation of the fragments which would prevent healing and necessitate a reduction in the weight used.

Open (compound) fractures
The patient with an open fracture requires special treatment as soon after the accident as possible. The site is potentially infected, and there is usually a greater amount of soft tissue damage and destruction. Infection and necrosis impede union and may result in serious crippling. As soon as the patient's general condition permits, the surgeon examines and cleanses the open fracture wound. Gross contaminants and foreign material are removed, and the open wound is covered. The surrounding skin is then cleansed thoroughly with an antiseptic solution. The open wound may then be irrigated with sterile normal saline. The surgeon explores the wound and a debridement[3] is performed, if neces-

---

[3] *Debridement* is the removal of foreign material and excision of devitalized tissue.

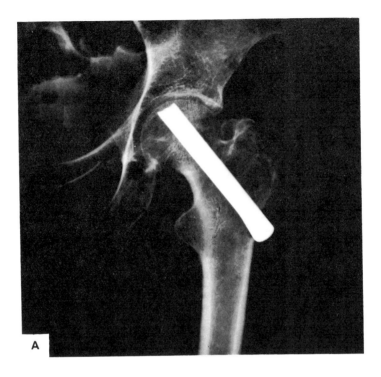

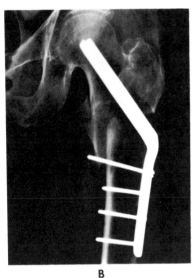

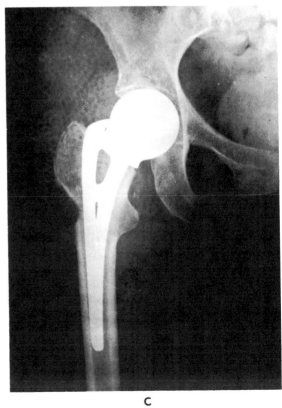

Fig. 25.16 X-rays showing: *A*, Smith-Petersen nail; *B*, McLaughlin nail and plate; *C* a femoral head prosthesis.

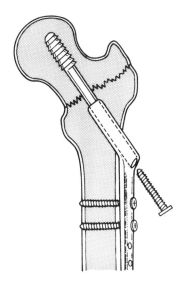

Fig. 25.17 Compression hip screw for trochanteric fracture.

sary. The repair of severed or torn tendons or nerves may be necessary. The fracture is reduced and then immobilized. If there has been gross contamination, the wound may be packed and left open until the danger of infection is past. Drains are inserted in the wound (e.g. Redivac drainage system). Antibiotic therapy may be prescribed.

Before the administration of the anaesthetic, it is determined if the patient has had previous immunization for tetanus. If he has, a booster dose of tetanus toxoid may be ordered. If he has not been immunized, human tetanus immunoglobulin is given.

Care of the patient in a cast

The care of the patient following the application of a cast requires the following considerations.

Drying of the cast
Complete drying of a plaster cast following its application may take several hours or days, depending on the material used, its thickness and the temperature, humidity and circulation of the air. During this period, support of the cast and handling are very important, since the cast is vulnerable to pressure and cracking which could alter its shape, cause indentations that result in undue pressure on an area of the body or make it ineffective. When the part must be lifted, it is supported on the palms of the hands to avoid making indentations by the finger tips. In the case of a body or long leg cast, firm support along the line of the cast is ensured. Pillows with plastic or rubber undercovers are placed under the part encased in plaster so that the cast is not subjected to pressure by the firm mattress. Since it is moulded to the contours of the part to which it is applied,

support by an extra pillow or folded flannelette sheet may be necessary under such regions as the lumbar or popliteal area.

Drying is promoted by exposure to dry, warm circulating air which evaporates the moisture from the cast. The bedding is arranged so that the cast is left uncovered. A fan may be placed approximately 45 cm (18 in) from the cast. Unless otherwise indicated, the patient is turned every 4–6 hours to facilitate drying of the complete cast. He is turned toward his uninjured side and, if it is a large or body cast, two or three persons act in unison and pillows are used to avoid strain on any part of the plaster. A moist cast has a dull grey appearance and produces a dull sound on percussion. When dry, it appears white and shiny and produces a resonant sound on percussion. If a walking cast has been applied, weight-bearing is not permitted for at least 48 hours.

ASSESSMENT

Following the application of the cast, the patient's general condition is noted at frequent intervals and recorded; occasionally, a patient develops delayed shock manifested by sudden weakness, fainting, pallor and weak pulse as a result of the initial injury. During the first 24–48 hours, swelling in the area of the fracture may occur, resulting in constriction by the cast. A frequent check is made of the parts distal to the cast (e.g. fingers, toes) for any indication of inteference with circulation or pressure on a nerve. Any blanching, discoloration, coldness, swelling, oedema, or loss of sensation or motion is reported immediately. Any complaint of pressure or pain at any time must be reported and recorded.

A daily inspection is made of the complete cast for softened areas, and the skin at the cast edges and over pressure areas is examined frequently for any signs of irritation or abrasion. The patient is questioned as to whether he is suffering any irritation or discomfort under the cast, as such symptoms indicate the possible development of a pressure sore and should be reported to the doctor. If a pressure sore is suspected, a 'window' is cut in the plaster to allow inspection of the skin. The window should then be replaced and taped into position, as oedema may otherwise occur in the exposed area causing pressure on the skin around the 'window' edges. After a few days, if the cast appears to have become loose and less effective, it is drawn to the surgeon's attention. This may occur as a result of reduced swelling or loss of weight. The nurse is alert for any odour arising from the cast. In some instances, the only indication of a pressure sore having developed under a cast is the offensive, musty odour characteristic of tissue necrosis. If there is a known surgical or accidental wound under the cast, the area is checked frequently for signs of bleeding, infection and drainage. Infection may be detected by an odour or suspected because of an elevation of temperature.

Protection of the cast

Care must be taken during bathing to prevent wetting of the plaster cast. If it approximates the buttocks and perineal area, it requires protection from soiling and wetting when the patient uses the bedpan. Sheets of plastic or other waterproof material may be tucked in well under the edges of the cast, turned back over the outside and secured with adhesive tape. When the patient is placed on the bedpan, pillows are placed under the shoulders and back so that the upper part of the body is level with or slightly higher than the hips and bedpan. The nurse makes sure the patient is thoroughly cleansed and dried following voiding or defecation and that the protective plastic is changed when it becomes soiled. If the cast edges are so close to the perineum that they interfere with adequate care, the cast may be trimmed to provide greater exposure.

A coat of plastic spray may be applied to the total cast when it is dry to help keep it dry and clean. Superficial soil may be removed with a damp cloth and abrasive powder. Newer cast materials are not harmed by water; however the cast should not be immersed in water as the padding under the cast will become waterlogged.

Skin care

If the patient is confined to bed, frequent skin care, especially of pressure areas, is necessary. The bed is kept free of wrinkles and crumbs. If it is a leg that is in a cast it is supported on a pillow to prevent constant pressure on the heel. The crumbling of cast edges can be a source of much discomfort and irritation; the binding may require changing or reinforcing from time to time. The fingers or toes distal to a cast may become irritated by dry, scaly skin: they are bathed, lightly oiled and massaged at least once daily, and frequent active exercise is encouraged.

Nutrition

The patient is encouraged to take a regular, well-balanced diet to provide the essentials for tissue healing as well as to maintain normal physiological processes. If activity is restricted, the roughage content may have to be increased to control bowel elimination. If, in the case of a hip spica or jacket cast, intestinal distension becomes troublesome, gas-forming foods may have to be avoided. If the discomfort keeps recurring, the surgeon may cut a 'window' in the cast over the abdominal region.

Exercise

Exercise is important in the care of the fracture patient to stimulate circulation and to prevent muscle atrophy, loss of strength, stiffness of uninvolved joints and promote healing of bone. Inactivity and immobilization promote the movement of calcium out of the bones, predisposing the person to hypercalcaemia and renal calculi. The purpose and details of the exercises are explained to the patient. Uninvolved joints are put through their full range of motion several times daily, and he is encouraged to exercise the unaffected limbs and use them in self-care, turning and raising as much as possible. An overhead trapeze is provided so he can move and lift himself. A schedule of deep breathing and coughing is established for inactive and older persons who are predisposed to pulmonary complications.

The muscles of the immobilized limb are exercised by instructing the patient to contract those muscles immediately above and below the fracture (isometric exercise) frequently, without moving the limb. These exercises may be demonstrated on the unaffected limb so that the patient sees that the muscles can be contracted without moving the limb. For quadriceps setting, the nurse places her hand under the knee and instructs the patient to push down. If it is an arm that is encased in plaster, isometric exercise of the arm muscles is done by instructing the patient to make a fist. The fingers or toes distal to the cast should be exercised several times daily. As soon as the cast is dry, use of the affected limb is encouraged.

Home management with a cast

Providing the patient is able to maintain his own safety, he is usually allowed to go home as soon as the cast is dry. The patient and his family are advised that the limb should be elevated for the first 24–48 hours. Instructions are given to examine the toes and fingers frequently and to report to the surgeon or the clinic or accident and emergency department immediately any swelling, blueness, coldness, numbness or inability to move the digits. Persisting pain of the limb or any crack or softening of an area in the cast should also be reported.

The arm with the cast may be supported in a sling when the patient is up. It is important that the sling supports the hand to prevent strain and pressure on the wrist. The knot of the sling at the back of the neck is placed lateral to the cervical vertebrae, and a pad may be placed between the sling and the neck to prevent pressure and irritation.

The patient who is discharged with a cast on his leg must know whether or not he may bear any weight on the limb. If he has a walking cast, he is advised as to when he may start to bear weight on it, how to protect the cast and to elevate the limb when sitting and the necessary precautions to avoid falls. If the patient is to use crutches, they are selected according to the patient's height, and instructions are given in their use and the patient is observed to ensure he is able to mobilize with them safely.

An appointment is usually made for the patient to have the limb and cast checked in 2 or 3 days and then to return in approximately 10–12 days for an x-ray to determine if the callus formation and healing are progressing favourably.

Removal of the cast

When the cast is taken off, the rigid support to joints which have been immobilized for a considerable period of time is removed. The patient is likely to be discouraged by the stiffness, instability and weakness which he encounters and requires reassurance that with exercise and progressive use function will be restored.

The cast is removed by special cast cutters or a plaster saw. The limb must be handled gently and with support under the joints. The skin is bathed gently, and an application of oil or lanolin is made to soften the accumulation of dry, scaly skin. Vigorous rubbing is discouraged to avoid skin irritation and abrasions.

A regimen of passive and active exercises and massage is established to restore joint and muscle function. Weight-bearing and activities are gradually resumed. When the cast is removed and the limb becomes dependent, oedema and swelling are likely to occur. The patient is advised to elevate the limb when sitting and lying, and an elastic or crêpe bandage or tubigrip may be applied when he is ambulatory to control the oedema which gradually becomes less troublesome as muscle tone improves and there is increasing activity.

Nursing the patient with external skeletal fixation

Preoperative preparation

The length of time that elapses between the time of injury and surgery varies and is dependent on the patient's general state of health and associated injuries. Forms of treatment, such as traction, may be employed temporarily to immobilize the fracture prior to surgery. The care of the patient in the accident and emergency department and following admission to the ward includes observations of vital signs to detect signs of haemorrhage and shock, and observations of colour, temperature, sensation, movement of digits and pulse are made of the injured limb to detect impaired circulation or nerve damage; any abnormal signs are reported to the doctor immediately. Intravenous infusion or a blood transfusion may be required depending on the extent of blood loss. The patient will require a strong analgesic, such as papaveretum, to control pain. Skin wounds are covered by sterile dressings; directions are obtained from the surgeon on the cleansing of wounds. If surgery is to be performed within a few hours of admission to hospital, the wounds may first be thoroughly cleansed in the operating theatre. Debridement of wounds may also be required to allow satisfactory healing to take place. Preoperative preparation includes blood tests and an electrocardiogram if it is indicated. If the period between the accident and the operation is more than a few hours the patient is asked to breathe deeply and to cough every hour to aid in the prevention of chest infection.

He is also encouraged to perform active exercises of unaffected limbs to maintain muscle tone, joint function and aid venous return. Regular, frequent skin care will also be required to assist in the prevention of pressure sores. Cleansing of the skin prior to surgery is important because of the bone's susceptibililty to infection.

The operation is explained to the patient by the surgeon, and the external skeletal fixation system is briefly described so as to alleviate some of the problems which could otherwise occur postoperatively, associated with altered body image. The nurse should make herself available to the patient to enable him to discuss any fears or worries he may have and to assist the patient in coming to terms with his injuries and the chosen method of treatment.

Postoperative care

The general principles of postoperative care are applicable (see Chapter 11). Observations of vital signs are monitored to detect signs of haemorrhage or shock. If the external skeletal fixation system has been applied to a fractured limb, the limb is elevated by means of suspension cords to a frame attached to a Balkan beam, or the limb is elevated on a frame supported on the bed (Braun frame) in cases of fracture of the tibia. Elevation of the limb assists in the reduction of swelling. The limb is observed for signs of impaired circulation and nerve compression or damage.

The external skeletal fixation system must be checked daily to ensure that the clamps and nuts are tight. The pin sites are observed for bleeding or leakage of exudate; however the pin sites should be dry approximately 48 hours after surgery. Dressings to the pin sites are renewed when they become soiled or when the pin site requires close inspection. Strict asepsis is adhered to when dressing the pin sites and when dressing any skin wounds. Pain, tenderness, erythema, swelling and increased skin temperature at a pin site must lead the nurse to suspect pin site infection. Any of these clinical features must be reported to the doctor, and a wound swab should be taken and sent for microscopy, culture and sensitivity. Antibiotic therapy is prescribed and the pin may be removed by the surgeon. Any loosening of a pin must also be reported as this increases the risk of pin tract infection; the offending pin is usually removed. Any exposed pin tips must be covered by metal or plastic caps or corks to prevent damage by the sharp ended pin to the other limb or body or to the nursing staff.

The patient will usually require a strong analgesic at regular intervals during the first 48 hours following surgery. If severe or moderate pain persists after this time the surgeon must be informed as it may be an indication of infection. The patient is confined to bed until skin wounds have healed. Exercises of all joints, including those of the affected limb, are commenced as soon as possible to maintain muscle tone, strength and mass and to maintain joint movements, to aid the patient to make a successful recovery. The patient with a lower limb fracture is at high risk of the formation of deep vein thrombosis. Foot and leg exercises are commenced on the day after the application of the fixation device and observations are made to detect any signs of this complication.

Some patients may be upset on seeing their injured limb and the fixation system. The nurse needs to show patience and understanding and should encourage the patient to express his anxieties and fears. By encouraging the patient to take part in the planning of his care and to take an interest in the care of the fixation system and his rehabilitation programme, the nurse may assist the patient in coming to terms with his altered body image.

The patient with a lower limb fracture is taught to mobilize with the aid of crutches: he is not permitted to put any weight on the affected limb until callus formation is detected by x-ray examination. Once callus has formed the patient may be taught to partial-weight bear through the affected limb.

The external skeletal fixation device is removed once fracture union has occurred, as diagnosed by radiograph. After removal of the fixation system (from a lower limb) the patient is generally not permitted to fully weight bear for a further 2 weeks.

Care of the patient in traction

It is important that the nurse is familiar with the purpose of the traction and that she understand how the appliances being used are designed and applied to achieve their purpose.

Assessment of the patient in traction
Traction must be constant to be effective in the treatment of fractures. The complete traction system is inspected frequently as well as after any movement or treatment of the patient to detect possible interference with the traction or the direction of its pull. Traction must be taut, ride freely over pulleys and be kept free of the bedding. Knots are examined frequently for security, and the weights, which must never be lifted or changed, unless directed by the doctor, are checked for free suspension.

Areas that may be subjected to irritation by adhesive tapes, constriction by circular bandages, or pressure or friction by contact with a part of the appliance are examined several times daily, and any interference with circulation or skin irritation is reported and recorded promptly. Distal portions of the extremity are checked for discoloration, coldness, swelling, oedema, and loss of sensation or movement. The nurse is alert for any sign of discharge or a musty odour that might indicate skin necrosis in an area covered by adhesive tapes or bandages. Any change in the alignment of the limb,

such as outward rotation, hyperextension or foot-drop, is brought to the doctor's attention. Any complaint of pain or discomfort deserves investigation and reporting.

Countertraction is maintained by elevation of the bed under the part to which the traction is applied and by preventing a change of position. For example, the patient should not be allowed to slide down so that the foot plate or bar rests against the foot of the bed or a crossbar. The heel, which is so vulnerable to pressure, must remain suspended, and the foot is supported to prevent plantar flexion (footdrop). If the limb is supported in a Thomas' splint, the ring should not cause undue pressure in the groin. The skin under the ring is bathed frequently, thoroughly dried and lightly powdered. If the patient keeps 'sliding into the ring' or if skin irritation occurs, the weights may require adjustment by the doctor or the splint may need to be changed if the ring has become too large once the swelling of the thigh has subsided. When the Pearson attachment is used with a Thomas' splint in suspension traction to support the leg from the knee down, the patient's knee should rest over the point of attachment of the Pearson knee flexion piece. When traction is applied to the neck with tongs in the skull (skeletal traction) or a halter, the head of the bed is elevated to provide countertraction.

When skeletal traction is used, the wounds are covered with small sterile dressings. The surrounding skin is inspected daily for any redness or discharge that may indicate infection. The protruding ends of the wire or pin are covered with cork or metal pin covers.

Positioning, skin care and exercises
The patient in traction is required to remain on his back; this becomes tiresome and is a source of discomfort for the patient. An explanation is made to the patient of the reason the dorsal position is necessary, and he is told that turning would prevent immobilization of the fracture area which is essential to healing. Directions are obtained from the doctor as to how much movement is permitted and if the patient may or may not use a monkey pole. Good body alignment is important; a firm mattress on a fracture board is used. The upper part of the body is kept straight; if the patient lies diagonally, it may alter the desired position of the affected limb and the direction of the pull on it. The patient in lower limb traction frequently has a tendency to keep his unaffected leg in flexion. He may need to be reminded to extend it for intervals to prevent shortening of the flexor muscles.

Frequent skin care (at least every 2–3 hours) of the back, buttocks, elbows and the heel of the unaffected leg is very important to prevent pressure sores, especially in elderly persons. Inspection of these areas and alteration of position within confines of the traction should be carried out. An occasional light application of lanolin or oil may be necessary to prevent excessive drying and possible cracking of the skin. Squares of synthetic sheepskin or foam pads are placed under the vulnerable areas. Thorough cleansing and drying following the use of the bedpan and keeping the bedding clean, dry and free of wrinkles and crumbs are important nursing measures. Vulnerable areas are carefully inspected frequently for any discoloration, mottling, oedema or break in the skin. A second person is necessary to assist with the raising of the patient while back care is given and the lower bed linen is changed. If the patient cannot be raised, the person assisting pushes down on the mattress, permitting the nurse to slide her hand in to give the necessary care. The patient may be permitted to raise himself slightly by pulling on a trapeze suspended from the overhead frame. Linen changes are made by working from the unaffected side toward the affected side or from the top of the bed toward the foot. The method which proves easier and least disturbing for the patient is used. The top bedding is arranged to avoid interference with the traction. Small lightweight blankets may be used over the limb in traction for warmth. If suspension traction is used, the patient usually has greater freedom of movement and can be raised with less danger of disturbing the fracture site. *When slight turning of the trunk is permitted for care, the turning is toward the leg in traction.*

The patient is required to practise deep breathing and coughing every 1–2 hours to prevent pulmonary complications. To stimulate his circulation and prevent muscle atrophy and joint stiffness, active exercises of uninvolved limbs are carried out several times daily. Self-care activities are encouraged and an explanation of their role in his progress is made to the patient. He is also taught to practise static exercises (isometric contractions or muscle setting) of the abdominal and gluteal muscles.

Nutrition

A well-balanced diet is provided, and the patient is advised of the need for adequate nutrition to provide the essential materials for healing of the fracture and to maintain resistance. The protein and vitamin C (ascorbic acid) intake receive special attention; a deficiency of these elements predisposes the skin to pressure sores. The reduced activity and subsequent constipation may necessitate increased dietary roughage. Immobilization causes some decalcification of the bones, predisposing to the formation of renal and bladder calculi as calcium is excreted by the kidneys. The patient is encouraged to take 2500–3000 ml of fluid daily (unless contraindicated) to promote elimination of the excessive blood calcium. The nurse makes sure that the food is within easy reach of the patient and that he receives the necessary assistance in cutting his meat, buttering bread, pouring coffee, etc.

Elimination

The use of the bedpan by the patient in traction frequently presents some difficulty, mainly because of the elevation of the foot of the bed for countertraction. Unless contraindicated, the patient assists in raising himself onto the bedpan by using the trapeze and unaffected leg. A pillow may be placed under the back and shoulders so that the patient is more level with the bedpan. A 'slipper' pan may be easier to use and more comfortable for the patient. The nurse must see that the patient and bed are left clean and dry.

As cited previously, the enforced inactivity may give rise to constipation and flatulence. If the problem is not corrected, faecal impaction may develop, necessitating manual evacuation of faeces and cleansing enemas, which are distressing and exhausting for the patient. Dietary adjustments and a mild laxative may prevent this problem.

Diversion

The patient is usually in traction for several weeks; time passes slowly, and he is likely to be discontented, depressed and unable to sleep. The provision of diversion and some form of occupation is an essential part of the nursing care plan. The patient's need for socialization, interest and occupation may be discussed with his family and friends. It may be suggested that they plan their visits so that he is not alone for several days and then visited by everyone at the same time. The patient's interests should be determined; reading material, a radio or television and small handicrafts frequently prove helpful. In the case of a housewife and mother, her family might be encouraged to have her participate in planning and decision-making regarding home matters so that she feels that she is still active in family affairs. Similarly, it is psychologically beneficial to the father or businessman to be consulted. Mental and purposeful physical activity help to produce normal fatigue; the patient is likely to sleep and rest better at night and will require less sedation.

Convalescence and rehabilitation

When the traction is removed, the patient will probably be surprised and depressed by the weakness, joint stiffness and joint instability in the limb. Before he is allowed up, the head of the bed is elevated so he may adjust to having his head and trunk in an upright position after being flat and in the countertraction position for so long. The elevation is gradual; otherwise he may experience faintness.

Appropriate passive, active and resistive exercises of the affected limb are introduced. These may be planned and supervised by a physiotherapist, but the nurse must be familiar with the plan so that the necessary assistance is provided when the therapist is not at the bedside. In the case of a lower limb, arm and shoulder exercises are continued to strengthen the upper limbs in preparation for the use of a walking frame or crutches. Specific orders are received from the doctor as to when weight-bearing and ambulation may begin. Depending on the strength and age of the patient, a walking frame may be used before crutches or sticks are introduced. It is usually used with elderly and debilitated patients because there is less danger of falls and they feel more secure. Firm, low-heeled walking shoes should be worn, preferably with a non-skid rubber heel.

When the patient's ability and confidence increase, he may then progress through crutch walking to sticks. When relearning to walk, he may need prompting to maintain an erect posture (avoid bending forward) and to increase the degree of flexion of his thigh and leg when raising a foot off the floor to take a step in order to overcome the tendency to shuffle (see gait assessment p. 963). Most patients require a good deal of encouragement and reassurance from the nurse. Physical assistance and support are gradually withdrawn, but the nurse remains with the patient when he is getting in and out of the bed or a chair until it is evident that he can safely manage on his own.

Before the patient is discharged, it is important to know the home situation in order to suggest necessary adjustments. Will he have to use stairs to get to the apartment or to the bathroom? Will there be someone there with him all the time? The necessary information may be obtained from the patient or family, or a visit may be made by an occupational therapist to assess the situation and suggest adjustments in the environment and arrangements for care. When he goes home, a referral may be made to the primary health-care team so that he receives regular assistance and supervision by a community nurse or health visitor. Resumption of his former occupation and activities will depend on his progress in relation to mobility and independence. He is seen at frequent intervals in the clinic or by his doctor until fully rehabilitated.

Nursing the patient with internal (surgical) fixation

Preoperative preparation
How soon the operation for internal fixation is performed after a fracture has occurred depends on the patient's condition and whether there are associated injuries or health problems. It is usually done as soon as possible to minimize soft tissue injury and before any fibroblasts develop, but may have to be delayed because of shock or because the patient has eaten recently and as a result should not have a general anaesthetic until the stomach empties. During the preoperative period, some temporary form of immobilization may be applied to the injured part (e.g. sandbags, splint or Buck's extension). It must be handled as little as possible to prevent movement of the fragments and further tissue damage. An analgesic such as morphine, papaveretum, pethidine or codeine may be ordered for relief of pain. Older

patients may not tolerate these drugs and, if given, must be observed closely, especially for respiratory depression, shock and disorientation. Cot-sides may be placed on their beds as a precautionary measure, and their condition may necessitate constant attendance at the bedside. The patient's blood is grouped and cross-matched, and blood is given to counteract shock or haemorrhage. If the patient manifests dehydration, intravenous infusions of electrolyte and glucose solutions are administered. If the patient is elderly, as so many are who have internal fixation, intravenous solutions (including blood) are given slowly to avoid an excessive demand on the heart caused by a rapid increase in the circulating intravascular volume. The urinary output and fluid intake are measured, and the balance is determined so that any renal insufficiency may be detected and reported. The preoperative assessment includes blood tests and an electrocardiogram may be performed. If the period between the accident and the operation is more than a few hours, the patient is required to cough and breathe deeply every 1–2 hours. Frequent special skin care may also be necessary because of the immobility and constant dorsal position.

Because of bone tissue's susceptibility to infection and the difficulty in bringing it under control if it occurs, meticulous preoperative cleansing of the skin is very important. Specific directions are usually received from the surgeon. A large area is carefully prepared and cleansed with an antiseptic solution. The cleansing may be repeated, depending on the amount of time available. If the surgery is to be performed on a limb, special attention is paid to the skin between digits and to the nails.

Postoperative care
Following internal reduction and fixation, the general principles of postoperative care are applicable (see Chapter 11).

Assessment. The patient is observed closely for any changes in colour, blood pressure, pulse and respirations that may reflect shock, haemorrhage or cardiac failure. If the surgery was performed on a limb, the extremity is elevated on pillows to prevent oedema. The operative site may be enclosed in a cast, making it difficult to detect early signs of bleeding. The area is checked for any staining of the cast or oozing from its edges. The initial area of staining may be encircled with a soft-nibbed pen mark so that continued bleeding may be recognized and assessed. As with any plaster application, the part of the limb distal to the cast is examined frequently for any nerve compression or interference with circulation.

Impairment of mobility. The limitations of positioning and activity are indicated by the surgeon. During thment to bed, exercises of uninvolved parts of the body and self-care activities are usually encouraged to maintain the normal range of joint movement and muscle tone and reduce the mobilization of calcium out of the bones. A trapeze attached to an over-the-bed bar (Balkan beam) allows the patient to move and shift his weight. He is instructed to cough and take eight to ten deep breaths every 2–3 hours if activity is restricted. When crutch walking is anticipated, exercises to strengthen the arms and shoulders are introduced. Frequent skin care, especially to susceptible pressure areas (scapular areas, sacrum, heels), is necessary. If turning is permitted, the patient is turned onto the unaffected side; the affected limb is supported during the process and is positioned on pillows to maintain good alignment and prevent strain. A cot-side on the side of the bed toward which he turns provides something for him to grasp when turning.

The patient may be allowed out of bed but, in the case of surgery on a lower extremity, he is not usually permitted to bear any weight on it for several days or weeks. He may be allowed the use of a wheelchair and is gradually introduced to the use of crutches. When sitting in either a stationary chair or a wheelchair, provision is made for elevation and support of the affected limb. Precautions against pressure sores and slumping posture are necessary when the patient is allowed up in a chair for long periods. Skin care is provided at regular intervals and he is taught to shift his weight frequently so that no one area is subjected to continuous pressure. Adjustments may also be necessary to avoid prolonged pressure on the popliteal area of the unaffected, dependent leg and to prevent forward sagging of the shoulders.

Exercises of the affected part are started as soon as the surgeon permits. They may be limited to isometric contractions for a period, followed by the gradual introduction of passive and active movements and resistive exercises. In the case of a lower extremity, weight-bearing is not introduced until roentgenograms indicate satisfactory healing. The overambitious patient is cautioned not to attempt standing or walking without the assistance of a physiotherapist or nurse. He should have a firm, non-skid pair of walking shoes and be assisted first to stand. The physiotherapist or nurse stands facing the patient and places her hands to the sides of his lower chest. She encourages him to stand erect, knees extended and head up. When he is sure of his balance in the upright position, he is then assisted with the next step, which may be the use of crutches, a walking frame or simply walking with only the assistance of one person. Support is given to the affected side.

Fracture of the hip

This refers to a fracture of the proximal extremity of the femur and may be classified as intracapsular or extracapsular. The *intracapsular fracture* occurs through the neck of the femur and is slower in healing because frequently there is an associated interruption of the blood vessels which supply the head of the bone. The *extracapsular hip fracture* may pass through either the greater or lesser trochanter or the intertrochanteric area. A fracture of the hip is usually treated by internal (surgical) reduction and fixation. A variety of metallic nails, plates and screws are available as fixation devices. The selection depends on the location and angle of the fracture. If the intracapsular fracture is comminuted, or if satisfactory reduction cannot be obtained, or if the surgeon suspects that avascular necrosis and non-union are likely to develop because of injury to blood vessels, the femoral head may be removed and replaced by a metal (vitallium) prosthesis. It has a ball-shaped head which fits into the hip socket (acetabulum) and a lower intramedullary rod which is fitted into the lower neck and upper part of the shaft of the femur.

The majority of patients who suffer a fracture of the hip are elderly persons. They do not tolerate the prolonged immobilization and bed rest imposed by traction and spica casts; under such treatment they are prone to develop pulmonary and circulatory complications, pressure sores and rapid debilitation. Internal fixation makes it possible for the patient to exercise and be out of bed much earlier than with traction, thus reducing the risk of serious complications.

Following the surgical reduction and fixation, constant nursing attention and close observation of the vital signs are necessary; the older person is more likely to develop shock, respiratory depression and cardiac failure. The patient is placed on a firm mattress on a fracture board to prevent sagging and flexion of the hips. When the patient is in the supine position, alignment can be maintained by sandbags placed along the lateral aspects of the limb. Occasionally, traction is applied for 2 or 3 days to overcome muscle spasm. A trapeze bar is installed over the bed to assist in mobility.

Postoperative disorientation and restlessness are common with elderly persons. Cot-sides are placed on the bed for protection. Analgesic drugs and sedatives are used judiciously; the patient must not be allowed to suffer unnecessarily, but the reduced tolerance of older persons for these drugs, especially opiates, may depress respirations and cause disorientation.

As soon as the patient regains consciousness, a schedule for frequent coughing and deep breathing is established. He is turned frequently as soon as possible to help prevent pulmonary congestion. Position is individualized according to the side and position which provides the most comfort for the patient, and the surgeon's wishes. Lamb found in a study of 53 elderly patients that 50% preferred lying on the operative side.[4] The affected limb is supported during the process, keeping the hip and knee

---

[4] Lamb (1979), p. 294.

in the same plane to prevent strain on the operative site.

Retention of urine or incontinence may be experienced in the early postoperative period. Intermittent catheterization may be necessary. A fluid intake of approximately 2500 ml is encouraged unless contraindicated by circulatory or renal insufficiency. Constipation is a common problem, and faecal impaction is prone to develop. A mild laxative may be ordered and the diet is adjusted to include increased roughage.

Exercises of the unaffected extremities are started as soon as possible, and the patient is encouraged to flex and extend the toes and ankle of the affected extremity alternately to stimulate circulation. The application of elastic or crêpe compression bandages or antiembolic stockings to the lower extremities helps to prevent venous stasis, which predisposes the patient to thrombophlebitis. Anticoagulant therapy may be prescribed to prevent the development of thromboemboli. Specific exercises are prescribed for the affected limb; passive movements may be introduced first, followed by active exercises. The patient is assisted or lifted out of bed into a chair as soon as possible following surgery. The affected leg is usually extended and supported the first few days unless otherwise indicated by the surgeon, and then lowered and observed for swelling and discoloration. The patient is taught to stand on the unaffected extremity and to transfer to a chair without bearing any weight on the affected limb. He may then be permitted early ambulation with a walking frame, sticks or crutches. In most instances, the elderly patient is not taught crutch walking because of the danger of his falling. If weight-bearing is permitted, the patient is supported and encouraged to ambulate; the older patient is usually taught to use a walking frame.

Continued pain or muscle spasm is reported and recorded; it may be due to unsatisfactory reduction or avascular necrosis of the head of the femur. When a prosthesis has been implanted, unless the limb is in traction, specific directions are received as to the positioning of the patient and the affected extremity as there is a risk of dislocation of the prosthesis. Positioning varies with the location of the operative approach through the joint capsule. If it has been posterior, the patient lies flat, and the leg is abducted and positioned in external rotation; if the approach through the capsule was anterior, the limb is internally rotated and abducted and the patient may be permitted to sit up.

Firm healing of the bone following a hip fracture and the resumption of walking is a long slow process. Periods of discouragement and depression are common. The patient requires a good deal of support. Self-care activities are promoted to reduce his feelings of dependence as well as to maintain muscle tone. Various forms of diversion in which he is interested are provided. The patient may be permitted to go home before weight-bearing is allowed. Adjustments in the home environment and care of the patient are discussed in detail with members of the family. A referral may be made to a community nurse or health visitor.

Complications

Complications that may occur with fractures include malunion, delayed healing and non-union of the fracture (see p. 970). The enforced immobilization associated with the treatment of some fractures predisposes the patient to hypostatic pneumonia, renal calculi and phlebothrombosis. It is important that a regimen of frequent deep breathing and coughing be established from the onset to prevent shallow respirations and the retention of secretions which readily become infected. Circulation and venous return are stimulated by exercising unaffected limbs regularly, encouraging as much movement by the patient as is permitted and promoting self-care. Movement of calcium out of the bones into the blood, which may lead to the formation of kidney or bladder stones, is reduced by patient movement and exercises. The patient is also encouraged to take 2500–3000 ml of fluid daily, unless contraindicated, to promote elimination of calcium by the urine.

Nerve compression and permanent damage may be incurred by prolonged pressure on the nerve by a part of a traction appliance or a plaster cast, or by direct injury to the nerve by a fracture fragment. Frequent observation and prompt reporting of the patient's complaint of pain and pressure may result in an adjustment or correction being made before permanent damage occurs, with consequent loss of function.

The patient with a lower extremity in traction should have the foot supported in the normal position (almost at a right angle to the leg) to prevent prolonged stress on the peroneal nerve which could result in a permanent footdrop.

A fat embolus may occur due to the liberation of fat into the blood from the marrow of the injured bone. The embolus is most often carried to the pulmonary arteries and eventually occludes a vessel, causing fat embolism of the lungs or brain. Commonly there is unexplained deterioration of the patient a few days after injury. There may be pyrexia, tachycardia, dyspnoea and a petechial rash may appear on the patient's back, chest and conjunctival folds. The patient may become confused, aggressive or comatose.

Infection of the fracture site develops most often because of the contamination associated with a compound fracture. It may occasionally follow open reduction and fixation.

AMPUTATION OF A LIMB

The incidence of amputation of a part of a limb increases sharply in the over-55 age group as a result of peripheral vascular disease.[5] Amputation of a limb is a very multilating procedure and an extremely devastating experience for the individual but it provides a positive step in function restoration.

For those for whom an amputation is a necessity, the loss of the limb has become less obvious and less disabling nowadays as a result of improved prostheses and rehabilitation programmes. A lower extremity is more frequently involved, and amputation occurs more often in males.

Reasons for amputation

An amputation is performed to preserve the patient's life or may be undertaken to improve function and usefulness. The conditions which necessitate amputation include: (1) insufficient blood supply to the part and resulting gangrene; (2) severe, uncontrollable infection such as gas gangrene (*Clostridium welchii* infection) or chronic osteomyelitis in which there is marked bone destruction; (3) malignant neoplasm (e.g. osteosarcoma); (4) an injury that has resulted in irreparable crushing of the limb or laceration of arteries and nerves; and (5) a handicapping deformity (e.g. flail limb).

Level and types of amputation

Occasionally an amputation is an emergency surgical procedure performed because of irreparable traumatic damage to a part. But, when possible, the level of the amputation is decided before operation so that the patient may be informed of the anticipated extent of the loss. The decision as to the level is based on achieving (1) complete removal of the diseased tissue, (2) viable tissue and an adequate blood supply to the remaining part of the limb, and (3) a stump that will allow for a satisfactory fitting and functional movement of a prosthesis. Adequate soft tissues (skin, subcutaneous tissue and muscle) are preserved so that the end of the bone is well padded and covered. If possible, the stump should be the optimum length for adequate leverage on the prosthesis. Too long a stump may interfere with the function of the prosthesis joint below. In amputation of the lower extremity the knee joint is maintained, if at all possible, since mobility and agility are more readily acquired. The prosthesis for the above knee amputation limits the person, especially if elderly, because of the high energy demands for locomotion.

Two types of operative procedures are used, the closed or flap type of amputation and the guillotine or open amputation.

In the *flap type* of procedure, fascia, probably muscle, and full-thickness skin flaps are brought over the end of the bone. In an above knee or through knee amputation, the anterior flap is usually longer in order to bring the suture line well to the posterior aspect. In a below knee or in a Syme's amputation, the posterior flap is usually longer, with the suture line situated on the anterior aspect of the stump. This arrangement prevents direct pressure on the scar by the prosthesis in weight-bearing. When it is an upper limb that is involved, the anterior and posterior flaps are generally equal in length, producing a terminal scar. The skin flaps are dissected to provide a smooth surface over the end of the stump, free of wrinkles and folds, and the skin edges are sutured in apposition with a minimum of tension.

A *guillotine or open amputation* is reserved for emergency cases in which the limp has been severely traumatized and contaminated or in which an infection such as gas gangrene has already developed. The skin and other soft tissues are severed at the same level as the bone. The wound is left open to promote adequate drainage and closed later when infection is brought under control. Traction may be applied to the skin while it remains open to prevent retraction of the soft tissues.

Traumatic amputation implies the loss of a whole or part of a limb in an accident. This is frequently a life-threatening situation because of the concomitant haemorrhage. A second problem incurred by such circumstances is contamination of the wound. Immediate emergency care is directed toward arrest of the bleeding and getting the person to where blood replacement may be instituted. Precautions are taken to handle and transport the amputated part with the patient carefully, since efforts may be made to reattach the separated unit.

Disarticulation is the term used when the amputation is at the level of a joint.

Preoperative nursing intervention

Psychological preparation
When the amputation is an elective procedure, the surgeon and the rehabilitation team work together to inform the patient and family of the need for the operation and the level at which the limb will be removed and what functional restoration can be anticipated. The loss may not be very important functionally, or it may prove a serious handicap. For example, an individual can readily adjust to the loss of a second, third or fourth finger but, if it is a thumb, the ability to pick up or grasp an object is seriously impaired. However, when the patient is first advised of the loss of a part of the body, regardless of how functionally insignificant, the information is still likely to be a shock, causing considerable emotional disturbance. The patient's body image and independence are seriously threatened, and he needs the support of an understanding nurse. He is encouraged to talk about his feelings and, through listening, the nurse identifies his particular fears and concerns. These and the reactions vary among

---

[5] Banerjee (1982), p. 4.

patients, depending on their personality, life situation and ability to handle crises. For example, the wage earner is likely to be greatly distressed about a loss of earning power to support his family. For another, an amputation may mean a complete change in his accustomed activities and occupation.

The patient and family receive explanations of how the problems associated with the loss of a limb may be handled through a planned rehabilitation programme. The knowledge that the interest and assistance of specialists in this area are available helps the patient to develop a hopeful and positive attitude toward overcoming the handicap. Opportunities are provided for questions and discussions about what is likely to take place before and after the operation. The patient may derive support from a visit by someone who has had a similar amputation and has been successfully rehabilitated.

Physical preparation
During the preoperative period the patient is taught deep breathing and coughing. If his condition permits, exercises are introduced which will facilitate his postoperative mobilization and rehabilitation. These include active exercises of the unaffected limbs to prevent loss of muscular strength. If the use of walking aids is anticipated, arm strengthening exercises using weight-lifting and push-ups may be introduced to strengthen the shoulder and arm muscles. Frequent skin care and change of position may be necessary for the patient confined to bed or a wheelchair to prevent pressure sores, since he often tends to remain immobile to reduce pain. Over-protection of an affected lower limb usually results in continuous flexion of the hip and knee joints, leading to contractures. This is discouraged by lying the patient in a prone position several times a day.

Attention is directed toward promoting optimum nutritional and hydrational status. The importance of adequate protein, vitamins and fluids in postoperative progress is explained to the patient. If the patient is overweight, the calorie intake may be moderately reduced, since excess weight may retard postoperative mobilization and rehabilitation. Too restricted a calorie intake (below 1000–1200 kcal) and a rapid weight loss are avoided because of the danger of causing acidosis, especially postoperatively. Blood grouping and cross-matching are performed, and compatible blood is made available; haemorrhage is always a hazard during and following an amputation. A transfusion may be given during the preoperative period, as well as during and following the operation, to improve the patient's general condition. The blood pressure and the pulse rate and volume are noted to serve as a base-line in postoperative care.

Preoperative preparation of the skin involves the usual thorough cleansing and may include shaving above and below the anticipated level of amputation.

Preparation to receive the patient after amputation

In preparing the postoperative bed, a fracture board is placed beneath a firm mattress to assist in maintaining good body alignment, facilitate postoperative exercises and, in the case of a leg amputation, prevent sagging of the bed at hip level which predisposes to flexion contracture. Obviously, amputation necessitates the severing and ligation of large blood vessels. Provision is also made for elevation of the foot of the bed in case of haemorrhage or shock. Blood, fluids and equipment are made available for prompt intravenous infusion.

Postoperative nursing intervention

The patient's problems following an amputation are listed in Table 25.3.

Assessment
The blood pressure, pulse and respirations are recorded, colour noted and the stump examined at frequent, regular intervals for the first 48 hours for early signs of shock and haemorrhage. The patient is observed for psychological distress following the amputation. Even though he was prepared for and consented to the operation, the actual loss of the body part may cause severe depression. The nurse is also alert for any indications of infection such as pyrexia, raised pulse, increased pain, erythema and wound discharge.

1. Promotion of healing
The stump is usually enclosed in a thick soft dressing and elasticated bandages. Rigid dressings of plaster are used in some hospitals. The disadvantage of their use is that they hinder close observation of the circulation to the stump; they are therefore infrequently used in patients who required amputation due to vascular disease. If the amputation is through the knee, below the knee or Syme's amputation and a rigid plaster has been applied, a metal socket may be implanted to accommodate a pylon or early training prosthesis when the patient is permitted to bear weight on the stump (Fig. 25.18). Straps may be incorporated into the cast which attach to a belt around the patient's waist while he is in bed to prevent the cast from moving or slipping off. When he is up, the straps extend over the shoulder. Immediate postoperative fitting of a prosthesis to a rigid plaster dressing is not advocated for the above knee amputee, due to problems in suspension of the prosthesis; however, a rigid plaster dressing without a prosthesis may be fitted. The rigid dressing application controls swelling and oedema; prevention of oedema favours more rapid healing. There is also less danger of haemorrhage with the steady pressure and immobilization. The inclusion of the knee in the cast prevents flexion contracture. The rigid dressing permits earlier ambulation which encourages and motivates

Table 25.3 Identification of patients' problems following amputation.

Problem	Causative factors	Goals
1 Potential for injury	Surgical construction of a residual limb (stump) Altered balance Possible disorientation in the post-operative period Phantom limb phenomenom	1 To promote wound healing 2 To achieve a residual limb that will support activity with a prosthesis 3 To prevent physical injury
2 Discomfort/pain	Surgical intervention Phantom pain phenomenon	1 To control the pain 2 To understand and minimize the experience of phantom sensations
3 Disturbance in body image	Amputation of a body part	1 To express feelings about the loss of a body part 2 To attain an acceptable level of social and physical functioning
4 Nutritional intake lower than body requirements	Surgery and anaesthesia	1 To maintain nutritional and fluid status
5 Impaired mobility	Surgery and loss of a body part	1 To prevent complications of immobility 2 To increase physical activity and ambulation
6 Inadequate knowledge about the care of the residual limb and the prosthesis, application and use of the prosthesis and follow-up care	Lack of information, skill and resources	1 To develop self-care skills 2 To develop a plan for follow-up health management

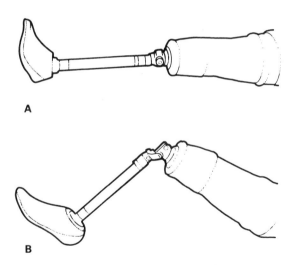

Fig. 25.18 Rigid plaster dressing with extension tube and foot, through knee level.

the patient. A disadvantage with the enclosure of the stump in a rigid plaster dressing is that the condition of the wound cannot be visualized and readily assessed. The cast must be examined frequently and any stain appearing on the cast is reported, outlined with a pencil and the time noted so that continued bleeding or drainage may be recognized. Any complaint of pain in the stump, offensive odour from the area or elevation of temperature must be reported promptly. These symptoms may indicate infection or pressure and tissue necrosis.

When a soft dressing is used, any blood staining is reported immediately. If serious drainage soaks through the dressing, it is promptly reinforced and pressure is applied until the bleeding is brought under control, if necessary, by the surgeon. Continuous closed wound suction drainage may be established to prevent haematoma formation. The wound dressing, providing it is comfortable, is generally left undisturbed until the wound drain is removed, thus reducing the risk of introduction of infection. The wound drain is removed 2–4 days following surgery and the sutures are left in place for 10–12 days for an above knee amputation and 3–4 weeks for a below knee wound, in order to ensure firm healing.

Unless the surgeon instructs otherwise, the patient should lie in a supine position with the stump resting flat on the bed. Following an amputation above the knee, the patient must be guarded against shortening of the hip flexors and abductors. In an amputation below the knee, the patient is encouraged to maintain extension of the knee to avoid contracture of the hamstrings (posterior thigh muscles). With an arm amputation, precautionary measures are used to prevent contracture of the shoulder adductor and inward rotator muscles.

When a rigid cast is not used and the wound has healed, a compression bandage (elastic or crêpe) is applied to the stump to reduce oedema and promote firming of the tissue in preparation for a prosthesis. The bandage is applied with the stump in extension whenever possible. Even tension is maintained during the applications made in 'figure-of-eight' turns. Circular turns are avoided as they tend to impair circulation. Tape is used to secure the bandage (*metal clips are avoided*) (see Fig. 25.19). The bandage must be sufficiently firm to compress the soft, flabby tissue, but one must guard against any interference with the blood supply by excessive tightness. The bandage is removed and reapplied when it becomes loose. The stump is always bandaged except when the prosthesis is on. While it is off, gentle massage of the tissue may be prescribed to stimulate circulation and prevent adherence of the scar tissue to the bone. The patient or a member of the family is taught the care of the stump and the correct application of the bandage. The stump is bathed as necessary with a mild soap and rinsed and dried thoroughly. Lanolin

may be applied if the skin is dry and flaky. The patient is taught to inspect the stump twice daily, using a mirror, for redness, swelling, irritation and calluses. If any symptoms develop, weight-bearing on the stump is avoided and the doctor or clinic consulted. Stump bandaging is resumed if the prosthesis is not worn during this time. Certain activities may be ordered which apply pressure to the stump in preparation for the use of a prosthesis and weight-bearing. Contact is first made with something quite soft and, as tolerance is developed, the firmness and resistance of the contact surface and pressure are progressively increased. If the patient complains of muscular spasms and discomfort, massage to the stump may provide relief. Fig. 25.20 illustrates points the patient is taught 'not to do' with the stump in order to prevent injury and promote healing.

When the rigid dressing is used, it remains for approximately 2 weeks unless there is some indication of bleeding or infection. The sutures are

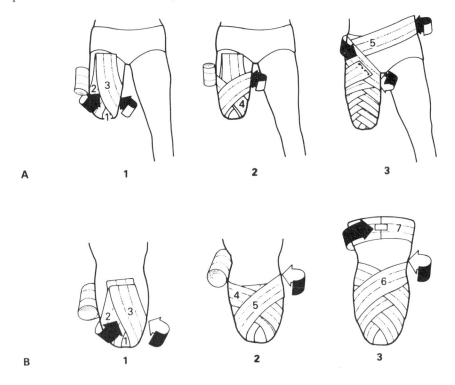

Fig. 25.19A Above knee stump bandaging. **1** (1) Using a 14 cm crêpe bandage, begin at the anterior aspect at the level of the inguinal ligament. (2) Take the bandage over the stump centrally and up to the gluteal fold. (3) Return to the starting point, covering the lateral aspect of the stump, then return bandage to gluteal fold, covering the medial aspect of the stump's extremity. **2** (4) Bandage from the 'outside in' with oblique figure-of-eight turns, covering the corners of the extremity and up the stump to the groin. Decrease the tension of the bandage as the bandage continues towards the groin. **3** (5) The bandage is secured by a full turn around the waist.

Fig. 25.19B Below knee stump bandaging. **1** (1) Start with the bandage at the level of the tibial plateau with the roll facing up. (2) Take the bandage firmly lengthwise over the centre of the stump extremity and up to the level of the fibular head. (3) Cover the medial and lateral aspects of the stump extremity. **2** (4) Bring the bandage in an oblique turn across the front of the stump. (5) Figure-of-eight turns are commenced to cover the sides of the extremity. **3** (6) Bandaging is continued (gradually reducing the tension to avoid constriction of the tissues) until the stump is covered. (7) The bandage is completed by two circular turns above the knee, ensuring the knee joint is left free.

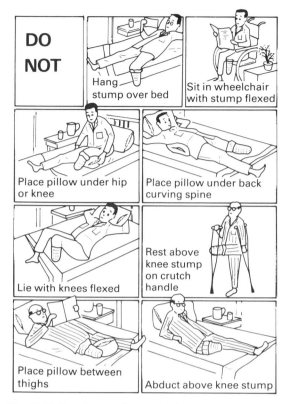

DO NOT

Hang stump over bed

Sit in wheelchair with stump flexed

Place pillow under hip or knee

Place pillow under back curving spine

Lie with knees flexed

Rest above knee stump on crutch handle

Place pillow between thighs

Abduct above knee stump

Fig. 25.20 Positions to be avoided by lower extremity amputee during the immediate postoperative period.

removed and a second cast applied which is changed again in 2 weeks.

2. Prevention of physical injury

Cot-sides on the bed may be a necessary precaution, especially with the older patients. They may become disoriented or, in turning, may readily lose their balance and fall out of bed. The most common cause of falls is that the patient forgets momentarily that he has only one leg. He may experience the sensation that his limb is still present; this phenomenon is known as *phantom limb*. The majority of amputees experience this phenomenon, which is strongest immediately following surgery. Good pain control, firm bandaging of the stump and wearing of a prosthesis tend to lessen the sensations of phantom limb. Awareness that it is a common experience following amputation helps to decrease the patient's anxiety.

3. Control of pain

A narcotic analgesic is usually required by the patient at regular intervals during the first 48 hours after surgery. Persistent pain 24–72 hours after surgery may indicate haematoma formation. This must be reported to the surgeon immediately, as breakdown of the wound could occur if the haematoma is not evacuated. If pain occurs later in the postoperative recovery period it may be due to wound infection or to the formation of a neuroma. If infection is suspected the wound is inspected, a wound swab is taken for microscopy, culture and sensitivity and the relevant antibiotic is prescribed. Some patients experience pain which is interpreted as originating in the portion of the limb which has been removed. This is referred to as phantom pain (see Chapter 8). It varies in severity and may be temporary, but if it persists, treatment in the form of local nerve blocks in the stump, transcutaneous nerve stimulation, ultrasound, relaxation training or drug therapy including the use of anticonvulsant agents (e.g. carbamazepine) may prove effective. No single method of treatment has shown itself to be consistently successful. Research continues and other therapies are in use.

4. Adjustment to altered body image

Acknowledgement by the nurse of the patient's feelings of depression, anger and frustration and provision of opportunities for the patient and family members to discuss feelings help the patient to accept the situation. An understanding of the meaning of the loss to him is necessary for the health professional to provide constructive support. The nurse and other health care workers set expectations that the patient will increase mobilization, socialization and self-care activities. Support and encouragement are provided as the patient attempts new activities. Early mobilization and patient participation in decision-making promote the development of a more positive attitude. A temporary prosthesis is worn as soon as possible so the patient only briefly experiences an empty sleeve or empty trouser leg. The permanent prosthesis (Fig. 25.21) is fitted within a few weeks for most patients. As the patient's functional capacity increases, feelings of self-worth and tolerance of the change in body image begin to emerge. Friends and relatives are encouraged to visit and opportunities for the patient to go home for an evening or weekend are created whenever possible.

Involvement of members of the rehabilitation team prior to surgery and during the postoperative period enables them to provide information about the expectations for functional restoration, develop plans for rehabilitation and establish a trusting relationship with the patient and family. Rehabilitation centres usually provide both individual and group sessions to allow patients to share experiences, gain support and learn new and effective coping strategies.

The patient is encouraged to discuss with the limb fitter how the artificial limb will look as well as function. Help is provided in selecting shoes, trousers, skirts, shirts and blouses to promote a favourable and acceptable appearance.

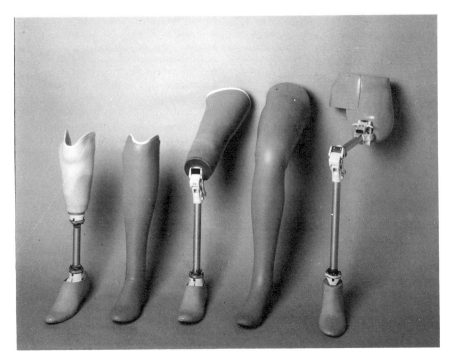

Fig. 25.21 Examples of leg prostheses.

Psychological adjustment is generally a longer process than is the relearning of physical functioning.

Specific therapy needs to be planned when the use of some unacceptable response is prolonged or interferes with health and safety. Plans are made to provide continuing support when the patient returns to the community and to encourage reintegration into community recreational, social and employment activities.

5. Maintenance of fluid and nutritional status

Intravenous fluid may be necessary during the first 24–48 hours to maintain an adequate intake. Oral fluids are given freely, and the patient progresses to a regular diet as soon as it is tolerated. An explanation is made, if necessary, of the importance of adequate nutrition in maintaining and promoting his muscular strength for the exercises that will assist in rehabilitation.

6. Promotion of mobility exercise

An hourly routine of coughing and deep breathing and frequent change of position are necessary until the patient is allowed up and becomes sufficiently active to prevent limited ventilation and circulatory stasis.

As soon as he is well enough, a daily regimen of exercises is introduced to maintain and promote the muscular strength and joint mobility that are needed for rehabilitation. The tone of the trunk muscles, as well as that of the limb muscles, receives attention since adjustments and compensation are necessary for the amputee to maintain his balance. If the lower limb has been amputated above the knee, the hip extensors and adductors play an important role in remobilization, as hip flexion and abduction deformity can occur. The patient should be taught active stump exercises to maintain and improve joint mobility and muscle strength. To prevent flexion contracture of a thigh stump, the patient lies in the prone position for a minimum of ½ hour two to three times a day (Fig. 25.22). While in the prone position, he is encouraged to do push-up exercises to strengthen the shoulder and arm muscles. If the leg has been amputated below the knee, particular attention is given to quadriceps exercises. Following the amputation of an arm, the shoulder muscles of that limb are exercised to prevent adduction and rounding of the shoulder.

7. Rehabilitation

The patient is allowed out of bed as soon as possible. Assistance must be available until he can maintain his balance and is able to manoeuvre safely. In the case of a lower limb, the patient first learns to stand and gain his balance, to transfer safely from bed to chair and from wheelchair to toilet. Some hospitals use pneumatic postamputation mobility aids (PPAM aid) (Fig. 25.23). The PPAM aid is made up of inflatable plastic envelops attached to a metal frame which suspends from the stump and has a rocker at the

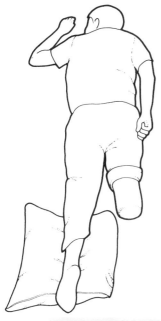

Fig. 25.22 The correct position for prone lying. The patient should be lying comfortably with his head turned toward his good side and both hips completely flat on the bed. His stump should be laid flat with the knee straight.

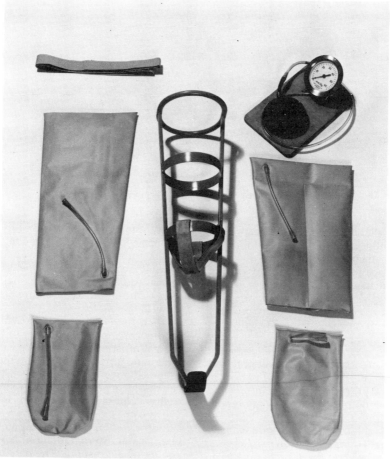

A

Fig. 25.23 The pneumatic postamputation mobility aid. *A,* The equipment. *B,* The equipment in use.

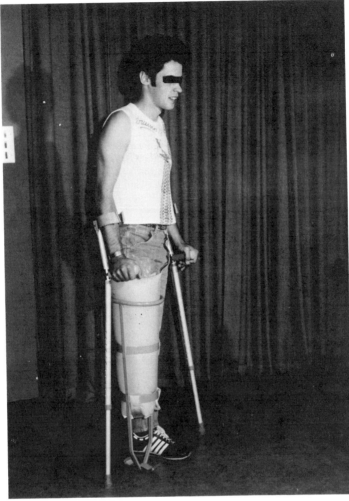

Fig. 25.23 The pneumatic postamputation mobility aid. *A*, The equipment. *B*, The equipment in use.

distal end. The aid allows early mobilization prior to referral to a limb-fitting centre for fitting of the first prosthesis. The patient is first taught to walk between parallel bars and then progresses to walking with the aid of crutches. The PPAM aid is a partial weight-bearing prosthesis; therefore walking sticks are not used. When fitted with a temporary prosthesis (pylon) the patient mobiizes using a walking aid such as a stick. A walking frame may be used by those unable to manage sticks, but it is generally not recommended as there is a risk of the patient falling backwards and also the frame limits the patient in various activities and pursuits because of its size and shape. Crutches should not be used as they hinder the patient in learning how to weight-bear. To ensure the patient is able to walk safely with walking sticks, he is first taught to walk between parallel bars, one hand holding a bar and the other a stick. The patient progresses to walking with the aid of two sticks, he is first taught to walk between parallel bars, one hand holding a bar and the other a stick. The patient progresses to walking with the aid of two sticks. If the patient has satisfactory gait and balance, he may walk with one stick, held in the opposite hand to the amputation, before his permanent prosthesis is fitted.

When the stump has sufficiently shrunk and is conditioned, measurements are taken, and a permanent prosthesis is made.

If a hand has been removed at the wrist or there is a below elbow amputation, a prosthesis can be provided which permits supination and pronation as well as voluntary opening and closing for grasping. The prosthesis used following an elbow disarticulation or mid-upper arm amputation is capable of internal and external rotation, flexion and extention and terminal grasping. The patient who has an arm disarticulation at the shoulder is more handicapped, units comparable to the upper arm, forearm and hook-hand, but they are more difficult in operation.

Following a below knee amputation, the patient is fitted for a prosthesis. It may involve a patellar tendon weight-bearing socket which suspends the prosthesis. It is lightweight and held in place by a strap around the thigh. A more commonly used type is a suction socket which negates the need for the strap. This model also eliminates the need for knee hinges and provides for greater freedom and agility by the wearer. With an above knee amputation a full-length prosthesis is necessary, and is supported by a pelvic band or corset-like arrangement. The knee is hinged and the upper portion is quadrilateral in shape. The development of the total surface-bearing self-suspending above-knee socket is a great improvement on previous models where weight-bearing was on the ischial tuberosity. The individual with this type of prosthesis uses considerably more energy in getting around than the person with a patellar tendon weight-bearing prosthesis.

Research in prosthetics has led to the artificial limb being designed to meet the needs and life-style of the individual. Currently, efforts are being made to develop limbs which permit the gait of runners and joggers as well as meet the needs of the elderly who require prostheses.

When learning to use a permanent lower limb prosthesis, the patient uses one or two walking sticks for support. When he achieves a satisfactory stable gait, he is encouraged to discontinue the use of a stick. All of this takes considerable time and perseverence; the amputee will require encouragement and support from his family and those working with him in rehabilitation. An elderly patient may feel more secure if he begins with a walking frame when he is instructed in wheelchair activities or the fitting of an appropriate prosthesis for weight-bearing is not possible.

8. Inadequate knowledge
Following an amputation, the patient and his family are taught to care for the stump and to inspect it several times daily for oedema, redness, drainage or breaks in the skin and to note any changes in sensation or tenderness. When the prosthesis is fitted, they are taught how to care for it, to assess for proper fit, what to do if the fit alters and when to return to the limb fitter for reassessment. The physiotherapist helps the patient develop a plan for continuing the exercise and activity programme at home. The nurse helps the patient and family plan how they may incorporate the recommended health care measures and activity programme into the daily routine of the patient. Referrals to a community nurse or resettlement officer are made as indicated. Arrangements are made for follow-up visits to the surgeon's clinic in the outpatient department.

The patient and family are also taught how to apply the 'stump socks' worn with the prosthesis (except when a suction suspension prosthesis is worn); these are changed daily or more often if the patient perspires excessively and the socks are washed after each use.

EXPECTED OUTCOMES

1 The skin over the stump is clean, dry and intact.
2 The patient indicates understanding of the phenomenon of phantom limb and phantom pain, if present.
3 The patient and family are able to express feelings regarding the loss of a body part and the change in body image.
4 The patient is able to apply the prosthesis and wear it with comfort.
5 The patient follows the planned exercise regimen to maintain and/or increase muscle tone and strength and joint function in all limbs.
6 The patient moves about safely.
7 Suitable body weight to aid mobilization is maintained or achieved.
8 The patient is able to assess the condition of the skin over the stump.
9 The patient knows how to contact his limb-fitting centre should problems occur.
10 The family takes part in the rehabilitation programme and is able to give assistance to the patient if required.

OSTEOMYELITIS

When bone tissue becomes infected the condition is known as osteomyelitis. The pathogenic organisms may be introduced directly through an open fracture or from infected contiguous tissue but are more commonly carried by the blood to the bone from a distant primary focus such as boils (furuncles), an abscessed tooth or infected tonsils. When the infection is bloodborne, the condition is referred to as *haematogenous osteomyelitis*. The most common bacterial offender is *Staphylococcus aureus*, but the disease may also result from the invasion of streptococci, pneumococci or other strains of staphylococci.

Growing bone is more susceptible to haematogenous osteomyelitis and, as a result, the incidence is highest in children and adolescents. The infection usually develops in long bones at the diaphyseal side of the growth plate. In adults the pelvis and vertebrae are more often affected. The bone marrow is affected first. Unless it is checked at the onset, the inflammatory process forms a purulent exudate that collects in the minute canals and spaces of the bone tissue. The pressure of the exudate builds up because of the resistant, rigid bone and compresses the blood vessels, causing thrombosis and occlusion. The accumulation under pressure eventually breaks through the cortex of the bone into the subperiosteal space. The periosteum at that site becomes elevated and stripped from the bone, interrupting the blood vessels that lead into the bone, Interference with the blood supply results in an area of dead bone tissue, which is called a *sequestrum*. The periosteum may rupture, and the infection may then extend into the adjacent soft tissues, forming a sinus tract that discharges onto the skin surface. Small sequestra, separated from the living bone tissue, may escape with the exudate through the sinus. The infection may destroy the growth plate (epiphyseal plate), leading to reduced growth of the limb, or it may extend into the adjacent joint with ensuing permanent loss of joint function. The periosteum initiates the formation of new bone tissue around the affected area. The new tissue is called the *involucrum*[6] and may enclose and trap sequestra and infecting organisms. These organisms continue to grow in the confined area and the osteomyelitis becomes chronic, characterized by recurring abscess formation and sequestration.

Signs and symptoms

The onset of acute osteomyelitis may be manifested by a chill, pyrexia and rapid pulse. The patient has the appearance of being acutely ill; he perspires freely, is restless and irritable and may be nauseated and vomit. Severe pain develops in the limb as a result of the pressure by the accumulating exudate and the destruction of bone. The pain is aggravated by slight movement or jarring of the bed. The patient protects the limb by avoiding weight-bearing and movement and usually holds the adjacent joint in flexion. The local area is very tender on slight pressure and becomes red and swollen when the infective process reaches the subperiosteal area and surrounding soft tissues. If the infection is near a joint, the joint may become swollen and tender and the infection may spread into the joint.

There is a marked increase in the leucocyte count, and the erythrocyte sedimentation rate is elevated. After 1–2 weeks, roentgenograms reveal destructive bone changes and periosteal elevation and reaction.

Treatment and nursing intervention

Antimicrobial drug therapy and rest in the early stage of osteomyelitis may bring the infection under control with minimal bone damage and before a sinus is formed. In more advanced cases, surgery may be necessary to provide drainage to relieve the pressure within the bone and periosteum and to remove dead bone tissue.

Efforts are made to identify the infecting organism

by making cultures of the blood, nose and throat secretions and discharge from any skin lesions (e.g. boils). If a positive culture is obtained, sensitivity tests may then be made to determine the most effective antibiotic therapy.

Large doses of antibiotic are given, usually by parenteral channels. If the response is favourable and the infective process controlled, antimicrobial therapy is generally continued for several weeks to ensure destruction of the organisms.

The patient is placed at rest, and the affected limb is handled very gently. It is positioned and supported to prevent contractures and deformities. A splint may be used to immobilize the adjacent joint or skin traction may be applied if a lower limb is affected. The patient tends to remain in one position because of fear of pain. He must be assisted to turn at frequent intervals to guard against pressure sores and respiratory complications. Good body alignment is necessary at all times. Fluids are given liberally because of the fever and blood infection. A high-calorie, well-balanced diet is encouraged to increase the patient's resistance. If nausea and vomiting are a problem, intravenous infusions of parenteral fluids may be necessary.

If surgical drainage or a sequestrectomy is performed, the wound is packed and allowed to heal by granulation from within toward the surface. Antibiotic or sulphonamide preparations may be introduced locally into the wound. The dressing is changed often enough to keep the wound clean and to prevent the development of an offensive odour that may become very distressing to the patient and those in his environment. Precautions must be taken to observe aseptic technique when dressing or treating the wound to prevent the introduction of secondary infection and to prevent the transmission of the patient's infection to others.

When the patient is allowed up, he must be protected against falls and injury to the limb. The loss of bone substance may weaken the bone structure, predisposing it to fracture when subjected to even slight injury or pressure. In the case of a lower extremity, weight-bearing may be contraindicated for many weeks while new bone tissue is being formed. The patient may then have to be taught to use crutches. He may be discharged from the hospital but is likely to require guidance and supervision for a considerable period of time.

As cited earlier, haematogenous osteomyelitis is seen most often in children as a result of infection in some area of the body and, unless treated early, it may lead to a long illness and serious crippling. Nurses (especially those visiting in homes and schools) and parents must be constantly alert to the possible significance of focal and recurring infections, such as boils. Medical treatment should be sought for the child. Any complaint of tenderness or pain in a limb, especially if it is associated with fever or general malaise, requires prompt attention.

---

[6] *Involucrum* is a covering or sheath, such as contains the sequestrum of a necrosed bone.

OSTEOPOROSIS

Osteoporosis is a metabolic bone disorder characterized by decreased density and atrophy due to an increase in calcium reabsorption in combination with a reduction in compensatory bone formation.[7] There is a diminished production of the collagenous matrix in which calcium and phosphorus are deposited; as a result, bone tissue is worn down more rapidly than it is replaced. The trabeculae are fewer, and the tissue is rarefied as compared to normal bone. The calcium and phosphorus levels of the blood are normal or may be elevated if the intake is normal.

The weight-bearing vertebrae (lower thoracic and lumbar) and pelvis are usually the first bones to be involved. As the disease becomes more advanced, the long bones, ribs and skull are affected. Osteoporosis has a higher incidence in females, especially after menopause, and is commonly seen in elderly persons.

Cause

Osteoporosis may be attributed to the decreased demand and strain that is associated with immobilization or sedentary life which reduces the stimulation of osteoblastic activity, a diminished secretion of anabolic sex hormones (e.g. oestrogen) (as occurs after the climacteric and in senility), a negative calcium balance or a deficient protein intake. In some instances, the disorder is secondary to some endocrine disturbances such as hyperthyroidism and Cushing's syndrome (adrenocortical hyperfunction) or may be the result of prolonged administration of large doses of corticoids. Others at risk are small women, nulliparous women, those with a family history of osteoporosis and persons suffering from alcoholism or who are heavy smokers. Evidence suggests that bone density is decreased in people with diabetes.

Signs and symptoms

The initial symptom in most patients is usually back pain due to a flattening or collapse or vertebrae and resulting pressure on spinal nerves. Muscle spasm and limited movement may also develop. Remissions occur and, frequently, exacerbations are precipitated by lifting or stooping. Kyphosis (forward curvature of the spine), loss of the normal lumbar curve and loss of stature may become apparent. The bones fracture more readily and osteoporosis contributes to the high incidence of fracture of the hip in older persons. Spontaneous compression fractures are common in vertebrae of the thoracolumbar region. In many instances, the condition goes unrecognized until the person receives a fracture in a simple fall and the x-rays reveal a loss of density in bone tissue.

Treatment and nursing intervention

During an acute episode, the patient is placed on bed rest and given analgesics to relieve pain. Application of ice or moist heat packs, intermittently, to areas of pain and administration of muscle relaxants may also be included in the early treatment programme. A firm mattress on a fracture board is important. As soon as the pain and muscle spasm are reduced the patient is mobilized, as prolonged bed rest only contributes to further weakening of the bone structure and muscles. For comfort and mobility, the patient may require a brace or corset to support the spine.

A diet high in calcium with vitamin D supplement is usually recommended. Since excessive protein from meat sources and phosphorus intake predisposes to bone reabsorption, protein from dairy products is encouraged and sources of phosphorus such as soft drinks discouraged. A liberal daily fluid intake is taken to reduce the possibility of hypercalciuria and ensuing renal or bladder calculus formation. The calorie intake is controlled to avoid obesity, which places added strain on the weakened bone structure. Activity is encouraged to stimulate osteoblastic activity, and a daily exercise regimen is frequently prescribed.

Medications that may be prescribed include a preparation of calcium (e.g. calcium gluconate), oestrogen (e.g. ethinyloestradiol) and progesterone, calcitonin or anabolic steroids [e.g. nandrolone (Deca-Durabolin)]. In the case of a female receiving oestrogen therapy, progesterone must be given if the patient still has her uterus; close observations are made for any sign of vaginal bleeding, which is reported promptly as the incidence of uterine carcinoma is known to increase in patients on this therapy. Any woman with abnormal vaginal bleeding should have a gynaecological assessment, including cervical smear and dilatation and curettage.

The patient is instructed to avoid lifting heavy objects and to keep his spine straight and flex his thighs and knees when he wants to reach something at floor level. Patients, especially older persons, are cautioned against falls. Scatter rugs, foot-stools or other objects in the environment that might lead to a fall are removed. A firm supportive shoe with a walking heel should be worn.

Currently, emphasis is being placed on the prevention of osteoporosis, especially in women past menopause. Controversy exists as to the use of oestrogen replacement therapy to prevent a disorder that is part of the ageing process. Oestrogen therapy has also been connected with an increased incidence of cervical cancer in females. There is growing agreement based on controlled studies that calcium intake should be increased in women during the pre- and postmenopausal periods. The recommended daily dietary calcium intake is 1200–1500 mg for women[8].

---

[7] Lukert (1982), p. 346.

[8] Heaney, Gallagher, Johnston et al (1982), p. 986.

Calcium supplements may be given if the recommended amount cannot be taken in a dietary form. Regular, weight-bearing exercise such as walking is recommended at all ages, but especially for the elderly, to decrease bone loss.

OSTEOMALACIA

Osteomalacia is an adult disorder comparable to rickets in children, and, for this reason, it is occasionally referred to as adult rickets. It is characterized by an insufficient plasma concentration of calcium and inorganic phosphate for normal calcification of bone tissue. The bones become soft and weak. The person complains of tenderness and an aching pain in the bones. Some bowing of long bones and deformities may develop. A loss of weight and muscular strength may be manifested and, if the calcium deficiency is marked, tetany may be exhibited (see p. 656).

Osteomalacia may be the result of an insufficient amount of calcium reaching the plasma or an excessive urinary excretion of the mineral. In the first instance, the deficiency of calcium may be due to a lack of calcium-containing foods in the diet, insufficient absorption of the mineral from the intestine (caused by steatorrhoea or prolonged diarrhoea), or a deficiency of vitamin D in the diet or as a result of renal failure, which is necessary for normal absorption of calcium and its deposition in bone tissue. Osteomalacia may also occur during pregnancy if the woman does not receive additional calcium to meet the increased demand incurred by the developing fetus.

The second major cause of the disease—that is, an excessive urinary excretion of calcium—is usually the result of acidosis associated with renal failure or of renal tubular damage and malfunction.

The treatment consists mainly of the administration of calcium, phosphorus and vitamin D. If the serum calcium concentration is markedly low, calcium (e.g. calcium gluconate 10%) may be given intravenously.

PAGET'S DISEASE (OSTEITIS DEFORMANS)

Paget's disease is a chronic bone disease of unknown aetiology characterized by structural changes. These are due to accelerated and excessive abnormal bone destruction (osteolysis) and regeneration together with the laying down of vascular fibrous tissue. The disorder seldom occurs in persons younger than 50 and the incidence increases in the later years.

Symptoms

The patient complains of skeletal pains and headache. Softening of the bones results in deformities; anterior bowing of the tibia and kyphosis become apparent. An x-ray shows thickening of the bones and an irregularity in their contour. There is a marked increase in the vascularity of the affected bones. The changes in bone structure begin at one end of the bone and spread progressively toward the other end. The blood calcium and phosphorus levels are normal, but the alkaline phosphatase concentration is elevated. The disorder seems to be a predisposing factor in the development of osteosarcoma, since some patients with Paget's disease develop this malignancy. Pathologic fractures are a common complication.

Treatment

Treatment and nursing care are supportive and symptomatic; there is no specific or curative treatment. Calcitonin or mithramycin may be given to decrease the alkaline phosphatase level and decrease bone reabsorption. Disodium etidronate is an alternative drug which reduces the rate of bone turnover and relieves pain. A high-calcium, high-protein diet with vitamin C and D supplements is recommended. A supervised exercise and activity programme is important. Aids such as a corset and brace are used to provide support for ambulation. Lifting, twisting and strenuous activities are avoided.

BONE NEOPLASMS

Primary and secondary neoplasms may develop in bone tissue. Primary newgrowths may be benign or malignant; secondary bone neoplasms are metastases from malignant disease in another area of the body and have a much higher incidence than primary neoplasms. Primary sites that frequently cause bone metastases are the breast, prostate, lung, thyroid and kidney. The bones that are the most common sites of metastases are the vertebrae, pelvic bones, femora and humeri.

Most primary bone neoplasms develop in children and adults younger than 40 years. They may be classified by the type of cell from which they originate, whether they are benign or malignant, and whether the tissue response is osteolytic or reactive. The neoplasm may cause a breakdown of the bone structure, with loss of calcium from the tissue; this type of reaction is referred to as osteolytic. The response of bone tissue to some types of neoplastic cells is the formation of dense bone tissue around the lesion, which may be referred to as a nidus. This type of reaction is called reactive bone formation.

The more common primary bone neoplasms are listed in Table 25.4.

Manifestations

Neoplasms of bones may be asymptomatic for a period of time and may only be discovered when the person has an x-ray for some other reason (e.g. sustained injury) or has a pathologic fracture. Persis-

Table 25.4 Common primary bone neoplasms.

Cell of origin	Neoplasm	Benign/malignant	Comments
Osteocyte	Osteoid osteoma	Benign	Small, reactive lesion. Femur and tibia common sites. Especially painful at night. Treatment involves surgical removal
	Osteochondroma	Benign	Commonest benign bone neoplasm; a hamartoma* consisting of bony outgrowth with a cartilage cap. Distal end of femur, proximal end of tibia and proximal end of humerus are common sites. Symptoms depend upon impingement on surrounding tissues
	Osteogenic sarcoma (osteosarcoma)	Malignant (rapid spread)	Destroys medullary and cortical bone tissue. Usually develops in end of long bone; almost 50% involve the knee joint. Severe pain and tenderness; area may be hot and swollen. Treatment consists of amputation and chemotherapy, or chemotherapy and endoprosthetic replacement
	Osteoclastoma (giant cell tumour)	Benign—may become malignant	Develops most often in epiphyseal region of femur, tibia or humerus of young adults. Rarefaction of bone occurs. It causes pain, swelling and rarely pathological fracture. Treated by curettage or by resection of the bone and replacement with a bone graft. If malignant, the limb is amputated, or chemotherapy and endoprosthetic replacement
Chondrocyte	Endochondroma	Benign	Growth of tumour cells of the hyaline cartilage may cause a pathological fracture. Treatment is by curettage
	Chondroblastoma	Benign	Develops toward end of adolescence. Common sites are femur, tibia and humerus. Highest incidence in males. Causes pain and swelling in epiphyseal area. Treatment is curettage and bone grafts
	Chondrosarcoma	Malignant (slower spread than osteosarcoma)	Age group most often affected 30–60 years. Common sites are scapula, pelvis, humerus and femur. Treatment involves radical excision, amputation, or chemotherapy and endoprosthetic replacement
Fibrocyte	Non-osteogenic fibroma	Benign	Most common site is end of diaphysis of long bone. If asymptomatic, it may be left untreated. If painful, it is excised
	Fibrosarcoma	Malignant	Rare. Usually in adults. Treated by amputation if in a limb or chemotherapy plus endoprosthetic replacement
Uncertain; reticulocyte suggested	Ewing's tumour or sarcoma	Malignant	May involve ilia, ribs, vertebrae and shafts of long bones. Begins in marrow cavity and gradually erodes the bone tissue. Manifestations include severe pain, swelling, fever and leucocytosis. Treatment is combination of irradiation, chemotherapy and surgery, including endoprosthetic replacement

*A *hamartoma* is a benign tumour formed by an overgrowth of normal mature cells characteristic of the area.

ting pain, progressively increasing in severity, and limitation of activity of the affected part are common characteristics. Local tenderness, swelling and warmth may be present. If the neoplasm is malignant, systemic symptoms such as weight loss and anaemia develop.

Diagnostic procedures

Investigation of the patient with the symptoms mentioned may include x-rays, bone scan, blood tests (haematocrit, leucocyte count, microscopy, sedimentation rate and serum alkaline phosphatase level) and biopsy.

Bone scanning is very useful in detecting early primary lesions or metastatic lesions. A radioisotope is administered that is normally picked up by bone. Examples of radioactive materials used are technetium-99m-tagged phosphate, fluoride-18, gallium-67 and strontium-85. When technetium, fluoride or gallium is used, the scan is made about 3 hours after its administration; if strontium is administered, a period of 2–3 days usually elapses before scanning.

Treatment

Benign bone neoplasms are treated by excision or curettage. The bone structure may have to be reinforced following the removal of the lesion by filling in the space with bone chips or small grafts. Treatment of primary malignant neoplasms involves a combination of surgery and chemotherapy. Radical excision is done if the lesion is accessible or, in the case of an extremity, the limb is amputated. Development has occurred in the preservation of mobility of many patients by the use of custom-made joint and bone replacement (endoprosthetic replacement).[9] Suitable cases may be those where there is no diffuse spread of the tumour into surrounding secondary deposits. Extending prostheses have been developed in the last decade. They can be used in the tibia, femur and humerus of the growing child or adolescent. For nursing care of the patient, the reader is referred to Nursing Intervention in Amputation, described earlier in this chapter, and Nursing Intervention of the Patient Receiving Chemotherapy in Chapter 9.

The treatment of the patient with skeletal metastases depends principally on the origin of the primary malignant disease. Chemotherapy, hormones and/or irradiation may be used. Irradiation may be used to reduce the severity of the pain experienced by the patient. Analgesics are prescribed to keep the patient comfortable; a small dose is used at first but usually has to be increased as the condition worsens and the patient develops a tolerance for the drug. Precautions are taken to prevent possible falls or injury because of the weakened bone structure; a pathologic fracture is a common complication. The nurse should show caring and understanding and should provide support. When the condition restricts movement and persisting pain is being experienced many simple nursing measures can mean much to the patient, and indicate understanding and caring. Examples are frequent gentle change of position, placing a support under a part, turning pillows, bathing and providing essential hygienic care, adherence to a pain control programme developed for the individual (see Management of the Patient with Chronic Progressive Pain, Chapter 8), provision of fluids and nourishment and merely remaining with the patient frequently for even a few minutes.

---

[9] *Endoprosthetic replacement* was pioneered at the Department of Biomedical Engineering, Institute of Orthopaedics at Stanmore Royal National Orthopaedic Hospital.

References and Further Reading

BOOKS

Banerjee SN (ed) (1982) *Rehabilitation Management of Amputees*. Baltimore: Williams & Wilkins.

Behs Symonds GW (1984) *Fracture Care and Management*. London: Macmillan.

Fields WL & McGinn-Campbell KM (1983) *Introduction to Health Assessment*. Reston, Virginia; Reston Publishing. Chapter 17.

Hart LK, Reese JL & Fearing MO (1981) *Concepts Common to Acute Illness*. St Louis: CV Mosby. Chapter 5.

Humm W (1977) *Rehabilitation of the Lower Limb Amputee*, 3rd ed. London: Ballière Tindall.

McRae R (1981) *Practical Fracture Treatment*. Edinburgh: Churchill Livingstone.

Miller M & Miller JH (1985) *Orthopaedics and Accidents Illustrated*. London: Hodder & Stoughton.

Monk CJE (1981) *Orthopaedics for Undergraduates*, 2nd ed. Oxford: Oxford University Press. Chapters 1 & 2.

Owens R, Goodfellow J & Bullogh P (eds) (1980) *Scientific Foundations of Orthopaedics and Traumatology*. Philadelphia: WB Saunders.

Powell M (1982) *Orthopaedic Nursing and Rehabilitation*, 8th ed. Edinburgh: Churchill Livingstone.

Robbins S, Angell M & Kumar V (1981) *Basic Pathophysiology*, 3rd ed. Philadelphia: WB Saunders. pp. 622–631.

Sabiston DC Jr (ed) (1986) *Davis–Christopher: Textbook of Surgery*, 13th ed. Philadelphia: WB Saunders. Chapter 43.

Sevitt S (1981) *Bone Repair and Fracture Healing in Man*. Edinburgh: Churchill Livingstone.

Smith LH & Thier SO (1986) *Pathophysiology*, 2nd ed. Philadelphia: WB Saunders. Section 9.

Stewart JDM & Hallett JP (1983) *Traction and Orthopaedic Appliances*. Edinburgh: Churchill Livingstone.

Troup IM & Wood MA (1982) *Total Care of the Lower Limb Amputee*. London: Pitman.

PERIODICALS

Anderson JT & Gustelo RB (1980) Immediate internal fixation in open fracture. *Orth. Clin. N. Am.*, Vol. 11 No. 3, pp. 569–578.

Andrew R & Pudner P (1985) Fractures. (Nursing Second Series). *Orth. Sports Inj.*, Vol. 44 No. 2, pp. 1293 & 1294.

Bailey M (1982) Emergency! first-aid for fractures. *Nurs. '82*, Vol. 12 No. 11, pp. 72–81.

Beasley RW (1981) General considerations in managing upper limb amputations. *Orth. Clin. N. Am.*, Vol. 12 No. 4, pp. 743–749.

Chamings PA & Stephenson CM (1982) Retrospective analysis of nursing care for a patient with hemipelvectomy. *Crit. Care Nurse*, Vol. 2 No. 2, pp. 18–23.

Courpron P (1981) Bone tissue mechanisms underlying osteoporosis. *Orth. Clin. N. Am.*, Vol. 12 No. 3, pp. 513–545.

Crowther H (1982) New perspectives on nursing lower limb amputees. *J. Adv. Nurs.*, Vol. 7 No. 5, pp. 453–460.

Dalinka M, Aronchick JM & Haddad JG Jr. (1983) Paget's disease. *Orth. Clin. N. Am.*, Vol. 14 No. 1, pp. 3–19.

Gill KP & Laflamme D (1984) External fixation: the erector sets of orthopedic nursing. *Can. Nurse*, Vol. 80 No. 5, pp. 29–31.

Heaney RP, Gallagher JC, Johnston CC, Neer R, Parfitt AM, Chir B & Whedon GD (1982) Calcium nutrition and bone health in the elderly. *Am. J. Clin. Nutr.*, Vol. 36 No. 5, pp. 986–1013.

Jaworski ZFG (1981) Physiology and pathology of bone remodelling. *Orth. Clin. N. Am.*, Vol. 12 No. 3, pp. 485–512.

Lamb K (1979) Effects of positioning of postoperative fractured hip patients as related to comfort. *Nurs. Res.*, Vol. 28 No. 5, pp. 291–294.

Lentz M (1981) Selected aspects of deconditioning secondary to immobilization. *Nurs. Clin. N. Am.*, Vol. 16 No. 4, pp. 729–737.

Lukert BP (1982) Osteoporosis—A review and update. *Arch. Phys. Med. Rehab.*, Vol. 63 No. 10, pp. 480–487.

MacPherson KI (1985) Osteoporosis and menopause: a feminist analysis of the social construction of a syndrome. *Adv. Nurs. Sci.*, Vol. 7 No. 4, pp. 11–22.

Mines A (1985) Osteoporosis: a detailed look at the clinical manifestations and goals for nursing care. *Can. Nurs.*, Vol. 81 No. 1, pp. 45–48.

Newman JC, Hurson B & Lane JM (1983) Osteogenic sarcoma. *Hosp. Med.*, Vol. 19 No. 12, pp. 113–114, 116, 119–126.

Palmason D (1985) Osteoporosis: catching the silent thief. *Can. Nurs.*, Vol. 81 No. 1, pp. 42–44.

Pashley J & Wahlstrom ML (1981) Polytrauma: the patient, the family, the nurse and the health team. *Nurs. Clin. N. Am.*, Vol. 16 No. 4, pp. 721–727.

Recker RR (1981) Continuous treatment of osteoporosis: current status. *Orth. Clin. N. Am.*, Vol. 12 No. 3, pp. 611–626.

Rice V (1983) Magnesium, calcium and phosphate imbalance; their clinical significance. *Crit. Care Nurs.*, Vol. 3 No. 3, pp. 88–112.

Rodts MF (1983) An orthopedic assessment you can do in 15 minutes. *Nurs. '83*, Vol. 13 No. 5, pp. 65–73.

Smith AG (1982) Common problems of lower extremity amputees. *Orth. Clin. N. Am.*, Vol. 13 No. 3, pp. 569–578.

Spencer H (1982) Osteoporosis: goals of therapy. *Hosp. Pract.* Vol. 17 No. 3, pp. 131–151.

Thompson JW (1985) Alleviating phantom-limb pain. *Mims magazine* (1st May), p. 91–93.

Tile M (1980) Pelvic fractures: operative versus nonoperative treatment. *Orth. Clin. N. Am.*, Vol. 13 No. 3, pp. 423–463.

Turner P (1982) Caring for emotional needs of orthopedic trauma patients. *AORN J.* Vol. 36 No. 4, pp. 566–570.

Wassell A (1981) Nursing assessment of injuries to the lower extremity. *Nurs. Clin. N. Am.*, Vol. 16 No. 4, pp. 739–748.

Wassel A (1983) Using prosthetics to aid independence. *Patient Care*, Vol. 17 No. 1, pp. 45, 47, 50, 55–56, 60–61, 64–65, 68–70.

Webb JT (1985) Orthopaedic conditions affecting children. (Nursing Second Series.) *Orth. Sports Inj.*, Vol. 44 No. 2, p.1309.

26

Nursing in Joint and Connective Tissue Disorders

Joint Structure and Function

A joint or articulation is formed at the junction of two bones. Joints may be classified according to their structures or the degree of movement they permit. *Synarthroses*, or fibrous joints, are immovable and have a layer of connective tissue which unites the bones. The cranial bones form synarthroses. *Amphiarthroses*, or cartilaginous joints, are slightly movable; the bones are separated by a layer of fibro-cartilaginous tissue which allows a limited amount of bending or twisting. The symphysis pubis of the pelvis and the joints between the vertebral bodies form amphiarthroses.

Most of the articulations of the skeleton are *diarthroses* or synovial joints, which are freely movable (Fig. 26.1). The bones are separated by a small cavity enclosed in a tough fibrous capsule which is continuous with the periosteum of the bones. This arrangement serves to stabilize the joint and keep the bones in normal apposition. The joint may be further reinforced by ligaments extending from one bone to the other. The capsule is lined with a synovial membrane (synovium) and the joint surfaces of the bones in diarthroses are covered by a layer of cartilage. The capsule contains synovial fluid which bathes the

cartilage, supplying nutrients to it in addition to functioning as a lubricant to promote smooth movement. Most of the fluid is a transudate of plasma which escapes from the vasculature of the synovium. Some constituents of synovial fluid are secreted by the synovial membrane. Some diarthrotic joints have flat, crescent-shaped pieces of cartilage lying in the cavity between the ends of the bones. These and the layer of cartilage on the joint surfaces buffer the impact of the rigid bone and cushion and protect the bone tissue. For example, in the knee joint, between the condyles of the femur and tibia, are semilunar cartilages referred to as menisci (singular—meniscus) (See Fig. 26.2). The medial and lateral menisci are frequent sites of internal joint derangement.

The shapes of the articulating surfaces vary with the particular type(s) of movement required of that area of the skeleton. For instance, the shoulder and hip joints are ball-and-socket in structure to allow all types of movement. The elbows and knees are hinge-like, allowing movement in one direction only.

Joint Disorders

NURSING PROCESS

Assessment

Assessment of the patient with disorders of joints includes a complete *history*, *physical examination* and a variety of *diagnostic tests* since these disorders are often part of a systemic disease. Although the following discussion focuses on the collection of data specific to joint function, the examiner must remember to assess other associated body systems when symptoms indicate systemic involvement. Assessment of the patient's gait is an important part of the physical assessment of joint function, (see Chapter 25).

HISTORY

The health history includes detailed data on the *presenting problems* which may be local only or both general and local. Joint pain, stiffness, swelling or

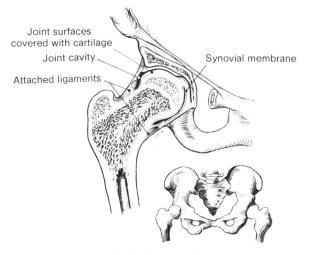

Joint surfaces covered with cartilage
Joint cavity
Attached ligaments
Synovial membrane

Fig. 26.1 Diagram of a freely moveable joint (diarthrosis).

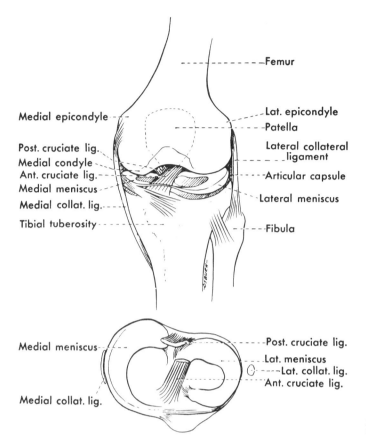

Fig. 26.2 Knee joint, showing supporting ligaments and medial and lateral menisci.

general fatigue or loss of strength may have led the patient to seek help. A description of joint pain indicates: the severity, duration, pattern and location of the pain, factors which cause or aggravate the pain, involvement of surrounding structures, and the effect of the pain on joint movement and function.

The pattern and degree of any joint swelling are determined. It may be more apparent at different times of the day or following certain activities or inactivity.

The degree and duration of joint stiffness are identified. Stiffness may be more apparent in the morning and last for varying lengths of time before activity can be undertaken.

The degree of impairment in joint movement may vary. The patient is asked to identify factors such as inactivity or specific activities which aggravate the stiffness and what alleviates the symptom and facilitates movement.

Generalized weakness, fatigue and listlessness are symptoms the patient may experience. Weight loss, anorexia and muscle wasting may also occur.

Environmental and occupational factors which affect joint functioning are identified: Does dampness, cold, warmth, or change in the weather influence symptoms? What physical activities are required as

part of job performance and is the patient at risk of musculo-skeletal injury? How the patient responds to the usual and unusual stresses of daily living is determined, as well as the effects of emotional stress on symptoms and mobility.

The patient's usual daily activity, ability to perform self-care and work-related activities and changes in usual physical functioning are noted. The patient is asked how his symptoms have affected his life-style and what they mean to him.

Past history includes information about musculo-skeletal injuries and surgery, nutritional state, metabolic disorders, infections and neurological problems. The patient's medication history is obtained in detail, including 'over-the-counter' as well as prescribed drugs. The use of muscle relaxants and salicylate preparations are particularly noted.

Any non-medical or folk medicine practices used by the patient are also identified. Many practices are handed down from relatives and neighbours; others are advertised in magazines and newspapers. It is important to identify what the patient is using and the importance he places on such practices. While the wearing of a copper bracelet may have no effect on the disease process, it may be very significant to the patient. Such practices may be relatively harmless or they may interfere with the patient receiving more effective treatment or cause economic hardships.

The *family history* includes information as to the incidence of arthritis and gout; these disorders have a familial predisposition.

PHYSICAL EXAMINATION

Vital signs. The patient's temperature, pulse and blood pressure are recorded.

General appearance. The patient is asked to stand, walk, bend, sit, lie down, grasp and to perform common daily activities such as combing the hair, putting on and removing various articles of clothing and feeding movements. While performing these activities, observations are made of general posture, symmetry, the ease and efficiency of movement and muscle strength.

Examination of individual joints. Knowledge of which joints are affected and the degree of impairment of motion is necessary to plan nursing intervention relevant to the needs of the individual patient. Individual joints or groups of joints and their surrounding tissues are observed, palpated and their range of motion determined. Table 26.1 cites tests for active range of motion of the major body joints. Fig. 26.3 illustrates common normal joint movements. Each joint movement is evaluated for any limitation or increase from the normal range.

Following active range of motion, joint mobility is assessed by passive range of motion. Painful joints are supported by the examiner's hands and movements are performed gently and slowly; movement should never be forced. Joint function and muscle strength may be appraised also by using resistance. This involves the examiner applying pressure against which the patient actively performs a specific movement (for example, the examiner's hands are placed on the patient's lower arm, pressure is applied and the patient is asked to flex his forearm). Illustrations of the human body may be used to record joint assessment and provide an overview of involved joints (see Fig. 26.4). A goniometer, which measures angles, may be used to measure degrees of movement of a joint. For example, the normal range of flexion of an elbow is 135–150°, and tension 0–5°; hip abduction varies from 45–50°, with hip adduction being approximately 20–30°. Some decrease in mobility of joints occurs with age.

Each joint is examined for swelling, tenderness, redness, warmth, physical deformity and crepitation. It is compared to the corresponding joint for symmetry and degree of change. Any discoloration, scar, discharge and subcutaneous nodule are noted. The adjoining muscles are observed for signs of atrophy, palpated for tone and tested for strength and symmetry of movement; the bones of involved joints and the tendons are palpated.

DIAGNOSTIC PROCEDURES

Roentgenograms are made of the joint(s) and may

Table 26.1 Tests for active range of motion.*

Joint	Motion	Test
Cervical spine	Flexion	The patient is instructed to bend the head forward and touch the chin to the chest
	Extension	The patient is instructed to bend the head backward and look at the ceiling
	Lateral bending	The patient is instructed to tilt the head and try to touch the left ear to the left shoulder and the right ear to the right shoulder
	Rotation	The patient is instructed to turn the head and try to touch the chin to the right shoulder and then to the left shoulder
Lumbar spine	Flexion	The patient is instructed to bend forward and try to touch the toes
	Extension	The patient is instructed to bend backward as far as possible with the examiner's hand supporting the lower spine
	Lateral bending	The patient is instructed to bend as far to the right and as far to the left as possible
	Rotation	The patient is instructed to twist the shoulders to the right and then to the left
Shoulder	Abduction and external rotation	The patient is instructed to reach behind and touch the superior, medial (upper, inner) angle of the opposite scapula with fingers
	Internal rotation and abduction	The patient is instructed to reach across chest and touch the opposite shoulder joint. Then client is asked to reach behind and touch the inferior, medial (lower, inner) angle of the opposite scapula with fingers
Elbow	Flexion	The patient is instructed to bend the elbows and touch the hands to the front of the shoulders
	Extension	The patient is instructed to straighten out elbows as much as possible

Table 26.1—*continued*

Joint	Motion	Test
	Supination	The patient is instructed to bend the elbows to 90° and hold them tightly against the waist. The client is asked to hold a pencil in each fist, palms facing downward, and then turn the fists until the palms are facing upward
	Pronation	The patient is instructed to bend the elbows to 90° and hold them tightly against the waist. The client is asked to hold a pencil in each fist, palms facing upward, and then turn the fists until the palms are facing downward
Wrist	Flexion	The patient is instructed to bend the wrist, moving the palmar surface of the hand down
	Extension	The patient is instructed to bend the wrist, moving the dorsal surface of the hand upward
	Ulnar deviation	The patient is instructed to bend the wrist toward the little finger side of the hand
	Radial deviation	The patient is instructed to bend the wrist toward the thumb side of the hand
	Supination	The patient is instructed to turn the forearm so the palm of the hand is facing upward
	Pronation	The patient is instructed to turn the forearm so the palm of the hand is facing downward
Hand	Finger flexion	The patient is instructed to make a tight fist
	Finger extension	The patient is instructed to open the hand and extend the fingers
	Finger abduction	The patient is instructed to spread the fingers apart as far as possible
	Finger adduction	The patient is instructed to close the fingers together tightly
	Thumb flexion	The patient is instructed to move the thumb over to the base of the little finger
	Thumb extension	The patient is instructed to bend the thumb away from the rest of the fingers
	Palmar abduction	The patient is instructed to move the thumb upward, away from the palm of the hand
	Palmar adduction	The patient is instructed to move the thumb back to touch the palm of the hand
	Opposition	The patient is instructed to touch the tips of each of his four fingers with the thumb
Hip	Flexion	The patient is instructed to bring the knees as far as possible toward the chest without bending the back
	Extension	While the patient is sitting, he is instructed to fold the arms across the chest, keep the back straight, and get up from the chair
	Abduction	While the patient is standing, the patient is instructed to spread the legs as far apart as possible
	Adduction	With the legs spread apart, the patient is instructed to bring them back together and then cross the right leg over the left and the left leg over the right
	External rotation	The patient is instructed to place the lateral side of the foot on the opposite knee. Repeat this for both sides
	Internal rotation	There are no adequate active tests
Knee	Flexion	The patient is instructed to do a deep knee bend
	Extension	The patient is instructed to stand up from a deep knee bend or to sit on the edge of the examining table and extend the leg out straight
	External rotation	The patient is instructed to rotate the foot outward (laterally)
	Internal rotation	The patient is instructed to rotate the foot inward (medially)
Ankle	Dorsiflexion	The patient is instructed to walk on the heels
	Plantar flexion	The patient is instructed to walk on the toes
Foot	Inversion	The patient is instructed to walk on the outer (lateral) borders of the feet
	Eversion	The patient is instructed to walk on the inner (medial) aspects of the feet
	Adduction	The patient is instructed to move the foot inward without twisting it
	Abduction	The patient is instructed to move the foot outward without twisting it
	Toe flexion	The patient is instructed to walk on the toes
	Toe extension	The patient is instructed to extend the toes

* Fields & McGinn-Campbell (1983).

include *arthography*. In the latter, a radiopaque substance is injected into the joint cavity to provide a contrast medium so that the soft tissue components may be visualized. This is generally done with investigation of a knee.

Aspiration of synovial fluid may be performed to obtain a specimen for laboratory examination for the presence of blood, pus, organisms, sodium urate crystals or malignant cells. A local anaesthetic is used and strict asepsis must be observed.

An *arthroscopy* may be done to provide endoscopic examination of a joint. It is used most often in knee disorders. The doctor is able to visualize and assess the synovium, articular surfaces, menisci and ligaments, and a biopsy may also be done.

The examination is performed in the operating

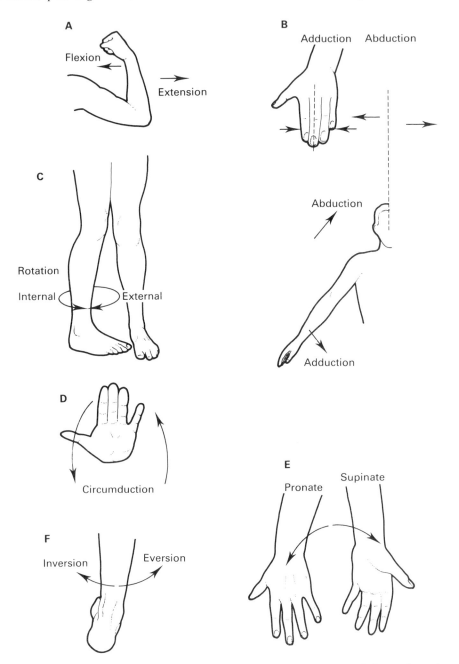

Fig. 26.3 Joint movements. *A*, Flexion and extension. *B*, Abduction and adduction. *C*, Internal rotation and external rotation, *D*, Circumduction. *E*, Pronation and supination. *F*, Inversion and eversion.

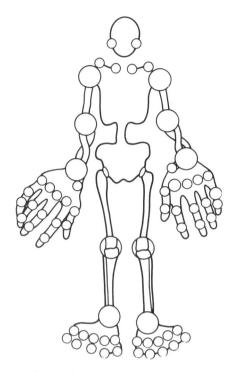

Fig. 26.4 Figure which may be used in joint assessment.

theatre under strict aseptic conditions. A local or general anaesthetic may be administered; the latter is used if surgical intervention is anticipated and is to follow the arthroscopy immediately.

The general and local preparations are the same as for surgery (see Chapter 11). A large-bore needle is introduced into the joint following anaesthesia and normal saline is introduced to 'fill out' the cavity. The arthroscope, which is a fibreoptic instrument, is then introduced. Following the examination, if no surgery is performed, the puncture area is sealed and a compressive bandage applied. Activity is usually limited for approximately 3 days.

The *electromyograph (EMG)* measures and records the electrical activity of skeletal muscles. Needle electrodes are placed in the muscle and the muscle is made to contract. The electrical activity is recorded on an oscilloscope and graph. Normal voluntary muscle is electrically inactive when at rest. Information is provided about the strength of the muscle's response. No physical preparation of the patient is necessary but the patient receives an explanation of the procedure beforehand.

Laboratory *blood and serum tests* that may be used in joint investigation include: (1) erythrocyte and leucocyte counts; (2) determination of haemoglobin, erythrocyte sedimentation rate (ESR), serum alkaline phosphatase, calcium and phosphorus concentrations and blood uric acid level; and (3) examination for rheumatoid (Rh) factors, antinuclear antibodies

(ANA), lupus erythematosus cells (LE prep), anti-DNA and complement fixation.

The blood cell counts, haemoglobin and ESR are used to determine the presence of anaemia, infection or tissue destruction. The serum phosphatase level is elevated in malignant disease, as is the ESR. The phosphorus and calcium concentrations are significant in bone disease, and the blood uric acid level is increased in gout. The presence of rheumatoid factors and autoimmune antibodies in serum occurs in 85% of people with late stage rheumatoid arthritis. The *latex fixation test* is most commonly used to identify rheumatoid factor IgG. Antinuclear antibodies and lupus erythematosus cells are usually present in patients with acute, active systemic lupus erythematosus. The anti-DNA test detects antibodies which react with DNA and is considered a specific test for systemic lupus erythematosus. Complement, a normal body protein associated with immune and inflammatory responses, may become fixed in rheumatoid arthritis and systemic lupus erythematosus.

Manifestations
Joint disorders may manifest local signs and symptoms only or both local and systemic disturbances. The local symptoms involve principally one or more joints.

Local manifestations
- *Pain.* Joint pain may be due to the inflammatory process, muscle spasm, adjoining soft tissue involvement or distension of the joint capsule by the disease process. It may develop suddenly or gradually, may radiate to another part and is aggravated by movement or weight-bearing.
- *Stiffness.* Joint stiffness develops following a period of inactivity and usually decreases with movement of the joint. It may be localized or generalized. The incidence increases with age and is most common in weight-bearing joints due to degenerative changes. Stiffness also occurs with an inflammatory disease process along with pain and muscle spasm. The duration of morning stiffness corresponds to the severity of disease activity; more than 1½ hours of morning stiffness may indicate acute inflammatory activity.
- *Swelling.* The inflammatory process resulting from injury or disease of a joint may cause an increase in synovial fluid; swelling, warmth, redness, pain and stiffness develop. Swollen joints are tender on palpation and the synovial membrane feels boggy or doughy. The range of motion is limited. Adjoining tissue may become oedematous.
- *Heat and redness.* An inflamed joint feels warm to the touch and the overlying skin may be red.
- *Crepitation.* This is a grating sound that occurs in a joint on movement when the joint surfaces are rough or denuded of cartilage.
- *Deformity.* Joint deformity is most commonly

associated with a dislocation, reactive bony overgrowth or joint disease.

Dislocation occurs when the bones of a joint are displaced and are no longer in the normal anatomical position. A partial dislocation is referred to as a subluxation. The cause of a dislocation may be trauma, unusual or sudden effort or movement, rheumatoid arthritis or degenerative joint disease.

Bony overgrowth, causing joint enlargement and deformity, develops when the ends of the bone are denuded of cartilage as occurs in the degenerative disease osteoarthrosis. Bony spurs or nodules may form; the latter are commonly seen in distal interphalangeal joints (Heberden's nodes).

- *Decreased range of motion.* Limitations in range of motion without pain or discomfort usually indicate previous damage to a joint. Pain on movement indicates trauma or an active disease process. Inactivity is a major contributor to loss of motion of joints. Functional limitations resulting from decreased range of motion depend on the joints involved and the severity of the loss. Ambulation is impaired when weight-bearing joints are involved, and the ability to perform activities of daily living is impaired when ambulation, upper extremity mobility and hand dexterity are affected.
- *Contracture* of a muscle results in limitation of range of motion and usually is caused by disuse of the joint and adjoining muscles. The muscle fibres shorten and atrophy, limiting the range of motion of the joint. The degree of resulting disability depends on the joints that are involved and the severity of the contracture. Knee and hip flexion contractures cause the greatest disability.
- *Muscle weakness and fatigue.* Muscular weakness and fatigue may be episodic, constant and generalized or localized. Muscle fatigue increases with the inflammatory activity of arthritis. Muscular weakness and wasting result from immobility. Weakness and decreased muscle mass develop around a chronically diseased joint. Generalized muscle weakness and wasting results with widespread joint involvement in patients with severe chronic rheumatoid arthritis, but may also occur with other diseases due to immobility. With muscle weakness, increased effort is required to perform activities.

Generalized symptoms. Systemic manifestations of widespread joint and connective tissue disorders include fatigue, weakness, anorexia, loss of weight, pallor and fever. A skin rash or subcutaneous nodules may also develop.

IDENTIFICATION OF PATIENT PROBLEMS

1 Impaired physical mobility related to limitations in range of motion of joints

2 Inflammation, pain and deformity of joints
3 Muscle weakness and wasting

Impaired mobility associated with joint and connective tissue disorders is a major problem for the individual, his family and society. The independence, security and total life-style of the patient and family are threatened; their productive role in society may be lost and they become dependent on others.

The *goals* are to maintain existing joint mobility, prevent or minimize further impairment of joint function and promote optimal functional mobility.

NURSING INTERVENTION

Maintenance of joint mobility and the promotion of optimal joint function are achieved through a combination of planned rest and exercise, and by protecting the joints from unnecessary stress. Planning and implementation of care requires cooperation between the nurse, physio- and occupational therapists, doctor, patient and family.

Rest

Rest is necessary for the patient with impaired joint mobility; it helps to control fatigue, inflammation and pain. The patient with limitation of joint function expends excessive energy in movement because of the limitations and pain. More sleep and several rest periods throughout the day are recommended; periods of activity are followed by periods of rest. Relaxation techniques may also be used by the patient to promote body relaxation and decrease emotional stress.

Joint rest may involve the use of splints to support and protect involved joints. The type of splint which may be applied depends on the purpose to be achieved (see Fig. 26.5). Resting splints are used to immobilize inflamed and painful joints and are worn continuously during periods of acute inflammation. They are removed for short intervals for essential activities such as eating and cleansing of the skin. During chronic or inactive phases of joint disease, rest splints are worn only at night. Functional splints are designed to stabilize and support a joint during activity. Corrective or dynamic splints are used to immobilize an involved joint, realign soft tissues or correct contractures or deformities. Splints are usually made of a lightweight thermoplastic material which is pliable when heated. They are moulded to the affected part and held in place with velcro straps. The patient's skin is protected from the splint by a layer of cloth material. The protective layer is either placed on the patient (e.g. a tube stocking) or is incorporated into the splint.

Assessment of the splint for proper fit is done when it is first applied. The skin under the splint is checked frequently during the first 24–48 hours and the splint is assessed for fit and achievement of the intended goal of immobility or functional

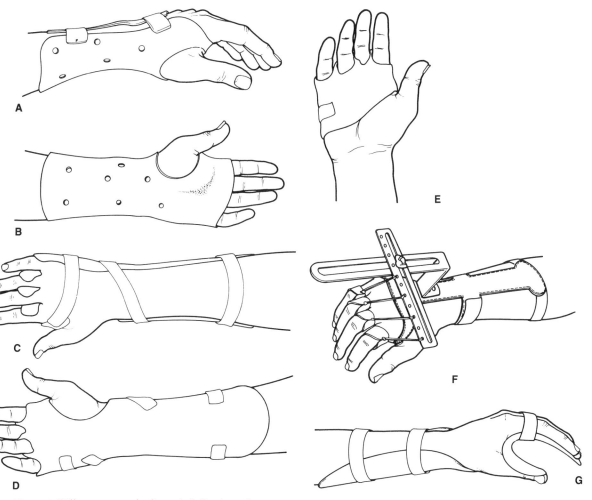

Fig. 26.5 Different types of splints. *A–E*, Resting splints to immobilize joints. *F*, Example of a functional splint used to stabilize and support a joint during activity. *G*, A corrective (dynamic) splint used to immobilize an involved joint, realign soft tissue or correct contractures or deformities.

movements. The patient and family are taught the application of the splints and to check for pressure points. A demonstration may be given to illustrate the pressure points that are created if the splint is not applied correctly. The patient is taught to inspect the skin under the splint for redness and tenderness each time it is removed. Splints require reassessment and possible replacement following acute illness, when the oedema has abated, and at regular intervals when used for long periods of time. Splints may be used on the fingers, hands, wrists, knees or ankles. Cervical collars may be used to restrict movement of the head and neck.

Heat and cold applications
Various forms of heat and cold applications are used to reduce muscle spasm, pain, joint stiffness and swelling. Moist heat is considered more effective than dry heat and may be applied in the form of

warm baths or pools, hot packs, or warm liquid par-affin wax.

Paraffin wax immersion consists of the application of several layers of melted paraffin wax to the affected extremity. The extremity is then wrapped in plastic to retain the heat.

Dry heat may be applied in the form of hot water bottles wrapped in towels, electric heating pads or infrared lamps. Short-wave diathermy and ultra-sound equipment provide deep (dry) heat and should be applied by a physiotherapist. Deep heat application is usually contraindicated for acutely inflamed joints. Table 26.2 describes home methods that may be used to apply heat or cold. Whatever form of heat is used, precautions must be used against burning the skin over the affected joints.

Applications of cold in the form of ice packs may be more or equally as effective as heat in relieving discomfort and spasm for some patients. Selection of either heat or cold is usually based on patient preference and perceived effectiveness of the modality in relieving pain and spasm.

Exercise
General exercise and therapeutic exercises contribute to the maintenance and promotion of joint function.
    Exercises may be classified as:
1 *Range-of-movement exercises.*   Normally, each joint is capable of a certain range of movement. In a joint

disorder, that range of movement may become limited and the muscle fibres shorten. Range-of-movement exercises involve the movement of a limb or part through its maximal potential range of movement to maintain or increase joint function. They may be passive, active, active assisted, functional or isotonic.
2 *Passive exercises.* In this type of exercise movement of the limb or part is carried out by some force or person other than the patient. Passive exercise is used to maintain joint mobility and

Table 26.2 Safe methods for heat or cold therapy at home.

Method	Suggestions/precautions
Heat	
General safety measures: never apply heat for more than 20–30 minutes; heat should not be used if the patient has poor circulation, decreased sensation, or if he is overly sensitive to heat	
Bath or shower: easy, allows some exercise during use but full range of motion is not possible; shower provides gentle massage	If the patient has trouble getting in and out of the bath he may need bath rails or a bathtub seat; showering may be easier
	If standing in the shower is stressful to the patient's legs or back, suggest showering sitting down on a stool
	A rubber bath mat should be used at all times
	To avoid burns, cold water should be turned on first and off last
Hand or foot bath: soak hands in the sink or feet in the bath	Encourage exercises that can be performed while soaking
Standard heating pad: easy method for one or two joints, but not as effective as moist heat in relieving pain and stiffness	Patient should not go to sleep with the heating pad on
	Standard heating pad should not come into contact with anything wet
Electric moist heating pad: a water-proof pad with a plastic cover; a flat sponge provides moist heat; holds heat well	Patient should not go to sleep with the heating pad on
	Check the pad regularly to make sure plastic cover is intact
Hot water bottle: easy method for heating one or two joints, but cools off quickly; less likely to cause burns	Follow general safety measures
Hot pack: commercially available pack that soaks up water and provides moist heat	
Cold	
General safety measures: never apply any method to one area for more than 15–20 minutes; remove when numbness is achieved; do not place ice between part being cooled and a firm surface; check skin during and after treatment for any signs of injury; dry skin thoroughly after treatment; do not use if overly sensitive to cold or if circulation is impaired (vasculitis, Raynaud's)	
Ice water bath: for one body part; especially good for hands and feet; surrounds joints with cold	Patient can exercise part while soaking
Plastic bag pack: does not surround joints with cold	Patient cannot exercise
Fill double plastic bag with ice	
Wrap bags in *warm*, wet towel; helps adjust to cold	
Commercially available packs can be kept in freezer	
Slush Pack:	
Line a bowl with two heavy plastic bags	
Fill bags with 2–3 cups water and 1 cup denatured alcohol (more water gives firmer slush)	
Fasten top of bags	
Place bowl in freezer until slush forms	
Wrap bags in warm, wet towel	
Return pack to bowl and place in freezer; bowl prevents possible leak of alcohol onto food	
Ice massage:	
Use either a large ice cube or freeze water in a paper cup and peel off paper	Use a rubber glove or some other protection for the hand holding the ice
Rub ice directly over area until skin feels numb (usually 10–15 minutes)	Some patients cannot tolerate intensity of cooling

prevent muscle contracture. Muscle strength is not increased.

3 *Active exercises.* These involve movements that are performed by the individual unassisted. Active exercises maintain or increase joint mobility and muscle strength and stimulate circulation and respiratory function as well as promote a sense of well-being.

4 *Active assistive exercises.* This type of exercise is carried out by the patient with the assistance of the physiotherapist or a device such as an overhead pulley and rope with a sling to provide support for the limb (sling suspension). The purpose is to increase muscle strength and maintain or increase joint range of motion.

5 *Functional exercises.* The activities of daily living (e.g. personal hygiene, dressing, etc.) provide exercises which maintain or promote muscle strengthening, joint mobility and help to achieve or maintain functional independence.

6 *Isometric (static) exercises.* These involve active, alternating maximal contraction and relaxation of muscles without movement of the respective joint and part. The length of the muscle remains the same.

7 *Isotonic exercises.* This type of exercise involves active contraction and shortening of muscles to produce movement with a minimal force of contraction. The purpose of isotonic exercises is to maintain or promote joint mobility; they are not used if the joint is inflamed since it increases pain and may further the inflammatory process.

Principles for planning and implementing exercise programmes include the following:

1 Range-of-movement exercises are planned to meet the needs of the individual patient at a specific time.

2 The purpose and importance of the exercises should be understood by the patient.

3 The exercises are carried out daily at regular intervals.

4 An exercise programme should be supervised by a qualified therapist.

5 Measures such as heat applications to promote muscle relaxation and decrease pain should precede exercise.

6 Indiscriminate movements and overstretching may cause a dislocation or torn tendons, and increase pain and inflammation.

7 During movement, support is provided above and below damaged, inflamed or painful joints.

8 A balance must be achieved between rest and exercise.

9 The exercise programme is modified if excessive fatigue or increased pain occurs.

10 Active or active-assistive range-of-movement exercises are carried out whenever possible.

11 The exercise programme is incorporated into activities of daily living as soon as possible.

12 Quadricep exercises are initiated as soon as possible, as muscle strength must be maintained or increased for walking and weight-bearing.

Protection of joints

Table 26.3 lists guidelines which help a patient to protect a damaged, inflamed or painful joint from further injury. The patient learns new ways to perform activities to decrease stress on affected joints. Conditions and unnecessary movements which cause pain and discomfort are avoided and the person learns to perform tasks with the least effort and greatest efficiency to minimize joint stress.

Table 26.3 Guidelines for joint protection.

Maintain good posture and body alignment at all times
Change position frequently
Use the largest muscles and strongest joints available for any task
Distribute weight of objects over several joints
Perform activities slowly and smoothly
Limit repetitive movements
Minimize use of swollen, painful joints
Stop activity when pain occurs
Space activities to provide frequent rest periods
Use assistive devices in the environment to eliminate unnecessary stress

Body positioning is important to prevent contractures and deformity. The patient tends to flex a painful joint to decrease pain, providing an initial decrease in pressure and relief of pain. As the flexed, and thus enlarged, joint space accumulates more fluid, pain returns and the patient is unable then to extend the parts. Knees are positioned in extension. A pillow may be used under the full length of the leg to maintain extension of the knee when the patient is supine. When the patient is turned to the side, he will automatically bend his knee; care is taken to change his position frequently. Rigid posterior splints (backslabs) are used if needed.

Good posture is maintained at all times. The bed should have a firm mattress or a board under the mattress. A straight-backed chair of the height which allows the feet to rest flat on the floor with the knees positioned at 90° angles and the spine straight, is used for sitting.

The patient is taught correct body mechanics and to distribute the weight over several joints. For example, a handbag worn over the shoulder distributes the weight over a larger joint in contrast with a handbag carried by a strap in the patient's hand which places stress on the smaller finger joints. When a heavy object is supported by both arms against the chest, the weight is more widely distributed than when it is supported by extended arms or hands.

Movements should be slow and smooth and unnecessary repetitive movements avoided. The patient is taught to change position frequently and to stop activities if pain occurs.

Conservation of energy requires planning and skill. The patient is assisted in achieving balance between rest and activity by planning his daily schedule, providing for rest periods after activity and ensuring sufficient hours of sleep. Activities should be spread throughout the week as well as each day. Heavy tasks are delegated to others and when this is not possible, careful organization of the activity is necessary to utilize assistive devices which minimize the weight or movement required.

EXPECTED OUTCOMES

The patient:
1 Describes a plan to balance rest and activity.
2 Demonstrates ability to carry out the prescribed exercise programme.
3 States techniques to protect joints.
4 Demonstrates ability to perform activities of daily living safely and efficiently.

Common Joint Disorders

COMMON JOINT INJURIES

Bursitis

A bursa is a protective structure consisting of a small, flat, fibrous sac lined with synovial membrane. The walls of the sac are separated by a film of synovial fluid. Bursae are located in areas that are subjected to friction or pressure, such as between a bone and overlying tendon or skin. Although inflammation of a bursa is not an internal joint disorder, the affected bursa most frequently is very close to or lies over a joint and results in its impaired function. Bursitis may develop in response to injury or infection. The bursae most commonly encountered clinically in bursitis are those situated between the olecranon process of the ulna and the skin, patella and the skin, shoulder muscles or their tendons and the head of the humerus or scapula, and tendon of Achilles and the calcaneus (heel bone). Excess fluid accumulates within the bursa in response to injury or irritation, causing swelling, pain, tenderness and impaired function.

Treatment involves the administration of non-steroidal antiinflammatory drugs and analgesics to decrease pain. An intrabursal injection of a steroid preparation may be given. Movement is promoted and encouraged as the inflammation and pain subside to prevent the development of adhesions. Chronic recurrence of bursitis may necessitate surgical removal of the affected bursa.

Sprain

A sprain is the tearing of ligaments of a joint and overstretching of the joint capsule by twisting or wrenching. The injury may also involve damage to blood vessels, tendons and/or nerves in or around the joint. The person experiences pain, which worsens on movement or weight-bearing, and loss of joint movement. Swelling develops and, if blood vessels are ruptured, extravasation of blood into the tissues causes discoloration. An x-ray of the injured part is usually recommended to rule out a fracture. The ankle is the most frequent site of this type of injury.

Treatment includes rest and elevation of the part and the application of cold for 12–24 hours to control oedema, bleeding and swelling; heat may then be used for comfort. The joint is immobilized and supported by a crêpe bandage or adhesive strapping; rarely, a plaster cast or splint may be necessary. Weight-bearing may be restricted for a considerable period of time, necessitating the use of crutches for mobility.

Dislocation

In a dislocation the bones of a joint are displaced and are no longer in normal anatomic apposition. The dislocation may be caused by a fall, blow or an unusual effort or movement. Some injury is sustained by the soft tissues of the joint (joint capsule, ligaments, semilunar cartilages, nerves and/or blood vessels).

Manifestations of a traumatic dislocation include pain, deformity, loss of motion of the involved part, and swelling. The joints most commonly affected are the shoulder, finger, thumb, knee and mandible. Dislocation of a hip in an infant or child is usually due to congenital failure of normal joint development.

The patient with a dislocation should receive prompt treatment which involves closed or open reduction and immobilization. The area is x-rayed to assess the extent of the injury and the dislocation is reduced as soon as possible. The patient is usually given a general anaesthetic; reduction involves manual traction and possibly abduction and/or rotation. The joint is then immobilized by the application of adhesive strapping, splint or plaster cast. The immobilization period varies from 2–6 weeks, depending upon the extent of damage to the joint capsule and ligamentous structures. Severe tearing and stretching of soft tissues may necessitate surgical repair in order to restore joint stability.

Internal derangement of a joint

Injury to a joint may incur tearing of the joint capsule, supporting ligaments and/or semilunar cartilages, resulting in a painful and weak joint with impaired function. The knee is the most common site of internal joint derangement.

The medial meniscus is very vulnerable to injury when the knee is subjected to rotation while flexed and then quickly extended. Tears do not heal; cartilage is less vascular than other tissues and does not regenerate readily. The patient experiences pain which is worse when the limb is used. Displacement of a torn part of the cartilage may cause locking of the joint. The knee is x-rayed and an arthroscopy may be done to assess the damage. Injury to the lateral meniscus occurs much less often than tearing of the medial cartilage.

Resting the affected joint, heat application and the administration of non-steroidal antiinflammatory drugs such as acetylsalicylic acid (aspirin) may provide relief for the patient. Surgical excision of the meniscus is done (meniscectomy) if pain and disability persist.

Preoperative preparation is the same as for any bone surgery. Surgery is usually performed by arthroscopy; that is by the insertion of an arthroscope into the joint. This approach produces less trauma and disability than surgery that involves opening of the joint.

Postoperatively, the leg is elevated on pillows in slight flexion for 12–18 hours.

The patient is taught to contract the quadriceps muscles several times at intervals throughout the day. Ambulation with crutches is usually commenced on the second postoperative day; weight-bearing on the operative limb may be gradually increased. Exercises are introduced to attain satisfactory range of joint motion. Full activity is usually resumed in about 5–6 weeks.

DEGENERATIVE JOINT DISEASE

Osteoarthritis (osteoarthrosis)

Osteoarthritis is a common chronic joint disorder which is also known as osteoarthrosis or degenerative arthritis. The disorder is characterized by degenerative changes in articular cartilage and marginal bony overgrowth.

MANIFESTATIONS AND CAUSES

Early symptoms appear in the middle or later years of life. It may develop in both males and females, but has a higher incidence in women over the age of 45 years. The cartilage on the articular ends of the bones becomes thin and worn and gradually breaks down, leaving the underlying bone exposed. The reaction of the denuded bone is manifested in outgrowths of bone from the joint margins, resulting in thickening of the ends of the bones and protruding ridges and spurs (osteophytes) which impair joint movement. Spurs may break off and become loose in the joint, causing further impairment of movement and more pain.

The weight-bearing joints, such as the spinal, hip and knee, and the interphalangeal joints are most frequently the site of degenerative joint disease. It may occur in a single joint or may involve several. The principal cause is thought to be the cumulative strain and wear on the joints through the preceding years, and the ageing process. Trauma of the joint, obesity, and malalignment, probably due to poor posture, may be causative factors.

The patient complains of stiffness, soreness and pain in the affected joint(s), and crepitation may be felt or heard on movement. The range of motion becomes increasingly limited because of pain, muscle spasm and the bony outgrowths. Joint enlargement and instability develop. The joints feel hard and irregular. Bony outgrowths on the dorsal surface of affected interphalangeal joints give the knuckles a knobby or gnarled appearance; these knobby protrusions are referred to as *Heberden's nodes*. Systemic manifestations do not occur.

CARE OF THE PATIENT

Most patients are treated conservatively but, if the pain becomes intractable and the disability severe, partial or total replacement arthroplasty may be used in selected instances.

In conservative treatment, strain on the affected joints is kept to a minimum. A full explanation of the nature of the disorder should be made to the patient in terms he can understand. This may be supplemented by providing the patient with a booklet that describes the disorder and care. Reduced use of the joints and living within the tolerance of the involved parts are stressed. The use of a walking stick or crutches is encouraged, if necessary, to reduce weight-bearing and keep the patient ambulatory. The patient may have to change his occupation and give up any strenuous sport or other form of recreation. If overweight, the patient is urged to lose weight. During periods of acute pain, a brief period of bed rest, heat applications and medication may be necessary.

Medications used in treating the patient with osteoarthrosis are prescribed primarily to control pain. They include aspirin and other analgesics, or regular medication with a non-steroidal antiinflammatory drug such as indomethacin.

Appropriate exercises are prescribed to maintain muscle tone and movement and promote good alignment and joint stability. The patient is encouraged to be posture-conscious and to review his regular daily activities and posture. Work should be interspersed with short intervals of rest, and unnecessary walking, climbing stairs, lifting and bending should be eliminated. A fitted corset may be helpful to immobilize and provide support in the case of degenerative changes in the spine. A firm mattress with a 'fracture' board between it and the bedsprings is recommended to promote good alignment and support for the affected joints.

The application of heat usually contributes to the relief of pain. It promotes circulation through the part and relaxation of the muscles. Precautions are observed to prevent burns.

SURGICAL THERAPY IN OSTEOARTHROSIS

When an arthritic or deformed joint causes intractable pain and severe disability, surgical intervention may be undertaken. The operative procedures used are osteotomy, arthrodesis, or total replacement arthroplasty.

Osteotomy is the reshaping of the bone by cutting or curettement to correct deformity and promote normal joint motion.

Arthrodesis is the surgical fusion of a joint, which results in loss of joint movement..It is done to provide relief from pain or to correct joint instability. In this surgery, the articular cartilage is removed and bone grafts are implanted across the joint surface.

An *arthroplasty* is a reconstructive procedure that may entail replacement of part of the joint or of the whole joint with a prosthesis. It is done to relieve pain and permit patient mobility.

Total hip replacement
Total hip arthroplasty is being used frequently with patients with degenerative joint disease and involves surgical replacement of both articulating surfaces of the joint. The femoral head and neck are removed.

The cartilage is removed from the acetabulum and a polyethylene cup is fitted into the socket. Surgical bone cement may be used to secure the plastic cup to the surface of the acetabulum or a porous, noncemented prosthesis is used. The head and neck of the femur are then replaced by a metal prosthesis consisting of a spherical head and stem (see Fig. 26.6). The latter is implanted and cemented into the proximal portion of the femoral shaft. The ball part of the prosthesis is fitted into the acetabulum and tested for a range of motions to make sure it does not dislocate on movement. Other types of prostheses may be used and require different surgical techniques. It is important that the nurse caring for the patient is familiar with the postsurgical position to be maintained and when movement may be resumed. If surgical cement is not used, the period of immobility is longer. When the wound is closed, a closed drainage system is established to promote drainage of accumulating secretions and decrease the potential for infection, as blood is an excellent medium for the growth of microorganisms. The extremity is placed in a position of abduction which must be maintained until it is assessed by the surgeon and other members of the team so that adduction may be resumed gradually. This is determined by the type of components used in the replacement, the stability of the ligaments, tendons and muscles and the patient's ability to understand and comply with instructions.

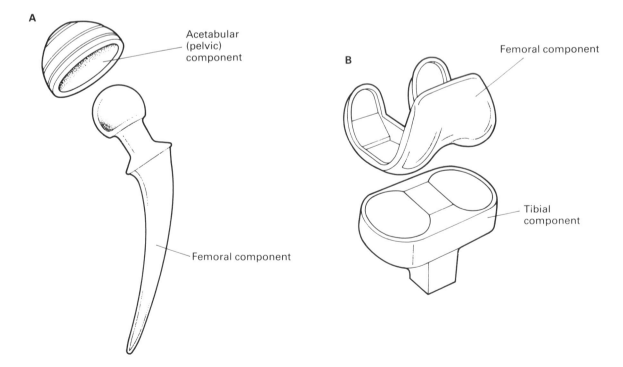

Fig. 26.6 *A*, Total hip arthroplasty prosthesis. *B*, Knee replacement prosthesis.

Preoperative preparation.   In preparing the patient for a replacement arthroplasty, the patient is told what to expect both preoperatively and postoperatively, and is informed about his role in self-care. A complete physical investigation is made during this period and includes an electrocardiogram, chest x-ray and blood examination (e.g. blood cell counts and determination of haemoglobin, serum electrolyte levels and prothrombin time). The patient's blood is typed and cross-matched and blood is made available for blood replacement during the surgery, and postoperatively if necessary.

An overhead bed frame with a pole or pulley is used to demonstrate how the patient may help with raising himself off the bed after the operation. Instruction is given in deep breathing, coughing and the exercises that will be required. The importance of these is explained while they are being taught. The exercises include isometric quadriceps and gluteal contractions, flexion and extension of toes and ankles and of the non-operative leg at the knee.

During the preoperative period, an anticoagulant and antibiotic may be prescribed. The anticoagulant is administered to reduce the risk of thrombophlebitis and ensuing embolism, and to promote microcirculation in the operative site. Because infection is a very serious postoperative complication, the surgeon may commence antibiotic therapy before the surgery as a prophylactic measure.

Local preparation will be indicated by the surgeon. Other general preoperative measures (as cited in Chapter 11) are applicable.

Postoperative nursing intervention.   Table 26.4 lists nursing diagnoses relevant for the patient following total hip replacement and goals for care. The major concerns during the postoperative period are dislocation and infection. If a total hip arthroplasty was done, weight-bearing is a concern until the replaced trochanter has fused. The postoperative regimen following a hip replacement varies with surgeons and with individual patients. For example, an elderly, weak and debilitated patient may require a different plan of care than that used for a younger person.

As with all postoperative patients, the plan of care includes the concerns cited in Chapter 11 (vital signs, ventilation, coughing, fluid balance, diet, elimination, hygienic care and comfort) as well as the following specific considerations.

● *Positioning.*   The patient's bed is prepared in the operating theatre so that the patient is moved only once because of the potential for dislocation, until the soft tissue is stable. The surgeon positions the operative limb in abduction. The desired position may be maintained by placing a special hard, triangular abduction pillow between the knees, which are secured to the pillow by straps. The skin surface in contact with the pillow is protected by thick padding to prevent pressure on nerves and on the skin.

In some instances an abduction splint is applied to the operative limb to reduce muscle spasm and maintain abduction. An overhead frame is attached to the bed in both instances, and a pole is provided so that the patient can assist with raising himself off the bed for skin care and for using the bedpan. The latter should be a small, paediatric bedpan, or fracture pan to minimize the extent of elevation of the hips.

The patient with the abduction splint remains in the supine position until the surgeon indicates he may be turned. The legs remain attached to the pillow and a minimum of two nurses are required for the procedure. One nurse supports the limb, maintaining the abduction position, while the second person turns the patient almost completely over onto his non-operative side. Pillows are placed anteriorly and posteriorly to provide support in the tilted position. The period of bed rest required when the abduction splint is used is variable. Following the removal of the splint or traction, the patient must be cautioned against lying on the operative side and against putting weight on it to 'push up in bed' until advised that he may do so.

Table 26.4 Identification of problems relevant to the patient following total hip replacement.

Problem	Causative factors	Goals
1 Impaired physical mobility	Surgical intervention Restrictions on positioning and activity	1 To maintain the hip in position 2 To follow a prescribed exercise plan
2 Alteration in comfort: pain	Surgical intervention Restricted mobility	To control the pain
3 Potential impairment of skin integrity	Restricted mobility	To maintain skin integrity
4 Potential for injury	Decreased mobility Increased potential for infection Potential for dislocation of hip	1 To maintain cardiovascular and respiratory function 2 To prevent infection 3 To promote healing
5 Anxiety	Surgery Fear of injury Pain and dependency	1 To be able to talk about his anxieties 2 To participate in treatment plan
6 Inadequate knowledge about the therapeutic plan and alterations in daily living	Lack of knowledge and skill	To develop a plan for home management

● *Assessment.* The position, circulation and nerve function of the operative limb are monitored hourly for the first 24 hours then 2 hourly. The amount and characteristics of the Redivac drainage are noted; if it contains fresh blood or excessive drainage it is reported promptly.

The temperature, pulse and respirations are recorded regularly—for example three times daily even though they remain normal; it is important that any elevation which might indicate infection of the wound or chest be recognized immediately. Patient complaints of pain and/or discomfort are recorded. If the patient complains of sudden severe pain in the hip, or if numbness or a tingling or burning sensation develops, dislocation should be suspected. A firm palpable mass may be felt in the operative area.

● *Exercises and ambulation.* Active foot and ankle exercises and gentle flexion and extension of the good knee are started the first or second postoperative day, if approved. The patient is reminded to do the isometric exercises that were taught preoperatively several times a day after the order has been given to start them. A limited range and slow flexion of the operative hip are introduced and then gradually increased in range and frequency under the supervision of the nurse or physiotherapist. The patient is usually assisted out of bed on the first postoperative day, but this varies considerably with the individual surgeon. The patient is assessed for weight-bearing and, if appropriate, crutches should be used for weight support. Walking is commenced using crutches or a walking frame. The patient usually remains in hospital for 5–10 days.

● *Wound care.* A closed (Redivac) drainage system is established at the time of operation. The length of time the drain is left in the wound depends upon the amount of drainage: it is usually removed the first or second day after operation. The large pressure dressing may be replaced on the second day with a smaller, lighter one so that the wound is kept dryer. Strict asepsis is very important in wound care; infection is disastrous in arthroplasty as infection results in destruction of bone and failure of the prosthesis to stabilize and fuse. Good healing is essential for a successful functioning prosthesis.

● *Pain.* The patient usually requires an analgesic for pain relief during the first day or two. Frequently, the hip replacement patient is an older person and narcotics may cause respiratory depression. Precautions are necessary to check the respirations before repeating a dose and again at intervals following administrations.

The patient's response to pain is assessed carefully. Experiences with severe, uncontrolled pain prior to surgery, may alter the patient's perception. He may feel relief and that pain is minimal even in the immediate postoperative period. The patient with rheumatoid arthritis may find non-steroidal antiinflammatory agents such as aspirin more effective in relieving pain than narcotic analgesics.

Analgesia should be provided regularly and consistently to control the pain, prevent complications of shock, promote movement and early ambulation and enable the patient to receive adequate rest.

● *Skin care.* Since the patient must remain in the supine position, dorsal pressure areas (sacral areas, buttocks, shoulders, elbows and knees) require attention every 2 hours. A full length synthetic sheepskin is placed under the patient. One nurse helps the patient raise himself with the pole while a second gives back care. The lower bedding is changed, working from the top of the bed towards the foot.

● *Prevention of complications.* The administration of a prophylactic antibiotic which was commenced 1 or 2 days before operation may be continued for several days. Close observations are made for early signs of infection (elevation of temperature and pulse rate, elevation of white blood cell count, complaints of pain and pressure in the affected hip, headache and general malaise).

The immobility of the lower limbs and probably the patient's age predispose to thrombus formation. Preventive measures include the prescribed exercises and possibly the use of elasticated stockings.

The required position and restricted movement also predispose the patient to hypoventilation and pneumonia. Frequent deep breathing and coughing are very important with this patient. Any sputum expectorated is inspected for signs of infection.

● *Anxiety.* When activity and ambulation are commenced, the nurse should be aware of the patient's need for considerable support. Having experienced so much pain and instability before the operation when he walked, the patient is likely to require repeated reassurance that he can now walk comfortably—that he can depend on the new joint. Early attempts with the frame or crutches are anxiety-producing experiences; the patient needs someone close by. Use of a Zimmer frame or crutches also requires tremendous energy and strength. Progress is made gradually according to the patient's physical status and ability. The support is very gradually withdrawn so that when he has sufficient control to be safe, he will have gained confidence and independence.

● *Patient teaching.* To prepare for going home and becoming as independent as possible, the patient gradually takes over self-care and is instructed in 'getting around' and walking up and down stairs. The patient is advised that he should continue to avoid lying on the affected side for at least 2 months, as well as avoid sitting in low chairs. A firm, straight-backed chair and a raised toilet seat are recommended. The importance of continuing the exercises and walking is stressed; distance should be increased gradually.

A referral is made to the community nurse and/or occupational therapist. A visit is made to the home before the patient is discharged to assess the situation and suggest, if necessary, any adaptations that would facilitate the person's independence, progress and safety. When the patient goes home, regular visits may be needed to the home to supervise the care and exercises and to assess progress. Assistance may be necessary in arranging a visit to the outpatient department for the postoperative appointment with the surgeon.

Expected outcomes:
1 The patient's skin is clean, dry and intact.
2 The patient's body temperature is within the normal range 1 week postoperatively.
The patient is able to:
3 State limitations placed on joint movement, activity and weight bearing.
4 Demonstrate the prescribed exercise programme.
5 Demonstrate safe ambulation with assistive devices or support.
6 Demonstrate deep-breathing and leg exercises to prevent complications.
7 Express anxieties and concerns.
8 Describe a plan for home management.
9 State the community resources available.

Knee replacement
Surgical implantation of a knee prosthesis may be done for the patient whose degenerative disease (e.g. osteoarthrosis) is causing intractable pain and severe incapacity. Various types of prostheses have been introduced but many were discarded because they did not provide sufficient joint stability. The device consisted of two parts—a metal femoral unit and a tibial unit. The components of the prosthesis were secured by bone cement. Patients were able to walk on level surfaces but their gait patterns were abnormal. Newer designs of total knee joint prostheses consist of three components: a patella, tibial component and a complex femoral component with a channel in which the patella moves. These artificial joints allow for flexion and extension movement of the knee. The prostheses are secured by bone cement or by bony ingrowths through a porous base. Some devices combine the two methods to obtain firmer fixation to bone.

Preoperatively the patient is taught and practises quadriceps, hamstring and gluteal setting exercises to maintain optimum strength. These exercises are performed hourly postoperatively. The patient is also taught to transfer from bed to chair and may practise with a Zimmer frame or crutches prior to surgery.

Postoperatively, during the first 24–48 hours, a drain is left in place in the wound to promote drainage. The closed-drainage system is checked regularly to ensure it is draining and is not clogged. Postoperative leg exercises are started early.

The nurse must be familiar with the type of prosthesis inserted and the method used for fixation. Porous-coated cementless devices require longer periods of immobilization. The underlying disease will also influence postoperative care. The patient with rheumatoid arthritis will require frequent rest periods and support and assistance in the early postoperative period to initiate movement and activity following the immobility experienced during surgery. Skin care is important because of the patient's age and immobility. The patient is turned every 2–4 hours and repositioned. The skin is kept clean and dry and special attention is given to heels to prevent breakdown.

Care of the patient following total knee replacement is similar to that following total hip replacement. Infection and dislocation are the major complications. Patient participation in the postoperative exercise regimen is very important to the success of the surgery. Preoperative teaching helps increase motivation and to prepare the patient for the postoperative regimen. Failure to exercise the knee and to strengthen quadricep muscles can result in a fused knee with less function than existed preoperatively. Ambulation begins with the use of the frame or crutches and the gradual introduction of partial weight-bearing on the operative knee. As the patient progresses only a walking stick will be required for support.

INFLAMMATORY JOINT DISEASES

Rheumatoid arthritis

Rheumatoid arthritis is a chronic inflammatory disease of connective tissues; the dominant site is the joints.

The disease is a major health problem, being responsible for much of the existing chronic illness and crippling incapacity of adults. The incidence is three times higher in women than in men. It may have its onset at any age but most commonly begins between the ages of 30 and 60.

The cause of rheumatoid arthritis remains obscure. Several aetiological factors, such as heredity, infection and nutritional deficiencies, have been suspected from time to time but none have been substantiated. In recent years, attention has been focused on an autoimmune reaction being the causative factor. Antibodies called rheumatoid factors are found in the blood of 70–80% of persons with rheumatoid arthritis. These antibodies interact with antigens in various connective tissues but the reaction is greatest in the synovium.

CLINICAL COURSE AND FEATURES

The onset is usually insidious; the person experiences a period of general fatigue, non-specific illness, and morning stiffness and tenderness in some joints. The small joints of the hands or feet or the wrists, elbows or knees are generally the first to be involved. The disease develops symmetrically and, as it progresses, the affected joints become swollen, painful, red and increasingly difficult to move. Their range of motion is reduced. The overlying skin may take on a stretched, smooth glossy appearance.

The severity of the disease varies in different people, and remissions and exacerbations may occur. Physical or psychological stress may be a precipitating factor or may aggravate the disease.

Muscle weakness and spasm are common in the early stages and are frequently followed by marked muscular atrophy. Unless early treatment is instituted, progressive joint tissue destruction and deformities develop, leading to permanent disability. Partial dislocation (subluxation) and flexion contractures occur. Deformities commonly seen include hyperextension of the distal phalanges, flexion contracture or ulnar deviation of the fingers due to metacarpal–phalangeal joint involvement and flexion contraction of the wrists, knees and hips. Subcutaneous nodules (*rheumatoid nodules*) appear principally on extensor surfaces or areas subjected to pressure. These are composed mainly of fibrinoid material (degenerative tissue cells) and granulation tissue.

The initial pathological changes within the joints are inflammation, effusion and swelling of the synovial membrane and joint capsule. The process is reversible in the early stage, and the joint may be left undamaged and functional. As the inflammation continues the synovium proliferates and, with the fibrin of the inflammatory exudate, forms a thick spreading membrane of granulation tissue known as a *pannus*. It spreads over the joint surfaces, gradually eroding the cartilage, and may even destroy the denuded bone surfaces. An x-ray may show rarefaction of the ends of the involved bones. Instability and irritation of the joint may cause muscle contraction with a resulting flexion or extension deformity or subluxation of the joint. Fibrous scar tissue and adhesions develop between the opposing joint surfaces, leading to fibrous ankylosis of the joint. The exposed, roughened ends of bone tissue may eventually proliferate bone cells into the joint cavity, resulting in calcification and bony ankylosis.

The patient with rheumatoid arthritis may also have diffuse involvement of non-articular connective tissue. Degenerative lesions of the collagen component of the connective tissue may develop in muscles, tendons, blood vessels, pleura, heart or lungs.

General constitutional disturbances are manifested; the patient is pale and looks ill. He experiences anorexia, loss of weight and energy, and mental depression. Low-grade fever, tachycardia, anaemia and a mild leucocytosis may be present. Later, leucopenia may develop. The erythrocyte sedimentation rate is usually elevated (normal: Westergren 3–5 mm in one hour for males and 4–10 mm in one hour for females) and, later in the disease, a blood examination may reveal the presence of the rheumatoid factor. When rheumatoid arthritis develops in children, it may be referred to as *Still's disease*. In addition to the symptoms mentioned for adults, children usually have some enlargement of the lymph nodes (lymphadenopathy).

CLASSIFICATION

The disorder may be classified according to the pathological changes (clinical stages) and the loss of functional capacity (functional classification) (see Table 26.5).

TREATMENT

The care of the patient with rheumatoid arthritis is directed toward the suppression of the inflammatory process, the prevention of deformities, and the maintenance and promotion of joint function. The earlier treatment is instituted, the less advanced and less crippling the disease is likely to be.

The patient may be hospitalized during the initial investigative and therapeutic periods and is then supervised by the rheumatologist, nurse and remedial therapists in the outpatient department. Bed rest may be prescribed for a brief period when many joints are acutely inflamed and when systemic dis-

Table 26.5 Classification of rheumatoid arthritis.

| | **By clinical stages** | | **By functional classification** | |
Stage	Manifestations	Class	Manifestations	
1 (Early)	No evidence of joint destruction or osteoporosis	1	No loss of functional capacity	
2 (Moderate)	Evidence of some destruction of cartilage and probably of subchondral bone. No deformity but full range of motion may be limited. Adjacent muscle atrophy present	2	Able to carry out usual activities despite some discomfort and limited joint mobility	
3 (Severe)	Cartilage and bone destruction quite evident. Muscle atrophy and joint deformities such as hyperextension, flexion contracture, ulnar deviation and subluxation present	3	Functional capacity impaired; occupational and self-care activities quite limited	
4 (Terminal)	Criteria of Stage 3 plus fibrous or bony ankylosis present	4	Confined to a wheelchair or bed; not able to carry out self-care. Dependent	

turbances such as fever, anaemia and severe fatigue are manifested.

Drug therapy. Various drugs are used in the treatment of rheumatoid arthritis, including non-steroidal antiinflammatory drugs, gold salts, antimalarial preparations, corticosteroids, cytotoxins and immunosuppressive preparations.

The non-steroidal antiinflammatory agent most commonly used is *acetylsalicylic acid* (aspirin). It is prescribed in relatively large doses and must be taken regularly at the intervals stated in order to maintain effective plasma salicylate levels. Salicylates may produce some adverse effects for which the nurse must be alert. The patient may complain of gastrointestinal disturbances, tinnitus (a ringing or roaring in the ears) and loss of auditory acuity. Since they frequently cause gastrointestinal irritation, the prescribed salicylate is likely to be tolerated better if taken with or soon after meals or with milk or some bland food between meals. Enteric-coated tablets may be used if the patient cannot tolerate the plain forms. Gastric or intestinal bleeding is not an uncommon side-effect, and patients with any history of peptic ulcer do not usually receive salicylate therapy.

Ibuprofen (Brufen) is an antiinflammatory, analgesic drug also used in the treatment of arthritis. The principal side-effects that develop with some patients are nausea, vomiting, diarrhoea and dizziness.

Indomethacin (Indocin) may be prescribed for its antiinflammatory, analgesic and antipyretic effects. Some patients cannot tolerate it because of side-effects, which may be gastrointestinal irritation and ulceration, nausea, headache, depression, dizziness and a sense of detachment.

Other non-steroidal antiinflammatory drugs are also available and are usually prescribed for patients who cannot tolerate aspirin. They include: naproxen (Naprosyn), fenoprofen (Fenopron), piroxicam (Feldene) and sulindac (Clinoril).

A *gold compound* may be given in addition to a non-steroidal agent. When a preparation of *gold salts* such as sodium aurothiamalate (Myocrisin) is given, the patient is observed closely for signs of toxic reactions. The initial dose is small to test the patient for adverse reactions. Such reactions may be seen as stomatitis (inflammation of the oral mucous membrane), dermatitis, renal damage and bone marrow depression leading to severe anaemia, leucopenia (agranulocytosis) and thrombocytopenia. Gold therapy usually involves an intramuscular injection given each week for a period of 4–6 months. Most responses occur during the first 16 weeks of treatment. Once a response has been obtained, maintenance theapy should be continued. Urine analysis and blood cell counts are done weekly, and the patient is checked for possible signs or symptoms of adverse side-effects.

The *antimalarial drugs* such as chloroquine (Niva-quine) and hydroxychloroquine (Plaquenil) may be prescribed over a period of several months for some patients. Toxic effects that may develop include skin eruptions, headache, anorexia, nausea, vomiting and auditory or visual disturbances. Frequent blood cell counts are done because occasionally bone marrow depression occurs, and frequent eye examinations are required to check for keratopathy which is reversible or a serious irreversible retinopathy.

Adrenal corticosteroids are now usually reserved for patients whose rheumatoid arthritis is rapidly progressing, is very painful and has not responded to therapeutic courses of other antirheumatic drugs. Examples of oral preparations used are prednisone, prednisolone and hydrocortisone. The dosage is individualized and kept to a minimum because of the unfavourable side-effects which may develop. It is important that the patient understand that the drug will be given only for a limited period. The dosage is gradually reduced and then completely withdrawn. Adverse side-effects which are likely to develop with overdosage or prolonged therapy include reduced lymphocyte and antibody production, leading to increased susceptibility to infection, sodium and water retention, excessive potassium excretion, mood swings or euphoria, restlessness or overactivity, hyperglycaemia and glucosuria, fullness or rounding of the face (moon face) and growth of hair on the face in the case of a female. The patient who has experienced increased appetite, a marked sense of well-being and some remission of the disease while receiving a corticosteroid may feel quite depressed and let down when the drug is withdrawn, and will require considerable emotional support from the nurse.

When only one or two joints are affected, intra-articular injections of a corticosteroid may be made to arrest the inflammatory process.

Immunosuppressive drugs such as azathioprine (Imuran) and cyclophosphamide have been used in treating the patient with rheumatoid arthritis, using the rationale that the cause is an antigen–antibody reaction. These drugs are prescribed for patients who are unresponsive to any of the drugs mentioned previously in this section. The suppression of leucocyte and antibody formation makes the patient very susceptible to infection. The rheumatoid arthritic patient is frequently debilitated and already has a lowered resistance. Precautions are necessary to protect him from exposure to infection; recognition of early symptoms is reported promptly so an antibiotic may be prescribed. The patient should be fully informed of the major side-effects which can occur with these drugs.

D-Penicillamine is an oral antiinflammatory agent that produces effects similar to those of gold. Benefits are not apparent for several months. It is used in patients with severe rheumatoid arthritis whose disease process has not responded to other medications. Side-effects include anorexia, nausea, vomiting, skin eruption, thrombocytopenia and nephritis.

Rest.   Bed rest may be prescribed for a brief period when many joints are acutely inflamed and when systemic disturbances such as fever, anaemia and severe fatigue are manifested. Rest periods through-out the day are scheduled for several weeks. During the acute inflammatory stage, the affected joints may be placed at rest and immobilized in a neutral posi-tion by the application of splints.

Exercise and activity.   As soon as possible, a daily exercise schedule is introduced to preserve as complete range of motion as possible and to increase and maintain muscle strength. Exercises are planned and prescribed on an individual basis and carried out under the supervision of a physiotherapist until well established.

Surgical treatment.   Various surgical procedures may be used with arthritic patients to facilitate joint func-tion and mobility, retard disease progress or correct a deformity. These include the following:
• *Synovectomy.* The removal of the thickened inflamed synovium is carried out rarely to retard joint destruction. Its use is limited to patients with intractable pain in a joint.
• *Joint replacement.* Total replacement of the hip, knee, ankle or shoulder may be done with advanced disease that has led to deformity or loss of function and mobility.
• *Arthroplasty,* which consists of realignment and reconstruction of the joint, may be used on the knees, wrists and small joints of the hands.
• *Arthrodesis* is the surgical fixation or fusion of a joint. It is rarely used when the joint is severely damaged and the patient is experiencing intractable pain or the joint is a distinct handicap.

NURSING PROCESS

Actual and potential problems, causes of problems and *goals* for the patient with rheumatoid arthritis are listed in Table 26.6.

Nursing intervention

1. Impaired physical mobility.   Assessment of joint mobility is discussed at the beginning of this chapter.
• *Positioning and the application of splints.* During the acute inflammatory stage, the affected joints are especially painful on movement. The involved part usually assumes the flexed position because of spasm of the dominant flexor muscles, and contrac-ture deformity is likely to develop. Limb joints may be placed at rest and immobilized in a neutral posi-tion by the application of splints to reduce the sever-ity of pain and prevent contractures and deformities. At first, these may only be removed during the daily

Table 26.6 Identification of problems relevant to the patient with rheumatoid arthritis.

Problem	Causative factors	Goals
1 Impaired physical mobility	Limitations in range of motion of joints Inflammation, pain and deformity of joints Muscle weakness and atrophy	1 To maintain existing joint mobility 2 To promote optimal functional mobility 3 To prevent or minimize further impairment of joint function
2 Alteration in comfort: pain	Inflammation Muscle spasm Stiffness	To control the pain during the acute phase and on a long-term basis
3 Alteration in nutrition: intake lower than body requirements and/or intake greater than body requirements	Loss of appetite Lack of physical dexterity and mobility to prepare and eat food Gastrointestinal side-effects of medications Use of folk remedies Obesity, causing increased stress on weight-bearing joints	1 To receive a well-balanced diet 2 To control weight 3 To avoid harmful dietary folk remedies
4 Inability to cope	Reduced energy and mobility resources Physical deformity Fear of dependency Uncertainty and unpredictability of daily functional ability	1 To express feelings about the effects of the disease on physical and social functioning, role change and independence 2 To identify coping patterns and the implications of resulting behaviour
5 Inadequate knowledge about alter-ations in life-style and activities of daily living and health management	Lack of knowledge of rheumatoid arthritis and its management Decreased dependence Decreased mobility Altered financial status and changes in family process	To acquire knowledge and skill neces-sary to achieve an acceptable life-style

passive exercise or heat therapy periods. Later, as the muscle spasm lessens, the splints are left off for most of the day and may only be necessary during the night.

To prevent hip and spinal flexion, a fracture board is placed under the mattress and the patient is encouraged to use only a small pillow to maintain good cervical alignment. If the patient is confined to bed for a period longer than 24 hours, he is instructed to change his position frequently. Two or three periods of ½ hour or more should be spent in the prone position to prevent flexure contraction at the hips. A footboard is provided to keep the feet at almost right angles while in the dorsal position. When positioning or assisting the patient, the affected parts must be handled very gently, and support is given to the joints. Jarring and quick, jerky movements are avoided. Independence and active movements are encouraged as acute inflammation subsides; the patient moves slowly and the nurse and family must learn to be patient and allow him the necessary time.

When the patient with arthritis is up, attention is paid to posture. He is encouraged to stand erect and 'sit straight' to avoid forward flexion of the trunk and drooping of the shoulders.

• *Heat and cold applications.* Various forms of heat and cold applications are used to help reduce muscle spasm, pain, joint stiffness and swelling (see p. 1009).

• *Exercises and activity.* As soon as possible, a daily exercise schedule is introduced to achieve and preserve the most complete range of motion possible, as well as to maintain muscle strength. Exercises are planned and prescribed on an individual basis and are carefully supervised by a physiotherapist or nurse until they are understood and are familiar to the patient. Indiscriminate movements or overstretching may cause a dislocation or torn tendons (see principles cited on p. 1011).

When acute inflammation, swelling and severe pain preclude joint movements, isometric exercises are recommended. Joint exercises may be passive or active-assisted to start with and are gradually progressed to active and resistive exercises within the limits set by the doctor. The exercises are only of value if carried out at regular intervals. The patient's reaction to the exercises is noted; excessive fatigue or increased pain necessitates some modification in the exercise programme. A balance must be struck between rest and exercise. The exercises may be performed with less difficulty if preceded by some form of heat application which promotes muscle relaxation. Special shoes, frames, crutches or a walking stick may be recommended to assist with weight-bearing and mobility.

Self-care and the activities of daily living are encouraged. If the range of motion is limited because of joint destruction or ankylosis, self-help devices may be provided to promote maximum indepen-dence in such activities as dressing, grooming and feeding. Good grooming and taking pride in appearance are encouraged by providing the essentials and commending the patient. Table 26.7 illustrates a home exercise programme for an arthritic patient.

Some activities which previously seemed very simple and were taken for granted may become quite a chore and time-consuming. Adjustments in the daily routine may be made to allow more time for such tasks. Many of the patients afflicted with rheumatoid arthritis are in what are referred to as the most productive years. Restricted employment, reduced earning capacity and limited social and recreational activities add considerable stress to the situation and are frequently a source of great concern for the patient and his family.

2. Alteration in comfort: pain. Assessment of the patient's pain involves identification of the involved joints, the degree of swelling, redness, warmth and range of motion of the joints, the degree and dur-ation of stiffness in the morning and following periods of inactivity, and the intensity, frequency and character of the pain.

Pain and discomfort become the more important aspects of the arthritic patient's life. New areas of pain may occur, signifying a flare-up of the disease process. Family and friends have difficulty under-standing why the patient is able to participate in acti-vities one day and then be dependent or withdrawn on the next day. Patients require assistance in learn-ing to cope with the pain and discomfort and to adapt their life-styles to incorporate measures to prevent and relieve pain. Activity and exercise should not be avoided but rather planned and incorporated with pain-relieving measures.

Regular administration of the prescribed antiin-flammatory drugs to maintain a therapeutic serum level of the drugs is important in pain control.

The patient's daily routine is planned to provide adequate rest and exercise. Morning care activities are delayed to accommodate the patient's morning stiffness. A warm bath or shower or the application of heat or cold prior to activity may help to relieve stiffness and muscle spasm. Splinting of the inflamed joints while at rest and the later application of functional splints may provide relief of local pain.

3. Alterations in nutrition. A well-balanced diet, similar to that essential to the health of all persons, is recommended for the arthritic patient. The total calo-rie intake may require some adjustment with a view to achieving or maintaining the person's normal weight. Overweight increases the strain on joints and may also reduce motivation in exercise.

The dietitian assists the patient in planning easily prepared meals. Breakfast should be easily available and simple to prepare to accommodate the patient's morning stiffness. The occupational therapist teaches methods of protecting joints while preparing foods and recommends utensils and dishes adapted for the arthritic patient. Padded handles on cutlery make them easier to grip; hand supports on cutlery eliminate the need for fine finger movements; special handles on cups and glasses are easier and safer in handling; suction cups stop dishes from sliding; and high edges on dishware prevent food from spilling.

Numerous diets for the treatment of rheumatoid arthritis have been proposed over the years. The patient is cautioned to guard against fads and folklore and to ensure that his diet contains a balance of all essential nutrients.

4. Inability to cope. *Assessment* of how the patient is coping with rheumatoid arthritis and its effects on life-style and daily functioning includes identification of the patient's feelings and how he perceives

Table 26.7 Example of home exercise programme for the patient with rheumatoid disease.

Note: Perform exercises on the bed.

Foot and ankle exercises
1 Move your ankles up and down 10 times
2 Make a circle with your ankles 10 times
3 Squeeze your toes 10 times

Leg exercises (hip and knee joints)
1 Place a padded soft-drink can under your right knee. Press knee into the can. Lift heel off the bed. Bring toes towards you. Count to three—relax. Repeat 10 times. Move the can to the left knee and repeat 10 times
2 Bend right knee up towards your chin. Straighten onto the bed. Bend left knee up towards your chin. Straighten onto the bed. Repeat 5 times each leg
3 Keeping your right leg straight, slide the leg out to the side and back to the centre. Repeat with left leg. Repeat 5 times each leg
4 (Do *not* perform the following exercise if neck *or* shoulders are in a flare up.)
   Lie on stomach for 5 minutes. Lift your right leg off the bed, keeping knee straight. Count to 3 and lower leg. Repeat with left leg. Repeat 5–10 times each leg

Shoulder exercises
1 Lift arms straight up above your head—5 times
2 Lift your elbows out to the side—5 times
3 With hands behind your neck with your fingers touching, move your elbows forward and back 5 times

Elbow exercises
Bend your elbows; touch your shoulders with your fingers; straighten your elbows out in front. 5 times

Neck exercises
1 Lift your head up and look at the ceiling; bend your head and look at the floor. Repeat 3–5 times
2 Turn your head to look over your right, then your left shoulder. Repeat 3–5 times

Hand exercises (perform sitting at a table)
1 Stretch thumb web space: With elbows into your sides, grasp the left web space with right thumb and fingers. Gently take thumbs out and away from fingers. Repeat with other hand. Perform 5 times each hand
2 Proper alignment of wrists and fingers: With elbows on the table, take your wrist out to the side, then gently 'walk' your fingers back to the middle. Keep wrists and fingers in a straight line. Repeat using the other hand. Perform 10 times each hand
3 To maintain movement of all joints of the fingers and thumbs: Working on one finger at a time, move each joint separately forwards and back holding below each joint at the same time. Repeat 3–5 times each hand
4 Stretching the intrinsic muscles: Place your right hand on its side with the palm facing you. Place the thumb of your left hand just below the knuckle to fully straighten the finger, then gently bend the next joint of the finger forward. Repeat with each finger. Repeat using the left hand. Perform 3–5 times each hand

Isometric exercises
Lying on back
Exercises 1 and 2 are responsible for strengthening hip and knee muscles which are needed for walking
1 Keep legs straight—push right leg into the bed, hold for the count of three, rest, push left leg into the bed, hold for the count of three. Repeat 10 times
2 Legs straight, squeeze legs together, hold for count of three. Repeat 10 times
Exercises 3 and 4 are responsible for strengthening the shoulder and arm muscles
3 Arms straight, squeeze arms into your side, hold for count of three. Repeat 10 times
4 Arms straight at side, push arms into bed, hold for the count of three. Repeat 10 times
Exercise 5 is responsible for strengthening the abdominal muscles (stomach muscles) to aid you in sitting up
5 Lift head and shoulders to look at feet, hold for count of three. Repeat 5 times
Lying on side
This exercise strengthens hip muscles responsible for sliding the leg out to the side
6 Keep legs straight, push bottom leg into bed, hold for count of three. Turn onto other side and push bottom leg into bed; hold for count of three. Repeat 10 times

his life has been affected by his arthritis. What functional deficits does the patient perceive as being most important and what is his perception of the importance of the strengths and functions he has maintained? Physical appearance, physical symptoms, emotional status and cognitive functioning provide objective data on the coping status.

An assessment is made of factors influencing coping, as well as of the individual's present coping pattern.[1] Wiener describes the arthritic patient as being caught between two imperatives: 'the inner or physiological world, monitored for pain and disability readings by day and sometimes the hour, and (2) the outer world of activity of maintaining what is perceived as a normal existence.'[2] Five coping strategies used by arthritic patients are cited by this same author. 'Covering up' is the principal strategy employed. Concealment of disability and pain are demonstrated by such responses as 'If anyone asks me how I am, I say fine.' The patient focuses on hiding the social significance of his handicap by making efforts to walk as normally as possible and to carry his weight in office or household tasks. This is termed 'keeping up'. 'Justifying inaction' results from use of the previous strategies and the fact that symptoms of arthritis are unpredictable. Some days the patient is successful in participating in daily activities while the next day he hurts and his energy is drained from the previous efforts. He reacts by justifying his inaction, leaving family and friends confused. 'Pacing' involves planning activities around periods of rest and accounting for the fact that it takes the patient longer to complete daily tasks. The ability to 'elicit help' from others varies with the individual and the person being asked for help. It may be relatively easy for a wife to ask her husband to open a jar but it may be very difficult for a single person to ask a neighbour to perform the same task. A husband may feel his role is threatened if he has to ask his wife or child to carry a heavy object.

Nursing intervention involves helping the patient to identify his feelings about his illness situation and what it means. By identifying how he copes in certain situations, the patient develops insight into his behaviour and looks at the consequences of that behaviour and the alternatives open to him. Does he ask for help or do without? Is social interaction worth the cost of occasional embarrassment and/or excessive fatigue? The patient is supported in lowering his expectations and establishing a new set of norms for action that are realistic for and acceptable to him. Covering up and keeping up drain the patient's energy, and asking for help may reinforce fears of being dependent. Hope may be a positive factor that motivates the patient to comply with therapy and learn to control symptoms. It may also

be a negative force, prompting the patient to self-treatment, use of home remedies and the quackery he may be exposed to. The patient and family need opportunities to discuss such ideas to help in making decisions about what is best for the patient. Family members and friends also need the opportunity to express their feelings and develop understanding of the patient's illness, limitations and potentials and how to respond to the daily or even hourly fluctuations in the patient's behaviour.

5. Insufficient knowledge about alterations in life-style and activities of daily living and disease management. It is important for the patient and family to understand the nature of rheumatoid arthritis and that much of the disability and deformity commonly associated with the disease can be prevented if early treatment is instituted and the prescribed regimen followed. The nurse's explanation can be reinforced by providing booklets especially prepared for patients and the public.[3]

● *Rehabilitation* depends largely on the severity of the patient's disease and whether or not the pathological process in the joints is arrested. Obviously, if the disease is severe and more and more joints are progressively involved, the patient is less likely to be well enough to return to his former occupation and will require a more active and closely supervised care programme. Many patients are well enough to go to work and adjust their daily life to provide for extra rest as well as continuance of a daily physical exercise regimen. Some find it necessary after the onset of arthritis to change their former type of work. This may necessitate assistance in finding suitable employment or in interpreting the patient's condition to the employer, who may be persuaded to employ him in another type of job. A period of vocational training or assessment by the Disablement Resettlement Officer (DRO) may be necessary before the arthritic patient can be re-employed.

Before leaving the hospital or clinic, the patient is given a written outline of his exercises (see Table 26.7). These are reviewed and discussed with him and a family member. If there is some restriction in the range of motion of some joints which interferes with self-care activities, arrangements are made for the provision of self-help devices. The family members are made aware of the importance of encouraging the patient to do things for himself. They are advised that he may be very slow in achieving various activities which seem very simple to them. They should appreciate the need for additional patience and for planning that will provide the required extra time.

If the patient is sufficiently handicapped to require physical care, a referral will be made to the community nurse. The community nurse and the

---

[1] Wiener (1984), pp. 88–98.
[2] Wiener (1984), p. 89.

[3] The Arthritis and Rheumatism Council, 41 Eagle Street, London WC1 R4AB.

occupational therapist can be of assistance in assessing the home situation and making recommendations for adjustments that will simplify the care of the patient and will increase mobility and independence. For example, suggestions may be made for reorganizing the kitchen in order to make equipment more readily available and lessen the demands on the worker. Such recommendations for simplification of household chores may enable a woman with arthritis to carry on the care of her home. The patient is taught to perform activities of daily living in new ways so as to protect the joints from unnecessary stress (see p. 1011).

The importance of maintaining good body alignment is stressed; in addition to fracture boards and footboards for the bed, a comfortable straight chair of appropriate height and good walking shoes are needed. Education of the patient about his drug therapy will be started in hospital.

The patient and his family are acquainted with the societies and organizations which are concerned with rheumatic disease and with publications that may be helpful. Transportation is frequently a problem for the arthritic. If he is required to go regularly to a physical therapy clinic or rehabilitation unit, the society will usually provide transportation, if requested.

In discussing the necessary care, emphasis is placed on the avoidance of becoming overtired, emotionally upset about things that cannot be corrected and exposure to cold. The patient is also reminded to minimize as much as possible the strain and pressure normally placed on the affected joints. He and his family are cautioned against quack and folk remedies and the taking of unprescribed drugs. Regular attendance at the outpatient department is essential for repeated ongoing evaluation and appropriate adjustments in treatment.

The nurse is alert for economic problems that may be imposed by the illness, and a referral is made, when necessary, to a welfare agency for assistance.

Expected outcomes
The patient:
1 Describes what rheumatoid arthritis is.
2 Describes a plan to balance rest and activity.
3 Demonstrates an ability to carry out the prescribed exercise plan.
4 States techniques to protect joints.
5 Demonstrates an ability to perform activities of daily living safely and efficiently.
6 Describes the type, frequency, intensity and location of pain and discomfort.
7 Describes measures that provide pain relief.
8 Describes a plan to safely use heat and cold therapy at home.
9 Describes a meal plan that is nutritionally balanced.
10 States the implications of over- and undernutrition and quack diets on his health.
11 Expresses feelings about the effects of arthritis on his life-style.
12 Indicates awareness of coping strategies used and the implications of resulting behaviour.
13 Describes the signs and symptoms of a flare-up of the disease process.
14 States the action, dose, method of administration and side-effects of each prescribed medication.
15 Describes the daily medication schedule.
16 Describes a plan to utilize available community resources.

Ankylosing spondylitis

This is a chronic disorder characterized by inflammation and ensuing ankylosis of the sacroiliac joints and spinal articulations. The pathological process is similar to that seen in rheumatoid arthritis, but there is a greater tendency toward calcification. In most instances the disease remains confined to the joints cited above but occasionally does spread to peripheral joints.

The highest incidence is in young men, the onset occurring most often in the late teens or the twenties. The cause is unknown, but heredity is suspected of having a role, since a large majority of those afflicted have a family history of some form of inflammatory arthritis.

CLINICAL FEATURES

The onset of this disease is usually insidious; the patient first complains of stiffness of the back in the morning or following a period of inactivity. Progressively, this becomes more noticeable; limitation in the range of spinal flexion develops, chest expansion is reduced and there is low back pain radiating to the buttocks and thighs along the sciatic nerve pathways. General systemic symptoms are usually absent or are limited to unusual fatigue and probably some weight loss.

Laboratory examinations indicate an increase in the erythrocyte sedimentation rate, but in most cases the rheumatoid factor is absent. Recently it has been recognized that the histocompatibility antigen HLA-B27 is present in 90% of these patients; this has become a confirming diagnostic factor of ankylosing spondylitis. Leucocytosis and anaemia may be present and the protein concentration of the cerebrospinal fluid is frequently increased.

Remissions and exacerbations of the acute disease are common. In most advanced stages, some patients develop some peripheral rheumatoid arthritis. A few develop circulatory complications due to aortitis and aortic valvular insufficiency. Uveitis[4] is also seen in about 25% of the patients.

---

[4] *Uveitis* is inflammation of the iris, ciliary body and choroid of the eye.

Progressive involvement of spinal segments may continue over a period of years and eventually leave the patient with practically the whole spine firmly ankylosed, producing what may be referred to as a poker back or poker spine. Rarely, rheumatoid spondylitis has an abrupt, acute onset and spreads rapidly through the lumbar, thoracic and cervical segments, leaving the patient with a poker spine in a relatively short period.

TREATMENT AND NURSING CARE

Care of the patient with ankylosing spondylitis is directed toward the relief of pain, maintenance of good spinal alignment and preservation of maximum spinal function.

During acute phases, the patient usually receives a non-steroidal antiinflammatory agent such as indomethacin (Indocid) (see p. 1019 for side-effects).

Rest and good posture at all times are extremely important so that ankylosis of the affected joints occurs while they are in the normal neutral position, thus preventing deformity and handicap. The patient is advised of the need for constant attention to good posture when he is up, with emphasis on contraction of the buttock and lower abdominal muscles and keeping the chest up, shoulders back and head erect. In some instances, he is fitted with a back brace to maintain optimum alignment of the affected joints. A fracture board and a firm mattress are placed on his bed, and it is suggested that he does not use a pillow or, if necessary, only a very small one. The patient is advised to sleep straight and flat on the back or in the prone position to discourage possible flexion of the spine.

A daily physical exercise programme is prescribed with the objective of strengthening the muscles which help to support the spine, maintain good alignment and promote the patient's functional capacity. Since ankylosis of the costovertebral joints may occur and reduce the ventilatory capacity, breathing exercises are also included in the suggested exercise regimen.

Heavy lifting and activities which place strain upon the back are restricted. The patient assists in determining his level of tolerance of physical activity; that which produces pain or exhaustion should be avoided; additional rest is important. The disease may necessitate a change of occupation and vocational retraining before suitable employment can be found.

If hip and spinal deformities develop, surgical correction may be undertaken to facilitate the patient's mobility and rehabilitation. The commonest deformity is fixed flexion of the spine (kyphosis).

METABOLIC JOINT DISEASE

Gout

Gout is a disorder of uric acid metabolism, char-acterized by recurring episodes of acute inflammation, pain and swelling in a joint. Any joint may be affected, but those of the foot are more susceptible; the condition usually develops first in the great toe. Gout occurs more commonly in men over 40 years of age and is rarely seen in females.

The disorder is thought to occur as the result of a genetic defect in the metabolism of purine. It causes an excessive concentration of uric acid in the plasma (hyperuricaemia) which may be brought about by an over-production or faulty disposal of the kidneys. Urate crystals may be precipitated and deposited within joint tissues, setting up irritation and a local inflammatory response. The small masses of crystals, which are called *tophi* may also form in cartilage, the kidneys or soft tissues in other areas of the body.

Secondary gout may develop in disorders such as blood dyscrasias in which there is a marked breakdown of cellular nucleic acid. When the urate crystals are deposited in joints and produce inflammation, the condition may be referred to as *gouty arthritis*.

SIGNS AND SYMPTOMS

Acute episodes are characterized by the sudden onset of excruciating pain in the affected joint. It becomes very tender, red, hot and swollen. Veins in the area stand out because of congestion and distension. The patient may also experience anorexia, headache, fever and constipation. The blood uric acid concentration is elevated (normal: 0.18–0.42 mmol/l). Subcutaneous tophi are frequently apparent in the ears or over joints or knuckles. Precipitations of urates may occur in kidney tissue, leading to impaired renal function. In some patients, the excessive concentration of uric acid results in the formation of kidney stones.

The acute attack usually subsides in a few days, and in the early stages of the disease the joint returns to normal. Remissions may gradually become shorter, and the disease may become chronic. More joints become involved, and there are irreversible changes, leading to deformity and loss of function.

TREATMENT AND NURSING INTERVENTION

During an acute attack of gout, the patient may be placed on bed rest and the affected part immobilized. Drug therapy is promptly instituted. The preparation that has proved most effective to date and is most commonly used is colchicine. It may be administered orally or intravenously. If it is given intravenously, precautions are taken to avoid any of the drug being deposited in the subcutaneous or extravascular tissues because of its local irritating effect. Side-effects include nausea, vomiting, abdominal discomfort and diarrhoea. The drug generally relieves the pain fairly quickly but does not lower the hyperuricaemia. If the patient cannot tolerate or does not respond to colchicine a non-steroidal antiinflammatory agent may be prescribed.

Hot or cold applications to the affected joint(s) may provide some relief, but frequently the patient cannot tolerate either. Discomfort is usually less when the part is protected as much as possible from any direct contact with applications and bedding.

A fluid intake of 2500–3000 ml is encouraged to promote dilution and renal elimination of the uric acid. The urinary output is recorded, and the fluid balance is determined.

Rigid dietary restrictions are usually not necessary. The patient is instructed to limit foods high in purines such as organ meats (liver, kidneys, heart, sweetbreads), shellfish, sardines and meat extracts and to limit also the intake of alcoholic beverages. If the patient is overweight, the caloric intake is adjusted to promote a gradual reduction to the optimum weight. The importance of a high fluid intake is explained to the patient, and a minimal daily intake of 2000–2500 ml is continued during remissions.

Patients who are having frequent and severe attacks may receive a uricosuric drug routinely. This type of preparation promotes the urinary excretion of uric acid and lowers the serum uric acid level by inhibiting renal tubular reabsorption. The patient must have a high fluid intake, and an effort is made to keep the urine alkaline. The patient is taught to take alkaline-producing foods and fluids or sodium bicarbonate tablets and to test the pH of the urine. The uricosuric drug that may be prescribed for the patient with chronic gout is allopurinol (Zyloric) or probenecid (Benemid). Salicylate, thiazide and frusemide preparations are not administered when the patient is receiving a uricosuric agent, since they counteract the desired effect.

Connective Tissue (Collagen) Disease

Systemic lupus erythematosus (SLE) (disseminated lupus erythematosus)

This disorder is a multisystem disease which is characterized by diffuse inflammation and biochemical and structural changes in the collagen fibres of connective tissues in organs and tissues throughout the body. Originally, lupus erythematosus, dermatomyositis and scleroderma comprised the collagen diseases. In recent years, some references include rheumatoid arthritis, rheumatic fever and polyarteritis nodosa in the classification of connective tissue disease.

Systemic lupus erythematosus is an autoimmune disorder characterized by antibodies which develop against cells' nuclear components. A sensitivity to the individual's own DNA develops and the antigen–antibody complexes damage the vasculature, structure and functions of tissues and organs. Several factors are suspected of having a role in precipitating the onset or an acute exacerbation of the disease; these include exposure to the sun's rays, emotional stress, infection and drugs (e.g. sulphonamide, penicillin, procainamide, isoniazid). The incidence is increasing and many patients are diagnosed with mild forms of lupus. The 15-year survival rate for patients with mild disease, is over 90%. Prognosis depends on the age of the patient (it is usually more severe in children; in the elderly it may be mild and respond well to treatment), severity of the disease, the organs affected, and the patient's response to treatment and willingness to comply with the prescribed treatment plan.

SIGNS AND SYMPTOMS

The disease may begin at any age in either sex, but is seen most often in young women. The signs and symptoms, especially at the onset, vary greatly from one person to another, depending upon the systems and organs involved. Those most commonly seen include fever, general malaise, excessive fatigue, weakness, anorexia, weight loss and joint pain. An erythematous rash may be evident on the face, neck and/or extremities. If the disorder is confined to the skin it is referred to as *discoid lupus erythematosus*. The lesions on the face typically spread over the nose and cheeks to form a butterfly pattern. Angioneurotic oedema[5] with burning or itchy sensations, patchy vitiligo or areas of hyperpigmentation, mucosal ulceration and alopecia may develop.

In the systemic type of lupus erythematosus, generalized lymphadenopathy occurs. The patient may complain of impaired vision as a result of corneal involvement and retinopathy. Raynaud's phenomenon may be troublesome, especially if the patient is exposed to even slight cold. As the disease progresses, serious visceral involvement and ensuing dysfunction are likely to develop. Impaired pulmonary, cardiovascular and kidney function are common. Clinical renal involvement occurs in many patients with systemic lupus erythematosus. Central nervous system involvement is also common.

The erythrocyte sedimentation rate is elevated (normal: Westergren, 3–5 mm in one hour for males and 4–10 mm in one hour for females), and anaemia is a frequent development. The presence of the lupus erythematosus cell factor and other antinuclear antibodies in the serum facilitates diagnosis. The haematocrit falls and thrombocytopenia may be manifested in petechiae and purpura.

---

[5] *Angioneurotic oedema* is the temporary appearance of large oedematous areas in the skin or mucous membrane due to a disturbance in the innervation of the vasomotor system.

TREATMENT

The care of the patient is mainly supportive and symptomatic; at present, no therapy is considered curative. In remissions, the patient is advised against exposure to sunlight, infection and excessive fatigue which are thought to predispose or precipitate an exacerbation of the disease process. Lotions may be used to screen out the ultraviolet sun rays when the person has to be exposed. Cold should be avoided because of the vascular reaction (Raynaud's).

Medications which may be prescribed include aspirin to control fever and joint involvement, an antimalarial drug such as hydroxychloroquine (Plaquenil) for the patient with skin and joint involvement if the condition is unresponsive to salicylates, and an adrenocorticosteroid preparation. The latter is used for the more severe stage of systemic lupus erythematosus when there is renal, central nervous system, cardiovascular and haemopoietic involvement. The steroid drug is given in relatively large doses during an acute exacerbation, and then gradually reduced to a maintenance dose or withdrawn completely. If hydroxychloroquine is given, frequent ophthalmological examinations are necessary since the drug may precipitate retinopathy. Cyclophosphamide (Endoxana) or azathioprine (Imuran) may be used when the patient with severe disease is unresponsive to the more conservative drugs.

Dialysis may be necessary when the disease attacks the kidneys. Infection is treated promptly with antibiotics. Emotional stress should be minimized and fatigue avoided.

New treatments, such as plasmapheresis, the use of monoclonal antibodies and pulse therapy which involves the intravenous administration of corticosteroids over a short period, are being used with some success.

NURSING INTERVENTION

Systemic lupus erythematosus is a serious chronic disease that is unpredictable in nature. The patient experiences remissions and exacerbations. Nursing intervention focuses on assisting the patient to manage the disease and adapt his life-style to his altered functional level. Emphasis is placed on the patient's strengths and the positive aspects of his functional ability. The patient is helped to identify factors which precipitate flare-ups or exacerbation of symptoms and to create an environment free of stress. His daily routine is planned to provide adequate rest.

The following points are emphasized in teaching patients and their families about the disease and self-management:

1 Knowledge of the disease process, its management and signs and symptoms of disease activity.
2 Actions, dosage and possible side-effects of the prescribed drug(s) and adjustment of medication dosage in response to symptom changes.
3 The importance of carrying an identification card if the patient is receiving corticosteroid therapy.
4 Awareness of expected weight gains with corticosteroid therapy and measures to minimize and cope with the weight gain.
5 The necessity of regular medical supervision so that tissue changes can be detected early by laboratory tests and prompt adjustment made in drug therapy to help control tissue damage. (Regular medical supervision enables the doctor to keep medication dosages to a minimal level, preventing or decreasing harmful side-effects of drug therapy.)
6 The importance of prompt identification of infection and the action to take if infection develops.
7 The importance of regular rest, sleep and good nutrition.
8 Methods of decreasing physical and emotional stress.
9 Knowledge of community resources and 'lupus self-help' groups.
10 Avoidance of over-exposure to sunlight.

Dermatomyositis (polymyositis)

In this form of connective tissue disease, the skin and voluntary muscles are the principal focal sites of the pathological inflammatory process. The incidence is higher in females. The onset is insidious and may be manifested by an erythematous skin rash, subacute fever, and tenderness, oedema and weakness of the muscles. Contracture of the skin and muscles due to the fibrous scar tissue may lead to tightly drawn skin in the affected areas, muscle contracture and loss of function. Involvement of the respiratory muscles may cause respiratory insufficiency and frequently is the cause of death. In some instances the condition is confined to muscle tissue and is referred to as *chronic polymyositis*; the skin is not involved. Diagnosis includes an electromyogram, muscle and/or skin biopsy and blood determination of enzyme levels. The serum levels of muscle enzymes, especially creatinine phosphokinase (CPK), are elevated.

This collagen disease may be treated with an adrenocorticosteroid preparation, but the outlook is generally unfavourable.

Scleroderma (progressive systemic sclerosis)

This is a chronic disorder in which the collagen component of the skin undergoes degenerative changes and becomes sclerotic. The dermal changes and contraction produce deformities and restricted movement. The pathologic sclerosing process may spread to viscera, causing systemic disturbances and organ dysfunction similar to those that may occur in systemic lupus erythematosus. The rate of progress varies with patients; some survive many years, while the disease may prove fatal to others in a few months.

Polyarteritis nodosa

This disorder is characterized by diffuse inflammatory and necrotizing lesions in the walls of smaller arteries with resultant fibrosis of vascular walls, thrombosis and infarction. The vessel wall is weakened at the site of the lesion and an aneurysm may develop. In other instances, thrombosis within the lumen of the vessel may lead to occlusion.

The incidence of polyarteritis nodosa is greater in males. Vague and varying signs and symptoms occur, as with other collagen diseases, and are referable to multiple systems and organs. Although any organ may be affected, those most commonly involved are the kidneys, muscles, heart, lungs, liver and gastrointestinal tract. If the arteries in vital organs such as the kidneys and heart are attacked, essential life-supporting functions may be threatened.

As with other connective tissue diseases, there is no specific treatment; adrenocorticosteroids may be administered and may provide a temporary remission. An immunosuppressive drug such as cyclophosphamide is administered along with the corticosteroid preparation but the response is slow. Care is symptomatic and supportive.

References and Further Reading

BOOKS

Anderson SVD & Bauqens EE (eds) (1981) *Chronic Health Problems*. St Louis: CV Mosby. Chapter 10.

Bluestone R (ed) (1980) *Rheumatology*. Boston: Houghton Mifflin.

Braunwald E et al (eds) (1987) *Harrison's Principles of Internal Medicine*. New York: McGraw-Hill. Chapters 273–278.

Ehrlich GE (ed) (1980) *Rehabilitation Management of Rheumatic Conditions* Baltimore: Williams & Wilkins.

Fields WL & McGinn-Campbell KM (1983) *Introduction to Health Assessment*. Reston, Virginia: Reston Publishing. Chapter 17.

Golding DN (1982) *A Synopsis of Rheumatic Diseases*, 4th ed. Bristol: Wright.

Kinash RG (1981) *Expressed Needs and Experiences of Patients with Systemic Lupus Erythematosus in Saskatchewan*. Saskatoon, Saskatchewan: University of Saskatchewan.

Krupp MA & Chatton MJ (eds) (1983) *Current Medical Diagnosis and Treatment*. Los Altos, CA: Lange Medical.

Moskowitz RW (1982) *Clinical Rheumatology*, 2nd ed. Philadelphia: Lea & Febiger.

Pigg JS, Driscoll PW & Caniff R (1985) *Rheumatology Nursing: A Problem-oriented Approach*. Chichester: Wiley Medical.

Scott JT (1982) *Arthritis and Rheumatism: The Facts*. Oxford: Oxford University Press.

Strauss AL, Corbin J, Fargerhaugh S, Glaser BG, Maines D, Suczek B & Weiner CL (1984) *Chronic Illness and the Quality of Life*, 2nd ed. St Louis: CV Mosby. Chapter 8.

Tresler KM (1982) *Clinical Laboratory Tests—Significance and Implications for Nursing*. Englewood Cliffs, NJ: Prentice-Hall. Chapter 13.

Weiner CL (1984) The burden of rheumatoid arthritis. In: AL Strauss et al (eds), *Chronic Illness and the Quality of Life*, 2nd ed, St. Louis: CV Mosby.

PERIODICALS

Banwell BF (1984) Exercise and mobility in arthritis. *Nurs. Clin. N. Am.*, Vol. 19 No. 4, pp. 605–616.

Blake SA (1985) Noncemented femoral prosthesis: intraoperative focus. *Orth. Nurs.*, Vol. 4 No. 4, pp. 40–42.

Brooks PM, Dougan MA, Mugford S & Meffin E (1982) Comparative effectiveness of 5 analgesics in patients with rheumatoid arthritis and osteoarthritis. *J. Rheumatol.*, Vol. 9 No. 5, pp. 723–726.

Clark CC (1983) Women and arthritis: holistic/wellness perspectives. *Top. Clin. Nurs.*, Vol. 4 No. 4, pp. 45–55.

Coles LS, Fries JF, Kraines RG & Roth SH (1983) From experiment to experience—side-effects of nonsteroidal antiinflammatory drugs. *Am. J. Med.*, Vol. 74 No. 5 pp. 820–827.

Derscheid G (1981) Rehabilitation of common orthopedic problems. *Nurs. Clin. N. Am.*, Vol. 16 No. 4 pp. 709–720.

Dickinson GR & Gorman TK (1983) Adult arthritis: the assessment. *Am. J. Nurs.*, Vol. 83 No. 2, pp. 262–265.

Doheny MO'B (1985) Porous coated femoral prosthesis: concepts and care considerations. *Orth. Nurs.*, Vol. 4 No. 1, pp. 43–45.

Gardner DL (1983) The nature and causes of osteoarthritis. *Brit. Med. J.*, Vol. 286, No. 6363, pp. 418–423.

Grace E (1983) Gold therapy and rheumatoid arthritis. *Can. Nurse*, Vol. 79 No. 11, pp. 40–42.

Hochberg MC (1984) Osteoarthritis: pathophysiology, clinical features, management. *Hosp Pract.*, Vol. 19 No. 12, pp 41–53.

Hughes GR (1982) The treatment of SLE: the care for conservative management. *Clin. Rheum. Dis.*, Vol. 8 No. 1, pp. 294–313.

Johnson J & Repp EC (1984) Nonpharmacologic pain management in arthritis. *Nurs. Clin. N. Am.*, Vol. 19 No. 4, pp. 583–591.

Koener ME & Dickinson GR (1983) Adult arthritis: a look at some of its forms. *Am. J. Nurs.*, Vol. 83 No. 2, pp. 254–262.

Lorig K, Laurin J & Gines GES (1984) Arthritis self-management: a five-year history of a patient education program. *Nurs. Clin. N. Am.*, Vol. 19 No. 4, pp. 637–645.

Mooney NE (1983) Coping with chronic pain in rheumatoid arthritis: patient behaviour and nursing interventions. *Rehab. Nurs.*, Vol. 8 No. 2, pp. 20–25.

Neuberger GB (1984) The role of the nurse with arthritis patients on drug therapy. *Nurs. Clin. N. Am.*, Vol. 19 No. 4, pp. 593–604.

Notwotny ML (1980) If your patient's joints hurt, the reason may be osteoarthritis. *Nurs. '80*, Vol. 10 No. 9, pp. 39–41.

Porter SF, Dapper MJ & Foran C (1983) Adult arthritis: hand splints. *Am. J. Nurs.*, Vol. 83 No. 2, pp. 276–278.

Potts M & Brandt KD (1983) Analysis of education support groups for patients with rheumatoid arthritis. *Patient Couns. Health Educ.*, Vol. 4 No. 3, pp. 161–166.

Programmed Instruction (1981) Patient assessment: examining joints of the upper and lower extremities. *Am. J. Nurs.*, Vol. 81 No. 4, pp. 763–786.

Simpson CF (1983) Adult arthritis: heat, cold or both. *Am. J. Nurs.*, Vol. 83 No. 2, pp. 270–273.

Simpson CF & Dickinson GR (1983) Adult arthritis: exercise. *Am. J. Nurs.*, Vol. 83 No. 2, pp. 273–275.

Strand CV & Clark SR (1983) Adult arthritis: drugs and remedies. *Am. J. Nurs.*, Vol. 83 No. 2, pp. 266–270.

Walsh CR & Wirth CR (1985) Total knee arthroplasty: biomechanical and nursing considerations *Orth. Nurs.*, Vol. 4 No. 1, pp. 29–34 & 70.

Wolfe F (1984) Arthritis and musculoskeletal pain. *Nurs. Clin. N. Am.*, Vol. 19 No. 4, pp. 565–574.

Ziegler GC (1984) Systemic lupus erythematosus and systemic sclerosis. *Nurs. Clin. N. Am.*, Vol. 19 No. 4, pp. 673–695.

27

Nursing in Skin Disorders and Burns

Structure and Functions of the Skin

The skin (integument) is the largest vital organ in the body. It is composed of a thin, avascular layer of epithelial cells called the epidermis, and a supporting layer of connective tissue (on which the epidermis rests) called the dermis or corium (Fig. 27.1). Beneath the dermis is a layer of subcutaneous fatty cells, called the panniculus adiposus, which acts as a cushion.

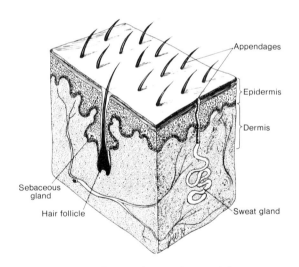

Fig. 27.1 Section showing layers of skin.

The *epidermis* has several layers of cells which differ in shape and composition from layer to layer. The cells are produced in the basal (germinating) layer and then gradually move through the other layers to the surface. As they ascend, they progressively undergo degenerative changes. The nuclei disintegrate, the cell substance changes to a water-repellent, waxy, protein-like substance called *keratin*, and the cells become flat. They are continuously reproduced in the basal layer and cast off from the surface. It is thought that normally they reach the surface in approximately 27–30 days. The cells that are shed disintegrate, leaving their keratin on the

surface; this keratin helps to protect the skin. The epidermis contains no blood vessels. The cells are nourished by intracellular fluid from the dermis, from which nutrients are diffused.

The thickness of the epidermis varies in different areas of the body, being thickest on the soles of the feet and palms of the hands and thinnest on the lips and eyelids. This provides maximum 'wear and tear' qualities for areas of maximum stress.

The *dermis*, consisting of fibrous and elastic connective tissue, contains many blood and lymphatic vessels, nerves and their end-organs, sebaceous and sweat glands, ducts and hair follicles. The undersurface merges with the loose, *fatty subcutaneous tissue*.

Lying between the epidermal germinating layer and the dermis are the melanocytes, which produce the pigment melanin and deliver it to the epidermal cells. The amount of pigment is mainly determined by the person's genetic inheritance. The activity of the pigment-producing cells may also be influenced by the melanocyte-stimulating hormone (MSH), which is released by the pituitary gland, and by exposure to sunlight and friction.

The *panniculus adiposus* or subcutaneous tissue is composed primarily of fat cells and functions as a heat insulator, a cushion against mechanical pressure and a caloric energy store. The subcutaneous tissue is distributed in varying thicknesses over the entire body surface. Its thickness is influenced by sex and age.

The sebaceous glands secrete an oily substance (sebum) which reaches the skin surface via the hair follicles. The secretion prevents drying of the hair and skin and helps to keep the skin soft and pliable. Blackheads (comedones; singular, comedo) are discoloured accumulations of sebum in hair follicles and frequently provide a medium for organisms, causing pimples or the condition acne. Sebaceous gland activity increases at puberty and decreases in later life due to the influence of gonadal hormones on the output of sebum. The growth of hair on certain areas of skin is also stimulated by gonadal hormones, principally the androgens.

The skin has many important functions, for example, protection, sensation, heat regulation, absorption and storage. By its continuity the skin protects the internal structures from injury, acts as a barrier to keep vital fluids and chemicals from leaking out, and prevents invasion of organisms. Its protective functions are enhanced by the water-repellent, waxy nature of the surface cells, desquamation (separation of the superficial cells) and the acid pH (4.5–6.5) of the secretion on the surface; this secretion has a bactericidal effect on many organisms.

The abundance of sensory receptors and nerves in the skin function in the sensations of touch, pressure, pain and temperature. These sensations serve as an important protective mechanism for the body and also convey impulses that contribute information about the external environment. For example, through touch we can appreciate shape, composition and texture.

The skin plays an important role in regulating body temperature by varying the calibre of its blood vessels and the activity of the sweat glands. These controlled mechanisms may promote the dissipation of the body heat or conserve it according to the need indicated by the heat-regulating centre in the hypothalamus. For further details of temperature regulation, see Chapter 7.

The fluid sweat lying on the surface of the skin cools the body by the process of evaporation, which requires energy in the form of heat; thus evaporation of sweat results in heat loss, so reducing body temperature. Sweat contains traces of albumin and urea; therefore sweating helps to remove these waste products from the body.

There are two types of *sweat glands; eccrine* glands which are distributed over the body surface and function to control body temperature and *apocrine* glands found mainly in the axillary and perineal areas which do not become functional until puberty. The latter are stimulated by stress and produce an odour.

Hair is a cylinder of keratinized cells. Distribution over the body varies with human groups, and with age and sex within each group. Hair serves primarily psychological functions.

The absorptive function of the skin is mainly limited to the absorption of ultraviolet rays from the sun or special lamps; it then converts sterol substances in the skin to vitamin D. A few drugs which may be included in ointments or lotions may be absorbed in small amounts.

The dermis and subcutaneous tissue may act as a storage area for water and fat. For instance, when an excess of water is retained in the body, the accumulation in these tissues becomes evident as oedema. The subcutaneous tissue serves as one of the main fat depots and acts as a pad over muscle and bone, cushioning them from mechanical forces.

With advancing years, the sebaceous and sweat glands become less active as a result of the decreased production of hormones, and the skin becomes dry. Degenerative changes occur in the elastic tissue and collagenous component of fibrous tissue, and the skin becomes wrinkled. Frequently, areas of melanocytes produce more pigment, and 'brown spots' characteristic of ageing skin appear.

Disorders of the Skin

Skin disorders may be primary or may be secondary to a systemic disease or reaction. It is not the author's intention to present an all-inclusive discussion of many specific skin disorders but, rather, to offer a brief description of common manifestations, general principles of nursing care of patients with skin disorders, and a discussion of a few conditions that are encountered frequently.

For more detailed information relating to skin diseases, the reader is referred to dermatology texts; several are listed in the references at the end of this chapter.

NURSING PROCESS

Assessment

HEALTH HISTORY

A skin disorder cannot be examined 'in isolation'; information about the patient's total health can reveal very significant diagnostic factors and influence the therapeutic plan. The social and occupational history as well as the health history are significant.

In taking the patient's history, particular attention is given to eliciting information about:
1 Any previous skin disorders, their nature, the patient's age, the season of the year at which they occurred and the treatment
2 Any known allergy or drug reactions
3 Drugs being taken, and for what reason
4 Known food(s), fluid(s) or contact substances (e.g. soap, certain material) that worsen the condition
5 Substances that are brought in contact with the skin throughout daily activities (e.g. cosmetics, chemicals at work)
6 Dietary habits
7 Recreational customs or hobbies
8 Family history, especially in relation to skin disorders, allergy and systemic disease; for example, a history of asthma may lead the doctor to suspect that heredity may have a role in the patient's disorder
9 Emotional stress resulting from job, interpersonal relations and other situations are identified. Stress and anxiety may influence the severity of skin disorders and the patient's responses to treatment.

In questioning the patient about the present skin condition, it is necessary to determine:
10 When it was first observed
11 Whether the lesion(s) persist or come and go, or change in appearance
12 The extent to which it has spread

13 Whether it itches or hurts
14 Whether the lesions are dry, moist or dis-
    charging.

PHYSICAL EXAMINATION

The history-taking is followed by an examination of
the skin. This involves inspection and palpation. A
good light is essential and the skin must be clean.
Care is taken to prevent unnecessary exposure of the
patient and to respect his dignity by closing curtains
or doors and protecting the patient with a gown or
sheet.

A general survey of the skin is done, noting: *colour*
(redness, palor, cyanosis, yellowness or brownness);
vascularity (any evidence of bruising or bleeding);
moisture (dryness, sweating, oiliness); *temperature*;
texture (roughness and smoothness); *thickness*; and
turgor (the rate at which it returns into place when a
section is pinched and lifted).[1]

Lesions are inspected and palpated; the nature of
the lesion (e.g. macule, papule, ulcer, etc.) is established and its characteristics recorded according to
size, shape, colour and whether is has a dry or wet
surface. It should be noted if an odour is associated
with the affected areas. The entire skin surface of the
body is examined to determine the general condition
of the total skin in addition to the distribution and
grouping of the affected areas. The latter is of assistance in diagnosis since certain disorders are known
to develop more frequently in certain areas. For
example, acne, impetigo, contact dermatitis, herpes
simplex and discoid lupus erythematosus develop
most commonly on the face. The oral mucosa is
usually included in an examination of the entire skin.
The fingernails and toenails are observed and palpated for colour, shape and the presence of lesions.
The quantity, texture and distribution of hair is also
noted.

DIAGNOSTIC TESTS

Many skin lesions can be diagnosed by physical
examination and history. If the lesions are moist or
discharging, a swab of the exudate may be obtained
for culture. If the affected areas are dry or scaly,
scrapings may be taken for cytological examination
and/or culture. Other laboratory tests may be done,
such as leucocyte and thrombocyte counts, examination for the lupus erythematosus (LE) cell, anti-D
test for SLE and erythrocyte sedimentation rate
determination. A biopsy of a lesion may be done if
malignancy is suspected or if the lesion is longstand-
ing and obscure in nature. If the condition is dermatitis, patch, intracutaneous or scratch tests may be
done during a remission to identify the allergen or
substance to which the person is sensitive. The

substances are administered intracutaneously or
applied to the skin on the back and observed at intervals over 48 hours. If positive, the reaction is manifested by inflammation and papules or vesicles.
Immunofluorescent tests may be done in certain skin
diseases to identify antinuclear antibodies.

Although the skin lesions prompted the patient to
seek medical assistance, the disorder may have internal or systemic components. This may necessitate
other investigative procedures, such as urinalysis,
x-rays, pulmonary function tests or further blood
studies.

MANIFESTATIONS OF SKIN DISORDERS

Lesions
Various changes in areas of the skin may occur, and
the exact nature of these is important in diagnosis
and treatment.

Primary lesions. Characteristic primary lesions in
which the skin is usually intact include the following:

Erythema—an area in which the blood vessels
become dilated, causing redness, warmth and
increased firmness of the skin.

Macule—a circumscribed, smooth, flat, discoloured area up to 1 cm in size.

Papule—a small circumscribed elevated area which
may or may not be discoloured and is not more than
1 cm in diameter.

Vesicle—an elevated area which contains clear
fluid.

Pustule—a small elevation of the skin which contains pus.

Nodule—a solid elevation larger than a papule,
usually involving both the skin and subcutaneous
layers.

Wheal—a localized, elevated, oedematous area
that is red at the margins with a blanched centre.

Bulla—an elevation larger than 1 cm of superficial
skin layers containing serous or purulent fluid.

Comedo (blackhead)—a plug of sebum and keratin
within a hair follicle.

Telangiectasia—a lesion composed of a group of
small blood vessels that are abnormally dilated.

Secondary lesions are those that develop as a result of a
break in the skin and destruction of cells. These
include:

Crust (scab)—a rough, dry area formed by the
coagulation and drying of plasma and exudate over a
primary lesion.

Scales—thin, flat, minute plates of dried epidermal
cells which have not completely undergone the
normal keratinization process before being separated. Desquamation is the term which refers to the
separation of scales or patches of cells.

Fissure—a split or crack in the surface, extending
through the epidermal layers and possibly into the

---
[1] Bates (1983), p. 46.

dermis. If it extends into the dermis, bleeding occurs. This type of lesion is most likely to occur in a natural skin or surface crease such as those located over knuckles, at the angles of the mouth, in the groin, between the buttocks and behind the ears.

Erosion (excoriation)—loss of the epidermis producing a superficial, reddened, weeping lesion.

Ulcer—a denuded area of irregular size and shape extending into the dermis or subcutaneous tissue due to necrosis of superficial tissue.

Lichenification—the thickening and hardening of skin as a result of continued irritation.

Atrophy—the skin is thin and wrinkled resembling tissue paper. Atrophy is seen with ageing.

Corn, callus (hyperkeratotic plaque)—an excessive thickness of the epidermis caused by chronic pressure and/or friction. In the case of a corn, the hyperkeratosis is sharply circumscribed.

Leucoplakia—a white plaque which is seen most commonly on the lips or mucous membranes of the oral cavity or tongue. About 10% of patients subsequently develop carcinoma in the lesions.

Scar (cicatrix)—an area of fibrous tissue replacing tissue destroyed by trauma or disease.

Hypertrophic scars. Normally a scar becomes paler and flatter as it matures. Hypertrophic scars become increasingly raised, red and itchy for several months after injury, due to excessive formation of fibrous tissue within the scar. The scar is then classified as hypertrophic. Over the next few years these scars usually flatten and lose their vascularity, thus becoming paler. The hypertrophy is confined to the site of injury. If these scars are excised there is some tendency for the hypertrophy to recur. It may be very difficult to determine if a scar is hypertrophic or keloid (see below).

Keloids. Histologically keloids are similar to hypertrophic scars, but keloids behave differently. Fibrous tissue formation is sometimes so excessive that the keloid has the appearance of a tumour, and the initial injury which produces the keloid may be so small as to appear insignificant, for example ear piercing, or an insect bite. Unlike hypertrophic scars, the keloid extends into surrounding uninjured skin and persists for many years. There is a high tendency to recur after excision. The incidence of keloid is highest in negroid skins.

It appears that tension within a scar encourages hypertrophy and keloid formation, therefore redistribution of the tension by use of elastic pressure garments usually produces some improvement in scar quality.

Pruritus

Generalized or localized itching is a common complaint in skin disorders. The sensory nerve endings or end-organs are irritated, giving rise to the desire to scratch. The patient is hard-pressed to refrain from scratching which further irritates the area and is frequently responsible for fissures, abrasions and subsequent secondary infection. Itching does not occur if the whole thickness of the skin has been removed as in a full-thickness burn.

Pain

The pain associated with skin lesions may be described as prickly or burning. It may be caused by chemical, mechanical or pressure irritation of the cutaneous sensory nerves, actual cellular damage or exposure of the nerve endings due to tissue destruction and erosion.

Redness

Erythema or redness of the skin indicates vasodilation and hyperaemia in the area. Erythematous lesions are initially macular but frequently become papular because of the oedema or developing exudate in the affected tissues.

Swelling

A puffy swollen area of the skin is usually due to localized oedema, resulting from increased permeability of the capillaries, or to localized inflammatory reaction.

Systemic disturbances

The skin reflects the individual's general physical and emotional status. Skin lesions are frequently manifestations of a systemic disorder (e.g. measles, systemic lupus erythematosus) or a systemic or emotional disturbance may be secondary to primary skin lesions. An elevated temperature is likely to be present if the skin disorder involves infection.

General principles in nursing patients with skin disorders

The nursing care varies greatly with these patients. The extent of the skin involvement as well as the nature of the condition determines whether or not the patient continues activities, is ambulatory and is treated at home. The patient's reaction to the disease also influences the plan of care and progress. The following are general considerations which will require adaptation and modification according to the individual; this, of course, is true of all nursing.

Psychological support

The patient with skin lesions is likely to be quite sensitive about the condition. Many are self-conscious about their appearance, worry constantly and tend to withdraw, believing that a skin disease carries a stigma. The disease may be such that it persists over a long period, interfering with the patient's ability to work or go out socially. Many skin diseases are aggravated by emotional stress. The understanding nurse helps the patient identify any emotional factors which may contribute to the skin condition and carefully assesses her own responses to the patient. Expression of revulsion at the patient's appearance add to his distress. The nurse should make a conscious effort to touch the patient's skin, thus reassuring him that his appearance and the texture of his skin are both accepted. The patient is advised whether or not the disorder is contagious, and there should be no hesitation on the part of the nurse to touch the affected parts when giving care. An effort is made to convey to the patient an appreciation of his feelings, to have him aware that he is accepted and to provide the necessary support and care which will help to reduce the patient's anxiety.

Local care

Cleansing. Cleansing of the skin or affected areas is determined for each patient. In some instances the application of soap and water may be contraindicated, and an alternative method of cleansing is necessary. For example, cleansing the skin with a vegetable oil may be necessary. If soap is permitted, it should be mildly alkaline and used very sparingly. A soft flannel is preferable, and the surface is washed lightly and gently to avoid injury and erythema. If there are open, discharging lesions, sterile gauze or a disposable absorbent cloth may be used in place of a flannel.

Special local or general therapeutic baths may be prescribed. These may be used to relieve itching, remove scales or crusts, or apply medications as well as for cleansing purposes. Caution is used against having the water or solution hot; a temperature higher than 35–38 °C (95–100 °F) is likely to be too hot for the sensitive areas. Also, higher temperatures are likely to promote hyperaemia and itching. Various preparations may be added to the bath according to its purpose. The patient is usually encouraged to remain in the prescribed bath for 10–20 minutes, and an attendant remains with the patient or close by, depending on his condition and age. Measures are taken to prevent the patient from slipping whilst getting into and out of the bath, since many of the preparations used (e.g. oatmeal, bran or emollients) make the surface of the bath especially slippery.

Moist compresses. Wet dressings may be applied over lesions, especially if they are open and discharging. The compresses are generally left uncovered and dry out very quickly, necessitating frequent changing or resoaking. The prescribed solution is usually used at room temperature. Wet dressings are not usually applied to dry or scaly lesions; an ointment or creamy lotion is more appropriate.

Topical applications. Many different drug preparations are used in treating skin diseases. Topical applications may be in powder, lotion, oil, cream, paste or ointment form. They may be classified according to their effect.
- *Antipruritic preparations* are applied to relieve itching. Examples are calamine lotion and corticosteroid cream or ointment.
- *Keratolytic agents* soften and remove scales and the horny layer. An example is salicylic acid ointment.
- *Antieczematous agents* are applied to relieve itching and remove the vesicular drainage. Examples are corticosteroid lotion or spray and coal tar solution.
- *Keratoplastic preparations* stimulate the epidermis, increasing its thickness. An example is a weak salicylic (1–2%) acid ointment.
- *Antimicrobial agents* destroy or inhibit the reproduction of bacteria and fungi. Examples are antibiotic ointments such as neomycin and gentamicin.
- Zinc undecylenate is a common *antifungal* agent.
- *Antiparasitic preparations* destroy or inhibit parasites. Examples are benzyl benzoate lotion and gamma benzene hexachloride.
- *Emollients* are used to soften the skin. Examples commonly used are lanolin, petroleum jelly and Alpha Keri bath oil.

Frequently, topical preparations are a combination of two or more agents which have been selected for their specific effect.

Assessment. Following each cleansing and before each local therapeutic application, the lesions are examined carefully. Any increase or spread, or change in size, colour or appearance is noted and reported. The nurse is constantly alert for factors in the patient's environment (e.g. contacts, diet, drugs) with which exacerbations of the condition may be associated. The patient's reaction to the disease and progress are noted.

Physical agents. Ultraviolet rays may be prescribed in the treatment of psoriasis, acne and seborrhoeic dermatitis. Irradiation is used if the lesion is malignant. Electrosurgery or cautery may be employed in the removal of warts, leucoplakia and seborrhoeic or senile keratoses (areas of horny thickening of epidermis).

Systemic therapy
If the skin disorder is secondary to a systemic disease, treatment is directed principally toward the primary condition.

Systemic drugs. The treatment of primary skin disorders may include the administration of systemic drugs. The drug will depend upon the nature of the disorder and the patient's general health and response to his condition. An oral corticosteroid (e.g. prednisone) is frequently prescribed in dermatitis, urticaria and pemphigus. If the skin lesions are infected, an antibiotic (e.g. tetracycline) may be ordered to be given orally. An antihistamine such as chlorpheniramine maleate (Piriton) may be used in urticaria. Vitamins may be given to improve the patient's appetite, general condition and resistance.

Concern about the condition and fear of disfigurement and rejection as well as itching may result in a considerable loss of sleep for the patient. A sedative may be necessary to provide rest, which plays an important part in the patient's recovery.

Nutrition
Attention is paid to the patient's nutritional status and to whether he is taking sufficient food. Frequently severe anorexia is a problem with the dermatological patient because of the skin irritation he experiences as well as the emotional disturbance. Dressings, ointments, lotions or similar applications on the hands may preclude his feeding himself.

Patient education
In the clinic or during preparation for discharge from the hospital, the patient and a family member are advised of the day-to-day care required and precautionary measures applicable to the prevention of an exacerbation of the skin disorder. Verbal and written directions are given about the local applications and taking of medicinal preparations. For example, adrenocorticosteroid preparations in the form of an ointment or cream are used topically to suppress inflammation and reduce sensitivity of the tissues. The patient must be cautioned to apply the corticoid preparation sparingly. If compresses or therapeutic baths are to be continued, specific details of the preparation, temperature and application are outlined and demonstrated if necessary. In the case of contact dermatitis, the patient may not be able to return to his former occupation. Referral to a rehabilitation or disablement resettlement officer may be helpful in finding a suitable job.

PRURITUS (ITCHING)

Pruritus is the sensation that arouses a desire to scratch. It is a symptom of many common skin disorders and may be generalized or localized. It may be associated with an internal disorder or excessive dryness as occurs with overbathing, dry atmosphere and the ageing process. Physiologically it is considered to be a modified form of pain; the impulses are carried on slow-transmitting sensory nerve fibres. Pruritus is extremely irritating and difficult to tolerate.

Assessment includes identification of the subjective sensation of itching by the patient. Objective data include: evidence of redness and scratch-marks on the skin, the presence of a rash or lesions, and observation or restlessness and irritability. Causative and contributing factors are identified. Local treatment varies with the cause and specific lesions if present, and also depends on whether the skin is dry or moist. Measures that may contribute to the relief of pruritus include:
1 The application of lotions, ointments, or creams which contain an antipruritic drug (e.g. calamine, corticosteroid)

2 The application of moist drying agents (wet compresses) or powders if the skin is moist
3 Dry skin is lubricated lightly with oil or cream applications
4 A *lukewarm* bath (15 minutes, two or three times daily) if the pruritus is generalized. After bathing excessive rubbing to dry the skin is avoided; the mosture is simply blotted gently with a towel
5 The suggestion that fewer baths should be taken. For elderly persons, and if the skin is dry, a bath only once or twice weekly is recommended. Excessively hot water should be avoided
6 The avoidance of soaps and detergents
7 A simple, adequate diet without rich and spicy foods
8 Cold applications cause vasoconstriction and decrease sensitivity and itching
9 Woollens and other irritating clothing are avoided

The patient is advised to refrain from scratching because of the danger of infection as well as the damage to the skin. The fingernails are kept short and clean. A systemic antipruritic drug may be prescribed (e.g. an antihistamine preparation, such as chlorpheniramine maleate) and, if the patient is very distressed and agitated, a sedative may be necessary.

URTICARIA

Urticaria is a skin disorder which is characterized by itching wheals of varying size which may develop very rapidly and become widespread. The lesions are a reaction to an external agent or to an irritating substance reaching the skin via the bloodstream. The reaction consists of dilatation and increased permeability of the capillaries and arteriolar dilatation. The combination of these is referred to as the triple response. The patient may experience general malaise and fever, especially if the urticaria is over an extensive area. The lesions frequently disappear in a few hours when the blood vessels return to normal.

A severe and possibly life-threatening form of this disorder is known as angioneurotic oedema. Very large wheals develop rapidly on the skin and mucous membranes. The commonest cause is a severe allergic reaction to a drug, food or insect bite. The patient is observed closely for respiratory distress due to laryngeal obstruction. Total obstruction of the airway may ensue with alarming speed. If laryngeal stridor is present, the patient should be prepared immediately for emergency laryngostomy or tracheostomy. Prompt action is necessary. A corticosteroid preparation such as hydrocortisone is given intravenously; this usually reverses the reaction rapidly.

Causes
Urticaria may be a manifestation of an allergic reaction to a food, drug, vaccine or serum, or it may be caused by insect bites, contact with certain plants

or chemicals or prolonged exposure to heat, cold, physical pressure or sunlight. It may also be associated with a systemic infection or internal disorder such as hepatitis.

Treatment
Urticaria is treated by the administration of an antihistamine preparation or, if it is widespread and causing considerable irritation, adrenalin 1:1000 may be ordered subcutaneously and usually provides immediate relief. The application of calamine lotion or a cream of calamine, diphenhydramine and camphor (Caladryl), or a corticosteroid preparation may be used in reducing the itching and local response. Unless the cause is definitely known, an investigation is made to identify the offending substance. Intracutaneous, patch or scratch sensitivity tests may be done (see p. 1032).

ACNE VULGARIS

This is a disorder of the sebaceous glands in which there is an increase in keratin, sebum and bacteria which accumulate in the follicular duct, forming a comedo (blackhead) or mila (whitehead). The lesions, which appear commonly on the face, progressively form comedones, papules and pustules or cysts. Rupture of the follicle releases the comedonal material into the surrounding skin, producing an inflammatory reaction and subsequent scarring in severe cases.

The incidence is greatest in adolescents after puberty. The increased sebaceous gland activity is associated with the increased production of sex hormones. Stress is also considered a contributing factor in acne.

Treatment is directed toward preventing obstruction of the follicles by which the sebum escapes onto the skin surface, and avoiding those factors, such as certain foods, which aggravate the condition; these foods include fatty foods, chocolate and pork. Thorough washing of the face three or four times daily with soap and warm water is recommended. The hair should be shampooed at least twice weekly. The comedones should be removed with a comedo expressor and young persons should be discouraged from squeezing the lesions and using unprescribed medicated preparations. Exposure to sunlight is beneficial because of the drying effects and slight scaling produced.

Topical medications such as the vitamin A derivative tretinoin (Retin-A) may be applied nightly over the affected area. During treatment caution is taken to avoid the area around the eyes and to prevent exposure of the eyes to sunlight. Other topical applications include benzoyl peroxide. Oral tetracycline or other systemic bacterial treatment may also be prescribed.

Relaxation techniques are taught to patients to decrease the physiological responses to stress.

CONTACT DERMATITIS

Contact dermatitis is a very common inflammatory disease of the skin and, according to the cause, may be referred to as primary irritant dermatitis or allergic contact dermatitis.

Causes
The former type is caused by contact of the skin with a substance (primarily irritant) that results in inflammation upon initial contact. Examples of primary irritants are strong soaps and some acids or alkalis. Allergic contact dermatitis is the result of an inflammatory reaction to a substance by a hypersensitive or allergic skin. The causative agent does not irritate the skin of a non-allergic or non-sensitized person. The person may not develop dermatitis with the first several contacts but repeated skin exposures sensitize him. The number of contacts with the substance before sensitization occurs varies with individuals. Examples of allergens which cause contact dermatitis are poison ivy, cosmetics, hair dye, soaps, and certain types of clothing material and dyes, plastic and insecticides. Dyes, flour, mineral dust, metal, industrial chemicals and enzymes used in 'biological' detergents and modern processing of cheese are examples of sensitizers.

Any causative agent can affect any area of the body, but because certain substances are commonly in contact with only certain areas, they become suspect. For example, lesions on the head, neck and face may be caused by cosmetics, soap, hair dye, or nickel (earrings). If the lesions are confined to the trunk, soaps, dusting powder, detergents and clothing may be suspect. Knowledge of the distribution of the dermatitis caused by different agents facilitates identification of the cause.

Manifestations
The lesions in contact dermatitis usually progress through various forms, beginning with an erythematous area on which small papules develop and rapidly progress to vesicles. The vesicles may rupture and discharge their contents. Those vesicles which do not rupture dry and form crusts or scales. The affected areas may become denuded, leaving a red glazed surface which probably oozes a serous discharge, giving rise to what is referred to as 'weeping eczema'. As the denuded areas are recovered by regenerated epidermis, more lesions may develop so that various stages (papular, vesicular, scaly, weeping, healing) exist at one time unless the reaction is corrected in the early stages. The patient experiences itching and burning, and scratching may result in infected lesions. The affected areas may remain localized to certain parts of the body or become disseminated.

Treatment
Local applications such as cold wet compresses, lotions, creams and ointments are used to reduce the

itching and tissue response and provide protection. If lesions are extensive, involving large areas of the body, therapeutic baths are used. An antibiotic ointment may be prescribed if there is infection.

A systemic drug may also be ordered for the relief of itching (e.g. diphenhydramine), and a corticosteroid (e.g. prednisone) may be administered to reduce the tissue response and inflammation. The patient is advised of the importance of avoiding scratching and the fingernails are kept short and clean. The application of mittens may be necessary to control scratching in children.

The patient undergoes investigation to determine the precipitating factor or allergen when the episode is controlled (see p. 1036). When the causative agent is identified, contact must be avoided. It should be remembered that dermatitis may be aggravated by emotional disturbances. Kind, sincere attention by the nurse may reduce the patient's tension or lead to discussions that reveal his concerns and disturbances.

Dermatitis is sometimes classified as: drug dermatitis, because of the obvious cause; exfoliative dermatitis, characterized by extensive scaling and thickening of the skin; infantile dermatitis, or eczema; or infective dermatitis because infection has been superimposed.

PSORIASIS

Psoriasis is a relatively common, chronic inflammatory skin disorder characterized by remissions and exacerbations and dry, scaly lesions. The lesions develop initially as dull, red papules on which silvery white, waxy scales accumulate in layers due to rapid, uncontrolled cell proliferation of the epidermis. Normally, the epidermis is replaced in 28 days; in psoriasis, it is reproduced in 4 days.[2] The lesions gradually increase in size, and several may coalesce, forming large, prominent, scaly plaques. Removal of the scale produces small, pinpoint bleeding areas.

The patient may or may not experience itching. Any skin area, including the nails, may be involved, but common sites are the extensor surfaces of the arms and legs (especially pressure areas such as the knees and elbows), the scalp, and the lumbar and sacral regions. The amount of involvement varies from one attack to another, and chronic patch areas vary in individuals; that is, it may always appear first on the fronts of the knees, on the elbows or on the back. If the nails become affected, they usually manifest pitting, discoloration and separation from the underlying tissue, which tends to become thick, dry and hard (keratosis).

The onset may be gradual or sudden. The lesions may persist for weeks or months and then may disappear spontaneously.

---

[2] North & Weinstein (1976), p. 410.

Cause

The cause of psoriasis is not known, but there is general agreement that heredity plays a role. Males and females are equally affected, and the incidence is much higher in temperate climates. The onset of the disease may be at any age but most commonly begins in adolescence. Psoriasis may be associated with rheumatoid arthritis. Exacerbations are more prevalent in winter months. Patients who move from a cold, wintry climate to a warm, sunny one have found that their psoriasis usually clears spontaneously and quickly. Many persons with the disease indicate knowing of someone in their family who is or was affected. The disorder is frequently precipitated by trauma, infections and psychological stress.

Treatment

The treatment consists principally of local applications, baths and exposure to ultraviolet rays. One preparation may prove effective for one patient and not for another. The treatment is individualized—this must be impressed on the patient. Various preparations in the form of ointments, creams or pastes are used and include salicylic acid, derivatives of coal tar, or dithranol. Topical and systemic corticosteroids should be treated with great caution and given only under specialist supervision.

The patient has a daily therapeutic bath, remaining in it for 20–30 minutes to soften and promote separation of the scales. The lesions may be scrubbed, gently, using a soft brush or rough flannel. If the scalp is affected, daily shampooing is also necessary. Following the bath the patient is exposed to ultraviolet light. Dark glasses are worn during the ultraviolet ray therapy. The period of exposure is very brief at first (1 minute) and then is increased very gradually. An application of the prescribed ointment or cream is applied. A coal tar preparation is generally used for the patient receiving ultraviolet therapy; it is considered to increase the effectiveness of the ultraviolet rays.

Dithranol paste is used less often than coal tar and corticosteroid preparations and only for severe psoriasis. It is an irritant, and precautions are taken to avoid getting it on unaffected skin. A protective substance such as petroleum jelly is applied around the lesions. The affected areas to which the dithranol is applied are left uncovered.

Methotrexate given orally may be used rarely for severe psoriasis that is not improving with local treatment. It is a chemotherapeutic antimetabolite (a folic acid antagonist) and has proved effective with some patients.

A more recent plan of care involves the administration of a psoralen before exposure to a high intensity ultraviolet light of a long wavelength (PUVA). The treatment is given 3 or 4 days weekly over a 1-month period on an outpatient basis.

The psychological impact of psoriasis for the patient and family is very great. Although it is non-infectious and not contagious, the appearance of the lesions frequently results in associates and even family members avoiding the person, especially personal skin contact. The patient who experiences rejection and isolation may withdraw, seek inappropriate emotional outlets and undergo personality changes. The nurse uses every opportunity available to provide support, especially understanding and willingness to help foster acceptance and encourage the person to cope with his problems. A full explanation of the disorder is made to the family (and employer, if necessary). A plan is developed with the patient and family for self-management of the treatment plan and coping with the resulting psychosocial problems.

SCABIES

Scabies is a contagious parasitic infestation caused by *Acarus scabiei* (itch mite). The disease is associated with overcrowding; it is transmitted by personal contact with an infested person.

The parasite burrows under the skin and lays eggs which hatch in 3–4 days. On the skin surface greyish-white, slightly elevated, zigzag lines appear and the patient experiences severe itching which is worse at night, resulting in loss of rest and sleep. Secondary lesions in the form of vesicles, papules, pustules and encrustations develop. Common infestation sites are the flexor surfaces of the wrist, palms, between the fingers and toes, groins and the areolae of the breasts.

Treatment
The patient takes a hot bath, vigorously scrubbing the affected areas to open the infested burrows. Following the bath, a benzyl benzoate preparation (Ascabiol) or Monosulfiram (Tetmosol) is applied over the entire skin surface. All clothing and bed linen are changed following the bath. The bath and application are repeated once, usually the next morning. Linen and clothing are washed in boiling water or pressed with a very hot iron. All close contacts of the patient are examined for scabies and treated if necessary.

TINEA (RINGWORM)

Ringworm is a contagious, fungal infection of the skin which may develop on any part of the body. Common forms are designated according to the location; for example, ringworm of the feet (athlete's foot), ringworm of the scalp (tinea capitis), ringworm of the nails (tinea unguium) and ringworm of the body (tinea corporis).

The lesions vary with the area of the body infected. For example, ringworm of the scalp is manifested by round, grey scaly patches. In athlete's foot, the primary lesions appear on the soles and between the toes in the form of itching, burning vesicles which

lead to secondary moist lesions and then to scaly areas. The lesions in tinea corporis may have an advancing peripheral ring of vesicles and a pustular or scaly centre. The area heals from the centre. The diagnosis of tinea is made by the microscopic examination of scrapings from the lesions. The specimen is placed in 10% potassium hydroxide.

Topical preparations include clotrimazole (Canestren), econazole (Ecostatin) and miconazole (Daktarin), as well as compound benzoic acid ointment (Whitfield's ointment). The drug commonly used in the treatment of tinea is griseofulvin, an antibiotic, and is administered orally. Toxic reactions include headache, dizziness, drowsiness, urticaria and gastrointestinal distress. It is least effective with ringworm of the hands and athlete's foot.

CANCER OF THE SKIN

Malignant tumours of the skin may or may not metastasize, and initially may appear quite innocuous. Carcinoma of the skin is readily discovered; therefore, provided the patient is aware of the significance of such skin lesions and seeks early treatment the prognosis is usually quite favourable compared to some other forms of cancer.

Causative factors include long periods of exposure to sunlight, radiation, chronic irritation (e.g. scars of poor quality, which frequently break down) and long standing contact with chemicals (e.g. oil, tar or paraffin).

Incidence of skin cancer is highest in people with blond or red hair, and lowest in Negroes.

The nurse should be alert for lesions that frequently indicate malignant changes. Most significant of these are moles which have changed in size or appearance, leucoplakia (white patches) on the lips or mucosa of the mouth and a sore which does not heal.

Bowen's disease is a brownish scaly thickening of the dermis which eventually progresses to carcinoma.

Basal cell carcinoma (rodent ulcer) may manifest as: a sore which does not heal and slowly enlarges; a nodule, which slowly enlarges; or a nodule which ulcerates. It spreads locally, destroying tissue, but does not metastasize. It rarely causes death unless it erodes some vital structure such as a major blood vessel or the brain, but if untreated may erode very extensive areas—for example the whole of a nose, cheek and/or orbit. Treatment may be by radiation, cryotherapy, electrodesiccation or excision.

Squamous cell carcinoma (epithelioma) may be present in various guises, including nodular lesions, open sores and long-standing scars which repeatedly break down. This type of skin cancer does metastasize by penetration into lymphatics and blood vessels. Rate of spread varies with different lesions, but generally the younger the patient the poorer the prognosis. Treatment is by excision and radiation.

Malignant melanoma are usually clearly pigmented

lesions which may arise from an existing mole which changes in size and/or colour, or present as a new 'mole'. Three types of melanoma are described as Lentigo maligna (Hutchinson's freckle), superficial spreading malignant melanoma and nodular malignant melanoma. All malignant melanoma metastasize, some with alarming speed, so that a lesion which appears as a small mole may represent an inoperable carcinoma. Generally the older the patient, the greater the chance of survival. There is increasing evidence that there is a close association with prolonged exposure to sunlight and the incidence of this type of tumour.

Identification of patient problems

POTENTIAL IMPAIRMENT OF SKIN INTEGRITY

Impairment of skin integrity is related to the presence of one or more risk factors (see Table 27.1):

- *Internal factors*: alterations in nutrition, metabolism, circulation, sensation, immune system, mental status, skin turgor, pigmentation, body fat and moisture, thickness and texture of the skin, the presence of infection, and actions of medications
- *External or environmental factors*: mechanical forces including pressure and shearing, chemical substances, radiation, temperature extremes, moisture and physical immobilization

Environmental and internal factors interact, influencing the condition and integrity of the skin.

Table 27.1 Factors contributing to impairment of skin integrity.*

External (environmental)
  Hyperthermia or hypothermia
  Chemical substance
  Mechanical factors
    Shearing forces
    Pressure
    Restraint
  Radiation
  Physical immobilization
  Humidity

Internal (somatic)
  Medication
  Altered nutritional state: obesity, emaciation
  Altered metabolic state
  Altered circulation
  Altered sensation
  Altered pigmentation
  Skeletal prominence
  Developmental factors
  Immunological deficit
  Alterations in turgor (change in elasticity)
  Excretions/secretions
  Psychogenic
  Oedema

* Kin, McFarland & McLane (1984), pp. 53 & 54.

The *goal* is to maintain the integrity of the skin. The underlying principles of the protective measures used to prevent a break in the skin and the development of a decubitus ulcer (pressure sore) are cited in Table 27.2. The protective measures include the following considerations.

Table 27.2 Nursing intervention to maintain skin integrity.

1 Maintain circulation
2 Maintain cleanliness and hygiene
3 Prevent mechanical, physical and chemical injury
4 Adequate nutrition and hydration
5 Control of incontinence
6 Good body alignment and proper positioning
7 Inspect the skin several times a day
8 Promote mental alertness and orientation to time, place and person
9 Educate the patient, family and those caring for the patient in skin care measures

Assessment
Assessment of the patient at risk for impairment of skin integrity includes identification of causative factors and internal and environmental factors which contribute to skin breakdown (see Table 27.1). The patient's age, nutritional status, circulatory status, degree of mobility and dependence, ability to exercise, voluntary control (continence), sensory awareness, mental awareness and degree of alertness are assessed.

Norton, McClaren and Exton-Smith[3] developed an assessment tool that assists in estimating the degree of risk of a skin breakdown for the patient (see Table 27.3). The maximum score used is 20; patients with high scores are least likely to develop a breakdown of their skin while those with lower scores are at greater risk.

The skin is inspected at frequent intervals; areas subjected to weight-bearing and friction should receive special attention. The vulnerable areas are the sacral region, buttocks, ischial tuberosity areas, spinal processes, scapular areas, occipital area, ears, elbows, knees and heels. The patient's body position is observed; the patient may favour one position, for example the dorsal recumbent or a lateral position, resulting in prolonged pressure on the respective vulnerable areas. In a lateral position, the area over the anterior iliac spine, greater trochanter, shoulder and malleoli become vulnerable. Fig. 27.2 illustrates the areas receiving greater pressure in different body positions.[4]

Body weight also influences the areas receiving greatest pressure. In the underweight individual, areas are more vulnerable in both the lying and sitting positions. In obese individuals pressure is distributed over larger areas. Casts, braces, restraints and

[3] Norton, McLaren & Exton-Smith (1975).
[4] Berecek (1975a) p. 161.

Table 27.3 The Norton scale for identifying the patient at risk of developing pressure sores.

A General physical condition		B Mental state		C Activity		D Mobility		E Incontinence	
Good	4	Alert	4	Ambulant	4	Full	4	Not	4
Fair	3	Apathetic	3	Walk with help	3	Slightly limited	3	Occasionally	3
Poor	2	Confused	2	Chairbound	2	Very limited	2	Usually urinary	2
Very bad	1	Stuporous	1	Bed-fast	1	Immobile	1	Double	1

underlying tubing are additional causes of pressure; the skin under these areas should be inspected regularly.

The skin over each pressure point should be carefully examined at frequent, regular intervals for redness, swelling, warmth, flaking and erosion.

Nursing intervention

Table 27.2 lists principles for nursing intervention directed at *maintaining skin integrity* and *preventing skin breakdown*. Nursing interventions include the following measures.

1 Promote ambulation and range-of-motion activities
2 Have the patient change his position frequently. If the patient is immobile, change his position every 2 hours throughout the day and night according to an established schedule. If redness is present, increase the frequency of the turning schedule

1 Supine position

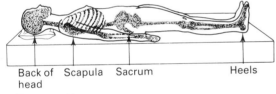

Back of head   Scapula   Sacrum   Heels

2 Prone position

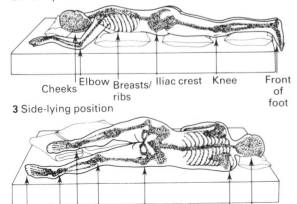

Cheeks   Elbow   Breasts/ribs   Iliac crest   Knee   Front of foot

3 Side-lying position

Toe   Ankle   Knee   Hip   Shoulder   Ear
Heel

Fig. 27.2 Risk areas for pressure sores.

3 Provide regular bathing and good perineal care twice daily and immediately following incontinence
4 Keep the patient's fingernails and toenails trimmed and clean, and dry well between toes after bathing
5 Establish a programme to control or manage incontinence
6 Encourage consistent intake of a nutritionally balanced diet with adequate fluid intake
7 Use a mattress that distributes body weight over a large area and/or alternates pressure such as a foam mattress, or alternating pressure mattress
8 Keep sheets dry and free of wrinkles and crumbs. Flannelette sheets or pads provide protection from any underlying plastic or rubber covers
9 Use devices to support specific pressure areas, such as foam pads, gel flotation pads, sheepskins and splints or pads over heels and elbows to relieve pressure on vulnerable areas and to decrease friction
10 Use a footboard or cradle to prevent pressure on toes
11 Provide space between the footboard and mattress for heels when the patient is lying supine, or the anterior part of the foot when lying in the prone position
12 Use pillows and trochanter rolls in positioning the patient to maintain good body alignment and to relieve pressure on known risk areas (see Fig. 27.2)
13 Keep connectors, tubes, pins and clamps from under the patient's body
14 Low Fowler's or reclining position are avoided because of the shearing forces caused by the patient sliding or slumping
15 Protect the patient with impaired sensation and mobility from injury by using devices such as clip-on ashtrays and drink holders on wheelchairs
16 Those caring for the patient should keep their nails trimmed and remove rings, watches or other jewellery that might scratch or injure the patient during turning or care activities
17 Teach patients to inspect their skin regularly using a long-handled mirror
18 Teach patients to shift their body weight and change position every 15–30 minutes while sitting
19 Do not use air rings which shift pressure to the area surrounding the pressure point or lesion

20 Avoid the use of bedpans when possible for patients with sensory loss and paralysis. If the use of a bedpan is unavoidable, a slipper pan should be used

21 Avoid the use of tight restraints or straps on urinary drainage leg-bags

22 Tape indwelling catheters to the thigh on male patients to prevent pressure on the penile–scrotal junction

23 Care is taken when applying external urinary devices to avoid excessive pressure on the penis.

DEVELOPMENT OF A PRESSURE SORE (DECUBITUS ULCER)

A frequent result of impairment of skin integrity is decubitus ulcer which is an area of inflamed and necrotic tissue. It develops as a result of sustained, localized pressure which compresses the blood vessels in the area causing ischaemia of the skin and underlying tissues. The area may appear blanched and cool at first followed by redness, warmth and a breakdown of the skin. Tissue underlying the skin may also be destroyed. As the necrotic tissue is sloughed off, an open, moist, inflamed excavation (ulcer) develops which is open to infection and is slow to heal by granulation (see Fig. 27.3).

Predisposing and causative factors include the following (see Table 27.1).

1 *Systemic disorders* such as:
   (a) Malnutrition (e.g. nutritional deficiency, obesity)
   (b) Metabolic disorder (e.g. diabetes mellitus, (hypo- or hyperthyroidism)
   (c) Cardiovascular disease
   (d) Neurological disorders that impair sensation and cause immobility (e.g. cerebral haemorrhage, brain tumour, spinal cord injury, multiple sclerosis)
   (e) Severe infection and fever
   (f) Debilitation (such as occurs in cancer and anaemia for example)
2 *External factors* such as:
   (a) Mechanical force (e.g. pressure, friction, shearing)
   (b) Moisture (e.g. excessive perspiration, incontinence of urine and faeces)
   (c) Temperature extremes
   (d) Chemicals
   (e) Radiation
   (f) Immobilization
3 *Skin characteristics*:
   (a) Thickness and texture of skin which vary in different areas of the body and are influenced by the person's genetic code and age
   (b) Turgor. Dehydration and oedema reduce the resistance of the skin
4 *Age*. The older person's skin is drier, less elastic and less turgid, predisposing it to breakdown when subjected to pressure or other mechanical forces or irritants.

Assessment

The pressure sore area is examined closely to determine the extent and depth of tissue involvement and must be described accurately. The size of the lesion is measured in centimetres and is recorded at the onset and at frequent intervals until healing takes place. Fig. 27.3 illustrates four different grades of decubitus ulcers according to the depth of the ulceration and involvement of underlying tissues. The pressure sore may be a reddened, slightly indurated area with only the epidermis sloughed off, forming a grade 1 decubitus ulcer. Grade 2, 3 and 4 indicate necrosis of progressively deeper tissues. The grading scale is useful for identifying the severity of tissue damage and changes that occur and in planning treatment. The lesion is examined for inflammation, bleeding, sloughing, infection and fibrous scar tissue formation. The area surrounding the lesion is inspected for discoloration, oedema and inflammation which may signify extension of tissue damage.

Pressure sores may develop in underlying tissue as a result of internal pressure exerted by the bony prominences on the deep tissues adjacent to the bone. Such deep tissue necrosis may occur without any initial signs of damage to the overlying skin. Subsequently there is an area of swelling and tension and the skin becomes shiny and/or cyanosed. Erythema and a sinus develop at a later stage. If a sinus has formed, its depth and path may be determined

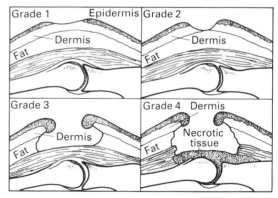

Fig. 27.3 Classification of decubitus ulcers (pressure sores). *Grade 1*: Involvement of epidermis with some extension into the dermal layer, producing redness, induration, warmth and slight erosion of the epidermis. The reddened area blanches to the touch. *Grade 2*: Involvement of the epidermis and dermis with extension into the subcutaneous layer. The shallow ulceration shows induration, redness and heat and does not blanch to the touch. *Grade 3*: Involvement of epidermis and subcutaneous layers with extension down to and including muscle. The ulceration is deep, foul-smelling with a necrotic base and undermining of tissue. The borders are hyperpigmented. *Grade 4*: The ulcer involves all layers of the skin, the underlying muscles and communicates with bone or joint. The ulcer is deep; the tissue is necrotic and foul-smelling. Undermining is extensive. Borders are darkly pigmented.

by gently introducing a sterile probe; a sinogram may be ordered to define the length, size and exact location of the sinus and underlying tissue damage.

The patient with a pressure sore is at risk of developing further lesions; vulnerable areas are inspected every 2 hours when his position is changed.

Nursing intervention
The number and variety of therapeutic measures and topical preparations used in the prevention and managment of pressure sores indicate an urgent need for further controlled research studies. Multiple patient variables contribute to the complexity of the problem. Nursing intervention for a patient with a decubitus ulcer has to be individualized, and is based on a detailed assessment of the patient as well as of the pressure sore; his general condition is important as well as the grade of the pressure sore. Consistency in carrying out the treatment plan is essential. The measures cited for the preventive care in the preceding pages are also applicable.

Further considerations include:
- Measures to correct existing health problems
- The use of mechanical devices
- Care of the lesion and the application of topical preparations
- Physical activity
- The control of injurious factors in the environment
- Surgical intervention

Control of existing health problems.   Optimal control of health problems is essential to promote healing as well as prevent a break in the skin. The reader is referred to the predisposing and causative factors cited on p. 1039. Management of these problems requires the cooperative efforts of the patient, doctor, nurse and other individuals caring for the patient.

A high protein, high vitamin diet is important to combat the tendency toward a negative nitrogen balance associated with inactivity and to provide the essentials for healing and tissue resistance.

Mechanical devices.   Berecek divides the mechanical devices used in the prevention and treatment of pressure sores into three categories:
1 Those designed to support specific pressure areas of the body such as heels, sacrum, buttocks or elbows. These devices include gel flotation pads, sheepskins, casts and splints.
2 Those designed to aid in turning and moving a patient such as turning frames, rotating beds and hydraulic lifts.
3 Those designed to support the entire body surface by minimizing or equalizing pressure. Alternating pressure mattresses, foam mattresses, water beds and air-fluidized beds are examples of these devices.[5]

Berecek found that no one device was solely efficient and effective in the treatment and/or prevention of pressure sores. Certain devices saved time in turning patients; others such as water beds have design problems for hospital and often home use. The gel flotation pad was found to be efficient and effective but pads large enough to support the entire body surface would be extremely heavy to handle.[6]

Care of the decubitus ulcer.   Aseptic care of the lesion is necessary to reduce the infection potential of the open area. Gentleness is required when cleansing the area and when removing paste or ointment to avoid tissue damage. An initial culture is made from material taken from the ulcer and should be repeated at intervals. If there is a firm eschar on the surface of the ulcer, the scar may be scored with a scalpel to allow topical applications to penetrate.

A large variety of topical preparations are available for application in the prevention and treatment of decubitus ulcers (see Table 27.4). They are categorized according to their action and include: cleansing and antiseptic agents; protective preparations; debriding agents; and agents which promote granulation and epithelial tissue formation.
1 *Cleansing and antiseptic* agents are used to remove necrotic tissue, 'old' blood and exudate as well as inhibit the growth of organisms.
2 *Protective agents* provide a protective covering for the skin surrounding the lesion and may also be applied to the ulcerated area to protect granulation and new epithelial tissue. They are especially useful to protect surrounding skin when moist applications and a debriding agent are being used on the ulcer.
3 *Debriding agents* may be enzymatic, keratolytic, autolytic or absorptive in action.

The enzymatic preparations used in debridement may be collagenic, fibrinolytic or proteolytic, according to the tissue component that reacts to the respective enzymatic agent.

A keratolytic agent promotes separation of the epidermal tissue and may also be antimicrobial and have a stimulating effect on granulation.

Autolytic preparations promote liquefaction of necrotic tissue by endogenous enzymes and keep the ulcer moist. A transparent adhesive dressing such as Op-Site is applied to seal the wound or a hydroactive dressing (a transparent occlusive dressing with an underlying layer of gel) may be used (see Table 27.5 for a list of dressings for pressure sores).

Absorptive agents absorb the products of tissue breakdown. They are prepared in granular or bead-like forms and, sprinkled into the area, can absorb copious amounts of exudate and debris.

---

[5] Berecek (1975b), pp. 171–172.

[6] Berecek (1975b), p. 190

The antiseptic sodium hypochlorite solution may also be used to debride the area in strengths of 1:20 to 1:12. It is usually applied in compresses and requires renewal every 2 hours to be effective.

Water used as a soak, bath or compress is an effective and inexpensive debriding agent. If softens and washes out necrotic and crusting tissues and exudate.

4 *Agents which promote granulation and epithelial tissue formation* are used initially on grade I and II pressure sores and on a deeper pressure sore following the removal of exudate and necrotic tissue.

Physical activity. Pressure on the area is removed as much as possible by having the patient change his position frequently. If the patient cannot turn himself, he is turned every 2 hours throughout the day and night. When turning or transferring a patient, precautions are observed to prevent further damage to the skin; the patient is gently lifted clear of the bed or chair to avoid dragging and a shearing force.

Patient activity is encouraged; it stimulates metabolism as well as circulation. A programme of regular exercises adapted to the patient's ability to actively participate is established as soon as possible.

Control of environmental factors. A frequent assessment is made of the patient's environment for possible sources of pressure and injury to his skin. Again, the reader is referred to the measures cited in the prevention of a decubitus ulcer. The bedding, wheelchair, bedpan or commode, clothing and appliances such as a prosthesis and drainage tubes or bags are examples of factors in the patient's environment that could be a source of pressure or injury.

Surgical treatment. Surgical debridement of a pressure sore may be done on the ward. Overgranulation of an ulcer may require removal of some of the excess tissue with scissors or by the use of a silver nitrate stick. Grade III and IV ulcers may require surgical excision and repair by skin flaps. For care of the patient following surgery see Chapter 11.

Selection of the treatment and nursing care for the patient with a decutibus ulcer should be a cooperative effort by all members caring for the patient and

Table 27.4 Topical agents used in the management of pressure sores.

Types of agent	Example	Comments
Cleansing and antiseptic agents	Soaps and detergents	Use sparingly as they tend to dry and irritate tissue If used, the skin should be rinsed well
	Antibacterial (topical)	Used *only* when sensitive organisms have been cultured from the ulcer Resistant strains of the organism may develop Should be avoided
	Antiseptics– Povidone iodine Chlorhexidine solution	Used to inhibit the growth of microorganisms as well as for cleaning
Protective agents	Silicone cream Zinc oxide cream	When incontinence is a problem and frequent washing of skin necessary, barrier cream can help replace natural skin oils
Debriding agents	Enzyme preparation Varidase topical streptokinase-streptodornase	Wound is cleansed with normal saline before application of debriding agent
	Absorptive agents: dextranomer beads (Debrisan) + starch gel micro beads + iodine (Iodasorb) Sodium hypochlorite solution (eusol)	A protective agent may be applied to wound edges and surrounding area of skin
Agents used to promote granulation and epithelial tissue formation	Human amniotic membrane	The amniotic membrane is cleaned and the chorionic surface (dull side) is applied to the ulcerative area Gold leaf has been useful in resistant ulcers
	Insulin	Insulin enhances protein synthesis by the dermal cells
	Benoxyl peroxide (Benoxyl) Ultraviolet light rays	Precautions necessary against burning when heat and ultraviolet light are used
	Vegetable gums (Karaya powder, paste or solids and Stomahesive)	Absorb moisture, keeping the wound moist to protect granulation
	Occlusive dressings (e.g. Op-site)	Keep the ulcer moist and promote healing

should take into consideration the patient's needs, overall status and resources. For example, if frequent dressing changes cause discomfort for the patient, consideration is given to a treatment method that requires dressing changes about every 5–7 days; an occlusive dressing (Op-Site) has additional advantages of being easier for the patient to manage at home, interfering less with daily activities and enabling the patient to have a bath without interfering with the dressing. A variety of interventions are usually required; selection is based on evaluation of the effectiveness of care and assessment of the individual patient.

Expected outcomes

The expected outcomes for the patient with potential for an actual skin breakdown include the following.
1 The skin is clean, dry and intact
2 The patient knows factors contributing to skin breakdown
3 The patient and family participate in the plan of care to maintain and promote integrity of the skin.

Nursing the Burned Patient

Burns continue to be a major cause of suffering, disfigurement, disability and death. A large proportion of those that occur are due to carelessness and are therefore preventable. More emphasis on safety measures, especially in the home, seems necessary. Through increased public education by the use of such aids as mass media and printed pamphlets, we have been able to alert the public to the danger signals of cancer and the importance of early treatment. A comparable programme relating to burn statistics, causes of fire and safety measures might produce greater caution in the home and elsewhere.

Causes of burns

A burn may be inflicted by dry or moist heat, irradiation, electrical current or chemicals. The burn that is caused by dry or moist heat may be referred to as a thermal burn and is the type of greatest incidence. The most frequent type of burn in young children is from hot liquid scalds occurring in the kitchen. Fabric ignition occurring in the home is the most common cause of burn injury in the elderly.[7]

Classification and assessment of burns

Burns are classified according to cause (thermal, electrical, chemical or irradiation), the extent of the

---

[7] Feller, James & Jones (1982), p. 285.

Table 27.5 Summary chart of representative dressings for pressure sores.

Classification	Examples	Comments	Frequency of change	Ulcer type
Foams	Silastic Synthaderm Lyofoam Coraderm	The surface that is applied directly to the wound is water-permeable while the back is non-absorbent Provide protection and a thermal effect Associated with a marked increase in exudate in the early stages Lyofoam is not very absorbent	2–10 days	Those that are not exudative with little slough and poor formation of granulation tissue
Polysaccharides	Debrisan	Can act as a cleaning or or debriding agent Can stick to the wound if not enough moisture An additional dressing is needed on top	Daily preferred	Offensive and sloughy ulcer
Hydrogels and hydrolloids	Vigilon Geliperm Scherisorb Comfeel Ulcus Granuflex	Absorb exudate from the wound and reduce smell Do not adhere to wound Some need additional dressing on top Various formulations are available	Vigilon, Geliperm, Scherisorb—Daily to every 3 days Comfeel Ulcus, Granuflex—up to every 7 days	Offensive and exudative wounds
Alginates	Sorbsan Kaltostat	Seaweed products which gel in contact with wound exudate	Daily to alternate days	Offensive and exudative wounds

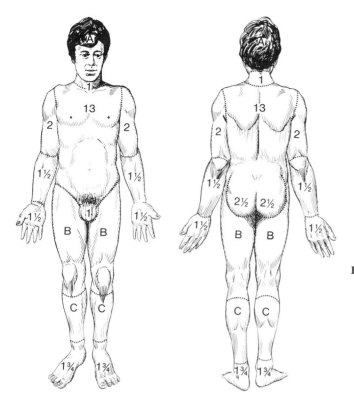

Fig. 27.4 The Lund and Browder burn chart.

body surface burned, and the depth of tissue damaged or destroyed. The assessment of the severity of a burn is made principally on the last two factors. The seriousness is also influenced by the patient's age, sex, health at the time of the accident and whether or not any other injury was incurred at the same time. Other variables which may be considered in estimating severity include the presence of inhalation injury and the parts of the body burned.

The most accurate estimation of the percentage of body surface burned may be based on the Lund and Browder chart (see Fig. 27.4). The chart assigns a certain percentage to various parts of the body and includes a table indicating the adjustments necessary for different ages, since the head and trunk represent relatively larger proportions of body surface in children. Copies of these charts should be kept available in the emergency department or intensive care unit so that the burned areas can be mapped out when the patient is examined and the percentage estimated.

If the Lund and Browder chart is not available, a quick approximate estimate of the percentage of body surface burned may be made using the Rule of Nines (see Fig. 27.5). The body is divided into areas, each of which represents 9%. The apportionment is as follows: the whole of the upper limb is 9%, a thigh 9%, a leg (below the knee) 9%, the anterior chest 9%, the posterior chest 9%, the abdomen 9%, the lower

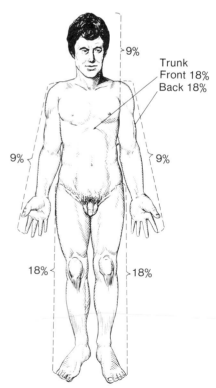

Fig. 27.5 Rule of Nines; used for estimating the percentage of body surface burned.

half of the back (lumbar and sacral regions) 9%, the head and neck 9%, and the perineum 1%. It should be remembered that in infants and children the head represents a relatively large percentage, but the extremities compose a smaller portion of the body surface.

If approximately *10% or more of the body surface of a child or 15% or more of that of an adult is burned, the injury is considered to be a major burn*. The patient requires hospitalization and fluid replacement.

The depth of tissue damage and destruction in a burn is indicated by the classification as superficial, partial thickness or full-thickness (see Fig. 27.6). This classification was established by the International Burn Association to replace the older terms—first degree, second degree and third degree.

A *superficial* burn involves destruction of only superficial epidermal tissue. It is characterized by a bright red appearance (erythema), the return of capillary circulation following compression, and spontaneous healing within 2–10 days without scarring.

A *partial-thickness* burn involves the epidermis and upper layers of dermal cells; lower dermal cells remain undamaged and viable (capable of regeneration of the cells to replace those burned). This type of burn is usually painful. Blisters form due to separation of epidermal tissue by the collection of fluid. The capillary circulation returns following compression. Healing takes place spontaneously within 10–14 days.

A *full-thickness* burn is characterized by the destruction of the full thickness of the skin and its appendages. Underlying tissues such as the subcutaneous fat, muscles, tendons and bone may also be burned. The appearance is white and waxy or charred and does not change with capillary compression. Burns of partial-thickness and superficial occur marginally. A full-thickness burn is not painful because of the destruction of sensory nerve endings, but the patient may complain of pain due to the marginal tissue burns of lesser depth. Spontaneous regeneration and replacement of the skin is not possible following a full-thickness burn. The area may be slowly filled in with granulation tissue and the fibrous scar tissue, proliferated from marginal or underlying connective tissue. In order to avoid the contracture disability that occurs with the fibrous scar tissue, the area may be covered with a skin graft.

The age of the patient is an important factor in the seriousness of a burn. The severity of the burn increases with age. A person of 20 withstands a burn better than a 40-year-old, and the patient of 40 has a much better chance of survival than a 60-year-old, even though the percentage of body surface burned and the depth are the same. Infants and young children also tolerate burns less well than young adults.

Pathophysiological effects of burns

The patient who suffers a major burn manifests shock which, in some cases, may be irreversible. Immediately following the injury, the pain and fear which may be experienced by the injured person are considered to be responsible for widespread vasodilation and subsequent hypotension and impaired circulation (see Fig. 15.1, Chapter 15). This phase may be referred to as *neurogenic shock* or *nervous compensation*. The duration varies; it may be brief or may persist to become a part of the *hypovolaemic (oligaemic)*

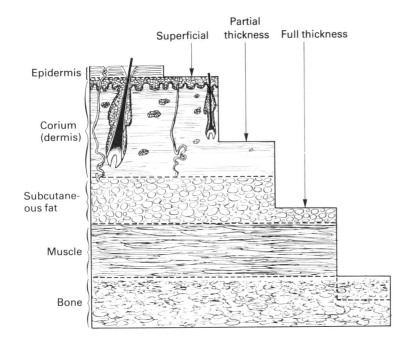

Fig. 27.6 Classification of burns according to depth.

shock that develops rapidly as a result of the loss of fluid from the circulating blood volume. Increased permeability and dilation of the capillaries in the burn area result in a shift of protein-rich fluid out of the vascular compartment into the interstitial spaces, causing the formation of blisters and oedema. Large volumes of the fluid, which is similar in composition to plasma, may seep into the tissues. Some is carried away via the lymphatics, but an amount in excess of what can be drained into the lymphatic system accumulates. The oedema is also promoted by the loss of blood proteins with the fluid and the ensuing reduction of the intravascular colloidal osmotic pressure. As a result oedema also occurs in non-burned tissue, resulting in generalized oedema. Oedema of the lungs from this cause can be life-threatening, even in the absence of any respiratory injury. In a full-thickness burn the fluid loss is extensive and, in areas of greater vascularization, such as the face, the oedema and swelling may be very severe.

The intravascular volume diminishes, the blood pressure falls, the cardiac output is reduced, and the blood flow through the tissues is reduced. *Hypovolaemic shock* develops unless there is adequate fluid replacement. The reduction in the intravascular volume produces a corresponding haemoconcentration, evidenced by an increase in the haematocrit and haemoglobin levels. (Normal haematocrit: males, 40–50%; females, 37–47%. Normal haemoglobin: males, 13–18 g/dl; females 12–15 g/dl.) The greater concentration of cellular elements in the blood increases the demand on the heart and predisposes to thrombosis and circulatory insufficiency.

An actual decrease in the number of red blood cells occurs especially in deep burns, due to trapping and heat injury of those blood cells in the skin capillaries at the time of the injury. Often red cells, including transfused cells, may also be destroyed in the immediate post-burn period; blood transfusion may be delayed for at least 48 hours. Normal red blood cell production may also be reduced because of depression of the bone marrow.

Inhalation of smoke and chemical fumes can seriously impair ventilatory function; irritation of the mucosa may cause laryngeal oedema and airway obstruction or pulmonary oedema and severe respiratory insufficiency.

The urinary output is decreased as a result of the decreased intravascular volume and subsequent hypotension. If the blood supply is markedly reduced in the shock phase, renal tubular damage may also result. Providing intravenous fluid replacement is adequate and shock is reversible a fluid shift occurs in the opposite direction from the initial stage. Oedema decreases and blood volume increases, producing haemodilution and diuresis. Diuresis and increased sodium excretion occurring in 3–5 days are favourable signs. When there is massive red blood cell destruction, large quantities of haemoglobin are released. These blood pigments may block the renal tubules, causing renal shutdown. Another cause of renal failure in the burn injured patient is due to the breakdown of protein from damaged tissue, especially muscle, and the release of these products (e.g. myoglobin) into the renal tubules.

The appearance of brownish black urine indicates the presence of free haemoglobin and/or myoglobin; this is an ominous sign which requires urgent action to achieve diuresis.

In severe burns gastrointestinal peristalsis is depressed; nausea, vomiting and abdominal distension may occur. Haematemesis or melaena may develop, indicating the presence of stress ulcers (Curling's ulcers).

Toxaemia may develop in 3–5 days, especially with a large surface area burn. This is attributed to absorption of the decomposition products of dead tissue.

Electrolyte imbalances develop because of the burn oedema, loss of fluid through the open wound, impaired renal function in the associated shock, and excessive release of potassium by the damaged tissue cells and erythrocytes. The disturbances are also influenced by the adrenocortical response (increased secretions) to the stress (see Fig. 15.2, Chapter 15), which results in sodium retention and increased potassium excretion by the kidneys (if they are functioning satisfactorily). The adrenocortical hyperactivity also accelerates protein catabolism, resulting in a negative nitrogen balance.

The effects of the heat at the site of the burn depend on the intensity of the heat and the length of exposure to it. The layer of burned tissues may form a dry, charred, coagulated surface, called an *eschar*, or a soft, moist non-coagulated area. Inflammation and oedema develop at the wound margins and below the layers of dead tissue. Many small blood vessels below the devitalized tissue may be thrombosed, promoting further cellular destruction. The decomposition of dead tissue and sloughing produce a favourable culture medium for organisms and the development of serious infection. Most major burns are mixed in depth; some areas will have partial-thickness skin loss while other areas suffer full-thickness destruction.

Treatment and nursing intervention

Treatment and care are directed toward the following:
1 The prevention of shock, or its reversal should it occur
2 The prevention of wound contamination and the treatment of infection
3 The alleviation of pain
4 The prevention of contractures and deformities
5 Maximum rehabilitation of the patient

Care of the patient who is severely burned can be divided into that necessary throughout the initial *emergent period*, the *acute phase* and the *rehabilitation period*. The patient may be gravely ill for many weeks requiring intensive and prolonged care.

Care during the emergent period includes first aid at the site of the injury and the initial medical and nursing care. This initial care is directed toward establishing and maintaining an airway if necessary, reversing hypovolaemic shock and cleansing and assessing the severity of the burned areas. The emergent period may last for 2–7 days.

The acute phase of burn care involves wound care to promote healing and recovery of skin, physical and psychological support, the prevention of complications and the treatment of complications, if they occur.

The rehabilitation period is the phase of regaining function and resuming a normal, active and useful pattern of life.

FIRST AID (see Table 27.6)

In the case of burning due to flames, smother the fire if possible or remove the victim from exposure to it. If his clothes are on fire, he should remain stationary because movement fans the flames, and lie down on the floor or ground. This position may prevent the igniting of his hair and the inhalation of flames, with subsequent respiratory damage. He is quickly rolled in a rug, blanket or something comparable to smother the flames or is doused freely with water. If nothing is quickly available, the flames may be extinguished if he rolls on the ground. Breathing is assessed and resuscitation measures are instituted immediately. Bleeding and shock are then evaluated and associated injuries determined.

Table 27.6 First aid: at the accident scene for the burned patient.

1 Stop the burning process
2 Maintain airway—resuscitation measures may be necessary
3 Assess for other injuries and check for any bleeding
4 Cool applications may be made to burn area to reduce the pain and effect of heat on the tissues
5 Protect wounds from further trauma
6 Provide emotional support—have someone remain with patient. Explain that assistance will be available
7 Transport the patient to where he can obtain medical care

Immediate cooling of the burn area by holding the part under cool running water, immersion, or the application of cold, moist towels or compresses is recommended as a valuable first aid measure. Cooling reduces pain and decreases the effect of heat transmission through the tissues. Ice is avoided because of the sudden vasoconstriction that it produces.

Oils, ointments, lotions and other preparations *should not* be applied, and no attempt is made to remove clothing that is adherent. The burn area is covered with a moist, sterile or clean material to exclude air (which stimulates pain) and to reduce contamination. Non-burned areas are covered with warm, dry covers. While awaiting transportation, the patient is kept at rest. A minimal amount of movement and handling is important, but any constricting shoes, clothing and jewellery are loosened or removed.

In the case of chemical burns, the area is washed with generous amounts of water. The patient's clothing is removed, since it is most likely holding some of the offending substances.

The patient with severe burns is conscious unless other injuries interfere with awareness. Simple explanations of what is being done should be provided and repeated frequently. Someone remains with the patient and he is calmly reassured that help is being provided.

Most superficial burns involving approximately *less than 10%* of body surface are treated at home or in the accident and emergency department. Systemic effects in such cases are minimal and are not considered sufficiently significant to require hospitalization. However, it should be remembered that there are variables; concomitant disease or injuries, if the patient is under 18 months of age or over 60 years, the patient's reactions and the availability of home care are a few factors which may influence the decision as to whether hospitalization is required.

The severely burned patient is transported as soon as possible by ambulance and/or helicopter to a centre with a burn unit.

PRE-ADMISSION PREPARATION

Once notified of the imminent admission of a severely burned patient, activities include assembling equipment and preparation of the area or room for the patient. The patient will be admitted to a burn unit or to intensive care. Emergency equipment should be on hand as well as central venous pressure monitoring equipment, burn dressings, topical ointments and solutions, catheterization tray, intravenous solutions, and sterile gowns, gloves and bed linen. If a special bed such as the air-fluidized system (Clinitron) or a turning frame (Circolectric or Stryker) is to be used, it is prepared for the patient; patients with major trunk, posterior or circumferential burns benefit most from these devices.

CARE ON ADMISSION (see Table 27.7)

An immediate *assessment* of the patient's general condition is made before attention is directed to the burn wound. A history as to how the burn was sustained is obtained from the patient or the person who accompanied him; this may indicate the need to search for other injuries. The burn patient is usually sufficiently alert to provide information; if drowsy,

Table 27.7 Treatment of the severely burned patient on admission.

1 Maintain an airway and administer oxygen if necessary
2 Assess severity of injuries and degree of shock
3 Initiate fluid replacement—establish an intravenous line
4 Insert an indwelling catheter
5 Insert a nasogastric tube
6 Control pain
7 Provide emotional support
8 Provide initial wound care
9 Initiate protective isolation measures
10 Administer tetanus prophylaxis

confused or comatose, other disorders or injuries are suspected (e.g. hypoxia, head injury, cerebral aneurysm or stroke).

Respiratory function
Damage to the respiratory tract and respiratory insufficiency demand prompt attention. Respiratory impairment is frequently associated with burns of the face or neck and may be the result of the inhalation of smoke, a gaseous chemical or flames. The presence of singed nasal hair or blackened oral or nasal mucosa are suggestive of inhalation burns. To assess ventilatory function, observe respiratory effects and listen for inspiratory wheezes, check odour of breath (a smoky or chemical odour may be detected which indicates inhalation of smoke or fumes), listen for hoarseness, and examine any sputum for blood and carbon particles. Humidified oxygen is administered, if necessary, and suctioning may be helpful to clear the airway of secretions. Intubation may be performed if respiratory embarrassment increases. If there is marked insufficiency, a mechanical ventilator may be used in conjunction with the endotracheal tube. Frequent estimations of the blood gases and expiratory or tidal volume may be done. See Chapter 16 for the care required in respiratory insufficiency and endotracheal intubation.

Respiratory insufficiency may develop later in circumferential or severe chest burns due to restricted respiratory excursion as a result of a firm unyielding coagulum or eschar. The doctor may have to make several incisions in the eschar to relieve the thoracic restriction. Following the initial assessment and treatment, the patient is required to breathe deeply and cough hourly if intubation or a tracheostomy is not necessary.

When satisfactory ventilation is established, attention is directed toward fluid therapy and assessment of the extent and severity of the burn and any other injuries.

Fluid replacement
The control of shock resulting from the loss of intravascular volume in a severe burn is dependent upon prompt, adequate fluid replacement. The extent and depth of burn and the patient's age and health status determine the need for fluid therapy. A reliable intravenous route is established by the insertion of a polyethylene cannula or catheter immediately on admission. The intravascular fluid shift commences immediately after burning but signs of shock may not appear for a few hours. Solutions that may be administered include colloidal solutions[8] such as plasma, whole blood and a plasma expander (e.g. dextran), or a solution of electrolytes (e.g. lactated Ringer's solution) and glucose 5% in distilled water. The volume, composition and rate of flow of the intravenous fluids are based on the percentage body surface burned, the weight of the patient, the hourly urinary output, arterial blood pressure, haematocrit, and serum electrolyte concentrations, especially potassium and sodium. Haematocrit determinations are usually done every 4–6 hours. An adult may require as much as 500–1000 ml per hour intravenously to maintain a urinary output of 30–60 ml per hour. Close monitoring and frequent adjustment of the intravenous flow rate is essential. If oral fluids are permitted, the amounts ingested are recorded accurately.

Generally, after the first 24–36 hours, fluid extravasation into the tissues lessens and the intravascular volume tends to stabilize gradually. The intravenous fluid therapy is gradually reduced and may be discontinued when laboratory studies indicate satisfactory concentrations and the patient is able to take adequate amounts of fluid orally. He is observed closely for signs of circulatory overload, since much of the fluid in the interstitial spaces is reabsorbed into the intravascular compartment as capillary integrity is re-established. Overloading of the circulatory system may be manifested by a urinary output greater than 100 ml per hour within the first 48 hours, pulmonary oedema, a central venous pressure in excess of 13 cm of water and a weak pulse. If renal function is satisfactory, the excessive amount is controlled by diuresis. A blood transfusion may be necessary later if the red blood cell count indicates anaemia.

Indwelling urinary cathether
An indwelling (Foley) catheter is passed as soon as the patient is admitted so that the hourly urinary output may be noted. This serves as a guide in determining intravenous fluid requirement and also provides information about the patient's general circulatory status and renal function. The urinary output should be at least 25–30 ml per hour for an adult, 20–25 ml per hour for a child and 10–20 ml per hour for an infant. A volume below the normal minimum is reported promptly. Urine specimens are tested hourly for specific gravity and sugar, acetone and protein and blood. Dark urine, indicating the presence of haemoglobin and myoglobin, is brought to

---

[8] A *colloidal solution* contains large non-diffusible particles of solutes which will not leak out of the capillaries.

the doctor's attention promptly. The intravenous fluid volume is increased, and a diuretic such as mannitol or frusemide (Lasix) may be prescribed to dilute the globins and produce diuresis.

The catheter is removed as soon as the patient's condition is stable and shock is reversed, since the indwelling catheter predisposes to bladder infection and loss of bladder tone.

Dialysis may be initiated if the urine output drops below 400 ml in 24 hours. Haemodialysis is usually the treatment of choice to remove toxic wastes and excessive body fluids.

Assessment

The patient is observed closely during the early post-burn period for symptoms of shock. The blood pressure, pulse and level of consciousness are noted every 15–30 minutes and the urinary output per hour is recorded. A diminishing intravascular volume and subsequent circulatory failure may be reflected by a fall in blood pressure, weak pulse, abnormal drowsiness, disorientation and a urinary output of less than 30 ml per hour.

Frequent haemoglobin and haematocrit determinations are made; abnormal elevations indicate haemoconcentration due to loss of intravascular fluid into the tissues. After 2 or 3 days a deficiency of erythrocytes and haemoglobin may indicate the need for a blood transfusion. Serum protein and electrolyte concentrations are also determined frequently; these help in selecting the type of intravenous solutions required. An accurate record of the fluid intake (oral and intravenous) and the output is of paramount importance. The patient is weighed daily. A gain is manifested at first because of the increased extracellular fluid and the intravascular infusion. Then a marked weight loss accompanies the diuresis that corresponds with the recovery from shock. Much of the fluid which escaped into the interstitial spaces is reabsorbed into the blood vessels. During this period, the patient is observed for any signs of overhydration. If the intravenous infusion is continued at the previous rate of administration at this time the vascular system may become overloaded, placing an excessive demand on the heart and causing pulmonary oedema. The reabsorption of the tissue fluid can usually be recognized by a marked increase in the urinary output.

After the emergent period the nurse is alert for an elevation of temperature, rapid pulse, leucocytosis and odour and discharge from the burned area which may indicate infection.

The patient's position, especially that of the burned parts of the body, is checked frequently during the day and night for optimum alignment. Flexion contracture may develop very quickly and preclude restoration of function.

Control of pain and discomfort

Unless contraindicated by respiratory impairment or depression, the patient is usually given an analgesic on admission to relieve pain and reduce anxiety, since both contribute to shock. A small dose of morphine, or codeine may be given. The intravenous route is used because the circulatory disturbance, shock and oedema reduce absorption of subcutaneous injections.

An analgesic may be necessary at frequent intervals for 2–3 days to keep the patient reasonably comfortable. Some patients require the administration of the prescribed narcotic only before the burn areas are dressed. Pain assessment and control of the pain experience are on-going from admission through rehabilitation.

Frequent mouth care helps to reduce the discomfort of thirst and dryness, especially in the early stage.

Emotional support

Following a severe burn, the patient and family experience considerable emotional disturbance. As with any severe stress, the reactions and adaptive mechanisms may vary markedly from one person to another, depending mainly on the particular situation and past experiences of each person. Factors which generate fear and anxiety in both the patient and family include the actual threat to life, permanent incapacity and disfigurement, the prolonged period of treatment necessitating dependence as well as separation, and the uncertain future. An understanding of the problems of the patient and family should be appreciated by the nurse in order to convey understanding support and to help the patient work through the loss and develop a more positive outlook. He may have guilt feelings about the accident, especially at first. Withdrawal, depression and resentment are commonly manifested. Long periods of the patient being alone should be avoided; family members and close friends are encouraged to visit regularly. The patient is always referred to by name and health-care personnel should introduce themselves by name. The patient is included in all discussions about his care. Talk to the patient, not about him, while performing long, tedious care procedures or assessing wound healing. Listen to the patient's concerns and provide opportunities for him to express his feelings. Reading material and a radio or television usually help and, as he improves, constructive activities in which he may be interested are gradually introduced by the occupational therapist.

It is important that the patient be given honest, realistic explanations of progress and of the plans for treatment (e.g. skin grafting) and rehabilitation. It is more supportive when the patient and family can relate to one or two key persons in the therapeutic team throughout the entire course of the illness. Constant change of personnel can be very disconcerting and may undermine the patient's confidence.

Wound care

Infection is a serious hazard in severe burns and is the major complication in burned patients. The skin, which is damaged or destroyed, is the normal protective barrier against environmental organisms as well as those commonly found on the skin, in hair follicles and in sweat and sebaceous ducts. Thrombosis and damage of local vessels and stasis of circulation in the burn area create an environment for bacterial growth. At the same time the patient's immune system is depressed.

Various forms of local treatment are used to prevent further wound contamination and tissue destruction, suppress the growth of bacteria in the area, and promote separation of the devitalized tissue and its replacement with skin. Staff members providing direct care wear sterile gowns, caps, mask and gloves. Placement of the patient receives consideration; if there is no special burn care unit the patient is placed in a single room where protective isolation technique can be used to reduce the risk of infection. If there is a burn care ward in the hospital or a regional burn centre, the patient is transferred there from the accident and emergency department.

Initially, the burn is cleansed of dirt, foreign substances and detached epithelium, using gauze and a mild soapy solution, water or normal saline. The temperature of the burn bath solution is kept at 37–38°C (99°F) to approximate body temperature. If a hydrotherapy bath is not available, the cleansing is done on the stretcher or in the patient's bed. The entire burned area is bathed during the admission procedure. Loose, sloughing skin and debris are removed with sterile forceps and the doctor removes the skin from blisters. The cleansing must be *very gentle* to avoid damage of exposed viable tissue and the area is rinsed with generous amounts of water or saline.

Following the cleansing, the patient is placed on a fresh sterile sheet and an estimate is made of the extent and depth of the burns.

Superficial, partial-thickness burns may be left exposed or may receive an application of an ointment. The ointment frequently contains a local anaesthetic for the relief of pain; an example is cinchocaine hydrocloride ointment (Nupercain). Cool moist applications for the first few hours will provide relief of the pain of superficial burns.

In *deep, partial-thickness burns*, opinion differs as to whether blisters are better left intact or should be opened and the overlying devitalized tissue removed. It is suggested that the dead tissue and the fluid encourage the development of infection. There is a consensus, however, that blisters on the palms of the hands, where the skin is thick and not easily ruptured, should be left intact.

The more common, current methods of local treatment of *major* and *full-thickness burns* include open treatment, closed treatment methods and skin grafting.

Open or exposure treatment. In this method of treatment the wound (with or without topical application) is exposed to the air; no dressings are applied. The exposure results in drying and the formation of a protective coagulum of serum. A cradle is used over the patient to support a sterile sheet and blanket to reduce body heat loss. Exposure is the preferred form of treatment for facial, neck, head and perineal burns. If infection develops under the coagulum, it is removed and baths and topical antimicrobials used. This method of treatment is useful when care is necessary for a large number of casualties.

Closed treatment. In the closed method the burned areas may be covered with a topical antimicrobial preparation and gauze. The topical applications commonly used include silver sulphadiazine, mafenide (Sulfamylon), povidone-iodine (Betadine) and gentamicin (Garamycin cream). The cream or ointment is applied in a thin layer, using a sterile gloved hand. Povidone-iodine and antimicrobial ointments are also available in the form of single-thickness gauze, impregnated with the ointment. The dressings are usually changed once daily and the wound cleansed, preferably in a bath. Contraindications to using the hydrotherapeutic bath include a fall below normal of the patient's blood pressure, or a sudden elevation in the blood pressure or pulse, fever of 39.4°C (103°F), electrolyte imbalance, extensive oedema, endotracheal intubation or tracheostomy, other injuries and for 3–5 days following skin grafting or until the graft has taken.

Further destruction of tissues and infection may lead to conversion of partial-thickness wounds to full-thickness wounds and skin loss.

Healing. In a partial-thickness burn, healing (i.e. re-epithelialization) occurs under the coagulum, which gradually separates. When a full-thickness burn is sustained, the non-viable tissue changes in 3–5 days to a hard, tough black layer called the *eschar*. The eschar eventually sloughs off, liquefies and detaches from the viable tissue. There may be considerable drainage before there is complete separation. The wound will not granulate until the eschar has been sloughed off, therefore treatment in wound care is directed towards the promotion of this process. Alternatively, the wound may be debrided surgically. If a patient has a circumferential burn on a limb, close observations are made for signs of interference with the circulation as a result of the constricting effect of the dry, shrinking eschar. In the case of a circumferential eschar of the trunk, the constriction may restrict chest excursion and embarrass respiratory function. If signs of constriction appear, an escharotomy is done immediately under aseptic conditions.

Infection may develop under the eschar as a result of organisms that were present deep in ducts or on adjacent areas which were not destroyed at the time of the burn. As the eschar is removed (by slough or debridement) granulation tissue consisting of fibroblasts and capillaries is gradually formed. If the granulation tissue is allowed to mature to fibrous scar tissue, the natural shortening of the collagenous fibres results in contracture of the area and possible deformity or loss of function, depending upon the location. Some marginal growth of epithelium may take place but, unless the burn is very small, this is usually insignificant.

The usual procedure is to apply split-thickness skin grafts to the area as soon as possible.

The patient's general condition and the size of the burn area determine whether the grafting will require several stages. Priority is given to areas where scarring and contraction produce loss of movement and marked deformity. The grafts may be laid or sutured or stapled, depending on their thickness. They are dressed with a pressure dressing or may be left exposed. If the grafts are around or over a joint surface, a splint or plaster cast may be applied to immobilize the part.

Split-thickness grafts may also be usually applied to deep partial-thickness burns since they produce a much better scar with improved wear and tear tolerance. Further information is offered about skin grafts at the end of this discussion on the care of the burned patient.

Control of infection
If the patient with a deep burn has been immunized within the preceding 5 years for tetanus, a booster dose of toxoid is given. The patient with no tetanus immunization is given a prophylactic dose of human tetanus immunoglobulin. This necessitates questioning the patient or family as to whether he has ever had asthma, eczema or any known drug reaction or allergy.

Infection of the burn area may originate with bacteria that were present in the patient before the burn. Special protective measures are used to minimize the possibility of contamination from outside sources. Protective isolation is used. Strict aseptic technique is observed in providing wound care and changing dressings. Protective clothing and gloves are worn by those participating in direct care. The patient may be moved to a special dressing room or to a small operating room for dressing changes. Obviously, personnel with infection (e.g. cold, sore throat, skin infection) are not allowed to care for the patient. Visitors are restricted in number and are given an explanation of their role in protecting the patient. They are required to wear protective clothing while with him.

When changing the dressing, the inner layers of gauze are removed very gently to prevent tissue bleeding and damage. Moistening of the gauze with a sterile solution or in a bath may be necessary to prevent trauma. The dressing procedure is likely to be painful and anxiety-producing for the patient,

especially in the early stages; an analgesic may be ordered for administration 15–30 minutes before the burn is dressed.

One of the most serious complications in burns is septicaemia; this generally develops during the second or third week, but can develop at any stage until complete skin cover is achieved. It may have a sudden onset, ushered in by rigors and a rapid elevation of temperature, or it may develop gradually over 2–3 days. It is characterized by high fever which may fluctuate, rapid pulse, drowsiness and disorientation. Paralytic ileus is a common concomitant, and petechiae, ecchymoses and oozing from the burn areas frequently appear, since a bleeding tendency develops. Blood cultures are made to identify the organism(s) which have invaded the blood stream. Common offenders are *Staphylococcus aureus*, haemolytic streptococcus and *Pseudomonas aeruginosa*.

Treatment of septicaemia includes massive doses of antibiotics intravenously, promotion of the separation of the eschar to permit drainage, the application of a topical antimicrobial preparation and supportive therapy. Intravenous fluids are given to sustain the patient. Blood transfusions may be given and, if the patient's condition deteriorates, which may be manifested by a subnormal temperature and shock, a corticosteroid preparation such as hydrocortisone may be given intravenously.

Positioning and exercises
The patient is turned every 2–3 hours to prevent respiratory congestion and circulatory stasis. If the back is burned or the involvement is circumferential, care is facilitated if the patient is nursed on an airfluidized support system (Clinitron bed), a Stryker frame or Circolectric bed. Because of the oedema, burned extremities are elevated on pillows or another form of support during the initial phase. Frequent attention is paid to body alignment; flexion contractures, outward rotation of thighs and footdrop must be prevented.

Splints may be applied to limbs if the closed wound care procedure is used. They may be used for immobilization to promote healing and to prevent contracture and deformity. The splint used must be non-supportive to bacterial growth, fit the contour of the part to which it is applied and be secured well enough to provide stability but not cause pressure or interfere with circulation.

Burned parts which involve joints are moved through their range of motion as soon as possible and as indicated by the doctor. Early skin grafting permits the patient to be mobile earlier and prevents contractures. The physiotherapist usually supervises the exercise programme. If the patient is placed in a bath, he is encouraged to exercise while soaking. As healing occurs, the activity programme is progressively increased to preserve normal range of motion and function.

Nutrition

In addition to fluid therapy, nutrition plays an important role in the recovery of the burned patient. In the initial shock period in severe burns the patient is sustained mainly by intravenous fluids. Oral food and fluids are usually restricted for 24–48 hours for patients with severe burns. The initial hypovolaemic shock produces depression of gastric motility. A nasogastric tube is inserted and connected to intermittent suction. The tube is removed in 2–3 days when bowel sounds have returned and a clear fluid diet initiated. Oral intake is carefully monitored in relation to the patient's fluid balance. The intake is progressively increased from fluids, through soft foods, to a full normal diet.

The patient develops a negative nitrogen balance as a result of tissue catabolism which increases susceptibility to infection and debilitation and delays healing. A high-calorie, high-protein (150–200 g per day for an adult) and high-vitamin diet is recommended to provide the essentials for tissue repair and the production of antibodies and blood cells. Vitamin C is essential in the synthesis of corticosteroids and in tissue repair, and the vitamin B complex is needed in the many cellular enzyme systems essential to normal cellular responses.

Ingenuity and resourcefulness are necessary on the part of the nurse to have the patient take the essential food. He should be advised of the important role of nutrients in his diet, and small frequent feedings of high-calorie foods are offered. Supplements of protein concentrates may be added to fluids or given through a fine bore nasogastric tube. Likes and dislikes are determined and respected, and the family is encouraged to bring in favourite foods. Adequate assistance is provided so that taking meals does not require too great an effort. A close check is made of the patient's daily intake, and the weight is also recorded daily.

Rehabilitation

Rehabilitation of the burned patient is fostered throughout the acute stages by conscientious attention to good body alignment, the prevention of infection and contractures, and the maintenance of joint and limb mobility as much as possible. Following recovery from the burn, the patient may require considerable reconstructive surgery and retraining before he can resume independent and self-supportive functioning. Rehabilitation is a lengthy process for many, and they and their families may require social guidance and financial assistance as well as psychological support throughout. Retraining for a different occupation may be necessary. In some instances the patient finds it very difficult to resume social contacts and to take his place in society because of scarring and gross disfigurement.

Expected outcomes

Following rehabilitation, the patient describes or demonstrates:

1 Absence of infection.
2 Intact skin.
3 Range-of-movement exercises and functional movement in involved joints.
4 A plan to continue the prescribed exercise programme.
5 A diet plan to obtain adequate protein, vitamins, minerals and calories.
6 Understanding of prescribed skin care routine.
7 Independence in personal care.
8 Return to social activities.
9 Return to employment or plans for job retraining.
10 Plans for continuing health care.

Grafts

A graft implies the placement of body tissue or other material in an area of the body where it becomes a part of the local structure, substituting for absent or damaged tissue.

Types of grafts

Various terms are used to describe grafts and are defined as follows:

Autograft or autogenous graft. The autograft is obtained from the recipient's own body and may be skin, vein, artery, fascia, tendon or bone, depending on the particular recipient site and correction to be made. No tissue rejection is involved.

Isograft or isologous graft. This is a graft between identical twins. Because of the same germ cell origin, the graft is biologically compatible with the recipient's tissue, and there is no tissue rejection.

Homograft (homologous graft or allograft). The donor and recipient of the graft are of the same species. It may be obtained from a living person or taken from a body shortly after death. Homografts of skin do not survive indefinitely because the tissue is recognized as 'unlike self' and rejected. The rejection phenomenon is an immunological reaction in which the graft is an antigen and antibodies are formed by the host in response to it. The tissue is attacked, and an inflammatory process ensues, ending in a breakdown of the graft. The graft must receive nutrients and oxygen from a blood supply; therefore, donor tissue which does not require a direct blood supply, such as the cornea, withstands rejection. Homografting of skin may be used in extensive burns as a temporary means of providing a covering to protect the patient against massive infection and excessive loss of fluid. In donor selection, the person most closely related to the patient is selected if possible. The survival period for the graft varies, but it is usually 1–3 weeks. By this time, the patient's condition may have improved sufficiently for a series of autogenous grafting to be done.

Heterograft. This implies the transfer of tissue between species and results in rapid rejection. Pig skin may be used to cover granulation tissue or following excision in massive burn injuries for temporary protection.

Synthetic grafts. Artificial skin provides temporary cover over excised areas or to protect granulation tissue or autografts.

Skin grafting

A large proportion of reconstructive surgery and the correction of cutaneous defects involves skin autografts. As indicated in the preceding discussion on the care of the burned patient, skin grafting is necessary following many burns to prevent handicapping and disfiguring contractures.

A skin graft may be classified as a *free graft* when it is completely separated from the donor site and is transferred to another area of the body. If the graft remains attached at one end to the donor site in order to maintain a blood supply, it may be referred to as a *flap*. The detached end is moved to the recipient area and, when sufficient blood vessels form to establish an adequate circulation between the graft and the surrounding tissue, the flap is then separated from the donor area. The thickness of skin grafts varies. The graft may be of *split thickness*, which consists of the epidermis and a portion of the dermis. A *full-thickness* graft includes the epidermis and complete dermis.

Types of free grafts include: the Ollier-Thiersch grafts, which are thin strips or sheets of partial thickness; stamp grafts which are split-thickness skin grafts applied as squares or rectangles; mesh grafting which involves passing a split thickness graft through a mesh dermatoma to produce small slits and cuts in the graft allowing it to be expanded for application over a larger surface area. The donor sites most commonly used for free autografts are the thighs and trunk. The donor site for a flap must be within reach of the recipient site, since one end is attached to each site. When grafts are placed in position, they may be held in place by dressings or may be sutured and left exposed.

Nursing intervention

The donor area is shaved and cleansed. The recipient site may receive frequent moist antiseptic dressings or the application of a topical antimicrobial preparation to render it as free of organisms as possible. If a thick layer of granulation tissue has developed, it may be pared down by the surgeon before the application of a graft.

The patient's blood is typed and cross-matched, and blood is made available for transfusion. Debridement (the removal of dead tissue, together with copious bleeding from the donor site) may result in a considerable loss of blood.

Following the operation, unless the graft is sutured, the area is covered with fine mesh, petroleum jelly gauze, dressing pads and elastic or crêpe bandages. Mesh grafts are usually covered with a biological dressing (frozen allograft or pigskin). If the recipient site involves or is adjacent to a joint, a splint or plaster cast is applied to immobilize the part. The dressing remains undisturbed for 4–6 days unless infection is suspected because of fever, leucocytosis, or there is an offensive odour and discharge from the area. Elastic support is worn over the area as soon as a pressure garment can be fitted. Pressure garments are usually worn for 12–18 months following grafting.

The donor site may be covered with petroleum jelly gauze or polyurethane film and left intact for 10 days. This area may be painful and is usually a greater source of discomfort than the recipient area.

References and Further Reading

BOOKS

Artz CT, Moncrief JA & Pruitt BA (1979) *Burns: A Team Approach*. Philadelphia: WB Saunders.

Bates B (1983) *A Guide to Physical Examination*, 3rd ed. Philadelphia: JB Lippincott.

Browne B & Robertson A (1985) *Skin Care Guidelines*. Dundas, Ontario: Anderson Inc.

Calnan JS (ed) (1976) *Recent Advances in Plastic Surgery*, Vol. 1. Edinburgh: Churchill Livingstone.

Cason JS (1981) *Treatment of Burns*. London: Chapman & Hall.

Epstein E (1983) *Common Skin Disorders*, 2nd ed. Oradell, NJ: Medical Economic Books.

Feller I, Archambeault-Jones C & Richards KE (1977) *Emergency Care of the Burn Victim*. Ann Arbor, MI: The National Institute for Burn Medicine.

Feller I & Grabb WC (1979) *Reconstruction and Rehabilitation of the Burned Patient*. Ann Arbor, MI: The National Institute for Burn Medicine.

Harvey KJV & Lamb BE (1984) *Plastic Surgical and Burns Nursing*. London: Baillière Tindall.

Horsley J, Crane J, Haller KB & Bingle JD (1981) *Preventing Decubitus Ulcers: CURN Project*. New York: Grune & Stratton.

Hummel RP (ed) (1982) *Clinical Burn Therapy*. Bristol: John Wright.

Kin MJ, McFarland GK & McLane AM (eds) (1984) *Pocket Guide to Nursing Diagnoses*. St Louis: CV Mosby.

Kinney MR, Dear CB, Donna R, Voorman DM & Nagelhout (Eds) (1981) *AACN's Clinical Reference for Critical Care Nursing*. New York: McGraw-Hill. Chapter 30.

Krupp MA & Chatton MJ (1983) *Current Medical Diagnosis and Treatment*. Los Altos, CA: Lange. Chapter 3.

Muir IKF & Barclay TL (1974) *Burns and Their Treatment*, 2nd ed. London: Lloyd-Luke.

Norton D, McLaren R & Exton-Smith AN (1975) *An Investigation of Geriatric Nursing Problems in Hospital*. Edinburgh: Churchill Livingstone.

Vasarinish P (1982) *Clinical Dermatology*. Boston: Butterworths.

Wagner MW (ed) (1981) *Care of the Burn-Injured Patient*. London: Croom-Helm.

Willatts SM (1982) *Lecture Notes on Fluid and Electrolyte Balance*. Oxford: Blackwell Scientific.

PERIODICALS

Ahmed MC (1980) Choosing the best method to manage pressure ulcers. *Nurs. Drug Alert* (Special Report), Vol. 4 No. 15, pp. 113–120.

Ahmed MC (1982) Op-Site for decubitus care. *Am. J. Nurs.*, Vol. 82 No. 1, pp. 61–64.

Andberg MM, Rudolph A & Anderson TB (1983) Improving skin care through patient and family teaching. *Top. Clin. Nurs.*, Vol. 5 No. 2, pp. 45–54.

Anderson TF (1982) Psoriasis. *Med. Clin. N. Am.*, Vol. 66 No. 4, pp. 769–794.

Berecek KH (1975a) Etiology of decubitus ulcers. *Nurs. Clin. N. Am.*, Vol. 10 No. 1, pp. 157–170.

Berecek KH (1975b) Treatment of decubitus ulcers *Nurs. Clin. N. Am.*, Vol. 10 No. 1, pp. 171–210.

Christopher KL (1980) The use of a model for hemodynamic balance to describe burn shock. *Nurs. Clin. N. Am.*, Vol. 15 No. 3, pp. 617–627.

David JA (1982) Pressure sore treatment: a literature review. *Int. J. Nurs. Stud.*, Vol. 19 No. 4, pp. 183–191.

Delaney VL & North C (1983) Skin assessment. *Top. Clin. Nurs.*, Vol. 5 No. 2, pp. 5–10.

Demling RH (1982) Burn edema. Part 1: pathogenesis. *J. Burn Care Rehab.*, Vol. 3 No. 3, pp. 138–148.

Demling RH, Gunther RA, Harms B & Kramer G (1982) Burn edema. Part II: complications, prevention and treatment. *J. Burn Care Rehab.*, Vol. 3 No. 4, pp. 199–206.

Edlich RF, Rodeheaver GT, Carucci D, Olsen TL, Sando WC, Apesos J & Kenny JG (1982) Technical considerations in mesh grafting. *J. Burn Care Rehab.*, Vol. 3 No. 1, pp. 6–16.

Feller I, James MH & Jones CA (1982) Burn epidemiology: focus on youngsters and the aged. *J. Burn Care Rehab.*, Vol. 3 No. 3, pp. 285–288.

Feustel DE (1982) Pressure sore prevention: 'aye, there's the rub.' *Nurs. '82*, Vol. 12 No. 4, pp. 78–83.

Flynn ME (1982) Influencing repair and recovery. *Am. J. Nurs.*, Vol. 82 No. 10, pp. 1550–1558.

Flynn ME & Rovee DT (1982) Promoting wound healing. *Am. J. Nurs.*, Vol. 82 No. 10, pp. 1544–1550.

Fowler E (1980) Education and pressure sores. *J. Enterost. Ther.*, Vol. 7 No. 6, pp. 18, 19 & 24.

Heckel P (1981) Teaching patients to cope with psoriasis:

the unshared disease. *Nurs. '81*, Vol. 11 No. 6, pp. 49–51.

Helm PA, Kevorkian G, Lushbough M, Pullium G, Head MD & Cromes F (1983) Burn injury: rehabilitation management in 1982. *J. Burn Care Rehab.*, Vol. 4 No. 6, pp. 411–422.

Judd CO (1981) Selected topical agents used in the treatment of pressure sores. *Can. Nurs.*, Vol. 77 No. 7, pp. 32–33.

Kerr JC, Stinson SM & Shannon ML (1981) Pressure sores: distinguishing fact from fiction. *Can. Nurse*, Vol. 77 No. 7, pp. 23–27.

Kolman PBR (1983) The incidence of psychopathology in burned adult patients: a critical review. *J. Burn Care Rehab.*, Vol. 4 No. 6, pp. 430–436.

Lawlis GF & Achterberg J (1983) Acne: the disease and stress. *Top. Clin. Nurs.*, Vol. 5 No. 2, pp. 23–31.

Lutherman A, Kraft E & Bookless S (1980) Biologic dressings: an appraisal of current practices. *J. Burn Care Rehab.*, Vol. 1 No. 1, pp. 18–22.

Marks R (1981) Psoriasis—its diagnosis and treatment. *Geriat. Med.*, Vol. 11 No. 5, pp. 90–94.

Marvin JA & Einfeldt LE (1980) Infection control for the burn patient. *Nurs. Clin. N. Am.*, Vol. 15 No. 4, pp. 833–842.

McNairn N (1979) Cutaneous ulcers: treatment protocols in the home. *Can. Family Phys.*, Vol. 25, pp. 952–957.

Meissner JE (1980) Which patient on your unit might get a pressure sore? *Nurs. '80*, Vol. 10 No. 6, pp. 64–65.

Montgomery BA (1981) Techniques for use of a new dressing: a moisture vapor permeable film. *J. Enterostom. Ther.*, Vol. 8 No. 6, pp. 26–29.

Morley M (1981) 16 Steps to better decubitus ulcer care. *Can. Nurse*, Vol. 77 No. 7, pp. 29–31.

Natow AB (1983) Nutrition in prevention and treatment of decubitus ulcers. *Top. Clin. Nurs.*, Vol. 5 No. 2, pp. 39–44.

North C & Weinstein GD (1976) Treatment of psoriasis. *Am. J. Nurs.*, Vol. 76 No. 3, pp. 410–412.

Olsten TG (1982) Therapy of acne. *Med. Clin. N. Am.*, Vol. 66 No. 4, pp. 851–871.

Perry S, Heidrich G & Ramos E (1981) Assessment of pain by burn patients. *J. Burn Care Rehab.*, Vol. 2 No. 6, pp. 322–326.

Reuler JB & Cooney T (1981) The pressure sore: pathophysiology and principles of management. *Ann. Int. Med.*, Vol. 94 No. 5, pp. 661–665.

Schulmeister L (1981) Screening for skin cancer. *Nurs. '81*, Vol. 10 No. 11, pp. 42–45.

Tobiasen J, Hiebert JM & Edlich RF (1982) A practical burn severity index. *J. Burn Care Rehab.*, Vol. 3 No. 4, pp. 229–232.

Tudhope M (1984) Management of pressure ulcers with a hydrocolloid occlusive dressing: results in 23 patients. *J. Enterostom. Ther.*, Vol. 11 No. 3, pp. 102–105.

Welch LB (1983) Relatively painless wound debridement. *RN*, Vol. 46 No. 10, pp. 39–41.

28

Nursing in Disorders of the Eye

Structure and Function of the Eyes

Vision, like all other sensory mechanisms, requires receptors, an afferent pathway to carry the impulses into the central nervous system and an interpretive centre. The eyes serve as receptors which are sensitive to light rays, the pathway is formed by the optic nerves and tracts within the brain, and the interpretive centres are composed of groups of neurons localized in the cortex of the cerebral occipital lobes (visual centres). In addition, the visual apparatus includes intrinsic and extrinsic muscles which play an important role in vision. There are also several accessory structures which function to protect the eyes.

LOCATION OF THE EYE

Each eyeball rests in a cone-shaped cavity (the orbit) in the skull. The orbit is covered posteriorly by a fibrous sac lined with a smooth moist membrane which promotes smooth movement of the eye in its socket. The space between the intra-orbital structures contains fatty tissue which serves as a cushion for the eyeball.

The accessory structures include the eyelids, lacrimal system and extrinsic ocular muscles.

Eyelids (palpebrae)

The upper and lower eyelids are curtain-like structures lying in front of the eyeball. They serve as protective coverings by shutting out intense light, dust and foreign bodies. The space between them is referred to as the palpebral fissure; the angles or corners where the lids meet are known as the inner (medial) and outer (lateral) canthi. Each eyelid has an outer layer of skin, a layer of firm fibrous tissue (tarsal plate), sebaceous-like glands (meibomian glands) which secrete an oily substance onto the free margins of the lids, and a mucous membrane lining called the conjunctiva. The conjunctiva is reflected over the anterior portion of the eyeball forming the bulbar conjunctiva, and is continuous with the corneal epithelium. The secretion of the meibomian glands prevents adherence of the lids when the eyes are closed and also prevents the overflow of normal amounts of lacrimal secretion. The eyelashes emerge from the free borders of the eyelids to protect the eye from dust and perspiration.

Lacrimal system

The lacrimal apparatus protects the eye by continuously secreting a fluid that 'washes' over the anterior surface of the eyeball, keeping it moistened and cleansed. The system of each eye consists of a gland, ducts and a drainage system (Fig. 28.1).

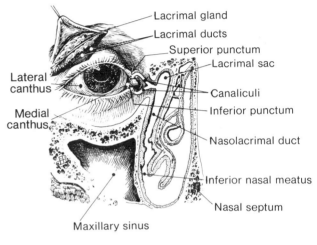

Fig. 28.1 The lacrimal system.

The lacrimal gland lies in a slight depression in the outer superior portion of the orbit. Several ducts carry the secretion of the gland onto the inner surface of the upper eyelid. The secreted fluid is distributed over the anterior surface of the eye and then drains through two small openings (puncta) in the medial canthus into two short canals (lacrimal canaliculi). The canals drain into a small sacular structure, the lacrimal sac, which narrows to form the nasolacrimal duct. The latter carries the secretion into the nasal cavity.

A volume of lacrimal secretion in excess of what the drainage system can handle results in fluid overflowing the eyelids and forming tears. Increased lacrimal secretion (lacrimation) occurs in response to irritation of the conjunctiva or to certain emotions. If there is excessive tear flow due to the blockage of the canaliculi or nasolacrimal duct, it may be referred to as *epiphora*.

Extrinsic ocular muscles

Several external muscles have their origin in orbital structures and insert on the eyeball to provide movement of the eye within its socket. There are four straight muscles (*recti muscles*); each is named for the direction in which it moves the eye. The superior rectus turns the eye up, the inferior rectus turns it downward, the medial rectus turns it in, and the lateral moves it in the reverse direction. In addition to the recti muscles, two *oblique muscles* (a superior and an inferior) provide rotation and modification of straight movements. For most movements, more than one external ocular muscle generally operates; various combinations of recti and oblique muscle action are necessary (Fig. 28.2).

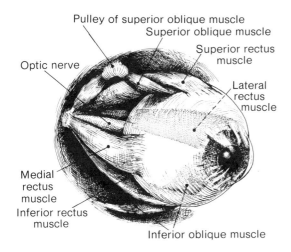

Fig. 28.2 Extraocular muscles of the eye.

The external ocular muscles include the levator palpebrae superioris muscle which inserts in the upper eyelid. It is responsible for raising the upper eyelid (opening the eye). The muscle responsible for closing the eye is the *orbicularis oculi*. This is a circular muscle situated in the eyelids.

EYEBALL

The eyeball is spherical with a slight anterior bulge. It is composed of three layers of tissue which enclose the iris and special transparent, refracting structures (Fig. 28.3). The tough, outer coat forms the sclera and cornea. The *sclera*, which covers the posterior five-sixths of the eyeball, is white, opaque fibrous tissue. The *cornea* is a continuation of the sclera over the anterior portion of the eye. It consists of transparent, special connective tissue that is devoid of blood vessels. The corneoscleral junction is referred to as the *limbus*.

Underlying and attached to the sclera is a thin, heavily pigmented, vascular coat, the *choroid*, which extends forward to what is referred to as the ciliary body. The pigmentation prevents the reflection of the light rays.

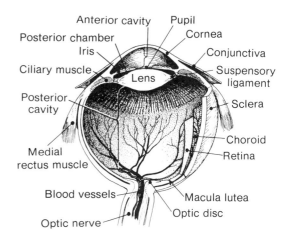

Fig. 28.3 Parts of the eyeball.

The *ciliary body* consists mainly of muscle tissue which takes its origin at the corneoscleral junction and inserts in the suspensory ligaments that are attached to the lens, holding it suspended in position. The action of the ciliary muscle influences the curvature, and thus the refractive power, of the lens.

The second layer of the eyeball continues forward and inward beyond the ciliary muscle to form the iris. The *iris* is composed of circular and radial muscles and pigmented cells and is perforated centrally, creating the opening referred to as the *pupil*. Contraction of the circular muscle fibres (sphincter pupillae) constricts the pupil; dilation is controlled by the radial fibres. The iris, ciliary body and choroid are known as the uvea or uveal tract.

The *retina* is the innermost and neural coat of the posterior two-thirds of the eyeball. It consists of several strata of cells through which light rays pass before reaching the outer layer of cells, which are light-sensitive receptors that convert luminous energy into nerve impulses. There are two types of receptor cells—the rods and cones. The rods have a lower response threshold, making them more sensitive to lower levels of illumination. The cones have a higher response threshold and, as a result, function in bright light and provide colour and detailed vision.

In the centre of the retina, a small area occurs in which the inner layers of cells are absent and only cones are concentrated. Light rays falling on this site strike the cones directly and produce the greatest visual acuity. This area is referred to as the *fovea centralis* and occurs as a slight depression in a small, elevated, yellowish area called the macula lutea, or yellow spot. Slightly medial to the macula there is a pale papillary area called the *optic disc*, or *fundus oculi*. It is at this point that the optic nerve and the central retinal vein and artery leave and enter the eyeball. The disc is a blind spot, since the area is devoid of rods and cones.

The eyeball is 'filled out' by contents composed of fluids (aqueous humour), a biconvex disc (lens) and a jelly-like mass (vitreous humour).

The *lens* is elastic and crystal-clear and is suspended just behind the iris by ligaments (suspensory ligaments or zonules) which attach to the ciliary body. Its shape varies with age; it is spherical in infancy, gradually flattening to a disc shape with age. In the elderly, the lens tends to flatten and become less elastic.

Divisions of the interior of the eyeball

The interior of the eyeball is divided into the anterior and posterior cavities. The *anterior cavity* is the space between the cornea and lens and is subdivided into the *anterior and posterior chambers*, which are areas frequently referred to in clinical work. The anterior chamber lies posterior to the cornea and in front of the iris. The posterior chamber is situated posterior to the iris and anterior to the lens. The content of the two chambers is *aqueous humour*.

The posterior cavity lies posterior to the lens and is the remainder of the interior of the eyeball. It is filled with the *vitreous humour*, or *vitreous body*.

Fluid system of the eye and intraocular pressure

The interior of the eyeball is filled by the aqueous and vitreous humours and the crystalline lens. The vitreous humour is a clear, jelly-like mass enclosed in a hyaloid membrane. The vitreous humour fills out the larger and posterior portion of the eyeball that lies behind the lens.

The anterior and posterior chambers are filled with a clear fluid, the aqueous humour. There is a continuous flow into and out of the eye. The fluid originates from capillaries contained in processes of the ciliary body. After circulating around the posterior chamber, it flows through the pupil into the anterior chamber. From here, a small amount of the aqueous humour continuously drains into the canal of Schlemm, from which it is carried into the venous circulation. The canal of Schlemm is a channel that circles the eye in the region of the corneoscleral junction. Small spaces (spaces of Fontana) in the trabecular mesh at the angle formed by the junction of the cornea with the anterior surface of the iris allow the fluid to pass into the canal of Schlemm. This area may be referred to as the filtration angle. The aqueous humour carries nutrients to the lens and cornea and removes waste products. This is necessary because both structures are avascular; the presence of blood vessels would alter their transparent nature. The production of aqueous humour and its drainage are constant in order to maintain a normal intraocular pressure, which is 16–21 mmHg. Any interference with normal drainage of the fluid from the anterior chamber raises the pressure, leading to decreased blood supply, pain and impaired vision.

VISUAL IMPULSE PATHWAY

Impulses generated by the rods and cones synapse through several neurons to ganglionic cells whose axons course toward the site of the optic disc where they unite to form the optic nerve. This nerve differs from most nerves in that it has no neurilemma; thus, it is even less capable of regeneration if damaged or destroyed. At the base of the brain, the nerve fibres from the medial half of the retina of each eye cross, going to the opposite sides of the brain. The fibres from the lateral halves of the retinae do not cross but continue on to the corresponding side of the brain. This arrangement forms the optic chiasma (see Fig. 28.4). Within the brain, the fibres from the lateral half of the right eye and those from the medial half of the left eye continue on as the right optic tract. The fibres of each tract synapse with the lateral geniculate in the thalamus on the corresponding side. From there, the impulses are transmitted along the postsynaptic fibres (optic radiations) to the visual centre in the occipital cerebral cortex of the same side, where they are interpreted as sensations of light, colour and form. Other cerebral areas are necessary for normal vision; correlation with information stored as memory in association areas has to occur in order to give meaning to what is seen. For example, a written word or an object may be seen but, unless the person has heard or experienced its meaning, he is unable to interpret it.

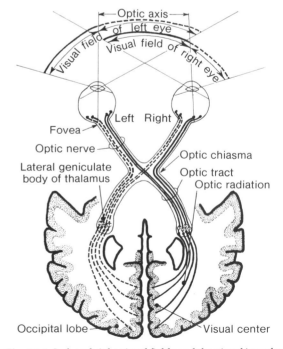

Fig. 28.4 Left and right visual fields and the visual impulse pathway.

VISUAL FIELDS

The retinae of both eyes receive light rays at the same time from an object within the field of vision (binocular vision). Light rays from an object in the left outer visual field are received on the medial, or nasal, side of the left retina and on the lateral, or temporal, side of the right retina. The ensuing impulses are carried over fibres of the left and right optic nerves but, with the crossing of fibres in the chiasma, the impulses will travel along the right optic tract to the visual centre in the right occipital lobe for interpretation. Conversely, rays from objects in the outer right visual field will fall on the lateral area of the left retina and nasal area of the right retina, with the resulting impulses ending up in the visual centre of the left occipital lobe. There is some overlapping between the two halves of each retina and, as a result, the central half of each is represented in each hemisphere.

If the optic nerve of one eye is destroyed, blindness occurs in that eye, but destruction of fibres of the optic tract (i.e. beyond the optic chiasma) causes blindness to occur in half of each retina, limiting the field of vision. The term for this blindness is *hemianopia*.

EYE REFLEXES

The eye reflexes are used frequently in assessing the patient's condition. Some fibres of each optic tract terminate in a group of neurons referred to as the superior colliculus (superior colliculus quadrigeminae) in the midbrain. From here, efferent impulses originate, resulting in blinking of the eyelids, movement of the head, or dilation or constriction of the pupil.

The conjunctival and corneal reflex of blinking is a protective response elicited by touching the conjunctival surface.

The pupils are normally round and of equal size. They adjust to light by constricting, and to darkness or dim light by dilating. A second reflex that may be noted is the accommodation reflex. The pupils are observed while the person shifts his gaze from a distant to a near object. The normal response is constriction of the pupils. In some pathological conditions (e.g. syphilis), the response of the pupil to light may be absent while the accommodation reflex is present. This type of response is referred to as an Argyll Robertson pupil.

REFRACTION, ACCOMMODATION, PUPILLARY MODIFICATION AND CONVERGENCE

Several processes may be necessary to focus the light rays on the retina in order to form a clear image.

Refraction

When light rays pass obliquely from one medium to another of a different density their velocity is altered, and they are bent or deflected. The process is referred to as refraction (Fig. 28.5). If the rays pass into a medium of greater density, they are deflected toward the perpendicular; conversely, in a medium of lesser density the rays are bent away from the per-

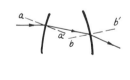

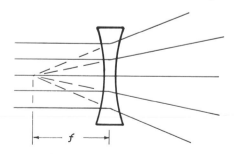

a. A double convex lens focuses light.

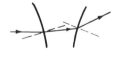

b. A double concave lens causes light to diverge.

Fig. 28.5 Diagram showing refraction. *a*, Refraction of light rays by a double convex lens (convergence). *b*, Refraction of light rays by a double concave lens.

pendicular. Parallel rays striking a surface at right angles are not refracted. Parallel light rays striking the centre of the cornea and lens pass through unrefracted. At either side of the centre of the convex surfaces of the cornea and lens, light rays enter at an angle to the surface and are refracted toward the perpendicular. The greater the curvature or convexity of the surface, the greater is the degree of refraction.

The cornea and lens are the principal refractive media in the eye; the lens is particularly significant in that its curvature and degree of refraction can be varied by the ciliary body, according to the amount required to focus the light rays on the retina. The aqueous and vitreous humours also contribute to refraction but the degree, as with the cornea, remains the same. Without strain or modification, the normal eye will refract light rays from an object 6 or more metres away sufficiently to focus them on the retina. For objects that are near, refraction must be increased, and for distant objects, the eye must decrease its refraction. When greater refraction is necessary, the ciliary muscles contract and the suspensory ligaments, which are attached to the lens and the ciliary body, move forward, reducing their pull on the lens. As a result, the lens increases its convexity and thickness and, thus, its refractive power. When light rays reflected by distant objects enter the eye, the ciliary muscles relax, and the suspensory ligaments exert greater tension on the lens. This reduces convexity, thickness and refractive power of the lens, and focus of the light rays on the retina is achieved.

Various errors of refraction occur which interfere with the ability of the eye to focus light rays on the retina, resulting in impaired vision.

Emmetropia implies normal refraction.

Shortsightedness, called *myopia*, is the result of light rays from an object at 6 metres or more being focused at a point in front of the retina. Close objects can be seen, but distant objects are blurred. Correction may be made by use of a concave lens, since a concave lens produces divergence of light rays (see Fig. 28.6A).

Long-sightedness (*hypermetropia*) is due to insufficient refraction and, as a result, light rays from an object at 6 metres or less are focused at a point behind the retina. The person sees distant objects more clearly than close ones. Correction may be made by use of a convex lens, since a convex lens focuses light rays by convergence (see Fig. 28.6B). In the later years of life, as part of the ageing process, the lens loses its elasticity and becomes thinner and flatter. This lessens the normal degree of refraction and the person becomes farsighted, a refractive error referred to as *presbyopia*.

In some persons, the horizontal and vertical curvatures of the cornea are uneven, producing differences in the degree of refraction. This results in different focal points; some light rays may be focused on the retina, but others may fall short or be carried to a point beyond the retina. This type of refractive error is known as *astigmatism*.

Accommodation
This is the process by which the degree of refraction by the lens is changed in order to focus rays from objects at various distances. This is made possible by the elastic nature of the lens and the action of the ciliary muscles on the suspensory ligaments, as explained under refraction (Fig. 28.7).

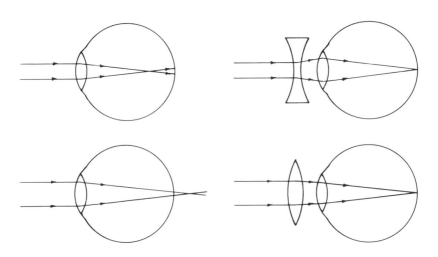

The use of lenses to correct common eye defects.

Fig. 28.6 Diagram showing: (top) myopia and correction by concave lens; (bottom) hypermetropia and correction by convex lens.

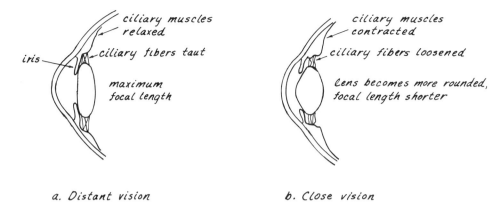

a. Distant vision   b. Close vision

Fig. 28.7 Diagram showing the ciliary body, suspensory ligaments and lens and the changes in accommodation.

Pupillary modification
The pupillary aperture is varied to control the amount of light entering the eye. For clear vision of near objects, the iris constricts the pupil of each eye to prevent divergent rays from entering. The opening is also reduced to restrict the entrance of excessively bright light, which may harm the retina. The iris constricts the pupil through parasympathetic innervation; sympathetic nervous stimulation produces dilation of the pupil. In dim light and when focusing on a distant, wider visual field, the iris dilates the pupil to admit more light rays.

Convergence
Although light rays from the same object(s) fall on both retinae, only single vision is experienced. This is due to light rays from the object falling on corresponding points of the two retinae. This is brought about by convergence, which involves the extrinsic muscles (recti and oblique). The movements of the two eyes must be coordinated accurately. As an object is brought closer to the eyes, convergence of their axes occurs as they turn inward. For distant objects convergence is not necessary; the eyes remain parallel. *Strabismus* (squint) is a defect which interferes with coordination of the eye movements, and the light rays do not fall on corresponding points of the two retinae. It is usually due to an abnormal extrinsic muscle, or to an undiagnosed refractive error. Two images result and the person 'sees double'; this is termed *diplopia*.

LIGHT AND DARK ADAPTATION

Light adaptation. When exposed to intense light, adaptation takes place by constriction of the pupils and lowering the eyebrows, eyelids and head; the visual purple (rhodopsin) within the rods is bleached which reduces their sensitivity and responses.

Dark adaptation
When a person goes from a light to a dark area, he cannot see immediately; then gradually he sees outlines of objects. This vision in dim light is due to an increased sensitivity of the rods as they produce a chemical pigment, visual purple or rhodopsin. Vitamin A is essential for the formation of the chemical; if it is deficient, the person experiences night blindness. At the same time that the rods increase their sensitivity, the pupils dilate to admit more light.

Nursing Patients with Eye Disorders

Assessment

It is necessary, in most instances,[1] that a thorough assessment is carried out before a diagnosis is made and, if appropriate, treatment prescribed. This includes a history of the patient's ocular disorder, general health, life-style, and an examination of the eyes. The latter involves inspection, palpation and the use of special equipment. The eye examination may require complex electrophysiological studies which are done by specialists in the field of ophthalmology.

HEALTH HISTORY

1 *Age.* The age of the person in relation to developmental changes and effects of ageing on the eyes is important.

---

[1] *Immediate* action would be required if the patient's eye is damaged by accidental instillation of chemicals.

2 Occupation and life-style. Information is obtained as to the demands for visual acuity, potential for eye injury and the use of protective devices. What are the patient's recreational activities; does he participate in sports that have a potential for head or eye injury or exposure to bright sunlight? Are sunglasses worn?

3 *Family history.* Since many eye disorders are inherited, it is significant to learn of any family history of eye disorders, diabetes mellitus, cardiovascular disease and thyroid disease.

4 *Past health.* Any childhood and adult illnesses, injuries and previous eye problems should be noted and the treatment and responses elicited. Ocular changes may be secondary to a disorder such as hypertension, diabetes mellitus, renal disease, hyperthyroidism and brain injury or tumour. Degenerative disease in the elderly is frequently the cause of their loss of vision.

It is determined whether corrective lenses are used, in what form and when the last eye examination was carried out.

CURRENT SYMPTOMS

What prompted the patient to seek health care? Has he experienced:
- Changes in visual acuity
- Blurring of vision
- Halos
- Flashes of light
- Spots before the eyes (floaters)
- Excessive lacrimation or epiphora
- Double vision (diplopia)
- Light sensitivity (photophobia)
- Night blindness
- Recurring headache
- Discomfort, burning sensation or itching of the eyes?

What events led to or just preceded the symptom(s)? When did the symptoms begin and are there measures that provide relief?

EXAMINATION OF THE EYES

Inspection and palpation, tests for ocular motility and measurement of visual acuity are usually performed before the examination of internal structures of the eye or tests which involve the touching of normally sensitive eye structures.

Assessment by inspection and palpation
Initial observations of the eyes include noting: general appearance; symmetry of visual axes and physical features; any discharge and its characteristics; excessive or deficient lacrimal secretion; swelling or discoloration of extraocular structures or surrounding tissues; and the presence of a foreign body. The size and equality of the pupils are recorded. The

medial canthi are examined for swelling and redness and *gently* palpated for tenderness.

The eyelids, lashes and brows are inspected for: redness or any discoloration; crusting; eversion or inversion of the lids; complete and equal opening and closing of the lids; swollen areas or oedema. The areas are very gently palpated for tender areas and nodules. The inner surface of the lower eyelid is examined by placing the index finger on the cheek and gently pulling down. The interior surface of the upper eyelid is examined by everting the lid over a cotton-tipped applicator; the lid is pulled gently downward by the eyelashes and then flipped upward over the applicator which is held against the outer surface of the lid. The colour of the conjunctiva of the lids is noted as are any swollen or raised areas.

Assessment of extrocular muscle function
The patient sits facing the examiner, holding his head in a fixed position. The neuromuscular balance or straightness of the eyes is assessed by shining a light directly on the patient's eyes. The patient is asked to focus on the light which should be reflected in corresponding positions in the pupillary corneas. If there is deviation of one eye, asymmetrical reflection occurs.

Movements of the eyes by the extrocular muscles are examined by having the patient in the position cited above; the examiner moves a light through several different positions while observing the eye movements. The patient is asked to fix his vision on the light and the movements of both eyes should be coordinated and symmetrical. Abnormal response may indicate paralysis of one or more extraocular muscles, muscular imbalance or injury.

Assessment of eye reflexes
Pupillary reflexes are observed in a dimly lit room by shining a light from the side on to the pupil of one eye at a time. Both pupils are observed; the normal response is constriction of both pupils when the light is shone in one. This is referred to as consensual pupil reaction.

The accommodation reflex is elicited by having the patient focus on a light held about 150 cm (20 in) from his nose. As the light is moved toward the patient, the eyes normally converge and the pupils constrict.

Measurement of visual acuity
Visual acuity implies the ability to distinguish details of objects and is measured as a means of evaluating ocular function. Each eye is tested separately; the eye not being examined is completely covered, but without any pressure being applied directly to the eye. A standard wall chart (Snellen chart) with rows of letters of gradually decreasing size is used and placed 6 metres from the patient and is well lit. The person is required to read the chart through to the line of smallest letters that he can see. The distance from which the normal eye can read each line is

known. The top line of the Snellen chart is perceived by the normal eye at 60 metres, the second line at 36 metres, the third at 24 metres, the fourth at 18 metres, the fifth at 12 metres, the sixth at 9 metres, the seventh at 6 metres, and the eighth line at 4 metres. Visual acuity is expressed as a fraction; the numerator represents the distance between the chart and the patient, and the denominator is the distance from which a person with normal vision could read the same line. Visual acuity recorded as 6/6 means normal vision. If the patient 6 metres from the chart can only read the line that the normal eye could read at 12 metres, the visual acuity is expressed as 6/12. The larger the denominator recorded, the poorer is the vision. In a person with severe impairment who can only see a hand moving in front of his face, the visual acuity may be recorded as HM (hand movements). If the person can only distinguish between light and dark, the recording is PL (perception of light) and if there is no light perception it is expressed as NPL (no perception of light). A recording of 3/60 or less in the better eye when wearing glasses or contact lenses indicates that the person is legally blind.

Near vision is assessed by also having the individual hold a card about 32 cm (13 in) from the eyes. The print on the card is sized proportionately to the 6 metres.

Refraction

The testing of the eyes' ability to focus the light rays on the retina is done by using a series of trial lenses as well as by assessing the person's visual acuity. In doing a refraction test in young children the doctor may require the instillation of a cycloplegic drug, such as atropine 0.5–2.0% which temporarily inhibits ciliary muscle action and dilates the pupil.

Visual field measurement (perimetry)

A special semicircular instrument, called a perimeter, which is marked in degrees, is used to determine if the patient's visual fields are normal or restricted. Defects in the visual fields are frequently associated with intracranial lesions or damage to an optic nerve.

Each eye is tested singly. Normal figures for perimetry evaluation are:

Lateral or temporal vision—90°
Looking up—50°
Looking down—70°
Medial—60°

Estimation of the visual fields may also be made by the confrontation test. The patient faces the examiner (approximately 60–90 cm away) and has one eye covered. The examiner covers his opposite eye and holds an object which is moved slowly from beyond the patient's peripheral vision towards the central line of vision. The patient is asked to indicate when the object first comes into view and this is compared with when it was first seen by the examiner. The difference is recorded, taking for granted the examiner's vision is normal. The test is made using lateral, upper and lower fields.

Ophthalmoscopic examination

With an ophthalmoscope, the posterior, internal surface (fundus) of each eye is magnified and observed. The lens, vitreous body, blood vessels, retina, optic nerve and disc are viewed. In order to get a wider view, the pupil is dilated by the instillation of a mydriatic such as cyclopentolate hydrochloride (Mydrilate) 0.5–1% or tropicamide 0.5–1%. Ophthalmoscopy is valuable in the recognition of some systemic disorders, as well as in the assessment of ocular function. The optic blood vessels and disc may reflect a disorder such as hypertension, renal disease and increased intracranial pressure.

Measurement of intraocular pressure

The detection of increased intraocular pressure is important; an excessive pressure may be very painful and progressively causes permanent damage within the eye, leading to loss of vision. The pressure is measured by an instrument called a tonometer. A few drops of a local anaesthetic (e.g. amethocaine 0.5–1%; oxybuprocaine 0.3%) are instilled in each eye. The tonometer is then placed on the corneal surface, causing indentation; the extent of the indentation reflects the intraocular pressure. If the pressure is high, the cornea resists indentation. The calibrated scale of the tonometer records the pressure in millimetres of mercury (mmHg). The normal intraocular pressure is approximately 16–21 mmHg.

A second instrument that is now generally employed to measure the ocular tension is the applanometer. This is an electronic device which is considered to provide a more accurate measurement of the intraocular pressure.

The patient with elevated intraocular pressure is at risk of serious impairment of vision due to ischaemic neuropathy.

Slit-lamp microscopy (biomicroscopy)

A more detailed examination of the internal structures of the eye can be made by the use of a slit-lamp microscope. This instrument provides much clearer viewing and magnification of the tissues within the eye than obtained with the ophthalmoscope because of its intense light along with the increased magnification. It is helpful in locating foreign bodies in the eye and identifying ulcer erosion as well as degenerative and inflammatory conditions.

Fluorescein staining

A fluorescein strip, which is a sterile strip of paper that has been impregnated with a solution of sodium flurorescein, is moistened at one end and lightly applied to the lower conjunctival sac. The dye flows over the eye and abrasions and corneal ulcers readily stain a yellowish-green.

Following the examination, the eye is irrigated with a sterile saline solution to remove the dye.

Fluorescein angiography
This test is done to assess vascular structures and blood circulation within the eye and the condition of the retina. Photographs are taken of the intraocular area and then a small dose (5 ml) of sodium fluorescein 10% is given intravenously and a series of photographs are taken at timed intervals.

The patient may experience a brief period of nausea and should be advised that the sclerae and possibly facial tissues will likely be a yellowish-green colour for a few hours as a result of the injection of the dye. The dye is eliminated in the urine which will be deeply coloured for approximately 24 hours.

Ultrasonography (echo-ophthalmography)
Ultrasound waves of very high frequency are directed into the eye and the echoes vary with the density of the tissues from which the sound waves are reflected. This test may be used to examine the fundus when the medium which transmit light rays becomes opaque (as in cataract), to detect retinal detachment or a tumour or to locate a foreign body.

Assessment of the retina
An electroretinogram may be done to record the extent of the electrical response made by the retina to light stimulation.

Gonioscopy
This involves the examination of the angle of the anterior chamber by means of an optical instrument (gonioscope) with an intense light.

Manifestations of disorders of the eyes (characteristics)

IMPAIRMENT OF VISION

The development of significant signs and symptoms of impaired visual function varies greatly. The onset of changes may be insidious in some cases, but in others, the onset may occur suddenly and be acute. One or both eyes may be involved. The manifestations may be principally subjective or may be objective only, with the abnormal structure or function being noted by an observer. In some instances manifestations may be recognized without tests or the aid of instruments.

The signs and symptoms of eye disorders include the following characteristics.

Subjective manifestations
1 Difficulty in reading and seeing objects clearly, blurred vision or headaches when reading or doing close work. These symptoms may be caused by simple refractive errors or by cataract, glaucoma, inflammation of the cornea (keratitis) and ulceration leading to scarring and opacity, degenerative changes, detachment of the retina or a systemic disease such as hypertension, diabetes mellitus and arteriosclerosis.
2 Photophobia (sensitivity to light) may be associated with inflammation of the conjunctiva, cornea or iris.
3 Excessive tear flow may indicate trauma, chemical irritation, allergy, inflammation of ocular tissue or obstruction of the tear duct.
4 Dryness of the conjunctival surface due to decreased lacrimal secretion which may be incurred by severe dehydration or cerebral trauma or disease (e.g. rheumatoid arthritis). It is frequently a problem in an abnormally dry environment and in the elderly. Some drugs may suppress lacrimal secretion.
5 Ocular pain may be due to irritation from a foreign body, infection, inflammation of eye tissues or accessory structures, or increased intraocular pressure (glaucoma).
6 Diplopia (double vision) is most frequently experienced by patients with a head injury or cerebral disorder (e.g. brain tumour) that incurs a paralysis or functional imbalance of the extraocular muscles.
7 Spots before or floaters in the eyes, single and occasional, are common and of no clinical significance. Frequent or sudden development of numerous spots or floaters may signify an intraocular haemorrhage or threatening of the retina. In the latter, the patient may experience flashing lights followed by a clouding across the eye.
8 Scotoma or blind spot develops as a result of damage to an area of the retina or optic nerve. It may be caused by an inflammatory disease process within the eye or a degenerative disorder. If the scotoma occurs in the same area in each eye, the aetiology may be intracranial, affecting the fibres in the visual pathway.
9 Halos around lights are usually associated with increased intraocular pressure and glaucoma.
10 Extensive loss of visual acuity of 3/60 or less in the better eye with correction, or a restriction of the visual field to 20° or less indicates blindness according to the legal definition.

Objective manifestations
1 The person is observed holding reading material or an object nearer than 30 cm (12 in) to the face or beyond the distance of approximately 40 cm (16–18 in).
2 A strained expression or scowl may be noted when an effort to see is being made.
3 The younger person may fail to develop at a normal rate, make normal progress at school or relate normally to peers.

4 Errors are made because of misread information or directions.

5 Deviation of one eye (the visual axis of one eye differs from that of the other eye) indicates impaired extraocular muscle structure or function. The latter may be due to a disorder involving the oculomotor (third cranial) nerve.

6 Discoloration of the eyelid or surrounding tissue. Redness of the eyelids suggests infection, allergy or injury. Redness of the exposed area of the eye may be caused by conjunctival irritation by a foreign body, infection, or trauma or may be incurred by a subconjunctival haemorrhage associated with trauma, hypertension or inflammatory disease of intraocular structures.

Yellow sclerae occur when the patient has an excessive concentration of bile pigment in the blood (jaundice) which may be due to a liver or gallbladder disease or a blood dyscrasia, but many are idiopathic and resolve spontaneously.

Discoloration of surrounding tissue may be the result of extravasation of blood related to an eye or facial injury.

7 Discharge (serous or purulent) or crusting may indicate infection, chemical irritation, allergy or trauma of the eyelid or eye.

8 Swelling or oedema may develop with local trauma, infection or cyst, or may be associated with renal or cardiac failure, a cerebral disorder or head injury.

9 Abnormal pupillary shape or reaction. Constriction, asymmetry, or failure of normal reaction to light is most often due to some cerebral disorder or iris collapse. A greyish white colour of the pupil suggests an opacity of the lens (cataract).

10 Exophthalmos or proptosis (prominence or bulging of the eyes) is usually caused by hyperthyroidism or brain tumour.

11 Ptosis or a lag in the closing of eyelid may indicate some oculomotor (third cranial) nerve involvement. The drooping of both eyelids is also characteristic of myasthenia gravis.

Visual Impairment

Man is very dependent upon his sense of vision, since most of his knowledge of his environment is obtained through his eyes. The eyes are also used in expressing emotions. Any impairment or loss of vision is a serious threat. In many instances the ability to freely move about safely and the privilege of enjoying colour, form, depth, beauty and distance are lost. Loss of vision results in reduced sensory input and stimulation; this may lead to boredom and reduced responsiveness and disorientation to time and place on the part of the person unless stimuli by other channels (e.g. hearing and touch) are increased and the person's interest maintained.

The nurse should appreciate the incalculable value of sight and the natural anxiety and concern of the patient when it is threatened. Reduced vision affects his whole way of life socially, physically, economically and emotionally. Effective nursing care can only be planned if the nurse has an understanding of the causes of visual impairment as this will allow her to identify appropriate goals for the individual.

CAUSE

Visual impairment may be due to a primary eye disorder or may be secondary to a neurological or systemic disorder. The causes include:

● Structural or functional defect in the eye or extraocular structures (e.g. malfunction of the extraocular muscles causing deviation of one or both eyes)
● Ageing (e.g. the lens becomes less spherical with age, may become opaque and the nucleus hardens)
● Infection
● Trauma (chemical or mechanical)
● New growth
● Impaired innervation of the eyes due to a neurological disorder (e.g. brain tumour or injury)
● Systemic disease (e.g. hypertension, diabetes mellitus, cardiovascular disease)
● Inadequate knowledge about the factors which contribute to the preservation of good vision (e.g. nutritional requirements, protection of eyes in potentially hazardous situations)

The *goals* are to:
1 Preserve vision
2 Identify factors contributing to visual impairment
3 Ensure the patient receives meaningful sensory input
4 Prevent the development of, or decrease the severity of, disorientation
5 Prevent injury or complications
6 Initiate retraining in performing daily activities if visual impairment is permanent

Once the goals have been identified, appropriate nursing intervention can be planned and implemented.

PRESERVATION OF VISION

The maintenance of vision and prevention of loss of sight includes consideration of the following:

Good general health
There is a tendency to consider vision as being independent of general health. It remains good in

some serious bodily disorders, while others may have a serious effect on visual acuity. Occasionally, general body disease is discovered because of changes in the eyes and vision (e.g. hypertension, diabetes, brain tumour).

Optimum diet
A well-balanced diet contributes to good eye health as well as to good general health. Vitamins A, B complex and C are considered important; a deficiency of vitamin A may cause drying and changes of the cornea and conjunctiva and a decreased production of the retinal pigment, rhodopsin, leading to night blindness. A deficiency in the vitamin B complex may predispose to retinal changes. Vitamin C plays a role in resistance to infection.

Protection of infants' and children's eyes
Babies' eyes should be observed regularly after birth so that signs of infection (e.g. gonorrhoea) may be detected early. Failure to treat an infection could lead to corneal scarring and blindness. Congenital cataracts and blindness occur most often in infants whose mothers have a history of a viral infection, especially rubella, during the first trimester. Immunization for German measles is encouraged for women of child-bearing age. The nurse has an important role in preventing blindness in premature and underweight newborn infants by maintaining the prescribed level of oxygen. Administration of high concentrations of oxygen to these infants causes retrolental fibroplasia. A child's eyes are not fully developed until he is at least 7 years of age. Toys and play-things should be selected to avoid broken, sharp and pointed parts that predispose to injury. Children are taught to keep dirty fingers and other objects away from their eyes and are also instructed in the necessary precautions when old enough to play with such things as arrows, catapults, guns and fireworks.

It is sensible to ensure that, when working, the light is adequate and that intensive detailed work is broken up by frequent rest periods. Close work should be avoided when fatigued.

Regular periodical eye examination
Some eye diseases and changes develop insidiously without markedly reducing vision or causing pain until they are well advanced. Regular eye examination may reveal early signs, and a serious disease may be checked before it progresses to loss of vision and blindness. If glasses are necessary, only those which have been properly prescribed should be used. Lenses are individually ground for each eye according to the testing and examination findings (see Table 28.1 for a list of terms which relate to eye examinations and errors of refraction.)

If glasses are worn, the importance of protecting the lens from scratches and maintaining good alignment is stressed. If glasses are not straight or if the distance between the eyes and lenses is not equal,

Table 28.1 Terminology and abbreviations.

Term	Meaning
RE	Right eye
LE	Left eye
BE	Both eyes
Emmetropia	Normal vision (normal refraction)
Myopia (M)	Short-sightedness
Hypermetropia (hyperopia; H)	Long-sightedness
Presbyopia	Reduced accommodation associated with the ageing process
Astigmatism	Uneven curvature of the cornea; results in different focal points
Diplopia	Perception of two images of a single object (double vision)
Hemianopia	Loss of vision in one half of the visual field
Entropion	Turning in of the eyelid
Ectropion	Turning out of the eyelid
Ptosis	Drooping of the upper eyelid
Aphakia	Absence of the lens of an eye
Hyphaema	Haemorrhage into the anterior chamber of the eye
Hypopyon	White blood cells in the anterior chamber
Photophobia	Hypersensitivity to light
Ophthalmologist (oculist)	A doctor who specializes in the treatment of eye disorders
Optometrist	A person who examines the eyes to assess vision and prescribes corrective spectacles or lenses
Optician	A specialist who prepares spectacles or lenses according to prescription
Mydriasis	Dilatation of the pupil
Mydriatic	Drug that dilates the pupil
Miosis	Contraction of the pupil of the eye
Miotic	Drug that contracts the pupil
Proptosis (exophthalmos)	Bulging forward of the eyes
Epiphora	Excessive lacrimal secretion (tears)

the degree of refraction is altered. Lenses in spectacles are safer if made of impact-resistant material.

The correct care and application of contact lenses are extremely important in preventing eye disorders (e.g. infection and ulceration) and reduced vision. When the person receives his prescribed fitted lenses, he must receive detailed instruction about the handling, wearing and cleaning of them. The patient should be able to describe and demonstrate the necessary techniques and precautions to ensure correct and safe use.

Prevention of trauma

The loss of vision due to exposure to chemicals, dust, wind, glaring light or direct sun rays and eye injury by mechanical objects (e.g. flying pieces of metal or wood) is preventable in most instances by the use of standard safety measures and devices. The use of legislated safety regulations, such as helmets, shatter-proof goggles or shields in potentially hazardous situations should be observed. Sunglasses may be necessary to protect the eyes from bright sun rays. The use of adequate protective equipment as well as observance of established safety rules in sports where there is a potential for injury should be promoted.

Rubbing of the eyes should be avoided because of the possibility of trauma and the introduction of infection, especially if wearing contact lenses. Cautious use of sprays and caustic solutions and the wearing of protective goggles when doing so should be emphasized.

Prompt treatment

No 'eyedrops' or ointment should be instilled in the eyes unless prescribed by a doctor. In the event of a persisting foreign body which cannot be gently washed or wiped away, inflammation or any other disturbance in an eye, early treatment by a doctor or oculist (ophthalmologist) should be secured.

If a chemical spray or irritating solution accidentally gets into the eye, immediate and extended irrigation with water or saline is recommended and prompt medical treatment sought to avoid potential ulceration and blindness.

Principles to be observed in giving eye care procedures

1 The patient receives a full explanation of the procedure and is advised that it is important that he holds his head steady—not jerk or pull away.
2 Hands are washed thoroughly before and after doing any eye procedure.
3 Precautions are used to protect the unaffected eye from possible injury and cross-infection from one eye to another. Irrigation solution or eye drops being used in the affected eye must not be permitted to enter the unaffected eye. Similarly,

dressings from the affected eye should not touch the unaffected eye. Dressings and swabs are used only once.
4 Pressure on the eyeball is avoided.
5 When irrigating the eye, the solution is directed on to the nasal side of the eyeball. The eye is gently wiped from the inner canthus to the outer canthus.
6 Solutions and drugs should always be fresh; they are dated as to preparation and expiry.
7 Frequent, regular assessment of the eye and the patient's vision is made. The eye is examined before and after each procedure; alteration in comfort, change in colour, discharge, dryness, oedema or swelling is brought to the attention of the doctor.
8 If both eyes are involved, separate sterile equipment and solutions are used for each eye. In the case of infection, the eye manifesting less inflammation and discharge is treated before the other eye.
9 A separate sterile eye dropper is used for each drug used in the eye.
10 If the eyelid does not close, precautions are necessary when handling articles such as bed-linen, towels and clothing to avoid abrasions and injury of the conjunctiva and cornea. An exposed (open) eye may become dry and susceptible to ulceration; the instillation of artificial tears may be prescribed as a prophylactic measure, as may ointment applied to the exposed conjunctiva.
11 It is important that the patient is warned of any effect the eye drops may have; for example cycloplegic agents will paralyse the muscles of accommodation, and cause blurring of vision.
12 Eye dressings are normally applied to protect, to absorb lacrimal secretions or exudate or to apply pressure. The skin around the eye should always be supported gently when the dressing is removed.
13 Drops are instilled at the *lateral* aspect of the inner lower lid, with the patient looking up, so that direct corneal contact is avoided and reflex squeezing of the eye prevented.
14 In order to keep the affected eye at rest, the unaffected eye may be covered. Adaptation to light is resumed gradually; the unaffected eye may first be exposed by wearing a shield with a small central opening. This minimizes eye movement. A similar shield may also be used later on the affected eye; however, it is more usual for the patient to wear dark glasses. Extreme gentleness is used when changing a dressing or doing any treatment; caution is used to avoid pressure on the eyeball.
15 Great care should be taken to prevent the eye opening under the dressing as this can cause corneal abrasion. The dressing should be secured firmly.

CARE OF THE VISUALLY HANDICAPPED PATIENT

MAINTENANCE OF ORIENTATION AND REDUCTION OF ANXIETY

Impairment and threatened loss of vision arouse considerable fear, insecurity and emotional reactions. All the implications which impaired vision may have in the present and future 'crowd in' on the patient. Fears and worry may be greatly exaggerated, and the patient becomes panicky and loses control. The patient's behavioural responses must be assessed frequently; with reduced or no vision, the patient (especially if elderly) may become disoriented, particularly if not in a familiar environment.

Individuals deprived of visual input become more dependent on other senses such as hearing and touch. The understanding of the nurse as to what the patient may be experiencing, the provision of emotional support and the use of communication techniques which promote the use of other senses contribute greatly to the care of this patient.

Factors which help to reduce the patient's anxiety include the following suggestions. The patient is carefully oriented to any new environment; if confined to bed, the orientation is by a verbal description. If he is allowed up, the verbal description is combined with helping him to explore it. An explanation is made of how the usual daily needs will be met.

The patient is given the opportunity and encouragement to express concerns and to ask questions. The person who cannot see is spoken to as he is approached and is advised who is speaking. Anything that is going to be done for him is outlined (e.g. treatment, investigative procedure). It means a great deal to the patient to always have the call-button within reach; it reassures him that help is always at hand. He should not be left alone for long periods; he may not require a lot of physical care but still requires support and contacts. The nurse should take time to talk to the patient and, as required, indicate the time and describe the place and current situation, the flowers and cards that he has received and details of the environment. He has visual memory from which he can recall sufficiently to form a mental picture of what is being described. Some appropriate form of diversion, such as a radio and visitors to chat with the patient or read to him, is encouraged to provide sensory input. Noisy, confusing situations are avoided; the visually handicapped patient is usually more sensitive to sounds and voice inflections. An effort is made to anticipate the patient's needs.

MAINTENANCE OF A SAFE ENVIRONMENT

Adequate orientation and frequent observations are important to prevent accidents when the patient's vision is seriously impaired. Cot-sides may be required on the bed. If the patient is disoriented, it may be necessary to have someone with him to ensure his safety. The environment must be checked carefully for any hazards for the unseeing, ambulatory person. He should be escorted around the area until he becomes familiar with it and encouraged to move about alone if his condition permits. Stools, rugs or other such articles over which he might trip should be removed. Furniture is not moved from its original position, and doors are kept closed or wide open. The person is cautioned about nearby stairs and radiators. All members of the staff—medical, nursing, paramedical and ancillary—should be made aware of the individual's degree of visual handicap.

CONTINUOUS ASSESSMENT

Prompt recognition of change in the eye, visual acuity and orientation is very important, as failure to do so can lead to an increase in the amount of impairment. The nurse is required to be familiar with any specific observations that are important in certain eye disorders. Generally, significant factors that should be brought promptly to the doctor's attention include elevation of temperature, discharge, unrelieved pain, headache, retraction of the eyelid, any evidence of disturbance in the unaffected eye, drying of the cornea, and signs of bleeding in the anterior chamber.

POSITIONING AND ACTIVITY

The position which the patient with an acute eye disorder is to assume varies with different conditions and is usually indicated by the doctor. Prolonged restriction of activity is rare; patients worry less and have fewer complications when allowed up as soon as possible. If the patient is required to remain in bed, lying flat with the head immobilized, the arms and lower limbs are moved through a range of motion, and active exercises of the legs are begun as soon as the doctor permits.

EATING AND DRINKING

The patient frequently experiences anorexia due to anxiety and because of the difficulty with taking food when he cannot see. The necessary assistance is provided and, when feeding him, the food is described; only small amounts are offered to avoid choking and coughing, since coughing raises the intraocular pressure. As soon as the patient is well enough, he is encouraged to start feeding himself and to become independent. Assistance is withdrawn gradually, not all at once.

The position of different foods on the plate may be described using the clock analogy. Aids such as plate guards and non-slide mats may also be useful.

Some visually handicapped patients are reluctant

to socialize at meal-times in case they cause embarrassment; the use of aids can help them overcome this. Drinks should be offered regularly and poured out if necessary; it is often difficult for the patient to do this, and they may just not drink.

COMMUNICATION

Verbal communication should be clear and concise and may need frequent repetition. Touch and tone are very important, as they offer a form of non-verbal and verbal reinforcement of which the patient can be aware.

REHABILITATION OF THE BLIND

There are two official categories of visual handicap in the United Kingdom: (1) blindness, and (2) partial sight.
1 *Blindness*
(a) 'So blind as to be unable to perform *any* work for which eyesight is essential'
(b) Visual acuity of below 3/60
(c) Visual acuity of 6/60 and below if there is considerable contraction of the visual field
2 *Partial sight*. A visual acuity of 6/60 or less, the individual being substantially or permanently handicapped by defected vision. The category to which the person is assigned (according to the amount of visual impairment) dictates how much help he is eligible to receive.

The patient with marked visual impairment or with total loss of vision needs a great deal of assistance in adjusting to the situation. He must be persuaded that life still holds something for him. Emphasis is placed on what he can do. He still has visual memory of form, colour, and space and can learn that other senses can be put to greater use.

The development of independence is started as soon as possible, beginning with self-care (feeding, bathing, dressing and hair). He is assisted with moving about the room and then from room to room, locating furniture and necessary articles by touch. The environment is organized to provide safety. Furniture is left in the same place unless he is advised and oriented to its new position; rugs, foot-stools and other such hazardous objects are removed. Doors are kept wide open or closed.

Anyone walking with a blind person allows him to take an arm rather than grasping his and pushing. Writing is practised, beginning with the signing of his name. Differentiation by touch is also tested and practised. The person learns to tell the time by using a specially designed watch.

Various forms of diversion and recreation are introduced (records of books and music, radio, games). The patient is referred to the Social Services and the Royal National Institute for the Blind,[2] which provide vocational training, assistance in learning Braille and in finding a job, recreation, transportation, and financial assistance when necessary. The use of the white cane is introduced and the necessary guidance given on excursions beyond the house until the person is capable of safely getting around alone.

The patient and family are advised of the financial assistance available for the blind and are assisted in making application for it. The family may require help in accepting the blind patient and in organizing the home environment in the interest of his safety and independence.

COMMON EYE DISORDERS

Refractive errors

Various errors of refraction occur which interfere with the ability of the eye to focus light rays on the retina, normally resulting in impaired vision. (See p. 1061 for a discussion of short-sightedness, long-sightedness, presbyopia and astigmatism.)

Blepharitis

This is an inflammation of the eyelid; it is usually bilateral and affects the marginal area of the lids.

Manifestations
The patient may complain of itching or irritation. The margins of the lids are reddened and develop crusts or scales. It may be associated with seborrhoea (excessive sebaceous gland secretion) of the scalp and eyebrows.

Treatment
Therapeutic measures include gentle removal of the crusts once or twice daily with warm water, the application of the prescribed antibacterial ointment and if the cause is seborrhoea, a daily shampoo with an antiseborrhoeic shampoo is recommended.

Conjunctivitis

Inflammation of the conjunctiva may be caused by bacteria, viruses, chemicals or an allergic reaction and may be acute or chronic. Sources of eye infection include foreign bodies, dust, hands, infected neighbouring structures (nose, face, sinus) or contaminated equipment or solutions used in treatment. Infection by the Koch–Weeks bacillus causes a very contagious form of conjunctivitis called pink eye and

---

[2] Royal National Institute for the Blind (RNIB), 224–228 Great Portland Street, London W1N 6AA. The RNIB publishes a comprehensive dictionary of agencies for the blind.

occurs most often in children. Prompt isolation precautions and therapeutic measures are necessary to prevent its rapid spread to others. Infection may begin in the conjunctival lining of the eyelids and spread or remain confined to that area.

Manifestations
The inflammation is manifested by irritation, feeling of grittiness, pain, redness, encrustations and excessive lacrimation or serous and purulent discharge. The patient may complain of photophobia. When infection is present a culture may be made from a swab of the discharge for identification of the invading organism; this should be carried out before instilling an antimicrobial agent.

Treatment
Frequent gentle cleansing of the lid margins is necessary to prevent encrustations. Precautions must be observed to treat each eye separately so that infection is not transferred from one to the other. The patient is usually more comfortable in dim light or darkness and dark glasses ease the discomfort in the early stages. A specific antimicrobial ointment or solution may be prescribed for instillation. In severe infection, an antibiotic may be prescribed for systemic administration. In an allergic reaction, an antihistamine preparation may be prescribed to relieve the irritation. The patient is advised to keep his hands away from the eyes and, if responsible for instilling medications, the patient must be cautioned to wash his hands thoroughly under running water before starting and after completing the medication procedure. The affected eye may be left uncovered.

If the conjunctivitis is due to allergy, efforts are made to identify the allergen so that it can be avoided if possible; it may be air-borne or transferred by the person's hands or by towels. A topical corticosteroid preparation may be prescribed to provide relief.

Hordeolum (stye)

A hordeolum, or stye, is a small abscess that develops within a marginal sebaceous gland or hair follicle of an eyelash. A small, red, swollen tender area appears. Spontaneous drainage of pus may be hastened by a broad-spectrum antibiotic such as chloramphenicol, which should be instilled regularly. If necessary, the offending eyelash is removed. Rarely, a small incision is necessary to drain the abscess. The patient with a stye is cautioned not to squeeze the area, as this may 'break down' the localization and lead to cellulitis.

Chalazion

A chalazion is a cyst that forms in a meibomian (sebaceous) gland. It may remain as a small, firm, painless swelling in the lid for a long period. Eventually it may become infected and irritate the palpe-

bral conjunctiva. Application of an antibiotic preparation is usually prescribed. Recurrence frequently necessitates a small incision in the eyelid for drainage and curettage.

Glaucoma

This disorder is characterized by an increase in the intraocular pressure above the normal, which causes damage to the optic disc and visual field loss. Normal pressure is generally maintained by a balance between the production of aqueous humour by the ciliary body and its drainage from the anterior chamber through the trabecular meshwork of the filtration angle into the canal of Schlemm. If an imbalance occurs between production and drainage, the pressure increases, compressing the retina and the blood vessels within the eye (Fig. 28.8). Permanent optic nerve damage leading to blindness results unless there is early recognition and treatment of the disease.

Glaucoma is usually due to some interference with the outflow of aqueous humour from the anterior chamber into the canal of Schlemm. It may be classified as *primary or secondary* and as *chronic or acute*. The acute form may be referred to as *acute angle-closure glaucoma*; the chronic type is called *open-angle* or simple chronic glaucoma.

Secondary glaucoma may be associated with infection, inflammation, trauma or a tumour within the eye.

OPEN-ANGLE (CHRONIC) GLAUCOMA

This chronic and more common type develops very gradually; the cause is not understood but the frequency of familial incidence points to hereditary aetiology that results in degenerative changes in the

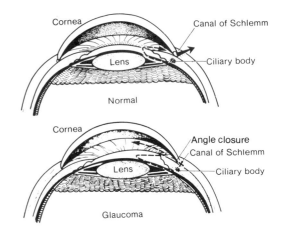

Fig. 28.8 This diagram shows how a disturbance in the balance of fluid within the eyeball increases pressure in the eye and can result in glaucoma.

trabecular meshwork of the filtration angle. It is usually bilateral and has a high incidence in persons over the age of 35 or 40 years; this emphasizes the importance of regular eye examinations which include the measurement of intraocular pressure.

Manifestations.
Because of the insidious onset of open-angle glaucoma, the central field of vision is not lost for some time. The disorder is frequently well advanced before the person seeks assistance. The visual field progressively diminishes, and the individual may become aware that something is wrong when he learns of objects on either side of him that he 'missed', or if he persistently sees halos around artificial lights. The condition may be discovered during a routine examination. As the condition progresses, the person may complain of some pain in the eye(s), especially in the morning on awakening. If chronic glaucoma is not recognized and treated in the early stage, the person eventually experiences symptoms similar to those cited for acute glaucoma.

Treatment of chronic (open-angle) glaucoma
In the early stages, treatment of open-angle glaucoma consists of instillation of a miotic 2–4 times a day which causes contraction of the ciliary body and constriction of the pupil. Preparations are available now which have a more prolonged effect, requiring instillation only twice in 24 hours. An example of such a preparation is timolol maleate (Timoptol), a beta-blocker which has the advantage of lowering the intraocular pressure, but does not constrict the pupil. Acetazolamide (a carbonic anhydrase inhibitor) is a diuretic which may be prescribed orally to lessen the formation of aqueous humour. Surgical treatment may become necessary. A trabeculectomy, an iridectomy, iridencleisis or cyclodialysis or cyclocryotherapy may be done. These promote drainage of the aqueous humour from the anterior chamber. *Iridencleisis* creates an opening between the anterior chamber and subconjunctival space; aqueous fluid is absorbed into the conjunctival tissues. *Cyclodialysis* involves the establishment of a communication between the anterior chamber and the suprachoroidal space. *Cyclodiathermy*, which involves destruction of part of the ciliary body by diathermy, or *cyclocryotherapy* (freezing of the ciliary body) is now replacing cyclodialysis as a method for treatment. The procedure is used mostly for patients with advanced glaucoma which does not respond to previously cited methods of treatment, and particularly when intractable pain is a problem.

ACUTE ANGLE-CLOSURE GLAUCOMA

This form of glaucoma is characterized by rapid marked increase in intraocular pressure as a result of a complete block in the outflow of the aqueous humour. The iris appears to have been pushed forward, narrowing the peripheral angle between it and the cornea (see Fig. 28.8), and, with dilatation of the pupil and the concomitant thickening of the iris, the openings in the filtration angle which lead into the canal of Schlemm become occluded. The condition demands prompt emergency care because rapid compression of the retinal blood vessels develops, and destruction of the optic nerve cells and fibres occurs, with resultant loss of vision.

Manifestations and treatment
The patient with acute glaucoma experiences severe pain, nausea and vomiting, halos or rainbows around artificial lights and blurring of vision. On examination, the pupil is seen to be dilated, and there is evidence of congestion and a marked increase in intraocular pressure. The cornea becomes oedematous and may eventually lose its lustre and transparency.

Prompt treatment is necessary to prevent blindness. A miotic preparation such as pilocarpine hydrochloride is instilled to constrict the pupil; this effects an increase in the peripheral angle by moving the iris away from the cornea. A drug such as acetazolamide (Diamox) may be administered orally or intravenously to reduce the formation of aqueous humour; or, an osmotic agent, such as intravenous urea or mannitol, or glycerol is given to reduce intraocular pressure. The latter can be unpalatable and sometimes an antiemetic is required.

A quiet environment is provided and the patient is helped to relax. He is positioned with the head and shoulders elevated; analgesia is prescribed to relieve the pain.

If an immediate, satisfactory response to drug therapy does not occur, surgical intervention is undertaken. A small section of the iris is removed (iridectomy) to prevent it from being imposed on the drainage system. Newer techniques include the use of a laser beam to make a hole through the iris. *Laser irodotomy* may be done on an outpatient basis.

Postoperative management. An important nursing responsibility is the instillation of eye drops: a mydriatic and a corticosteroid are usually prescribed and the eye kept at rest. A topical antibiotic may also be prescribed, and in some instances the ophthalmologist may require the alternate instillation of a mydriatic and miotic to produce alternating periods of dilatation and constriction of the pupil to guard against the formation of adhesions between the iris and the cornea and lens. It is important that the cycloplegic effect of some mydriatics is explained to the patient *before* instillation, as this may cause a decrease in visual acuity which can be very frightening for them. Reassurance should be given that this alteration is temporary.

Because glaucoma accounts for such a large proportion of blindness, more effort has been directed toward informing the general public about the disease and the significance of early recognition.

Glaucoma cannot be cured, but blindness can be prevented by continuous use of a miotic as prescribed, by surgery and by medical supervision, if it is begun early in the disease.

An important nursing responsibility is to alert the patient to activities and situations that predispose to a rise in intraocular pressure. The condition is explained to the patient and family, and emphasis is placed upon the need for some precautions to prevent visual damage. Emotional and stressful situations are avoided as much as possible; the patient must learn to tolerate and live with what cannot be changed.

The patient and family must appreciate the importance of regularly scheduled visits to the ophthalmologist for measurement of the intraocular pressure and visual field and acuity testing. They are taught the correct method of instilling the prescribed miotic, and cautioned against the use of any solution or medication that is not prescribed by the doctor. An identification card or Medic-Alert pendant indicating that the person suffers from glaucoma is recommended. He is encouraged to continue his occupation unless it is visually impossible. Some job modification or change may be made by encouraging the patient to consult with his employer and the occupational health programme in his place of work. Patients with advanced glaucoma and loss of vision are referred to the Royal National Institute for the Blind or another appropriate agency.

Cataract

A cataract is a clouding of the crystalline lens, resulting in opacity. It may be classified as a *degenerative* or *developmental* (congenital or juvenile) cataract; the latter type of cataract occurs most often in infants whose mothers have a history of a viral infection (e.g. German measles) during the first trimester of pregnancy, or is associated with a genetic defect, which, for example, causes an inborn error of metabolism.

The degenerative cataract has a high incidence in persons over 50 years of age and may be referred to as a senile cataract. The cause is not known; metabolic changes in the lens substance are considered to be a major factor. It is also suggested that an inherited predisposition to develop the characteristic lens changes plays a role. Some deficiencies in nutrients, such as vitamins C and B, have also been suggested as possible aetiological factors. Degenerative cataract is frequently associated with diabetes mellitus. Opacity of the lens may also be secondary to eye trauma or to exposure to radiation or extreme heat. It may develop following uveitis or the prolonged use of the miotic echothiopate or a topical corticosteroid preparation.

Manifestations. The opacity develops very gradually and may be localized to the centre of the lens, incurring early impairment of vision, or it may start in the periphery. A cataract, even in its early stage, is readily recognized through the pupil, using an ophthalmoscope. As it matures, the examiner is not able to visualize the fundus or optic disc and the pupillary area appears grey or whitish because of the opaque lens behind it.

The loss of the normal refractive ability of the lens prevents light rays from being focused on the retina. Vision becomes blurred, objects may appear distorted and colour perception decreases. Visual loss is very gradual and is directly proportional to the degree of opacity of the lens. Cataract may be unilateral or bilateral; if bilateral the opacity does not usually develop at the same rate in both lenses.

Treatment

Cataract is irreversible but as loss of transparency of the lens develops, visual acuity and distant vision can usually be improved by increasing the correction of lens in the person's spectacles. Eventually, the opacity increases to the point that no light rays pass through the lens to reach the retina.

When the person's visual impairment becomes a handicap and interferes with his usual life-style and activities, surgical treatment is undertaken. The operative procedure used may be classified as extracapsular or intracapsular cataract extraction.

In the *extracapsular extraction*, the anterior portion of the capsule and the lens content may be removed, or the procedure may involve phacoemulsification (a small incision is made in the anterior capsule and the lens content is aspirated). Phacoemulsification uses ultrasonic vibrations to fragment the lens content which prepares it for aspiration. The extracapsular extraction leaves the posterior part of the capsule intact and the vitreous body undisturbed. If the posterior capsule of the lens has lost its transparency, a small opening (a capsulotomy) may be made in it with a laser beam several weeks or months following the initial surgery.

In *intracapsular cataract extraction*, the lens is removed, complete with its capsule, usually by cryoextraction in which a probe-like instrument is introduced so that it lies against the lens and is cooled to −30°C to −35°C. The lens and its capsule freeze to the probe, and are removed when the probe is withdrawn. To make the zonules (attaching fibres) more readily detachable, an enzymatic preparation of chymotrypsin (Zonulysin) may be instilled behind the iris a few minutes before the lens is removed, especially in younger patients.

Following either an extracapsular or intracapsular extraction, an *intraocular lens implant* may be placed in the anterior or posterior chamber.

Usually cataract extraction is done in only one eye at a time; if both eyes are affected, they are treated (in most cases) in separate operations several weeks or months apart.

MANAGEMENT BEFORE AN OPERATION IS NECESSARY

During the period through which the lens is progressively losing its transparency, a nurse usually has contact with the patient only at the clinic, the surgery or on home visits that are for some other purpose. During such contacts, the nurse assesses the person in relation to the visual impairment.

Potential patient problems
1 Anxiety due to the visual impairment and fear of blindness and dependency
2 Potential for injury
3 Decreased mobility, usually due to a fear of moving about, especially outside the immediate familiar environment
4 Alteration in self-image due to limitations

Nursing intervention

1. Anxiety. The nurse explains cataract to the patient and family and reassures them that it is a common problem. They should be advised that vision can be improved by corrective lenses in glasses for a period of time and that eventually the cataract can be treated by surgery. Details should then be given about what this will entail.

2. Potential for injury. Advice should be given to the patient and his family about adjustments within the patient's environment that may be necessary to prevent accidents. Improved lighting may help and other aids, such as stair rails can be installed. Direct vision into sunlight and bright lights is avoided. The patient should be asked whether he drives and advised that the advisability of continuing to do so depends on the degree of visual impairment and that he should discuss the matter with his ophthalmologist.

3. Decreased mobility. Because of the fear of falling, of making errors and being unable to read signs, price tags, etc., the patient becomes reluctant to venture beyond his own immediate familiar environment, and activity within that may gradually decrease. Socialization decreases. The patient is encouraged to go out with family members and friends, not to hesitate to ask for assistance when alone and to turn his head to the side when looking at something, since peripheral vision is usually decreased. The patient and family are informed that books in large print are available to them in public libraries. They are advised also of the services of the local branch of the Royal National Institute for the Blind. For example, when the patient is unable to

read and watch television, recordings may be obtained. He may be registered as blind or partially sighted so that help is available until he has surgery.

4. Alteration in self-image. The person with loss of vision may become depressed and lose self-esteem as his activities and participation progressively become restricted and he becomes more dependent upon others. He is helped to recognize the positive factors, and to use accessible forms of diversion. Unless there is some existing complication that contraindicates surgery, the patient is reassured that this is a temporary problem that will be relieved when he has the surgery.

IMMEDIATE PREOPERATIVE CARE (see Table 28.2)

Nursing intervention
The patient is alerted to any furniture or articles over which he might trip or stumble. Preoperative medication usually includes a sedative so that the patient is drowsy and less apprehensive. Cot sides are kept up on the bed and on the stretcher when transferring the patient to the operating theatre. Contact lenses must be removed before leaving the ward, as must dentures, prostheses and hairclips. Spectacles and hearing aids can be removed in the anaesthetic room.

The nurse should check that the correct eye has been marked by the surgeon and that the consent form has been signed.

An example of a care plan for a patient about to undergo intraocular surgery is given in Table 28.2. This describes potential problems, full nursing intervention and expected outcomes.

POSTOPERATIVE CARE (see Table 28.3)

Potential eye injury and complications are the major concern following cataract extraction. The period of bedrest and hospitalization varies considerably. The patient is usually allowed out of bed the day of or day after surgery and may be discharged home the first or second postoperative day.

Identification of patients' problems and *nursing intervention* are discussed in Table 28.3.

Spectacles and contact lenses
When the dressing is removed, dark glasses are worn because the patient may experience discomfort in the eye with exposure to light; gradual adaptation is necessary. If an intraocular lens has not been implanted at the time of the surgery, the patient may be fitted with a contact lens. The lens may be of the type which has to be removed each night, or an extended-wear type which can be left in the eye for several weeks. With the latter, the patient returns to the clinic or ophthalmologist at regular intervals (approximately 90–120 days) to have the lens removed, cleansed and replaced.

Table 28.2 Preoperative care* of patients undergoing intraocular surgery.

Problem	Goal	Nursing intervention	Expected outcomes
1 Anxiety related to the unfamiliar environment and lack of knowledge about the surgical procedure and local anaesthetic; and fear of an undesirable outcome	1 Alleviate anxiety 2 Acquire an understanding of what will be done, what to expect and the patient's role	**a** Orient the patient to his environment and staff **b** Encourage the patient and family to express their fears and concerns **c** Identify specific fears, misconceptions and learning needs relevant to the disorder, surgery, postoperative care and the patient's future **d** Provide the necessary information; answer their questions **e** Preoperative medication may be prescribed	Anxiety is reduced, as evidenced by decreased restlessness and conversation that indicates understanding and acceptance of the situation and what may be expected
2 Inadequate knowledge about anticipated postoperative care	Awareness of the activities and restrictions to be expected after surgery	**a** The anticipated restrictions in positioning and activities in the postoperative period and their significance are explained. **b** The patient is informed about the following. If nauseated he should notify the nurse promptly so an antiemetic can be given to avoid vomiting. The eye should not be squeezed closed and sudden jerky movements, bending over, pushing, lifting and constipation are avoided. **c** If both eyes are likely to be covered, explain the reason for this and assure the patient that assistance will be readily available to meet his needs	The patient indicates understanding of anticipated procedures
3 Alteration in nutrition: intake of less than body requirements	Prevent nausea and vomiting	Food and fluid may be withheld for 4–6 hours preceding surgery	Nausea and vomiting are absent
4 Bowel elimination: potential for constipation	Prevent constipation and straining at stool postoperatively	A rectal suppository or small cleansing enema may be ordered, especially if the patient's activity is to be restricted after surgery	Bowel movements are soft, regular and are evacuated without strain
5 Potential for injury related to infection and surgical intervention	Prevent infection of the eye	**a** Inspect the eyes for irritation, redness, discharge and excessive lacrimation **b** A routine culture of the conjunctival sacs may be required **c** Specific directions are given by the surgeon; the eyelids and area around the eye are cleansed. If the eyelashes are to be cut, the blades of the scissors used are coated with chloramphenicol ointment to prevent lash remnants dropping into the eye **d** Some marking should be used to ensure identification of the eye to receive surgery **e** A prophylactic antibiotic may be instilled in the eye before surgery, as prescribed	The patient is free of infection
6 Alteration in comfort: pain related to surgical procedure	Pain and discomfort are absent	Instil drops prescribed by the surgeon (e.g. Mydrilate) prior to surgery and give any appropriate prescribed systemic premedication	1 The patient's eye is at rest; the pupil is dilated or constricted as indicated 2 Patient is relaxed and free of pain and discomfort

*Therapeutic measures and care vary with the disorder, surgery to be performed and the surgeon. Specific requirements are cited with the discussion of the various disorders.

Table 28.3 Postoperative care of patients following intraocular surgery.

Problem	Goal	Nursing intervention	Expected outcomes
1 Alteration in comfort: pain	Prevent pain and discomfort	a The patient may experience some burning or smarting sensation which may be relieved by a mild analgesic. Severe pain, particularly if it develops suddenly or if the patient expresses a 'feeling of pressure within the eye' is reported promptly to the surgeon b Temperature, pulse, and respirations are recorded at regular intervals; an elevation in temperature may indicate infection c The patient is usually allowed to use the bathroom on the first postoperative day and walking is progressively increased, or he may be discharged on the second postoperative day d If the patient is on bedrest for several days or longer, deep breathing at regular intervals is encouraged; secretions are less likely to be retained and cause infection and coughing e Lower limb and arm exercises are introduced for the bed patient to promote circulation but the patient is cautioned against moving his head while doing them	1 The patient feels no pain or discomfort. However, if an episode of severe pain develops, it is identified promptly 2 The patient's temperature remains within normal limits
2 Potential for injury related to surgical intervention	1 Promote healing 2 Prevent intraocular haemorrhage, increased intraocular pressure and rupture of the incision line	a The head is held steady and supported during transfer from the operating theatre table to his bed b If confined to bed, the patient is assisted to change position c After the initial dressing, prescribed drops or ointment are instilled 3 or 4 times daily. A pad may be reapplied or dark glasses worn, except at night when a dressing and protective shield should be worn d Restrictions in positioning and activity are indicated by the ophthalmologist and should be made familiar to staff and family members e The patient is sat up when the surgeon allows; the head is well supported and the patient is discouraged from lying on the affected side f The patient is reminded: to avoid straining at stool, to avoid any pressure on the eye, not to lean over the side of the bed or make sudden movements, to try to avoid coughing by taking a deep breath and if it cannot be avoided to cough with mouth open (lessens intracranial pressure), as these actions may increase intraocular pressure which may cause intraocular haemorrhage or prolapse of the iris, and to inform the nurse promptly of pain in the eye; severe pain should be brought to the surgeon's attention immediately, since it may indicate intraocular haemorrhage	The patient does not experience intraocular haemorrhage, increased intraocular pressure or rupture of incision line

Table 28.3—*continued*.

Problem	Goal	Nursing intervention	Expected outcomes
2 Potential for injury (continued)		**g** Nausea and vomiting should also be controlled because of the associated strain; an antiemetic is prescribed if necessary	
3 Potential for infection	To prevent infection	**a** The length of time a dressing is kept on depends on the surgery and the surgeon **b** The daily instillation of topical antibiotics may be prescribed; aseptic technique is observed **c** The patient's temperature is recorded regularly and any elevation above the normal is recorded **d** Each time the eye is uncovered it is inspected for inflammation and discharge **e** If infection is suspected or present, prompt antibiotic therapy is prescribed (topical and systemic). A culture is usually made to identify the organism and determine its sensitivity **f** A topical corticosteroid preparation may be instilled in the eye to reduce the effects of the inflammation on intraocular structures	The eye is free of infection
4 Potential for injury related to sensory deprivation or disorientation	**1** Prevent injury **2** Orient the patient to his surrounding	**a** Reorient the patient on his return from the operating theatre (location, staff and time) and reassure him as to assistance and care **b** Cot-sides are kept up and the call-button always ready within the patient's reach **c** Do not leave the patient alone for long periods; frequent communication reduces sensory deprivation, especially if both eyes are covered or the room is darkened. On each visit, the person's orientation is assessed **d** An effort is made to anticipate the patient's needs so he is not tempted to over-reach or get up. It may be helpful to have a family member or friend remain with the patient **e** Articles that the patient is likely to want are placed within reach and always in the same place **f** The affected eye is protected by a shield; a plastic one is always used at night **g** When ambulatory, the patient is assisted until familiarity with the environment is indicated. The environment is cleared of hazardous articles such as foot-stools, loose rugs and anything which he may bump into or trip over. When ambulatory, furniture should remain in its original position and doors kept wide open or closed **h** If the patient becomes confused restraints on the arms may be necessary to prevent his interference with the eye	**1** The patient is free from injury **2** The patient is oriented to time, place and person **3** The environment is free of physical hazards

Table 28.3—*continued.*

Problem	Goal	Nursing intervention	Expected outcomes
4 Potential for injury related to sensory deprivation (continued)		dressing. The use of body restraints are avoided because the resistance to them may increase intraocular pressure. Someone (e.g. a family member) may have to remain with him to ensure his safety. **i** Sedation may be prescribed	
5 Alteration in nutrition: less than body requirements	Nutritional and fluid intake is progressively increased to normal as tolerated	**a** The restoration of a balanced diet will aid healing. The patient should be given sips of water on return from theatre. Then a light easily digestible diet should gradually be introduced the following day. Fluid intake should be encouraged unless the patient complains of nausea in which case an antiemetic should be given. Fluid intake and output should be recorded until the patient is capable of taking control of his own eating and drinking. He should be advised to choose a high-fibre diet in order to prevent straining at stool **b** It is important that the necessary assistance is available for the person with severely impaired vision. Assistance is also necessary for the patient whose movement is restricted. The food is described and the patient fed slowly to avoid possibility of aspiration and coughing	The patient's usual body weight is maintained
6 Inadequate knowledge about post-hospitalization care and rehabilitation	The patient requires knowledge and skill essential to follow-up care	**a** The patient's home situation should be determined and the patient and a family member assisted to develop an appropriate plan of care. Instruction and/or demonstrations are given relevant to: • Restrictions to prevent intraocular haemorrhage and increased intraocular pressure (bending over, lifting, pushing, falls and bumps) • The prescribed therapeutic eye procedures (dressing, and how to clean away discharge and the instillation of drops or ointment) **b** Emphasis is placed on: • The need for the washing of hands and careful handling of dressings • Securing the dressing so it does not abrade the eye • The wearing of dark glasses when the dressing is removed and the subsequent wearing of corrective spectacles or contact lenses (see text for details) • The wearing of the eye shield at night for 2–3 weeks • The avoidance of rubbing the eye • The restriction on reading and driving for the period indicated by the ophthalmologist	The patient and family: **1** Indicate an awareness of the importance of compliance with the recommended restrictions **2** Demonstrate ability to perform the prescribed eye procedures safely **3** Express an awareness of the: need for an eye shield and dark glasses; symptoms that require prompt medical attention; and the correct care of corrective lenses **4** Describe plans for follow-up care and demonstrate awareness of community resources

Table 28.3—*continued.*

Problem	Goal	Nursing intervention	Expected outcomes
6 Inadequate knowledge (continued)		• The care of corrective glasses or lenses. If an enucleation was done, the application, removal and care of the artificial eye • The symptoms that indicate the need to promptly contact the ward (pain in the eye, increased redness and discharge, loss of vision) • Subsequent appointments with the ophthalmologist or clinic	

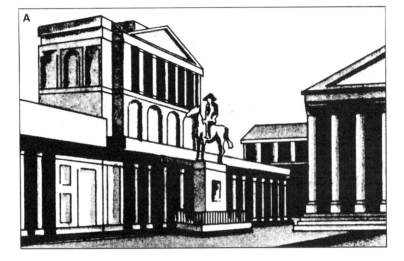
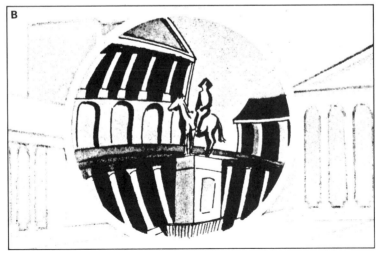

Fig. 28.9 The Bank of England. *A*, As seen normally. *B*, Illustrates the loss of peripheral vision as seen through the eyes of a patient wearing cataract glasses. The central vision appears larger and nearer than it is. The side vision is bowed and outside this there is a ring area of no vision at all.

When only one eye has had cataract extraction, spectacles are not useful since the thick biconvex lens that would be necessary magnifies considerably and would not produce binocular vision. When both eyes have had cataract surgery without intraocular lens implant, the patient is fitted for spectacles with thick biconvex lenses which are used for a few weeks or months before permanent glasses or contact lenses are provided. With spectacles, peripheral vision is restricted (see Fig. 28.9).

Implantation of an intraocular lens at the time of the cataract extraction is becoming more common. The advantages are the provision of greater depth perception, full visual field, and binocular vision (less magnification than glasses).

Teaching patients in preparation for discharge
This includes the following considerations:

* The avoidance of lifting, bending over and straining at stool for about 3 weeks is stressed. The patient is cautioned against squeezing the eye closed or applying pressure on the eye. A shield is worn at night for 2–3 weeks to avoid pressure and unconscious rubbing.
* A family member and the patient are instructed how to care for the eye following discharge (dressings and the instillation of drops and ointment).
* If redness, oedema or pain develops in the eye, the surgeon should be contacted promptly.
* If glasses are to be worn an explanation is made about the reduced peripheral vision. The patient is advised that in order to see, he must learn to look straight-on; this necessitates turning the head when making a side-on peripheral observation. Because of the magnification and difference in spatial judgement, the patient is advised of the necessary precautions when using stairs and handling objects.
* Once the dressing is removed permanently, the eye is protected by a shield or sunglasses until non-implant contact lenses or glasses are provided.
* When the patient receives a contact lens, detailed instructions and demonstrations are necessary. A contact lens is a thin plastic disc shaped to fit the anterior surface of the eye. The outer surface is ground to meet the patient's visual need. The patient is taught the daily procedure of putting in and removing the lens, the cleansing and care of it and the prevention of complications. Meticulous care is necessary to prevent complications, which are painful and could cause loss of vision. Washing the hands thoroughly with soap under running water before handling the lens is emphasized. If worn in both eyes, on removal each lens is stored separately in containers marked for right and left; the correction in one may be quite different to that of the other. Directions for cleansing are provided in writing. Before applying the lenses, they are rinsed free of any chemical

that may have been used for cleansing and a wetting solution may be used. Solutions must be fresh and are not reused.

The patient is advised to use the lens for brief periods at first, progressively increasing the length of time until the eye is comfortable with it. Unless the lenses are of the extended-wear type, they are removed at the end of each day; they are *not* worn during sleep. If the eye is inflamed or painful or if there is excessive lacrimal secretion (tearing), the lens is not applied. The most common complications that develop are conjunctivitis, corneal abrasion and keratitis.

Complications
Complications that may occur following cataract extraction include the following.

Haemorrhage into the anterior chamber (hyphaema) is a serious complication that may occur in the early postoperative period. The patient experiences sharp pain in the eye and on examination, blood can be seen in the eye. The patient is placed at rest, his head is elevated and the ophthalmologist is notified immediately. A mydriatic preparation is usually ordered to dilate the pupil and rest the eye.

Wound rupture and iris prolapse occurs rarely and is manifested by a mis-shapen iris and bulging in the incision area. It requires prompt surgical treatment to avoid serious visual impairment. Mydriatics must not be instilled if a prolapse is suspected.

Infection may develop; the eye becomes red, swollen and painful. It is treated by topical and parenteral antibiotics. Extreme precautions are necessary to avoid the spread of the infection to the other eye.

A severe infection may manifest itself as a hypopyon: white cells in the anterior chamber. Intensive instillation of eye drops may be supplemented by a subconjunctival injection of a broad-spectrum antibiotic such as gentamicin or methicillin.

Retinal detachment occurs rarely as a result of the formation of adhesions within the eye—usually between the retina and the vitreous. (See treatment of retinal detachment p. 1081).

Glaucoma may also develop as a result of adhesions forming between the iris and the cornea, blocking the filtration angle, and secondary to a hyphaema.

Expected outcomes
The patient:

1 Does not experience discomfort in the affected eye.
2 Indicates understanding of the importance of avoiding activities which may cause increased intraocular pressure and, if pain or discomfort is experienced, the need for prompt contact with the ophthalmologist or clinic.
3 Is able to see because of the intraocular lens, contact lens or glasses.

4 The patient and/or a family member has satisfactorily demonstrated the necessary procedures to care for his eyes and his contact lenses.

5 The patient is free from post-cataract extraction complications.

Detachment of the retina

Retinal detachment is separation of the pigmented epithelium of the retina from the layer of rods and cones; the pigmented layer remains attached to the choroid. The separation occurs as a result of tears or holes in the retina. These openings permit fluid from within the eye to leak through and accumulate in the retina, incurring the separation.

The cause may be degenerative retinal changes associated with the ageing process, aphakia (absence of the lens), trauma or tumour. The trauma may be directly to the eye (e.g. penetrating foreign body) or may be associated with a head injury. Retinal detachment may occur as a complication following cataract extraction or an inflammatory intraocular disorder. There is a higher incidence in those who have myopia and are over 50 years of age. The damaged areas are usually toward the periphery of the retina but may occur in the area of the macula, causing severe visual impairment.

Manifestations
Manifestations of a detached retina appear suddenly and include flashes of light, blurred vision, floating particles in the line of vision, the sensation of a curtain coming in front of a part of the eye, restricted visual field and eventual loss of vision.

Treatment
The patient is placed at rest and both eyes may be covered. A mydriatic and cycloplegic drug such as cyclopentolate hydrochloride (Mydrilate) may be prescribed for instillation to dilate the pupils and arrest accommodation by depressing ciliary action. The ophthalmologist indicates the position the patient is to assume—left or right lateral or on the back (never prone). The position is such that the detached area of the retina will approximate the underlying layers. A sedative or tranquillizer may be prescribed to reduce the patient's fear and apprehension and promote immobility. The patient is advised of the importance of maintaining the recommended position and of avoiding sudden movements, bending over, coughing, sneezing and rubbing the eye. He is informed that assistance is close at hand and how it is summoned.

Surgical intervention is usually undertaken fairly early. Various procedures are used, but the underlying principle is scarring of the area. As the scar tissue forms, it fills in the retinal hole and provides attachment to the underlying sclera. The surgical procedures include electrodiathermy, encirclement plombage, cryosurgery (the application of extreme cold), photocoagulation which involves the application of heat by means of directing a very intense light into the eye (laser beam), and scleral buckling. In scleral buckling, the accumulated fluid is removed, the area is treated to produce scar tissue, and a fold is then made in the underlying sclera, which buckles the overlying choroid and retina bringing them in contact.

After the operation, a patch is placed over the eye for 24 hours. Dilating and antimicrobial eye drops may then be ordered. In some hospitals cold moist compresses may be applied to the operative eye to decrease swelling. The patient is instructed to ask for assistance when ambulating and not to bend or strain. The light in the room is kept low to decrease light sensitivity when the patch is removed and dark glasses may be worn. Because of the amount of oedema within a confined space (the orbit) pain can be a problem and may be for 6–8 weeks postoperatively. A full explanation of the cause of pain and regular analgesia may be given. Analgesia to take home should also be prescribed.

Prior to discharge the patient is taught to instil the eye drops and is given written instructions about activity limitations. No heavy lifting or heavy work is undertaken for at least a period of 5–6 weeks. Appointments are made for follow-up care. The patient must be cautioned against bumping the head, rapid eye movements, reading and close work.

Uveitis

Inflammation due to injury or infection may develop in the uveal tract, which includes the choroid, iris and ciliary body. It may also be associated with collagen disease (e.g. rheumatoid arthritis, sarcoidosis).

Manifestations
The eye is reddened and the patient complains of pain, photophobia, and impaired vision in the affected eye. The pupil usually remains constricted.

Treatment
Treatment may include rest of the eyes, the application of heat and the administration of an antimicrobial drug if infection is suspected as being the cause. A mydriatic (e.g. atropine, cyclopentolate, tropicamide) is instilled to dilate the pupil and prevent adhesions from developing between the iris and the lens. A corticoid preparation may be given systemically and also instilled in the eye(s) to arrest the inflammatory process and scar formation; scar formation is likely to cause loss of vision.

Keratitis

This term is used for inflammation of the cornea, which is a serious condition. It may be due to infection or trauma and is likely to lead to ulceration and scarring. The affected areas lose their transparency, diminishing the light rays entering the eye.

Debilitated persons and those with vitamin A deficiency and allergies develop corneal ulceration more readily with an eye infection or trauma. The inflammation may be superficial or deep and in some instances becomes chronic.

Manifestations

Keratitis is manifested by irritation, discharge if the cause is infection, redness of the eye due to injection of the peripheral areas of the cornea by blood vessels, photophobia and lacrimation. Ulcerated areas may be identified by the instillation of fluorescein which outlines the lesions.

Treatment

Prompt medical treatment is necessary to prevent perforation of the cornea and serious visual damage. Keratitis frequently may be prevented by early removal of foreign bodies as well as early treatment of injuries and infection.

Treatment includes rest, the use of antimicrobial drugs, the instillation of a mydriatic and the administration of a systemic analgesia to relieve pain. The eyes may be covered to protect them from light and to limit eye movement. If ulcers develop and are complicated by corneal perforation the aqueous humour escapes, the anterior chamber collapses and there may be intraocular bleeding. The patient is placed on complete bedrest, a mydriatic is instilled in the affected eye to dilate the pupil, and a pressure dressing is applied. Sometimes a soft contact lens called a protective membrane or bandage lens is applied.

If a cornea appears to be in danger of perforating, the lids may be closed over it, either by closure by tape or actually sutured shut—a tarsorrhaphy.

Vitreous haemorrhage

The most common cause of vitreous opacity is bleeding from adjacent papillary, retinal or ciliary vessels. With minimal bleeding the patient may be conscious of floaters or 'small black dots'; more serious bleeding causes a sudden flood of floaters and subsequent loss of visual acuity so that the patient is only able to perceive light.

The haemorrhage may be associated with trauma, retinal tears and detachment, hypertension or diabetes mellitus. Many diabetics develop diabetic retinopathy, which is a common cause of blindness; increased vascular permeability, microaneurysms and atheroma (fatty plaques in the walls of the arteries) develop in the ocular blood vessels in diabetic retinopathy.

Loss of vitreous transparency may also be incurred by uveitis in which the inflammatory exudate and debris are carried into the vitreous and cause opacity.

Minor haemorrhages into the vitreous resolve fairly quickly. In more severe bleeding, which causes a serious visual impairment or where there is a loss of vitreous transparency due to other aetiological factors, a *vitrectomy* may be undertaken. This involves the removal of vitreous content and opacities with a special instrument to which there is a fibreoptic light attached. The vitreous is replaced with a saline solution such as Ringer's solution.

Keratoconus

This is a rare degenerative disorder of the cornea that is seen in young persons, usually young men. There is a degenerative thinning and protrusion of the central cornea, usually of both eyes. Severe astigmatism develops, causing visual impairment.

An excessive amount of fluid collects posterior to the protruding cornea, and scar tissue develops as a result of the damage to tissue by stretching and rupture. The person experiences blurring of vision in the early stages but progressive changes may eventually lead to complete loss of vision. The patient may be helped at first by the wearing of hard contact lenses but may finally required keratoplasty.

Keratoplasty (cornea transplantation)

Loss of vision due to destruction of the cornea, keratoconus or loss of transparency may be corrected by a cornea transplantation. The central portion of the affected cornea is removed and replaced with a cornea obtained from a cadaver. The period between death and removal of the graft should not exceed 6–8 hours, and the transplant must be performed within 24–48 hours. During the interval following enucleation the donor eye is refrigerated at 4°C to minimize degenerative changes. Rejection is less of a problem with corneal transplantation than with other types of organ transplantation. It is suggested that this is due to the avascularity of the cornea. In the absence of blood vessels, donor tissue antigens do not get into the recipient's blood to initiate the formation of antibodies and sensitized lymphocytes.

Preoperative preparation

A detailed discussion of all that is involved in a keratoplasty occurs between the surgeon and the patient and family. The patient is informed that several weeks will elapse following the transplant before the results can be evaluated. If the patient elects to have the transplant, he is placed on a waiting list and should be prepared to go to the hospital on very short notice when a donor cornea becomes available.

The immediate preoperative period is as brief as possible. Blood specimens are collected for the usual preoperative blood studies, and the surgeon usually prescribes the instillation of a miotic (e.g. pilocarpine 2–4%) in the affected eye to constrict the pupil so that the lens is protected during surgery. Acetazolamide (Diamox) or mannitol may be prescribed intravenously to reduce the intraocular fluid volume and tension (see Table 28.2).

Types of keratoplasty

The operative procedure may be a penetrating keratoplasty or a lamellar transplant. The penetrating transplant involves a full-thickness removal of the central portion of the affected cornea and replacement with an equivalent full-thickness section of the donor cornea. In a lamellar keratoplasty, a partial-thickness piece of the donor cornea replaces superficial layers of the recipient's cornea.

Postoperative management (See Table 28.3)

Both eyes may be covered for a few days. This increases sensory deprivation so it is not to be recommended for more than a minimum of time. During this period the patient may require a good deal of support and assistance. The nurse observes him closely and anticipates his needs since he may be somewhat confused and unable to express his needs and feeling of distress. The patient experiences some pain, not severe, and a mild analgesic or sedative may be prescribed. The main cause of discomfort, is the presence of the sutures giving a continuous 'foreign body' sensation. The sutures stay in for 3–9 months, but his eyes usually become more comfortable, as the epithelium grows over the sutures.

The patient may be allowed up to use the bathroom on the first postoperative day and, by the second or third day, he is allowed up as much as he wishes.

The eye is protected by a dressing. Sunglasses are worn during the day; at night a shield (usually of plastic) is applied.

Topical medications prescribed for instillation for a period of time may include, in addition to a mydriatic (e.g. Mydrilate), a corticosteroid preparation to suppress inflammation which would reduce the clearness and transparency of the cornea. A prophylactic topical antibiotic may also be used for a few days. When instilling ointments or drops, as always, precautions are observed to avoid any pressure on the eye and having the dropper or the tube applicator touch the eye.

During the weeks and months following the transplantation, the patient has alternating periods of optimism and discouragement. It is important for the patient to be informed before leaving the hospital that healing will be slow because a transparent cornea does not have blood vessels.

A family member and the patient receive demonstrations and instruction in the care of the eye and the instilling of medications in preparation for leaving the hospital. If a family member or the patient is not able to undertake the care safely, a referral may be made to the district nurse. The patient is followed closely by frequent visits to the clinic or surgeon.

Injury to the eye

An eye may be traumatized by a foreign body, laceration or chemical. The patient may experience the discomfort associated with 'something in the eye', excessive lacrimation, pain, redness and sensitivity to light. Persisting pain, loss of vision and bleeding usually manifest a serious injury. With any type of injury, contact lenses should be removed promptly.

A *foreign body* may lodge on the conjunctiva or may be embedded in the conjunctival or corneal tissue, causing inflammation and possible ulceration. In some accidents, the injury may penetrate the lens or even the retina. If a foreign body is not easily and lightly wiped off or washed out, the patient is promptly referred to his general practitioner or ophthalmologist. Fluorescein dye may be used in the eye during the assessment to localize the foreign body. Deep metal foreign bodies may be removed by the use of a strong electric magnet. If the foreign body has caused an abrasion or was penetrating, an antibiotic ointment is instilled and a dressing may be applied.

Lacerations of the eyeball seriously threaten vision because of the formation of scar tissue in healing and by predisposing the eye to infection. Prompt treatment and strict asepsis are very important.

Various *chemicals*, acids and alkalis may cause serious irritation or burns of the conjunctiva and cornea. Emergency treatment consists of washing the eye with copious amounts of water or saline. The lids must be wide open and assistance may have to be provided in order to keep the eye open during the flushing. The person is referred to an ophthalmologist as quickly as possible. A local anaesthetic may be instilled to provide relief and facilitate examination of the eye(s). Both eyes are covered to limit eye movement.

Strabismus (squint)

Normally, both eyes perform an equal range of movement and assume corresponding lines of position when focusing on an object. Strabismus ('cross eyes') is characterized by the deviation of one eye from the position of the other. One eye (the normal or fixing eye) focuses directly on the object, but the other one (the deviating eye) appears to be focused on a different object or area.

The inequality in the movement of the eyes is due to an imbalance in the function of one or more extrinsic ocular muscles. The defect may result in the eye being turned medially, producing a convergent strabismus (*esotropia*). If the eye is turned laterally, the condition is referred to as divergent strabismus (*exotropia*). The result of the unequal movement and two points of focus is double vision (*diplopia*). Two images are formed on the retinae and the visual centres in the brain receive two sets of impulses, each producing a separate picture.

Strabismus may also be classified as being non-paralytic or paralytic and monocular or alternating. Non-paralytic strabismus (the more common) is the result of a congenital abnormality. The defect is in the central nervous system mechanism which co-ordinates the movements of the eyes in order to bring them into the positions that will focus the light rays from an object on corresponding areas of the two retinae. The person may be able to focus the right eye on an object of attention but the left deviates, presenting a second image. If the person has alternating strabismus, he may be able to focus first with one eye on the object, then with the other. The eye that is in the correct position is referred to as the fixing eye; the other is called the deviating eye. If it is always the same eye, the strabismus is said to be monocular.

The person with strabismus develops single vision over a period of time, seeing only what the fixing or non-deviating eye perceives by involuntarily suppressing the confusing image presented by the deviating eye. Non-paralytic strabismus is generally recognized in early childhood.

Paralytic strabismus is due to the inability of the extraocular muscles to move the eye into the position corresponding to that of the other eye. As a result the person experiences diplopia. The cause of paralytic strabismus may be a defect in the muscle itself or a disturbance in the muscle innervation. The condition may be a manifestation of a disorder within the brain or orbit that interferes with the transmission of impulses by the third (oculomotor), fourth (trochlear) or sixth (abducens) cranial nerve.

Treatment
Strabismus requires medical treatment; unfortunately, in some instances parents think it will correct itself as the child becomes older. A delay may result in permanent damage; constant suppression of the image presented by the deviating eye may lead to loss of vision in that eye (amblyopia). The form of treatment will depend on the cause and severity of the strabismus. Obviously, if it is secondary to a lesion that is interrupting nerve impulses, the primary condition is surgically treated, if possible. Strabismus in the child may be corrected by the wearing of prescribed glasses. The unaffected eye may be covered for periods to enforce the use of the deviating (or so-called 'lazy') eye. Special eye exercises may be ordered (*orthoptics*).

If the condition does not respond to these conservative forms of treatment, surgical correction may then be undertaken. The procedure may involve shortening or lengthening of one or more extrinsic eye muscles. Following the surgery, exercise and the wearing of glasses may still be necessary for a period of time. The patient requires continual medical supervision.

Neoplasms of the eye and accessory structures

Tumours that develop in the skin on other parts of the body may also occur on the skin of the eyelids. Neoplasms of the external structures are usually discovered in the early stages since they are visible.

Neoplasms of the eye may be benign or malignant and the latter may be primary or secondary. Secondary malignancies in the eye are rare. A biopsy is done if the neoplasm is accessible. Malignant melanoma is the most common intraocular tumour. It usually originates in the choroid, ciliary body or iris. Retinoblastoma which develops in both eyes is attributed to a genetic defect that is considered hereditary.

Early symptoms of an intraocular neoplasm depend on its location. As it enlarges and spreads, pain is experienced because of the increased intraocular pressure; retinal detachment, intraocular haemorrhage and loss of vision occur. Primary malignant tumours may be treated by radiotherapy or enucleation.

Enucleation

Enucleation is the removal of an eyeball and may be necessary because of a malignant neoplasm, deep infection, severe trauma or persisting pain in a blind eye. Rarely, an enucleation is done to remove a disfiguring blind eye. When an eyeball is removed, the extrinsic muscles are severed close to their insertion, and the Tenon's capsule is retained. These may be arranged around a plastic ball to provide support and movement for an artificial eye. A plastic shell is inserted as soon as possible to maintain lid tone and prevent adhesions developing between the layers of conjunctiva which would make the fitting of a prosthesis difficult. The prosthesis is made as soon as the incision has healed and the oedema has subsided.

The patient should not be discharged until he or another member of the family can clean the socket and handle the shell proficiently. A district nurse may be asked to visit.

Occasionally, the operation performed is an evisceration in which the contents of the eyeball are removed, leaving the sclera.

A more radical procedure may be necessary in malignancy or severe trauma. The operation performed is called exenteration and involves the removal of the eyeball and the surrounding structures. These operations can be psychologically very distressing as they alter the individual's body image. The patient should be given time to express his feelings.

Sympathetic ophthalmia

Following an eye injury, especially a deep penetrating one, the patient may develop uveitis (inflammation of the ciliary body, choroid and iris) in the uninjured eye. This response is not understood; it has been suggested that it may be an allergic reaction to the pigment released by the damaged eye. Any redness or tearing of the uninjured eye and any complaint of photophobia, pain or loss of vision must be reported promptly. The condition may develop soon after the injury or several months or years later. Unless the inflammatory reaction is checked promptly, loss of vision results. Corticoid preparations are used locally and generally. Rarely, the injured eye is removed to prevent sympathetic ophthalmitis from developing.

References and Further Reading

BOOKS

Gaston H & Elkington AE (1986) *Ophthalmology for Nurses*. London: Croom-Helm.

Glasspool M (1984) *Eyes—Their Problems and Treatment*. London: Martin Dunitz.

Krupp MA & Chatton MJ (eds) (1983) *Current Medical Diagnosis and Treatment*. Los Altos, CA: Lange. Chapter 4.

Nave CR & Nave BC (1985) *Physics for the Health Sciences*, 3rd ed. Philadelphia: WB Saunders. Chapter 20.

Newell FW (1982) *Ophthalmology: Principles and Concepts*, 5th ed. St Louis: CV Mosby.

Phillips CI (1984) *Basic Clinical Ophthalmology*. London: Pitman.

Roper-Hall JJ (ed) (1980) *Stallard's Eye Surgery*, 6th ed. Bristol: John Wright & Sons.

Trevor-Roper PD (1980) *Lecture Notes on Ophthalmology*, 6th ed. Oxford: Blackwell Scientific.

Vale JM & Cox B (1985) *Drugs and The Eye*, 2nd ed. London: Butterworths.

Vaughan D & Ashbury T (1980) *General Ophthalmology*, 9th ed. Los Altos, CA: Lange.

PERIODICALS

Anonymous (1983) Cataract surgery: providing total patient care' *Nurs. '83*, Vol. 13 No. 4, pp. 65–69.

Belmont O (1981) Some common visual symptoms: what they mean and what to do about them. *Occup. Health Nurs.*, Vol. 29 No. 6, pp. 21–24.

Boyd-Monk H (1981) Practical methods of how to examine the external eye. *Occup. Health Nurs.*, Vol. 29 No. 6, pp. 10–14.

Boyd-Monk H (1979) Screening for glaucoma. *Nurs. '79*, Vol. 9 No. 8, pp. 42–45.

Boyd-Monk H (1980) Examining the eye: part 2. *Nurs. '80*, Vol. 10 No. 6, pp. 58–63.

Boyd-Monk H (1981) Retinal detachment and vitrectomy: nursing care. *Nurs. Clin. N. Am.*, Vol. 16 No. 3, pp. 433–451.

Bryant WM (1981) Common toxic effects of systemic drugs on the eye. *Occup. Health Nurs.*, Vol. 29 No. 6, pp. 15–17.

Cavalier JP (1981) When moments count: The two eye emergencies that demand constant intervention. *R.N.*, Vol. 44 No. 11, pp. 41–43.

Ellis RA (1981) Advances in cataract surgery. *Occup. Health Nurs.*, Vol. 29 No. 7, pp. 34–38.

Gaston NC (1981) Kerato refractive surgery: new horizon. *AORN J.*, Vol. 33 No. 6, pp. 1068–1074.

Gillin SE (1981) Simple nursing procedures for the occupational health nurse. *Occup. Health Nurs.*, Vol. 29 No. 6, pp. 18–20.

Hayes PL (1981) Treatment and nursing care of corneal disease. *Nurs. Clin. N. Am.*, Vol. 16 No. 3, pp. 383–392.

King RC (1982) Taking a close look at the eye. *R.N.*, Vol. 45 No. 2, pp. 48–56.

Levenson L & Levenson J (1977) Corneal transplantation. *Am. J. Nurs.*, Vol. 77 No. 7, pp. 1160–1163.

Jeglum EL (1981) Ocular therapeutics. *Nurs. Clin. N. Am.*, Vol. 16 No. 3, pp. 453–477.

McCoy K (1981) Cataracts and intraocular lenses: from cloudy to clear. *Nurs. Clin. N. Am.*, Vol. 16 No. 3, pp. 405–414.

Norman S (1982) The pupil check. *Am. J. Nurs.*, Vol. 82 No. 4 pp. 588–591.

O'Cauaghan B & Wright M (1983) Structure and function of the eye. *Nurs. 2*, No. 17, pp. 485–512.

Pearce V (1981) Sensory changes in old age. *Nurs. 1*, No. 25, pp. 1111.

Rowley RS (1981) Chemical and thermal burns of the eye. *Occup. Health Nurs.*, Vol. 29 No. 6, pp. 28–30.

Schneeman YT & Taylor JA (1981) A technical look at vitrectomy. *AORN J.*, Vol. 33 No. 5, pp. 867–872.

Shreeve C (1985) Understanding glaucoma. *Nurs. Mirror*, Vol. 160 No. 17, pp. 18–19.

Stern EJ (1980) Helping the person with low vision. *Am. J. Nurs.*, Vol. 80 No. 10, pp. 1788–1790.

Sullivan N (1983) Vision in the elderly: coping with declining visual function. *J. Gerontol. Nurs.*, Vol. 9 No. 4, pp. 228–235.

Watkinson S (1985) Dry eye syndrome. *Nurs. Times*, Vol. 80 No. 43, pp. 32–35.

Wolf MA (1981) The management of corneal abrasions and corneal foreign bodies. *Occup. Health Nurs.*, Vol. 29 No. 6, pp. 32–33.

29

Nursing in Disorders of the Ear

Structure and Functions of the Ear

The ear is concerned with the special sense of hearing as well as with the maintenance of equilibrium. It has three divisions: the external and middle ears for the collection and conduction of sound waves and the inner ear, which actually serves as the receptor. The eighth cranial (auditory or acoustic) nerve provides the afferent impulse pathway of the sensory unit. Part of its fibres carry imulses to the interpretive centres for sound in the temporal lobes, and the others transmit impulses to areas of the brain stem and cerebellum associated with control of body posture.

EAR STRUCTURE (Fig. 29.1)

External ear
The outer ear consists of the *auricle (pinna)* and the external auditory meatus. The auricle is an immobile cartilaginous framework covered with skin and may contribute slightly to the collection of sound waves. The external auditory meatus is an S-shaped tube approximately 2.5 cm (1 in) long. The tube ends at the tympanic membrane (eardrum), which separates the external and middle ears. The skin lining the canal is covered with fine hairs near the opening and has special glands which produce a yellow waxy secretion called *cerumen* for protection against insects and dust particles. The *tympanic membrane* is a thin, semitransparent membrane covered externally with skin and internally with mucous membrane which is continuous with that which lines the middle ear cavity. The middle layer is composed of thin elastic and fibrous tissue. A white streak is normally seen extending from the periphery towards the centre; this is the handle of the malleus in the middle ear (Fig. 29.2).

Middle ear
This portion of the ear is contained within a small cavity in the temporal bone. the cavity communicates with the nasopharynx by means of the *auditory or Eustachian tube* and with the mastoid cells. The auditory tube permits the entrance of air into the middle ear; this equalizes the pressure on the internal surface of the eardrum with atmospheric pressure (that which is exerted on the external surface of the drum). The cavity is lined with mucous membrane which is continuous with that of the auditory tube and mastoid cells. The *mastoid cells* are small air spaces within the posterior portion of the temporal bone, just behind the middle ear. Obviously the continuity of the lining membrane provides a ready means for the spread of infection from the throat to the middle ear and from the middle ear to the mastoid.

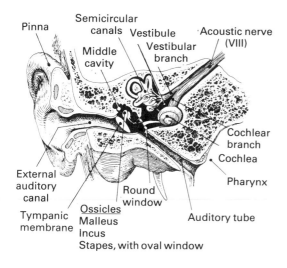

Fig. 29.1 The parts of the ear.

Pinna
Semicircular canals Vestibule Acoustic nerve (VIII)
Middle cavity Vestibular branch
External auditory canal
Tympanic membrane
Ossicles
Malleus
Incus
Stapes, with oval window
Round window
Cochlear branch
Cochlea
Pharynx
Auditory tube

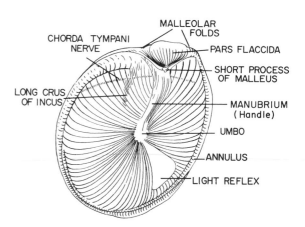

Fig. 29.2 Diagram of a tympanic membrane (eardrum).

CHORDA TYMPANI NERVE
MALLEOLAR FOLDS
PARS FLACCIDA
SHORT PROCESS OF MALLEUS
LONG CRUS OF INCUS
MANUBRIUM (Handle)
UMBO
ANNULUS
LIGHT REFLEX

The middle ear cavity contains three small bones called the auditory ossicles, which are movable for the purpose of transmitting sound vibrations. The first ossicle, the *malleus*, is attached to the eardrum and articulates with the second ossicle, the *incus*. The incus articulates with the third ossicle, the *stapes*, which is attached to the membranous oval window (fenestra ovalis) that leads into the inner ear. The middle ear also has two small muscles; one, the tensor tympani, is inserted on the malleus and the other, the stapedius, is inserted on the foot plate of the stapes. Contraction of these muscles reduces the amplitude of the sound waves entering the middle ear and cochlea.

Inner ear (labyrinth)
The inner ear consists of a system of irregularly shaped cavities which contain fluid and complex membranous structures which initiate nerve impulses as a result of sound waves or change of position. The *bony (osseous) labyrinth* is divided into a series of channels—the cochlea, vestibule and semicircular canals. Within the bony labyrinth is a membranous labyrinth which conforms fairly closely to the shape of the bony-walled cavities (Fig. 29.3). The fluid contained within the osseous cavities is called *perilymph*, and that within the membranous cavities is known as *endolymph*.

The complex snail-shaped structure, the *cochlea*, consists of three tubes wound two to three times around a central column called the modiolus. The channels formed by the tubes are called the scala vestibuli, scala media (cochlear duct) and scala tympani (Fig. 29.4). The scala vestibuli is closed at one end by the membrane of the oval window. As a result, vibrations transmitted to the membrane by the stapes set up waves in the fluid within the scala vestibuli. The scala vestibuli communicates with the scala tympani at the apex of the cochlea so that when the fluid within the scala vestibuli is set in motion,

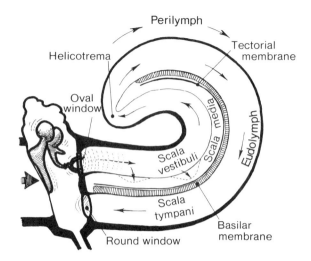

Fig. 29.4 Schematic drawing of the cochlea.

the fluid in the scala tympani is similarly affected. The base of the scala tympani is closed off by the membrane covering an opening into the middle ear which is known as the *round window (fenestra rotunda)*.

The scala media is walled off from the scala vestibuli by Reissner's membrane and from the scala tympani by the basilar membrane. On the surface of the basilar membrane are special cells with hair-like projections which collectively are known as the organ of Corti. Contained within the organ of Corti are receptor cells which produce auditory nerve impulses when stimulated by vibrations of the basilar membrane (see Fig. 29.5).

The *vestibule* lies between the cochlea and the semicircular canals. The bony-walled cavity contains perilymph. The suspended membranous portion is divided into two sacs, called the utricle and the saccule, which contain endolymph. Within these cavities are hair-like projections and calcium carbonate concretions (otoliths) which respond to movements of the head by giving rise to neural impulses concerned with the maintenance of equilibrium.

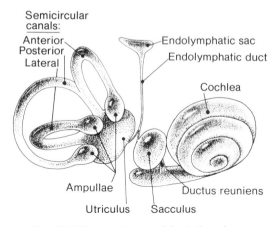

Fig. 29.3 The membranous labyrinth in the ear.

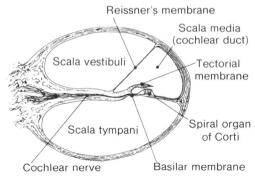

Fig. 29.5 Cross-section of the cochlea.

The third division of the inner ear consists of three *semicircular canals* hollowed out of the temporal bone at right angles to each other. They communicate with the osseous vestibule and contain perilymph. Three semicircular membranous ducts suspended within the osseous canals contain endolymph and communicate with the utricle. Each membranous semicircular canal has a dilated portion at one end, called the ampulla, which contains special sensory hair cells, forming the *crista acustica*, or crista ampullaris. The crista is sensitive to movement of the endolymph within the ampulla and initiates neural impulses that are transmitted by the vestibular portion of the acoustic (eighth cranial) nerve to the central nervous system.

AUDITORY PATHWAY

Sound waves passing into the external ear strike the tympanic membrane, causing it to vibrate with the same frequency as the sound waves. This in turn results in vibrations of the ossicles in the middle ear. The stapes, being attached to the oval window, causes its membrane to move in and out. The ossicles serve as amplifiers but, if the amplitude of the waves is excessive, producing excessive loudness, the vibrations may be modifed by contraction of the tensor tympani and the stapedius. The tensor tympani decreases tympanic membrane contractions and the stapedius pulls the stapes away from the oval window, reducing the force of the vibrations which strike the oval window. The vibrations are transferred into the perilymph of the scala vestibuli of the inner ear and in turn through the Reissner's membrane and through the endolymph in the scala media to the basilar membrane. Movements of the endolymph and basilar membrane stimulate the receptor cells of the organ of Corti, initiating neural impulses which are transmitted via nerve fibres to a ganglion in the central core (the modiolus) of the cochlea. The axons of the ganglionic neurons form the cochlear branch of the acoustic (eighth cranial) nerve. The cochlear branch synapses with a group of neurons in the medulla (cochlear nucleus). The impulses are then transmitted to the inferior colliculi which are the centres for auditory startle reflexes, through the thalami and eventually reach a cortical area of the temporal lobe (auditory centre) where they are interpreted as sound. Each ear delivers impulses to both auditory centres.

The movements of the perilymph, initiated by the vibrations of the oval window, are transmitted through the helicotrema (communicating channel between the scalae at the apex of the cochlea) to the scala tympani and subsequently to the membrane of the fenestra rotunda (round window).

PITCH AND INTENSITY OF SOUND

The pitch of a sound depends upon the frequency of the vibrations (number per second). The number of vibrations or cycles per second (cps) are expressed as a unit of frequency referred to as a hertz (Hz) which is used in measuring the pitch of sound. The fibres of the basilar membrane vary in length. It is thought that different frequencies stimulate selective areas of fibres and cells of the membrane—that is, each place on the basilar membrane is sensitive to sound waves of a certain frequency.

The intensity, or loudness, of a sound depends upon the amplitude or force of movement of the vibrations. The louder the sound, the greater is the displacement back and forth.

PHYSICAL EQUILIBRIUM

When the head moves, neural impulses originate in the crista acustica of the semicircular canals and the maculae acusticae of the utricle and saccula and are transmitted by nerve fibres which form the vestibular branch of the acoustic nerve. The vestibular nerve fibres pass to groups of neurons (vestibular nuclei) in the brain stem from which impulses may be delivered to the cerebellum, reticular formation, down the vestibulospinal tracts to motor neurons which innervate skeletal muscle, the oculomotor centre and the thalami. The principal purpose of these impulses is to orient the person in space, and reflexly stimulate muscles so that he may assume an upright position or maintain the position that has been assumed against gravity.

Nursing Process

Assessment

A HEALTH HISTORY

Illness history. A nursing assessment of a patient with an ear disorder involves collecting information regarding previous ear disease or surgery that may have altered the normal architecture of the ear, history of ear infections, trauma and complications including perforation of the eardrum and aural discharge.

Any history of associated symptoms is recorded [i.e. upper respiratory tract infections, dizziness, (vertigo) tinnitus, hearing loss].

Medications. Information is obtained about exposure to ototoxic drugs that may produce hearing loss, dizziness or tinnitus. Common examples of such drugs are acetylsalicylic acid (aspirin) and aminoglycosides.

Family history of hearing loss and the type of hearing loss is obtained; congenital malformation of the auditory system and sensorineural damage may account for the loss of hearing.

Present disorder. The reason for seeking health care is identified. The manifestations being experienced and the duration and severity of the smyptoms are determined. It is important to identify what the patient perceives as the problem and if someone else prompted him to seek care.

SOCIAL HISTORY AND BEHAVIOURAL CHANGES

Behavioural clues are often important indicators of hearing loss. Does the patient avoid social or work situations where several persons are talking at the same time? Have friends, relatives or the patient noticed evidence of inattentiveness, strained facial expressions, frequent requests to repeat instructions, increased volume of the radio or television, complaints about others mumbling, or postural change such as leaning forward or turning the head to one side to hear? Language development and school record are assessed if the patient is a child.

Use of hearing aids. It is important to document the use of a hearing aid and to communicate this to all health-care personnel working with the patient.

PHYSICAL EXAMINATION

Physical examination of the ear may include inspection of the external ear, tests for Eustachian tube patency, evaluation of hearing, labyrinth tests, 'mastoid x-rays', blood tests and cultures. Obviously, the selection of investigational procedures depends upon the presenting signs and symptoms.

Inspection of the external ear
The ear is inspected inside and outside. The pinna (auricle) is examined for size, position, symmetry and lesions, and the mastoid process is palpated, especially if infection of the middle ear is suspected. The entrance of the ear canal is inspected for presence of debris or pus. The inside of the auditory canal is inspected with an auriscope (otoscope) which has a magnifying lens in addition to a light. The canal is inspected for lesions, foreign bodies and the amount and characteristics of the cerumen (wax). The tympanic membrane is viewed and the colour and tension noted (normal: light pearl-grey). It is examined for retraction or bulging, increased vascularity and perforation(s). During examination of the tympanic membrane, the patient is asked to take a breath and then to try to exhale forcibly through the nose with it tightly pinched and the lips closed. The normal Eustachian tube opens to admit air into the middle ear and the tympanic membrane may be seen to move outward. This latter procedure is referred to as Valsalva's manoeuvre (autoinflation) for testing the patency of the Eustachian tube.

HEARING EVALUATION

In hearing evaluation, the examiner assesses the degree of hearing loss and establishes whether it is due to conductive or sensorineural impairment. Conductive deafness results from failure of the conducting mechanism to transmit sound impulses from the external ear to the inner ear fluids. Sensorineural deafness can be a result of disease of the sensor organ (the cochlea), auditory nerve or auditory cerebral centre.

Hearing screening. A quick evaluation of hearing acuity can be made using whispered and spoken voice tests[1] and watch ticking. The patient occludes one ear while the examiner is positioned to the side with the lips 1 metre (3 feet) from the patient's unoccluded ear. The examiner exhales and softly whispers numbers which the patient is asked to repeat. A medium and then a loud whisper are used, and then, if necessary, a soft, medium and louder voice until the patient hears. The ability to hear high-frequency sounds is estimated by slowly moving a watch away from the patient's unoccluded ear and indicating when the ticking sound is no longer heard. The patient's hearing acuity is compared to that of the examiner which is presumed to be within normal range.

Tuning fork tests. These are used to differentiate the type of deafness. The tuning fork may produce a frequency of 512 or 1024 cycles per second (cps). The tests should be made in a room free of noise.
- *Rinne test.* A tuning fork of 512 Hz is struck and held 2.5–5.0 cm (1–2 in) in front of the patient's external auditory canal. It is then placed firmly on the mastoid process and the patient is asked to state whether it is heard better by bone conduction (BC) or air conduction (AC).

  A more accurate method of performing the Rinne test is to hold the tuning fork 2.5–5.0 cm (1–2 in) in front of the external auditory meatus; the patient is asked to say when he can no longer hear it. It is then placed on the mastoid process and the patient states whether or not he can still hear it; if he cannot, air conduction is better than bone conduction—a positive Rinne. Conversely if the tuning fork can be heard by bone conduction, then bone conduction is better than air conduction—a negative Rinne.

  In the normal ear air is a better conductor than bone (i.e. positive Rinne).
- *Weber's test.* This test is used to compare the degree of impaired hearing in the two ears. The tuning fork is set in vibration; the stem is held

---

[1] *Voice tests.* The patient's ability to hear the normal speaking voice and then the whispered voice is tested in a room free of sounds. The ear opposite to the one being tested is covered. The normal ear can hear the spoken word at 7 m (20 feet) and the whisper at 5 m (15 feet).

against the middle of the forehead or the vortex and the patient is asked if he hears the sound better in one ear than the other. Normally, the sound appears to be in the midline, being heard equally by both ears. If conductive deafness is present the sound is greater in the affected ear. If the sound is heard equally well in both ears, the hearing loss is the same in both ears.

In sensorineural loss of hearing, the sound will be localized in the normal ear.

Thus, if the sound is louder in one ear there may be conductive loss of hearing in that ear or there may be a sensorineural deafness in the other ear.

• *Schwabach test*. This test compares the patient's bone conduction with that of the examiner, whose hearing is normal. The tuning fork is set in vibration and the stem is placed against the patient's mastoid process. The patient is instructed to indicate when the sound becomes inaudible. The stem of the tuning fork is then transferred to the mastoid bone of the examiner. If the sound is still audible to the latter, the patient has some sensorineural loss of hearing.

Audiometric tests. These tests provide information as to the degree of hearing loss. The unit used to express the intensity (or loudness) of sound is the *decibel (dB)*. The audiometer is operated to produce sounds of known intensity and frequency (cps). Hearing is evaluated by recording the minimum intensity of sounds of various frequencies that are just audible to the patient. A normal adult ear is most sensitive to frequencies of 500–4000 Hz or cps. The normal ear in a child and young adult is sensitive to frequencies much lower and much higher. A soft whisper suggests about 20 dB; speech in normal conversation ranges from 55–60 dB.

Audiometric tests are conducted in a soundproof room and the patient wears earphones. The audiometric methods of assessing hearing that are commonly used are the pure-tone and speech tests.

• *Pure-tone audiometry*. The audiometer produces a range of pure tones of varying frequencies (cps or Hz). The intensity is adjusted in 5-decibel steps. The procedure is explained to the patient before the earphones are put on, and he is instructed as to when and how to signal. The test commences with a sound of high intensity which is gradually reduced to below the patient's threshold of hearing sound. The patient signals when the sound disappears. The intensity then is increased very slowly until the patient signals that the tone is just discernible. A range of frequencies is used, and the threshold intensity for each frequency is recorded on a chart called an audiogram. This indicates any hearing loss and the range of tones most affected. The test may be made of bone or air conduction. The greater the number of decibels recorded at which sound is perceived, the greater is the degree of defective hearing.

• *Speech audiometry*. In this test, a recording of lists of words representing normal vocabulary sound is played at varying volumes. The patient indicates the words he hears. The percentage of words correctly heard for each intensity is recorded.

TESTS FOR VESTIBULAR FUNCTION[2]

Tests used to assess the function of the vestibular system of the internal ear involve observing responses to certain stimuli. Strong stimulation normally produces vertigo or the falling to one side, nystagmus (involuntary, rhythmic eye movement) and nausea.

Rotation test. The patient is seated in a chair that can be rotated, with the head tilted forward and the eyes closed. The chair is rotated quickly for ten full turns and stopped suddenly. The patient is asked to look at the doctor's finger which is held in front of the patient. Nystagmus is a normal response and its duration is timed. It should continue for about 25–40 seconds.

Caloric test. This test is also used in neurological investigation of the vestibular portion of the acoustic (VIII) nerve (see p. 786). The patient lies recumbent with the head raised at 30°. Water at 7°C above or below body temperature is injected into the external auditory canal and the patient observed for nystagmus. The nystagmus is timed, and past-pointing and testing for swaying to one side may be done. The test is carried out in each ear. The normal response to cold water is rotary nystagmus away from the ear being tested. If hot water is used, the normal movement of the eyes is toward the ear being irrigated. Pathological disturbances in the labyrinth may result in an absence of responses or excessive reaction.

Electronystagmography. This is an electroencephalographic recording of the eye movements in nystagmus. A study is made of the frequency, speed and amplitude of the eye movements. The recording is carried out in darkness or with the eyes closed to prevent fixation which suppresses nystagmus.

RADIOLOGICAL EXAMINATION

Mastoid x-rays may be done to determine if mastoiditis has developed.

---

[2] *Note*: Since the vestibular function tests may cause vertigo, nausea and vomiting, the nurse remains with the patient, prepared to provide the necessary support and assistance. Precautions are taken to prevent possible falls when the patient moves or attempts to walk.

Blood examinations
Leucocyte and differential cell counts may be ordered if acute infection of the middle ear or labyrinthitis is suspected. In the case of acute infection and inflammation, the leucocyte count is usually above normal, the increase being principally in neutrophils.

Culture
Any discharge from the ear is usually cultured as soon as observed in order to identify the causative organism. Sensitivity tests to antibiotics may also be done.

Manifestations of disorders of the ear

LOSS OF HEARING

The incidence of loss of hearing in varying degrees is very high and, in many instances, the person is unaware of it until it is well advanced. Hearing limitations interfere with the ability to communicate with others, which is extremely important. It may also result in the individual not being alerted to a threatening object or situation. Obviously, the effects and problems vary with the degree of loss and the age at which it developed. In the child, it retards development, affecting the learning of speech and normal adjustment within society. It creates physical, emotional and socioeconomic problems for both the person and family.

The degree of loss of hearing may be indicated by classifying those affected as 'hard of hearing' or 'deaf'. The hearing is defective in those who are hard of hearing but is not totally absent. They have sufficient hearing, either with or without the use of a hearing aid, to cope with ordinary activities. Persons who are described as deaf have a marked or total loss of hearing that makes it very difficult, if not impossible, to function normally.

Manifestations of impaired hearing
Indications of a hearing deficit may include failure to respond when addressed, frequent requests for repetition, and misinterperetation of what was said, especially of words that sound alike. A short attention span or lack of attention, lack of interest, a strained confused expression, turning of the head to direct the 'good' ear to the source of sound, irritability and fatigue because of the strain and withdrawal from the group may be manifested. The person who is hard-of-hearing may hesitate to acknowledge the handicap and may feign hearing when actually he does not hear. In some instances the person may talk continuously to avoid the situation of someone else speaking and his not being able to hear what is said. Changes in speech, such as a lack of inflections, and

a low or excessive volume, may also develop. A person with conductive deafness tends to speak softly; the person with nerve deafness usually speaks loudly.

In the case of a child, impaired hearing may be suspected if there is a failure in the development of speech, a lack of normal progress in school, no response to voice or sound, or no interest in noise-making toys. The severity of the speech defect depends on when the hearing deficit developed and the degree of loss. If the person is partially deaf with loss for high frequency (high pitched) sounds, he may hear vowels but not consonants. The deaf child responds more readily to movements than to sound and, when in need of comfort and reassurance, responds to cuddling or touch rather than to verbal expressions. He may develop and persistently use gestures to indicate needs or wishes rather than producing vocal expressions.

Classification and causes of loss of hearing
A hearing deficit may be congenital or acquired and may be classified as conductive, sensorineural, central or combined.

In a *conductive hearing loss*, sound waves fail to reach the internal ear as a result of some disturbance in the external ear, middle ear or the oval window (fenestra ovalis).

The person with conductive deafness tends to speak softly as he can hear himself.

In *sensorineural deafness*, which may also be called *nerve or perceptive deafness*, the disorder is located in the organ of Corti, cochlear division of the acoustic nerve, or auditory impulse pathway or centre within the brain.

The person with nerve deafness cannot hear anything, so he tends to shout, hoping to hear himself.

Central hearing loss denotes a hearing deficit resulting from disturbances within the brain, principally the auditory centre in the temporal lobe.

Combined hearing loss occurs because of impairment within both the conductive and neural auditory mechanisms.

Congenital loss of hearing may be due to a prenatal malformation or lack of development of a part of the auditory apparatus. Heredity may play a role, or it may be the result of a viral infection in the mother during the first trimester of the pregnancy, the effect of a toxic drug taken by the mother during pregnancy, hypoxia or a birth injury.

Acquired impairment of hearing may be caused by obstruction of the external auditory canal by a foreign body or impacted cerumen, infection (e.g. otitis media, labyrinthitis, meningitis), a neoplasm (e.g. acoustic neuroma), an ototoxic drug (e.g. streptomycin, quinine), trauma associated with a skull fracture or excessively loud noise, obstruction of the Eustachian tube, or degenerative changes in the auditory pathway frequently associated with the ageing process (presbycusis).

TINNITUS

Tinnitus or ringing in the ears may be unilateral or bilateral and constant or intermittent. It may be of high or low pitch and vary in quality from a humming, buzzing, hissing, roaring, popping or pulsating sound. The sound sensation experienced by the patient is without a relevant external stimulus. It is usually heard only by the patient and rarely by others. Tinnitus is not a disease but a symptom. It may be a symptom of any abnormal condition of the ear, may be associated with deafness, or it may be drug-related.

VERTIGO

Vertigo is a disturbance of equilibrium characterized by a sensation of movement or rotation of one's self or of one's surroundings. The patient experiences feelings of dizziness, light-headedness, falling or spinning. It may be accompanied by staggering or falling, clumsiness, nausea, vomiting and nystagmus which produces blurring of vision. It may occur suddenly, be transient in nature or recur as with Menière's syndrome. Disorders of the labyrinth are the most common cause. Disturbances in the pathways in the central nervous system may also produce vertigo.

OTALGIA (EARACHE)

Ear pain is usually severe and may be caused by infection, a neoplasm of the external or middle ear or may be referred pain from more distant disease processes. Inflammation of the middle ear produces pressure on the tympanic membrane and may lead to rupture. Obstruction of the Eustachian tube which is produced or aggravated by sudden changes in atmospheric pressure causes pain when the tympanic membrane is suddenly retracted.

OTORRHOEA

Otorrhoea is the term used for a discharge from an ear which may develop suddenly or gradually. It may be purulent, sanguineous, serous, waxy or mucoid in nature and may be associated with pain, vertigo, tinnitus and/or hearing loss. Causes include trauma and infection.

Identification of patient problems

The problem is a *sensory–perceptual alteration*; that is, an *auditory* deficit due to a disorder of one or both ears or the central nervous system.
The *goals* are to:
1 Preserve or maintain hearing
2 Identify factors contributing to hearing loss
3 Maintain or develop ability to communicate with others.

PRESERVATION OF HEARING

Nurses, especially those working with industrial workers and schoolchildren, have an important role in the prevention of hearing loss. The public requires education about the causes and early signs of impaired hearing and significant preventive measures.

Good prenatal care and the avoidance of contact with persons with measles or other viral infections are important in preventing congenital deafness. Immunization against measles should be promoted. Prompt treatment of respiratory infection and infectious diseases may allay the complication of otitis media. Prompt medical treatment and follow-up are urged for persons with an ear disorder.

The danger of introducing foreign objects into the external ear canal should be emphasized; for example, cleansing the ear with applicators, matches and hairpins is dangerous, as accidental perforation of the eardrum may occur. If the wax (cerumen) becomes dry and impacted or an insect or foreign body becomes lodged in the canal, a few drops of warm oil or sodium bicarbonate may be instilled and followed by a warm water or sodium bicarbonate irrigation in a few minutes. If this does not remove the foreign object or impacted wax, the person is advised to go to the doctor for advice.

Routine tests of schoolchildren's hearing are important so that early recognition may be made of any impairment. Teachers and school nurses must be familiar with manifestations of a hearing deficit.

The nurse caring for a patient receiving a preparation of streptomycin, kanamycin or other ototoxic drugs and quinine must be alert for early signs of damage to the hearing.

The occupational health nurse, especially in an industry in which there is prolonged, intense noise in the work environment, must be cognizant of the possibility of noise-induced hearing loss. Frequently the employees tend to accept noise simply as a necessary part of the occupation and do not realize that hearing damage may be insidiously developing. Gradual loss of hearing usually involves, first, failure of response to high frequency sounds. Later, areas of the cochlea which respond to lower frequencies become damaged. In order to protect persons exposed to noise that endangers hearing, protective devices in the form of earmuffs, ear plugs or a special helmet should be provided. Employees should receive regular hearing tests and be exposed to an active educational programme.

High intensity music such as 'rock' music is another source of noise pollution. Frequent exposure to the noise of firearms may also lead to hearing loss. Public education about the effects of noise pollution and the importance of the use of ear plugs or earmuffs to decrease the intensity of the noise is necessary and should be directed to high-risk groups.

- Do not speak until you have the person's attention. The speaker's face should be in full view of the listener so that he has the opportunity to observe lip movement.
- Determine which is the better ear and go to that side if possible. Look directly at the listener.
- Speak slowly, enunciate clearly and avoid raising the pitch of voice. The volume is increased, but actual shouting is avoided. Guard against running words together. The natural form of conversation is used rather than broken statements and incomplete sentences.
- Exaggerated lip movement only confuses the listener.
- If repetition is necessary, rephrasing the communication may be helpful; remember that vowels are heard more readily than consonants.
- Patience, tact and understanding are needed. Avoid any irritation or annoyance; such reactions on the part of the speaker only discourage the listener.
- Do not prolong a conversation unnecessarily, since the listener tires under the strain.
- If a hearing aid is used, give the person time to adjust it. Do not get within 4–5 feet of the aid and use natural volume and tone.
- A misinterpretation must not be ridiculed or treated as a joke.
- When a deaf person enters a room, an effort is made to draw him into the group. He is advised of the topic of conversation and is encouraged and given the opportunity to participate. Otherwise, he tends to withdraw and become isolated.
- If it is not possible to communicate verbally, write the message. In hospital it is necessary to go to the patient's room in response to a call-button; sounds transmitted by the intercommunication system are distorted to the hard-of-hearing.
- If a patient is totally deaf and does not lip-read, pictures or symbols that represent objects may be helpful to orient the patient and for use during hospitalization.

SUGGESTIONS TO THOSE WHO ARE HARD OF HEARING

- Look directly at the speaker (preferably in a good light) since observation of lip movements proves helpful.
- Concentrate on the speaker.
- Observe the total situation, since this may give a lead to the topic of conversation.
- Acknowledge your hearing deficit; do not guess at things rather than ask for repetition.
- Indicate understanding of the speaker.

HEARING AIDS

Some persons with a hearing deficit may be helped by using a hearing aid, which is a small, battery-operated instrument which amplifies sounds. Aids are helpful to persons who have reduced conduction of sound waves into the inner ear. Few of those with sensorineural loss of hearing receive help from hearing aids; amplification of sound does not assist with the distortion and impaired discrimination resulting from impairment of the neural elements of the auditory apparatus. Before purchasing a hearing aid, the person with a hearing deficit should be examined by a doctor for evaluation of the residual hearing and identification of the type of hearing loss. The selection of the aid is based on the patient's particular type of hearing loss. If an aid is recommended, it should be worn for a trial period to determine if it does help.

AUDITORY AND SPEECH TRAINING

Auditory training is intended to help the individual utilize residual hearing effectively and improve communication skills. The process helps the patient develop good listening skills and increases his awareness of sounds and other clues.

Lip-reading or speech reading is the process of interpreting spoken words through the study of lip movements, facial expressions, body movements and gestures used in speech. Training helps the individual consciously and effectively use these cues.

Speech training is provided to maintain existing speech skills which deteriorate when the usual monitoring mechanism of hearing is lost. Hearing is necessary to assess loudness, clarity, tone and rate of speech. The congenitally deaf child requires a different type of programme to develop speech and language skills.

COMMUNITY RESOURCES

Those who are deaf or hard of hearing and their families should be familiar with the Royal National Institute for the Deaf and Hard Of Hearing.[3] Assistance may be provided in the form of procuring medical examination and treatment, counselling as to the type of hearing aid that would be helpful, obtaining vocational training and employment, arranging for special classes (e.g. speech) and obtaining printed advice in pamphlets.

Expected outcomes

The patient should:
1 Understand the factors which contribute to hearing impairment.
2 Describe health practices to preserve hearing.
3 Understand how to obtain a hearing aid (if relevant).

---

[3] The Royal National Institute for the Deaf and Hard Of Hearing, 105 Gower Street, London WC1E 6AH.

4 Understand how to use and care for his hearing aid.

5 Understand that he may need an auditory or speech training programme (if relevant).

6 Apply acquired skills in communicating with others if he so wishes.

7 Be informed about the local branch of the Royal National Institute for the Deaf and Hard Of Hearing.

Common Disorders of the Ear

Impacted cerumen

The normal secretion of the external auditory canal (cerumen) may accumulate and become hard and dry. The retention may be due to abnormal narrowness of the canal, dryness of the skin or excess hair in the canal or misguided attempts to clean the ear with cotton-wool buds. It may also be associated with the person's occupation; it is a common problem for those working in a dusty or dry environment.

Symptoms develop with the obstruction of the canal; the person may experience a sense of fullness, noises, loss of hearing, irritation or, rarely, a cough. The latter is a reflex response to stimulation of the vagus nerve. Examination of the ear with an otoscope reveals a firm yellow or dark mass.

Removal of the mass may be by irrigation with warm water. It is important that any solution introduced into the ear be warmed to approximately 38°C (100°F); cold or hot solutions may stimulate the labyrinth and cause nystagmus, vertigo and nausea. It may be necessary to soften the wax prior to syringing. Instillation of sodium bicarbonate ear drops are recommended. If the mass cannot be removed by irrigation, the doctor may remove it with a Jobson–Horne probe.

Otitis externa

This is a generalized inflammation of the external ear that may vary in severity from a mild dermatitis to cellulitis. The tympanic membrane may be affected. The causative factor is usually bacteria but, in some instances, may be a fungus (otomycosis). A predisposing factor is moisture in the ear. The incidence is higher in summer and may result from swimming in contaminated water (swimmer's ear). The infection is more likely to develop in a warm moist atmosphere or if the person swims frequently. It may be secondary to trauma inflicted by efforts to remove wax. External otitis may also be due to allergic dermatitis. Some people are prone to otitis externa because of a narrow external canal.

Symptoms

The patient may complain of pruritus if the disorder is dermatitis, and the skin may be dry and scaly at first. If the cause is infection, the ear is painful and examination may reveal redness, swelling, oedema of the walls of the auditory meatus and often the tympanic membrane and purulent lesions. An elevation of temperature and increased leucocyte count indicate a serious infection.

Treatment

Scrupulous aural cleansing is performed, and a swab obtained for culture; the topical application of an antibiotic preparation is prescribed in the case of infection of the canal. If allergic dermatitis is the cause a corticosteroid ointment or solution may be prescribed. Inflammation of the auricle (pinna) may be treated by warm compresses.

The patient with severe infectious otitis which has extended beyond the skin receives an oral or parenteral antimicrobial preparation as well as local treatment. An analgesic may also be necessary to provide relief from the pain. The patient should be advised to keep the ear dry and not to touch the ear. Antihistamines may be indicated to relieve irritation in dermatitis, especially at night.

Acute otitis media

This is an inflammation of the middle ear and is frequently a complication of an upper respiratory tract infection or an infectious disease in measles. Often the organisms gain access through the auditory tube and, less frequently, through a perforation in the tympanic membrane. The disorder is usually acute but may become chronic.

The initial inflammatory response causes congestion and swelling of the mucous membrane lining of the middle ear, and the cavity fills with exudate. The tympanic membrane bulges externally and, unless the infection is checked, the exudate generally becomes purulent. If the cavity is not surgically drained, the tympanic membrane may rupture spontaneously.

Manifestations

The patient with otitis media experiences a sensation of fullness in the ear and dullness of hearing at first, then severe pain, and increasing loss of hearing because of failure of the conduction of sound waves through the middle ear. The temperature and leucocyte count are elevated, and the patient feels generally ill. Examination of the eardrum by means of an auriscope reveals redness, hyperaemia and external bulging due to the pressure of the collection of exudate in the middle ear, or rupture and discharge in the advanced stage.

Treatment

The patient is given an antibiotic and a nasal vaso-constrictor is administered to dilate the auditory tubes. A mild analgesic may be taken to alleviate pain. The eardrum may occasionally be surgically opened to permit drainage if the exudate is producing excessive pressure on the eardrum and there is danger of spontaneous rupture. The operative procedure is referred to as a *myringotomy*. Incision and drainage is preferable to leaving the condition until there is spontaneous rupture of the tympanic membrane. Delayed treatment of acute otitis media may predispose to mastoiditis, chronic otitis media and permanent hearing loss.

The patient having a myringotomy receives a local anaesthetic. Fluid is aspirated from the middle ear cavity through the incision, and a culture is taken. Absorbent cotton may be placed loosely in the outer ear to absorb the drainage. The patient is encouraged to lie on the affected side to promote drainage. A persistent elevation of temperature, pain and deep tenderness in the region of the mastoid, headache, drowsiness or disorientation is reported to the doctor. These may indicate the onset of a serious complication such as mastoiditis, meningitis or brain abscess.

Serous otitis media

Serous otitis media is characterized by an accumulation of fluid in the middle ear. The effusion is usually caused by obstruction of the Eustachian tube incurred by enlarged adenoids, severe nasopharyngitis or an allergic reaction. It may also develop following acute otitis media that has not been completely resolved. Rarely, the condition may be associated with a benign or malignant neoplasm of the nasopharynx or pharynx which blocks the Eustachian tube.

The fluid is a thin and watery transudate. Blockage of the Eustachian tube results in a negative pressure in the middle ear cavity which promotes movement of fluid out of the mucous membrane capillaries.

Manifestations

The patient experiences loss of hearing and discomfort in the affected ear. Examination of the eardrum reveals its immobility and an air-fluid level in the middle ear. The nasopharyngeal area is investigated for disease that is the likely primary cause.

Treatment

Any nasopharyngeal disorder is corrected; for example, if hypertrophied adenoids are found to be the cause, an adenoidectomy is performed. The allergic reaction is treated if it is found to be the problem. If nasopharyngitis due to infection is obstructing the auditory tube, the patient receives antibiotic therapy.

A myringotomy is done and the fluid aspirated.

This may be followed by repeated Valsalva manoeuvres to clear the Eustachian tube (see p. 1089) and ventilate the middle ear. Following the myringotomy, a plastic indwelling tympanostomy tube (grommet) may have to be inserted via the external auditory canal. This permits continuous ventilation and drainage of the middle ear (see Figs. 29.6 and 29.7). The tube is left in position until patency of the auditory tube is re-established; this may be a period of several weeks or months. The patient is closely supervised following the surgery. Usually he is seen in the outpatient department 6 weeks postoperatively, then every 3 months, when the tube and the patient's hearing are checked.

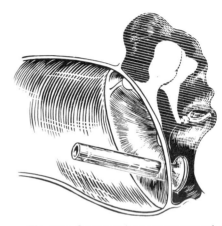

Fig. 29.6 Grommet (tympanostomy tube).

When the tube is inserted the nurse instructs the patient, and the parents if the patient is a child, about the care of the affected ear and the restrictions on activities. If the doctor prescribes the instillation of drops, an explanation and demonstration are given to the parents, and an opportunity provided for one of them to carry out the procedure under supervision. They are cautioned that if the medication causes pain following the instillation, the procedure is discontinued and the surgeon contacted promptly. The surgeon is also notified immediately of any increase or change in the fluid drainage, increasing deafness or pain. The patient must guard against getting water into the ear. During a bath or shower, a cotton ball coated with petroleum jelly is placed in the entrance to the ear canal. Swimming is allowed after the first 6 weeks and with the surgeon's consent. The ear should be prepared as for a bath or shower, and the patient is cautioned against diving.

Chronic otitis media

This chronic inflammatory disorder of the ear is associated with a permanent perforation of the tympanic membrane. It usually is a sequela of repeated episodes of acute otitis media that were not treated or

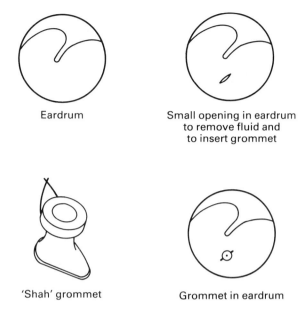

Eardrum

Small opening in eardrum
to remove fluid and
to insert grommet

'Shah' grommet

Grommet in eardrum

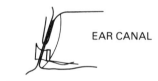

EAR CANAL

Grommet tube seen in cross section

Fig. 29.7 The grommet tube.

were caused by virulent or antibiotic-resistant organisms. The perforation may also be the result of mechanical trauma or blast injury.

The location of the perforation is an important factor in the seriousness of the disease. If it is central or at least does not involve the margin of the eardrum, the perforation is less serious and can be treated more effectively. This type of perforation is categorized as *tubotympanic*. If the perforation involves the tympanic margin in the posterior-superior area, the disorder is a more serious and life-threatening problem. There are usually several perforations and, because of their location, may be referred to as *attic perforations*.

Manifestations
The otitis media associated with a central perforation is manifested by purulent discharge with an offensive odour. The discharge may be greatly increased during periods of acute upper respiratory infections or if water gets into the ear during bathing or swimming. Over a period of time, middle ear structures are damaged by the infection and necrosis. There is usually some impairment of hearing which worsens during exacerbations.

Treatment
The initial treatment of the patient with a *tubotympanic perforation* is directed towards eliminating any upper respiratory tract infection as well as that in the ear. An antibiotic is administered orally or parenterally. The ear is cleansed by suction and dry mopping, followed by the instillation of an antimicrobial solution. If the exudate is excessive, it may be removed by daily aspiration by the doctor. When the infection is cleared up, the perforated area very occasionally fills in with scar tissue. If the perforation persists, a tympanoplasty may be done to improve the patient's hearing and reduce the risk of reinfection by establishing a barrier between external and middle ears. The type of surgical procedure used depends upon whether there is damage to the middle ear structures or not and, if so, the extent of the involvement. Tympanoplastic surgery is only undertaken if infection is controlled.

Tympanoplasty Type I indicates a myringoplasty in which a graft is used to repair the perforated eardrum when the middle ear structures are intact and functional. Epithelium from the ear canal, skin from the postauricular area, fascia stripped from the temporal muscle or a section of a vein may be used as a graft. Tympanoplasty Types II, III, IV, and V operative procedures involve plastic correction of the perforated eardrum and repair of damaged middle ear structures. The operations progressively increase in complexity, involving more extensive surgery and structural replacement. The reparative and/or reconstructive procedures are directed toward re-establishing a conductive system from the eardrum through the ossicles and the oval window and providing sound protection for the round window. Re-establishing ossicular continuity may necessitate the replacement of ossicles by a graft or a prosthesis.

Postoperatively, the pressure dressing is left undisturbed for 48 hours. If necessary, the outer part may be reinforced. Dressings are changed and the packing is removed by the surgeon. Precautions are taken to avoid wetting the dressing during bathing. The patient is asked not to blow his nose and to avoid coughing and sneezing to prevent air being forced through the Eustachian tube into the middle ear. When he first gets up, a nurse assists and remains with him for a while since he may experience dizziness and nausea.

In *marginal (attic) perforations*, the disease involves the bony rim of the tympanic membrane and the mastoid cells as well as the middle ear structures. An invasive *cholesteatoma* may develop; this is a mass that forms in the middle ear as a result of the growth of epithelial tissue implanted in the mddle ear from the collapsed and invaginated parts of the eardrum when it perforates. The inflammation causes hyper-activity of the basal layer of the epidermis. The epidermal tissue encloses sebum and desquamated epidermal cells; these serve as a good culture medium for organisms. The mass compresses middle ear structures and mastoid cells, causing necrosis and bone erosion. The presence of the cholesteatoma predisposes to the serious complications of labyrnthitis and brain abscess. Marginal perforation and the development of a cholesteatoma are treated by radical surgery. A mastoidectomy is done, the cholesteatoma and middle ear debris are removed and reconstruction undertaken to provide a conductive channel. The surgery is done in two stages; the first operation removes the cholesteatoma and clears out the infected and necrotic tissue. The patient receives antibiotic therapy and, when the area is free of infection and there is no drainage, the reconstructive plastic surgery is undertaken.

Mastoiditis

The small spaces (air cells) in the mastoid communicate with the middle ear cavity and are lined with mucous membrane which is continuous with that of the middle ear. As a result, infection may spread readily to the mastoid in acute or chronic otitis media. The patient experiences tenderness over the mastoid process, headache and fever. Mastoid x-rays show a cloudiness in the mastoid cells.

Treatment and nursing intervention
Generally, early treatment with antibiotics checks the infection and no residual damage to hearing occurs. Rarely, if the infection is neglected or is virulent and unresponsive to the antibiotic given, bone tissue of the mastoid becomes infected, necessitating surgery. A myringotomy and a simple mastoidectomy are done. A simple mastoidectomy involves an incision behind the auricle and the removal of the diseased bone by curettage.

If the patient develops chronic otitis media and chronic mastoiditis, more extensive surgery may be undertaken. A radical mastoidectomy involves the removal of the diseased mastoid tissue and the incus, malleus and remainder of the tympanic membrane, leaving the mastoid and middle ear as one large cavity. This surgery on the middle ear results in loss of hearing.

Preoperative preparation for a mastoidectomy is the same as that for any patient who is to have a general anaesthetic (see Chapter 11). The scalp is shaved 2 cm around the affected ear, and the long hair is combed toward the opposite side and secured.

Postoperatively, the pressure bandage remains intact for 48 hours. The meatal pack is left undisturbed until it is removed by the surgeon in the out-patient clinic 2 weeks postoperatively.

The patient is observed closely for nystagmus or any sign of facial paralysis. Facial paralysis is a threat in mastoidectomy because of the facial (seventh cranial) nerve's proximity to the operative site. Persisting headache, stiffness of the neck, elevation of temperature or disorientation is brought to the surgeon's attention, since it may indicate a complicating brain abscess or meningitis. Fluids are given freely and a regular diet is served as soon as it is tolerated.

The patient is generally allowed up on the evening of surgery or the following morning; someone remains with him at first in case of dizziness and nausea that may develop as a result of labyrinth disturbance, especially following a radical mastoidectomy.

If the patient suffers some hearing loss, he is reassured that assistance is available. The nurse advises him how he may help himself in trying to communicate with others and may also refer him to the Royal National Institute for the Deaf and Hard Of Hearing.

Otosclerosis

This is a chronic ear disease in which the stapes becomes immobilized because of progressive growth of bone tissue over the oval window and fixation of the stapes, interfering with the transmission of vibrations into the inner ear. Both ears are affected eventually.

The disease appears to be hereditary and has a higher incidence in females. The ability of the stapes to vibrate progressively decreases, and the loss of hearing usually becomes apparent in the teens or twenties, and during pregnancy. The person may complain of tinnitus as the deafness becomes more marked. The testing of hearing with a tuning fork reveals that the person has good bone conduction of sound but none by air.

Treatment
A hearing aid may be of some help for a period of time, but a stapedectomy has proved to be the treatment of choice at present. By means of a surgical microscope, the surgeon works through the external auditory canal and the middle ear. The stapes is removed, and a prosthesis introduced to transfer the vibrations of the incus through the oval window into the inner ear. Various forms of prostheses have been used and include a wire or teflon tube with a section of vein, a 'pad' of fat or Gelfoam. The teflon prosthesis is attached to the incus with its distal end in the oval window. The oval window niche is sealed using a free graft of fat or vein, and protected with Gelfoam. Only one ear is done at a time.

Postoperatively, dizziness and nausea may be troublesome because of the disturbance of the labyrinth. A specific directive is received from the surgeon about the position in which the head is to be maintained as practices vary in different hospitals. A close check is made for any sign of infection (elevation of temperature and leucocyte count, discharge and pain); if it is suspected, an antimicrobial drug is prescribed. The patient is instructed not to blow his nose to prevent air from being forced through the Eustachian tube to the middle ear. The patient is cautioned to move slowly and not to stoop over. If vertigo is experienced, ambulation may have to be delayed. The patient requires assurance that the dizziness is temporary. The patient should be observed closely for nystagmus or any sign of facial palsy.

Packing is placed in the ear upon completion of the surgery; this is removed by the surgeon in approximately 7–9 days. When the packing is removed, the patient may find the noise in the environment very confusing and disturbing. A nurse or family member should accompany him to provide support and reassurance.

Menière's disease or syndrome

This is a disorder of the internal ear characterized by recurrent attacks of severe vertigo, nausea, vomiting, tinnitus and a progressive loss of hearing. The cause is not known but an excess of endolymph (endolymphatic hydrops) resulting in increased pressure and dilation of the canals develops. Vascular spasm and allergic reaction have been suggested as possible aetiological factors. The disorder usually makes its appearance between the ages of 40 and 60 years, and occurs more often in males.

The episodes have a sudden onset, and the patient is generally prostrated by the dizziness and nausea. The duration of an attack varies from hours to days.

During an attack the patient remains in bed in a quiet environment. Cot-sides may be necessary for safety because of the vertigo. An antiemetic such as dimenhydrinate (Dramamine) and a sedative may provide some relief. Diphenhydramine hydrochloride (Benadryl) given intravenously may arrest an acute attack. In an effort to offset episodes, the patient is placed on a low-sodium diet and receives ammonium chloride; a diuretic such as hydrochlorothiazide (Esidrex) may also be prescribed to reduce the formation of endolymph. A vasodilator (e.g. nicotinic acid) to discourage vasospasm may be helpful. Recent usage of betahistine has provided good evidence that it is effective in Menière's disease, by increasing cochlear circulation. Although the acute attacks are episodic, the hearing loss tends to be permanent.

The condition can be very incapacitating and may necessitate surgery. The procedure entails the destruction of the membranous labyrinth. More recently, ultrasonic waves have been used. This form of treatment requires a mastoidectomy to permit the application of the probe. If the patient still has considerable hearing in the affected ear, ultrasonic treatment is used because it is thought to be less hazardous for the hearing.

References and Further Reading

BOOKS

Articles from the British Medical Journal (1981) *ABC of Ear Nose and Throat*. London: British Medical Association. pp. 1–28.

Ballantyne J (1977) *Deafness*. Edinburgh: Churchill Livingstone.

Ballantyne J & Groves J (eds) (1979) *Scott Brown's Diseases of the Ear Nose and Throat. Vol. 2: The Ear*, 4th ed., London: Butterworths.

Birrell JF (ed) (1982) *Logan Turner's Diseases of the Nose Throat and Ear*. Bristol: John Wright. pp. 286–443.

Browning GG (1982) *Updated ENT*. London: Butterworths. pp. 1–68.

Doyle J (ed) (1981) *No Need to Shout*. London: ITV.

Fields WL & McGinn-Campbell KM (1983) *Introduction to Health Assessment*. Reston, Virginia: Reston Publishing. Chapter 8.

Ganong WF (1985) *Review of Medical Physiology*, 11th ed., Los Altos, CA: Lange. Chapter 9.

Hawke M et al (1984) *Clinical Otoscopy*. Edinburgh: Churchill Livingstone.

Krupp MA & Chatton MJ (1983) *Current Medical Diagnosis and Treatment*. Los Altos, CA: Lange. pp. 93–100.

Marshall KG & Attia EL (1983) *Disorders of the Ear*. Boston: John Wright.

Miles EH (1980) *Lecture Notes on Diseases of the Ear Nose and Throat*. Oxford: Blackwell. pp. 1–85.

Nash & Nash (1981) *Deafness in Society*. Massachusetts: Lexington Books.

Nave CR & Nave BC (1985) *Physics for the Health Sciences*, 3rd ed., Philadelphia: WB Saunders. Chapter 18.

Smith LH & Thier SO (1985) *Pathophysiology*, 2nd ed. Philadelphia: WB Saunders. pp. 1113–1121.

PERIODICALS

Broder MI, Busis SN, Dewesse D, Friedman A & Lau FY (1981) Probing physical causes of dizziness. *Patient Care*, Vol. 15 No. 11, pp. 41–44, 49–51, 55–57, 61, 62, 64, 66–71, 75–79, 82–84, 86, 89, 90, 91, 95, 99–102.

Burton RC, Frederic MW, Pulec JL & Rubin W (1981) Evaluating complaints of dizziness. *Patient Care*, Vol. 15 No. 10, pp. 23–25, 28, 29, 33, 36, 43, 47, 54–56, 59–61.

Hanawalt A & Troutman K (1984) If your patient has a hearing aid. *Am. J. Nurs.*, Vol. 84 No. 7, pp. 900–901.

Hayes C (1981) Ergonomics: the body's reaction to noise. *Occup. Health*, Vol. 33 No. 1, pp. 75–83.

Heller BR & Gaynor EB (1981) Hearing loss and aural rehabilitation of the elderly. *Top. Clin. Nurs.*, Vol. 3 No. 1, pp. 21–29.

Holder L (1982) Hearing aids. *Nurs. '82*, Vol. 12 No. 4, pp. 64–67.

Malkiewicz J (1982) How to assess the ears and test hearing acuity. *R.N.*, Vol. 45 No. 3, pp. 56–63.

Morgan RH (1983) Breaking through the sound barrier. *Nurs. '83*, Vol. 13 No. 6, pp. 112–114.

Useful Addresses

Accept Clinic
200 Seagrave Road
London SW6

Age Concern England
60 Pitcairn Road
Mitcham
Surrey CR4 3LL

Al-Anon Family Groups UK
61 Dover Street
London SE1 4YF

Alcohol Concern
3 Grosvenor Crescent
London SW1 6LD

Alcoholics Anonymous
PO Box 514
11 Redcliffe Gardens
London SW10

Alzheimer's Disease Society
3rd Floor
Bank Building
Fulham Broadway
London SW6 1EP

Anorexia Aid
The Priory Centre
11 Priory Road
High Wycombe

Anorexic Family Aid
Sackville Place
44–48 Magdalen Street
Norwich
Norfolk NR3 1JE

Arthritis Care
6 Grosvenor Crescent
London SW1X 7ER

ASH
Margaret Pike House
5–11 Mortimer Street
London W1

Association for All Speech-Impaired
  Children
347 Central Markets
Smithfield
London EC1A 9NH

Association for Improvement in the
  Maternity Services
67 Lennard Road
London SE20 7LY

Association for Research into
  Restricted Growth
2 Mount Court
81 Central Hill
London SE19 1BS

Association for Spina Bifida and
  Hydrocephalus
Tavistock House North
Tavistock Square
London WC1H 9HJ

Association for the Prevention of
  Addiction
11 Grosvenor Street
Cardiff CF5 1NH

Association for the Promotion of
  Preconception Care
The Old Vicarage
Church Lane
Witley, Godalming
Surrey GU8 5PN

Association of British Adoption and
  Fostering Agencies
4 Southampton Row
London WC1B 4AA

Association of British Paediatric
  Nurses
c/o Central Nursing Office
The Hospital for Sick Children
Great Ormond Street
London WC1

Association of Carers
First Floor
21–23 New Road
Chatham
Kent ME4 4JQ

Association of Parents of
  Vaccine-Damaged Children
2 Church Street
Shipston-on-Stour
Warwickshire CV36 4AP

Birth Centre
16 Simpson Street
London SW11

British Association for Cancer United
  Patients (BACUP)
121 Charterhouse Street
London EC1

British Association for Counselling
37a Sheep Street
Rugby
Warwickshire CV21 3BX

British Council for the Rehabilitation of
  the Disabled
Tavistock House South
Tavistock Square
London WC1H 9LB

British Deaf Association
38 Victoria Place
Carlisle CA1 1HU

British Diabetic Association
10 Queen Anne Street
London W1M 0BD

British Epilepsy Association
3–6 Alfred Place
London WC1E 7EE

British Guild for Sudden Infant Death
  Study
Pathology Department
Royal Infirmary
Cardiff CF2 1SZ

British Heart Foundation
57 Gloucester Place
London W1H 4DH

British Medical Association
BMA House
Tavistock Square
London WC1

British Pregnancy Advisory Service
Austry Manor
Wootton Wawen
Solihull
West Midlands B95 6DA

British United Provident Association
24/27 Essex Street
London WC2

Brittle Bone Society
63 Byron Crescent
Dundee DD3 6SS

Brook Advisory Centre
233 Tottenham Court Road
London W1P 9AE

Canadian Nurses' Association
50 The Driveway
Ottawa
Canada K2P 1EA

Catholic Nurses' Guild of Great Britain
Bevendean Hospital
Brighton
East Sussex

Central Midwives Board
39 Harrington Gardens
London SW7 5JY

Central Midwives Board for Scotland
24 Dublin Street
Edinburgh EH1 3PU

Chest and Heart Association
Tavistock House North
Tavistock Square
London WC1H 9HJ

Children's Chest Circle
Tavistock House North
Tavistock Square
London WC1

Cleft Lip and Palate Association
Dental Department
The Hospital for Sick Children
Great Ormond Street
London SW1U 1PB

Coeliac Society
PO Box 220
High Wycombe
Bucks HP11 2HY

Colostomy Welfare Group
38–39 Eccleston Square
London SW1V 1PB

Committee on Safety of Drugs
Finsbury Square House
33/37a Finsbury Square
London EC2

Compassionate Friends
2 Norden Road
Blandford

Council for the Education and Training
   of Health Visitors
Clifton House
Euston Road
London NW1 2RS

Cruse
Cruse House
126 Sheen Road
Richmond
Surrey TW9

Cystic Fibrosis Trust
5 Blythe Road
Bromley
Kent BR1 3RS

Department of Health and Social
   Security
Alexander Fleming House
Elephant and Castle
London SE1 6BY

Depressives Associated
19 Merley Ways
Wimborne Minster
Dorset BH21 12N

Down's Syndrome Association
12–13 Clapham Common Southside
London SW4 7AA

Drink Watchers
200 Seagrave Road
London SW6

Emergency Bed Service
24 Nutsford Place
London W1H 6AN

English National Board for Nursing,
   Midwifery and Health Visiting
Victory House
170 Tottenham Court Road
London W1P 0HA

Families Anonymous
88 Caledonian Road
London N1

Family Planning Association
Margaret Pyke House
27–35 Mortimer Street
London W1

Family Welfare Association
501–505 Kingsland Road
Dalston
London E8 4AU

Federated Superannuation Scheme for
   Nurses and Hospital Officers
Rosehill
Park Road
Banstead

Florence Nightingale House
173 Cromwell Road
London SW5 0SE

The Foundation for the Study of Infant
   Deaths
15 Belgrave Square
London SW1X 8PS

Gamblers Anonymous
17/23 Blantyre Street
Cheyne Walk
London SW10

General Medical Council
44 Hallam Street
London W1

General Nursing Council for England
   and Wales
23 Portland Place
London W1A 1BA

General Nursing Council for Scotland
5 Dunaway Street
Edinburgh EH3 6DP

Gingerbread
Minerva Chambers
35 Wellington Street
London WC2E 7BN

Guild of St Barnabas for Nurses
St Helena's Retreat House
Drayton Green
London W13

Haemophilia Society
PO Box 9
16 Trinity Street
London SE1 1DE

Health Education Council
78 New Oxford Street
London WC1A 1AH

Health Services Superannuation
   Division
Hesketh House
200–220 Broadway
Fleetwood
Lancs FL7 8LG

Health Visitors' Association
36 Eccleston Square
London SW1

Help the Aged
16–18 St James's Walk
London EC1R 0BE

Her Majesty's Prisons and Borstal
   Institutions Nursing Service
Her Majesty's Prison
Holloway
London N5 1PL

Hospital Savings Association
30 Lancaster Gate
London W2 3LT

Hysterectomy Support Group
11 Henryson Road
London SE4 1HL

Imperial Cancer Research Fund
Lincoln's Inn Fields
London WC2

Institute for the Study of Drug
    Dependence
1–4 Hatton Place
Hatton Garden
London EC1N 8ND

International Confederation of
    Midwives
57 Lower Belgrave Street
London SW1W 0LR

International Council of Nurses
37 rue Vermont
1202 Geneva
Switzerland

Invalid Children's Aid Association
126 Buckingham Palace Road
London SW1W 9SB

King's Fund Centre
126 Albert Street
London NW1 7NF

Lady House Trust for Physically
    Disabled Children
7 North Street
Midhurst
West Sussex GU29 9DJ

Let Live Association
56a Kyverdale Road
London N16

Leukaemia Research Fund
61 Great Ormond Street
London WC1

Leukaemia Society
28 Eastern Road
London N2

London University
Department of Extramural Studies
26 Russel Square
London WC1B 5DQ

Margaret Pyke Centre
27–35 Mortimer Street
London W1A 4QW

Marie Curie Memorial Foundation
28 Belgrave Square
London SW1X 8QG

Marie Stopes Clinic
Well Woman Centre
108 Whitfield Street
London W1P 6BE

Medical Council on Alcoholism
31 Bedford Square
London WC1

Medical Defence Union Ltd
3 Devonshire Place
London W1

Medic-Alert Foundation
11–13 Clifton Terrace
London N4 3JP

Medical Protection Society Ltd
50 Hallam Street
London W1

Medical Research Council
20 Park Crescent
London W1

Midwife Teachers Training College
High Coombe
Warren Road
Kingston Hill

MIND (National Association for
    Mental Health)
22 Harley Street
London W1

Miscarriage Association
18 Stoneybrook Close
West Bretton
Wakefield
West Yorkshire WF4 4TP

Motor Neurone Disease Association
61 Derngate House
Northampton
NN1 1UE

Multiple Sclerosis Society
4 Tachbrook Street
London SW1

Muscular Dystrophy Group of Great
    Britain and Northern Ireland
Nattrass House
35 Macaulay Road
London SW4 0QP

Narcotics Anonymous
PO Box 246
London SW10

National Association for Colitis and
    Crohn's Disease (NACC)
98a London Road
St Albans
Herts AL1 1NX

National Association for Deaf/Blind
    and Rubella Children
164 Cromwell Lane
Coventry
Warwickshire CV4 8AP

National Association for Gifted
    Children
1 South Audley Street
London W1

National Association for Limbless
    Disabled (NALD)
134 Martindale Road
Hounslow
Middlesex TW4 7NQ

National Association for Maternal and
    Child Welfare
1 South Audley Street
London W1Y 6JS

National Association for the Education
    of the Partially Sighted
Joseph Clark School
Vincent Road
Higham Park
London E4

National Association for the Welfare of
    Children in Hospital (NAWCH)
7 Exton Street
London SE1 8VE

National Association of State Enrolled
    Nurses
1 Vere Street
London W1

National Autistic Society
276 Willesden Lane
London NW2

National Board for Nursing,
    Midwifery and Health Visiting for
    Northern Ireland
123/137 York Street
Belfast BT15 1JB

National Board for Nursing,
    Midwifery and Health Visiting for
    Scotland
Trinity Park House
South Trinity Road
Edinburgh EH5 3SF

National Childbirth Trust
9 Queensborough Terrace
London W2 3TB

National Council for One-Parent
    Families
255 Kentish Town Road
London NW5 2LX

National Council for Special Education
1 Wood Street
Stratford on Avon

National Deaf Children's Society
31 Gloucester Place
London W1H 4EA

National Eczema Society
Mary Ward House
5–7 Tavistock Place
London WC1

National Federation of Kidney
  Patients' Associations
Acorn Lodge
Woodsets
Nr. Worksop
Notts S81 8AT

National Fund for Nurses
1 Henrietta Place
Cavendish Square
London W1M 0AB

National Marriage Guidance Council
Herbert Gray College
Little Church Street
Rugby

National Schizophrenia Fellowship
79 Victoria Road
Surbiton

National Society for Autistic Children
1a Golders Green Road
London NW11

National Society for Cancer Relief
Michael Sobell House
30 Dorset Square
London NW1

National Society for Epilepsy
Chalfont Centre
Chalfont St Peter
Bucks SL9 0RJ

National Society for the Prevention of
  Cruelty to Children
1 Riding House Street
London W1

National Society for Mentally
  Handicapped Children
117 Golden Lane
London EC1Y 0RT

National Society of Phenylketonuria
  and Allied Disorders
6 Rawdon Close
Palace Fields
Runcorn

New Life Foundation Trust
The Red House
Kelham
Newark NG23 5QP

New Zealand Nurses' Association
GPO Box 2128
504/505 Brandon House
Featherston St
Wellington
New Zealand

Northern Ireland Council on
  Alcoholism
36/40 Victoria Street
Belfast

Nuffield Foundation
Nuffield Lodge
Regent's Park
London NW1

Nuffield Provincial Hospitals Trust
3 Prince Albert's Road
London NW1

Nursing and Hospital Careers
  Information Centre
121 Edgware Road
London W2 2HX

Nursing Education Research Unit
Chelsea College Road
London SW3 6LX

Nursing Practice Research Unit
Northwick Park Hospital
Watford Road
Harrow
Middlesex HA1 3UJ

Office of Population Censuses and
  Surveys
St Catherine's House
10 Kingsway
London WC2B 6TP

Open Door Association
447 Pensby Road
Heswall
Wirral

Open University
Milton Keynes

Parkinson's Disease Society
36 Portland Place
London W1N 3DG

Partially Sighted Society
40 Wordsworth Street
Hove
E. Sussex BN3 5BH

Phobias Confidential
1 Clovelly Road
Ealing
London W5 5HF

Phobics Society
4 Cheltenham Road
Chorlton-cum-Hardy
Manchester M21 1QN

Pregnancy Advisory Service
13 Charlotte Street
London W1P 1HD

Princess Mary's Royal Air Force
  Nursing Service
Ministry of Defence
First Avenue House
High Holborn
London WC1V 6HE

Psoriasis Association
7 Milton Street
Northampton
NN2 7JG

Queen Alexandra's Royal Army
  Nursing Corps
Ministry of Defence
First Avenue House
High Holborn
London WC1V 6HD

Release
1 Elgin Avenue
London W9

Renal Society
64 South Hill Park
London NW3 2SJ

Royal Australian Nursing Federation
132–6 Albert Road
South Melbourne
Australia

Royal British Nurses Association Club
194 Queen's Gate
London SW7 3DL

Royal College of General Practitioners
14 Princes Gate
Hyde Park
London SW7

Royal College of Midwives
15 Mansfield Street
London W1M 0BE

Royal College of Nursing and National
  Council of Nurses of the United
  Kingdom
1 Henrietta Place
Cavendish Square
London W1M 0AB

Royal College of Nursing and National
  Council of Nurses of the United
  Kingdom (Scotland)
44 Heriot Row
Edinburgh EH3 6EY

Royal College of Nursing and National
  Council of Nurses of the United
  Kingdom (Welsh Board)
Tŷ Maeth
King George V Drive
East Cardiff CF4 4XZ

Royal College of Obstetricians and
  Gynaecologists
27 Sussex Place
Regent's Park
London NW1

Royal College of Physicians
11 St Andrew's Place
London NW1

Royal College of Physicians of
    Edinburgh
9 Queen Street
Edinburgh EH2

Royal College of Psychiatrists
17 Belgrave Square
London SW1

Royal College of Surgeons of England
Lincoln's Inn Fields
London WC1

Royal National Institute for the Blind
224 Great Portland Street
London W1Y 6AA

Royal National Institute for the Deaf
105 Gower Street
London WC1E 6BR

Royal National Pension Fund for
    Nurses
Burdett House
15 Buckingham Street
Strand
London WC2N 6ED

Royal Society of Medicine
1 Wimpole Street
London W1

Samaritans
17 Uxbridge Road
Slough
Berkshire SL1 1SN

Schizophrenia Association of Great
    Britain
International Schizophrenia Centre
Bryn Hyfryd, The Crescent
Bangor
Gwynedd LL57 2AG

Scottish Association for Counselling
14 Caiystane Hill
Edinburgh EH10 6SL

Scottish Association for Mental Health
40 Shandwick Place
Edinburgh EH2 4RT

Scottish Association for the Deaf
158 West Regent Street
Glasgow G2

Scottish Council for Health Education
21 Landsdowne Crescent
Edinburgh EH12

Scottish Council for the Care of
    Spastics
Rhuemore
Corstorphine Road
Edinburgh EH12

Scottish Council for the Unmarried
    Mother and Her Child
44 Albancy Street
Edinburgh EH1

Scottish Council on Alcoholism
147 Blythswood Street
Glasgow G2 4EN

Scottish Epilepsy Association
48 Govan Road
Glasgow G51

Scottish Home and Health Department
St Andrew's House
Edinburgh EH1

Scottish National Federation for the
    Welfare of the Blind
39 St Andrew's Street
Dundee

Scottish Society for the Mentally
    Handicapped
69 West Regent Street
Glasgow G2 2AN

Sickle Cell Society
Green Lodge
Barretts Green Road
London NW10 7AP

Society for Registered Male Nurses
38 Marland Avenue
Oldham

Society of Apothecaries
Blackfriars Lane
Queen Victoria Street
London EC4

Spastics Society
12 Park Crescent
London W1N 4EQ

SPOD (Association to Aid the Sexual
    and Personal Relationships of
    People with a Disability)
286 Camden Road
London N7 0BJ

Stillbirth and Neonatal Death Society
Argyle House
29–31 Euston Road
London NW1 2SD

Stillbirth Association
15a Christchurch Hill
London NW3

Student Nurses Association
Royal College of Nursing
1 Henrietta Place
Cavendish Square
London W1M 0AB

Terrence Higgins Trust
BM Aids
London WC1N 3XX

Toy Libraries Association
Seabrooke House/Wyllyots Manor
Darkes Lane
Potters Bar
Hertfordshire EN6 5HC

Trained Nurses' Association of India
L–16 Green Park
New Delhi 10016
India

Trained Nurses' Association of
    Pakistan
c/o The College of Nursing
Jinnah Postgraduate Medical School
Karachi 35
Pakistan

Tranquillizer Withdrawal Support
160 Tosson Terrace
Heaton
Newcastle NE6 5EA

United Kingdom Central Council for
    Nursing, Midwifery and Health
    Visiting
23 Portland Place
London W1N 3AH

United Nursing Services Club
40 South Street
London W1

United States Information Service
24 Grosvenor Square
London W1

VAD Ladies Club
44 Great Cumberland Place
London W1H 8BS

Welsh Board of Health
Cathays Park
Cardiff

Welsh National Board for Nursing,
    Midwifery and Health Visiting
13th Floor, Pearl Assurance House
Greyfriars Road
Cardiff CF1 3AG

Womens Royal Voluntary Service
17 Old Park Lane
London W1Y 4AJ

World Health Organization
Geneva
Switzerland

Index